Critical Care Nursing

Diagnosis and Management

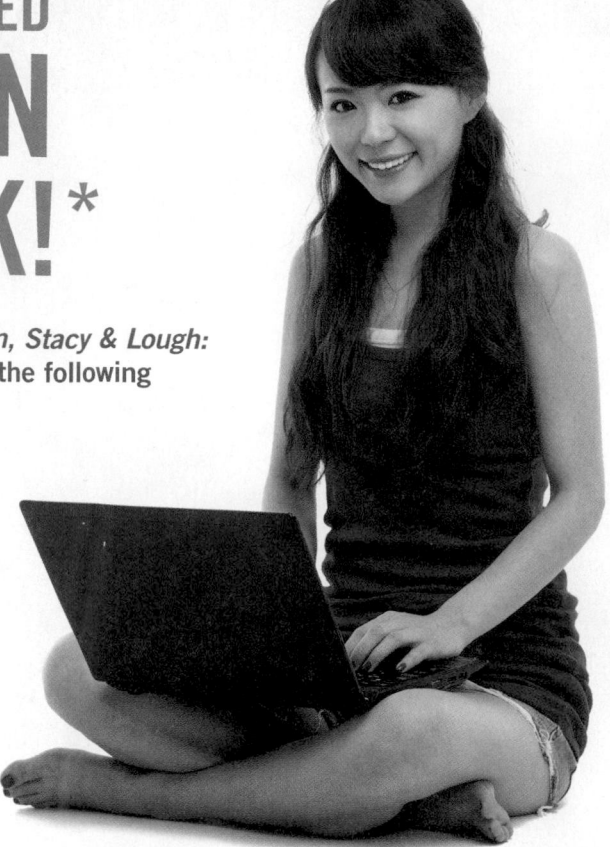
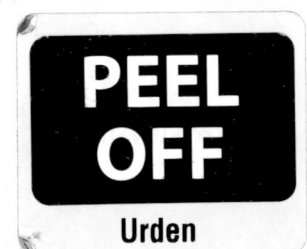

Critical Care Nursing

seventh editon

Diagnosis and Management

Linda D. Urden, DNSc, RN, CNS, NE-BC, FAAN
Professor and Director
Master's and International Nursing Programs
University of San Diego
San Diego, California

Kathleen M. Stacy, PhD, RN, CNS, CCRN, PCCN, CCNS
Clinical Nurse Specialist–Pulmonary/Medicine PCU
Palomar Medical Center
Escondido, California;
Clinical Associate Professor
Hahn School of Nursing and Health Science
University of San Diego
San Diego, California

Mary E. Lough, PhD, RN, CNS, CCRN, CNRN, CCNS
Clinical Nurse Specialist–Critical Care
Stanford Hospital and Clinics
Stanford, California;
Clinical Professor
Department of Physiological Nursing
University of California, San Francisco (UCSF)
San Francisco, California

ELSEVIER

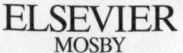

3251 Riverport Lane
St. Louis, Missouri 63043

CRITICAL CARE NURSING: DIAGNOSIS AND MANAGEMENT ISBN: 978-0-323-09178-7

Notices

ISBN: 978-0-323-09178-7

Executive Content Strategist: Tamara Myers
Senior Content Development Specialist: Linda Thomas
Publishing Services Manager: Deborah L. Vogel
Project Manager: Bridget Healy
Design Direction: Amy Buxton

Printed in Canada

Last digit is the print number: 9 8 7 6 5 4 3 2 1

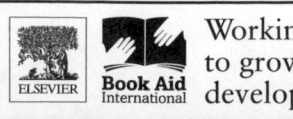

Working together
to grow libraries in
developing countries

www.elsevier.com • www.bookaid.org

Linda D. Urden, DNSc, RN, CNS, NE-BC, FAAN

Linda Urden received her diploma in nursing from Barnes Hospital School of Nursing, St. Louis, Missouri; her BSN from Pepperdine University, Malibu, California; her MN, Cardiovascular Clinical Nurse Specialist, from UCLA; and her DNSc from the University of San Diego. She is doubly credentialled as a clinical nurse specialist and in Executive Nursing by the American Nurses Credentialing Center and is a Fellow in the American Academy of Nursing. Linda has held a variety of clinical and administrative positions, with accountabilities for quality, evidence-based practice, research, education, and advanced practice. In her various positions she has striven to create cultures that are sensitive to differentiated practice and ensure healthy work environments supporting excellence in nursing practice. In addition to this text, Linda coauthored *Priorities in Critical Care Nursing*. Other publications are in the areas of heart failure, ethics, research, outcomes measurement, management and care delivery redesign, executive decision support databases, and collaborative practice models, clinical nurse practice outcomes, and Magnet environments. In addition, she is a member of editorial boards and is a peer reviewer for several nursing journals. Her research is focused on clinical, fiscal, quality, and behavioral outcomes of care delivery and services.

Kathleen M. Stacy, PhD, RN, CNS, CCRN, PCCN, CCNS

Kathleen Stacy has been a nurse for 34 years, the majority of which she has spent working in critical care. She graduated in 1978 with a BS in nursing from the State University of New York at Plattsburgh, in 1989 with an MS in critical care nursing from San Diego State University, and in 2010 with a PhD in nursing from University of San Diego. She has held a variety of positions, including staff nurse, clinical educator, outcomes manager, and nurse manager. Currently Kathleen is the Clinical Nurse Specialist for the Pulmonary/Medicine Progressive Care Unit at Palomar Medical Center. As an advanced practitioner, Kathleen collaborates with the health care team to facilitate the achievement of optimal outcomes for the critically ill patient. As a consultant, she facilitates change to improve patient care. As an educator, Kathleen develops and implements programs to assist the staff with acquisition of the skills and knowledge needed to care for the critically ill patient. As a researcher, she conducts nursing research with a focus on patient safety and end-of-life care. Kathleen also holds a faculty position at the Hahn School of Nursing and Health Science at University of San Diego and an adjunct faculty position at San Diego State University School of Nursing. In addition to this text, Kathleen coauthored *Priorities in Critical Care Nursing*.

Mary E. Lough, PhD, RN, CNS, CCRN, CNRN, CCNS

Mary Lough is a critical care nurse with more than 30 years of experience as a staff nurse, educator, and Clinical Nurse Specialist. Mary received her BSN from the University of Manchester in England and her MS and PhD from the University of California, San Francisco (UCSF). Mary is the Clinical Nurse Specialist for the medical/surgical/neuroscience/trauma ICU at Stanford Hospital and Clinics in Palo Alto, California. She is also a Clinical Professor in the Department of Physiological Nursing at her alma mater, UCSF.

Mary has been involved with all seven editions of *Critical Care Nursing: Diagnosis and Management*, and she also has published many other articles and research abstracts. As a clinician, Mary appreciates the benefits of a clinically grounded textbook because when she began her career as a critical care nurse so little information was available.

CONTRIBUTORS

Caroline Arbour, BSc, RN, PhD (c)
PhD Candidate
School of Nursing
McGill University
Montreal, Quebec
Canada
Chapter 9, Pain and Pain Management

Jamie D. Blazek, MPH, APRN, FNP-C
Nurse Practitioner
Ochsner Multi-Organ Transplant Center
Ochsner Clinic
New Orleans, Louisiana
*Chapter 37, Organ Donation and
    Transplantation*

Barbara Buesch, MSN, RN, CNS
District Stroke Coordinator
Palomar Health
Escondido, California
*Chapter 24, Neurologic Disorders and
    Therapeutic Management*

Darlene M. Burke, MS, MA, RN
Adjunct Nursing Faculty
MiraCosta College
Oceanside, California;
Consultant and Educator
Professional Source Nursing Consulting
Carlsbad, California
*Chapter 23, Neurologic Clinical Assessment
    and Diagnostic Procedures*

Beverly Carlson, PhD, RN, CNS, CCRN
Lecturer and Graduate Advisor
School of Nursing
San Diego State University
San Diego, California
*Chapter 35, Shock, Sepsis, and Multiple
    Organ Dysfunction Syndrome*

Kelly Dineen, BSN, JD
Assistant Dean for Academic Affairs and
    Instructor of Health Law
Saint Louis University School of Law
St. Louis, Missouri
Chapter 3, Legal Issues

Joni L. Dirks, MS, RN-BC, CCRN
Manager, Clinical Educators
Nurse Educator
Adult Intensive Care Units
Providence Urban Hospitals
Spokane, Washington
*Chapter 16, Cardiovascular Therapeutic
    Management*

**Caroline Etland, PhD, RN, CNS, AOCN,
ACHPN**
Director of Education, Research and
    Professional Practice
Department of Nursing
Bioethics Consultant
Sharp Chula Vista Medical Center
Chula Vista, California
Chapter 11, End-of-Life Issues

**Lorraine Fitzsimmons, PhD, APRN, FNP,
ANP-BC**
Chair, Advanced Practice Nursing of Adults
    and Elderly
School of Nursing
San Diego State University
San Diego, California
*Chapter 35, Shock, Sepsis, and Multiple
    Organ Dysfunction Syndrome*

Céline Gélinas, PhD, RN
Assistant Professor
Ingram School of Nursing
McGill University;
Researcher
Centre for Nursing Research and Lady Davis
    Institute for Medical Research
Jewish General Hospital
Montreal, Quebec
Canada
Chapter 9, Pain and Pain Management

Christine Hartley, MS, RN, ACNP-BC
Nurse Practitioner
Critical Care Services
Stanford Hospital and Clinics
Stanford, California
*Chapter 37, Organ Donation and
    Transplantation*

Annette Haynes, MS, RN, CNS, CCRN
Cardiology Clinical Nurse Specialist
Stanford Hospital and Clinics
Stanford, California
Chapter 15, Cardiovascular Disorders

Susie Hutchins, DNP, RN, CNE
Associate Clinical Faculty
Coordinator of Standardized Patient and
    Simulation Lab
Department of Nursing
University of San Diego
San Diego, California
Chapter 39, The Obstetric Patient

**Lourdes Januszewicz, MSN, RN, CNS,
CCRN**
Clinical Nurse Specialist
Intensive Care/Intermediate Care
Palomar Health
Poway, California
*Chapter 24, Neurologic Disorders and
    Therapeutic Management*

Elaine Bishop Kennedy, EdD, RN
Salisbury, Maryland
Concept Map Illustrator

**Sheryl Leary, MS, RN, CCNS, CCRN,
PCCN, PhD**
Clinical Nurse Specialist
San Diego VA Healthcare System
San Diego, California
*Chapter 30, Gastrointestinal Disorders and
    Therapeutic Management*

Cynthia A. Lewis, RN, MS, CNS, CPN
Pediatric Clinical Nurse Specialist
Medical Unit
Rady Children's Hospital San Diego
San Diego, California
Chapter 40, The Pediatric Patient

**Mary E. Lough, PhD, RN, CNS, CCRN,
CNRN, CCNS**
Clinical Nurse Specialist–Critical Care
Stanford Hospital and Clinics
Stanford, California;
Clinical Professor
Department of Physiological Nursing
University of California, San Francisco
    (UCSF)
San Francisco, California
*Chapter 4, Genetics and Genomics in Critical
    Care*
*Chapter 10, Sedation, Agitation, Delirium:
    Assessment and Management*
*Chapter 12, Cardiovascular Anatomy and
    Physiology*
Chapter 13, Cardiovascular Clinical Assessment
*Chapter 14, Cardiovascular Diagnostic
    Procedures*
Chapter 25, Kidney Anatomy and Physiology
*Chapter 26, Kidney Clinical Assessment and
    Diagnostic Procedures*
*Chapter 27, Kidney Disorders and
    Therapeutic Management*
Chapter 31, Endocrine Anatomy and Physiology
*Chapter 32, Endocrine Clinical Assessment
    and Diagnostic Procedures*
*Chapter 33, Endocrine Disorders and
    Therapeutic Management*
*Chapter 37, Organ Donation and
    Transplantation*

Jeanne M. Maiden, PhD, RN, CNS-BC
Associate Dean and Professor
Director, MSN Program
School of Nursing
Point Loma Nazarene University
San Diego, California
Chapter 19, Pulmonary Diagnostic Procedures

Mary Martel, MSN, RN, FNP-BC
Nurse Practitioner
Physical Medicine & Rehabilitation
Stanford Medicine Outpatient Center
Red Wood City, California
*Chapter 37, Organ Donation and
   Transplantation*

Kasuen Mauldin, PhD, RD
Assistant Professor
Department of Nutrition, Food Science, and
   Packaging
San José State University
San José, California
*Chapter 8, Nutrition Alterations and
   Management*

Barbara Mayer, MS, RN, CNS, PhD (c)
Director of Professional Practice
Nursing Administration
St. Vincent Medical Center
Los Angeles, California
Chapter 5, Patient and Family Education

**MaryAlice McCubbins, RN, MSN,
CPCP-PC, TNS, LtCol USAF(ret)**
Trauma Nurse Practitioner
Department of Pediatric Surgery, Trauma
   Services
Washington University—St. Louis
St. Louis Children's Hospital
St. Louis, Missouri
Chapter 36, Burns

**Denise O'Brien, DNP, RN, ACNS-BC,
CPAN, CAPA, FAAN**
Perianesthesia Clinical Nurse Specialist
Department of Operating Rooms/Post-
   anesthesia Care Unit
University of Michigan Hospitals and
   Health Centers;
Adjunct Clinical Instructor
School of Nursing
University of Michigan
Ann Arbor, Michigan
Chapter 42, The Perianesthesia Patient

**Mary Russell, MSN, RN, CNS, CCRN,
FNP (c)**
Clinical Nurse Specialist
Acute Surgical Unit
Surgical Progressive Unit
Trauma Intensive Care Unit
Palomar Pomerado Health
Escondido, California
*Chapter 38, Hematologic Disorders and
   Oncologic Emergencies*

**Elizabeth Scruth, MN, MPH, RN, CCRN,
CCNS, PhD (c)**
Clinical Practice Consultant
Department of Quality and Regulatory
   Services
Kaiser Permanente
Oakland, California
Chapter 15, Cardiovascular Disorders

Jennifer Seigel, RN, CPNP, CWCN
Pediatric Nurse Practitioner
Pediatric Surgery/ Pediatric Acute Wound
   Service
Washington University—St. Louis
St. Louis Children's Hospital
St. Louis, Missouri
Chapter 36, Burns

Teresa J. Shafer, MSN, RN, CPTC
Executive Vice President and Chief
   Operating Officer
LifeGift
Fort Worth, Texas
*Chapter 37, Organ Donation and
   Transplantation*

Kara A. Snyder, MS, RN, CCRN, CCNS
Clinical Nurse Specialist
Surgical Trauma Critical Care Department
University of Arizona Medical Center
Tucson, Arizona
Chapter 34, Trauma

**Kathleen M. Stacy, PhD, RN, CNS,
CCRN, PCCN, CCNS**
Clinical Nurse Specialist–Pulmonary/
   Medicine PCU
Palomar Medical Center
Escondido, California;
Clinical Associate Professor
Hahn School of Nursing and Health Science
University of San Diego
San Diego, California
Chapter 7, Sleep Alterations and Management
*Chapter 17, Pulmonary Anatomy and
   Physiology*
Chapter 18, Pulmonary Clinical Assessment
*Chapter 22, Neurologic Anatomy and
   Physiology*
Chapter 20, Pulmonary Disorders
*Chapter 21, Pulmonary Therapeutic
   Management*
*Chapter 28, Gastrointestinal Anatomy and
   Physiology*
*Chapter 29, Gastrointestinal Clinical
   Assessment and Diagnostic Procedures*

**Carol A. Suarez, MSN, RN, CNS, PHN,
FNP (c)**
Clinical Nurse Specialist
Orthopaedic Medical/Surgical Acute Care
   and NeuroSciences Progressive Care Unit
Palomar Pomerado Health
Escondido, California
*Chapter 38, Hematologic Disorders and
   Oncologic Emergencies*

**Christine Thompson, MS, RN, CNS,
CCRN, CHFN**
Clinical Nurse Specialist
Department of Cardiovascular Health
Stanford Hospital and Clinics
Stanford, California
*Chapter 14, Cardiovascular Diagnostic
   Procedures*

**Linda D. Urden, DNSc, RN, CNS, NE-BC,
FAAN**
Professor and Director
Master's and International Nursing
   Programs
University of San Diego
San Diego, California
Chapter 1, Critical Care Nursing Practice
Chapter 2, Ethical Issues

Julie M. Waters, MS, RN, CCRN
Clinical Nurse Educator
Critical Care Department
Providence Sacred Heart Medical Center
Spokane, Washington
*Chapter 16, Cardiovascular Therapeutic
   Management*

Schawnté Williams-Taylor, BSN, RN, CCRN, CPTC
Managing Director
Life Gift
Lubbock, Texas
Chapter 37, Organ Donation and Transplantation

Carrie M. Wilson, MSN, RN, CPNP-PC, CPNP-AC, WCC
Pediatric Nurse Practitioner
Pediatric General Surgery
Washington University—St. Louis
St. Louis, Missouri
Chapter 36, Burns

Fiona Winterbottom, MSN, RN, APRN, ACNS-BC, CCRN
Clinical Nurse Specialist for Critical Care
Ochsner Medical Center—New Orleans
New Orleans, Louisiana
Chapter 41, The Older Adult Patient

Valerie J. Yancey, PhD, RN, CHPN, HNC
Associate Professor
Department of Nursing
Southern Illinois University—Edwardsville
Edwardsville, Illinois
Chapter 6, Psychosocial and Spiritual Alterations and Management

Collin Bowman-Woodall, MS, RN
Assistant Professor
Samuel Merritt University
San Francisco Peninsula Learning Center
San Mateo, California

Marylee Bressie, DNP, RN, CCRN, CCNS, CEN
Assistant Professor
Department of Nursing
Capella University
Minneapolis, Minnesota;
University of Arkansas—Fort Smith
Fort Smith, Arkansas

Gloria Brummer, MS, RN, CEN, CNE
Assistant Professor
Department of Nursing
St. John's College
Springfield, Illinois

Teresa Burkhalter, MSN, RN, BC
Nursing Faculty
Technical College of the Lowcountry
Beaufort, South Carolina

Deborah K. Drummonds, RN, MN, CCRN, CEN
Assistant Professor
Abraham Baldwin Agricultural College
School of Nursing and Health Sciences
Tifton, Georgia

Rebecca Hickey, BA, RN
Adjunct Instructor
Allied Health
University of Cincinnati—Blue Ash
Blue Ash, Ohio

Julene B. Kruithof, MSN, RN, CCRN
Adult Critical Care Nurse Educator
Spectrum Health
Grand Rapids, Michigan

Adisa Kudumovic, MSN, ARNP, CNE, NP-C
Associate Professor
Allen College
Waterloo, Iowa

Robert E. Lamb, PharmD
REL & Associates, LLC
Downington, Pennsylvania

Kristine Hart L'Ecuyer, RN, MSN, CCNS, CNL
Associate Professor of Nursing
Saint Louis University
St. Louis, Missouri

Jennifer Manning, MN, RN, CNS
Instructor of Nursing and Adult Health
Clinical Nurse Specialist
School of Nursing
Louisiana State University Health Sciences
    Center
New Orleans, Louisiana

Michaelynn Paul, RN, MS, CCRN
Assistant Professor of Nursing
School of Nursing
Walla Walla University
College Place, Washington

Brenda Sloan, MA, RN, ACNS-BC
Assistant Professor
School of Nursing
Indiana Wesleyan University
Marion, Indiana

Michelle D. Smeltzer, MSN, RN, CEN
Clinical Nurse Specialist
Emergency Services
Einstein Medical Center
Philadelphia, Pennsylvania

Lisa A. Webb, MSN, RN, CEN
Instructor of Nursing
Derry Patterson Wingo School of Nursing
Charleston Southern University
Charleston, South Carolina

Kathleen S. Whalen, PhD, RN, CNE
Associate Professor
Loretto Heights School of Nursing
Regis University
Denver, Colorado

Shirley K. Woolf, MSN, MA, RN, CNE, CCRN
Clinical Assistant Professor
Department of Adult Health
School of Nursing
Indiana University
Indianapolis, Indiana

We are most grateful to the many students and nurses who made the previous editions of this book successful. This success has validated our commitments to proclaiming the outstanding contributions of critical care nurses and to promoting evidence-based nursing practice in the complex critical care environment. We actively solicited feedback from users of the previous editions and eagerly incorporated their comments and suggestions regarding format, content, and organization. And so, with this seventh edition, we again present to you a book that is thorough in all that is most pertinent to critical care nurses in a format that is organized for clarity and comprehension.

ORGANIZATION

The book's nine units and two appendices are again organized around alterations in dimensions of human functioning that span biopsychosocial realms.

The content of Unit I, "Foundations of Critical Care Nursing," forms the basis of practice, regardless of the physiologic alterations of the critically ill patient. Although chapters in the book may be studied in any sequence, we recommend that Chapter 1, "Critical Care Nursing Practice," be studied first because it clarifies the major assumptions on which the entirety of the book is based. Chapter 2, "Ethical Issues," delineates theories and strategies for dealing with the ethical dilemmas that arise on a daily basis in critical care. Chapter 3, "Legal Issues," provides a base of information to help the critical care nurse be cognizant of practice issues that may have legal implications.

Chapter 4, "Genetics and Genomics in Critical Care," provides information of the biological basis of genetics, descriptions of the different types of *genetic* and *genomic* studies are included, plus examples of genetic diseases and pharmacogenetic syndromes already encountered in critical care. The genomic arena mandates a new range of clinical and ethical competencies for nursing practice, and this list is included in the chapter.

Teaching and learning theory and strategies to best meet the learning needs of critical care patients are delineated in Chapter 5, "Patient and Family Education." Chapter 6, "Psychosocial and Spiritual Alterations and Management," examines the theoretic basis and nursing process for alterations in self-concept, spiritual practices, and coping. Chapter 7, "Sleep Alterations and Management," addresses a perennial problem in critical care. Chapter 8, "Nutrition Alterations and Management," examines the nutritional needs of the critically ill patient and provides specific recommendations for different disorders. The concepts of pain and pain management in the critically ill are discussed in Chapter 9, "Pain and Pain Management." "Sedation, Agitation, Delirium: Assessment and Management" are described in Chapter 10. Chapter 11, "End-of-Life Issues," delineates special needs for dealing with end-of-life and palliative care.

Unit II, "Cardiovascular Alterations," and Unit III, "Pulmonary Alterations," are each structured with the following chapters:

- Anatomy and Physiology
- Clinical Assessment
- Diagnostic Procedures
- Disorders
- Therapeutic Management

This organization permits easy retrieval of information for students and clinicians and provides flexibility for the instructor to individualize teaching methods by assigning chapters that best suit student needs. Unit IV, "Neurologic Alterations"; Unit V, "Kidney Alterations"; Unit VI, "Gastrointestinal Alterations"; and Unit VII, "Endocrine Alterations," are organized similarly. However, in these units, the assessment parameters, such as clinical and diagnostic procedures, are discussed in one chapter. In addition, disorders and therapeutic management are combined into one chapter.

Unit VIII, "Multisystem Alterations," covers disorders that affect multiple body systems and necessitate discussion as a separate category. Unit VIII consists of five chapters: "Trauma," "Shock, Sepsis, and Multiple Organ Dysfunction Syndrome," "Burns," "Organ Donation and Transplantation," and "Hematologic Disorders and Oncologic Emergencies."

Unit IX, "Special Populations," addresses the needs of the critically ill pediatric, obstetric, and older adult in the critical care unit, as well as the management of the recovery of the perianesthesia patient.

Appendix A, "Nursing Management Plans of Care," contains management plans organized alphabetically by nursing diagnosis for easy access by students and practitioners.

Finally, Appendix B, "Physiologic Formulas for Critical Care," features commonly encountered hemodynamic, pulmonary, and other calculations and is presented in easily understood formulas. Recommendations for nutritional supplements also are included.

NURSING DIAGNOSIS AND MANAGEMENT

A dominant theme of the book continues to be nursing diagnosis and management, reflecting the strength of critical care nursing practice. Wherever possible, evidence-based critical care practice is incorporated into nursing interventions. To foster critical thinking and decision making, a boxed "menu" of nursing diagnoses complete with specific etiologic or related factors accompanies each medical disorder and major medical treatment discussion and directs the learner to Appendix A, where appropriate nursing management is detailed. To facilitate student learning, the nursing management plans of care incorporate nursing diagnosis definition, etiologic or related factors, clinical manifestations, and interventions with rationale. The nursing management plans are liberally cross-referenced throughout the book for easy retrieval by the reader.

NEW TO THIS EDITION

- **QSEN boxes** highlight the quality and safety issues for nurses that are key to the care of critically ill patients. Boxes devoted to this material are identified with the QSEN icon.
- **Internet Resources Boxes** are located at the end of chapters, as appropriate, and contain references for the reader to search the source directly for further information.
- **Glossary** has been added to the Evolve website for quick reference regarding definition of concepts in the text.

Special Features

- **Concept Maps** appear in the disorders chapters. Eighteen concept maps portray the nursing care and treatment for complex medical conditions. Eight maps are new to this edition; ten are carried over from the 6th edition. The map design has been updated from the last edition. A key explaining the components and shapes of the maps is included on each one. Maps are provided for the following conditions: Acute Coronary Syndrome, Acute Kidney Injury, Acute Lung Failure, Anaphylactic Shock, Cardiogenic Shock, Diabetes Insipidus (DI), Diabetic Ketoacidosis, Gastrointestinal Hemorrhage, Heart Failure, Hyperglycemic Hyperosmolar State (HHS), Hypovolemic Shock, Inappropriate Secretion of Antidiuretic Hormone (SIADH), Intracranial Hypertension, Neurogenic Shock, Septic Shock, Shock, and Stroke.
- The maps portray the *outcome* approach to nursing care, depicting how the nursing interventions will alter a nursing diagnosis once they are implemented. The diagnosis is substantiated by the pathophysiology, by the things that are known to exist within the patient. The illustrations provide an additional learning tool for users to understand the complexity of the various conditions.
- **Case Studies** promote student learning and critical thinking by illustrating the clinical course of a patient experiencing the history, clinical assessment, diagnostic procedures, and diagnoses discussed in the related unit or chapter. All Case Studies include critical thinking questions to facilitate discussion. Answers to the questions are available on the Evolve website as a special resource for instructors.
- **Evidence-Based Practice** special feature highlights important research-based articles on key topics in critical care nursing.
- **Nursing Interventions Classification (NIC)** feature appears in the therapeutic management chapters and lists the important nursing actions for a variety of nursing interventions that would be commonly incorporated in the management of a critically ill patient requiring a specific therapeutic treatment, such as mechanical ventilation
- **Pharmacologic Management** tables are also found in the therapeutic management chapters; these tables outline the common medications, along with any special considerations, used in treatment of the different disorders presented in the text.

- **Patient Education** boxes are placed in the disorders chapters and list the special topics that should be taught to the patient and family to prepare them for discharge.
- **Data Collection** boxes located in the clinical assessment chapters contain information that should be included as part of the patient's history.
- **Nursing Diagnoses** boxes display the diagnoses associated with particular disorders in a summary format with references to the corresponding nursing management plans in Appendix A.

EVOLVE RESOURCES FOR *CRITICAL CARE NURSING*

We are pleased to offer additional new and updated resources for students and instructors on our companion site, Evolve Resources for *Critical Care Nursing*.

STUDENT RESOURCES

Student Resources are available at http://evolve.elsevier.com/Urden/criticalcare/ and include the following:
- Self-assessment opportunities, including:
  - NCLEX® Review Questions
  - CCRN Review Questions
  - PCCN Review Questions
- A selection of assessment animations and video clips for specific chapters
- Procedures from the most recent edition of *Mosby's Nursing Skills* with corresponding animations

INSTRUCTOR RESOURCES

Instructor Resources, available at http://evolve.elsevier.com/Urden/criticalcare/, provide a variety of aids to enhance classroom instruction. Instructors have access to all of the Student Resources listed above, as well as the following:
- TEACH for Nurses—a brand new feature that replaces the Instructor Manual. TEACH for Nurses consist of detailed lesson plans that offer:
- Objectives and Teaching Focus
- Nursing Curriculum Standards (QSEN, BSN Essentials, Concepts from Concept-Based Curriculum, CCRN, and PCCN)
- List of all student and instructor chapter resources found on Evolve
- Teaching Strategies that present a chapter outline, content highlights, and learning activities
- New Case Study for select chapters
- Answers to the textbook Case Study provided for select chapters
- Test Bank of approximately 1200 questions
- PowerPoint presentation by chapter, consisting of a total of approximately 1500 lecture slides. New to the presentations for this edition are lecture notes on most slides, more images from the book, 2-3 audience response questions for each chapter, and a progressive Case Study in 3 therapeutic management chapters.
- Image Collection containing all of the images from the text

Critical Care Nursing: Diagnosis and Management, seventh edition, represents our continued commitment to bringing you the finest in all things a textbook can offer: the best and brightest contributing and consulting authors, the latest scientific research befitting the current state of health care and nursing, an organizational format that exercises diagnostic reasoning skills and is logical and consistent, and outstanding artwork and illustrations that enhance student learning. We pledge our continued commitment to excellence in critical care education.

Linda D. Urden
Kathleen M. Stacy
Mary E. Lough

ACKNOWLEDGMENTS

A project of this book's magnitude is never merely the work of its authors. The concerted talent, hard work, and inspiration of a multitude of people have produced *Critical Care Nursing: Diagnosis and Management*, seventh edition, and have helped to make it the state-of-the-science text we affirm it to be. A "tradition of publishing excellence" has been evident throughout our partnership with Elsevier. We deeply appreciate the assistance of Tamara Myers, Executive Content Strategist, and Linda Thomas, Senior Content Development Specialist, who have helped us document and refine our ideas and transform our book into a reality. Their creativity, expertise, availability, and generosity of time and resources have been invaluable to us throughout this endeavor. We are also grateful to Bridget Healy, Project Manager, for her scrupulous attention to detail.

Finally, we wish to thank those authors who contributed work to the first six editions of this book. Without the foundation they provided, a seventh edition would not have been born. We continue to be proud of our partnership with Elsevier, the teamwork and mutual respect among the three co-editors, and the final published book.

Linda D. Urden
Kathleen M. Stacy
Mary E. Lough

CONTENTS

UNIT II   CARDIOVASCULAR ALTERATIONS

Critical Care Nursing Practice

Linda D. Urden

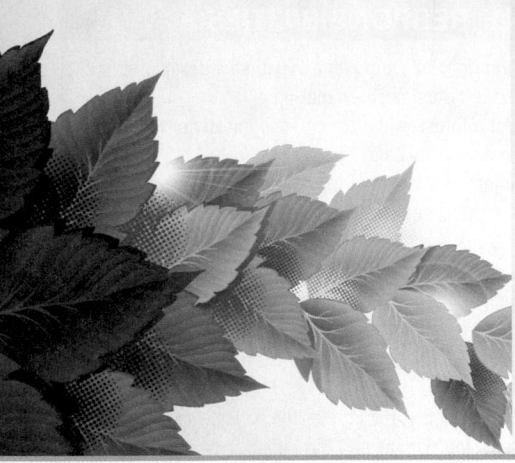

OVERVIEW

Health care is undergoing dramatic change at a speed that makes it almost impossible to remain current and be proactive. The chaos and many challenges facing health care providers and consumers are evident in critical care, in which new treatment modalities and technology interface with the continuing effort to strive for quality care and positive outcomes. Efficiency and cost-effectiveness in relation to health care services are frequently discussed and are emphasized to all health care providers. To some, it appears that quality patient care has taken a back seat to the emphasis on cost containment and that quality and cost-effectiveness are not congruent. It is incumbent on all critical care health care providers to face these challenges from their individual discipline's scope of practice and collectively from collaborative and interdisciplinary approaches.

The ever-changing health care environment creates many challenges for providers and consumers of care. Sensitivity to the appropriate time to eliminate or modify practices and adopt innovations is key to maintaining quality, cost-effective care delivery. Willingness to step outside of traditional structures and roles is the first step in making necessary changes. Change is constant. Flexibility and adaptation to change are essential to maintaining personal and organizational balance and to surviving in today's health care environment.

This chapter provides an overview of the evolution of critical care and describes the trends and current issues affecting critical care nurses and interdisciplinary team. The information in this chapter serves as the framework for the remainder of the book in the areas of professional nurse decision making, holistic care, interdisciplinary collaboration, evidence-based practice (EBP), quality, and safety.

HISTORY OF CRITICAL CARE

Critical care evolved from the recognition that the needs of patients with acute, life-threatening illness or injury could be better met if the patients were organized in distinct areas of the hospital. In the 1800s, Florence Nightingale described the advantages of placing patients recovering from surgery in a separate area of the hospital. A three-bed postoperative neurosurgical intensive care unit was opened in the early 1900s at Johns Hopkins Hospital in Baltimore. This was soon followed by a premature infant unit in Chicago.[1]

Major societal issues have affected the development of intensive care as a specialty. During World War II, shock wards were established to care for critically injured patients. The nursing shortage after the war forced the grouping of postoperative patients into designated recovery areas so that appropriate monitoring and care could be provided. The technologies and combat experiences of health care providers during the wars of the 20th century also provided an impetus for specialized medical and nursing care in the civilian setting. The 1950s brought the new technology of mechanical ventilation and the need to group patients receiving this new therapy in one location.

CRITICAL CARE NURSING

Critical care nursing was organized as a specialty less than 60 years ago; before that time, critical care nursing was practiced wherever there were critically ill patients. The development of new medical interventions and technology prompted recognition that nursing was important in the monitoring and observation of critically ill patients. Physicians depended on nurses to watch for critical changes in the condition of patients in the physicians' absence, and they sometimes depended on the nurses to initiate emergency medical treatment.

As sophisticated technology began to support more elaborate medical interventions, hospitals began to organize separate units to make more efficient use of equipment and specially trained staff. Postoperative care, once provided by private duty nurses on general nursing wards throughout the hospital, was moved into recovery rooms, where nurses with specialized knowledge regarding anesthesia recovery provided the patient care. Medical and surgical intensive care units segregated the most critically ill patients in locations where they could be cared for by nurses with specialized knowledge in those areas of care. By the 1960s, nurses had begun to consolidate their knowledge and practice into focused areas such as coronary care, nephrology, and intensive care. In the hospital units established for patients needing such specialized care, nurses assumed many functions and responsibilities formerly reserved for physicians, and they assumed a new authority by virtue of their knowledge and expertise.

CONTEMPORARY CRITICAL CARE

Modern critical care is provided to patients by a multidisciplinary team of health care professionals who have in-depth education in the specialty field of critical care. The team consists of physician intensivists, specialty physicians, nurses, advanced practice nurses and other specialty nurse clinicians, pharmacists, respiratory therapy practitioners, other specialized therapists and clinicians, social workers, and clergy. Critical care is provided in specialized units or departments, and importance is placed on the continuum of care, with an efficient transition of care from one setting to another.

Critical care patients are at high risk for actual or potential life-threatening health problems. Those who are more critically ill require more intensive and vigilant nursing care. There are more than 500,000 nurses in the United States who care for critically ill patients.

These nurses practice in a variety of settings: adult, pediatric, and neonatal critical care units; step-down, telemetry, progressive, or transitional care units; cardiac catheterization laboratories; and postoperative recovery units.[2] Nurses are now considered to be knowledge workers because they are highly vigilant and use their intelligence and cognition to go past tasks in order to quickly pull together multiple data to make decisions regarding subtle and/or deteriorating conditions. Nurses work technically with theoretical knowledge.[3]

A growing trend in acute care settings is the designation of progressive care units, considered to be part of the continuum of critical care. In past years, patients who are placed on these units would have been exclusively in critical care units. However, with the use of additional technology and monitoring capabilities, newer care delivery models, and additional nurse

BOX 1-1 AACN CRITICAL CARE NURSE ROLE RESPONSIBILITIES

- Respect and support the right of the patient or patient's designated surrogate to autonomy and informed decision making.
- Intervene when the best interest of the patient is in question.
- Help the patient obtain necessary care.
- Respect the values, beliefs, and rights of the patient.
- Provide education and support help to the patient or patient's designated surrogate to make decisions.
- Represent the patient in accordance with the patient's choices.
- Support the decisions of the patient or patient's designated surrogate or transfer care to an equally qualified critical care nurse.
- Intercede for patients who cannot speak for themselves in situations that require immediate attention.
- Monitor and safeguard the quality of care that the patient receives.
- Act as a liaison between the patient and the patient's family and other health care professionals.

From *American Association of Critical-Care Nurses*. Fact sheet: about critical care nursing (press room). http://www.aacn.org. Accessed December 2008.

education, these units are considered the best environment. The patients are less complex, more stable, have a decreased need for physiologic monitoring, and more self-care capabilities. They can serve as a bridge between critical care units and medical-surgical units, while providing high quality and cost effective care at the same time.[4] Additionally, these progressive units can be found throughout the acute care setting, thus leaving critical care unit beds for those who need the highest level of care and monitoring.[5]

CRITICAL CARE NURSING ROLES

Nurses provide and contribute to the care of critically ill patients in a variety of roles. The most prevalent role for the professional registered nurse is that of direct care provider. The American Association of Critical-Care Nurses (AACN) has delineated role responsibilities important for the critical care nurse[5] (Box 1-1).

Expanded-Role Nursing Positions

Expanded-role nursing positions interact with critical care patients, families, and the health care team. Nurse case managers work closely with the care providers to ensure appropriate, timely care and services and to promote continuity of care from one setting to another. Other nurse clinicians, such as patient educators, cardiac rehabilitation specialists, physician office nurses, and infection control specialists, also contribute to the care. The specific types of expanded-role nursing positions are determined by patient needs and individual organizational resources.

Advanced Practice Nurses

Advanced practice nurses (APNs) have met educational and clinical requirements beyond the basic nursing educational requirements for all nurses. The most commonly seen APNs in the critical care areas are the clinical nurse specialist (CNS) and the nurse practitioner (NP) or acute care nurse practitioner

(ACNP). APNs have a broad depth of knowledge and expertise in their specialty area and manage complex clinical and systems issues. The organizational system and existing resources of an institution determine what roles may be needed and how the roles function.

CNSs serve in specialty roles that use their clinical, teaching, research, leadership, and consultative abilities. They work in direct clinical roles and systems or administrative roles and in various other settings in the health care system. CNSs work closely with all members of the health care team, mentor staff, lead quality teams, and consult on complex patients. They are instrumental in ensuring that care is evidence-based and that safety programs are in place. They may be organized by specialty, such as cardiovascular care, or by function, such as cardiac rehabilitation. CNSs also may be designated as case managers for specific patient populations.

NPs and ACNPs manage direct clinical care of a group of patients and have various levels of prescriptive authority, depending on the state and practice area in which they work. They also provide care consistency, interact with families, plan for patient discharge, and provide teaching to patients, families, and other members of the health care team.[6]

CRITICAL CARE PROFESSIONAL ACCOUNTABILITY

Professional organizations support critical care practitioners by providing numerous resources and networks. The Society of Critical Care Medicine (SCCM) is a multidisciplinary, multispecialty, international organization. Its mission is to secure the highest quality, cost-efficient care for all critically ill patients.[1] Numerous publications and educational opportunities provide cutting-edge critical care information to critical care practitioners.

The organization most closely associated with critical care nurses is the AACN. It is the world's largest specialty nursing organization and was created in 1969. AACN is focused on "creating a healthcare system driven by the needs of patients and their families, where acute and critical care nurses make their optimal contribution."[7] The top priority of the organization is education of critical care nurses. AACN publishes numerous materials, evidence-based practice summaries, and practice alerts related to the specialty and is at the forefront of setting professional standards of care.

AACN serves its members through a national organization and many local chapters. The AACN Certification Corporation, a separate company, develops and administers many critical care specialty certification examinations for registered nurses. The examinations are provided in specialties such as neonatal, pediatric, and for those who practice in diverse settings, such as critical care, progressive care, "virtual" ICU, or remote monitoring (e-ICU). Certification is considered one method to maintain high quality of care and to protect consumers of care and services. Research has demonstrated more positive outcomes when care is delivered by health care providers who are certified in their specialty.[8] AACN also recognizes critical care and acute care units who achieve a high level of excellence through its

Beacon Award for Excellence. The unit that receives this award has demonstrated exceptional care through improved outcomes and greater overall satisfaction. It reflects on a supportive overall environment, teamwork and collaboration, and distinguishes itself with lower turnover and higher morale.[9]

CRITICAL CARE NURSING STANDARDS

AACN has established nursing standards that provide a framework for critical care nurses. Nursing practice varies depending on the setting in which the nurse is employed and the patients cared for in that setting. The standards set forth by AACN describe the practice of the nurse who cares for an acutely or critically ill patient in the health care environment. The standards are authoritative statements that describe the level of care and performance by which the quality of nursing care can be judged. They serve as descriptions of the expected roles and responsibilities, describing the standards of care and the standards of professional practice.

EVIDENCE-BASED NURSING PRACTICE

Much of early medical and nursing practice was based on non-scientific traditions, intuition, and traditions. These traditions and rituals, which were based on folklore, gut instinct, trial and error, and personal preference, were often passed down from one generation of practitioner to another. Examples of non–scientific-based critical care nursing practice include Trendelenburg positioning for hypotension, use of rectal tubes to manage fecal incontinence, gastric residual volume and aspiration risk, accuracy of assessment of body temperature, and suctioning artificial airways every 2 hours—to name a few. In order to deliver the highest quality of care, EBP is essential and must be embraced by all nurses.[10]

The dramatic and multiple changes in health care and the ever-increasing presence of managed care in all geographic regions have placed greater emphasis on demonstrating the effectiveness of treatments and practices on outcomes. Emphasis is on greater efficiency, cost-effectiveness, quality of life, and patient satisfaction ratings. It has become essential for nurses to use the best data available to make patient care decisions and carry out the appropriate nursing interventions.[10-11] By using an approach employing a scientific basis, with its ability to explain and predict, nurses are able to provide research-based interventions with consistent, positive outcomes. The content of this book is research-based, with the most current, cutting-edge research abstracted and placed throughout the chapters as appropriate to topical discussions.

The increasingly complex and changing health care system presents many challenges to creating an EBP. Appropriate research studies must be designed to answer clinical questions, and research findings must be used to make necessary changes for implementation in practice. Multiple EBP and research utilization models exist to guide practitioners in the use of existing research findings. One such model is the *Iowa Model of Evidence-Based Practice to Promote Quality Care*, which incorporates evidence and research as the bases for practice.[12] Cullen and Adams describe a framework with four key phases to implement EBP: 1) create awareness and interest; 2) build knowledge and commitment; 3) promote action and adoption; and 4) pursue integration and sustained use. Each step has multiple strategies that will facilitate successful progression to the next phase. The authors indicate that this model is particularly suited to complex static organizations.[11]

Just as there has been such an exponential growth of EBP literature, reports, publications and acceptance, others are posing the question, "But at what cost?" Newhouse describes this as a complex issue to address and states that economists would go beyond the costs of human labor and materials in their analysis. Another way to evaluate this is to examine "whose" cost is being considered.[13] More recently, a published article reported estimates of costs per event for several health-acquired conditions (HACs). The estimated cost of care for one catheter-associated urinary tract infection (CAUTI) was $758. A patient fall was estimated to be $4,233 per fall; and a surgical "never event" cost $62,000 per event. These are most likely underestimated; but it is easy to realize the tremendous impact of situations that should not occur because there is sufficient evidence to prevent such outcomes.[14] Thus, inquisitive practitioners who strive for best practices using valid and reliable data will demonstrate quality outcomes-driven care and practices.

Evidence-based nursing practice considers the best research evidence on the care topic, along with clinical expertise of the nurse, and patient preferences. For instance, when determining the frequency of vital sign measurement, the nurse would use available research, nursing judgment (stability, complexity, predictability, vulnerability, and resilience of the patient),[15] along with the patient's preference for decreased interruptions and the ability to sleep for longer periods of time. At other times the nurse will implement an evidence-based protocol or procedure that is based on evidence, including research. An example of an evidence-based protocol is one in which the prevalence of indwelling catheterization and incidence of hospital-acquired catheter-associated urinary tract infections in the critical care unit can be decreased.[16]

The AACN has promulgated several EBP summaries in the form of a "Practice Alert." These alerts are short directives that can be used as a quick reference for practice areas (e.g., oral care, noninvasive blood pressure monitoring, ST segment monitoring). They are succinct, supported by evidence, and address both nursing and multidisciplinary activities. Each alert includes the clinical information, followed by references that support the practice.[17] An example of one of the alerts is found on in Box 1-2.

HOLISTIC CRITICAL CARE NURSING

Caring

The high technology–driven critical care environment is fast paced and directed toward monitoring and treating life-threatening changes in patients' conditions. For this reason, attention is often focused on the technology and treatments necessary for maintaining stability in the physiologic

functioning of the patient. Great emphasis is placed on technical skills and professional competence and responsiveness to critical emergencies. Concern has been voiced about the diminished emphasis on the caring component of nursing in this fast-paced, highly technologic health care environment.[18,19] Nowhere is this more evident than in areas in which critical care nursing is practiced. It has been said that keeping the *care* in nursing care is one of our biggest challenges.[19] The critical care nurse must be able to deliver high-quality care skillfully, using all appropriate technologies, while incorporating psychosocial and other holistic approaches as appropriate to the time and condition of the patient.

The caring aspect between nurses and patients is most fundamental to the relationship and to the health care experience. The literature demonstrates that nurse clinicians focus on psychosocial aspects of caring, whereas patients place more emphasis on the technical skills and professional competence.[20] Physical and emotional absence, inhumane and belittling interactions, and lack of recognition of the patient's uniqueness indicate noncaring. Holistic care focuses on human integrity and stresses that the body, the mind, and the spirit are interdependent and inseparable. All aspects need to be considered in planning and delivering care.[21]

Individualized Care

The differences between nurses' and patients' perceptions of caring point to the importance of establishing individualized care that recognizes the uniqueness of each patient's preferences, condition, and physiologic and psychosocial status. It is clearly understood by care providers that a patient's physical condition progresses at fairly predictable stages, depending on the presence or absence of comorbid conditions. What is not understood as distinctly is the effect of psychosocial issues on the healing process. For this reason, special consideration must be given to determining the unique interventions that can positively affect each person and help the patient progress toward the desired outcomes.

An important aspect in the care delivery to and recovery of critically ill patients is the personal support of family members and significant others. The value of patient- and family-centered care should not be underestimated.[22,23] It is important for families to be included in care decisions and to be encouraged to participate in the care of the patient as appropriate to the patient's personal level of ability and needs.

Cultural Care

Cultural diversity in health care is not a new topic, but it is gaining emphasis and importance as the world becomes more accessible to all as the result of increasing technologies and interfaces with places and peoples. Diversity includes not only ethnic sensitivity but also sensitivity and openness to differences in lifestyles, opinions, values, and beliefs. More than 28% of the U.S. population is made up of racial and ethnic minority groups.[24] The predominant minorities in the United States are Americans of African, Hispanic, Asian, Pacific Island, Native American, and Eskimo descent. Significant differences exist

BOX 1-2 AACN PRACTICE ALERT

Family Presence During Resuscitation and Invasive Procedures

Expected Practice:

- Family members* of all patients undergoing resuscitation and invasive procedures should be given the option of presence at the bedside. [Level B]
- All patient care units should have an approved written practice document (i.e., policy, procedure, or standard of care) for presenting the option of family presence during resuscitation and bedside invasive procedures. [Level D]

Family members are those individuals who are relatives or significant others with whom the patient shares an established relationship.

Scope and Impact of the Problem:

Evidence is mounting that family presence during resuscitation and invasive procedures is beneficial to patients, families, and staff. Meeting psychosocial needs in a time of crisis exemplifies care driven by the needs of patients and families.

Supporting Evidence:

- Research[1-11] and public opinion polls[12-14] have found that 50% to 96% of consumers believe family members should be offered the opportunity to be present during emergency procedures and at the time of their loved one's death.
- Despite support by professional organizations and critical care experts,[15-24] only 5% of critical care units in the U.S. have written policies allowing family presence.[25] Surveys of nurses' practice find that most critical care nurses have been requested by family members to be present during resuscitation and invasive procedures and have brought families to the bedside, despite the lack of formal hospital policies.[25-27]
- Studies find the following benefits of family presence:
  - For patients: Almost all children want their parents present during medical procedures[28-30]; and adult patients report that having family members at the bedside comforted and helped them.[3,31-32]
  - For family members: Their presence at the bedside helped in removing doubt about the patient's condition by witnessing that everything possible was being done.[8,9,32-35] It decreased their anxiety and fear about what was happening to their loved one.[7,10,29,32,36-37] It facilitated their need to be together[8,10] and the need to help and support their loved one.[8-11,33-4,36] They experienced a sense of closure[3,8,11,34] and their presence facilitated the grief process should death occur.[3,5,11,32-36]
- Studies show that 94% to 100% of families involved in family presence events would do so again.[3,7,8,9,33,36]
- Studies also find that there are no patient-care disruptions, no negative outcomes during family presence events,[8,9,32-34,38-39] and no adverse psychologic effects among family members who participated at the bedside.[8,10,32,40]

AACN Evidence Leveling System

Level A Meta-analysis of quantitative studies or metasynthesis of qualitative studies with results that consistently support a specific action, intervention, or treatment.

Level B Well-designed, controlled studies with results that consistently support a specific action, intervention, or treatment.

Level C Qualitative studies, descriptive or correlational studies, integrative review, systematic reviews, or randomized controlled trials with inconsistent results.

Level D Peer-reviewed professional organizational standards with clinical studies to support recommendations.

Level E Multiple case reports, theory-based evidence from expert opinions, or peer-reviewed professional organizational standards without clinical studies to support recommendations.

Level M Manufacturer's recommendations only.

Actions for Nursing Practice:

- Ensure that your health care facility has written policies and procedures that support family presence during resuscitation and invasive procedures.
- Policies and procedures, and educational programs for professional staff should include the following components:
  - Benefits of family presence for the patient and family.[23]
  - Criteria for assessing the family to ensure uninterrupted patient care.[9,20,23]
  - Role of the family facilitator in preparing families for being at the bedside and supporting them before, during, and after the event, including handling the development of untoward reactions by family members.[21-22,34,41] Family facilitators may include nurses, physicians, social workers, chaplains, child life specialists, respiratory care practitioners, family therapists, and nursing students.[20,23,41]
  - Support for patient's or family members' decision not to have family members present.[23]
  - Contraindications to family presence (for example, family members who demonstrate combative or violent behaviors; uncontrolled emotional outbursts; behaviors consistent with an altered mental state from drugs or alcohol; or those suspected of abuse).[9,20,22-23]
- Develop proficiency standards for all staff involved in family presence to ensure patient, family, and staff safety.
- Determine your unit's rate of compliance in offering families the option of family presence during resuscitation and invasive procedures. If compliance is ≤90%, develop a plan to improve compliance:
  - Consider forming a multidisciplinary task force (e.g., nurses, physicians, chaplains, social workers, child life specialists) or a unit core group of staff to discuss approaches to improve compliance.
  - Re-educate staff about family presence; discuss the intervention as a component of family-centered care and evidence-based practice.
  - Incorporate content into orientation programs as well as initial and annual competency verifications.
  - Develop a variety of communications strategies to alert and remind staff about the family presence option.
- Develop documentation standards for family presence and include rationale for when family presence would not be offered as an option to family members.

Need More Information or Help?

- Go to www.aacn.org and select Practice Resource Network.
- The guidelines for "Presenting the Option for Family Presence,"[23] developed by the Emergency Nurses Association and endorsed by AACN, are suitable for adaptation to critical care units and include educational slides and handouts, a family presence department assessment tool, a staff assessment tool, an educational needs assessment tool, a sample family presence guideline, and other supporting documents. This resource (Product #120632) is available online at www.aacn.org or by calling (800) 899-2226.
- AACN endorses the American College of Chest Physician's Critical Care Family Assistance Program. This toolkit empowers you and your team to create a family-friendly critical care environment at your hospital. This resource (Product #120631) is available online at www.aacn.org or by calling (800) 899-2226.

Continued

BOX 1-2   AACN PRACTICE ALERT
Family Presence During Resuscitation and Invasive Procedures—cont'd

References:

1. Bauchner H, Waring C, Vinci R. Parental presence during procedures in an emergency room: Results from 50 observations. *Pediatrics*. 1991;87(4):544.
2. Sacchetti A, Lichenstein R, Carraccio CA, et al. Family member presence during pediatric emergency department procedures. *Pediatr Emerg Care*. 1996;12(4):268.
3. Belanger MS, Reed S. A rural community hospital's experience with family-witnessed resuscitation. *J Emerg Nurs*. 1997;23(3):238.
4. Barratt F, Wallis DN. Relatives in the resuscitation room: their point of view. *J Accid Emerg Med*. 1999;16(1):109.
5. Meyers TA, Eichhorn DJ, Guzzetta CE. Do families want to be present during CPR? A retrospective survey. *J Emerg Nurs*. 1998;24(5):400.
6. Boie ET, Moore GP, Brommett C, et al. Do parents want to be present during invasive procedures performed on their children in the emergency department? A survey of 400 parents. *Ann Emerg Med*. 1999;34(1):70.
7. Powers KS, Rubenstein JS. Family presence during invasive procedures in the pediatric intensive care unit: a prospective study. *Arch Pediatr Adolesc Med*. 1999;153(9):955.
8. Meyers TA, Eichhorn DJ, Guzzetta CE, et al. Family presence during invasive procedures and resuscitation: the experiences of family members, nurses, and physicians. *Am J Nurs*. 2000;100(2):32.
9. Mangurten J, Owens J, Vinson L, et al. *Family presence during resuscitation interventions and invasive procedures in a pediatric emergency department: attitudes and experiences of healthcare providers and family members*. Unpublished data. Dallas: Children's Medical Center of Dallas; 2004.
10. Mangurten J, Scott SH, Guzzetta CE, et al. Effects of family presence during resuscitation and invasive procedures in a pediatric emergency department. *J Emerg Nurs*. 2006;32(3):225.
11. Tinsley C, Hill JB, Shah J, et al. Experience of families during cardiopulmonary resuscitation in a pediatric intensive care unit. *Pediatrics*. 2008;122(4):e799.
12. NBC Dateline Poll. *Should family members of patients be allowed in the emergency department during emergency procedures?* Available at: http://www.nbc.com. Accessed August 17, 1999.
13. USA Today Poll. *Would you want to be in the emergency department while doctors worked on a family member?* USA Today. Available at: http://www.usatoday.com. Accessed March 7, 2000.
14. Mazer MA, Cox LA, Capon A. The public's attitude and perception concerning witnessed cardiopulmonary resuscitation. *Crit Care Med*. 2006;34(12):2925.
15. Eckle N, Haley K, Baker P, eds. *Emergency Nursing Pediatric Course: Provider Manual*. 2nd ed. Park Ridge, IL: Emergency Nurses Association; 1998.
16. Jacobs BB, Hoyt KS, eds. *Trauma Nursing Core Course: Provider Manual*. 5th ed. Park Ridge, IL: Emergency Nurses Association; 2000.
17. Royal College of Nursing. *Witnessed resuscitation: guidance for nursing staff*. London: The College; 2002.
18. Guzzetta GE. Critical Care Research: Weaving a Body-Mind-Spirit Tapestry. *Am J Crit Care*. 2004;13(4):320.
19. 2005 American Heart Association Guidelines for Cardiopulmonary Resuscitation and Emergency Cardiovascular Care. Part 2 Ethical Issues and Part 12 Pediatric Advanced Life Support. *Circulation*. 2005;112(24 Suppl):IV6 and IV167.
20. Clark AP, Aldridge MD, Guzzetta CE, et al. Family presence during cardiopulmonary resuscitation. *Crit Care Nurs Clin North Am*. 2005;17(1):23.
21. Davidson JE, Powers K, Hedayat KM, et al. Clinical practice guidelines for support of the family in the patient-centered intensive care unit: American College of Critical Care Medicine Task Force 2004-2005. *Crit Care Med*. 2007;35(2):605.
22. Henderson DP, Knapp JF. Report of the national consensus conference on family presence during pediatric cardiopulmonary resuscitation and procedures. *J Emerg Nurs*. 2006;32(1):23.
23. Emergency Nurses Association. *Presenting the Option for Family Presence*. 3rd ed. Des Plaines, IL: Emergency Nurses Association; 2007 (www.ena.org).
24. Moons P, Norekval TM. European nursing organizations stand up for family presence during cardiopulmonary resuscitation: A joint position statement. *Prog Cardiovasc Nurs*. 2008;23(3):136.
25. MacLean SL, Guzzetta CE, White C, et al. Family presence during cardiopulmonary resuscitation and invasive procedures: practices of critical care and emergency nurses. *Am J Crit Care*. 2003;12(3):246-257 and *J Emerg Nurs* 2003;29(3):32.
26. Fallis WM, McClement S, Pereira A. Family presence during resuscitation: a survey of Canadian critical care nurses practices and perceptions. *Dynamics*. 2008;19(3):22.
27. Twibell RS, Siela D, Riwitis C, et al. Nurses' perceptions of their self-confidence and the benefits and risks of family presence during resuscitation. *Am J Crit Care*. 2008;17(2):101.
28. Wolfram RW, Turner ED. Effects of parental presence during children's venipuncture. *Acad Emerg Med*. 1996;3(1):58.
29. Gonzalez JC, Routh DK, Saab PG, et al. Effects of parent presence on children's reactions to injections: behavioral, physiological, and subjective aspects. *J Pediatr Psychol*. 1989;14(3):449.
30. Fiorentini SE. Evaluation of a new program: Pediatric parental visitation in the postanesthesia care unit. *J Post Anesth Nurs*. 1993;8(4):249.
31. Eichhorn DJ, Meyers TA, Guzzetta CE, et al. Family presence during invasive procedures and resuscitation: hearing the voice of the patient. *Am J Nurs*. 2001;101(5):26.
32. Robinson SM, Mackenzie-Ross S, Campbell-Hewson GL, et al. Psychological effect of witnessed resuscitation on bereaved relatives. *Lancet*. 1998;352(9128):614.
33. Doyle CJ, Post H, Burney RE, et al. Family participation during resuscitation: an option. *Ann Emerg Med*. 1987;16(6):673.
34. Hanson C, Strawser D. Family presence during cardiopulmonary resuscitation: Foote Hospital emergency department's nine-year perspective. *J Emerg Nurs*. 1992;18(2):104.
35. Timmermans S. High touch in high tech: the presence of relatives and friends during resuscitation efforts. *Sch Inq Nurs Pract*. 1997;11(2):153.
36. Powers KS, Rubenstein JS. Family presence during invasive procedures in the pediatric intensive care unit. *Arch Pediatr Adolesc Med*. 1999;153(9):955.
37. Shapira M, Tamir A. Presence of family member during upper endoscopy. What do patients and escorts think? *J Clin Gastroenterol*. 1996;22(4):272.
38. O'Connell KJ, Farah MM, Spandorfer P, et al. Family presence during pediatric trauma team activation: an assessment of a structured program. *Pediatrics*. 2007;120(3):e565.
39. Sachetti A, Paston C, Carraccio C. Family members do not disrupt care when present during invasive procedures. *Academic Emergency Medicine*. 2005;12(5):463.
40. Maxton FJ. Parental presence during resuscitation in the PICU: the parents' experience. Sharing and surviving the resuscitation: a phenomenological study. *J Clin Nurs*. 2008;17(23):3168.
41. Clark AP, Calvin AO, Meyers TA, et al. Family presence during cardiopulmonary resuscitation and invasive procedures: a research-based intervention. *Crit Care Nurs Clin North Am*. 2001;13(4):569.

among their cultural beliefs and practices and the level of their acculturation into the mainstream American culture.[25]

Unless cultural differences are taken into account, optimal health care cannot be provided. More attention has been directed recently at determining the physiologic differences and those of disease development and progression among various ethnic groups. An increased sensitivity to the health care needs and vulnerabilities of all groups must be developed by care providers.

Cultural competence is one way to ensure that individual differences related to culture are incorporated into the plan of care.[26-27] Nurses must possess knowledge about biocultural, psychosocial, and linguistic differences in diverse populations to make accurate assessments. Interventions must then be tailored to the uniqueness of each patient and family.

COMPLEMENTARY AND ALTERNATIVE THERAPIES

Consumer activism has increased, and consumers are advocating for quality health care that is cost-effective and humane. They are asking whether options other than traditional Western medical care exist for treating various diseases and disorders. The possibilities of using centuries-old practices that are considered alternative or complementary to current Western medicine have been in demand.[28-29] These types of therapies can be seen in all health care settings, including the critical care unit. Complementary therapies offer patients, families, and health care providers additional options to assist with healing and recovery.[30]

Two terms, alternative and complementary, have been in the mainstream for several years. *Alternative* denotes that a specific therapy is an option or alternative to what is considered conventional treatment of a condition or state. The term *complementary* was proposed to describe therapies that can be used to complement or support conventional treatments.[30] The remainder of this section includes a brief discussion about nontraditional complementary therapies that have been used in critical care areas.

Spirituality and Prayer

As persons search for meaning and guidance in critical, emergent, and unexpected tragic circumstances, spirituality becomes more important.[31] Likewise, health care practitioners turn to their own spirituality to manage stress and find answers to the health care issues that they face on an intense, daily basis. Spiritual practices consist of meditation, prayer, and spiritual materials and are based on personal values and beliefs.[32] Holt-Ashley[31] describes how to incorporate prayer into the critical care unit, concentrating on patients, their families, and the nurse. The study author also offers strategies for creating an environment that is conducive to spiritual well-being for patients and staff.

Guided Imagery

One of the most well-studied complementary therapies is guided imagery, a mind-body strategy that is frequently used to decrease stress, pain, and anxiety.[33] Additional benefits of guided imagery are: 1) decreased side effects; 2) decreased length of stay; 3) reduced hospital costs; 4) enhanced sleep; and 5) increased patient satisfaction.[33] Guided imagery is a low-cost intervention that is relatively simple to implement. The patient's involvement in the process offers a sense of empowerment and accomplishment and motivates self-care.

Massage

Back massage as a once-practiced part of routine care of patients has been eliminated for various reasons, including time constraints, greater use of technology, and increasing complexity of care requirements. However, there is a scientific basis for concluding that massage offers positive effects on physiologic and psychologic outcomes.

A comprehensive review of the literature revealed that the most common effect of massage was reduction in anxiety, with additional reports of a significant decrease in tension. There was also a positive physiologic response to massage in the areas of decreased respiratory and heart rates and decreased pain. The effects on sleep were inconclusive. The study authors concluded that massage was an effective complementary therapy for promoting relaxation and reducing pain, and they thought it should be incorporated into nursing practice.[34]

Animal-Assisted Therapy

The use of animals has increased as an adjunct to healing in the care of patients of all ages in various settings. Pet visitation programs have been created in various health care delivery settings,[35] including acute care, long-term care, and hospice. In the acute care setting, animals are brought in to provide additional solace and comfort for patients who are critically or terminally ill. Fish aquariums are used in patient areas and family areas, because they humanize the surroundings. Scientific evidence indicates that animal-assisted therapy results in positive patient outcomes in the areas of attention, mobility, and orientation. Other reports have shown improved communication and mood in patients.[36]

NURSING'S UNIQUE ROLE IN HEALTH CARE

Today's health care environment necessitates a nursing framework that is flexible and responsive to the needs of the public that is served. The American Nurses Association (ANA) has defined nursing as the "protection, promotion, and optimization of health, and abilities, prevention of illness and injury, alleviation of suffering through the diagnosis and treatment of human response, and advocacy in the care of individuals, families, communities, and populations."[37] Although nursing has independent and dependent nursing actions, it is essential that an interdependence with all health care professionals is actualized.

CRITICAL CARE NURSING PRACTICE

Researchers have studied critical care nurses to better understand their clinical judgment and interventions and the link

---

BOX 1-3   CATEGORIES OF CRITICAL CARE NURSING THOUGHT, ACTION, AND PRACTICE

Thought and Action
- Clinical grasp and clinical inquiry: problem identification and clinical problem solving
- Clinical forethought: anticipating and preventing potential problems

Practice
- Diagnosing and managing life-sustaining physiologic functions in unstable patients
- Managing a crisis by using skilled know-how
- Providing comfort measures for the critically ill
- Caring for patients' families
- Preventing hazards in a technologic environment
- Facing death: end-of-life care and decision making
- Communicating and negotiating multiple perspectives
- Monitoring quality and managing breakdown
- Exhibiting the skilled know-how of clinical leadership and the coaching and mentoring of others

---

between the two. They identified two major categories of thought and action and nine categories of practice that illustrate clinical judgment and the clinical knowledge development of critical care nurses.[38] These major categories are delineated in Box 1-3.

The Nursing Process

The nursing process is a method for making clinical decisions. It is a way of thinking and acting in relation to the clinical phenomena of concern by nurses. The nursing process is a systematic decision-making model that is cyclic, not linear. By virtue of its evaluation phase, the nursing process incorporates a feedback loop that maintains quality control of its decision-making outputs. The nursing process is a method for solving clinical problems, but it is not merely a problem-solving method. Similar to a problem-solving method, the nursing process offers an organized, systematic approach to clinical problems. Unlike a problem-solving method, the nursing process is continuous, not episodic.

Nursing Diagnosis

The North American Nursing Diagnosis Association (NANDA) has supported the continued development and evolution of research-based nursing diagnoses.[39] With nursing diagnosis as a component of the decision-making method, there is a more systematic collection and interpretation of data. The most essential and distinguishing feature of any nursing diagnosis is that it describes a health condition *primarily resolved by nursing interventions or therapies.*

Nursing Interventions

Also known as *nursing orders* or *nursing prescriptions*, nursing interventions constitute the treatment approach to an identified health alteration. Interventions are selected to satisfy the outcome criteria and prevent or resolve the nursing diagnosis.

It is important to link diagnostic labels with interventions and nurse-sensitive outcomes so that a consistent framework is available for evaluating nursing interventions and outcomes.

Intervention strategies that consist solely of monitoring, measuring, checking, obtaining physician orders, documenting, reporting, and notifying do not completely fulfill criteria for the treatment of a problem. Nursing interventions for nursing diagnoses designate therapeutic activity that assists the patient in moving from one state of health to another. Medically delegated actions, such as administering medications and initiating ventilator setting changes, are included in the interventions but with the emphasis placed squarely on the assessments and judgments the nurse makes in evaluating their effectiveness, patient tolerance, safety, dosage, titration, and discontinuance.

The Nursing Interventions Classification (NIC) framework contains 544 nursing interventions that are categorized into 30 classes and 7 domains.[40] Many nursing interventions are directly linked with NANDA nursing diagnoses. *Nurse-initiated treatments* are interventions initiated by the nurse in response to a nursing diagnosis. The use of the NIC framework facilitates clinical decision making and provides a standardized language that describes the core of essential nursing interventions. An example of an NIC nursing intervention on surveillance is presented in Box 1-4. The research base provides a method to link diagnoses with outcomes in the evaluation of care and services.[40]

Outcomes Evaluation

Evaluation of attainment of the expected patient outcomes occurs formally at intervals designated in the outcome criteria. Informal evaluation occurs continuously. The evaluation phase and the activities that take place within it are perhaps the most important dimensions of the nursing process. Evaluation of a patient's progress against a standard of nursing care management incorporates accountability into the process—accountability to the standard of care. Lack of progress in outcome attainment or lack of progress in problem solving is readily identified and kept in check, and alternate solutions can then be proposed.

TECHNOLOGY IN CRITICAL CARE

The growth in technologies has been seen throughout health care, especially in critical care settings. All providers are challenged to learn new equipment, monitoring devices, and related therapies that contribute to care and services. Take, for example, the evolving electronic health record (EHR) that was originally designed to capture data for clinical decision making and to increase the efficiency of health care providers. There are complexities inherent in providing a "user-friendly" EHR. Thus, one that meets the needs and reflects the thought processes and actual work flow of diverse clinicians has been greatly lacking. Add to that the fact that staff-created "work-arounds" to some of the software/procedures have not significantly reduced errors or increased productivity. There is a tremendous amount of data, but those data are not turned into meaningful information

◎ BOX 1-4   NIC

Surveillance

Definition

Purposeful and ongoing acquisition, interpretation, and synthesis of patient data for clinical decision making

Activities

Determine patient's health risks, as appropriate

Obtain information about normal behavior and routines

Ask patient for her or his perception of health status

Select appropriate patient indices for ongoing monitoring, based on patient's condition

Determine presence of patient trigger areas for immediate response (e.g., change in vital signs, low or elevated heart rate, low or elevated blood pressure, difficulty breathing, low oxygen saturation despite increasing oxygen delivery, change in level of consciousness, repeated or prolonged seizures, chest pain, acute changes in mental status, or when nurse or patient "just feels something is wrong")

Activate the rapid response team if indicated by presence of trigger areas per agency protocol

Ask patient about recent signs, symptoms, or problems

Establish the frequency of data collection and interpretation, as indicated by status of the patient

Monitor unstable or critically ill stable patients (e.g., patients who require frequent neurologic assessments, patients experiencing cardiac dysrhythmias, patients receiving continuous intravenous infusions of medications such as nitroglycerine or insulin)

Facilitate acquisition of diagnostic tests, as appropriate

Interpret results of diagnostic tests, as appropriate

Retrieve and interpret laboratory data

Contact physician, as appropriate

Explain diagnostic test results to patient and families

Involve patient and family in monitoring activities, as appropriate

Monitor patient's ability to do self-care activities

Monitor neurological status

Monitor behavior patterns

Monitor cognitive ability

Monitor emotional state

Monitor vital signs, as appropriate

Collaborate with physician to institute invasive hemodynamic monitoring, as appropriate

Collaborate with physician to institute ICP monitoring, as appropriate

Monitor comfort level, and take appropriate action

Monitor coping strategies used by patient and family

Monitor changes in sleep patterns

Monitor oxygenation and initiate measures to promote adequate oxygenation of vital organs

Initiate routine skin surveillance in high-risk patient

Monitor for signs and symptoms of fluid and electrolyte imbalance

Monitor tissue perfusion, as appropriate

Monitor for infection, as appropriate

Monitor nutritional status, as appropriate

Monitor gastrointestinal function, as appropriate

Monitor elimination patterns, as appropriate

Monitor for bleeding tendencies in high-risk patient

Note type and amount of drainage from tubes and orifices and notify the physician of significant changes

Troubleshoot equipment and systems to enhance acquisition of reliable patient data

Compare current status with previous status to detect improvements and deterioration in patient's condition

Initiate and/or change medical treatment to maintain patient parameters within the limits ordered by the physician, using established protocols

Facilitate acquisition of interdisciplinary services (e.g., pastoral services or audiology), as appropriate

Obtain a physician consult when patient data indicates a needed change in medical therapy

Institute appropriate treatment, using standing protocols

Prioritize actions, based on patient status

Analyze physician orders in conjunction with patient status to ensure safety of the patient

Obtain consultation from the appropriate health care worker to initiate new treatment or change existing treatments

Provide proper environment for desirable patient outcomes (e.g., match nurse competency to patient care needs; provide required patient to nurse ratio; provide adequate auxiliary staffing; ensure continuity of care)

From Bulechek GM, et al, eds. *Nursing Interventions Classification (NIC).* 6th ed. St. Louis: Mosby; 2013.

on which to make decisions.[41] For this reason, it is important that critical care nurses are involved in the selection, trial, education, and evaluation of any health care informatics technologies that are being considered for their practice areas. Nurse informaticians, clinical nurse specialists, educators, and managers are also essential in the selection processes so that all aspects are considered.[42] Another area for critical care nurse involvement is in assessing new products that come into the system. Often, there are numerous "avenues" that products enter, such as product fairs, individual physicians, vendors, and supply departments, to name a few. It is important that all proposed new products are overseen by a central committee or group who establishes criteria by which to select, pilot, evaluate, adopt, and communicate about the new product. Some criteria that can be used in the initial assessment are: 1) clinical relevance; 2) clinical void; 3) cost; 4) extra costs; and 5) safety.[43] This type of process ensures consistency and the same standards regarding product selection across the organization.

A more recent opportunity for critical care nurses is working in a role that encompasses the Tele-ICU. Telemedicine was initially employed in outpatient areas, remote, rural geographic locations, and areas where there was a dearth of medical providers. Currently, there are Tele-ICUs in areas where there are limited resources on site. However, there are experts (critical care nurses, intensivists) located in a central distant site. Technologies relay continuous surveillance with monitoring information and communication among care providers. Each Tele-ICU varies in size and location; the key component is the availability of back-up experts. Goran describes competencies for critical care nurses who practice in a Tele-ICU.[44]

INTERPROFESSIONAL COLLABORATIVE PRACTICE

The growing managed care environment has placed emphasis on examining methods of care delivery and processes of care by all health care professionals. Collaboration and partnerships have been shown to increase quality of care and services while containing or decreasing costs.[45-50] It is more important than ever to create and enhance partnerships, because the resulting interdependence and collaboration among disciplines is essential to achieving positive patient outcomes. A recent article reported a study in which physician-nurse relationships improved collaboration after meeting together to create a method to change the unit culture. They met together to examine collaboratively on what the issues were and create strategies to resolve them. There were higher scores on openness of communication within groups, between groups, accuracy between groups, and overall collaboration.[51]

The Interprofessional Education Collaborative (IEC) published their *Core Competencies for Interprofessional Collaborative Practice* in 2011. The IEC sponsors include the American associations of nursing, dentistry, medicine, osteopathy, public health, and pharmacy. Their goal was to establish a set of competencies to serve as a framework for professional socialization of health care professionals. They also intended to assess the relevance of the competencies and develop an action plan for implementation.[52] These competencies are especially important at this time as we move forward with health care reform and explore innovative care delivery models using the skill sets of all health care providers in the most effective and efficient manner. Box 1-5 delineates the four core competencies.

INTERDISCIPLINARY CARE MANAGEMENT MODELS AND TOOLS

Several models of care delivery and care management are used in health care. An overview of the various terms and models are presented in this chapter, but it is a good idea to seek additional resources and consultation for a more in-depth explanation of the models.

Care Management

Care management is a system of integrated processes designed to enable, support, and coordinate patient care throughout the continuum of health care services. Care management takes place in many different settings; care is delivered by various professional health care team members and nonlicensed providers, as appropriate.

Coordination of care and services may be done by the health care staff or the insurance or payer staff. Care management must be patient focused, continuum driven, and results oriented, and it must employ a team approach. Another term associated with this model of care is *disease state management*, which connotes the process of managing a population's health over a lifetime. In disease state management, however, there is a focus on managing complex and chronic disease states, such as diabetes or heart failure, over the entire continuum.

Case Management

Case management is the process of overseeing the care of patients and organizing services in collaboration with the patient's physician or primary health care provider. The case manager may be a nurse, allied health care provider, or the patient's primary care provider. Case managers are usually assigned to a specific population group and facilitate effective coordination of care services as patients move in and out of different settings. Ideally, the case manager oversees the care of the patient across the continuum of care.

Care Management Tools

Many quality improvement tools are available to providers for care management. The three evidence-based tools addressed in this chapter are clinical algorithm, practice guideline, and protocol.[53] All of these tools may be embedded in the EHR.

Algorithm

An *algorithm* is a stepwise decision-making flowchart for a specific care process or processes. Algorithms guide the clinician through the "if, then" decision-making process, addressing patient responses to particular treatments. Well-known examples of algorithms are the advanced cardiac life support (ACLS) algorithms published by the American Heart Association. Weaning, medication selection, medication titration, individual practitioner variance, and appropriate patient placement algorithms have been developed to give practitioners additional standardized decision-making abilities.

Practice Guideline

A *practice guideline* is usually created by an expert panel and developed by a professional organization (e.g., AACN, Society of Critical Care Medicine, American College of Cardiology, government agencies such as the Agency for Health Care Research and Quality [AHRQ]). Practice guidelines are generally written

---

BOX 1-5 **CORE COMPETENCIES FOR INTERPROFESSIONAL COLLABORATIVE PRACTICE**

Values/Ethics for Interprofessional Practice
- Work with individuals of other professions to maintain a climate of mutual respect and shared values.

Roles/Responsibilities for Collaborative Practice
- Use the knowledge of one's own role and the role of other professions to appropriately assess and address the health care needs of the patients and populations served.

Interprofessional Communication
- Communicate with patients, families, communities, and other health professionals in a responsive and responsible manner that supports a team approach to maintaining health and treatment of disease.

Interprofessional Teamwork and Team-Based Care
- Apply relationship-building values and principles of team dynamics to perform effectively in different team roles to plan and deliver patient/population-centered care that is safe, timely, efficient, effective, and equitable.

in text prose style rather than in the flowchart format of algorithms.

Protocol

A *protocol* is a common tool in research studies. Protocols are more directive and rigid than guidelines, and providers are not supposed to vary from a protocol. Patients are screened carefully for specific entry criteria before being started on a protocol. There are many national research protocols, such as those for cancer and chemotherapy studies. Protocols are helpful when built-in *alerts* signal the provider to potentially serious problems. Computerization of protocols assists providers in being more proactive regarding dangerous medication interactions, abnormal laboratory values, and other untoward effects that are preprogrammed into the computer.

Order Set

An *order set* consists of preprinted provider orders that are used to expedite the order process after a standard has been validated through analytic review of practice and research. Order sets complement and increase compliance with existing practice standards. They can also be used to represent the algorithm or protocol in order format.

Managing and Tracking Variances

All variances must be addressed and managed in a timely manner by the health care team members. All of the previously described tools provide methods to track variances. Whether variance coding is included in the EHR or is tracked by another quality improvement method, the individual and aggregate data must be assessed and analyzed. Except for protocols, which are more rigid and research based, algorithms and guidelines can be used according to the practitioner's discretion. Tracking variances from the expected standard is one method to determine the utility of the tools in particular settings and patient populations. There must be a link between the care management system and the quality improvement program so that changes, as appropriate, can be made to positively affect the outcomes of care and services.

QUALITY, SAFETY, AND REGULATORY ISSUES IN CRITICAL CARE

Quality and Safety Issues

Patient safety has become a major focus of attention by health care consumers, providers of care, and administrators of health care institutions. The Institute of Medicine (IOM) publication *Crossing the Quality Chasm: A New Health System for the 21st Century* was the impetus for debate and actions to improve the safety of health care environments. In this seminal report, information and details were given indicating that health care harms patients too frequently and routinely fails to deliver its potential benefits.[54] Often, the definitions of medical errors and approaches to resolving patient safety issues differ among nurses, physicians, administrators, and other health care providers.[55] Subsequently through its use of expert panels, the IOM

has published numerous other important reports related to quality, safety, and the nursing environment.

Patient safety has been described as an ethical imperative, and one that is inherent in health care professionals' actions and interpersonal processes.[56] In critical care units errors may occur because of the hectic, complex environment, where there is little room for error and safety is essential.[56-57] In this environment, patients are particularly vulnerable because of their compromised physiologic status, multiple technologic and pharmacologic interventions, and multiple care providers who frequently work at a fast pace. It is essential that care delivery processes that minimize the opportunity for errors are designed and that a "safety culture" rather than a "blame culture" is created.[58] One author discussed results of a research study in which nurses were hesitant to report medication errors or unsafe practices so that they would not be ridiculed or "talked about" by their peer nurses. This uncivil behavior was thought to continue to contribute to an unsafe environment and one in which true error or unsafe practices and systems were greatly unreported.[59]

Medication administration continues to be one of the most error-prone nursing interventions for the critical care nurse.[60] Many medication errors are related to system failures, with distraction as a major factor. Various interventions have been created in an attempt to decrease medication errors. One article reported establishing a "no interruption zone" for medication safety in a critical care unit. In this pilot study, there was a 40% decrease in interruptions from the baseline measurement. Although researchers questioned the feasibility of sustaining this decrease in interruptions in the future,[61] this is an example of an approach that could be used to increase medication safety in the critical care unit.

When an injury or inappropriate care occurs, it is crucial that health care professionals promptly give an explanation of how the injury or mistake occurred and the short- or long-term effects on the patient and family. They should be informed that the factors involved in the injury will be investigated so that steps can be taken to reduce or prevent the likelihood of similar injury to other patients.

It has been shown that intimidating and disruptive clinician behaviors can lead to errors and preventable adverse patient outcomes. Verbal outbursts, physical threats, and more passive behaviors such as refusing to carry out a task or procedure are all under this category. Unfortunately, these types of behavior are not rare in health care organizations. If these behaviors go unaddressed, it can lead to extreme dissatisfaction, depression, and turnover. There also may be systems issues that lead to or perpetuate these situations, such as push for increased productivity, financial constraints, fear of litigation, and embedded hierarchies in the organization.[58]

Technologies are both a solution to error-prone procedures and functions, and another potential cause for error. Consider bar-code medication administration procedures, multiple bedside testing devices, computerized medical records, bedside monitoring, computerized physician order entry (CPOE), and many other technologies now in development. Each in itself can be a great assistance to the clinician, but must be monitored for effectiveness and accuracy to ensure the best in outcomes as intended for specific use.[60]

Quality and Safety Regulations

There are numerous regulations governing health care, including local, state, national, Medicare/Medicaid, and payer requirements. However, for purposes of this chapter, key regulations and accreditation standards impacting the majority of critical care areas will be discussed.

The Joint Commission (TJC) is an independent, not-for-profit organization that certifies more than 19,000 health care organizations in the United States. Its goal is to evaluate these health care entities using their pre-established standards of performance to ensure high levels of care are provided in these entities. Annually, it establishes National Patient Safety Goals (NPSGs)[62] that are to be implemented in health care organizations (Box 1-6).

The Safe Medical Device Act (SMDA) requires that hospitals report serious or potentially serious device-related injuries or illness of patients and/or employees to the manufacturer of the device, and if death is involved, to the U.S. Food and Drug Administration (FDA). In addition, implantable devices must be documented and tracked.[63-] This reporting serves as an early warning system so that the FDA can obtain information on device problems. Failure to comply with the act will result in civil action.

Quality and Safety Resources

The Institute for Safe Medication Practices (ISMP) is a not-for-profit organization dedicated to medication error prevention and safe medication use. It has numerous tools to assist care providers, including newsletters, education programs, safety alerts, consulting, patient education materials, error reporting system, and more. One newsletter is devoted specifically to nurses. It offers a very comprehensive array of tools.[64]

The Institute for Healthcare Improvement (IHI) is an interdisciplinary organization focused on quality that also offers many tools and resources: educational materials, conferences, case studies, publications, white papers, quality measure tools, plus many more. IHI developed the "bundle" concept, which consists of EBPs on specific high-risk quality issues as determined by a multidisciplinary group. There are many bundles published by IHI, such as central line, ventilator, and sepsis.[65] The National Quality Forum (NQF) is also a not-for-profit

organization that facilitates consensus-building with multiple partners to establish national priorities and goals for performance improvement. They also establish common definitions and consistent measurement. In addition, their goal is that all health care providers and stakeholders are educated regarding quality, priorities, and outcomes.[66] The Healthcare Information and Management Systems Society (HIMSS) is an interdisciplinary organization focused on patient safety and quality of care. They specifically focus on integration of patient safety tools and practices to enhance communication, quality, efficiency, productivity, and clinical support systems.[67] A national quality database devoted entirely to nursing is the National Database of Nursing Quality Indicators (NDNQI). The program provides ongoing nurse-sensitive indicator consultation and research-based expertise. Their mission is to aid the registered nurse in patient safety and quality improvement efforts. It is the only nursing national quality measurement program that provides hospitals with unit-level quality performance comparison reports.[68]

The Quality and Safety Education for Nurses (QSEN) project established standards for educating registered nurses at the baccalaureate and master' levels of academic education. In this model, the knowledge, skills, and attitudes (KSAs) were created so that nurses would be able to continuously improve the quality and safety of the health care systems for which they work. There are six major categories that delineate the KSAs for each section (Box 1-7).[69] Boxes that address one of the QSEN competencies will be presented throughout the book, with the QSEN icon **QSEN** appearing in them. Box 1-8, Internet

---

BOX 1-6 2012 HOSPITAL NATIONAL PATIENT SAFETY GOALS

- Identify patients correctly
- Improve staff communication
- Use medications safely
- Prevent infection
- Identify patient safety risks
- Prevent mistakes in surgery

From the *Joint Commission Accreditation Program*. Hospital national patient safety goals. Oak Brook Terrace, IL: 2012; The Joint Commission.

BOX 1-7 QUALITY AND SAFETY EDUCATION FOR NURSES (QSEN) COMPETENCIES

QSEN
- Patient-Centered Care
  - Recognize the patient or designee as the source of control and full partner in providing compassionate and coordinated care based on respect for patient's preferences, values, and needs.
- Teamwork and Collaboration
  - Function effectively within nursing and interprofessional teams, fostering open communication, mutual respect, and shared decision-making to achieve quality patient care.
- Evidence-Based Practice
  - Integrate best current evidence with clinical expertise and patient/family preferences and values for delivery of optimal health care.
- Quality Improvement
  - Use data to monitor the outcomes of care processes and use improvement methods to design and test changes to continuously improve the quality and safety of health care systems.
- Safety
  - Minimizes risk of harm to patients and providers through both system effectiveness and individual performance.
- Informatics
  - Use information and technology to communicate, manage knowledge, mitigate error, and support decision making.

From Cronenwett L, Sherwood G, Barnsteiner J, et al. Quality and safety education for nurses. *Nursing Outlook.* 2007;55(3):122.

BOX 1-9   HEALTHY WORK ENVIRONMENT STANDARDS

Standard I: Skilled Communication
Nurses must be as proficient in communication skills as they are in clinical skills.

Standard II: True Collaboration
Nurses must be relentless in pursuing and fostering true collaboration.

Standard III: Effective Decision Making
Nurses must be valued and committed partners in making policy, directing and evaluating clinical care, and leading organizational operations.

Standard IV: Appropriate Staffing
Staffing must ensure the effective match between patient needs and nurse competencies.

Standard V: Meaningful Recognition
Nurses must be recognized and must recognize others for the value each brings to the work of the organization.

Standard VI: Authentic Leadership
Nurse leaders must fully embrace the imperative of a healthy work environment, authentically live it, and engage others in its achievement.

From *American Association of Critical-Care Nurses (AACN). Standards for establishing and sustaining healthy work environments. Aliso Viejo, CA: 2005; AACN.

Resources, lists the website addresses of all of the quality, safety, and regulatory resources detailed above.

PRIVACY AND CONFIDENTIALITY

A landmark law was passed to provide consumers with greater access to health care insurance, promote more standardization and efficiency in the health care industry, and protect the privacy of health care data.[70] The Health Insurance Portability and Accountability Act of 1996 (HIPAA) has created additional challenges for health care organizations and providers because of the stringent requirements and additional resources needed to meet the requirements of the law. Most specific to critical care clinicians is the privacy and confidentiality related to protection of health care data. This has implications when interacting with family members and others, and the oftentimes very close work environment, tight working spaces, and emergency situations. Clinicians are referred to their organizational policies and procedures for specific procedures for their organizations.

HEALTHY WORK ENVIRONMENT

The health care environment is stressful, and increasing challenges in the areas of financial constraints, regulatory requirements, consumer scrutiny, quickly changing technologies and treatment regimens, and workforce diversity contribute to conflicts and difficulties on a daily basis. In this environment, it is essential to offer support for health care providers that can mitigate these challenges and ensure a healthy place to work.

There is an increasing amount of evidence that unhealthy work environments lead to medical errors, suboptimal safety monitoring, ineffective communication among health care providers, and increased conflict and stress among care providers. Synthesis of research in the area of work environment has demonstrated that a combination of leadership styles and characteristics contributes to the development and sustainability of healthy work environments.[71]

The AACN has formulated standards for establishing and sustaining healthy work environments (HWE).[72] The intent of the standards is to promote creation of environments that will have a positive impact on nursing and patient outcomes. Evidence-based and relationship-centered principles were used to create the standards of professional performance. A summary of the six standards is provided in Box 1-9. Figure 1-1 illustrates the interdependence of each standard, and the ultimate impact on optimal patient outcomes and clinical excellence.

Everyone has a role in creating and sustaining a healthy work environment. Although the manager has a major role in establishing the culture, it is the staff who greatly impact the culture by mentoring new staff, role modeling behaviors, and leading interdisciplinary teams. It is this peer pressure that has the most impact on all other staff.[73-74] Bylone discussed her experience of talking with many staff members about how they think that they can influence the work unit culture. She recommends asking them how they influence each of the HWE standards, thus making it a personal experience and journey in achieving the HWE.[75] Kupperschmidt and colleagues posed a five-factor model for becoming a skilled communicator: 1) becoming aware of self-deception; 2) becoming authentic; 3) becoming candid; 4) becoming mindful; and 5) becoming reflective; all of which lead to being a skilled communicator, thus creating a healthy work environment.[76] An additional approach for implementing the HWE model was offered by Blake, who suggested five steps: 1) rallying the team; 2) surveying the team; 3) establishing work groups; 4) setting goals and developing action steps; and 5) celebrating successes along the way.[77] Whatever approach taken will depend on the passion and commitment of the team.

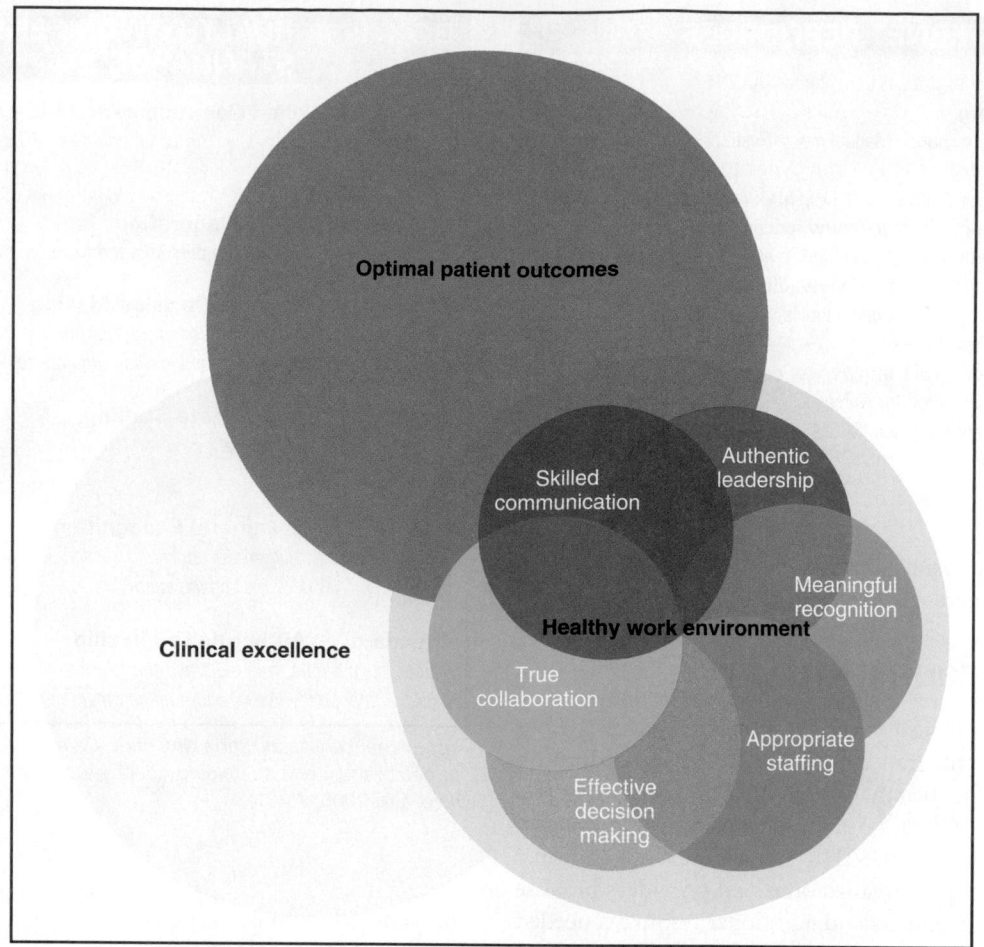

FIGURE 1-1 Interdependence of Healthy Work Environment, Clinical Excellence, and Optimal Patient Outcomes. (From *American Association of Critical-Care Nurses [AACN]*. Standards for establishing and sustaining healthy work environments. Aliso Viejo, CA: AACN; 2005.)

SUMMARY

- Sensitivity to appropriate times to eliminate or modify practices and adopt innovations is key to maintaining quality, cost-effective care delivery.
- It is essential for nurses to use the best data available to make patient care decisions and to carry out the appropriate interventions.
- The critical care nurse must be able to deliver high-quality care skillfully, using all appropriate technologies while incorporating psychosocial and other holistic approaches as appropriate to the time and condition of the patient.
- Nurses must possess knowledge about biocultural, psychosocial, and linguistic differences in diverse populations to make accurate assessments and plan interventions.

- Although nursing has independent and dependent nursing actions, it is essential that an interdependence with all health care providers is actualized.
- Multiple quality indicators have been developed for critical care; nurses are pivotal in quality monitoring and improvement.
- AACN Practice Alerts are succinct, evidence-based directives for critical care nurses and other health care providers to ensure that the most current evidence is used to provide safe care.
- A healthy work environment is essential for establishing a collaborative, trusting, and safe environment for the delivery of patient care.

REFERENCES

1. *Society of Critical Care Medicine. About SCCM: History of critical care.* http://www.sccm.org. Accessed June 2012.
2. *American Association of Critical Care Nurses. About critical care nursing.* http://www.aacn.org. Accessed June 2012.
3. Jost SG, Bonnell M, Chako SJ, Parkinson DL. Integrated primary nursing: a care delivery model for the 21st-century knowledge worker. *Nurs Admin Q.* 2010;34(3):208.
4. Stacy KM. Progressive care units: different but the same. *Crit Care Nurse.* 2011;31(3):77.

5. *American Association of Critical Care Nurses.* Progressive care unit fact sheet.. http://www.aacn.org. Accessed June 2012.

6. *American Association of Critical Care Nurses.* About critical care nursing. http://www.aacn.org. Accessed June 2012.

7. *American Association of Critical Care Nurses.* AACN Fact Sheet. http://www.aacn.org. Accessed June 2012.

8. *American Association of Critical Care Nurses.* Value of certification resource center. http://www.aacn.org. Accessed June 2012.

9. *American Association of Critical Care Nurses.* Welcome to the beacon award for excellence. http://www.aacn.org. Accessed June 2012.

10. Makic MB, VonRueden KT, Rauen CA, Chadwick J. Evidence-based practice habits: putting more sacred cows out to pasture. *Crit Care Nurse.* 2011;31(2):38.

11. Cullen L, Adams SL. Planning for implementation of evidence-based practice. *JONA.* 2012;42(4):222.

12. Titler MG, et al. The Iowa model of evidence-based practice to promote quality care. *Crit Care Nurs Clin North Am.* 2001;13(4):497.

13. Newhouse R. Do we know how much the evidence-based intervention cost? *JONA.* 2010;40(7/8):296.

14. Schifalacqua MM, Soukup M, Kelley W, Mason AR. Does evidence-based nursing increase ROI? *Am Nurse Today.* 2012;7(1):32.

15. Schulman CS, Staul L. Standards for frequency of measurement and documentation of vital signs and physical assessments. *Crit Care Nurse.* 2010;30(3):74.

16. Gray M. Reducing catheter-associated urinary tract infection in the critical care unit. *AACN Adv Crit Care.* 2010;21(3):247.

17. *American Association of Critical Care Nurses.* Practice alert. http://www.aacn.org. Accessed Sept 2012.

18. Panting K. Intensive care/intensive cure: the future of critical care? *Crit Care Nurse.* 1995;15(12):100.

19. Miller KL. Keeping the care in nursing care: our biggest challenge. *J Nurse Adm.* 1995;25(11):29-32.

20. Patistea E, Siamanta H. A literature review of patients' compared with nurses' perceptions of caring: implications for practice and research. *J Prof Nurs.* 1999;15(5):302.

21. Mariano C. Holistic ethics. *AJN.* 2001;101(1):24A.

22. Warren NA. The phenomenon of nurses' caring behaviors as perceived by the critical care family. *Crit Care Nurs Q.* 1994;17(3):67.

23. Powers PH, et al. The value of patient- and family-centered care. *Am J Nurs.* 2000;100(5):84.

24. Collins KS, Hall A. *US Minority Health: A Chart Book.* Commonwealth Fund; 1999.

25. Bushy A. Social and cultural factors affecting health care and nursing practice. In: Lancaster J, ed. *Nursing: Issues in Leading and Managing Change.* St. Louis: Mosby; 1999.

26. Gonzales R, et al. Eliminating racial and ethnic disparities in health care. *Am J Nurs.* 2000;100(3):56.

27. Leonard B, Plotnikoff GA. Awareness: the heart of cultural competence. *AACN Clin Issues.* 2000;11(1):51.

28. Lindquist R, Kirksey K. Preface. *AACN Clin Issues.* 2000;11(1):1.

29. Lindquist R, et al. Challenges of implementing a feasibility study of acupuncture in acute and critical care settings. *AACN Adv Crit Care.* 2008;19(2):202.

30. Kreitzer MJ, Jensen D. Healing practices: trends, challenges, and opportunities for nurses in critical care. *AACN Clin Issues.* 2000;11(1):7.

31. Holt-Ashley M. Nurses pray: use of prayer and spirituality as a complementary therapy in the intensive care setting. *AACN Clin Issues.* 2000;11(1):60.

32. Eldridge CR. Meeting your patients' spiritual needs. *Am Nurse Today.* 2007;2(10):51.

33. Tusek DL, Cwynar RE. Strategies for implementing guided imagery program to enhance patient experience. *AACN Clin Issues.* 2000;11(1):68.

34. Richards KC, et al. Effects of massage in acute and critical care. *AACN Clin Issues.* 2000;11(1):77.

35. McKenney C, Johnson R. Unleash the healing power of pet therapy. *Am Nurse Today.* 2008;3(5):29.

36. Cole K, Fawlinski A. Animal-assisted therapy: the human-animal bond. *AACN Clin Issues.* 2000;11(1):139.

37. American Nurses Association. *Nursing's Social Policy Statement.* 2nd ed. Washington, DC: The Association; 2008.

38. Benner P, et al. *Clinical Wisdom and Interventions in Critical Care.* Philadelphia: Saunders; 1999.

39. NANDA International. *Nursing Diagnoses: Definitions & Classification, 2012-2014.* Des Moines: Wiley Blackwell; 2012.

40. Bulechek GM, et al, eds. *Nursing Interventions Classification (NIC).* 6th ed. St. Louis: Mosby; 2013.

41. Harrington L, Kennerly D, Johnson C. Safety issues related to the electronic medical record (EMR): synthesis of the literature from the last decade, 2000-2009. *J Healthcare Management.* 2011;56(1):31.

42. McLane S, Turley JP. Informaticians: how they may benefit your healthcare organization. *JONA.* 2011;41(1):29.

43. Tottle J. Applying a systematic approach to new-product assessment. *Am Nurse Today.* 2008;3(9).

44. Goran SF. A new view: Tele-intensive care unit competencies. *Crit Care Nurse.* 2011;31(5):17.

45. Wheelan SA, et al. The link between teamwork and patients' outcomes in intensive care units. *Am J Crit Care.* 2003;12(6):527.

46. Boyle DK, Kochinda C. Enhancing collaborative communication of nurse and physician leadership in two intensive care units. *J Nurs Adm.* 2004;34(2):60.

47. Falise JP. True collaboration: interdisciplinary rounds in nonteaching hospitals—it can be done! *AACN Adv Crit Care.* 2007;18(4):346.

48. Golanowski M, et al. Interdisciplinary shared decision-making—taking shared governance to the next level. *Nurs Admin Q.* 2007;31(4):341.

49. Reina ML, et al. Trust: the foundation for team collaboration and healthy work environments. *AACN Adv Crit Care.* 2007;18(2):103.

50. Manojlovich M, Antonakos C. Satisfaction of intensive care unit nurses with nurse-physician communication. *JONA.* 2008;38(5):237.

51. Tschannen D, et al. Implications of nurse-physician relations: report of a successful intervention. *Nurs Economics.* 2011;29(3):127.

52. Interprofessional Education Collaborative Expert Panel. *Core competencies for interprofessional collaborative practice.* Association of American Medical Colleges, 2011.

53. D'Arcy Y. Practice guidelines, standards, consensus statements, position papers: what they are, how they differ. *Am Nurse Today.* 2007;2(10):23.

54. Institute of Medicine. *Crossing the Quality Chasm: A New Health System for the 21st Century.* Washington, DC: National Academy Press; 2001.

55. Cook A, et al. An error by any other name. *AJN.* 2004;104(6):32.

56. White GB. Patient safety: an ethical imperative. *Nurs Economics.* 2002;20(4):195.

57. Henneman EA, et al. Strategies used by critical care nurses to identify, interrupt, and correct medical errors. *AJCC.* 2010;19(6):500.

58. The Joint Commission. Behaviors that undermine a culture of safety. *Sentinel Event Alert.* 2008;(40). http://www.jointcommission.org/sentinel_event.aspx. Accessed September 19, 2010.

59. Covell CL. Can civility in nursing work environments improve medication safety? *JONA.* 2010;40(7/8):300.

60. Henneman EA. Patient safety and technology. *AACN Adv Crit Care.* 2009;20(2):128.

61. Anthony K, et al. No interruptions please: impact of a no interruption zone on medication safety in intensive care units. *Crit Care Nurse.* 2010;30(3):21.

62. *The Joint Commission.* 2012 Hospital National Patient Safety Goals. http://www.jointcommission.org. Accessed June 2012.

63. *Medical Device Reporting (MDR).* http://www.fda.gov/MedicalDevices/Safety/ReportaProblem/default.htm. Accessed September 9, 2012.

64. *Institute for Safe Medication Practices.* About ISMP. http://www.ISMP.org. Accessed June 2012.

65. *Institute for Healthcare Improvement.* Using Bundles to Improve Health Care Quality. http://www.ihi.org. Accessed June 2012.

66. *National Quality Forum.* About NQF. http://www.NQF.org. Accessed June 2012.

67. *Healthcare Information and Management Systems Society.* Patient safety and quality outcomes. http://www.HIMSS.org. Accessed June 2012.

68. American Nurses Association (ANA). *National Database Nursing Quality Indicators (NDNQUI).* http://www.nursingquality.org. Accessed June 2012.

69. Quality Safety Education for Nurses. http://www.QSEN.org. Accessed June 2012.

70. *Centers for Medicare and Medicaid Services.* The HIPAA law and related information. http://www.cms.gov/Regulations-and-Guidance/HIPAA-Administrative-Simplification. Accessed September 10, 2012.

71. Pearson A, et al. Comprehensive systematic review of evidence on developing and sustaining nursing leadership that fosters a healthy work environment in healthcare. *Int J Evidence-Based Health.* 2007;5:208-253.

72. *American Association of Critical-Care Nurses (AACN).* AACN standards for establishing and sustaining healthy work environments. http://www.aacn.org. Accessed June 2012.

73. Bylone M. Healthy work environments: whose job is it anyway? *AACN Adv Crit Care.* 2009;20(4):325.

74. Bylone M. I think they are talking about me!! *AACN Adv Crit Care.* 2009;20(2):137.

75. Bylone M. Health work environment 101. *AACN Adv Crit Care.* 2011;22(1):19.

76. Kupperschmidt B, et al: *A healthy work environment: it begins with you.* The Online Journal of Issues in Nursing. 2010;15(1)manuscript 3. http://nursingworld.org/mainmenucategories/ANAMarketplace/ANAPeriodicals/OJIN. Accessed February 17, 2010.

77. Blake N. Practical steps for implementing healthy work environments. *AACN Adv Crit Care.* 2012;23(1):14.

Ethical Issues

Linda D. Urden

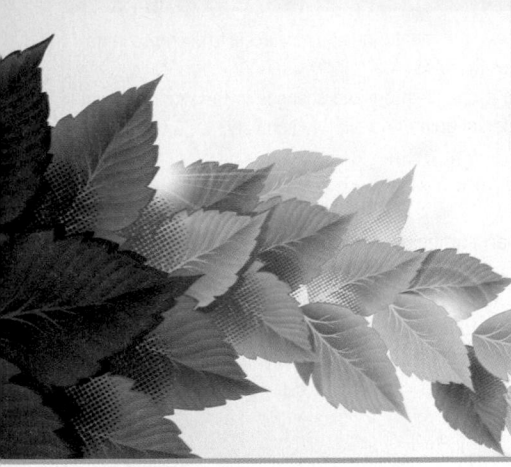

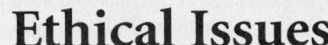
It is essential that critical care nurses have an understanding of professional nursing ethics and ethical principles and that they are able to use a decision-making model to guide nursing actions. This chapter provides an overview of ethical principles and professional nursing ethics. An ethical decision-making model is described and illustrated, and recommendations are given concerning methods to use when confronting ethical issues in the critical care setting.

DIFFERENCES BETWEEN MORALS AND ETHICS

Morals are the "shoulds," "should nots," "oughts," and "ought nots" of actions and behaviors, and they are related closely to cultural and religious values and beliefs that govern our social interactions. Morals form the basis for action and provide a framework for the evaluation of behavior.[1]

Ethics are concerned with the basis of the action rather than whether the action is right or wrong, good or bad. Imposition of ethics implies that an evaluation is being made that is based on or derived from a set of standards. It refers to what rules are required to prevent harm to persons and to the collective beliefs and values of a community or profession.[1]

Moral Distress

Recently, moral distress has been a topic widely discussed in the literature as a serious problem for nurses.[2-5] Nurses face multiple challenges on a daily basis: emergency situations, tension from conflict with others, complex clinical cases, new technologies, increasing regulatory requirements, acquisition of new skills/knowledge, staffing issues, financial constraints,

workplace violence, to name a few. This care environment has led to increasingly complex moral and ethical dilemmas.[5] In addition, they frequently may experience emotional outbursts from patients, families, co-workers, and feel a lack of control and "burnt out."[2,5] Moral distress occurs when a person knows the ethically appropriate action to take but cannot act on it. It also manifests when a nurse acts in a manner contrary to personal and professional values. As a result, there can be significant emotional and physical stress that leads to feelings of loss of personal integrity and dissatisfaction with the work environment. Relationships with co-workers and patients are affected, and the quality of care can be negatively affected. There is also a great impact on personal relationships and family life; nurses experiencing moral distress may resign their position or leave the profession entirely.[3]

It is therefore important that nurses recognize moral distress and actively seek strategies to address the issue through institutional, personal, and professional organizational resources. Knowledge and application of ethical principles and guidelines can assist the nurse in daily practice when ethical dilemmas occur. Box 2-1 provides a position statement on moral distress, promulgated by the American Association of Critical-Care Nurses (AACN).[6] The document is evidence-based, providing additional references for the reader. There is also a reference to ensuring that support to alleviate moral distress is present in a healthy work environment (see Chapter 1). Actions are listed for direct care staff nurses as well as employers.

The AACN has created a framework—*The 4A's to Rise Above Moral Distress*—to support nurses who are experiencing moral distress (Figure 2-1). ASK, the first stage, is a self-awareness and

BOX 2-1   AACN POSITION STATEMENT: MORAL DISTRESS

Issue

Moral distress is a serious problem in nursing. It results in significant physical and emotional stress, which contributes to nurses' feelings of loss of integrity and dissatisfaction with their work environment. Studies demonstrate that moral distress is a major contributor to nurses leaving the work setting and profession. It affects relationships with patients and others and can affect the quality, quantity, and cost of nursing care.

Definition

Moral distress occurs when:

- You know the ethically appropriate action to take, but are unable to act upon it.
- You act in a manner contrary to your personal and professional values, which undermines your integrity and authenticity.

Evidence

Compelling evidence indicates that moral distress has a negative impact on the healthcare work environment. In one study, 1 in 3 nurses experienced moral distress.[1] In another, nearly half the nurses studied left their units or nursing altogether because of moral distress.[2]

Additional studies have shown:

- Among 760 nurses, nearly 50% had acted against their consciences in providing care to terminally ill patients.[3]
- Nurses lose their capacity for caring, avoid patient contact, and fail to give good physical care as a result of moral distress.[1]
- Nurses experience physical and psychological problems as a result of moral distress.[4-10]
- Nurses physically withdraw from the bedside, barely meeting the patient's basic physical needs, or they leave the profession altogether.[1-2,4-5,11-12]

Summary

Moral distress is a key issue affecting the workplace environment. Research demonstrates that moral distress is a significant cause of emotional suffering among nurses and contributes to loss of nurses from the workforce. Further, it threatens the quality of patient care. In recognition of these harmful effects, the provision of education and tools to address and manage moral distress in the work environment is imperative and will lead to essential improvements in patient care and outcomes.

AACN Policy Position

Moral distress is a critical, frequently ignored, problem in healthcare work environments. Unaddressed, it restricts nurses' ability to provide optimal patient care and to find job satisfaction. AACN asserts that every nurse and every employer is responsible for implementing programs to address and mitigate the harmful effects of moral distress in the pursuit of creating a healthy work environment.

AACN Calls to Action

For Nurses

Every nurse must:

- Recognize and name the experience of moral distress (moral sensitivity).
- Affirm the professional obligation to act and commit to addressing moral distress.
- Be knowledgeable about and use professional and institutional resources to address moral distress, such as:
  - American Nurses Association *Code of Ethics for Nurses*
  - International Council of Nurses *Code of Ethics for Nurses*
  - AACN *4 A's to Rise Above Moral Distress Handbook*
  - AACN *4 A's to Rise Above Moral Distress Facilitators Toolkit*
- Actively participate in professional activities to expand knowledge and understanding of the impact of moral distress.

- Develop skill, through the use of mentoring and resources, to decrease moral distress.
- Implement strategies to accomplish desired changes in the work environment while preserving personal integrity and authenticity.

For Employers

Every organization must:

- Implement interdisciplinary strategies to recognize and name the experience of moral distress.
- Establish mechanisms to monitor the clinical and organizational climate to identify recurring situations that result in moral distress.
- Develop a systematic process for reviewing and analyzing the system issues enabling situations that cause moral distress to occur and for taking corrective action.
- Create support systems that include:
  - Employee assistance programs
  - Protocols for end-of-life care
  - Ethics committees
  - Critical stress debriefings
  - Grief counseling
- Create interdisciplinary forums to discuss patient goals of care and divergent opinions in an open, respectful environment.
- Develop policies that support unobstructed access to resources such as the ethics committees.
- Ensure nurses' representation on institutional ethics committees with full participation in all decision making.
- Provide education and tools to manage and decrease moral distress in the work environment.

References

1. Redman B, Fry ST. Nurses' ethical conflicts: what is really known about them? *Nurs Ethics.* 2000;7(4):360.
2. Millette BE. Using Gilligan's framework to analyze nurses' stories of moral choices. *West J Nurs Res.* 1994;16(6):660.
3. Solomon M, O'Donnell L, Jennings B, et al. Decisions near the end of life: professional views on life sustaining treatments. *Am J Public Health.* 1993;83:14.
4. Kelly B. Preserving moral integrity: a follow-up study with new graduate nurses. *J Adv Nurs.* 1998;28:1134.
5. Wilkinson JM. Moral distress in nursing practice: experience and effect. *Nurs Forum.* 1987-1988;23(1):16.
6. Perkin RM, Young T, Freier MC, et al. Stress and distress in pediatric nurses: lessons from Baby K. *Am J Crit Care.* 1997;6:225.
7. Fenton M. Moral distress in clinical practice: implications for the nurse administrator. *Can J Nurs Adm.* 1988;1:8.
8. Davies B, Clarke D, Connaughty S, et al. Caring for dying children: nurses' experiences. *Pediatr Nurs.* 1996;22:500.
9. Krishnasamy M. Nursing, morality, and emotions: phase I and phase II clinical trials and patients with cancer. *Cancer Nurs.* 1999;22:251.
10. Anderson SL. Patient advocacy and whistle-blowing in nursing: help for the helpers. *Nurs Forum.* 1990;25:513.
11. Hefferman P, Heilig S. Giving "moral distress" a voice: ethical concerns among neonatal intensive care unit personnel. *Cambridge Q Healthc Ethics.* 1999;8:173.
12. Corley MC. Moral distress of critical care nurses. *Am J Crit Care.* 1995;4:280.

Bibliography

Corley MC, Elswick RK, Gorman M, et al. Development and evaluation of a moral distress scale. *J Adv Nurs.* 2001;33(2):250.

BOX 2-1   AACN POSITION STATEMENT: MORAL DISTRESS—cont'd

Corley MC, Minick P. Moral distress or moral comfort. *Bioethics Forum.* 2002;18(1-2):7.

Cronqvist A, Theorell T, Burns T, et al. Caring about–caring for: moral obligations and work responsibilities in intensive care nursing. *Nurs Ethics.* 2004;11(1):63.

Erlen JA, Sereika SM. Critical care nurses, ethical decision making and stress. *J Adv Nurs.* 1997;26:953.

Jameton A. Dilemmas of moral distress: moral responsibility and nursing practice. *Clin Issues Perinat Womens Health Nurs.* 1993;4:542.

Jameton A. Nursing Practice: *The Ethical Issues.* Englewood Cliffs, NJ: Prentice-Hall; 1984.

Kalvemark S, Hoglund AT, Hansson MG, et al. Living with conflicts: ethical dilemmas and moral distress in the health care system. *Soc Sci Med.* 2004;58(6):1075.

Liaschenko J. Artificial personhood: nursing ethics in a medical world. *Nurs Ethics.* 1995;2:185.

Penticuff JH, Waldren M. Influence of practice environment and nurse characteristics on perinatal nurses' responses to ethical dilemmas. *Nurs Res.* 2000;49(2):64.

Raines ML. Ethical decision making in nurses: relationships among moral reasoning, coping style, and ethics stress. *JONAS Healthc Law Ethics Regul.* 2000;2(1):29.

Rushton CH. The Baby K case: ethical challenges of preserving professional integrity. *Pediatr Nurs.* 1995;21:367.

Storch JL, Rodney P, Pauly B, et al. Listening to nurses' moral voices: building a quality health care environment. *Can J Nurs Leadersh.* 2002;15(4):7.

Sundin-Huard D, Fahy K. Moral distress, advocacy and burnout: theorizing the relationships. *Int J Nurs Pract.* 1999;5(1):8.

U.S. General Accounting Office. *Nursing Workforce: Emerging Nurse Shortages Due to Multiple Factors* [Report to the Chairman, Subcommittee on Health, Committee on Ways and Means, House of Representatives]. Washington, DC: US General Accounting Office.

From American Association of Critical-Care Nurses. *Position Statement: Moral Distress.* Aliso Viejo, CA: American Association of Critical-Care Nurses; 2008.

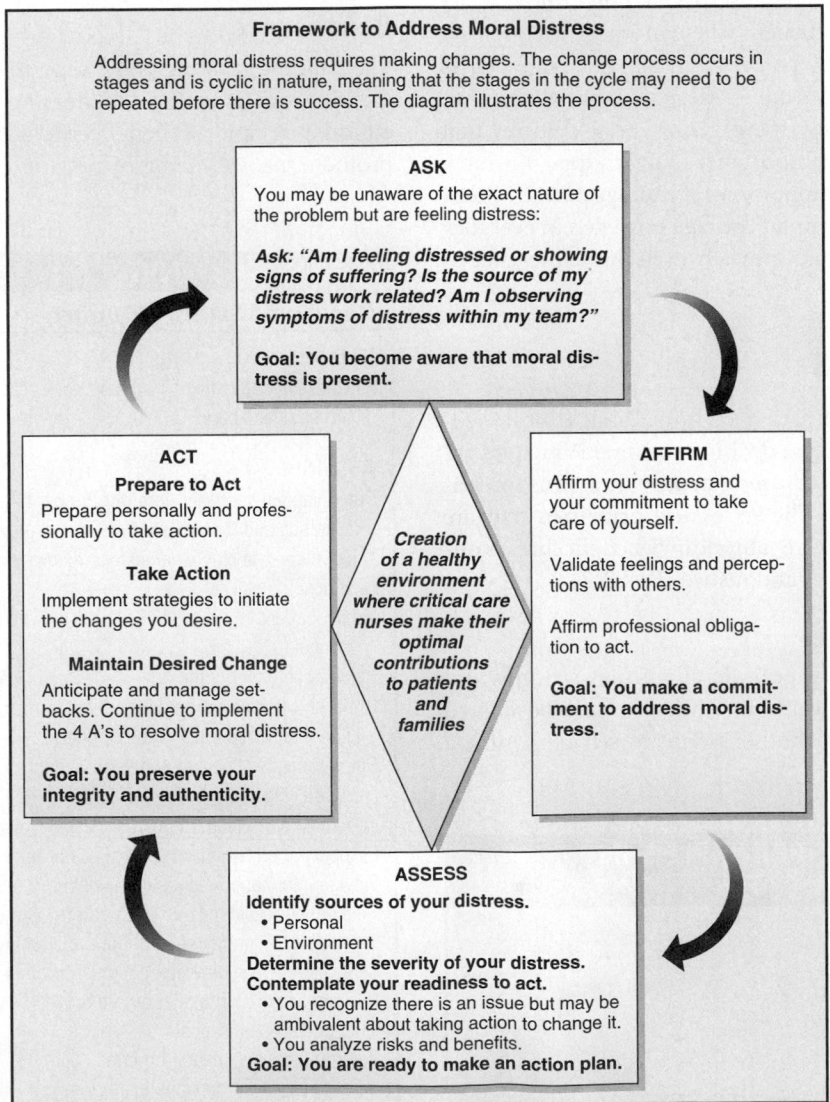

Framework to Address Moral Distress

Addressing moral distress requires making changes. The change process occurs in stages and is cyclic in nature, meaning that the stages in the cycle may need to be repeated before there is success. The diagram illustrates the process.

ASK

You may be unaware of the exact nature of the problem but are feeling distress:

Ask: "Am I feeling distressed or showing signs of suffering? Is the source of my distress work related? Am I observing symptoms of distress within my team?"

Goal: You become aware that moral distress is present.

ACT
Prepare to Act

Prepare personally and professionally to take action.

Take Action

Implement strategies to initiate the changes you desire.

Maintain Desired Change

Anticipate and manage setbacks. Continue to implement the 4 A's to resolve moral distress.

Goal: You preserve your integrity and authenticity.

Creation of a healthy environment where critical care nurses make their optimal contributions to patients and families

AFFIRM

Affirm your distress and your commitment to take care of yourself.

Validate feelings and perceptions with others.

Affirm professional obligation to act.

Goal: You make a commitment to address moral distress.

ASSESS

Identify sources of your distress.
• Personal
• Environment
Determine the severity of your distress.
Contemplate your readiness to act.
   • You recognize there is an issue but may be ambivalent about taking action to change it.
   • You analyze risks and benefits.
Goal: You are ready to make an action plan.

FIGURE 2-1   The ACCN 4 A's to Rise Above Moral Distress. (From American Association of Critical-Care Nurses. *Position Statement: Moral Distress.* Aliso Viejo, CA: AACN; July 8, 2004.)

reflection period in which one becomes more aware of the distress and its effects on oneself. Specific areas to address are physical, spiritual, emotional, and behavioral responses. During stage two, AFFIRM, one affirms the distress and makes a commitment to take care of oneself. In stage three, ASSESS, one needs to identify the timing and context of when the stressors occur; determine the severity of the distress; and examine one's readiness to act. The final stage, ACT, consists of preparation, the action itself, and maintaining the desired change. Although the model was created by AACN, it is a framework that can be used in diverse settings and by various health care professionals.[7] McCue[8] reported using this model as a resource for resolving an issue between a chief nurse executive and chief executive officer. In this case, the impact of the outcome was at the organizational level.

Moral Courage

In order to avoid moral distress, nurses must feel free to advocate for themselves, their patients, co-workers, and a safe and effective work environment. Lachman and colleagues describes moral courage as "the willingness to stand up for and act according to one's ethical beliefs when moral principles are threatened, regardless of the perceived or actual risks (such as stress, anxiety, isolation from colleagues, or threats to employment)".[9,p24] They describe organizational cultures that support moral courage, the importance of peer support, education, and policies that can support moral courage of staff. Other authors have reported that moral courage is needed in everyday practice and that one must act ethically even in the presence of risk.[4,10]

ETHICAL PRINCIPLES

Certain ethical principles were derived from classic ethical theories that are used in health care decision making. Principles are general guidelines that govern conduct, provide a basis for reasoning, and direct actions. The six ethical principles that are discussed in this chapter are autonomy, beneficence, nonmaleficence, veracity, fidelity, and justice (Box 2-2).

Autonomy

The concept of autonomy appears in all ancient writings and early Greek philosophy. In health care, autonomy can be defined as an agreement to respect another's right to self-determine a

---

BOX 2-2 ETHICAL PRINCIPLES IN CRITICAL CARE

- Autonomy
- Beneficence
- Nonmaleficence
- Veracity
- Fidelity
- Confidentiality
- Privacy
- Justice or allocation of resources

---

course of action and the support of independent decision making[11] without coercion or interference from others. Autonomy is a freedom of choice or a self-determination that is a basic human right. It can be experienced in all human life events.

The critical care nurse is often "caught in the middle" in ethical situations, and promoting autonomous decision making is one of those situations. As the nurse works closely with patients and families to promote autonomous decision making, another crucial element becomes clear. Patients and families must have all of the information about a particular situation before they can make a decision that is best for them. They should be given all the pertinent information and facts, and they must have a clear understanding of what was presented. This is where the nurse is a most important member of the health care team—as patient advocate, the nurse provides more information as needed, clarifies points, reinforces information, and provides support during the decision-making process. Box 2-3 presents the Nursing Interventions Classification (NIC) feature on nursing intervention activities that facilitate decision making.

Beneficence

The concept of doing good and preventing harm to patients is the sine qua non for the nursing profession. However, the ethical principle of beneficence—which requires a nurse to promote the well-being of patients—points to the importance

---

◎ BOX 2-3 NIC

Decision-Making Support

Definition

Providing information and support for a patient who is making a decision regarding health care

Activities

Determine whether there are differences between the patient's view of own condition and the view of health care providers

Assist patient to clarify values and expectations which may assist in making critical life choices

Inform patient of alternative views or solutions in a clear and supportive manner

Help patient identify the advantages and disadvantages of each alternative

Establish communication with patient early in admission

Facilitate patient's articulation of goals for care

Obtain informed consent, when appropriate

Facilitate collaborative decision making

Be familiar with institution's policies and procedures

Respect patient's right to receive or not to receive information

Provide information requested by patient

Help patient explain decision to others, as needed

Serve as a liaison between patient and family

Serve as a liaison between patient and other health care providers

Use interactive computer software or web-based decision aides as an adjunct to professional support

Refer to legal aid, as appropriate

Refer to support groups, as appropriate

From Bulechek GM, et al: *Nursing Interventions Classification (NIC)*. 6th ed. St. Louis: Mosby; 2013.

of this duty for the health care professional. The principle of beneficence presupposes compassion; taking positive action to help others; desire to do good. It is the core principle of patient advocacy.[11] Harms and benefits are balanced, leading to positive or beneficial outcomes. In approaching issues related to beneficence, conflict with another principle, that of autonomy, is common. Paternalism exists when the nurse or physician makes a decision for the patient without consulting the patient.

Traditional health care has been based on a paternalistic approach to patients. Many patients are still more comfortable in deferring all decisions about care and treatment to their health care provider. Active involvement by various organizations, agencies, and consumer groups in regard to health care has demonstrated a trend toward the public's need and desire for more information about health care in general and more information about alternative treatments and providers. Paternalism may always be a possibility in the health care setting, but enlightened consumers are causing a change in this practice.

In the critical care setting, many instances of and possibilities for paternalistic actions by the nurse exist. Postoperative care, which is designed to assist the patient with achieving a quick recovery, is a good example. Encouraging the patient to turn, cough, and deep breathe and increasing the patient's activity in the form of dangling, sitting in a chair, and ambulating are all paternalistic actions when the patient is experiencing pain and sleep deprivation and wanting to be left alone. However, the benefits and harms sometimes must be balanced. In these instances, the duty to do no harm—which is the next principle to be discussed—takes precedence over the need to avoid paternalistic actions. When ethical principles are in conflict, the nurse must weigh all the benefits and choose the best principle to follow.

Nonmaleficence

The ethical principle of nonmaleficence, which dictates that the nurse prevent harm and correct harmful situations, is a prima facie duty for the nurse. Thoughtfulness and care are necessary, as is balancing risks and benefits, which was discussed earlier. Beneficence and nonmaleficence are on two ends of a continuum and are often adhered to differently, depending on the views of the practitioner.

A practitioner may consider long-term consequences and the good to society as a whole, or the principle and its effect on the single individual in the situation. Such complex problems as quality of life versus sanctity of life are always difficult to analyze in the critical care setting, as well as in noncritical care settings.

Veracity

Veracity, or truth-telling, is an important ethical principle that underlies the nurse-patient relationship. Veracity is important when soliciting informed consent, because the patient needs to be aware of all potential risks and benefits to be derived from specific treatments or their alternatives. The critical care nurse can be in the middle of a situation in which all of the facts and information about a particular treatment option are not disclosed.

Sometimes, information has been given accurately to the patient and family but has been delivered with bias or in a way that is misleading. Veracity must guide all areas of practice for the nurse—that is, colleague relationships and employee relationships, as well as the nurse-patient relationship.

Fidelity

Another ethical principle that is closely related to autonomy and veracity is fidelity. Fidelity, or faithfulness and promise-keeping to patients, is an essential aspect of nursing. The American Nurses Association (ANA) states that this principle requires loyalty, fairness, truthfulness, advocacy, and dedication to our patients. It involves an agreement to keep our promises. Fidelity refers to the concept of keeping a commitment and is based on the virtue of caring.[11] It forms a bond between individuals and is the basis of all professional and personal relationships. Regardless of the amount of autonomy that patients have in critical care areas, they still depend on the nurse for many types of physical care and emotional support. A trusting relationship that establishes and maintains an open atmosphere is one that is positive for all involved.

Like all of the other principles, fidelity extends to the family of the critical care patient. When a promise is made to family members that they will be called if an emergency arises or that they will be informed of any other special events concerning the patient, the nurse must make every effort to follow through on the promise. Fidelity upholds the nurse-family relationship and reflects positively on the nursing profession as a whole and on the institution in which the nurse is employed.

Confidentiality is one element of fidelity that is based on traditional health care professional ethics. Confidentiality is described as a right whereby patient information may be shared only with those involved in the care of the patient. An exception to this guideline might occur if the welfare of others would be put at risk by keeping patient information confidential. In this situation, the nurse must balance ethical principles and weigh risks and benefits. Special circumstances, such as the existence of mandatory reporting laws, guide the nurse in certain situations.

Privacy also has been described as being inherent in the principle of fidelity. It may be closely aligned with confidentiality of patient information and a patient's right to privacy of his or her person, as in maintaining privacy for the patient by pulling the curtains around the bed or making sure that he or she is adequately covered. The ANA summary and principle on privacy and confidentiality are found in Box 2-4.

Justice

The principle of justice is often used synonymously with the concept of allocation of scarce resources. According to the ANA, it is based on analysis of benefits and burdens of decisions. Justice implies that all have equal rights and that there be a fair and equal distribution of resources to all.[11] Contrary to the belief of many people, health care is not a right guaranteed by the Constitution of the United States. Rather, it is the *access* to health care that should be provided to all people. With escalating health care costs, expanded technologies, an aging

BOX 2-4 ANA STATEMENT ON PRIVACY AND CONFIDENTIALITY

Summary: Advances in technology, including computerized medical databases, the Internet, and telehealth, have opened the door to potential, unintentional breaches of private/confidential health information. Protection of privacy/confidentiality is essential to the trusting relationship between health care providers and patients. Quality patient care requires the communication of relevant information between health professionals and/or health systems. Nurses and other health professionals who regularly work with patients and their confidential medical records should contribute to the development of standards, policies, and laws that protect patient privacy and the confidentiality of health records/information.

Background

Recent developments in technology have changed the delivery of health care and the system used to record and retrieve health information. In addition to using paper medical records, health professionals, hospitals and insurers routinely use computers, phones, faxes, and other methods or recording and transferring information. In many instances, this information—which could include medical diagnoses, prescriptions, or insurance information—is readily available to anyone (including clerical and other staff) who walks by a fax machine or logs on to a computer. This lack of privacy has the potential to undermine patients' relationships with providers and adversely affect the quality of care. Patients may also fear that the exposure of personal health information, including the results of genetic tests that are becoming increasing available, could result in the loss or denial of health insurance, job discrimination or personal embarrassment.

In keeping with the nursing profession's commitment to patient advocacy and the trust that is essential to the preservation of the high quality of care patients have come to expect from registered nurses, the American Nurses Association supports the following principles with respect to patient privacy and confidentiality:

- A patient's right to privacy with respect to individually identifiable health information, including genetic information, should be established statutorily. Individuals should retain the right to decide to whom, and under what circumstances, their individually identifiable health information will be disclosed. Confidentiality protections should extend not only to health records, but also to all other individually identifiable health information, including genetic information, clinical research records, and mental health therapy notes.
- Use and disclosure of individually identifiable health information should be limited.
- A patient should have the right to access his or her own health information and the right to supplement such information so that they are able to make informed health care decisions, to correct erroneous information, and to address discrepancies that they perceive.

- Patients should receive written, easily understood notification of how their health records are used and when their individually identifiable health information is disclosed to third parties.
- The use or disclosure of individually identifiable health information absent an individual's informed consent should be prohibited. Exceptions should be permitted only if a person's life is endangered, if there is a threat to the public, or if there is a compelling law enforcement need. In the case of such exceptions, information should be limited to the minimum amount necessary.
- Appropriate safeguards should be developed and required for the use, disclosure and storage of personal health information.
- Legislative or regulatory protections on individually identifiable health information should not unnecessarily impede public health efforts or clinical, medical, nursing, or quality of care research.
- Strong and enforceable remedies for violations of privacy protections should be established, and health care professionals who report violations should be protected from retaliation.
- Federal legislation should provide a floor for the protection of individual privacy and confidentiality rights, not a ceiling. Federal legislation should not preempt any other federal or state law or regulation that offers greater protection.

References

Aronovitz L. *Testimony before the House Ways and Means Subcommittee on Health, Hearing on Confidentiality of Health Information.* July 20, 1999.

Badzek L, Gross L. Confidentiality and privacy: at the forefront for nurses. *Am J Nurs.* 1999;99(6):52-54.

Foerstel K. Protecting medical records: privacy vs. 'progress'. *CQ Weekly.* 1999;593-595.

Goldman J. Protecting privacy to improve health care. *Health Affairs.* 1998;17(5):47-60.

Hamburg M. *Testimony before the House Ways and Means Subcommittee on Health, Hearing on Confidentiality of Health Information.* July 20, 1999.

Hash M. *Testimony before the House Ways and Means Subcommittee on Health, Hearing on Confidentiality of Health Information.* July 20, 1999.

Health Privacy Project. *Best principles for health privacy, a report of the Health Privacy Working Group.* Institute for Health Care Research and Policy, Georgetown University; 1999.

Hodge J, Gostin L, Jacobson P. Legal issues concerning electronic health information, privacy, quality, and liability. *JAMA.* 1999;282(15):1466.

Koyanagi C. *Testimony before the U. S. Senate Committee on Health, Education, Labor, and Pensions on the Confidentiality of Medical Information.* April 27, 1999.

Serafini M. Open Secrets. *National Journal.* 1999;2878.

From *American Nurses Association.* Privacy and confidentiality. Approved December 8, 2006. http://gm6.nursingworld.org/MainMenuCategories/Policy-Advocacy/Positions-and-Resolutions/ANAPositionStatements/Position-Statements-Alphabetically/PrivacyandConfidentiality.html. Accessed July 9, 2012.

population with its own special health care needs, and in some instances a scarcity of health care personnel, the question of how to allocate health care becomes even more complex.

SCARCE RESOURCES IN CRITICAL CARE

Major factors influencing health care ethics are rapid health care cost inflation and the shrinking allocation of public funds for both primary and secondary care. As health care resources become increasingly scarce, allocation of resources to certain programs and rationing of resources within programs may become more evident. Allocation of resources creates ethical challenges for health care practitioners facing the daily clinical realities of providing increasingly complex care with growing technologies and treatment modalities.

Technologies and Treatments

Limitations of resources force society and critical care health professionals to reexamine the goals of critical care for patients. The application of new or experimental treatments and procedures needs to be carefully analyzed for each case, with particular attention paid to the expected outcome.

Quality of life is an issue that should be considered carefully when examining the use of technologies. This issue is personal and value laden; it is different for each individual involved and depends on the various aspects of the case. Quality of life has the dual dimensions of objectivity and subjectivity. Objectivity examines the person's ability to function, whereas subjectivity analyzes his or her psychosocial state. Patients' treatment preferences reflect the values they place on various health outcomes and may be very different from those of health care providers.

Health Care Personnel

Critical care nurses are faced with rationing of critical care beds and nursing staff on a daily basis. Strengths and weaknesses of the staff must be balanced with the needs of the patient. Orientation and other special circumstances—such as designation of a charge nurse, trauma nurse, or code nurse—must be considered when scheduling staff and making assignments. Any inexperienced staff, float staff, or registry staff must be given appropriate orientation and backup during the shift.

Commonly, a triage system for critical care units is called on when there are more admissions than available beds. The critical care nurse is instrumental in assisting the medical director to determine patient selection for transfer, if appropriate. Hospitals establish a set of standards, criteria, or guidelines for determining patient admission and transfer to and from critical care areas.

WITHHOLDING AND WITHDRAWING TREATMENT

The technologic support of life at all costs has been questioned by health care professionals and health care consumers. Physicians and nurses who are closest to the issues have debated the moral and ethical implications and have looked to ethicists for guidance and legal opinions. Medical and nursing associations have developed guidelines for their practitioners concerning withholding and withdrawing treatments. The decision to not employ aggressive measures or to discontinue treatments that have been in place is always difficult and stressful for all involved in the decision, particularly those who continue to care for the patient on a daily basis.

There may be reluctance to withdraw treatments, reflecting the ethical and moral conflicts within each practitioner. Withholding usually means that there is no hope for success from the onset, whereas withdrawing means surrendering hope. Difficult discussions must take place between the health care professionals and the family, and such communication is especially difficult when families are faced with choices about forgoing life-sustaining treatment. This is a time when families most need timely information, honesty, and care providers who are clear regarding treatment options. Care providers need to listen to the families and be informed about their loved one's wishes.

In order to accomplish a positive outcome for the patient, family, and health care providers, a plan for this complex and difficult process must be established. Stacy reported a case study that described nursing management of an adult patient undergoing withdrawal of mechanical ventilation as part of an end-of-life protocol. The clinical nurse specialist was instrumental in coordinating a patient care conference that included all involved members of the health care team along with family members. Key to the process that followed was symptom management, clear communication among health care team and family, determining the procedure for withdrawal of mechanical ventilation, and documentation of the care. Another key component is bereavement debriefing for the health care team, which ideally occurs several days after the event.[12]

MEDICAL FUTILITY

The concept of medical futility has resulted in various discussions and proposed criteria or formulas to predict outcomes of care.[13-14] Medical futility has a qualitative and a quantitative basis and can be defined as "any effort to achieve a result that is possible but that reasoning or experience suggests is highly improbable and that cannot be systematically reproduced."[13] Quantitative futility was based on statistical calculations and assumed to be objective. However, there is no agreement regarding statistical thresholds for treatments to be considered futile.[15] Qualitative futility is subjective and has no consistency in agreement.[14] Hofmann and Schneiderman indicate that "Death is not necessarily a medical failure; a bad death is not only a medical failure, but also an ethical breakdown".[16]

Therapy or treatment that achieves its predictable outcome and desired effect is, by definition, effective, but effect must be distinguished from benefit. If that predictable and desired effect is of no benefit to the patient, the treatment is nonetheless futile. It is suggested that when physicians conclude from personal experience or that of colleagues or from empiric data that a particular treatment has proved to be useless in the most recent 100 cases, the treatment should be considered futile. It is incumbent on health care practitioners to make optimal use of health-related resources in a technically appropriate and effective manner.

ETHICS AS A FOUNDATION FOR NURSING PRACTICE

Traditional theories of professions include a code of ethics on which the practice of the profession is based. It is by adherence to a code of ethics that the professional fulfills an obligation to provide quality practice to society.

A professional ethic forms the framework for any profession[17] and is based on three elements: 1) the professional code of ethics; 2) the purpose of the profession; and 3) the standards of practice of the professional. The code of ethics developed by the profession is the delineation of its values and relationships with and among members of the profession and society. The need for the profession and its inherent promise to provide certain duties form a contract between nursing and society. The professional standards describe specifics of practice in a variety of settings and subspecialties. Nursing professionals must stay consistent with their values and ethics, and ensure that the ethical environment is maintained wherever nursing care and services are performed.[18-19] Each element is dynamic, and ongoing evaluations are necessary as societal expectations change, technologies increase, and the profession evolves.

Nursing Code of Ethics

The ANA *Code of Ethics for Nurses*[20] provides the major source of ethical guidance for the nursing profession. The nine statements of the code are found in Box 2-5. Further delineation of each of the provisions along with in-depth discussion and examples of application can be found on the ANA website, www.nursingworld.org.

The code was first adopted by the ANA in 1950 and has undergone revisions over the years. It provides a framework for the nurse to follow in ethical decision making and provides society with a set of expectations of the profession. When the requirements of the code are not in concert with the law, it is the nurse's obligation to uphold the code because of the societal commitment inherent in nursing.

ETHICAL DECISION MAKING IN CRITICAL CARE

The Nurse's Role

Benner[21] described the concept of the relational ethics of comfort, touch, and solace and questioned whether it is an endangered art lost to times past. However, she and her colleagues did find that there are still many examples of such comforting in daily practice, despite the overwhelming emphasis on using technologies in treating critically ill patients. Voice and touch are described as being central for the patient recovering from anesthesia. Critical decisions such as the conservative uses of restraints are another example related to comfort and ethical care of patients. Lachman described the ethics of caring to nursing practice. Through the very decision to become a nurse, one makes a moral commitment to provide care and services for patients, and that indicates a focus on meeting all the needs of patients.[22] Acknowledging the importance of the nurse-patient relationship and establishing time to listen, explain, and comfort can assist the nurse in determining unmet needs of patients. Box 2-6 presents the NIC feature on values clarification.

As discussed earlier, the critical care nurse encounters ethical issues on a daily basis. Pavlish and colleagues studied nurses' ethically difficult situations, their early indicators and risk factors, nurse actions, and outcomes. From this study, they derived risk factors for patients, families, health care providers,

---

BOX 2-5 ANA CODE OF ETHICS FOR NURSES

1. The nurse, in all professional relationships, practices with compassion and respect for the inherent dignity, worth, and uniqueness of every individual, unrestricted by considerations of social or economic status, personal attributes, or the nature of health problems.
2. The nurse's primary commitment is to the patient, whether an individual, family, group, or community.
3. The nurse promotes, advocates for, and strives to protect the health, safety, and rights of the patient.
4. The nurse is responsible and accountable for individual nursing practice and determines the appropriate delegation of tasks consistent with the nurse's obligation to provide optimum patient care.
5. The nurse owes the same duties to self as to others, including the responsibility to preserve integrity and safety, to maintain competence, and to continue personal and professional growth.
6. The nurse participates in establishing, maintaining, and improving health care environments and conditions of employment conducive to the provision of quality health care and consistent with the values of the profession through individual and collective action.
7. The nurse participates in the advancement of the profession through contributions to practice, education, administration, and knowledge development.
8. The nurse collaborates with other health professionals and the public in promoting community, national, and international efforts to meet health needs.
9. The profession of nursing, as represented by associations and other members, is responsible for articulating nursing values, for maintaining the integrity of the profession and its practice, and for shaping social policy.

From American Nurses Association. *Guide to the Code of Ethics for Nurses.* Washington, DC: ANA; 2008.

BOX 2-6 NIC

Values Clarification

Definition
Assisting another to clarify her/his own values in order to facilitate effective decision-making

Activities
Consider the ethical and legal aspects of free choice, given the particular situation, before beginning the intervention
Create an accepting, nonjudgmental atmosphere
Encourage consideration of issues
Encourage consideration of values underlying choices and consequences of the choice
Use appropriate questions to assist the patient in reflecting on the situation and what is important personally
Assist patient to prioritize values
Use a value sheet clarifying technique (written situation and questions), as appropriate
Pose reflective, clarifying questions that give the patient something to think about
Avoid use of cross-examining questions
Encourage patient to make a list of what is important and not important in life and the time spent on each
Encourage patient to list values that guide behavior in various settings and types of situations
Develop and implement a plan with the patient to try out choices
Evaluate the effectiveness of the plan with the patient
Provide reinforcement for actions in the plan that support the patient's values
Help patient define alternatives and their advantages and disadvantages
Help patient to evaluate how values are in agreement with or conflict with those of family members/significant others
Support the patient in communicating own values to others
Avoid use of the intervention with persons with serious emotional problems

From Bulechek GM, et al. *Nursing Interventions Classification (NIC).* 6th ed. St. Louis: Mosby; 2013.

BOX 2-7 EARLY INDICATORS FOR ETHICAL DILEMMAS

- Signs of conflict among health care (HC) team members, family members, and HC team and family
- Signs of patient suffering
- Signs of nurse distress
- Signs of ethics violation
- Signs of unrealistic expectations
- Signs of poor communication

BOX 2-9 STRATEGIES FOR NURSING SHIFT REPORT

- Monitor language and tone
- Challenge assumptions
- Be alert to the presence of gossip
- Develop professional norms
- Hold yourself and one another accountable
- Use a standard framework
- Adopt a "need-to-know" policy

BOX 2-8 SAMPLE QUESTIONS TO TRIGGER PREVENTATIVE ETHICS INTERVENTION

1. Is the patient able to contribute to decisions about his or her care?
2. Is the patient still in critical condition 48 hours after admission?
3. Has the patient's family visited in the last 48 hours?
4. Are the patient and family non-English speaking, or are they members of a cultural group that is unfamiliar to most providers on this unit?
5. Has the family been updated by the team in the past 24 hours?
6. Has today's bedside nurse cared for this patient before?
7. Has the bedside nurse established rapport with this patient and family?
8. How many different nurses have cared for this patient in the past week?
9. Has the family stated strong religious beliefs that could potentially conflict with medical treatment?
10. Is there consensus among the team members with regard to this patient's prognosis and treatment plan?
11. Are there any unit routines or procedures that negatively affect this patient's care?
12. Is this patient's situation ethically challenging at present?

From Epstein EG. Preventative ethics in the intensive care unit. *AACN Adv Crit Care.* 2012;23(2):217.

and health care organizations. Additionally, they delineated early indicators for ethical dilemmas in six areas (Box 2-7).[23]

Health care organizations and authors have emphasized that responding to individual ethical issues is not enough and that there must be a plan in place that asserts a systematic approach for proactively addressing ethical situations.[24-25] This program should identify, prioritize, and address concerns about ethics at an organizational level. Thus, measurable improvements will be able to demonstrate reduced disparities between current practices and ideal practices.[24] Epstein described an intervention in which the role of the critical care nurse is essential in early identification of potential ethical issues, i.e., preventative ethics.[25] Sample questions to consider are listed in Box 2-8.

One common practice for nurses on a daily basis is their oncoming and "hand-off" patient report. Rushton reports that nurses may overlook common issues and potential ethical violations. She offers several strategies to ensure an ethically grounded nursing shift report[26] (Box 2-9). Another patient care issue that arises is when the critically ill patient needs a surrogate decision maker. Especially difficult is when that patient has no family member or is otherwise from a vulnerable and/or marginalized population. There are major concerns when clinicians serve as

both the clinical and the surrogate for the patient. The decision must be made by someone other than the treating clinician, considering procedural fairness for the situation.[27]

Ethical conflicts occur frequently in the health care setting. Negative outcomes of such conflicts are in the areas of staff morale, operational and legal costs, and public relations. It is essential that the health care organization has methods in place to address ethical issues. Because the nurse is on the front line with issues such as do not resuscitate (DNR) orders, response to treatments, and application of new technologies and protocols, he or she may be the one person who best knows the patient's and family's wishes about treatment prolongation or cessation. It is therefore important that the nurse be included as a member of the health care team that determines ethical dilemma resolution. Box 2-10 presents a sample of ethics-related resources.

What Is an Ethical Dilemma?

In general, ethical cases are not always clear-cut. An ethical dilemma exists if there are two (or more) morally correct actions that cannot be followed. The result is that both something right and something wrong occur. In these situations, there are both ethical conflict and ethical conduct issues.[28] The most common ethical dilemmas encountered in critical care are forgoing treatment and allocating the scarce resource of critical care, but how does the health care worker know that a true ethical dilemma exists?

Before any decision model is applied, it must be determined whether a true ethical dilemma exists. Criteria for defining moral and ethical dilemmas in clinical practice are threefold: 1) an awareness of the various options; 2) an issue that has options; and 3) two or more options with true or "good" aspects, with the choice of one option compromising the option not chosen. One must pause, expand group consciousness about the issue, validate assumptions, look for patterns of thoughts or behaviors, and facilitate reflection and inquiry prior to making any decision.[29]

Steps in Ethical Decision Making

To facilitate the ethical decision-making process, a model or framework must be used so that all involved will consistently and clearly examine the multiple ethical issues that arise in critical care. There are various ethical decision-making models in the literature.[30-31] Box 2-11 lists steps in an ethical decision-making model that will be briefly discussed in this chapter.

BOX 2-10 ETHICS RESOURCES

American Association of Critical-Care Nurses (AACN): www.aacn.org
- Joint Position Statement on ICU Overflow Patients
- Acute and Critical Care Choices—Guide to Advanced Directives
- Clinical Practice Guidelines for Quality Palliative Care
- Clinical Practice Guideline on Shared Decision Making in the Appropriate Initiation of Withdrawal from Dialysis
- Last Acts: Precepts of Palliative Care
- Pain Assessment in Nonverbal Patients

American Nurses Association (ANA): www.nursingworld.org
- Position Statements
  - Nursing Care and Do Not Resuscitate (DNR) and Allow Natural Death Decisions
  - Reduction of Patient Restraint and Seclusion in Health Care Settings
  - Forgoing Nutrition and Hydration
  - Registered Nurse' Roles and Responsibilities in Providing Expert Care and Counseling at End of Life
  - The Nurses' Role in Ethics and Human Rights: Protecting and Promoting Individual Worth, Dignity, and Human Rights in Practice Settings

- Assuring Patient Safety: The Employers' Role in Promoting Healthy Nursing Work Hours for Registered Nurses in All Roles and Settings
- Assuring Patient Safety: Registered Nurses' Responsibility in All Roles and Settings to Guard Against Working When Fatigued
- Risk and Responsibility in Providing Nursing Care
- Active Euthanasia
- Cultural Diversity in Nursing Practice

The Hastings Center: www.thehastingscenter.org
- Independent, nonpartisan, nonprofit bioethics research institute
- Provides educational resources and conferences, publications, and ethics consultation

International Council of Nurses (ICN): www.icn.org
- International Code of Ethics for Nurses

United States Department of Veterans Affairs: www.ethics.va.gov
- Created ISSUES Preventative Ethics Model
- Preventative Ethics tools, educational resources, and toolkit for implementing the model
  - Integrated Ethics Program materials available

BOX 2-11 STEPS IN ETHICAL DECISION MAKING

1. Identify the health problem.
2. Define the ethical issue.
3. Gather additional information.
4. Delineate the decision maker.
5. Examine ethical and moral principles.
6. Explore alternative options.
7. Implement decisions.
8. Evaluate and modify actions.

Step One

The major aspects of the medical and health problems must be identified. In other words, the scientific basis of the problem, potential sequelae, prognosis, and all data relevant to the health status must be examined.

Step Two

The ethical problem must be clearly delineated from other types of problems. *Systems problems* result from failures and inadequacies in the health care facility's organization and operation or in the health care system as a whole and are often misinterpreted as ethical issues. *Social problems* arising from conditions in the community, state, or country as a whole also are occasionally confused with ethical issues. Social problems can lead to *systemic problems,* which can constrain responses to ethical problems.

Step Three

Although categories of necessary additional information vary, whatever is missing in the initial problem presentation should be obtained. If not already known, the health prognosis and potential sequelae should be clarified. Usual demographic data—age, ethnicity, religious preference, and educational and economic status—may be considered in the decision-making process. The role of the family or extended family and other support systems must be examined. It is essential to ascertain any desires the patient might have expressed about the treatment decision in writing or in conversation.

Step Four

The patient is the primary decision maker and autonomously makes these decisions after receiving information about the alternatives and sequelae of treatments or lack of treatments. However, in many ethical dilemmas the patient is not competent to make a decision, such as when the patient is comatose or otherwise physically or mentally unable to make a decision. It is in these situations that surrogates are designated or appointed by a court if the urgency of the situation requires a quick decision.

Others who are involved in the decision, such as the family, nurse, physician, social worker, clergy, and members of other disciplines having close contact with the patient, need to be identified at this time. The role of the nurse must be examined. It may not be necessary for the nurse to make a decision at all; rather, the nurse's role may be simply to provide additional information and support to the decision maker.

Step Five

Personal values, beliefs, and moral convictions of all involved in the decision process need to be known. Whether actually achieved through a group meeting or through personal introspection, values clarification facilitates the decision process. See the NIC feature on values clarification in Box 2-6.

The professional ethical codes of the nurse and physician will serve as a foundation for future decisions. At this time, legal constraints or previous legal decisions regarding circumstances at hand need to be assessed and acknowledged.

General ethical principles must be examined in regard to the case at hand. For instance, are veracity, informed consent, and autonomy being promoted? Beneficence and nonmaleficence should be analyzed as they relate to a patient's condition and desires. Close examination of these principles may reveal any compromise of ethical or moral principles for the patient or the health care provider and can assist in decision making.

Step Six

After the identification of alternative options, the outcome of each action must be predicted. This analysis helps the nurse to select the option with the best fit for the specific situation or problem. The short-range and long-range consequences of each action must be examined, and new or creative actions must be encouraged. Consideration also must be given to the "no action" option, which is another choice.

Step Seven

A decision is reached, usually after much thought and consideration, and the decision is implemented. Close attention to detail of the agreed-upon plan is essential. All members of the health care team must be updated, along with the family. It is important that there be one family member designated as the "liaison" between the team and all family members. Ongoing frequent, accurate communication is essential, as well as support for the family and caregivers.

Step Eight

Evaluation of an ethical decision assesses the decision at hand and provides a basis for future ethical decisions. If outcomes are not as predicted, it may be possible to modify the plan or to use an alternative that was not originally chosen. The case can then be reviewed for implications in future ethical interventions and education of the health care team.

STRATEGIES FOR PROMOTION OF ETHICAL DECISION MAKING

The complexity of health care and ethical dilemmas encountered frequently in clinical practice demand the establishment of mechanisms used to address ethical issues in hospitals and health care facilities. Four types of mechanisms are discussed briefly here: institutional ethics committees, inservice and education programs, nursing ethics committees, and ethics rounds and conferences.

Institutional Ethics Committees

Although they are not required by law, many health care facilities have developed institutional ethics committees (IECs) as a way to review ethical cases that are problematic for the practitioner. Major functions of IECs are education, consultation, and recommendation to policy-making bodies. An IEC may function in a variety of ways. The committee may serve as consultants and make recommendations that are not binding. In other situations, health care providers may be required to consult with the committee when there is an ethical problem, with recommendations again not being binding. The third approach requires that ethical dilemmas be presented to the committee and that the recommendations made by the committee must be followed. Regardless of the type of IEC, ethics consultations can help to resolve conflicts that may otherwise prolong unwanted or nonbeneficial treatments.

IECs very often comprise executive medical staff. Membership may include staff physicians, administrators, legal counsel, nurses, social workers, clergy, and community public volunteers. To fulfill its requirement for consultation, the committee must include members who not only have expertise but also are representative of various groups. Regardless of the type of committee model, the IEC provides consultation and support to the practitioners.

Inservice and Education Programs

Basic education about ethical principles and decision making is an important first step in facilitating ethical decision making among nursing staff in the critical care area.[32-33] It is important for nurses to examine their own values, beliefs, and moral convictions. Nurses need to know and use the ANA *Code for Nurses* in their daily clinical practice. Treatment choices for patients and ethical issues involving patients, nurses, and medical colleagues must be explored and discussed in the classroom setting, where no time constraints or extraneous distractions exist to interrupt the decision-making process. Use of the nursing process as a framework can be a teaching strategy for understanding ethical issues[1] (Box 2-12).

Nursing Ethics Committees

Nursing ethics committees provide a forum in which nurses can discuss ethical issues that are pertinent to nurses at the individual, the unit, or the department level.[32-33] Unlike the IEC, which involves treatment choices for patients, the nursing committee may or may not address a patient situation. Depending on the specific goals of the committee, it can also serve as a resource to nursing staff, make recommendations to a policy-making body about a variety of professional issues, or actually formulate policies. It also may serve to educate the department on ethical and professional issues. Membership usually comprises representatives from all major clinical areas or divisions, educators, clinical nurse specialists, administrators, and other specialty staff. Some departments, such as critical care, may have their own unit or division committee.

Ethics Rounds and Conferences

Ethics rounds at the unit level regarding patients in the unit can be done by nurses on a weekly or other established basis. Rounds educate the staff about problems and can have preventive effects when facilitated appropriately. During the discussion, potential problems may be identified early, and actions may be taken to decrease or prevent the incidence of a problem. An individual patient ethics conference may be scheduled to include only the nursing staff or to include a multidisciplinary group to discuss unit issues.[32-33] A patient ethics conference may function as a liaison with the IEC or as an end in itself.

BOX 2-12 ETHICS AND THE NURSING PROCESS

Initial Steps: Clarify and Define the Nature of the Problem
- What is the crisis (or dilemma) requiring a decision?

Assessment: Identify Key Facts and Values That Are Applicable
- What are the crucial facts of the case?
- What moral principles are at issue here?
- What decision-making procedure is appropriate?

Planning: Explore Available and Best Means to Reach Our Goal
- What is the primary aim or good for which we are acting?
- What objectives, benefits, and moral goals are achievable?
- What previous cases or contingencies should we take into account?

Implementation: Take Decisive and Effective Action to Implement Plan
- How do we begin, continue, and finish the process of intervention?
- How do we assess costs/benefits of the intervention?
- How do we monitor success/failure in the overall process?

Evaluation: Evaluate Progress and Outcomes with Planned Objectives
- What means have we set up for debriefing and feedback?
- Have we used the "right" means to a "good" end?
- How do we review the pros/cons for the action taken?

Final Steps: In Retrospect, Apply the Following Tests
- Could I/we provide a reasonable ethical justification for the course of action taken?
- Can I/we identify what we have learned from applying this model to decision making?
- How do we integrate this learning into the next decision-making cycle?

From Thompson IE, et al. *Nursing Ethics*. 5th ed. London: Churchill Livingston; 2006.

BOX 2-13 CASE STUDY

Patient with Ethical Dilemma

Brief Patient History

Mr. X is a 67-year-old obese male. He has a 2-year history of emphysema (100 packs/year history of tobacco abuse in the past) with two recent hospitalizations for pneumonia that required ventilatory support. Mr. X states that he does not want to be placed on a ventilator again but does not want to suffer either. He was involved in a motor vehicular accident (MVA) and sustained blunt trauma to his trunk and lower extremities, with bilateral femur fractures. Although his condition is critical, he is expected to recover. Mr. X received morphine 5 mg by intravenous push in the emergency department, with minimal pain relief; however, he has experienced new-onset confusion. Mr. X's spouse and children express concern about the risk of respiratory depression due to pain medication. They state that they would rather Mr. X experience pain than have him placed on the ventilator again.

Clinical Assessment

Mr. X is admitted to the critical care unit from the emergency department with blood transfusions in progress. Buck's traction (5 pounds) has been applied to both lower extremities. He is awake, alert, and oriented to person, time, place, and situation. Mr. X is breathing through his mouth, taking shallow breaths. He complains of right upper quadrant abdominal pain when taking a deep breath. His skin is warm and dry. Mr. X is able to move his toes on command, and lower extremity sensation to touch is intact; however, he is complaining of severe bilateral lower extremity pain with restlessness.

Diagnostic Procedures

Arterial blood gases: PaO_2, 55 mm Hg; $PaCO_2$, 28 mm Hg; pH, 7.35; HCO_3^-, 24 mEq/L; O_2 saturation, 88%.

Hematocrit, 24%; hemoglobin, 8 g/dL. Patient reports pain as a 10 on the Baker-Wong Faces Scale. Riker Sedation-Agitation Scale score = 5.

Medical Diagnosis

Mr. X is diagnosed with a hepatic hematoma and bilateral femur fractures from an MVA.

Questions

1. What major outcomes do you expect to achieve for this patient?
2. What problems or risks must be managed to achieve these outcomes?
3. What interventions must be initiated to monitor, prevent, manage, or eliminate the problems and risks identified?
4. What interventions should be initiated to promote optimal functioning, safety, and well-being of the patient?
5. What possible learning needs would you anticipate for this patient?
6. What cultural and age-related factors might have a bearing on the patient's plan of care?

SUMMARY

- Ethical dilemmas are encountered daily in the practice of critical care.
- The AACN statement on moral distress and framework to address moral distress provide insight and guidelines for critical care nurses who experience moral distress.
- The critical nature of the situation and the speed that is required to make decisions often prevent practitioners from gaining insight into the desires, values, and feelings of patients.
- By assuming a solely technologic approach, practitioners violate the rights of patients and their professional codes of ethics.

- By using an ethical decision-making process, practitioners protect the rights of the patient, and logical analysis of the case leads to a decision that is made in the best interests of the patient.
- It is through moral reasoning and examining, weighing, justifying, and choosing ethical principles that patient's rights and individuality are upheld.
- The practice of nursing is built on a foundation of moral and ethical caring; the critical care nurse is pivotal in identifying patient situations with an ethical component and can participate in the decision-making process to address the issues.

REFERENCES

1. Thompson IE, Melia KM, Boyd KM, Horsburgh D. *Nursing Ethics*. 4th ed. London: Churchill Livingston; 2006.
2. Cummings CL. Moral distress and the nursing experience. *Nurse Leader*. 2010.
3. Epstein EG, Delgado S. Understanding and addressing moral distress. *OJIN*. 2010;15(3), Manuscript 1.
4. Gallagher A. Moral distress and moral courage in everyday nursing practice. *OJIN*. 2010;16(2).
5. LaSala CA, Biarnason D. Creating workplace environments that support moral courage. *OJIN*. 2010;15(3).
6. *AACN* Position statement: moral distress. http://www.aacn.org. Accessed July 9, 2012.
7. *AACN*. The 4A's to rise above moral distress. http://www.aacn.org. Accessed July 7, 2012.
8. McCue C. Using the AACN framework to alleviate moral distress. *OJIN*. 2010;16(1).
9. Lachman VD, Murray JS, Iseminger K, Ganske KM. Doing the right thing: pathways to moral courage. *American Nurse Today*. 2012;7(5):24.
10. Murray JS. Moral courage in healthcare: acting ethically even in the presence of risk. *OJIN*. 2010;15(3), Manuscript 2.
11. *ANA*. Short definitions of ethical principles and theories. http:// www.nursingworld.org. Accessed July 7, 2012.
12. Stacy KM. Withdrawal of life-sustaining treatment. *Critical Care Nurse*. 2012;32(3):1
13. Schneiderman LJ, et al. Medical futility: its meaning and ethical implications. *Ann Intern Med*. 1990;112(12):949.
14. McIntosh B. Medical futility: *DCMS Online, Northeast Florida Supplement*, January 2008, accessed July 9, 2010.
15. Bernat JL. Medical futility: definition, determination, and disputed in critical care. *Neurocrit Care*. 2005;2(2):198.
16. Hofmann PB, Schneiderman LJ. Physicians should not always pursue a good clinical outcome. Hastings Center Report 2007. May-June, 37(3), inside back cover.
17. Lachman VD. Practical use of the nursing code of ethics: part I. *Medsurg Nurs*. 2009;18(1):55.
18. Curtin L. Ethics for nurses in everyday practice. *American Nurse Today*. 2010;5(2).
19. Murray JS. Creating ethical environments in nursing. *American Nurse Today*. 2007;2(10):48.
20. Fowler DM, ed. *Guide to the Code of Ethics for Nurses*. Silver Springs, MD: American Nurses Association; 2008.
21. Benner P. Relational ethics of comfort, touch, and solace—endangered arts? *Am J Crit Care*. 2004;13(4):346.
22. Lachman VD. Applying the ethics of care to your nursing practice. *MEDSURG Nursing*. 2012;21(2):112.
23. Pavlish C, Brown-Saltzman K, Hersh M, Shirk M, Nudelman O. Early indicators and risk factors for ethical issues in clinical practice. *Image: J Nursing Scholarship*. 2011;43(1):13.
24. *United States Department of Veterans Affairs*. Preventative ethics. http://www.ethics.va.gov. Accessed July 12, 2010.
25. Epstein EG. Preventative ethics in the intensive care unit. *AACN Advanced Critical Care*. 2012;23(2):217.
26. Rushton CH. Ethics of nursing shift report. *AACN Advanced Critical Care*. 2010;21(4):380.
27. White DB, Jonsen A, Lo B. Ethical challenge: When clinicians act as surrogates for underrepresented patients. *AJCC*. 2012;21(3):202.
28. Purtilo RB, Doherty RF. *Ethical Decisions in the Health Professions*. 5th ed. St. Louis: Saunders; 2011.
29. Rushton CH. Ethical discernment and action: the art of pause. *AACN Adv Crit Care*. 2009;20(1):108.
30. Rushton CH, Penticuff JH. A framework for analysis of ethical dilemmas in critical care nursing. *AACN Adv Crit Care*. 2007;18(3):323.
31. Clark AP. A model for ethical decision making in cases of patient futility. *Clin Nurse Spec*. 2010;24(4):189.
32. Pavlish C, Brown-Saltzman K, Hersh M, Shirk M, Rounkle AM. Nursing priorities, actions, and regrets for ethical situations in clinical practice. *Image: J Nursing Scholarship*. 2011;43(4):385.
33. Robichaux C. Developing ethical skills: From sensitivity to action. *Critical Care Nurse*. 2012;32(2):65.

CHAPTER

3

Legal Issues

Kelly K. Dineen

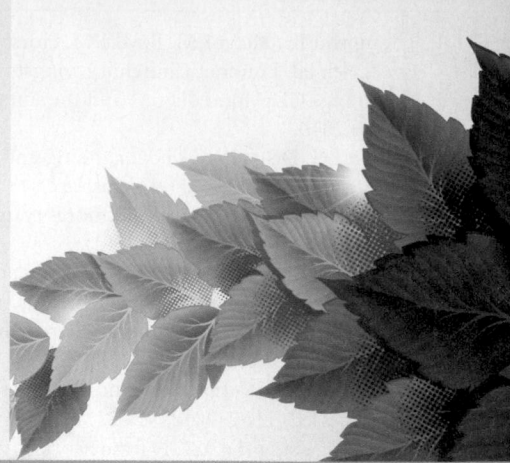

OVERVIEW

The law routinely influences and intersects with the practice of nursing and with health care in general. This influence extends far beyond the common notion of malpractice and the trial system. Legal systems operate at the local, state, and federal level and range from matters handled through the courts to those handled through administrative agencies to agreements between private individuals or organizations. Regardless of the setting, the law, in general, is concerned with minimum standards rather than best practices or even ethical practice. In other words, practice that meets legal criteria is often far less than what meets ethical criteria or criteria for best practices. Nursing licensure is one such example as it indicates that the nurse has demonstrated the basic competencies to safely practice as an entry-level nurse.

Of course, effective nursing is about much more than minimal competencies. The National Council of State Boards of Nursing (NCSBN), an organization that works to develop policy and consistent standards throughout the state licensing boards, defines nursing as: 1) a scientific process founded on a professional body of knowledge; 2) a learned profession based on an understanding of the human condition across the lifespan and the relationship of a client with others and within the environment; and 3) an art dedicated to caring for others.[1] The NCSBN further describes nursing as a "dynamic discipline that increasingly involves more sophisticated knowledge, technologies and client care activities." As nurses practice in this increasingly complex and rapidly evolving health care system, it is critical to understand some basic principles of law, the differences between legal thresholds and quality and scope of practice, and the ways in which practice is impacted by law and the ability of nurses to impact health law and policy.

This chapter will highlight some of the laws and legal systems that figure prominently in nursing practice, including 1) administrative law (illustrated by the regulation of the profession by state boards of nursing); 2) tort law (lawsuits brought by patients for the actions or inactions of nurses); 3) constitutional law (illustrated through a discussion of the legal rights of patients to make decisions to accept or refuse treatment); and 4) federal and state health care statutory laws (illustrated through self-determination laws and select federal laws).

ADMINISTRATIVE LAW: PROFESSIONAL REGULATION

For most nurses, the first professional interaction with a legal system is through the process of licensure. The very ability to practice as a licensed professional nurse is a privilege granted by the state and is a function of each state's authority to promote and protect the health and welfare of its citizens. State boards of nursing (BON) are administrative bodies created by—and that operate under—state statutes, or more generally written state laws created by state legislatures and signed by the governor. In turn, the BONs develop more specific rules (or regulations) for obtaining and maintaining licensure.

This process is consistent throughout every administrative system, whether federal or state. Administrative bodies are created and granted power under statutes written and passed by legislatures and signed by the governor (in the case of state law) or the president (in the case of federal law). Administrative agencies, in turn, develop, propose and effectuate specific regulations in their areas. These regulations can be changed by the administrative agencies through a process of rulemaking that allows the agencies to adapt to changes in their relative areas without requiring the action of the legislature. For example, state nurse practice acts (NPAs) are statutes that established the scope of practice in each state. BONs, state administrative agencies, create more specific rules or regulations further defining the scope of practice, delineating the standards of practice or criteria for licensure and may change them through the same rulemaking process. The work of the BONs is just one tangible example of an administrative system, but perhaps the most important to nurses, as BONs control the very ability to practice.

Functions of Boards of Nursing

The regulation of nursing practice is intended to protect the health and safety of citizens by: 1) regulating the conditions of licensure; 2) regulating the scope of practice; 3) establishing a framework of standards of nursing practice; 4) removing incompetent or unsafe practitioners through disciplinary actions; and 5) prohibiting unlicensed persons from providing services reserved for licensed individuals. In addition, the regulation of nursing can enhance the professional status and public's trust of nurses.

Scope of Practice

BONs maintain expectations for and limits of nursing practice in each state through the licensure of nurses and also through challenges to non-nurses engaged in professional activities that intrude upon the nursing scope of practice. The scope of practice generally refers to the broad range of activities that nurses perform and manage in the delivery of care. The scope of practice activities is framed broadly to account for the many professional nursing settings and roles but also to account for activities that are reserved for professional nurses or, as appropriate, their delegatees with nursing supervision. Scope of practice provisions are also intended to prevent unlicensed professionals from providing services that are reserved to licensed professionals.

Yet, the absolute outside limits of the scope of practice are sometimes a bit difficult to define. As such, the scope and limits of nursing practice have often been the subject of disciplinary action and legal challenges through the court system. In some cases, these challenges arise from other professional licensing boards, such as state medical boards, in response to circumstances within their state. The importance of the scope of practice has been demonstrated by several important legal cases. In *Sermchief v Gonzales,*[2] the Supreme Court of Missouri heard a case involving two nurses who worked with several physicians in rural Missouri to provide women's health care services. The nurses engaged in health counseling, routine pelvic exams and testing such as pap smears, as well as community education under standing orders from physicians. All of the parties were in agreement that the nurses had provided excellent care and

that the patients were satisfied. The issue was strictly whether they were practicing within the scope of nursing practice or if they were infringing upon the scope of medical practice (practicing medicine without a license). The court held in favor of the nurses because their work was within the boundaries of the then-existing NPA and within the limits of the physicians' orders.

The field of obstetrics has commonly served as an example for scope of practice issues. A case in Ohio, *Marion Ob/Gyn v State Med. Bd.,*[3] established that delivering infants was beyond the scope of physician assistant practice in Ohio. At the same time, nurses could deliver infants as the scope of nursing practice allowed licensed nurses to practice midwifery. In Kansas, lay midwives can deliver infants without infringing on the scope of nursing or medical practice. In *State Board of Nursing v Ruebke,*[4] the Kansas Supreme Court held lay midwifery was a common and longstanding exception to the prohibition against the unauthorized practice of medicine if the midwife is working under the supervision of a physician.

Standards of Practice

NPAs establish the scope of nursing practice while BONs usually develop standards of practice at the state level through administrative rulemaking. These standards of practice communicate the expectations of safe and effective nursing practice within the scope of practice. State standards of practice also assist BONs in evaluating the ongoing practice of nursing. Thus, to fully understand the expectations for and limits of nursing in any particular state, it is necessary to review both the NPA and the rules or regulations of the BON.

In addition to standards developed by BONs, many specialty nursing organizations have developed standards of practice. While the BON standards establish broad expectations of safety and efficacy, specialty standards are more targeted and aimed at fostering excellence in the specialized field. An example of specialty standards are those developed by the American Association of Critical-Care Nurses (AACN).[5]

The Model Nursing Act (Model Act) and Model Administrative Rules (Model Rules) developed by the NCSBN serve as example NPAs and standards of practice for individual states in regulating nursing practice.[6] Actual state laws governing professional nursing practice vary from state to state in the degree to which they have adopted all or part of the current or previous model acts and rules. Nonetheless, the Model Act scope of practice provisions (Box 3-1) and the Model Rules for standards of practice (Box 3-2) are useful in illustrating the differences between scope and standards. For example, the seventh activity listed within the scope of practice is "advocating the best interest of clients." Within the standards of practice in Box 3-2, standard 3 lists eight specific obligations or expectations of nurses in advocating for clients.

In addition, nursing standards developed by professional and specialty nursing organizations complement BON standards, provide detail and specificity, and are typically drafted to promote excellence in clinical practice. Foundational organizations such as the American Nurses Association (ANA) and the AACN publish standards of practice and standards of care.[7] The

BOX 3-1   SCOPE OF PRACTICE (ACTIVITIES OF PROFESSIONAL NURSES)

Model Nursing Act, Scope of Nursing Practice (Model Statutory Law)

1. Providing comprehensive nursing assessment of the health status of clients.
2. Collaborating with health care team to develop an integrated client-centered health care plan.
3. Developing a strategy of nursing care to be integrated within the client-centered health care plan that establishes nursing diagnoses; sets goals to meet identified health care needs; prescribes nursing interventions; and implements nursing care through the execution of independent nursing strategies and regimens requested, ordered or prescribed by authorized health care providers.
4. Delegating and assigning nursing interventions to implement the plan of care.
5. Providing for the maintenance of safe and effective nursing care rendered directly or indirectly.
6. Promoting a safe and therapeutic environment.
7. Advocating the best interest of clients.
8. Evaluating responses to interventions and the effectiveness of the plan of care.
9. Communicating and collaborating with other health care providers in the management of health care and the implementation of the total health care regimen within and across care settings.
10. Acquiring and applying critical new knowledge and technologies to the practice domain.
11. Managing, supervising and evaluating the practice of nursing.
12. Teaching the theory and practice of nursing.
13. Participating in development of policies, procedures, and systems to support the client.
14. Other acts that require education and training as prescribed by the BON commensurate with the RN's continuing education, demonstrated competencies, and experience.

Modified from National Council of the State Boards of Nursing (NCSBN). *NCSBN Model Nursing Practice Act and Model Nursing Administrative Rules.* Chicago: NCSBN; 2011.

AACN standards appear in Box 3-3. These specialty standards are helpful in establishing and measuring quality care and often reflect a consensus opinion of experts in the particular specialty of appropriate nursing care.

The extent to which specialty standards are introduced in a legal context varies widely from state to state. It is critical to understand that the legal term of art, "standard of care," is not the same as the standards of practice. In some cases, specialty standards of practice or care have been introduced in court to help establish a legal "standard of care," but not all courts will consider these. The legal standard of care and the use of specialty standards will be discussed further in the Tort Law section.

TORT LAW: NEGLIGENCE AND PROFESSIONAL MALPRACTICE, INTENTIONAL TORTS

Many civil lawsuits for injuries fall under the legal heading of torts. Anyone can find themselves as a party in such a lawsuit. Torts are civil lawsuits based on unintentional acts (failure to act or negligence that results in harm) or intentional acts, such as assault, battery, or defamation. For the lay public, the standard for behavior for negligence is based on reasonableness, or what a reasonably prudent person would do in the same situation. This is also known as ordinary negligence.

In a professional capacity, individuals are judged based on their professional standard of care. Nurses caring for acutely and critically ill patients may be alleged to have acted in a manner that is inconsistent with standards of care or standards of professional practice and may find themselves involved in civil litigation that focuses in whole or in part on the alleged failure. This is professional malpractice or negligence law applied to professional behavior.

There are many types of cases based in tort law but this chapter will focus on negligence and professional malpractice, intentional torts of assault and battery, and some cases based on specific clinical circumstances. These include the respiratory management of acutely and critically ill patients, as well as liability associated with blood transfusions, infection control, and informed consent.

Ordinary Negligence

Generally, the standard for negligence is failing to act as a reasonably prudent person would under similar circumstances. There are four criteria or elements for all negligence cases: 1) duty to another person; 2) breach of that duty; 3) harm that would not have occurred in the absence of the breach (causation); and 4) damages that have a monetary value. All four elements must be satisfied for a case to go forward. For example, suppose a grocery store employee mops the floor but fails to block off the area or put up a wet floor sign and a customer walks in the area, falls and breaks a hip, and is left with hospital bills and lost wages. The grocery store has a duty to its customers to provide a reasonably safe environment and warn customers of areas of danger. Warning customers and/or blocking off the wet area is what a reasonably prudent grocery store would do. Failing to warn customers was a breach of that duty. Because the customer had no warning, she walked on the wet floor, fell, and suffered the harm of a broken hip. She would not have suffered the broken hip if the area had been blocked off. Finally, there are monetary damages in the form of hospital bills and lost wages. This is an example of ordinary negligence in which any person could make a determination of what is reasonable in a given circumstance. A juror need not hear from a professional to determine what is a reasonably prudent practice for the grocery store (standard for non-negligent behavior) in this case. On the other hand, negligence in the professional health care context differs in that expert testimony is needed to establish the standard of care. These cases are referred to as professional negligence or professional malpractice.

Professional Malpractice

Whereas negligence claims may apply to anyone, malpractice requires the alleged wrongdoer to have special standing as a

BOX 3-2 STANDARDS OF PRACTICE*

Model Nursing Administrative Rules, Standards of Nursing Practice (Model Regulations or Administrative Rules)

1. Standards Related to Registered Nurse (RN) Professional Accountability

The RN:

a. Practices within the legal boundaries for nursing through the scope of practice authorized in the NPA and rules governing nursing.

b. Demonstrates honesty and integrity in nursing practice.

c. Bases professional decisions on nursing knowledge and skills, the needs of clients, and the expectations delineated in professional standards.

d. Accepts responsibility for judgments, individual nursing actions, competence, decisions, and behavior in the course of nursing practice.

e. Maintains continued competence through ongoing learning and application of knowledge in the client's interest.

2. Standards Related to RN Responsibility for Nursing Practice Implementation

The RN:

a. Conducts a comprehensive nursing assessment that is an extensive data collection (initial and ongoing) regarding individuals, families, groups, and communities.

b. Detects faulty or missing patient/client information.

c. Applies nursing knowledge effectively in the synthesis of the biologic, psychologic, and social aspects of the client's condition.

d. Uses this broad and complete analysis to plan strategies of nursing care and nursing interventions that are integrated within the client's overall health care plan.

e. Provides appropriate decision making, critical thinking, and clinical judgment to make independent nursing decisions and nursing diagnoses.

f. Seeks clarification of orders when needed.

g. Implements treatment and therapy, including medication administration and delegated medical and independent nursing functions.

h. Obtains orientation/training for competence when encountering new equipment and technology or unfamiliar care situations.

i. Demonstrates attentiveness and provides client surveillance and monitoring.

j. Identifies changes in client's health status and comprehends clinical implications of client signs, symptoms, and changes as part of expected and unexpected client course or emergent situations.

k. Evaluates the impact of nursing care, the client's response to therapy, the need for alternative interventions, and the need to communicate and consult with other health team members.

l. Documents nursing care.

m. Intervenes on behalf of client when problems are identified and revises care plan as needed.

n. Recognizes client characteristics that may affect the client's health status.

o. Takes preventive measures to protect client, others, and self.

3. Standards Related to RN Responsibility to Act as an Advocate for Client

The RN:

a. Respects the client's rights, concerns, decisions, and dignity. *(This standard includes respecting the client's concerns regarding end-of-life care.)*

b. Identifies client needs.

c. Attends to client concerns or requests.

d. Promotes safe client environment.

e. Communicates client choices, concerns, and special needs with other health team members regarding:

1. Client status and progress.
2. Client response or lack of response to therapies.
3. Significant changes in client condition.

f. Maintains appropriate professional boundaries.

g. Maintains client confidentiality.

h. Assumes responsibility for nurse's own decisions and actions.

4. Standards Related to RN Responsibility to Organize, Manage, and Supervise the Practice of Nursing

The RN:

a. Assigns to another only those nursing measures that fall within that nurse's scope of practice, education, experience, and competence or unlicensed person's role description.

b. Delegates to another only those nursing measures for which that person has the necessary skills and competence to accomplish safely.

c. Matches client needs with personnel qualifications, available resources, and appropriate supervision.

d. Communicates directions and expectations for completion of the delegated activity.

e. Supervises others to whom nursing activities are delegated or assigned by monitoring performance, progress, and outcomes; and assures documentation of the activity.

f. Provides follow-up on problems and intervenes when needed.

g. Evaluates the effectiveness of the delegation or assignment.

h. Intervenes when problems are identified and revises plan of care as needed.

i. Retains professional accountability for nursing care as provided.

5. Standards Related to RN Responsibilities as a Member of an Interdisciplinary Health Care Team

The RN:

a. Functions as a member of the health care team, collaborating and cooperating in the implementation of an integrated client-centered health care plan.

b. Respects client property and the property of others.

c. Protects confidential information.

*Methods by which nurses safely and effectively deliver care within the scope of practice.
Modified from National Council of the State Boards of Nursing (NCSBN). *NCSBN Model Nursing Practice Act and Model Nursing Administrative Rules.* Chicago: NCSBN; 2011.

professional. If a nurse caring for acutely and critically ill patients is accused of failing to act in a manner consistent with the standard of care, that nurse is subject to liability for professional malpractice (negligence applied to a professional). Just as in ordinary negligence, the person bringing the lawsuit must prove the elements of negligence. In the health care context,

patient/plaintiffs (person[s] bringing the lawsuit) must prove: 1) that the nurse had a duty to care for the patient; 2) that the nurse breached that duty by deviating from the standard of care; 3) that the breach caused harm that would not have occurred in the absence of negligence; and 4) that the plaintiff should be compensated for the resulting damages.

BOX 3-3 STANDARDS FOR ACUTE AND CRITICAL CARE NURSING

STANDARDS OF CARE FOR ACUTE AND CRITICAL CARE NURSING PRACTICE

Standard 1: Assessment

The nurse caring for the acutely and critically ill patient collects relevant data pertinent to the patient's health or situation.

Measurement Criteria

1. Data are collected from the patient, family, other health care providers, and the community, as appropriate, to develop a holistic picture of the patient's needs.
2. The priority of data collection activities is driven by the patient's characteristics related to immediate condition and anticipated needs.
3. Pertinent and sufficient data are collected using appropriate evidence-based assessment techniques and instruments.
4. Analytical models and problem-solving tools are used.
5. Relevant data are documented.
6. Relevant data are communicated to other healthcare providers.

Standard 2: Diagnosis

The nurse caring for the acutely and critically ill patient analyzes the assessment data in determining diagnosis and care issues.

Measurement Criteria

1. Diagnoses and care issues are derived from the assessment data.
2. Diagnoses and care issues are validated throughout the nursing interactions with the patient, family, other health care providers, the community, and across the healthcare system when possible and appropriate.
3. Diagnoses and care issues are prioritized and documented in a manner that facilitates prioritizing outcomes and developing or modifying the plan.

Standard 3: Outcomes Identification

The nurse caring for the acutely and critically ill patient identifies outcomes for the patient or the patient's situation.

Measurement Criteria

1. Outcomes are derived from actual or potential diagnoses and care issues.
2. Outcomes are formulated in collaboration with the patient, family, and other health care providers, in relation to the level of participation in care and decision making.
3. Outcomes recognize, appreciate, and incorporate differences.
4. Outcomes are attainable in relation to resources available; outcomes consider associated risks, benefits, current evidence, clinical expertise, and cost.
5. Outcomes provide direction for continuity of care.
6. Outcomes are modified on the basis of changes in patient characteristics or evaluation of the situation.
7. Outcomes are documented as measurable goals.

Standard 4: Planning

The nurse caring for the acutely and critically ill patient develops a plan that prescribes interventions to attain outcomes.

Measurement Criteria

1. The plan is individualized and considers patient characteristics and the situation.
2. The plan is developed collaboratively with the patient, family, and healthcare providers in a way that promotes each member's contribution toward achieving the outcomes.
3. The plan reflects current best evidence.
4. The plan provides for continuity of care and matching the nurse's competencies with the patient's characteristics.

5. The plan establishes priorities for care.
6. The plan includes strategies for promotion and restoration of health and prevention of further illness, injury, and disease.
7. The plan considers economic impact and resources available.

Standard 5: Implementation

The nurse caring for the acutely and critically ill patient implements the plan, coordinates care delivery, and employs strategies to promote health and a safe environment.

Measurement Criteria

1. Interventions are delivered in a manner that minimizes complications and life-threatening situations.
2. The patient and family participate in implementing the plan according to their level of participation and decision-making capabilities.
3. Interventions are responsive to the uniqueness of the patient and family and create a compassionate and therapeutic environment, with the aim to promote comfort and prevent suffering.
4. The implemented plan and modifications are documented.
5. Collaboration to implement the plan occurs with the patient, family, healthcare providers, and the healthcare system.
6. The plan facilitates learning for patients, families, nursing staff, other members of the healthcare team, and the community including but not limited to health teaching, health promotion, and disease management according to patient characteristics.

Standard 6: Evaluation

The nurse caring for the acutely and critically ill patient evaluates progress toward attaining outcomes.

Measurement Criteria

1. Evaluation is systematic and ongoing using evidence-based techniques and instruments.
2. The team of patient, family, and healthcare providers is involved in the evaluation process as appropriate.
3. Evaluation of the effectiveness of interventions toward achieving the desired outcome occurs.
4. Evaluation occurs within an appropriate time frame after interventions are initiated.
5. Ongoing assessment data are used to revise the diagnoses, outcomes, and plan as needed.
6. Results of the evaluation are documented.

STANDARDS OF PROFESSIONAL PERFORMANCE

Standard 1: Quality of Practice

The nurse caring for the acutely and critically ill patient systematically evaluates and seeks to improve the quality and effectiveness of nursing practice.

Measurement Criteria

1. The nurse participates in clinical inquiry through quality improvement activities.
2. The nurse uses systems thinking to initiate changes in nursing practice and the healthcare delivery system.
3. The nurse ensures that quality improvement activities incorporate the patient's and family's beliefs, values, and preferences as appropriate.
4. The nurse questions and evaluates practice in an ongoing process, providing informed practice and innovation through research and experiential learning.
5. The nurse identifies organizational systems barriers to quality care and patient outcomes.

BOX 3-3 STANDARDS FOR ACUTE AND CRITICAL CARE NURSING—cont'd

6. The nurse collects data to monitor the quality and effectiveness of nursing practice.
7. The nurse develops, implements, evaluates, and updates policies, procedures, and/or guidelines to improve the quality and effectiveness of nursing practice.

Standard 2: Professional Practice Evaluation
The nurse caring for the acutely and critically ill patient evaluates his or her own nursing practice in relation to professional practice standards, institutional guidelines, relevant statutes, rules, and regulations.

Measurement Criteria
1. The nurse engages in a self-assessment and/or formal performance appraisal on a regular basis, identifying areas of strength as well as areas where professional development would be beneficial.
2. The nurse seeks and reflects on constructive feedback regarding his or her own competencies from the team of patient, family, and other healthcare providers.
3. The nurse takes action to achieve performance goals.

Standard 3: Education
The nurse acquires and maintains current knowledge and competency in the care of acutely and critically ill patients.

Measurement Criteria
1. The nurse participates in ongoing learning activities to acquire and refine knowledge and skills needed to care for acutely and critically ill patients and their families.
2. The nurse seeks learning opportunities that reflect evidence-based practice in order to maintain clinical skills and competencies needed to care for acutely and critically ill patients and their families.
3. The nurse participates in ongoing learning activities related to professional practice.
4. The nurse maintains professional records that provide evidence of competency and lifelong learning.

Standard 4: Collegiality
The nurse caring for the acutely and critically ill patient interacts with and contributes to the professional development of peers and other healthcare providers as colleagues.

Measurement Criteria
1. The nurse shares knowledge, skills, and experiences with peers and colleagues.
2. The nurse provides peers and colleagues with constructive feedback regarding their practice.
3. The nurse interacts with peers and colleagues to enhance his or her own professional practice and promote optimal patient outcomes.
4. The nurse contributes to a supportive and healthy work environment that is conducive to the education of healthcare professionals.
5. The nurse contributes to a healthy work environment by working with others in a way that promotes mutual respect and meaningful recognition of each person's contribution.

Standard 5: Ethics
The nurse's decisions and actions are carried out in an ethical manner in all areas of practice.

Measurement Criteria
1. The nurse's practice is guided by the ANA Code of Ethics for Nurses with Interpretive Statements, the AACN Ethic of Care, and ethical principles.
2. The nurse maintains patient confidentiality within legal and regulatory parameters.
3. The nurse works on another's behalf and represents the concerns of patients, their families, and the community.
4. The nurse delivers care in a nonjudgmental and nondiscriminatory manner that meets the diverse needs, strengths, and weaknesses of the patient and preserves patient autonomy, dignity, and rights.
5. The nurse uses available resources in formulating ethical decisions.
6. The nurse demonstrates a commitment to self-care and self-advocacy.
7. The nurse reports illegal, incompetent, or impaired practices.

Standard 6: Collaboration
The nurse caring for the acutely and critically ill patient uses skilled communication to collaborate with the team of patient, family, and healthcare providers in providing patient care in a safe, healing, humane, and caring environment.

Measurement Criteria
1. The nurse uses skilled communication to foster true collaboration.
2. The nurse partners with others to effect change and generate optimal outcomes through knowledge of the patient or situation.
3. The nurse commits to establishing and maintaining a healthy work environment.
4. The nurse initiates referrals as appropriate to promote continuity of care.
5. The nurse collaborates with the patient's family and significant others to promote effective transition across care settings.

Standard 7: Research/Clinical Inquiry
The nurse caring for the acutely and critically ill patient uses clinical inquiry and integrates research findings into practice.

Measurement Criteria
1. The nurse continually questions and evaluates practice and uses best available evidence, including research findings, to guide practice decisions.
2. The nurse participates in activities to support clinical inquiry as appropriate to the nurse's skills, knowledge, and experience.

Standard 8: Resource Utilization
The nurse caring for the acutely and critically ill patient considers factors related to safety, effectiveness, cost, and impact in planning and delivering nursing services.

Measurement Criteria
1. The nurse considers factors related to safety, effectiveness, availability, cost, and impact on outcomes when choosing among practice options.
2. The nurse assists the patient and family in identifying and securing appropriate and available services to address health-related needs according to resource availability.
3. The nurse assigns or delegates aspects of care as defined by the state nurse practice acts, based on an assessment of the needs and condition of the patient, the potential for harm, the stability of the patient's condition, the predictability of the outcome, the availability and competence of the healthcare provider, and the availability of resources.
4. The nurse assists the patient and family to become informed consumers by facilitating learning of the options, alternatives, risks, benefits, and costs of treatment and care.

Modified from American Association of Critical-Care Nurses. *Standards for Acute and Critical Care Nursing Practice.* Aliso Viejo, CA: AACN; 2008.

In civil cases alleging wrongdoing by health care professionals, the terms "malpractice" and "negligence" are used interchangeably, although there are courts that distinguish between the two causes of action. The malpractice-negligence distinction was addressed in *Candler General Hospital Inc. v McNorrill.*[8] In that case, the court concluded that malpractice was merely a negligence action applied to a professional.

The legal standard of care for nurses is established by expert testimony and is generally "the care that an ordinarily prudent *nurse* would perform under the same circumstances."[9] The standard of care determination focuses more on accepted practice of competent nurses rather than best practice of excellent nurses (which may be reflected in some specialty standards of practice). In addition to expert testimony, courts may rely on multiple types of evidence to establish the standard of care.

In *Gould v NY City Health and Hospital,*[10] the court looked more closely at the standard of care and determined that there were three obligations inherent in a malpractice cause of action. The nurse should 1) possess the requisite knowledge and skill possessed by an average member of the profession; 2) exercise reasonable and ordinary care in the application of professional knowledge and skill; and 3) use best judgment in the application of professional knowledge and skill.

Duty

Duty to the injured party is the first element of a malpractice case and is premised on the existence of a nurse-patient relationship. Nurses assume a duty to the patient to provide care that is consistent with the standard of care when the nurse-patient relationship is established. Cases from a number of states recognize the nurse-patient relationship as a separate and distinct relationship[11] and as a prerequisite for determining whether a nurse owes the patient a duty to provide care in accordance with the requisite standard of care. If a nurse shows that he or she 1) was not assigned to that particular patient on the date that the negligence allegedly occurred or 2) was not working on the day or at the time the negligence allegedly occurred, no duty will be imposed on the nurse. Because no duty is imposed on the nurse, negligence allegations will fail.[12]

Although courts have been willing to construct parameters around a nurse's duty to his or her patient, if the patient establishes that a specific nurse actually rendered care, the nurse will be found to have assumed a duty to provide reasonable care for the patient. This duty cannot be waived or overridden by the instructions of a physician or hospital administrator. A nurse's failure to provide reasonable care subjects the nurse to civil liability for negligence provided the patient proves that the failure caused damage or injury.

Lunsford v Board of Nurse Examiners[13] illustrates this principle. In this case, Donald Floyd arrived at an emergency department in Texas complaining of chest pain and pressure that radiated down his left arm. Mr. Floyd was accompanied by Francis Farrell, who attempted to have Mr. Floyd examined by a physician who was sitting at the nurses' station in the emergency department. The physician told Ms. Farrell that Mr. Floyd would need to first be seen by a nurse. The physician then instructed Nurse Lunsford to transfer Mr. Floyd to a neighboring hospital located 24 miles away because the equipment that would likely be needed to treat Mr. Floyd was already in use by another patient.

Lunsford interviewed Mr. Floyd and suspected cardiac involvement. Because of the transfer instruction that she received from the physician, Lunsford instructed Ms. Farrell to drive with her flashers on and to speed to get to the neighboring hospital. Reportedly, Lunsford also asked Ms. Farrell if she knew cardiopulmonary resuscitation (CPR) and suggested that she might need to perform CPR at some point on the way. Unfortunately, within approximately 5 miles of the Harlingen emergency department, Mr. Farrell died from cardiac arrest.

An administrative complaint was subsequently filed with the Texas Board of Nurse Examiners alleging negligence and challenging Lunsford's nursing licensure. After a hearing on the matter, the Texas Board of Nurse Examiners suspended the license of Lunsford for 1 year. Lunsford appealed the decision and the court determined that Lunsford, as well as other nurses who are similarly situated, have a duty to evaluate the status of persons who are ill and seeking professional help. The court also determined that Lunsford, as well as other nurses, have a duty to implement care needed to stabilize a patient's condition and to prevent complications. According to this Texas Court of Appeals, Lunsford failed to act reasonably and breached her duty to Mr. Floyd when she failed to 1) assess him; 2) inform the physician of the life-and-death nature of his condition; 3) take appropriate action to stabilize him and prevent his death. The court also pointed out that hospital policy or physician orders do not relieve a nurse of his or her duty to a patient.

Breach

Breach is the failure to act consistently within applicable standards of care. For a nurse to be found negligent, the patient-plaintiff must establish that the nurse had a duty to provide care and that the nurse failed to provide care consistent with those standards. Moreover, the nurse's failure, or breach, must have caused the damages about which the patient-plaintiff seeks redress. A breach of duty does not exist if the standard of care is met.

In *Sparks v St. Luke's Regional Medical Center,*[14] the family of Thomas Sparks sued St. Luke's Regional Medical Center and treating physicians, alleging that their negligence resulted in Thomas Sparks sustaining brain damage after he was extubated. The case reached the Idaho Supreme Court. The court concluded that although Mr. Sparks suffered severe harm, no breach of duty existed and the evidence established that the standard of care regarding extubation and subsequent hospital care was met by the St. Luke's personnel.

Sparks demonstrated that some courts will consider many sources of evidence in determining the standard of care. These may include applicable NPAs, specialty practice standards, job descriptions, and organizational policies, procedures, protocols, and pathways, together with other reference sources including case law, journal articles, textbooks, and other manuscripts.

Actions that are consistent with professional practice standards may be used as evidence that the nurse did not breach his or her duty to patients. Even if not used as evidence for the standard of care, these standards provide guidance on quality nursing care. Nurses caring for acutely and critically ill patients should practice in accordance with the practice specialty standards issued by the AACN (Box 3-3). These standards provide guidance for nurses, and they increasingly provide definitive guidance in courtrooms.

For example, in *Koeniguer v Eckrich*[15] standards promulgated by the ANA were used in a case in which the plaintiff alleged that standards of care were breached. In *Koeniguer*, Winnifred Scoblic was admitted to Dakota Midland Hospital for surgical correction of incontinence. Two days later, J.A. Eckrich performed the surgery. After surgery, Ms. Scoblic had a temperature that fluctuated. On the day of discharge, Ms. Scoblic's temperature was 100.2° F. Despite her temperature, Ms. Scoblic was discharged. Sixteen days after her original surgery, Ms. Scoblic was readmitted because of a fever and severe abdominal pain. She was diagnosed with septicemia. Two days later, Ms. Scoblic was transferred to the University of Minnesota Hospital. She died from multiple organ failure several weeks later.

On behalf of Ms. Scoblic, her daughter, Patricia Koeniguer, filed a malpractice cause of action contending that the care rendered to her mother deviated from the standard of care. An expert retained by Koeniguer used the standards published by the ANA and other general nursing treatises to conclude that the nursing staff failed to adhere to standards of care applicable to Ms. Scoblic as a postoperative urologic patient.

Documents or policies specific to the nurse's employer or practice setting may also be used to inform the appropriate standard of care. For example, a nurse's job description or employment contract may contain provisions that require a nurse to act or to refrain from acting in a specific manner and within a specific period of time. Failure to adhere to those provisions could give rise to negligence causes of action wherein the patient-plaintiff asserts that the nurse failed to act in accordance with his or her job description or employment contract. Accordingly, job descriptions and employment contracts must be reflective of the standard of care, and expectations must be articulated in a manner that is reasonable.

Nurses caring for acutely and critically ill patients are required to act in a manner that is consistent with organizational policies, procedures, protocols, and clinical pathways. Failure to do so may result in liability if a patient is harmed because of the failure. For example, in *Teffeteller v University of Minnesota*,[16] a nurse's failure to follow a protocol resulted in a critically ill pediatric patient's death from narcotic toxicity.

Harm Caused by the Breach

Patient-plaintiffs must prove that the nurse breached his or her duty to the patient and that the breach caused the patient to sustain injuries or damages for which he or she seeks monetary remuneration. Causation of the harm is a pivotal element in civil cases filed against nurses. If patient-plaintiffs fail to establish that some act or omission directly resulted in the harm or if something else can be shown to have caused the harm, recovery will be denied.

McMullen v Ohio State University Hospitals[17] dealt with the causation issue and was ultimately decided by the Ohio Supreme Court. In *McMullen*, a patient had been intubated and placed on a ventilator. Three days after she was intubated, her oxygen saturation level suddenly dropped, as did her blood pressure, and she became cyanotic and dyspneic. The patient also developed a squeak, which the nurse thought was a cuff leak on the endotracheal tube. The nurse believed that the patient was dying and made a "stat" page so that on-call physicians would be notified. Before the arrival of the physicians, the nurse removed the patient's endotracheal tube. When the physicians arrived, they attempted to reintubate the patient. It took more than twenty minutes for their reintubation attempts to be successful. The patient never resumed consciousness and died seven days later.

The patient's estate brought a wrongful death cause of action against the Ohio State University Hospitals. The case went to trial, through several appeals and eventually to the Ohio Supreme Court. The court held the nurse's actions caused the harm. The removal of the patient's endotracheal tube was negligent and set into motion a chain of events that directly caused the patient to die.

Damages

The fourth element of negligence is damages. Damages are derived from the harm or injury suffered by the acutely or critically ill patient and are calculated as a dollar amount. In order for liability to be imposed against a nurse caring for an acutely or critically ill patient, that patient must prove that something the nurse did or failed to do was inconsistent with the standard of care and that the inconsistency caused harm or injury for which the patient should be *compensated*. Patient-plaintiffs in a malpractice case can usually point to additional medical bills associated with their injuries to satisfy this element.

The number of nurses being named defendants in these cases is increasing, and this is especially true for advanced practice nurses. Accordingly, nurses caring for acutely and critically ill patients need to carefully consider whether to purchase professional liability insurance and, if so, the amount and type of coverage that is needed. Most institutions will provide some level malpractice insurance coverage for nurses, but the amount and circumstances under which each nurse is covered are important considerations.

Professional Malpractice and the Nursing Process

Malpractice claims may be premised on care delivered at any point from the moment a nurse-patient relationship is established to patient discharge. What constitutes reasonable care has been the focus of many cases filed against health care professionals and the hospitals in which they practice. For nurses, there seems to be an emerging trend. If the nurse reasonably executes every component of the nursing process by assessing, planning, implementing, and evaluating the care in accordance with the requisite standard of care, reasonable care will have been provided. However, if the nurse fails with regard to a single component of the nursing process, care provided to an acutely or critically ill patient will be deemed insufficient, unreasonable, and negligent. The following cases are examples of malpractice resulting from failures in particular stages of the nursing process.

Assessment Failure: Failure to Assess and Analyze the Level of Care Needed by the Patient.

Nurses caring for acutely and critically ill patients have a duty to assess and analyze the level of care needed by their patients. Where a nurse allegedly fails to fulfill this responsibility, liability for negligence may be threatened. *Brandon HMA, Inc. v Bradshaw*[18] demonstrates how courts handle failure to assess and analyze the level of care needed by acutely and critically ill patients.

In *Brandon*, Dawn Bradshaw contended that, while hospitalized at Rankin Medical Center (RMC) to be treated for bacterial pneumonia, she sustained permanent injuries because of negligence on the part of the nursing staff. The case was tried before a jury, and the jury agreed that Ms. Bradshaw sustained permanent, severe, oxygen deprivation–related brain damage because of the negligence of the nursing staff. They awarded her $9,000,000 in damages.

The alleged failure occurred after a chest tube had been inserted; on the night shift, a nurse allegedly failed to take vital signs between 11:00 PM and 3:30 AM until Ms. Bradshaw's condition had significantly worsened. At 3:30 AM, Ms. Bradshaw was found to be nauseated, disoriented, sweating profusely, and unable to follow verbal commands. Approximately 10 minutes later, she stopped breathing and had no pulse. A code was called, and CPR was administered. The code team arrived, and Ms. Bradshaw was revived. Subsequently, she was transferred to a rehabilitation facility specializing in the treatment of brain injury and filed this negligence cause of action against RMC.

To withstand allegations of failure to assess and analyze, it is important for nurses not only to assess and analyze the level of care needed by patients but also to document their assessment findings, as well as all actions taken to properly care for patients. Failure to assess and analyze the situation and to document the assessment findings, the interventions, and the patient's response to those interventions exposes the nurse and, as in the case of *Brandon*, the hospital to liability for negligence.

Assessment Failure: Failure to Ascertain a Patient's Wishes with Regard to Self-Determination.

Nurses caring for acutely and critically ill patients have a legal and ethical obligation to act in accordance with a patient's wishes with regard to self-determination. The patient's rights are discussed further in the Constitutional Law section below but nurses must determine and abide by those wishes or risk facing disciplinary action and civil liability.

Anderson v St. Francis-St. George Hospital[19] demonstrated how self-determination issues were dealt with in Ohio. In this case, Edward H. Winter was admitted to the hospital because he was having chest pain and was fainting. After discussing treatment options with Mr. Winters, his physician, Dr. Russo, entered a "no code" order in Mr. Winter's chart. Three days later, Mr. Winter began having ventricular tachycardia and a nurse defibrillated Mr. Winter. After he regained consciousness, he thanked the nurse for saving his life. When Russo was informed of Mr. Winter's condition, he ordered that lidocaine be administered. Two hours later, Mr. Winter experienced another ventricular tachycardia episode, but it resolved spontaneously.

The next day, Russo ordered the discontinuation of lidocaine and heart monitor. The day after that, Mr. Winter suffered a stroke that paralyzed his right side. Mr. Winter was eventually discharged, but his right side paralysis persisted until his death almost 2 years after his admission to St. Francis-St. George Hospital. Before his death, Mr. Winter sued the hospital, alleging that it was negligent in failing to obey the "no code" order that had been issued. The Ohio Supreme Court eventually heard the case and concluded that the failure to honor Mr. Winter's wishes constituted a breach of care.

Planning Failure: Failure to Appropriately Diagnose.

Nurses caring for acutely and critically ill patients must plan effective courses of treatment. Such a course of treatment depends on a proper diagnosis. Historically, cases of failure to diagnose have been filed against physicians, rather than nurses. However, nurses who diagnose patient conditions may find themselves the target of a failure to diagnose case and need to be aware that liability may be imposed if the plan of care is based on an erroneous diagnosis.

Implementation Failure: Failure to Timely Communicate Patient Findings.

Nurses spend more time with patients than any other health care professionals do, and this is especially true for nurses caring for acutely and critically ill patients. As a result, these nurses are in the best position to promptly detect changes in a patient's condition. Detection, however, is only the first step. Nurses caring for acutely and critically ill patients must promptly communicate troublesome patient findings. Failure to properly communicate patient findings can be devastating for patients and can be the reason that patients file malpractice causes of action. *Denesia v St. Elizabeth Community Health Center*[20] exemplifies how courts handle these kinds of cases.

In *Denesia* it was alleged that the death of Lucille Denesia was the result of the nursing staff's administering anticoagulation therapy and failure to timely notify the physician of an alarmingly high partial thromboplastin time (PTT). Initially, Lucille Denesia was thought to be suffering a transient ischemic attack because of her history of atrial fibrillation. As a result, anticoagulation therapy was ordered which included an injection of heparin, a heparin drip, and the administration of oral Coumadin. After this treatment regimen commenced, a PTT test was ordered and obtained. The lab notified the nurse 90 minutes later that the PTT was greater than 200 seconds. The nurse caring for Ms. Denesia called the primary treating physician to report the values, but the answering service that the nurse called never contacted the physician. Approximately 70 minutes after the nurse first called the answering service, Ms. Denesia was alert but had symptoms including a headache, vomiting, and ECG changes of six seconds of atrial beats with no corresponding ventricular response. Approximately seven minutes later, the nurse called and spoke with Ms. Denesia's cardiologist, although the nurse could not recall what she told the cardiologist. The nurse stated that her practice would be to report the patient's headaches, the vomiting, and the results of the PTT test. However, the cardiologist contended that the nurse only reported that the PTT test had been done and that the nurse was waiting on the primary treating physician to return her call.

Approximately 75 minutes after the telephone conversation with the cardiologist, the nurse spoke with the primary treating physician. Again, she could not remember what she told him but said that her practice would be to report the PTT test result and the nausea and vomiting, as well as the headache Ms. Denesia was having. The primary treating physician testified that he was not informed of the PTT result but that he ordered the IV infusion of heparin to be reduced. Twenty minutes after this conversation, Ms. Denesia vomited again. Antinausea medication was administered, but Ms. Denesia vomited again about 45 minutes later.

After these two vomiting episodes, Ms. Denesia rested comfortably for approximately 2 hours and 5 minutes. When she awoke, she vomited again, became lethargic, could not sit up, and her right hand grasp was found to be stronger than her left. The nurse called the primary treating physician again. The heparin infusion was discontinued. It was at this point, the primary treating physician testified, that he learned of the abnormal PTT result. Twenty-five minutes later, Ms. Denesia was transferred to the critical care unit because of continuing neurologic impairment. Two hours and 45 minutes later, her PTT was down to 27 seconds. However, Ms. Denesia lapsed into a coma and died from a massive cerebral hemorrhage.

The case was appealed to the Supreme Court of Nebraska, where the justices ordered that the case be retried because prejudicial jury instructions were given during the first trial. The results of the subsequent trial are not available, likely because the parties settled. Nonetheless, the case provides a cautionary tale on the importance of monitoring patient status, communicating changes, and documenting those communications. For nurses caring for acutely and critically ill patients, it is imperative that interactions with physicians be documented, whether in person or over the telephone, as well as the information conveyed during those interactions. Had the nurse taken the time to document what she told the cardiologist and the primary treating physician, this litigation might have been avoided.

Implementation Failure: Failure to Take Appropriate Action.
Cases from across the country continue to affirm that it is the nurse's responsibility to take affirmative action when action is indicated. *Garcia v United States*[21] is one such case. In *Garcia*, Candido Garcia was admitted to a Veterans Administration Medical Center for removal of a subdural hematoma. After surgery, he began making snorting noises and emitting white bubbles at his mouth. Mr. Garcia's wife reported the occurrence to the nurse caring for him. The nurse, Margaret John, reportedly told the Mrs. Garcia that the extent of her responsibility was to ensure that the surgically inserted drainage tubes were kept clear. Doctors from a neighboring hospital were eventually called but were not informed of the emergency nature of the situation. The result was that Mr. Garcia did not receive proper medical assistance for a period of about 45 to 50 minutes. Following medical intervention, including a return trip to the operating room, Mr. Garcia was quadriplegic. At trial, the hospital was found to be negligent and liable for the damages sustained by Candido Garcia; more than $2.3 million in damages, interest, and the cost of litigation was awarded to Mr. Garcia and his wife. In reaching its decision, the court found

that the nursing staff should have recognized the emergency nature of the situation and taken proper steps to notify the attending physician.

Failure to take appropriate action in cases involving acutely and critically ill patients has included not only physician-notification issues but also failure to follow physician orders,[22,23] failure to properly treat,[24] and failure to appropriately administer medication.[24-26] To avoid allegations of failure to take appropriate action, nurses caring for acutely and critically ill patients need to recognize signs and symptoms of complications and patient compromise. Nurses must also ensure that those signs and symptoms are timely communicated to the physician and take other affirmative action that is authorized and appropriate. Patient findings, interventions and actions taken, and patient responses to those interventions must be documented.

Implementation Failure: Failure to Document.
Nurses caring for acutely and critically ill patients are required not only to take appropriate action but also to accurately document their findings, interventions performed, and patients' response to those interventions. Failure to thoroughly and accurately document any aspect of care gives rise to negligence causes of action.

Haney v Alexander,[27] a case from North Carolina, demonstrates how courts and juries deal with a nurse's failure to properly document. In *Haney*, a nurse caring for a patient who was experiencing atrial fibrillation failed to take, record, and communicate all of the patient's vital signs, failed to properly document the order for Librium, and failed to document the administration of Librium. Reportedly, Librium had already been administered, but the on-call physician was told that Librium had not been administered based on the lack of documentation. Therefore, the physician ordered another dose, a nurse gave the medication, and 45 minutes later, the patient was found dead. The court of appeals concluded that the nurse was negligent in several respects, including that the events that led to the double administration of Librium could have prevented the patient from being able to communicate his worsening condition and receiving lifesaving medical assistance.

Haney and *Denesia* are indicative of the need for nurses caring for acutely and critically ill patients to thoroughly document the care that is given, interventions and actions taken, and the response of the patient to those interventions and actions. Failure to thoroughly document opens the door for patient-plaintiffs to allege that the absence of documentation signals a breach of the standard of care.

Implementation Failure: Failure to Preserve Patient Privacy.
Nurses have a duty to preserve patient privacy. State and federal statutes and case law affirm this duty. *Doe v Ohio State University Hospital and Clinics*[28] explores the issue. In *Doe*, a nurse taking care of a patient who was positive for the human immunodeficiency virus (HIV) wrote his HIV status on a laboratory requisition slip in the "other test" section of the form. This was done so that laboratory personnel could be alerted to the patient's HIV status. The patient was to have a complete blood count and potassium level drawn prior to a lithotripsy to remove kidney stones. The laboratory staff interpreted the notation made by the nurse as an instruction to perform an HIV screen, and not a message regarding the patient's HIV status.

The patient found out that the HIV screen had been done and was outraged that the HIV testing had been done without his consent. This facility had a policy that prohibited HIV testing without informed consent being obtained by the physician.

The case was ultimately dismissed, but it serves as a reminder to guard the privacy of every patient. Nurses can ensure that the privacy of acutely and critically ill patients is protected by following privacy-related regulations, such as state privacy laws and the privacy provisions of the Health Insurance Portability and Accountability Act (HIPAA),[29] as well as institutional policies and procedures in place to protect patient privacy.

Nurses should also refrain from having discussions about specific patients with anyone except other health care professionals involved in the care of the patient. When discussing specific patients with other health care professionals, it is imperative that patient-specific discussions occur in non-public settings. Discussions about specific patients are never appropriate in public areas such as elevators, cafeterias, gift shops, and parking lots.

Evaluation Failure: Failure to Act as a Patient Advocate. From admission to discharge, nurses have a duty to act as a patient advocate. For nurses caring for acutely and critically ill patients, this duty imposes the responsibility to evaluate the care that is being given to patients. The landmark failure to advocate case was *Darling v Charleston Community Memorial Hospital*,[30] a case decided by the Illinois Supreme Court in 1965.

In this case, Dorrence Darling II was an 18-year-old athlete who broke his leg playing football. He was taken to Charleston Community Memorial Hospital for treatment. Dorrence was placed in traction, and his broken leg was placed in a plaster cast. A heat cradle was used to dry the cast. Shortly after the cast was applied, Dorrence began to complain of severe pain in the broken leg. Dorrence's toes that protruded from the cast became swollen and dark in color and eventually became cold and insensitive to tactile stimulation.

The day after Dorrence was admitted, his treating physician, John R. Alexander, notched the cast around Dorrence's toes. The next day, Alexander cut the cast approximately 3 inches from the foot toward Dorrence's knee. The day after that, Alexander used a Stryker saw to split the sides of the cast and cut both sides of Dorrence's broken leg. By this time, blood and other drainage had been noted by the nursing staff. The room in which Dorrence was staying became filled with a noxious odor.

Fourteen days after his admission to Charleston Community Memorial Hospital, Dorrence was transferred to Barnes Hospital in St. Louis, Missouri. There he was cared for by surgeon Fred Reynolds. After multiple attempts to save the leg of Dorrence Darling, Reynolds finally had to amputate the lower leg approximately 8 inches below the knee.

Subsequently, Charleston Community Hospital and John R. Alexander were sued. The hospital, through the actions of the nursing staff and John R. Alexander, was alleged to have failed to treat Dorrence consistently with the requisite standard of care. With regard to the nursing staff, Darling alleged that they were negligent in assessing his deteriorating circulatory condition in accordance with hospital policy and procedure and that

they failed to report the developments to the medical staff or hospital administration. A settlement was reached with the doctor, John R. Alexander, so the case against the hospital was presented to an Illinois jury. After listening to the evidence, the jury returned a verdict against the hospital for $150,000. The hospital appealed the decision, and the Supreme Court of Illinois eventually heard the appeal. In affirming the jury verdict, the Illinois Supreme Court justices determined that a jury could have reasonably concluded that the nurses involved in the care and treatment of Dorrence Darling were negligent in assessing his circulatory status. According to the court, if the nursing staff had promptly recognized that circulatory compromise was occurring, steps could have been taken to prevent the irreversible effects of prolonged inadequate circulation. Had they recognized the significance of the symptoms they were seeing, the nursing staff could have exercised their duty to inform hospital authorities so that appropriate action could be taken. Because they failed to act as patient advocate, Dorrence lost his leg, and the hospital was liable for their failure.

Although the *Darling* case was decided in 1965, courts continue to hold that all nurses, including those caring for acutely and critically ill patients, have a nondelegable duty to act as patient advocate. Failure to act as patient advocate exposes the nurse to substantial liability and, more importantly, exposes patients to life-altering and life-ending complications that could have been avoided.

Wrongful Death

Wrongful death cases are a variation of negligence action in which the harm is the actual death of the individual. Like ordinary negligence, wrongful death claims can also be brought against non-professionals. However, in the professional health care context, these claims are a form of professional negligence and are filed by the survivors of patients who allege that the patient died because of the negligence of health care organizations or health care professionals. *Manning v Twin Falls Clinic & Hospital*[31] provides insight into how courts handle wrongful death cases.

In *Manning*, the trial court determined that the nurse failed to exercise reasonable care, and the nurse was deemed negligent in the death of Daryl Manning, a 67-year-old man. Mr. Manning had been admitted to the hospital in the last stages of chronic obstructive pulmonary disease, hypoxemia, and increased carbon dioxide retention and was receiving continuous supplemental oxygen by a nasal cannula. On his admission to the hospital, Mr. Manning was classified as a "no code." His condition steadily deteriorated, and the nurse discontinued Mr. Manning's supplemental oxygen and began to transfer him to a private room. The family requested that oxygen be administered during the move, but the nurse declined to apply it, citing the proximity between the patient's current location and the private room. After the bed had been moved approximately 15 feet, Mr. Manning stopped breathing. Resuscitation was attempted, but when the physician who was aware of Mr. Manning's "no code" status arrived, resuscitative measures were discontinued. The jury determined that the nurse was negligent in transferring Mr. Manning without using supplemental oxygen.

For families and health care professionals, wrongful death cases are among the most traumatic. It is in these cases that the life-and-death nature of the health care experience is exposed. In reviewing these kinds of cases, one learns that what is at issue is rarely the use, misuse, or malfunction of sophisticated, cutting-edge technology or the miscalculation of a complex formula. On the contrary, a review of wrongful death cases suggests that the alleged failures at issue are typically foundational matters of patient care and critical thinking. For instance, failure to thoroughly assess a patient, to take vital signs, to properly administer medication, or to administer portable oxygen to a respiratory-compromised patient has been the focus of most of the wrongful death cases discussed in this chapter. To avoid wrongful death liability, it is imperative that nurses caring for acutely and critically ill patients remain vigilant, recognize the signs and symptoms of complications and compromise, and take affirmative action to advocate for the best interest of the patient.

Assault and Battery

Assault and battery are examples of intentional torts that are frequently brought against health care providers. Although they are often used together, they are actually two separate torts. Assault is any intentional act that creates reasonable apprehension of immediate harmful or offensive contact with the plaintiff. With assault, no actual contact is necessary. Battery, on the other hand, is any intentional act that brings about actual harmful or offensive contact with the plaintiff.

In health care cases, patient consent is a defense to these claims. Assault occurs if a patient fears harmful or offensive touching. Assault may be alleged if a patient was aware that he or she was going to be touched in a manner not authorized by informed consent. For example, the act of telling a patient that they will be restrained may be assault. Battery occurs if the health care professional actually touches the patient in an unauthorized manner. The act of restraining a patient without consent is battery. Another defense to assault and battery is an emergency situation. Thus, cutting a patient's throat to create an emergency tracheostomy to create an airway may be justified while cutting a patient's neck on the wrong side in opposition to the informed consent may be battery.

Special Clinical Circumstances and Professional Malpractice

Although the issues discussed in this section could have been inserted and discussed as examples of negligence or malpractice, the nature of these cases is such that special attention is warranted. These issues include the respiratory management of acutely and critically ill patients, liability associated with blood transfusions, needlestick injuries, infection control, and informed consent.

Respiratory Management

The management of an acutely or critically ill patient's respiratory status gives rise to more litigation than does the management of any other physiologic system.

In *Allman v Holleman*,[32] Linda Allman was a 28-year-old patient who had been hospitalized because of a ruptured spleen. After surgery, Ms. Allman's endotracheal tube (ETT) became dislodged, and she was reintubated. Subsequently the ETT became dislodged again, and efforts to revive her were unsuccessful. This case was filed, and a jury returned a verdict in favor of Ms. Allman.

In a 1993 case, *Dixon v Taylor*,[33] Willie L. Dixon was admitted to Watauga County Hospital for treatment of pneumonia. Later that day, she was transferred to the critical care unit because her condition began to deteriorate. In the early morning hours, just after she was transferred to the critical care unit, a Code Blue was called because Mrs. Dixon was in cardiac and respiratory arrest. During the code, she was intubated and her physiologic condition stabilized. Approximately 17.5 hours after she was intubated, a critical care nurse and respiratory therapist extubated Mrs. Dixon. Nasal prongs were applied initially, but an oxygen mask was needed, so the respiratory therapist left the room to get the mask. When the respiratory therapist returned to the room, he realized that the patient was not breathing normally. The respiratory therapist examined her and found no air movement. Reintubation activities commenced.

However, bed rails had to be removed, the bed rolled down, and the restraints placed on Mrs. Dixon removed. In the process, Mrs. Dixon's heart stopped beating, and a Code Blue was called. During the second code, the nurse recording events on the Code Sheet noted that the respiratory therapist was unsuccessful at attempting to reintubate Mrs. Dixon. The issue was that the laryngoscope blade he was using was too small, and an appropriately sized blade could not be found in the crash cart. The crash cart had not been restocked after the first code, so the blade had to be obtained from the cardiac care unit across the hall.

When the appropriately sized blade was found and taken to her room, Mrs. Dixon was quickly reintubated by a physician. She was placed on a ventilator but never regained consciousness. After the second code, Mrs. Dixon was found to be brain-dead secondary to suffocation. She was eventually discharged from the hospital to a nursing home, where she died approximately 10 months later.

This cause of action was subsequently filed and tried before a jury. The jury returned a verdict in the amount of $900,000 to the estate of Mrs. Dixon, citing that the hospital, because of the actions of the respiratory therapist and nurse, was negligent in failing to adequately assess Mrs. Dixon as a candidate for extubation, failing to communicate concerns about her readiness for extubation to the physician before extubation, failing to stock the crash cart, and failing to properly position Mrs. Dixon after extubation for possible reintubation.

Five years later, *Moon v St. Thomas Hospital*[34] was published. In this case, a portion of Mr. Moon's ETT had to be extricated from his airway after he transected it by biting through it. The family of Mr. Moon alleged that permitting him to bite on the ETT to the extent that it was transected was negligent and that a bite block should have been inserted or the ETT repositioned to avoid the transection.

At the trial court level, the transection of this ETT was determined to be not reasonably foreseeable, and the court dismissed the case. That decision was appealed, and, 1 year later, the appellate court ordered the case to trial, concluding that a jury should determine whether inserting a bite block or repositioning the ETT was consistent with the standard of care.

In *Owensboro Mercy Health System v Payne*,[35] a jury awarded a man $2,270,000 in damages for the negligent transfer of Mr. Payne from the operating room to the critical care unit. Mr. Payne had been involved in a motor vehicle accident and, because of extensive internal injuries, had spent between 8 and 8.5 hours in the operating room. At the conclusion of surgery, he was transferred to the critical care unit without supplemental oxygen being administered. This failure caused Mr. Payne to sustain a serious brain injury, resulting in a persistent vegetative state.

A year after *Owensboro*, a verdict for the defense was rendered in *Martin v St. Vincent Medical Center*.[36] In *Martin*, the family alleged that a certified registered nurse anesthetist (CRNA) punctured Mr. Martin's trachea while inserting an internal jugular line during a quadruple coronary artery bypass graft procedure. After surgery, Mr. Martin developed mediastinitis and died. His family filed this wrongful death cause of action, but the defense verdict was affirmed on appeal, citing in part the inability of Mr. Martin's family to affirmatively establish causation.

As in *Martin*, the patient-plaintiff in *Kent v Baptist Memorial Hospital*[37] was denied a verdict in her favor. The patient in Kent was a 16-year-old person with diabetes who experienced a diabetic seizure and went into septic shock. On arrival at the hospital, she was unresponsive and had to be intubated. After she was intubated, she was transferred to another hospital. She was eventually extubated and filed this cause of action, contending that she sustained vocal cord damage at intubation because the ETT was too large for her height and weight.

In *Miller v Marymount Medical Center*,[38] a 31-year-old pregnant woman, Mrs. Miller, was admitted to Marymount Medical Center to give birth. Two days later, she gave birth via cesarean section to a healthy baby girl. After the C-section, respiratory problems began. A chest radiograph obtained on the morning after the C-section revealed that Mrs. Miller had pneumonia. A blood gas analysis done that same morning indicated that her Po_2 was 64.4 mEq/L. Antibiotic therapy was started, and a nasal cannula was applied to improve oxygenation. Mrs. Miller was also treated for pain and stress with Demerol and Vistaril injections. Throughout the day, respiratory distress continued.

At 9:45 that same night, her physician told the Miller family that a pulmonologist was going to be called. Five minutes later, the nurse administered Demerol and Vistaril injections. Ten minutes after the injections, Mrs. Miller's physician returned to her room to find Mrs. Miller unresponsive and in respiratory arrest. A code was called, and 5 minutes later Mrs. Miller was intubated, placed on an oxygen bag delivering 100% oxygen, and transferred to the critical care unit. After she was intubated, another blood gas determination was made, and the Po_2 was 90 mEq/L. Twelve minutes after she was intubated and transferred to the critical care unit, Mrs. Miller was breathing without assistance. However, she never regained consciousness. She was eventually transferred to a nursing home, where she remains in a comatose state.

Mrs. Miller's family filed this case. With regard to the nursing care rendered to Mrs. Miller, they alleged that the nursing staff failed to furnish treating physicians with up-to-date information about Mrs. Miller's symptoms and to obtain repeat blood gas analyses as required by an order entered by Mrs. Miller's physician. They also contended that the administration of Demerol 10 minutes before her respiratory arrest was negligent, because Demerol accelerates the progression of acute respiratory distress syndrome (ARDS). ARDS is the condition the experts retained by the family concluded that Mrs. Miller had on the morning the chest radiograph was obtained.

The trial lasted 7 days, and the jury returned a defense verdict because they were unable to definitively determine that negligence was the proximate cause of Mrs. Miller's injuries. This verdict was affirmed by the Court of Appeals and the Kentucky Supreme Court.

In a 2008 case from Philadelphia, *Small v Temple Univ. Hosp.*,[39] a patient in the critical care unit died after his ETT became obstructed by mucous and the nurses failed to suction the tube or act based on patient reports. Hours before he died, the patient wrote a note to his daughters saying he could not breathe. The daughters informed the nurses, who failed to communicate this information to the physicians. Later, when the man's breathing struggles worsened, he became agitated and tried to remove the tube. The physician, thinking he was suffering from critical care unit psychosis, gave him sedatives and had him restrained.

Regardless of the verdict rendered, these cases serve as a stark reminder of the life-altering and life-ending implications associated with management of the respiratory status of an acutely or critically ill patient. Consequently, nurses caring for patients with respiratory compromise must diligently assess, plan, implement care, and evaluate these patients with laser-like precision. The life of the acutely or critically ill patient depends on it.

Blood Transfusions

Tobin v Providence Hospital[40] serves as a reminder that blood transfusions carry with them considerable risks. In *Tobin*, Rollin Tobin underwent hip replacement surgery but died from sepsis and disseminated intravascular coagulation. The wife of Mr. Tobin asserted that he died because blood contaminated with *Yersinia* bacteria was administered to him during surgery.

Before surgery, Mr. Tobin donated three units of his own blood, and all three of those units were transfused in the operating room, as well as an additional, allogeneic unit. After Mr. Tobin's death, the American Red Cross and the Centers for Disease Control and Prevention investigated the situation and determined that the fourth unit administered to Mr. Tobin was contaminated with *Yersinia* bacteria.

Mr. Tobin's family filed a wrongful death cause of action, contending that failure to monitor or record his temperature before, during, and after the operation caused his death. This case went to trial, and the jury returned a verdict in the amount of $6,485,681.06 in favor of the estate of Mr. Tobin. However, because there was an absence of testimony asserting failure to monitor or record the patient's temperature before, during, and after the operation and because of other evidentiary errors, the Michigan Court of Appeals ordered a new trial.

Like managing a patient's respiratory status, the administration of blood and blood products, although routine in critical care settings, is a high-risk intervention that can prove to be deadly. *Tobin* is an example. To avoid liability associated with administration of blood and blood products, nurses must carefully follow organizational procedures and protocols that govern these interventions. They must then take the time to thoroughly document the care that was taken to protect the patient.

Infection Control

In *Carroll v Sisters of St. Frances Health Services*,[41] Bessie Mae Carroll was visiting her sister, who was a patient in the critical care unit at St. Joseph Hospital, when, after washing her hands, she attempted to remove a paper towel from the container located adjacent to the wash basin she was using. She thought the container was a paper towel dispenser and inserted her right hand into the opening at the top of the container. When she did so, three of her fingers were stuck by sharp objects. After she told a nurse that she hurt her fingers on the paper towel dispenser, the nurse told Ms. Carroll that the container was not a paper towel dispenser but a receptacle for contaminated needles.

Ms. Carroll developed a fear of contracting acquired immunodeficiency syndrome (AIDS) and filed this negligence-based cause of action, contending that the container had been placed too close to the wash basin and that a warning should have been placed on the container indicating its purpose and contents.

At the trial court level the case was dismissed, but on appeal a trial was ordered so that the jury could determine whether Ms. Carroll's fear of acquiring AIDS was reasonable.

The case of *Piedmont Hospital v Reddick*,[42] like *Carroll*, arose out of an allegation that appropriate infection control standards were not followed. In *Piedmont*, James Davis died after contracting a fungal infection. His estate filed this cause of action, contending that construction work performed in or near the critical care unit where Mr. Davis was being treated caused the *Aspergillus* fungus to become airborne and transmitted to him.

The complaint asserted that construction work was performed without proper safeguards and that this failure led to a breach of industry standards. Although a number of issues were addressed by the Georgia Court of Appeals Second Division, the court ordered the case be tried as to the alleged negligence of the construction company and hospital.

Carroll and *Piedmont* demonstrate that infection control issues find their way to courtrooms across America. To minimize risks associated with alleged infection control failures, sharps containers must be clearly labeled and positioned away from wash basins and paper towel dispensers. Before remodeling or other construction begins, the environment must be safeguarded from the airborne spread of deadly microorganisms.

CONSTITUTIONAL LAW: PATIENT DECISION MAKING

The right of competent adult patients to refuse treatment is well established. This right has evolved from the common law doctrine of informed consent, the laws of assault and battery (the right to be free from fear of harm and unwanted touching), and the common law right to "possession and control of his own person, free from all restraint or interference of others, unless by clear and unquestionable authority of law."[43]

A competent adult patient has the right to refuse even life-sustaining treatment for any reason, without regard for that individual's motivations. *Bouvia v Superior Court*[44] is representative of this principle. In *Bouvia*, a young woman with significant mobility disabilities refused to eat and accept treatment. The facility in which she resided subjected her to countless competency and psychiatric evaluations, all of which indicated she was fully competent (or had decision-making capacity). The court held that because she was a competent adult who understood the consequences of her decisions, she could not be compelled to accept even food against her wishes.

In general, American law values individual autonomy to such a degree that a competent patient's wishes can almost never be legally overruled. It is important to note that no constitutional right is absolute and there are legal frameworks for determining when a competing right or obligation may outweigh an individual right. For example, the right to refuse unwanted touching can be compromised by considerations such as the health and safety of citizens, as is the case with mandatory vaccinations. Even within that example, there are exceptions based on constitutional considerations such as religious freedom. In practice, there have been no legally justified reasons to override the wishes of a competent patient to refuse medical treatment.

Critical care nurses will participate in the withholding or withdrawing of treatment. This is difficult whether or not the patient has decision-making capacity, and it is important for nurses to keep in mind that there are times when the legal rights of patients and ethical decisions will match and times when these will seem at odds. Health care decisions become most complex when patients lose the capacity to make their own decisions personally. These decisions can also be difficult in patients who were never competent to make their own decisions. Navigating the law surrounding the right to refuse treatment in patients who do not have decision-making capacity is much more legally complicated than for those with capacity.

Patients Without Decision-Making Capacity

Patients without decision-making capacity include individuals who were previously competent (those who reached adulthood but lost competence), those who were never competent (those born with severe to profound cognitive disabilities), those who are not yet competent (primarily children under 18), and those with fluctuating competence, such as individuals with cyclical disorders such as the manic phase of bipolar disorder that can seriously impair decision making. The law also imposes standards of judgment for surrogate decision makers to guide and evaluate decisions.

A number of legal mechanisms exist that can simplify at least the legal issues surrounding decision making for patients without decision-making capacity (admittedly, the ethical and emotional issues are much more nuanced). These include state probate laws that may allow courts to appoint guardians for all or some decisions. There are also a variety of state law based procedures for individuals with decision-making capacity to direct their future care through documents and/or the appointment of a surrogate decision maker in the event they should lose capacity. These include living wills, advance directives, durable powers of attorney, and physician orders for life-saving treatment (POLSTs). The legal requirements and analyses are more stringent for decisions that may directly impact life, including decisions to forgo or withdraw treatment at the end of life.

Never and Not Yet Competent Patients

Competent adults can refuse treatment for any reason, even if others believe it is in opposition to their best interests. On the other hand, in the absence of a competent adult decision maker or their documented wishes, the law imposes a best interest standard. The standard is self-explanatory; parents and legal guardians of children have a legal obligation to make informed decisions based on the best interests of the patient. As a child matures, there are increased legal obligations to involve the patient in health care decision making based on what is developmentally and situationally appropriate.

It is inevitable that on occasion a parent or guardian's judgment will clash with that of the provider or the maturing child. Every effort should be made by the nurse and the extended health care team to facilitate discussion, understanding, and resolution without resorting to the courts. However, there are procedures in every state to petition the court on an emergent basis to evaluate and rule on what is in the best interest of the patient. The majority of legal authority surrounds cases that involve a decision to withdraw or forgo life-sustaining treatment in patients without decisional capacity and who have not specified their wishes at an earlier time when they had capacity.

Previously Competent Patients

Several highly publicized cases beginning in the 1970s concerned the withdrawal of treatment in young women who were previously competent. In each of these cases, the patient had sustained devastating neurologic injury and a legal challenge was presented to their families' ability to withdraw treatment, including nutrition and hydration.[45-47] In each case, those same family members were entrusted for years with medical decisions for complex and life-threatening procedures on behalf of the patients, but the request to withdraw care or artificial nutrition or hydration was met with years of struggle in the legal system. This was, in part, because of a state's right to establish high standards for evidence of what the patient herself would have wanted in regard to those decisions likely to ultimately result in death when the patient had not clearly communicated their wishes before their incapacity. In addition to affirming the states' ability to set high evidence standards in favor of preserving life, these cases established that in the absence of specific directions from the patient, surrogate decision makers should make a substituted judgment standard. This means that decision makers must base their decisions on the patient's preferences and values and what the patient would have done if then competent. The surrogate decision maker's own judgment about what should be done may differ from what the law requires. He or she must abandon personal values and preferences and instead assume the preferences and values of the patient in making the decision. Obviously, this is an enormous responsibility as well as a difficult task. To the extent patients can make their wishes known, in advance, the agony already associated with these difficult decisions can by lessened.

These decisions, beginning with *In re Quinlan* in 1976, initiated the slow process of state-by-state legislation to provide competent adults with a way to legally direct their care in the event of future incapacity. Today, there are a wide variety of state law-based procedures for individuals with decision-making capacity to direct their future care through documents and/or the appointment of surrogate decision makers in the event they should lose capacity. These include, but are not limited to, living wills, advance directives, durable powers of attorney, and POLSTs.

Advance Directives

Patients themselves can provide clear direction by preparing in advance written documents that specify their wishes. These documents are termed *advance directives* and include the living will and the durable power of attorney for health care. The *living will* specifies that if certain circumstances occur, such as terminal illness, the patient will decline specific treatments, such as cardiopulmonary resuscitation and mechanical ventilation. It has proven to be of limited value because it does not cover all treatments; in some states, for example, nutritional support may not be declined through a living will. Advance directives include the ability to appoint a *durable power of attorney for health care*. These are legally binding documents that allow individuals to specify a variety of preferences, particular treatments they want to avoid, and circumstances in which they wish to avoid them. The *durable power of attorney for health care* is a directive through which a patient designates an "agent," someone who will make decisions for the patient if the patient becomes unable to do so. Recall, the agent is obligated to use the patient's values and preferences to make the decision the patient would make if he or she were able to do so. This is not an easy task and individuals are urged to carefully consider their choice of agent. Each state has requirements for advance directives and how they must be created to be validly executed. Once a patient creates an advance directive in their own state, other states will honor it under the full faith and credit doctrine. Nurses may care for critically ill patients in one state who have executed an advance directive in another. The fact that it was drafted in another state does not negate its validity.

The Patient Self-Determination Act of 1990 is an example of a federal statute that impacts practice. It was designed to encourage competent patients to consider what they would want in the event of serious illness and to facilitate them to complete advance directives.[48] The statute requires that all adults must be provided written information regarding an individual's rights under state law to make medical decisions, including the right to refuse treatment and the right to formulate advance directives.

The law mandates that providers of health care services under Medicare and Medicaid must comply with requirements relating to patient advance directives, which are written instructions recognized under state law for provision of care when persons are incapacitated. Providers may not be reimbursed for the care they provide unless the requirements of this provision are met.

Providers must have written policies and procedures 1) to inform all adult patients at initiation of treatment of their right to execute an advance directive and of the provider's policies on the implementation of that right; 2) to document in the medical record whether an individual has executed an advance directive; 3) *not* to condition care and treatment or otherwise discriminate on the basis of whether a patient has executed an advance directive; 4) to comply with state laws on advance directives; and 5) to provide information and education to staff and the community on advance directives.

Futile Treatment and Orders Not to Resuscitate

It is important to distinguish the reality that it is at times appropriate to stop aggressive treatment from the need to continue care; this may mean that supportive care and comfort are the best actions for the patient. Any critical care nurse will observe and even deliver care at some point that seems useless, unnecessary, and even unkind. Nurses play an incredibly valuable role in the health care team by advocating for the best interest of the patient in a holistic way. This is incredibly valuable in an area where providers focus heavily on particular disease processes. Nurses may be responsible for reminding the team of the "big picture" and the need to provide quality of life and compassionate care to the patient.

Many providers have reported feeling obligated to continue treating patients in the absence of any reasonable chance of improvement. There is no legal obligation to provide care that

is not, in the provider's judgment, reasonably calculated to improve the patient's condition or symptoms. Although patients have a legal right to refuse treatment, there is no corresponding right to receive treatment. Nonetheless, some states have recently created state statutes that provide protection from liability for providers refusing to provide futile care. The Texas Futile Care Act[49] even creates a specific process for providers withdrawing or refusing to provide futile care, even over the objections of the patient.

Institutional policies in regard to do not resuscitate (DNR) orders should be well established and tested after decades of implementation. Policies that address orders to withhold or withdraw treatment should exist in all critical care units. Policies surrounding DNR orders should include, but are not limited to, the following:

1. DNR orders should be entered in the patient's record with full documentation by the responsible physician about the patient's prognosis and the patient's agreement (if he or she is capable) or, alternatively, the family's consensus.
2. DNR orders should require concurrence of another physician as standard policy (depending upon state law).
3. Policies should specify that orders are reviewed periodically (some policies require daily review).
4. Patients with capacity must give their informed consent.
5. For patients without capacity, that incapacity must be thoroughly documented, along with the diagnosis, prognosis, and family consensus.
6. If applicable, DNR orders should be consistent with advance directives, or if not, the reasons for those differences should be documented and explained.

Other orders to withhold or withdraw treatment may involve any intervention. These may include mechanical ventilation, oxygen, IV vasoactive agents or other medications, serial labs, imaging tests, pulmonary artery catheters, and other invasive monitoring. The legal and ethical implications of these orders for each patient must be carefully considered. Hospital policies should exist to guide the withdrawal of care in light of state and federal legal constraints. In addition, hospital ethicists and ethics committees can play a valuable role to providers negotiating the complexities of these decisions.

LEGAL ISSUES LOOKING FORWARD

This chapter could not begin to cover the labyrinth of legal issues affecting nursing practice. Each year brings new developments in legislation, case law, and administrative law that can change nursing practice. Most recently, the Patient Protection and Affordable Care Act of 2010 (ACA),[50] upheld by the United States Supreme Court in 2012,[51] instituted sweeping changes in areas ranging from eligibility for health care coverage to funding of medical and nursing research to numerous workplace programs that are to enhance to supply of advanced practice nurses. Of particular interest to nurses, many aspects of the ACA enhance the value and reimbursement of APRNs.

BOX 3-4   CASE STUDY

Patient with Legal Issues

Brief Patient History

Mr. A is an 87-year-old man. He has a history of aortic stenosis; however, he has been relatively healthy until recent episodes of syncope. Mr. A lives in an assisted living facility because of forgetfulness but was independent in activities of daily living before this hospitalization.

Clinical Assessment

Mr. A. was admitted to the critical care unit yesterday, after undergoing aortic valvuloplasty. Mr. A. has not received any opioids or benzodiazepines since yesterday's interventional procedure. The night nurse reported that Mr. A was confused to place when awakened during the night but commented that this is normal for an 87-year-old. This morning, Mr. A was oriented to person, time, place, and situation. He is easily aroused but dozes off and on when unstimulated. Although Mr. A is able to follow simple commands, he requires repeated instructions. The nurse failed to document or report the patient's mental status change or the abnormal serum electrolyte findings to the physician.

Diagnostic Procedures

Mr. A's baseline vital signs are blood pressure, 110/62 mm Hg; heart rate, 82 beats/min (sinus rhythm); respiratory rate, 18 breaths/min; and temperature,

98.4° F. The chest radiograph is normal; O_2 saturation (pulse oximetry) is 96% on room air. Results from serum electrolyte analysis include the following: sodium, 120 mmol/L; potassium, 4.1 mmol/L; chloride, 95 mmol/L; CO_2, 25 mEq/L; blood urea nitrogen, 60 mg/dL; and creatinine, 2 mg/dL.

Medical Diagnosis

Mr. A is diagnosed with delirium secondary to hyponatremia.

Questions

1. What major outcomes do you expect to achieve for this patient?
2. What problems or risks must be managed to achieve these outcomes?
3. What interventions must be initiated to monitor, prevent, manage, or eliminate the problems and risks identified?
4. What interventions should be initiated to promote optimal functioning, safety, and well-being of the patient?
5. What possible learning needs would you anticipate for this patient?
6. What cultural and age-related factors might have a bearing on the patient's plan of care?

▌ S U M M A R Y

- Nursing is 1) a scientific process founded on a professional body of knowledge; 2) a learned profession based on an understanding of the human condition across the lifespan and the relationship of a patient with others and within the environment; and 3) an art dedicated to caring for others.
- The ability to practice professional nursing is a privilege granted by state law and under the direction of BONs, state administrative agencies charged with protecting the health and welfare of state citizens by limiting nursing practice to qualified individuals who have demonstrated at least minimal competencies.
- Nursing scope of practice is defined by state NPAs. Standards of practice are delineated by BONs and are used as a basic measure of safe and effective nursing practice.
- Standards of practice and standards of professional performance, such as those promulgated by the ANA and AACN, further delineate expectations of nurses in providing quality nursing care and may help inform the standard of care in the legal context.
- Common legal theories based in civil litigation include professional negligence, wrongful death, and assault and battery. Nurses have a duty to their patients to provide care that is consistent with what a reasonably prudent nurse in the same situation would provide. This is the legal standard of care.

- The risk of liability can be diminished by taking affirmative action that is responsive to the patient's condition.
- Thorough documentation regarding actions taken to protect the patient is essential.
- Nurses can minimize the risk of liability by remaining true to the professional obligations to advocate for the best interests of the patients, attending to the patient's status, including carefully listening to and acting on patient reports or changes in status, and documenting all of these issues.
- A competent patient has a constitutional right to refuse even lifesaving treatment.
- States may require additional procedural protections when a decision maker wishes to withdraw care from patients who are not competent.
- Judicial intervention in decision making is an option but should be seen as a last step. Interdisciplinary cooperation, discussion, and collaboration between providers and decision makers should be fully explored first.
- Providers of health care must comply with requirements relating to patient advance directives.
- Any orders to withdraw or withhold treatment, including DNR orders, should be entered into the patient's medical record with full documentation by the responsible physician about the patient's prognosis and the patient's agreement or, alternatively, the family's consensus. These should be done in compliance with institutional policy.

REFERENCES

1. National Council of the State Boards of Nursing (NCSBN). *NCSBN Model Nursing Practice Act and Model Nursing Administrative Rules.* Chicago: NCSBN; 2011.
2. *Sermchief v Gonzales*, 660 SW2d 683 (Mo 1983).
3. *Marion Ob/Gyn v State Med. Bd.*, 137 Ohio App. 3d 522 (Ohio Ct. App., Franklin County 2000).
4. *State Bd. of Nursing v Ruebke*, 259 Kan. 599 (Kan. 1996).
5. American Association of Critical-Care Nurses (AACN). *Standards for Acute and Critical Care Nursing Practice.* Aliso Viejo, California: AACN; 2008.
6. National Council of the State Boards of Nursing (NCSBN). *NCSBN Model Nursing Practice Act and Model Nursing Administrative Rules.* Chicago: NCSBN; 2011.
7. American Nurses Association (ANA). *Nursing: Scope and Standards of Practice.* Washington, DC: ANA; 2004.
8. *Candler General Hospital Inc. v McNorrill*, 354 SE2d 872 (Ga. 1987).
9. Painter L, Dudjak L, Kidwell K, et al. The nurse's role in the causation of compensable injury. *Journal of Nursing Care Quality.* 2011;26(4):311-319.
10. *Gould v New York City Health and Hospital Corp.*, 490 NYS.2d 87 (1985).
11. For example, California: *Ybarra v Spangard*, 154 P.2d 687 (Cal. 1944); Colorado: *Wood v Rowland*, 592 P.2d 1332 (Colo. 1978); Delaware: *Larrimore v Homeopathic Hospital Association*, 176 A.2d 362 (Del. 1962); Minnesota: *Plutshack v University of Minnesota Hospital*, 316 NW2d 1 (Minn. 1982); Montana: *Hunsaker v Bozeman Deaconess Foundation*, 588 P.2d 493 (Mont. 1978); Pennsylvania: *Baur v Mesta Machine Co.*, 176 A.2d 684 (Pa. 1962); Texas: *Childs v Greenville Hospital Authority*, 479 S.W.2d 399 (Tx. 1972); and Washington: *Stone v Sisters of Charity of the House of Providence*, 469 P.2d 229 (Wash. 1970).
12. *Clough v Lively*, 387 SE2d 573 (Ga. 1989).
13. *Lunsford v Board of Nurse Examiners*, 648 SW2d 391 (Tx. App. 1983).
14. *Sparks v St. Luke's Regional Medical Center*, 768 P.2d 768 (Idaho 1989).
15. *Koeniger v Eckrich*, 422 NW2d 600,601(S.D. 1988).
16. *Teffeteller v University of Minnesota*, 645 NW2d 420 (Minn. 2002).
17. *McMullen v Ohio State University Hospitals*, 725 NE2d 1117 (Ohio 2002).
18. *Brandon HMA, Inc. v Bradshaw*, 809 So.2d 611 (Miss. 2001).
19. *Anderson v St. Francis-St. George Hospital*, 671 NE2d 225 (Ohio 1996).
20. *Denesia v St. Elizabeth Community Health Center*, 454 NW2d 294 (Neb. 1990).
21. *Garcia v United States*, 697 F.Supp. 1570 (Colo. 1988).
22. *Keyser v Garner*, 922 P.2d 409 (Idaho 1996).
23. *Long v Methodist Hospital of Indiana*, 699 NE2d 1164 (Ind. 1998).
24. *Richardson v Miller*, 44 SW3d 1 (Tenn. 2000).
25. *Ginsberg v St. Michaels Hospital*, 678 A.2d 271 (N.J. 1996).
26. *G.S. v Dep't of Human Servs., Div. of Youth & Family Servs.*, 723 A.2d 612 (N.J. 1999).
27. *Haney v Alexander*, 323 SE2d 430 (1984).
28. *Doe v Ohio State Univ. Hosp. & Clinics*, 663 NE2d 1369 (Ohio 1995).
29. The Health Insurance Portability and Accountability Act of 1996 (HIPAA), Public Law 104-191, enacted on August 21, 1996.
30. *Darling v Charleston Comm. Mem. Hosp.*, 211 NE2d 614 (Ill. 1965).
31. *Manning v Twin Falls Clinic & Hospital*, 830 P.2d 1185 (Id. 1992).
32. *Allman v Holleman*, 667 P.2d 296 (Ks. 1983).
33. *Dixon v Taylor*, 431 SE2d 778 (N.C. 1993).
34. *Moon v St. Thomas Hospital*, 983 SW2d 225 (Tenn. 1998).
35. *Owensboro Mercy Health System v Payne*, 24 SW3d 675 (Ky. 1999).
36. *Martin v St. Vincent Medical Center*, 142 Ohio App. 3d 347 (2001).
37. *Kent v Baptist Memorial Hospital*, 853 So.2d 873 (Miss. 2003).
38. *Miller v Marymount Medical Center*, 125 SW3d 274 (Ky. 2004).
39. *Small v Temple Univ. Hosp.*, 2008 Phila. Ct. Com. Pl. LEXIS 258 (Pa. C.P. 2008).
40. *Tobin v Providence Hospital*, 624 NW2d 548 (Mich. 2001).
41. *Carroll v Sisters of St. Francis*, 868 SW2d 585 (Tenn. 1993).
42. *Piedmont Hospital, Inc. v Reddick*, 599 SE2d 20 (Ga. 2004).
43. *Cruzan v Director*, Missouri Department of Mental Health, 497 U.S. 261 (1990).
44. *Bouvia v Superior Court*, 179 Cal. App. 3d 1127, 225 Cal. Rptr. 297, 1986 Cal. App. LEXIS 1467 (Cal. App. 2d Dist. 1986).
45. *In re Quinlan*, 70 N.J. 10 (N.J. 1976).
46. *Cruzan v Director, Missouri Department of Mental Health*, 497 U.S. 261 (1990).
47. *In re Schiavo*, 851 So.2d 182 (Fla. Ct. App. 2003).
48. *Patient Self Determination Act, Omnibus Budget Reconciliation Act of 1990*, Pub.L. 101-508 (1990).
49. For example, the *Texas Futile Care Law*, Texas Health and Safety Code, Section 166 (1999).
50. *Patient Protection and Affordable Care Act and Reconciliation Act* (2010).
51. See, *National Federation of Independent Business v Sebelius*, U.S. (2012).

Genetics and Genomics in Critical Care

Mary E. Lough

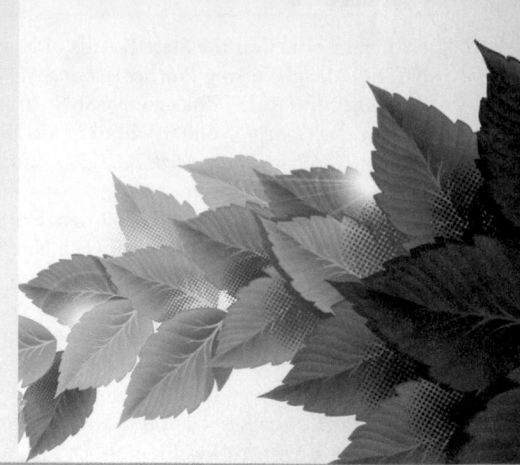

evolve WEBSITE

http://evolve.elsevier.com/Urden/criticalcare/

Evolve features:

- NCLEX Review Questions
- CCRN Review Questions
- PCCN Review Questions
- Mosby's Nursing Skills Procedures
- Animations
- Video Clips
- Glossary

The field of genetics and genomics continues to expand and affect crucial aspects of health care. Genetic testing does not yet have a large role in the critical care unit, but given the exponential growth of knowledge in this field, and the decreasing costs of genomic sequencing, the day when *personalized health care* will include a genetic screen to tailor treatment to individual biology is on the horizon.[1] This chapter includes an overview of the biologic basis of genomics, a description of the different types of genetic and genomic studies, and the growing impact of pharmacogenetics. It also incorporates some examples of genetic diseases and pharmacogenetic syndromes in critical care. A list of genetic and genomic terms is provided at the end of the chapter.

GENETICS AND GENOMICS

Genetics is the study of heredity, particularly as it relates to the ability of individual genes to transfer heritable physical characteristics. *Genes* are specific sequences of *deoxyribonucleic acid* (DNA) located on chromosomes within the nucleus of each cell (Fig. 4-1). Genes contain the blueprint for protein production that results in the physical characteristics of each individual. The pioneering work in human genetics has focused on single-gene variants that are rare in the population but have a large effect for the affected individual and follow classic inheritance patterns. About 6,000 rare disorders have been identified, and while single-gene conditions are relatively rare in the population, cumulatively they affect about 25 million people.[1,2] Single-gene disorders include Huntington's disease, Tourette syndrome, cystic fibrosis, and Duchenne muscular dystrophy.[2]

In single-gene variant disorders the influence of genetics is strong and the environmental effect is very weak.

Genomics refers to the study of all of the genetic material within the cell and encompasses the environmental interaction and impact on biologic and physical characteristics. Thus, genomics is a much larger and more complex area of study. The *genome* is the complete set of DNA in an organism. Each human nucleated somatic cell contains a copy of the complete genome. The exceptions are reproductive cells (oocytes and sperm), which contain only one half of the paired chromosomes, and red blood cells, because they do not have a nucleus. The human genome contains between 20,000 and 25,000 protein-coding genes, which represent less than 2% of the total genome.[3]

Many disease conditions that are commonly seen in the modern world result from a confluence of both environmental and genomic influences. These are described as *complex traits* or *polygenic* conditions.[4] Furthermore, environmental conditions can alter the expression of different genes and consequently enhance the signs and symptoms associated with a disease. This represents a relatively new field of research known as *epigenetics*.[5] Coronary artery disease is an example of a widespread disease that has both a strong environmental component (diet, obesity, diabetes, smoking) and a genomic effect that alters risk of developing the condition.[4] Whole genome sequencing methods and genome wide association studies (GWAS) are employed to examine multiple genes simultaneously. As the cost of genomic sequencing plummets, this will increasingly become a viable clinical option.[6] Nowhere is the genomic influence more evident than in pharmacogenomics, or the unique

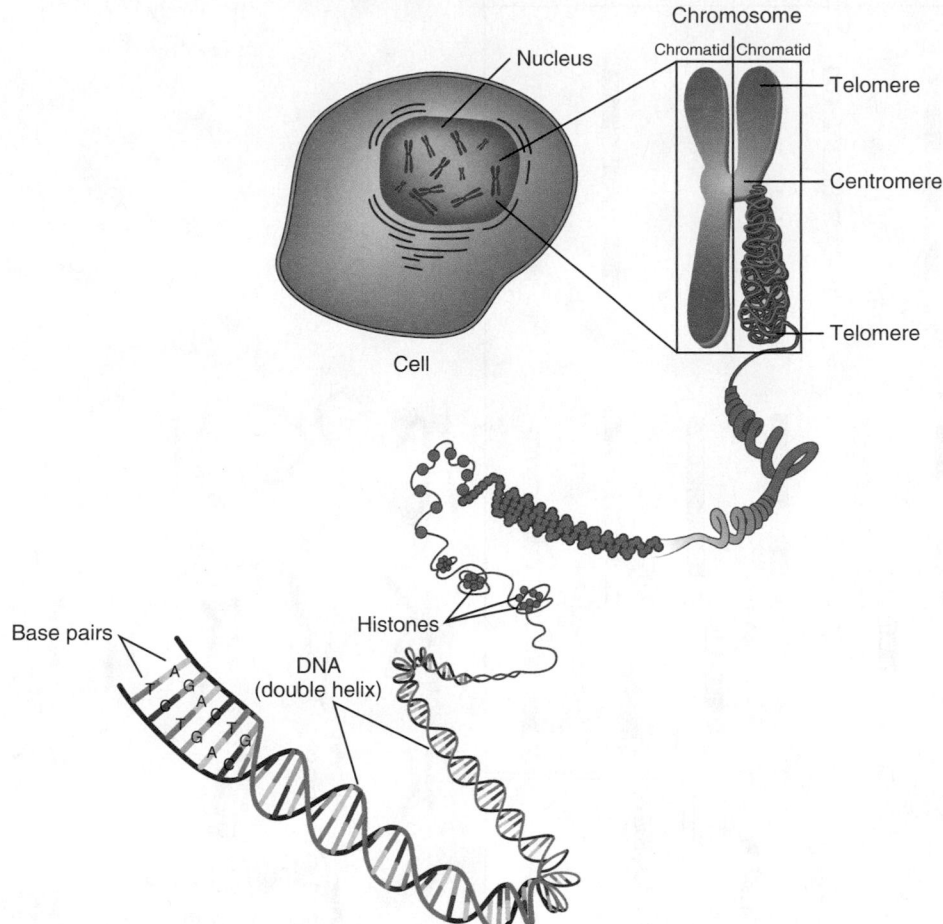

FIGURE 4-1 Chromosomes are tightly packed with DNA and reside in the nucleus of the cell.

individual response to medications (environmental impact) based upon gene expression (genomic impact).[7]

GENETIC AND GENOMIC STRUCTURE AND FUNCTION

Chromosomes

The nucleus inside each human cell contains each person's full genetic blueprint of 23 pairs of chromosomes—22 pairs of autosomes and 1 pair of sex chromosomes—making the total 46. A number system is used to identify each chromosome. The chromosomes are traditionally arranged in order of size, starting with the largest (chromosome 1) to the smallest (chromosome 22), with the sex chromosomes placed last or to the side. A schematic of this chromosome arrangement to show the variation in size is shown in Figure 4-2A; the chromosomes are obviously not arranged this way inside the cell. A *karyotype* is the arrangement of human chromosomes from largest to smallest, as shown in the sequence in Figure 4-2B.

Each chromosome consists of an unbroken strand of DNA. To fit all of this genetic material inside the cell nucleus, the DNA is tightly coiled inside the chromosomes in a hierarchical order of compact structures. A specialized class of proteins called *histones* organizes the double-stranded DNA into what looks like a tightly coiled telephone cord (see Fig. 4-1).

Each somatic chromosome, also called an *autosome*, is made of two strands, called *chromatids*, which are joined near the center (see Fig. 4-1). This central region is called the *centromere*, and the ends of the chromatids are called *telomeres*. The segments of the chromosome separated by the centromere are called *arms*. The shorter arm of each chromosome is called *p* (for *petit*, or small), and the longer arm is called *q*. Differential staining of chromosomes produces alternating dark and light transverse *bands*. The bands are labeled p1, p2, p3, and so forth on the p arm and q1, q2, q3, and so forth on the q arm, counted from the centromere toward the telomeres.

The p and q labels and bands are used to specify the location of specific DNA sections on the chromosome. There are also subbands within the major bands. This series of letters and numbers is the equivalent of an address for the location of a gene on a chromosome. For example, the cystic fibrosis gene *CFTR* (cystic fibrosis transmembrane conductance regulator) is located at 7q31.2, which indicates it is on chromosome 7, q arm, band 3, subband 1, and sub-subband 2.

DNA and the Double Helix

DNA is foundational to genetics. Within the nucleus of the cell, within each chromosome, DNA is arranged like a ladder, with two long strands of sub-units twisted around each other to form the double-stranded three-dimensional helix.

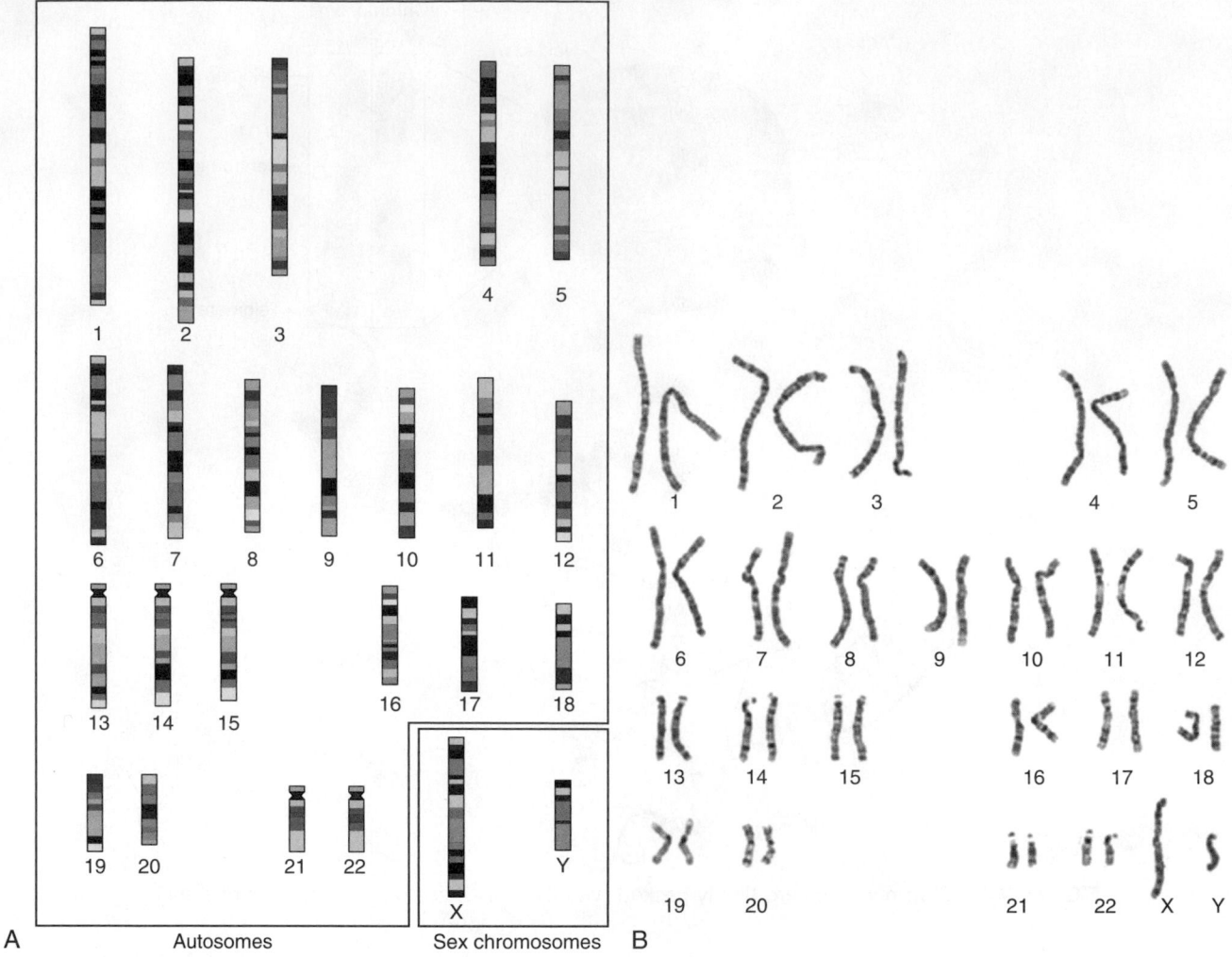

FIGURE 4-2 *A*, Schematic of the standard chromosomal arrangement used for classification of chromosomes by number, arranged from the largest (chromosome 1) to the smallest (chromosome 22). Chromosomes 1 to 22 are known as autosomes. Autosomal chromosomes are present in two identical copies, which are the same in males and females. The sex chromosomes are X (female) and Y (male). *B*, This is a male karyotype because the sex chromosome arrangement is XY. The striped bands that appear on the chromosomes are achieved by use of specialized staining techniques.

DNA Base Pairs

The subunits within each DNA strand are called *nucleotides* or *bases*, and they are combined in pairs to form the rungs of the DNA ladder. Four nucleotide bases—adenine (A), thymine (T), guanine (G), and cytosine (C)—comprise the "letters" in the genetic DNA "alphabet." Each nucleotide base is attached to a phosphorylated molecule of the 5-carbon sugar deoxyribose that forms the backbone of the DNA chain and can be visualized as the two sides of a ladder that have been twisted around (Fig. 4-3). The bases in the double helix are paired T with A, and G with C. The nucleotide bases are designed so that only G can pair with C and only T can pair with A to achieve a consistent distance across the width of the DNA strand. The TA and GC combinations are known as *base pairs* (see Fig. 4-3). There are approximately three billion bases in the human genome, based on findings from the Human Genome Project.[3]

The two DNA strands are orientated in opposite directions. Each DNA strand has a specific direction that is labeled as the 3′ end or the 5′ end (pronounced 3 prime, and 5 prime) (see Fig. 4-3). Because the DNA strands face in opposite directions, the 3′ end of one strand is always matched to the 5′ end of the other strand. This fact becomes important for replication (discussed next). The 3′ end is described as the *leading strand* because new nucleotides can be added only at the 3′ end.

DNA Replication

Before a cell divides, it needs to make a second copy of the entire DNA content within the cell. This process is called *DNA replication*. Sections of the DNA double helix separate longitudinally, creating openings between base pairs, known as *replication bubbles*, and mirror-image copies are made from the original strands. Stated another way, the original DNA strands provide

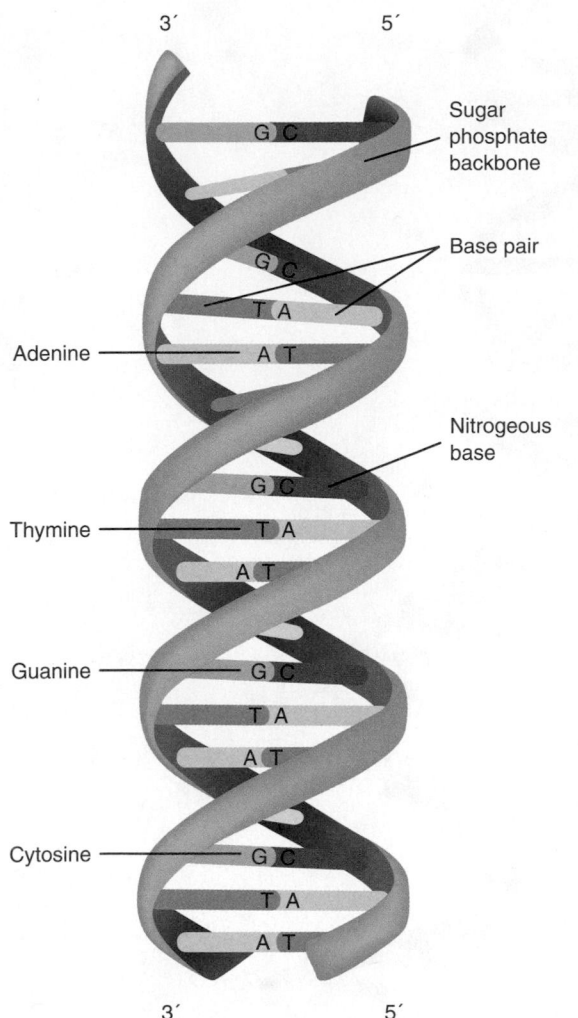

FIGURE 4-3 Deoxyribonucleic Acid (DNA) Double Helix.

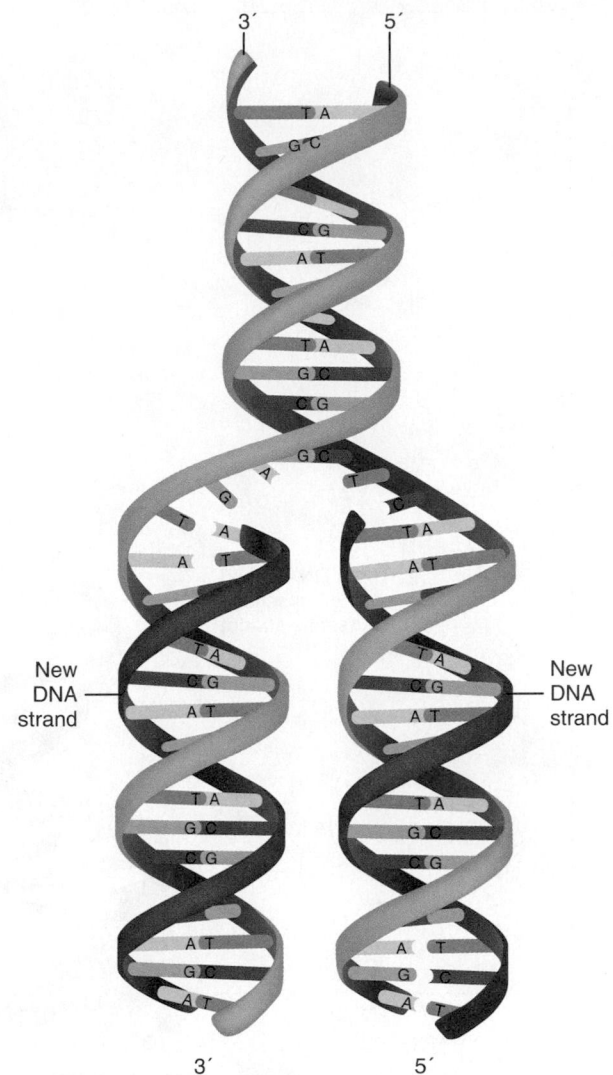

FIGURE 4-4 DNA replication occurs before the cell divides. The template is provided by the original DNA strand (colored blue). The mirror-image DNA strand (colored red) is adding nucleotides to elongate the new DNA strand.

a template that will be copied. The original is called the *parent strands* and the mirror-image copies are described as the *daughter strands*. In Figure 4-4 the parent strand is illustrated by the color blue with the 5′ and 3′ ends of each parent strand labeled. The daughter strands are colored in red. The replication process is facilitated by *DNA polymerase*, an enzyme that lengthens the DNA strand by the addition of new nucleotide bases at the 3′ end of the daughter strand (Fig. 4-4). After DNA replication is accomplished, the cell uses a sophisticated mechanism for identifying and fixing errors in the replicated strand.[8] After this procedure, the cell is ready to divide, and each new cell will contain a copy of the original DNA code.

DNA Alphabet

The nucleotides A, T, C, and G can be thought of as "letters" of a genetic alphabet that are combined into three-letter "words" that are transcribed (written) by the intermediary of *ribonucleic acid* (RNA). The RNA translates the three-letter words into the amino acids used to make the polypeptide chains that constitute proteins. This process may be written as DNA → RNA → protein.[9]

Transcription

The process of making an RNA strand from a DNA strand is known as *transcription*. The strand with the genetic code that is to be transcribed is labeled as the *sense* strand or sometimes as the *coding strand*. The other strand, which is the RNA mirror image, is called the antisense or non-coding strand (Fig. 4-5). The reason there are two strands oriented in opposite directions is to facilitate replication of a DNA strand during cell division (see Fig. 4-4), or when proteins are needed (see Fig. 4-5) without compromising the original genetic material. To visualize how the process of transcription works, it may be helpful to study Figure 4-5 and locate the names of the different strands; the DNA strand is colored blue, the RNA strand is colored green to make the distinction clear.

Transcription occurs under the guidance of the enzyme RNA *polymerase*, sections of the DNA double helix unfold and separate into two single strands within the length of the double helix

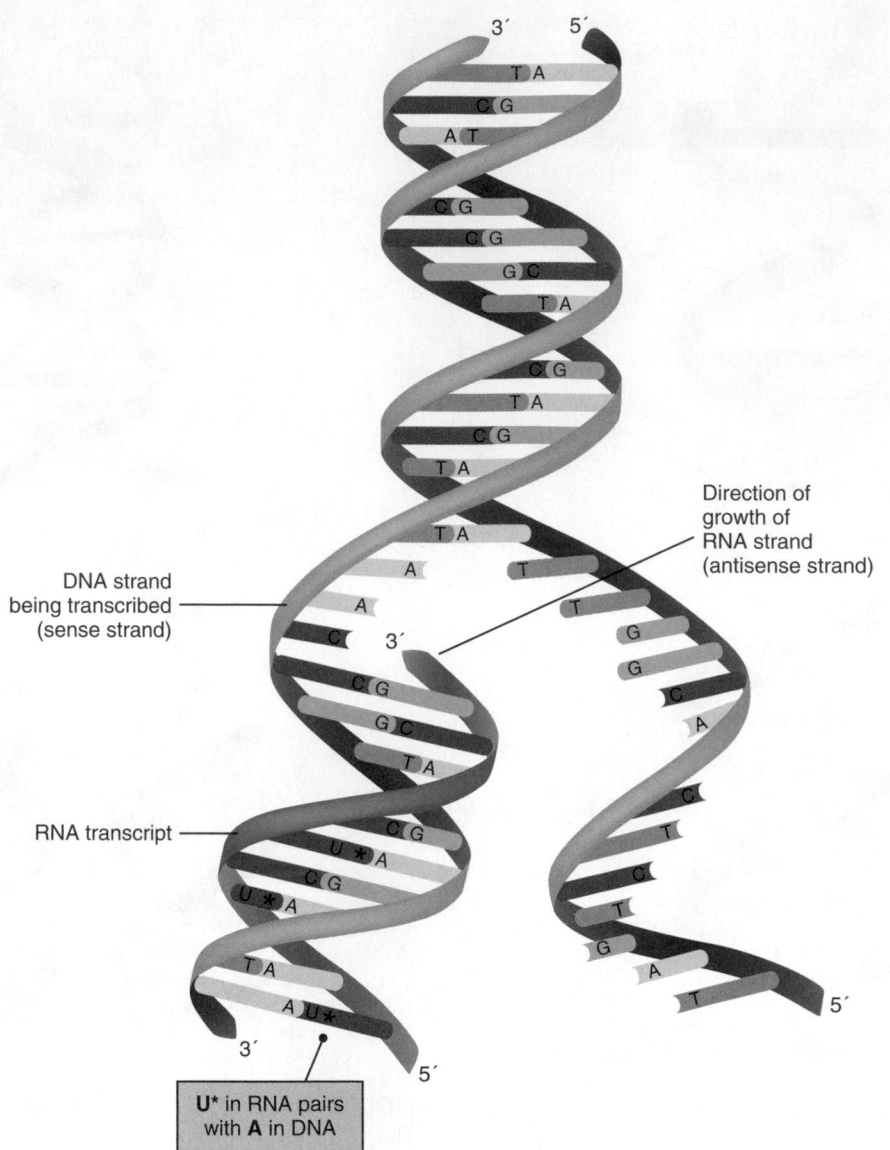

FIGURE 4-5   DNA transcription and production of a complementary RNA strand. The template DNA strand is colored blue. The RNA nucleotide uracil *(U)* pairs with the DNA nucleotide adenine *(A)* in the growing RNA strand (colored green).

(see Fig. 4-5). The mirror-image DNA strand (shown in red in Fig. 4-4) serves as a template for the synthesis of a complementary, mirror-image strand of RNA (shown in green in Fig. 4-5). The purpose of transcription is to have the RNA mirror strand replicate the genetic code in the original DNA sense strand.

When RNA transcribes DNA nucleotides, one significant change occurs. The adenosine (A) DNA base is paired with a uracil (U) base in the RNA transcript (see Fig. 4-5). Each RNA strand also has a 3′ end (can be conceptualized as a head) and a 5′ end (conceptualized as a tail), and the growing RNA strand adds bases only at the 3′ leading end. The RNA strand, called *messenger RNA*, then leaves the nucleus of the cell, and the next action takes place in the cytoplasm.

Translation

The next step is to translate the RNA bases into three-letter words (e.g., AUC, UGA) called *codons* that can be used to specify an amino acid. The 3-base RNA codons are designed to code for one of 20 amino acids. Some codons signal to stop the sequence; these termination sequences are UAA, UAG, and UGA. The three-letter codons are not unique; for example, both UAU and UUC code for the amino acid *phenylalanine*. Most amino acids can be made from more than one codon. This can be appreciated by an examination of the list of three-letter codons, the corresponding three-letter amino acid abbreviation, the single-letter abbreviation, and the name of the amino acid in Table 4-1. The process by which proteins are made from instructions encoded in DNA is called *gene expression*.

Only a brief review of how DNA contributes to the genetic code is possible in this chapter. The volume of information that underpins genetics and genomics reflects the work of many scientists who performed research to advance this knowledge, and it may take some individual study or additional classes to master the content. An excellent and free online tutorial called

TABLE 4-1 THE GENETIC CODE: AMINO ACIDS*

First nucleotide in codon		Second nucleotide in codon				Third nucleotide
		U	C	A	G	
U		UUU Phe F *Phenylalanine*	UCU Ser S *Serine*	UAU Tyr Y *Tyrosine*	UGU Cys C *Cysteine*	U
		UUC Phe F *Phenylalanine*	UCC Ser S *Serine*	UAC Tyr Y *Tyrosine*	UGC Cys C *Cysteine*	C
		UUA Leu L *Leucine*	UCA Ser S *Serine*	UAA Termination	UGA Termination	A
		UUG Leu L *Leucine*	UCG Ser S *Serine*	UAG Termination	UGG Trp W *Tryptophan*	G
C		CUU Leu L *Leucine*	CCU Pro P *Proline*	CAU His H *Histidine*	CGU Arg R *Arginine*	U
		CUC Leu L *Leucine*	CCC Pro P *Proline*	CAC His H *Histidine*	CGC Arg R *Arginine*	C
		CUA Leu L *Leucine*	CCA Pro P *Proline*	CAA Gln Q *Glutamine*	CGA Arg R *Arginine*	A
		CUG Leu L *Leucine*	CCG Pro P *Proline*	CAG Gln Q *Glutamine*	CGG Arg R *Arginine*	G
A		AUU Ile I *Isoleucine*	ACU Thr T *Threonine*	AAU Asn N *Asparagine*	AGU ser S *Serine*	U
		AUC Ile I *Isoleucine*	ACC Thr T *Threonine*	AAC Asn N *Asparagine*	AGC ser S *Serine*	C
		AUA Ile I *Isoleucine*	ACA Thr T *Threonine*	AAA Lys K *Lysine*	AGA Arg R *Arginine*	A
		AUG Met M *Methionine*	ACG Thr T *Threonine*	AAG Lys K *Lysine*	AGG Arg R *Arginine*	G
G		GUU Val V *Valine*	GCU Ala A *Alanine*	GAU Asp D *Aspartic acid*	GGU Gly G *Glycine*	U
		GUC Val V *Valine*	GCC Ala A *Alanine*	GAC Asp D *Aspartic acid*	GGC Gly G *Glycine*	C
		GUA Val V *Valine*	GCA Ala A *Alanine*	GAA Glu E *Glutamic acid*	GGA Gly G *Glycine*	A
		GUG Val V *Valine*	GCG Ala A *Alanine*	GAG Glu E *Glutamic acid*	GGG Gly G *Glycine*	G

Codon ⟶ Three-letter and single-letter abbreviations

*Amino acids are the building blocks of proteins. The 20 amino acids are constructed from information contained in the DNA blueprint that is translated and transcribed by RNA. This transfer of information from DNA to amino acids is called the genetic code. Triple sets of bases (codons) are transcribed into the 20 amino acids. Sixty-four combinations of codons are possible, and several codons code for the same amino acids. The amino acids are connected in long polypeptide chains that form proteins. Three combinations signal the end of a protein chain: UAA, UAG, and UGA. Each three-letter codon also has a single-letter abbreviation, which is shown in the table.

"DNA from the Beginning" is available through the Cold Spring Harbor Laboratory website.[10] The 41 modules use animation, video interviews, and text to present an interesting and informative introduction to the history and science of genetics.[10]

Genetic Variation, Mutation and Polymorphism
Variation

Genetic variation is common to all species. It means that individuals do not have the same nucleotides (A, C, T, G) in exactly the same position on the DNA strand. Some nucleotide differences result in the expression of different proteins and physical traits. Many nucleotide changes produce no visible external alteration, although those that have health-related consequences are of great interest to clinicians, patients, and researchers. Genetic variation can result from a variety of changes. It can be a single-letter substitution of one nucleotide base for another that can produce an inappropriate stop codon or produce a codon for a different amino acid. The amino acid codes are shown in Table 4-1. An example of a single-letter switch that results in an increased risk for disease is the G-to-A substitution at nucleotide 1691 in the coagulation factor V gene. This is also an example of a relatively rare single-gene variant that alters the protein product and increases the incidence of deep vein thrombosis (DVT), as described in Box 4-1.

Genetic material in the chromosome can also be deleted (Fig. 4-6A), new information from another chromosome can be inserted (Fig. 4-6B), or a *tandem repeat* (multiple repeats of the same sequence) may produce duplicate genetic material within the chromosome (Fig. 4-6C).

Translocation of genetic material describes a process in which chromosomes break and genetic material is moved from one chromosome to another. For example, the *Philadelphia Chromosome*, or *Philadelphia translocation*, is a specific chromosomal abnormality associated with chronic myelogenous leukemia (CML). It results from a reciprocal translocation between chromosomes 9 and 22, in which parts of these two chromosomes switch places, producing the oncogenic Philadelphia Chromosome and development of dysregulated tyrosine kinase. CML represents 20% of all adult cases of leukemia.[11]

Mutation

The term *genetic mutation* refers to a change in the DNA genetic sequence that can be inherited. The term *mutation* typically is used to describe alterations that occur in less than 1% of a population. This use of the word *mutation* does not have the negative connotation of being more deadly than other genetic changes. It just means the incidence is rare.

Single-Nucleotide Polymorphisms

When a genetic variant occurs frequently and is present in 1% or more of the population, it is described as a *genetic polymorphism*. The most common change is the substitution of one

BOX 4-1 GENETIC CONDITIONS IN CRITICAL CARE: DEEP VEIN THROMBOSIS AND FACTOR V LEIDEN

Clinical Presentation

Carriers of the coagulation factor V Leiden polymorphism are at increased risk for venous thromboembolism (VTE), identified by deep vein thrombosis (DVT) or pulmonary embolism (PE). The phenotype (clinical signs and symptoms) is defined by an increased incidence of DVT. Factor V Leiden thrombophilia is suspected in individuals with a history of DVT or PE and in people with first-degree family members who have experienced recurrent thromboemboli. Assessment is warranted for women who experience DVT during pregnancy or DVT while on oral contraceptives or hormone replacement therapy (HRT).[12] Factor V Leiden is found in up to 25% of patients with VTE, and in 50% of patients with familial thrombophilia.[12]

Genetic Evidence

The factor V (F5) gene is located on chromosome 1 on the long arm at position 23 (1q23). The Factor V Leiden polymorphism refers to the specific G-to-A substitution at nucleotide 1691 in the coagulation factor V gene (genotype). This causes a single amino acid replacement at position 506 from arginine to glutamine. The resultant nonfunctional gene protein is called factor V Leiden.[12]

Normal factor V circulates in plasma as an inactive cofactor. Activation by thrombin results in the formation of factor Va, which serves as a cofactor in the conversion of prothrombin to thrombin. To express its anticoagulant function, normal factor Va must be cleaved by activated protein C (APC) at arginine in the 506 position and then at other sites within the factor Va molecule. Factor Va Leiden cannot be cleaved by APC because there is a glutamine at the 506 position. Factor Va Leiden therefore is inactivated more slowly than normal factor Va. This leaves more factor Va available within the prothrombin complex, which increases coagulation because of ongoing generation of thrombin.

The term *Leiden* in the name refers to the town in the Netherlands, where the gene was initially discovered. Factor V Leiden is also the most common cause of APC resistance, which may additively increase the risk of thrombosis.

Several large studies have examined the association between factor V Leiden and venous thrombosis. The Longitudinal Investigation of Thromboembolism Etiology (LITE) study was a prospective cohort study involving 335 men and women in the United States who developed a venous thromboembolism during 8 years of follow-up. This was a case-control study nested within a much larger cardiovascular trial. The LITE study evaluated genetic risk factors for future DVT or PE. The occurrence of VTE, adjusted for age, was 3.67-fold higher in carriers of factor V Leiden than in noncarriers.

Gene-Environment Interactions

The standard risk factors for DVT also apply to patients with factor V Leiden. The risk for DVT is increased by smoking, obesity, immobility, and trauma. Several additional genetic defects in the factor V gene have been identified as possible risk factors for thrombosis. One study identified seven other single-nucleotide polymorphisms (SNPs) associated with DVT occurrence. Individuals with two or more genetic risk factors (gene-gene interactions) are at much higher risk for DVT. Studies to more clearly evaluate this risk are ongoing.

Inheritance

The factor V Leiden allele is inherited in an autosomal dominant pattern.[12] This means the person needs only one copy (allele) of the factor V Leiden gene (heterozygous) to be at increased risk for DVT. People who are homozygous have two copies of the variant gene, (one from each parent) and have an even greater risk of DVT. The average age for first venous thrombosis is reported as 44 years for factor V Leiden heterozygotes and 31 years for factor V homozygotes.[68]

Who Should Undergo Genetic Testing?

Genetic testing is reserved for those in high-risk groups who have experienced a first DVT before age 50 years; a first, unprovoked (no environmental stimuli) DVT at any age; a history of recurrent DVT; and thromboembolism in unusual venous locations, such as the cerebral, mesenteric, portal, and hepatic veins.[12]

There is no recommendation to test asymptomatic family members unless they have additional risk factors such as taking hormone replacement therapy.[12,69]

To test for factor V Leiden, the first step is to do an APC-resistance assay. If the blood test shows APC resistance, it is likely the individual carries the factor V Leiden variant, and genetic testing is undertaken as a secondary analysis.[12]

---

single-nucleotide base. A single-letter switch is known as a *single-nucleotide polymorphism* (SNP), commonly abbreviated and pronounced "snip" (Fig. 4-7). This is significant when the SNP occurs in a region of DNA that codes for an amino acid. If the SNP change alters the amino acid product that is produced, it is called a *nonsynonymous SNP*, or *missense SNP*. If a nonsynonymous SNP occurs in a coding region, it may affect protein structure and lead to alterations in phenotype (disease manifestation). An example is the G-to-A coding SNP at the 1691 site of the factor V gene associated with blood coagulation.[12] This polymorphism leads to the substitution of an arginine (A) by glutamine (G) at amino acid position 506, which alters one of the cleavage sites for *activated protein C*. Factor Va inactivation is delayed because the cleavage site is atypical. This change in one amino acid reduces the anticoagulant activity of factor V, creates a hypercoagulable state, and consequently increases the risk for DVT[12] (see Box 4-1).

Alleles

Another name for a variant of a gene that occurs at a single locus is an *allele*. Allele symbols consist of the gene symbol, an asterisk, and the italicized allele designation. For example, the apolipoprotein E gene (APOE) has three major alleles (APOE*E2, APOE*E3, APOE*E4), and each allele codes for a different isoform of the ApoE protein.[13] Apolipoprotein E is involved with cholesterol metabolism, and expression of the APOE*E4 allele is associated with the development of hyperlipidemia. APOE*E4 expression also is associated with late-onset Alzheimer's disease and with a less favorable outcome after traumatic brain injury and brain hemorrhage.[13]

Not all changes in the DNA sequence have deleterious effects. Most SNPs have no effect because they are *synonymous SNPs*, variants that code for the same amino acid (see Table 4-1), or because they are located in non-coding genomic region.

GENETIC INHERITANCE

Genetic Disorders

All genetic and genomic disorders do not have the same cause. The categories of disorders are chromosome disorders, single-gene disorders, complex gene and multifactorial disorders, and mitochondrial disorders.

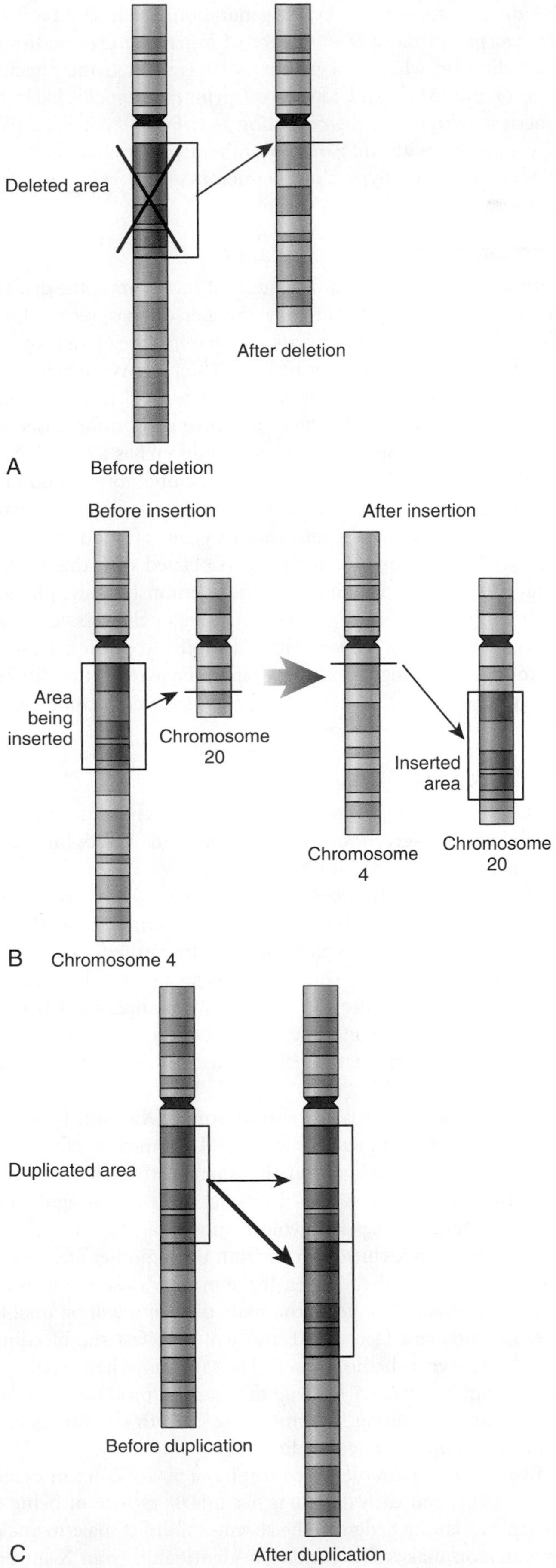

Deleted area

After deletion

A Before deletion

Before insertion

After insertion

Area being inserted

Chromosome 20

Inserted area

Chromosome 4

Chromosome 20

B Chromosome 4

Duplicated area

Before duplication

C After duplication

FIGURE 4-6 *A,* Deletion of chromosomal genetic material. *B,* Insertion of genetic material from one chromosome to another. *C,* Duplication of chromosomal genetic material.

Chromosome Disorders

In chromosome disorders, the entire chromosome or very large segments of the chromosome are damaged, missing, duplicated, or otherwise altered. Down syndrome (trisomy 21), in which there is an extra copy of chromosome 21, is an example of a chromosome disorder.

Single-Gene Disorders

In single-gene disorders, a single gene is altered. Single-gene disorders can result from inheritance of one dominant gene or two recessive genes. Cystic fibrosis, sickle cell disease, hemophilia A, and Marfan syndrome are examples of single-gene disorders. Single-gene disorders may also be described as monogenetic or *Mendelian gene* disorders. Single-gene disorders are rare in the population but have a significant physical impact on the affected individual.

Complex Gene and Multifactorial Disorders

In some disorders, many genes interact to produce the condition, or there must be an interaction between vulnerable genes and the environment. Cardiovascular atherosclerotic diseases and type 2 diabetes are examples of complex gene disorders that result from an interaction of genetic and environmental factors.[4] Pharmacogenetic syndromes are also in this category, resulting from the interactions of genes and medications.

Mitochondrial Disorders

Some diseases are caused by alterations in the DNA of the mitochondria, which are intracellular organelles found in the

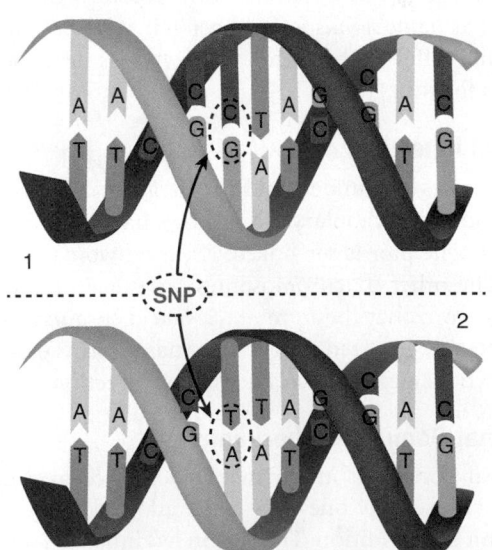

FIGURE 4-7 A single-nucleotide polymorphism (SNP) where one nucleotide base letter is replaced by a different base letter.

cytoplasm. Mitochondrial DNA is totally different and separate from the double-helix DNA found in the nucleus. Mitochondrial DNA is transferred to offspring by maternal transmission only, because mitochondria occur in oocytes but not in sperm. Most mitochondrial genetic diseases are associated with disorders of enzyme function that disrupts mitochondrial energy production. Tissues and organs that have high energy requirements such as skeletal muscles, the heart, and the central nervous system are most often affected.[14]

Genotype and Phenotype

The *genotype* refers to the genetic makeup at a particular *locus* or location on a specific chromosome within the genome; this is conceptually similar to a unique street address. The *phenotype* refers to the signs and symptoms that are clinically associated with a particular genetic condition; this is conceptually similar to describing the defining characteristics of the house, apartment, boat, dorm room, or castle at this particular address.

Genetic History and Family Pedigree

One of the tools used to determine whether a disease has a genetic component is construction of a family pedigree.[15] For nurses, it is important to develop the skills to ask questions to elucidate which family members are affected and which are unaffected and then to identify the individuals who may carry the gene in question but do not have symptoms (carriers). Standardized symbols are used in the construction of a pedigree.[15] The use of a legend to explain what the symbols mean prevents misinterpretation. The *proband* is the name given to the first person diagnosed in the family pedigree. Examples of three simple pedigrees that illustrate the single-gene inheritance patterns and the symbols used to construct a pedigree are shown in Figure 4-8 with examples described below.

Homozygous versus Heterozygous

Each individual inherits genetic material from his or her father and mother. If an individual inherits the same gene at a specific locus (genetic address) from both parents, the person is described as *homozygous* for that gene. If the genes donated by the parents differ at that locus, the person is described as *heterozygous* for that gene.

Modes of Inheritance

One of the keys to understanding the genetics literature is to understand the vocabulary. All humans have 23 pairs of chromosomes. One pair is sex linked: XX for a woman and XY for a man. The other 22 chromosomes are called *autosomes*. It is from this word that the term *autosomal inheritance* is derived. The differences between some of the major forms of autosomal inheritance are described in the following sections.

Autosomal Dominant Inheritance

Autosomal dominant inheritance is described as a dominant pattern because only one copy of an affected gene is required to transmit the condition. The person has inherited one affected gene from one parent and one healthy gene from the other parent, and is described as heterozygous for that gene. Typically, the disease appears in every generation. Each child of an affected parent has a 50% chance of inheriting the condition, depending on whether a parent has transmitted the affected gene or not. Male and female offspring are equally likely to inherit and transmit the condition (see Fig. 4-8A). Examples of conditions with autosomal dominant inheritance patterns include familial hypercholesterolemia (FH) and Marfan syndrome.

Autosomal Recessive Inheritance

With an autosomal recessive pattern of inheritance, the disease or condition manifests only if the person has received an affected gene from both parents. The parents are *carriers* of the gene but are not themselves affected. The parents are heterozygous, because they have one copy of a normal gene and one copy of an affected gene. The inheritance pattern for this situation is slightly complex. Any of their children has a 25% chance to inherit in the following combinations: one normal and one affected gene (heterozygous carrier), two normal genes (unaffected), or two affected genes (homozygous affected). Persons who are homozygous for the gene associated with the disease always are affected, which means they demonstrate the phenotype of the disease (see Fig. 4-8B). In autosomal recessive inheritance, the phenotype associated with the condition is seen more often in siblings (sibships) than in the parents. Conditions associated with autosomal recessive inheritance include cystic fibrosis and sickle cell disease.

Sex-Linked Inheritance

Traits controlled by genes located on the sex chromosomes are sex-linked. Red-green color blindness and hemophilia are examples of X-linked conditions.

Hemophilia A and Hemophilia B. Some diseases are inherited through an X-linked pattern of inheritance. A classic example is the *F8* gene, which codes for the protein that makes coagulation factor VIII. The *F8* gene is located on the X chromosome.[16] Of note, the inheritance of hemophilia B is also sex-linked because the *F9* gene, which codes for the protein that makes coagulation factor IX, is also located on the X chromosome.[16]

Women always have two X chromosomes (XX), one from the mother and one from the father. Even if the mother carried an affected *F8* gene, the gene on the unaffected X chromosome from the father confers the ability to make the coagulation factor and female offspring avoid hemophilia. However, males (XY) inherit one X chromosome from their mother and one Y chromosome from their father. If the mother's X chromosome carries the affected *F8* gene, the male offspring will be unable to make sufficient factor VIII and will manifest the bleeding disorder known as hemophilia A. The same inheritance pattern occurs with an affected *F9* gene that cannot produce coagulation factor IX resulting in hemophilia B. Both conditions can result in life-threatening bleeding.

In an *X-linked disorder*, each son has a 50% chance of being hemophiliac, and each daughter has a 50% chance of being a carrier. In a family pedigree, the absence of direct male-to-male transmission makes this condition identifiable as an X-linked disorder. Hemophilia A is an example of a single-gene disorder. Figure 4-8C illustrates an X-linked family pedigree for hemophilia A; a male who is affected (generation I) may pass the X-linked *F8* gene only to his daughters (generation II), who may pass the gene to sons who will be affected, or to daughters who will be carriers (generation III). A female will only be affected if she receives a defective X-linked gene from both her father and mother as occurs in generation IV.

Complex Gene-Gene and Gene-Environment Disorders

Many genomic disorders are complex, and multiple factors are thought to contribute to manifestation of disease phenotypes. They result from *gene-gene* interactions or *gene-environment* interactions. Many patients who are admitted to the critical care unit may exhibit the phenotype of a complex genomic condition if they are obese or have type 2 diabetes.

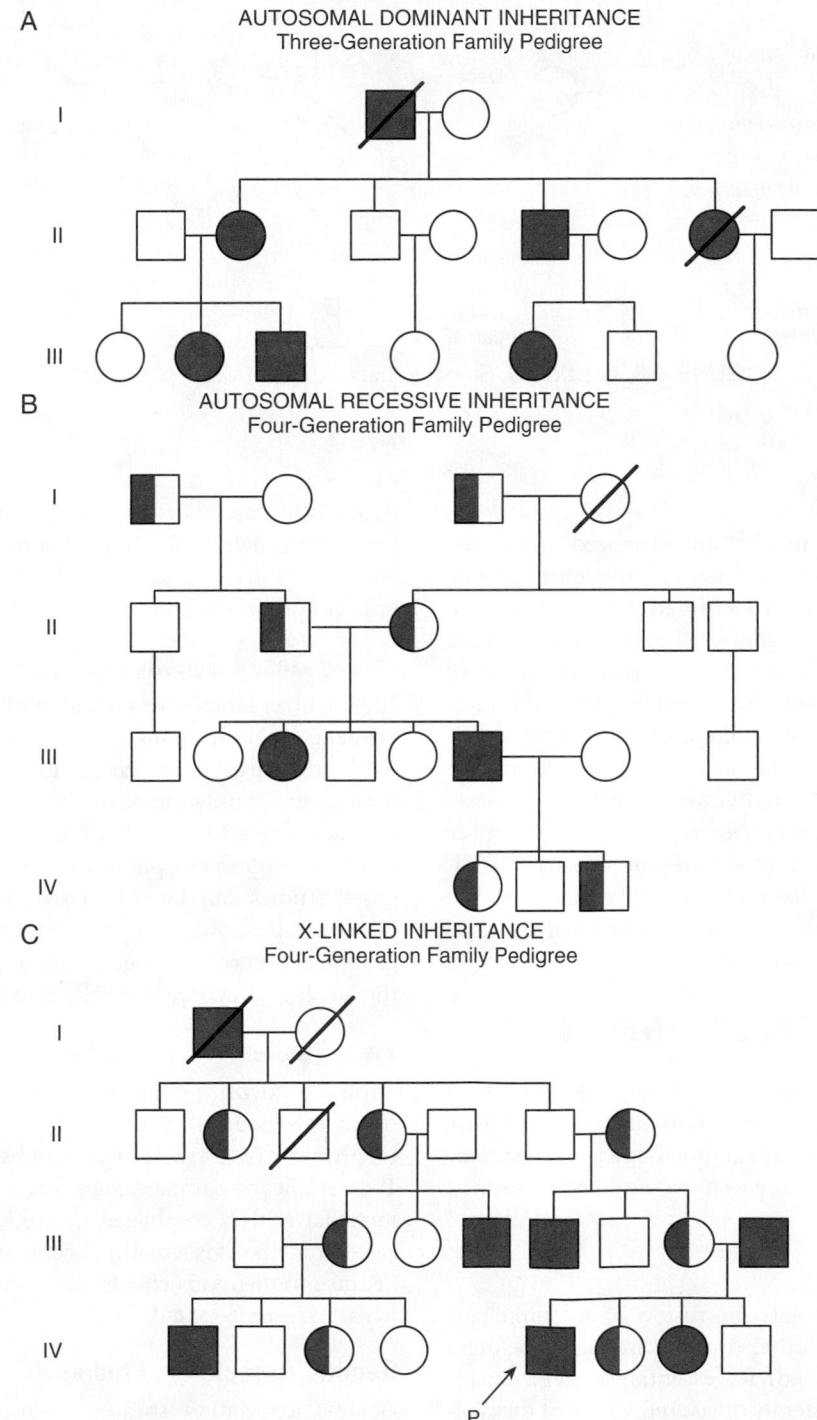

FIGURE 4-8   *A,* Pedigree of a dominant mode of inheritance. *B,* Pedigree of a recessive mode of inheritance. *C,* Pedigree of an X-linked mode of inheritance. See text for further information.

Continued

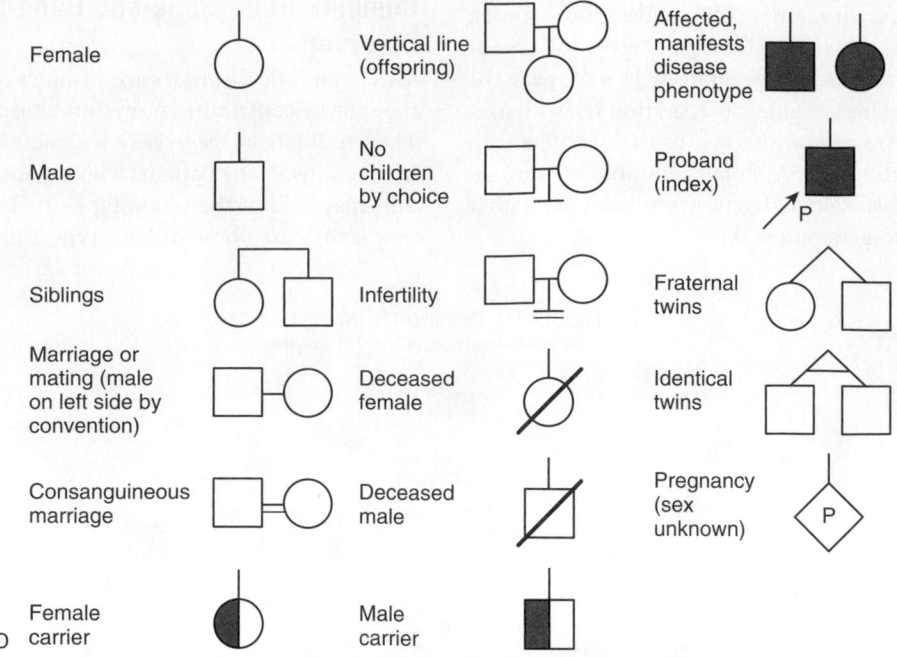

Female

Male

Siblings

Marriage or
mating (male
on left side by
convention)

Consanguineous
marriage

D Female
carrier

Vertical line
(offspring)

No
children
by choice

Infertility

Deceased
female

Deceased
male

Male
carrier

Affected,
manifests
disease
phenotype

Proband
(index)

Fraternal
twins

Identical
twins

Pregnancy
(sex
unknown)

FIGURE 4-8, cont'd   *D,* Symbols used to construct a pedigree.

Obesity and the *FTO* Gene

The pandemic of obesity in the industrialized world has entrained higher rates of cardiovascular atherosclerotic disease and type 2 diabetes. GWAS have identified polymorphisms in the *fat mass and obesity-associated gene (FTO)* on chromosome 16 that are linked to obesity.[17] A patient who is overweight or obese may blame it on "my bad genes," and this raises the question of whether the presence of an altered *FTO* gene automatically means the individual will be obese. From the results of a GWAS analysis of over 38,000 individuals, the 16% who were homozygous for the FTO gene carried about 3 kilograms more weight, with an increased risk of developing obesity.[17] Additional genes are now being identified that will further increase our understanding of the shared genetic and environmental contribution to the obesity epidemic.[18]

HOW INFORMATION ABOUT GENETICS IS OBTAINED

Genetic information can be collected in many ways. Often, when a gene is selected, all of the methods described here may be used to link the phenotype, genotype, and environmental effects.

Genetic Epidemiology

Genetic epidemiology represents the fusion of epidemiologic studies and genetic and genomic research methods. Before a gene can be mapped (genotyped), it is essential to have a reliable phenotype that can be consistently measured.[19] One of the challenges in applying genetics to the critical care arena is that the genotype is stable but the phenotype is dynamic. Phenotypes are different at different stages of a disease and are influenced by medications, environmental factors, and gene-gene interactions.[19] It is helpful to discuss the methods used outside of the critical care unit as a way of understanding the challenges in the application of genomics in this arena.

Family-Based Genetic Studies

In genetic epidemiologic research of a rare disease, it can be a challenge to find enough people to study. One method is to work with large, extended families, known as *kinships*, which have several family members affected with the disease. Genetic testing is done to construct a genetic linkage map of the area close to the polymorphic gene found in that family. Family-based studies can identify a significant phenotype-genotype relationship. Subsequently, it is important to do studies of other groups to determine whether the original finding is unique to the kinship or can be generalized to people outside the family.

Twin Studies

Studies of identical twins offer a unique opportunity to investigate the association of genetics, environment, and health. Identical twins are *monozygotic* and share an identical genome. Twin studies to compare the effects of genetics versus environment have been conducted by studying identical twins separated at birth. This situation occurs much less frequently today because tremendous efforts are made to keep siblings together when they are adopted.

Genetic Association Studies

Genetic association studies are usually conducted in large, unrelated groups based on demonstration of a phenotype (disease trait or symptoms) and associated genotype. In genetic association studies, it is important to recruit a diverse group of individuals to determine whether a trait is universal or found only in selected groups. Genetic studies can be conducted in isolated populations, in which *population stratification* is expected, or in highly mixed groups. It is important to collect information about ancestral and racial heritage to enable linkage of phenotypic and genotypic data. Diverse populations are sometimes called *admixed populations*, indicating that many different heritage groups have been included in the mix of people. The purpose of these different kinds of studies is to make a clear phenotype-genotype match and to identify which genetic conditions are associated with specific racial or ethnic groups and which genetic conditions are universal.

Case-Control Studies

In case-control studies, individuals are identified with the phenotypic and genotypic traits of a disease (cases). These cases are then matched to nonrelated controls by age, race, sex, and sometimes other associated disease factors.

Candidate Gene Studies

Candidate gene studies usually are exploratory studies in which a gene is suspected as a contributor to a phenotype or disease. Unrelated individuals with the phenotype are then tested for presence of the gene. These usually are smaller studies, and there is a strong biologic rationale for investigating the association between genotype and phenotype.

Genome-Wide Association Studies

GWAS examine the breadth of the human genome and typically use very large samples. The intent is to use genetic microarray technology and statistical computational power to find SNPs associated with a disease. Some GWAS are conducted with the intent of finding additional genes. However, one of the strengths of the GWAS model is that it does not have to begin with a biologic model in mind as long as the disease of interest is sufficiently common in the population, and by testing thousands of SNPs, the researchers may find associations that have not been detected by other methods. A classic example is a GWAS of 14,000 individuals (cases) with 3000 shared controls genotyped to find SNPs associated with seven common diseases.[20] Significant new SNPs were found for five of seven diseases: type 1 diabetes, type 2 diabetes, rheumatoid arthritis, Crohn's disease, and coronary artery disease.[20] New GWAS are published every month, and the National Human Genome Research Institute (NHGRI) maintains an online catalog of published studies that can be searched by disease trait, chromosomal region, gene, or SNP.[21]

Genome Mapping Projects
The Human Genome Project

The Human Genome Project was a huge, internationally collaborative project that began in 1990 with the goal of making a map of all the human genes (the genome). The final genome sequence was published in 2003. Big discoveries came out of the Human Genome Project, including a map of the human genome and a wealth of new clinical and computational tools that could be used for future studies.

The human genome map was created from the DNA of only a few people.[22] One of the surprising discoveries was that the number of genes possessed by humans was not as large as expected. The number of protein-coding genes in the chromosome is estimated to be between 20,000 and 25,000.[3] Although researchers were initially surprised that the gene number was not higher, it has become apparent than many posttranscriptional alterations occur to actively change the protein product. The ongoing research agenda is to understand all of these additional sequence elements.

ENCODE Project

The *ENCyclopedia Of DNA Elements* (ENCODE) pilot project involved a detailed analysis of 1% of the human genome using cell lines.[23] The goal was to elucidate all of the functional elements that enable relatively few human genes to produce such a wide variety of biologic products (e.g., proteins). The second phase of the ENCODE project examined the entire genome in 147 different cell types. The focus was on the regulatory role of RNAs in modulating cellular functions directly as biologically active molecules or indirectly by encoding other active molecules.[23,24] Across coding and non-coding areas, 80% of the human genome is involved in at least one biochemical RNA or chromatin-associated event in the cell-types examined.[24] Other areas of research focus on epigenetics histone modification, DNA methylation, and on the transcriptional regulatory elements that control gene expression.[24] This database will be a rich resource for future biomedical genomic research.

HapMap Project

The International HapMap Project database[25] contains over 4 million SNPs from 270 individuals representing four populations: African (Yoruba, Nigeria), European Americans (Utah), Japanese (Tokyo), and Han Chinese. HapMap displays short linear sections of genetic loci on the same chromosome known as *haplotypes* or *haplotype blocks*. Loci are grouped as a haplotype if they are close to each other on a chromosome and are inherited as a linear group. Genetic epidemiologists call this grouped pattern *linkage disequilibrium*. It means that the loci are linked due to shared ancestry, where genetic information was inherited by offspring in "chunks" or "blocks" rather than as individual genes. The mixing of sections of different chromosomes that are inherited from each parent is called *recombination*. The resultant linked genetic loci are called *haplotypes*. The edges of the haplotypes are conceptualized as *recombination hotspots*, where little ancestral relationship remains.[22] More than 32,000 hotspots have been identified. Hotspots account for approximately 60% of recombination in the human genome and represent about 6% of the genomic sequence.[26] An example of the expected haplotype change over 150,000 years from African ancestral chromosomes to modern chromosomes is shown in Figure 4-9. The biologic rationale for recombination is to increase genetic diversity.

1000 Genomes Project

The *1000 Genomes Project* builds on the information gained in the HapMap project because it greatly increases the number of

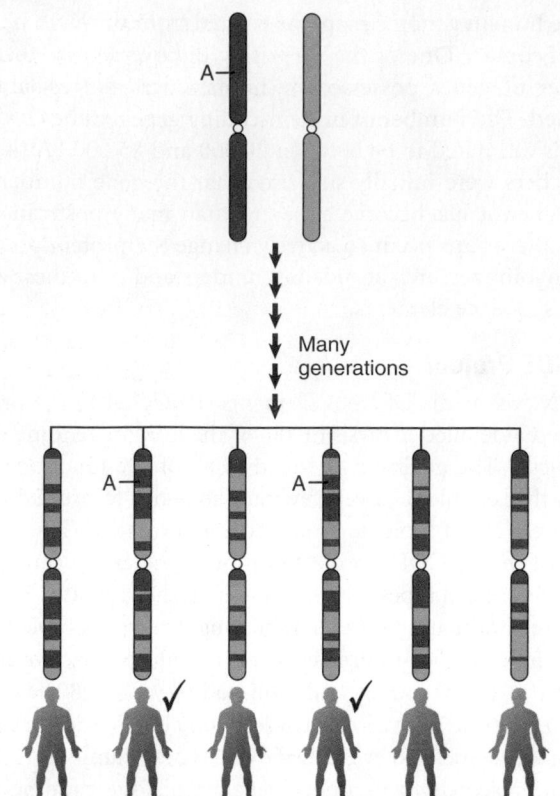

FIGURE 4-9 Effect of recombination on ancestral chromosomes. A gene is labeled **A** on the red ancestral chromosome. It is an example of a gene that has been conserved in modern chromosomes in one-third of cases. The gene (A) is associated with a specific phenotype or trait (shown as a checkmark). Because of recombination of chromosomes over thousands of generations, two-thirds of modern chromosomes no longer carry this gene.

included genomes. Scientific goals of the *1000 Genomes Project* were to produce a catalog of human genomes identifying genetic variants that occur at 1% or greater frequency in the human population across most of the genome, and down to 0.5% frequency or lower, within genes.[22] The 1000 Genomes Project did not collect any health-related phenotypic information.

Personal Genome Project

The *Personal Genome Project* (PGP) is in the process of enrolling 100,000 individual volunteers from the general public, with the goal of creating a reference database, to ultimately make individual genome sequencing more affordable.[27] The purpose is to create a diverse catalog of the human genome linked to phenotypes such as medical records and medical history. This will provide a reference database against which individual genomes can be compared. As of May 12, 2012, over 1800 participants have enrolled.[28] Even with only a small percentage of the intended individuals yet enrolled, the number of new genomic variants being identified with each new genome entered into the database (i.e., not seen in a previously entered genome) has dropped dramatically.[26] As the number of participants increases, the researchers plan to examine the genotype-phenotype relationships of specific diseases.[26]

The Human Microbiome Project

In the healthy human body, microbial cells vastly outnumber human cells sometimes being described as our second genome.[29] The human body is host to many microbial communities (human microbiome) located on the skin and in the nose, mouth, gastrointestinal, and urogenital tracts.[30] The spectrum of these microbial communities was previously almost entirely unknown. The Human Microbiome Project is designed to identify the core human microbiome, and to determine whether changes in the human microbiome can be correlated with changes in human health.[29,31] The human microbiome project is highly relevant to critical care because so many patients are admitted with sepsis or experience disruption of the gastrointestinal tract with diarrhea. The interaction of host bacteria, pathologic bacteria, critical care environment, and pharmacogenetics has the potential to bring novel insights to our current understanding of critical illness.

Genetic Diversity

The oldest human genetic lineages originate from the continent of Africa. The migration of a subset of humans out of Africa resulted in loss of genetic diversity. Numerous studies have shown higher levels of nucleotide and haplotype diversity of nuclear and mitochondrial genomes in Africans than in non-Africans.[32,33] Large-scale autosomal studies of African genetic diversity are being conducted.

Copy Number Variation

Copy number variation (CNV) adds another level of variation to the human genome. CNV describes structural changes of DNA, larger than 1 kilobase, that include insertions, deletions, and inversions. The impact of CNVs on frequently seen diseases appears to be negligable,[34] but when rare DNA loci associated with a disease state are inserted, the "dose" of affected DNA can alter disease expression. Examples include familial Parkinson's disease[35] and schizophrenia.[36] CNVs can be either associated with a Mendelian gene inheritance or appear *de novo*, as a new variant, in the genome.[37]

Individual Genome Sequences

It was stratospherically expensive to sequence the genome of an individual. However, the price is dropping dramatically and the goal of a $1000 individual genome may soon be a reality. One of the many challenges is how to use all of the data provided by genome analysis.[38] Another issue is personal privacy. These issues will require serious legal and ethical discussion at both individual and societal levels.

GENETICS IN CRITICAL CARE

The next step in the genomics revolution will be to connect the growing amounts of research data to clinical interventions that may help patients. The areas of clinical practice in which this has received most attention are cancer,[39] cardiovascular disease,[40] and pharmacogenomics.

Cancer Genetics

Somatic Mutations

The word *somatic* means "related to the body." Somatic mutations are changes within a specific group of body tissues that are not heritable. Often, somatic changes are related to changes in genetic markers associated with cancer or cardiovascular disease.

The Cancer Genome Atlas

There is strong evidence that many forms of cancer are caused by epigenetic alterations; one mechanism is the addition of methyl groups to specific genes to block their effect, a process sometimes referred to as *gene silencing*. Epigenetic changes can disrupt the normal balance in cell proliferation, cell survival, and cell differentiation. The Cancer Genome Atlas (TCGA) project was established to accelerate understanding of the molecular basis of human cancers. The large-scale genome sequencing techniques, first developed in the Human Genome Project, are used to sequence genes associated with lethal and common cancers.[41] The goal is to document all cancer genetic changes from chromosomal rearrangements to DNA mutations to epigenetic changes (chemical modifications of DNA that can turn genes on or off without altering the DNA sequence). TCGA is an international research initiative that has demonstrated it may be more important to identify and target specialized biologic pathways in many lethal cancers than single genes. Biologic pathway disruptions result in multiple gene rearrangements of gene clusters, which at first appear to be unrelated but are connected by cellular signaling systems orchestrated by complex biologic pathways.[42-44]

Cardiovascular Genetics

Genetic markers are being included in many cardiovascular research studies.[45] A classic example is the Framingham Heart Study. This longitudinal, multigenerational study was started in 1948 to identify the common factors that contribute to cardiovascular disease.[46] The researchers have phenotypic and pedigree data for several generations, and they have added genetic markers to their investigation of biologic and epidemiologic factors.[47] These cardiac genomic research studies will improve understanding of the interactions between genomic and environmental factors that underpin cardiovascular disease.

Long QT Syndrome

Long QT syndrome (LQTS) is a hereditary cardiac channelopathy with several different genotypes (LQTS 1-10), and a phenotype that manifests as a prolongation of the corrected QT interval (QTc) on the electrocardiogram (ECG); affected individuals incur an increased risk of sudden cardiac death (SCD)[48] (Box 4-2). Not all patients who have the LQTS genotype are

---

BOX 4-2   GENETIC CONDITIONS IN CRITICAL CARE: LONG QT SYNDROME

Clinical Presentation

Long QT syndrome (LQTS) is a cardiac genetic disorder identified by prolongation of the QT interval. This is defined as a corrected QT interval (QTc), longer than 500 milliseconds on the resting electrocardiogram (ECG). LQTS is estimated to affect 1 in 5000 individuals and is one of the primary causes of sudden cardiac death (SCD) in the young.[70] In children it is often called Congenital LQTS.

Frequently patients are identified following a syncopal episode, a life-threatening dysrhythmia such as torsades de pointes, or SCD. Treatment regimens include beta-blockers.[48,71] For LQTS patients at high risk of cardiac arrest, insertion of a pacemaker/internal cardioverter defibrillator (ICD) is warranted.[48,71]

Critically ill patients with undiagnosed LQTS are vulnerable to additional prolongation of their QT interval from a variety of medications. The American Heart Association recommends monitoring of the QTc interval.[49]

Genetic Evidence

Several genes have been identified for LQTS 1-10, and the three most common are listed below.

All encode protein components of the cardiac ion channels, and modulate ionic flow. Sometimes these disorders are described as "channelopathies."[48]

- **LQTS1** is caused by a mutation in the *KCNQ1* gene (also known as the *KvLQT1* gene), which encodes a potassium channel protein active in phase 3 of the cardiac action potential (the I_{ks} current). It is seen in 35%-50% of LQTS cases.
- **LQTS2** is caused by a mutation in the *KCNH2* gene (also known as the *HERG* gene), which encodes a potassium channel protein that normally terminates the cardiac action potential (the I_{Kr} current). It is seen in 25%-30% of cases.
- **LQTS3** is caused by a mutation in the *SCN5A* gene, which encodes a sodium channel protein in phase 0 of the cardiac action potential (the NaV15 current). It is seen in 5%-10% of cases.

Gene-Environment Interactions

Gene environment interactions are significant for LQTS patients and vary by genotype and by individual[72,73]:

- LQTS1 have a higher incidence of ventricular dysrhythmias and SCD events during exercise, especially swimming (physical exertion trigger).
- LQST2 have a higher incidence of ventricular dysrhythmias and SCD events during sleep and are very sensitive to sudden loud noises that cause a startle reflex (auditory trigger).
- LQST3 have a higher incidence of ventricular dysrhythmias and SCD events during sleep and rest.

Inheritance

Both autosomal dominant and autosomal recessive patterns of inheritance occur. LQTS1, LQTS2, and LQTS3 all have an autosomal dominant pattern of inheritance.[74]

Not all individuals have the same phenotype even with the same genotype.[74] This is thought to be due to the influence of additional genes acting in concert with the primary gene to alter the cardiac action potential, to cause QTc prolongation.

Who Should Undergo Genetic Testing?

Clinical genetic testing is available for LQTS. Genetic testing is very helpful within families of patients with LQTS. If the family member has a prolonged QTc interval the reasonable assumption during the cardiac and genetic work-up is that they have the mutation. It is also important to test family members with a normal QTc interval, as up to 50% have "concealed" LQTS, meaning they have a positive genotype and negative phenotype (normal QTc on the resting ECG).[48] This is because of a genetic concept termed *penetrance*, where the same gene does not have the same phenotypic effect on everyone who is affected. If a person carries the genetic mutation, but has a normal QTc interval at rest, he or she may still be vulnerable during exercise or physiologic stress.

aware of their condition, and not all have a prolonged QTc at rest.[48] In the critical care unit these patients are at high risk of gene-environment or gene-medication interactions that can lengthen the QTc interval and entrain *polymorphic ventricular tachycardia,* also known as *torsades de pointes*[49]; see torsades de pointes in Chapter 14.

Cardiomyopathy

There is a very wide spectrum of cardiomyopathy genotypes and phenotypes. Some are single-gene disorders (inherited), and some are complex trait disorders with a strong environmental component where cardiomyopathy has resulted from ischemic or valvular heart disease (see cardiomyopathy in Chapter 15).

Hypertrophic Cardiomyopathy. Hypertrophic cardiomyopathy is the most frequently encountered inherited cardiomyopathy.[50] It is both genetically and phenotypically heterogeneous with documented mutations in more than 11 genes that encode for cardiac sarcomere proteins.[50] Most mutations are missense SNPs in which the normal nucleotide is replaced; this alters the resultant protein. The risk of sudden cardiac death (SCD) is high for patients who manifest the phenotype of a hypertrophied ventricle or hypertrophied ventricular septum. To identify other members of the family who may be affected, construction of a three-generation pedigree and genetic testing is recommened.[50]

Dilated Cardiomyopathy. Familial dilated cardiomyopathy is associated with mutations in more than 14 genes. The phenotype is left ventricular enlargement with systolic dysfunction with more than two affected family members.[51] In patients over 40 years of age a diagnosis of idiopathic dilated cardiomyopathy can be made based upon the phenotype when other structural causes have been ruled out. Genetic testing is rarely performed in older adults, although the falling costs of genomic sequencing may make this feasible in the future.[52]

Restrictive Cardiomyopathy. Familial restrictive cardiomyopathy is the least common inherited cardiomyopathy. The condition is usually not identified until the patient is symptomatic and the restrictive disease is at an advanced stage.[53]

Pharmacogenetics

Pharmacogenetics is the study of gene-medication interactions. Pharmacogenetics is likely to be the most visible impact of genetics encountered in the adult critical care unit in the immediate future, particularly in relation to the cytochrome P450 family of enzymes involved in medication metabolism.

Cytochrome P450 Family and Medication Metabolism

The cytochrome P450 (CYP450) enzymes are a superfamily of heme-containing enzymes that are vital for medication metabolism. The CYP450 family contains 57 genes that code for enzymes involved in medication metabolism.[54] The isoenzymes CYP3A4 and CYP3A5 metabolize about 50% of currently marketed medications, and they constitute approximately 60% of the total hepatic CYP450 enzyme content.[55] The metabolism of more than 90% of the most clinically important medications

can be accounted for by seven CYP isozymes: 3A4, 3A5, 1A2, 2C9, 2C19, 2D6, and 2E1.[55]

CYP3A4 can be used to understand what the abbreviations represent. *CYP* represents the symbol for all cytochrome P450 proteins, *3* denotes the gene family, *A* designates the subfamily, and *4* represents the individual gene.[55] The U.S. Food and Drug Administration (FDA) requires that new medications undergo testing for interactions with the CYP450 pathway before release.

Warfarin

Warfarin (Coumadin) is a frequently prescribed anticoagulant for patents with atrial fibrillation, mechanical cardiac valves, or thrombotic disorders. Variants in the cytochrome P450 enzyme *CYP2C9* gene and in the vitamin K epoxide reductase complex subunit 1 gene *(VKORC1)* contribute to the considerable dose variation seen with this anticoagulant.[56,57] The vitamin K epoxide reductase (VKOR) enzyme activates the vitamin K–dependent clotting factors (II, VII, IX, X). Warfarin is used to inhibit the VKOR complex to prevent clot formation.

Several prospective studies showed that up to 30% of dose variability during the initiation phase of warfarin anticoagulation could be explained by *CYP2C9* and *VKORC1* polymorphisms. Genetic testing is not currently recommended for everyone who takes warfarin. Laboratory tests to detect the *CYP2C9* and *VKORC1* variants are available only at specialized reference laboratories. The FDA has added a warning label on the package to alert clinicians about *CYP2C9* and *VKORC1* polymorphism interactions and their effects on warfarin dosing.[58]

Malignant Hyperthermia

Malignant hyperthermia is a rare inherited genetic disorder that negatively affects skeletal muscle upon exposure to volatile anesthetics and depolarizing muscle relaxants. It may be unexpectedly discovered during general anesthesia. In malignant hyperthermia, calcium is released from the muscle sarcoplasmic reticulum and induces life-threatening muscle contracture with skeletal muscle rigidity, acidosis, and elevated temperature. The first gene to be identified was the ryanodine receptor 1 gene *(RYR1)* associated with calcium release in the sarcoplasmic reticulum.[59-61] Malignant hyperthermia is described in more detail in Box 4-3.

GENETICS, GENOMICS, AND NURSING

As genetics and genomics exert more influence in clinical practice, it will have implications for the knowledge base of nurses and other professionals in health care. The learning curve may be steep. The addition of genetics also introduces new ethical and legal dilemmas into health care discussions. Genetics and genomics will have a big impact on how health and illness are conceptualized in the future. This is already required content for baccalaureate nursing education, and is now recommended for nurses with graduate degrees.[62] Essential competencies for nursing practice have been developed by the American Nurses Association (ANA), and examples are listed in Table 4-2.[63] It is

BOX 4-3 GENETIC CONDITIONS IN CRITICAL CARE: MALIGNANT HYPERTHERMIA

Clinical Presentation

Malignant hyperthermia (MH) is a pharmacogenetic syndrome. MH is a disorder of skeletal muscle calcium regulation. On exposure to volatile anesthetics and depolarizing muscle relaxants, susceptible patients experience life-threatening symptoms, including sustained muscle contracture with skeletal muscle rigidity, which causes metabolic acidosis, tachycardia, and fever. The symptoms result from an abnormally high release of intracellular calcium in skeletal muscle.

Genetic Evidence

Genetic linkage studies associated the MH phenotype with the ryanodine receptor 1 gene *(RYR1)* at chromosome 19q13.1 in several families. Calcium transport from muscle sarcoplasmic reticulum through the ryanodine receptor into the sarcoplasm occurs during muscular excitation and contraction. A biologic model also supported *RYR1* as a candidate gene. Other candidate genes exist, but none is as well characterized as the *RYR1* gene variants. The *RYR1* gene is highly polymorphic, with more than 170 variants in the gene, although not all are causative. Currently, 29 *RYR1* mutations are known to cause MH. Presence of any of these mutations is diagnostic for MH susceptibility. A genetic analysis exists to test for causative *RYR1* gene mutations.[60,61]

Another gene *(CACNAIS)* that encodes a receptor involved in muscle excitation-contraction has now been identified.[75]

Gene-Environment Interactions

MH is an example of a gene-environment interaction. It is not an allergy, and it occurs under the specific environmental condition of general anesthesia with inhalation anesthetics (e.g., chloroform, desflurane, enflurane, halothane, isoflurane, methoxyflurane, sevoflurane, trichloroethylene) and depolarizing muscle relaxants (e.g., succinylcholine).

Inheritance

MH is inherited in an autosomal dominant pattern. This means that only one affected allele is needed to have the condition, and that children of an affected person have a 50% chance of inheriting the mutated *RYR1* gene.

Who Should Undergo Genetic Testing?

MH crisis under general anesthesia is rare. The genetic test for *RYR1* is not recommended as a general screening test. Genetic testing is recommended only for people who have experienced an MH crisis, those who are first-degree relatives of a person with known MH, or individuals who have had a positive result from a muscle biopsy. The value of the genetic test is that when a mutation is discovered, family members with the same mutation are considered susceptible to MH and can avoid a diagnostic muscle biopsy. The major advantage of being aware of the diagnosis is that high-risk anesthetics can be avoided for general anesthesia in MH-susceptible individuals.[60,61]

Online Resources

European Malignant Hyperthermia Group: **http://www.emhg.org**

Malignant Hyperthermia Association of the United States:
   http://www.mhaus.org

Online Mendelian Inheritance in Man (OMIM), ryanodine receptor 1 gene *(RYR1)*: **http://omim.org/entry/180901**

---

always demanding to embrace a new model of health care delivery, and that is the challenge for all health care professionals in the coming decades. The tsunami of genetic information that is now flowing into research journals will rapidly make its way into clinical practice, including into critical care. This flood of new and relevant information will mandate that nurses understand genetic terms, incorporate genetic pedigree information into the history and physical examination, and be knowledgeable about pharmacogenetic interventions. Genetics and genomics constitute a complex area of study, made more so by the rapid evolution of scientific knowledge. One way to begin is to look at some of the free, internet-based, interactive educational tutorials listed in Box 4-4 and to become familiar with the genetic and genomic vocabulary in the key terms list at the end of the chapter.

Ethical and Legal Issues in Genetics and Genomics

One of the paramount concerns in the genomic era is to protect the privacy of individuals' unique genetic information. Many countries have established biobanks as repositories of genetic material, and many tissue samples are stored in medical center tissue banks. Because all of the individual's genome is contained within the cell, genomic identity or susceptibility to diseases can easily be determined from a small sample. It is essential to ensure that ethical and legal protections keep pace with technical innovation. Key issues are who *owns* the genetic material and *consent* as to who has access to the genetic information. Debate about these issues is expected to continue as new advances push the technical limits of what can be discovered from a few drops of blood, a muscle biopsy sample, or a cheek swab.

Direct-to-Consumer Tests

A new frontier in genomics testing is the ability of any individual to voluntarily undergo genetic testing. Several private companies advertise this service on the internet. Patients send a sample of their DNA, usually a swab from the inside of the cheek (buccal swab), to check for selected genetic risks. Other websites offer paternity testing from buccal swabs of the child and father. Many countries are now enacting laws to ensure individuals' genomic information is protected. Genetic counselors caution that the results may be hard to understand or misleading for some individuals but clearly this is of great interest to many people.[64]

The Genetic Information Nondiscrimination Act

The Genetic Information Nondiscrimination Act (GINA) of 2008 is an essential piece of legislation designed to prevent abuse of genetic information in employment and health insurance decisions in the United States.[65] The purpose of GINA is to protect individuals who may have the gene for a disorder—but do not manifest the phenotype—from being penalized. Some people who may be at risk for a disorder disease will not be tested because they fear that a positive result may affect their employability. GINA also mandates that genetic information about individuals and their families has the same protections as health information. It is important that clinicians understand

TABLE 4-2 ESSENTIAL GENETICS AND GENOMICS COMPETENCIES FOR NURSES

DOMAIN	COMPETENCIES OF THE REGISTERED NURSE
Professional Responsibilities	
Competent nursing incorporating genetic and genomic knowledge and skills	Recognizes when one's own attitudes and values related to genetic and genomic science may affect care provided to patients
	Advocates for patients' access to desired genetic or genomic services and resources, including support groups
	Examines competency of practice on a regular basis, identifying areas of strength and areas in which professional development related to genetics and genomics would be beneficial
	Incorporates genetic and genomic technologies and information into registered nurse practice
	Demonstrates in practice the importance of tailoring genetic and genomic information and services to patients based on their culture, religion, knowledge level, literacy, and preferred language
	Advocates for the rights of all patients for autonomous, informed genetic and genomic related decision making and voluntary action
Professional Practice and Assessment	
Application and integration of knowledge	Demonstrates an understanding of the relationship of genetics or genomics to health, prevention, screening, diagnostics, prognostics, selection of treatment, and monitoring of treatment effectiveness
	Demonstrates an ability to elicit a minimum of three generations of family health history information
	Constructs a pedigree from collected family history information using standardized symbols and terminology
	Collects personal, health, and developmental histories that consider genetic, environmental, and genomic influences and risks
	Conducts comprehensive health and physical assessments that incorporate knowledge about genetic, environmental, and genomic influences and risk factors
	Critically analyzes the history and physical assessment findings for genetic, environmental, and genomic influences and risk factors
	Assesses patients' knowledge, perceptions, and responses to genetic and genomic information
	Develops plan of care that incorporates genetic and genomic assessment information
Identification of needed information	Identifies patients who may benefit from specific genetic and genomic information or services based on assessment data
	Identifies credible, accurate, appropriate, and current genetic and genomic information, resources, services, and technologies specific to given patients
	Identifies ethical, ethnic or ancestral, cultural, religious, legal, fiscal, and societal issues related to genetic and genomic information and technologies
	Defines issues that undermine the rights of all patients for autonomous, informed genetic and genomic-related decision making and voluntary action
Assistance with referrals	Facilitates referrals for specialized genetic and genomic services for patients, as needed
Provision of education, care, and support	Provides patients with interpretation of selective genetic and genomic information or services
	Provides patients with credible, accurate, appropriate, and current genetic and genomic information, resources, services, and technologies that facilitate decision making
	Uses health promotion and disease prevention practices that consider genetic and genomic influences on risk with personal and environmental risk factors
	Incorporates knowledge of genetic or genomic risk factors (e.g., patient with a genetic predisposition for high cholesterol levels that can benefit from a change in lifestyle to decrease the likelihood that the genotype will be expressed)
	Uses genetic and genomic based interventions and information to improve patients' outcomes
	Collaborates with health care providers in providing genetic and genomic health care
	Collaborates with insurance providers or payers to facilitate reimbursement for genetic and genomic health care services
	Performs interventions and treatments appropriate to patients' genetic and genomic health care needs
	Evaluates impact and effectiveness of genetic and genomic technology, information, interventions, and treatments on patients' outcome

From Consensus Panel on Genetic/Genomic Nursing Competencies. *Essentials of Genetic and Genomic Nursing: Competencies, Curricula Guidelines, and Outcome Indicators.* 3rd ed. Silver Spring, MD: American Nurses Association; 2009.

BOX 4-4   INTERNET RESOURCES

Genomic Databases and Reference
- GeneReviews, University of Washington, Seattle, WA:
  http://www.genetests.org/
- Online Mendelian Inheritance in Man (OMIM), Johns Hopkins University:
  http://www.ncbi.nlm.nih.gov/omim/
- Genome-wide association studies (GWAS) catalog maintained by NHGRI:
  http://www.genome.gov/gwastudies/
- The Cancer Genome Atlas (TCGA): **http://cancergenome.nih.gov/**
- The International HapMap Project: **http://www.hapmap.org/**
- The 1000 Genomes Project: **http://www.1000genomes.org/**
- Encyclopedia of DNA Elements (ENCODE):
  http://genome.ucsc.edu/ENCODE/
- Personal Genome Project: **http://www.personalgenomes.org**

Organizations
- International Society of Nurses in Genetics (ISONG):
  http://www.isong.org/
- National Coalition of Health Professional Education in Genetics (NCHPEG):
  http://www.nchpeg.org/

Tutorials and Education
- Learn Genetics, The University of Utah:
  http://gslc.genetics.utah.edu/
- Educational materials about genetics and genomics from the NHGRI:
  http://www.genome.gov/Education/
- Current Topics in Genome Analysis 2012, NHGRI:
  http://www.genome.gov/12514288
- DNA Learning Center, Cold Spring Harbor Laboratory:
  http://www.dnalc.org/home.html

NHGRI, National Human Genome Resource Institute.

---

that the GINA legislation does not cover all categories of insurance. It offers no protection against discrimination for life insurance, disability insurance, or long-term care insurance. The GINA legislation does not cover members of the military, the Veteran's Affairs Service, or Indian Health Service.[66,67]

HUMAN GENETICS KEY TERMS

Allele: one of several alternative gene variants that can exist at a single locus (location) on a chromosome. The term *allele* may also be used when referring to SNP variants. The most frequently found allele in a population is called the *wild-type allele.*

Candidate gene: a gene that is believed to cause or contribute to a disease. This term is typically used when the gene will be included in a research study.

Chromosomes: structures made of DNA and proteins and located in the nuclei of cells. Chromosomes come in pairs, and a normal human cell contains 46 chromosomes: 22 pairs of autosomes and a pair of sex chromosomes. Chromosomes are composed of genes, regulatory sequences, and non-coding DNA segments.

Codon: three-sequence nucleotide bases that code for an amino acid.

DNA: deoxyribonucleic acid is made up of four nucleotide bases: adenine (A), guanine (G), cytosine (C), and thymine (T). DNA is heritable genetic information that resides in chromosomes inside each cell nucleus.

Epigenetic: chemical modifications of DNA that can turn genes on or off without altering the DNA sequence. Epigenetic changes are not heritable.

Gene: a unit of inheritance; a working subunit of DNA. Each of the 20,000 to 25,000 genes in the body contains the code for a specific product, typically a protein such as an enzyme, and other specific tissue cells.

Gene expression: the process by which the coded information of a gene is translated into the structures present and operating in the cell (proteins or ribonucleic acid [RNA]).

Gene map: a description of the relative positions of genes on a chromosome and the distance between them.

Genetic linkage maps: DNA maps that assign relative chromosomal locations to genetic locations—either genes for known traits or distinctive sequences of DNA on the basis of how frequently they are inherited together.

Genetics: the scientific study of heredity, which is how particular qualities or traits are transmitted from parents to offspring. Traditionally, the focus has been on individual genes and their impact on uncommon single-gene disorders. Today the study of genetics also involves multi-gene disorders and gene-environment interactions.

Genomics: the expansive study of all the genes in the human genome, including gene-gene interactions, gene interactions with the environment, and the influence of other psychosocial and cultural factors.

Genotype: the genetic code sequence carried by an individual.

Haplotype: closely linked loci on a chromosome. Haplotype blocks denote chromosomal regions where SNPs are in strong linkage disequilibrium, and they are mapped in the HapMap Project database.

HapMap Project: a map of haplotype blocks that researchers use when searching for candidate genes. Haplotypes are cataloged according to racial and ethnic group in the HapMap database.

Heterozygous: possessing two different sequences (alleles) of a particular gene, with one inherited from each parent.

Homozygous: possessing two identical sequences of a particular gene, with one inherited from each parent.

Linkage: the association of genes or markers that lie very near each other on a chromosome. Linked genes and markers tend to be inherited together.

Linkage analysis: a gene-mapping technique that finds patterns of heredity in large, high-risk families to locate a disease-causing gene mutation by identifying traits that are co-inherited with the gene.

Linkage disequilibrium (LD): the nonrandom association between alleles at different loci. These alleles at loci occur together on the same section of a chromosome more often than would be predicted by chance alone. This technique has been used to determine which genes are linked and therefore inherited together.

Locus and loci: the place on a chromosome where a specific gene is located, similar in concept to a street address for the gene. The singular term is locus, and the plural is loci.

Mendelian diseases: single-gene disorders that appear in families in dominant or recessive inheritance patterns.

Mutation: a change, deletion, or rearrangement in an individual's DNA sequence that may lead to the synthesis of an altered protein or the inability to produce the protein. The term *mutation* is used when the variant occurs in less than 1% of the population.

Nucleotide: a building block of DNA or RNA that consists of one nitrogenous base, one phosphate molecule, and one glucose molecule.

Pedigree: a graphic multigenerational family health history that uses standardized symbols.

Pharmacogenomics: the study of genetically determined responses to medications, genetic variation in medication metabolizing enzymes, and consequent alteration in medication effectiveness across the genome.

Phenotype: the observable manifestation of a genetic trait that results from a specific genotype or gene-environment interaction. These are physical characteristics such as the signs and symptoms associated with a disease.

Polymorphism: a common variation in the sequence of DNA that occurs in more than 1% of the population. The most frequent sequence is referred to as the *wild type*, and less common variants are called *polymorphisms*.

Proband: the first person diagnosed with a condition in a family pedigree. An arrow in the family pedigree identifies the proband.

Single-nucleotide polymorphism (SNP): a change in the DNA nucleotide sequence caused by replacement of a single-nucleotide base. If the change of nucleotide results in a different protein product, it is called a *non-synonymous SNP*. If the protein product is not changed, it is called a *synonymous SNP*.

Somatic cells: all body cells, except the reproductive cells.

Transcription: the process used by DNA to code for messenger RNA.

Translation: the process used by RNA to code for a protein.

SUMMARY

- DNA is arranged inside the nucleus of the cell. DNA resembles a ladder with two long strands twisted around each other to form a double-stranded helix. The rungs of the ladder are made up of nucleotide base pairs. There are 20,000 to 25,000 genes in the human genome.
- Several conditions seen in critical care have a genetic component, including factor V Leiden thrombosis, hemophilia A, LQTS, and cardiomyopathy. Pharmacogenetic syndromes represent medication-gene interactions; examples include malignant hyperthermia owing to *RYR1* polymorphisms, and warfarin dosage affected by *CYP2C9* and *VKORC1* polymorphisms.
- The GINA legislation is designed to prevent the use of an individual's genetic risk profile in employment and insurance decisions in the United States.
- Genetic and genomic competency is recommended for all registered nurses.

REFERENCES

1. Salari K, Watkins H, Ashley EA. Personalized medicine: hope or hype? *European Heart Journal*. 2012;33(13):1564-1570.
2. Rare Diseases Act of 2002. Public Law 107–280—NOV.6, 2002. http://history.nih.gov/research/downloads/PL107-280.pdf Accessed August 1, 2012.
3. International Human Genome Sequencing Consortium. Finishing the euchromatic sequence of the human genome. *Nature*. 2004;431(7011):931-945.
4. Damani SB, Topol EJ. Emerging genomic applications in coronary artery disease. *JACC: Cardiovascular interventions*. 2011;4(5):473-482.
5. Baccarelli A, Ghosh S. Environmental exposures, epigenetics and cardiovascular disease. *Current Opinion in Clinical Nutrition and Metabolic Care*. 2012;15(4):323-329.
6. Ashley EA, Butte AJ, Wheeler MT, et al. Clinical assessment incorporating a personal genome. *Lancet*. 2010;375(9725):1525-1535.
7. Madian AG, Wheeler HE, Jones RB, Dolan ME. Relating human genetic variation to variation in drug responses. *Trends in Genetics*. 2012; EPub ahead of print.
8. Odell ID, Wallace SS, Pederson DS. Rules of engagement for base excision repair in chromatin. *Journal of Cellular Physiology*. 2012; EPub ahead of print.
9. Feero WG, Guttmacher AE, Collins FS. Genomic medicine–an updated primer. *The New England Journal of Medicine*. 2010;362(21):2001-2011.
10. Cold Spring Harbor Laboratory. DNA from the Beginning. 2012. http://www.dnaftb.org/dnaftb/. Accessed August 1, 2012.
11. Radich JP. Measuring response to BCR-ABL inhibitors in chronic myeloid leukemia. *Cancer*. 2012;118(2):300-311.
12. Kujovich JL. Factor V Leiden thrombophilia. *Genetics in Medicine*. 2011;13(1):1-16.
13. Verghese PB, Castellano JM, Holtzman DM. Apolipoprotein E in Alzheimer's disease and other neurological disorders. *Lancet Neurology*. 2011;10(3):241-252.
14. Schapira AH. Mitochondrial diseases. *Lancet*. 2012;379(9828):1825-1834.
15. Bennett RL, French KS, Resta RG, Doyle DL. Standardized human pedigree nomenclature: update and assessment of the recommendations of the National Society of Genetic Counselors. *Journal of Genetic Counseling*. 2008;17(5):424-433.

16. Jayandharan GR, Srivastava A. Role of molecular genetics in hemophilia: from diagnosis to therapy. *Seminars in Thrombosis and Hemostasis.* 2012;38(1):64-78.

17. Frayling TM, et al. A common variant in the FTO gene is associated with body mass index and predisposes to childhood and adult obesity. *Science.* 2007;316(5826):889-894.

18. Razquin C, Marti A, Martinez JA. Evidences on three relevant obesogenes: MC4R, FTO and PPARgamma. Approaches for personalized nutrition. *Molecular Nutrition & Food Research.* 2011;35(1):136-149.

19. Wojczynski MK, Tiwari HK. Definition of phenotype. *Adv Genet.* 2008;60:75-105.

20. Wellcome Trust Case Control Consortium. Genome-wide association study of 14,000 cases of seven common diseases and 3,000 shared controls. *Nature.* 2007;447(7145):661-678.

21. Hindorff LA, et al. A Catalog of Published Genome-Wide Association Studies. 2012. http://www.genome.gov/gwastudies. Accessed August 1, 2012.

22. Collins A, Tapper WJ. Genome variation: a review of Web resources. *Methods in molecular biology.* 2011;713:129-139.

23. The ENCODE Project Consortium. Identification and analysis of functional elements in 1% of the human genome by the ENCODE pilot project. *Nature.* 2007;447(7146):799-816.

24. The ENCODE Project Consortium. An integrated encyclopedia of DNA elements in the human genome. *Nature.* 2012; 489(7414):57-74.

25. International HapMap Project. http://www.hapmap.org. Accessed August 1, 2012.

26. The International HapMap Consortium. A second generation human haplotype map of over 3.1 million SNPs. *Nature.* 2007;449(7164):851-861.

27. Personal Genome Project. 2012; http://www.personalgenomes.org/. Accessed August 1, 2012.

28. Ball MP, et al. A public resource facilitating clinical use of genomes. *Proceedings of the National Academy of Sciences of the United States of America.* 2012;109(30):11920-11927.

29. Grice EA, Segre JA. The human microbiome: our second genome. *Annual Review of Genomics and Human Genetics.* 2012;13:1151-1170.

30. A framework for human microbiome research. *Nature.* 2012;486(7402):215-221.

31. Segata N, et al. Composition of the adult digestive tract bacterial microbiome based on seven mouth surfaces, tonsils, throat and stool samples. *Genome Biology.* 2012;13(6):R42.

32. Campbell MC, Tishkoff SA. African genetic diversity: implications for human demographic history, modern human origins, and complex disease mapping. *Annu Rev Genomics Hum Genet.* 2008;9:403-433.

33. Tishkoff SA, et al. The genetic structure and history of Africans and African Americans. *Science.* 2009;324(5930):1035-1044.

34. The Wellcome Trust Case Control Consortium. Genome-wide association study of copy number variation in 16,000 cases of eight common diseases and 3,000 shared controls. *Nature.* 2010;464(7289):713-720.

35. Pankratz N, et al. Copy number variation in familial Parkinson disease. *PLoS One.* 2011;6(8):e20988.

36. Grozeva D, et al. Independent estimation of the frequency of rare CNVs in the UK population confirms their role in schizophrenia. *Schizophrenia Research.* 2012;135(1-3):1-7.

37. Kirov G, et al. De novo CNV analysis implicates specific abnormalities of postsynaptic signalling complexes in the pathogenesis of schizophrenia. *Molecular Psychiatry.* 2012;17(2):142-153.

38. Johansson AC, Feuk L. Characterizing and interpreting genetic variation from personal genome sequencing. *Methods in Molecular Biology.* 2012;838:343-367.

39. Robson ME, et al. American Society of Clinical Oncology policy statement update: genetic and genomic testing for cancer susceptibility. *Journal of Clinical Oncology.* 28(5):893-901.

40. Ashley EA, et al. Genetics and Cardiovascular Disease: A Policy Statement From the American Heart Association. *Circulation.* 2012;126(1):142-157.

41. The Cancer Genome Atlas. 2012. http://cancergenome.nih.gov. Accessed August 1, 2012.

42. The Cancer Genome Atlas Research Network. Integrated genomic analyses of ovarian carcinoma. *Nature.* 2011;474(7353):609-615.

43. The Cancer Genome Atlas Research Network. Comprehensive genomic characterization defines human glioblastoma genes and core pathways. *Nature.* 2008;455(7216):1061-1068.

44. The Cancer Genome Atlas Network. Comprehensive molecular characterization of human colon and rectal cancer. *Nature.* 2012;487(7407):330-337.

45. O'Donnell CJ, Nabel EG. Genomics of cardiovascular disease. *The New England Journal of Medicine.* 2011;365(22):2098-2109.

46. Framingham Heart Study. http://www.framinghamheartstudy.org/. Accessed August 1, 2012.

47. Govindaraju DR, et al. Genetics of the Framingham Heart Study population. *Advances in Genetics.* 2008;62:33-65.

48. Goldenberg I, Moss AJ. Long QT syndrome. *Journal of the American College of Cardiology.* 2008;51(24):2291-2300.

49. Drew BJ, et al. Prevention of torsade de pointes in hospital settings: a scientific statement from the American Heart Association and the American College of Cardiology Foundation. *Circulation.* 2010;121(8):1047-1060.

50. Maron BJ, Maron MS, Semsarian C. Genetics of hypertrophic cardiomyopathy after 20 years: clinical perspectives. *Journal of the American College of Cardiology.* 2012;60(8):705-715.

51. Hershberger RE, Morales A, Siegfried JD. Clinical and genetic issues in dilated cardiomyopathy: a review for genetics professionals. *Genetics in Medicine.* 2010;12(11):655-667.

52. Hershberger RE, Siegfried JD. Update 2011: clinical and genetic issues in familial dilated cardiomyopathy. *Journal of the American College of Cardiology.* 2011;57(16):1641-1649.

53. Daneshvar DA, Kedia G, Fishbein MC, Siegel RJ. Familial restrictive cardiomyopathy with 12 affected family members. *The American Journal of Cardiology.* 2012;109(3):445-447.

54. Zhou SF, Liu JP, Chowbay B. Polymorphism of human cytochrome P450 enzymes and its clinical impact. *Drug Metabolism Reviews.* 2009;41(2):89-295.

55. Mann HJ. Drug-associated disease: cytochrome P450 interactions. *Crit Care Clin.* 2006;22(2):329-345, vii.

56. Cooper GM, et al. A genome-wide scan for common genetic variants with a large influence on warfarin maintenance dose. *Blood.* 2008;112(4):1022-1027.

57. Rieder MJ, et al. Effect of *VKORC1* haplotypes on transcriptional regulation and warfarin dose. *N Engl J Med.* 2005;352(22):2285-2293.

58. Schwarz UI, et al. Genetic determinants of response to warfarin during initial anticoagulation. *N Engl J Med.* 2008;358(10):999-1008.

59. Hirshey Dirksen SJ, et al. Special article: Future directions in malignant hyperthermia research and patient care. *Anesthesia and Analgesia.* 2011;113(5):1108-1119.

60. Girard T, Litman RS. Molecular genetic testing to diagnose malignant hyperthermia susceptibility. *J Clin Anesth.* 2008;20(3):161-163.

61. Robinson R, et al. Mutations in *RYR1* in malignant hyperthermia and central core disease. *Hum Mutat.* 2006;27(10):977-989.

62. Greco KE, Tinley S, Seibert D. *Essential genetic and genomic competencies for nurses with graduate degrees.* Silver Spring, MD: American Nurses Association and International Society of Nurses in Genetics; 2011.

63. Jenkins J, American Nurses Association. *Essentials of Genetic and Genomic Nursing Competencies, Curricula Guidelines and Outcome indicators (2nd Edition).* 2nd ed. Silver Spring, MD: American Nurses Association; 2009.

64. McBride CM, Wade CH, Kaphingst KA. Consumers' views of direct-to-consumer genetic information. *Annual Review of Genomics and Human Genetics.* 2010;11:427-446.

65. Health law—genetics—Congress restricts use of genetic information by insurers and employers.—Genetic Information Nondiscrimination Act of 2008, Pub. L. No. 110-233, 122 Stat. 881 (to be codified in scattered sections of 26, 29, and 42 U.S.C.). *Harvard Law Review.* 2009;122(3):1038-1045.

66. Steck MB, Eggert JA. The need to be aware and beware of the genetic information nondiscrimination act. *Clinical Journal of Oncology Nursing.* 2011;15(3):E34-41.

67. Laedtke AL, O'Neill SM, Rubinstein WS, Vogel KJ. Family physicians' awareness and knowledge of the Genetic Information Non-Discrimination Act (GINA). *Journal of Genetic Counseling.* 2012;21(2):345-352.

68. Bezemer ID, et al. Gene variants associated with deep vein thrombosis. *JAMA.* 2008;299(11):1306-1314.

69. Evaluation of Genomic Applications in Practice and Prevention (EGAPP) Working Group. Recommendations from the EGAPP Working Group: routine testing for Factor V Leiden (R506Q) and prothrombin (20210G>A) mutations in adults with a history of idiopathic venous thromboembolism and their adult family members. *Genetics in Medicine.* 2011;13(1):67-76.

70. Collins KK, Van Hare GF. Advances in congenital long QT syndrome. *Current Opinion in Pediatrics.* 2006;18(5):497-502.

71. Goldenberg I, et al. Beta-blocker efficacy in high-risk patients with the congenital long-QT syndrome types 1 and 2: implications for patient management. *Journal of Cardiovascular Electrophysiology.* 2010;21(8):893-901.

72. Sauer AJ, et al. Long QT syndrome in adults. *Journal of the American College of Cardiology.* 2007;49(3):329-337.

73. Schwartz PJ. The congenital long QT syndromes from genotype to phenotype: clinical implications. *Journal of Internal Medicine.* 2006;259(1):39-47.

74. Nannenberg EA, et al. Mortality of inherited arrhythmia syndromes: insight into their natural history. *Circulation: Cardiovascular Genetics.* 2012;5(2):183-189.

75. Carpenter D, et al. The role of *CACNA1S* in predisposition to malignant hyperthermia. *BMC Medical Genetics.* 2009;10:104.

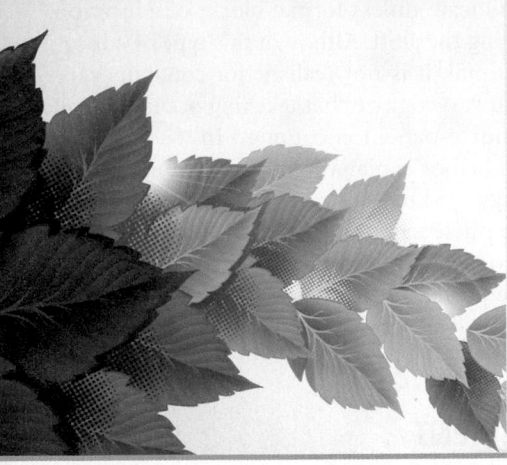

Patient and Family Education

Barbara Mayer

evolve WEBSITE

http://evolve.elsevier.com/Urden/criticalcare/

Evolve features:
- NCLEX Review Questions
- CCRN Review Questions
- PCCN Review Questions
- Mosby's Nursing Skills Procedures
- Animations
- Video Clips
- Glossary

CHALLENGES OF PATIENT AND FAMILY EDUCATION

At no other point in history has the availability of information within the general population been so great. Televisions are practically in every home, computers with wireless access to the Internet are available for use anywhere at any time, and cell phones are clipped to the waistbands of the young and old. It seems as if this century's population of adults cannot tolerate a lack of information. The ease of access to the world's library of information meets a compulsive need to satisfy a desire for immediate gratification. Gathering information in bits and pieces from various sources allows people to collect information at their own pace and to gather as much or as little information as they desire. These "knowledge bites" are sorted and stored on an individual's "cerebral hard drive." The "file" is retrieved and "opened" whenever the situation warrants.

When alterations in health arise in daily life, people use all available resources to discover information to help them cope and adapt to the new experience. This type of consumerism has developed a populace that is more educated in health matters than ever before. It is our duty as health professionals to assist patients and families with information gathering and self-care management skills so they can lead lives of the best quality possible. According to The Joint Commission, patients must receive "sufficient information to make decisions and to take responsibility for self-management activities related to their needs."[1] The goals of patient and family education are to improve health outcomes by promoting healthy behavior and involvement in care and care decisions.[1]

Admission to a critical care unit usually is an unexpected event in anyone's life. The seriousness of the situation and unfamiliarity of the hospital or unit environment evokes a stress response in patients and their families. Nursing care is focused on improving the patient's physiologic stability and promoting end-organ tissue perfusion. Promoting the most basic human physiologic survival need for cellular oxygenation is the priority. Alterations in normal functioning related to disease-process progression, sedation, assist devices, or mechanical ventilation contribute to the possibility of mental alterations in the patient. Sleep deprivation and sensory overload add to the complexity of the issues that affect the patient's ability to receive and understand medical information. Mental alterations may limit the effectiveness of the teaching-learning encounter. These physical and cognitive limitations prevent patients from receiving or understanding information related to their care and impair their ability to make an informed decision.[2] At these times, critical life-or-death care decisions are transferred to a proxy, usually an immediate family member. The designated proxy has the responsibility to make informed treatment decisions for the patient. These types of situations present the nurse with special challenges in the education of patients and families.

Critical illness disrupts the normal patterns of daily life. Stress and crisis can develop within the family unit and stretch its members' coping resources.[3] These many emotional factors build barriers to the teaching-learning process and can become frustrating for the learner and the nurse. Amid the chaos, how do bedside nurses effectively provide patient and family education that can optimize outcomes and deliver quality, cost-effective care? It is the nurse's responsibility to educate himself or herself about concepts that provide insight into the framework for patient and family education. Adult educational concepts such as adult learning principles, types of educational needs, barriers to learning, stress and coping strategies, and evidence-based interventions must be used to develop an individualized education plan to meet the identified learning needs of the patient and family.

EDUCATION

Definition

Patient education is a process that includes the purposeful delivery of health-related information to promote changes in behavior that will optimize health practices and assist the individual in attaining new skills for living.[4,5] This concept can be overwhelming in the fast-paced, technology-rich setting of the critical care environment. The bedside nurse must incorporate the abundant educational needs of the patient or family into the education plan and be aware of the requirements of regulatory agencies and the legalities of documenting the teaching-learning encounter.

Benefits

Studies have documented that quality education shortens hospital length of stay, reduces readmission rates, and improves self-care management skills.[4-6] Complications associated with the physiologic stress response may be prevented if the patient or family perceives the education encounter as positive. Positive encounters decrease the stress response, relieve anxiety, promote individual growth and development, and increase patient and family satisfaction.[4-6] The following are examples of positive outcomes associated with a structured teaching-learning process.[7,8]

- Clarification of patients' understanding and perceptions of their chronic illness and care decisions
- Improved health outcomes relative to self-management techniques, such as symptom management
- Promotion of informed decision making and control over the situation
- Diminished emotional stress associated with an unfamiliar environment and unknown prognosis
- Improved adaptation to stressful situations
- Improved satisfaction with the care received
- Improved relationship with the health care team
- Promotion of self-concept

The Education Process

The education process follows the same framework as the nursing process: assessment, diagnosis, goals or outcomes, interventions, and evaluation.[4] Although this chapter discusses these steps individually, in practice, they may occur simultaneously and repetitively. The teaching-learning process is a dynamic, continuous activity that occurs throughout the entire hospitalization and may continue after the patient has been discharged. This process is often envisioned by the nurse as a time-consuming task that requires knowledge and skills to accomplish. Whereas knowledge and skills can be obtained,

time in the critical care unit is a scarce commodity. Many nurses believe they cannot educate unless formal blocks of education time are planned during the shift. Although this type of education encounter is optimal, it is not realistic for contemporary nursing. The nurse must recognize that teaching occurs during every moment of a nurse-patient encounter.[9] Instructions for how to use to the call bell or explanations of events and sensations to expect during a bed bath can be considered an education session. It is the nurse's role to recognize that education, no matter how brief or extensive, affects the daily lives of each person with whom he or she comes in contact. By following the nursing process, the physical assessment and education assessment can occur simultaneously.

STEP 1: ASSESSMENT

According to The Joint Commission, education provided should be appropriate to the patient's condition and should address the patient's identified learning needs.[1] The assessment is an important first step to providing need-targeted patient and family education. It begins on admission and continues until the patient is discharged. A formal, comprehensive, initial education assessment produces valuable information; however, it can take the nurse hours to complete. The nurse must focus the initial and subsequent education assessments on identifying gaps in knowledge related to the patient's current health-altering situation.

Learning needs can be defined as gaps between what the learner knows and what the learner needs to know, such as survival skills, coping skills, and ability to make a care decision. Identification of actual and perceived learning needs directs the health care team to provide need-targeted education. Need-targeted or need-to-know education is directed at helping the learner to become familiar with the current situation. Educational needs of the patient and family can be categorized as 1) information only (environment, visitation hours, get questions answered); 2) informed decision making (treatment plan, informed consent); or 3) self-management (recognition of problems and how to respond).[5,10] Patient education to be included in the education plan should address the plan of care, health practices and safety, safe and effective use of medications, nutrition interventions, safe and effective use of medical equipment or supplies, pain, and habilitation or rehabilitation needs.[1]

Learning needs may change from day to day, shift to shift, or minute to minute. Educational needs are influenced by how the patient or the family perceives or interprets the critical illness.[11] Perceptions of experiences vary from person to person, even if two people are involved in the same event. This intense internal feeling affects the desire to learn and understanding of the current situation. Satisfaction with the learning encounter is often judged to be positive if the nurse meets the expected learning needs of the patient and family. Congruency between nurse-identified needs and patient-identified needs brings about more positive learning experiences and encourages the learner to seek further information. The nurse must actively listen, maintain eye contact, seek clarification, and pay attention to verbal and nonverbal cues from the patient and the family to gather relevant information concerning perceived learning needs. The nurse should seek to first understand the learning need from the patient's point of view and then seek to be understood.

Strategic questioning provides an avenue for the nurse to determine whether the patient or family has any misconceptions about the environment, their illness, self-management skills, or the medication schedule. Health care providers use the term *noncompliant* to describe a patient or family members who do not modify behaviors to the meet the demands of the prescribed treatment regimen, such as following the rules of a low-fat diet or medication dosing. However, the problem behind noncompliance may not be a conscious desire to defy the treatment plan but instead be a misunderstanding of the importance of the medication or how to take the medication. The technique of asking open-ended questions ("Can you tell me what you know about your medication?") can elicit more information about the patient's knowledge base than asking closed-ended questions ("You know this is your water pill, right?"). Open-ended questions provide the nurse an opportunity to assess actual knowledge gaps rather than assume knowledge by obtaining a yes-or-no response. These types of questions also assist the patient and family to tell their story of the illness and communicate their perceptions of the experience,[5] allowing the adult learner to feel respected and involved in the treatment process. Questions that elicit a yes-or-no response close off communication and do not provide an interactive teaching-learning session. Box 5-1 contains sample questions the nurse can use in an assessment to obtain needed information. Generally, with practice and effort, it can be determined what educational information is needed in a brief period without much disruption in the routine care of the patient. Patients and families are multidimensional. Even with good questioning skills, the nurse cannot assess many aspects of the learner during the initial contact or even during the hospital stay.

BOX 5-1 ASSESSMENT QUESTIONS

- Why have you come to the hospital today?
- What problem are you having?
- How can we help you today?
- When did these problems start?
- Have you had these problems before?
- Have you been hospitalized for these problems before?
- Who is your doctor for this problem? Who is your family doctor?
- What medications are you taking?
- Can you tell me why you take each medication?
- How do you care for yourself at home? Do you have help?
- Are any family or friends with you today?
- Are these people your main support system?
- Are there any special needs, religious or otherwise, that we need to be aware of while you are in the hospital?
- What is your goal for coming to the hospital today?
- How can we help you reach this goal?
- Is there any information that I can give you right now that would help you understand more about why you are here or about your plan of care?
- What information have you received from other members of the health care team today?

Learner Identification

Identifying learner characteristics benefits the nurse and results in optimal communication and the patient's understanding of information. Certain factors can affect the education process. Culture or ethnicity, age, and adult learning principles influence the manner in which information is presented and concepts are understood.[5,12]

Family

A family can be defined as a group of individuals who are bonded by biologic, legal, and social relationships.[3] The modern family is diverse in ethnic backgrounds, sexual orientation, age, gender, work experience, physical or mental challenges, communication skills, educational backgrounds, work experience, geographic location, lived experiences, and religious beliefs.[13-15] A picture of the modern family would resemble that of a large patchwork quilt. Patches of different sizes, ethnicities, religions, cultures, attitudes, stages of development, and lived experiences would overlap and occupy their own individual spaces within the quilt framework. Bedside practitioners are expected to provide culturally competent care to each individual in the critical care setting. Culturally competent care is the delivery of sensitive, meaningful care to patients and families from diverse backgrounds.[15] This implies that the practitioner must value diversity and become knowledgeable concerning the cultural strengths and abilities of those for whom they care.[16] Communication and understanding impact the education process. Provision of language-appropriate literature and translation services and recognition of cultural or religious differences in the perception of illness and treatment influence the education encounter.[15]

Age-Specific Considerations

The critical care patient population differs culturally and by age and stages of human development. Older adult patients may have more difficulty reading patient educational materials or the label on the bottle of prescription medication than younger adults. Printed materials with larger fonts may be needed for these patients. Older adults were not exposed to technology during their youth and may find it difficult to navigate the fragmented maze of modern health care. Because of advanced age, this population of adults may have prescriptions for multiple drug therapies. Education to prevent adverse drug reactions may be required because of the prevalence of multiple drug therapies.[17] Older adults may also be coping with end-of-life issues and are in need of information to make informed decisions. Young adults may struggle with the issue of how to incorporate intimacy into their lives without feeling isolated from the mainstream social scene. The need for privacy and peer support may be required to assist the young adult in coping with the current situation. The practitioner must recognize these age-specific issues and incorporate them into the education plan.[1]

Adult Learners

Adults learn in large part through lived experiences. The motivation to learn is internal and problem-oriented, focusing on life events. Malcolm Knowles described these principles of adult learning in a model known as *andragogy*. Adult learning theory stresses concepts of individualism, self-assessment, self-direction, motivation, experience, and autonomy. Adults tend to have a strong sense of self-concept, are goal-oriented learners, and like to make their own decisions.[18] They take responsibility and accountability for their own learning and want to be respected as individuals, as well as recognized for accomplished life experiences. Adults have individualized learning styles and often lack confidence in their ability to learn. Education is resisted when the information given is perceived to be in conflict with the individual's self-image.

The learning process generally involves altering some part of current behavior to produce changes in lifestyle, incorporating the new or chronic illness into daily living. Coping mechanisms such as anger, disbelief, and denial affect the willingness of the patient or family to learn. The unwillingness to change behavior to manage health needs adds to the complexity of the critical care teaching-learning encounter. The nurse must provide need-to-know information in easy, understandable terms and in short bursts. Positive feedback and repetition of information may also be required before health education is incorporated into the patient's or family's bank of experiences.[18] Adults are sensitive about making mistakes and tend to view mistakes as failures. Learning situations that the patient and family interpret as belittling or embarrassing or that are perceived as insurmountable will be avoided or disregarded. The nurse should act more as a coach or facilitator of information instead of a didactic instructor.[12] The teacher can only show the learner to the door; the learner must decide to walk through that door. Learning is an active process that occurs internally over time and cannot be forced. Bedside nurses are obliged to be proactive and to have a good understanding of adult learning theory and to incorporate its concepts into the assessment of learning needs, development of an education plan, implementation of the plan, and evaluation of the outcomes of the education encounter.

Factors Affecting the Learning Process

Information must also be gathered on factors that affect the education process and impair the ability of the patient or family to respond. These factors include 1) desire and motivation; 2) physical or cognitive limitations; 3) cultural and religious views of illness or health; 4) emotional barriers; and 5) barriers to effective communication.[1]

Readiness, Willingness, Ability

For teaching to be successful and learning to be achieved the patient or family must be ready, willing, and able to learn. The ability to learn is the capacity of the learner to understand, pay attention, and comprehend the material being taught. Willingness to learn describes the learner's openness to new ideas and concepts. Readiness to learn is the motivation to try out new concepts and behaviors.[5] Even if the inventive teaching methods, well-considered education materials, and amounts of time are unlimited, learning cannot take place if the patient or family is not ready, willing, and able to learn.[19] Several factors affect the ability, willingness, and readiness to learn, as well as the ability

to cope and adapt to the current situation. These factors include physiologic, psychologic, sociocultural, financial, and environmental aspects.[5,12]

Physiologic Factors

The need for oxygen and survival predominates over all other human needs. This need is described by a theory known as Maslow's hierarchy of human needs. It is a concept in which lower-level, physiologic needs must be satisfied before an individual can move on to higher-level, self-esteem–building issues. The motivation to meet the need to survive and to feel safe and secure predominates over the need to learn a lifestyle change such as smoking cessation. Only when lower-level needs are met can the patient be open to learning new concepts and skills. There is an instinctive need to decrease the effects of stressors and reestablish a normal daily routine. A physical assessment can supply the nurse with information concerning the patient's response to the stressors.

Physiologic alterations in heart rate and blood pressure can be measured and taken into consideration during the teaching-learning encounter.[3] Sources of physiologic stress in the critically ill include medications, pain, hypoxia, decreased cerebral and peripheral perfusion, hypotension, fluid and electrolyte imbalances, infection, sensory alterations, fever, and neurologic deficits.[12] Experiencing one or more of these stressors may completely consume all the patient's available energy and thoughts, affecting his or her ability to interact, comprehend, and respond to teaching.

Health Literacy

Patients and families may be ready and willing to learn but lack the ability to comprehend and act upon the information presented to them. In its report *Health Literacy: A Prescription to End Confusion* the Institute of Medicine (IOM) states that nearly half of adult Americans struggle to understand and follow the health information they are provided. The IOM defines health literacy as "the degree to which individuals have the capacity to obtain, process and understand basic health information and services needed to make appropriate health decisions." However, health literacy goes beyond the individual. Practitioners must develop the ability to present information and instructions in a way that patients and families can best understand.[20]

Assessing health literacy is not an easy task, but knowing what to look for can make it easier. Several tools are available to assist health care professionals to screen for low literary skills. Generally, these tools fall into four categories: 1) word recognition; 2) reading comprehension; 3) functional health literacy; and 4) informal methods.[21,22] Each tool has both positive and negative aspects to its use.

Word recognition tests consist of lists of health care terms that patients are asked to read. The patient is given a time limit and scoring is based on how many words the patient can correctly pronounce. Examples of word recognition tests include the Rapid Estimate of Adult Literacy in Medicine (REALM), Wide Range Achievement Test-Revised (WRAT-R), Short Assessment of Health Literacy for Spanish Adults (SAHLSA-50), and

Medical Terminology Achievement Test (MART). Although these tests can often be administered in 5-10 minutes, they only test the reading abilities of the individual, not comprehension or interpretation.

Reading comprehension tests assess understanding of health care information presented but do not demonstrate the individual's ability to apply this information. Reading comprehension tests are extremely time consuming and are not often used in the clinical setting.

Functional health literacy tests assess the individual's level of comprehension and ability to put into action what they have learned. Examples of these tests include the Test of Functional Health Literacy in Adults (TOFHLA)[4] and the Newest Vital Sign (NVS).[21-22] The TOFHLA requires the individual to complete missing sections of written statements to assess the ability to read and comprehend directions for taking medications, monitoring blood glucose, and keeping appointments.[23] The tool takes 20-30 minutes to administer and score, making it undesirable for use in the critical care setting. An abbreviated version, the S-TOFHLA, is now available. It takes approximately 10-12 minutes to complete and score. Figure 5-1 shows the NVS tool and scoring sheet.

Informal methods include identifying socioeconomic characteristics, observation of behaviors, and direct questioning. A common misconception among health care providers is that reading and comprehension levels are directly related to wealth and level of education; the implication is that someone with a graduate-level education has a higher reading level than someone who completed only grade school. This is not true; wealth and education levels do not necessarily correlate with the ability to read and comprehend health care information.

Shame has been cited as one of the most common emotions associated with low health literacy.[24] Behaviors such as handing a form to a family member to complete, claiming to be too tired,

Nutrition Facts

Serving Size			½ cup
Servings per container			4
Amount per serving			
Calories	250	Fat Cal	120
			%DV
Total Fat 13g			20%
Sat Fat 9g			40%
Cholesterol 28mg			12%
Sodium 55mg			2%
Total Carbohydrate 30g			12%
Dietary Fiber 2g			
Sugars 23g			
Protein 4g			8%

*Percentage Daily Values (DV) are based on a 2,000 calorie diet. Your daily values may be higher or lower depending on your calorie needs.

Ingredients: Cream, Skim Milk, Liquid Sugar, Water, Egg Yolks, Brown Sugar, Milkfat, Peanut Oil, Sugar, Butter, Salt, Carrageenan, Vanilla Extract.

The Newest Vital Sign™
A Health Literacy Assessment Tool

Score Sheet for the Newest Vital Sign
Questions and Answers

READ TO SUBJECT:
This information is on the back of a container of a pint of ice cream.

ANSWER CORRECT? yes / no

1. If you eat the entire container, how many calories will you eat?
Answer: 1,000 is the only correct answer

2. If you are allowed to eat 60 grams of carbohydrates as a snack, how much ice cream could you have?
Answer: Any of the following is correct: 1 cup (or any amount up to 1 cup), half the container. Note: If patient answers "two servings," ask "How much ice cream would that be if you were to measure it into a bowl?"

3. Your doctor advises you to reduce the amount of saturated fat in your diet. You usually have 42 g of saturated fat each day, which includes one serving of ice cream. If you stop eating ice cream, how many grams of saturated fat would you be consuming each day?
Answer: 33 is the only correct answer

4. If you usually eat 2,500 calories in a day, what percentage of your daily value of calories will you be eating if you eat one serving?
Answer: 10% is the only correct answer

READ TO SUBJECT:
Pretend that you are allergic to the following subtances: penicillin, peanuts, latex gloves, and bee stings.

5. Is it safe for you to eat this ice cream?
Answer: No

6. (Ask only if the patient responds "no" to question 5): Why not?
Answer: Because it has peanut oil.

Number of correct answers:

Interpretation

Score of 0–1 suggests high likelihood (50% or more) of limited literacy.
Score of 2–3 indicates the possibility of limited literacy.
Score of 4–6 almost always indicates adequate literacy.

Pfizer Working together for a healthier world™ February 2011

FIGURE 5-1 The Newest Vital Sign (NVS) health literacy test tool and scoring sheet. (Courtesy Pfizer, New York, NY.)

BOX 5-2 BEHAVIORAL CUES INDICATING LOW HEALTH LITERACY

- Requests family to always be present
- Opens a medication bottle to identify a medicine
- Makes excuses:
  I forgot my glasses.
  I want my son to read it first.
  I'll take it home with me.
- Refers to medications by shape or color rather than name
- Cannot teach-back
- Frequently misses appointments
- Postpones decision making
- Watches or mimics behavior or responses of others
- Pretends to read material—eyes wander over page, slow to read
- Does not complete forms or asks staff or family to complete

or "forgetting" their glasses are a few behaviors that may be used by individuals to hide their limitations. Other behaviors that may also provide clues to a patient's health literacy are listed in Box 5-2.

In some cases, asking a direct question can elicit an individual's level of health literacy. For example, how the individual answers questions such as "How comfortable are you in reading medicine labels?" or "How well do you understand your disease process?" may help the practitioner gain insight into the level of health literacy and plan appropriate educational interventions.

Sociocultural Factors

Variables such as culture, ethnicity, values, beliefs, lifestyle, and family role influence the way an individual perceives illness, pain, and healing.[15] Culturally sensitive educational strategies should be developed to communicate specific needs to other members of the health care team and achieve optimal learning outcomes.[1]

Financial Factors

Patients and families often worry about financial issues related to the hospitalization and the possibility of long-term disability. Examples of financial concerns are 1) fear of income loss related to time away from work or possible long-term disability; 2) how health care expenses will be paid; and 3) complex insurance coverage issues. Patients may be more concerned with the amount of out-of-pocket expenses they will have to pay for this illness rather than receiving information on symptom management strategies. The nurse must recognize these issues as patient concerns and mobilize resources to calm financial anxiety. Practitioners in other disciplines, especially social work, are available to assist patients and families obtain community resources to help cover expenses such as medication costs.

Psychologic Factors

When confronted with life-altering situations such as admission to a critical care unit, patients and families may experience anxiety and emotional stress. Anxiety and fear disrupt the normalcy of daily life. Sources of emotional stress include fear of death, uncertain prognosis, role change, self-image change, social isolation, disruption in daily routine, financial concerns, and unfamiliar critical care environment.[3,20] These intense emotions can lead to a crisis situation and alter the ability of the patient and family to cope.[25,26] During the critical illness, an individual's ability to process or retain information and ability to participate in the treatment plan could be altered.[2] If the disease process or physiologic stressors impair the patient's ability to make decisions, the burden of decision making will transfer to the family. Gender differences affect a patient's reaction to stress. For example, women who have experienced a myocardial infarction report higher anxiety levels than men at all points during the hospital stay.[27] Physiologic alterations caused by anxiety negatively impact the recovery process and the long-term prognosis.[27] In critical situations, the nurse may find it necessary to repeat information or limit teaching sessions to short bursts rather than one long encounter. Medical jargon should be limited and replaced by terms that are easy to understand. Provision of honest and accurate disease state information may decrease the effects of stressors and alleviate anxiety and fear.

Coping

Coping refers to the way a person manages stressful events that are straining or exceeding personal resources.[5,28] The stressful event is appraised according to the level of threat to the individual and is managed by focusing on the problem at hand or the emotions felt at the moment.[29] Critical illness disrupts the normalcy of daily routines. Coping strategies are used by the patient and family to help maintain control over the situation and encourage hope and stability in life. Disbelief and denial may be present any time during the hospitalization. Phrases such as "Why me" and "I can't believe this is happening" are common in the critical care setting. Other coping mechanisms, such as denial and anger, hamper the ability of the patient or family to problem solve and cope with the situation. All are barriers to the ability of the patient to receive information and incorporate it into the self-concept. Adults must be physically ready and emotionally willing to learn. Teaching new skills or self-management techniques to the adult learner therefore presents a special challenge to the nurse in critical care. For example, until the patient accepts the diagnosis of heart failure as part of who he or she is, he or she will not make appropriate changes in lifestyle to avoid an exacerbation of the disease.

Adaptation

A stressor can be any condition, situation, or perception that requires an individual to adapt.[30] All situations in a critical care facility may well be considered stressful. The capacity of an individual to adapt is paramount in breaking down emotional barriers that affect willingness and readiness for learning. Culture, beliefs, attitudes, and ability to mobilize resources affect a person's ability to respond to a crisis situation.[28] General characteristics of the stages of adaptation to illness are outlined in Table 5-1 with corresponding applications for the teaching-learning process. Patients and families move through these stages on an individual timeline and at a variable pace. A person

TABLE 5-1	TEACHING-LEARNING PROCESS IN ADAPTATION TO ILLNESS	
STAGE OF ADAPTATION	**CHARACTERISTIC PATIENT RESPONSE**	**IMPLICATIONS FOR TEACHING-LEARNING PROCESS**
Disbelief	Denial	Orient teaching to present. Teach during other nursing activities. Reassure patient about safety. Explain all procedures and activities clearly and concisely.
Developing awareness	Anger	Continue to orient teaching to present. Avoid long lists of facts. Continue to foster development of trust and rapport through good physical care.
Reorganization	Acceptance of sick role	Orient teaching to meet patient. Teach whatever patient wants to learn. Provide necessary self-care information; reinforce with written material.
Resolution	Identification with others with same problem; recognition of loss	Use group instruction. Use patient support groups and visits by recovered patients with same problem.
Identifying change	Definition of self as one who has undergone change and is now different	Answer the patient's questions as they arise. Recognize that as basic needs are met, more mature needs will arise.

may move back and forth between stages and may skip one altogether. The patient and each member of the family may be experiencing different stages in the adaptation process at the same time. The education encounter may need to be modified to meet the needs of the patient and family.

Environmental Factors

The critical care environment can be considered a source of stress to the learner. Although sounds, people, and state-of-the-art equipment are familiar and mundane for the nurse, this environment may appear foreign and intimidating to the patient and family. Prior exposure to a critical care unit is a double-edged sword. Depending on whether the outcome of the experience was positive or negative, it may help alleviate or heighten anxiety. The nurse must pay attention to the perceptions of the environment by the patient and family and alter the teaching-learning encounter accordingly. Sleep cycle alterations caused by sleep deprivation or sensory overload related to continuous noise from machines or people affect the patient's ability to concentrate and comprehend information. Allowing frequent uninterrupted rest periods assists the patient in obtaining structured sleep.[30]

For patients and families to value education, they must believe the information source is reliable. The bedside nurse is the most available source of information in the critical care unit. It is important for him or her to develop a rapport and establish a sense of trust within the nurse-patient relationship. These positive characteristics are recommended for a supportive learning environment. Assignment of multiple caregivers may negatively affect the ability of the patient and family to form a trusting relationship with the nursing staff. Arranging consistency in the assigned caregivers can help promote rapport and

trust, as well as decrease anxiety and enhance comfort level with the environment.[5,28]

STEP 2: EDUCATION PLAN DEVELOPMENT

Education must be ongoing, interactive, and consistent with the patient's plan of care and education level.[1] The nurse must analyze information gathered from the assessment to prioritize the educational needs of the patient and family. The nursing diagnosis for deficient knowledge and accompanying interventions can be applied to any situation. The nurse must also consider the patient's physical and emotional status when setting education priorities. Ability, willingness, and readiness to learn are factors that impair acceptance of new information and add to the complexity of teaching-learning encounter. These factors should be recognized by the nurse before implementation of teaching. The written teaching plan should identify the learning need, goals or expected outcome of the teaching-learning encounter, interventions to meet that outcome, and appropriate teaching strategies.

Research and accepted national guidelines or standards can be used to assist the practitioner in developing an evidence-based plan for education. Examples of organizations that offer education standards are the American Association of Critical-Care Nurses, American Heart Association Guidelines for Practice, and the Society of Critical Care Medicine. A database for nursing interventions and outcomes has been developed from research that began in the 1980s. This research is known as the IOWA Project. It can be used in daily practice and can be found in two books: *Nursing Interventions Classification (NIC)* and *Nursing Outcomes Classification (NOC)*. These evidence-based interventions and outcomes assist the nurse in providing consistent outcomes and interventions from nurse to nurse, shift to shift, and discipline to discipline.

Determining What to Teach

It can be difficult to prioritize the multitude of learning needs that practitioners are required to address during a period in critical care. Learning needs in the critical care unit, the progressive care, or the telemetry setting can be separated into four different categories to help set teaching priorities in each phase of the hospitalization (Table 5-2). Learning needs during the initial contact or first hours of hospitalization can be predicted. Education during this time frame should be directed toward the reduction of immediate stress, anxiety, and fear rather than future lifestyle alterations or rehabilitation needs. Interventions are targeted to promote comfort and familiarity with the environment and surroundings.[31] The plan should focus on survival skills, orientation to the environment and equipment, communication of prognosis, procedure explanations, and the immediate plan of care.

Three learning domains are considered when developing an individualized education plan: knowledge, attitude, and skills. The knowledge domain is centered on the acquisition of information or facts by the patient about a given topic, such as listing the signs and symptoms of hypoglycemia and knowing what to do if he or she becomes symptomatic. A patient who has had diabetes for years has life experiences with his or her disease process that are different from those of the newly diagnosed patient. Even though two patients have the same diagnosis, educational needs differ. The attitude domain includes the incorporation of new values, beliefs, or attitudes into patients' behavior, such as believing smoking is bad for them and then exerting a conscious effort to stop. The skills domain is involved with the acquisition of skills that enable a person to perform a new technique, such as endotracheal suctioning or dressing changes. The nurse may incorporate one or more of these domains into the education plan.

Patients and their families are attempting to cope with the seriousness of the current situation and need information continually to adapt their behavior accordingly. Leske and Molter's hallmark research in the area of needs of the families of critically ill patients has provided nursing with a scientific body of knowledge for identification of the learning needs of this population. Results of these studies found that families of critically ill patients needed to have their questions answered honestly and to have a feeling of hope.[32] The outcomes of this research can be used in developing interventions for the initial phase in the hospitalization process. Box 5-3 includes a sample listing of interventions that can be used to help meet the needs of the family. During this time of elevated stress, the nurse may have to refocus the patient and family to help concentrate efforts on coping with the present instead of dwelling on possibilities of the future. Not addressing these immediate concerns can result in further anxiety, affect the ability to cope, and prevent open and honest communication.[3]

As the hospital length of stay increases, patients and families begin to adapt to the situation, and learning needs change. The patient and family develop positive feelings of relief and happiness in the fact that survival has been achieved. Because lower-level, physiologic needs are met, the patient's efforts can be concentrated on modifying behavior to meet higher-level needs, such as self-concept and self-actualization. Teaching during the continuous phase of nursing care is aimed at answering the patient's or family members' questions about the treatment plan or how the critical illness will impact their daily lives. Education on lifestyle modification and self-management skills should be presented during this phase of nursing care.

Discharge planning is also part of the education process and should start with admission to the hospital. Instructions for home care, also known as aftercare, should be accomplished before the day of discharge to avoid decreased retention of education that occurs with information overload.

Patient Education boxes are placed in each Disorders chapter. Special topics that should be taught to patients and families in preparation for discharge are listed.

Writing Goals or Outcomes

An outcomes statement helps clarify to the teacher and the learner what is to be taught, what is to be learned, what is to be evaluated, and what is to be documented. When goals or expected outcomes of the education encounter are clearly stated, the teacher and the learner understand the expectations and will do their best to achieve them. These statements differ from interventions in that they reflect what the learner is to accomplish, not what the nurse is to teach.[33] Identifying and writing outcomes may be the most difficult aspect in the development of the education plan of care. The written outcomes provide direction for the teaching-learning process and should be straightforward, attainable, and include one task or learning domain.[33]

The three components in the outcomes statement are 1) the individual who will meet the objective; 2) a measurable or observable verb; and 3) the content to be evaluated or learned. Examples of measurable verbs include define, list, identify, perform, prepare, and demonstrate, whereas nonmeasurable, higher-level verbs include believe, value, and understand. Remember the KISS rule: *Keep It Simple, Simon.* Outcomes should include behavioral lifestyle changes for self-management, psychomotor skill acquisition, and acquisition of knowledge. This is an example of a clearly stated outcome: The patient and family will list the signs and symptoms of postoperative infection.

Developing Interventions

Interventions describe how a nurse will become involved in providing education to the patient or the family. Determining education interventions is part of clinical decision making.[34] Nurse-initiated interventions are based on clinical knowledge and judgment and have a direct impact on the outcome of the teaching encounter.[34] Although physiologic problems occupy most of the nursing plan of care, it is essential to incorporate teaching interventions into the daily plan to create positive patient outcomes. Nurses just entering the profession readily refer to education plans developed by experienced nurses to guide them in their new role of patient educator.[35] Carefully

TABLE 5-2 CATEGORIES OF EDUCATIONAL NEEDS IN CRITICAL CARE

PHASE	EDUCATIONAL NEEDS
Initial contact or first visit, with a focus on immediate needs	Preparation for the visit: patient representatives or nurses can prepare the family and patient for the first visit What to expect in the environment How long the visit will last What the patient may look like (e.g., tubes, IV lines) Orientation to the unit or environment: call light, bed controls, waiting rooms, unit contact numbers Orientation to unit policies and hospital policies HIPAA, advanced directives, visitation policies Equipment orientation: monitors, IV pumps, pulse oximetry, pacemakers, ventilators Medications: rationale, effects, side effects What to do during the visit: talk to the patient, hold the patient's hand, monitor length of visits (if applicable) Patient status: stable or unstable and what that terminology means What treatments and interventions are being done for the patient Upcoming procedures When the doctor visited or is expected to visit Disciplines involved in care and the services they provide Immediate plan of care (next 24 hours) Mobilization of resources for crisis intervention
Continuous care	Day-to-day routine: meals, laboratory visits, doctor visits, frequency of monitoring (VS), nursing assessments, daily weights, and shift routines Explanation of any procedures: expected sensations or discomforts (e.g., chest tube removal, arterial sheath removal) Plan of care: treatments, progress, patient accomplishments (e.g., extubation) Medications: name, why the patient is receiving them, side effects to report to the nurse or health care team Disease process: what it is and how it will affect life, symptoms to report to health care team How to mobilize resources to assist the patient and family in coping with stress and crisis: pastoral care, social workers, case managers, victim assistance, domestic violence counseling Gifts: When a loved one is ill, it is traditional to send flowers, balloons, or cards. If your unit has restrictions on gifts, make the family aware. Begin teaching self-management skills, and discuss aftercare information.
Transfer to a different level of care	**Sending Unit** Acknowledge positive move out of critical care When the transfer will occur Why the transfer is occurring What to expect in the different unit Name of the new caregiver Availability of care provider Visiting hours Directions for how to get there; the new room number and phone number **Receiving Unit** Orientation to environment, visitation policies, visitors Unit routine, meals shift changes, doctor visits Expectations about patient self-care; ADLs Medication and diagnostic testing routine times
Planning for aftercare, discharge planning	Self-care management: symptom management, medication administration, diet, activity, durable medical equipment, tasks or procedures What to do for an emergency What constitutes an emergency or when to call the physician How to care for incisions or procedure sites
Completed throughout the hospital stay	Return appointment: name of physician practice, practice phone numbers and contacts Obtaining medications: prescriptions, pharmacy, special medication ordering information Required lifestyle changes: mobility and safety issues for the paraplegic or stroke victim, activities of daily living issues relative to medications or symptoms Potential risk modifications: smoking cessation, diet modifications, exercise Resources: cardiac rehabilitation, support groups, home care agencies
End-of-life care	End-of-life care: participation in care, services available, mobilizing resources Palliative care Hospice

ADLs, Activities of daily living; *HIPAA*, Health Insurance Portability and Accountability Act; *IV*, intravenous; *VS*, vital signs.

planned and developed interventions support nurses, patients, and families focused on achievable outcomes. Education interventions are targeted toward information to be taught, such as how to care and use oxygen or how to recognize signs and symptoms of an infection. The following is an example of a clearly stated research-based intervention: Instruct the patient and family on proper name of prescribed diet.[34]

Standardized Education Plans

Standardized education plans provide the health care team with consistent outcomes and interventions. Even though standardized plans are easy to implement, they must be individualized to meet the specific needs of the patient or family. Examples of standardized plans of care include patient pathways, traditional nursing care plans for Deficient Knowledge, and the Nursing Interventions Classification (NIC) for Teaching: Disease Process, which is presented in Box 5-4. Examples of nursing management plans for Deficient Knowledge are included in Appendix A.

STEP 3: IMPLEMENTATION

After the assessment is completed and the education plan is developed, need-targeted education can commence. Beginning practitioners differ from experienced practitioners in their skills of implementing the education plan of care. Experienced practitioners use their intuition and knowledge base to anticipate learning needs and form a mental list of interventions and possible outcomes.[35] Those just starting in the profession need the concrete education plan that has been developed to guide the teaching-learning encounter.[35]

Setting up the Environment

The optimal environment for learning is one that is nonthreatening, comfortable, open, and honest. Many factors concerning the critical care environment can be threatening or anxiety producing. The practitioner must assess for these distractions and control them as much as possible. Providing the family with open visitation and access to the patient and health care providers can help decrease their anxiety level and improve satisfaction with care.[3] Current Health Insurance Portability and Accountability Act (HIPAA) requirements for patient confidentiality necessitate a need for privacy during the teaching-learning encounter. Bedside practitioner attention to this detail in open

---

BOX 5-3 INTERVENTIONS FOR IDENTIFIED PATIENT AND FAMILY NEEDS

- Answer questions openly and honestly.
- Give as much or as little realistic information as the patient and family members need to understand about the situation or the patient's physiologic condition.
- Provide specific facts about the patient's daily or hourly progress.
- Provide information that is understandable and given in simple terms.
- Use short sentences, and incorporate only a couple of pieces of information at one time.
- Provide emotional comfort to reduce anxiety and facilitate the feeling of hope.
- Prepare the patient and family for their first visit to the unit.
- Explain the possible appearance of the patient, purpose of the equipment, the family role in visitation, and the unit environment.
- Keep the family informed and involved in the daily plan of care.
- Explain what procedures will be done, why they are being done, and what information is hoped to be gained from each procedure.

BOX 5-4 NIC

Teaching: Disease Process

Definition

Assisting the patient to understand information related to a specific disease process

Activities

Appraise the patient's current level of knowledge related to a specific disease process

Explain the pathophysiology of the disease and how it relates to the anatomy and physiology, as appropriate

Review patient's knowledge about condition

Acknowledge patient's knowledge about condition

Describe common signs and symptoms of the disease, as appropriate

Explore with patient what she/he has already done to manage the symptoms

Describe the disease process, as appropriate

Identify possible etiologies, as appropriate

Provide information to the patient about condition, as appropriate

Identify changes in physical condition for patient

Avoid empty reassurances

Provide reassurance about patient's condition, as appropriate

Provide the family/significant other(s) with information about the patient's progress, as appropriate

Provide information about available diagnostic measures, as appropriate

Discuss lifestyle changes that may be required to prevent future complications and/or control the disease process

Discuss therapy/treatment options

Describe rationale behind management/therapy/treatment recommendations

Encourage the patient to explore options/get a second opinion, as appropriate or indicated

Describe possible chronic complications, as appropriate

Instruct the patient on measures to prevent/minimize side effects of treatment for the disease, as appropriate

Instruct the patient on measures to control/minimize symptoms, as appropriate

Explore possible resources/support, as appropriate

Refer the patient to local community agencies/support groups, as appropriate

Instruct the patient on which signs and symptoms to report to health care provider, as appropriate

Provide the phone number(s) to call if complications occur

Reinforce information provided by other health care team members, as appropriate

From Bulechek GM, et al, eds. *Nursing Interventions Classification* (NIC). 6th ed. St. Louis: Mosby; 2013.

environments such as critical care units, waiting rooms, and emergency departments is important in creating an environment of trust and reassurance. Supportive education promotes behaviors that facilitate motivation to learn and adherence to lifestyle changes.[36] The following is a list of strategies the practitioner can implement to facilitate learning[36]:

- Show empathy and concern. Actively listen to the learner and acknowledge lived experiences and ideas.
- Use language and nonverbal communication to enhance choice and promote problem solving.
- Reduce language that is controlling, criticizing, guilt provoking, judgmental, or punishing.
- Provide rationale for self-management behaviors: the importance of changing lifestyle to manage symptoms.

One example of the difference between supportive education and nonsupportive education is demonstrated by a patient diagnosed with chronic heart failure who is experiencing an exacerbation of symptoms related to dietary salt intake. Suppose the patient states that he or she is doing "okay" at adhering to the low-salt diet, but family members complain that he or she eats too many processed foods and too much take-out fast food. This is an example of a nonsupportive teaching phrase: "You know salt isn't good for you."[36] This phrase is judgmental, critical, and guilt provoking and makes an assumption of the patient's level of knowledge. By revising the wording in the phrase, the meaning of the information is changed. This is an example: "I know it is difficult not to eat all of your favorite foods. Adding salt is up to you. Do you understand that salt will affect your heart condition?"[36] This supportive statement transfers accountability of performing the self-management skill from the nurse to the patient and motivates the patient to make the conscious decision to limit salt intake.

Teaching Strategies

The nurse may be the first health care provider to initiate patient teaching. Bedside nurses are in a unique position to facilitate, mentor, and coach patients through the endless maze of information presented in the critical care arena. Information overload often occurs, and the information taught can easily be forgotten. Nurses may become frustrated when family members and patients ask the same questions repeatedly. Patience with repeated questioning is essential, because information taught may be lost within minutes after its presentation. Although health care providers would like patients and families to retain 100% of information given, in reality, learning does not take place in one session or may not occur at all. An individual may be able to remember only two to three pieces of information in one education session.

Nurses are continuously interacting with patients and discussing their progress, updating them on treatment plans, and describing procedures. With that in mind, every patient contact can be thought of as a brief teaching-learning encounter. The nurse must use every teachable moment and take advantage of the patient's readiness and willingness to learn. When educating adults, a combination of teaching strategies should be used to facilitate giving and receiving information. Each individual has

a different learning style: visual, auditory, or tactile. Common strategies include discussion, demonstration, and use of media.

Discussion

Informal discussion can take place anywhere and at any time. This strategy allows for interaction between the teacher and the learner. Discussion occurs one-on-one or in groups. Education sessions need to be adapted quickly, as they are occurring, to meet the ever-evolving needs of the patient and family. Although teaching through discussion is informal, the information given should promote the goals of the education plan. Focus on what the patient or family wants or *needs* to know at that moment, rather than on what might be *nice* to know. Obtaining and maintaining the learner's attention during the discussion may be challenging. The nurse must use different teaching strategies and techniques and modify them frequently according to the situation and the patient's or family's response to the education.

Several strategies are used to maintain a positive teaching-learning encounter:

- Addressing the patient and family members by name
- Clearly stating the purpose of the education encounter
- Getting and keeping them involved in the learning process
- Maintaining eye contact during the encounter
- Keeping the encounter brief and to the point
- Giving positive reinforcement
- Communicating with professionals in other disciplines about the progress and additional learning needs of the patient and family[4,5]

Demonstration and Practice

Demonstration and practice are the best strategies for teaching technical skills. Adults learn best when they are able to participate in the learning process. Involving the learner, providing consistent step-by-step instructions, and presenting a visual demonstration of the skill being performed are important strategies to achieve successful task acquisition. By allowing the patient or family to practice the skill in a simulated or real situation, the outcome of the teaching encounter can be evaluated. This strategy allows the nurse to offer positive reinforcement and constructive feedback during the learning encounter, thereby building learner confidence in performing the newly acquired skill. Many demonstration sessions and repetitive practice may be required for the patient or family to acquire and feel comfortable with the new skill.

Audiovisual Media

The use of media in mainstream patient education is becoming more prevalent as a first-line teaching strategy. Media are excellent tools to relay information to persons with any one of the three learning styles. Pamphlets, videos, and anatomic pictures or models are the most common types of audiovisual aids. This teaching strategy supplies the learner with a large amount of information in a relatively short period. Videos and written materials enable different nurses to distribute information that remains consistent from patient to patient and family to family. The use of media can assist practitioners to obtain informed consent and to communicate current and future prescribed treatment plans.

Media are used to educate patients on a variety of educational needs, such as medications, disease processes, procedures, symptom management, weight monitoring, laboratory tests, diet, surgery, and health maintenance issues. Patient education videos require the patient's attention for only a few minutes and supply the learner with "nice-to-know" and "need-to-know" information. Interactive video technology offers on-demand educational and health information video programs, which are delivered to the patient through television. Patients and families are able to access education videos anytime they desire during their hospital stay. The digital video system allows multiple TVs to show the same video at the same time. Bedside call systems are linked to the computer server, and the video is selected from the bedside. These video systems can be customized to meet the needs of specialty patient populations (e.g., cardiac, obstetrics). Individual reports can be generated to list all educational films viewed during the patient's stay. Evaluation of learning can be achieved through the system by administration of a pretest or posttest available on the system.

Viewing a video does not ensure retention of information or knowledge acquisition. Patient-education videos should not be used in place of patient-family interaction. After the patient watches the video, the nurse must review the content and reiterate key points of information. This postvideo encounter is also used to evaluate the outcome of the teaching-learning encounter. To review the content with the patient or family, the nurse must also watch the video and choose key points to discuss with the learner in the postvideo discussion. Video presentation should be used to assist the learner in meeting identified educational needs.

Written Materials

Written media, such as brochures, pamphlets, patient pathways, and booklets, are common in outpatient and inpatient areas of health care. They usually are inexpensive and offer opportunities for a wide range of education: disease process education, risk factor modification information, procedure education, medication education, and use of medical equipment in the home setting. Written materials address multiple learning styles and offer learner-centered teaching with concrete, basic information that can be placed at the learner's fingertips for immediate review, as well as future review anytime the learner desires. The practitioner must make sure that written materials are appropriate for the patient population as a whole and for a particular individual patient or family. Several factors should be considered when choosing printed materials for patient education: readability, cultural considerations, age-specific considerations, primary language, and literacy.[6]

Readability is an important factor in the consideration of printed educational materials. *Readability* refers to how easy or hard the literature is to read. Nearly 20% of the U.S. adult population have low literacy skills and read at or below the fifth-grade reading level.[37] Typical patient educational materials are written at or above the eighth- or ninth-grade reading level and may be out of reach for many readers.[5,38] If the patient or family is unable to read the material or understand its meaning, he or she cannot perform self-management tasks to maintain health. This sets the patient and the family up for failure and being labeled noncompliant.

Readability tools are designed to provide quick and easy assessment of the readability level of patient educational materials. However, it is important to know that these formulas do not assess the understandability of the material. Many formulas, such as the Simplified Measure of Gobbledygook (SMOG) and the Suitability Assessment of Materials (SAM) assessment tools, are available to assist practitioners in determining the readability of health educational materials. Selection of the appropriate readability formula is dependent on the type of information being presented. Additional tools maybe found at www.readabilityformulas.com.

Providing written educational materials at the appropriate reading level is important, if the information is to be easily read and understood by most patients and families. To assist the nurse in overcoming literacy-related barriers to health education, it is recommended that patient educational materials be printed at or below the fifth-grade reading level.[37,39] Samples of health-related instructions at different reading levels are provided in Box 5-5.

Several situations present special challenges with regard to the use of printed patient-education materials. The inability of a patient or family to read or understand the English language does not mean they cannot understand directions and treatment regimens. Multilingual, written educational materials are a necessity in any health care institution. Hodgdon states that "communication is 55% visual, 37% vocal, and 7% verbal or the actual message."[40] Including pictures, drawings, diagrams, charts, or tables in educational materials has been shown to enhance understanding and increase retention in patients with low literacy skills.[41] Materials translated into Braille or provided in audio format may be used for the blind patient.

Many vendors supply printed materials for patient education, often translated into multiple languages. Common vendors include HERC Publishing, Pritchett and Hull, and Krames. National associations such as the American Cancer Society, the American Lung Association, and the American Heart

---

BOX 5-5   **SAMPLES OF READING LEVELS**

College Reading Level
Consult your physician immediately at the onset of chest discomfort, shortness of breath, or increased perspiration.

Twelfth-Grade Reading Level
Call your physician immediately if you experience chest discomfort, shortness of breath, or increased sweatiness.

Eighth-Grade Reading Level
Call your doctor immediately if you start having chest pain or shortness of breath or you feel sweaty.

Fourth-Grade Reading Level
Call your doctor right away if you start having chest pain, cannot breathe, or feel sweaty.

Association also publish educational materials for patients. Each of these companies has a website for easy viewing of sample patient-education materials and pricing information. Prices for these materials vary from pennies per pamphlet to several dollars; some pamphlets by national organizations are available free of charge to the consumer. There are several items to consider when choosing standardize, printed educational materials. Read the entire pamphlet or booklet to determine appropriateness of the material for the desired patient population. Ask the vendor to supply the reading level of the material and the method used to determine it. Inquire about the frequency with which the printed material is updated to ensure that the patient or family members have the most recent edition.

Thoroughly read the document for inconsistent information or information that is incongruent with a specific unit's treatment plan. For example, if the nurse educates the patient on a low-fat diet, but the pamphlet teaches only a low-salt diet, the patient may become confused and frustrated and not be able to determine which diet to follow at home. Another point to consider is whether the material contains information required by the institution and regulatory agencies such as The Joint Commission. Core measures outlined by The Joint Commission include certain items that must be included in discharge education and tracked by the institution. Some materials may not properly fit with a unit's plan for education and therefore are not appropriate for that particular institution. Printed material should be an adjunct to patient and family education and match what is taught and practiced in a specific facility.

When predeveloped educational materials do not meet the needs of the institution's patient population, the decision is made to develop internal patient educational materials. Producing homegrown educational materials can be time consuming and difficult.[12] Time must be spent determining content, readability, and design. Some simple rules when designing written patient-education materials include 1) use a white background; 2) use pictures and graphics to illustrate major concepts; 3) use bullet points instead of paragraphs to reduce reading time and "word clutter"[42]; and 4) emphasize only key facts and desired behaviors, avoiding the addition of "nice to know" information that may distract the reader from the true message.

The practitioner must keep in mind that patients and families may receive a variety of educational materials during their hospital stay. Streamlining educational materials within an organization decreases inconsistency of information, increases the clarity of prescribed treatment, and helps to avoid duplication of efforts between disciplines and shifts. Although providing written materials may seem like a quick and easy educational method, the practitioner must still review the content with the patient or family to determine whether learning has occurred and whether there are any questions about the material.

Computer-Assisted Instruction

Computer-assisted instruction is a relatively new strategy for providing patient and family education. Even though personal computers have become common, they may not be suitable because comfort levels with the technical aspects of the computer vary from person to person. The learner should be able to pay attention to the material being presented and not be preoccupied with learning how to use the computer mouse. The costs of computers and new software development may prohibit institutions from considering them for their patient education programs. Software programs can be accessed through a single hard drive or through a server for multiple computer sites. The use of touch screen technology instead of the standard mouse opens up computer learning to many individuals who do not feel comfortable with standard systems. Touch screen technology is even available in local grocery stores for self-checkout. Computer screens may be placed in every patient's room at the bedside for easy access to education videos or the Internet. Bedside computers provide the patient and family with an avenue to receive education on demand whenever they are ready, willing, and able. Computers offer self-directed learning. Because adults are self-directed individuals, they can go through the program at their own pace and spend as much or as little time as desired in one area of content. Computers stimulate all aspects of the adult learner—visual, auditory, and tactile.

Internet Sites

Patients and families often use websites to research information about the illness or condition about which they are concerned.[43] Information on the Internet is generally presented on an eighth-grade reading level.[9] Websites contain a wealth of information. However, the information is not regulated or controlled for reliability or validity,[43] and not all information provided on every website is accurate. The nurse must advise the patient and family about this concern and ask them to print out and bring in such material so it can be discussed. Government websites and those of professional organizations, reputable health care organizations, and consumer health groups offer trustworthy information for the practitioner and the public.[43]

Communication

Communicating effectively is essential to obtaining positive outcomes for patient education. Speaking slowly, clearly, and avoiding the use of slang or medical jargon is essential. Even when the patient and family speak English, the stress of hospitalization, fear of health outcomes, and difficulty speaking of personal issues with a stranger can present a challenge to providing patient education. When the patient or family has limited English proficiency (LEP) the challenge becomes even greater. In many instances a family member is called upon to serve in the role of interpreter. Although this may seem like an ideal solution, the family member may not have any better comprehension of the material being taught, and thus is unable to adequately relay the information. The use of professional interpreter services is preferable when the message is vital to a patient's health and well-being. Interpreter services are available through a variety of modes.[44] Some hospitals employ professional interpreters or provide special training for multilingual staff in effective interpretation. Telephonic interpretive services are offered by many vendors and special phones with dual handsets are available for use. Emerging technology has given rise to video-on-demand interpretive services such as those offered through the Language Access Network. Whichever

BOX 5-6 TIPS FOR USING AN INTERPRETER

- Speak directly to the patient, not the interpreter
- Position yourself so that you can maintain eye contact with the patient
- Introduce the interpreter and clarify roles of others in the room
- Nothing should be said that the patient shouldn't hear
- Pause after each complete thought to give interpreter time to translate
- Plan ahead, let the interpreter know exactly the content and purpose of the session
- Use the teach-back method to evaluate learning
- Listen to the interpreter, who may identify cultural practice or norms that impede understanding

From Techniques for educating with the aid of an interpreter. *Patient Education Management.* 2007;7:77.

method is used, interpretation can be a frustrating process. Box 5-6 describes helpful techniques to enhance the experience.[45]

All patients and families desire to be understood and have their concerns validated. This can be difficult for patients who are critically ill and whose ability to communicate to family and health care providers is impaired. Communication aids such as picture cards, picture boards, or word boards enhance the ability of the nurse to understand educational needs and communicate information. Augmentative and alternative communication (AAC) systems may be considered for temporarily nonspeaking patients in the critical care unit. Technology that has been available in the outpatient setting to help persons who cannot speak is becoming available in the critical care environment. This technology is known as an electronic voice output communication aid (VOCA). VOCA is a prerecorded, human or digitized computer-generated voice message.[46] It can be beneficial for patients who are awake and alert but are unable to talk for reasons such as mechanical ventilation through an endotracheal tube or tracheostomy tube. Whole phrases, as opposed to pictures or single words, are communicated to the health care team; for example, "I am having pain."[46] This technology can assist the patient to communicate comfort needs, anxiety, and fears and to ask questions concerning care or progress. Intubated patients describe the inability of families and caregivers to effectively understand their needs as an extremely stressful part of being in the critical care unit.[30] AACs can also assist the nurse to evaluate more effectively the outcome of education. Use of verbal, whole-sentence communication rather than traditional, nonverbal picture board communication has been found to decrease the guesswork in interpreting patient needs.[46]

Special Considerations
The Older Adult

As individuals age, cognitive, physiologic, and psychologic changes occur that must be considered when planning and implementing a teaching plan. It is the nurse's responsibility to understand the effects of aging and adjust teaching strategies to accommodate them.[47]

Cognitive Effects of Aging. Cognitive effects include processing information more slowly, a decrease in the ability to take in multiple messages, and difficulty understanding the abstract.

When teaching the older adult, nurses should provide information slowly and deliberately to allow the patient time to process each concept. Information should be presented in two to three essential points and reviewed frequently. Nurses should avoid using vague terms such as "several times a day" or "until better." Instead, they must be very specific with amounts, times, and frequencies.

Physical Effects of Aging. Presbyopia, cataracts, glaucoma, and macular degeneration affect the vision of many older adults. Although additional lighting is necessary, it is also necessary to avoid direct sunlight, harsh lights, and using glossy paper. Colors in the blue end of the spectrum are difficult for the older adult to distinguish because of yellowing of the lens of the eye. When using written instructions or color-coded dosing, blues, greens, and purples should not be used.

High-pitched tones become more difficult to hear as an individual ages. Female nurses will need to make an effort to modulate their voices into the lower register so the older adult can hear better. In addition, careful enunciation of words containing higher-pitched sounds like "f", "s", "k", and "sh" may be necessary. Providing audio and video recordings will help reinforce learning.

Aging and associated co-morbidities may result in fatigue, joint pain, or decreased dexterity. Learning can be facilitated by scheduling teaching sessions early in the day, keeping sessions short, and managing pain prior to learning.

Psychologic Effects of Aging. Older adults often suffer from depression. Learning can be enhanced by selecting content that holds value and relevance to the individual. Nurses should choose content that is perceived by the learner as important in maintaining quality of life, and should try to relate what they are teaching to the individual's previous life experiences.

Sedated and Unconscious Patients

Patient education should not be reserved for the conscious and coherent patient only; it should be provided to the unconscious or sedated patient as well. Addressing the learning needs of this critically ill population of patients is challenging. These patients cannot communicate their educational needs, nor can they interact and participate in the learning process. Although it is truly not known what the unconscious or sedated patient hears or remembers, it is known that some sedated patients undergoing surgery remember discussions that took place among physicians and staff during the procedure. Therefore, one should not ignore unconscious or sedated patients during the education process. These patients may not be able to respond or participate, and the effectiveness of the teaching process cannot be evaluated, but providing information regarding environment, procedures, sensations, and time of day is benevolent and may help to decrease immediate physiologic stress.

The Noncompliant Patient

Noncompliance, or an unwillingness to learn, does not necessarily mean that the patient is consciously choosing not to participate in their care or follow medical instructions. There are many other issues that can lead to noncompliance. The nurse must be alert for barriers that may prevent a willing patient

BOX 5-7	CONTRIBUTING FACTORS TO NONCOMPLIANCE

- Limited English Proficiency (LEP)
- Lack of education
- Cultural or ethnic beliefs
- Financial constraints
- Lack of adequate tools or supplies
- Lack of family support

from being compliant. Box 5-7 lists factors that may contribute to noncompliance or unwillingness to learn.[48]

STEP 4: EVALUATION

Evaluation is the final component in the patient- and family-education process. The intent of evaluation is to determine the effectiveness of the educational interventions. The nurse must use his or her clinical judgment and knowledge of adult-learning principles to determine how well the learner has met the expected outcomes and objectives. The evaluation process is continual and assesses the entire teaching-learning interaction, including the level of learner interest in the session, willingness to learn the content, and level of participation during the encounter. Evaluation should be completed at the end of each teaching-learning encounter. This allows the nurse to immediately present positive and constructive feedback to the patient and family, as well as revise the education plan to accommodate ongoing learning needs. It is also important to assess the response to teaching and determine whether follow-up education is required.

How to Evaluate

How does the nurse know if learning has occurred? Techniques such as verbalization of information, return demonstration, and physiologic measurement are common evaluation methods to determine the effectiveness of a teaching-learning encounter. Evaluation of knowledge retention can be completed by verbally questioning the learner. This method is known as teach-back. Teach-back is an interactive process that assists the nurse in determining whether the learner has retained the information taught. The nurse may ask the patient if he or she is able to list signs and symptoms of heart failure. Verbal questioning should occur immediately after the teaching event and throughout the hospitalization to assess knowledge retention. For example, the physician orders a new medication for the patient today, and the nurse educates that patient on the effects and side effects; the next day, the nurse may assess retention by asking the patient if he or she remembers the reason for taking the new medication. Common items that patients and families are asked to verbalize are reportable signs and symptoms, how to manage symptoms at home, when to take medication, how often the medication should be taken, and who to call for questions or concerns.

Changes in attitude, beliefs, or lifestyle are often difficult to evaluate, because learners can say they have changed their attitude when actually they have not. In this learning domain, the nurse must use his or her detective skills to assess whether the individual has accepted the prescribed treatment plan and modified behavior accordingly. Sometimes, the best way to evaluate a change in attitude is by observation and verbal questioning. An example is a patient who has been asked to comply with a low-cholesterol diet; a food diary the patient has kept as requested provides some evidence about what the patient has eaten. A wealth of information can also be obtained from the family concerning the patient's exhibited changes.

Physiologic evidence of the effectiveness of education can also be measured. Indicators such as blood cholesterol levels, blood pressure, heart rate, blood sugars, and weight can lead the practitioner to the conclusion that the patient and family may be having difficulties understanding or following through with the identified plan of care.[36] Adults generally want to comply with new expectations but often cannot for various reasons, such as a lack of money for medications or an inability to understand what is expected of them. These barriers must be explored and included in the education plan.

Observation and return demonstration is the evaluation of choice for the skills-learning domain. For the patient and family members to be "checked off" on a particular skill, they should be able to perform it independently, using the nurse only as a resource for questions. Endotracheal suctioning, placing condom catheters, and performing dressing changes are examples of common tasks that patients and families may be asked to learn. Because of the increasingly complex care that patients require at home after discharge, these skills may be the entire focus of teaching before discharge. Not every teaching moment is a success, and the nurse need not feel guilty or like a failure when the learner has not achieved the desired objective. Revisiting and revising the goals and objectives during the teaching-learning session may be necessary to meet the ever-changing needs of the patient or family.

STEP 5: DOCUMENTATION

Documentation of education is necessary to communicate educational efforts to members of the health care team, patients and families, and regulatory agencies. The nurse should recognize that informal teaching at the bedside is education. It is important to record any information given to the patient on formal documents approved for use by each health care institution. In most institutions, formal education records are used to document education rendered by practitioners of any discipline involved in the care of a particular patient and family. These forms are communication tools used to indicate progress in the teaching-learning process from shift to shift, day to day, and discipline to discipline.[49] Documentation should include education from admission to discharge on topics ranging from orientation to the environment to acquisition of self-management skills for home care.

What Should Be Documented?

The complexity of information, demand by governing agencies, lawsuits, and the sheer volume of patients in and out of a unit are driving nurses to provide quality documentation of the education encounter.[49] Documentation of the teaching-learning process is multifaceted. The documentation form should "tell the story" of the education encounter from assessment to evaluation. Documentation of the education assessment should include learning preferences; factors that impair ability, readiness, and willingness to learn; and actual or perceived learning needs. Information should be recorded on the interaction, material taught, supplemental materials distributed, response to the education, achievement of outcome, and any follow-up education or resources needed.

FACTORS THAT AFFECT THE TEACHING-LEARNING PROCESS

Many factors can produce barriers to a successful teaching-learning process. The physiologic, psychologic, sociocultural, financial, and environmental factors previously discussed are known to affect the patient's and family's ability, willingness, and readiness to learn. Physical disabilities, impaired vision, and hearing loss affect the learner's ability to read materials, listen to instructions, or perform a technical task.[50] If a technical task is required, ensure that the patient or family member has the physical ability or manual dexterity to perform the required skill. Provision of eyeglasses and hearing aids is essential to improving participation in learning. Several other factors have an impact on the teaching-learning process[5,12]:

- Lack of an accurate assessment
- Setting unrealistic goals
- Not involving the patient or the family in the process
- Overloading the learner with information
- Relying too heavily on resources
- Haphazard and nondirected teaching; lack of an education plan of care
- Teaching at the wrong time, hurried teaching, not paying attention to the learner
- Lack of trust and rapport between the teacher and learner
- Lack of communication among health care providers
- Language-related communication barriers

Although this list may seem overwhelming, it is important to be proactive and to remove as many of these barriers as possible. It takes less time and fewer resources to start with a structured education plan than it does to start over after the teaching-learning process has begun.

Barriers to the teaching-learning process exist for the patient or family and for the bedside nurse. Time constraints, decreased length of stay, and daily routines interrupt or impair the nurse's ability to communicate information to the patient and the family. Table 5-3 includes common barriers to the education process experienced by nurses. The patient's positive interactions and relationships with health care providers, as well as a clear understanding of his or her illness, symptoms, and medications, will promote adherence to the patient education plan.[51]

INFORMATIONAL NEEDS OF FAMILIES IN CRITICAL CARE

Family members and significant others of critically ill patients are integral to the recovery of their loved ones. When planning

TABLE 5-3	**NURSING BARRIERS TO EDUCATION**	
BARRIER	**EXAMPLE**	**SOLUTION**
Interruptions	Daily routines	Use all available teachable moments.
Distractions	Tasks; medication administration Phone calls TV or other noise in patient's room	Turn TV off; minimize noise.
Night shift	Sleeping patients	Plan education before bedtime.
Sedation or pain medications	Narcotic analgesic	Teach before administering the medication.
Nurse unaware of what to teach	Diabetic education	Educate self.

Data from London F. *No Time to Teach*. Philadelphia: JB Lippincott; 1999; Rankin S, Stallings K. *Patient Education: Principles and Practice*. 4th ed. Philadelphia: JB Lippincott; 2001.

for the overall care of patients, nurses and other caregivers need to consider the informational and emotional support needs of this group.[52] Families of critically ill patients report their greatest need is for information.[52] Flexible visiting hours and informational booklets regarding the critical care experience are recommended to meet this need.[54]

PREPARATION OF THE PATIENT AND FAMILY FOR TRANSFER FROM CRITICAL CARE

When patients are more stable, requiring less hemodynamic monitoring and close observation, they are frequently transferred to another level of care in a different geographic hospital setting. They may be transferred to an intermediate care unit (i.e., step-down unit, intermediate care area, or telemetry). While on these units, patients receive optimal care to their level of requirement, a lower nurse-to-patient ratio, and less expensive technologic monitoring in a quieter environment.[55-56]

Transferring a patient from the critical care unit to a step-down unit may result in anxiety and stress. Patients and families have become dependent on the monitors, equipment, constant nursing attention, and abundant information received while in the critical care unit. The patient has become secure knowing that immediate physiologic and emotional needs are being met. A strong bond has often developed between the staff and the family. Many patients and families are reluctant to give up that bond and believe that their needs will not be met as well on a step-down unit. To avoid anxiety and provide the patient and family with some control over the event, nurses need to prepare them for the transfer process.

Preparation for transfer should start after the patient has been stabilized and the life-threatening event that resulted in hospitalization has subsided. The stressor at this point is no longer the critical care environment but has become the unfamiliar step-down environment. Explanations about where the patient will be transferred, the reason for transfer, and the name of the nurse who will be providing care should be offered as soon as known. Before transfer, information about changes in care, expectations for self-care, and visiting hours should be provided to the patient and family. Family members should be contacted concerning exactly when the patient will be transferred so they can be present during the transfer or made aware of the patient's new location (Box 5-8).

The education plan of care and tips learned by the critical care staff about that particular patient and family should be communicated to the step-down unit staff. Most of the patient transfers made from the critical care unit to a step-down unit are planned events. However, unplanned or unexpected transfers sometimes occur, usually when the critical care unit requires bed space for a more seriously ill patient. In this situation, the transfer occurs quickly during the day or often at night. Families may be present in the hospital or may have gone home for the evening. This sudden need to transfer the patient can produce as much anxiety as the initial event, primarily because the patient and family may not feel ready for the transfer or may think they have lost control of the situation. Providing the patient and family with concrete evidence of improvement, such as more favorable vital signs or the need for fewer medications or tubes, can assure them about improvement in the patient's condition before unplanned transfers occur. Increasing communication and providing consistent information to patients and families also increases satisfaction with care and services.[57]

BOX 5-8 EDUCATION COMPONENTS FOR PATIENT TRANSFER TO ANOTHER UNIT

Sending Unit
- Acknowledge positive move out of critical care
- When the transfer will occur
- Why the transfer is occurring
- What to expect in the different unit
- Name of the new caregiver
- Availability of care provider
- Visiting hours
- Directions for how to get there; the new room number and phone number

Receiving Unit
- Orientation to environment, visitation policies, visitors
- Unit routine, meals, shift changes, doctor visits
- Expectations about patient self-care, activities of daily living
- Medication and diagnostic testing routine times

BOX 5-9 CASE STUDY

Patient and Family Education

Brief Patient History
Mr. S is a 30-year-old Vietnamese-American man who is employed as a fisherman. Mr. S is married and has three children younger than 5 years. He was diagnosed a few months earlier with type 1 diabetes mellitus after a 30-pound weight loss and a change in visual acuity. He has had two admissions for diabetic ketoacidosis in the past month.

Clinical Assessment
Mr. S was admitted to the critical care unit with diabetic ketoacidosis 2 days ago. His condition has been stabilized, and he is ready to be transferred to a nursing unit today. Mr. S states that he does not understand why "this keeps happening" because he takes his insulin if he plans on eating but does not always eat. Mr. S's wife states that his blood sugar seems to be okay when he is at home but that he gets into trouble when offshore.

Diagnostic Procedures
These laboratory results were obtained on admission: blood glucose level of 620 mg/dL, carbon dioxide concentration of 11 mEq/L, and pH of 7.25. Ketones were identified in the urine and blood.

Assessment of learning needs identified a deficit in understanding regarding glucose monitoring and insulin requirements while away from home.

Medical Diagnosis
Mr. S is diagnosed with diabetic ketoacidosis resulting from noncompliance.

Questions
1. What major outcomes do you expect to achieve for this patient?
2. What problems or risks must be managed to achieve these outcomes?
3. What interventions must be initiated to monitor, prevent, manage, or eliminate the problems and risks identified?
4. What interventions should be initiated to promote optimal functioning, safety, and well-being of the patient?
5. What possible learning needs do you anticipate for this patient?
6. What cultural and age-related factors may have a bearing on the patient's plan of care?

SUMMARY

- A collaborative, well-organized, need-targeted education plan of care is essential to improving health outcomes and decreasing lengths of stay.
- The teaching-learning process is a dynamic, continuous activity that occurs throughout the entire hospitalization and may continue after the patient has been discharged.
- Information must be gathered on many factors that may affect the education process: cultural or religious views of illness or death, emotional barriers, desire and motivation, physical or cognitive limitations, and barriers to effective communication.
- The learner's needs can be defined as gaps between what the learner knows and what the learner needs to know

(e.g., survival skills, coping skills, ability to make a care decision).

- Standardized education plans provide consistent interventions and outcomes; however, they must be individualized to meet the unique needs of the patient and family.
- The optimal environment for learning is one that is non-threatening, comfortable, open, and honest.
- Determination of an appropriate teaching strategy is essential to meet the needs of the patient.

- Providing information regarding the environment, procedures, sensations, and time of day is important for patients who are unconscious and may help to decrease immediate physiologic stress.
- When planning for the overall care of patients, nurses must consider the informational needs and emotional support of family members.
- It is important to prepare patients and families for transfers to other units to decrease stress and anxiety related to going to a less intensively monitored environment.

REFERENCES

1. The Joint Commission. *2012 Comprehensive Accreditation Manual for Hospitals.* Oakbrook Terrace, IL: The Joint Commission; 2004.
2. Davis N, et al. Improving the process of informed consent in the critically ill. *JAMA.* 2003;289(15):1963.
3. Leske J. Comparison of family stresses, strengths, and outcomes after trauma surgery. *AACN Clin Issues Crit Care.* 2003;14(1):33.
4. Bastable S. *Nurse as Educator: Principles of teaching and learning for nursing practice.* 3rd ed. Boston: Jones and Bartlett Publishers; 2008.
5. Rankin S, Stallings K, London F. *Patient Education in Health and Illness: Issues, Principles and Practice.* 5th ed. Philadelphia: JB Lippincott; 2005.
6. Wei H, Camargo C. Patient education in the emergency department. *Acad Emerg Med.* 2000;7(6):710.
7. Briggs L, et al. Patient-centered advance care planning in special patient populations a pilot study. *J Prof Nurs.* 2004;20(1):47.
8. Moorhead S, et al, eds. *Nursing Outcomes Classification (NOC).* 4th ed. St Louis: Mosby; 2012.
9. Burkhead V, et al. Enter: a care guide for successfully educating patients. *J Nurses Staff Dev.* 2003;19(3):143.
10. London F. *No Time to Teach.* Philadelphia: JB Lippincott; 1999.
11. Gentz C. Perceived learning needs of the patient undergoing coronary angioplasty: an integrative review of the literature. *Heart Lung.* 2000;29(3):161.
12. Phillips LD. Patient education: understanding the process to maximize time and outcomes. *J Intraven Nurs.* 1999;22(1):19.
13. Glittenburg J. A transdisciplinary, transcultural model for health care. *J Trans Nurs.* 2004;15(1):6.
14. Walsh S. Formulation of a plan of care for culturally diverse patients. *Int J Nurs Terminol Classif.* 1999;15(1):17.
15. Giger JM. *Transcultural Nursing: Assessment and Interventions.* 6th ed. St. Louis: Mosby; 2012.
16. Suh EE. The model of cultural competence through an evolutional concept analysis. *J Trans Nurs.* 2004;15(2):93.
17. Blount KA, Moore LA. Medications and the elderly. *Crit Care Nurs Clin North Am.* 2002;14(1):111.
18. Knowles MS. *The Modern Practice of Adult Education: From Pedagogy to Andragogy.* New York: Cambridge Books; 1976.
19. Ruzicki D. Realistically meeting the educational needs of hospitalized acute and short stay patients. *Nurs Clin North Am.* 1989;24(3):629.
20. Institute of Medicine. *Health literacy: a prescription to end confusion.* Washington, DC: National Academies Press; 2004.
21. Egbert M, Nanna KM. Health literacy: challenges and strategies. http://nursingworld.org/MainMenuCategories/ANAMarketplace/ANAPeriodicals/OJIN/TableofContents/Vol142009/No3Sept09/Health-Literacy-Challenges.html. Accessed April 28, 2012.
22. Glassman P. Health literacy. http://nnlm.gov/outreach/consumer/hlthlit.html. Accessed April 28, 2012.
23. Wilson J. The crucial link between literacy and health. *Ann Intern Med.* 2003;139(10):875.
24. Moore, V. Assessing health literacy. *J Nurse Practitioners.* 2012;8(3):243.
25. Leske JS. Protocols for practice: applying research at the bedside. *Crit Care Nurs.* 1998;18(4):92.
26. VanHorn E, et al. Family interventions during the trajectory of recovery from cardiac event: an integrative literature review. *Heart Lung.* 2002;31(3):186.
27. An K, et al. A cross-sectional examination of changes in anxiety early after acute myocardial infarction. *Heart Lung.* 2004;33(2):75.
28. Leske JS. Family stresses, strengths, and outcomes after critical injury. *Crit Care Nurs Clin North Am.* 2000;12(2):237.
29. Lazarus RS, Folkman S. *Stress, Appraisal, and Coping.* New York: Springer; 1984.
30. Thomas L. Clinical management of stressors perceived by patients on mechanical ventilation. *AACN Clin Issues Crit Care.* 2003;14(1):73.
31. Laubach E. How to communicate with seriously ill patients. *Nurs Manage.* 2000;31(4):24H.
32. Leske J. Overview of family needs after critical illness: from assessment to intervention. *AACN Clin Issues Crit Care.* 1991;2(2):220.
33. Saunders R. Constructing a lesson plan. *J Nurses Staff Dev.* 2003;19(2):70.
34. Bulechek GM, et al, eds. *Nursing Interventions Classification (NIC).* 6th ed. St. Louis: Mosby; 2013.
35. Benner C, et al. *From Beginner to Expert: Excellence and Power in Clinical Nurse Practice.* Menlo Park: Addison-Wesley; 1984.
36. Clark P, Dunbar S. Family partnership intervention: a guide for family approach to care of patients with heart failure. *AACN Clin Issues.* 2003;14(4):467.
37. Doak C, et al. Improving comprehension for cancer patients with low literacy skills: strategies for clinicians. *CA Cancer J Clin.* 1998;38(3):151.
38. Falvo D. *Effective Patient Education: A Guide to Increased Adherence.* Boston: Jones and Bartlett Publishing; 2011.
39. Kingbeil C, et al. Readability of pediatric patient education materials. *Clin Pediatr.* 1995;34(2):96.
40. Hodgdon, L. *Visual Strategies for Improving Communication: Supports for School and Home.* Troy, MI: QuirkRoberts Publishing; 2001.

41. Houts P, et al. The role of pictures in improving health communication: a review of research on attention. *Patient Educ Couns*. 2006;61:173.

42. Peregrin T. Picture this: visual cues enhance health education messages for people with low literacy skills. *J ADA*. 2010;110(5):S28.

43. Jones J. Patient education and the use of the Internet. *Clin Nurs Spec*. 2003;17(6):281.

44. Mikkelson H. The art of working with interpreters: a manual for health care professionals. http://www.acebo.com/papers/artintrp.htm. Accessed April 28, 2012.

45. Techniques for educating with the aid of an interpreter. *Patient Educ Manag*. 2007;77.

46. Happ MB, et al. Electronic voice-output communication aids for temporarily non-speaking patients in a medical intensive care unit: a feasibility study. *Heart Lung*. 2004;33(2):92.

47. Speros C. More than words: promoting health literacy in older adults. *Online J Issues Nurs*. 2009;14(3).

48. Thomas M, ed. Lack of compliance may mean patients don't understand. *Case Management Advisor*. 2009;20(8):85.

49. Russell C, Freiburghaus M. Heart transplant patient teaching documentation. *Clin Nurs Spec*. 2004;17(5):249.

50. Bruccoliere T. How to make patient teaching stick. *RN*. 2000;63(2):34.

51. Wu JR, et al. Factors influencing medication adherence in patients with heart failure. *Heart Lung*. 2008;37(1):8.

52. Doering LV, et al. Recovering from cardiac surgery: what patients want to know. *Am J Crit Care*. 2002;11(4):333.

53. Henneman EA, et al. An evaluation of interventions for meeting the information needs of families of critically ill patients. *Am J Crit Care*. 1993;1(3):85.

54. Miracle VA, Hovenkamp G. Needs of families of patients undergoing invasive cardiac procedures. *Am J Crit Care*. 1994;3(3):155.

55. White SK, Edwards RJ. Visitation guidelines promote safe satisfying environments. *Nurs Manage*. 2006;37(8):21.

56. Radtke A. Telemetry monitoring: a preferred solution for intermediate care. *Nurs Manage*. 2006;37(12):52.

57. Mages ME. Helping patients, helping families. *Healthc Exec*. 2006;11(4):40.

6

Psychosocial and Spiritual Alterations and Management

Valerie Yancey

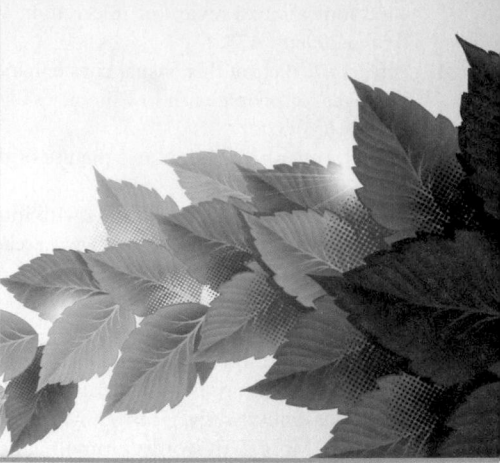

Patients are admitted to critical care units because they need physiologic rescue. Life or death depends on restoring physiologic homeostasis through the use of highly technical interventions carried out by a competent critical care team. When a person is seriously ill or injured, however, it is not just the body that suffers. An experience of critical illness impacts the whole person—body, mind, and spirit. While not as readily measured as physical parameters, psychologic and spiritual variables significantly impact outcomes in physically compromised and vulnerable patients. Psychologic and spiritual interventions have the power to engage a patient's hope, energy, will to survive, and his or her ability to meet life's challenges.[1] This chapter provides a discussion of the psychosocial-spiritual challenges encountered by critically ill patients and offers holistic nursing interventions for helping patients and family members cope effectively and thrive during a stressful experience.

Nursing diagnoses related to psychologic, social, and spiritual health are discussed. Relevant nursing diagnoses include stress overload, risk for post-trauma syndrome, anxiety, compromised individual or family coping, disturbed body image, situational low self-esteem, hopelessness, powerlessness, risk for compromised human dignity, and spiritual distress.[2] The chapter also provides an overview of holistic nursing responses to the psychosocial and spiritual needs of critically ill patients. Critical care nurses provide psychosocial-spiritual care by communicating with compassion and understanding, practicing dignity-enhancing care, supporting patient coping, using a family-centered focus, and engaging spiritual resources. In a problem-oriented environment like a critical care unit, nurses should remember that acute events also have the

potential to surface patient strengths and trigger a readiness for spiritual well-being and enhanced hope. Finally, providing meaningful person-to-person psychologic and spiritual care also depends, in part, on the nurse's own psychologic health and spiritual well-being. It is not possible to give what one does not have. A discussion of critical care nurses' self-care concludes the chapter.

STRESS AND PSYCHONEUROIMMUNOLOGY

The term "stress" is often used to indicate a negative experience or internal tension. While living with chronic stress can contribute to numerous health problems over time,[3,4,5] an acute stress response is an essential, protective, inherent reaction to a stressor, designed to mobilize the body's response to threats, actual or perceived, for purposes of survival. Stress is a nonspecific response to any demand placed on a person to adapt or change, and can come from physical, emotional, social, spiritual, cultural, chemical, or environmental sources.[6,7]

The nursing diagnosis "stress overload" refers to excessive amounts and types of demands that require action. The stressors are experienced as a problem and contribute to the development of other problems.[8] Stress overload should be differentiated from other stress-related nursing diagnoses discussed in this chapter—anxiety, fear, low self-esteem, hopelessness, powerlessness, spiritual distress, or ineffective coping. Stress overload does not occur because the patient or family members have coping deficits or psychologic disorders. Rather, the stressors of critical illness are so numerous and severe, people become overwhelmed. The appropriate nursing response to patients at risk

---

for stress overload is to reduce the number or types of stressors that patients experience.

To respond appropriately to patients at risk for stress overload, nurses must first become aware of the many stressors faced by critical care patients (Box 6-1). Normal life patterns are disrupted and patients experience alterations in their bodily functions, social roles, job status, and finances. They are in strange, frightening, and restrictive environments. Critically ill patients report distressing bodily reactions, deprivation of control, fear of medical equipment, loss of meaning, and relationship disturbances during and after treatment in a critical care unit.[9] They are subjected to painful procedures, abrupt or continual noises, loss of privacy, sleep interruptions, pain, medications, isolation, and minimal contact with loved ones.[10,11] Lack of sleep and interrupted sleep-wake cycles depress mood and immune functions.[12] Sources of stress overload described in the literature include worry about life events, illness, social factors, low educational level or lack of education, poverty, severe emotional responses, lack of resources, and environmental threats.[8]

Stress Response

Stress of any type—whether positive or negative, biologic, psychologic, spiritual, or social—elicits the same physical responses.[7] Classic stress theorists describe stress as a stimulus, a response, and a transaction.[13-16] Selye, in his pioneering work,[13] described the body's responses to a stressor the "general adaptation syndrome" (GAS), characterized by three stages: alarm reaction, resistance, and exhaustion. An alarm reaction is initiated by the hypothalamus, which upon receiving sensory and chemical information regarding the presence of a stressor signals the release of corticotrophin-releasing factor (CRF). The pituitary gland, signaled by CRF, releases stress hormones: cortisol and aldosterone. The sympathetic nervous division of the autonomic nervous system (ANS) releases neurotransmitters and endocrine hormones associated with an acute stress response. Known as the "fight or flight" response, an alarm reaction triggers highly integrated cardiovascular and endocrine changes, evidenced by elevations in blood pressure, respiratory rate, heart rate, systemic vascular resistance, and glucose production, sweating, tremors, and nausea. During the resistance stage, the person's systems fight back, leading to adaptation and a return of normal functioning. If the stressors continue, exhaustion occurs, a stage in which reserves have been depleted. Reversal of stress exhaustion can be accomplished by restoration of one's reserves through the use of medications, nutrition, and other stress-reduction measures.

Nuerberger[16] first described the process of "shutting down," a person's eventual emotional response to a stressor that results from overstimulation of the parasympathetic nervous system. He labeled this survival tactic the general inhibition syndrome (GIS), or the "possum response." Defense mechanisms such as withdrawal, avoidance, and detachment are typical behaviors associated with this type of response.[14,17] Both sympathetic and parasympathetic nervous system responses are innate and protective, but prolonged stimulation or imbalances in either response can be detrimental. Sustained or frequent sympathetic nervous system arousal places added physiologic burdens on a compromised critical care patient. Similarly, an exhausted patient lacks the reserves necessary to recover from the demands of illness or injury.

Psychoneuroimmunology

The idea of complex, multifactorial interactions between persons and their internal and external environments first described by stress theorists has led to an area of multidisciplinary study known as psychoneuroimmunology (PNI). PNI research verifies, measures, and explicates the intricate interactions between a person's psyche, and his or her neural, endocrine, and immune systems.[18,19,20] PNI is based on the understanding that health and well-being are not simply physiologic processes, but rather are expressions of a person's emotions, personality traits, social connections, health behaviors, social environments, and spiritual life. Instead of thinking of the mind being located in the brain, PNI theory posits that the whole human organism "knows," has a memory, and reacts to sensory input and interpretations of life in every cell of the body. Psychologic stressors and emotional states, experienced in the mind (consciousness), trigger a series of physiologic reactions. Sensory input and environmental cues are interpreted and appraised in the prefrontal cortex of the brain, association areas, and the hippocampus. The content of the appraisal of the threat generates specific emotional states, which initiate autonomic and endocrine responses and outflow. The autonomic responses also send feedback to the cortex and limbic systems.[6]

Behavior and emotions profoundly impact the immune system. Negative psychologic states are associated with decreased lymphocyte proliferation, natural killer cell activity, and the number of white blood cells, and change the amount of antibodies in circulation and antibody produced after exposure to a harmful substance.[21] The multiple stressors faced by critical care patients become bodily chemistry, impacting their cardiovascular, neurologic, endocrine, and immune systems. An interpretation of words a patient hears, or the anticipation of a procedure can generate a stress response as if it were actually happening. PNI theory posits that actions to promote psychologic and spiritual well-being have healing potential and profoundly impact a person's immune system.[19,22] PNI posits a world view that serves as a foundation for holistic critical care nursing based on interpersonal connection, empathy, and compassion.

POST-TRAUMATIC STRESS REACTIONS

Increasingly, clinicians and researchers have begun to describe the frequency and nature of acute stress reactions, panic attacks, or post-traumatic stress disorder (PTSD) experienced by patients after discharge from critical care units.[23,24,25] Even though post-traumatic reactions occur from several weeks to years after an event, critical care nurses should be aware of the possibility of PTSD reactions after critical care for purposes of recognizing and reducing all unnecessary stressors during a patient's stay, being alert to patients at higher risk for developing PTSD, and by using psychosocial-spiritual interventions to reduce the occurrence of PTSD in the critical care patient population. A patient may survive a critical illness, only to face an even greater challenge on the road to recovery after leaving the critical care unit.

The actual incidence and nature of PTSD symptoms in the critical care population has not yet been fully determined. The problem is serious enough, however, to demand the attention of critical care professionals. Published studies report a wide range, from 5%-63%, of critical care patients experiencing PTSD symptoms of varying degrees.[26] Numerous studies indicate that patients with PTSD are at risk for developing other mental health problems and physical illnesses.[26,27]

Labeling post-traumatic stress reactions a "disorder" misrepresents the true nature of the phenomenon. As with stress overload, PTSD is not a disordered response to stress resulting from a failure of a person's will, strength, endurance, or courage. The stress response is automatic and essential for survival. If threats to survival are multiple and relentless, without adequate time for recovery time, it is difficult for brain and body chemistry to quickly adjust. PTSD should be thought of as a "normal" response to abnormal and impossible demands. Post-traumatic stress responses, however, manifest as multiple distressing symptoms.

Classified often as an anxiety disorder, post-traumatic stress reactions involve a wide range of cardiovascular, neuromuscular, gastrointestinal, cognitive, emotional, mood, and memory responses.[25,28] After an exposure to a traumatic event of any sort, people may experience unbidden, intrusive recall of the distressing event often triggered by a noise, sound, sight, smell, event, or memory that produces an acute stress response. Nightmares and delusional memories, during which a trauma is re-experienced, provoke intense psychologic and physiologic distress. People with PTSD can also exhibit numbing responses, including detachment, isolation, restricted affect, and depression. States of hyperactivity lead to sleep disturbances, hypervigilance, nervous, and repetitive behaviors. Cognitively, stress reactions lead to difficulty concentrating, poor executive function, and impaired decision making.

Griffiths and Jones, summarizing 20 years of follow-up with critical care unit survivors, discuss the importance of the quality and types of patients' memories of their critical care experience.[28] Even though most critical care patients have poor factual recall or amnesia related to their stay, they often live with delusional, paranoid, or nonfactual memories or create false substitute interpretations and experiences. Nightmares and delusional recall result in PTSD symptoms for a significant number of patients and can cause problems as they attempt to construct a realistic understanding of their recovery.[29]

Family members are also at risk for developing post-traumatic stress reactions[30-31] related to prolonged periods of uncertainty, anxious waiting, disrupted sleep patterns, financial concerns, witnessing emergency interventions, and confronting fears of loss and death. Koss et al[32] report both depression and higher rates of PTSD in family members of patients who die during a critical care admission. Also at higher risk are family members of younger patients and those for whom mechanical ventilation is not withdrawn.

Critical care nurses can engage in health-promotion activities related to preventing post-traumatic stress reactions in patients and family members. Being aware of the possibility for stress overload in critical care settings is the first step. Care providers should then take steps to manage or eliminate as many of those stressors as possible. Often patients are unaware or uncertain of what has happened to them and their bodily function. Nurses should engage in encouraging but realistic discussions of the patient's experiences, explain events carefully, and talk openly about recovery timelines and the gradual process of regaining strength. Certain populations are at greater risk for developing PTSD. Independent of case mix or illness severity, researchers identify patients of younger age, those with delusional memories, pre-existing mental health problems, and physical restraints without sedation as conditions known to increase risk for PTSD symptoms.[25,28] While inconclusive, research into the relationship between PTSD symptoms and the duration and degree of sedation used in critical care highlights the need to consider the impact of all critical care practices on long-term outcomes.[33,34] Another study notes that pessimism is a predictor of post-discharge stress reactions.[35] Although the process of identifying PTSD risk and symptoms is complex and multidimensional, screening questionnaires have been developed and tested for initially evaluating risk for PTSD soon after discharge.[36]

Patient and family members usually recall and interpret the events, decisions, and time sequences involved in a critical care stay differently. Keeping a diary with photographs taken during a patient's stay in the critical care unit can help patients and family members reach a degree of shared common ownership of the experience. Journal review helps patients understand what happened so they can better come to terms with their illness and their recovery process.[37,38] In learning to live with the memories of critical care, patients benefit when they can construct a meaningful story.[39] The interventions described in this chapter not only support patients while they are in the unit, they are also designed to support patients' well-being over time, preparing them for the challenges of rehabilitation and recovery.

ANXIETY

Anxiety is a normal and common subjective human response to a perceived or actual threat, which can range from a vague, generalized feeling of discomfort to a state of panic and loss of control. Feelings of anxiety are common in critically ill patients but are often undetected by care providers.[40] In a study of 171 patients with high risk for dying in critical care units, 58% reported feeling anxiety of a moderate level of intensity.[41] Anxiety and agitation in critical care patients can complicate patient recovery due to unplanned extubations,[42] shortness of breath episodes, and behavioral changes.

The physiologic effects of anxiety can produce negative effects in critically ill patients by activating the sympathetic nervous system and hypothalamic-pituitary-adrenal axis. Anxiety elicits changes in the neurohumoral release patterns involving the neurotransmitters in the brain that regulate mood—including acetylcholine, norepinephrine, dopamine, and serotonin and gamma-aminobutyric acid (GABA)—and their corresponding receptors. The neurotransmitters' complex and elusive integration of these responses within the central nervous system relies on communication among the cerebral cortex, limbic system, thalamus, hypothalamus, pituitary gland, and the reticular activating system. The cortex is involved with cognition, attention, and alertness, whereas emotional responses to stress are located in the limbic system. Corticotropin-releasing factor (CRF) controls the endocrine response and the norepinephrine pathway that is active in regulating the sympathetic branch of the ANS. A positive feedback loop between the CRF and the ANS occurs when increased activation in one system influences the other system. It is also proposed that large amounts of circulating CRF can accelerate behavioral responses (i.e., anxiety and hypersensitivity) to stressful stimuli.[17] As anxiety levels increase, a patient experiences the physiologic effects of sympathetic nervous system stimulation with feelings of excitement and heightened awareness, followed by a diminishment of his or her perceptual field, problem-solving abilities, and coping skills. Panic attacks, a manifestation of severe anxiety not uncommon in critical care patients, can produce an acute stress response with tachycardia, hyperventilation, and dyspnea. Pharmacologic interventions for acute anxiety include the use of benzodiazepines, antihistamines, noradrenergic agents, antidepressants, and anxiolytics.[17]

The stressful experiences of having an acute or chronic illness, facing a real or anticipated loss, being admitted or discharged from a critical care unit, or requiring mechanical ventilation can trigger high degrees of patient anxiety.[43,44,45] Research also suggests that women, patients with less social support, and those with longer critical care length of stay are at higher risk for developing anxiety upon transfer out of the unit to a less intense level of care.[45,46] Whether the causes of anxiety are biochemical, genetic, emotional, or driven by the threats inherent in the situation, the critical care nurse should consider all contributing factors if interventions are to be effective.

Although rates of moderate to high anxiety exist in critical care patients, leading to higher complication rates,[47] valid and reliable methods to assess anxiety have not been put into practice. Critical care nurses most often rely on behavioral indicators such as agitation and restlessness and physiologic parameters such as increased heart rate and blood pressure.[48] Behavioral or vital sign changes do not provide consistently reliable indicators of anxiety and may lead to underestimation of the extent of anxiety in critical care patients.[46] The literature on anxiety in critical care patients cites over 50 clinical indicators, many of which are nonspecific or can be associated with multiple causes.[48] Using valid scales for evaluating patients' self-perceived anxiety levels can be helpful in determining the level and extent of anxiety.[40,47,48] See also Appendix A, Nursing Management Plan: Anxiety.

Anxiety and Pain

Of particular importance in the critical care setting is the cyclic relationship between levels of anxiety and perceptions and tolerance of pain. Pain triggers anxiety, and increased anxiety intensifies pain experiences. This reciprocal relationship varies, depending on whether pain is produced by disease processes or invasive procedures, is acute or chronic in nature, or if the pain is anticipated. In critical care, pain experiences arise from many sources, including injured tissues, immobility, pre-existing and chronic pain conditions, intubation, diagnostic or treatment procedures, bright lights, excessive noise, and interrupted sleep. When pain or a discomfort such as nausea is severe enough, patients try to conserve energy and focus inwardly to gain control of their pain and anxiety. They may startle easily, become irritable, display anger, be vigilant and wary of caregivers, or may be perceived as demanding. An overwhelmed patient often withdraws from interpersonal contact.[17,49] In situations of pain-induced anxiety, the nurse must identify the source of the pain, validate observations with the patient, and initiate pain-management strategies. Medications such as theophylline, anticholinergics, dopamine, levodopa, salicylates, and steroids can also contribute to feelings of anxiety[49,50] (see Chapter 9).

ALTERATIONS IN SELF-CONCEPT

The stressors imposed by serious illness, trauma, and surgical procedures can cause disturbances in the self-concept. Self-concept can be defined as the values, beliefs, and ideas that form a person's self-knowledge and influence relationships with others. One's self-concept is unique to the individual and is developed through perceptions of his or her own characteristics and abilities, goals, and ideals, interactions with others and the environment, and how those interactions are valued. One's self-concept also includes body image, self-esteem, and self-identity.[17,51]

People must make adjustments to their self-concept or role limitations when life circumstances necessitate change. Patients admitted to critical care settings may experience self-concept challenges, perceiving themselves to be viewed by others as a problem, as only their disease, or as a patient instead of as a person.[51] Patients in critical care units usually do not have time to adjust to their altered health status. They may exhibit early signs of a response to loss or disability, including shock, numbness, and avoidance of reality and they may be unable to clearly understand the implications of the situation.[17,52] Self-concept constructs of particular relevance for critical care patients include body image, self-esteem, and identity disturbance.

Body Image

One's body is central to self-concept. Body image is the mental picture an individual has of his or her body and its physical functioning at a given time. Body image includes attitudes and feelings about one's appearance, body build, health, performance, ability, and gender. A person's body image develops over time, influenced by contact with people and the environment, emotional experiences, and fantasies. Body image is dynamic and changes based on present and past perceptions and experiences.[17,53]

When ill, inevitably a person knows that experience as a body. In their classic description of the impact of stress and coping on health and illness, Benner and Wrubel[54] note that a person does not just *have* a body; rather he or she *is* a body. The experiences of being ill are "embodied" and are stored in bodily memory. Often bodily sensations in a state of illness do not make sense to the patient, which creates a cascade of stress responses.[9] Patients in critical care units are subjected to prolonged periods of lying in bed, position disorientation, sensory deprivation, muscle atrophy, changed metabolic patterns, mechanical ventilation, pain, profound weakness,[28] nutritional alterations, and medication-induced physical symptoms. Disturbances in body image in critical care arise when the person fails to perceive or adapt to the changes that are imposed by the situation. In some instances, the person may feel betrayed by his or her body, which no longer seems normal. Body image issues, of course, often emerge and resolve over time, but critical care nurses begin the process of helping the patient live with a change in bodily appearance or function. A more keen awareness of the embodied nature of a patient's experiences will help nurses attune to the patient's bodily perceptions of all nursing activities. See Appendix A, Nursing Management Plan: Disturbed Body Image.

Self-Esteem

Self-esteem refers to how well one's behavior correlates with a sense of the ideal self and is most closely linked to one's sense of self-worth.[17] Maslow, one early theorist of human flourishing, identified self-esteem and actualization as an important component in his hierarchy of human needs.[55] Having high self-esteem helps a person deal with maturational and situational life crises more easily.

Self-esteem has been studied in a variety of contexts. Because nurses interact with patients so intimately and frequently, it is important that nurses develop a deeper appreciation of the impact of self-esteem on a patient's energy, recovery, and sense of self-efficacy. Illness robs a person of perspective, often leading to low self-esteem and feelings of powerlessness, helplessness, and depression.[56] Low self-esteem impairs one's ability to adapt. A patient may refuse to participate in self-care, exhibit self-destructive behavior, or become too compliant—asking no questions and permitting others to make all decisions.[52,56] A comprehensive approach to recovery includes the provision of ongoing supportive measures designed to help patients maintain self-esteem and a healthy body image. See Appendix A, Nursing Management Plan: Situational Low Self-Esteem.

Identity Disturbance

A personal identity disturbance, as a type of altered self-concept, is defined as an inability of a person to differentiate the self as a unique and separate human being from others within a social environment. The sense of depersonalization that accompanies identity disturbance engenders a high level of anxiety. Personal identity disturbance can result from the effects of psychoactive medications, biochemical imbalances in the brain, and organic brain disorders, dementia, traumatic brain injury, amnesia, or delirium (see Chapter 10). A careful nursing assessment, including the use of psychiatric or neurologic consultation, is essential in cases of identity disturbance. Disorientation and confusion, common in patients in critical care settings, are influenced by several factors, including the severity of the physical problem, chemical imbalances, sensory overload or deprivation, and previous illness or health care experiences.

RISK FOR COMPROMISED HUMAN DIGNITY

A sense of the dignity of the person underlies considerations of self-concept, body image, and self-esteem. The underlying purpose of all interactions with patients and family members is to bring them to restored health. When people are treated with dignity and respect, they are put in the best position to recover their health and well-being.[57]

When patients enter the health care system, including critical care units, they bring with them their diseases, defects, inadequacies, and shortcomings. Their bodily or psychologic "failures" have brought them into relationship with health care providers. During a health care encounter, patients are subjected to intense physical, psychologic, and lifestyle scrutiny. They feel literally and figuratively exposed. Patients' own disappointment and regrets are magnified when they experience the concern, effort, and emphasis placed on their failing health, leading to self-critical feelings.

Lazare's[58] insightful description of the shame and humiliation patients experience in medical encounters has provoked an analysis of health care culture. Moral philosophers point to the "rules of cultural systems" as a source for the unintended but distressing experiences of shame, embarrassment, and humiliation experienced by patients and providers when giving and receiving medical care. The rules of cultural systems are notably present in critical care environments: objectification of the person (for more precise physiologic management), disempowerment, distancing the self from the experience of others, indifference, and dissociation. The authority of the medical model supersedes patient experiences, interpretations, and meanings.[59] The rules of cultural systems determine, in part, the behaviors of the people within a culture. Although health care providers do not intend to humiliate patients, they become accustomed to the cultural attitudes and circumstances that diminish patients' dignity on a daily basis.

A sense of dignity includes a person's positive self-regard, an ability to invest in and gain strength from one's own meaning in life, feeling valued by others, and how one is treated by caregivers. Chochinov's[60] model for dignity-conserving care identifies sources of threats to dignity inherent in health care contexts, including the level of a person's independence and his or her symptom distress. Patients in most acute care settings, especially critical care, must by necessity give up those things that give them a sense of self: clothing, daily habits, and privacy. Their bodies are frequently exposed to people who inspect them for their pathology and irregularities. Often patients cannot communicate their preferences, or give permission for assessments, tests, or interventions. Family members and friends have restricted access to patients due to environmental constraints. Stripped of everything that communicates personal identity, patients are known as their pathologies instead of as a person with a history and hopes for a future. When caregivers become more aware of their own feelings and humanity in an exchange, they are less often to unintentionally minimize patients' emotions and experiences.[59]

SPIRITUAL CHALLENGES IN CRITICAL CARE

Many of the psychosocial issues already discussed—stress, anxiety, self-concept, body image, self-esteem, coping, dignity, and relationships with others—are rooted in the spiritual dimension of life, the seat of a person's deepest meanings and ground of being. One's spiritual dimension encompasses those elements of life that provide meaning, purpose, hope, and connectedness to others and a higher power.[56,61,62] Providing spiritual care is essential for patient recovery in critical care units.

Spiritual Distress

Spiritual distress has been defined as a disruption in the life principle that pervades a person's entire being and that integrates and transcends one's biologic and psychosocial nature.[56] Threats of physiologic or psychologic illness, prolonged pain, and suffering can challenge a person's spirituality. Separation from one's meaningful religious or spiritual practices and rituals, coupled with intense suffering, can induce spiritual distress for patients and their families. Patients experiencing spiritual distress may question the meaning of suffering and death in relation to their personal belief system. They may wonder why the illness or injury has happened to them or may fear that what they have believed in has failed them in the time of greatest need. Some individuals in spiritual despair may question their existence, verbalize their wish to die, or display anger toward

religious traditions. Unresolved spiritual distress is interpreted in the body as a stressor. Prolonged spiritual distress may lead to a sense of hopelessness, unwillingness to seek further treatment, or consent to therapeutic interventions or regimens.[56]

Hope and Hopelessness

Hope is a subjective, dynamic internal process essential to life. Considered to be a spiritual process, hope is an energy that arises out of a sense of being meaningfully connected to one's self, others, and powers greater than the self. With hope, a person is able to transition from a state of vulnerability to a point of being able to live as fully as possible.[63] The need for hope is stimulated by a demand to adapt or change in unexpected situations, as is the case for people who are critical ill. The desire to maintain hope underlies many coping mechanisms. When people have hope and belief in their goals, they are empowered to engage in their own recovery with a sense of internal peace and freedom. While hope has a future orientation, it also has a present orientation that impacts people in the here and now.[64] We have come to understand, through observations of people in extreme circumstances, that an element of hope must be maintained for survival[65] and is an essential component in the successful treatment of illness.[66]

By contrast, hopelessness is a subjective state in which an individual sees extremely limited or no alternatives and is unable to mobilize energy on his or her own behalf.[49,56] Feelings of hopelessness can greatly hinder recovery. Conditions that increase a person's risk for feeling hopeless include a loss of dignity, long-term stress, loss of self-esteem, spiritual distress, and isolation, all of which can be present in a critical care experience. Patients who feel hopeless may be less involved in their recovery, may withdraw from the support of others, and lack the energy and initiative to engage in increasing degrees of self-care.[56]

Loss of Control and Powerlessness

Many patients admitted to a critical care unit have experienced a rapid onset of illness or an injury and have not had time to adjust to the limits of their changed circumstances. They have to adapt quickly to a loss of control. The loss of control in critical care hospitalization can be as minor as not getting a preferred food or as serious as experiencing a radical loss of a sense of self. Control, a person's ability to determine the use of time, space, and resources, becomes compromised in the critical care unit. On admission to a hospital, people forfeit much of their independence as they become patients. Choice of clothing and use of other personal belongings are usually restricted in a critical care unit. Patients cannot decide who enters the room, who provides personal care, or who intrudes with painful treatments. Hospital rules are usually not open to modification.

Rotter's early research[67] on human behavior and perception of control has been helpful in explaining the wide range of responses people have in situations in which they must give up control. Rotter suggests that a person's locus of control is internally or externally focused. Individuals who have an internal locus of control perceive themselves to be responsible for the outcome of events. Individuals with an external locus of control believe that their actions will have no effect on the outcome of a situation. Furthermore, as with any highly individualized concept, people vary in the amount of control they prefer.

Patients who have a pervasive sense that they can do nothing to change or control their circumstances are at risk for feeling powerless.[52,56] Critically ill people can experience powerlessness due to the constraints of their health and the care environment, a loss of meaningful interpersonal interactions with their usual support system, inability to maintain cultural or religious beliefs and practices, or by adopting a helpless coping style. The degree of powerlessness a person experiences depends on his or her perceived sense of control, the type of loss that was experienced, and the availability of social support. Powerlessness can be manifested by a refusal to participate in decision making, disengagement from plan of care, expressions of self-doubt, or a seeming lack of interest in recovery. Frustration, anger, and resentment over being dependent on others often occur and are exhibited in verbal expressions regarding dissatisfaction with care.[56] Poor interactions with health care providers who are perceived as imposing restrictions can make the situation worse. Patients may react aggressively, may try bargaining, or may refuse to comply with diagnostic and treatment regimens. Patients may lose sight of those areas of life over which they still maintain some influence because so much control has been taken from them. See Appendix A, Nursing Management Plan: Powerlessness.

COPING WITH STRESS AND ILLNESS

Coping mechanisms are intentional processes used to adjust, adapt, and successfully meet life stressors. Each patient's response to stress is unique and depends on a variety of environmental factors and individual differences, including cognitive variables, one's place in the life cycle, degree of social support, and the person's perception of the nature of the stressor or loss.[17]

If a patient is coping effectively, he or she appears relatively comfortable with self and others, is able to form a valid appraisal of stressors, makes decisions consistent with his or her own preferences and values, and has access to needed resources. Effective coping mechanisms help a person maintain a perception of an acceptable degree of control, empower him or her to take necessary actions, share concerns, use healthy denial, and manage troublesome life challenges and uncertainties (see Chapter 11). Most people have a repertoire of coping mechanisms to manage stressful situations and life challenges. Coping mechanisms are learned and practiced over a lifetime and are based on the person's sense of the effectiveness of any given strategy for adapting to the stressor.[53]

Ineffective coping is defined as the impairment of a person's adaptive behaviors and problem-solving abilities when meeting life's demands and necessary roles. Manifestations of ineffective coping in critical illness include verbalization of an inability to cope, anxiety, and being unable to meet basic needs. The patient exhibits inappropriate use of defense mechanisms and has diminished problem-solving abilities. The patient may display apathy or destructive behavior toward self and others.

A person's coping mechanisms may or may not be effective, depending on the nature and seriousness of the challenge being faced, his or her prior experience with a similar situation, or the extent to which the coping mechanism can be used in given situation. For example, a person may ordinarily cope with a distressing situation by careful problem analysis, information gathering, talking things over, and getting some refreshing sleep. That person will likely have a sense of ineffective coping when facing the lack of control characteristic of acute illness and critical care environments: inability to speak or process information, sleep interruptions, diminished access to resources, or limited time to make careful deliberations. Common effective coping responses can be problem focused, cognitively focused, or emotionally focused. Coping methods include physical exercise, meditation, prayer, healthful foods, social support, positive self-talk, reframing, time management, counseling, new skill-building, and the use of spiritual and religious rituals.[17,53]

Use of Psychologic Defense Mechanisms

The overuse of psychologic defense mechanisms may give evidence of ineffective patient or family coping. Defense mechanisms are automatic self-protective measures developed in response to an internal or external stressor and may be evident when patients or family members feel out of control and unable to cope.[64] Unrelenting anger, excessive protectiveness, distrust of others, extreme dependence or regression, psychologic withdrawal, denial, or apathy concerning treatment goals may suggest that the stressors of the critical care experience have outstripped a person's coping abilities. Use of maladaptive measures may temporarily minimize anxiety but does not effectively or permanently resolve the conflict. Two common defense mechanisms especially evident in critical care settings include regression and denial.

Regression

Regression is an unconscious defense mechanism characterized by a retreat, in the face of stress, to behaviors characteristic of an earlier developmental level.[17] Regression allows a patient to give up his or her usual role, autonomy, and privacy to become the passive recipient of medical and nursing care. Admittedly, patients in critical care settings are expected to relinquish control and rely on others for even the most basic needs. To resist the care that others provide can jeopardize a patient's outcome. On the other hand, favorable patient outcomes and a speedy recovery can be threatened when patients regress to the point of relinquishing all control and responsibility for themselves to others and become excessively dependent on others. Behaviors such as whining, clinging to staff, needing the nurse constantly at the bedside, and giving evidence of an inability to self-modulate feelings of anxiety or fear can interfere with patient recovery and negatively affect nurse-patient relationships.

When expectations related to patient or family participation in self-care must be challenged or changed, patients are best served when limits and responsibilities are mutually determined and set in a supportive manner. Responses to patients will be more understanding when nurses recall that regression has been encouraged and expected at certain phases of a critical care stay, fear and anxiety have been reinforced in critical care experiences, and usual coping mechanisms have been abandoned. Although regressive behaviors can be frustrating to caregivers, avoid confrontations or reprimands. Threatening responses from staff may worsen a situation in which the patient is already struggling with issues of dependence, autonomy, and self-worth.

Denial

Denial is defined as the "conscious and unconscious attempts to disavow knowledge or the meaning of an event to reduce anxiety and fear."[2] Critically ill patients or their family members may use denial as a defense mechanism to protect against and manage an overwhelming sense of threat brought on by illness, injury, or impending death. As Weisman[69] notes in his classic work denial has both protective and potentially detrimental functions.

The degree to which denial is used varies from person to person or may vary in the same person at different times. An inability to face the realities of a potential health problem leads some people to deny various aspects of their illness or the significance of potentially serious symptoms. Denial can lead to delayed treatment or lack of awareness of the danger of a symptom. Family members, unable to cope with a loved one's serious, irreversible illness, may focus only on the possibility of a full recovery. They resist having realistic discussions concerning goals of care, insist on repeated resuscitation attempts, or invest in home remodeling in anticipation of a homecoming. They may regard caregivers who try to discuss anything other than a full recovery as being negative or untrustworthy people.

While it is common to be alert to the potentially negative aspects of ineffective denial, denial can serve as a valuable defense mechanism for people unable to absorb the full force of a loss or significant life change at a given time. Denial is protective, in that sense, and gives a person the psychologic space and time needed to process and accept the realities of a highly distressing loss.

Nurses may find it particularly difficult to communicate with people who seem to be using denial to their own detriment. It may seem to the caregiver that the person would cope better by facing the realities of a situation and by taking the steps needed to go on with life. Depending on the need people have to protect against their changing realities, they may or may not be readily influenced by information that contradicts their beliefs. Patients or family members who give evidence of firm or fixed denial are best supported by caregivers who understand that their denial is protective at this time, and who watch for cues that indicate a readiness to accept the reality of their situation.

Witnessing or responding therapeutically to problematic behavior can be challenging and uncomfortable, especially when the behavior seems to be directed at the caregiver. Critical care nurses should carefully evaluate their own response to what seems to be maladaptive behavior. Patients and family members are usually doing the best they can, under very stressful circumstances, and rely on the insight and understanding of caregivers who appreciate the complexities of stress, coping styles, and use of defensive mechanisms. A patient's stay in the critical care unit is only one phase in an often long journey to recovery from a serious health threat. Patients and family members need time to work through their experiences and often do so more effectively when they are given the support and encouragement they need during the acutely stressful events of being in a critical care unit. See Appendix A, Nursing Management Plan: Compromised Family Coping.

HOLISTIC PSYCHOSOCIAL-SPIRITUAL CARE

In addition to having sophisticated knowledge of anatomy and physiology, the pathophysiology of disease processes, and appropriate nursing interventions, the holistic critical care nurse also needs the knowledge, wisdom, and skills to interpret the internal human responses to experiences of serious illness or injury. Attention to the whole patient is the ultimate goal of nursing care, and is vitally important for critical care patients, families, and nurses. Nightingale believed that it was "unthinkable to consider sick humans as mere bodies who could be treated in isolation from their minds and spirits."[70] Essential skills that underlie nursing interventions for psychosocial-spiritual care include using communication patterns based on compassion and care, practicing dignity-enhancing care, supporting patient coping, using a family-centered focus, and engaging spiritual resources.

COMMUNICATE WITH COMPASSION AND CARE

Caring, compassionate verbal and nonverbal communication patterns give substance to nursing activities that promote expert psychosocial-spiritual care interventions. Nelson et al[71] describe the top challenges to providing care in the critical areas, especially for the very seriously ill. None of the top challenges had to do with technical issues of medical management. Instead, the top challenges include inadequate patterns of communication between the critical care team and family members, insufficient staff knowledge of effective communication, unrealistic family and provider expectations, family disagreements, lack of advance directives, voiceless patients, and suboptimal space for having meaningful conversations. Patients and family members rank their needs for communication with health care providers as one of the most important aspects of feeling cared for in the critical care setting,[72] especially in nonspeaking patients.[73,74] Interviews with patients after critical care revealed that they believed that a nurse's caring attitude led to more positive memories of their experience. Patients also reported less stress when they perceived nurses to be caring, warm, and competent, and when they communicated respect.[75] Many patients interpret a nurse's expressions of empathy and physical contact as evidence of caring and support.[76]

Many times sharing concerns with a caring and understanding listener can relieve emotional or spiritual distress. Patients are consoled knowing that they are not alone and when they sense that someone knows and cares about their feelings and experiences. Although the patient may share concerns with family members, she or he may be reluctant to upset loved ones and find that talking to a nurse seems more appropriate and emotionally safer. A patient who copes by talking to others will benefit from a nurse who recognizes when the patient needs to talk and who knows how to listen.[57,77]

Nurses should not avoid difficult conversations. Many patients need to talk about their fears and prefer conversations that balance their needs for honesty with their need to maintain hope.[76,78] It is also important to remember cultural differences in communicating with patients and family members. Many people in Western and American culture expect and value honesty and truth-telling in difficult situations. Patients and family members from other cultures may have taboos surrounding what should be discussed regarding the diagnosis and prognosis in serious illness.[79,80] Careful medical and nursing assessments, use of family and team conferences to foster communication, and enlisting the assistance of a spiritual counselor lead to more fruitful, understanding conversations in crisis and decision-making situations. Patients and family members in critical care areas need careful nurse-patient communication strategies (Box 6-2).

Trust

Effective verbal and nonverbal communication is essential for the development of trust in a nurse-patient relationship.[57] Trust manifests itself in critical care patients' belief that the people they depend on will get them through the illness and will be able to manage any untoward event that might occur. A patient needs to trust the nurse's competence in the physical and technical aspects of care and rely on what the nurse says. Patients are keen observers of their caregivers and read them well. Trust and hope are easily lessened when inappropriate information is given or nurses do not follow through on what they say. See also Appendix A, Nursing Management Plan: Impaired Verbal Communication.

PRACTICE DIGNITY-ENHANCING CARE

"The capacity to give one's attention to a sufferer is a very rare and difficult thing; it is almost a miracle; it is a miracle."[81] The practice of dignity-enhancing care is anchored in authentic human presence, the giving of one's whole attention and being to another person in a given moment. When authentically present, the nurse is able to go beyond relying only on scientific information and attunes him- or herself to patient needs, experiences, and emotions in a way that facilitates the patient's healing.[82]

Dignity-enhancing perspectives include the need a person has to maintain a continuity of the self, one's roles and legacy, and a sense of pride, hopefulness, control, acceptance, and resiliency. Dignity-enhancing care has four components: attitude, behaviors, compassion, and dialogue.[84] Caregivers' first step in providing dignity-conserving care involves reflecting on the attitudes and assumptions they hold about other people and their situations. The nurse's attitudes, worldviews, and beliefs about a patient or family member influence his or her openness and ability to develop a trusting relationship.

Dignity-enhancing care is manifest in behaviors. Attending to the patient's physical appearance affirms the person's self-esteem and a healthy body image. Cleanliness and absence of body odors give patients a sense of worth. When providing physical care, provide privacy, respect social boundaries, and ask permission before touching when possible. Validate the patient by giving importance to the things that he or she cares about. Spending time with patients as they share their life stories helps the nurse know the patient better and facilitates the development of individualized interventions. Show respect for patients by calling them by their preferred names or titles to help reinforce the patient's self-concept and identity. Obtain the patient's permission to include others in private conversations.

Compassion refers to the awareness of another person's suffering, coupled with a sincere intention to alleviate the suffering. In compassion, caregivers are able to identify with another person and recognize a shared humanity. Showing compassion can be quite simple, in acts of consideration, kindness, or a simple touch. Critical care nurses frequently touch people in the completion of procedures and caregiving activities. Keeping in mind individual and cultural differences, nurses should include nonprocedural touch in their care. The use of touch intended to communicate care and comfort can be an important part of patient healing and interpersonal connection. Compassion is also evidenced in dialogue, the fourth element of dignity-conserving care. At the most basic level, patients and family members need timely updates, explanations, repetition of unfamiliar information, and thorough information sharing. At a

---

BOX 6-2 STRATEGIES FOR COMMUNICATING WITH PATIENTS AND FAMILY MEMBERS

- Be patient. What is routine for caregivers can be stressful and new to patients and family members.
- Repeat information as many times as necessary. Stress reduces concentration, memory, and comprehension, especially in unfamiliar situations.
- Assess patient and family knowledge level and prior experience with critical care.
- Use understandable language and interpret medical terms, without talking down.
- Asking clarifying questions to help validate understanding.
- Use a welcoming, open communication style. Critical care units can feel intimidating to people unfamiliar with the environment.
- Offer frequent updates regarding patient's condition, even if not asked.
- Engage in conversations of meaning with patients and family members, even if brief. Often critical care conversations are reduced to conveying only technical aspects of care.
- Honor privacy and provide space for family conferences.
- Speak to patients, even if they are unconscious. This conveys caring to family and words may comfort the patient, even if there is no response.
- Use communication boards or other devices with patients unable to speak.
- Give patients time to respond and ask questions patient can likely answer easily.
- Speak slowly and look at patients when communicating. Gestures, lip movements, and facial expressions convey important messages.

deeper level, patients need to feel that they are heard by their caregivers and know that their personhood is valued and respected.[84]

SUPPORT PATIENT COPING

A goal of expert psychosocial-spiritual care is to promote patient and family flourishing, empowering them to experience as much control and predictability as possible. As noted above, coping is a dynamic process involving cognitive and behavioral efforts to manage specific internal or external demands that are perceived to exceed the person's resources. The key to effective coping is to encourage the use of the best mix of strategies appropriate for a given situation.

Most adults cope by relying on their previously developed conscious and unconscious coping strategies and defense mechanisms, which are automatically triggered in a stressful situation. Teaching new coping skills to people who are experiencing acute psychologic stress may be unrealistic. However, by using active listening skills and initiating conversations with patients and family members, the nurse can identify those coping resources, skills, and preferences that may be most helpful.

Helping Patients Maintain Control

Research suggests that one of the most effective ways to decrease the stress of being in a critical environment is give patients as much control over their care and the environment as possible.[75] Allow patients to make decisions as they are able, such as how and when to administer personal hygiene, diet preferences, and the timing of nursing interventions. Inform patients and family members about daily activities, tests, or therapies, their purpose, and anticipated effects. Critical care patients are often unable to see or turn around to witness what is going on in their environments. During treatments and procedures, provide the patient with explanations, brief discussions on what to expect, the anticipated time of a procedure, and descriptions of what is happening during an intervention. The patient for whom control is important should be helped to maintain control in as many areas of his or her life as possible. On the other hand, a patient must be given the opportunity to not exercise control if having too many choices provokes even greater stress.

Support Patient Preferred Complementary Therapies

Patients and families enter health care settings with well-established practices and beliefs about managing stress, maintaining wellness, balance, and harmony in their lives, and knowing what methods best facilitate their bodies' own healing responses. Integrative health care practices involve a blending of allopathic medical health care methods with patient-identified complementary therapies.[86]

The type of complementary or integrative therapies used depends on a patient's preferences, coping style, physical capabilities, and personality type. Music therapy, relaxation, guided imagery, therapeutic massage, visualization, prayer, biofeedback, and mindfulness meditation are potentially useful for critical ill patients.[21,87] Significant decreases in anxiety and symptom distress have been attributed to tactile touch. Although more research is needed to support the value of complementary therapies on selected outcomes in critically ill hospitalized patients, early studies support their potential as therapeutic nursing interventions (see Chapter 1).

Creating Healing Environments

People are continuous with their environments. Alterations in the physical environment of critical care units can provide a sense of calm, enhance patient coping, and facilitate healing.[88] Nurses can make changes in care environments to give patients a greater sense of comfort and familiarity while they are in the unit.

Visiting Policies

While practices vary among critical care units, a more relaxed visitation policy humanizes the environment and facilitates healing. The American Association of Critical-Care Nurses' AACN Practice Alert[89] recommends giving unrestricted access of hospitalized patients to a chosen support person. Giving family members access to their loved ones enhances patient and family satisfaction and improves safety of care. Family members have insight into the patient's behaviors and preferences, especially with patients who are unable to communicate. Interactions with family members reduces patient anxiety and enhances a sense of control.[90] Including patients and family members in critical care interdisciplinary rounds has been shown to improve perceptions of accessibility and communication.[91]

Physical Environment

Critical care areas are bright, loud, and busy. Close patient doors to adjacent areas, use sound dampening panels, turn off unnecessary noisy equipment, and decrease noise at workstations. Nurse call interruptions can be minimized with the use of smart phones. Music can be used to produce therapeutic sound in critical care areas. Control lighting for individual patient preference, allow for natural sunlight if possible, and position patients so that they can see out of windows.[88] Within the limits of unit policy, familiarize patient rooms by displaying photographs, cards, drawings, and favored items. Sleep deprivation is a serious concern in critical care environments. To prevent light exposures that awaken patients, nurses should group care activities to limit nighttime interruptions and collaborate with lab personnel to decrease sleep interruptions.[75,92]

PROVIDE FAMILY-CENTERED CARE

Family-centered care, endorsed by the AACN as a practice standard for critical care, formalizes the patient and family as the unit of care. Family-centered care is based on the belief that patients and families should participate in decisions together and that patients need their families for love, understanding, and support while coping with critical illness.[93] The nurse's observable support of family members at the bedside gives the patient comfort.

The elements essential to family-centered care include respect, collaboration, and support. Research had demonstrated that family members of critical care patients want information, reassurance, and proximity to their loved ones. They also want accurate information, communicated in an understandable manner, and they need room for hope.[78] A majority of family members who helped in acts of caregiving had a more positive outlook.

Family members, themselves in a time of crisis, are particularly sensitive to a nurse's words and actions, making it essential that the nurse convey understanding and acceptance. Although the critical care nurse rarely has the time or opportunity to perform a full family assessment or give ongoing support to all family members, he or she can observe the quality of the patient-family interaction and formulate interventions that will aid the family in supporting the patient.[84] The patient determines who counts as "family." Regard non-biologic or non-legal partners as full members of the patient's family or support system if that is the nature of the patient's relationships. The critical care nurse provides interventions aimed at supporting family members throughout the patient's stay in the unit (Box 6-3).

ENGAGE SPIRITUAL RESOURCES

A time of crisis can also lead to a time of positive spiritual renewal and readiness for an enhanced spiritual life. Spiritual and religious beliefs and practices often give patients and family members some measure of acceptance of an illness, a sense of mastery and control, strength to endure the stressors of illness, and a source of hope and trust beyond what medical interventions can provide.

Transformative spiritual care strategies are particularly helpful in times of crisis and uncertainty. When faced with significant life challenges, people need resources to transcend their circumstances and know that no matter what happens, they will endure. Spiritual resources include faith in a higher power, support communities, a sense of hope and meaning in life, and religious practices. Patient and family spirituality affects their ability to cope with loss.[94]

Cutcliffe's[95] qualitative research on critically ill patients' perspective on hope reveals that hope is perceived as being directly related to help. That is, when patients know there is help, they feel more hopeful. They also described hope as closely interwoven with care. To feel cared for and cared about brings hope to critically ill patients. Hope was related to patients' sense of their personal future and was used as a coping resource. In each patient description of hope in Cutcliffe's study, the nurse plays a pivotal, potentially inspirational role. Nursing interventions that engender hope can be quite simple, quiet, and informal. Listening to patients' concerns, offering support, being present, enhancing dignity, and developing caring, trusting relationships with patients gives hope.[96] People hope for different things over the course of an illness. Listen for shifts in what patients hope for and find ways to help them meet their desired goals.[60]

◎ BOX 6-3 NIC

Family Support

Definition
Promotion of family values, interests, and goals

Activities
Assure family that best care possible is being given to patient
Appraise family's emotional reaction to patient's condition
Determine the psychological burden of prognosis for family
Foster realistic hope
Listen to family concerns, feelings, and questions
Facilitate communication of concerns/feelings between patient and family or between family members
Promote trusting relationship with family
Accept the family's values in a nonjudgmental manner
Answer all questions of family members or assist them to get answers
Orient family to the health care setting, such as hospital unit or clinic
Provide assistance in meeting basic needs for family, such as shelter, food, and clothing
Identify nature of spiritual support for family
Identify congruence between patient, family, and health professional expectations
Reduce discrepancies in patient, family, and health professional expectations through use of communication skills
Assist family members in identifying and resolving a conflict in values
Respect and support adaptive coping mechanisms used by family
Provide feedback for family regarding their coping
Counsel family members on additional effective coping skills for their own use

Provide spiritual resources for family, as appropriate
Provide the family with information about the patient's progress frequently, according to the patient preference
Teach the medical and nursing plans of care to family
Provide necessary knowledge of options to family that will assist them to make decisions about patient care
Include family members with patient in decision making about care, when appropriate
Encourage family decision making in planning long-term patient care affecting family structure and finances
Acknowledge understanding of family decision about postdischarge care
Assist family to acquire necessary knowledge, skills, and equipment to sustain their decision about patient care
Advocate for family, as appropriate
Foster family assertiveness in information seeking, as appropriate
Provide opportunities for visitation by extended family members, as appropriate
Introduce family to other families undergoing similar experiences, as appropriate
Give care to patient in lieu of family to relieve them and/or when family is unable to give care
Arrange for ongoing respite care, when indicated and desired
Provide opportunities for peer group support
Refer for family therapy, as appropriate
Tell family members how to reach the nurse
Assist family members through the death and grief processes, as appropriate

From Bulechek GM, et al, eds. *Nursing Interventions Classification (NIC)*. 6th ed. St. Louis: Mosby; 2013.

While distinctions between spiritual and religious concerns are important to highlight,[62] many people find spiritual strength in their adherence to a particular religious tradition. They get inspiration to endure, hope, comfort, assurance, and confidence from the texts, rituals, and beliefs of their faith communities. Facilitate patient access to religious rituals, prayer, and scripture reading as hope-sustaining activities and help patients make connections to their spiritual or cultural communities. Collaborate with the hospital's spiritual care department when you sense that a person has unmet or unaddressed spiritual questions or needs. Often a professional spiritual care provider is the best person to assess spiritual needs and plan helpful interventions. Spiritual and religious leaders can also provide valuable insights when discussing ethical decisions that may have implications for the person's values and beliefs. Religious, spiritual, or philosophical practices can also directly inform diet, hygiene practices, and rituals surrounding birth, death, and medical interventions.

PATIENTS WITH MENTAL HEALTH CO-MORBIDITIES

Not infrequently, patients admitted to critical care settings have a pre-existing mental health conditions. Chronic depression, bipolar disorders, substance addiction, and self-destructive behaviors, including suicide attempts, can also be the primary cause of a critical care hospitalization. The critical care team should make every effort to continue medications for mental health conditions during the critical care stay unless medically contraindicated. If the patient is unable to take oral medications, attempt to find an alternative route if possible. If psychotropic medications have been discontinued for medical reasons, discuss the need to resume those medications with the health care providers receiving the patient after discharge from the critical care unit.

Alcohol Withdrawal in Critical Care Settings

Nurses in any acute care setting must be alert to the symptoms of withdrawal from chemical substances, including alcohol, which can complicate recovery from the admitting diagnosis. Not infrequently, in emergency admissions to a critical care unit, a full patient history of substance use has not been elicited. Investigators estimate that 1 in 4 patients admitted to general hospitals meet criteria for alcohol dependence.[97] Withdrawal progresses to delirium tremens without treatment and can occur from three hours up to 7 days after the last alcohol consumption. Peak withdrawal time is 48-72 hours after last alcohol consumption in a person with alcohol addiction.[98]

The signs and symptoms of alcohol withdrawal syndrome (AWS) are easily confused with other conditions. Patient with AWS exhibit altered concentration, tremulousness, autonomic hyperarousal, hallucinations, disorientation, psychosis, tachycardia, hypertension, low-grade fever, agitation, diaphoresis, and delirium tremens.[99] Critical care nurses can quickly and accurately assess a patient's risk for AWS by using the Clinical Institute Withdrawal Assessment for Alcohol, revised (CIWA-Ar).[100] This 10-item scale assesses for nausea and vomiting, tremors, paroxysmal sweats, anxiety, agitation, tactile, auditory, and visual disturbances, headache, and orientation. Treatment protocols for AWS depend on the severity of the patient's symptoms. Commonly used medications include chlordiazepoxide and lorazepam for withdrawal symptoms, and ondansetron and promethazine for nausea. Thiamine, folic acid, and multivitamins should be added to intravenous fluids.[99] (See also Chapter 34, Alcohol Screening Questionnaire, Box 34-1.)

Caring for Patients After Attempted Suicide

Nurses in critical care settings not infrequently care for patients who have attempted suicide. It is especially important to practice dignity-enhancing care in these situations. Nurses should carefully consider their own attitudes concerning self-destructive behaviors. Patients who have attempted suicide are often stigmatized, and caregivers can resent caring for a person whose critical condition is self-inflicted. A suicide attempt indicates, however, that the patient was experiencing personal and spiritual distress to the point of wanting to end his or her life. A suicidal behavior resides at the extreme, maladaptive end of a continuum of self-protective responses to life's challenges.[17] Usually a person who has attempted suicide is quickly transferred out of the unit for further evaluation and mental health care when they are medically stable. While the patient is in the unit, however, primary nursing interventions include validating the patient's worth and self-esteem, helping him or her regulate emotional states and behaviors, and mobilizing the patient's social support, necessary for long-term recovery.[17,53]

Nurses also care for family members of persons who have attempted suicide. They are often undergoing a significant family crisis and can have feelings of shame, guilt, or anger concerning the suicide attempt. Talk to family members in a private setting, and establish an atmosphere of interested concern for their loved one. Before the patient is discharged from the unit or hospital, gather assessment data from family members, including information about the patient's medical and psychiatric history, history of previous suicide attempts, presence of a trigger for self-destructive behavior (recent disagreement with someone, or anniversary of a loss), presence of acute stressors, and availability of support systems. Family members should be encouraged to inform health care providers if the patient has stopped taking prescribed psychotropic medications or seeing a mental health provider and begin to make a plan for immediate follow-up care after discharge from the unit.[101]

NURSE SELF-CARE

Critical care nurses do amazing, life-giving work. In the words of poet John O'Donohue, nurses "stand like a secret angel between the bleak despair of illness and the unquenchable light of spirit that can turn the darkest destiny towards dawn."[102] Critical care nurses possess the knowledge, wisdom, and power to help others in situations of uncertainty and suffering.

Remembering always critical care nurses' life-giving work, it is also important to recognize the need for consistent, intentional self-care. A nurse cannot give fully engaged, compassionate care to others when he or she feels depleted or does not feel cared for him- or herself. In critical care settings, nurses rarely have time to recover from one emotionally draining situation before they are called upon to respond to another. They often witness prolonged, concentrated suffering on a daily basis, leading to feelings of frustration, anger, guilt, sadness, or anxiety. Frequent, intense, or prolonged exposure to grief and loss places nurses at risk for developing compassion fatigue, a physical, emotional and spiritual exhaustion accompanied by emotional pain. The stressors of caregiving can lead to a decreased capacity to show compassion or empathize with suffering people.[103] Nurses, too, are at risk for developing PTSD reactions to the relentless stress and psychologically difficult work of caring for others in extreme situations.[104,105]

To avoid the extremes of either becoming overly involved in patients' suffering or detaching from them, nurses can use self-care activities to maintain balance. Nurses should first use self-reflection when they feel overwhelmed, considering the possible reasons for their feelings. There are often multiple causes for feeling overwhelmed: sadness about a particular patient, overwork, lateral hostility at work,[106] and disruptions in one's personal life. Reflection is an important first step because without awareness, it is difficult to identify possible solutions. Talking with friends, a spiritual care provider, or a close colleague can help the nurse recognize his or her own grief and reflect on the meaning of work.

Stress-management techniques help to restore energy and enjoyment in caring for patients. In some instances, nurses choose to work temporarily in less emotionally stressful settings. Nurses who practice self-care are more likely to experience professional and personal growth and find much meaning in their work. Maintain physical health by eating well, exercising, engaging in relaxing activities, laughing, and by getting enough sleep. Promote emotional health by participating in calming activities such as meditation, daily gratitude reflections, deep breathing, walking, or listening to music.[107,108] Use self-transcendence (spiritual awareness) activities, such as journal writing, sharing stories, recognizing one's own positive contributions and unique gifts, and connecting with one's self.[109] Given the ongoing demands of critical care nursing, balance time at work with time for recreation and relaxation. Invest time in those people and activities that nurture the spirit. Learn from the courage exhibited by patients and family members, and with good self-care, find joy and fulfillment in being a critical care nurse.

BOX 6-4 CASE STUDY

Patient with Psychosocial Needs

Brief Patient History
Ms. T is a 17-year-old woman who took an acetaminophen overdose after her boyfriend broke up with her. She states that she did not want to kill herself but just wanted to scare her boyfriend. Ms. T is having difficulty facing the need for a psychiatric evaluation and the potential for severe liver damage.

Clinical Assessment
Ms. T was admitted to the critical care unit from the emergency department in stable condition. She is awake, alert, and oriented to person, time, place, and situation. She is irritable, withdrawn, and wants to be left alone. Her parents stay at her bedside, and share with the nurse their intense feelings of fear, confusion, and uncertainty concerning their daughter's serious psychologic and physical condition.

Diagnostic Procedures
A psychiatric evaluation was completed, with the recommendation that Ms. T receive inpatient psychiatric care when medically stable.

Medical Diagnosis
Ms. T is diagnosed with acetaminophen toxicity and risk for hepatic failure.

Questions
1. What major outcomes do you expect to achieve for this patient?
2. What problems or risks must be managed to achieve these outcomes?
3. What interventions must be initiated to monitor, prevent, manage, or eliminate the problems and risks identified?
4. What interventions should be initiated to promote optimal functioning, safety, and well-being of the patient?
5. What possible learning needs do you anticipate for this patient?
6. What cultural and age-related factors may have a bearing on the patient's plan of care?

SUMMARY

- Critical care nurses consider connections between the body, mind, and spirit in providing holistic nursing care to critically ill patients.
- Patients in critical care settings must cope with many stressors. Each patient's response is unique and depends on a variety of environmental factors and individual differences.
- A person's perceptions of self and relationships with others, of spiritual values, and of self-competency in social roles play a role in how he or she responds to stress or illness.

- Anxiety is a normal subjective response to a perceived or actual threat to self-integrity, which can range from a vague, generalized feeling of discomfort to a state of panic and loss of control.
- Disturbances in self-concept, body image, and self-esteem often accompany experiences of critical illness or injury.
- Spiritual distress, hopelessness, and powerlessness in critically ill patients can complicate recovery and should be addressed by critical care nurses.

- Each person has a preferred set of coping strategies for meeting life stressors.
- Dignity-enhancing care includes elements of attitude, behaviors, compassion, and dialogue.
- Supportive family members and friends provide a source of strength and hope for patients facing the stressors of a critical illness or injury.

- Spirituality provides patients with transcending practices for accepting what cannot be changed, and for fostering hope and trust in self, others, and the transcendent.
- Critical care nurses should engage in self-care practices for their own wellness and to sustain meaning in their work with critically ill people and their families.

REFERENCES

1. Chochinov H. Dignity-conserving care- a new model for palliative care: helping the patient feel valued. *JAMA*. 2002;287(17):2253.
2. NANDA International. *Nursing diagnosis: definitions and classification 2012-2014*. Philadelphia: Wiley-Blackwell; 2011.
3. Cropley M, Steptoe A. Social support, life events and physical symptoms: a prospective study of chronic and recent life stress in men and women. *Psychology, Health Med*. 2005;10:317.
4. Lloyd C, et al. Stress and diabetes: a review of the links. *Diabetes Spectrum*. 2005;18:121.
5. Neilsen N, et al. Self reported stress and risk of breast cancer. *British Med J*. 2005;331:548.
6. Lovallo W. *Stress and Health: Biological and Psychological Interactions*. Thousand Oaks, CA: Sage; 2005.
7. Seaward BL. *Managing Stress: Principles and Strategies for Health and Wellbeing*. 5th ed. Sudbury, MA: Jones and Bartlett; 2009.
8. Lunney M. Stress overload: a new diagnosis. *Internat J Nurs Term Classif*. 2006;17(4):165.
9. Fredriksen ST, Ringsberg K. Living the situation stress-experiences among intensive care patients. *Internat Crit Care Nurs*. 2007;23:124.
10. Pang P, Suen L. Stressors in the ICU: a comparison of patients' and nurses' perception. *J Clin Nurs*. 2008;17:2681.
11. Rattray J, et al. Patients' perceptions of and emotional outcome after intensive care: results from a multicenter study. *Nurs Crit Care*. 2010;15(2):86.
12. Ganz F. Sleep and immune function. *Crit Care Nurs*. 2012;32(2):19.
13. Selye H. *Stress in health and disease*. Boston: Butterworth; 1976.
14. Lazarus R, Lazarus B. *Passion and reason: making sense of emotions*. New York: Oxford University; 1994.
15. Lazarus R, Folkman S. *Stress, Appraisal, and Coping*. New York: Springer; 1984.
16. Neurberger P. *Freedom from Stress: A Holistic Approach*. Honesdale, PA: The Himalayan International Institute of Yoga Science and Philosophy; 1981.
17. Stuart G. *Principles and Practices of Psychiatric Nursing*. 9th ed. St. Louis: Mosby; 2009.
18. DeKeyser F. Psychoneuroimmunology in critically ill patients. *AANC Clinical Issues*. 2003;14(1):25.
19. Halldorsdottir S. A psychoneueoimmunological view of the healing potential of professional caring in the face of human suffering. *Intern J Human Caring*. 2007;11(2):32.
20. McCain NL, et al. Implementing a comprehensive approach to the study of health dynamics using the psychoneuroimmunology paradigm. *Adv Nurs Sci*. 2005;28(4):320.
21. Caine R. Psychological influences in critical care: perspectives from psychoneuroimmunology. *Crit Care Nurs*. 2003;23(2):60.
22. Langley P, et al. Psychoneuroimmunology and health from a nurse perspective. *Brit J Nurs*. 2006;15(20):126.
23. Davydow D, et al. Posttraumatic stress disorder in general intensive care unit survivors: a systematic review. *Gen Hosp Psychiatry*. 2008;30:421.
24. Tedstone J, Tarrier N. Posttraumatic stress disorder following medical illness and treatment. *Clin Psych Rev*. 2003;23:409.
25. Wallen K, et al. Symptoms of acute posttraumatic stress disorder after intensive care. *Am J Crit Care*. 2008;17(6):534.
26. Jackson JC, et al. Posttraumatic stress disorder and posttraumatic stress symptoms following critical illness in medical ICU patients: assessing the magnitude of the problem. *Criti Care*. 2007;11:R27.
27. Jones C, et al. Precipitants of post-traumatic stress disorder following intensive care: a hypothesis generating study of diversity in care. *Intensive Care Med*. 2007;33:978.
28. Griffiths R, Jones C. Seven lessons from 20 years' of follow-up intensive care unit survivors. *Curr Opin Crit Care*. 2007;13:508.
29. Kiekkas P, et al. Psychological distress and delusional memories after critical care: a literature review. *Internat Nurs Rev*. 2010;57:288.
30. Azoulay E, et al. Risk of post-traumatic stress symptoms in family members of intensive care patients. *Am J Resp Crit Care Med*. 2005;171:987.
31. Pillai L, et al. Can we predict intensive care relatives at risk for posttraumatic stress disorder? *Indiana J Crit Care Med*. 2010;14(2):83.
32. Kross E, et al. ICU care associated with symptoms of depression and posttraumatic stress disorder among family members of patients who died in the ICU. *Chest*. 2011;139(4):795.
33. Luks A. Are we causing PTSD with our current sedation practices? *Crit Care Alert*. 2009;17(1):49.
34. Samuelson K, et al. Stressful experiences in relation to depth of sedation in mechanically ventilated patients. *Nurs Crit Care*. 2007;12(2):93.
35. Myhren H, et al. Posttraumatic stress, anxiety and depression symptoms in patients during the first year post intensive care unit discharge. *Crit Care*. 2010.
36. Twigg E, et al. Use of a screening questionnaire for post-traumatic stress disorder (PTSD) on a sample of UK ICU patients. *ACTA Anaesthesiol Scand*. 2007;52:202.
37. Combe D. The use of patient diaries in the intensive care unit. *Nurs Crit Care*. 2005;10:31.
38. Phillips C. Use of patient diaries in critical care. *Nurs Stand*. 2011;26(11):35.
39. Williams S. Recovering from the psychological impact of intensive care: how constructing a story helps. *Nurs Crit Care*. 2009;14(6):281.

40. Perpina-Galvan J, Richart-Martinez M. Scales for evaluating self perceived anxiety levels in patients admitted to intensive care units: a review. *Am J Crit Care*. 2009;18(6):571.

41. Puntillo K, et al. The prevalence, intensity and distress of symptoms in high-risk ICU patients, 2008 (abstract). National Meeting of the American Association of Critical Care Nurses.

42. Jaber S, et al. A prospective study of agitation in a medical-surgical ICU: incidence, risk facors, and outcomes. *Chest*. 2005;128(4):2749.

43. Khalaila R, et al. Communication difficulties and psychoemotional distress in patients receiving mechanical ventilation, *Am J Crit Care*. 2011;20(6):470.

44. Chlan L, Savik K. Patterns of anxiety in critically ill patients receiving mechanical ventilator support. *Nurs Res*. 2011;60(3S):S50.

45. Brodsky-Israeli M, Ganz F. Risk factors associated with transfer anxiety among patients transferring from the intensive care unit to the ward. *J Adv Nurs*. 2011;67(3):510.

46. Moser D. The rust of life: impact of anxiety on cardiac patients. *Am J Crit Care*. 2007;16(4):361.

47. Ruz M, et al. Evidence that the brief symptom inventory can be used to measure anxiety quickly and reliably in patients hospitalized for acute myocardial infarction. *J Cardiovascular Nurs*. 2010;25(2):117.

48. Frazier S, et al. Critical care nurses' assessment of patients anxiety: reliance on physiological and behavioral parameters. *Am J Crit Care*. 2002;11(1):57.

49. Doenges ME, Murr A, Moorhouse MF. *Nurse's Pocket Guide: Diagnoses, Interventions, and Rationales*. 12th ed. Philadelphia: FA Davis; 2010.

50. Pasacreta JV, Minarik P, Nield-Anderson L. Anxiety and depression. In: Ferrell B, Coyle N, eds. *Textbook of Palliative Nursing*. 3rd ed. New York: Oxford University Press; 2010.

51. Fortinash KM. The nursing process. In: Fortinash KM, Holoday-Worret PA, eds. *Psychiatric Mental Health Nursing*. 5th ed. St. Louis: Mosby; 2012.

52. Newfield S, et al, eds. *Cox's Clinical Applications of Nursing Diagnosis*. 5th ed. Philadephia: F.A. Davis; 2007.

53. Varacarolis E, Halter M, eds. *Foundations of Psychiatric Mental Health Nursing: A Clinical Approach*. 6th ed. St. Louis: Elsevier; 2010.

54. Benner P, Wrubel J. *The Primacy of Caring: Stress and Coping in Health and Illness*. Menlo Park, CA: Addison-Wesley Publishing Co; 1989.

55. Maslow H. *Motivation and Personality*. New York: Harper & Row; 1954.

56. Ackley B, Ladwig G, eds. *Nursing Diagnosis Handbook: An Evidence Based Guide to Planning Care*. St. Louis: Mosby; 2011.

57. Watson J. *Caring Science as Sacred Science*. Philadelphia: F A Davis; 2005.

58. Lazare A. Shame and humiliation in the medical encounter. *Arch Intern Med*. 1987;147:1653.

59. Malterud K, Hollnagel H. Avoiding humiliations in the clinical encounter. *Scan J Prim Health Care*. 2007;25:69.

60. Chochinov H, et al. Dignity in the terminally ill: a developing empirical model. *Soc Sci Med*. 2006;54(3):3433.

61. Griffin A, Yancey V. (2009). Spiritual dimensions of the perioperative experience: theoretical and practical concerns. *J AORN*. 2009;89(5):875.

62. Puchalski C. Spirituality and the care of patients at the end of life: an essential component of care. *Omega*. 2007-2008;56(1):33.

63. Arnaert A, et al. Stroke patients in the acute care phase: role of hope in self-healing. *Holist Nurs Prac*. 2006;20(3):137.

64. Cutcliffe J, Hearth K. The concept of hope in nursing 5: hope and critical care nursing. *Brit J Nurs*. 2002;11(18):1190.

65. Frankl V. *Man's Search for Meaning*. New York: Washington Square Press; 1959.

66. Miller JF. Hope: a construct central to nursing. *Nurs Forum*. 2007;42(1):12-19.

67. Rotter JB. Generalized expectancies for internal versus external control of reinforcement. *Psychol Monogr*. 1966;80(1):1.

68. Holoday-Worret P. Foundations of psychiatric mental health nursing. In: Fortinash K, Holoday-Worret P, eds. *Psychiatric Mental Health Nursing*. 5th ed. St. Louis: Mosby; 2012.

69. Weisman A. *On Dying and Denying: A Psychiatric Study of Terminality*. Mourning Heights, NY: Behavioral Publications; 1972.

70. Dossey B. Body-mind-spirit: attention to holistic care. *Am J Nurs*. 1998;98(8):35.

71. Nelson JE, et al. End of life care for the critically ill: a national intensive care unity survey. *Crit Care Med*. 2006;34:2547.

72. Batty S. Communication, swallowing and feeding in the intensive care unit patient. *Nurs Crit Care*. 2009;14(4):175.

73. Happ M, et al. Nurse-patient communication interactions in the intensive care unit. *Am J Crit Care Nurs*. 2011;20(2):e28.

74. Grossbach I. Promoting effective communication for patients receiving mechanical ventilation. *Crit Care Nurs*. 2011;31(3):46.

75. Lusk B, Lash A. The stress responses, psychoneuroimmunology, and stress among ICU patients. *Dim Crit Care Nurs*. 2005;24(1):25.

76. Stajduha K, et al. Patient perceptions of helpful communication in the context of advanced cancer. *J Clin Nurs*. 2010;19:2039.

77. Lowey S. Communication between the nurse and family caregiver in end of life care: a review of the literature. *J Hosp Pall Nursing*. 2008;10(1):35.

78. Verhaeghe S, et al. How does information influence hope in family members of traumatic coma patients in intensive care unit? *J Clin Nurs*. 2007;16:1488.

79. Johnstone L, Kanitsaki O. Ethics and advance care planning in a culturally diverse society. *J Transcult Nurs*. 2009;20(4):405.

80. Erichsen E, et al. A phenomenological study of nurses' understanding of honesty in palliative care. *Nurs Ethics*. 2010;17(1):39.

81. Lipson M, Lipson A. Psychotherapy and the ethics of attention. *Hast Cent Rep*. 1996;26(1):17.

82. Newman M. *Transforming Presence: The Difference that Nursing Makes*. Philadelphia: F.A. Davis; 2008.

83. Chochinov H. Dignity and the essence of medicine: the A B C and D of dignity conserving care. *Br J Med*. 2007;335:184.

84. Tulsky J. Inteventions to enhance communication among patients, providers, and families. *J Palliat Med*. 2005;8(S 1):S95.

85. Mariano C. Holistic integrative therapies in palliative care. In: Matzo M, Sherman D, eds. *Palliative Care Nursing: Quality Care to the End-of-Life*. 3rd ed. New York: Springer Publishing; 2010:39–63.

86. Henricson M, et al. The outcome of tactile touch on stress parameters in intensive care: a randomized controlled trial. *Compl Ther Clin Prac*. 2008;14:244.

87. Austin D. The psycholophysiological effects of music therapy in intensive care units. *Paediatric Nurs*. 2010;22(3):14.

88. Bazuin D, Cardon K. Creating healing intensive care unit environments: physical and psychological considerations in designing critical care areas. *Crit Care Nurs*. 2011;24(4):259.

89. AACN Practice alert. Family Visitation in the Adult ICU, AACN, 2011.
90. Black P, et al. The effect of nurse-facilitated family participation in the psychological care of the critically ill patient. *J Adv Nurs.* 2011;67(5):1091.
91. Jacobowski N, et al. Communication in critical care: family rounds in the intensive care unit. *Am J Crit Care.* 2010;19(5):421.
92. Dunn H, et al. Nighttime lighting in intensive care units. *Crit Care Nurs.* 2010;30(3):31.
93. Mitchell M, et al. Positive effects of a nusing intervention on family-centered care in adult critical care. *Am J Crit Care.* 2009;18(6):543.
94. Hermann C. The degree to which spiritual needs of patients near the end of life are met. *Onc Nurs Forum.* 2007;34(1):70.
95. Cutcliffe J. Critically ill patients' perspectives of hope. *Br J Nurs.* 1996;26(5):687.
96. Tanis S, DiNapoli P. Paradox of hope in patients receiving palliative care: a concept analysis. *Internat J Human Caring.* 2008;12(1):53.
97. Repper-DeLisi J, et al. Successful implementation of an alcohol withdrawal pathway in a general hospital. *Psychomatics.* 2008;39(4):292.
98. York L, Rayback S. Behavioral and psychological factors in critical care. In: Ahrens T, Prentice D, Kleinpell R, eds. *Critical Care Nursing Certification.* New York: McGraw Hill; 2010.
99. Nuss MA, et al. Utilizing CIWA-Ar to assess use of benzodiazepines in patients vulnerable to alcohol withdrawal syndrome. *W Virginia Med J.* 2004;99:21.
100. Sullivan JT, et al. Assessment of alcohol withdrawal: the revised Clinical Institute Withdrawal Assessment for Alcohol scale (CIWA-Ar). *Brit J Addiction.* 1989;84:1353.
101. National Suicide Prevention Lifeline. After attempt: a guide for talking care of your family member after treatment in the emergency department. http://www.suicidepreventionlifeline.org. Accessed September 20, 2012.
102. O'Donahue J. *To Bless the Space Between Us: A Book of Blessings.* New York: Doubleday; 2008.
103. Bush N. Compassion fatigue: are you at risk? *Onc Nurs Forum.* 2009;26(1):24.
104. Mealer M, et al. The prevalence and impact of post-traumatic stress disorder and burnout syndrome in nurses. *Depression Anxiety.* 2009;26:1118.
105. Mealer M, et al. Increased prevalence of post-traumatic stress disorder symptoms in critical care nurses. *Am J Respir Crit Care Med.* 2007;175:693.
106. Alspach G. Lateral hostility between critical care nurses: a survey report. *Crit Care Nurs.* 2008;28(2):13.
107. Showalter S. Compassion fatigue: what is it? why does it matter? recognizing the symptoms, acknowledging the impact, developing the tools to prevent compassion fatigue, and strengthen the professional already suffering from the effects. *Am J Hosp Palliat Med.* 2010;27(4):239.
108. Wilson L. Getting a self care tune-up. *Beginnings.* 2008;28(1):8.
109. Hunnibell L, et al. Self-transcendence and burnout in hospice and oncology nurses. *J Hosp Palliat Nurs.* 2008;10(3):172.

Sleep Alterations and Management

Kathleen M. Stacy

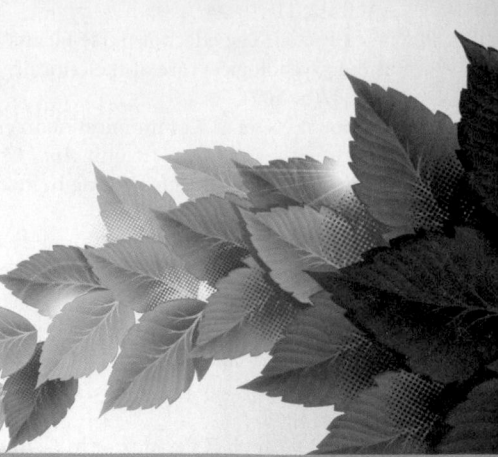

evolve WEBSITE

http://evolve.elsevier.com/Urden/criticalcare/

Evolve features:
- NCLEX Review Questions
- CCRN Review Questions
- PCCN Review Questions
- Mosby's Nursing Skills Procedures
- Animations
- Video Clips
- Glossary

Sleep is the only medication that gives ease.—Sophocles

Nurses who have an appreciation of the importance of sleep place a higher priority on protection of patients' sleep.[1] Health care providers interrupt patients' sleep for assessment, treatments, or interventions, and environmental noise, pain, or anxiety can also disturb it.[2] Although prioritizing care is essential, the consequence of sleep interruptions is not merely sleep-deprived patients; alterations in sleep patterns can result in chronic sleep problems, poor recovery, and decreased quality of life.[1] To facilitate sleep and healing, critical care nurses need to understand the essentials of sleep and chronobiology, the effect of pharmacologic therapy on sleep, and the consequences of disrupted sleep. The purpose of this chapter is to acquaint nurses with the characteristics of normal human sleep and chronobiology, changes in sleep associated with aging and pharmacologic treatment, and abnormal sleep patterns that may affect critically ill patients. Evidence-based nursing care for critically ill patients with sleep disturbances is discussed.

NORMAL HUMAN SLEEP

Sleep Physiology

Humans spend about one third of their lives engaged in a process known as *sleep*. Although little is now known about the physiologic process or the depths to which it affects us, researchers are learning more about sleep every day. The behavioral definition of sleep is a reversible behavioral state of perceptual disengagement from and unresponsiveness to the environment.[3] Sleep is a basic human need, just as food and water are. For patients to regain and maintain their optimal physical and emotional health, they must be able to get adequate amounts of quality sleep. To help patients obtain their optimal amount of sleep, a nurse must first understand what constitutes normal sleep and how the nursing plan of care can contribute to accomplishing this goal.

Polysomnography (PSG) is the collection of multiple channels of physiologic data to assess sleep and its disorders using various electrodes.[4] Electroencephalographic (EEG) electrodes are attached to the patient's scalp to measure brain waves. Changes in the EEG frequency (number of waveforms) and amplitude (height of waveform) over the course of the study allow the sleep to be scored into stages. Sleep stages are distinguished primarily by the EEG waveforms they produce. Sleep is scored by each 30-second epoch or segment of the tracing. The criteria for scoring sleep in infants differ from those used for adults.[4]

Electrooculography (EOG) measures eye movement activity. The study can help to determine when the patient is in rapid eye movement (REM) sleep; it also can establish when sleep onset occurs as reflected by slow, rolling eye movements.[4] Electromyography (EMG) involves leads placed over various muscle groups. When placed over the chin, the leads can help detect muscle atonia associated with REM sleep. Intercostal leads detect respiratory effort, whereas leads over the anterior tibialis detect leg movements that may be causing the patient to arouse. The electrocardiogram (ECG) shows any cardiac abnormalities, oximetry monitors the oxygen saturation levels, and piezoelastic bands around the chest and abdomen detect respiratory disorders such as apnea. Thermocouples are used to monitor airflow through the nose and mouth.[4]

Sleep Stages

Humans experience three states of being. They are awake, in REM sleep, or in non–rapid eye movement (NREM) sleep. NREM sleep usually occupies 70% to 75% of the sleep cycle, with REM sleep comprising 20% to 25%.[5] Some theorize that NREM sleep is a restorative period that relieves the stresses of waking activities, whereas REM sleep serves to refuel creative brain stores.

Non-Rapid Eye Movement Sleep

NREM sleep can be further divided into stages 1 through 3 (N1-N3), with each stage being a progressively deeper sleep state. Adults usually enter sleep through NREM stage N1 sleep, which is a transitional, lighter sleep state from which the patient can be easily aroused by light touch or by softly calling his or her name.

Stage N1 comprises 2% to 5% of a night's sleep and is demonstrated by an EEG pattern of low-voltage, mixed-frequency waveforms with vertex sharp waves.[5] The EOG during stage N1 may demonstrate slow, side-to-side eye movements. A patient with severely disrupted sleep may experience an increase in the amount of stage N1 sleep throughout the sleep cycle. As a patient makes the transition from awake to asleep, a brief memory impairment may occur.[4] As a result, the patient may not remember educational or care instructions given by the nurse during the transition between sleep and wake states. Stage N2 sleep occupies about 45% to 55% of the night, with sleep deepening and a higher arousal threshold being required to awaken the patient. Changes seen in the EEG pattern include sleep spindles and K complexes.[5] As stage N2 continues, high-voltage, slow-wave activity begins to appear.[4] When these slow waves represent 20% of the EEG activity per page, the criteria are met for stage N3 sleep, which constitutes 15% to 20% of the cycle.[5] In stage N3 sleep, slow waves continue to develop until 50% of the EEG waveforms are slow wave. This stage of sleep is often referred to as *slow-wave sleep*.[5]

NREM sleep is dominated by the parasympathetic nervous system. The body tries to maintain a homeostatic regulation, and this causes a decreased level of energy expenditure. Blood pressure, heart and respiratory rates, and the metabolic rate return to basal levels. EMG levels are lower in NREM as opposed to wake states but not as low as in REM sleep. Sweating or shivering that a patient may experience with temperature extremes occurs during NREM sleep but ceases during REM sleep.[3] During slow-wave sleep, 80% of the total daily growth-stimulating hormone is released, which works to stimulate protein synthesis while sparing catabolic breakdown. The release of other hormones, such as prolactin and testosterone, suggests that anabolism is occurring during slow-wave sleep. Cortisol release peaks during early morning hours, whereas melatonin is released only during darkness, and thyroid-stimulating hormone is inhibited during sleep. The activities associated with stage N3 sleep include protein synthesis and

tissue repair, such as the repair of epithelial cells and specialized cells of the brain, skin, bone marrow, and gastric mucosa.[6]

Rapid Eye Movement Sleep

REM sleep occupies about 20% to 25% of the night in healthy young adults and is sometimes known as the *dream stage*. However, dreaming is not the exclusive property of any one stage. REM can be viewed as a highly active brain in a paralyzed body and is frequently referred to as a *paradoxic sleep*. The paradox is that some areas of the brain remain very active, whereas others are suppressed. EEG waveforms are relatively slow voltage and sawtooth waves are present. Increased cortical activity occurs, with the EEG pattern resembling those of the wake state. Synchronized bursts of rapid, side-to-side eye movements with suppressed EMG activity (muscle atonia) are seen, indicating functional paralysis of the skeletal muscles.[7]

The sympathetic nervous system predominates during REM sleep. Oxygen consumption increases, and blood pressure, cardiac output, and respiratory and heart rates become variable. The body's response to decreased oxygen levels and increased carbon dioxide levels is lowest during REM sleep. Cardiac efferent vagus nerve tone is generally suppressed during REM sleep, and irregular breathing patterns can lead to oxygen reduction, particularly in patients with pulmonary or cardiac disease. An increase in premature ventricular contractions and tachydysrhythmias may be associated with respiratory pauses during REM sleep. Arterial pressure surges and increases in heart rate, coronary arterial tone, and blood viscosity may cause the combination of plaque rupture and hypercoagulability in persons with cardiac disease.[7]

Sleep Cycles

NREM and REM sleep cycles alternate (Fig. 7-1) throughout the night. Sleep onset usually occurs in stage 1 sleep, progressing through stages 2 and 3, then going back to stage 2, at which time the person usually enters REM. This first cycle typically takes about 70 to 100 minutes, with later cycles lasting 90 to 120 minutes. Four to five cycles are completed during normal adult sleep. NREM sleep predominates during the first third of the night, whereas REM is more prominent during the last third. Brief episodes of wakefulness (usually less than 5%) tend to intrude later into the night and are usually not remembered the next morning.[5]

The amount of sleep required is uncertain. No set number of hours has been established, and sleep length may be determined by many factors, including genetic predisposition. A sufficient amount of sleep has been achieved when one awakens without external stimuli and gets through the day without feeling sleepy.

Chronobiology

Sleep is not merely a response to fatigue. A complex group of interacting systems determines the timing and depth of sleep. The following section reviews circadian and homeostatic processes and theories of sleep regulation.

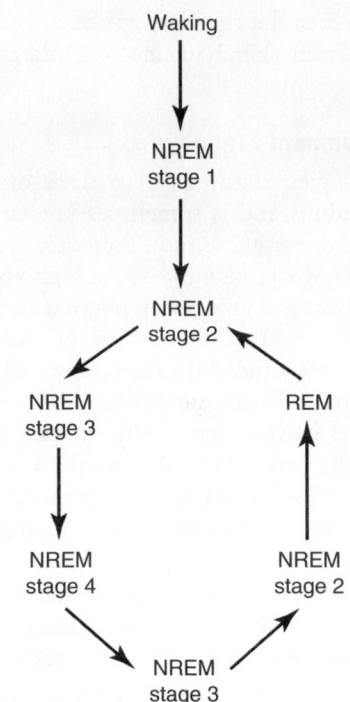

FIGURE 7-1 The cyclic nature of sleep.

Circadian System

Many body systems cycle with approximately a 24-hour period, hence the name circadian rhythm (from *circa* ["about"] and *dies* ["day"]).[8] Among these systems is the sleep-wake rhythm. A bundle of cells in the anterior hypothalamus, known as the *suprachiasmatic nucleus*, functions as the pacemaker for these rhythms. The circadian system facilitates cycling of the pre-scribed functions within a predictable period, but the functions are also influenced by other conditions, such as social activity, posture, and physical environment.[8]

Under normal conditions, a person's rhythms interact and influence one another. For example, when body temperature is becoming lower, a person is more likely to sleep, and as the body temperature rises in early morning hours, people awaken. Another example is the melatonin cycle, which tends to run in synchrony with the sleep-wake cycle.[8]

External influences such as posture, exercise, and light also influence the sleep circadian rhythm. These external influences, known as *zeitgebers*, can shift the rhythm, causing it to peak at different times, or fragment it. Light is the most influential zeitgeber for sleep[8]; critical care nurses therefore need to limit the light in the environment during nocturnal hours to facilitate sleep and circadian continuity in their patients.[9]

Homeostatic Mechanism

The recent history of the sleep obtained by an individual also influences timing and depth of sleep. Known as the *homeostatic process of sleep regulation*, this determinant of sleep is linked to how much sleep the individual has had previously. Essentially, someone who is sleep-deprived will sleep more readily, regard-less of circadian phase, whereas someone who is well rested will not fall asleep readily.[10,11] The amount of slow-wave sleep (stage N3) reflects sleep intensity, and individuals recovering from sleep deprivation have increased amounts of slow-wave sleep.[11]

Circadian and Homeostatic Interaction

Circadian and homeostatic processes function together to ensure optimal sleep for an individual. In essence, these studies have shown that homeostatic processes primarily regulate slow-wave activity and that the ratio of REM to NREM sleep is pri-marily regulated by the interaction of circadian and homeostatic processes.[11]

PHARMACOLOGY

It is essential that nurses understand the relationship between various medications and the sleep of patients in the critical care unit. Pathophysiology and age may profoundly affect not only medication absorption and elimination but also how patients cope with their illness and their ability to maintain health.

Hypnotic benzodiazepines remain the medications of choice to treat insomnia. Insomnia is a patient complaint of inability to initiate or maintain sleep, and prescriptions for treatment of insomnia cost more than $1 billion annually.[12] Acute stress, such as admission to a critical care unit, may cause some patients to experience acute sleep-onset insomnia. Hypnotics tend to promote lighter sleep stages and have a higher lipophilicity, which can cause the elderly to experience an increased drug half-life.[12] Care should be used in the administration and dosage of hypnotics in the elderly. This age group may experience night terrors, nightmares, and increased agitation. The metabolism of hypnotics in elderly patients can be inhibited by the use of steroids, or it can be accelerated in those who smoke. Hypnotics may also produce anterograde amnesia, which is a memory failure of information processed after the medication is con-sumed. Patients with normal ventilation should not be affected by the mild respiratory depression caused by hypnotics, although patients with chronic obstructive pulmonary disease (COPD) or sleep-disordered breathing may be affected.[13]

Wake-promoting medications produce increased arousal, behavioral activation, and alertness. They can be divided into three classes: direct-acting sympathomimetics (e.g. phenyleph-rine), indirect-acting sympathomimetics (e.g., methylpheni-date, amphetamine, mazindol), and stimulants that are not sympathomimetics (e.g., caffeine). Common side effects can include irritability and sweating, with talkativeness, anorexia, gastrointestinal complaints, dyskinesias, insomnia, and palpita-tions occurring less frequently.[14] Wake-promoting medications can be used for patients who experience disabling symptoms of sleepiness resulting from narcolepsy, idiopathic central nervous system hypersomnia, or sleep deprivation. Wake-promoting medications should be used only when sustained alertness is required for the individual or for reasons of public safety.

Wake-promoting medications possess a high abuse poten-tial. A sequence of euphoria, dysphoria, paranoia, and psychosis can occur after a single exposure, and sustained use can lead to cognitive and behavioral disorders. Proper dosing and a struc-tured management plan are recommended for wake-promoting medication use. This includes providing patient education with treatment goals, beginning with low doses, emphasizing good sleep hygiene such as naps, and adjusting the dosage according to clinical information. Wake-promoting medications should be included as part of a treatment plan only to decrease excessive somnolence. Sustained use of high-dose wake-promoting medications can lead to cognitive and behavioral disorders.[15] Effective sleep hygiene and attention to other substances or medications that can affect sleep may be beneficial for patients who want to avoid the abuse potential.

Many people use alcohol to assist them in falling asleep. Alcohol is a central nervous system sedative and will cause suppression of REM sleep. More than two alcoholic drinks may cause an increase in NREM stages 1 and 2 and decrease the onset of slow-wave sleep. Alcohol also may cause shallow, fragmented sleep and may precipitate or aggravate an existing obstructive sleep apnea (OSA) condition. In the 2008 National Sleep Foundation survey, 8% reported self-medicating for insomnia with alcohol. Of those polled, 20% reported using alcohol, over-the-counter medications (7%), prescription sleep medications (3%), or alternative therapy or herbal supplements (2%).[16]

Some persons who suffer from sleep problems have turned to alternative therapies or herbs for treatment. Because these are not considered prescription medications, patients do not always inform their caregivers that they are using them. Some herbs are considered effective hypnotics, whereas others may be used as stimulants. It is the responsibility of the nurse to inquire about all medications used, whether prescription or over-the-counter.

Patients with illness may respond differently to medications than do healthy patients. Patients may come to the critical care unit with impaired sleep or poor cognitive function. Beta-blockers, a commonly used class of medications in critical care, are known to produce nightmares and have disruptive effects on sleep quality in some individuals.[17] The effect of various drug combinations are not well known.

The critical care nurse should assess the patient's need for sedative and analgesic medications. The nurse has a responsibility to administer these medications in the most efficient manner to promote sleep and to monitor effectiveness. This can be achieved through assessment, including a medication history, diagnostic test results, and review of the patient's medical history. Information from that assessment assists the nurse in formulating a nursing diagnosis with outcome criteria and interventions. Evaluation of the patient ensures attainment of the desired outcomes.[18]

SLEEP PATTERN DISTURBANCE

Description

Sleep disturbance in critically ill patients is defined as insufficient duration or stages of sleep that results in discomfort and interferes with quality of life. When ill, most people need more sleep than usual, and sleep seems to promote recovery. Studies have demonstrated that the nocturnal sleep of patients in critical care units is severely disturbed, even though many receive medications to promote sleep.[1,19,20]

Etiology and Pathophysiology

Normal sleep is a period of decreased physiologic workload for the cardiovascular system. Insufficient sleep in acutely and critically ill patients has been associated with physiologic and psychologic exhaustion and may delay recovery from illness. These effects include mental status changes resulting in delirium.[21] A general consensus among sleep experts and researchers is that sleep deprivation results in psychologic alterations such as changes in mood and performance, fatigue, increased irritability, and feelings of persecution.[1,22]

The intensification of pain related to sleep disturbance is a significant problem in acutely and critically ill patients. Sunshine and colleagues related a potential theory for pain alleviation from massage therapy that is linked to quiet or restorative sleep. During deep sleep, somatostatin is normally released. Without this substance, pain is experienced. Substance P is released when an individual is deprived of deep sleep, and substance P is noted for causing pain. When people are deprived of deep sleep, they may have less somatostatin and increased substance P, which results in greater pain and more sleep disruption.[23]

Sleep disturbance in critically ill patients may stem from psychologic stress associated with critical illness and the critical care environment, surgical stress, noise, interruptions for care, painful procedures or physiologic processes, excessive bright light, and muscular and joint discomfort resulting from bed rest.[22] Of 84 patients' recollections about sleep-disturbing factors in the critical care unit, the most frequently mentioned factors included an inability to get comfortable or lie comfortably (recalled by 70% of patients), inability to perform one's usual routine before going to sleep (57%), anxiety (55%), and pain (54%).[24] The stressful nature of the critical care environment and uncertainty and worry regarding the outcomes of a critical illness may explain why some patients have such difficulty sleeping while hospitalized. These concerns are not culturally isolated. A Swedish study identified pain, anxiety, and environmental noise among factors that interfered with sleep.[25] However, perhaps because of staffing issues and general work flow, nurses tend to provide labor-intensive tasks during early morning hours.[2] This trend is clearly counterproductive and should be discouraged. Another source of sleep disturbance in critically ill patients is surgical stress. A general inflammatory response caused by the heart-lung machine or the incisions, altered endocrine neurometabolism control, and the effects of medications such as benzodiazepines, barbiturates, scopolamine, and systemic opioids may disturb sleep.[26]

Bright nocturnal light, excessive noise, and frequent interruptions for care procedures also may disturb sleep in critically ill patients. In a study of light and sound levels and interruptions to sleep in medical and respiratory critical care units, light levels maintained a day-night rhythm, with peak levels dependent on window orientation. Peak sound levels were extremely high in all areas and exceeded recommendations of the Environmental Protection Agency as acceptable for a hospital. Patient interruptions for care procedures tended to be variable but ubiquitous, leaving little time for condensed sleep.[1,2,22] However, one group determined that noise and nursing interventions explained fewer than 30% of sleep interruptions.[27] Identifying additional factors that create these sleep disruptions remains an area of potential research.

Not surprisingly, mechanical ventilation and the required care associated with it contribute to sleep disturbances. Cooper and colleagues studied 20 subjects who were receiving mechanical ventilation and classified as critically ill; based on PSG-accepted criteria, none of these patients had normal sleep. Twelve did not experience sleep at all, and the remaining eight demonstrated PSG findings consistent with severely disrupted sleep. The magnitude of sleep disruption found in the latter group was similar to the excessive daytime sleepiness and cognitive impairment of patients with untreated OSA.[28] Ventilatory modes may also influence sleep patterns. Bosma and associates compared the effects of pressure support and proportional assist ventilation (PAV) on sleep. PAV resulted in greater patient-ventilator synchrony and therefore improved sleep.[29] A comparison of assist control ventilation (AC) and low levels of pressure support also found that use of AC improved sleep quality. The authors suggested that ventilating patients at night may improve weaning outcomes. However, additional evidence suggests that sleep disturbances associated with prolonged mechanical ventilation do not resolve with extubation and discharge.[30] These findings emphasize the nursing responsibility to promote and protect the sleep of all patients in the critical care environment.

Assessment and Diagnosis

Assessment of the patient on admission to the critical care unit includes a description of multiple sleep-related factors: the normal sleep pattern, including awakenings, naps, normal bedtime, and waking time; customary habits that enhance sleep (e.g., number of pillows, extra blankets, bedtime rituals, medications); any recent changes in the patient's normal sleep pattern resulting from the acute illness; recent history of difficulty falling asleep or staying asleep, snoring, gasping for breath at night, stopping breathing at night, or excessive daytime sleepiness; frequency and duration of daytime naps; and the severity, duration, and history of chronic illnesses and disturbances that may disrupt sleep, such as COPD, arthritis, nocturnal angina, reflux esophagitis, or nocturia.

The patient's psychologic response to admission to the critical care unit needs to be assessed, along with the noise level in the patient's immediate environment. The critical care nurse needs to elicit any history of snoring because of its relationship to sleep apnea and sleep disturbances. One effective way to assess the quality of the patient's sleep is for the nurse to ask the patient how his or her sleep in the hospital compares with sleep at home. Because individuals differ in their sleep behaviors and requirements, a flexible, individualized plan of care must be formulated to promote rest and sleep.

Compiling a record of a patient's sleep for 48 to 72 hours may assist in assessing actual quantity of sleep as well as necessary and unnecessary awakenings. The sleep record includes the date and time, whether the patient was awake or asleep, and any procedures that necessitated waking the patient. A 24-hour flow sheet, commonly used in critical care units, could include an area for documentation of sleep. Just as nurses document other data relevant to the patient's recovery, sleep periods of more than 90 minutes in duration, number and length of awakenings, and total possible sleep time should be recorded and evaluated.

Medical Management

Medical management of sleep pattern disturbance in critically ill patients consists of the administration of sedative-hypnotics. The nonbenzodiazepine short-acting hypnotics zolpidem and zaleplon have few side effects and little effect on sleep architecture. Because of their short half-life, they may be repeated once during the night. Although hypnotics may assist the patient in falling asleep, it is a nursing responsibility to provide an environment and care procedures that promote sleep and allow patients to stay asleep.

Nursing Management

If one of the primary causes of the sleep pattern disturbance for a patient hospitalized in the critical care unit is a state of heightened anxiety and discomfort,[31] nursing interventions, such as massage, that promote relaxation and comfort may be effective. In a review of 22 articles investigating the effects of massage on relaxation, comfort, and sleep, massage consistently reduced anxiety and pain.[33] Another research-based intervention is playing audio of ocean sounds or other relaxing auditory sounds. Williamson found that an audiotape of the ocean or the rain significantly increased sleep quality in patients in a progressive care unit.[34] Providing a relaxed, caring environment that encourages confidence in care providers may also assist the patient to relax. Allowing close family members to sit quietly at the bedside while the patient rests may comfort the family and the patient and allow the patient to rest better. Stanchina and colleagues found that white noise machines in patient rooms decreased the variance in peak noises and increased arousal thresholds for patients.[35]

Nurses should limit interruptions for care procedures and should coordinate the care among other disciplines to allow patients time for consolidated nocturnal sleep and a daytime nap. Draperies or blinds should be opened during the day to allow patients to receive bright natural light and to help orient them to time of day, with lights dimmed at night. Noise from staff, squeaky carts, alarms, televisions, slamming doors, and ringing phones should be minimized. Offering the patient earplugs may help decrease noise and promote sleep. Outcomes of these nursing interventions can be assessed and documented on the 24-hour flow sheet. One group reported that an enforced afternoon quiet time resulted in benefits for patients as well as the multidisciplinary team.[36]

SLEEP APNEA SYNDROME

Description

Sleep apnea syndrome, sometimes called *sleep-disordered breathing*, occurs when airflow is absent or reduced. Apnea during sleep can be divided into three types: 1) obstructive; 2) central; and 3) mixed. In obstructive apnea, the absence of

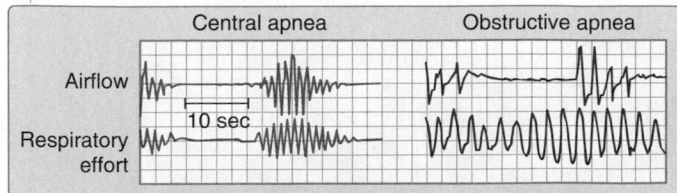

FIGURE 7-2 Comparison of airflow and respiratory effort in obstructive sleep apnea (OSA) and central sleep apnea (CSA). (From Kryger MH, et al, eds. *Principles and Practice of Sleep Medicine.* 5th ed. St. Louis: Saunders; 2011.)

◎ BOX 7-1 NURSING DIAGNOSES

Sleep Apnea

- Ineffective Breathing Pattern related musculoskeletal fatigue or neuromuscular impairment, p. 1149
- Decreased Cardiac Output related to alterations in preload, p. 1128
- Disturbed Sleep Pattern related to fragmented sleep, p. 1137
- Disturbed Body Image related to functional dependence on life-sustaining technology, p. 1136
- Deficient Knowledge related to lack of previous exposure to information, p. 1134 (see Patient Education, Box 7-2)

airflow is caused by an obstruction in the upper airway. Complete obstruction lasting 10 seconds or longer is referred to as an *obstructive apnea*, whereas a partial obstruction is known as a *hypopnea* (Fig. 7-2). In central apnea, airflow is absent because of lack of ventilatory muscle effort. The third type of sleep apnea syndrome, mixed apnea, occurs when a combination of obstructive and central patterns occurs in a single apneic event. An apnea-hypopnea index (the number of apneas and hypopneas per hour divided by the hours of sleep) of 5 or greater is diagnostic of sleep apnea syndrome. With new understandings of alterations in ventilatory effort, researchers have developed the respiratory distress index (RDI). To calculate the index, the total number of apneas and hypopneas plus the number of respiratory effort–related arousals (RERAs) or other respiratory events is divided by the hours of sleep. An RDI greater than 5 in addition to reports of daytime sleepiness supports a diagnosis of sleep apnea.[37]

All types of sleep apnea syndrome are accompanied by arterial desaturation and potentially by hypoxemia, which may cause pulmonary vasoconstriction and an increased systemic vascular resistance. However, desaturation and hypoxemia are most severe in the obstructive type. Although the pathophysiology of OSA is unclear, hypotheses suggest that the various types of sleep apnea are all part of a disease continuum. Failure of the central respiratory rhythm control center to generate a stable rhythm is thought to be the basic defect responsible for sleep apnea syndrome. Cyclic oscillations occur with greater frequency at night and are further exacerbated by mouth breathing.[38]

Nursing management of the patient with sleep apnea incorporates a variety of diagnoses (Box 7-1). Nursing interventions include optimizing oxygenation and ventilation, providing comfort and emotional support, maintaining surveillance for complications, and educating the patient and family (Box 7-2).

BOX 7-2 PATIENT EDUCATION

Sleep Apnea

- Pathophysiology of the disease specific to the patient and type of apnea
- Modification of risk factors, such as weight loss, abstaining from alcohol, establishing a program of sleep hygiene, lateral body positioning during sleep
- Importance of compliance with continuous positive airway pressure (CPAP)
- Consequences of untreated apnea, such as vascular hypertension, coronary artery disease, cerebrovascular disease, arrhythmias, pulmonary hypertension, diabetes, daytime sleepiness, death

Obstructive Sleep Apnea
Etiology and Pathophysiology

OSA syndrome occurs when at least five apnea or hypopnea events per hour of sleep occur as the result of an obstruction in the upper airway. In the general population, between 3% and 7% of people have severe OSA.[39] The incidence of OSA is believed to increase with age. Consequences include chronic hypoventilation syndrome; arousals that fragment sleep; cardiovascular changes such as hypertension, stroke, ischemic heart disease, insulin resistance, ventricular hypertrophy, and nocturnal angina.[40] Because of the cardiovascular complications and accidents caused by sleepiness, OSA is a significant condition that should be effectively evaluated.

The cause of OSA is not entirely understood; however, upper airway structure, hormonal balance, and neural control are implicated. Factors that contribute to OSA are: 1) anatomic narrowing of the upper airway; 2) increased compliance of the upper airway tissue; 3) reflexes affecting upper airway caliber; and 4) pharyngeal inspiratory muscle function.[41] Computed tomographic studies of awake subjects have shown that patients with OSA have narrower airways than normal subjects do. The narrower the airway, the more easily it may become obstructed (Fig. 7-3).

Upper airway patency is also affected by upper airway function, which is under the control of the respiratory motor neurons. During sleep, this control varies and causes decreased neural activity, thereby narrowing the airway. This effect is especially prevalent during REM sleep, when the motor neurons are hypotonic. Unstable control of the respiratory nerves of the diaphragmatic, intercostal, and upper airway muscles can cause sleep apneas.[41] Hypothyroidism can alter respiratory controls and thereby contribute to OSA. Other contributing disorders are exogenous obesity, kyphoscoliosis, and autonomic dysfunction.[42]

The patient with OSA develops cycles of hypoxemia, hypercapnia, and acidosis with each episode of apnea until he or she is aroused and airflow resumes. Alveolar hypoventilation accompanies each episode of apnea and results in hypercapnia. Between episodes, alveolar ventilation improves so that overall there is no retention of carbon dioxide (CO_2).

With obstruction, inspiratory subatmospheric intrathoracic pressures are abnormally elevated. This leads to a tendency for airways to collapse, resulting in hemodynamic and electrocardiographic changes. The extremely elevated pressures that occur in individuals with OSA who have apneic episodes i

Midsagittal MRI

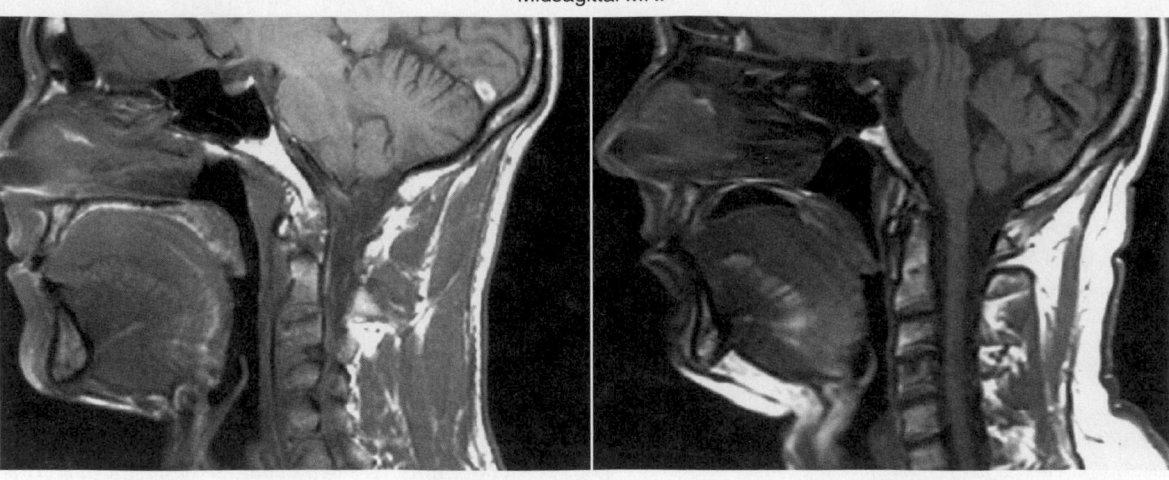

Normal   Apneic

FIGURE 7-3 Midsagittal magnetic resonance imaging of a normal subject *(left)* and a subject with sleep apnea *(right)*. Notice the narrowing of the trachea and the elongated soft palate. (From Kryger MH, et al, eds. *Principles and Practice of Sleep Medicine.* 5th ed. St. Louis: Saunders; 2011.)

REM and NREM stages cause systemic and pulmonary hypertension. Systemic pressures of 200/120 mm Hg (awake control: 130/80 mm Hg) and pulmonary artery pressures of 80/54 mm Hg (awake control: 30/20 mm Hg) have been reported.[43] Cardiac dysrhythmias associated with obstructive apnea include bradycardias, sinus arrest, and occasionally, second-degree heart blocks. After resumption of airflow, tachycardias commonly occur. Bradycardia-tachycardia syndrome is associated with OSA.[44]

Assessment and Diagnosis

Careful monitoring of oxygen saturation and breathing patterns can help the critical care nurse identify patients with this syndrome and assist in its diagnosis and treatment. Patients at risk for OSA may have the following symptoms: snoring; obesity; short, thick neck circumference; cardiovascular disease; systemic hypertension; pulmonary hypertension; sleep fragmentation; gastroesophageal reflux; and an impaired quality of life. Apneas may occur in people whose throats are abnormally small or collapsible. Muscles that would normally hold the throat open relax while the patient is asleep. Snoring is caused when those soft tissues in the throat vibrate. Snoring often precedes the complaint of daytime sleepiness, and the intensity increases with weight gain and alcohol ingestion.[42] Men with a collar size of 17 or greater and women with a size 16 or greater are thought to have an increased incidence of apnea. Friedman and others showed a clinical correlation between Modified Mallampati grade (MMP), tonsil size, body mass index, and the severity of apnea. These assessments are used by anesthesiologists to determine intubation difficulty.[42] There is an increased incidence of sleep apnea among African Americans as well as Mexican Americans, and an increased incidence is observed among those with metabolic syndrome.

OSA episodes frequently end in brief EEG arousals. Patients may experience hundreds of arousals and not even realize they

awaken hundreds of times during the night. These arousals cause sleep fragmentation and daytime sleepiness, which can lead to irritability, poor job performance, troubled relationships, depression, and impaired quality of life.

The definitive diagnosis of OSA syndrome is made with PSG during an overnight sleep study. PSG is used to determine the number and length of apnea episodes and sleep stages, number of arousals, airflow, respiratory effort, and oxygen desaturation.

Medical Management

For patients with mild OSA (apnea-hypopnea index of 5 to 10), weight loss, sleeping on the side if apneas are associated with sleeping on the back, avoidance of sedative medications and alcohol before bedtime, and avoidance of sleep deprivation may be all that is necessary. Oral appliances may be prescribed to stabilize the jaw or retain the tongue. These devices must be fitted by a dentist and are not always as effective as continuous positive airway pressure (CPAP). Moderate to severe levels of apnea may be treated with mechanical, surgical, or pharmacologic therapy. Treatment can vary depending on the type and severity of illness.

CPAP via nasal mask is the treatment of choice. CPAP machines are simply pressure generators with the effective pressure being determined during the titration part of the PSG. This holds the airway open and prevents collapse. The patient wears a small, triangle-shaped mask over the nose or uses nasal pillows if the mask is not tolerated. CPAP treats the obstruction and the snoring, choking, and gasping that accompany it, and it provides cardiovascular benefits. Although CPAP is the treatment of choice, it is only effective if the patient is compliant with therapy. If a patient cannot tolerate the continuous pressure of CPAP, bimodal positive airway pressure (BiPAP), which provides separate pressures for inspiration and expiration, may be tried.[45]

Various surgical interventions are available for the treatment of apnea and snoring. Patients with mild OSA or snoring alone may undergo an outpatient procedure called *laser uvulopalatopharyngoplasty (LAUP)*, which uses lasers to remove excess tissue at the soft palate level. For patients who snore but do not have apnea, somnoplasty may provide relief. Somnoplasty involves inserting a small electrode into the soft palate and heating the tissue, causing the area to shrink and tighten.[46]

Uvulopalatopharyngoplasty (UPPP) was one of the earlier surgeries used to treat OSA. Essentially, a large tonsillectomy is performed and all redundant tissue is removed (Fig. 7-4). Reports of success from UPPP vary widely, with 40% to 80% of patients experiencing sleep apnea improvement.[47] Complications include speech impairment, inability to eat, postoperative bleeding, and infection. Severe pain after UPPP is documented and may continue well into the postoperative period.[47] UPPP patients are not usually admitted to critical care areas, because the postoperative recovery does not require critical care.

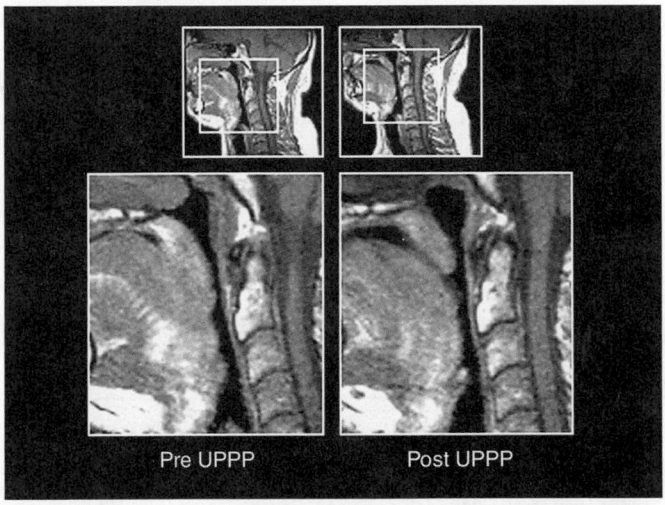

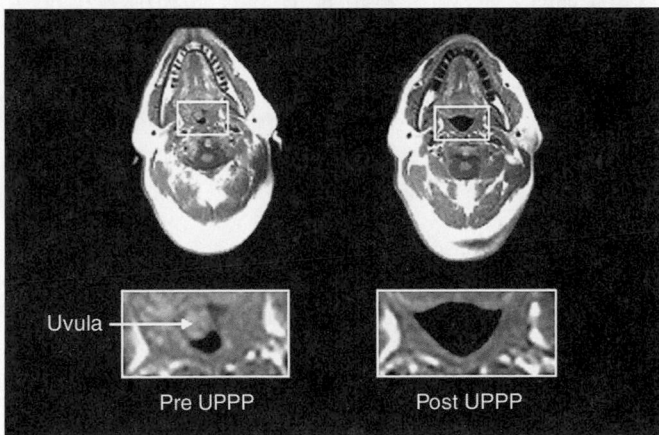

FIGURE 7-4 *A,* Midsagittal images of a patient before and after uvulopalatopharyngoplasty (UPPP). Notice the shortened uvula. Because the soft palate was not resected, the tracheal lumen remains narrow. *B,* Axial images at the level of the uvula; notice the significant increase in the diameter of the airway. (From Kryger MH, et al, eds. *Principles and Practice of Sleep Medicine.* 5th ed. St. Louis: Saunders; 2011.)

Although tracheostomy was the original surgery procedure used to treat OSA, it is now used only in the most severe cases of apnea that do not respond to other treatments. Bariatric surgery is an effective means to facilitate weight loss and subsequent improvement in OSA.[48]

Treatment of OSA with medication is usually a last resort and has proved to be very disappointing. Protriptyline has been shown to decrease apnea and reduce excessive daytime sleepiness by decreasing sleep apnea frequency that increases during REM sleep. Oxygen may be used to lower hypoxemia and nocturnal desaturations.

Nursing Management

The nurse's role in the management of sleep apnea includes educating the patient and family about the syndrome and the consequences of noncompliance with treatment regimens. This education may also include preoperative teaching for any surgery procedures such as UPPP. Monitoring of patients with OSA while in critical care should include assessment of the breathing patterns, hours of sleep, and pulse oximetry. Cautious administration of narcotics to patients with sleep apnea is suggested because of the potential for respiratory depression, although the concern regarding adequate pain relief is not well studied.

Nasal CPAP is most effective when patients are properly fitted with the nasal mask and have clear instructions regarding its use. Several types and sizes of masks are available, including one type called a *nasal pillow*, which does not cover the nose but instead fits into the nostrils. If patients are admitted to the critical care unit with a history of OSA, they need to use their home CPAP mask and equipment as part of their regular sleep routine. The nurse can enhance compliance with the CPAP system. Nursing care includes ensuring proper fit of the CPAP mask, with no air blowing into the patient's eyes, correct airway pressure, no pressure sores from the mask, and no gastric insufflation.

Central Sleep Apnea
Etiology and Pathophysiology

Central sleep apnea (CSA) can be seen on PSG as an absence of airflow and respiratory effort for at least 10 seconds. A complete loss of electromyographic activity by the respiratory muscles would be expected, because CSA is defined as a pause in respiration without ventilatory effort.[49]

A chemoreceptor sensitive to the levels of CO_2 resides within the brain. When CO_2 levels become excessive, ventilatory efforts are increased to blow off the excess CO_2. This negative-feedback loop exists to provide a homeostatic balance in the carbon dioxide and oxygen levels of the body. Whereas OSA results from an obstructed or collapsed airway, patients with CSA suffer from a lack of ventilatory effort. This can be observed in patients with cardiopulmonary disease (e.g., COPD) or heart failure, because their chemoreceptors have become adjusted to an increased CO_2 level.[50] However, the uniting factor is cessation of breathing momentarily during sleep due to the transient withdrawal of central nervous system drive to the muscles of respiration.[51] It is not uncommon for a patient who experiences CSA to also have some obstructive events.

CSA may result from many physiologic or pathophysiologic events.[51] Possible causes of nonhypercapnic CSA include periodic breathing at high altitude, renal or metabolic disturbances, and idiopathic central apnea seen at sea level. Hypercapnic CSA can occur in many neuromuscular conditions such as spinal cord or brain injury, encephalitis, brainstem neoplasm or infarcts, muscular dystrophy, myasthenia gravis, bulbar poliomyelitis, and postpolio syndrome.

Assessment and Diagnosis

Clinical characteristics of hypercapnic CSA include respiratory failure, cor pulmonale, peripheral edema, polycythemia, daytime sleepiness, and snoring. Patients with nonhypercapnic CSA have clinical features very similar to those of OSA. Nonhypercapnic CSA characteristics include daytime sleepiness, insomnia or poor sleep, mild or intermittent snoring, and awakenings accompanied by choking or feeling short of breath; frequently, the patients are of normal body weight. Diagnosis is made by overnight PSG or sleep study, which will determine the respiratory and sleep patterns of the patient.[51]

Medical Management

Because there are two types of CSA, there are two therapeutic approaches depending on the cause of the apnea. The hypercapnic patient who has worsening hypoventilation during sleep is best served by nocturnal ventilation. Most such patients experience some respiratory muscle failure. One treatment for the nonhypercapnic or heart failure patients is nasal CPAP, which also may provide a beneficial cardiovascular effect. Nocturnal oxygen supplementation may be effective as well. If CPAP is not tolerated, pharmacologic management may be tried. Medroxyprogesterone, a respiratory stimulant, may improve ventilation in selected patients. Acetazolamide, a carbonic anhydrase inhibitor that can result in metabolic acidosis, also may decrease the frequency of apneic episodes. Several studies have reported the development of obstructive apnea in patients successfully treated for central apnea.[52]

Nursing Management

For the nurse caring for a patient with CSA, patient and family education about the patient's condition and treatment regimen can help to ensure patient compliance. The nurse needs to address any fear or anxiety about going to sleep. Nurses also need to caution patients to avoid alcohol and sedative medications. Weight loss is recommended if the patient is obese. The nurse needs to carefully monitor and assess the respiratory status of the patient. For more information, see the Case Study on Sleep Alterations (Box 7-3).

BOX 7-3   CASE STUDY

Patient with Sleep Alterations

Brief Patient History

Mr. D is a 43-year-old, severely obese, self-employed man. His medical history includes excessive daytime sleepiness, hypertension, and sinus dysrhythmia. He received a diagnosis of obstructive sleep apnea (OSA) 2 years ago, and his health care provider prescribed nasal continuous positive airway pressure (CPAP) for use at night. However, Mr. D has been, for the most part, noncompliant because of reported discomfort and interference with his sex life. Mr. D's hypertension has required increasing medication, and he has begun to develop cardiomegaly. His business suffers from his inability to stay awake and focus. He and his wife have started sleeping in separate rooms because of his snoring. These circumstances have prompted Mr. D's physician to recommend surgical correction of Mr. D's airway. He refused to consider a tracheostomy but agreed to uvulopalatopharyngoplasty (UPPP) despite the 50% chance of success. Mr. D and his spouse understand that endotracheal intubation may be necessary for 24 to 48 hours because of the severity of his condition.

Clinical Assessment

Mr. D is admitted to the surgical critical care unit after a very complicated surgical procedure with an oral endotracheal tube connected to supplemental oxygen with spontaneous respiration. He is awake and follows commands; however, he is having periods of restlessness and pulling at tubes.

Diagnostic Procedures

Mr. D's vital signs include blood pressure of 160/72 mm Hg, heart rate of 120 beats/min (sinus tachycardia), respiratory rate of 20 breaths/min, and temperature of 97.8° F. The chest radiograph is clear. Arterial blood gases were obtained: pH of 7.38, PaO_2 of 90 mm Hg, $PaCO_2$ of 35 mm Hg, HCO_3^- level of 24%, and O_2 saturation of 98%. Mr. D indicates that his pain is a 5 on the Baker-Wong faces scale by pointing. The Riker Sedation-Agitation Scale score is 5.

Medical Diagnosis

Mr. D is diagnosed with OSA.

Questions

1. What major outcomes do you expect to achieve for this patient?
2. What problems or risks must be managed to achieve these outcomes?
3. What interventions must be initiated to monitor, prevent, manage, or eliminate the problems and risks identified?
4. What interventions should be initiated to promote optimal functioning, safety, and well-being of the patient?
5. What possible learning needs do you anticipate for this patient?
6. What cultural and age-related factors may have a bearing on the patient's plan of care?

SUMMARY

Normal Human Sleep

- The behavioral definition of sleep is a reversible behavioral state of perceptual disengagement from and unresponsiveness to the environment.
- Humans experience three states of being: awake, REM sleep, or NREM sleep.
- A sufficient amount of sleep has been achieved when one awakens without external stimuli and gets through the day without feeling sleepy.
- Circadian and homeostatic processes function together to ensure optimal sleep for an individual.

Pharmacology

- Hypnotic benzodiazepines remain the medications of choice to treat insomnia.
- Wake-promoting medications produce increased arousal, behavioral activation, and alertness.
- Patients with illness may respond differently to medications than do healthy patients.
- The nurse has a responsibility to administer these medications in the most efficient manner to promote sleep and to monitor effectiveness.

Sleep Pattern Disturbance

- Sleep disturbance in critically ill patients is defined as insufficient duration or stages of sleep that results in discomfort and interferes with quality of life.

- Insufficient sleep in acutely and critically ill patients has been associated with physiologic and psychologic exhaustion and may delay recovery from illness.
- Sleep disturbance in critically ill patients may stem from psychologic stress associated with critical illness and the critical care environment, surgical stress, noise, interruptions for care, painful procedures or physiologic processes, excessive bright light, and muscular and joint discomfort that result from bed rest.
- Medical management of sleep pattern disturbance in critically ill patients consists of the administration of sedative-hypnotics.

Sleep Apnea Syndrome

- Sleep apnea syndrome, sometimes called sleep-disordered breathing, occurs when airflow is absent or reduced and can be divided into three types: 1) obstructive; 2) central; and 3) mixed.
- All types of sleep apnea syndrome are accompanied by arterial desaturation and potentially by hypoxemia, which may cause pulmonary vasoconstriction and an increased systemic vascular resistance.
- Medical management focuses on correcting the underlying cause, supporting ventilation with CPAP, and evaluating for the patient for surgery.
- Nursing interventions include optimizing oxygenation and ventilation, providing comfort and emotional support, maintaining surveillance for complications, and educating the patient and family.

REFERENCES

1. Matthews EE. Sleep disturbances and fatigue in critically ill patients. *AACN Adv Crit Care.* 2011;22:204.
2. Boyko Y, et al. Sleep disturbances in critically ill patients in ICU: how much do we know? *Acta Anaesthesiol Scand.* Epub ahead of print. 2012.
3. Carskadon MA, Dement WC. Normal human sleep: an overview. In: Kryger MH, et al, eds. *Principles and Practice of Sleep Medicine.* 5th ed. St Louis: Saunders; 2011.
4. Jafari B, Mohsenin V. Polysomnography. *Clin Chest Med.* 2010;31:287.
5. Collop NA, et al. Normal sleep and circadian processes. *Crit Care Clin.* 2008;24:449.
6. Ganz FD. Sleep and immune function. *Crit Care Nurse.* 2012;32(2):e19.
7. Siegel JM. REM sleep. In: Kryger MH, et al, eds. *Principles and Practice of Sleep Medicine.* 5th ed. St Louis: Saunders; 2011.
8. Czeisler CA, Buxon OM. The human circadian timing system and sleep-wake regulation. In: Kryger MH, et al, eds. *Principles and Practice of Sleep Medicine.* 5th ed. St Louis: Saunders; 2011.
9. Hardin KA. Sleep in the ICU: potential mechanisms and clinical implications. *Chest.* 2009;136:284.
10. Brandon SL, Zee PC. Neurobiology of sleep. *Clin Chest Med.* 2010;31:309.
11. Achermann P, Borbely AA. Sleep homeostasis and models of sleep regulation. In: Kryger MH, et al, eds. *Principles and Practice of Sleep Medicine.* 5th ed. St Louis: Saunders; 2011.
12. Mendelson W. Hypnotic medications: mechanisms of action and pharmacologic effects. In: Kryger MH, et al, eds. *Principles and Practice of Sleep Medicine.* 5th ed. St Louis: Saunders; 2011.
13. Roux FJ, Kryger MH. Medication effects on sleep. *Clin Chest Med.* 2010;31:397.
14. Nishino S, Mignot E. Wake-promoting medications: basic mechanisms and pharmacology. In: Kryger MH, et al, eds. *Principles and Practice of Sleep Medicine.* 5th ed. St Louis: Saunders; 2011.
15. Malley MB, et al. Wake-promoting medications: efficacy and adverse effects. In: Kryger MH, et al, eds. *Principles and Practice of Sleep Medicine.* 5th ed. St Louis: Saunders; 2011.
16. *National Sleep Foundation.* 2008 Sleep in America Poll. Washington, DC: National Sleep Foundation; 2008. http://www.sleepfoundation.org. Accessed June 2012.
17. Schweitzer PK. Drugs that disturb sleep and wakefulness. In: Kryger MH, et al, eds. *Principles and Practice of Sleep Medicine.* 5th ed. St Louis: Saunders; 2011.
18. Ahmed AQ. Effects of common medications used for sleep disorders. *Crit Care Clin.* 2008;24:493.
19. Nicolas A, et al. Perception of nighttime sleep by surgical patients in an intensive care unit. *Nurs Crit Care.* 2008;13:25.

20. Ugras GA, Oztekin SD. Patient perception of environmental and nursing factors contributing to sleep disturbances in a neurosurgical intensive care unit. *Tohoku J Exp Med.* 2007;212:299.

21. Stuck A, et al. Preventing intensive care unit delirium. *Dimen Crit Care Nurs.* 2011;30:315.

22. Salas RE, Gamaldo CE. Adverse effects of sleep deprivation in the ICU. *Crit Care Clin.* 2008;24:461.

23. Sunshine W, et al. Massage therapy and transcutaneous electrical stimulation effects on fibromyalgia. *J Clin Rheumatol.* 1997;2:18.

24. Simpson T, et al. Patients' perceptions of environmental factors that disturb sleep after cardiac surgery. *Am J Crit Care.* 1996;5:173.

25. Frisk U, Nordstrom G. Patients sleep in an intensive care unit: patients' and nurses' perception. *Intens Crit Care Nurs.* 2003;19:342.

26. Redeker NS, et al. Sleep patterns in women after coronary artery bypass surgery. *Appl Nurs Res.* 1996;9:115.

27. Gabor JY, et al. Contribution of the intensive care unit environment to sleep disruption in mechanically ventilated patients and health subjects. *Am J Respir Crit Care Med.* 2003;167:708.

28. Cooper AB, et al. Sleep in critically ill patients requiring mechanical ventilation. *Chest.* 2000;117:809.

29. Bosma K, et al. Patient-ventilator interaction and sleep in mechanically ventilated patients: pressure support versus proportional assist ventilation. *Crit Care Med.* 2007;35:1048.

30. Toublan B, et al. Assist-control ventilation vs. low levels of pressure support ventilation on sleep quality in intubated ICU patients. *Intensive Care Med.* 2007;33:1148.

31. Combes A, et al. Morbidity, mortality, and quality-of-life outcomes of patients requiring >14 days of mechanical ventilation. *Crit Care Med.* 2003;31:1373.

32. Bihari S, et al. Factors affecting sleep quality of patients in Intensive Care Unit. *J Clin Sleep Med.* 2012;8:301.

33. Richards KC, et al. Effects of massage in acute and critical care. *AACN Clin Issues.* 2000;11:77.

34. Williamson JW. The effects of ocean sounds on sleep after coronary artery bypass graft surgery. *Am J Crit Care.* 1992;1:91.

35. Stanchina JL, et al. The influence of white noise on sleep in subjects exposed to ICU noise. *Sleep Med.* 2005;6:423.

36. Lower J, et al. High-tech high-touch: mission possible? *Dimens Crit Care Nurs.* 2002;21:201.

37. Cao MT, et al. Clinical features and evaluation of obstructive sleep obstructive sleep apnea and upper airway resistance syndrome. In: Kryger MH, et al, eds. *Principles and Practice of Sleep Medicine.* 5th ed. St Louis: Saunders; 2011.

38. Naughton MT. Common sleep problems in ICU: heart failure and sleep-disordered breathing syndromes. *Crit Care Clin.* 2008;24:565.

39. Punjabi NM. The epidemiology of adult obstructive sleep apnea. *Proc Am Thorac Soc.* 2008;5:136.

40. Krieger S, Caples SM. Obstructive sleep apnea and cardiovascular disease: implications for clinical practice. *Cleve Clin J Med.* 2007;74:853.

41. Yaggi HK, Strohl KP. Adult obstructive sleep apnea/hypopnea syndrome: definitions, risk factors, and pathogenesis. *Clin Chest Med.* 2010;31:179.

42. Ulualp SO. Snoring and obstructive sleep apnea. *Med Clin N Am.* 2010;94:1047.

43. Young T, et al. Systemic and pulmonary hypertension in obstructive sleep apnea. In: Kryger MH, et al, eds. *Principles and practice of sleep medicine.* 5th ed. St Louis: Saunders; 2011.

44. Somers VK, Javaheri S. Cardiovascular effects of sleep-related breathing disorders. In: Kryger MH, et al, eds. *Principles and Practice of Sleep Medicine.* 5th ed. St Louis: Saunders; 2011.

45. Freedman N. Treatment of obstructive sleep apnea syndrome. *Clin Chest Med.* 2010;31:187.

46. Friedman M, Wilson MN. Surgical therapy for sleep breathing disorders. *Sleep Med Clin.* 2010;5:153.

47. Carpenter JM, LaMear WR. Uvulopalatopharyngoplasty: results of a patient questionnaire. *Ann Otol Rhinol Laryngol.* 2008;117:24.

48. Buchwald H, et al. Bariatric surgery: a systematic review and meta-analysis. *JAMA.* 2004;292:1724.

49. Wellman A, White DP. Central sleep apnea and periodic breathing. In: Kryger MH, et al, eds. *Principles and Practice of Sleep Medicine.* 5th ed. St Louis: Saunders; 2011.

50. Javaheri S. Central sleep apnea. *Clin Chest Med.* 2010;31:235.

51. Ekhert DJ, et al. Central sleep apnea: pathophysiology and treatment. *Chest.* 2007;131:595.

52. Buysse DJ, et al. Clinical pharmacology of other drugs used as hypnotics. In: Kryger MH, et al, eds. *Principles and Practice of Sleep Medicine.* 5th ed. St Louis: Saunders; 2011.

Nutrition Alterations and Management

Kasuen Mauldin

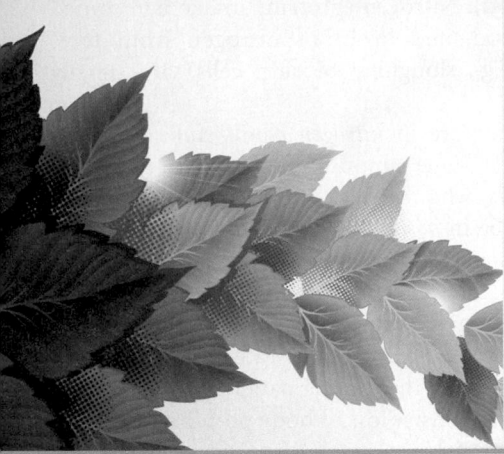

Nutrition support is an essential component of providing comprehensive care to the critically ill patient. Nutrition screening must be conducted on every patient, and a more thorough nutrition assessment completed on any patient screened to be nutritionally at risk. Malnutrition can be related to any essential nutrient or nutrients. A serious type of malnutrition found frequently among hospitalized patients is protein-calorie malnutrition (PCM). Malnutrition is associated with a variety of adverse outcomes, such as wound dehiscence, infections, pressure ulcers, respiratory failure requiring ventilation, longer hospital days, and death. The purpose of this chapter is to provide an overview of nutrient metabolism, nutritional status assessment, and implications of undernutrition for the sick or stressed patient. Specifically, nutrition for each of the system alterations will be discussed along with nursing management.

NUTRIENT METABOLISM

Nutrients are chemical substances found in foods that are needed for human life, growth, maintenance, and repair of body tissues. The main nutrients in foods are carbohydrates, proteins, fats, vitamins, minerals, and water. The process by which nutrients are used at the cellular level is known as *metabolism*. The energy-yielding nutrients or macronutrients are carbohydrates, proteins, and fats. For proper metabolic functioning, adequate amounts of micronutrients, such as vitamins, minerals (including electrolytes), and trace elements also must be supplied to the human body.

Energy-Yielding Nutrients
Carbohydrates

Through the process of digestion, carbohydrates are broken down into glucose, fructose, and galactose. After absorption from the intestinal tract, fructose and galactose are converted to glucose, the primary form of carbohydrate used by the cells. Glucose provides the energy needed to maintain cellular functions, including transport across cell membranes, secretion of specific hormones, muscle contraction, and synthesis of new substances. Most of the energy produced from carbohydrate metabolism is used to form adenosine triphosphate (ATP), the principal form of immediately available energy within all body cells. One gram of carbohydrate provides approximately 4 kcal of energy. For example, if a food contains 10 grams of carbohydrates, then 40 kcal (10 g × 4 kcal/g) of the total calories for that food comes from carbohydrates.

Inside the cell, glucose can be stored as glycogen or metabolized in a process called *glycolysis* for the subsequent release of energy. Liver and muscle cells have the largest glycogen reserves. In addition to glucose obtained from glycogen, glucose can be formed from lactate, amino acids, and glycerol. This process of manufacturing glucose from non-glucose precursors is called *gluconeogenesis*. Gluconeogenesis is carried out at all times, but it becomes especially important in maintaining a source of glucose in times of increased physiologic need and limited supply. Only the liver and, to a lesser extent, the kidney are capable of producing significant amounts of glucose for release into the blood for use by other tissues.

Proteins

Proteins are made up of chains of amino acids. Each amino acid consists of carbon, hydrogen, and oxygen, and nitrogen in the form of one or more amine groups ($-NH_2$). Amino acids are the protein components that can be used by cells.

Proteins have important structural and functional duties within the body. Proteins provide the structural basis of all lean body mass, such as the vital organs and skeletal muscle. Proteins are important for visceral (cellular) functions, such as initiation of chemical reactions (e.g., hormones, enzymes), transportation of other substances (e.g., apoproteins, albumin), preservation of immune function (e.g., antibodies), and maintenance of osmotic pressure (e.g., albumin) and blood neutrality (e.g., buffers). Some amino acids are used for energy, providing approximately 4 kcal per gram.

Proteins are synthesized continuously, broken down into amino acids, and then resynthesized into new protein. This three-step process is called *protein turnover*. The rate of turnover is fastest (often only a few hours) in enzymes and hormones involved in metabolic activities. In very active tissues—such as those of the liver, kidney, and gastrointestinal mucosa—protein turnover occurs every few days. If necessary, 90% of the amino acids released by tissue breakdown can be reused, with the diet providing the remaining 10% of the amino acids needed for protein synthesis. In the injured or undernourished individual, many of the amino acids released by tissue breakdown may be used for gluconeogenesis. To preserve lean body mass, adequate energy must be supplied by the diet so that most of the amino acids from the diet and from tissue breakdown can be used for tissue synthesis, rather than gluconeogenesis.

Proteins, which often consist of hundreds or thousands of amino acids, are too large to be absorbed intact under normal circumstances. Through digestion, the proteins are broken down into amino acids and *dipeptides* or *tripeptides* (composed of two or three amino acids, respectively) that can be absorbed across the intestinal wall. Certain amino acids are *essential*; they cannot be produced by the body and must be supplied through the diet. Essential amino acids include valine, leucine, isoleucine, lysine, phenylalanine, tryptophan, threonine, and methionine, as well as histidine and arginine in infants. Other amino acids are nonessential and can be manufactured by the body under normal circumstances if the essential amino acids are in adequate supply. Some amino acids that may be nonessential in healthy adults become essential during illness. For example, histidine is an essential amino acid for adults with renal failure, and glutamine may be essential for individuals with trauma, sepsis, or other physiologic types of stress.

The amine group is essential for protein synthesis, but the nonamine portion of the molecule (ketoacid) is used in gluconeogenesis. If a ketoacid is used for gluconeogenesis, the amine group can be excreted in the urine as ammonia or urea. If the rate of gluconeogenesis rises, urinary nitrogen excretion also increases. In assessing protein nutrition, it is common to measure nitrogen balance, or the amount of nitrogen excreted compared with that consumed. Normally, most of the body's nitrogen losses are in the urine, and in determining nitrogen balance, urinary nitrogen excretion is measured (preferably over a 24-hour period). Nitrogen (protein) intake is recorded over the same period, and losses of nitrogen from feces and other routes (e.g., sloughing of skin cells) are usually estimated.

Most healthy adults are in *nitrogen equilibrium*, meaning that they excrete the same amount of nitrogen that they consume. Individuals who excrete less nitrogen than they consume are said to be in *positive nitrogen balance*; this occurs during growth, pregnancy, and healing. Individuals who excrete more nitrogen than they consume are in *negative nitrogen balance*. Negative nitrogen balance is common in the early period after trauma or surgery. When the rate of gluconeogenesis is high, as may occur in the trauma patient who is initially too unstable to be fed, extensive loss of body proteins can occur. Losses include structural (e.g., muscle) and visceral proteins. Visceral proteins, including immunoglobulins, albumin, and complement, are critical for survival. Preservation of body protein is therefore a key goal of nutrition support of critically ill patients.

Lipids (Fats)

Lipids include fatty acids, triglycerides (three fatty acids bound to a glycerol backbone), phospholipids (lipids containing phosphate groups), cholesterol, and cholesterol esters. Aside from their involvement in functions such as the maintenance of cell membranes and the manufacture of prostaglandins, lipids—primarily in the form of triglycerides—provide a stored source of energy. They are calorically dense molecules, providing more than twice the amount of energy (9 kcal) per gram as protein and carbohydrates.

Most dietary lipids—consisting primarily of triglycerides—are too large to be absorbed intact and are partially broken down (hydrolyzed) in the intestine to form monoglycerides and diglycerides, which contain one or two fatty acids, respectively, bound to glycerol.

Bile salts produced in the liver are detergents, and they promote the formation of micelles, which are emulsions of fatty acids, monoglycerides, and bile salts. Long-chain fatty acids, which contain more than 12 carbon atoms, are very insoluble in water; they are found mainly in the interior of the micelle. The external portion of the micelle, which includes the glycerol part of the triglycerides, is more water soluble than the interior portion. This allows the micelle to cross the unstirred water layer that coats the intestinal absorptive surface.

Inside the intestinal cells, monoglycerides and long-chain fatty acids rejoin to form triglycerides, and they are surrounded by phospholipids and specific proteins to form chylomicrons. These chylomicrons are transported out of the intestine through the lymphatic system, finally entering the blood circulation through the thoracic duct. Some of the chylomicrons are taken up by the liver, but most are directly transported to other tissues. Short-chain fatty acids (less than 8 carbon atoms long) and medium-chain fatty acids (8 to 12 carbon atoms long) are more water soluble than longer fatty acids; triglycerides containing these fatty acids can be absorbed without hydrolysis and are soluble enough to be transported to the liver through the portal vein, without chylomicron formation. Short- and medium-chain fatty acids have advantages in nutritional care of patients who have insufficient bile salt formation or inadequate intestinal surface area for absorption of long-chain fatty acids.

With the aid of the enzyme lipoprotein lipase, triglyceride-containing chylomicrons are broken down outside the cell and enter the cell as fatty acids and glycerol. Heparin stimulates lipoprotein lipase, and low doses of heparin are sometimes given to patients receiving intravenous lipid emulsions to improve lipid use. Insulin also stimulates the cellular uptake of triglycerides. Inside the cell, the fatty acids are oxidized (metabolized for energy) or reformed into triglycerides for storage. During an overnight fast, prolonged starvation, or metabolic stress when the carbohydrate supply is limited, the blood glucose level declines, and consequently, insulin levels decrease. In response, a process called *lipolysis* causes the breakdown of intracellular triglycerides, which provides fatty acids for energy production and glycerol for gluconeogenesis.

The fatty acids released from adipose tissue can be used by the liver, heart, or other tissues. In the liver, fatty acids are broken down to ketones (beta-hydroxybutyrate, acetoacetate, and acetone). In the absence of glucose, fatty acid breakdown and ketone production are increased. Ketones can be directly oxidized by skeletal muscle and used for energy. During prolonged starvation, the brain—which normally uses glucose—converts to using ketones as its primary energy source. This is a body defense mechanism to ensure a supply of energy when carbohydrate intake is low.

ASSESSING NUTRITIONAL STATUS

In the United States, The Joint Commission mandates nutrition screening be conducted on every patient within 24 hours of admission to an acute care center.[1] A brief questionnaire to be completed by the patient or significant other, the nursing admission form, or the physician's admission note usually provides enough information to determine whether the patient is at nutritional risk (Box 8-1). Any patient judged to be nutritionally at risk needs a more thorough nutrition assessment. The nutrition assessment process is continuous, with reassessments as a part of the overall nutrition care plan, as shown in Figure 8-1.[2]

Nutrition assessment involves collection of four types of information: 1) anthropometric measurements; 2) biochemical (laboratory) data; 3) clinical signs (physical examination); and 4) diet and pertinent health history. This information provides a basis for 1) identifying patients who are malnourished or at risk of malnutrition; 2) determining the nutritional needs of individual patients; and 3) selecting the most appropriate methods of nutrition support for patients with or at risk of developing nutritional deficits. Nutrition support is the provision of specially formulated or delivered oral, enteral, or parenteral nutrients to maintain or restore optimal nutrition status.[3] The nutrition assessment can be performed by or under the supervision of a registered dietitian or by a nutrition care specialist (e.g., nurse with specialized expertise in nutrition).

BOX 8-1   PATIENTS WHO ARE AT RISK FOR MALNUTRITION

Adults Who Exhibit Any of the Following:
- Involuntary loss or gain of a significant amount of weight (>10% of usual body weight in 6 months, >5% in 1 month), even if the weight achieved by loss or gain is appropriate for height
- Chronic disease
- Chronic use of a modified diet
- Increased metabolic requirements
- Illness or surgery that may interfere with nutritional intake
- Inadequate nutrient intake for >7 days
- Regular use of three or more medications
- Poverty

Infants and Children Who Exhibit Any of the Following:
- Low birth weight
- Small for gestational age
- Weight loss of 10% or more
- Weight-for-length or weight-for-height <5th percentile or >95th percentile
- Increased metabolic requirements
- Impaired ability to ingest or tolerate oral feedings
- Inadequate weight gain or a significant decrease in an individual's usual growth percentile
- Poverty

Figure 8-2 shows the route of administration of specialized nutrition support.

Anthropometric Measurements

Height and current weight are essential anthropometric measurements, and they should be measured rather than obtained through a patient or family report. The most important reason for obtaining anthropometric measurements is to be able to detect changes in the measurements over time (e.g., track response to nutritional therapy). The patient's measurements may be compared with standard tables of weight-for-height or standard growth charts for infants and children. Another simple and reliable tool for interpreting appropriateness of weight for height for adults and older adolescents is the body mass index (BMI).

$$BMI = weight \div height^2$$

Weight is measured in kilograms and height in meters. BMI values are independent of age and gender and are used for assessing health risk. BMI can be classified as shown in Table 8-1.[4,5] Evidence that the associations between BMI, percent of body fat, and body fat distribution differ across populations suggests the possible need for developing different BMI cut-off values for different ethnic groups.[6] For example, alternate BMI classification cut-off values exist for Asians, who are at risk for obesity-related co-morbidities at lower BMI.[6]

It may be impossible to measure the height of some patients accurately. Total height can be estimated from arm span length or knee height.[7,8] To measure knee height, bend the knee 90 degrees, and measure from the base of the heel to the anterior surface of the thigh.

Admission
Not At Risk
Patient Screening
Not At Risk
Periodic Re-screening
At Risk
Patient Assessment
Development of Nutrition Care Plan
Implementation of Nutrition Care Plan
Yes
Continued Inpatient Care?
No
Discharge Planning/ Continuity of Care
Patient Monitoring
Goals Achieved
Change in Status
Patient Re-assessment and Updating of Nutrition Care Plan
Termination of Therapy

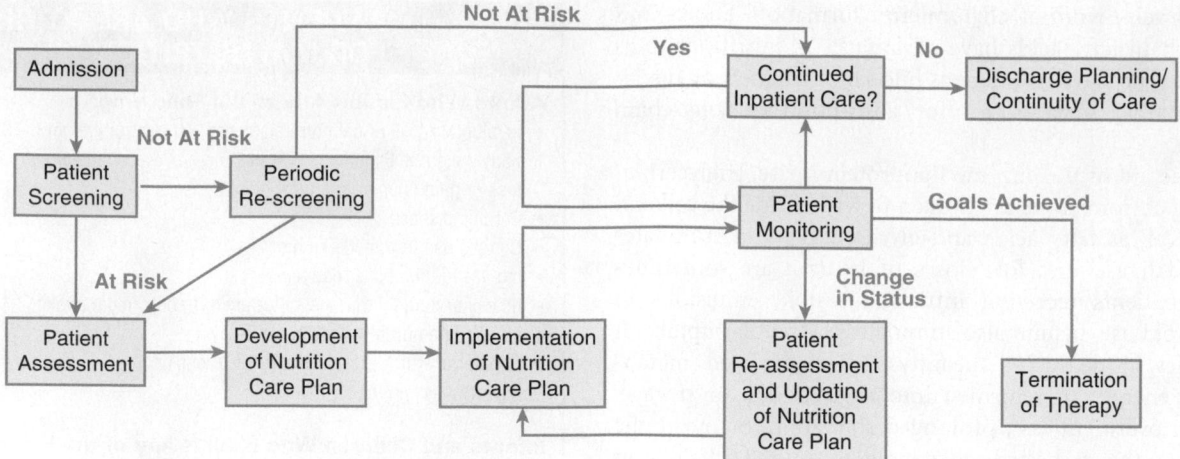

FIGURE 8-1 Nutrition Care Process. (Redrawn from Mueller C, et al. A.S.P.E.N. Clinical guidelines, nutrition screening, assessment, and intervention in adults. *JPEN J Parenter Enteral Nutr.* 2009;33[1]:16.)

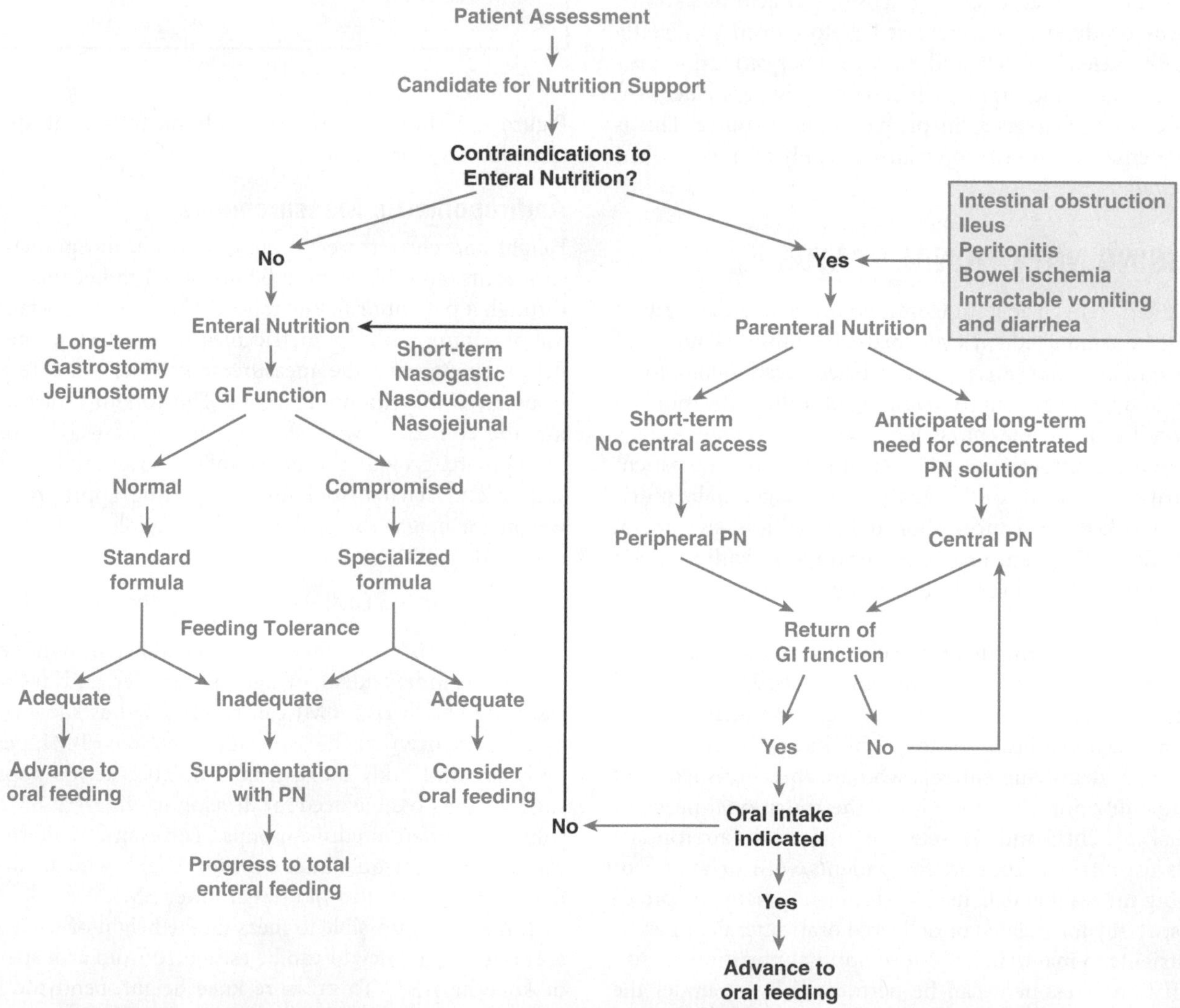

Patient Assessment
Candidate for Nutrition Support
Contraindications to Enteral Nutrition?
No
Yes
Intestinal obstruction
Ileus
Peritonitis
Bowel ischemia
Intractable vomiting and diarrhea
Enteral Nutrition
Long-term
Gastrostomy
Jejunostomy
GI Function
Short-term
Nasogastic
Nasoduodenal
Nasojejunal
Normal
Compromised
Standard formula
Specialized formula
Feeding Tolerance
Adequate
Inadequate
Adequate
Advance to oral feeding
Supplimentation with PN
Consider oral feeding
Progress to total enteral feeding
Parenteral Nutrition
Short-term
No central access
Anticipated long-term need for concentrated PN solution
Peripheral PN
Central PN
Return of GI function
Yes
No
Oral intake indicated
No
Yes
Advance to oral feeding

FIGURE 8-2 Route of Administration of Specialized Nutrition Support. (Redrawn from Ukleja A, et al. Standards for nutrition support. *Nutrition in Clinical Practice.* 2010;25[4]:403.)

TABLE 8-1   ADULT BMI CLASSIFICATIONS

CLASSIFICATION	BMI (kg/m²)
Underweight	<18.5
Normal	18.5-24.99
Overweight:	≥25
Pre-obese	25-29.99
Obese class I	30-34.99
Obese class II	35-39.99
Obese class III	≥40

From World Health Organization. Obesity: preventing and managing the global epidemic. Report of a WHO Consultation. *WHO Technical Report Series 894.* Geneva: World Health Organization; 2000.

For men:

$$\text{height (cm)} = 64.19 - (0.04 \times \text{age in years}) + (2.02 \times \text{knee height [cm]})$$

For women:

$$\text{height (cm)} = 84.8 - (0.24 \times \text{age in years}) + (1.83 \times \text{knee height [cm]})$$

During critical illness, changes in anthropometric measures such as weight are more likely to reflect changes in body water and its distribution. Good judgment must be used in interpreting anthropometric data. For example, edema may mask significant weight loss or underweight. Despite these limitations, weight remains an important measure of nutritional status, and any recent weight change must be evaluated. A woman who was obese 4 months earlier and has lost 15 kg (33 lb) since then may be at nutritional risk even if her current weight is appropriate for her height.

In addition to height and weight data, other measurements such as arm muscle circumference, skin fold thickness, and body composition (proportion of fat and lean tissue, determined by bioelectric impedance or other methods) are sometimes performed, but these measurements are of limited use in assessing critically ill patients.[9]

Biochemical Data

A wide range of laboratory tests can provide information about nutritional status. Those most often used in the clinical setting are described in Table 8-2. No diagnostic tests for evaluation of nutrition are perfect, and care must be taken in interpreting the results of the tests.[10]

Clinical or Physical Manifestations

A thorough physical examination is an essential part of nutrition assessment. Box 8-2 lists some of the more common findings that may indicate an altered nutritional state. It is especially important for the nurse to check for signs of muscle wasting, loss of subcutaneous fat, skin or hair changes, and impairment of wound healing.

Diet and Health History

Information about dietary intake and significant variations in weight is a vital part of the history. Dietary intake can be

TABLE 8-2   COMMON BLOOD AND URINE TESTS USED IN NUTRITION ASSESSMENT

TEST	COMMENTS AND LIMITATIONS
Serum Proteins Albumin or prealbumin	Levels decrease with protein deficiency and in liver failure. Albumin levels are slow to change in response to malnutrition and repletion. Prealbumin levels fall in response to trauma and infection.
Hematologic Values Anemia	
Normocytic (normal MCV, MCHC)	Common with protein deficiency
Microcytic (decreased MCV, MCH, MCHC)	Indicative of iron deficiency (can be from blood loss)
Macrocytic (increased MCV)	Common in folate and vitamin B_{12} deficiency
Lymphocytopenia	Common in protein deficiency

MCH, Mean corpuscular hemoglobin; *MCHC,* mean corpuscular hemoglobin concentration; *MCV,* mean corpuscular volume.

BOX 8-2   CLINICAL MANIFESTATIONS OF NUTRITIONAL ALTERATIONS

Manifestations That May Indicate Protein-Calorie Malnutrition
- Hair loss; dull, dry, brittle hair; loss of hair pigment
- Loss of subcutaneous tissue; muscle wasting
- Poor wound healing; decubitus ulcer
- Hepatomegaly
- Edema

Manifestations Often Present in Vitamin Deficiencies
- Conjunctival and corneal dryness (vitamin A)
- Dry, scaly skin; follicular hyperkeratosis, in which the skin appears to have gooseflesh continually (vitamin A)
- Gingivitis; poor wound healing (vitamin C)
- Petechiae; ecchymoses (vitamin C or K)
- Inflamed tongue, cracking at the corners of the mouth (riboflavin [vitamin B_2], niacin, folic acid, vitamin B_{12}, or other B vitamins)
- Edema; heart failure (thiamine [vitamin B_1])
- Confusion; confabulation (thiamine [vitamin B_1])

Manifestations Often Present in Mineral Deficiencies
- Blue sclerae; pale mucous membranes; spoon-shaped nails (iron)
- Hypogeusia, or poor sense of taste; dysgeusia, or bad taste; eczema; poor wound healing (zinc)

Manifestations Often Observed with Excessive Vitamin Intake
- Hair loss; dry skin; hepatomegaly (vitamin A)

evaluated in several ways, including a diet record, a 24-hour recall, and a diet history. The diet record, a listing of the type and amount of all foods and beverages consumed for some period (usually 3 days), is useful for evaluating the patient's intake in the critical care setting if the adequacy of intake is questionable. However, such a record reveals little about the patient's habitual intake before the illness or injury. The 24-hour recall of all food and beverage intake is easily and quickly performed, but it also may not reflect the patient's usual intake and has limited usefulness. The diet history consists of a detailed interview about the patient's usual intake, along with social, familial, cultural, economic, educational, and health-related factors that may affect intake. Although the diet history is time consuming to perform and may be too stressful for the acutely ill patient, it does provide a wealth of information about food habits over a prolonged period and a basis for planning individualized nutrition education if changes in eating habits are desirable. Other information to include in a nutrition history is listed in Box 8-3.

BOX 8-3 NUTRITION HISTORY INFORMATION

Inadequate Intake of Nutrients
- Alcohol abuse
- Anorexia, severe or prolonged nausea or vomiting
- Confusion, coma
- Poor dentition
- Poverty

Inadequate Digestion or Absorption of Nutrients
- Previous gastrointestinal operations, especially gastrectomy, jejunoileal bypass, and ileal resection
- Certain medications, especially antacids and histamine H_2-receptor antagonists (reduce upper small bowel acidity), cholestyramine (binds fat-soluble nutrients), and anticonvulsants

Increased Nutrient Losses
- Blood loss
- Severe diarrhea
- Fistulas, draining abscesses, wounds, decubitus ulcers
- Peritoneal dialysis or hemodialysis
- Corticosteroid therapy (increased tissue catabolism)

Increased Nutrient Requirements
- Fever
- Surgery, trauma, burns, infection
- Cancer (some types)
- Physiologic demands (pregnancy, lactation, growth)

Evaluating Nutrition Assessment Findings

A key part of the nutrition assessment process is using gathered patient information to estimate nutrient, specifically calorie or energy, needs. In the in-patient setting, estimated energy needs can be measured or calculated as described below.

Determining Nutritional Needs

A variety of methods can be used in clinical practice to estimate caloric requirements. Indirect calorimetry, a method by which energy expenditure is calculated from oxygen consumption (Vo_2) and carbon dioxide production (Vco_2), is the most accurate method for determining caloric needs.[11,12] Indirect calorimetry is useful in those patients suspected to have a high metabolic rate. This test can also analyze substrate use, which can be extrapolated from V_{O2} and V_{CO2} during a steady state of respiration. The respiratory quotient (RQ) is equal to the V_{CO2} divided by the Vo_2. Fat, protein, and carbohydrates each have a unique RQ, thus RQ identifies which substrate is being preferentially metabolized and may provide target goals for calorie replacement.[12] For example, the RQ for the metabolism of fats is about 0.7 while the RQ for the metabolism of carbohydrates is 1.0. A mixed fuel diet results in an RQ of approximately 0.8.[12] The test can be performed on spontaneously breathing patients and on those who require mechanical ventilation. Some ventilators are constructed so that they can perform indirect calorimetry. However, for most patients, indirect calorimetry requires the use of a metabolic cart, which is not available in all institutions. To maintain accuracy and reliability of measurement, several testing criteria must be met.[12] Information received from the metabolic cart is limited; measurements are conducted over a relatively brief period (often 20 to 30 minutes) and may not be representative of energy expenditure over the whole day.

Calorie and protein needs of patients are often estimated using formulas that provide allowances for increased nutrient use associated with injury and healing. Although indirect calorimetry is considered the most accurate method to determine energy expenditure, estimates using formulas have demonstrated reasonable accuracy.[13-15] Commonly used formulas for critically ill patients can be found in Appendix B. Some rules of thumb are available to provide a rough estimate of caloric needs so that nurses and other caregivers can quickly determine if patients are being seriously overfed or underfed (Table 8-3).

TABLE 8-3 ESTIMATING ENERGY NEEDS

CATEGORY	DESCRIPTION	CALORIES/kg	CALORIES/lb
Obese	More than 40% over ideal body weight or BMI >30	21	9.5
Sedentary	Relatively inactive individual without regular aerobic exercise; hospitalized patient without severe injury or sepsis	25-30	11-13.5
Moderate activity or injury	Individual obtaining regular aerobic exercise plus routine activities; patient with trauma or sepsis	30-35	13.5-16
Very active or severe injury	Manual laborer or athlete in very active training; patient with major burns or trauma	40	18

The goal of nutrition assessment is to obtain the most accurate estimate of nutritional requirements. Underfeeding and overfeeding must be avoided during critical illness. Overfeeding results in excessive production of carbon dioxide, which can be a burden in the person with pulmonary compromise. Overfeeding increases fat stores, which can contribute to insulin resistance and hyperglycemia. Hyperglycemia increases the risk of postoperative infections in diabetic and nondiabetic individuals.[16]

IMPLICATIONS OF UNDERNUTRITION FOR THE SICK OR STRESSED PATIENT

As many as 40% of hospitalized patients are at risk for malnutrition.[17-20] Although illness or injury is the major factor contributing to development of malnutrition, other possible contributing factors are lack of communication among the nurses, physicians, and dietitians responsible for the care of these patients; frequent diagnostic testing and procedures, which lead to interruption in feeding; medications and other therapies that cause anorexia, nausea, or vomiting and thereby interfere with food intake; insufficient monitoring of nutrient intake; and inadequate use of supplements, tube feedings, or parenteral nutrition to maintain the nutritional status of these patients.

Nutritional status tends to deteriorate during hospitalization unless appropriate nutrition support is started early and continually reassessed. Malnutrition in hospitalized patients is associated with a wide variety of adverse outcomes. Wound dehiscence, pressure ulcers, sepsis, infections, respiratory failure requiring ventilation, longer hospital stays, and death are more common among malnourished patients.[21-23] Decline in nutritional status during hospitalization is associated with higher incidences of complications, increased mortality rates, increased length of stay, and higher hospital costs.

It is rare for a patient to exhibit a lack of only one nutrient. Nutritional deficiencies usually are combined, with the patient lacking adequate amounts of protein, calories, and possibly vitamins and minerals.

Energy Deficiency
Protein-Calorie Malnutrition

Malnutrition results from the lack of intake of necessary nutrients or improper absorption and distribution of them, as well as from excessive intake of some nutrients. Malnutrition can be related to any essential nutrient or nutrients, but a serious type of malnutrition found frequently among hospitalized patients is protein-calorie malnutrition (PCM). Poor intake or impaired absorption of protein and energy from carbohydrate and fat worsens the debilitation that may occur in response to critical illness. In PCM, the body proteins are broken down for gluconeogenesis, reducing the supply of amino acids needed for maintenance of body proteins and healing. Malnutrition can be caused by simple starvation—the inadequate intake of nutrients (e.g., in the patient with anorexia related to cancer). It also can result from an injury that increases the metabolic rate beyond the supply of nutrients (hypermetabolism). In the

seriously ill patient, if malnutrition occurs, usually it is the result of the combined effects of starvation and hypermetabolism. Two types of PCM are kwashiorkor and marasmus.

Kwashiorkor results in low levels of the serum proteins *albumin, transferrin,* and *prealbumin;* low total lymphocyte count; impaired immunity; loss of hair or hair pigment; edema resulting from low plasma oncotic pressure caused by a loss of plasma proteins; and an enlarged, fatty liver. Marasmus is recognizable by weight loss, loss of subcutaneous fat, and muscle wasting. In the marasmic person, creatinine excretion in the urine is low, an indication of reduced muscle mass. Because PCM weakens muscles, increases vulnerability to infection, and can prolong hospital stays, the health care team should diagnose this serious disorder as quickly as possible so that an appropriate nutrition intervention can be implemented.

Metabolic Response to Starvation and Stress

To understand the development of malnutrition in the hospitalized patient, the nurse must understand the metabolic response to starvation and physiologic stress. Changes in endocrine status and metabolism together determine the onset and extent of malnutrition. Nutritional imbalance occurs when the demand for nutrients is greater than the exogenous nutrient supply. The major difference between a person who is starved and one who is starved and injured is that the latter has an increased reliance on tissue protein breakdown to provide precursors for glucose production to meet increased energy demands. Although carbohydrate and fat metabolism are also affected, the main concern is about protein metabolism and homeostasis.

During an acute, nonstressed fast, blood levels of glucose and insulin fall, and glucagon levels rise. Glucagon stimulates the liver to release glucose from its glycogen reserves, which become exhausted within a few hours. Glucagon also stimulates gluconeogenesis, and skeletal muscle provides a large amount of the substrates required for gluconeogenesis. As fasting progresses, fat becomes the primary source of fuel, and the blood ketone levels begin to increase. After the circulating ketone level rises, the brain is able to use ketones for 70% of its energy, thereby decreasing the total body's reliance on glucose as an energy source. As gluconeogenesis from protein precursors decreases, protein breakdown and nitrogen excretion also slow. Some tissues, such as red blood cells, the renal medulla, and 30% of brain cells, are obligatory glucose users, and they continue to require a small amount of amino acids for gluconeogenesis. However, endogenous protein stores are spared from use for gluconeogenesis to a major extent, and protein homeostasis is partially restored.

Critically ill patients are at risk for a combination of starvation and the physiologic stress resulting from injury, trauma, major surgery, or sepsis. Starvation occurs because the person must have nothing by mouth (NPO) for surgical procedures, is unable to eat because of disease-related factors, or is hemodynamically too unstable to be fed. The physiologic stress causes an increased metabolic rate (hypermetabolism) that results in increased oxygen consumption and energy expenditure.

The hypermetabolic process results from increased catabolic hormone changes caused by the stressful event. The sympathetic nervous system is stimulated, causing the adrenal medulla to release catecholamines (epinephrine and norepinephrine). Other hormones released in response to stress include glucagon, adrenocorticotropic hormone (ACTH), antidiuretic hormone (ADH), and glucocorticoids and mineralocorticoids (e.g., cortisol, aldosterone). Cytokines are peptide messengers secreted by macrophages as part of the inflammatory response, and they serve as hormonal regulators of the immune system. Cytokine levels increase in response to sepsis and trauma. Important cytokines include tumor necrosis factor (TNF), cachectin, interleukin 1 (IL-1), and interleukin 6 (IL-6). All of these hormonal changes cause nutrient substrates, primarily amino acids, to move from peripheral tissues (e.g., skeletal muscle) to the liver for gluconeogenesis.

Unfortunately, this mobilization of substrates occurs at the expense of body tissue and function at a time when the needs for protein synthesis (e.g., wound healing, acute-phase proteins) also are high. Hyperglycemia results from the effects of increased catecholamines, glucocorticoids, and glucagon. The body relies on its protein stores to provide substrates for gluconeogenesis, because glucose becomes the major fuel source. Loss of protein results in a negative nitrogen balance and weight loss. Catabolism may be unresponsive to nutrient intake.

NUTRITION SUPPORT

Nursing Management of Nutrition Support

Nutrition support is an important aspect of the care of critically ill patients. Maintenance of optimal nutritional status may prevent or reduce the complications associated with critical illness and promote positive clinical outcomes.[3] Critical care nurses play a key role in the delivery of nutrition support and must work closely with dietitians and physicians in promoting the best possible outcomes for their patients.

Nutrition support is the provision of oral, enteral, or parenteral nutrients. It is an essential adjunct in the prevention and management of malnutrition in critically ill patients.[3] The goal of nutrition support therapy is to provide enough support for body requirements, to minimize complications, and to promote rapid recovery. Critical care nurses must have a broad understanding of nutrition support, including the indications, prevention, and management of associated complications.

Oral Supplementation

Oral supplementation may be necessary for patients who can eat and have normal digestion and absorption but cannot consume enough regular foods to meet caloric and protein needs. Patients with mild to moderate anorexia, burns, or trauma sometimes fall into this category. To improve intake and tolerance of supplements, there are several steps for the critical care nurse to take:

1. Collaborate with the dietitian to choose appropriate products and allow the patient to participate in the selection process, if possible. Milk shakes and instant breakfast preparations are often more palatable and economical than commercial supplements. However, lactose intolerance is common among adults. Many disease processes (e.g., Crohn's disease, radiation enteritis, human immunodeficiency virus [HIV] infection, severe gastroenteritis) can cause lactose intolerance. Individuals with this problem require commercial lactose-free supplements or milk treated with lactase enzyme.

2. Offer to serve commercial supplements well chilled or on ice, because this improves flavor.

3. Advise patients to sip formulas slowly, consuming no more than 240 mL over 30 to 45 minutes. These products contain easily digestible carbohydrates. If formulas are consumed too quickly, rapid hydrolysis of the carbohydrate in the duodenum can contribute to dumping syndrome, characterized by abdominal cramping, weakness, tachycardia, and diarrhea.

4. Record all supplement intake separately on the intake-and-output sheet so that it can be differentiated from intake of water and other liquids.

Enteral Nutrition

Enteral nutrition or tube feedings are used for patients who have at least some digestive and absorptive capability but are unable or unwilling to consume enough by mouth. When possible, the enteral route is the preferred method of feeding over total parenteral nutrition (TPN). The proposed advantages of enteral nutrition over TPN include lower cost, better maintenance of gut integrity, and decreased infection and hospital length of stay.[3] A review of the literature comparing enteral nutrition and TPN indicates that enteral nutrition is less expensive than TPN and is associated with a lower risk of infection.[3,24]

The gastrointestinal (GI) tract plays an important role in maintaining immunologic defenses, which is why nutrition by the enteral route is thought to be more physiologically beneficial than TPN. Some of the barriers to infection in the GI tract include neutrophils; the normal acidic gastric pH; motility, which limits GI tract colonization by pathogenic bacteria; the normal gut microflora, which inhibit growth of or destroy some pathogenic organisms; rapid desquamation and regeneration of intestinal epithelial cells; the layer of mucus secreted by GI tract cells; and bile, which detoxifies endotoxin in the intestine and delivers immunoglobulin A (IgA) to the intestine. A second line of defense against invasion of intestinal bacteria is the gut-associated lymphoid tissue (GALT).[25] The systemic immune defenses in the GI tract are stimulated by the presence of food within it. In animal models, resting the GI tract by providing TPN contributes to *bacterial translocation*, whereby bacteria normally found in the GI tract cross the intestinal barrier, are found in the regional mesenteric lymph nodes, and give rise to generalized sepsis. However, there is insufficient evidence in humans that TPN causes atrophy of the intestinal mucosa or that enteral nutrition prevents bacterial translocation.[26,27]

Patients who are experiencing severe stress that greatly increases their nutritional needs (caused by major surgery, burns, or trauma) often benefit from tube feedings. Table 8-4 lists different enteral formula types and the nutritional indications for using each one. Individuals who require elemental formulas because of impaired digestion or absorption or the specialized formulas for altered metabolic conditions usually

TABLE 8-4 ENTERAL FORMULAS

FORMULA TYPE	NUTRITIONAL USES	CLINICAL EXAMPLES	EXAMPLES OF COMMERCIAL PRODUCTS (MANUFACTURER)
Formulas Used When GI Tract Is Fully Functional			
Polymeric (standard): Contains whole proteins (10%-15% of calories), long-chain triglycerides (25%-40% of calories), and glucose polymers or oligosaccharides (50%-60% of calories); most provide 1 calorie/mL	Inability to ingest food Inability to consume enough to meet needs	Oral or esophageal cancer Coma, stroke Anorexia resulting from chronic illness Burns or trauma	Ensure (Ross) NuBasics (Nestlé) IsoSource (Novartis) PediaSure (Ross), for children 1-10 years old Boost (Mead Johnson)
High-nitrogen: Same as polymeric except protein provides >15% of calories	Same as polymeric plus mild catabolism and protein deficits	Trauma or burns Sepsis	IsoSource HN (Novartis) Osmolite HN (Ross) Ultracal (Mead Johnson)
Concentrated: Same as polymeric except concentrated to 2 calorie/mL	Same as polymeric but fluid restriction needed	Heart failure Neurosurgery COPD Liver disease	Deliver 2.0 (Mead Johnson) TwoCal HN (Ross) Nutren 2.0 (Nestlé)
Formulas Used When GI Function Is Impaired			
Elemental or predigested: Contains hydrolyzed (partially digested) protein, peptides (short chains of amino acids), and/or amino acids, little fat (<10% of calories) or high MCT, and glucose polymers or oligosaccharides; most provide 1 calorie/mL	Impaired digestion and/or absorption	Short bowel syndrome Radiation enteritis Inflammatory bowel disease	Criticare HN (Mead Johnson) Vital High Nitrogen (Ross) Reabilan HN (Nestlé)
Diets for Specific Disease States*			
Renal failure: Concentrated in calories; low sodium, potassium, magnesium, phosphorus, and vitamins A and D; low protein for renal insufficiency; higher protein formulas for dialyzed patients	Renal insufficiency Dialysis	Predialysis Hemodialysis or peritoneal dialysis	Suplena (Ross) Renalcal (Nestlé) Nepro (Ross) Magnacal Renal (Mead Johnson)
Hepatic failure: Enriched in BCAA; low sodium	Protein intolerance	Hepatic encephalopathy	NutriHep (Nestlé) Hepatic-Aid II (B Braun/McGaw)
Pulmonary dysfunction: Low carbohydrate, high fat, concentrated in calories	Respiratory insufficiency	Ventilator dependence	NutriVent (Nestlé) Pulmocare (Ross)
Glucose intolerance: High fat, low carbohydrate (most contain fiber and fructose)	Glucose intolerance	Individuals with diabetes mellitus whose blood sugar is poorly controlled with standard formulas	Glucerna (Ross) Choice DM (Mead Johnson) Diabetisource (Novartis) Glytrol (Nestlé)
Critical care, wound healing: High protein; most contain MCT to improve fat absorption; some have increased zinc and vitamin C for wound healing; some are high in antioxidants (vitamin E, beta-carotene); some are enriched with arginine, glutamine, and/or omega-3 fatty acids	Critical illness	Severe trauma or burns Sepsis	Immun-Aid (B Braun/McGaw) Impact (Novartis) Perative (Ross) Crucial (Nestlé) TraumaCal (Mead Johnson)

*These diets may be beneficial for selected patients; costs and benefits must be considered.
BCAA, Branched chain–enriched amino acid; *COPD,* chronic obstructive pulmonary disease; *GI,* gastrointestinal; *MCT,* medium-chain triglyceride.

require tube feeding because the unpleasant flavors of the free amino acids, peptides, or protein hydrolysates used in these formulas are very difficult to mask if taken in orally.

Immune-enhancing formulas (IEFs) have emerged as a means to protect and stimulate the immune system. Some of the enterally delivered nutrients that may benefit critically ill patients include fiber, the amino acids glutamine and arginine, the omega-3 (n-3) fatty acids, and the nucleotide ribonucleic acid (RNA).[28] Fiber is not digested by humans but can be metabolized by gut bacteria to yield short-chain fatty acids, the primary fuel of the colon cells. Glutamine is the major fuel of the small intestinal cells. It is considered a nonessential amino acid, but it becomes conditionally essential in illness. It has been shown to improve mortality and infectious morbidity in critically ill patients.[29-31] Arginine is involved in protein synthesis and is a precursor of nitric oxide, a molecule that stimulates vasodilation in the GI tract and heart and mediates hepatic protein synthesis during sepsis.[28] The omega-3 fatty acids, derived primarily from fish oils, are involved in synthesis of eicosanoids (molecules with hormone-like activity)—prostaglandins, prostacyclin, and leukotrienes—and may modulate the inflammatory response.

There are a variety of commercial enteral feeding products, some of which are designed to meet the specialized needs of the critically ill. Products designed for the stressed patient with trauma or sepsis are usually rich in glutamine, arginine, branched amino acids (a major fuel source, especially for muscle), and antioxidant nutrients, such as selenium and vitamins C, E, and A.[32] The antioxidants help to reduce oxidative injury to the tissues (e.g., from reperfusion injury). Despite the fact that IEFs may reduce the incidence of infectious complications, the efficacy and safety of these formulas in critically ill patients have not been clearly demonstrated.[33-36]

Early enteral nutrition, administered with the first 24 to 48 hours of critical illness, has been advocated as a way to reduce septic complications and improve feeding tolerance in critically ill patients. Although studies[37] have shown a lower risk of infection and decreased length of stay with early enteral nutrition, the benefit of early enteral nutrition compared with enteral nutrition delayed a few days remains controversial.[3,38] Current guidelines support the initiation of nutrition support in critically ill patients who will be unable to meet their nutrient needs orally for a period of 5 to 10 days.[3] To avoid complications associated with intestinal ischemia and infarction, enteral nutrition must be initiated only after fluid resuscitation and adequate perfusion have been achieved.[39,40]

Critically ill patients may not tolerate early enteral feeding because of impaired gastric motility, ileus, or medications administered in the early phase of illness. This is particularly true for patients receiving gastric enteral feeding.[41] The assessment of enteral feeding tolerance is an important aspect of nursing care. Monitoring of gastric residual volume is a method used to assess enteral feeding tolerance. However, evidence suggests that gastric residuals are insensitive and unreliable markers of tolerance to tube feeding.[42] There is little evidence to support a correlation between gastric residual volumes and tolerance to feedings, gastric emptying, and potential aspiration. Except in selected high-risk patients, there is little evidence to support holding tube feedings in patients with gastric residual volumes less than 400 mL.[42] The gastric residual volume should be evaluated within the context of other gastrointestinal symptoms. Prokinetic agents, including metoclopramide and erythromycin, have been used to improve gastric motility and promote early enteral nutrition in critically ill patients.[43-45]

Enteral Feeding Access. Achievement of enteral access is the cornerstone of enteral nutrition therapy. Several techniques can be used to facilitate enteral access. These include surgical methods, bedside methods, fluoroscopy, endoscopy, air insufflation, and prokinetic agents.[9] Placement of feeding tubes beyond the stomach (postpyloric) eliminates some of the problems associated with gastric feeding intolerance. However, placement of postpyloric feeding tubes is time-consuming and may be costly. Tubes with weights on the proximal end are available; they were originally designed for postpyloric feeding in the belief that that they would be more likely than unweighted

tubes to pass spontaneously through the pyloric sphincter. However, randomized trials with the two types of tubes have shown that unweighted tubes are more likely to migrate through the pylorus than weighted tubes.[46] The weights sometimes cause discomfort while being inserted through the nares. Unweighted tubes therefore may be preferable.

After the tube is placed, correct location must be confirmed before feedings are started and regularly throughout the course of enteral feedings. Radiographs are the most accurate way of assessing tube placement, but repeated radiographs are costly and can expose the patient to excessive radiation. After correct placement has been confirmed, marking the exit site of the tube to check for movement is helpful. Alternative methods for confirming tube placement have been researched that attempt to verify placement in the stomach or small intestine. An inexpensive and relatively accurate alternative method involves assessing the pH of fluid removed from the feeding tube; some tubes are equipped with pH monitoring systems. Assessing the pH and the bilirubin concentration in fluid aspirated from the feeding tube is a newer method for confirming tube placement.[47]

Location and Type of Feeding Tube. Decisions regarding enteral access should be determined based on gastrointestinal anatomy, gastric emptying, and aspiration risk.[3] Nasal intubation is the simplest and most commonly used route for enteral access. This method allows access to the stomach, duodenum, or jejunum. Tube enterostomy—a gastrostomy or jejunostomy—is used primarily for long-term feedings (6 to 12 weeks or more) and when obstruction makes the nasoenteral route inaccessible. Tube enterostomies may also be used for the patient who is at risk for tube dislodgment because of severe agitation or confusion. A conventional gastrostomy or jejunostomy is often performed at the time of other abdominal surgery. The percutaneous endoscopic gastrostomy (PEG) tube has become extremely popular because it can be inserted at the bedside without the use of general anesthetics. Percutaneous endoscopic jejunostomy (PEJ) tubes are also used.

Postpyloric feedings through nasoduodenal, nasojejunal, or jejunostomy tubes are commonly used when there is a high risk of pulmonary aspiration, because the pyloric sphincter theoretically provides a barrier that lessens the risk of regurgitation and aspiration.[48] However, some studies have demonstrated that gastric feeding is safe and not associated with an increased risk of aspiration.[49-51] Postpyloric feedings have an advantage over intragastric feedings for patients with delayed gastric emptying, such as those with head injury, gastroparesis associated with uremia or diabetes, or postoperative ileus. Delivery of enteral nutrition into the small bowel is associated with improved tolerance,[52] higher calorie and protein intake,[53] and fewer gastrointestinal complications.[41] Small bowel motility returns more quickly than gastric motility after surgery, and it is often possible to deliver transpyloric feedings within a few hours of injury or surgery.[48] Figure 8-3 shows the locations of tube feeding sites.

Assessment and Prevention of Feeding Tube Complications. Nursing care of patients receiving enteral nutrition involves prevention and management of complications associated

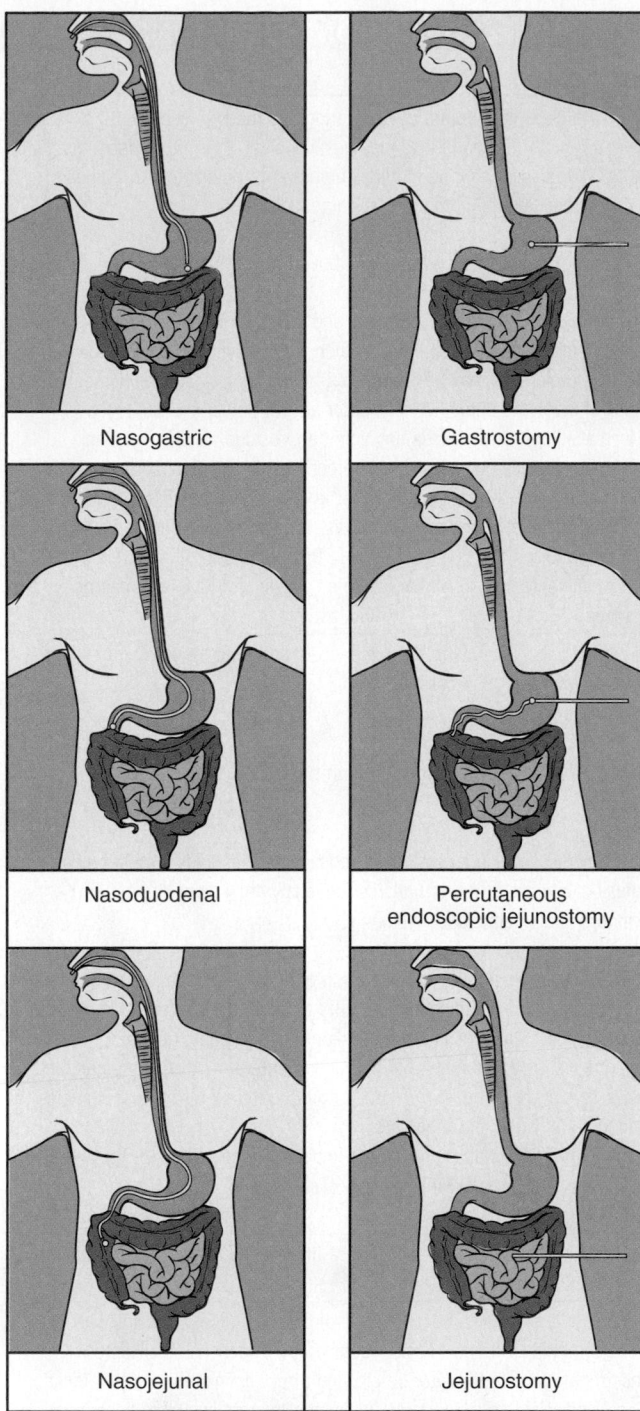

Nasogastric

Gastrostomy

Nasoduodenal

Percutaneous
endoscopic jejunostomy

Nasojejunal

Jejunostomy

FIGURE 8-3   Tube Feeding Sites.

with the use of feeding tubes. Nursing management of these problems is summarized in Table 8-5. The skin around the feeding tube should be cleaned at least daily and the tape around the tube replaced whenever loosened or soiled. Secure taping helps to prevent movement of the tube, which may irritate the nares or oral mucosa or result in accidental dislodgment. The tube must be taped in the dependent position to prevent unnecessary pressure and prevent necrosis. Commercially available attachment devices may be used to avoid inadvertent dislodgment.

To prevent mouth dryness, the patient is encouraged to breathe through the nose as much as possible. Frequent mouth care can clear the palate of unpleasant flavors from the formula and clean the teeth, tongue, and oral mucous membranes.

Dressings are used initially around gastrostomy insertion sites. The dressing is changed daily and the skin cleansed with soap and water. If leakage of gastric fluid occurs around a gastrostomy tube, the integrity of the gastrostomy balloon should be evaluated.[54] Karaya powder can be used to protect the peristomal skin from leakage. Fever, redness, purulent drainage, foul odor, or pain at the insertion site may indicate infection. Treatment may include application of a topical antibiotic ointment and daily cleansing with soap and water. Buried bumper syndrome may occur when the gastrostomy device disk, or bumper, is pulled tight against the abdominal wall. To prevent this, it is necessary to minimize tension on the disk. The tube may also become dislodged. A new gastrostomy tube needs to be reinserted within hours to prevent closure of the stoma.

Feeding Tube Occlusion. Regular irrigation helps to prevent feeding tube occlusion. Usually, 20 to 30 mL of warm water every 3 to 4 hours during continuous feedings and before and after intermittent feedings and medication administration can maintain patency.[3] The volume of irrigant may have to be reduced for fluid restriction. Automatic enteral flush pumps are also available. Although cranberry juice or cola beverages are sometimes used in an effort to reduce the incidence of tube occlusion, water is the preferred irrigant because it has been shown to be superior in maintaining tube patency.[55] Tube occlusion may occur as a result of stagnant formula, inadequately crushed pills, or medication interactions with formula. Enteral infusion pumps should be used, and tubes should be flushed before feeding infusions are paused. Liquid medications or elixirs should be used when possible to avoid tube occlusion with pill fragments. The use of pancreatic enzymes in the feeding tube appears to reduce the risk of tube clogging and may be successful in removing a clog after it has formed.[55,56]

Aspiration. Pulmonary aspiration of enteral formulas and subsequent pneumonia is a serious complication of enteral feeding in critically ill patients. Risk factors for aspiration of enteral feeding include decreased level of consciousness, supine position, and swallowing disorders.[57] Figure 8-4 shows the risk factors for aspiration in patients on tube feeds. To reduce the risk of pulmonary aspiration of formula during enteral feeding, the nurse must keep the head of the bed elevated unless contraindicated; temporarily stop feedings when the patient must be supine for prolonged periods; position the patient in the right lateral decubitus position when possible to encourage gastric emptying; use postpyloric feeding methods; keep the cuff of the endotracheal tube inflated as much as possible during enteral feeding, if applicable; and be alert to any increase in abdominal distention.

Two bedside methods have been used in the past to detect pulmonary aspiration of enteral feeding. One is the addition of blue dye to the enteral formula and observation of the patient for any dye-tinged tracheal secretions, and the other is glucose testing of tracheal secretions to detect the presence of the

TABLE 8-5   NURSING MANAGEMENT OF ENTERAL TUBE FEEDING COMPLICATIONS

COMPLICATION	CONTRIBUTING FACTORS	PREVENTION OR CORRECTION
Pulmonary aspiration (signs and symptoms include tachypnea, shortness of breath, hypoxia, and infiltrate on chest radiographs)	Feeding tube positioned in esophagus or respiratory tract Regurgitation of formula	Confirm proper tube placement before administering any feeding; check tube placement at least every 4-8 hr during continuous feedings; consider intermittent feedings. Elevate head to 30-45 degrees during feedings unless contraindicated; if the head cannot be raised, position the patient in lateral (especially right lateral, which facilitates gastric emptying) or prone position to improve drainage of vomitus from the mouth. Consider giving feeding into small bowel rather than stomach in high-risk patients. Metoclopramide may improve gastric emptying and decrease the risk of regurgitation. Evaluate feeding tolerance every 2 hr initially, then less frequently as condition becomes stable. Intolerance may be manifested by bloating, abdominal distention and pain, lack of stool and flatus, diminished or absent bowel sounds, tense abdomen, increased tympany, nausea and vomiting, residual volume >200 mL aspirated from an NG tube or >100 mL aspirated from a gastrostomy tube, although a high residual volume in the absence of other abnormal findings may not be grounds for stopping feedings (measuring residual volumes is a controversial practice; see the section on tube occlusion that follows below in this Table 8-5). If intolerance is suspected, abdominal radiographs may be done to check for distended gastric bubble, distended loops of bowel, or air-fluid levels.
Diarrhea	Medications with GI side effects (e.g., antibiotics, digitalis, laxatives, magnesium-containing antacids, quinidine, caffeine, many others)	Evaluate the patient's medications to determine their potential for causing diarrhea, and consult the pharmacist if necessary.
	Predisposing illness (e.g., short bowel syndrome, inflammatory bowel disease)	Use continuous feedings; consider a formula with MCT and/or soluble fiber.
	Hypertonic formula or medications (e.g., oral suspensions of antibiotics, potassium, other electrolytes), which can cause dumping syndrome	Evaluate formula administration procedures to ensure that feedings are not being given by bolus infusion; administer the formula continuously or by slow intermittent infusion. Dilute enteral medications well.
	Bacterial contamination of the formula	Use scrupulously clean technique in administering tube feedings; prepare formula with sterile water if there are any concerns about the safety of the water supply or if the patient is seriously immunocompromised; keep opened containers of formula refrigerated, and discard them within 24 hr; discard enteral feeding containers and administration sets every 24 hr; hang formula no more than 4-8 hr unless it comes prepackaged in sterile administration sets.
	Fecal impaction with seepage of liquid stool around the impaction	Perform a digital rectal examination to rule out impaction; see guidelines for prevention of constipation that follow below in this table (Table 8-5).
	Lactose intolerance	Use lactose-free formula.
Constipation	Low-residue formula, creating little fecal bulk, lack of fiber	Consider using a fiber-containing formula; ensure fluid intake is adequate; stool softeners may be beneficial.
Tube occlusion	Medications administered by tube that physically plug the tube or coagulate the formula, causing it to clog the tube Sedimentation of formula	If medications must be given by tube, avoid use of crushed tablets; consult with the pharmacist to determine whether medications can be dispensed as elixirs or suspensions. Irrigate tube with water before and after administering any medication; never add any medication to the formula unless the two are known to be compatible. Irrigate tube every 4-8 hr during continuous feedings and after every intermittent feeding. If residuals are measured, flush the tube thoroughly after returning the formula to the stomach, since gastric juices left in tube may cause precipitation of formula. Instilling pancreatic enzymes into the tube can remove or prevent some occlusions.
Gastric retention	Delayed gastric emptying related to head trauma, sepsis, diabetic or uremic gastroparesis, electrolyte balance, or other illness	The cause must be corrected if possible. Consult with the physician about use of postpyloric feedings or prokinetic agents to stimulate gastric emptying. Encourage the patient to lie in the right lateral position frequently, unless contraindicated.

Modified from Moore MC. *Pocket Guide to Nutritional Assessment and Care.* 6th ed. St. Louis: Mosby; 2009.
GI, Gastrointestinal; *NG,* nasogastric.

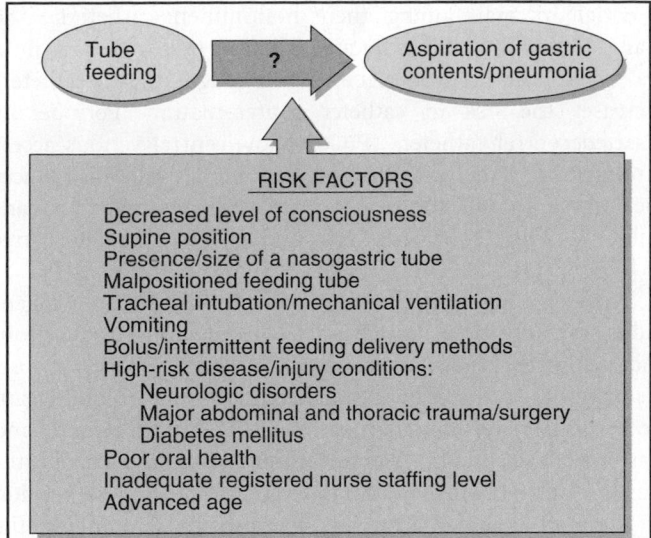

FIGURE 8-4 Factors that Influence Aspiration in Tube-Fed Patients. (From Metheny NA. Risk factors for aspiration. *JPEN J Parenter Enteral Nutr.* 2002;26[6 suppl]:S26.)

glucose-containing enteral formula. The glucose oxidase method may cause false-positive reactions if blood is present. It has a low sensitivity when low-glucose formulas are used, and it has questionable specificity.[58] There is no established protocol for blue dye testing. Although it has been used routinely in clinical practice for several years, there is no evidence to support its efficacy or safety. It lacks sensitivity and specificity in ruling out aspiration. Numerous clinical reports of systemic absorption of blue dye and adverse outcomes have been described.[59,60] Glucose oxidase testing and blue food coloring are not recommended as appropriate methods for detecting aspiration of enteral feedings.[59,61]

Gastrointestinal Complications. Diarrhea is common in patients receiving enteral nutrition, with an incidence of 2% to 70%.[62] No single definition has been established for diarrhea. Current definitions include various stool frequencies, volumes, and weights.[63] Diarrhea in enterally fed critically ill patients has many factors. Common causes include medications, malabsorption, formula contamination, or low-fiber formulas. While the cause of diarrhea is being determined, nurses must provide adequate fluid and electrolyte replacement, maintain skin integrity, and administer antidiarrheal agents. To prevent complications, stool must be checked for infection, especially *Clostridium difficile*, before antidiarrheal medications can be administered.[64] Constipation is a complication of enteral feeding that may result from dehydration, bed rest, opioid administration, or lack of adequate fiber in enteral formulas. Pasty stools are normal in enterally fed patients. Bowel movements should be assessed daily. The nurse must ensure adequate fluid and fiber intake, promote optimal mobility, and administer laxatives and stool softeners as necessary.[65]

Formula Delivery. Careful attention to administration of tube feedings can prevent many complications. Very clean or aseptic technique in the handling and administration of the formula can help prevent bacterial contamination and a resultant infection. When using cans of formula transferred to a feeding container, wash hands and tops of cans before opening, hang enough formula for just 8 hours of infusion, and do not add new formula to formula already hanging. Closed systems that use a prefilled sterile container that can be spiked with the enteral tube are also available.

Tube feedings may be administered intermittently or continuously. Bolus feedings, which are intermittent feedings delivered rapidly into the stomach or small bowel, are likely to cause distention, vomiting, and dumping syndrome with diarrhea. Instead of using bolus feedings, nurses can gradually drip intermittent feedings, with each feeding lasting 20 to 30 minutes or longer, to promote optimal assimilation. The question of which feeding schedule—continuous or intermittent—is superior for critically ill patients remains unanswered.

Adequacy of Enteral Nutrition. Critically ill patients have so many needs for care that it is easy to overlook the importance of nutrition. Many studies have shown that critically ill patients receive considerably less enteral nutrition than required.[66-69] This is a complication unique to enteral nutrition not observed with TPN. The discrepancy in nutritional intake has a variety of causes, including patient factors (e.g., high residual volumes, emesis, abdominal distention), tube-related factors (e.g., occlusion, malposition), and treatment-related factors (e.g., interruptions caused by procedures, airway management, and medications).[67] Inadequate enteral nutrition delivery is also related to physicians' prescribing practices in the critical care unit.[69] The enteral delivery practices in the critical care unit and clinicians' concerns about aspiration may lead to inappropriate and prolonged interruptions in enteral feeding. Chest physiotherapy, suspicion of formula in the tracheobronchial secretions, and excessive gastric retention of formula are examples of appropriate reasons for stopping feedings. Enteral nutrition delivery practices that are evidence-based are necessary for optimal nutritional outcomes in critically ill patients.

Tubing and Catheter Misconnections. Tubing and catheter or Luer connector (small device used in the connection of many medical components and accessories) misconnection errors have gain recent attention with The Joint Commission issuing a *Sentinel Event Alert* in April 2006.[70] Examples of misconnection errors include misconnecting an enteric feeding tube into an intravenous catheter or injection of an intravenous fluid into a tracheostomy cuff inflation tube. These misconnection errors are potentially life threatening, and increased awareness as well as precautions can improve patient safety. The following strategies should be followed to minimize risk for tubing and catheter misconnections[71]:

- Label all tubes and catheters, especially arterial, epidural, and intrathecal catheters.
- Trace lines back to their origins when initiating any new device or infusion.
- Standardize a line reconciliation process with patient handoffs.
- Consider routing tubes and catheters with different purposes in different, standardized directions.
- Never use a standard Luer syringe for oral medications or enteric feedings.

Total Parenteral Nutrition

TPN refers to the delivery of all nutrients by the intravenous route. It is used when the GI tract is not functional or when nutritional needs cannot be met solely through the GI tract. Likely candidates for TPN include patients who have a severely impaired absorption (e.g., short bowel syndrome, collagen vascular diseases, radiation enteritis), intestinal obstruction, peritonitis, or prolonged ileus. Some postoperative, trauma, or burn patients may need TPN to supplement the nutrient intake that they are able to tolerate by the enteral route.

Types of Parenteral Nutrition. TPN involves administration of highly concentrated dextrose (25% to 70%), providing a rich source of calories. These highly concentrated dextrose solutions are hyperosmolar, as much as 1800 mOsm/L, and therefore must be delivered through a central vein.[72] Peripheral parenteral nutrition (PPN) has a glucose concentration of 5% to 10% and may be delivered safely through a peripheral vein. PPN solution delivers nutrition support in a large volume that cannot be tolerated by patients who require fluid restriction. It provides short-term nutrition support for a few days to less than 2 weeks.

Regardless of the route of administration, PPN and TPN provide glucose, fat, protein, electrolytes, vitamins, and trace elements. Although dextrose–amino acid solutions are commonly thought of as good growth media for microorganisms, they actually suppress the growth of most organisms usually associated with catheter-related sepsis, except yeasts. However, because the many manipulations required to prepare solutions increase the possibility of contamination, TPN solutions are best used with caution. They should be prepared under laminar flow conditions in the pharmacy, with avoidance of additions on the nursing unit. Solution containers need to be inspected for cracks or leaks before hanging, and solutions must be discarded within 24 hours of hanging. An in-line 0.22-micron filter, which eliminates all microorganisms but not endotoxins, may be used in the administration of solutions. Use of the filter, however, cannot be substituted for good aseptic technique.

Nursing Management of Potential Complications. Nursing management of the patient receiving TPN includes catheter care, administration of solutions, prevention or correction of complications, and evaluation of patient responses to intravenous feedings. Table 8-6 describes nursing management of TPN complications. Evaluation of the patient's response is discussed later in this chapter.

Because TPN requires an indwelling catheter in a central vein, it carries an increased risk for sepsis and potential insertion-related complications such as pneumothorax and hemothorax. Air embolism is also more likely with central vein TPN. Patients requiring multiple intravenous therapies and frequent blood sampling usually have multilumen central venous catheters, and TPN is often infused through these catheters.

Some clinical studies have reported that catheter-related sepsis is higher with multilumen catheters; others have found no difference compared with single-lumen catheters.[73] Patients requiring multilumen catheters are likely to be very ill and immunocompromised, and scrupulous aseptic technique is essential in maintaining their multilumen catheters. The manipulation involved in frequent changes of intravenous fluid and obtaining blood specimens through these catheters increases the risk of catheter contamination. Peripherally inserted central catheters (PICC) allow central venous access through long catheters inserted in peripheral sites. This reduces the risk of complications associated with percutaneous cannulation of the subclavian vein and provides an alternative to PPN.[74]

The indwelling central venous catheter provides an excellent nidus for infection. Catheter-related infections arise from endogenous skin flora, contamination of the catheter hub, seeding of the catheter by organisms carried in the bloodstream from another site, or contamination of the infusate. Good hand washing and scrupulous aseptic technique in all aspects of catheter care and TPN delivery are the primary steps for prevention of catheter-related infections. Other measures to reduce the incidence of catheter-related infections include using maximal barrier precautions (e.g., cap, mask, sterile gloves, sterile drape) at the time of insertion, tunneling the catheter underneath the skin, use of a 2% chlorhexidine preparation for skin cleansing, no routine replacement of the central venous catheter for prevention of infection, and use of antiseptic- or antibiotic-impregnated central venous catheters.[75]

Metabolic complications associated with parenteral nutrition include glucose intolerance and electrolyte imbalance. Slow advancement of the rate of TPN (25 mL/hr) to goal rate allows pancreatic adjustment to the dextrose load. Capillary blood glucose should be monitored every 4 to 6 hours. Insulin can be added to the TPN solution or can be infused as a separate drip to control glucose levels. Rapid cessation of TPN may not lead to hypoglycemia; however, tapering the infusion over 2 to 4 hours is recommended.[76]

Serum electrolytes are obtained on starting TPN. During critical illness, levels should be monitored and corrected daily and then weekly or twice weekly after the patient is more stable. The refeeding syndrome is a potentially lethal condition characterized by generalized fluid and electrolyte imbalance. It occurs as a potential complication after initiation of oral, enteral, or parenteral nutrition in malnourished patients. During chronic starvation, several compensatory metabolic changes occur. The reintroduction of carbohydrates and amino acids leads to increased insulin production. This creates an anabolic environment that increases intracellular demand for phosphorus, potassium, magnesium, vitamins, and minerals.[77] These metabolic demands result in severe shifts from the extracellular compartment. Increased insulin levels also result in fluid retention. Severe hypophosphatemia, hypokalemia, and hypomagnesemia result in altered cardiac, gastrointestinal, and neurologic function. In particular, hypophosphatemia causes a decrease in 2,3-diphosphosoglycerate (2,3-DPG) and limits the many reactions that require ATP. Hypophosphatemia and other electrolyte deficiencies may lead to respiratory failure, congestive heart failure, and dysrhythmias.

It is important to anticipate refeeding syndrome in patients who may be at risk. Patients with chronic malnutrition or underfeeding, chronic alcoholism, or anorexia nervosa or those

TABLE 8-6	NURSING MANAGEMENT OF TOTAL PARENTERAL NUTRITION COMPLICATIONS	
COMPLICATION	**CLINICAL MANIFESTATIONS**	**PREVENTION OR CORRECTION**
Catheter-related sepsis	Fever, chills, glucose intolerance, positive blood culture	Use aseptic technique when handling catheter, IV tubing, and TPN solutions. Hang a bottle of TPN no longer than 24 hr, lipid emulsion no longer than 12-24 hr. Use an in-line 0.22-micron filter with TPN to remove microorganisms. Avoid drawing blood, infusing blood or blood products, piggybacking other IV solutions into TPN IV tubing, or attaching manometers or transducers through the TPN infusion line, if possible. If catheter-related sepsis is suspected, remove the catheter or assist in changing the catheter over a guidewire and administer antibiotics as ordered.
Air embolism	Dyspnea, cyanosis, apnea, tachycardia, hypotension, "millwheel" heart murmur; mortality estimated at 50% (depends on quantity of air entering)	Use Luer-Lok connections; use an in-line air-eliminating filter. Have the patient perform a Valsalva maneuver during tubing changes; if the patient is on a ventilator, change tubing quickly at end expiration. Maintain occlusive dressing over catheter site for at least 24 hr after removing catheter to prevent air entry through catheter tract. If an air embolism is suspected, place the patient in left lateral decubitus and Trendelenburg positions (to trap air in the apex of the right ventricle, away from the outflow tract) and administer oxygen and CPR as needed; immediately notify physician, who may attempt to aspirate air from the heart.
Pneumothorax	Chest pain, dyspnea, hypoxemia, hypotension, radiographic evidence, needle aspiration of air from pleural space	Thoroughly explain the catheter insertion procedure to the patient, because when a patient moves or breathes erratically, he or she is more likely to sustain pleural damage. Perform x-ray examination after insertion or insertion attempt. If pneumothorax is suspected, assist with needle aspiration or chest tube insertion, if necessary.
Central venous thrombosis	Edema of neck, shoulder, and arm on same side as catheter; development of collateral circulation on chest; pain in insertion site; drainage of TPN from the insertion site; positive findings on venography	Follow measures to prevent sepsis; repeated or traumatic catheterizations are most likely to result in thrombosis. If thrombosis is confirmed, remove the catheter, and administer anticoagulants and antibiotics, as ordered.
Catheter occlusion or semi-occlusion	No flow or a sluggish flow through the catheter	If the infusion is stopped temporarily, flush the catheter with saline or heparinized saline. If the catheter appears to be occluded, attempt to aspirate the clot; if this is ineffective, the physician may order a thrombolytic agent such as streptokinase or alteplase (tPA) instilled in the catheter.
Hypoglycemia	Diaphoresis, shakiness, confusion, loss of consciousness	Infuse TPN within 10% of the ordered rate; monitor blood glucose until stable. If hypoglycemia is present, administer oral carbohydrate; if the patient is unconscious or oral intake is contraindicated, the physician may order an IV bolus of dextrose.
Hyperglycemia	Thirst, headache, lethargy, increased urinary output	Administer TPN within 10% of the ordered rate; monitor blood glucose level at least daily until stable. The patient may require insulin added to the TPN if hyperglycemia is persistent; sudden appearance of hyperglycemia in a patient who was previously tolerating the same glucose load may indicate the onset of sepsis.
Hypertriglyceridemia	Serum triglyceride concentrations elevated (especially serious if >400 mg/dL); serum may appear turbid	Monitor serum triglycerides at baseline, 6 hr after lipid infusion, and at least 3 times weekly until stable in patients receiving lipid emulsions; reduce lipid infusion rate or administer low-dose heparin with lipid emulsions as ordered if elevated levels are observed.

Modified from Moore MC. *Pocket Guide to Nutritional Assessment and Care.* 6th ed. St. Louis: Mosby; 2009.
CPR, cardiopulmonary resuscitation; *IV*, intravenous; *TPN*, total parenteral nutrition.

maintained NPO for several days with evidence of stress are at risk for refeeding syndrome.[78] In high-risk patients, nutrition support should be started cautiously at 25% to 50% of required calories and slowly advanced over 3 to 4 days as tolerated. Close monitoring of serum electrolytes before and during feeding is essential. Normal values do not always reflect total body stores. Correction of pre-existing electrolyte imbalances are necessary before initiation of feeding. Continued monitoring and supplementation with electrolytes and vitamins are necessary throughout the first week of nutrition support.[78]

Lipid Emulsion. Lipids or fat emulsions provide calories for energy and prevent essential fatty acid depletion. In contrast to dextrose–amino acid solutions, intravenous lipid emulsions provide a rich environment for the growth of bacteria and fungi, including *Candida albicans.* Lipid emulsions cannot be filtered through an in-line 0.22-micron filter, because some particles in the emulsions have larger diameters than this. Lipids may be infused into the TPN line downstream from the filter. No other medications should be infused into a line containing lipids or TPN. Lipid emulsions are handled with strict asepsis, and they must be discarded within 12 to 24 hours of hanging. There is a trend toward mixing lipid emulsions with dextrose–amino acid TPN solutions; these are called 3-in-1 solutions or total nutrient admixtures (TNAs). Consolidating the nutrients in one container is more economical and saves nursing time, although TNA solutions may be less stable.[72]

Monitoring and Evaluation of Nutrition Support

A multidisciplinary approach is required in evaluating the effects of nutrition support on clinical outcomes. Assessment of response to nutrition support is an ongoing process that involves anthropometric measurements, physical examination, and biochemical evaluation. Daily monitoring of nutritional intake is an important aspect of critical care and is a key element in preventing problems associated with underfeeding and overfeeding. Daily weights and the maintenance of accurate intake-and-output records are crucial for evaluating nutritional progress and the state of hydration in the patient receiving nutrition support. Serum levels of electrolytes, calcium, phosphorus, and magnesium serve as a guide to the amount of these nutrients that must be supplied. Blood urea nitrogen (BUN) and creatinine levels reflect the adequacy of renal function to handle nutrition support. Blood glucose is an indicator of the patient's tolerance of the carbohydrate, and prealbumin is an indicator of the adequacy of nutrition support. Serum triglyceride concentrations (in patients receiving intravenous lipid emulsions) reflect the ability of the tissues to metabolize the lipids.

Recently, the Society of Critical Care Medicine (SCCM) and the American Society for Parenteral and Enteral Nutrition (A.S.P.E.N.) published *The Guidelines for the Provision and Assessment of Nutrition Support Therapy in the Adult Critically Ill Patient.* The publication is based on an extensive review of 307 articles and is intended for the care of critically ill adults who require a stay of greater than 3 days in the critical care area. All practitioners who care for this target population are encouraged to become familiar with these evidence-based guidelines.[3]

It is within the scope of practice for critical care nurses to calculate caloric requirements and analyze daily caloric delivery, advocate for early nutrition support, and minimize feeding interruptions through careful patient assessment and interruption analysis. In addition to monitoring changes in weight and laboratory values, the nurse is the health care team member who has the most constant contact with the patient and who is therefore highly qualified to evaluate feeding tolerance and adequacy of delivery.

NUTRITION AND CARDIOVASCULAR ALTERATIONS

Diet and cardiovascular disease may interact in a variety of ways. Excessive nutrient intake—manifested by overweight or obesity and a diet rich in cholesterol and saturated fat—is a risk factor for development of arteriosclerotic heart disease. However, the consequences of chronic myocardial insufficiency can include malnutrition.

Nutrition Assessment in Cardiovascular Alterations

A nutrition assessment provides the nurse and other members of the health care team the information necessary to plan the patient's nutrition care and education. Common findings in the nutrition assessment of the cardiovascular patient are summarized in Box 8-4. The major nutritional concerns relate to appropriateness of body weight and the levels of serum lipids and blood pressure.

Nutrition Intervention and Education in Cardiovascular Alterations
Myocardial Infarction

Short-Term Interventions. In the early period after a myocardial infarction (MI), nutrition interventions and education are designed to reduce angina, cardiac workload, and risk of dysrhythmia. Meal size, caffeine intake, and food temperatures are some of the dietary factors that are of concern. Small, frequent snacks are preferable to larger meals for patients with severe myocardial compromise or postprandial angina.

If caffeine is included in the diet, its effects should be monitored. Because caffeine is a stimulant, it may increase heart rate and myocardial oxygen demand. In the United States and in most industrial nations, coffee is the richest source of caffeine in the diet, with about 150 mg of caffeine per 180 mL (6 fluid oz) of coffee. In comparison, the caffeine content of the same

---

BOX 8-4 **COMMON FINDINGS IN THE NUTRITION ASSESSMENT OF THE PATIENT WITH CARDIOVASCULAR DISEASE**

Anthropometric Measurements
- Overweight or obesity; underweight (cardiac cachexia)
- Abdominal fat: increased risk of cardiovascular disease with waist measurement >102 cm (>40 inches) for men and >88 cm (>35 inches) for women

Biochemical (Laboratory) Data
- Elevated total serum cholesterol, low-density lipoprotein (LDL) cholesterol, and triglycerides

Clinical Findings
- Wasting of muscle and subcutaneous fat (cardiac cachexia)

Diet or Health History
- Sedentary lifestyle
- Excessive intake of saturated fat, cholesterol, salt, or alcohol
- Angina, respiratory difficulty, or fatigue during eating
- Medications that impair appetite (e.g., digitalis preparations, quinidine)

volume of tea or cola is approximately 50 mg or 20 mg, respectively. Very hot or very cold foods should be avoided because they can potentially trigger vagal or other neural input and cause cardiac dysrhythmias.

Long-Term Changes

The focus of nutritional and lifestyle interventions for the person who has had one MI or is at increased risk for heart disease are directed at primary and secondary prevention strategies. These strategies include weight reduction if the person is overweight and control of cholesterol, fat, and saturated fat intake. Most of the education regarding these changes takes place in the rehabilitation period. However, during the acute phase of recovery, the patient and family may have an interest in learning more about risk reduction.

For the individual who is overweight or obese, gradual loss of weight (0.45 to 0.9 kg [1 to 2 lb] per week) is the goal.[79] Weight loss can be achieved through moderate exercise (with the physician's approval) and reduction of dietary intake by 500 to 1000 kcal/day. Dietary guidelines for the National Cholesterol Education Program (NCEP) Adult Treatment Panel III (ATP III) support lipid-lowering therapy through adoption of a low-saturated-fat and low-cholesterol diet, maintenance of a healthy weight, and regular physical activity.[80] Recommendations include low-density lipoprotein (LDL) cholesterol levels of 100 mg/dL or less as optimal and increased focus on the metabolic syndrome.[81,82] Metabolic syndrome is a group of risk factors (Table 8-7) associated with increased risk for

cardiovascular disease and diabetes. The primary target for patients with metabolic syndrome is weight reduction reinforced with increased physical activity, as it is expected that lipid parameters and insulin resistance will be improved with a decrease in obesity.[83,84]

Elevated plasma levels of homocysteine, derived from the essential amino acid *methionine*, are a risk factor for heart disease. Homocysteine can damage the endothelium of the blood vessels, cause proliferation of smooth muscle in the vessel walls, and activate platelets and the coagulation cascade, contributing to thrombus formation. Adequate amounts of folic acid and vitamins B_6 and B_{12} are known to reduce homocysteine levels. Although elevated homocysteine levels remain a risk marker for heart disease, current research does not support treatment with folic acid, B_6 and B_{12} in lowering homocysteine levels to prevent risk of death from cardiovascular disease.[85]

For hypertensive cardiac disease, sodium chloride restriction is recommended. Some individuals have been shown to be more salt sensitive than others, and this salt sensitivity contributes to hypertension. Adoption of a healthy lifestyle is critical for the prevention of high blood pressure and is an indispensable part of the management of those with hypertension.[86] Weight loss of as little as 10 pounds reduces blood pressure. Adoption of the Dietary Approaches to Stop Hypertension (DASH)[87] eating plan also benefits blood pressure. DASH comprises a diet rich in fruits, vegetables, and low-fat dairy products with a reduced content of dietary cholesterol and reduced levels of saturated and total fat. It is rich in potassium and calcium content. Dietary sodium should be reduced to no more than 100 mmol per day (2.4 g of sodium). Alcohol intake should be limited to no more than 1 ounce (30 mL) of ethanol per day in men and no more than 0.5 ounce of ethanol in women.

Heart Failure

Nutrition intervention in heart failure is designed to reduce fluid retained within the body and therefore reduce the preload. Because fluid accompanies sodium, limitation of sodium is necessary to reduce fluid retention. Specific interventions include limiting salt intake, usually to 2 g a day or less, and limiting fluid intake as appropriate.[88] If fluid is restricted, the daily fluid allowance is usually 1.5 to 2 L/day, which includes fluids in the diet and those given with medications and for other purposes (see "Heart Failure" in Chapter 15).

Cardiac Cachexia

Malnutrition is common in patients with heart failure. The term *cachexia* is derived from the Greek words *kakos*, meaning "bad," and *hexis*, meaning "condition." It is characterized by weight loss, anorexia, weakness, early satiety, and edema.[89] Cachexia is seen in a variety of disorders, including cancer and heart failure. It is well recognized as an independent predictor of higher mortality in patients with heart failure.[90] Sodium and fluid restriction are appropriate interventions. It is important to concentrate nutrients into as small a volume as possible and to serve small amounts frequently, rather than three large meals daily, which may overwhelm the patient. The individual

TABLE 8-7	METABOLIC SYNDROME* DEFINITION
RISK FACTOR	**DEFINING LEVEL**
Elevated waist circumference	
Men	≥40 in (≥102 cm)
Women	≥35 in (≥88 cm)
Elevated triglycerides	≥150 mg/dL (≥1.7 mmol/L)
	or on medication treatment for elevated triglycerides
Reduced HDL cholesterol	
Men	<40 mg/dL (<1.03 mmol/L)
Women	<50 mg/dL (<1.3 mmol/L)
	or on medication treatment for reduced HDL cholesterol
Elevated blood pressure	≥130 mm Hg systolic or ≥85 mm Hg diastolic
	or on antihypertensive medication treatment in a patient with a history of hypertension
Elevated fasting glucose	≥100 mg/dL (≥5.6 mmol/L)
	or on medication treatment for elevated glucose

Adapted from Grundy SM, et al. Diagnosis and management of the metabolic syndrome: an American Heart Association/National Heart, Lung, and Blood Institute scientific statement. *Circulation.* 2005;112:2735.
*Metabolic Syndrome diagnosed when 3 of 5 of the listed risk factors are present.

should be encouraged to consume calorie-dense foods and supplements.

Because the patient is likely to tire quickly and to suffer from anorexia (lack or loss of appetite), enteral tube feeding may be necessary. Most commonly used tube feeding formulas provide 1 calorie per milliliter, but more concentrated products are available to provide adequate nutrients in a smaller volume. The nurse must monitor the fluid status of these patients carefully when they are receiving nutrition support. Assessing breath sounds and observing for presence and severity of peripheral edema and changes in body weight are performed daily or more frequently. A consistent weight gain of more than 0.11 to 0.22 kg (0.25 to 0.5 lb) per day usually indicates fluid retention rather than gain of fat and muscle mass.

NUTRITION AND PULMONARY ALTERATIONS

Malnutrition has extremely adverse effects on respiratory function, decreasing surfactant production, diaphragmatic mass, vital capacity, and immunocompetence. Patients with acute respiratory disorders find it difficult to consume adequate oral nutrients and can rapidly become malnourished. Individuals who have an acute illness superimposed on chronic respiratory problems are also at high risk. Nearly three fourths of patients with chronic obstructive pulmonary disease (COPD) have had weight loss.[91] Patients with undernutrition and end-stage COPD, however, often cannot tolerate the increase in metabolic demand that occurs during refeeding. They also are at significant risk for development of cor pulmonale and may fail to tolerate the fluid required for delivery of enteral or parenteral nutrition support. Prevention of severe nutritional deficits, rather than correction of deficits after they have occurred, is important in nutritional management of these patients (see "Acute Respiratory Failure" and "Long-Term Mechanical Ventilator Dependence" in Chapter 20).

Nutrition Assessment in Pulmonary Alterations

Common findings in nutrition assessment related to pulmonary alterations are summarized in Box 8-5. The patient with

---

BOX 8-5	COMMON FINDINGS IN THE NUTRITION ASSESSMENT OF THE PATIENT WITH PULMONARY DISEASE

Anthropometric Measurements
Underweight

Biochemical (Laboratory) Data
Elevated PCO_2 related to overfeeding

Clinical Findings
Edema, dyspnea, signs of pulmonary edema related to fluid volume excess

Diet or Health History
Poor food intake related to dyspnea, unpleasant taste in the mouth from sputum production or bronchodilator therapy; endotracheal intubation preventing oral intake

---

respiratory compromise is especially vulnerable to the effects of fluid volume excess and must be assessed continually for this complication, particularly during enteral and parenteral feeding.

Nutrition Intervention and Education in Pulmonary Alterations
Prevent or Correct Undernutrition and Underweight
The nurse and dietitian work together to encourage oral intake in the undernourished or potentially undernourished patient who is capable of eating. Small, frequent feedings are especially important, because a very full stomach can interfere with diaphragmatic movement. Mouth care should be provided before meals and snacks to clear the palate of the taste of sputum and medications. Administering bronchodilators with food can help to reduce the gastric irritation caused by these medications.

Because of anorexia, dyspnea, debilitation, or need for ventilatory support, however, many patients will require enteral tube feeding or TPN. It is especially important for the nurse to be alert to the risk of pulmonary aspiration in the patient with an artificial airway. To reduce the risk of pulmonary aspiration during enteral tube feeding, keep the patient's head elevated at least 45 degrees during feedings, unless contraindicated; keep the cuff of the artificial airway inflated during feeding, if possible; monitor the patient for increasing abdominal distention; and check tube placement before each feeding (if intermittent) or at least every 4 to 8 hours if feedings are continuous.

Avoid Overfeeding
Overfeeding of total calories or of carbohydrate or lipid alone can impair pulmonary function. The production of carbon dioxide (VCO_2) increases when carbohydrate is relied on as the primary energy source. This is unlikely to be significant in the patient who is eating foods. Instead, it is an iatrogenic complication of TPN, in which glucose is often the predominant calorie source, or occasionally of tube feeding in a patient with a very high carbohydrate formula. Excessive calorie intake can raise $PaCO_2$ sufficiently to make it difficult to wean a patient from the ventilator. A balanced regimen with lipids and carbohydrates providing the nonprotein calories is optimal for the patient with respiratory compromise, and the patient needs to be reassessed continually to ensure that caloric intake is not excessive.[3]

Excessive lipid intake can impair capillary gas exchange in the lungs, although this is not usually sufficient to produce an increase in $PaCO_2$ or decrease in PaO_2.[92] However, the patient with severe respiratory alteration may be further compromised by lipid overdose. If lipid intake is maintained at no more than 2 g/kg/day, lipid excess is rarely a problem. Serum triglyceride levels greater than 400 mg/dL may indicate inadequate lipid clearance and a need to decrease the lipid dosage.

Prevent Fluid Volume Excess
Pulmonary edema and failure of the right side of the heart, which may be precipitated by fluid volume excess, further worsen the status of the patient with respiratory compromise. Maintaining careful intake and output records allows for

accurate assessment of fluid balance. Usually the patient requires no more than 35 to 40 mL/kg/day of fluid. For the patient receiving nutrition support, fluid intake can be reduced by using 20% lipid emulsions as a source of calories, by using tube feeding formulas that provide at least 2 calories/mL (the dietitian can recommend appropriate formulas), and by choosing oral supplements that are low in fluid. Additionally, powdered glucose polymers or powered protein products can be used to increase caloric intake without increasing volume. The nurse plays a valuable role in continually reassessing the patient's state of hydration and alerting other team members to changes that may indicate the need for an increase or decrease in fluid intake.

NUTRITION AND NEUROLOGIC ALTERATIONS

Because neurologic disorders such as stroke and closed head injury tend to be long-term problems, they necessitate good nutritional care to prevent nutritional deficits and promote well-being.

Nutrition Assessment in Neurologic Alterations

Nutrition-related assessment findings vary widely in the patient with neurologic alterations, depending on the type of disorder present. Some common assessment findings are listed in Box 8-6.

Nutrition Intervention and Education in Neurologic Alterations
Prevention or Correction of Nutritional Deficits

Oral Feedings. Patients with dysphagia or weakness of the swallowing musculature often experience the greatest difficulty in swallowing foods that are dry or thin liquids, such as water, that are difficult to control. For these patients, the nurse, the dietitian, and the speech therapist can work together to plan suitable meals and evaluate patient acceptance and tolerance (see "Stroke" in Chapter 24).

Soft, moist foods are usually easier to swallow than dry ones. An upright sitting position is preferable during meals, if possible, to allow gravity to facilitate effective swallowing. Water and other thin liquids may be especially difficult for the person with swallowing dysfunction to manage. Beverages may be thickened with commercial thickening products, with infant cereal, or with yogurt if the patient has difficulty swallowing thin fluids. Fruit nectars may be better tolerated than thinner juices.

The patient should not be rushed while eating because this may increase the risk of pulmonary aspiration. Providing small amounts of food at frequent intervals rather than larger amounts only at mealtimes may help the patient feel less need to hurry. Suction equipment should be kept available in case aspiration occurs. Dysphagia is frustrating and frightening for the patient and requires much understanding and patience by the family and caregivers.

Tube Feedings or Total Parenteral Nutrition. Patients who are unconscious or unable to eat because of severe dysphagia, weakness, ileus, or other reasons require tube feedings or TPN. Prompt initiation of nutrition support must be a priority in the patient with neurologic impairments. Needs for protein and calories are increased by infection and fever, as may occur in the patient with encephalitis or meningitis. Needs for protein, calories, zinc, and vitamin C are increased during wound healing, as occurs in the trauma patient and the patient with pressure ulcers.

Patients with neurologic deficits are at increased risk for certain complications (particularly pulmonary aspiration) during tube feeding and therefore require especially careful nursing management. Patients of most concern are 1) those with an impaired gag reflex, such as some patients with cerebral vascular accident; 2) those with delayed gastric emptying, such as patients in the early period after spinal cord injury and patients with head injury treated with barbiturate coma; and 3) patients likely to experience seizures. To help prevent pulmonary aspiration, the patient's head is kept elevated at an angle of 30 to 45 degrees, if not contraindicated; when elevation of the head is not possible, administering feedings with the patient in the prone or lateral position allows free drainage of emesis from the mouth and decreases the risk of aspiration (see "Aspiration Pneumonitis" in Chapter 20).

Administering phenytoin with enteral formulas decreases the absorption of the medication and the peak serum level achieved. A problem arises when a patient is receiving continuous enteral feedings and requires anticonvulsant therapy. One way to deal with the problem is stop the feeding for 1 to 2 hours before and after phenytoin administration.[93] Even when this practice is followed, the patient may require a higher phenytoin dosage than normal to maintain therapeutic serum concentrations. When continuous feedings are discontinued and the patient resumes eating meals or receives intermittent enteral feedings, the phenytoin dosage must be adjusted appropriately. Phenytoin levels should be monitored carefully in patients receiving enteral feedings. The infusion rate may need to be increased to account for the time that the enteral feeding is held for phenytoin administration.

Hyperglycemia is a common complication in patients receiving corticosteroids. Regular monitoring of blood glucose levels

---

BOX 8-6   COMMON FINDINGS IN THE NUTRITION ASSESSMENT OF THE PATIENT WITH NEUROLOGIC ALTERATIONS

Biochemical (Laboratory) Data
- Hyperglycemia (with corticosteroid use)

Clinical Findings
- Wasting of muscle and subcutaneous fat related to disuse or to poor food intake

Diet or Health History
- Poor food intake related to altered state of consciousness, dysphagia or other chewing or swallowing difficulties, or ileus resulting from spinal cord injury or use of pentobarbital
- Hypermetabolism resulting from head injury
- Pressure ulcers

is an important part of care of such patients. They may require insulin to control the hyperglycemia.

Prompt use of nutrition support is especially important for patients with head injuries because head injury causes marked catabolism, even in patients who receive barbiturates, which should decrease metabolic demands. Head-injured patients rapidly exhaust glycogen stores and begin to use body proteins to meet energy needs, a process that can quickly lead to PCM. The catabolic response is partly a result of corticosteroid therapy in head-injured patients. However, the hypermetabolism and hypercatabolism are also caused by dramatic hormonal responses to this type of injury.[94] Levels of cortisol, epinephrine, and norepinephrine increase as much as seven times normal. These hormones increase the metabolic rate and caloric demands, causing mobilization of body fat and proteins to meet the increased energy needs. Head-injured patients undergo an inflammatory response and may be febrile, creating increased needs for protein and calories. Improvement in outcome and reduction in complications have been observed in head-injured patients who receive adequate nutrition support early in the hospital course[94,95] (see Traumatic Brain Injuries in Chapter 34).

Prevention of Overweight and Obesity. Many stable patients with neurologic disorders are less active than their healthy counterparts and require fewer calories. They may become overweight or obese if given normal amounts of calories for their age and gender. Within 1 or 2 months after spinal cord injury, substantial amounts of muscle atrophy and loss of body mass begin to occur as a result of denervation and disuse. Consequently, body weight and caloric needs decline. Ideal body weights for paraplegics and quadriplegics are less than those for healthy adults of the same height.[96] Stable, rehabilitating paraplegics need approximately 27.9 calories/kg/day, and quadriplegics need approximately 22.7 calories/kg/day.[96,97] Patients with dysphagia or extreme swallowing musculature weakness may rely on very soft, easy-to-chew foods that are usually more dense in calories than are bulky, high-fiber foods. They also may gain unneeded weight that will hamper their care and impede mobility. For these reasons, nutrition education of the patient and family coping with a spinal cord injury should include instruction about prevention of undesirable weight gain. Decreased use of high-fat foods (e.g., milk—such as shakes, ice cream, butter, margarine, pastries) can help to reduce calorie intake. Fruits and vegetables without added fat or sauces are good choices because they are generally low in fat and supply fiber needed to help maintain regular bowel habits.

NUTRITION AND RENAL ALTERATIONS

Providing adequate nutrition care for the patient with renal disease can be extremely challenging. Although renal disturbances and their treatments can markedly increase needs for nutrients, necessary restrictions in intake of fluid, protein, phosphorus, and potassium make delivery of adequate calories, vitamins, and minerals difficult. Thorough nutrition assessment provides the basis for successful nutrition management in patients with renal disease.

BOX 8-7 COMMON FINDINGS IN THE NUTRITION ASSESSMENT OF THE PATIENT WITH RENAL FAILURE

Anthropometric Measurements
- Underweight (may be masked by edema)

Biochemical (Laboratory) Data
- Electrolyte imbalances
- Hypoalbuminemia related to protein restriction and amino acid losses in dialysis
- Anemia related to inadequate erythropoietin production and blood loss with hemodialysis
- Hypertriglyceridemia related to use of glucose as osmotic agent in dialysis and use of carbohydrates to supply needed calories

Clinical Findings
- Wasting of muscle and subcutaneous tissue (may be masked by edema)

Diet or Health History
- Poor dietary intake related to protein and electrolyte restrictions and alterations in taste

---

Nutrition Assessment in Renal Alterations

Some common assessment findings in individuals with renal disease are listed in Box 8-7.

Nutrition Intervention and Education in Renal Alterations

Nutritional needs of patients with renal disease are complex. The goal of nutrition intervention is to balance adequate calories, protein, vitamins, and minerals, while avoiding excesses of protein, fluid, electrolytes, and other nutrients with potential toxicity.

Protein

The kidney is responsible for excreting nitrogen from amino acids or proteins in the form of urea. When urinary excretion of urea is impaired in renal failure, BUN rises. Excessive protein intake may worsen uremia. However, the patient with renal failure often has other physiologic stresses that increase protein or amino acid needs: losses because of dialysis, wounds, and fistulas; use of corticosteroid medications that exert a catabolic effect; increased endogenous secretion of catecholamines, corticosteroids, and glucagon, all of which can cause or aggravate catabolism; metabolic acidosis, which stimulates protein breakdown; and catabolic conditions, such as trauma, surgery, and sepsis.[98] Patients with acute kidney injury need adequate amounts of protein to avoid catabolism of body tissues.

Patients with stable acute kidney injury without evidence of fluid overload or electrolyte or acid-base disturbances can often be managed conservatively without dialysis. However, when renal function worsens, some form of renal replacement therapy (RRT) is required to maintain homeostasis and prevent metabolic complications. Types of RRT include peritoneal dialysis, intermittent hemodialysis, and continuous arteriovenous (AV) hemofiltration.[98] During hemodialysis, amino acids are freely filtered and lost, but proteins such as albumin and immunoglobulin are not. Proteins and amino acids are removed during peritoneal dialysis, creating a greater nutritional requirement for protein.[99,100] Protein needs may be higher, depending on the level of stress.[101] To limit catabolism, patients with acute kidney injury on dialysis therapy should receive approximately 1.5 to 2.0 g of protein/kg/day (with a maximum of 2.5 g of protein/kg/day), depending on catabolic rate, renal function, and dialysis losses.[3,102]

Fluid

The patient with renal insufficiency usually does not require a fluid restriction until urine output begins to diminish. Patients receiving hemodialysis are limited to a fluid intake resulting in a gain of no more than 0.45 kg (1 lb) per day on the days between dialysis. This generally means a daily intake of 500 to 750 mL plus the volume lost in urine. With the use of continuous peritoneal dialysis, hemofiltration, or hemodialysis, the fluid intake can be liberalized.[103] This more liberal fluid allowance permits more adequate nutrient delivery by oral, tube, or parenteral feedings. Enteral formulas containing 1.5 to 2 calories/mL or more provide a concentrated source of calories for tube-fed patients who require fluid restriction. Intravenous lipids, particularly 20% emulsions, can be used to supply concentrated calories for the TPN patient. Intradialytic TPN can be given during hemodialysis sessions to some malnourished patients; it supplies an additional source of nutrients at a time when the fluid can be rapidly removed in dialysis.[99]

Energy (Calories)

Energy needs are not increased by renal failure, but adequate calories must be provided to avoid catabolism.[98,103] It is essential that the renal patient receive an adequate number of calories to prevent catabolism of body tissues to meet energy needs. Catabolism reduces the mass of muscle and other functional body tissues, and it releases nitrogen that must be excreted by the kidney. Adults with renal insufficiency need about 30 to 35 calories/kg/day to prevent catabolism and ensure that all protein consumed is used for anabolism rather than to meet energy needs.[103] After renal transplantation, when the patient usually receives large doses of corticosteroids, it is especially important to ensure that caloric intake is adequate (usually 25 to 35 calories/kg/day) to prevent undue catabolism.

Glucose in the peritoneal dialysate may be a significant calorie source and a contributing factor in hypertriglyceridemia. Approximately 70% of the glucose instilled during peritoneal dialysis to serve as an osmotic agent may be absorbed, and this must be considered part of the patient's carbohydrate intake. The glucose monohydrate, dextrose, used in intravenous and dialysate solutions supplies 3.4 calories/g. If the patient receives 4.25% glucose (4.25 g glucose/100 mL solution) in the dialysate, he or she receives the following:

$$42.5 \text{ g/L} \times 70\% \times 3.4 \text{ Calories/g}$$
$$= 101 \text{ Calories/L of dialysate}$$

To help control hypertriglyceridemia, only about 30% to 35% of the patient's calories should come from carbohydrates, including glucose from the dialysate, with the major portion of dietary carbohydrate coming from complex carbohydrates.

Consuming at least 20 to 25 g of fiber daily can help to control triglyceride levels. Sources of dietary fiber include cooked dried beans and peas (5 to 7 g of fiber/0.5 cup); cereals containing whole grains (not 100% bran); berries, apples, oranges, pears, corn, and peas (3 to 5 g/serving); whole-grain breads; and most fruits and vegetables other than those listed previously (1 to 2 g/serving). Wheat bran is a good source of fiber (5 to 10 g/oz), but it is also a good source of phosphorus and therefore may cause renal failure to progress more rapidly. For the tube-fed patient, a formula containing dietary fiber can be chosen. To help control hypertriglyceridemia and to provide concentrated calories in minimal fluid, fat may need to supply as much as 40% of the patient's calories.

Hypercholesterolemia is commonly found in patients with renal failure, and unsaturated fats and oils (corn, soybean, sunflower, safflower, cottonseed, canola, and olive) are preferred over saturated fats (primarily from meats and dairy products), which tend to raise cholesterol levels. The necessary restriction of meat, milk, and other protein foods in the diet helps lower intake of cholesterol and saturated fat. Intravenous lipids and the long-chain fats found in most commercial enteral formulas are primarily polyunsaturated.

Other Nutrients

Certain nutrients such as potassium and phosphorus are restricted because they are excreted by the kidney. The patient has no specific requirement for the fat-soluble vitamins A, E, and K, because they are not removed in appreciable amounts by dialysis and restriction generally prevents development of toxicity. Patients with end-stage renal disease may have decreased clearance of vitamin A, and levels should be monitored.[102] The needs for several water-soluble vitamins and trace minerals are increased in the dialysis patient because they are small enough to pass freely through the dialysis filter. Vitamin and minerals should be supplemented as necessary.[103]

NUTRITION AND GASTROINTESTINAL ALTERATIONS

Because the GI tract is inherently related to nutrition, it is not surprising that impairment of the GI tract and its accessory organs has a major impact on nutrition. Two of the most serious GI-related illnesses seen among critical care patients are hepatic failure and pancreatitis, and the following discussion focuses on these disorders.

Nutrition Assessment in Gastrointestinal Alterations

Some common assessment findings in individuals with GI disease are listed in Box 8-8.

BOX 8-8   COMMON FINDINGS IN THE NUTRITION ASSESSMENT OF THE PATIENT WITH GASTROINTESTINAL DISEASE

Anthropometric Measurements

- Underweight related to malabsorption (from inadequate production of bile salts or pancreatic enzymes), anorexia, or poor intake (because of pain caused by eating)

Biochemical (Laboratory) Data

- Hypoalbuminemia (may result primarily from liver damage and not malnutrition)
- Hypocalcemia related to steatorrhea
- Hypomagnesemia related to alcohol abuse
- Anemia related to blood loss from bleeding varices

Clinical Findings

- Wasting of muscle and subcutaneous fat
- Confusion, confabulation, nystagmus, or peripheral neuropathy related to thiamine deficiency caused by alcohol abuse (Wernicke-Korsakoff syndrome)

Diet or Health History

- Steatorrhea

Nutrition Intervention and Education in Gastrointestinal Alterations

Hepatic Failure

The liver is the most important metabolic organ, and it is responsible for carbohydrate, fat and protein metabolism, vitamin storage and activation, and detoxification of waste products. Liver failure is associated with a wide spectrum of metabolic alterations. Because the diseased liver has impaired ability to deactivate hormones, levels of circulating glucagon, epinephrine, and cortisol are elevated. These hormones promote catabolism of body tissues and cause glycogen stores to be exhausted. Release of lipids from their storage depots is accelerated, but the liver has decreased ability to metabolize them for energy. Moreover, inadequate production of bile salts by the liver results in malabsorption of fat from the diet. Body proteins are used for energy sources, producing tissue wasting. The branched-chain amino acids (BCAAs)—leucine, isoleucine, and valine—are especially well used for energy, and their levels in the blood decline. Conversely, levels of the aromatic amino acids (AAAs)—phenylalanine, tyrosine, and tryptophan—increase as a result of tissue catabolism and impaired ability of the liver to clear them from the blood. BCAAs are not as dependent on liver metabolism as the AAAs are.[104] The AAAs are precursors for neurotransmitters (serotonin and dopamine) within the central nervous system. Rising levels of AAAs cause encephalopathy by promoting synthesis of false neurotransmitters that compete with endogenous neurotransmitters. The damaged liver cannot clear ammonia from the circulation adequately, and ammonia accumulates in the brain. The ammonia may contribute to the encephalopathic symptoms and to brain edema.[3,104]

Monitoring Fluid and Electrolyte Status. Ascites and edema are caused by a combination of factors. Colloid osmotic pressure in the plasma decreases because of the reduction of production of albumin and other plasma proteins by the diseased liver, increased portal pressure caused by obstruction, and renal sodium retention from secondary hyperaldosteronism. To control the fluid retention, restriction of sodium (usually 2000 mg) and fluid (1500 mL or less daily) usually is necessary in conjunction with the administration of diuretics. Patients are weighed daily to evaluate the success of treatment. Physical status and laboratory data must be closely monitored for deficiencies of potassium, phosphorus, zinc, and vitamins A, D, E, and K.[3]

Provision of a Nutritious Diet and Evaluation of Response to Dietary Protein. PCM and nutritional deficiencies are common in patients with liver failure. The causes of malnutrition are complex and usually are related to decreased intake, malabsorption, maldigestion, and abnormal nutrient metabolism. Nutrition intervention is individualized and based on these metabolic changes. A diet with adequate protein helps to suppress catabolism and promote liver regeneration. Stable patients with cirrhosis usually tolerate 0.8 to 1 g of protein/kg/day. Patients with severe stress or nutritional deficits have increased needs—as much as 1.2 to 2 g of protein/kg/day.[104] Aggressive treatment with medications, including lactulose, neomycin, or metronidazole, is considered first-line therapy in the management of acute hepatic encephalopathy. Chronic protein restriction, which could lead to PCM, is not recommended as a long-term management strategy for patients with liver disease.[3,104]

Anorexia may interfere with oral intake, and the nurse may need to provide much encouragement to the patient to ensure intake of an adequate diet. Prospective calorie counts may need to be instituted to provide objective evidence of oral intake. Small, frequent feedings are usually better tolerated by the anorexic patient than are three large meals daily. Soft foods are preferred because the patient may have esophageal varices that may be irritated by high-fiber foods. If patients are unable to meet their caloric needs, they may require oral supplements or enteral feeding. Small-bore nasoenteric feeding tubes can be used safely without increasing risk of variceal bleeding.[104] TPN should be reserved for patients who are absolutely unable to tolerate enteral feeding.[3] Diarrhea from concurrent administration of lactulose should not be confused with feeding intolerance.

A diet adequate in calories (at least 30 calories/kg daily) is provided to help prevent catabolism and to prevent the use of dietary protein for energy needs.[105] In cases of malabsorption, medium-chain triglycerides (MCTs) may be used to meet caloric needs. Pancreatic enzymes may also be considered for malabsorption problems.

BCAA-enriched products have been developed for enteral and parenteral nutrition of patients with hepatic disease. These products may be used in patients with acute hepatic encephalopathy who do not tolerate standard diets or enteral formulas or who are unresponsive to lactulose. However, no substantial evidence exists showing BCAAs are superior to standard formulas in regard to nitrogen balance or as treatment for encephalopathy.[3,104] The patient who undergoes successful liver transplantation is usually able to tolerate a regular diet with few restrictions. Intake during the postoperative period must be adequate to support nutritional repletion and healing; 1 to 1.2 g of protein/kg/day and approximately 30 calories/kg/day are usually sufficient. Immunosuppressant therapy (corticosteroids and cyclosporine or tacrolimus) contributes to glucose intolerance. Dietary measures to control glucose intolerance include 1) obtaining approximately 30% of dietary calories from fat; 2) emphasizing complex sources of carbohydrates; and 3) eating several small meals daily. Moderate exercise often helps to improve glucose tolerance.

Pancreatitis

The pancreas is an exocrine and endocrine gland required for normal digestion and metabolism of proteins, carbohydrates, and fats. Acute pancreatitis is an inflammatory process that occurs as a result of autodigestion of the pancreas by enzymes normally secreted by that organ. Food intake stimulates pancreatic secretion, increasing the damage to the pancreas and the pain associated with the disorder. Patients usually present with abdominal pain and tenderness and with elevations of pancreatic enzymes. A mild form of acute pancreatitis occurs in 80% of patients requiring hospitalization, and a severe form of acute pancreatitis occurs in the other 20%.[106] Patients with the mild form of acute pancreatitis do not require nutrition support and generally resume oral feeding within 7 days. Chronic pancreatitis may develop, and it is characterized by fibrosis of pancreatic cells. This results in loss of exocrine and endocrine function because of the destruction of acinar and islet cells. The loss of exocrine function leads to malabsorption and steatorrhea. In chronic pancreatitis, the loss of endocrine function results in impaired glucose intolerance.[106]

Prevention of Further Damage to the Pancreas and Preventing Nutritional Deficits. Effective nutritional management is a key treatment for patients with acute pancreatitis or exacerbations of chronic pancreatitis. The concern that feeding may stimulate the production of digestive enzymes and perpetuate tissue damage has led to the widespread use of TPN and bowel rest. Recent data suggest that for patients with severe pancreatitis, providing enteral nutrition support is more beneficial than prolonged bowel rest and provision of TPN.[3,107] Enteral nutrition infused into the distal jejunum bypasses the stimulatory effect of feeding on pancreatic secretion and is associated with fewer infectious and metabolic complications compared with TPN.[108,109]

The results of randomized studies comparing TPN with total enteral nutrition (TEN, or enteral tube feeding) indicate that TEN is preferable to TPN in patients with severe acute pancreatitis, reducing costs and the risk of sepsis and improving clinical outcome.[108-110] Patients unable to tolerate TEN should receive TPN, and some patients may require a combination of TEN and TPN to meet nutritional requirements.[111,112] Low-fat enteral formulas and those with fat provided by MCTs are more readily absorbed than formulas that are high in long-chain triglycerides (e.g., corn oil, sunflower oil).

When oral intake is possible, small, frequent feedings of low-fat foods are least likely to cause discomfort,[109] though the level of fat restriction should depend on the level of steatorrhea

and abdominal pain the patient experiences.[107] For patients with chronic pancreatitis, pancreatic enzyme replacement therapy may be indicated.[107] Guidelines for the treatment of diabetes (discussed later) are appropriate for the care of the person with glucose intolerance or diabetes related to pancreatitis.

NUTRITION AND ENDOCRINE ALTERATIONS

Endocrine alterations have far-reaching effects on all body systems and affect nutritional status in a variety of ways. One of the most common endocrine problems in the general population and among critically ill patients is diabetes mellitus.

Nutrition Assessment in Endocrine Alterations

Because of the prevalence of patients with non–insulin-dependent diabetes mellitus (type 2 diabetes) among the hospitalized population and the association of type 2 diabetes with overweight, the nutritional problems most commonly identified in patients with endocrine alterations are overweight and obesity. Hyperglycemia and hyperlipidemia are other common findings in the individual with diabetes.

Nutrition Intervention in Endocrine Alterations
Nutrition Support and Blood Glucose Control

Patients with insulin-dependent diabetes mellitus (type 1 diabetes) or endocrine dysfunction caused by pancreatitis often have weight loss and malnutrition as a result of tissue catabolism because they cannot use dietary carbohydrates to meet energy needs. Although patients with type 2 diabetes are more likely to be overweight than underweight, they also may become malnourished as a result of chronic or acute infections, trauma, major surgery, or other illnesses.[113] Nutrition support should not be neglected simply because a patient is obese, because PCM can develop in these patients. When a patient is not expected to be able to eat for at least 5 to 7 days or inadequate intake persists for that period, initiation of tube feedings or TPN is indicated. No disease process benefits from starvation, and development or progression of nutritional deficits may contribute to complications, such as pressure ulcers, pulmonary or urinary tract infections, and sepsis, which prolong hospitalization, increase the costs of care, and may even result in death.

Blood glucose control is especially important in the care of surgical patients. Poorly controlled diabetes reduces immune function by impairing granulocyte adherence, chemotaxis, and phagocytosis.[114,115] In surveys of critically ill patients undergoing a variety of elective operations and coronary artery surgery,[114] glucose levels of 206 to 220 mg/dL or higher during the first 24 to 36 postoperative hours were associated with higher rates of nosocomial infection than lower glucose levels.[114,116] To maintain tight control of blood glucose, glucose levels are monitored regularly, usually several times a day, until the patient is stable. Patients unable to tolerate oral diets or enteral feeding may require TPN to meet nutritional requirements during acute illness.[117] Regular insulin added to the solution is a common method of managing hyperglycemia in the patient receiving TPN. The dosage required may be larger than the patient's usual dose because some of the insulin adheres to glass bottles and plastic bags or administration sets. Multiple injections or, preferably, a continuous infusion of regular insulin may be used to maintain tight control of blood glucose in the enterally fed patient.[118] Although further study is needed, the following glucose goals are recommended: 80 mg/dL to 120 mg/dL in critically ill patients in the critical care unit and 100 mg/dL to 150 mg/dL for stable patients on the wards.[117]

In patients receiving enteral tube feedings, the postpyloric route (through a nasoduodenal, nasojejunal, or jejunostomy tube) may be the most effective, because gastroparesis may limit tolerance of intragastric tube feedings.[119] Postpyloric feedings are given continuously because dumping syndrome and poor absorption may occur if feedings are given rapidly into the small bowel. Continuous enteral infusions are associated with improved control of blood glucose. Fiber-enriched formulas may slow the absorption of the carbohydrate, producing a more delayed and sustained glycemic response. Most standard formulas contain balanced proportions of carbohydrate, protein, and fats appropriate for diabetic patients. Specialized diabetic formulas have not shown improved outcomes compared with standard formulas.[118]

Severe Vomiting or Diarrhea in the Patient with Type 1 Diabetes Mellitus

When insulin-dependent patients experience vomiting and diarrhea severe enough to interfere significantly with oral intake or result in excessive fluid and electrolyte losses, adequate carbohydrates and fluids must be supplied. Nausea and vomiting should be treated with antiemetic medication.[119] Delayed gastric emptying is common in diabetes and may improve with administration of prokinetic agents.[119] Small amounts of food or liquids taken every 15 to 20 minutes usually are the best tolerated by the patient with nausea and vomiting. Foods and beverages containing approximately 15 g of carbohydrate include ½ cup of regular gelatin, ½ cup of custard, ¾ cup of regular ginger ale, ½ cup of a regular soft drink, and ½ cup of orange or apple juice. Blood glucose levels should be monitored at least every 2 to 4 hours.

Nutrition Education in Diabetes

Optimal control of blood glucose in type 1 and type 2 diabetes is associated with a decreased risk of development of retinopathy, neuropathy, and other long-term complications.[113] Self-monitoring of blood glucose is essential in maintaining diabetic control, and nutrition is considered the most critical component of diabetes care in achieving blood glucose goals.[120] Meals are based on heart-healthy diet principles, according to which saturated fat and cholesterol are limited and protein accounts for 15% to 20% of total calories. Most carbohydrate foods should be whole grains, fruits, vegetables, and low-fat milk.[121] Evidence-based medical nutrition therapy supports hospitals implementing a consistent carbohydrate meal plan for diabetic patients.[122] The meal plan is based on the amount of carbohydrate that is consistent from meal to meal each day. Although exact calorie levels are not specified, a typical daily menu provides approximately 1500 to 2000 calories with a range of three to five carbohydrate foods at each meal, each containing 15 g of carbohydrate.[121]

Careful monitoring of dietary intake and blood glucose levels is essential during critical illness to meet nutritional needs and maintain glucose control. Avoidance of overfeeding limits hyperglycemia and associated complications. Insulin can be adjusted to maintain blood glucose control based on frequent monitoring. Intensive insulin therapy has been shown to reduce mortality rates for critically ill surgical patients.[114] It is vital for the dietitian to work closely with the interdisciplinary team to determine feeding methods, appropriate enteral formulas, and the amounts of protein, lipid, and carbohydrate supplied in parenteral nutrition.[122]

BOX 8-9   **CASE STUDY**

Patient with Nutritional Issues

Brief Patient History

Mrs. S is a 49-year-old woman with end-stage cardiomyopathy. She and her husband have been restaurant owners for many years. She is anorexic and finds it difficult to eat solid foods, which is emotionally distressing for her and her family. She has lost 10 pounds in the past month. Mrs. S was placed on the heart transplant list 6 months ago. She has agreed to hospitalization to optimize her medical management and nutritional status.

Clinical Assessment

Mrs. S is admitted to the critical care unit. A central line has been inserted for dobutamine therapy. A nutritional assessment has been completed by the dietitian that includes recommendations for frequent, small, calorie-dense, low-sodium feedings.

Diagnostic Procedures

Mrs. S is 5 feet 2 inches tall and weighs 90 pounds. Her vital signs are as follows: blood pressure of 100/60 mm Hg, heart rate of 80 beats/min (sinus rhythm), respiratory rate of 20 breaths/min, and temperature of 98.2° F. Serum laboratory findings are as follows: hemoglobin level of 8.3 g/dL, prealbumin level of 14 mg/dL, sodium level of 125 mmol/L, potassium level of 3.3 mmol/L, chloride level of 94 mmol/L, carbon dioxide concentration of 26 mEq/L, calcium level of 8 mg/dL, magnesium level of 1.5 mg/dL, and B-type natriuretic peptide concentration of 500 pg/mL.

Medical Diagnosis

Mrs. S is diagnosed with cachexia resulting from end-stage cardiomyopathy.

Questions

1. What major outcomes do you expect to achieve for this patient?
2. What problems or risks must be managed to achieve these outcomes?
3. What interventions must be initiated to monitor, prevent, manage, or eliminate the problems and risks identified?
4. What interventions should be initiated to promote optimal functioning, safety, and well-being of the patient?
5. What possible learning needs do you anticipate for this patient?
6. What cultural and age-related factors may have a bearing on the patient's plan of care?

SUMMARY

Nutrient Metabolism

- The major purposes of metabolism of the energy-yielding nutrients are the production of energy and the formation and preservation of lean body mass.

Assessing Nutritional Status

- Nutrition screening should be conducted on every patient, and a more thorough nutrition assessment should be completed on any patient screened to be nutritionally at risk.

Implications of Undernutrition for the Sick or Stressed Patient

- Malnutrition can be related to any essential nutrient or nutrients, but a serious type of malnutrition found frequently among hospitalized patients is protein-calorie malnutrition (PCM). It is usually the result of the combined effects of starvation and hypermetabolism.
- The hypermetabolic process results from increased catabolic changes caused by a stressful event.
- Malnutrition is associated with a variety of adverse outcomes: wound dehiscence, pressure ulcers, infections, respiratory failure requiring ventilation, longer hospital stays, and death.

Nursing Management of Nutrition Support

- Whenever possible, the enteral route is the preferred method of feeding because of lower cost, better maintenance of gut integrity, and decreased infection and hospital stay.
- Oral supplementation may be necessary for patients who can eat and have normal digestion and absorption.
- Early enteral nutrition (within the first 24 to 48 hours of critical illness) reduces septic complications and improves feeding tolerance in critically ill patients.
- It is essential to check tube placement before feedings and regularly throughout the course of enteral feedings.
- Continued oral care is provided during the course of the enteral feedings.

Nutrition and Cardiovascular Alterations

- In the early period after an MI, interventions are aimed at reducing angina, cardiac workload, and the risk of dysrhythmia; meal size, caffeine intake, and food temperatures are monitored closely.
- Interventions in heart failure are designed to reduce fluid retention, thereby reducing the preload.
- Calorie-dense foods and supplements are provided to the patient with cardiac cachexia.

Nutrition and Pulmonary Alterations

- Malnutrition has adverse effects on respiratory function, decreasing surfactant production, diaphragmatic mass, vital capacity, and immunocompetence.
- Because of anorexia, dyspnea, debilitation, or the need for ventilatory support, many patients require tube feeding or TPN.

- It is especially important to be alert to the risks of pulmonary aspiration in the patient with an artificial airway, keeping the hob elevated 45 degrees during feedings, unless contraindicated, and keeping the cuff of the artificial airway inflated during feedings.

Nutrition and Neurologic Alterations

- Patients with dysphagia or weakness of the swallowing musculature often experience the greatest difficulty in swallowing foods that are dry or thin liquids, such as water, which are difficult to control.
- Beverages may be thickened with commercial thickening products, infant cereal, or yogurt; fruit nectars may be better tolerated than fruit juices.
- Prompt use of nutrition support is important for patients with head injuries because head injuries cause marked catabolism, and patients undergo an inflammatory response and may be febrile, increasing the need for proteins and calories.

Nutrition and Renal Alterations

- The goal of intervention is to balance adequate calories, protein, vitamins, and minerals while avoiding excesses of proteins, fluid, electrolytes, and other nutrients with potential toxicities.
- Patients with acute kidney injury need adequate amounts of protein to avoid catabolism of body tissues.
- With the use of continuous peritoneal dialysis, hemofiltration, or hemodialysis, the fluid intake can be liberalized. This allows for more adequate nutrient delivery through oral, tube, or parenteral feedings.
- The need for several water-soluble vitamins and trace minerals is increased in dialysis patients because these nutrients are small enough to pass through the dialysis filter.

Nutrition and Gastrointestinal Alterations

- Ascites and edema in the patient with liver failure have many causes. There is decreased colloid osmotic pressure in the plasma because of reduced production of albumin and other plasma proteins; increased portal pressure caused by obstruction; and renal sodium retention from secondary hyperaldosteronism.
- Causes of malnutrition in liver failure are complex and related to decreased intake, malabsorption, maldigestion, and abnormal nutrient metabolism.
- In the patient with pancreatitis, concern that feeding may stimulate the production of digestive enzymes and perpetuate liver damage has led to the use of TPN and bowel rest.

Nutrition and Endocrine Alterations

- Blood glucose control is especially important in the care of surgical patients.
- Poorly controlled diabetes reduces immune function by impairing granulocyte adherence, chemotaxis, and phagocytosis.

REFERENCES

1. Joint Commission on Accreditation of Healthcare Organizations. *Comprehensive Accreditation Manual for Hospitals.* Chicago, IL: Joint Commission on Accreditation of Healthcare Organizations; 2007.
2. Mueller C, et al. A.S.P.E.N. Clinical guidelines, nutrition screening, assessment, and intervention in adults. *JPEN J Parenter Enteral Nutr.* 2009;35(1):16.
3. McClave SA, Martindale RG, Vanek VW, et al. Society of Critical Care Medicine (SCCM) and American Society for Parenteral and Enteral Nutrition (ASPEN): Guidelines for the provision and assessment of nutrition support therapy in the adult critically ill patient. *J Parenter Enteral Nutr.* 2009;33(3):277.
4. WHO. *Physical status: the use and interpretation of anthropometry. Report of WHO Expert Committee. WHO Technical Report Series 854.* Geneva: World Health Organization; 1995.
5. WHO. *Obesity: preventing and managing the global epidemic. Report of a WHO Consultation. WHO Technical Report Series 894.* Geneva: World Health Organization; 2000.
6. WHO expert consultation. Appropriate body-mass index for Asian populations and its implications for policy and intervention strategies. *Lancet.* 2004;363:157.
7. Prins A. Nutritional assessment of the critically ill patient. *South African Journal of Clinical Nutrition.* 2010;23(1).
8. Berger MM, Cayeux MC, Schaller MD, et al. Stature estimation using the knee height determination in critically ill patients. *e-SPEN, the European e-Journal of Clinical Nutrition and Metabolism.* 2008;3(2):e84.
9. Ravasco P, et al. A critical approach to nutritional assessment in critically ill patients. *Clin Nutr.* 2002;21(1):73.
10. Raguso C, et al. The role of visceral proteins in the nutritional assessment of intensive care unit patients. *Curr Opin Nutr Metab Care.* 2003;6:211.
11. Academy of Nutrition and Dietetics. Evidence Analysis Library. What is the most accurate method for determination of resting metabolic rate (RMR) in critically ill patients? http://www.adaevidencelibrary.com. Accessed April 25, 2012.
12. Satchell MA. Nutrition in critical illness: calorimetry. *Pediatric Critical Care Study Guide.* 2012;452.
13. Academy of Nutrition and Dietetics. Evidence Analysis Library. Estimating RMR with predictive equations: what does the evidence tell us? http://www.adaevidencelibrary.com. Accessed April 24, 2012.
14. Academy of Nutrition and Dietetics. Evidence Analysis Library. If indirect calorimetry is unavailable or impractical, what is the best way to estimate resting metabolic rate (RMR) in obese adult critically ill patients? http://www.adaevidencelibrary.com. Accessed April 24, 2012.
15. Academy of Nutrition and Dietetics. Evidence Analysis Library. If indirect calorimetry is unavailable or impractical, what is the best way to estimate resting metabolic rate (RMR) in non-obese adult critically ill patients? http://www.adaevidencelibrary.com. Accessed April 24, 2012.
16. Ramos M, et al. Relationship of perioperative hyperglycemia and postoperative infections in patients who undergo general and vascular surgery. *Ann Surg.* 2008;248(4):585.
17. Pirlich M, et al. Prevalence of malnutrition in hospitalized medical patients: impact of underlying disease. *Dig Dis.* 2003;21(3):245.
18. Kyle UG, et al. Prevalence of malnutrition in 1760 patients at hospital admission: a controlled population study of body composition. *Clin Nutr.* 2003;22(5):473.
19. Barker LA, Gout BS, Crowe TC. Hospital malnutrition: prevalence, identification and impact on patients and the healthcare system. *International Journal of Environmental Research and Public Health.* 2011;8(2):514.
20. Joosten KFM, Hulst JM. Malnutrition in pediatric hospital patients: current issues. *Nutrition.* 2011;27(2):133.
21. Braunschweig C, et al. Impact of declines in nutritional status on outcomes in adult patients hospitalized for more than 7 days. *J Am Diet Assoc.* 2000;100:1316.
22. Mathus-Vliegen EMH. Nutritional status, nutrition and pressure ulcers. *Nutr Clin Pract.* 2001;16:286.
23. Rubinson L, et al. Low caloric intake is associated with nosocomial bloodstream infections in patients in the medical intensive care unit. *Crit Care Med.* 2004;32:350.
24. Braunschweig CL, et al. Enteral compared with parenteral nutrition: a meta-analysis. *Am J Clin Nutr.* 2001;74(4):534.
25. Langkamp-Henken B. If the gut works, use it: but what if you can't? *Nutr Clin Pract.* 2003;18:449.
26. Jeejeebhoy KN. Total parenteral nutrition: potion or poison? *Am J Clin Nutr.* 2001;74(2):160.
27. Alpers DH. Enteral feeding and gut atrophy. *Curr Opin Nutr Metab Care.* 2002;5:679.
28. Schloerb PR. Immune-enhancing diets: products, components, and their rationales. *JPEN J Parenter Enteral Nutr.* 2001;25(2):S3.
29. Kelly D, Wischmeyer PE. Role of L-glutamine in critical illness: new insights. *Curr Opin Nutr Metab Care.* 2003;6:217.
30. Wernerman J. Glutamine and acute illness. *Curr Opin Crit Care.* 2003;9:279.
31. Boelens PG, et al. Glutamine alimentation in the catabolic state. *J Nutr.* 2001;131:2569S.
32. Preiser J-C, et al. Enteral feeding with a solution enriched with antioxidant vitamins A, C, and E enhances the resistance to oxidative stress. *Crit Care Med.* 2000;28(12):3828.
33. Heyland DK, et al. Should immunonutrition become routine in critically ill patients? A systematic review of the evidence. *JAMA.* 2001;286(8):944.
34. Heyland DK. Immunonutrition in the critically ill patient: putting the cart before the horse? *Nutr Clin Pract.* 2002;17:267.
35. Montejo JC, et al. Immunonutrition in the intensive care unit: a systematic review and consensus statement. *Clin Nutr.* 2003;22(3):221.
36. Stechmiller JK, et al. Arginine immunonutrition in critically ill patients: a clinical dilemma. *Am J Crit Care Nurs.* 2004;13(1):17.
37. Marik PE, Zaloga GP. Early enteral nutrition in acutely ill patients: a systematic review. *Crit Care Med.* 2001;29(12):2264.
38. Jeejeebhoy KN. Enteral feeding. *Curr Opin Clin Nutr Metab Care.* 2002;5:695.
39. Zaloga GP, Roberts PR, Marik PE. Feeding the hemodynamically unstable patient: a critical evaluation of the evidence. *Nutr Clin Pract.* 2003;18:285.
40. Moore FA, Weisbrodt NW. Gut dysfunction and intolerance to enteral nutrition in critically ill patients. *Nestle Nutr Workshop Ser Clin Perform Programme.* 2003;8:149.
41. Montejo JC, et al. Multicenter, prospective, randomized, single-blind study comparing the efficacy and gastrointestinal complications of early jejunal feeding with early gastric feeding in critically ill patients. *Crit Care Med.* 2002;30(4):796.

42. McClave SA, Snider HL. Clinical use of gastric residual volumes as a monitor for patients on enteral tube feeding. *JPEN J Parenter Enteral Nutr.* 2002;26(suppl 6):S43.

43. Berne JD, et al. Erythromycin reduces delayed gastric emptying in critically ill trauma patients: a randomized, controlled trial. *J Trauma.* 2002;53(3):422.

44. Booth CM, et al. Gastrointestinal promotility drugs in the critical care setting: a systematic review of the evidence. *Crit Care Med.* 2002;30(7):1429.

45. Doherty WL, Winter B. Prokinetic agents in critical care. *Crit Care.* 2003;7(3):206.

46. Lord LM, et al. Comparison of weighted vs. unweighted enteral feeding tubes for efficacy of transpyloric intubation. *JPEN J Parenter Enteral Nutr.* 1993;17(3):271.

47. Metheny NA, et al. pH and concentration of bilirubin in feeding tube aspirates as predictors of tube placement. *Nurs Res.* 1999;48:189.

48. Heyland DK, et al. Effect of postpyloric feeding on gastroesophageal regurgitation and pulmonary microaspiration: results of a randomized controlled trial. *Crit Care Med.* 2001;29(8):1495.

49. Esparza J, et al. Equal aspiration rates in gastrically and transpylorically fed critically ill patients. *Intensive Care Med.* 2001;27:660.

50. Neumann DA, DeLegge MH. Gastric versus small-bowel tube feeding in the intensive care unit: a prospective comparison of efficacy. *Crit Care Med.* 2002;30(7):1436.

51. Marik PE, Zaloga GR. Gastric versus postpyloric feeding: a systematic review. *Crit Care.* 2003;7(3):R46.

52. Davies AR, et al. Randomized comparison of nasojejunal and nasogastric feeding in critically ill patients. *Crit Care Med.* 2002;30(3):586.

53. Kearns PJ, et al. The incidence of ventilator-associated pneumonia and success in nutrient delivery with gastric versus small intestine feeding: a randomized clinical trial. *Crit Care Med.* 2000;28(6):1742.

54. Grant MJC, Martin S. Delivery of enteral nutrition. *AACN Clin Issues.* 2000;11(4):507.

55. Lord LM. Restoring and maintaining patency of enteral feeding tubes. *Nutr Clin Pract.* 2003;18:422.

56. Bourgault AM, et al. Prophylactic pancreatic enzymes to reduce feeding tube occlusions. *Nutr Clin Pract.* 2003;18:398.

57. Metheny NA. Risk factors for aspiration. *JPEN J Parenter Enteral Nutr.* 2002;26(6 suppl):S26.

58. Metheny NA, et al. A survey of bedside methods used to detect pulmonary aspiration of enteral formula in intubated tube-fed patients. *Am J Crit Care.* 1999;8:160.

59. Maloney JP, Ryan TA. Detection of aspiration in enterally fed patients: a requiem for bedside monitors of aspiration. *JPEN J Parenter Enteral Nutr.* 2002;26(6):S34.

60. Lucarelli MR, et al. Toxicity of food drug and cosmetic blue no. 1 dye in critically ill patients. *Chest.* 2004;125(2):793.

61. McClave SA, et al. North American summit on aspiration in the critically ill patient: consensus statement. *JPEN J Parenter Enteral Nutr.* 2002;26(6):S80.

62. Eisenberg P. An overview of diarrhea in the patient receiving enteral nutrition. *Gastroenterol Nurs.* 2002;25(3):95.

63. Wiesen P, et al. Diarrhoea in the critically ill. *Curr Opin Crit Care.* 2006;12(2):149.

64. Bernard AC, et al. Defining and assessing tolerance in enteral nutrition. *Nutr Clin Pract.* 2004;19(5):481.

65. Mostafa SM, et al. Constipation and its implications in the critically ill patient. *Br J Anaesth.* 2003;91(6):815.

66. Elpern EH, et al. Outcomes associated with enteral tube feedings in a medical intensive care unit. *Am J Crit Care.* 2004;13:221.

67. Engel JM, et al. Enteral nutrition practice in a surgical intensive care unit: what proportion of energy expenditure is delivered enterally? *Clin Nutr.* 2003;22(2):187.

68. Krishnan JA, et al. Caloric intake in medical ICU patients: consistency of care with guidelines and relationship to clinical outcomes. *Chest.* 2003;124:297.

69. DeJonghe B, et al. A prospective survey of nutritional support practices in intensive care unit patients: What is prescribed? What is delivered? *Crit Care Med.* 2001;29(1):8.

70. The Joint Commission. Sentinel Event Alert: Tubing misconnections – a persistent and potentially deadly occurrence. http://www.jointcommission.org/assets/1/18/SEA_36.PDF. Published April 2006. Accessed April 23, 2012.

71. Aust MP. Tubing misconnections. *American Journal of Critical Care.* 2011;20(4):346.

72. Worthington P, et al. Parenteral nutrition for the acutely ill. *AACN Clin Issues.* 2000;11(4):559.

73. Dobbins BM, et al. Each lumen is a potential source of central venous catheter-related bloodstream infection. *Crit Care Med.* 2003;31(6):1688.

74. Orr ME. The peripherally inserted central catheter: what are the current indications for its use? *Nutr Clin Pract.* 2002;17:99.

75. O'Grady NP, et al. Guidelines for the prevention of intravascular catheter-related infections. *Infect Control Hosp Epidemiol.* 2002;23(12):759.

76. Speerhas R, et al. Maintaining normal blood glucose concentrations with total parenteral nutrition: is it necessary to taper total parenteral nutrition? *Nutr Clin Pract.* 2003;18:414.

77. Crook MA, et al. The importance of the refeeding syndrome. *Nutrition.* 2001;17:632.

78. Hearing SD. Refeeding syndrome. *BMJ.* 2004;328(7445):908.

79. Academy of Nutrition and Dietetics. Nutrition Care Manual website. Nutrition Care > Weight Management > Overweight & obesity > Nutrition Intervention. http://nutritioncaremanual.org. Accessed April 24, 2012.

80. National Cholesterol Education Program (NCEP) Expert Panel on Detection, Evaluation, and Treatment of High Blood Cholesterol in Adults (Adult Treatment Panel III). Third Report of the NCEP Expert Panel on Detection, Evaluation, and Treatment of High Blood Cholesterol in Adults (ATP III) final report. *Circulation.* 2002;106:3143.

81. Lipsy RJ. The National Cholesterol Education Program Adult Treatment Panel III guidelines. *J Managed Care Pharm.* 2003;9(1 suppl):2.

82. Brewer HB. New features of the National Cholesterol Education Program Adult Treatment Panel III lipid-lowering guidelines. *Clin Cardiol.* 2003;26:19.

83. Grundy SM, et al. Diagnosis and management of the metabolic syndrome: an American Heart Association/National Heart, Lung, and Blood Institute scientific statement. *Circulation.* 2005;112:2735.

84. Ginsberg HN. Treatment for patients with the metabolic syndrome. *Am J Cardiol.* 2003;91(7):29.

85. Ebbing M, et al. Mortality and cardiovascular events in patients treated with homocysteine-lowering B vitamins after coronary angiography. *JAMA.* 2008;300:795.

86. Chobanian AV, et al. Seventh report of the Joint National Committee on Prevention, Detection, Evaluation, and Treatment of High Blood Pressure. *Hypertension.* 2003;42(6):1206.

87. Sacks FM, et al. Effects of blood pressure of reduced dietary sodium and the dietary approaches to stop hypertension (DASH) diet. *N Engl J Med.* 2001;344(1):3.

88. Academy of Nutrition and Dietetics. Nutrition Care Manual website. Nutrition Care > Cardiovascular Disease > Heart Failure > Nutrition Prescription. http://nutritioncaremanual.org. Accessed April 24, 2012.

89. Barber MD. The pathophysiology and treatment of cancer cachexia. *Nutr Clin Pract.* 2002;17:203.

90. Gerasimos S, et al. Leptin levels in cachectic heart failure patients. *Int J Cardiol.* 2000;76:117.

91. Cochrane WU, Afolabi OA. Investigation into the nutritional status, dietary intake and smoking habits of patients with chronic obstructive pulmonary disease. *J Hum Nutr Diet.* 2004;17(1):3.

92. Driscoll DF. Intravenous lipid emulsions: 2001. *Nutr Clin Pract.* 2001;16:215.

93. Dickerson RN, et al. Adverse effects from inappropriate medication administration via a jejunostomy feeding tube. *Nutr Clin Pract.* 2003;18:402.

94. Donaldson J, et al. Nutrition strategies in neurotrauma. *Crit Care Nurs Clin North Am.* 2000;12(4):465.

95. Taylor SJ, et al. Prospective, randomized, controlled trial to determine the effect of early enhanced enteral nutrition on clinical outcome in mechanically ventilated patients suffering head injury. *Crit Care Med.* 1999;27(11):2525.

96. Cox SA, et al. Energy expenditure after spinal cord injury: an evaluation of stable rehabilitating patients. *J Trauma.* 1985;25:419.

97. Aquilani R, et al. Energy expenditure and nutritional adequacy of rehabilitation paraplegics with asymptomatic bacteriuria and pressure sores. *Spinal Cord.* 2001;39:437.

98. Kapadi FN, et al. Special issues in the patient with renal failure. *Crit Care Clin.* 2003;19:233.

99. Charney P, Charney D. Nutrition support in renal failure. *Nutr Clin Pract.* 2002;17:226-236.

100. Case KO, et al. Nutrition support in the critically ill patient. *Crit Care Nurs Q.* 2000;22(4):75-89.

101. Scheinkestel CD, et al. Prospective randomized trial to assess caloric and protein needs of critically ill, anuric, ventilated patients requiring continuous renal replacement therapy. *Nutrition.* 2003;19:909.

102. Brown RO, Compher C, and the American Society for Parenteral and Enteral Nutrition (ASPEN) Board of Directors. A.S.P.E.N. Clinical guideline: nutrition support in adult acute and chronic renal failure. *J Parenter Enteral Nutr.* 2010;34(4):366.

103. Wiggins KL, Harvey KS. A review of guidelines for nutrition care of renal patients. *J Renal Nutr.* 2002;12(3):190.

104. Patton KM, Aranda-Michel J. Nutritional aspects in liver disease and liver transplantation. *Nutr Clin Pract.* 2002;17:332.

105. Florez DA, Aranda-Michel J. Nutritional management of acute and chronic liver disease. *Semin Gastrointest Dis.* 2002;13(3):169.

106. Khokhar AS, Seidner DL. The pathophysiology of pancreatitis. *Nutr Clin Pract.* 2004;19:5.

107. Academy of Nutrition and Dietetics. Nutrition Care Manual website. Nutrition Care > Gastrointestinal Disease > Liver, Gallbladder, and Pancreas Disease > Pancreatitis > Nutrition Intervention. http://nutritioncaremanual.org. Accessed April 27, 2012.

108. Avgerinos C, et al. Nutritional support in acute pancreatitis. *Dig Dis.* 2003;21(3):214.

109. Russell MK. Acute pancreatitis: a review of pathophysiology and nutrition management. *Nutr Clin Pract.* 2004;19:16.

110. Al-Omran M, et al. Enteral versus parenteral nutrition for acute pancreatitis. *Cochrane Database Syst Rev.* 2003;1:CD002837.

111. Dejong CH, et al. Nutrition in patients with acute pancreatitis. *Curr Opin Crit Care.* 2001;7(4):251.

112. Abou-Assi S, O'Keefe SJ. Nutrition support during acute pancreatitis. *Nutrition.* 2002;18:938.

113. Woolf SH, et al. Controlling blood glucose levels in patients with type 2 diabetes mellitus: an evidence-based policy statement by the American Academy of Family Physicians and American Diabetes Association. *J Fam Pract.* 2000;49(5):453.

114. Van den Berghe, G, et al. Intensive insulin therapy in critically ill patients. *N Engl J Med.* 2001;345:1359.

115. Rassias AJ, et al. Insulin increases neutrophil count and phagocytic capacity after cardiac surgery. *Anesth Analg.* 2002;94:1113.

116. Umpierrez GE, et al. Hyperglycemia: an independent marker of in-hospital mortality in patients with undiagnosed diabetes. *J Clin Endocrinol Metab.* 2002;87:978.

117. McMahon MM. Management of parenteral nutrition in acutely ill patients with hyperglycemia. *Nutr Clin Pract.* 2004;19:120.

118. Charney P, Hertzler SR. Management of blood glucose and diabetes in the critically ill patient receiving enteral feeding. *Nutr Clin Pract.* 2004;19:129.

119. Jones MP. Management of diabetic gastroparesis. *Nutr Clin Pract.* 2004;19:145.

120. Paul E. New interventions in diabetes with medical nutrition therapy. *Case Manager.* 2002;13(2):78.

121. American Diabetes Association. Nutrition recommendations and interventions for diabetes [position statement]. *Diabetes Care.* 2008;31(suppl 1):S61.

122. Clement S, et al. Management of diabetes and hyperglycemia in hospitals. *Diabetes Care.* 2004;27:553.

Pain and Pain Management

Céline Gélinas, Caroline Arbour

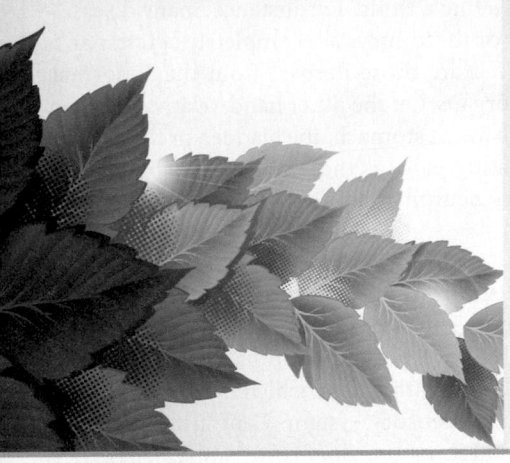

evolve WEBSITE

http://evolve.elsevier.com/Urden/criticalcare/

Evolve features:

- NCLEX Review Questions
- CCRN Review Questions
- PCCN Review Questions
- Mosby's Nursing Skills Procedures
- Animations
- Video Clips
- Glossary

Despite national and international efforts, guidelines, standards of practice, position statements, and many important discoveries in the field of pain management in the past three decades, critically ill patients suffer from moderate to severe pain that can be experienced at rest or during routine care.[1,2] For instance, chest tube removal, turning, drain removal, and wound care were identified as the most painful procedures by critically ill adults in previous studies.[2-4] Despite this situation, pain remains undertreated in most critically ill patients.[5] Poor treatment of acute pain may lead to the development of serious complications[6,7] and chronic pain syndromes,[8-10] which may seriously impact the patient's functioning, quality of life, and well-being. Such evidence reinforces the importance of providing attention to pain in this specific context of care.

IMPORTANCE OF PAIN ASSESSMENT

Appropriate pain assessment is the foundation of effective pain treatment. Because pain is recognized as a subjective experience, the patient's self-report is considered the most valid measure for pain and should be obtained as often as possible.[11] Unfortunately in critical care, many factors such as the administration of sedative agents, the use of mechanical ventilation, and altered levels of consciousness may impact communication with patients.[12,13] These obstacles make pain assessment more complex. Nevertheless, except for being unable to speak, many mechanically ventilated patients can communicate that they are in pain by using head nodding, hand motions or by seeking attention with other movements.[4] In such a situation, use of appropriate communication methods may reduce patients'

distress associated with the presence of the endotracheal tube by enabling them to report the presence of pain or discomfort in a comprehensive way.[14]

Self-report pain intensity scales have been used with postoperative mechanically ventilated patients who were asked to point on the scale.[2,15] However, in a study of mechanically ventilated adults with various diagnoses (trauma, surgical, or medical), only one third of mechanically ventilated patients were able to use a pain intensity scale.[15] With a greater degree of critical illness, providing a pain intensity self-report becomes more difficult because it requires concentration and energy. When the patient is unable to communicate in any way, observable behavioral indicators become unique indices for pain assessment and are part of clinical guidelines and recommendations developed in North America.[16,17] Pain is frequently encountered in critical care, and there is increased emphasis on the professional responsibility to manage the patient's pain effectively. The critical care nurse must understand the mechanisms, assessment process, and appropriate therapeutic measures for managing pain.

This chapter provides nurses with a better understanding of the physiology of pain. It also demonstrates indicators that can be used for pain assessment and several methods for pain management in critically ill patients.

DEFINITION AND DESCRIPTION OF PAIN

Pain is described as an unpleasant sensory and emotional experience associated with actual or potential tissue damage or described in terms of such damage.[18] This definition emphasizes the subjective and multidimensional nature of pain. More specifically, the subjective characteristic implies that pain is whatever the person experiencing it says it is and that it exists whenever he or she says it does.[19] This definition also suggests that the patient is able to self-report. However, in the critical care context, many patients are unable to self-report their pain. Some authors[20] have proposed an alternative definition for nonverbal patients, in this case infants, but the same principle applies to any non-verbal population, stating that changes in behaviors caused by pain are valuable forms of self-report and should be considered as alternative measures of pain. Based upon this, pain assessment must be designed to conform to the communication capabilities of the patient.

Components of Pain

The experience of pain includes sensory, affective, cognitive, behavioral, and physiologic components[21]:

The sensory component is the perception of many characteristics of pain, such as intensity, location, and quality.

The affective component includes negative emotions such as unpleasantness, anxiety, fear, and anticipation that may be associated with the experience of pain.

The cognitive component refers to the interpretation or the meaning of pain by the person who is experiencing it.

The behavioral component includes the strategies used by the person to express, avoid, or control pain.

The physiologic component refers to nociception and the stress response.

Types of Pain

Pain can be acute or chronic, with different sensations related to the origin of the pain.

Acute Pain

Acute pain has a short duration, and it usually corresponds to the healing process (30 days), but should not exceed 6 months. It implies tissue damage that is usually from an identifiable cause. If undertreated, acute pain may bring a prolonged stress response and lead to permanent damage to the patient's nervous system. In such instance, acute pain can become chronic.[8,9]

Chronic Pain

Chronic pain persists for more than 6 months after the healing process from the original injury, and it may or may not be associated with an illness.[22] It develops when the healing process is incomplete or, as described earlier, when acute pain is poorly managed.[23]

Both acute and chronic pain can have a nociceptive or neuropathic origin.[11]

Nociceptive Pain

Nociceptive pain arises from activation of nociceptors,[11] and it can be somatic or visceral. Somatic pain involves superficial tissues, such as the skin, muscles, joints, and bones. Its location is well defined. Visceral pain involves organs such as the heart, stomach, and liver. Its location is diffuse, and it can be referred to a different location in the body.[24] Interestingly, not all organs

are sensitive to pain and some can be damaged quite extensively without the patient feeling a thing. For instance, many diseases of the liver, the lungs or the kidneys are completely painless and the only symptoms felt are those derived from the abnormal functioning of these organs. On the other hand, relatively minor lesions in viscera such as the stomach, the bladder, or the ureters can produce excruciating pain, as these organs are abundantly innervated by sensory neurons that signal harmful events.[25]

Neuropathic Pain

Neuropathic pain arises from a lesion or disease affecting the somatosensory system.[11] The origin of neuropathic pain may be peripheral or central. Neuralgia and neuropathy are examples related to peripheral neuropathic pain, which implies a damage of the peripheral somatosensory system. Central neuropathic pain involves the central somatosensory cortex and can be experienced by patients after a cerebral stroke. Neuropathic pain can be difficult to manage and frequently requires a multimodal approach (i.e., the combinations of several pharmacologic and/or nonpharmacologic treatments).[24]

Physiology of Pain
Nociception

Nociception represents the neural processes of encoding and processing noxious stimuli necessary, but not sufficient, for pain.[11] Pain results from the integration of the pain-related signal into specific cortical areas of the brain associated with higher mental processes and consciousness. In other words, pain is the conscious experience that emerges from nociception.[26] Four processes are involved in nociception[24]:

1. Transduction
2. Transmission
3. Perception
4. Modulation

The four processes are shown in Figure 9-1, which integrates pain assessment with nociception, and in Figure 9-2.

Transduction

Transduction refers to mechanical (e.g., surgical incision), thermal (e.g., burn), or chemical (e.g., toxic substance) stimuli that damage tissues. In critical care, many nociceptive stimuli exist, including the patients' acute illness or condition, invasive technology used for patients, and multiple interventions that have to be done for them. These stimuli, also called stressors, stimulate the liberation of many chemical substances, such as prostaglandins, bradykinin, serotonin, histamine, glutamate, and substance P. These neurotransmitters stimulate peripheral nociceptive receptors and initiate nociceptive transmission.

Transmission

As a result of transduction, an action potential is produced and is transmitted by nociceptive nerve fibers in the spinal cord that reach higher centers of the brain. This is called transmission, and it represents the second process of nociception. The principal nociceptive fibers are the A-delta (Aδ) and C fibers. Large-diameter, myelinated Aδ fibers that transmit well-localized, sharp pain are involved in "first pain" sensation, which leads to

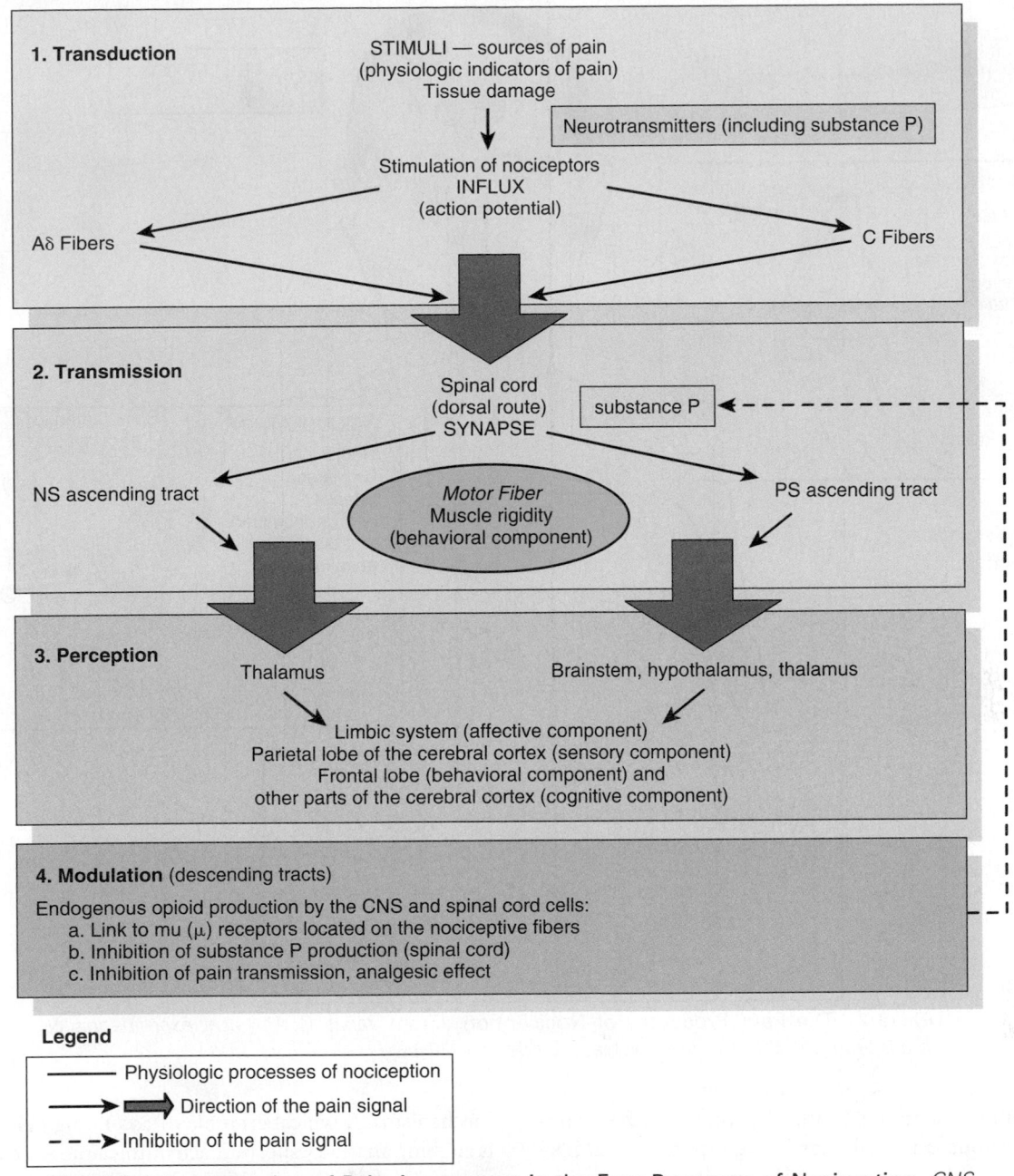

FIGURE 9-1 Integration of Pain Assessment in the Four Processes of Nociception. *CNS,* central nervous system; *NS,* neospinothalamic pathway; *PS,* paleospinothalamic pathway. (Courtesy Céline Gélinas, Ingram School of Nursing, McGill University, Canada.)

reflex withdrawal. Small-diameter, unmyelinated C fibers transmit diffuse, dull, aching pain, which is referred to as "second pain."[26] These fibers transmit the noxious sensation from the periphery through the dorsal root of the spinal cord. With the liberation of substance P, these fibers then synapse with ascending spinothalamic fibers to the central nervous system (CNS). These spinothalamic fibers are clustered into two specific pathways: neospinothalamic (NS) and paleospinothalamic (PS) pathways. Generally, the Aδ fibers transmit the pain sensation to the brain within the NS pathway, and the C fibers use the PS pathway.[27]

Through synapsing of nociceptive fibers with motor fibers in the spinal cord, muscle rigidity can appear because of a

reflex activity.[28] Muscle rigidity can be a behavioral indicator associated with pain. It can contribute to immobility and decrease diaphragmatic excursion. This can lead to hypoventilation and hypoxemia. Hypoxemia can be detected by a pulse oximeter (Spo_2) and by oxygen arterial pressure (Pao_2) monitoring. A ventilated patient's interaction with the machine (e.g., activation of alarms, fighting the ventilator) also may indicate the presence of pain.[29]

Perception

The pain message is transmitted by the spinothalamic pathways to centers in the brain, where it is perceived. Pain sensation transmitted by the NS pathway reaches the thalamus, and

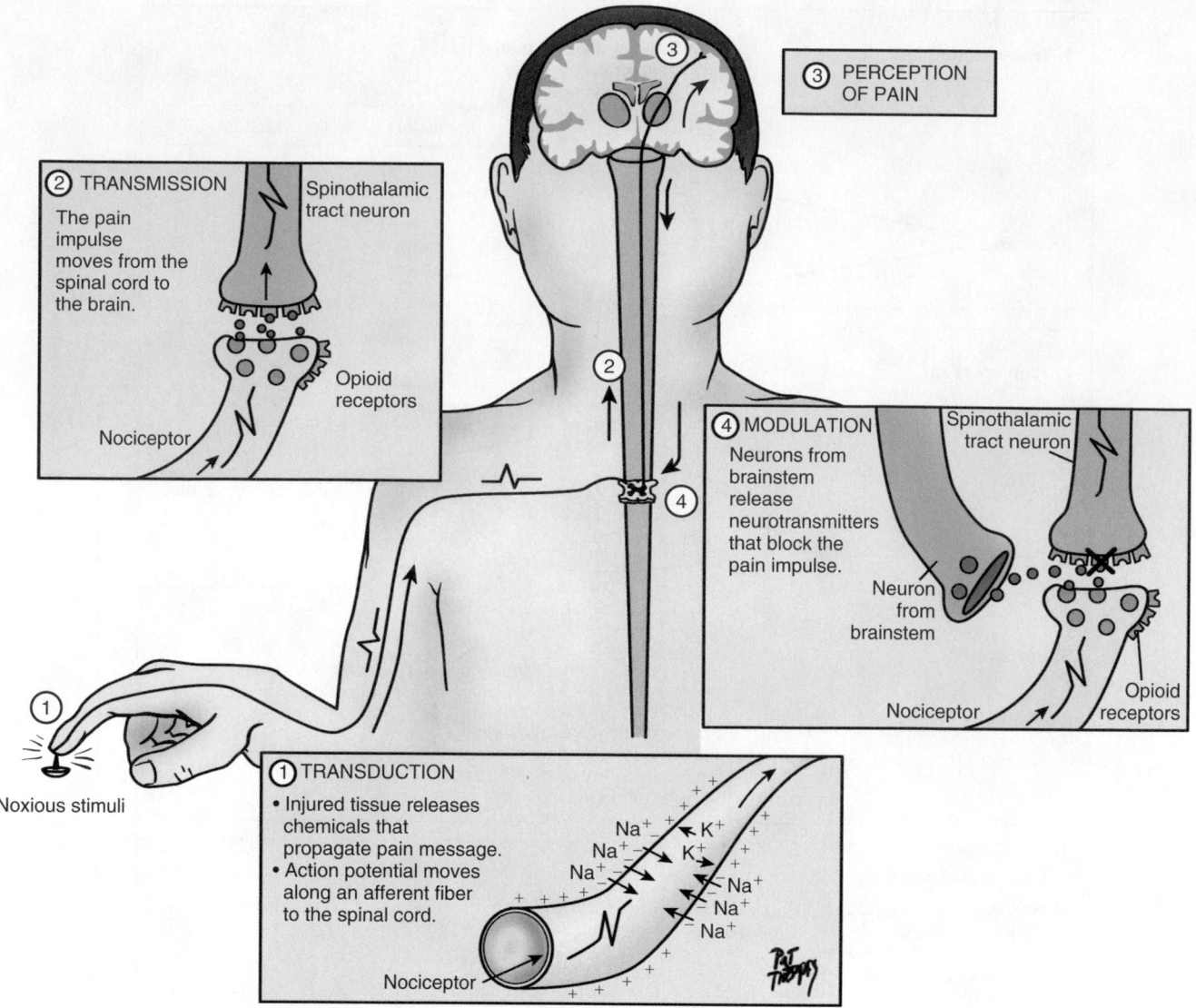

FIGURE 9-2   **The Four Processes of Nociception.** (From Jarvis C. *Physical examination & health assessment.* 6th ed. Philadelphia, Saunders; 2011.)

the pain sensation transmitted by the PS pathway reaches brainstem, hypothalamus, and thalamus.[27] These parts of the CNS contribute to the initial perception of pain. Projections to the limbic system and the frontal cortex allow expression of the affective component of pain.[30] Projections to the sensory cortex located in the parietal lobe allow the patient to describe the sensory characteristics of his or her pain, such as location, intensity, and quality.[30,31] The cognitive component of pain involves many parts of the cerebral cortex and is complex. These three components (affective, sensory, and cognitive) represent the subjective interpretation of pain. Parallel to this subjective process, certain facial expressions and body movements are behavioral indicators of pain occurring as a result of pain fiber projections to the motor cortex in the frontal lobe.

Modulation

Modulation is a process by which noxious stimuli that travel from the nociceptive receptors to the CNS may be enhanced or inhibited. Pain can be modulated by ascending and descending

mechanisms. A typical example of ascending pain modulation is rubbing an injury site, thus activating large A-beta (Aβ) fibers in the periphery. Stimulation of these fibers activates inhibitory interneurons in the dorsal horn of the spinal cord, effectively preventing nociceptive signal transmission from the periphery to the higher brain regions. The physiologic basis of this mechanism of pain modulation was elucidated by Melzack and Wall in 1965[32] and refers to the Gate Control Theory (GCT). Analgesia may also be produced at the level of the spinal cord and the brainstem (spinothalamic pathway) via the release of endogenous opioids and neurotransmitters. Endogenous opioids are naturally occurring morphine-like pentapeptides found throughout the nervous system and exist in three general classes: beta-endorphins, enkephalins, and dynorphins. These substances block neuronal activity related to nociceptive impulses by binding to opioid mu (μ) receptor sites in the central and peripheral nervous systems.[27] In the ascending pain modulation mechanism, endogenous opioids may be produced in the brainstem, and the dorsal horn or exogenous opioids may be introduced by administration of an opioid analgesic. The released or introduced opioids bind to the mu-opioid receptors on nociceptive nerve fibers, blocking the release of substance P. In the descending pain modulation mechanism, the efferent spinothalamic nerve fibers that descend from the brain can inhibit the propagation of the pain signal by triggering the release of endogenous opioids in the brain stem and in the spinal cord. Serotonin and norepinephrine are important inhibitory neurotransmitters that act in the CNS. These substances are also released by the descending fibers of the descending spinothalamic pathway.[33] The use of distraction, relaxation and imagery techniques can facilitate the release of endogenous opioids, and has been shown to reduce the overall pain experience.[34]

In summary, nociception is an important physiologic mechanism of pain that can integrate many components of pain for its assessment. In transduction, stimuli are sources of pain that trigger the liberation of neurotransmitters. In transmission, diffusion of the action potential along the NS pathway may lead to muscle rigidity—a reflex activity that can be observed as a behavioral indicator associated with pain. Muscle rigidity may also influence respiratory rate and amplitude, and cause decrease in Spo_2 and increase in Pao_2. In perception, the patient's self-report of affective, sensory, and cognitive information can be obtained, and behavioral responses to pain may also be observed. Finally, in modulation, pain sensation may be attenuated by ascending and descending mechanisms.

Biologic Stress Response

A biologic stress response is activated by pain, an obvious stressor.[29] This stress response involves the nervous, endocrine, and immune systems in the hypothalamic-pituitary-adrenal axis (HPA).[35] The biologic stress response includes a short-term direct response, a midterm response, and a long-term indirect response. Stress mechanisms are depicted in Figure 9-3.

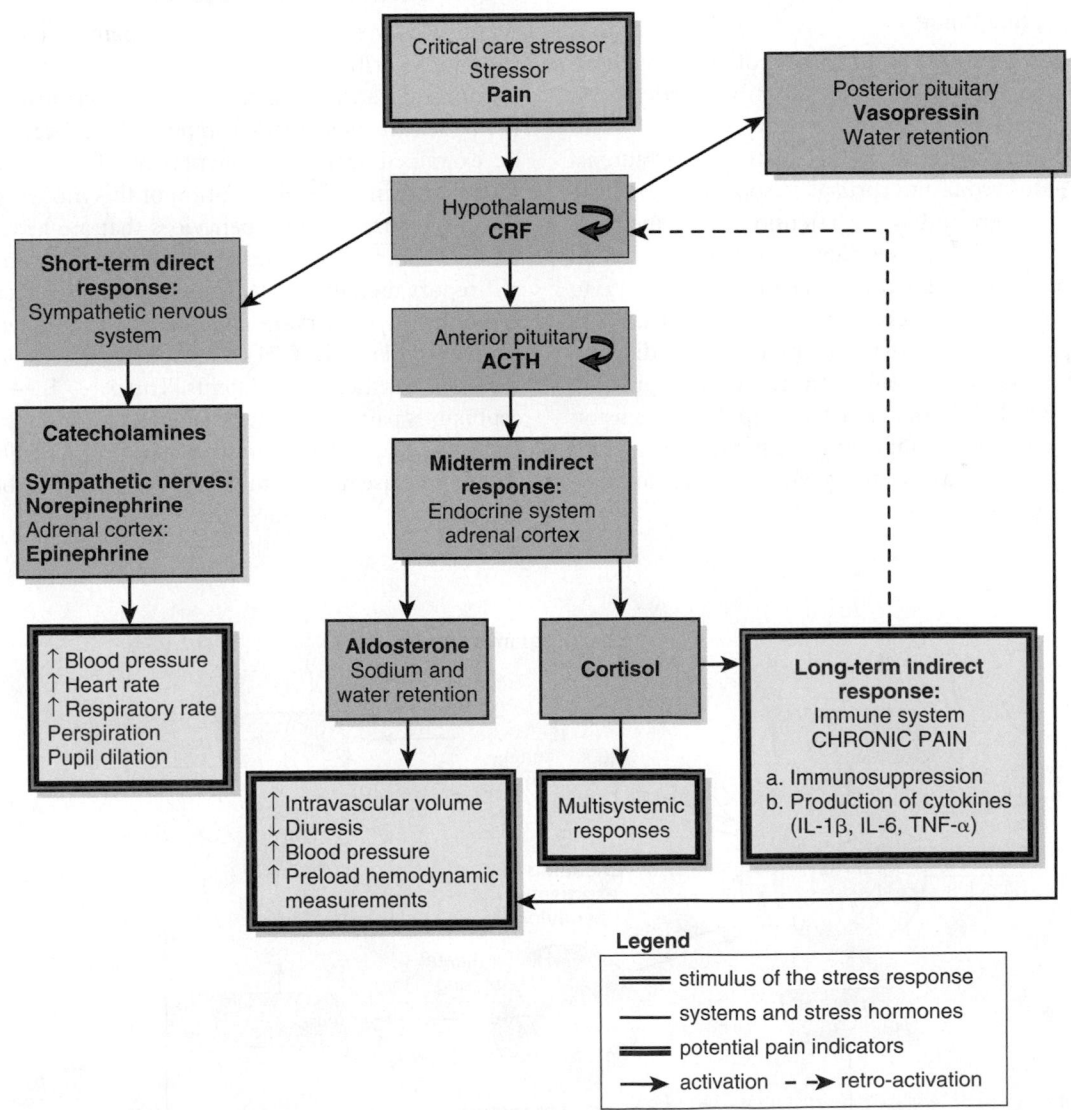

FIGURE 9-3 Integration of Potential Physiologic Pain Indicators in the Biologic Stress Response. *ACTH*, adrenocorticotropic hormone; *CRF*, corticotropin-releasing factor; *IL*, interleukin; *TNS*, tumor necrosis factor. (Courtesy Céline Gélinas, Ingram School of Nursing, McGill University, Canada.)

Short-Term Direct Response

In the presence of a stressor such as pain, the hypothalamus releases corticotropin-releasing factor (CRF), which activates the sympathetic nervous system (SNS). Norepinephrine is then released from the terminals of sympathetic nerves, and epinephrine is released from the adrenal cortex. This mechanism constitutes the short-term direct stress response. The effects of these stress hormones allow observation of physiologic responses associated with activation of SNS. For instance, increased blood pressure, increased heart rate, and increased respiratory rate are common signs of acute pain.[15,29,36] Moreover, pupil dilation can be observed.[37]

If pain persists over time or injuries are located in the bladder or the intestines, the parasympathetic nervous system (PNS) may be dominant. The blood pressure and heart rate may decrease rather than increase. The absence of pain-related indicators related to the activation of the SNS does not necessarily imply an absence of pain sensation.[38]

Midterm Indirect Response

At midterm, the CRF released from the hypothalamus stimulates the anterior pituitary to release adrenocorticotropic hormone (ACTH) and the posterior pituitary to release vasopressin, the antidiuretic hormone. ACTH activates the adrenal cortex to release aldosterone and cortisol. Vasopressin and aldosterone increase sodium and water retention. This increases intravascular volume and decreases diuresis and increases blood pressure and cardiac preload. Cortisol also may contribute to systemic responses such as infection and hyperglycemia.

At midterm, pain may be associated with decreased diuresis, increased blood pressure, increased central venous pressure (CVP), and increased pulmonary artery capillary occlusion pressure (PAOP). However, changes in these parameters are not specific to pain, and their associations with pain are not supported by empirical data.

Long-Term Indirect Response

Long term, the stress hormones, specifically cortisol, influence the immune system in two ways: immunosuppression and release of cytokines.[39] Cytokines may prolong by retroactivation the release of cortisol, which may exacerbate tissue damage, contributing to the chronic pain process.[23]

In summary, the biologic stress response allows observation of fluctuations in physiologic signs that represent a source of stress and may be associated with acute pain. The short-term signs are mainly related to SNS activation. Other signs, such as decreased diuresis and increased CVP and PAOP, relate to the midterm indirect stress response. The immune system is involved in the long-term indirect response of stress. No acute pain indicators have been associated with this process. All the indicators identified within the biologic stress response are not specific to pain because they can be attributed to other distress conditions, homeostatic changes, and medications.[16]

Framework for Pain Assessment and Definition

As previously stated, self-report of pain is not always possible to obtain in critically ill patients as many of them may be unable to communicate during their stay in the critical care unit. When the patient is unable to self-report, the expression of pain can be examined from the perspective of the Communications Model of Pain.[40] The foundation of this model is that observational measures capture behaviors that are less subject to voluntary control and more automatic in comparison with self-report measures that depend on higher mental processes. Consequently, observational measures should be used to assess pain when the individual's self-report is not available, as is often the case in critically ill patients. This A → B → C model conceptualizes pain as an internal state (A) that may be encoded in particular features of expressive behaviors (B), allowing observers (in this case nurses) to draw inferences (C) about the nature of the sender's experience (Fig. 9-4).

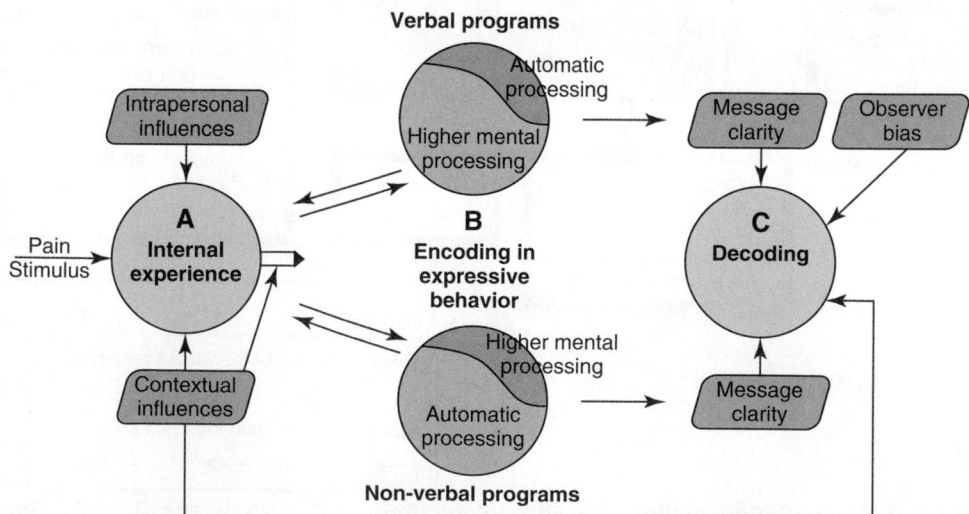

FIGURE 9-4   The Communications Model of Pain. (Redrawn from Hadjistavropoulos T, Craig KD. A theoretical framework for understanding self-report and observational measures of pain: a communications model. *Behav Res Ther.* 2002;40:551.)

More specifically, when an individual is exposed to a nociceptive stimulus known to be painful, information about real or potential tissue damage is transmitted and processed centrally into the brain. The processing of a nociceptive stimulus can be modulated by intrapersonal and/or contextual factors influencing the way information is integrated and consequently how pain is experienced in each individual. In critical care, intrapersonal factors that could potentially influence the processing of a nociceptive stimulus include the patient's sociodemographic characteristics, severity of critical illness/injury, level of sedation, and level of consciousness. Similarly, examples of contextual factors specific to the critical care unit environment that could influence the patient's pain experience include mechanical ventilation and administration of sedatives and opioids. Taking into account the various intrapersonal and contextual factors, critically ill patients may express their pain through different patterns of verbal and nonverbal expressive modalities. The depicted pattern will depend largely on the degree of impairment in the cortical areas of the brain associated with consciousness. Indeed, while some patients with a mild alteration of the level of consciousness may still have the capacity to self-report and/or express their pain with voluntary behaviors (e.g., localization of the pain site), others with a severe alteration of the level of consciousness might respond to pain only through autonomic reactions such as reflex or fluctuations in physiologic signs. Whether patients are able to express their pain through self-report, voluntary behaviors and/or autonomic reactions will undoubtedly affect the message clarity and the capacity of nurses to identify the specific nature of patients' pain. Because behaviors are difficult to decode, educational training of nurses is necessary to support them in developing the competence of adequately assessing pain behaviors using observational measures.

PAIN ASSESSMENT

Pain assessment is an integral part of nursing care. It is a prerequisite for adequate pain control and relief. As stated earlier, pain is a subjective, multidimensional concept that requires complex assessment. Many factors may alter verbal communication in critically ill patients, making pain assessment more difficult. This situation should not discourage nurses from assessing pain in these vulnerable patients because acute pain is a stressor that can exacerbate their conditions.

Pain assessment has two major components: 1) nonobservable or subjective and 2) observable or objective. The complexity of pain assessment requires the use of multiple strategies by critical care nurses. In the following sections, patient, health professional, and organizational barriers to pain assessment and management are addressed, and recommendations are proposed.

Pain Assessment: The Subjective Component

Pain is known as a subjective experience. The subjective component of pain assessment refers to the patient's self-report about his or her sensorial, affective, and cognitive experience of pain. Because it is considered the most valid measure of pain,

the patient's self-report must be obtained whenever possible.[16] A simple yes or no (presence versus absence of pain) is a valid self-report. Mechanical ventilation should not be a barrier for nurses to document patients' self-reports of pain. Many mechanically ventilated patients can communicate that they have pain or can use pain scales by pointing to numbers or symbols on the scale.[2,4,15] Attempts should be made before concluding that a patient is unable to self-report. More importantly, sufficient time should be allowed for the patient to respond with each attempt.[16]

If sedation and cognition levels allow the patient to give more information about pain, a multidimensional assessment can be documented. Multidimensional pain assessment tools including the sensorial, emotional, and cognitive components are available, such as the Brief Pain Inventory,[41] the Initial Pain Assessment Tool,[24] and the McGill Pain Questionnaire–Short Form.[42] However, because of the administration of sedative and analgesic agents in mechanically ventilated patients, the tool must be short enough to be completed. For instance, the McGill Pain Questionnaire–Short Form takes 2 to 3 minutes to complete and has been used to assess mechanically ventilated patients who were in a stable condition.[2]

The patient's self-report of pain can also be obtained by questioning the patient using the mnemonic PQRSTU[43]:

P: provocative and palliative or aggravating factors
Q: quality
R: region or location, radiation
S: severity and other symptoms
T: timing
U: understanding

P: Provocative and Palliative or Aggravating Factors

The P in the mnemonic indicates what provokes or causes the patient's pain, what he or she was doing when the pain appeared, and what makes the pain worse or better. For instance, deep breathing intensifying chest pain in the case of pericarditis is an illustration of an aggravating factor. Moderating factors that reduce/alleviate the pain or discomfort are also important findings and may include resting to diminish burning chest pain due to angina. Knowledge of any intensifying or alleviating conditions can contribute to the patient's plan of care throughout the continuum of care.

Q: Quality

The Q in the mnemonic refers to the quality of the pain or the pain sensation that the patient is experiencing. For instance, the patient may describe the pain as dull, aching, sharp, burning, or stabbing. This information provides the nurse with data regarding the type of pain the patient is experiencing (e.g., somatic or visceral). The differentiation between types of pain may contribute to the determination of cause and management. A patient who has had open-heart surgery may complain of chest pain that is shooting or burning.[4] This information can lead the nurse to investigate for cutaneous or bone injuries as a result of a sternotomy. Another patient may describe a sharp thoracic pain that may lead the nurse to consider visceral pain as a result of pulmonary embolism. A verbal description of pain

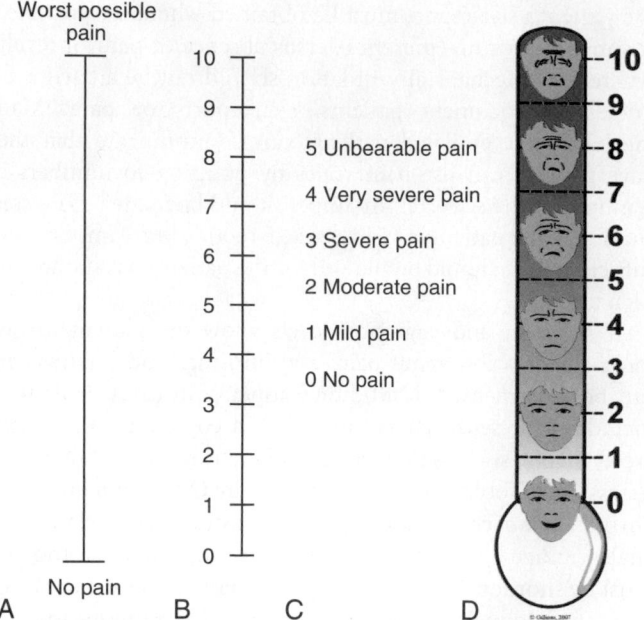

FIGURE 9-5 Pain Intensity Scales (Vertical Format). *A*, Visual analog scale (VAS). *B*, Numeric Rating Scale (NRS). *C*, Descriptive Rating Scale (DRS). *D*, Faces Pain Thermometer. (Courtesy Céline Gélinas, Ingram School of Nursing, McGill University, Canada.)

is important because it provides a baseline account, allowing the critical care nurse to monitor changes in the type of pain, which may indicate a change in the underlying pathology.

R: Region or Location, Radiation

R usually is easy for the patient to identify, although visceral pain is more difficult for the patient to localize.[24] If the patient has difficulty naming the location or is mechanically ventilated, ask the patient to point to the location on himself or herself or on a simple anatomic drawing.[44]

S: Severity and Other Symptoms

S, the severity or intensity of pain, is a measurement that has undergone much investigation. Many pain intensity scales are available, including the descriptive and numeric pain rating scales that are often used in the critical care environment (Fig. 9-5). Many critical care units use a specific pain intensity scale. The use of a single tool provides consistency of assessment and documentation. Employment of a pain intensity scale is useful in the critical care environment. Asking the patient to grade his or her pain on a scale of 0 to 10 is a consistent method and aids the nurse in objectifying the subjective nature of the patient's pain. However, the patient's tool preference should be considered.

The S in the mnemonic also refers to other symptoms accompanying the patient's pain experience, such as shortness of breath, nausea, and fatigue. Anxiety and fear are common emotions associated with pain.

T: Timing

The T in the mnemonic refers to documenting the onset, duration, and frequency of pain. This information can help to determine whether the origin of the pain is acute or chronic. Duration of pain can indicate the severity of the problem. For instance, chest pain of less than 15 minutes' duration may be angina, and pain lasting more than 15 minutes may indicate a myocardial infarction.

U: Understanding

The U in the mnemonic is the patient's perception of the problem or cognitive experience of pain. Patients with known cardiac problems can tell the nurse whether their pain is the same as they had during myocardial infarction. Patients with a cerebral hemorrhage often describe experiencing the worst headache they have ever had.

Because of the patient's change in communication, lack of concentration due to sedation therapies, and the life-or-death immediacy of most actions in the critical care environment, pain assessment is often reduced to minimal information. Begin by asking, "Do you have pain?" The use of a simple yes or no question allows the patient to answer verbally or to indicate his or her response by nodding the head or by other signs. It is easier for mechanically ventilated patients to communicate with nurses in this way because they cannot express themselves verbally. Pain intensity and location also are necessary for the initial assessment of pain.

Pain Assessment: The Observable or Objective Component

When the patient's self-report is impossible to obtain, nurses can rely on the observation of behavioral indicators, which are strongly emphasized in clinical recommendations and guidelines for pain management in nonverbal patients.[16,17] Fluctuations in vital signs should never be used alone but rather considered as a cue to begin further assessment for pain.

Pain-related behaviors have been described in critically ill patients and were also studied in the AACN Thunder Project II.[45] Patients who experienced pain during nociceptive procedures were three times more likely to have increased behavioral responses such as facial expressions, muscle rigidity, and vocalization than patients without pain. Similar observations were found in a study of 257 mechanically ventilated critically ill adults.[30] Patients who experienced pain during turning showed significantly more intense facial expressions (e.g., grimacing), muscle rigidity, and less compliance with the ventilator (e.g., fighting the ventilator) compared with patients without pain. Behavioral indicators are strongly recommended for pain assessment in nonverbal patients,[16] and several tools have been developed and tested in critically ill adults including the Behavioral Pain Scale (BPS),[46] the Critical-Care Pain Observation Tool (CPOT),[47] the NonVerbal Pain Scale (NVPS),[48] the Pain Behavioral Assessment Tool (PBAT),[46] and the Pain Assessment and Intervention Notation (PAIN) algorithm.[39] The BPS and the CPOT are supported by experts in critical care[49,50] and are suggested for use in medical, postoperative, and non-brain trauma critically ill adults unable to self-report in the clinical guidelines of the Society of Critical Care Medicine (SCCM).[17] Moreover, their implementation in critical care units has led to enhanced nursing practices of pain assessment and management,[51] and improved patient outcomes including

TABLE 9-1	BEHAVIORAL PAIN SCALE (BPS)	
ITEM	DESCRIPTION	SCORE
Facial expression	Relaxed	1
	Partially tightened (e.g., brow lowering)	2
	Fully tightened (e.g., eyelid closing)	3
	Grimacing	4
Upper limbs	No movement	1
	Partially bent	2
	Fully bent with finger flexion	3
	Permanently retracted	4
Compliance with ventilation	Tolerating movement	1
	Coughing but tolerating ventilation for most of the time	2
	Fighting ventilator	3
	Unable to control ventilation	4
Total		3 to 12

From Payen JF, et al. Assessing pain in the critically ill sedated patients by using a behavioral pain scale. *Crit Care Med.* 2001;29(12):2258.

shorter durations of mechanical ventilation and stay in the critical care unit.[52]

Behavioral Pain Scale

The BPS shown in Table 9-1 was tested mostly in nonverbal mechanically ventilated patients with altered levels of consciousness.[46,53-56] Its validity was supported with significantly higher BPS scores during nociceptive procedures (e.g., turning, endotracheal suctioning, peripheral venous cannulation) compared with rest or nonnociceptive procedures (e.g., arterial catheter dressing change, compression stocking applications, eye care). The authors of the BPS determined a cut-off score greater than 5 for the presence of pain. A positive association was found between nurses' BPS ratings and conscious sedated patients' self-report of pain intensity during turning.[54] Good interrater reliability of BPS scores between several raters including nurses was reached. The BPS can be used quickly (2 to 5 minutes), and most clinicians were satisfied with its ease of use.[46] However, some expressed concerns about the lack of conceptual clarity of certain items.[49] For instance, scores of 3 (i.e., fighting ventilator) and 4 (i.e., unable to control ventilation) for compliance with the ventilator category may be ambiguous. Similarly, movements with upper limbs category may be confused with muscle tension.

Critical-Care Pain Observation Tool

The CPOT shown in Table 9-2 was tested in verbal and nonverbal, critically ill adult patients.[15,29,47,57] Content validity was supported by critical care unit expert clinicians, including nurses and physicians.[58] Validity of the CPOT was supported with significantly higher CPOT scores during a nociceptive procedure (e.g., turning with or without other care) compared with rest or a nonnociceptive procedure (e.g., taking blood pressure). Positive associations were found between the CPOT scores and the patient's self-report of pain.[15,29,47] A cut-off score greater than 2 was established with the CPOT in postoperative critical

care unit adults.[59] Similarly to the BPS, good interrater reliability of CPOT scores was achieved with critical care nurses.[15,47] Feasibility and clinical utility of the CPOT were positively evaluated by critical care nurses.[60] Nurses agreed that the CPOT was quick enough to be used in the critical care unit, simple to understand, easy to complete, and helpful for nursing practice. An online teaching video to learn how to use the CPOT at the bedside is available (see Table 9-2).

Use of Cut-Off Scores

A cut-off score refers to the score on a specific scale associated with the best probability of correctly ruling in or ruling out a patient with a specific condition—in this case pain. The use of a cut-off score with behavioral pain scales can help to identify when pain is highly likely to be present, and guide nurses in determining whether an intervention to alleviate pain is required or not. Also, a cut-off score can help to evaluate the effectiveness of pain-management interventions. It is important to highlight that cut-off scores are established using a criterion (i.e., a gold standard in the field). As mentioned previously, in the case of pain, the patient's self-report is known as the gold standard criterion.[11] For a case example showing how a cut-off score can be used in practice, refer to Box 9-1.

Limitations Related to the Use of Behavioral Pain Scales

Behaviors have been validated for pain assessment in critically ill patients, but they present some limitations. In fact, they are impossible to monitor in patients unable to respond behaviorally to pain such as those suffering from paralysis or under the effects of neuromuscular blocking agents. Also, behavioral responses may be blurred with the administration of high doses of sedative agents.[15] Indeed, minimal behavioral responses to painful procedures were found in unconscious, mechanically ventilated critically ill adults who were more heavily sedated compared with conscious patients.[29] Similar results were found in previous studies in which patients who received a higher dose of midazolam obtained a lower score on the BPS.[56]

In addition, behavioral pain scales developed for nonverbal critically ill patients may not be applicable for those with a brain injury and an altered level of consciousness as they were found to exhibit atypical behavioral responses to pain.[29,61,62] Instead of frowning and grimacing, brain-injured patients with altered levels of consciousness seemed to react mostly by opening their eyes, showing tears, opening their mouth, and exhibiting repetitive movements of the lower limbs when exposed to pain. Further studies are needed to better understand how brain-injured patients react to painful procedures. Therefore existing behavioral pain scales may be inappropriate for this specific vulnerable group. When selecting a scale, nurses should make sure that is has been tested in a patient population and context in which they plan to use it. Indeed, a scale can only be shown to be valid with a specific group of people and in a given context.[63]

Physiologic Indicators

When patients cannot react behaviorally to pain, the only possible clues left for the detection of pain are physiologic

TABLE 9-2 CRITICAL CARE PAIN OBSERVATION TOOL (CPOT)

INDICATOR	SCORE		DESCRIPTION
Facial expression	Relaxed, neutral	0	No muscle tension observed
	Tense	1	Presence of frowning, brow lowering, orbit tightening and levator contraction or any other change (e.g., opening eyes or tearing during nociceptive procedures)
	Grimacing	2	All previous facial movements plus eyelid tightly closed (the patient may present with mouth open or biting the endotracheal tube)

Relaxed, neutral — 0   Tense — 1   Grimace — 2

INDICATOR	SCORE		DESCRIPTION
Body movements	Absence of movements or normal position	0	Does not move at all (doesn't necessarily mean absence of pain) or normal position (movements not aimed toward the pain site or not made for the purpose of protection)
	Protection	1	Slow, cautious movements, touching or rubbing the pain site, seeking attention through movements
	Restlessness/ Agitation	2	Pulling tube, attempting to sit up, moving limbs/thrashing, not following commands, striking at staff, trying to climb out of bed
Compliance with the ventilator (intubated patients)	Tolerating ventilator or movement	0	Alarms not activated, easy ventilation
	Coughing but tolerating	1	Coughing, alarms may be activated but stop spontaneously
or	Fighting ventilator	2	Asynchrony: blocking ventilation, alarms frequently activated
Vocalization (nonintubated patients)	Talking in normal tone or no sound	0	Talking in normal tone or no sound
	Sighing, moaning	1	Sighing, moaning
	Crying out, sobbing	2	Crying out, sobbing
Muscle tension	Relaxed	0	No resistance to passive movements
	Tense, rigid	1	Resistance to passive movements
	Very tense or rigid	2	Strong resistance to passive movements, incapacity to complete them
TOTAL		___ / 8	

1. The patient must be observed at rest for one minute to obtain a baseline value of the CPOT.
    1.1 Observation of patient at rest (baseline).
The nurse looks at the patient's face and body to note any visible reactions for an observation period of one minute. She gives a score for all items except for muscle tension. At the end of the 1-minute period, the nurse holds the patient's arm in both hands—one at the elbow, and uses the other one to hold the patient's hand. Then, she performs a passive flexion and extension of the upper limb and feels any resistance the patient may exhibit. If the movements are performed easily, the patient is found to be relaxed with no resistance (score 0). If the movements can still be performed but with more strength, then it is concluded that the patient is showing resistance to movements (score 1). If the nurse cannot complete the movements, strong resistance is felt (score 2). This can be observed in patients who are spastic.
2. Then the patient should be observed during painful procedures (e.g., turning, wound care) to detect any changes in the patient's behaviors.
    2.2 Observation of patient during a painful procedure.
While she's performing a procedure known to be painful, the nurse looks at the patient's face to note any reactions such as frowning or grimacing. These reactions may be brief or can last longer. The nurse also looks out for body movements. For instance, she looks for protective movements like the patient trying to reach or touching the pain site (e.g., surgical incision, injury site). In the mechanically ventilated patient, she pays attention to alarms and if they stop spontaneously or require that she intervenes (e.g., reassurance, administering medication). It is important that the nurse auscultates the patient to check for the position of the endotracheal tube and the presence of secretions as these factors may influence this item without being indicative of pain. According to muscle tension, the nurse can feel if the patient is resisting to the movement or not. A score 2 is given when the patient is resisting against the movement and attempts to get on his/her back.
3. The patient should be evaluated before and at the peak effect of an analgesic agent to assess whether the treatment was effective or not in relieving pain.
4. The patient should be attributed the highest score observed during the observation period.
5. The patient should be attributed a score for each behavior included in the CPOT and muscle tension should be evaluated last as it may lead to behavioral reactions not necessarily related to pain, but more to the actual stimulation. According to compliance with the ventilator, the nurse must check that the endotracheal tube is well positioned, and for the presence of secretions which could lead to higher scores for this item.

Modified from Gélinas C, et al. Validation of the Critical-Care Pain Observation Tool (CPOT) in adult patients. *Am J Crit Care*. 2006;15:420. Figure of facial expressions a courtesy of Caroline Arbour, RN, BSc, PhD candidate, McGill University, Canada, and redrawn by Elsevier.
An online teaching video funded and created by Kaiser Permanente Northern California Nursing Research (KPNCNR) to learn how to use the CPOT at the bedside is available at *http://pointers.audiovideoweb.com/stcasx/il83win10115/CPOT2011-WMV.wmv/play.asx*.

indicators (i.e., vital signs). Although vital sign values generally increase during painful procedures,[15,29,36,46,56] they are not consistently related to the patient's self-report of pain, nor are they predictive of pain.[15,29] For example, none of the monitored vital signs (heart rate, mean arterial pressure [MAP], respiratory rate, transcutaneous oxygen saturation [Spo_2], and end-tidal CO_2) predicted the presence of pain in critically ill patients.[29]

In the ASPMN recommendations and the SCCM guidelines, it is stated that vital signs should not be considered as primary indicators of pain because they can be attributed to other distress conditions, homeostatic changes, and medications. Changes in vital signs should instead be considered a cue to begin further assessment of pain or other stressors.[16,17] Physiologic measures other than vital signs can support the nurses in detecting the presence of pain in nonverbal critically ill patients especially when behavioral indicators are no longer available.

Cerebral Monitoring and Pain Assessment

Other than vital signs, human brain reactivity has been studied using brain imaging technology such as positron emission tomography (PET) and functional magnetic resonance imaging (fMRI) in healthy individuals and in patients with clinical pain conditions.[64] Many regions of the brain are involved in the perception of pain, including the somatosensory cortex, the frontal cortex, and the thalamus. The anatomic connections between these regions suggest that they function in an interactive way in encoding the different aspects of pain (sensory and affective components of pain). For instance, the somatosensory cortex plays a major role in processing the sensory component of pain, whereas the frontal cortex appears to reflect the affective component of pain.[26] A closer look into brain activity may elucidate how pain inputs are first received and processed within the cerebral cortex, offering a direct and more precise indicator of pain.

Electroencephalogram

Continuous electroencephalographic (cEEG) activity is being used more frequently in critical care units, especially in the brain-injured population, to detect epileptic activity and ischemia.[65] So far, few studies have examined the EEG reactivity of patients when exposed to pain. Frontal EEG activation was observed in 34 critically ill infants when exposed to a noxious stimulation (i.e. heelstroke).[66] In a recent study with 32 cardiac surgery patients in a critical care unit, EEG activation was observed over the somatosensory cortex during chest tube removal only in patients who did not receive preprocedural analgesics (i.e., morphine). Interestingly, self-reported pain intensity of patients who did not receive morphine was higher than those who were administered morphine prior to chest tube removal.[67]

Bispectral Index

Another innovative technology, the Bispectral Index (BIS), is being explored for its relevance in the pain assessment process of critically ill, sedated patients.[37,68] The primary utility of the BIS is as an objective measure of sedation levels during surgery in the operating room or during neuromuscular blocking in the critical care unit. This noninvasive monitor uses electrodes placed on the forehead, and displays a signal-processed electroencephalogram (EEG) with a digital number from 0 (flat EEG activity) to 100 (fully awake) that relates to the depth of sedation. An electromyographic (EMG) sensor that reflects muscle stimulation of the forehead is included to identify EMG artifact.

A study of 48 mechanically ventilated and sedated critically ill patients after cardiac surgery reported that the BIS value significantly increased when patients were exposed to a noxious stimulation (turning or endotracheal suctioning) instead of a nonnoxious procedure (gentle touch). However, the most commonly reported pain-related behaviors (e.g., facial expressions, body movements, tense posture, ventilator asynchrony) were not induced by the noxious stimulation in deeply sedated patients, highlighting the limitation of behaviors for pain assessment in heavily sedated critically ill patients. In a more recent study with nine sedated and mechanically ventilated critically ill patients,[68] the median BIS value increased from 20% to 30% between rest and the painful procedures (turning and endotracheal suctioning). As opposed to the previous study, behavioral responses were exhibited by the patients with an increase in the median CPOT score from 0 to 3 during the procedures.

The new bilateral BIS is an alternative option to the conventional BIS monitoring system. The bilateral BIS allows the recording of EEG and EMG information of both hemispheres separately (i.e., BIS-Left and BIS-Right). As a result, the bilateral BIS could be particularly useful for pain assessment in patients with suppression of unilateral brain function, such as those with a cerebral stroke or a traumatic brain injury (TBI). For instance, in a recent pilot study with 12 critically ill TBI with altered level of consciousness,[69] increases in BIS-Left (>6.6%) and BIS-Right (>7.2%) were observed in patients when exposed to turning compared with rest or a nonpainful procedure. Interestingly, the BIS increase was more pronounced on the noninjured side of the brain. Based on available study findings, the BIS may be an interesting technique to further study in critical care pain assessment because of its noninvasive nature and its suitability for use at the bedside.

Pain as a Vital Sign

Because pain is considered as another vital sign, including pain assessment with other routinely documented vital signs may help ensure that pain is assessed and controlled for in all patients on a regular basis. This approach can ensure that pain is detected and treatment implemented before the patient develops complications associated with unrelieved pain. The use of a pain flow sheet in critical care settings allows for a visible and ongoing pain assessment before and after an intervention for pain that is accessible to all clinicians involved in the assessment and management of pain.[51,70]

Patient Barriers to Pain Assessment and Management
Communication

The most obvious patient barrier to the assessment of pain in the critical care population is an alteration in the ability to communicate. The patient who is mechanically ventilated cannot verbalize a description of the pain. If the patient can communicate in any way, such as by head nodding or pointing, he or she may report the pain in that manner. If writing is possible, the patient may be able to thoroughly describe the pain. With patients unable to self-report, the nurse relies on behavioral indicators to assess the presence of pain.

The patient's family can contribute significantly in the assessment of pain. The family is intimately familiar with the patient's normal responses to pain and can assist the nurse in identifying clues. A family member's impression of a patient's pain should be considered in the pain assessment process of the critically ill patient.[16]

Altered Level of Consciousness and Unconsciousness

The patient either unconscious or with an altered level of consciousness presents a dilemma for all clinicians. Because pain relies on cortical response to provide recognition, the belief that the patient with a brain injury altering higher cortical function has no perception of pain may persist. Conversely, the inability to interpret the nociceptive transmission does not negate the transmission. Interviews by Lawrence[71] with 100 patients, who recalled their experiences from a time when they were unconscious in critical care, revealed that they could hear, understand, and respond emotionally to what was being said. Experts recommend assuming that patients who are unconscious or with an altered level of consciousness have pain and that they be treated the same way as conscious patients are treated when they are exposed to sources of pain.[16] It has been demonstrated that behavioral and physiologic indicators of pain can be observed in reaction to a painful procedure in critically ill patients, no matter what their level of consciousness.[29] Moreover, it has been shown that some cortical activation related to pain perception is still present in unconscious patients in a neurovegetative state.[72] Knowing this, the critical care nurse can initiate a discussion with the other members of the health care team to formulate a plan of care for the patient's comfort.

Older Adult Patients

Many older adult patients do not complain much about pain. Some misconceptions, such as believing that pain is a normal consequence of aging or being afraid to disturb the health care team, are barriers to pain expression for older adults.[24] Cognitive deficits or delirium present additional pain assessment barriers. Many older adult patients with mild to moderate cognitive impairments and even some with severe impairment are able to use pain intensity scales.[73,74] Vertical pain intensity scales are more easily understood by this group of patients and are recommended[16] (see Fig. 9-5). Older adult patients with cognitive deficits should receive repeated instructions and be given sufficient time to respond. When the self-report of pain is impossible to obtain, direct observation of pain-related behaviors is highly recommended in this population.[16,74] More than 24 behavioral tools have been developed for older adult patients with cognitive deficits.[75] The Pain Assessment Checklist for Seniors with Limited Ability to Communicate (PACSLAC),[76] Doloplus-2,[77] and the Pain Assessment in Advanced Dementia (PAINAD)[78] are promising tools that are recommended by experts.[75,79]

Delirium is a form of transient cognitive impairment that is highly prevalent among older adult patients in the critical care unit.[80] A major challenge with delirium is that there is overlap between delirium behaviors and pain-related behaviors. It remains unclear whether pain behavioral tools may assist the nurse in the detection of pain in older adult patients during episodes of delirium. Because pain is a modifiable factor of delirium, it can be controlled with adequate pain management.[81]

Neonates and Infants

Two-way verbal communication is impossible with critically ill infants, and this remains an important barrier to pain assessment. The misconception that preterm neonates were incapable of pain sensation has persisted for a long time. Evidence supports that term and preterm neonates have the anatomic and functional capacity for pain sensation at birth.[82] One critical review examined more than 35 instruments used to assess pain in neonates and infants.[83] The Premature Infant Pain Profile (PIPP)[84] is the most recommended valid tool for pain assessment of infants, and it has been implemented in many clinical settings. The PIPP includes behavioral and physiologic indicators. The emphasis in pain assessment should be on behavioral indicators. Physiologic indicators should be interpreted with caution because they are also affected by disease, medications, and physiologic status.[16]

Cultural Influences. Another barrier to accurate pain assessment is cultural influences on pain and pain reporting.[85] Cultural influences are compounded when the patient speaks a language other than that of the health team members. To facilitate communication, the use of a pain intensity scale in the patient's language is vital. The 0 to 10 numeric pain scales have been translated into many different languages.[24]

Although this chapter does not address specific cultural groups and their typical responses to pain, a few generalizations can be made. First, when assessing a patient from a cultural group different from your own, do not assume the patient will have a specific response to pain or exhibit a particular behavior because of his or her culture. Patients have individual responses to pain. The health care practitioner may wrongfully assign or expect behaviors that a patient will not exhibit. A second consideration that is commonly overlooked is the role of pain in the life of the patient. The nurse must communicate with the patient or the family to ascertain what that role is.

Some cultures believe that God's test or punishment takes the form of pain. Persons with these cultural backgrounds do not necessarily believe that the pain should be relieved. Other cultures perceive pain as being associated with an imbalance in life. Persons from these cultures believe they need to manipulate the environment to restore balance to control pain.[85]

The complexities and intricacies of cultural beliefs require more extensive discussion than is possible here. It is important for the nurse to support, whenever possible, the special beliefs and needs of the patient and his family to provide the most therapeutic environment for healing to occur.

Lack of Knowledge

A relatively overlooked patient barrier to accurate pain assessment is the public knowledge deficit regarding pain and pain management. Many patients and their families are frightened by the risk of addiction to pain medication. They fear that addiction will occur if the patient is medicated frequently or with sufficient amounts of opioids necessary to relieve the pain. This concern is so powerful for some that they will deny or deliberately underreport the frequency or intensity of pain. Another misconception held by some patients is the expectation that unrelieved pain is simply part of a critical illness or procedure.[86] Many patients have no memory of receiving an explanation of their pain-management plan.[87] With that in mind, it is important that the critical care nurse teach the family and the patient about the importance of pain control and the use of opioids in treating pain in the critically ill.

Health Professional Barriers to Pain Assessment and Management

The health professional's beliefs and attitudes about pain and pain management are frequently a barrier to accurate and adequate pain assessment. This can lead to poor management practices. Misconceptions or lack of knowledge regarding addiction, physiologic dependence, drug tolerance, and respiratory depression remain. Addiction rates for patients in acute pain who receive opioid analgesics are less than 1%. Some of the false beliefs that surround addiction result from a lack of knowledge about addiction and tolerance, and other concerns are related to the possible side effects of opioids.

Addiction and Tolerance

Addiction is defined by a pattern of compulsive drug use that is characterized by an incessant longing for an opioid and the need to use it for effects other than pain relief.

Tolerance is defined as a diminution of opioid effects over time. Physical dependence and tolerance to opioids may develop if the medication is given over a long period. Physical dependence is manifested by withdrawal symptoms when the opioid is abruptly stopped. If this is an anticipated problem, withdrawal may be avoided by weaning the patient from the opioid slowly to allow the brain to reestablish neurochemical balance in the absence of the opioid.[24]

Respiratory Depression

Another concern of the health care professional is the fear that aggressive management of pain with opioids will cause critical respiratory depression. Opioids can cause respiratory depression, but in the critically ill, this is a rare phenomenon. The incidence of respiratory depression is less than 2%.[88,89] Respiratory depression from the administration of opioids can be managed with diligent assessment practices, which are discussed later.

Organizational Barriers to Pain Assessment and Management

The organizational system influences pain and pain-management practices as well as associated outcomes. Failure to make pain management a priority is the initial barrier. Failure to adopt standard pain assessment tools or to provide staff with sufficient time to assess and document pain, and a lack of accountability for pain-management practices are observed in some organizations. Evidence has demonstrated the lack of documentation of pain assessment and the undertreatment of pain in critical care settings.[5,90,91] The lack of collaboration between physicians and nurses is identified as a barrier to effective pain management.[92]

Because unrelieved pain is harmful to patients and increases the cost of care, it must be a priority for the health organization. Every organization must analyze their pain-management issues and practices and provide education about pain and pain management to staff. Now that pain is considered as the fifth vital sign, pain assessment must be included in documentation systems as a standard. Pain has to be assessed in all critically ill patients, regardless of their clinical condition or their level of consciousness. The implementation of pain assessment tools is essential so that the health care team can establish a common language of communication. This can facilitate interprofessional collaboration. There is an increased commitment to clinical practice guidelines and standards for pain assessment and management by organizations such as The Joint Commission (http://www.jointcommission.org), which have considerable influence in health care institutions. In addition, strategies to enhance collaboration among health professionals may include interdisciplinary care rounds or case reviews.[92] Patients have the right to be consulted about their pain care plan and should be involved in making decisions. The organization must continually evaluate outcomes and work to improve the quality of pain management.

PAIN MANAGEMENT

The management of pain in the critically ill patient is as multidimensional as the assessment. It is a multidisciplinary task. The control of pain can be pharmacologic, nonpharmacologic,

BOX 9-2   SUMMARY OF PAIN AND ANALGESIA GUIDELINES

1. ICU patients routinely experience pain at rest and with ICU care. Pain in cardiac surgery patients, especially women, is poorly treated. Procedural pain is common in ICU patients.

2. Perform routine pain assessment in all patients. In motor intact patients unable to self report, we suggest using behavioral pain scales rather than vital signs to assess pain. The BPS and CPOT are the most valid and reliable behavioral pain scales. Vital signs should only be used as a cue for further pain assessment.

3. For non-neuropathic pain, use intravenous opioids as first line analgesic therapy; use non-opioid analgesics to reduce opioid side effects; and use either gabapentin or carbamazepine in conjunction with intravenous opioids for neuropathic pain.

4. Suggest preemptively treating procedural pain, especially chest tube removal.

5. Use thoracic epidural analgesia for abdominal aortic surgery, and suggest also using for traumatic rib fractures. No evidence guides the use of lumbar epidural analgesia for abdominal aneurysm surgery, or thoracic epidural analgesia for either intrathoracic or nonvascular abdominal surgical procedures. No evidence guides the use of regional vs. systemic analgesia in medical ICU patients.

From Barr J, Fraser G, Puntillo K, et al. Clinical practice guidelines for the management of pain, agitation, and delirium in adult ICU patients. *Critical Care Medicine.* In press.

or a combination of the two therapies. Pharmacologic pain management is predominantly used in critical care.

Pharmacologic Control of Pain

Pharmacologic management of pain has infinite variety in the critical care unit. Although this chapter is not an in-depth discussion of pharmacology, some commonly administered agents are discussed. Pain pharmacology is divided into three categories of action: opioid agonists, nonopioids, and adjuvants. Elements of the pain and analgesia clinical guidelines[17] of the Society of Critical Care Medicine (SCCM) for the treatment of pain in the critically ill adult are presented in Box 9-2. A care bundle for pain assessment and management in the critical care unit was created to facilitate the translation of the SCCM practice guidelines to the bedside and is shown in Figure 9-6. How pain is approached and managed is a progression or combination of the available agents, the type of pain, and the patient response to the therapy. Figure 9-7 illustrates the analgesic action sites in relation to nociception.

Opioid Analgesics

The opioids most commonly used and recommended as first-line analgesics are the agonists. These opioids bind to mu (μ) receptors (transmission process; see Fig. 9-7), which appear to be responsible for pain relief. Additional pharmacologic information is presented in Table 9-3. In the SCCM guidelines, opioids should be used as first line therapy for treatment of non-neuropathic pain.[17]

Morphine. Morphine is the most commonly prescribed opioid in the critical care unit. Because of its water solubility, morphine has a slower onset of action and a longer duration compared with the lipid-soluble opioids (e.g., fentanyl).

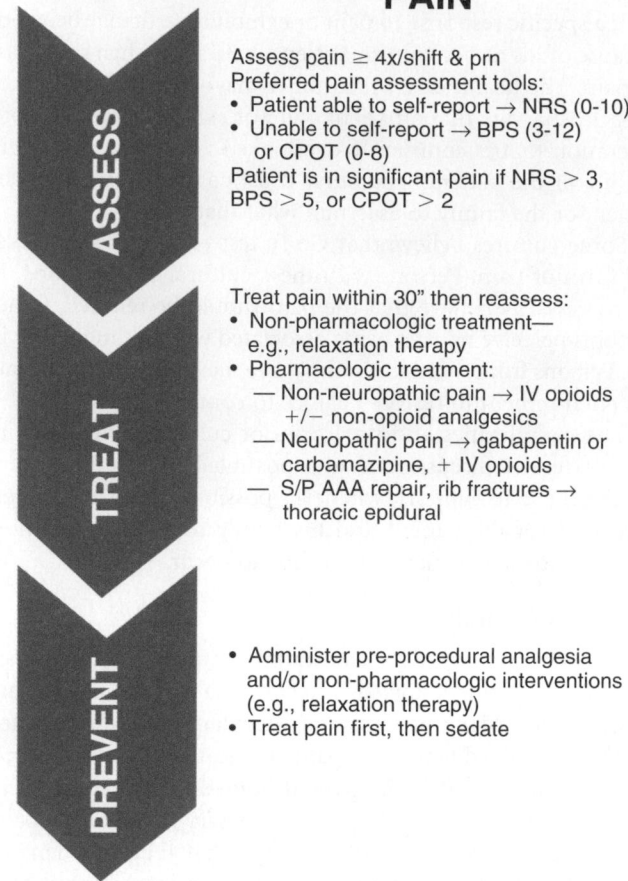

PAIN

ASSESS

Assess pain ≥ 4x/shift & prn
Preferred pain assessment tools:
- Patient able to self-report → NRS (0-10)
- Unable to self-report → BPS (3-12) or CPOT (0-8)
Patient is in significant pain if NRS > 3, BPS > 5, or CPOT > 2

TREAT

Treat pain within 30" then reassess:
- Non-pharmacologic treatment— e.g., relaxation therapy
- Pharmacologic treatment:
  — Non-neuropathic pain → IV opioids +/− non-opioid analgesics
  — Neuropathic pain → gabapentin or carbamazipine, + IV opioids
  — S/P AAA repair, rib fractures → thoracic epidural

PREVENT

- Administer pre-procedural analgesia and/or non-pharmacologic interventions (e.g., relaxation therapy)
- Treat pain first, then sedate

FIGURE 9-6 Pain Care Bundle. *BPS,* Behavioral Pain Scale; *CPOT,* Critical-Care Pain Observation Tool; *NRS,* Numeric Rating Scale; *S/P AAA,* status post abdominal aortic aneurysm.

Morphine has two main metabolites: morphine-3-glucuronide (M3G, inactive) and morphine-6-glucuronide (M6G, active). M6G is responsible for the analgesic effect but may accumulate and cause excessive sedation in patients with renal failure or hepatic dysfunction.[93] Morphine is available in a variety of delivery methods. It is the standard by which all other opioids are measured. It is also the agent that most closely mimics the endogenous opioids in the human pain modification system.

Morphine is indicated for severe pain. It has additional actions that are helpful for managing other symptoms. Morphine dilates peripheral veins and arteries, making it useful in reducing myocardial workload. Morphine is also viewed as an antianxiety agent because of the calming effect it produces.

Many side effects have been reported with the use of morphine (see Table 9-3). The hypotensive effect can be particularly problematic in the hypovolemic patient. The vasodilation effect is potentiated in the volume-depleted patient, and the hemodynamic status must be carefully monitored. Volume resuscitation restores blood pressure in the event of a prolonged hypotensive response.

A more serious side effect requiring diligent monitoring is the respiratory depressant effect. Opioids may cause this complication because they reduce the responsiveness of carbon dioxide chemoreceptors in the respiratory center located in the

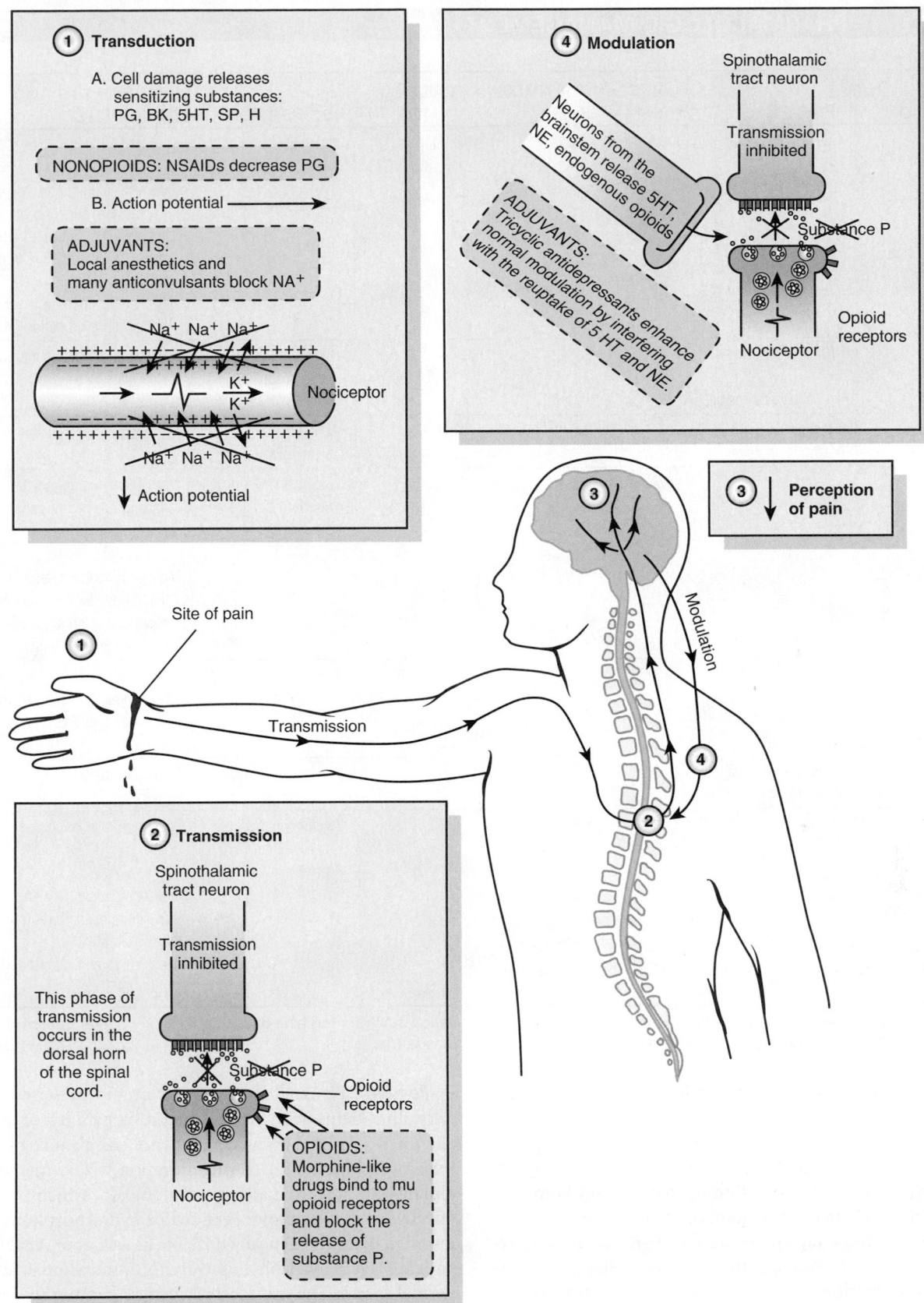

FIGURE 9-7 **Nociception and Analgesic Action Sites.** *BK*, Bradykinin; *H*, histamine; *PG*, prostaglandins; *SP*, substance P; *5HT*, serotonin. (From McCaffery M, Pasero C. *Pain: Clinical Manual for Nursing Practice*. 2nd ed. St. Louis: Mosby; 1999.)

TABLE 9-3 PHARMACOLOGIC MANAGEMENT

Pain

MEDICATION	DOSAGE	ONSET (min)	DURATION (hr)	AVAILABLE ROUTES	PROPERTIES	SIDE EFFECTS AND COMMENTS
Morphine	1-4 mg IV bolus 1-10 mg IV infusion	5-10	3-4	PO, SL, R, IV, IM, SC, EA, IA	Analgesia, antianxiety	Standard for comparison Side effects: sedation, respiratory depression, euphoria or dysphoria, hypotension, nausea, vomiting, pruritus, constipation, urinary retention M6G can accumulate in renal failure or hepatic dysfunction patients.
Fentanyl	25-100 mcg IV bolus 25-200 mcg IV infusion	1-5	0.5-4	OTFC, IV, IM, TD, EA, IA	Analgesia, antianxiety	Same side effects as morphine Rigidity with high doses
Hydromorphone (Dilaudid)	0.2-1 mg IV bolus 0.2-2 mg IV infusion	5	3-4	PO, R, IV, IM, SC, EA, IA	Analgesia, antianxiety	Same side effects as morphine
Codeine	15-30 mg IM, SC	10-20	3-4	PO, IM, SC	Analgesia (mild to moderate pain)	Lacks potency (unpredictable absorption; not all patients convert it to an active form to achieve analgesia) Most common side effects: light-headedness, dizziness, shortness of breath, sedation, nausea, and vomiting
Methadone (Dolophine)	5-10 mg IV	10	4-8	PO, SL, R, IV, SC, IM, EA, IA	Analgesia	Usually less sedating than morphine, but repeated doses can result in accumulation and can cause serious sedation (2-5 days).
Acetaminophen	650 mg maximum of 4 g/day	20-30	4-6	PO, R	Analgesia, antipyretic	Rare side effects Hepatotoxicity
Ketorolac (Toradol)	15-30 mg IV	<10	6-8	PO, IM, IV	Analgesia, minimum antiinflammatory effect	Short-term use (<5 days) Side effects: gastric ulceration, bleeding, exacerbation of renal insufficiency Use with care in older adult and renal failure patients.

EA, Epidural analgesia; *IA*, intrathecal analgesia; *IM*, intramuscular; *IV*, intravenous; *M6G*, morphine-6-glucuronide; *OTFC*, oral transmucosal fentanyl citrate; *PO*, oral; *R*, rectal; *SC*, subcutaneous; *SL*, sublingual; *TD*, transdermal.

medulla.[94] Although infrequent, this effect can have significant sequelae for the critically ill patient. Many risk factors for opioid-induced respiratory depression have been identified.[24] From these, advanced age, obesity, sleep apnea, impaired renal/pulmonary/hepatic/cardiac functioning, patients in whom pain is controlled after a period of poor control, patients who are opiate naïve (i.e., receiving opiates for less than a week), concurrent use of central nervous system depressants, and postoperative day 1 were described.[89] The critical care nurse must monitor the patient intensively to prevent this complication. Monitoring of patients receiving opioid analgesics is discussed in more detail later in this chapter. In addition to side effects common to all opioids, morphine may stimulate histamine release from mast cells, resulting in cardiac instability and allergic reactions.

Fentanyl. Fentanyl is a synthetic opioid preferred for critically ill patients with hemodynamic instability or morphine allergy. It is a lipid-soluble agent that has a more rapid onset than morphine and a shorter duration.[95] The metabolites of fentanyl are largely inactive and nontoxic, which makes it an effective and safe opioid. Fentanyl or hydromorphone are preferred in hemodynamically unstable as well as in renal impaired patients.[95] It is available in intravenous, intraspinal, and transdermal forms. The transdermal form is commonly referred to as the *Duragesic patch* or the *72-hour patch.*

Because the side effects of fentanyl are similar to those of morphine, the nurse must monitor carefully the hemodynamic and respiratory response. When fentanyl is given by rapid administration and at higher doses, it has been associated with the additional hazard of bradycardia and rigidity in the chest wall muscles.[93,96] The use of transdermal fentanyl is indicated rarely in the critically ill patient. The customary use of the "fentanyl patch" is for those experiencing chronic pain or cancer pain, and in critical care, it is used for the patient who requires extended pain control. Transdermal delivery requires 12 to 16 hours for onset of action, and it has a duration of 72 hours.[24] If this delivery method is used, the patient will require other opioid management until the transdermal fentanyl takes effect.

Hydromorphone. Hydromorphone is a semisynthetic opioid that has an onset of action and a duration similar to those of morphine.[96] It is an effective opioid with multiple routes of delivery. It is more potent than morphine. Hydromorphone produces an inactive metabolite (i.e., hydromorphone-3-glucuronide), making it the opioid of choice for use in patients with end-stage renal disease.[99] Studies have shown that some side effects (e.g., pruritus, sedation, nausea, vomiting) may occur less with hydromorphone than morphine.[97]

Meperidine. Meperidine (Demerol) is a less potent opioid with agonist effects similar to those of morphine. It is considered the weakest of the opioids, and it must be administered in large doses to be equivalent in action to morphine. Because the duration of action is short, dosing is frequent. A major concern with this medication is the metabolite *normeperidine*, which is a CNS neurotoxic agent. At high doses in patients with kidney failure or liver dysfunction or in older adult patients, it may induce CNS toxicity, including irritability, muscle spasticity, tremors, agitation, and seizures.[24] Although meperidine is useful in short-term specific conditions (e.g., treating postoperative shivering[98]), it should not be used routinely for analgesia in the critical care unit.[95,99,100]

Codeine. Codeine has limited use in the management of severe pain. It is rarely used in the critical care unit. It provides analgesia for mild to moderate pain. It is usually compounded with a nonopioid (e.g., acetaminophen). To be active, codeine must be metabolized in the liver to morphine.[24] Codeine is available only through oral, intramuscular, and subcutaneous routes, and its absorption can be reduced in the critical care patient by altered gastrointestinal motility and decreased tissue perfusion.

Methadone. Methadone is a synthetic opioid with morphine-like properties but less sedation. It is longer acting than morphine and has a long half-life. This makes it difficult to titrate in the critical care patient. Methadone lacks active metabolites, and routes other than the kidney eliminate 60% of the medication. This means that methadone does not accumulate in patients with kidney failure. Methadone can be used to treat chronic pain syndromes when patients experience tolerance with other opioids and may help facilitate the down-titration of opioid infusions in the critical care unit.[99] However, prolongation of the QT interval, which can lead to torsades de pointes, has been reported with its use.[93]

More Potent Opioids: Remifentanil and Sufentanil. Remifentanil and sufentanil are agonist opioids. The use of these potent medications has been studied in critically ill patients.

Remifentanil is 250 times more potent than morphine, and it has a rapid onset and predictable offset of action. For this reason, it allows a rapid emergence from sedation, facilitating the evaluation of the neurologic state of the patient after stopping the infusion.[101,102] As opposed to fentanyl, the use of remifentanil was associated with a lower incidence of postoperative delirium.[103]

Sufentanil is 7 to 13 times more potent than fentanyl and 500 to 1000 times more potent than morphine. It has more pronounced sedation properties than fentanyl and other opioids. Patients under sufentanil require minimal sedative agent doses to achieve an adequate sedation level. It has a rapid distribution and a high clearance rate, preventing accumulation when given for a long period.[104] Sufentanil has a longer emergence from sedation compared with remifentanil, but it allows a longer analgesic effect after stopping its administration.[102]

Preventing and Treating Respiratory Depression

Respiratory depression is the most life-threatening opioid side effect. The risk of respiratory depression increases when other medications with CNS depressant effects (e.g., benzodiazepines, antiemetics, neuroleptics, antihistamines) are concomitantly administered to the patient. While no universal definition of respiratory depression exists, it is usually described in terms of decreased respiratory rate (fewer than 8 or 10 breaths/min), decreased SpO_2 levels, or elevated ETCO2 levels.[94] A change in the patient's level of consciousness or an increase in sedation normally precedes respiratory depression.

Monitoring. Recent guidelines on monitoring for patients receiving opioid analgesia of ASPMN were established.[94] In addition to assessing pain intensity as a targeted outcome of analgesia, regular sedation and respiratory assessments should be done. Valid and reliable sedation scales developed for use in critically ill patients should be used. Respirations should be evaluated over 1 minute and qualified according to rate, rhythm, and depth of chest excursion. The use of technology-supported monitoring (e.g., continuous pulse oximetry and capnography) can be useful in high-risk patients. More vigilant monitoring should be performed when patients may be at greater risk, such as during the first 24 hours after surgery, after an increase in the dose of an opioid, or a change in opioid agent or route of administration. For instance, Pasero et al have suggested monitoring these parameters at least every 2 hours for the first 24 hours and every 4 hours thereafter in stable patients.[105]

Snoring is a warning sign. It can be a sign of respiratory depression associated with airway obstruction by the tongue, leading to hypoxemia and possibly to cardiorespiratory arrest.[24] A patient snoring after the administration of an opioid requires the critical care nurse to observe closely.

Opioid Reversal. Critical respiratory depression can be readily reversed with the administration of the opiate antagonist *naloxone*.[24] The usual dose is 0.4 mg, which is mixed with 10 mL of normal saline (for a concentration of 0.04 mg/mL). Naloxone is normally given intravenously very slowly (0.5 mL over 2 minutes) while the patient is carefully monitored for reversal of the respiratory signs. Naloxone administration can be discontinued as soon as the patient is responsive to physical stimulation and able to take deep breaths. However, the medication should be kept nearby. Because the duration of naloxone is shorter than most opioids, another dose of naloxone may be needed as early as 30 minutes after the first dose. The nurse must monitor sedation and respiratory status and remind the patient to breathe deeply every 1 to 2 minutes until he or she becomes more alert. The benefits of reversing respiratory depression with naloxone must be carefully weighed against the risk of a sudden onset of pain and the difficulty achieving pain relief. To prevent this from occurring, it is important to provide a nonopioid medication for pain relief. Moreover, the use of naloxone is not recommended after prolonged analgesia, because it can induce withdrawal and may cause nausea and cardiovascular complications (e.g., dysrhythmias).

New Sedative with Analgesic Properties: Dexmedetomidine

Dexmedetomidine (Precedex) is a short-acting alpha 2 agonist that is indicated for the short-term sedation (<24 hours) of mechanically ventilated patients in the critical care unit.[106] Its mechanism of action is unique and differs from those of other commonly used sedatives in critical care. Indeed, compared to midazolam (Versed) or lorazepam (Ativan)—whose hypnotic effects act mainly on the limbic system and/or the cortex—the effect of dexmedetomidine is located in the locus ceruleus section of the brainstem. As a result, patients receiving dexmedetomidine IV infusions are calm and sleepy, yet they remain easily arousable.[107] For this reason, dexmedetomidine is ideal for mild to moderate sedation, often referred to as conscious sedation. Refer to the *Sedation and Delirium Management* chapter for details on dosage and administration.

Dexmedetomidine also possesses an analgesic property. The analgesic effects of dexmedetomidine are principally due to spinal antinociception via binding to non-noradrenergic receptors (heteroreceptors) located on the dorsal horn neurons of the spinal cord.[105] Recently, dexmedetomidine was found to decrease postoperative opioid requirements in both adults and children.[109,110] These results suggest that dexmedetomidine could be of interest with respect to improving postoperative pain in critical care.

While dexmedetomidine is increasing in popularity for short-term sedation in the critical care unit, it is not without adverse effect. Indeed, inhibition of noradrenergic receptors in the brainstem and the spinal cord often causes hypotension and bradycardia.[107] Less common adverse effects include decreased salivation, decreased secretion, and decreased bowel motility in the gastrointestinal tract; contraction of vascular and other smooth muscle; inhibition of renin release, increased glomerular filtration, and increased secretion of sodium and water in the kidney; decreased intraocular pressure; and decreased insulin release from the pancreas.[108]

Nonopioid Analgesics

In the SCCM guidelines, the use of nonopioids in combination with an opioid is recommended to reduce opioid requirements and opioid related side effects.[17] This strategy provides greater analgesic effect through action at the peripheral and central levels. Pharmacologic information is presented in Table 9-3.

Acetaminophen. Acetaminophen is an analgesic used to treat mild to moderate pain. It inhibits the synthesis of neurotransmitter prostaglandins in the CNS, and this is why it has no antiinflammatory properties.[111] Acetaminophen is metabolized by two pathways: major (nontoxic metabolite) and minor (toxic metabolite that is rapidly converted into a nontoxic form by glutathione). In an acetaminophen overdose, a larger amount is processed by the minor pathway, and this results in a larger quantity of toxic metabolites and may cause damage to the liver. Side effects are rare at therapeutic doses (total daily dose should not exceed 4 g in 24 hours). Nonopioids are rarely used alone in critically ill patients. The nurse must consider the other products containing acetaminophen that the patient may receive when calculating the total daily dose of acetaminophen. Special care must be taken for patients with liver dysfunction, malnutrition, or a history of excess alcohol consumption, and their acetaminophen total dose should not exceed 2 g/day.[17]

Nonsteroidal Antiinflammatory Drugs. The use of NSAIDs in combination with opioids is indicated in the patient with acute musculoskeletal and soft tissue inflammation.[24] The mechanism of action of NSAIDs is to block the action of cyclooxygenase (COX, which has two forms: COX-1 and COX-2), the enzyme that converts arachidonic acid to prostaglandins. This inhibits the production of prostaglandins (transduction process; see Fig. 9-7). This action occurs in the PNS and the CNS components of pain. NSAIDs can be grouped as first-generation (COX-1 and COX-2 inhibitors, such as aspirin, ibuprofen, naproxen, and ketorolac) or second-generation (COX-2 inhibitors, such as celecoxib) agents. The inhibition of COX-1 is thought to be responsible for many of the side effects, such as gastric ulceration, bleeding as a result of platelet inhibition, and acute renal failure. In contrast, the inhibition of COX-2 is responsible for the suppression of pain and inflammation.[111] Second-generation NSAIDs are associated with minimal risks of serious adverse effects, but their role in critically ill patients remains unknown.[17]

Ketorolac is the most appropriate NSAID for use in the critical care setting. Research has shown that it is a safe and effective agent for postoperative pain.[112] Not all critically ill patients are candidates for ketorolac therapy because of its side effects. Caution is advised for using ketorolac in older adults or patients with kidney dysfunction because of their slower clearance rates. Because ketorolac is an NSAID, monitoring for clumping of platelets is of primary importance. Laboratory data should be evaluated for an increase in bleeding time, and the patient should be assessed for any signs of abnormal bleeding. Moreover, prolonged use of ketorolac for more than 5 days was associated with an increase in kidney failure and bleeding.[113,114] It is important to consider the concurrent use of opioids and NSAIDs to affect pain modification at both areas of transmission. This combination of agents often significantly reduces the amount of opioids required for effective pain management.

Other pharmacologic agents are used in the critical care unit. The most important factor to be considered in the management of pain with any pharmacologic agent is the careful assessment and reassessment of the patient's pain status during the administration of the medication. The need to adjust the dosage, increase the frequency, or change the agent is based on assessment findings. The use of a pain flow sheet allows ongoing pain assessment and complete documentation of pain management in the critical care setting.

Adjuvants. Although not widely mentioned in the critical care literature, adjuvants can be helpful for pain relief in patients with complex pain syndromes such as neuropathic pain or for other specific purposes (e.g., procedural pain). Anticonvulsants (e.g., carbamazepine, phenytoin, gabapentin, pregabalin) are first-line analgesics for lancing neuropathic pain. The use of gabapentin or carbamazepine, in addition to intravenous opioids, is recommended for treatment of neuropathic pain in the SCCM guidelines.[17] Even if the specific mechanism for pain relief is unknown, analgesia probably results from the suppression of sodium ion (Na^+) discharges, reducing the neuronal hyperexcitability (action potential) in the transduction process[24] (see Fig. 9-7). Antidepressants are also considered as analgesics in a variety of chronic pain syndromes, such as headache, fibromyalgia, low back pain, neuropathy, central pain, and cancer pain. The analgesic dose is often lower than that required to treat depression. Antidepressant adjuvant analgesics are usually divided into two main groups: tricyclic antidepressants (e.g., amitriptyline, imipramine, desipramine), and biogenic amine reuptake inhibitors (e.g., venlafaxine, paroxetine, sertraline). The mechanism of analgesia most widely accepted is the ability of antidepressants to block the reuptake of neurotransmitters serotonin and norepinephrine in the CNS.[24] This increases the activity of the modulation process (see Fig. 9-7).

Ketamine. Anesthetics may be used to treat pain in the critical care setting. Ketamine is a dissociative anesthetic agent that has analgesic properties. It was traditionally used intravenously for procedural pain in burn patients. It is also available in enteral routes. Compared with opioids, ketamine has the benefit of sparing the respiratory drive, but it has many side effects related to the release of catecholamines and the emergence of delirium. For this reason, ketamine is not recommended for routine therapy in critically ill patients.[96,112] Before administering ketamine, the dissociative state should be explained to the patient. *Dissociative state* refers to the feelings of separateness from the environment, loss of control, hallucinations, and vivid dreams. The use of benzodiazepines (e.g., midazolam) can reduce the incidence of this unpleasant effect.[24]

Lidocaine. Lidocaine is another anesthetic that can be used for procedural and acute pain or for some patients with chronic neuropathic pain.[24] When used locally, anesthetics act through the transduction process (see Fig. 9-7).

Delivery Methods

The most common route for medication administration is the intravenous route by means of continuous infusion, bolus administration, or patient-controlled analgesia (PCA). Traditionally, the choice has been intravenous bolus administration. The benefits of this method are the rapid onset of action and the ease of titration. The major disadvantage is the rise and fall of the serum level of the opioid, leading to periods of pain control with periods of breakthrough pain.[111]

Continuous infusion of opioids with an infusion pump provides constant blood levels of the ordered opioid. This promotes a consistent level of comfort. It is a particularly helpful method of administration during sleep because the patient awakens with an adequate level of pain relief. It is important that the patient be given the loading dose that relieves the pain and raises the circulating dose of the medication. After the basal rate is established, the patient maintains a steady state of pain control unless there is additional pain from a procedure, an activity, or a change in the patient's condition. In this situation, physician orders to administer additional boluses of opioid need to be available.

Patient-Controlled Analgesia

PCA is a method of medication delivery that uses the intravenous route and an infusion pump. It allows the patient to self-administer small doses of analgesics. Different opioids can be used, but the most extensively used is morphine. This method of medication delivery allows the patient to control the level of pain and sedation and to avoid the peaks and valleys of intermittent dosing by the health care professional. The patient can self-administer a bolus of medication the moment the pain begins, acting preemptively. Nursing management for the patient receiving analgesia medication via a PCA pump is described in the Nursing Interventions Classification (NIC) feature in Box 9-3.

Certain patients are not candidates for PCA. Alterations in the level of consciousness or mentation preclude the patient understanding the use of the equipment. Very elderly patients or patients with kidney failure or liver dysfunction may require careful screening for PCA.

Allowing the patient to self-administer opioid doses does not diminish the role of the critical care nurse in pain management. The nurse advises about necessary changes to the prescription and continues to monitor the effects of the medication and doses. The patient is closely monitored during the first 2 hours of therapy and after every change in the prescription. If the patient's pain does not respond within the first 2 hours of therapy, a total reassessment of the pain state is essential. The nurse monitors the number of boluses the patient delivers. If the patient is pressing the button to bolus medication more often than the prescription, the dose may be insufficient to maintain pain control. Naloxone must be readily available to reverse adverse opiate respiratory effects. Ideally, the patient undergoing an elective procedure requiring opioid analgesia postoperatively is instructed in the use of PCA during preoperative teaching. This allows the patient to become comfortable with the concept of self-medication before use.

Intraspinal Pain Control

Intraspinal anesthesia uses the concept that the spinal cord is the primary link in nociceptive transmission. The goal is to mimic the body's endogenous opioid pain modification system by interfering with the transmission of pain and providing an opiate receptor binding agent directly into the spinal cord. The hemodynamic status of the patient changes very little.

◎ **BOX 9-3 NIC**

Patient-Controlled Analgesia (PCA) Assistance

Definition
Facilitating patient control of analgesic administration and regulation

Activities
Collaborate with physicians, patient, and family members in selecting the type of narcotic to be used

Recommend administration of aspirin and nonsteroidal antiinflammatory drugs in conjunction with narcotics, as appropriate

Recommend discontinuation of opioid administration by other routes

Avoid use of meperidine hydrochloride (Demerol)

Ensure that patient is not allergic to analgesic to be administered

Instruct patient and family to monitor pain intensity, quality, and duration

Instruct patient and family to monitor respiratory rate and blood pressure

Establish nasogastric, venous, subcutaneous, or spinal access, as appropriate

Validate that the patient can use a PCA device (is able to communicate, comprehend explanations, and follow directions)

Collaborate with patient and family to select appropriate type of patient-controlled infusion device

Instruct patient and family members how to use the PCA device

Assist patient and family to calculate appropriate concentration of drug to fluid, considering the amount of fluid delivered per hour via the PCA device

Assist patient or family member to administer an appropriate bolus loading dose of analgesic

Instruct the patient and family to set an appropriate basal infusion rate on the PCA device

Assist the patient and family to set the appropriate lockout interval on the PCA device

Assist the patient and family in setting appropriate demand doses on the PCA device

Consult with patient, family members, and physician to adjust lockout interval, basal rate, and demand dosage, according to patient responsiveness

Instruct patient how to titrate doses up or down, depending on respiratory rate, pain intensity, and pain quality

Instruct the patient and family members the action and side effects of pain-relieving agents

Recommend a bowel regimen to avoid constipation

Consult with clinical pain experts for a patient who is having difficulty achieving pain control

From Bulechek GM, et al. *Nursing interventions classification (NIC)*. 6th ed. St. Louis: Mosby; 2013.

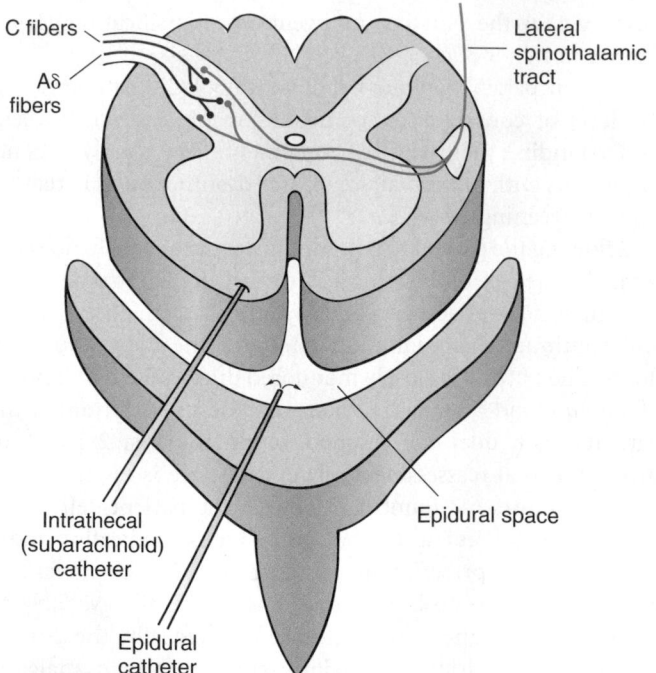

FIGURE 9-8 Intraspinal Catheter Placement in a Spinal Cord Cross Section.

Intraspinal anesthesia is particularly appropriate for pain in the thorax, upper abdomen, and lower extremities. The two intraspinal routes are intrathecal and epidural (Fig. 9-8). Regardless of the route, the effects of the opioid agonist used is the same, and assessment parameters are the same as those used for other routes. Nursing management of the patient receiving intraspinal analgesia is described in the Nursing Interventions Classification (NIC) feature in Box 9-4.

Intrathecal Analgesia

Intrathecal (subarachnoid) opioids are placed directly into the cerebral spinal fluid and attach to spinal cord receptor sites. Opioids introduced at this site act quickly at the dorsal horn. The dural sheath is punctured, eliminating the barrier for pathogens between the environment and the cerebral spinal fluid. This creates the risk of serious infections. The intrathecal route is usually reserved for intraoperative use. Single-bolus dosing provides short-term relief for pain that is short lived (the pain of labor and delivery is well managed using this regimen). Side effects of intrathecal pain control include postdural puncture headache and infection.

Epidural Analgesia

Epidural analgesia is commonly used in the critical care unit after major abdominal surgery, nephrectomy, thoracotomy, and major orthopedic procedures. Per the SCCM guidelines, its use should be considered in postoperative abdominal aortic aneurysm patients, and for those with traumatic rib fractures.[17] Certain conditions preclude the use of this pain control method: systemic infection, anticoagulation, and increased intracranial pressure. Epidural delivery of opiates provides longer-lasting pain relief with less dosing of opiates. When delivered into the epidural space, 5 mg of morphine may be effective for 6 to 24 hours, compared with 3 to 4 hours when delivered intravenously. Opioids infused in the epidural space are more unpredictable than those administered intrathecally. The epidural space is filled with fatty tissue and is external to the dura mater. The fatty tissue interferes with uptake, and the dura acts as a barrier to diffusion, making diffusion rate difficult to predict.

The type of medication used determines the rapidity of medication diffusion. Hydrophilic medications (e.g., morphine) are water soluble and penetrate the dura slowly, giving

◎ BOX 9-4 **NIC**

Analgesic Administration: Intraspinal

Definition

Administration of pharmacologic agents into the epidural or intrathecal space to reduce or eliminate pain

Activities

Check patency and function of the catheter, port, and/or pump

Ensure that intravenous access is in place at all times during therapy

Label the catheter, and secure it appropriately

Ensure that the proper formulation of the drug is used (e.g., high concentrating and preservation free)

Ensure narcotic antagonist availability for emergency administration and administer per physician order, as necessary

Start continuous infusion of analgesic agent after correct catheter placement has been verified, and monitor rate to ensure delivery of prescribed dosage of medication

Monitor temperature, blood pressure, respirations, pulse, and level of consciousness at appropriate intervals, and record on flow sheet

Monitor level of sensory blockade at appropriate intervals, and record on flow sheet

Monitor catheter site and dressings to check for a loose catheter or wet dressing, and notify appropriate personnel per agency protocol

Administer catheter site care according to agency protocol

Secure needle in place with tape and apply appropriate dressing according to agency protocol

Monitor for adverse reactions, including respiratory depression, urinary retention, undue somnolence, itching, seizures, nausea, and vomiting

Monitor orthostatic blood pressure and pulse before the first attempt at ambulation

Instruct patient to report side effects, alterations in pain relief, numbness of extremities, and need for assistance with ambulation if weak

Follow institutional policies for injection of intermittent analgesic agents into the injection port

Provide adjunct medications as appropriate (e.g., antidepressants, anticonvulsants, nonsteroidal antiinflammatory agents)

Increase the intraspinal dose based on a pain intensity score

Instruct and guide patient through nonpharmacologic measures (e.g., relaxation therapy, guided imagery, and biofeedback) to enhance pharmacologic effectiveness

Instruct patient about proper home care for external or implanted delivery systems, as appropriate

Remove or assist with removal of catheter according to agency protocol

From Bulechek GM, et al. *Nursing interventions classification (NIC)*. 6th ed. St. Louis: Mosby; 2013.

them a longer onset and duration of action. Lipophilic medications (e.g., fentanyl) are lipid soluble; they penetrate the dura rapidly and therefore have a rapid onset of action and a shorter duration of action.

The dura acts as a physical barrier and causes delay in diffusion of the medication. Compared with the intrathecal route, it allows more medication to be absorbed in the systemic circulation, requiring greater doses for pain relief. Medications delivered epidurally may be administered by bolus or continuous infusion. Epidural analgesia is being used more often in the critical care environment, and it requires careful monitoring.

The nurse must assess the patient for respiratory depression. This phenomenon may occur early in the therapy or as late as 24 hours after initiation. The epidural catheter also puts the patient at risk for infection. The efficiency of this pain control method and the increased mobility of the patient do not diminish the nurse's responsibility to monitor and evaluate the outcomes of the pain-management protocol in use.

Equianalgesia

When a modification of opioid is considered, the nurse must be aware of equianalgesic dosages. In doing any conversion, the goal is to provide equal analgesic effects with the new agents. This concept is referred to as *equianalgesia*. Morphine is the standard for the conversion of opioids. Prescribed dosages must take into account the patient's age and health status.[24] The critical care nurse must have access to a chart for easy referral on the unit to administer the correct dosages of opioids to critically ill patients. Because of the variety of agents and routes, the professional pain organizations have developed equianalgesia charts for use by the health care professional. All critical care units need to have an equianalgesic chart posted for easy

BOX 9-5 **A GUIDE TO USING EQUIANALGESIC CHARTS**

• Equianalgesic means approximately the same pain relief

• The equianalgesic chart is a guideline. Doses and intervals between doses are titrated according to the individual's response

• The equianalgesic chart is helpful when switching from one medication to another or when switching from one route of administration to another

• Dosages in the equianalgesic chart for moderate to severe pain are not necessarily starting doses. The doses suggest a ratio for comparing the analgesia of one medication with another

• For older adult patients, initially reduce the recommended adult opioid dose for moderate to severe pain by 25% to 50%

• The longer the patient has been receiving opioids, the more conservative the starting dose of a *new* opioid

The key to success with any of these therapies is a comprehensive understanding of their mechanism of action so that the therapy matches the needs of the patient. Most of the previously mentioned interventions require the patient's cooperation. There must be some commitment to the treatment on the part of the patient. When handled effectively, nonpharmacologic methods can assist in pain management.

reference. Box 9-5 presents a guide to using these charts. Table 9-4 provides the equianalgesic dose for different medications used in clinical practice. Table 9-5 presents an equianalgesic chart with PO nonopioid and opioid doses for mild to moderate pain.

Nonpharmacologic Methods of Pain Management

Although numerous methods of pain management other than medications appear in the critical care literature,[115] very few studies have been done to provide evidence of their effectiveness in the critical care settings. Nonpharmacologic methods can be

TABLE 9-4   EQUIANALGESIC CHART

Approximate Equivalent Doses of Opioids for Moderate-to-Severe Pain

ANALGESIC	PARENTERAL (IM, SC, IV) ROUTE[1,2] (mg)	PO ROUTE[1] (mg)	COMMENTS
Mu Opioid Agonists			
Morphine	10	30	Standard for comparison; multiple routes of administration; available in immediate-release and controlled-release formulations; active metabolite M6G can accumulate with repeated dosing in renal failure
Codeine	130	200 NR	IM has unpredictable absorption and high side-effect profile; used PO for mild-to-moderate pain; usually compounded with nonopioid (e.g., Tylenol No. 3)
Fentanyl	100 mcg/hr parenterally and transdermally ≅ 4 mg/hr morphine parenterally; 1 mcg/hr transdermally ≅ 2 mg/24 hr morphine PO	—	Short half-life, but at steady state, slow elimination from tissues can lead to a prolonged half-life (up to 12 hr); start opioid-naïve patients on no more than 25 mcg/hr transdermally; transdermal fentanyl NR for acute pain management; available by oral transmucosal route
Hydromorphone (Dilaudid)	1.5	7.5	Useful alternative to morphine; no evidence that metabolites are clinically relevant; shorter duration than morphine; available in high-potency parenteral formulation (10 mg/mL) useful for SC infusion; 3 mg rectal ≅ 650 mg aspirin PO; with repeated dosing (e.g., PCA), it is more likely than 2-3 mg parenteral hydromorphone =10 mg parenteral morphine
Levorphanol (Levo-Dromoran)	2	4	Longer-acting than morphine when given repeatedly; long half-life can lead to accumulation within 2-3 days of repeated dosing
Meperidine	75	300 NR	No longer preferred as a first-line opioid for the management of acute or chronic pain due to potential toxicity from accumulation of metabolite, normeperidine; normeperidine has 15-20 hr half-life and is not reversed by naloxone; NR in elderly or patients with impaired renal functions; NR by continuous IV infusion
Methadone (Dolophine)	10	20	Longer-acting than morphine when given repeatedly; long half-life can lead to delayed toxicity from accumulation within 3-5 days; start PO dosing on PRN schedule; in opioid-tolerant patients converted to methadone, start with 10%-25% of equianalgesic dose
Oxycodone	—	20	Used for moderate pain when combined with a nonopioid (e.g., Percocet, Tylox); available as single entity in immediate-release and controlled-release formulations (e.g., OxyContin); can be used like PO morphine for severe pain
Oxymorphone (Numorphan)	1	10 rectal	Used for moderate to severe pain; no PO formulation
Agonist-Antagonist Opioids: Not recommended for severe, escalating pain. If used in combination with mu agonists, may reverse analgesia and precipitate withdrawal in opioid-dependent patients.			
Buprenorphine (Buprenex)	0.4	—	Not readily reversed by naloxone; NR for laboring patients
Butorphanol (Stadol)	2	—	Available in nasal spray
Dezocine (Dalgan)	10	—	
Nalbuphine (Nubain)	10	—	
Pentazocine (Talwin)	60	180	

Duration of analgesia is dose dependent; the higher the dose, usually the longer the duration.

IV boluses may be used to produce analgesia that lasts approximately as long as IM or SC doses. However, of all routes of administration, IV produces the highest peak concentration of the medication, and the peak concentration is associated with the highest level of toxicity, e.g., sedation. To decrease the peak effect and lower the level of toxicity, IV boluses may be administered more slowly, e.g., 10 mg of morphine over a 15-minute period, or smaller doses may be administered more often, e.g., 5 mg of morphine every 1-1.5 hours.

FDA, U.S. Food and Drug Administration; *IM*, intramuscular; *IV*, intravenous; *M6G*, morphine-6-glucuronide; *MCG*, micrograms; *MG*, milligrams; *NR*, not recommended; *PCA*, patient-controlled analgesia; *PO*, by mouth; *PRN*, pro re nata (as needed); *SC*, subcutaneous.

Reference: Pasero C, McCaffrey M. *Pain Assessment and Pharmacologic Management*, St. Louis: Elsevier; 2011. Table 16-1, p. 444-445.

TABLE 9-5 EQUIANALGESIC CHART

Approximate Equivalent Doses of PO Nonopioids and Opioids for Mild to Moderate Pain

ANALGESIC	PO DOSAGE (mg)
Nonopioids	
Acetaminophen	650
Aspirin (ASA)	650
Opioids*	
Codeine	32-60
Hydrocodone[†]	5
Meperidine (Demerol)	50
Oxycodone[‡]	3-5
Propoxyphene (Darvon)	65-100

*Often combined with acetaminophen; avoid exceeding maximum total daily dose of acetaminophen (4000 mg/day).
[†]Combined with acetaminophen (e.g., Vicodin, Lortab).
[‡]Combined with acetaminophen (e.g., Percocet, Tylox); also available alone as controlled-release OxyContin and immediate-release formulations.
Selected references for more information: McCaffery M, Pasero C. Acetaminophen and NSAIDS: adult dosing information, p 211. In Pasero C, McCaffery M. *Pain Assessment and Pharmacologic Management*. St. Louis: Mosby; 2011; American Pain Society (APS). *Principles of Analgesic Use in the Treatment of Acute Pain and Cancer Pain*. 3rd ed. Glenview, IL: APS; 1992; Kaiko R, et al. Analgesic efficacy of controlled-release (CR) oxycodone and CR morphine. *Clin Pharmacol Ther*. 1996;59:130.
Modified from Pasero C, McCaffery M. *Pain Assessment and Pharmacologic Management*. St. Louis: Elsevier; 2011.

used to supplement analgesic treatment, but they are not intended to replace analgesics. In most instances, these therapies may enhance the pharmacologic management of the patient's pain. Per the SCCM guidelines, administration of preemptive analgesic therapy and/or non-pharmacological interventions, it is suggested to alleviate pain during invasive or potentially painful procedures in critically ill adults.[17]

Critical care nurses identify many barriers to the use of nonpharmacologic methods for pain management, including a lack of knowledge, training, and time.[116] Despite these problems, more than 60% of them are willing to use the methods to relieve their patients' pain. It is crucial that critical care nurses be provided with the appropriate training and equipment required to apply nonpharmacologic methods for pain management in the critically ill.

Physical Techniques

Stimulating other non–pain sensory fibers (Aβ) in the periphery modifies pain transmission. These fibers are stimulated by thermal changes as in the application of heat or cold, and simple massage.

Cold Application

Ice therapy was found to be helpful to reduce procedural pain in critically ill patients. In a study with 50 cardiac surgery patients in a critical care unit, a significant decrease in pain intensity was obtained after chest tube removal when ice packets were placed around the site for 10 minutes prior to removal.[117] The analgesic property of ice therapy was also studied by Demir and Khorshid[118] using a 20-minute application of cold packs before chest tube removal in the critical care unit. Pain intensity was significantly lower after chest tube removal in patients who received the cold packs and a dose of analgesic compared with a placebo and a control group.

Massage

The effect of massage on pain relief was explored in two studies with postoperative cardiac surgery patients after they have been transferred from the critical care unit.[119,120] In these two studies with a total of 171 patients, a significant decrease in pain intensity scores was obtained in patients who received a 20-minute massage intervention between postoperative day 2 and day 5 compared to a control group who received standard care and a 20-minute quiet time during the same period. Similar findings were found in the critical care unit. Indeed, in a recent pilot study[121] with 40 postoperative cardiac surgery patients, a decrease in pain intensity scores was observed in patients who were administered two to three 15-minute hand massage sessions during the first 24 hours after surgery compared to a control group who did not receive hand massage but had the nurse holding their hands and reported no change in pain intensity.

Cognitive-Behavioral Techniques

Using the cortical interpretation of pain as the foundation, several interventions can reduce the patient's pain report. These modalities include cognitive techniques such as relaxation, distraction, guided imagery, and music therapy.

Relaxation

Relaxation is a well-documented method for reducing the distress associated with pain. Although not a substitute for pharmacology, relaxation is an excellent adjunct for controlling pain. Relaxation decreases oxygen consumption and muscle tone, and it can decrease heart rate and blood pressure. Relaxation gives the patient a sense of control over the pain and reduces muscle tension and anxiety. Not all patients are interested in relaxation therapy. For those patients, deep-breathing exercises may be helpful. Indeed, in a recent study,[3] lower pain scores were found both after chest tube removal in 40 critically ill patients executing deep breathing and receiving an analgesic compared to those who solely received an analgesic. Excellent references for thorough techniques in relaxation therapy are available.[24]

Guided Imagery

Guided imagery is a technique that uses the imagination to provide control over pain. It can be used to distract or relax. Guiding a patient to a place that is pain free and relaxing takes a considerable time commitment on the part of the nurse. Although this may be difficult in the critical care environment, guiding a patient to a place in his or her imagination that is free from pain may be beneficial.[122]

Music Therapy

Music therapy is a commonly used intervention for relaxation. Music that is pleasing to the patient may have soothing effects, but its effects on reducing pain are controversial.[123] Ideally, the music should be supplied by a small set of headphones. It is important to educate the patient and family regarding the role of music in relaxation and pain control and to provide music of the patient's choice.

The patient and family may provide information about other sources of distraction for the patient. Determining what distraction therapies the patient normally uses may provide a clue to which one may work during the illness. Some persons are distracted by television; for others, television is a source of increased anxiety. Do not assume that the patient does or does not want to watch television until you determine whether it will be beneficial or harmful to the patient.

BOX 9-6   CASE STUDY

Patient with Pain

Brief Patient History

Ms. X is a woman with type 2 diabetes mellitus and peripheral arterial occlusive disease with neuropathy. Ms. X is disabled because of limited mobility and chronic pain associated with lower extremity claudication and neuropathic pain. She has been admitted for an elective right femoral to distal tibial bypass. Ms. X's chronic pain has been effectively managed with gabapentin (600 mg three times daily) and a 75-mcg fentanyl patch every third day. Ms. X reports that her pain patch is due to be changed the next day. Her diabetes mellitus has been effectively managed with diet and a combination of oral agents. Postoperatively, orders for pain management include her home regimen of gabapentin and fentanyl patch and an order for morphine for breakthrough pain.

Clinical Assessment

Ms. X is admitted to the critical care unit from the perianesthesia recovery room after an 8-hour surgical revascularization of the right lower extremity. She is awake, alert, and oriented to person, time, place, and situation. Ms. X is breathing through her mouth and taking shallow breaths. She complains of right lower extremity and bilateral foot pain. Her skin is warm and dry. Ms. X is able to move her toes on command, and lower extremity sensation to touch is intact; however, she is complaining of severe burning in both feet.

Diagnostic Procedures

Ms. X reports that her pain is a 10 on the Numeric Rating Scale. The Riker Agitation Sedation Scale score is 5.

Medical Diagnosis

The diagnosis is acute postoperative incisional pain superimposed on chronic neuropathic pain involving both lower extremities. Neuropathic pain is likely worsened because of missed doses of gabapentin.

Questions

1. What major outcomes do you expect to achieve for this patient?
2. What problems or risks must be managed to achieve these outcomes?
3. What interventions must be initiated to monitor, prevent, manage, or eliminate the problems and risks identified?
4. What interventions should be initiated to promote optimal functioning, safety, and well-being of the patient?
5. What possible learning needs do you anticipate for this patient?
6. What cultural and age-related factors may have a bearing on the patient's plan of care?

▌ SUMMARY

- Pain in the critically ill patient is difficult to assess and manage. There are many sources of pain in the critical care setting, and the effects of unrelieved acute pain can have a significant impact on the patient's recovery.

- When possible, the patient's self-report of pain must be obtained. A simple yes or no communicated by head nodding from a mechanically ventilated patient is considered a valid self-report of pain.

- When the patient's self-report is not available, behavioral indicators represent alternative measures of pain assessment, and assessment tools (e.g., BPS, CPOT) have been developed for assessment of pain in nonverbal critically ill patients.

- In some situations, behavioral indicators may be impossible to assess accurately. The use of physiologic indicators is then crucial. However, vital signs do not represent valid information for pain assessment. Innovative physiologic measures (e.g., BIS, EEG) are being explored and may support the nurses in the pain assessment process.

- The critical care nurse must collaborate with the multidisciplinary team to ensure a plan of care for management of the patient's pain is developed. To fully participate, the nurse must have extensive knowledge of nonpharmacologic and pharmacologic therapies designed to achieve effective pain relief.

REFERENCES

1. Chanques G, Sebbane M, Barbotte E, et al. A prospective study of pain at rest: incidence and characteristics of an unrecognized symptom in surgical and trauma versus medical intensive care unit patients. *Anesthesiology*. 2007;107:858.

2. Puntillo KA, et al. Patients' perceptions and responses to procedural pain: results from Thunder Project II. *Am J Crit Care*. 2001;10:238.

3. Friesner SA, Curry DM, Moddeman GR. Comparison of two pain-management strategies during chest tube removal: relaxation exercise with opioids and opioids alone. *Heart & Lung*. 2006;35:269.

4. Gélinas C. Management of pain in cardiac surgery ICU patients: have we improved over time? *Intensive Crit Care Nurs*. 2007;23:298.

5. Puntillo KA, et al. Practices and predictors of analgesic interventions for adults undergoing painful procedures. *Am J Crit Care*. 2002;11:415.

6. Dunwoody CJ, et al. Assessment, physiological monitoring, and consequences of inadequately treated acute pain. *Pain Manag Nurs.* 2008;9:S11.

7. Kehlet H. Surgical stress and postoperative outcome—from here to where? *Reg Anesth Pain Med.* 2006;31:47.

8. Joshi GP, Ogunnaike BO. Consequences of inadequate postoperative pain relief and chronic persistent postoperative pain. *Anesth Clin North Am.* 2005;23:21.

9. Kehlet H, et al. Persistent postsurgical pain: risk factors and prevention. *Lancet.* 2006;367:1618.

10. Nampiaparampil DE. Prevalence of chronic pain after traumatic brain injury: a systematic review. *JAMA.* 2008;300:711.

11. Loeser JD, Treede RD. The Kyoto protocol of IASP basic pain terminology. *Pain.* 2008;137:473.

12. Lome B. Acute pain and the critically ill trauma patient. *Crit Care Nurs Quart.* 2005;28:200.

13. Shannon K, Bucknall T. Pain assessment in critical care: what have we learnt from research. *Intensive Crit Care Nurs.* 2003;19:154.

14. Khalaila R, et al. Communication difficulties and psychoemotional distress in patients receiving mechanical ventilation. *Am J Crit Care.* 2011;20:470.

15. Gélinas C, Johnston C. Pain assessment in the critically ill ventilated adult: validation of the Critical-Care Pain Observation Tool and physiological indicators. *Clin J Pain.* 2007;23:497.

16. Herr K. Pain assessment strategies in older adults. *The Journal of Pain.* 2011;3(Suppl.1):S3-S13.

17. Barr J, Fraser G, Puntillo K, et al. Clinical practice guidelines for the management of pain, agitation, and delirium in adult ICU patients. *Critical Care Medicine.* In press.

18. International Association for the Study of Pain (IASP) Subcommittee on Taxonomy. Pain terms: a list with definitions and notes on usage. *Pain.* 1979;6:249.

19. McCaffery M. *Nursing Management of the Patient with Pain.* 2nd ed. Philadelphia: JB Lippincott; 1979.

20. Anand KJS, Craig, KD. New perspectives on the definition of pain. *Pain.* 1996;67:3.

21. McGuire D. Comprehensive and multidimensional assessment and measurement of pain. *J Pain Symptom Manage.* 1992;7:312.

22. International Association for the Study of Pain (IASP) Task Force on Taxonomy. *Classification of Chronic Pain.* Seattle: IASP Press; 1994.

23. Melzack R. Pain and stress: a new perspective. In: Gatchel RJ, Turk DC, eds. *Psychological Factors in Pain.* New York: Guilford Press; 1999.

24. Pasero C, McCaffery M. *Pain Assessment and Pharmacologic Management.* St Louis: Mosby; 2011.

25. Cervero F, Laird JMA. Visceral Pain. *Lancet.* 1999;353:2145.

26. Marchand S. The physiology of pain mechanisms: from the periphery to the brain. *Rheum Dis North Am.* 2008;34:285.

27. Melzack R, Wall PD. *The Challenge of Pain.* 2nd ed. London: Penguin Books; 1996.

28. Carr DB, Goudas LC. Acute pain. *Lancet.* 1999;353:2051.

29. Gélinas C, Arbour C. Behavioral and physiological indicators during a nociceptive procedure in conscious and unconscious mechanically ventilated adults: similar or different? *J Crit Care.* 2009;24:628.e7.

30. Rainville P. Brain mechanisms of pain affect and pain modulation. *Curr Opin Neurobiol.* 2002;12:195.

31. Derbyshire SW, Osborn J. Modeling pain circuits: how imaging may modify perception. *Neuroimaging Clin N Am.* 2007;17:485.

32. Melzack R, Wall PD. Pain mechanisms: a new theory. *Science.* 1965;150:171.

33. Marks DM, Shah MJ, Patkar AA, et al. Serotonin-norepinephrine reuptake inhibitors for pain control: premise and promise. *Current Neuropharmacology.* 2009;7:331.

34. Lorenz J, Minoshima S, Casey KL. Keeping pain out of mind: the role of the dorsolateral prefrontal cortex in pain modulation. *Brain.* 2003;126:5.

35. McCance KL, Huether SE. *Pathophysiology: the biologic basis for disease in adults and children.* 5th ed. St. Louis: Mosby; 2006.

36. Arbour C, Gélinas C. Are vital signs valid indicators for the assessment of pain in cardiac surgery ICU adults? *Int Crit Care Nurs.* 2010;26:83.

37. Li DT, et al. Evaluations of physiologic reactivity and reflexive behaviors during noxious procedures in sedated critically ill patients. *J Crit Care.* 2009;24:472.e9.

38. Puntillo KA, et al. Relationship between behavioral and physiological indicators of pain, critical care self-reports of pain, and opioid administration. *Crit Care Med.* 1997;25:1159.

39. Rabin BS, et al. Bidirectional interaction between the central nervous system and the immune system. *Crit Rev Immunol.* 1989;9:279.

40. Hadjistavropoulos T, Craig KD. A theoretical framework for understanding self-report and observational measures of pain: a communication model. *Behav Res Ther.* 2002;40:551.

41. Daut RL, Cleeland CS. The prevalence and severity of pain in cancer. *Cancer.* 1982;50:1913.

42. Melzack R. The short form McGill Pain Questionnaire. *Pain.* 1987;30:191.

43. Jarvis C. *Physical examination & health assessment.* 6th ed. Philadelphia: Saunders; 2011.

44. Puntillo KA. Pain management. In: Schell HM, Puntillo KA, eds. *Critical care nursing secrets.* 2nd ed. Philadelphia: Hanley & Belfus; 2006.

45. Puntillo KA, et al. Pain behaviors observed during six common procedures: results from Thunder Project II. *Crit Care Med.* 2004;32:421.

46. Payen JF, et al. Assessing pain in the critically ill sedated patients by using a behavioral pain scale. *Crit Care Med.* 2001;29:2258.

47. Gélinas C, et al. Validation of the Critical-Care Pain Observation Tool (CPOT) in adult patients. *Am J Crit Care.* 2006;15:420.

48. Odhner M, Wegman D, Freeland N, et al. Assessing pain control in nonverbal critically ill adults. *DCCN—Dimensions of Critical Care Nursing.* 2003;22:260.

49. Li D, et al. A review of objective pain measures for use with critical care adult patients unable to self-report. *J Pain.* 2008;9:2.

50. Sessler CN, et al. Evaluating and monitoring analgesia and sedation in the intensive care unit. *Crit Care.* 2008;12:S2.

51. Gélinas C, Arbour C, Michaud C, et al. The impact of the implementation of the Critical-Care Pain Observation Tool on pain assessment/management nursing practices in the intensive care unit with nonverbal critically ill adults. *International Journal of Nursing Studies.* 2011;48:1495.

52. Chanques G, Jaber S, Barbotte E, et al. Impact of systematic evaluation of pain and agitation in an intensive care unit. *Critical Care Medicine.* 2006;34:1691.

53. Ahlers S, et al. Comparison of different pain scoring systems in critically ill patients in a general ICU. *Crit Care.* 2008;12:1.

54. Ahlers S, et al. The use of the behavioral pain scale to assess pain in conscious sedated patients. *Anesth Anal*. 2010;110:127.

55. Aïssaoui Y, et al. Validation of a behavioral pain scale in critically ill sedated, and mechanically ventilated patients. *Anesth Analg*. 2005;101:1470.

56. Young J, et al. Use of a Behavioral Pain Scale to assess pain in ventilated, unconscious and/or sedated patients. *Intensive Crit Care Nurs*. 2006;22:32.

57. Marmo L, Fowler S. Pain assessment tool in the critically ill post-open heart surgery patient population. *Pain Manag Nurs*. 2010;11:134.

58. Gélinas C, et al. Item selection and content validity of the Critical-Care Pain Observation Tool: an instrument to assess pain in critically ill nonverbal adults. *J Adv Nurs*. 2009;65:203.

59. Gélinas C, et al. Sensitivity and specificity of the Critical-Care Pain Observation Tool for the detection of pain in intubated adults following cardiac surgery. *J Pain Symptom Manage*. 2009;37:58.

60. Gelinas, C. Nurses' evaluations of the feasibility and the clinical utility of the Critical Care Pain Observation Tool. *Pain Manag Nurs*. 2010;11:115.

61. Arbour C, Gélinas C. Behavioral and physiologic indicators of pain in nonverbal patients with a traumatic brain injury: an integrative review. *Pain Manag Nurs*. 2012, in press.

62. Le Q, et al. Description of behaviors in traumatic brain injury patients when exposed to common procedures in the intensive care unit: a pilot study. *Pain Manag Nurs*. 2012, in press.

63. Streiner DL, Norman GR. *Health Measurement Scales: a Practical Guide to Their Development and Use*. 4th ed. Oxford: Oxford University Press; 2008.

64. Apkarian AV, et al. Human brain mechanisms of pain perception and regulation in health and disease. *Eur J Pain*. 2005;9:463.

65. Kurtz P, et al. Continuous EEG monitoring: is it ready for prime time? *Curr Opin Crit Care*. 2009;15:99.

66. Fernandez M, et al. Sucrose attenuates a negative electroencephalographic response to an aversive stimulus for newborns. *Dev Behav Peds*. 2003;24:261.

67. Gélinas C, Gotman J, Arbour C, Zerouali Y, Choinière M, Johnston C, & Cervero F. Electroencephalogram (EEG) reactivity and self-reports of pain in post-operative cardiac surgery adults during mediastinal tube removal in the intensive care unit: Do they match? *Pain Research & Management*. 2012;17(3):203.

68. Gelinas C, Tousignant-Laflamme Y, Tanguay A, et al. Exploring the validity of the bispectral index, the Critical-Care Pain Observation Tool and vital signs for the detection of pain in sedated and mechanically ventilated critically ill adults: a pilot study. *Intensive & Critical Care Nursing*. 2011;27:46.

69. Arbour C, Gélinas C, Loiselle C, Bourgault P, Stone C, Razek T, Gursahaney A, & Choinière M. Detecting pain in nonvebal ICU patients with a traumatic brain injury and altered level of consciousness using the bilateral bispectral index (BIS): a pilot study. *Pain Research & Management*. 2012;17(3):203.

70. Gordon DB, et al. American Pain recommendations for improving the quality of acute and cancer pain management. *Arch Intern Med*. 2005;165:1574.

71. Lawrence M. The unconscious experience. *Am J Crit Care*. 1995;4:227.

72. Laureys S, Faymonville ME, Peigneux P, et al. Cortical processing of noxious somatosensory stimuli in the persistent vegetative state. *Neuroimage*. 2002;17:732.

73. Bjoro K, Herr K. Assessment of pain in the nonverbal or cognitively impaired older adult. *Clin Geriatr Med*. 2008;24:237.

74. Hadjistavropoulos T, et al. An interdisciplinary expert consensus statement on assessment of pain in older persons. *Clin J Pain*. 2007;23:S1.

75. Zwakhalen SM, et al. Pain in elderly people with severe dementia: a systematic review of behavioral pain assessment tools. *BMC Geriatr*. 2006;6:1.

76. Fuchs-Labelle S, Hadjistavropoulos T. Development and preliminary validation of the Pain Assessment Checklist for Seniors with Limited Ability to Communicate (PACSLAC). *Pain Manag Nurs*. 2004;5:37.

77. Wary B, Doloplus C. Doloplus-2, a scale for pain measurement. *Soins Gerontol*. 1999;19:25.

78. Warden V, Hurley AC, Volicer L. Development and psychometric evaluation of the Pain Assessment in Advanced Dementia (PAINAD) scale. *J Am Med Dir Assoc*. 2003;4:9.

79. Herr K, Bursch H, Ersek M, et al. Use of pain-behavioral assessment tools in the nursing home: expert consensus recommendations for practice. *J Gerontol Nurs*. 2010;36:18.

80. McNicoll L, et al. Delirium in the intensive care unit: occurrence and clinical course in older patients. *J Am Geriatr Soc*. 2003;51:591.

81. Graf C, Puntillo KA. Pain in the older adult in the intensive care unit. *Crit Care Clin*. 2003;19:749.

82. Anand KJS. The applied physiology of pain. In: Anand KJS, McGrath PJ, eds. *Pain in Neonates and Infants*. 3rd ed. Amsterdam: Elsevier; 2007.

83. Duhn LJ, Medves JM. A systematic integrative review of infant pain assessment tools. *Adv Neonatal Care*. 2004;4:126.

84. Stevens B, et al. Premature Infant Pain Profile: development and initial validation. *Clin J Pain*. 1996;12:13.

85. Davidhizar R, Giger JN. A review of the literature on care of clients in pain who are culturally diverse. *Int Nurs Rev*. 2004;51:47.

86. Ulmer J. Identifying and preventing pain mismanagement. In: Salerno E, Willens J, eds. *Pain Management Handbook: an Interdisciplinary Approach*. St Louis: Mosby; 1996.

87. Carroll KC, et al. Pain assessment and management in critically ill postoperative and trauma patients: a multisite study. *Am J Crit Care*. 1999;8:105.

88. Cashman JN, Dolin SJ. Respiratory and haemodynamic effects of acute postoperative pain management: Evidence from published data. *Br J Anaesth*. 2004;93:212.

89. Smith LH. Opioid safety: is your patient at risk for respiratory depression? *Clin J Oncol Nurs*. 2007;11:293.

90. Gélinas C, et al. Pain assessment and management in critically ill intubated patients: a retrospective study. *Am J Crit Care*. 2004;13:126.

91. Idvall E, Ehrenberg A. Nursing documentation of postoperative pain management. *J Clin Nurs*. 2002;11:734.

92. Pasero C, Puntillo K, Li D, et al. Structured approaches to pain management in the ICU. *Chest*. 2009;135:1665.

93. Devlin JW, Mallow-Corbett S, Riker RR. Adverse drug events associated with the use of analgesics, sedatives, and antipsychotics in the intensive care unit. *Crit Care Med*. 2010;38:S231.

94. Jarzyna D, Jungquist CR, Pasero C, et al. American Society for Pain Management Nursing guidelines on monitoring for opioid-induced sedation and respiratory depression. *Pain Manag Nurs*. 2011;12:118.

95. Brush DR, Kress JP. Sedation and analgesia for the mechanically ventilated patient. *Clin Chest Med.* 2009;30:131.

96. Liu LL, Gropper MA. Postoperative analgesia and sedation in the adult intensive care unit: a guide to drug selection. *Drugs.* 2003;63:755.

97. Sarhill N, et al. Hydromorphone: pharmacology and clinical applications in cancer patients. *Support Care Cancer.* 2001;9:84.

98. Ashley E, Given J. Pain management in the critically ill. *Br J Perioper Nurs.* 2008;18:504.

99. Devlin JW, Roberts RJ. Pharmacology of commonly used analgesics and sedatives in the ICU: benzodiazepines, propofol, and opioids. *Crit Care Clin.* 2009;25:431.

100. Erstad BL, Puntillo K, Gilbert HC, et al. Pain management principles in the critically ill. *Chest.* 2009;135:1075.

101. Cavalière F, et al. A low-dose remifentanyl infusion is well tolerated for sedation in mechanically ventilated, critically ill patients. *Can J Anaesth.* 2002;49:1088.

102. Soltész S, et al. Recovery after remifentanyl and sufentanyl for analgesia and sedation of mechanically ventilated patients after trauma or major surgery. *Br J Anaesth.* 2001;86:763.

103. Radtke FM, Lorenz M, Luetz A, et al. Remifentanyl reduces the incidence of post-operative delirium. *J Int Med Res.* 2010;38:1225.

104. Ethuin F, et al. Pharmacokinetics of long-term sufentanyl infusion for sedation in ICU patients. *Intensive Care Med.* 2003;29:1916.

105. Pasero C, et al. IV opioids range orders for acute pain management. *Am J Nurs.* 2007;107:62.

106. Bhana N, Goa KL, McClellan KJ. Dexmedetomidine. *Drugs.* 2000;59:263.

107. Abramov D, Nogid B, Nogid A. The role of dexmedetomidine (Precedex) in the sedation of critically ill patients. *P and T.* 2005;30:158.

108. Pestieau SR, Quezado ZM, Johnson YJ, et al. High-dose dexmedetomidine increases the opioid-free interval and decreases opioid requirement after tonsillectomy in children. *Can J Anaesth.* 2011;58:540.

109. Ohtani N, Yasui Y, Watanabe D, et al. Perioperative infusion of dexmedetomidine at a high dose reduces postoperative analgesic requirements: a randomized control trial. *J Anesth.* 2011;25:872.

110. Gertler R, Brown C, Mitchell DH, et al. Dexmedetomidine: a novel sedative-analgesic agent. *BUMC Proceedings.* 2001;14:13.

111. Lehne RA. *Pharmacology for Nursing Care.* 8th ed. Philadelphia: Elsevier; 2012.

112. Summer GJ, Puntillo KA. Management of surgical and procedural pain in a critical care setting. *Crit Care Nurs Clin North Am.* 2001;13:233.

113. Feldman HI, et al. Parenteral ketorolac: the risk for acute renal failure. *Ann Intern Med.* 1997;126:193.

114. Strom BL, et al. Parenteral ketorolac and risk of gastrointestinal and operative site bleeding. *JAMA.* 1996;275:376.

115. Faigeles B, Miaskowski C, Howie-Esquivel J, et al. Predictors and use of nonpharmacologic interventions for procedural pain associated with turning among hospitalized adults. *Pain Manag Nurs.* 2010.

116. Tracy MF, et al. Nurse attitudes towards the use of complementary and alternative therapies in critical care. *Heart Lung.* 2003;32:197.

117. Sauls J. The use of ice for pain associated with chest tube removal. *Pain Manag Nurs.* 2002;3:44.

118. Demir Y, Khorshid L. The effect of cold application in combinaison with standard analgesic administration on pain and anxiety during chest tube removal: a single-blinded, randomized, double-controlled study. *Pain Manag Nurs.* 2010;11:186.

119. Bauer BA, et al. Effect of massage therapy on pain, anxiety, and tension in cardiac surgical patients: a randomized study. *Comp Ther Clin Pract.* 2010;16:70.

120. Cutshall SM, et al. Effect of massage therapy on pain, anxiety, and tension in cardiac surgical patients: a pilot study. *Comp Ther Clin Pract.* 2010;16:92.

121. Gélinas C, Michaud C, Arbour C, et al. Evaluation of the feasibility and preliminary effectiveness of hand massage for pain relief in cardiac surgery ICU patients. 2012.

122. Good M, et al. Relief of postoperative pain with jaw relaxation, music and their combination. *Pain.* 1999;81:163.

123. Biley FC. The effects on patient well-being of music listening as a nursing intervention: a review of the literature. *J Clin Nurs.* 2000;9:668.

Sedation, Agitation, Delirium: Assessment and Management

Mary E. Lough

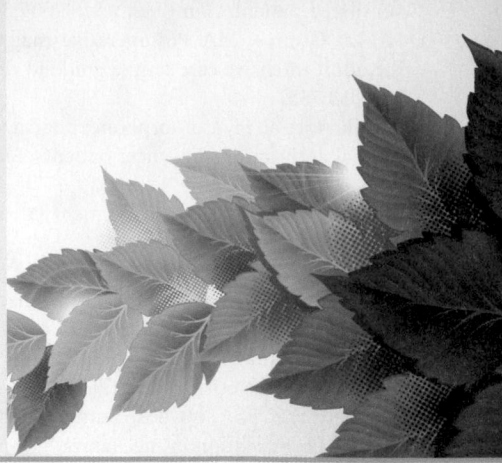

evolve WEBSITE

http://evolve.elsevier.com/Urden/criticalcare/

Evolve features:

- NCLEX Review Questions
- CCRN Review Questions
- PCCN Review Questions
- Mosby's Nursing Skills Procedures
- Animations
- Video Clips
- Glossary

One of the challenges facing clinicians is how to provide a therapeutic healing environment for patients in the alarm-filled, emergency-focused critical care unit. Many critical care patients demonstrate agitation and discomfort caused by painful procedures, invasive tubes, sleep deprivation, fear, anxiety, and physiologic stress. Clinical practice guidelines were developed by the Society of Critical Care Medicine (SCCM) to increase awareness of these issues in the critically ill. The initial guidelines were released in 2002[1] and substantially revised in 2013.[2]

SEDATION

Sedation and Agitation Assessment Scales

The use of scoring systems to assess and record levels of sedation and agitation is now strongly recommended.[1,2] Four frequently used scales are the Ramsay Scale,[3] the Riker Sedation-Agitation Scale (SAS),[4] the Motor Activity Assessment Scale (MAAS),[5] and the Richmond Agitation-Sedation Scale (RASS)[6,7] (Table 10-1). The two scales that are recommended for assessment of agitation and sedation in the adult critically ill patient are the SAS and the RASS.[2] Because individuals do not metabolize sedative medications at the same rate, the use of a standardized scale will ensure that continuous infusions of sedatives such as propofol or dexmedetomidine are titrated to a specific goal. Collaboratively, the critical care team must determine which level of sedation is most appropriate for each individual patient.

Pain Assessment Scales

The first step in assessing the agitated patient is to rule out any sensations of pain.[1,2] Clinical assessment is more challenging when the patient is obtunded or has an artificial airway in place. If the patient can communicate, the verbal pain scale of 0 to 10 is very useful. If the patient is intubated and cannot vocalize, pain assessment becomes considerably more complex. The Behavioral Pain Scale (BPS) and the Critical-Care Pain Observation Scale (CPOT) are the most reliable behavioral pain scales for monitoring of pain in critically ill adults.[2] These pain scales are shown in Table 9-1 (BPS) and Table 9-2 (CPOT) in Chapter 9. Pre-emptive analgesia should be provided before painful procedures.[2] The next step is to determine the minimum level of sedation required[1,2] (Box 10-1). The SCCM guidelines recommend that all critically ill, intubated, mechanically ventilated patients have stated goals for analgesia and sedation.[2] Assessment, treatment and prevention strategies for the management of pain are listed in Figure 9-6 in Chapter 9.

Complications of Sedation

Oversedation is recognized as a state of unintended patient unresponsiveness in which the patient resides in a state of suspended animation resembling general anesthesia. Prolonged deep sedation is associated with significant complications of immobility, including pressure ulcers, thromboemboli, gastric ileus, nosocomial pneumonia, and delayed weaning from mechanical ventilation.

Pharmacologic Management of Sedation

Several categories of sedatives are available. If the patient is experiencing pain, analgesia must be administered in addition to any sedative agents. Sedative agents include the benzodiazepines, sedative-hypnotic agents such as propofol, and the central alpha agonist dexmedetomidine (Table 10-2).[1] Currently

TABLE 10-1 SEDATION SCALES

SCORE	DESCRIPTION	DEFINITION
Riker Sedation-Agitation Scale (SAS)*		
7	Dangerously agitated	Pulls at endotracheal tube (ETT), tries to remove catheters, climbs over bed rail, strikes at staff, thrashes side to side
6	Very agitated	Does not calm despite frequent verbal reminding of limits, requires physical restraints, bites ETT
5	Agitated	Anxious or mildly agitated, attempts to sit up, calms down to verbal instructions
4	Calm and cooperative	Calm, awakens easily, follows commands
3	Sedated	Difficult to arouse, awakens to verbal stimuli or gentle shaking but drifts off again; follows simple commands
2	Very sedated	Arouses to physical stimuli but does not communicate or follow commands; may move spontaneously
1	Unarousable	Minimal or no response to noxious stimuli; does not communicate or follow commands
Motor Activity Assessment Scale (MAAS)†		
6	Dangerously agitated	No external stimulus required to elicit movement; is uncooperative, pulls at tubes or catheters, thrashes side to side, strikes at staff, tries to climb out of bed, does not calm down when asked
5	Agitated	No external stimulus required to elicit movement; attempts to sit up or move limbs out of bed, does not consistently follow commands (e.g., will lie down when asked but soon reverts back to attempts)
4	Restless and cooperative	No external stimulus required to elicit movement; picks at sheets or tubes or uncovers self; follows commands
3	Calm and cooperative	No external stimulus required to elicit movement; adjusts sheets or clothes purposefully; follows commands
2	Responsive to touch or name	Opens eyes, raises eyebrows, or turns head toward stimulus; or moves limbs when touched or when name loudly spoken
1	Responsive only to noxious stimulus	Opens eyes, raises eyebrows, or turns head toward stimulus; or moves limbs with noxious stimulus
0	Unresponsive	Does not move with noxious stimulus
Ramsey Scale‡		
1	Awake	Anxious; agitated and/or restless
2		Cooperative, oriented, and tranquil
3		Responds only to commands
4	Asleep	Brisk response to light glabellar tap or loud auditory stimulus
5		Sluggish response to light glabellar tap or loud auditory stimulus
6		No response to light glabellar tap or loud auditory stimulus

Richmond Agitation-Sedation Scale (RASS)§,‖

Score	Term	Description	
+4	Combative	Overtly combative, violent, immediate danger to staff	
+3	Very agitated	Pulls or removes tube(s) or catheter(s); aggressive	
+2	Agitated	Frequent nonpurposeful movement; fights ventilator	
+1	Restless	Anxious but movements not aggressive vigorous	
0	Alert and calm		
−1	Drowsy	Not fully alert, but has sustained awakening (eye-opening/eye contact) to *voice* (**≤10 seconds**)	Verbal stimulation
−2	Light sedation	Briefly awakens with eye contact to *voice* (<**10 seconds**)	
−3	Moderate sedation	Movement or eye opening to *voice* (**but no eye contact**)	
−4	Deep sedation	No response to voice, but movement or eye opening to *physical* stimulation	Physical stimulation
−5	Unresponsive	No response to *voice* or *physical* stimulation	

*Riker RR, et al. Prospective evaluation of the Sedation-Agitation Scale for adult critically ill patients. *Crit Care Med.* 1999;27:1325-1329.
†Devlin JW, et al. Motor Activity Assessment Scale: a valid and reliable sedation scale for use with mechanically ventilated patients in an adult surgical intensive care unit. *Crit Care Med.* 1999;27:1271-1275.
‡Ramsey MA, et al. Controlled sedation with aiphaxalone-alphadolone. *Br Med J.* 1974;2:656-659.
§Sessler CN, et al. The Richmond Agitation-Sedation Scale: validity and reliability in adult intensive care unit patients. *Am J Respir Crit Gate Med.* 2002;166:1338-1344.
‖Ely EW, et al. Monitoring sedation status over time in ICU patients: reliability and validity of the Richmond Agitation-Sedation Scale (RASS). *JAMA.* 2003;289:2983-2991.

BOX 10-1 LEVELS OF SEDATION

Light Sedation (Minimal Sedation, Anxiolysis)
Medication-induced state during which patients respond normally to verbal commands. Although cognitive function and coordination may be impaired, ventilatory and cardiovascular functions are unaffected.

Moderate Sedation with Analgesia (Conscious Sedation, Procedural Sedation)
Medication-induced depression of consciousness during which patients respond purposefully to verbal commands, alone or accompanied by light tactile stimulation. No interventions are required to maintain a patent airway, and spontaneous ventilation is adequate. Cardiovascular function is usually maintained.

Deep Sedation and Analgesia
Medication-induced depression of consciousness during which patients cannot be easily aroused but respond purposefully after repeated or painful stimulation. The ability to maintain ventilatory function independently is impaired. Patients require assistance in maintaining a patent airway, and spontaneous ventilation may be inadequate. Cardiovascular function is usually maintained.

General Anesthesia
Medication-induced loss of consciousness during which patients are not arousable, even by painful stimulation. The ability to maintain ventilatory function independently is impaired, and assistance to maintain a patent airway is required. Positive-pressure ventilation may be required because of depressed spontaneous ventilation or medication-induced depression of neuromuscular function. Cardiovascular function may be impaired.

Data from Joint Commission on Accreditation of Healthcare Organizations. *Comprehensive Accreditation Manual for Hospitals.* Oakbrook Terrace, IL: The Joint Commission; 2000; Jacobi J, et al. Clinical practice guidelines for the sustained use of sedatives and analgesics in the critically ill adult. *Crit Care Med.* 2002;30:119.

dexmedetomidine-based and propofol-based sedative regimens are recommended for routine sedation of mechanically ventilated adult patients.[2]

Targeted Sedation

All sedatives are to be administered to a specific target level identified by a RASS or SAS level appropriate to the patient's clinical condition (Figure 10-1).[2] A target level is specified every day and reevaluated whenever there is a change in sedation dosage or patient condition. One likely sedation goal is that the patient is awake and calm, specified as a target sedation level of RASS = 0, or SAS = 4. This describes a patient who follows simple verbal commands without agitation and who can sustain eye contact for at least 10 seconds, as described in Table 10-1. When the intent is to provide deep sedation, the target sedation level is specified as RASS = -3 to -5 or SAS = 1 to 2.[2] This describes a mechanically-ventilated patient who is not responsive to voice, but who may respond to physical stimulation (see Table 10-1).

Neuromuscular Blockade

Pharmacologic neuromuscular blockade (NMB) induces a state of physical paralysis. NMB is administered to achieve ventilator synchrony and improve oxygenation when this cannot be achieved by sedation and analgesia alone. Table 21-10 in Chapter 21 lists NMB medications, dosages, and management.

Because NMB causes a pharmacologic paralysis, the patient will not be able to respond to verbal or physical stimuli and additional monitoring methods are required. NMB is never administered unless adequate analgesia and sedation are also provided. This is because NMB paralyzes skeletal muscle but does not alleviate pain or confer sedation. It is vital that measures are in place to avoid a scenario where a patient who has received NMB cannot move, yet retains mental awareness.

Peripheral Muscle Monitoring. A peripheral nerve stimulator (PNS) is used to assess paralysis of skeletal muscle as described in the section on neuromuscular blocking agents in Chapter 21. A PNS stimulator is shown in Figure 21-17.

Brain Function Monitoring. Brain function monitoring is recommended to assess level of consciousness following NMB administration (see Figure 10-1).[2] In the operating room, brain function or activity is routinely monitored during anesthesia to ensure the patient does not have awareness during surgery. Similar monitoring technologies are now recommended for critically ill patients receiving NMB in addition to standard sedation assessments with RASS or SAS.[2] Various technologies are available that monitor the electrical activity of the brain frontal lobes and include electromyelogram (EMG) sensors to record forehead muscle movements.

Benzodiazepines

Benzodiazepines have powerful amnesic properties that inhibit reception of new sensory information.[1,7] Benzodiazepines do not confer analgesia. The most frequently used benzodiazepines are diazepam (Valium), midazolam (Versed), and lorazepam (Ativan). Once a mainstay of sedation, benzodiazepines are no longer recommended for sedation of the mechanically ventilated critically ill adult.[2] This is because benzodiazepine-based sedative regimens are associated with worse patient outcomes, including longer duration of mechanical ventilation and delirium.[8-10]

Short-acting benzodiazepines (midazolam) are still helpful for the treatment of acute short-term agitation,[2] because the intravenous (IV) onset of action is less than 3 minutes. However, when midazolam is administered for longer than 24 hours as a continuous infusion, the sedative effect is prolonged by its active metabolites.[1] Longer acting benzodiazepines (lorazepam and diazepam) also have a role in the management of delirium tremens (described later in the chapter) and seizures,[2] but these are different indications from routine sedation in critical illness.

The major unwanted side effects associated with benzodiazepines are dose-related respiratory depression and hypotension. If needed, flumazenil (Romazicon) is the antidote used to reverse benzodiazepine overdose in symptomatic patients. Flumazenil should be avoided in patients with

TABLE 10-2 **PHARMACOLOGIC MANAGEMENT**

Sedation

MEDICATION	DOSAGE	ACTION	SPECIAL CONSIDERATIONS
Benzodiazepines *Diazepam*	Loading Dose IV: 5-10 mg slowly Maintenance Dose IV: 0.03-01 mg/kg every 0.5-6.0 hr PRN	Anxiolysis Amnesia Sedation	*Onset:* 2-5 min after IV administration *Side effects:* hypotension, respiratory depression *Half-life:* long (20-120 hr); active metabolites also contribute to prolonged sedative effect *Tolerance:* physical tolerance develops with prolonged use, and higher doses of medication are required to achieve the same effect over time; slow wean required from diazepam after continuous prolonged use Phlebitis occurs with peripheral IV administration
Lorazepam	Loading Dose IV: 0.02-0.04 mg/kg (≤2 mg) slowly	Anxiolysis Amnesia Sedation	*Onset:* 15-20 min after IV administration *Side effects:* hypotension, respiratory depression, propylene glycol-related acidosis, nephrotoxicity *Half-life:* relatively long (8-15 hr)
	Intermittent maintenance IV every 2-6 hr: 0.02-0.6 mg/kg slowly Continuous IV maintenance infusion: 0.01-0.1 mg/kg/hr (≤10 mg/hr)		*Tolerance:* physical tolerance develops with use, and higher medication dosage is required to achieve the same effect over time; slow wean required from lorazepam after continuous prolonged use Solvent-related acidosis and kidney failure occur at high doses
Midazolam	Loading Dose IV: 0.01-0.05 mg/kg slowly over several minutes	Anxiolysis Amnesia Sedation	*Onset:* 2-5 min after IV administration *Side effects:* hypotension, respiratory depression *Half-life:* 3-11 hr; sedative effect is prolonged when midazolam infusion has continued for many days, due to presence of active sedative metabolites; sedative effect is also prolonged in kidney failure
	Continuous IV maintenance infusion: 0.02-0.1 mg/kg		*Tolerance:* physical tolerance develops with prolonged use, and higher medication dosages are required to achieve the same effect over time; slow wean required from midazolam after prolonged use
Sedative-Hypnotics *Propofol*	Loading Dose IV: 5 mcg/kg/min over 5 min Continuous IV maintenance infusion: 5-50 mcg/kg/min	Anxiolysis Amnesia Sedation	*Onset:* very rapid onset (1-2 min) after IV administration *Side effects:* hypotension, respiratory depression (patient must be intubated and mechanically ventilated to eliminate this complication), pain at the injection site if administered via peripheral IV; pancreatitis; hyper triglyceridemia, propofol related infusion syndrome (PRIS), allergic reactions *Half-life:* 1-2 min when used as a short-term agent *Half-life:* 3-68 hours with prolonged continuous IV infusion; effective short-term anesthetic agent, useful for rapid "wake-up" of patients for assessment; if continuous infusion is used for many days, emergence from sedation can take hours or days; sedative effect depends on dose administered, depth of sedation, and length of time sedated Change IV infusion tubing every 12 hr Requires a dedicated IV catheter and tubing (do not mix with other medications) Monitor serum triglyceride levels
Central Alpha-Adrenergic Receptor Agonists *Dexmedetomidine*	Loading Dose IV: 1 mcg/kg over 10 min	Anxiolysis Analgesia Sedation	*Onset:* 5-10 min *Side effects:* Bradycardia, hypotension, loss of airway reflexes *Half life:* 1.8-3.1 hr. No active metabolites Intermittent bolus dosing is not recommended
	Continuous IV maintenance infusion: 0.2-0.7 mcg/kg/min		Maintenance infusion is adjusted to achieve desired level of sedation

Barr J, et al. Clinical Practice Guidelines for the Management of Pain, Agitation, and Delirium in Adult Patients in the Intensive Care Unit. *Crit Care Med.* 2013;41(1):278.

AGITATION

ASSESS

Assess agitation, sedation ≥ 4 times/shift and prn
Preferred sedation assessment tools:
- RASS(−5 TO +4) or SAS (1 to 7)
- NMB → suggest using brain
  function monitoring

Depth of agitation, sedation defined as:
- *Agitated* if RASS = +1 to +4, or SAS = 5 to 7
- *Awake and calm* if RASS = 0, or SAS = 4
- *Lightly sedated* if RASS = −1 to −2, or SAS = 3
- *Deeply sedated* if RASS = −3 to −5, or SAS = 1 to 2

TREAT

Targeted sedation *(Goal: patient purposely follows commands without agitation):*
RASS = −2-0, SAS = 3-4
- If *under sedated* (RASS >0, SAS >4)
  assess/treat pain → treat with sedatives prn
  (non-benzodiazepines preferred, unless alcohol
  withdrawal or benzodiazepine withdrawal is
  suspected)
- If *over sedated* (RASS < −2, SAS <3) hold
  sedatives until at target, then restart at
  50% of previous dose

PREVENT

- Consider daily SBT, early mobility and exercise
  when patients are at goal sedation level, unless
  contraindicated

DELIRIUM

Assess delirium every shift and prn
Preferred delirium assessment tools:
- CAM-ICU (+ or −)
- ICDSC (0 to 8)

Delirium present if:
- CAM-ICU is positive
- ICDSC 4

- Treat pain as needed
- Reorient patients; familiarize
  surroundings; use patient's eyeglasses,
  hearing aids if needed
- Pharmacologic treatment of delirium:
  – Avoid benzodiazepines unless alcohol
    withdrawal or benzodiazepine withdrawal
    is suspected
  – Avoid rivastigmine
  – Avoid antipsychotics if increased risk of
    Torsades de pointes

- Identify delirium risk factors: dementia,
  HTN, alcohol abuse, high severity of illness,
  coma, benzodiazepine administration
- Avoid benzodiazepine use in those at
  increased risk for delirium
- Mobilize and exercise patients early
- Promote sleep (control light, noise; cluster
  patient care activities; decrease nocturnal
  stimuli)
- Restart baseline psychiatric medications,
  if indicated

FIGURE 10-1 **Agitation and Delirium Care Bundle.** *CAM-ICU,* Confusion Assessment Method for the Intensive Care Unit; *HTN,* hypertension; *ICDSC,* Intensive Care Delirium Screening Checklist; *NMB,* neuromuscular blockade; *RASS,* Richmond Agitation-Sedation Scale; *SAS,* Riker Sedation-Agitation Scale; *SBT,* spontaneous breathing trial. (From Barr J, Fraser GL, Puntillo KA, Ely WE, Gelinas C, Dasta JF, et al. Clinical practice guidelines for the management of pain, agitation, and delirium in adult patients in the intensive care unit. *Critical Care Medicine.* 2013, in press.)

benzodiazepine dependence, because rapid withdrawal can induce seizures.[11]

Sedative-Hypnotic Agents

Propofol is a powerful sedative and respiratory depressant used for sedation in mechanically ventilated patients in critical care. It is immediately identifiable by its white milky appearance, always in a glass container. At high doses (>100 to 200 mcg/kg/min), propofol is intended to produce a state of general anesthesia in the operating room.[12] In the critical care unit, propofol is prescribed as a continuous infusion at lower doses (5 to 50 mcg/kg/min) to induce a state of deep sedation.[12] Because propofol is lipid soluble it quickly crosses cell membranes, including the cells that comprise the blood-brain barrier. This allows rapid onset of sedation (about 30 seconds), with immediate loss of consciousness. In addition to a rapid onset of action propofol has very short half-life with initial use (2 to 4 minutes), is rapidly eliminated from the body (30 to 60 minutes), and does not have metabolites.[12,13] This makes it an ideal sedative for use when a patient needs to be quickly awakened for a spontaneous awakening trial (SAT) and spontaneous

breathing trial (SBT), or to assess neurologic status. This feature makes propofol an ideal medication to manage rapid ventilator weaning postsurgery. Propofol is both clinically effective and cost effective because it shortens time to extubation. It is important to add an opiate to ensure adequate pain control and amnesia. Propofol is not a reliable amnesic, and patients sedated with only propofol can have vivid recollections of their experiences.

Risks of unwanted complications increase when propofol is administered long term at high doses (>4.00 mg/kg/hr for longer than 48 hours). Propofol is delivered in a fat-based emulsion, and side effects may be related to disruption of fatty acid metabolism, muscle injury, and release of toxic intracellular contents. Complications have been collectively grouped under the term *Propofol Related Infusion Syndrome* (PRIS) including: metabolic acidosis, muscular weakness, rhabdomyolysis, myoglobinuria, acute kidney injury, and cardiovascular dysrhythmias. PRIS affects about 1% of all patients who receive propofol; almost one third of those affected will not survive.[8,13,14] Other secondary side effects related to the fat-emulsion carrier include hyperlipidemia, hypertriglyceridemia, and acute pancreatitis.

Nursing vigilance is required to monitor sedation levels, and to be alert for the rare but significant risk of propofol-related complications. Serum triglycerides should be measured on all patients who receive propofol for longer than 48 hours. For additional information see Table 10-2.

Central Alpha Agonists

Two central alpha-adrenergic agonists with sedative properties are available. *Clonidine* is often prescribed as a Catapres patch and *dexmedetomidine* (Precedex) as a continuous infusion. Clonidine may be prescribed for patients experiencing alcohol withdrawal syndrome (see later in chapter).

Dexmedetomidine is an alpha-2 agonist that is FDA approved for use as a short-term sedative (<24 hours) in mechanically ventilated patients. Sedation occurs when the medication activates postsynaptic alpha-2 receptors in the central nervous system in the brain. This activation inhibits norepinephrine release and blocks sympathetic nervous system (SNS) fight-or-flight functions, leading to sedation. SNS inhibition may cause hypotension and bradydysrhythmias, both well-known side effects of dexmedetomidine. Analgesic effects occur because dexmedetomidine binds to alpha-2 receptors in the spinal cord. These unique mechanisms of action allow patients to be sedated but still arousable, factors that are associated with a shorter time to extubation compared with traditional sedative regimens.

Dexmedetomidine is prescribed with a loading dose of 1.0 mcg/kg over 10 minutes, followed by a continuous infusion of 0.4 mcg/kg (range 0.2 to 0.7 mcg/kg/hr).[15] Dexmedetomidine has a short half-life (6 minutes) and is eliminated from the body in about 2 hours.[15] Elimination from the body is dramatically slowed if the patient has liver failure (see Table 10-2). Complications include bradycardia and hypotension.[16]

Many patients will have other sedatives or opiates infusing in addition to dexmedetomidine, and the combination may potentiate the overall sedative effect. Monitoring of sedation level, blood pressure, heart rate, respiratory rate, and pulse oximetry are mandatory. Dexmedetomidine confers sedation and analgesic effects without respiratory depression.[15] Consequently patients can be extubated while still on a dexmedetomidine infusion. This can be helpful for patients who are anxious during ventilator weaning. Dexmedetomidine has also been used for patients on noninvasive mask ventilation.[17] Because of this favorable profile many clinicians now use dexmedetomidine as a first-line sedative agent.[18]

Daily Sedation Interruption

One innovative strategy to avoid the pitfalls of sedative dependence and withdrawal is a planned strategy to turn off the sedative infusions once each day.[2] This intervention has been given several names, including *sedation vacation* and *spontaneous awakening trial* (SAT). At a scheduled time, all continuously infusing sedatives are stopped. Sometimes analgesics are also stopped, depending on the hospital's protocol. The patient is allowed to regain consciousness for clinical assessment using a standardized instrument such as the RASS or SAS (see Table 10-1).[19,20] The patient is carefully monitored, and when awareness is attained, an assessment of level of consciousness and

TABLE 10-3 SIGNS AND SYMPTOMS OF SEDATIVE OR ANALGESIC MEDICATION WITHDRAWAL*

SYSTEM	OPIATE WITHDRAWAL	BENZODIAZEPINE WITHDRAWAL[†]
Neurologic	Delirium, tremors, seizures	Agitation, anxiety, delirium, tremors, myoclonus, headache, seizures, fatigue, paresthesias, sleep disturbances
Sensory	Dilation of pupils, teary eyes, irritability, increased sensitivity to pain, sweating, yawning	Increased sensitivity to light/sound, sweating
Musculoskeletal	Cramps, muscle aches	Muscle cramps
Gastrointestinal	Vomiting, diarrhea	Nausea, diarrhea
Respiratory	Tachypnea	Tachypnea

*Data on propofol is limited, but withdrawal symptoms after prolonged use are similar to those of the benzodiazepines.[1]
[†]Not all symptoms are seen in all patients.[1]

neurologic function is performed. If the patient becomes agitated, it is essential that a protocol be in place for the nurse to restart the sedatives. One protocol scheduled the daily interruption of sedatives in the morning and recommended, after a full assessment, restarting the sedative and opiate infusions at 50% of the previous morning dose and adjusting upward until the patient was comfortable.[19]

An important nursing responsibility is to prevent the patient from coming to harm during sedative or analgesic medication withdrawal (Table 10-3). If the patient is seriously agitated, it is vital to consult with the physician and pharmacist to establish an effective treatment plan that will allow safe weaning from sedative medications (see Table 10-1).

AGITATION

Agitation describes hyperactive patient movements that range in intensity from slight restless hand and body movements, to pulling out lines and tubes, or physical aggression and self-harm. Agitation can be caused by, pain, anxiety, delirium, hypoxia, ventilator dyssynchrony, neurological injury, uncomfortable position, full bladder, sleep deprivation, alcohol withdrawal, sepsis, medication reaction, or organ failure, to name but a few frequently encountered causes. In the past, when a patient showed physical signs of agitation, a benzodiazepine sedative (lorazepam or midazolam) was quickly administered to reduce the patient's mental awareness (see Table 10-2). However, because benzodiazepines have been shown to induce delirium, it is now recommended that proactive assessments be conducted at least 4 times in a nursing shift (see Figure 10-1).[2]

Agitation is assessed using a validated scale such as the SAS or RASS (see Table 10-1).[2] Standardized assessment scales allow clinicians to identify agitation in its milder forms and to potentially ameliorate the patient's symptoms. The goal is to treat the

BOX 10-2 CAUSES OF DELIRIUM IN CRITICALLY ILL PATIENTS

Metabolic Causes
- Acid-base disturbance
- Electrolyte imbalance
- Hypoglycemia

Intracranial Causes
- Epidural or subdural hematoma
- Intracranial hemorrhage
- Meningitis
- Encephalitis
- Cerebral abscess
- Tumor

Endocrine Causes
- Hyperthyroidism or hypothyroidism
- Addison's disease
- Hyperparathyroidism
- Cushing's syndrome

Organ Failure
- Liver encephalopathy
- Kidney encephalopathy
- Septic shock

Respiratory Causes
- Hypoxemia
- Hypercarbia

Medication-Related Causes
- Alcohol withdrawal syndrome
- Benzodiazepines
- Heavy metal poisoning

Modified from Szokol JW, Vender JS. Anxiety, delirium, and pain in the intensive care unit. *Crit Care Clin.* 2001;17(4):821.

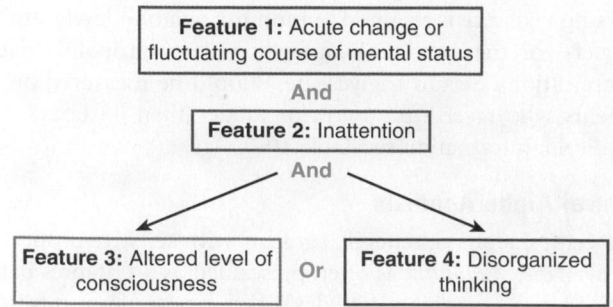

FIGURE 10-2 The Confusion Assessment Method for the ICU (CAM-ICU). Delirium is defined as positive in Feature 1 AND Feature 2 and EITHER Feature 3 OR Feature 4.

Checklist (ICDSC) (Fig. 10-4).[28,29] Both instruments are used in tandem with the RASS to exclude patients in coma and identify delirium. Coma is a known risk factor for development of delirium.[2] Both the CAM-ICU and ICDSC provide a structured format to evaluate delirium both for verbal patients and for nonverbal and mechanically ventilated patients.

Pharmacologic Management of Delirium

Pharmacologic treatment of delirium remains challenging.[2] The neuroleptic medication haloperidol (Haldol) has traditionally been administered to treat hyperactive delirium.[30] This antipsychotic agent stabilizes cerebral function by blocking dopamine-mediated neurotransmission at the cerebral synapses and in the basal ganglia. Electrocardiographic (ECG) monitoring is recommended, because haloperidol prolongs the QTc-interval, increasing the risk of ventricular dysrhythmias. Haloperidol and other antipsychotics should be avoided in patients who have a prolonged QTc or a history of torsades de pointes.[2]

Atypical antipsychotics are sometimes administered to treat delirium associated with critical illness. These are medications that were developed to treat another condition, such as schizophrenia or bipolar disorder, which are administered to shorten the duration of delirium in critical illness. In a small clinical trial of mechanically ventilated patients, quetiapine was associated with a faster resolution of delirium compared with placebo.[31,32] Other antipsychotics need to be subjected to the rigors of a clinical trial. This is needed because there is limited evidence on the efficacy and safety of atypical antipsychotics used to treat delirium in critical illness. The cholinesterase inhibitor medication rivastigmine should be avoided as it is associated with higher mortality.[33]

Haloperidol or other atypical antipsychotics are not to be administered prophylactically as prevention against delirium because there is no evidence that this reduces the incidence of delirium.[2]

Nonpharmacologic Interventions to Prevent Delirium

Delirium is frequently associated with critical illness.[2] Provision of adequate sleep and early mobilization are recommended to reduce the incidence of delirium.[2] The nonpharmacologic strategies used to prevent agitation and delirium are similar to those used as adjuncts to minimize pain.[2] These methods include

cause of the agitation rather than to over-medicate. Obviously, when a patient is dangerously agitated (SAS +7), is combative (RASS +4), or could endanger themselves or others, immediate sedation is warranted. In these extreme situations, a benzodiazepine is administered.[2]

DELIRIUM

Delirium represents a global impairment of cognitive processes, usually of sudden onset, coupled with disorientation, impaired short-term memory, altered sensory perceptions (i.e., hallucinations), abnormal thought processes, and inappropriate behavior. Routine monitoring for delirium is recommended.[2] Delirium is more prevalent than generally recognized; it is difficult to diagnose in the critically ill patient and represents acute brain dysfunction caused by sepsis, critical illness, or dysfunction of other vital organs (Box 10-2). Between 60% and 85% of mechanically ventilated patients experience delirium.[21] Delirium increases hospital stay and mortality rates for patients who are mechanically ventilated.[22] The increased mortality remains even after controlling for associated variables such as coma and administration of sedatives and analgesics.[22]

When patients are agitated, restless, and pulling at tubes and lines, they are often identified as being delirious. In this scenario, delirium may be described as "ICU psychosis" or "sundowner syndrome." However, the delirious patient is not always agitated, and it is much more difficult to detect delirium when the patient is physically calm.[1,23] Provision of adequate analgesia is an essential component of delirium prevention.[2]

Specific scoring instruments are available to assess delirium, and two have been validated for use with mechanically ventilated critical care patients.[2,24] They are the *Confusion Assessment Method for the Intensive Care Unit* (CAM-ICU) (Fig. 10-2 and Fig. 10-3)[25-27] and the *Intensive Care Delirium Screening*

RICHMOND AGITATION-SEDATION SCALE (RASS)

Step 1 Sedation Assessment

Scale	Label	Description	
+4	COMBATIVE	Combative, violent, immediate danger to staff	V
+3	VERY AGITATED	Pulls to remove tubes or catheters; aggressive	O
+2	AGITATED	Frequent non-purposeful movement, fights ventilator	I
+1	RESTLESS	Anxious, apprehensive, movements not aggressive	C
0	ALERT & CALM	Spontaneously pays attention to caregiver	E
−1	DROWSY	Not fully alert, but has sustained awakening to voice (eye opening & contact >10 sec)	
−2	LIGHT SEDATION	Briefly awakens to voice (eyes open & contact <10 sec)	
−3	MODERATE SEDATION	Movement or eye opening to voice (no eye contact)	

→ **If RASS is ≥−3 proceed to CAM-ICU (is patient CAM-ICU positive or negative?)**

			T
−4	DEEP SEDATION	No response to voice, but movement or eye opening to physical stimulation	O U
−5	UNAROUSABLE	No response to voice or physical stimulation	C H

→ **If RASS is −4 or −5 → STOP (patient unconscious), RECHECK later**

Confusion Assessment Method for the ICU (CAM-ICU)

Step 2 Delirium Assessment

1. Acute Change or Fluctuating Course of Mental Status:
- Is there an acute change from mental status baseline? **OR**
- Has the patient's mental status fluctuated during the past 24 hours?

— No → **CAM-ICU negative NO DELIRIUM**

↓ YES

2. Inattention:
- *"Squeeze my hand when I say the letter 'A'."*
  Read the following sequence of letters: S A V E A H A A R T
  ERRORS: No squeeze with 'A' & Squeeze on letter other than 'A'
- If unable to complete letters → Pictures

0–2 Errors → **CAM-ICU negative NO DELIRIUM**

↓ > 2 Errors

3. Altered Level of Consciousness
Current RASS level (think back to sedation assessment in Step 1)

RASS other than zero → **CAM-ICU positive DELIRIUM present**

↓ RASS = zero

4. Disorganized thinking:
1. Will a stone float on water?
2. Are there fish in the sea?
3. Does one pound weigh more than two?
4. Can you use a hammer to pound a nail?

Command: "Hold up this many fingers" (Hold up 2 fingers)
"Now do the same thing with the other hand" (Do not demonstrate)
OR "Add one more finger" (If patient unable to move both arms)

>1 Error → **CAM-ICU positive DELIRIUM present**

0–1 Error → **CAM-ICU negative NO DELIRIUM**

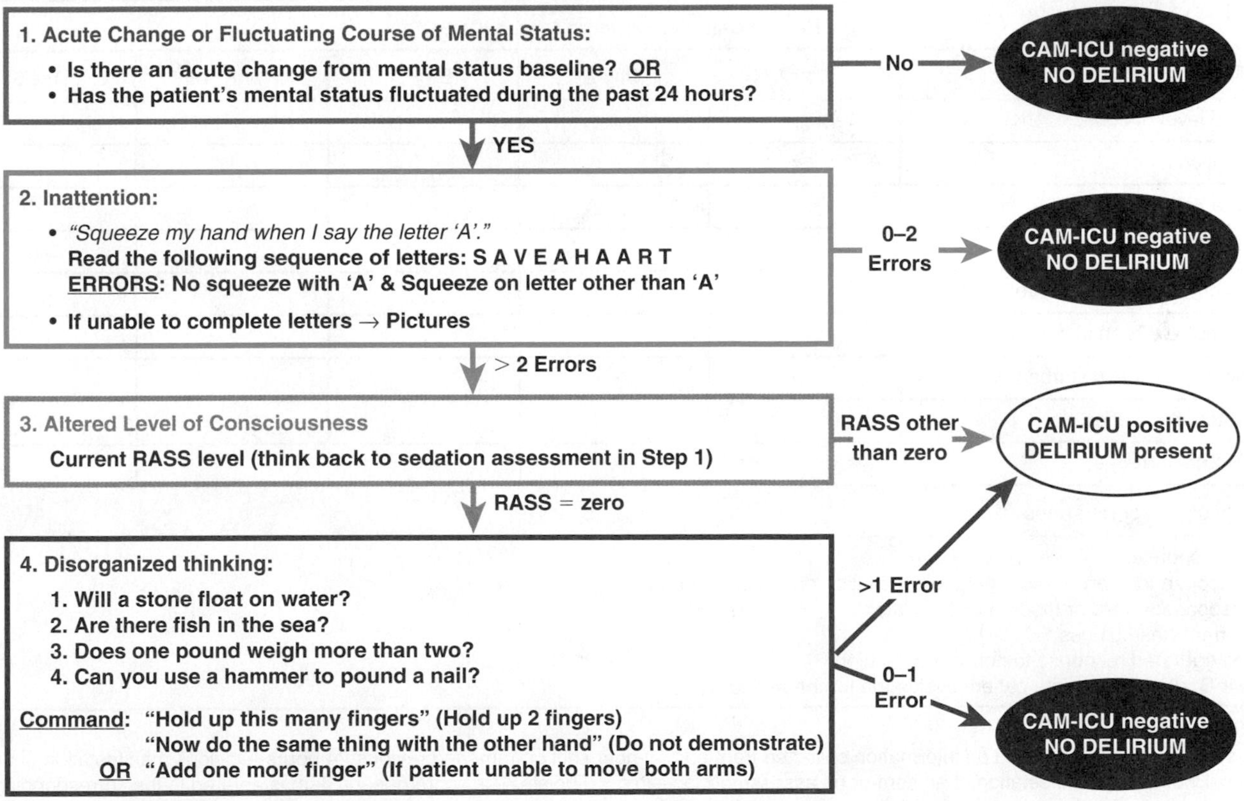

FIGURE 10-3 The Confusion Assessment Method for the ICU (CAM-ICU) Delirium Assessment. Step 1—Sedation Assessment; Step 2—Delirium Assessment. (Copyright 2002, E. Wesley Ely, MD, MPH and Vanderbilt University, all rights reserved.)

The Intensive Care Delirium Screening Checklist (ICDSC)

1. Altered level of consciousness

(A) No response or (B) the need for vigorous stimulation in order to obtain any response signified a severe alteration in the level of consciousness precluding evaluation. If there is coma (A) or stupor (B) most of the time period, then a dash (—) is entered and there is no further evaluation for that period.

(C) Drowsiness or response to a mild to moderate stimulation implies an altered level of consciousness and scores 1 point.

(D) Wakefulness or sleeping state that could easily be aroused is considered normal and scores zero points.

(E) Hypervigilance is rated as an abnormal level of consciousness and scores 1 point.

2. Inattention

Difficulty in following a conversation or instruction, easily distracted by external stimuli, or difficulty in shifting focus all score 1 point.

3. Disorientation

Any obvious mistake in time, place or person scores 1 point.

4. Hallucination, delusion or psychosis

The unequivocal clinical manifestation of hallucination or of behaviour probably due to hallucination (e.g., trying to catch a non-existent object) or delusion, or gross impairment in reality testing all score 1 point.

5. Psychomotor agitation or retardation

Hyperactivity requiring the use of additional sedative drugs or restraints in order to control potential danger (e.g., pulling out IV lines, hitting staff), hypoactivity or clinically noticeable psychomotor slowing all score 1 point.

6. Inappropriate speech or mood

Inappropriate, disorganized or incoherent speech, inappropriate mood related to events or situation all score 1 point.

7. Sleep/wake cycle disturbance

Sleeping less than four hours or waking frequently at night (do not consider wakefulness initiated by medical staff or loud environment), or sleeping during most of the day all score 1 point.

8. Symptom fluctuation

Fluctuation of the manifestation of any item or symptom over 24 hours (e.g., from one shift to another) scores 1 point.

How to Calculate a Score for the ICDSC*

Patient Evaluation	Day 1	Day 2	Day 3	Day 4	Day 5
Altered level of consciousness (A-E)*					
Inattention					
Disorientation					
Hallucination, delusion, psychosis					
Psychomotor agitation or retardation					
Inappropriate speech or mood					
Sleep-wake cycle disturbance					
Symptom fluctuation					
Total Score (0-8)					

*Level of Consciousness	Score
A: no response	–
B: response to intense and repeated stimulation (loud voice and pain)	–
C: response to mild or moderate stimulation	1
D: normal wakefulness	0
E: exaggerated response to normal stimulation	1
If **A** or **B**, do not complete patient evaluation for the period.	

Scoring System

The scale is completed based on information collected from each 8-hour shift or from the previous 24 hours. Obvious manifestation of an item = 1 point. No manifestation of an item or no assessment possible = 0 points. The score of each item is entered in the corresponding space and is 0 or 1. A total score of ≥4 on any given day has a 99% sensitivity for correlation with a psychiatric diagnosis of delirium.

*The ICDSC is also used in tandem with the RASS (see Table 10-1) to assess sedation-agitation in addition to delirium.

FIGURE 10-4 The Intensive Care Delirium Screening Checklist (ICDSC). The ICDSC is also used in tandem with the RASS scale (see Table 10-1) to assess sedation-agitation in addition to delirium. (From Bergeron N, et al. Intensive Care Delirium Screening Checklist: evaluation of a new screening tool. *Intensive Care Med.* 2001;27:859.)

back massage, music therapy, noise reduction, decreasing lights at night to promote sleep, clustering nursing care interventions to provide some uninterrupted rest, and speaking in a calm and gentle voice. Some pre-existing conditions increase the likelihood that a patient will experience delirium, including dementia, alcohol use disorder, and prior sedative/opiate dependence.

ALCOHOL WITHDRAWAL SYNDROME AND DELIRIUM TREMENS

Critically ill patients who are alcohol dependent and were drinking prior to hospital admission are at risk of *alcohol withdrawal syndrome* (AWS).[34] AWS is associated with an increased risk of delirium, hallucinations, seizures, increased need for mechanical ventilation, and death. When hyperactive agitated delirium is caused by alcohol withdrawal, it is termed *delirium tremens,* often verbally described as *DTs.*[34] Following hospital admission, as the alcohol-dependent patient's blood-alcohol concentration (BAC) falls, about 50% of patients will have AWS-related symptoms.[35] Fewer than 5% will experience severe complications such as DTs or a seizure.[34,35] Screening tools to identify alcohol dependence such as the *Alcohol Use Disorders Identification Test* (AUDIT) shown in Table 34-1 in the Trauma chapter are very helpful. Management of alcohol withdrawal involves close monitoring of AWS-related agitation, and administration of IV benzodiazepines, generally diazepam (Valium) or lorazepam (Ativan). Diazepam has the advantage of a longer half-life and high lipid solubility.[34] Lipid-soluble medications quickly cross the blood-brain barrier and enter the central nervous system to rapidly produce a sedative effect.[34,36] Benzodiazepines should be administered in response to increased signs of agitation associated with DTs, with dosage guided by a clinical protocol. This is described as an AWS symptom-triggered approach.[34] The severity of alcohol withdrawal can be assessed with a scale such as the Clinical Institute Withdrawal Assessment of Alcohol Scale (revised) (CIWA-Ar).[34,36] Multivitamins, including thiamine (Vitamin B_1), are administered prophylactically to prevent additional neurologic sequelae.[34-37] Delirium related to alcohol withdrawal is pharmacologically managed very differently than delirium from other causes. Long-acting benzodiazepines are the medications of choice in AWS.[34] In contrast; benzodiazepines are contraindicated for treatment of delirium from non–alcohol-related causes.[38]

COLLABORATIVE MANAGEMENT

Collaborative management of anxiety, agitation, sedation, and delirium is a responsibility shared by all members of the health care team, as indicated by the clinical practice guidelines summarized in Box 10-3. Recognition of the problem is the first step toward a solution to establish a more effective standard of patient care in sedation, analgesia, and delirium management.

BOX 10-3 EVIDENCE-BASED PRACTICE

Summary of Guidelines for Assessment and Treatment of Agitation and Delirium

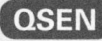 • Agitation in critically ill patients may result from inadequately treated pain, anxiety, delirium, and/or ventilator dysynchrony.
- Detection and treatment of pain, agitation, and delirium should be reassessed often in these patients.
- Patients should be awake and able to purposely follow commands in order to participate in their care unless a clinical indication for deeper sedation exists.

Agitation
- Depth and quality of sedation should be routinely assessed in all ICU patients.
- The RASS and SAS are the most valid and reliable scales for assessing quality and depth of sedation in ICU patients.
- Target the lightest possible level of sedation and/or use daily sedative interruption.
- Use sedation protocols and checklists to facilitate ICU sedation management.
- Suggest using analgesia-first sedation for intubated and mechanically-ventilated ICU patients.

- Suggest using non-benzodiazepines for sedation (either propofol or dexmedetomidine) rather than benzodiazepines (either midazolam or lorazepam) in mechanically-ventilated adult ICU patients.

Delirium
- Delirium assessment should be routinely performed in all ICU patients.
- The CAM-ICU and ICDSC delirium monitoring tools are the most valid and reliable scales to assess delirium in ICU patients.
- Mobilize ICU patients early when feasible to reduce the incidence and duration of delirium, and to improve functional outcomes.
- Promote sleep in ICU patients by controlling light and noise, clustering patient care activities, and decreasing stimuli at night.
- Avoid using rivastigmine to reduce the duration of delirium in ICU patients.
- Suggest avoiding the use of antipsychotics in patients who are at risk for torsades de pointes.
- Suggest not using benzodiazepines in ICU patients with delirium unrelated to alcohol/benzodiazepine withdrawal.

From Barr J, Fraser GL, Puntillo KA, Ely WE, Gelinas C, Dasta JF, et al. Clinical practice guidelines for the management of pain, agitation, and delirium in adult patients in the intensive care unit. *Critical Care Medicine.* 2013, in press.

BOX 10-4   CASE STUDY

Patient with Delirium

Brief Patient History

Mr. K is a 42-year-old, Asian, out-of-town businessman in your city. He is transported to your facility from his hotel because of a witnessed grand mal seizure. Paramedics administered lorazepam in the field. Mr. K's wife reports by phone that he is in good health and that she is not aware that he takes any medications regularly. However, she states that he recently quit drinking alcohol because of pressure from the family. She also comments that she thinks he takes alprazolam to calm his nerves once in a while.

Clinical Assessment

Mr. K is admitted to the critical care unit from the emergency department with hypertension, restlessness, mental confusion, paranoid ideations with rambling speech, and visual and auditory hallucinations. Mr. K's skin is warm and moist. Intravenous administration of thiamine, folic acid, multivitamins, and magnesium was begun in the emergency department. Physician orders were written for lorazepam every 6 hours and clonidine every 4 hours as needed for delirium-related symptoms.

Diagnostic Procedures

Mr. K's baseline vital signs are as follows: blood pressure of 190/92 mm Hg, heart rate of 130 beats/min (sinus tachycardia), respiratory rate of 26 breaths/min, and temperature of 98.8° F. Pulse oximetry O_2 saturation is 90% on 4 L/min oxygen using a nasal cannula. Confusion Assessment Method indicates presence of acute and fluctuating change in mental status, inattention, and disorganized thinking. The *Sedation-Agitation Scale* (SAS) score is 5. Serum and urine toxicology studies are negative for ethyl alcohol, cannabis, and opioids; urine is strongly positive for benzodiazepines. The sodium level is 135 mmol/L, potassium level is 4.3 mmol/L, chloride level is 84 mmol/L, carbon dioxide level is 26 mEq/L, calcium level is 8 mg/dL; magnesium level is 2.0 mg/dL, and gamma-glutamyl transpeptidase (GGT) level is 80 IU/L.

Medical Diagnosis

Mr. K is diagnosed with delirium tremens caused by alcohol and benzodiazepine withdrawal.

Questions

1. What major outcomes do you expect to achieve for this patient?
2. What problems or risks must be managed to achieve these outcomes?
3. What interventions must be initiated to monitor, prevent, manage, or eliminate the problems and risks identified?
4. What interventions should be initiated to promote optimal functioning, safety, and well-being of the patient?
5. What possible learning needs do you anticipate for this patient?
6. What cultural and age-related factors may have a bearing on the patient's plan of care?

■ SUMMARY

- Use a validated sedation instrument (RASS or SAS) and titrate sedation medications to achieve the lightest possible level of sedation to prevent immobility-associated problems and delirium.
- Benzodiazepines are not recommended for routine sedation of mechanically ventilated adult patients.
- Dexmedetomidine and propofol are recommended for sedation of mechanically ventilated adult patients.
- Daily interruption of sedation and a spontaneous breathing trial are recommended for patients who are mechanically ventilated.
- Delirium is a frequent complication of critical illness. Delirium can be hypoactive (withdrawn) or hyperactive (with agitation).

- Use a validated delirium assessment instrument (CAM-ICU or ICDSC) to identify delirium.
- Pharmacologic management of delirium includes treatment with haloperidol and sometimes atypical antipsychotics.
- Non-pharmacologic interventions to prevent delirium include provision of adequate sleep and early mobility.
- Delirium tremens is a complication of alcohol withdrawal syndrome.
- The benzodiazepines, diazepam (Valium) or lorazepam (Ativan) are used in the treatment of delirium tremens.

REFERENCES

1. Jacobi J, et al. Clinical practice guidelines for the sustained use of sedatives and analgesics in the critically ill adult. *Crit Care Med.* 2002;30:119-141.
2. Barr J, Fraser GL, Puntillo KA, Ely WE, Gelinas C, Dasta JF, et al. Clinical practice guidelines for the management of pain, agitation, and delirium in adult patients in the intensive care unit. *Critical Care Medicine.* 2013, in press.
3. Ramsay MA, et al. Controlled sedation with alphaxalone-alphadolone. *Br Med J.* 1974;2:656-659.
4. Riker RR, et al. Prospective evaluation of the Sedation-Agitation Scale for adult critically ill patients. *Crit Care Med.* 1999;27:1325-1329.
5. Devlin JW, et al. Motor Activity Assessment Scale: a valid and reliable sedation scale for use with mechanically ventilated patients in an adult surgical intensive care unit. *Crit Care Med.* 1999;27:1271-1275.
6. Ely EW, et al. Monitoring sedation status over time in ICU patients: reliability and validity of the Richmond Agitation-Sedation Scale (RASS). *JAMA.* 2003;289:2983-2991.
7. Sessler CN, et al. The Richmond Agitation-Sedation Scale: validity and reliability in adult intensive care unit patients. *Am J Respir Crit Care Med.* 2002;166:1338-1344.
8. Fong JJ, et al. Propofol associated with a shorter duration of mechanical ventilation than scheduled intermittent lorazepam: a database analysis using Project IMPACT. *Ann Pharmacother.* 2007;41:1986-1991.
9. Pandharipande P, et al. Lorazepam is an independent risk factor for transitioning to delirium in intensive care unit patients. *Anesthesiology.* 2006;104:21-26.

10. Pandharipande PP, et al. Effect of sedation with dexmedetomidine vs lorazepam on acute brain dysfunction in mechanically ventilated patients: the MENDS randomized controlled trial. *JAMA.* 2007;298:2644-2653.
11. Betten DP, et al. Antidote use in the critically ill poisoned patient. *J Intensive Care Med.* 2006;21:255-277.
12. Whitcomb JJ, et al. The use of propofol in the mechanically ventilated medical/surgical intensive care patient: is it the right choice? *Dimens Crit Care Nurs.* 2003;22:60-63.
13. Zaccheo MM, Bucher DH. Propofol infusion syndrome: a rare complication with potentially fatal results. *Crit Care Nurse.* 2008;28:18-26.
14. Corbett SM, et al. Propofol-related infusion syndrome in intensive care patients. *Pharmacotherapy.* 2008;28:250-258.
15. Lam SW, Alexander E. Dexmedetomidine use in critical care. *AACN Advanced Critical Care.* 2008;19:113-120.
16. Tan JA, Ho KM. Use of dexmedetomidine as a sedative and analgesic agent in critically ill adult patients: a meta-analysis. *Intensive Care Med.* 2010;36(6):926-939.
17. Akada S, et al. The efficacy of dexmedetomidine in patients with noninvasive ventilation: a preliminary study. *Anesth Analg.* 2008;107:167-170.
18. Pichot C, et al. Dexmedetomidine and clonidine: from second- to first-line sedative agents in the critical care setting? *J Intensive Care Med.* 2012;27(4):219-237.
19. Kress JP, et al. Daily interruption of sedative infusions in critically ill patients undergoing mechanical ventilation. *N Engl J Med.* 2005;342:1471-1477.
20. Girard TD, et al. Efficacy and safety of a paired sedation and ventilator weaning protocol for mechanically ventilated patients in intensive care (Awakening and Breathing Controlled trial): a randomised controlled trial. *Lancet.* 2008;371:126-134.
21. Pun BT, Ely EW. The importance of diagnosing and managing ICU delirium. *Chest.* 2007;132:624-636.
22. Ely EW, et al. Delirium as a predictor of mortality in mechanically ventilated patients in the intensive care unit. *JAMA.* 2004;291:1753-1762.
23. Roberts BL, et al. Patients' dreams in ICU: recall at two years post discharge and comparison to delirium status during ICU admission. A multicentre cohort study. *Intensive Crit Care Nurs.* 2006;22:264-273.
24. Plaschke K, et al. Comparison of the confusion assessment method for the intensive care unit (CAM-ICU) with the Intensive Care Delirium Screening Checklist (ICDSC) for delirium in critical care patients gives high agreement rate(s). *Intensive Care Med.* 2008;34:431-436.
25. Ely EW, et al. Evaluation of delirium in critically ill patients: validation of the Confusion Assessment Method for the Intensive Care Unit (CAM-ICU). *Crit Care Med.* 2001;29:1370-1379.
26. Ely EW, et al. Delirium in mechanically ventilated patients: validity and reliability of the confusion assessment method for the intensive care unit (CAM-ICU). *JAMA.* 2001;286:2703-2710.
27. Pun BT, et al. Large-scale implementation of sedation and delirium monitoring in the intensive care unit: a report from two medical centers. *Crit Care Med.* 2005;33:1199-1205.
28. Bergeron N, et al. Intensive Care Delirium Screening Checklist: evaluation of a new screening tool. *Intensive Care Med.* 2001;27:859-864.
29. Ouimet S, et al. Subsyndromal delirium in the ICU: evidence for a disease spectrum. *Intensive Care Med.* 2007;33:1007-1013.
30. Milbrandt EB, et al. Haloperidol use is associated with lower hospital mortality in mechanically ventilated patients. *Crit Care Med.* 2005;33:226-229.
31. Devlin JW, et al. Efficacy and safety of quetiapine in critically ill patients with delirium: a prospective, multicenter, randomized, double-blind, placebo-controlled pilot study. *Crit Care Med.* 2010;38:419-427.
32. Devlin JW, et al. Impact of quetiapine on resolution of individual delirium symptoms in critically ill patients with delirium: a post-hoc analysis of a double-blind, randomized, placebo-controlled study. *Crit Care.* 2011;15:R215.
33. van Eijk MM, et al. Effect of rivastigmine as an adjunct to usual care with haloperidol on duration of delirium and mortality in critically ill patients: a multicentre, double-blind, placebo-controlled randomised trial. *Lancet.* 2010;376:1829-8237.
34. Sarff M, Gold JA. Alcohol withdrawal syndromes in the intensive care unit. *Crit Care Med.* 2010;38(9 Suppl):S494-S501.
35. Schuckit MA. Alcohol-use disorders. *Lancet.* 2009;373:492-501.
36. Amato L, et al. Benzodiazepines for alcohol withdrawal. *Cochrane Database Syst Rev.* 2010;3:CD005063.
37. Repper-DeLisi J, et al. Successful implementation of an alcohol-withdrawal pathway in a general hospital. *Psychosomatics.* 2008;49(4):292-299.
38. Lonergan E, et al. Benzodiazepines for delirium. *Cochrane Database Syst Rev.* 2009;(4)CD006379.

End-of-Life Issues

Caroline Etland

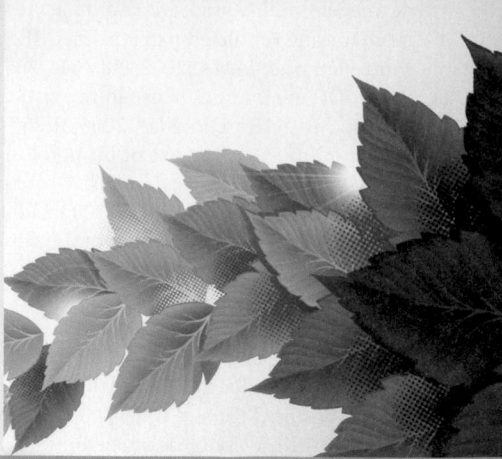

evolve WEBSITE

http://evolve.elsevier.com/Urden/criticalcare/
Evolve features:
- NCLEX Review Questions
- CCRN Review Questions
- PCCN Review Questions
- Mosby's Nursing Skills Procedures
- Animations
- Video Clips
- Glossary

End of life has become an important clinical topic in critical care, although requisite improvements in end-of-life care have been slow to follow. Because the primary purpose of admission of patients to a critical care unit is to provide aggressive, lifesaving treatment, the death of a patient is generally regarded as a failure. Because the culture emphasizes saving lives, the language that describes the end of life employs negative terms, such as "forgoing life-sustaining treatments," "do not resuscitate (DNR)," and "withdrawal of life support." Sometimes the phrase *withdrawal of care* is used, which can cause families to think there will be no comfort measures or assistance provided after a decision is made to discontinue mechanical ventilation and other life-sustaining treatments. This lack of end-of-life language has hampered literature searches until recently. The medical subject headings (MeSH) term for withdrawal of life support is *passive euthanasia*. Content on the end of life in medical[1] and nursing[2] critical care textbooks is minimal. The first textbook on end of life in critical care was published in 1998[3] and the second in 2001.[4] Recently, more accurate language has been used in health care and popular literature to describe end-of-life decision making and medical interventions, such as *allow natural death* instead of "do not resuscitate" and *withholding of non-beneficial treatment* in place of "futile care."[5,6] This shift toward more realistic descriptors reflects extensive recent research in health care, especially palliative care, and the effectiveness of goals-of-care discussions in people with serious illnesses prior to crisis events.

More attention is being given to the quality of the end-of-life experience of people with serious illnesses, particularly those who become critically ill. Recent studies suggest that "medical care for patients with advanced illness is characterized by inadequately treated physical distress; fragmented care systems; poor communication between doctors, patients, and families; and enormous strains on family caregiver and support systems."[7] In addition to health care system barriers to good end-of-life care, mainstream media has significantly influenced misconceptions among the American population about the success rate of medical interventions in seriously ill people. A familiar media presentation of life and death in the hospital is a critical event in a patient who is resuscitated and immediately awakens with full capacity. In reality, treatment options are usually explained in rapid technical language, followed by a frightening question, "Do you want us to keep going?" or "Tell us what you want us to do." This heavy burden placed on loved ones means they must choose between treatment options, one of which may result in loss of their loved one.

The emphasis on patient autonomy as a valued ethical principle is deeply embedded in the health care system of the United States. Expert medical recommendations are offered to patients and families and they must determine in a brief space of time whether those recommendations are aligned with their personal values. Most nurses are familiar with the scenario of families of critical care unit patients who are told how well one body organ is functioning being unable to understand why another physician communicates a poor prognosis. Less often, families are provided with a longer-term perspective that addresses the loss of functional status, decreased quality of life, and potential need for long-term care. Hope is a powerful influence on decision making, and a shift from hope for recovery to hope for a peaceful death should be guided by clinicians with exemplary communication skills. Strategies for communicating with critically ill patients and their families are further described in Chapter 6 (Box 6-2). Critical care nurses are often the interpreters of medical information and how it applies to personal preferences and values. The ability to respond realistically in accordance with the listener's values and culture is a learned skill. Fortunately, many resources are available to further develop the necessary skills to better support patients and families through a critical care unit admission to discharge. The American Association of Critical-Care Nurses (AACN) has recognized the importance of this aspect of care in the critical care unit by developing protocols for palliative and end-of-life issues in the critical care unit and by identifying palliative and end-of-life care as a major advocacy initiative.[8,9] Several key resources to enhance communication and elicit goals of care will be discussed throughout this chapter.

This chapter focuses on the evidence available for the care rendered to the dying critical care patient and his or her family through research reports and summaries of research and guidelines. One such report is from the National Consensus Project and the National Quality Forum,[10] in which the preferred practices of the imminently dying are discussed. This type of report can be used to make a checklist of indicators for quality improvement in end-of-life care. Other reports that are specific to the critical care unit have been written by groups headed by Teno,[11] Nelson,[12] Glavan,[13] Beckstrand,[14] and Mularski.[15] Curtis and Rubenfeld[4] have provided a "how to" guide for critical care quality improvement to outline the process that can be used with these indicators. More recently, the Center to Advance Palliative Care has created a resource site for implementing palliative care in the critical care unit.[16]

END-OF-LIFE EXPERIENCE IN CRITICAL CARE

Attention to the end of life of hospitalized patients has increased since the publication of the Study to Understand Prognoses and Preferences for Outcomes and Risks of Treatment (SUPPORT).[17] In this major report, more than 9000 seriously ill patients in five medical centers were studied. Despite an intervention to improve communication, shortcomings were found, aggressive treatment was common, only one half of physicians knew their patients' preferences to avoid cardiopulmonary resuscitation (CPR), more than one third of patients who died spent at least 10 days in a critical care unit, and for 50% of conscious patients, family members reported moderate to severe pain at least one half of the time.

Following closely after the publication of the SUPPORT study, the Institute of Medicine (IOM) released a report, *Approaching Death: Improving Care at the End of Life.*[18] The group detailed deficiencies in care and gave seven recommendations to improve care:

1. Patients with fatal illnesses and their family should receive reliable, skillful, and supportive care.
2. Health professionals should improve care for the dying.
3. Policymakers and consumers should work with health professionals to improve quality and financing of care.
4. Health profession education should include end-of-life content.

5. Palliative care should be developed, possibly as a medical specialty.
6. Research on end of life should be funded.
7. The public should communicate more about the experience of dying and options available.

In SUPPORT and in the IOM report, critical care patients were not distinguished from other hospitalized patients, preventing distinctions to be made between types of units. To describe the number of deaths in critical care units, Angus and colleagues[19] reviewed hospital discharge data from six states and the National Death Index. Of the more than 500,000 deaths studied, 38.3% were in hospitals, and 22% (59% of all hospital deaths) occurred after admission to the critical care unit. Terminal admissions associated with critical care accounted for 80% of all terminal hospitalization costs. The likelihood of dying in the hospital increased from age 25 to 74 years, and the likelihood of dying after critical care unit admission remained at 25% of all deaths for each age category.[19] Although 90% of people would prefer to die in their own homes,[18] more than 20% of those who died in this review received high-tech, aggressive care before they died.

An important shift in care of the terminally ill patient in the critical care unit has occurred with the growth of palliative care programs in the United States in the last decade. The rapid expansion of hospital-based palliative care programs has decreased the mortality rate in critical care units for patients followed by palliative care services through transfer to lower acuity, as well as decreased the costs associated with higher acuity critical care beds, pharmacy, laboratory, and diagnostic costs.[20,21] Studies by Morrison and colleagues reviewed hospital and Medicare data to demonstrate that hospitals with palliative care services had significant cost savings in comparison to patients receiving usual care.[21]

Advance Directives

Although advance directives, also known as a *living will* or a *health care power of attorney*, were intended to ensure that patients received the care they desired at end of life, their enactment has been less than desired. Like other preventive measures, advance directives are underused, even though they are inexpensive and potentially effective.[22] Completion rates in adults range from 16% to 36% overall with less than one half of seriously or terminally ill patients having documented their wishes.[23] Most patients have expressed a desire to avoid "general life support" if dying or permanently unconscious, and few have expressed preferences regarding specific life-sustaining treatments; however, only about one third of physicians are aware of the existence of advance directives in their patients.[24,25] Cook and others[25] found that factors differed for determining the establishment of directives for advanced life support more than for informing a decision to limit or withdraw that support after admission to a critical care unit. Care providers also reported discomfort because they believed interventions were excessive and not compatible with an acceptable future quality of life. Even when advance directives are present, the question arises about whether they are applicable for current care decisions; in other words, is this a terminal illness?

Physician Orders for Life Sustaining Treatment

The Physician Orders for Life Sustaining Treatment (POLST) initiative began in Oregon in the 1990s when medical leaders collaborated to address the problem of patients' advance directives not being honored.[26] Different from an advance directive, POLST forms are medical orders that are honored across all treatment settings and are especially important to emergency responders in the community. Also, they are completed by the patient and physician in the presence of a serious chronic illness and should be incorporated into medical orders upon admission to the hospital or skilled nursing facility. POLST forms are more easily read than an advance directive in that the format is one of check boxes with specific directions. States that have approved use of POLST forms through legislation or specific regulations have witnessed a shift in proactive discussions of patients' wishes for life-sustaining treatment.[27,28] Preventing unwanted life-sustaining treatment through ongoing communication between patient and provider impacts the critical care setting in several ways. Treatment decision making is supported when prior discussions have occurred between physicians, patients, and their loved ones regarding declining health and limits on intervention. Resource utilization is maximized when inappropriate critical care unit admissions are prevented. Finally, moral distress of nurses is decreased when care is congruent with patient autonomy. Critical care nurses in states that recognize POLST forms need to be aware whether a regulatory mandate requires health care providers to honor the patient's wishes documented on the form, or if the documentation is merely a guideline. Equally important is the need to identify the POLST form when it is presented and to communicate with medical staff to ensure that stated treatment wishes are incorporated into the plan of care.

Advance Care Planning

Cultural influences in the United States discourage discussion of death. Planning for decisions to be made at a later date if one is deemed incompetent is a difficult process, but this knowledge helps the family members left to make the treatment decisions. Advance care planning for those with chronic illness is advantageous for all involved.[29] When surrogates hear the patient's wishes for end-of-life care, they can be more congruent and knowledgeable about those wishes in future decision making. Significant effort has been expended on determining ideal interventions for the treatment and recovery from serious illnesses in the critical care setting. Currently, an equal amount of effort is being placed on providing adequate support and symptom management when recovery from illness is not likely to occur. This process may look different for individual patients or settings, but some guiding principles for a good death assist clinicians to identify what patients' individual values are and where gaps in care exist that may be resolved (Box 11-1).[30]

Communication of the patient's wishes between primary care providers and intensivists is critical. If patients have stated desires, they should be communicated when patients are transferred out of the critical care unit. If the patient has not specified his or her preferences, that information also is important and should be communicated to new health care providers; the level of care patients desire should be offered as appropriate.

BOX 11-1 PRINCIPLES OF A GOOD DEATH

- Anticipate and be able to prepare for a good death
- Retain some control
- Be afforded dignity and privacy
- Have symptom control including pain relief
- Choose place of death when possible
- Have access to information and expertise when necessary
- Have emotional and spiritual support
- Have access to hospice care
- Have control over who is present at death
- Respect the wishes of the dying through advance directives
- Have time to say good-bye
- Be able to die rather than pointlessly prolonging life

Adapted from Smith R. A good death. *BMJ*. 2000;320:129.

Families and care providers should be informed if patients decline aggressive care, so their families will not be left with difficult decisions in emergency situations. Emotional support for the patient and the family is important as they discuss advance care planning in the critical care setting and is described in the Nursing Interventions Classification (NIC) feature on Family Support in Box 6-3 in Chapter 6.

ETHICAL AND LEGAL ISSUES

Legal and ethical principles guide many of our decisions in caring for the dying patient and the family. The patient is respected as autonomous and able to make his or her own decisions. When the patient is unable to make decisions, however, the same respect should be accorded to surrogates. These wishes might have been put in writing by the patient as an advance directive and preferably discussed with the surrogate. The Patient Self-Determination Act supports the patient's right to control future treatment in the event the individual cannot speak for himself or herself.

Two of the basic principles underlying the provision of health care are beneficence and nonmaleficence. *Beneficence* is the principle of intending to benefit the other through one's actions. *Nonmaleficence* means to do no harm. Sometimes at end of life, these two principles are in conflict, such as when resuscitation is attempted under beneficence but causes harm to the patient, especially if resuscitation was not desired by the patient. An equally troubling situation exists when the fear of liability drives decision making from the clinician's perspective. Medical recommendations for limitation of life-sustaining treatment or comfort care often result in conflict with surrogate decision makers. When life-sustaining interventions are offered, even though they are likely to be unsuccessful, families are given hope that their loved one may respond and recover. In family conferences, a shift in language and dialogue to distinguish non-beneficial treatment from interventions that may produce long-lasting benefit after discharge should occur early in the critical care unit stay. Most physicians and nurses have not been taught how to conduct this type of dialogue in their training. Fortunately there are many more options to gain the training and experience necessary to shift the decision making from a purely clinical perspective to a more humanistic view. Programs such as Education in Palliative and End-of-life Care (EPEC), End of Life Nursing Education Consortium (ELNEC) and the Center to Advance Palliative Care's Palliative Care Leadership Center (PCLC) training are cost-effective methods to educate and support clinicians to more effectively communicate with patients and families at the end of life. Additional information on ethical and legal issues can be found in Chapter 2, Ethical Issues and Chapter 3, Legal Issues.

COMFORT CARE

The decision to withdraw life-sustaining treatments and switch to comfort care at end of life should be made with as much involvement of the patient as possible, including physical presence of the patient in decision making or procuring paper documents if the patient is not able to participate. If neither option is available, the patient's intent as understood from discussions or knowledge of the patient should guide the decision about whether to withdraw treatment. Withholding and withdrawing care are considered to be morally and legally equivalent.[31] However, because families experience more stress in withdrawing treatments than in withholding them,[32] treatments should not be started that the patient would not want or that would not benefit him or her.

The goal of withdrawal of life-sustaining treatments is to remove treatments that are not beneficial and may be uncomfortable. Any treatment in this circumstance may be withheld or withdrawn. After the goal of comfort has been chosen, each procedure should be evaluated to see if it is necessary or causes discomfort. Treatments that cause discomfort do not need to be continued. Another defining question is whether treatments are prolonging the dying process. When disagreements arise, ethics consultations have been found to resolve conflicts regarding inappropriately prolonged, non-beneficial, or unwanted treatments in the critical care unit, shifting the focus to more appropriate comfort care.[33]

Forgoing life-sustaining treatments is not the same as active euthanasia or assisted suicide. Killing is an action causing another's death, whereas allowing a person to die by withholding or withdrawing life-sustaining treatment is avoiding any intervention that interferes with a natural death after illness or trauma.[3]

Cardiopulmonary Resuscitation

CPR was originally developed for those with coronary artery disease, and they are the most likely to survive resuscitation to discharge, as well as those who suffer cardiac arrest in the critical care unit.[34] The benefits of resuscitation may be overestimated for survival and for the more relevant outcome of resumption of baseline functional status. In a meta-analysis of 51 studies, Ebell and colleagues[34] found that the rate of overall survival to discharge after in-hospital CPR was 13.4%. A decreased rate of immediate survival was found for patients with acquired immune deficiency syndrome, those with a hematocrit above 35%, and patients who were male. Decreased survival to discharge was related to sepsis on the day before resuscitation, cancer with or without metastasis, dementia, elevated serum creatinine level, African American race, and

dependent status. Brindley and colleagues[35] found the same rate for overall survival to hospital discharge (13.4%) in a retrospective study of hospital charts for inpatients who had undergone or experienced resuscitation. A study from Norway found that only 17% of older adult patients older than 75 years survived resuscitation to return home.[36] The survival rate for cancer patients has risen from 2% to 6.7% since 1990 perhaps because better treatment and support have transformed many cancers into chronic diseases.[37] It has also become evident that critical care unit patients don't survive CPR as often as ward patients and overall functional status declined 25% in all survivors.[37]

FitzGerald and others[38] found that functional status among almost half of the survivors of in-hospital CPR had deteriorated compared with their condition 2 months before the event. After 6 months, 30% of those patients had died, and two thirds continued to lose function. Despite these dismal statistics, CPR is offered as an option without fully informing patients or families of the low possibility of survival, the pain and suffering involved during and after the procedure, and the potential for decline in functional status.

Family members typically are asked to leave the room during resuscitation. The American Association of Critical-Care Nurses (AACN)[39] and the Emergency Nurses Association (ENA)[40] have issued position statements recommending that families be allowed to be present during CPR and invasive procedures. Family presence is a significant source of support for the patient, and there may be a benefit to the family in observing the resuscitation that can aid in the grieving process when resuscitation is not successful by knowing that all was done that could be done.

Impact of Do Not Resuscitate Orders

As death approaches, the decision to initiate a DNR order is frequently delayed.[41] A DNR order is intended to prevent the initiation of life-sustaining measures such as endotracheal intubation or CPR. In a review of the literature covering the 25 years since the DNR was established, Burns and colleagues[42] found that those with a DNR order sometimes received less care and that some treatments were withheld[43] without those changes being specified in the DNR order. Although acuity of illness and organ dysfunction consistently predicted mortality, only the medical history was positively associated with a DNR order for critically ill surgical patients.[44] Documentation of consent conversations for DNR is less than ideal because the reasons for the DNR order were documented in only 55% of cases, and a consent conversation was documented in only 69%.[45]

Chang et al[46] studied the effect of DNR orders in two critical care units in Taiwan and found that even though a DNR order was issued late in the clinical course, life-sustaining interventions were reduced through discussions and consent by surrogate decision makers. Nurses in Korea did not change their nursing activities substantially after receiving a DNR order, continuing to focus on maintenance, preventive, and hygiene tasks.[47] They reported becoming more passive with interventions such as CVP monitoring, fluid and electrolyte balance, and reporting the patient's condition. However, the nurses were more active in communicating with the family.

TABLE 11-1	SELECTED PROGNOSTIC SCALES		
PROGNOSTIC SCALE	**DISEASE/CLINICAL CONDITION**	**PROGNOSTIC SCALE**	**DISEASE/CLINICAL CONDITION**
Palliative Prognostic Scale (PPS)	Any hospice population; palliative care patients	Lung Cancer Prognostic Model (LCPM)	Terminal lung cancer patients
Palliative Prognostic Index (PPI)	Terminal cancer patients	Dementia Prognostic Model (DPM)	Demographic, diagnosis, laboratory, and functional data on dementia residents
Palliative Prognostic Score (PaP)	Terminal cancer patients	Prognostic Index for One-Year Mortality in Older Adults (PIMOA)	Adults >70 years of age with previous stay in hospital
Seattle Heart Failure Model; Heart Failure Risk Scoring System (HFRSS)	Acute heart failure	Cancer Prognostic Scale (CPS)	Terminal cancer patients in Progressive Care Unit
BODE Scale	COPD	Mortality Risk Index Score (MRIS)	New admission to nursing home

Adapted from Lau F, et al. A systematic review of prognostic tools for estimating survival time in palliative care. *J Palliat Care.* 2007;23(2):93.

DNR is sometimes perceived to mean "do not care," but that is not the intent. Families should be assured that patients will continue to receive care, including pain and symptom management, but that aggressive measures to extend life will not be employed. DNR orders should be written before withdrawal of life support is initiated; this documentation ensures that the patient is not subjected to unwanted interventions during the period between initiation of withdrawal and death.

Prognostication and Prognostic Tools

Why patients who are dying would have received life-prolonging therapy or aggressive interventions shortly before their death can be explained in part by a series of studies. It was found that physicians' ability to prognosticate the length of time before death is limited[48,49] and that the time to death usually is overestimated. Patients' wishes are often not known, can be vague even when they are known,[50] or change over the course of an illness.[51] Care may not be in accordance with patients' wishes, and this discrepancy is more prevalent when comfort care is desired over aggressive care.[52] Skills in communication and end-of-life care that would enable providers to better assess patient and family wishes are poorly developed and are not emphasized in medical curricula.[53,54]

Severity scoring systems belong to one of five classes: prognostic, disease-specific, single-organ failure, trauma scores, and organ dysfunction.[55] Two common tools for estimating critical care unit mortality are the Acute Physiology and Chronic Health Evaluation (APACHE) and multiple organ dysfunction score (MODS).[56] However, when these tools were compared with physicians' estimates of critical care unit survival of less than 10%, the physicians' estimates were associated with subsequent life-support limitation. A physician's estimate was more powerful in predicting mortality than illness severity, organ dysfunction, and use of inotropes or vasopressors.[57]

A majority of patients in the critical care unit have one or more chronic illnesses that greatly impact long-term recovery from major health events such as respiratory failure, myocardial infarction, or sepsis. In addition to use of prognostic tools specific to the critical care unit, it makes sense to incorporate prognostic tools for chronic illnesses into overall decision making and the communication process with patients and families. Scoring diagnoses with a traditionally poor prognosis or a consistent trajectory of functional decline can be helpful in comparing current health status with that which existed at the time of diagnosis. Loved ones of critically ill patients have witnessed the functional decline and may have hoped for improvement despite advancement of disease. Use of prognostic scales can add meaningful information to help patients and families make informed decisions. A summary of some of the more commonly used prognostic scales is listed in Table 11-1.[58]

Despite this information and these tools, uncertainty remains a major issue in decision making for physicians, patients, and families.[51] Because of uncertainty and because a few patients who were never thought likely to survive actually return to visit a critical care unit, professionals are not confident about issues of survivability. Moreover, many families cling to small hopes of survival and recovery.

COMMUNICATION AND DECISION MAKING

Communication with the patient and family is critical. White and colleagues[59] found that shared decision making about end-of-life treatment choices in physician-family conferences was often incomplete, especially among less educated families. Families were found to go through a process in their decision making in which they considered the personal domain (rallying support and evaluating quality of life), the critical care unit environment domain (chasing the doctors and relating to the health care team), and the decision domain (arriving at a new belief and making and communicating the decision).[60] Higher levels of shared decision making were associated with greater family satisfaction. Regardless of the health literacy of the patient or family, simple language explanations of life-sustaining treatments such as CPR, ventilation, and tube feedings are necessary to effectively communicate. Many patients and families experience a "data dump" during communication with health care providers who focus on reporting vital statistics and odds of success. Several organizations have made available education handouts—some in multiple languages—that explain life-sustaining treatments in realistic terms that are intended to be accompanied by health care provider discussion.[61,62] Focusing on improving critical care unit communication when patients are dying reduces lengths of stay and resource use.[63]

Patient Communication

Patients' capacity for decision making is limited by illness severity; they are too sick or are hampered by the therapies or medications used to treat them.[64] When decision making is required, the patient is the first person to be approached. Information that can assist the clinical team to facilitate and support health-related decision making is provided in the NIC feature on Decision-Making Support in Box 2-3 in Chapter 2. When the patient is not able to safely make health care decisions because of disease progression or the therapy used for treatment, written documents such as a living will or a health care power of attorney should be obtained when possible. Additional information on power of attorney for health care can be found in the section on "Advance Care Planning" earlier in this chapter. Without those documents, wishes of the patient should be ascertained from those closest to the patient. Some states have a legal order of priority for surrogates. Some patients have neither capacity nor surrogates to assist in decision making, accounting for up to 27% of deaths in one study.[65]

Family Communication

How questions are asked of surrogates is extremely important. The question is not "What do you want to do about (patient's name)?" but rather "What would (patient's name) want if he knew he were in this situation?" These two questions have vastly different meanings and consequences for the patient and the family. The former question has a greater likelihood of engendering guilt over "pulling the plug." The latter question provides a sense of fulfilling the patient's wishes and respecting choices. Sometimes, this discussion is held during the family meeting, in which a general sense of goals can be discussed. As families make decisions, they appreciate support for those decisions, because the support can reduce the burden they experience. There is some evidence from a French study that families are reluctant to participate in decision making.[66] This evidence reinforces the need to support families who are highly stressed and possibly exhausted while they are trying to make the most difficult decisions they have ever faced.

Family members have reported dissatisfaction with communication and decision making.[67] Increasing the frequency of communication and sharing concerns early in the hospitalization will make subsequent discussions easier for the patient, family, and health professional. Having the entire critical care unit team present for morning rounds is one method of improving communication.[68] Family members who understood the communication of staff were acknowledged and comforted by them; those who had difficulties drew back and received less adequate communication.[69] Families who reported increased understanding when communicating with staff also reported greater acknowledgment and comfort from staff members, whereas families who experienced a lack of understanding when communicating with staff tended to withdraw, further limiting the effectiveness in communication with the hospital staff.

Having to focus on understanding the professional is an unacceptable burden.

A publication from the Society of Critical-Care Medicine (SCCM) recommends supporting the families of critical care unit patients.[70] Forty-three recommendations are presented, including an endorsement of a shared decision-making model, family care conferencing, culturally appropriate requests for truth-telling and informed refusal, spiritual support, staff education and debriefing, family presence at rounds and resuscitation, open and flexible visitation, family-friendly signs, and family support before, during, and after a death. One use of this guideline is to assess the level of family support for each critical care unit so that the most deficient recommendations could be addressed with quality-improvement actions. The categories used in this guideline are for general support of critical care unit families. When cross-indexed with seven end-of-life domains,[71] the needs of a family with a dying patient are decision making; spiritual and cultural support; emotional and practical support of families, including visitation and family preparation for death; and continuity of care.[72]

Cultural and Spiritual Influences on Communication

Cultural and spiritual influences on attitudes and beliefs about death and dying differ dramatically. The cultures of the predominant religions commonly seen in the surrounding community should be familiar to the local health care team. These differences may affect how the health care team is viewed, how decisions are made, whether aggressive treatment is preferred, how death is met, and how grieving will occur.[73,74] Patients who do not follow a particular religion should be assessed for their individual spiritual beliefs, or lack thereof. Identifying sources of spiritual comfort strengthens the bond between caregivers, patients, or family. Satisfaction with critical care unit care has been associated with the extent to which the family is satisfied with their spiritual care, especially when the patient is near death.[75] Staff members' own attitudes about the specific practices of a culture should be carefully assessed[76] and should be tempered with respect and humility. Interpreters are necessary when the patient or the family members do not speak English. A cultural and religious assessment is warranted in all situations, because cultural or religious affiliation does not imply that patients or families follow all of the tenets of that group.

Hospice Information

Although hospice care has been available for many years, patients and families often consider this method of care only in the last weeks or months of a patient with end-stage illness, and they frequently view hospice care as "giving up." Health professionals can assist patients and families by providing information about the hospice benefit, particularly regarding the aggressive symptom management and family support. Some hospices are offering to partner with critical care units in the provision of end-of-life care and in the process of withdrawal of ventilatory support. Hospice care is an option that should be considered, especially in end-stage illness, and the benefit to surviving family should be emphasized.

WITHDRAWAL OR WITHHOLDING OF TREATMENT

Discussions about the potential for impending death are never held early enough. Usually, the first discussion about prognosis occurs in conjunction with the topic of the discontinuation of life support. The late timing of that first discussion is an issue, particularly because some families have arrived at the notion of withdrawal before physicians.[64,77] Equally important is that some family members dread such conversations but are grateful to discuss the uncertainty of their loved one's future. Physicians should give families time to adjust to this information and make preparations by providing discussions early about prognosis, goals of therapy, and the patient's wishes.[4]

Proactive Approach

After a poor prognosis is established, a period can elapse before end-of-life treatment goals are determined. Campbell and Guzman[78] recommended a proactive case-finding approach by palliative care personnel to decrease hospital length of stay for patients with multiorgan system failure and global cerebral ischemia. They shortened the time between identifying the poor prognosis and establishing comfort care goals, decreased length of critical care unit stay for patients with multisystem organ dysfunction, and reduced the cost of care. Proactive palliative care should occur when admission diagnoses trigger a consultation instead of after several avenues of treatment have been exhausted. Case managers and social workers can be particularly helpful in this regard.

When patients are admitted with serious illnesses and are likely to die, a proactive approach to palliative care has been found to shorten critical care unit stays without a significant difference in mortality rates or discharge disposition.[79] The use of nonbeneficial resources decreased, and prolonged dying was avoided.[78] Patients with assistive cardiac devices present a different challenge in discussion of withdrawal of life support. Many times, these patients are cognitively intact and consent to removal of technology that is keeping them alive. Weigand and Kalowes outlined issues surrounding discontinuation of cardiac devices as a preventive ethics approach with health care providers anticipating the need to shift goals of care and support patients and families through the process.[80]

Disagreement and Distress for Caregivers

Nurses and doctors frequently disagree about the futility of interventions. Sometimes, nurses consider withdrawal before physicians and patients do, and they then feel the care they are giving is unnecessary and possibly harmful. Nurses in one study were found to be more pessimistic but more often correct than physicians about the prognoses of dying patients, but the nurses also proposed treatment withdrawal for some very sick patients who survived.[81] This issue is a serious one for critical care nurses, because emotional and ethical distress can lead to burnout. Meltzer found that the score on the emotional exhaustion subscale of the Maslach Burnout Inventory and the score on the frequency subscale on the Moral Distress Scale correlated for a group of 60 critical care nurses.[82] Often, critical care nurses experience moral distress due to the severity of patients' illnesses as well as the requirement of technology to maintain vital organ function. Collaborative strategies for minimizing moral distress rely on the bedside nurse and critical care leadership to implement individual and organizational changes.[83]

Barriers to Dying

Ellershaw and Ward[84] identified a number of barriers to diagnosing dying: hope for the patient to improve, unclear diagnosis, pursuance of futile interventions, disagreement about the patient's condition, failure to recognize key signs and symptoms, poor ability to communicate, fears about foreshortening life, concerns about withdrawal and withholding, and medicolegal issues. Prognostic models are used to predict mortality rates for groups of critical care patients, not to guide specific decisions to forgo treatment.[85] This perspective is changing with the increased availability of end-of-life research recommendations, newer prognostic models, and the growth of palliative care services to support patients, families, and providers.

Steps Toward Comfort Care

If a series of interventions is to be withdrawn, dialysis usually is discontinued first along with diagnostic tests and vasopressors. Next, intravenous fluids, monitoring, laboratory tests, and antibiotics are stopped.[85] Withdrawal of specific treatments may have effects necessitating symptom management. Withdrawal of dialysis may cause dyspnea from volume overload, which may necessitate the use of opioids or benzodiazepines. Efforts to discontinue artificial feeding may be met with concern from the family, because offering food has great social significance. It is essential to share information with family and providers regarding the potential benefits of withholding food and fluids in the days immediately prior to death to prevent unnecessary suffering.[86]

PALLIATIVE CARE

The growth of palliative care programs in the United States has demonstrated the importance of this new health care specialty, with a 125% increase from 2000 to 2008.[20] Initiatives such as the IPAL-ICU have demonstrated that a focus on life-saving interventions can be integrated with palliative care concurrently, rather than one following the failure of another.[20] Evidence-based clinical, communication, and quality tools are available through the Center to Advance Palliative Care (CAPC). Resources include templates for

- Family conference documentation
- Quality of palliative care surveys
- Pocket reference cards on pain, family conferences, and communication
- Model policies for ventilator withdrawal and medical futility
- Palliative care triggers and brochures

Patients who are identified as being near the end of life require aggressive care for their symptom management, provided by a team of health professionals. The most relevant clinical goal is to palliate these unpleasant situations by assessing for them and implementing appropriate interventions.[3] Palliative care guidelines have been released by a consortium of organizations concerned with palliative care and end-of-life care, and they may provide guidance when the usual first-line treatments do not promote comfort for critically ill patients who are near death.[87] Strategies that are based on research evidence and expert opinion for specific conditions such as delirium, opioid dose escalation, and dyspnea at the end of life are outlined on the End of Life/Palliative Education Resource Center (EPERC) website.[88] Palliative care has been thought of as desirable only when the patient nears death or when several interventions have been tried for management of symptoms without success. However, publications such as these guidelines and the IOM report *Improving Palliative Care for Cancer*[89] have stated that palliative care ideally begins at the time of diagnosis of a life-threatening illness and continues through cure or until death and into the family's bereavement period.

Pain Management

Because many critical care patients are not conscious, assessment of pain and other symptoms becomes more difficult.[90] Gélinas and colleagues[91] recommended using signs of body movements, neuromuscular signs, facial expressions, or responses to physical examination for pain assessment in patients with altered consciousness (see Chapter 9). Foley,[92] while acknowledging the usual three-step approach of the World Health Organization, admitted that in critical care units, step 3 is frequently used because of the intensity of the pain.

Nonopioid medications are the first-line approach, followed by adding an opioid for additional analgesia when relief is not obtained. Because opioids provide sedation, anxiolysis, and analgesia, they are particularly beneficial in the ventilated patient. Morphine is the medication of choice, and there is no upper limit in dosing.[3] In nonventilated patients, sedation may cause respiratory depression,[92] and nonopioids or specific anesthetic agents may be more appropriate. In the sedated ventilated patient, especially those receiving neuromuscular blocking medications, there is no systematic, reliable method to determine presence or degree of pain.[93] The absence of the usual clinical indicators of pain, such as grimacing or guarding, makes it a challenge to determine whether pain is present. Titration of intravenous infusions to achieve maximum effect with minimum sedation is an inexact science. Sedation/agitation scales are one method of monitoring the effectiveness of medications but are not performed continuously with frequent titration, such as during surgery. Potential pain sources include prone position, endotracheal tube, wounds, and immobility, and should necessitate preventive analgesia administration.[93] Critical care nurses should assume pain is present in the immobile patient and administer routine analgesics to prevent suffering. Jacobi and others[94] published a guideline for the sustained use of sedatives and analgesia (see Chapter 10); it is also available on the SCCM's website (http://www.sccm.org).

Symptom Management

It has long been in question whether critical care patients can accurately report their symptoms because of the effects of sedating medications, severe illness, and organ dysfunction. Kalowes studied non-cancer critical care unit patients during a daily wake up and compared their report of symptoms with those of their family members.[95] Almost all patients had more than 10 symptoms, and there was 85.5% congruence between patient and family report of physiologic and psychologic symptoms. Overall, patients experienced significant symptom burden near the end of life but received limited treatment to alleviate suffering.

Campbell,[3] in her book chapter titled "Usual Care Requirements for the Patient Who Is Near Death," listed the following symptoms as necessary parts of the assessment: dyspnea, nausea and vomiting, edema and pulmonary edema, anxiety and delirium, metabolic derangements, skin integrity, and anemia and hemorrhage.

Dyspnea

Campbell published a review of terminal dyspnea and respiratory distress.[96] Dyspnea is best managed with close evaluation of the patient and the use of opioids, sedatives, and nonpharmacologic interventions (oxygen, positioning, and increased ambient air flow). Morphine reduces anxiety and muscle tension and increases pulmonary vasodilatation but is not effective when inhaled. Benzodiazepines may be used in patients who are not able to take opioids or for whom the respiratory effects are minimal. Benzodiazepines and opioids should be titrated to effect. Treatment efforts should be aimed at the patient's expression of dyspnea rather than at respiratory rates or oxygen levels.[97]

Nausea and Vomiting

Nausea and vomiting are common and should be treated with antiemetics. The cause of nausea and vomiting may be intestinal obstruction. Treatment for decompression may be uncomfortable in dying patients, and its use should be weighed using a benefit-to-burden ratio.

Fever and Infection

Fever and infection necessitate assessment of the benefits of continuing antibiotics so as not to prolong the dying process.[3] Management of the fever with antipyretics may be appropriate for the patient's comfort, but other methods such as ice or hypothermia blankets should be balanced against the amount of distress the patient may experience.

Edema

Edema may cause discomfort, and diuretics may be effective if kidney function is intact. Dialysis is not warranted at the end of life. The use of fluids may contribute to the edema when kidney function is impaired and the body is slowing its functions. In a Database of Abstracts of Reviews of Effectiveness (DARE) report,[98] little relationship was found between thirst and fluid therapy or fluid status.

Anxiety

Anxiety should be assessed verbally, if possible, or by changes in vital signs or restlessness. Benzodiazepines, especially midazolam with its rapid onset and short half-life, are frequently used. Minimizing noxious sounds and playing a patient's favorite music may help to soothe anxiety.

Delirium

Delirium is commonly observed in the critically ill and in those approaching death. Haloperidol is recommended as useful, and restraints should be avoided. In a review of the available literature, Kehl[99] concluded that despite the recommendations of most study authors to use neuroleptic medications as a treatment for restlessness, several studies demonstrated the effectiveness of other medications, such as benzodiazepines (notably midazolam and lorazepam) or phenothiazines, alone or in combination.

Metabolic Derangement

Treatments for metabolic derangements, skin problems, anemia, and hemorrhage should be tempered with concerns for the patient's comfort. Only interventions promoting comfort should be performed. Patients do not necessarily feel better "when the laboratory values are right."

Providing Comfort

The nursing interventions at end of life should focus on the provision of comfort care as an active, desirable, and important service. Unnecessary checks of vital signs, laboratory work, and any treatment that does not promote comfort should be avoided. Positioning the patient who is actively dying has as its purpose only comfort, not the schedule to promote skin integrity. Coordinating this care with the many members of the critical care team is important to ensure consistency across disciplines and across shifts. When symptom management is not successful in ensuring comfort, the services of the pain team or the palliative care service may be required.

Near-Death Awareness

Two hospice nurses have described a phenomenon of near-death awareness.[100] The same behaviors may be seen in conscious critical care patients near death. Having an awareness of the phenomenon enables more careful assessment of behaviors that may be interpreted as delirium, acid-base imbalance, or other metabolic derangements. These behaviors include communicating with someone who is not alive, preparing for travel, describing a place they can see, or even knowing when death will occur.[101] Family members may find these behaviors disturbing but find comfort in understanding the phenomenon and in sharing these experiences with their loved one.

Family Meetings

Although family meetings should be held within 72 hours of an admission,[102] they are frequently held to formulate a decision to withdraw life support. Lilly and colleagues[102] found that an earlier meeting led to shorter critical care unit stays for patients who eventually died, and allowed them earlier access to palliative care. These results held up in a 4-year evaluation of this intervention, and they found that they were providing advanced life support to patients with the potential to survive and an earlier withdrawal when ineffective.[103]

WITHDRAWAL OF MECHANICAL VENTILATION

A dramatic geographic variation in the prevalence of withdrawal of life-sustaining therapies has been found. Some evidence suggests this variation may be driven more by physicians' attitudes and biases than by factors such as patients' preferences or cultural differences.[104] This inconsistency in care further complicates a difficult process. From the clinical, ethical, and legal perspectives, standardized withdrawal from life-support order sets are recommended to direct and support nursing judgment in this complex and emotional clinical situation.

Selph et al taped end-of-life conversations between families and physicians and found that at least one supportive statement was provided 66% of the time during the discussion.[105] Recommendations for creating a supportive atmosphere during withdrawal discussions included
- Taking a moment at the beginning of the conversation to inquire about the family's emotional state
- Acknowledging verbal and nonverbal expressions of emotion and using that to support families
- Acknowledging that most family members face a significant emotional burden when a loved one is critically ill or dying

During the family meeting in which a decision to withdraw life support is made, a time to initiate withdrawal is usually established. For example, a distant family member may need to arrive, and then the procedure will occur. When appropriate, the patient should be moved to a separate or special room. It is helpful if other staff members are alerted to the fact that a withdrawal is occurring. A neutral sign hung on the door or use of a special room may caution staff to avoid loud conversations and laughter, which is quite upsetting to grieving families. Nurses can support the family by suggesting specific measures to modify the environment and minimize symptoms that the family might perceive as suffering of their loved one.[104]

After the decision to remove ventilatory support is made and the family is gathered, the family should be told what the impending death will be like. When the patient is dependent on ventilatory support or vasopressors and that support is removed, death typically follows in minutes. The patient appears as if sleeping, and the usual signs of color and skin temperature changes will not be seen before death. The opposite is true if the patient is not ventilator dependent. When the patient will be extubated at the beginning of the withdrawal process, the family should be prepared for respiratory noises and gasping respirations. These signs are less likely when the endotracheal tube is removed near the end of the withdrawal process, as is more commonly done. When assessing how prepared family members felt for what would happen during withdrawal of life support, Kirchhoff and colleagues[106] found that families who did not receive preparatory information before the withdrawal of life support requested this information during interviews 2 to 4 weeks after the patient's death. Family members who received this recommended information felt significantly more prepared. Providing information to families for the experience of withdrawal alerts them to what the patient may exhibit as death approaches, reducing the distress families may feel during the withdrawal process.

Pacemakers or implantable cardioverter-defibrillators should be turned off to prevent patient distress from their firing[107] and to avoid interfering with the pronouncement of death.[85] Wiegand and Kalowes[108] provide detailed information about the conversations that should be held with the patient[109] and how each of the specific devices are deactivated. Neuromuscular blocking agents should be discontinued, because paralysis precludes the assessment of the patient's discomfort and the means of the patient to communicate with loved ones. Time for clearance of the medication should be carefully considered in planning the withdrawal process.[85]

The removal of monitors is usually recommended.[110] However, physicians and nurses may use the monitor to assess the distress of the patient during the withdrawal process and to adjust the amount of medication needed for symptom management. Families may glance at the monitor to verify that electrical activity has ceased, because the appearance of death may be too subtle to detect. If not needed, monitors should be removed to make the room appear as normal as possible. It is important, however, to include family members in the decision-making process.

Opioids and Sedatives

Opioids and benzodiazepines are the most commonly administered medications, because dyspnea and anxiety are the usual symptoms related to ventilator withdrawal. Campbell[111] stated that brain-dead patients do not require sedation and that patients with brainstem activity only may not show signs of distress or need sedation. Von Gunten and Weissman[112] recommended sedating all patients, even those who are comatose. They recommend a bolus dose of morphine (2 to 10 mg IV) and a continuous morphine infusion at 50% of the bolus dose per hour. Midazolam (1 to 2 mg IV) is given, followed by an infusion at 1 mg/hr. The intent is to provide good symptom control so that doses accelerate until the patient's comfort is achieved. Additional medication should be available at the bedside for immediate administration if discomfort is observed in the patient. In one study, the use of opioids or benzodiazepines to treat discomfort after the withdrawal of life support did not hasten death in critically ill patients.[113]

Ventilator Settings

After the patient's comfort is achieved, ventilator settings are reduced. An experienced physician, a respiratory therapist, and a nurse should be present during this time. Ventilator alarms should be turned off. The method of withdrawal adopted is usually determined by the clinician's preference. The choice of terminal wean as opposed to extubation is based on considerations of access for suctioning, appearance of the patient for the family, how long the patient will survive off the ventilator, and whether the patient has the ability to communicate with loved ones at the bedside.

If terminal wean is used, positive end-expiratory pressure (PEEP) is reduced to normal, and then the mode is set to patient control. Next, the Fio_2 is reduced to 0.21 (21%). All of these steps are taken slowly while observing the patient for distress or anxiety. If extubation is performed immediately rather than at the end of the terminal wean, the family should be prepared for airway compromise and the appearance of the patient.

All patients do not require the same ventilator weaning or extubation protocols. For example, Campbell[111] recommended turning off the ventilator and extubating patients who are brain dead, placing patients who have brainstem-only injuries on a T-piece, and using terminal weaning for those with altered consciousness or those who are conscious. The terminal wean offers the most control over secretions, respiratory noises, and gasping.

PROFESSIONAL ISSUES

Health Care Settings

Professional issues surround the provision of palliative care within traditional acute and clinical settings. In critical care units, care may be managed by an intensivist or by a committee of specialists, but seldom by the family physician who knows the patient. The use of consultants may be limited. Palliative care specialists may be available at certain times, but they are often considered "outsiders" and are infrequently invited. How the consultation is arranged may vary by institution. Turf issues should not compromise patient care. Having a clear plan for withdrawal and better preparation of the family may assist the professionals involved in feeling more comfortable with the care provided.[114] Expert nurses should advocate for vulnerable patients by communicating the patient's wishes and presenting a realistic picture to family members.[115]

Some interventions have been found helpful for health professionals in improving patient care. Although it did not improve nurses' assessment of patients' dying experience, a standardized order form for withdrawal was found to increase the amount of medications nurses administered for sedation.[116] Death rounds for critical care unit medical residents were well received and recommended to be included in future rotations.[117]

Emotional Support for the Nurse

Nurses who care for the dying patient need to have their work as valued as other high-tech functions in the critical care unit. Critical care units usually have several nurses who are looked to by other staff to provide end-of-life care or to assist with withdrawal of life support. When several deaths occur close together, those nurses may be called on frequently. Some consideration in assignment should be given when a nurse has more than one death in a shift or a week. Taking a new admission is also difficult immediately after a death, and it can occur before the family has left the unit. Nurse administrators can provide some additional resources, debriefing, or time off when the burden has been high. Hearing supportive words from colleagues has been reported by critical care nurses as helpful in coping with the death of a patient.[118]

Nurses experience moral distress when aggressive care is offered to patients who are not expected to benefit from it. These levels of distress are high and have implications for retention of highly skilled nurses.[119] One study showed that nurses' experience of moral distress and a negative ethical environment is more severe than that of their physician colleagues.[120] Developing a consensus about care was found to be the most helpful approach.[121] Nurses in this study had a number of suggestions when questioned about what could be done to improve end-of-life care, such as facilitating dying with dignity, having someone with patients who are dying, managing patients' symptoms, knowing and then following patients' wishes for end-of-life care, and promoting earlier cessation of treatment or not initiating aggressive treatment at all.

Until recently, end-of-life content in nursing school curriculums and textbooks was sparse, and continuing education was limited for licensed nurses on this topic. The End of Life Nursing Education Consortium (ELNEC) was created in 2000 to address gaps in education for nurses caring for dying patients. Based on national reports, guidelines, recommendations, and research studies, ELNEC has grown into the premier source of end-of-life training for nurses all over the world. The Critical Care ELNEC course became available in 2006 and addressed topics focused on the critical care unit setting.[122]

ORGAN DONATION

Legal Issues

The Social Security Act Section 1138 requires that hospitals have written protocols for the identification of potential organ donors.[123] The Joint Commission (TJC) has a standard on organ donation and there is a variety of state legislation to direct health care providers and organ recovery agencies.[124] Although an impending death marks a difficult time for family members, the nurse must notify the organ procurement official to approach the family with a donation request. These individuals have training to make a supportive request and are the ones to decide whether a family should not be approached based on the patient's disease. Although organ donation may not be appropriate in some cases, tissue donation remains a consideration. More information is available in Chapter 37.

Brain Death

Death may be pronounced when the patient meets a list of neurologic criteria. However, there are differences among hospital policies for certification of brain death, which may permit differences in the circumstances under which patients are pronounced dead in different U.S. hospitals.[125] Families do not always understand the meaning of brain death, and they are less likely to donate organs when they believe the patient will not be dead until the ventilator is turned off and the heart stops.[126] How these conversations are held will determine families' understanding and positively affect donation. Campbell[3] recommended not suggesting that the organs are alive while the brain is dead, but rather that the organs are functioning as a result of the machines used. Chapter 37 provides more information on the specifics of brain death.

FAMILY CARE

In this chapter, the term *family* means whatever the patient states is the family. An integral part of the patient-family dyad, families expect a cure for any condition the patient may have; they do not expect to receive bad news. They look for the good news in any message received from caregivers and are surprised

when told that death is the only outcome possible.[106] Families need assistance in forming their expectations about outcomes. Ongoing communication about the patient's progress is preferable to waiting until the patient is near death and then communicating with the family. Most studies of families at this time are descriptive, and interventions need to be developed to help them.[127]

One intervention used with families at the end of life is the use of a grieving or comfort cart. In one critical care unit,[128] the cart has a top drawer with English and Spanish versions of the Bible, Koran, and Book of Mormon and pamphlets about grief and bereavement. The lower portion of the cart holds paper cups, napkins, and condiments. Fresh coffee and tea are brewed on the unit and served with muffins and cookies from the cafeteria. Family responses have been positive because they do not want to leave the bedside despite their hunger. Another strategy is to provide nursing units with supplies to support the emotional and spiritual needs of families at the end of life that include religious items and music.[129,130]

Communication Needs

Families have complained about infrequent physician communication,[131] unmet communication needs in the shift from aggressive to end-of-life care,[132] and lacking or inadequate communication.[133] Sometimes families are not ready to receive the prognosis and engage in decision making.[134] Communication seems to be the most common source of complaints in families across studies and should be at the center of efforts to improve end-of-life care.

The health care team can reinforce the legitimacy of the family expressing feelings of disappointment, sadness, and loss. It is important that the family is made aware that the patient was more than a clinical disease and that he or she was recognized as an individual while in the critical care unit. When relatives of critical care unit patients were provided with a brochure on bereavement and received a proactive communication, they had lower negative scores on the Impact of Event Scale and on the Hospital Anxiety and Depression Scale. Ways to address the cultural, social, and emotional issues surrounding the expression of grief are given in the NIC feature on Grief Work Facilitation (Box 11-2).[135]

Waiting for Good News

Patients and families do not come to the critical care unit with the expectation of death. Even those who have had previous admissions expect to be "saved." They tend to listen to imparted information looking for good news; even when bad news is given, they may initially deny it or have great difficulty taking it in.[133] Having this in mind while talking to families may assist professionals in interpreting families' responses.

Preparing families for changes in the patient as the health condition deteriorates helps them make plans. They need to know if other family members should be called, if someone should spend the night, or if financial arrangements should be changed before an impending death (e.g., to enable the widow to have access to funds). Anticipated changes can be described to prepare families. Emotional support and grieving can be facilitated through discussion of the dying patient and their

BOX 11-2 NIC

Grief Work Facilitation

Definition

Assistance with the resolution of a significant loss

Activities

Identify the loss

Assist the patient to identify the nature of the attachment to the lost object or person

Assist the patient to identify the initial reaction to the loss

Encourage expression of feelings about the loss

Listen to expression of grief

Encourage discussion of previous loss experiences

Encourage the patient to verbalize memories of the loss, both past and current

Make empathetic statements about grief

Encourage identification of greatest fears concerning the loss

Instruct in phases of the grieving process, as appropriate

Support progression through personal grieving stages

Include significant others in discussions and decisions, as appropriate

Assist patient to identify personal coping strategies

Encourage patient to implement cultural, religious, and social customs associated with the loss

Communicate acceptance of discussing loss

Answer children's questions associated with the loss

Use clear words, such as *dead* or *died*, rather than euphemisms

Encourage children to discuss feelings

Encourage expression of feelings in ways comfortable to the child, such as writing, drawing, or playing

Assist the child to clarify misconceptions

Identify sources of community support

Support efforts to resolve previous conflict, as appropriate

Reinforce progress made in the grieving process

Assist in identifying modifications needed in lifestyle

From Bulechek GM, et al. *Nursing Interventions Classification (NIC)*. 6th ed. St. Louis: Mosby; 2013.

unique qualities and families' memories. Interactive patient education television services provide healing music and videos that help to create a more comfortable environment for families as they wait for the next step in the dying process. Often, families will play the patient's favorite music or movies. Many services also provide access to the Internet through which family pictures or videos can be accessed. Even before the patient dies, provision of these services can be beneficial through visiting a shared past, making the most of the present, and hoping for an end to the patient's suffering and healing for loved ones.

Families may refuse to forgo life-supporting treatments and want "everything done" because of mistrust of health professionals, poor communication, survivor guilt, or religious or cultural reasons.[64] Effective communication throughout the hospitalization and information provided throughout the stay predispose the family to better acceptance of news as the patient deteriorates. Family satisfaction is increased when they feel supported during their decision making[136,137] or hear more empathic statements from physicians.[105]

Family Meetings

Families may experience a sense of crisis as emergencies occur or as the patient deteriorates and dies. Responses to the news

of the death vary. Family members may show anger or be quiet, exhibit emotions or stoicism. Culture or religious beliefs may affect their response to news. It is helpful to ask if they would like to see a chaplain or a social worker. Quiet and calm, some privacy, and support are always appreciated.

Family meetings in the presence of the critical care team have been one method used to arrive at a common understanding of the patient's prognosis and goals for future care.[138,139] An analysis of the amount of time families had to speak in these meetings revealed that when families had greater opportunity to talk, their satisfaction with physician communication increased and their ratings of conflict with the physician decreased. Abbott and colleagues[140] discussed families' descriptions, 1 year after decisions about withdrawal of life support, of conflict centering on communication and the behavior of the staff. After the patient's death, greater family satisfaction with withdrawal of life support was associated with the following measures[141]:

- The process of withdrawal of life support being well explained
- Withdrawal of life support proceeding as expected
- Patient appearing comfortable
- Family and friends being prepared
- Appropriate person initiating discussion
- Adequate privacy during withdrawal of life support
- A chance to voice concerns

Curtis and colleagues[142] have been studying the process of family meetings and how to improve them to promote better end-of-life care for critical care unit patients and their families. They found that the missed opportunities that occur during these meetings were occasions to listen to family, to acknowledge and address emotions, and to pursue key tenets of palliative care, such as patient preferences, surrogate decision making, and nonabandonment.

Family Presence During Cardiopulmonary Resuscitation

To be helpful, the family's presence during procedures or resuscitative attempts[40] should be coupled with staff support. Critical care nurses and emergency nurses have taken family members to the bedside for resuscitation or invasive procedures, but most did not have written policies for the family's presence.[143] Sometimes, these experiences provide opportunities for the family to be supportive of the patient. At other times, the family may become more aware of what is involved in decisions they have made on behalf of the patient. Seeing the steps of resuscitation may make clearer the impact of decisions made or delayed.

Visiting Hours

Visiting in critical care units continues to be restricted,[144] despite national calls for increases in patient or family control over the care.[145] Restricting visiting for dying critical care unit patients seems to be unconscionable. Providing the visiting time to help family members say good-bye is an important function. Family members may have difficulty in seeing the person they knew among all the tubes. Coaching can be provided about how to approach the patient and about how the patient may still be able to hear despite appearing to be nonresponsive. Visitors should be permitted to the extent possible, while not interfering with other patients' privacy or rest. Children, unless they represent a significant source of infection, should be allowed to say good-bye, but they may need adult assistance in understanding the situation. Families may have religious or cultural ceremonies that are important for them to perform before the patient dies or experiences withdrawal of life support. These practices should be encouraged and facilitated as much as possible. Continuity of care by the same nurse is important. As the patient nears death, nurses have sometimes stayed with the family after the end of a shift when death was imminent so that they would not need to adjust to another person at this difficult time.[118]

After Death

After the death, the family may wish to spend time at the bedside. The family members' time with the body should be unhurried and private. They need adequate room to sit and spend time. They can be asked if they need assistance or resources and whether they wish to be alone or have someone nearby. Frequently, the bed is needed for another patient, and juggling is required to ensure that the family has sufficient time even as another patient needs to be admitted. Supporting families after a death involves immediate bereavement support, information on what to do about the death, bereavement support for the future, contact with the family after death, and assessment of the quality of care the patient experienced.[146] Having material already prepared with the necessary after-death information is quite helpful at this time. Most hospices offer post-death bereavement support groups that are available to any member of the community free of charge, regardless of whether a loved one was enrolled in hospice. Nurses need to be aware of their own judgment on what is an appropriate response, because individuals respond differently to the same news, even within the same family.

COLLABORATIVE CARE

The ability to provide collaborative, compassionate end-of-life care is the responsibility of all clinicians who work with the critically ill. Interdisciplinary collaborative efforts are associated with improvement in care.[147] In 2008, the SCCM published a revised guideline, "Recommendations for End-of-Life Care in the Intensive Care Unit," to provide guidance for end-of-life care for the team.[148] The Evidence-Based Practice feature on end-of-life care provides a summary of the topics included (Box 11-3). The Robert Wood Johnson Foundation (RWJF) Critical Care End-of-Life Peer Workgroup[71] identified seven end-of-life care domains for use in the critical care unit:
1. Patient- and family-centered decision making
2. Communication
3. Continuity of care
4. Emotional and practical support
5. Symptom management and comfort care

BOX 11-3   EVIDENCE-BASED PRACTICE

Guideline for End-of-Life Care in the Critical Care Unit

QSEN The key topics of the guidelines for end-of-life care in the critical care unit, based on research and expert panel review, are categorized below.

Patient- and Family-Centered Care and Decision Making: The Comprehensive Ideal for End-of-Life Care
- Use the legal standards for decision making.
- Resolve conflict.
- Communicate with families.

Ethical Principles Related to Withdrawal of Life-Sustaining Treatment
- Withholding versus withdrawing
- Killing versus allowing to die
- Intended versus merely foreseen consequences

Practical Aspects of Withdrawing Life-Sustaining Treatments in the Critical Care Unit
- The procedure
- Specific issues
- Use of paralytics

Symptom Management in End-of-Life Care
- Pain and dyspnea
- Delirium
- Medications used

Considerations at the Time of Death
- Notification of death
- Brain death
- Organ donation
- Bereavement and support
- Needs of the interdisciplinary team

Research, Quality Improvement, and Education
- Develop interventions likely to improve the quality of care.
- Develop education programs.

Data from Truog RD et al. Recommendations for end-of-life care in the intensive care unit: a consensus statement by the American Academy of Critical Care Medicine. *Crit Care Med.* 2008;36(3):953.

---

6. Spiritual support
7. Emotional and organizational support for ICU clinicians

Individuals[149] and groups[150,151,152] have developed websites for online tools to improve end-of-life care. Critical care unit staff will be able to assess the quality of their care by assessing perceptions of families and staff, auditing documentation,[153] or making observations of care. The same attention should be placed on improving end-of-life care that is placed on skills of electrocardiogram interpretation or hemodynamic monitoring.

BOX 11-4   CASE STUDY

Patient at the End of Life

Brief Patient History

Mr. C is a 17-year-old, African American boy who was involved in a motor vehicle accident. He sustained a cervical fracture at the level of C2 that transected his spinal column and both vertebral arteries. Rescue breathing was begun in the field by bystanders, and he was intubated by paramedics en route to the hospital. Mr. C's parents state that they want everything possible done and that they have faith that God will heal their son.

Clinical Assessment

Mr. C is admitted to the critical care unit from the emergency department. He is ventilator dependent. His skin is warm and dry. He is unresponsive to verbal or painful stimuli, and there is no physical movement. Mr. C's family remains at the bedside 24 hours each day throughout the week. They converse with Mr. C, speaking about all the things they are going to do when he gets home.

Diagnostic Procedures

Mr. C's vital signs are as follows: blood pressure of 120/72 mm Hg, heart rate of 120 beats/min (sinus tachycardia), no spontaneous respiration, temperature of 97.8° F, and Glasgow Coma Scale score of 3. Computed tomography of the head showed a global ischemic infarct involving both ventricles, and electroencephalography revealed no detectable cortical activity.

Medical Diagnosis

Mr. C is diagnosed with brain death.

Questions

1. What major outcomes do you expect to achieve for this patient?
2. What problems or risks must be managed to achieve these outcomes?
3. What interventions must be initiated to monitor, prevent, manage, or eliminate the problems and risks identified?
4. What interventions should be initiated to promote optimal functioning, safety, and well-being of the patient?
5. What possible learning needs do you anticipate for this patient?
6. What cultural and age-related factors may have a bearing on the patient's plan of care?

■ SUMMARY

- End-of-life care requires knowledge and skill, similar to any other aspect of critical care unit care.
- Patient- and family-centered decision making is key.
- Communication skills are enhanced with additional training in end-of-life conversations.
- Family presence during procedures or resuscitative attempts should be coupled with staff support.
- Extended visiting times are needed to help family members say good-bye.
- Proactive control of symptoms is vital for the patient's comfort.

REFERENCES

1. Rabow MW, et al. End-of-life care content in 50 textbooks from multiple specialties. *JAMA.* 2000;283(6):771.
2. Kirchhoff KT, et al. Analysis of end-of-life content in critical care nursing textbook. *J Prof Nurs.* 2003;19(6):372.
3. Campbell ML. *Forgoing life-sustaining therapy: how to care for the patient who is near death.* Aliso Viejo, CA: AACN; 1998.
4. Curtis JR, Rubenfeld GD, eds. *Managing death in the intensive care unit: the transition from cure to comfort.* Oxford: Oxford University Press; 2001.
5. Siegel MD. End of life decision making in the ICU. *Clin Chest Med.* 2009;30:181.
6. Roche V. Do Not Resuscitate vs. Allow Natural Death, USA Today, 3/2/2009. 2009. http://www.usatoday.com/news/health/2009-03-02-DNR-natural-death_N.htm. Accessed April 22, 2012.
7. Morrison RS, et al. The growth of palliative care programs in United States hospitals. *J Palliat Med.* 2005;8(6):1127.
8. Medina J, Puntillo K, eds. *AACN Protocols for Practice: Palliative Care and End of Life Issues in Critical Care.* Boston: Jones & Bartlett; 2006.
9. *AACN.* Paliative and End of Life Advocacy Initiative. Available at http://aacn.org/WD/Palliative/Content/PalAndEOLInfo.content?menu=Practice&lastmenu=. Accessed April 15, 2012.
10. Lynch M, Dahlin C. The national consensus project and national quality forum preferred practices in care of the imminently dying: implications for nursing. *J Hosp Palliat Nurs.* 2007;9(6):316.
11. Teno JM, et al. Bereaved family member perceptions of quality of end-of-life care in U.S. regions with high and low usage of intensive care unit care. *J Am Geriatr Soc.* 2005;53(11):1905.
12. Nelson JE, et al. End-of-life care for the critically ill: a national intensive care unit survey. *Crit Care Med.* 2006;34(10):2547.
13. Glavan BJ, et al. Using the medical record to evaluate the quality of end-of-life care in the intensive care unit. *Crit Care Med.* 2008;36(4):1138.
14. Beckstrand RL, et al. Providing a "good death": critical care nurses' suggestions for improving end-of-life care. *Am J Crit Care.* 2006;15(1):38.
15. Mularski RA, et al. Quality of dying in the ICU: ratings by family members. *Chest.* 2005;128(1):280.
16. Mosenthal AC, et al. Integrating palliative care in the surgical and trauma intensive care unit: a report from the Improving

Palliative Care in the Intensive Care Unit (IPAL-ICU) Project Advisory Board and the Center to Advance Palliative *Care. Crit Care Med.* 2010;40(4):1199.

17. SUPPORT Investigators. A controlled trial to improve care for seriously ill hospitalized patients. The study to understand prognoses and preferences for outcomes and risks of treatments (SUPPORT). *JAMA.* 1995;274(20):1591.

18. Field MJ, Cassell CK, eds. *Approaching Death: Improving Care at the End of Life.* Washington, DC: National Academy Press; 1997.

19. Angus DC, et al. Use of intensive care at the end of life in the United States: an epidemiologic study. *Crit Care Med.* 2004;32(3):638.

20. *Center to Advance Palliative Care.* Palliative care programs continue rapid growth in U.S. hospitals becoming standard practice throughout the country. http://www.capc.org/news-and-events/releases/analysis-of-us-hospital-palliative-care-programs-2010-snapshot.pdf/file_view. Accessed March 4, 2012.

21. Morrison RS, et al. Cost savings associated with US hospital based palliative care programs. *Arch Intern Med.* 2008;168(16):1783.

22. Gillick MR. Advance care planning. *N Engl J Med.* 2004;350(1):7.

23. DHHS. Department of Health and Human Services. Advance directives and advance care planning: Report to Congress, August, 2008. Retrieved April 2, 2012.

24. Nishimura A, et al. Patients who complete advance directives and what they prefer. *Mayo Clin Proc.* 2007;82(12):1480.

25. Cook D, et al. Levels of care in the intensive care unit: a research program. *Am J Crit Care.* 2006;15(3):269.

26. Center for Ethics in Health Care. Oregon Health Sciences University. History of the POLST paradigm initiative, 2008. Retrieved April 26. 2012.

27. Hickman SE, et al. The consistency between treatments provided to nursing facility residents and orders on the Physician Orders for Life Sustaining Treatment form. *J Am Geriatr Soc.* 2011;59(11):2091.

28. Hickman SE, et al. A comparison of methods to communicate treatment preferences in nursing facilities: traditional practices versus the physician orders for life-sustaining treatment program. *J Amer Geriatr Soc.* 2010;58(7):1241.

29. Briggs LA, et al. Patient-centered advance care planning in special patient populations: a pilot study. *J Prof Nurs.* 2004;20(1):47.

30. Smith R. A good death. *BMJ.* 2000;320:129.

31. Rubenfeld GD. Principles and practice of withdrawing life-sustaining treatments. *Crit Care Clin.* 2004;20(3):435.

32. Tilden V, et al. Family decision-making to withdraw life-sustaining treatments from hospitalized patients. *Nurs Res.* 2001;50(2):105.

33. Gilmer T, et al. The costs of nonbeneficial treatment in the intensive care setting. *Health Aff (Millwood).* 2005;24(4):961.

34. Ebell MH, et al. Survival after in-hospital cardiopulmonary resuscitation: a meta-analysis. *J Gen Intern Med.* 1998;13(12):805.

35. Brindley PG, et al. Predictors of survival following in-hospital adult cardiopulmonary resuscitation. *CMAJ.* 2002;167(4):343.

36. Elshove-Bolk J, et al. In-hospital resuscitation of the elderly: characteristics and outcome. *Resuscitation.* 2007;74(2):372.

37. *EPERC.* Fast Facts #179 CPR survival in the hospital setting, 2009. http://www.eperc.mcw.edu/EPERC/FastFactsIndex/ff_179.htm.

38. FitzGerald JD, et al. Functional status among survivors of in-hospital cardiopulmonary resuscitation. SUPPORT investigators study to understand progress and preferences for outcomes and risks of treatment. *Arch Intern Med.* 1997;157(1):72.

39. American Association of Critical-Care Nurses. Family presence during CPR and invasive procedures, 2004. www.aacn.org/WD/Practice/Docs/Family_Presence_During_CPR_11-2004.pdf. Accessed January 2009.

40. Emergency Nurses Association. Family presence at the bedside during invasive procedures and cardiopulmonary resuscitation, 2005. http://www.ena.org/about/position/PDFs/5F118F5052C2479C848012F5BCF87F7C.PDF. Accessed January 2009.

41. Covinsky KE, et al. Communication and decision-making in seriously ill patients: findings of the SUPPORT project. The study to understand prognoses and preferences for outcomes and risks of treatments. *J Am Geriatr Soc.* 2000;48(5 suppl): S187.

42. Burns JP, et al. Do-not-resuscitate order after 25 years. *Crit Care Med.* 2003;31(5):1543.

43. Keenan CH, Kish SK. The influence of do-not-resuscitate orders on care provided for patients in the surgical intensive care unit of a cancer center. *Crit Care Nurs Clin North Am.* 2000;12(3):385.

44. Bacchetta MD, et al. Factors influencing DNR decision-making in a surgical ICU. *J Am Coll Surg.* 2006;202(6):995.

45. Sulmasy DP, et al. The quality of care plans for patients with do-not-resuscitate orders. *Arch Intern Med.* 2004;164(14):1573.

46. Chang Y, Huang CF, Lin CC. Do-not-resuscitate orders for critically ill patients in intensive care. *Nurs Ethics.* 2010;17(4):445.

47. Park YR, Kim JA, Kim K. Changes in how ICU nurses perceive the DNR decision and their nursing activity after implementing it. *Nurs Ethics.* 2011;18(6):802.

48. Christakis NA, Lamont EB. Extent and determinants of error in doctors' prognoses in terminally ill patients: prospective cohort study. *BMJ.* 2004;320 (7233):469.

49. Lynn J, et al. Prognoses of seriously ill hospitalized patients on the days before death: implications for patient care and public policy. *New Horiz.* 1997;5(1):56.

50. McDonald DD, et al. Communicating end-of-life preferences. *West J Nurs Res.* 2003;25(6):652; discussion 667-675.

51. Fried TR, Bradley EH. What matters to seriously ill older persons making end-of-life treatment decisions? A qualitative study. *J Palliat Med.* 2003;6(2):237.

52. Teno JM, et al. Medical care inconsistent with patients' treatment goals: association with 1-year Medicare resource use and survival. *J Am Geriatr Soc.* 2002;50(3):496.

53. Mularski RA, et al. Educational agendas for interdisciplinary end-of-life curricula. *Crit Care Med.* 2001;29(2 suppl):N16.

54. Wood EB, et al. Enhancing palliative care education in medical school curricula: implementation of the palliative education assessment tool. *Acad Med.* 2002;77(4):285.

55. Strand K, Flaatten H. Severity scoring in the ICU: a review. *Acta Anaesthesiol Scand.* 2008;52(4):467.

56. Marshall JC, et al. Multiple organ dysfunction score: a reliable descriptor of a complex clinical outcome. *Crit Care Med.* 1995;23(10):1638.

57. Rocker G, et al. Clinician predictions of intensive care unit mortality. *Crit Care Med.* 2004;32(5):1149.

58. Lau F, et al. A systematic review of prognostic tools for estimating survival time in palliative care. *J Palliat Care.* 2007;23(2):93.

59. White DB, et al. Toward shared decision making at the end of life in intensive care units: opportunities for improvement. *Arch Intern Med.* 2007;167(5):461.

60. Limerick MH. The process used by surrogate decision makers to withhold and withdraw life-sustaining measures in an intensive care environment. *Oncol Nurs Forum.* 2007;34(2):331.

61. *Coalition for Compassionate Care California.* Brochures and FAQs (CPR/DNR, Tube Feeding). http://capolst.org/?for=providers#brochures. 2012.

62. Family Caregiver Alliance. Facts Sheets (End of life choices: CPR/DNR, Ventilators/Tube Feedings), 2012. http://caregiver.org/caregiver/jsp/publications.jsp?nodeid=345&expandnodeid=384.

63. Ahrens T, et al. Improving family communications at the end of life: implications for length of stay in the intensive care unit and resource use. *Am J Crit Care.* 2003;12(4):317; discussion 324.

64. Prendergast TJ, Puntillo KA. Withdrawal of life support: intensive caring at the end of life. *JAMA.* 2002;288(21):2732.

65. White DB, et al. Decisions to limit life-sustaining treatment for critically ill patients who lack both decision-making capacity and surrogate decision-makers. *Crit Care Med.* 2006;4(8):2053.

66. Azoulay E, et al. Half the family members of intensive care unit patients do not want to share in the decision-making process: a study in 78 French intensive care units. *Crit Care Med.* 2004;32(9):1832.

67. Baker R, et al. Family satisfaction with end-of-life care in seriously ill hospitalized adults. *J Am Geriatr Soc.* 2000;48(5 suppl):S61.

68. Curtis JR. Communicating about end-of-life care with patients and families in the intensive care unit. *Crit Care Clin.* 2004;20(3):363.

69. Soderstrom IM, et al. Interactions between family members and staff in intensive care units—an observation and interview study. *Int J Nurs Stud.* 2006;43(6):707.

70. Davidson JE, et al. Clinical practice guidelines for support of the family in the patient-centered intensive care unit: American College of Critical Care Task Force 2004-2005. *Crit Care Med.* 2007;35(2):605.

71. Clarke EB, et al. Quality indicators for end-of-life care in the intensive care unit. *Crit Care Med.* 2003;31(9):2255.

72. Kirchhoff KT, Faas AI. Family support at end of life. *AACN Adv Crit Care.* 2007;18(4):426.

73. Degenholtz HB, et al. Race and the intensive care unit: disparities and preferences for end-of-life care. *Crit Care Med.* 2003;31(5 suppl):S373.

74. Lipson JG, et al. *Culture and nursing care: a pocket guide.* San Francisco: UCSF Nursing Press; 1996.

75. Wall RJ, et al. Spiritual care of families in the intensive care unit. *Crit Care Med.* 2007;35(4):1084.

76. Crawley LM. Racial, cultural, and ethnic factors influencing end-of-life care. *J Palliat Med.* 2005;8(suppl 1):S58.

77. Breen CM, et al. Conflict associated with decisions to limit life-sustaining treatment in intensive care units. *J Gen Intern Med.* 2001;16(5):283.

78. Campbell ML, Guzman JA. Impact of a proactive approach to improve end-of-life care in a medical ICU. *Chest.* 2003;123(1):266.

79. Norton SA, et al. Proactive palliative care in the medical intensive care unit: effects on length of stay for selected high-risk patients. *Crit Care Med.* 2007;35(6):1530.

80. Weigand DL, Kalowes PG. Withdrawal of cardiac medications and devices. *AACN.* 2007;18(4):415.

81. Frick S, et al. Medical futility: predicting outcome of intensive care unit patients by nurses and doctors-a prospective comparative study. *Crit Care Med.* 2003;31(2):456.

82. Meltzer LS, Huckabay LM. Critical care nurses' perceptions of futile care and its effect on burnout. *Am J Crit Care.* 2004;13(3):202.

83. *AACN.* Position Statement on Moral Distress. http://www.aacn.org/WD/Practice/Docs/Moral_Distress.pdf. Accessed March 26, 2012.

84. Ellershaw J, Ward C. Care of the dying patient: the last hours or days of life. *BMJ.* 2003;326(7379):30.

85. Faber-Langendoen K, Lanken PN. Dying patients in the intensive care unit: forgoing treatment, maintaining care. *Ann Intern Med.* 2000;133(11):886.

86. *National Hospice and Palliative Care Organization.* HPNA Position Statement: Artificial nutrition and hydration in advanced illness. http://www.hpna.org/pdf/Artifical_Nutrition_and_Hydration_PDF.pdf. Accessed January 14, 2012.

87. National Consensus Project. Clinical practice guidelines for quality palliative care, 2nd ed., 2009. http://www.nationalconsensusproject.org. Accessed April 2012.

88. EPERC. End of Life and Palliative Education Resource Center. Fast Facts. http://www.eperc.mcw.edu/EPERC/FastFactsandConcepts. Accessed April 2012.

89. Institute of Medicine. *Improving Palliative Care for Cancer: Summary and Recommendations.* Washington, DC: National Academy Press; 2001.

90. Mularski RA. Pain management in the intensive care unit. *Crit Care Clin.* 2004;20(3):381.

91. Gélinas C, et al. Pain assessment and management in critically ill intubated patients: a retrospective study. *Am J Crit Care.* 2004;13(2):126.

92. Foley KM. Pain and symptom control in the dying ICU patient. In Curtis JR, Rubenfeld GD, eds. *Managing Death in the Intensive Care Unit: the Transition from Cure to Comfort.* Oxford: Oxford University Press; 2001.

93. Weissman C. Sedation and neuromuscular blockade in the ICU. *Chest.* 2005;128(2):477.

94. Jacobi J, et al. Clinical practice guidelines for the sustained use of sedatives and analgesics in the critically ill adult. *Crit Care Med.* 2002;30(1):119.

95. Kalowes P. Symptom burden at the end of life in patients with terminal and life threatening illness in intensive care units. *University of San Diego.* doctoral dissertation. 2007.

96. Campbell ML. Terminal dyspnea and respiratory distress. *Crit Care Clin.* 2004;20(3):403.

97. Fabbro ED, et al. Symptom control in palliative care, part III: dyspnea and delirium. *J Palliat Med.* 2006;9(2):422.

98. Viola RA, et al. The effects of fluid status and fluid therapy on the dying, 2003 Database of Abstracts of Reviews of Effectiveness (DARE), NHS Centre for Reviews and Dissemination, University of York. http://www.crd.york.ac.uk/CRDWeb/ShowRecord.asp?ID=11998005105. Accessed January 2009.

99. Kehl KA. Treatment of terminal restlessness: a review of the evidence. *J Pain Palliat Care Pharmacother.* 2004;18(1):5.

100. Callanan M, Kelley P. *Final Gifts: Understanding the Special Awareness, Needs, and Communications of the Dying.* New York: Bantam Books; 1997.

101. Marchand L. Fast fact and concept #118: near death awareness, 2009. http://www.eperc.mcw.edu/FastFactPDF/Concept%20 118.pdf. Accessed March 18, 2012.

102. Lilly CM, et al. An intensive communication intervention for the critically ill. *Am J Med.* 2000;109(6):469.

103. Lilly CM, et al. Intensive communication: four-year follow-up from a clinical practice study. *Crit Care Med.* 2003;31(5 suppl): S394.

104. Curtis JR. Interventions to improve care during withdrawal of life-sustaining treatments. *J Palliat Med.* 2005;8(suppl 1):S116.

105. Selph RB, et al. Empathy and life support decisions. *JGIM.* 2008;23(9):1311.

106. Kirchhoff KT, et al. Preparing ICU families for withdrawal of life support: a pilot study. *Am J Crit Care.* 2008;17(2):113.

107. Mueller PS, et al. Ethical analysis of withdrawal of pacemaker or implantable cardioverter-defibrillator support at the end of life. *Mayo Clin Proc.* 2003;78(8):959.

108. Wiegand DL, Kalowes PG. Withdrawal of cardiac medications and devices. *AACN Adv Crit Care.* 2007;18(4):415.

109. Goldstein NE, et al. Management of implantable cardioverter defibrillators in end-of-life care. *Ann Intern Med.* 2004;141(11):835.

110. Rubenfeld GD, Crawford SW. Withdrawal of life-sustaining treatment. In: Curtis JR, Rubenfeld GD, eds. *Managing Death in the Intensive Care Unit: The Transition from Cure to Comfort.* Oxford: Oxford University Press; 2001.

111. Campbell ML. How to withdraw mechanical ventilation: a systematic review of the literature. *AACN Adv Crit Care.* 2007;18(4):397.

112. von Gunten C, Weissman DE. Fast fact and concept #034: symptom control for ventilator withdrawal in the dying patient (part II), 2009. http://www.eperc.mcw.edu/FastFactPDF/ Concept%20034.pdf. Accessed April 21, 2012.

113. Chan JD, et al. Narcotic and benzodiazepine use after withdrawal of life support: Association with time to death? *Chest.* 2004;126(1):286.

114. Rocker GM, et al. Canadian nurses' and respiratory therapists' perspectives on withdrawal of life support in the intensive care unit. *J Crit Care.* 2005;20(1):59.

115. Robichaux CM, Clark AP. Practice of expert critical care nurses in situations of prognostic conflict at the end of life. *Am J Crit Care.* 2006;15(5):480.

116. Treece PD, et al. Evaluation of a standardized order form for the withdrawal of life support in the intensive care unit. *Crit Care Med.* 2004;32(5):1141.

117. Hough CL, et al. Death rounds: end-of-life discussions among medical residents in the intensive care unit. *J Crit Care.* 2005;20(1):20.

118. Kirchhoff KT, et al. Intensive care nurses' experiences with end-of-life care. *Am J Crit Care.* 2000;9(1):36.

119. Elpern EH, et al. Moral distress of staff nurses in a medical intensive care unit. *Am J Crit Care.* 2005;14(6):523.

120. Hamric AB, Blackhall LJ. Nurse-physician perspectives on the care of dying patients in intensive care units: collaboration, moral distress, and ethical climate. *Crit Care Med.* 2007;35(2):422.

121. Badger JM. Factors that enable or complicate end-of-life transitions in critical care. *Am J Crit Care.* 2005;14(6):513.

122. Ferrell BR, Virani R, Malloy P. Evaluation of the end of life nursing education consortium in the USA. *Intl J Palliat Care.* 2006;12(6):269.

123. *Social Security Administration.* Hospital protocols for organ procurement and standards for organ procurement

agencies, 2004: compilation of the Social Security laws. http://www.ssa.gov/OP_Home/ssact/title11/1138.htm. Accessed January 1, 2009.

124. The Joint Commission. Approved: revisions to Standard LD.3.1.10, Element of Performance 12, for critical access hospitals and hospitals. *Joint Commission Perspectives.* 2007;27(6):14.

125. Powner DJ, et al. Variability among hospital policies for determining brain death in adults. *Crit Care Med.* 2004;32(6):1284.

126. Siminoff LA, et al. Families' understanding of brain death. *Prog Transplant.* 2003;13(3):218.

127. Wiegand DL. Families and withdrawal of life-sustaining therapy: state of the science. *J Fam Nurs.* 2006;12(2):165.

128. Whitmer M, et al. Caring in the curing environment. *J Hosp Palliat Nurs.* 2007;9(6):329.

129. Davidson J. Family-centered care: meeting the needs of patients' families and helping families adapt to critical illness. *Crit Care Nurse.* 2009;29(3):28.

130. Davidson J. Gap analysis of cultural and religious needs of hospitalized patients. *Crit Care Nurs Quar.* 2008;31(2): 119-126.

131. Heyland DK, et al. Family satisfaction with care in the intensive care unit: results of a multiple center study. *Crit Care Med.* 2002;30(7):1413.

132. Norton SA, et al. Life support withdrawal: communication and conflict. *Am J Crit Care.* 2003;12(6):548.

133. Kirchhoff KT, et al. The vortex: families' experiences with death in the intensive care unit. *Am J Crit Care.* 2002;11(3):200.

134. Murphy PA, et al. Under the radar: contributions of the SUPPORT nurses. *Nurs Outlook.* 2001;49(5):238.

135. Bulechek GM et al. *Nursing Interventions Classification (NIC).* 6th ed. St Louis: Mosby; 2013.

136. Gries CJ, et al. Family member satisfaction with end-of-life decision making in the ICU. *Chest.* 2008;133(3):704.

137. Stapleton RD, et al. Clinician statements and family satisfaction with family conferences in the intensive care unit. *Crit Care Med.* 2006;34(6):1679.

138. Ambuel B, Weissman D. Fast fact and concept #016: conducting a family conference, 2001. http://www.eperc.mcw.edu/fastFact/ ff_016.htm. Accessed January 2009.

139. Curtis JR, et al. The family conference as a focus to improve communication about end-of- life care in the intensive care unit: opportunities for improvement. *Crit Care Med.* 2001; 29(2 suppl):N26.

140. Abbott KH, et al. Families looking back: one year after discussion of withdrawal or withholding of life-sustaining support. *Crit Care Med.* 2001;29(1):197.

141. Keenan SP, et al. Withdrawal of life support: how the family feels, and why. *J Palliat Care.* 2000;16(suppl):S40.

142. Curtis JR, et al. Missed opportunities during family conferences about end-of-life care in the intensive care unit. *Am J Respir Crit Care Med.* 2005;171(8):844.

143. MacLean SL, et al. Family presence during cardiopulmonary resuscitation and invasive procedures: practices of critical care and emergency nurses. *Am J Crit Care.* 2003;12(3):246.

144. Kirchhoff KT, Dahl N. American association of critical-care nurses' national survey of facilities and units providing critical care. *Am J Crit Care.* 2006;15(1):13.

145. Berwick DM, Kotagal M. Restricted visiting hours in ICUs: time to change. *JAMA.* 2004;292(6):736.

146. Shannon S. Helping families cope with death in the ICU. In: Curtis JR, Rubenfeld GD, eds. *Managing Death in the Intensive*

Care Unit: The Transition from Cure to Comfort. Oxford: Oxford University Press; 2001.

147. Baggs JG, et al. The dying patient in the ICU: role of the interdisciplinary team. *Crit Care Clin.* 2004;20(3):525.

148. Truog RD, et al. Recommendations for end-of-life care in the intensive care unit: a consensus statement by the American Academy of Critical Care Medicine. *Crit Care Med.* 2008;36(3):953.

149. Curtis JR. End of life care research program. http://depts. washington.edu/eolcare/currentprojects. Accessed April 14, 2012.

150. Promoting Excellence in End-of-Life Care. Innovative models and approaches for palliative care. http://www. promotingexcellence.org. Accessed March 15, 2012.

151. *EPERC.* End of life/palliative education resource center. http://www.eperc.mcw.edu/EPERC. Accessed April 2, 2012.

152. *CAPC.* Center to Advance Palliative Care. http://capc.org. Accessed March 15, 2012.

153. Kirchhoff KT, et al. Documentation on withdrawal of life support in adult patients in the intensive care unit. *Am J Crit Care.* 2004;13(4):328.

12

Cardiovascular Anatomy and Physiology

Mary E. Lough

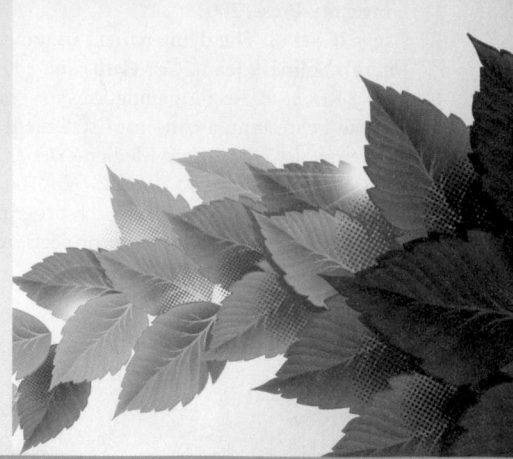

ANATOMY

Discussion of the anatomy of the heart and blood vessels in this text begins on a macroscopic level with a description of the major structures and then progresses to the cellular and molecular levels for each structure.

Macroscopic Structure

Structures of the Heart

The heart is situated in the anterior thoracic cavity, just behind the sternum (Fig. 12-1). Several important structures, including the esophagus, the aorta, the vena cava, and the vertebral column, are located behind the heart. The position of the heart within the chest cavity is such that the chambers normally described as "right" and "left" are, in fact, anterior and posterior.[1] The right ventricle constitutes the majority of the anterior surface (closest to the chest wall) and also the inferior surface (directly above the diaphragm). The left ventricle makes up the anterolateral (front and side) and posterior surfaces. The base of the heart is superior (atrial and great vessel level), and the tip (apex) is inferior (ventricular level), above the diaphragm. The base of the heart includes not only the superior portion of the heart itself but also the roots of the aorta, the vena cava, and pulmonary vessels.

The increasing use of thoracic computed tomography in critical care has highlighted the anatomic inaccuracy of the terms *right ventricle* and *left ventricle* because these terms do not relate to the position of the heart in the chest when described in the standard anatomic position (i.e., upright and facing the observer).[1-3] Despite discussion of these differences, the impetus to change the traditional nomenclature is lacking.

Size and Weight of the Heart

Generally, the size of an individual's heart is about the size of that person's clenched fist. In the adult, this averages 12 cm in length and 8 to 9 cm in breadth at the broadest part. In adult men, the weight of the normal heart averages 310 g, and in women averages 255 g. No significant differences exist in ventricular wall thickness between men and women. Body weight is a better predictor of healthy heart weight than is body surface area or height. Pathologic conditions such as hypertension increase the weight of the heart muscle because of ventricular hypertrophy.

Layers of the Heart

The four distinct layers of the heart are: 1) the pericardium, 2) the epicardium, 3) the myocardium, and 4) the endocardium.

Pericardium. The heart and the origins of the great vessels are surrounded and enclosed by the *pericardium*. The outermost *fibrous pericardium* is a thick envelope that is tough and inelastic. Ligaments anchor the outer pericardium to the diaphragm and the great vessels such that the heart is maintained in a fixed position within the thoracic cavity. The pericardium also provides a physical barrier to infection. Inside the fibrous layer is an inner, double-walled membrane described as the *serous pericardium*.[4] The two layers are labeled "parietal" and "visceral." The *parietal pericardium* adheres to the tough, outer pericardium. The *visceral pericardium* is flexible, adheres directly to the heart, and folds with the surface contours of the heart. The *pericardial cavity* is the potential space between the visceral and parietal layers.[4,5] The space between these two layers normally contains a small amount of pericardial fluid, which is

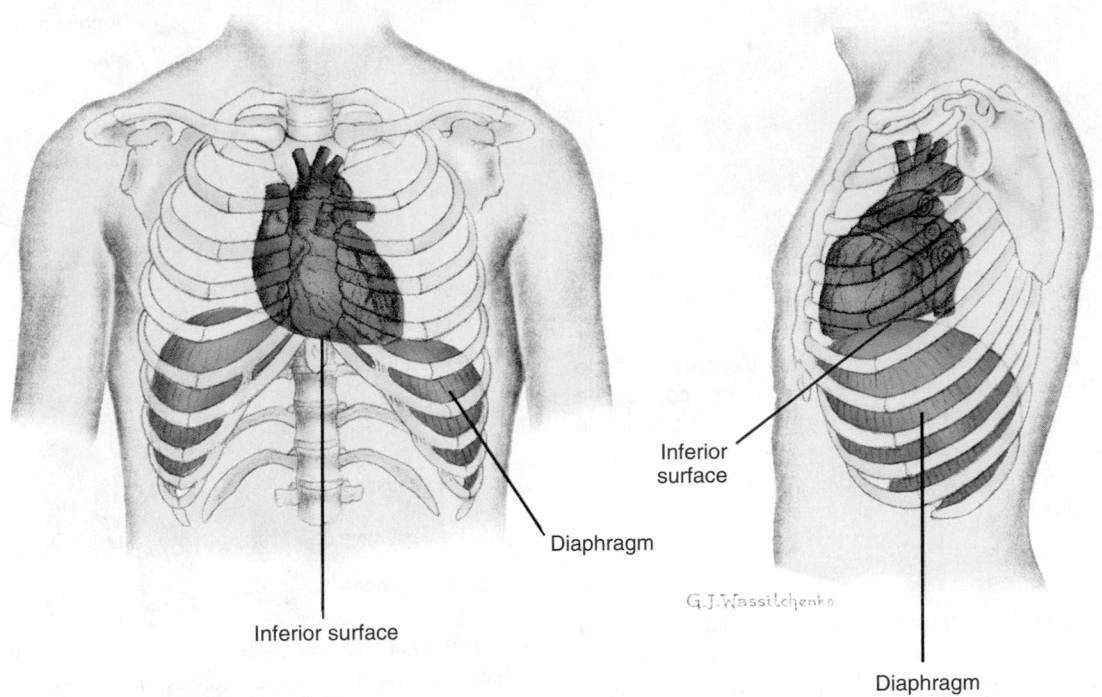

FIGURE 12-1 Anatomic Location of the Heart Within the Thoracic Cavity.

secreted, resorbed, and serves as a lubricant between the layers so that the heart can move without friction.[5] The fibrous, outer pericardial sac is noncompliant and unable to adapt to rapid increases in pericardial fluid.[5] For example, blood can collect in this sac in cardiac tamponade, or serum can collect in pericardial effusion. If the fluid collection in the sac impinges on ventricular filling, ventricular ejection, or coronary artery perfusion, removal of the excess pericardial fluid may be necessary, a procedure known as *pericardiocentesis*.[5] The phrenic nerve provides sensory fibers to the pericardium. The pain that accompanies pericardial effusion and cardiac tamponade is sensed via phrenic nerve innervation.[5]

Epicardial Fat. In adults, a layer of adipose tissue is typically present beneath the visceral pericardium and may surround the heart. This epicardial fat accumulates along the routes of the major coronary arteries and veins. Autopsy data indicate that epicardial fat increases until age 20 to 40 years, but thereafter, the quantity does not depend on age.[6] Epicardial fat covers 80% of the surface of the heart and constitutes about 20% of the total weight of the heart, with the largest quantity positioned over the right ventricle.[6] If a person is overweight or obese with a large quantity of visceral and subcutaneous adipose tissue, usually more epicardial fat is present.[7] Because obesity is endemic in modern society, epicardial fat is receiving more attention. Epicardial fat is hypothesized to increase the risk of coronary artery disease (CAD) because it contains smaller adipocytes compared with other fat deposits, has a different fatty acid composition, and has a higher protein content. This composition facilitates the infiltration of free fatty acids and adipokines into coronary arteries.[8] The fibrous, outer pericardium does not contain any fat deposits.

Epicardium. The epicardium is tightly adhered to the heart and the base of the great vessels as described earlier. The coronary arteries lie on the top of the visceral epicardium.

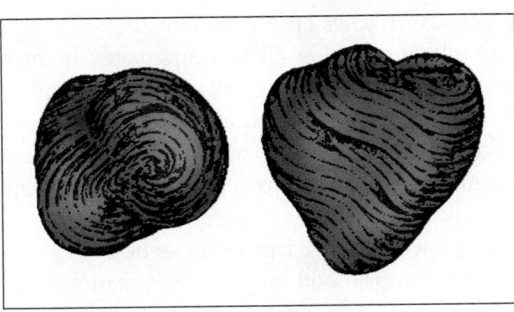

FIGURE 12-2 Macroscopic Structure of the Spiral Musculature of the Ventricular Walls.

Myocardium. The next layer of the heart is the myocardium, a thick, muscular layer. This layer includes all of the atrial and ventricular muscle fibers necessary for contraction. The fibers of the myocardium do not have the same thickness throughout the ventricular walls. The left ventricle is much thicker than the right ventricle or the atria. The fibers are organized in such a manner that the force of contraction is most efficient in ejecting blood toward the outflow tracts in a wringing motion from the apex toward the base (Fig. 12-2).[9] The myocardium is the muscle that is damaged by a "heart attack" or transmural myocardial infarction (MI).

Endocardium. The innermost layer is the endocardium, which is a thin layer of endothelium and connective tissue lining the inside of the heart. This layer is continuous with the endothelium of the great vessels to provide a continuous closed system. Disruption in the endothelium as a result of surgery, trauma, or congenital abnormality can predispose the endocardium to infection. This infective endocarditis is a devastating disease, which, if left untreated, can lead to massive valve damage or sepsis and death.

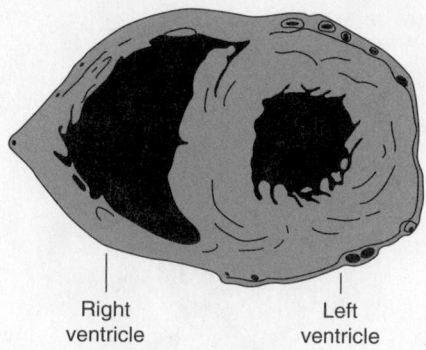

FIGURE 12-3 A Transverse Section of the Ventricles of the Adult Heart. The right ventricle forms the greater part of the anterior surface of the heart, and the wall of the left ventricle is three times as thick as the wall of the right ventricle. (From Quaal S. *Comprehensive Intraaortic Balloon Pumping.* 2nd ed. St. Louis, MO: Mosby; 1993.)

Cardiac Chambers

The human heart has four chambers: the left and right atria and the left and right ventricles. The atria are thin-walled and normally low-pressure chambers. They function to receive blood from the vena cavae and pulmonary arteries and to pump blood into their respective ventricles. Atrial contraction, also known as *atrial kick*, contributes approximately 20% of blood flow to ventricular filling; the other 80% occurs passively during diastole. The ventricles are the primary pumping chambers of the heart. The healthy left ventricle is about 10 to 13 mm thick, and the interior chamber appears round in cross-section.[10] The healthy right ventricle is approximately 3 mm thick, appears to have a triangular shape when viewed from the side, and has a crescent shape when viewed in cross-section (Fig. 12-3). The right ventricle pumps blood into the low-pressured pulmonary circulation, which has a normal mean pressure of approximately 15 mm Hg. The left ventricle must generate tremendous force to eject blood into the aorta (normal mean pressure of approximately 100 mm Hg). Because of left ventricular wall thickness and the large force it must generate, the left ventricle is considered the major pump of the heart. When the left ventricular muscle is damaged from cardiomyopathy or infarction, the effective pumping pressure is diminished, leading to increased left atrial pressure, pulmonary vasculature congestion, and ultimately, systemic venous congestion.

Cardiac Valves

Cardiac valves are composed of flexible, fibrous tissue. A normal valve has the translucent appearance of a rose petal. The valve structure allows blood to flow in only one direction. The opening and closing of the valves depends on the relative pressure gradients on either side of the valve. The four cardiac valves lie in an oblique plane of collagen described as the *fibrous skeleton.* Four adjacent rings of connective tissue contain and support the cardiac valves (Fig. 12-4).

Atrioventricular Valves. The two atrioventricular (AV) valves are named for their location between the atria and the ventricles. These are the tricuspid valve on the right and the mitral valve on the left. The mitral valve is described as having two leaflets, although the "leaflets" are a continuous,

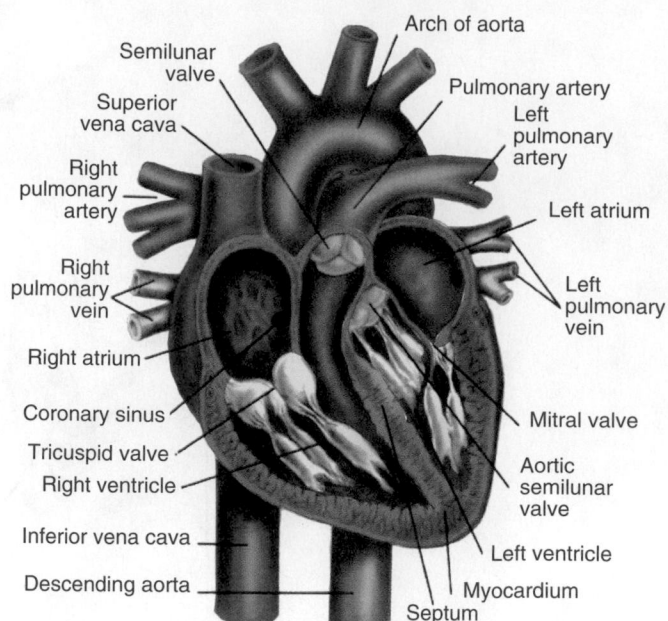

FIGURE 12-4 Cross-Sectional View of the Heart. Note the position of the four cardiac valves. (From Thompson JM, et al. *Mosby's Clinical Nursing.* 5th ed. St. Louis, MO: Mosby; 2002.)

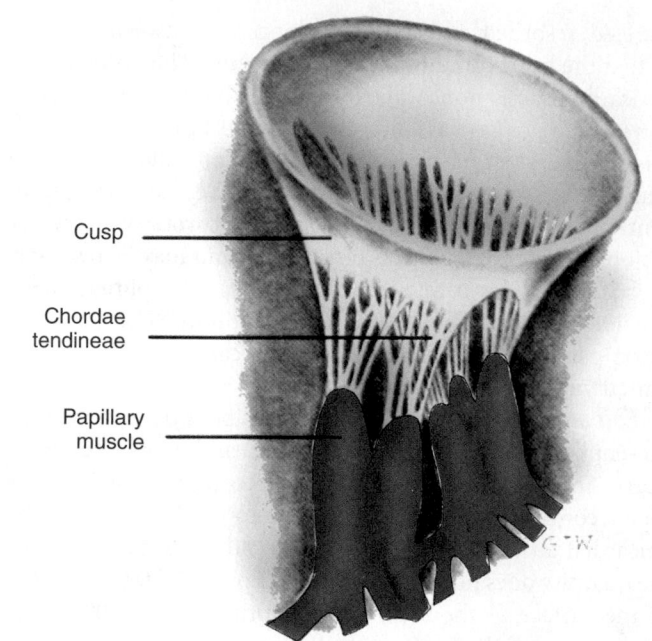

FIGURE 12-5 The mitral valve and the relationship of the cusps, chordae tendineae, and the papillary muscles.

noninterrupted structure.[11] The AV valves are open during ventricular diastole (filling) and prevent backflow of blood into the atria during ventricular systole (contraction). The *chordae tendineae* and *papillary muscles*, which attach to the tricuspid and mitral valves, give the valves stability and prevent valve leaflet eversion during systole (Fig. 12-5). Papillary muscles arise from the ventricular myocardium and derive their blood supply from the coronary arteries. Each papillary muscle gives rise to approximately 4 to 10 main chordae tendineae, which divide into increasingly finer cords as they approach and attach to the valve leaflets. The chordae tendineae are fibrous, avascular

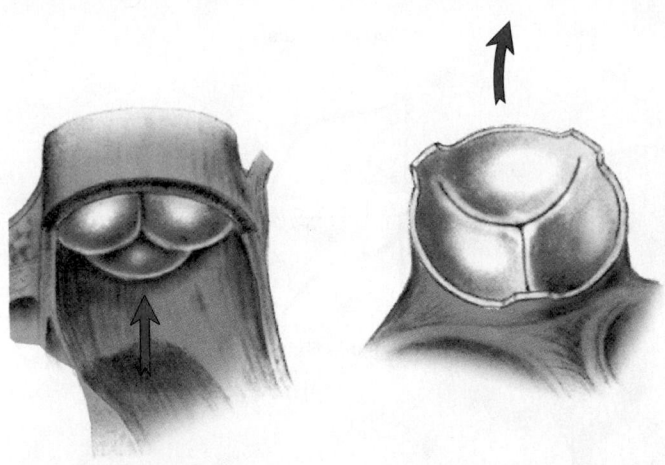

Inferior view   Superior view
FIGURE 12-6 The aortic valve and its cuplike leaflets.

TABLE 12-1 CARDIAC VALVES AND THEIR LOCATIONS

VALVE	TYPE	SITUATED BETWEEN
Tricuspid	Atrioventricular	Right atrium and right ventricle
Pulmonic	Semilunar	Right ventricle and pulmonary artery
Mitral	Atrioventricular	Left atrium and left ventricle
Aortic	Semilunar	Left ventricle and aorta

structures covered by a thin layer of endocardium. Dysfunction of the chordae tendineae or of a papillary muscle may cause incomplete closure of an AV valve, which results in backflow of blood into the atrium. Degenerative disease of the valve leaflets is another cause of regurgitation of blood into the atrium.[12] Valvular regurgitation produces a murmur that can be auscultated with a stethoscope.

Semilunar Valves. The semilunar valves are pulmonic and aortic valves. Each valve has three cuplike leaflets (Fig. 12-6). These valves separate the ventricles from their respective outflow arteries (Table 12-1). During ventricular systole (contraction), semilunar valves open, allowing blood to flow out of the ventricles. As systole ends and the pressure in the outflow arteries exceeds that of the ventricles, the semilunar valves close, preventing blood regurgitation back into the ventricles. In most individuals, the aortic valve has three leaflets. In less than 1% of the population, it is bicuspid (a two-leaflet valve), which increases susceptibility to aortic valve failure over time.[13,14] Aortic valve dysfunction, from any cause, not only affects the valve leaflets but also pathologically alters the shape of the left ventricle.

Conduction System

To analyze electrical activity within the heart, it is helpful to understand the three main areas of impulse propagation and conduction: 1) the sinoatrial (SA) node, 2) the AV node, and 3) the conduction fibers within the ventricle, specifically the bundle of His, the bundle branches, and the Purkinje fibers.[15]

Sinoatrial Node. The SA node is considered the natural pacemaker of the heart because it has the highest degree of

TABLE 12-2 INTRINSIC PACEMAKER RATES OF CARDIAC CONDUCTION TISSUE

LOCATION	RATE (BEATS/MIN)
Sinoatrial (SA) node	60-100
Atrioventricular (AV) node	40-60
Purkinje fibers	15-40

automaticity, producing the fastest intrinsic heart rate (Table 12-2). The node is a spindle-shaped structure located near the entrance of the superior vena cava, on the posterior aspect of the right atrium. Some normal variability in the position and shape of the node exists. The SA node is supplied from the right coronary system in 63% of people and from the left coronary system in 37%.[16] The SA node contains two types of cells, the *specialized pacemaker cells* found in the node center and the *border zone cells*. Both cell types have inherent pacemaker properties (they automatically depolarize 60 to 100 times per minute). The cells in the nodal center are responsible for the pace making of the heart, whereas the intrinsic depolarization capability of the fibers in the border zone is depressed by surrounding atrial tissue.

Once the center nodal cells depolarize, the impulse is conducted through the nodal border zone toward the atrium. Atrial depolarization occurs cell to cell. Some anatomists postulate that specialized conduction pathways exit the SA node (Fig. 12-7A). These *internodal pathways* are directed to the AV node.[17] An intra-atrial conduction pathway, known as *Bachmann's bundle*, travels from the right atrium to the left atrium.[18,19]

Atrioventricular Node. The AV node is located posteriorly on the right side of the interatrial septum, on the floor of the right atrium.[20] The AV node receives its blood supply from the first posterior septal branch of the right (90%) or left (10%) coronary artery.[16] Because the atria and ventricles are separated by nonconductive tissue, electrical impulses initiated in the atria are conducted to the ventricles only via the AV node. The AV node performs four essential functions to support cardiac conduction:

1. The AV node delays the conduction impulse from the atria (0.8 to 1.2 seconds) to provide time for the ventricles to fill during diastole.
2. The AV node controls the number of impulses that are transmitted from the atria to the ventricles. This prevents rapid irregular atrial heart rhythms from destabilizing the ventricular rhythm.
3. The AV node acts as a backup pacemaker if the faster SA node fails. Normally, the intrinsic AV nodal rate is slower than the SA nodal rate (see Table 12-2). When an impulse from the SA node arrives at the AV node, AV nodal tissue becomes depolarized, and the AV nodal pacemaker timing is reset (see Fig. 12-7B). This prevents the AV node from initiating its own pacemaker impulse that would compete with the SA node.
4. The AV node can conduct retrograde (backward) impulses through the node. If the SA and AV pacemaker cells fail to fire, an electrical impulse may be initiated in the ventricles

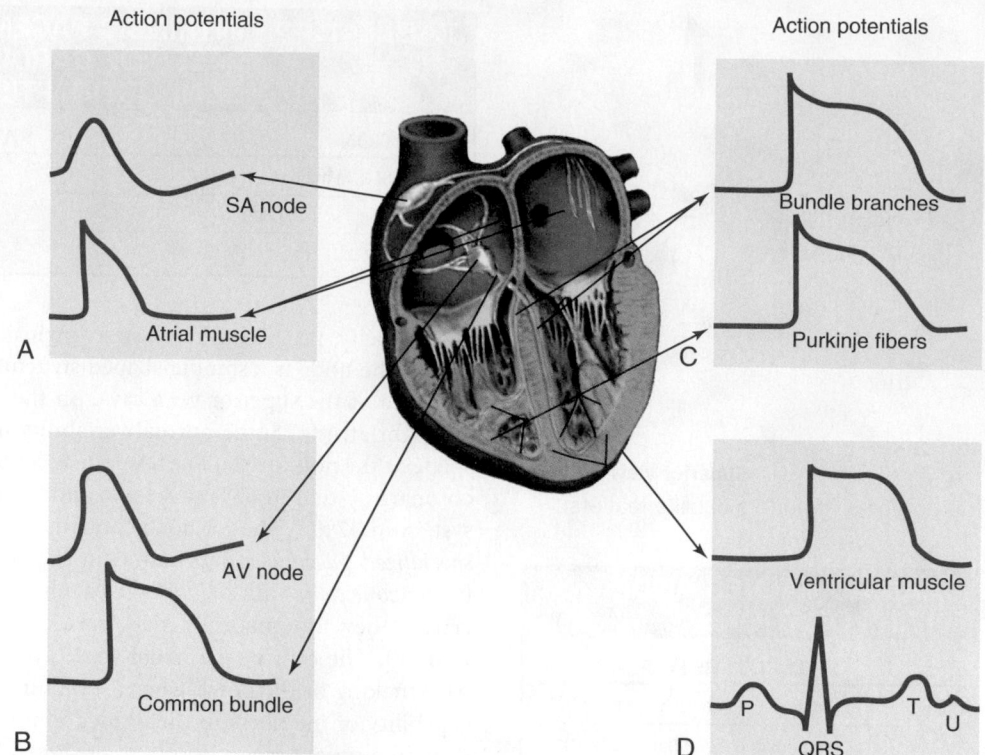

FIGURE 12-7   The heart with normal conduction pathways and transmembrane action potentials of sinoatrial (SA) node and atrial muscle *(A)*; atrioventricular (AV) node and common bundle *(B)*; bundle branches *(C)*; and ventricular muscle *(D)*. (From Thompson JM, et al. *Mosby's Clinical Nursing.* 5th ed. St. Louis, MO: Mosby; 2002.)

and conducted backward via the AV node. Retrograde conduction time is usually longer than antegrade (forward) conduction.

Bundle of His, Bundle Branches, and Purkinje Fibers. Electrical impulses are conducted in the ventricles through the bundle of His, the bundle branches, and the Purkinje fibers (see Fig. 12-7C). These structures run through the subendocardium, down the right side of the interventricular septum. About 12 mm from the AV node, the bundle of His divides into the right and left bundle branches. The right bundle branch continues down the right side of the interventricular septum toward the right apex. The left bundle branch is thicker than the right and takes off from the bundle of His at an almost right angle. It traverses the septum to the subendocardial surface of the left interventricular wall, where it divides into a thin anterior branch and a thick posterior branch. Functionally, when one of the left branches is blocked, it is referred to as a *hemiblock*. All of the bundle branches are subject to conduction defects (bundle branch blocks) that give rise to characteristic changes in the 12-lead electrocardiogram (ECG).

The right bundle branch and the two divisions of the left bundle branch eventually divide into the Purkinje fibers, which have the fastest conduction velocity of all heart tissue. Purkinje fibers divide many times, terminating in the subendocardial surface of both ventricles. This is followed by ventricular muscle depolarization (see Fig. 12-7D).

Coronary Blood Supply

The coronary circulation consists of those vessels that supply the heart structures with oxygenated blood (coronary arteries) and then return the blood to the general circulation (coronary veins). The right and left coronary arteries arise at the base of the aorta, immediately above the aortic valve (Fig. 12-8).[21] They then traverse the outside of the heart, above the epicardium, in the natural grooves (sulci) between the chambers. To perfuse the thick heart muscle, branches from these main arteries arise at acute angles, penetrating the muscular wall and eventually feeding the endocardium (Fig. 12-9).[21]

The right coronary artery (RCA) serves the right atrium and the right ventricle in most people. In 63% of the population, the sinus node artery, which supplies the SA node, arises from the RCA.[16] The AV node is supplied via the RCA in 90% of the population.[16] The term *dominant coronary artery* is used to describe the artery that supplies the posterior part of the heart. In most people, the RCA is dominant, supplying the posterior cardiac wall.[21]

The left coronary artery is a short but important artery that divides into two large arteries—the left anterior descending (LAD) and the circumflex (Cx) arteries. These vessels serve the left atrium and most of the left ventricle (Fig. 12-10). The LAD artery travels in the sulcus over the anterior intraventricular septum. Septal perforator branches branch off at right angles to provide blood supply to the intraventricular septum.[21]

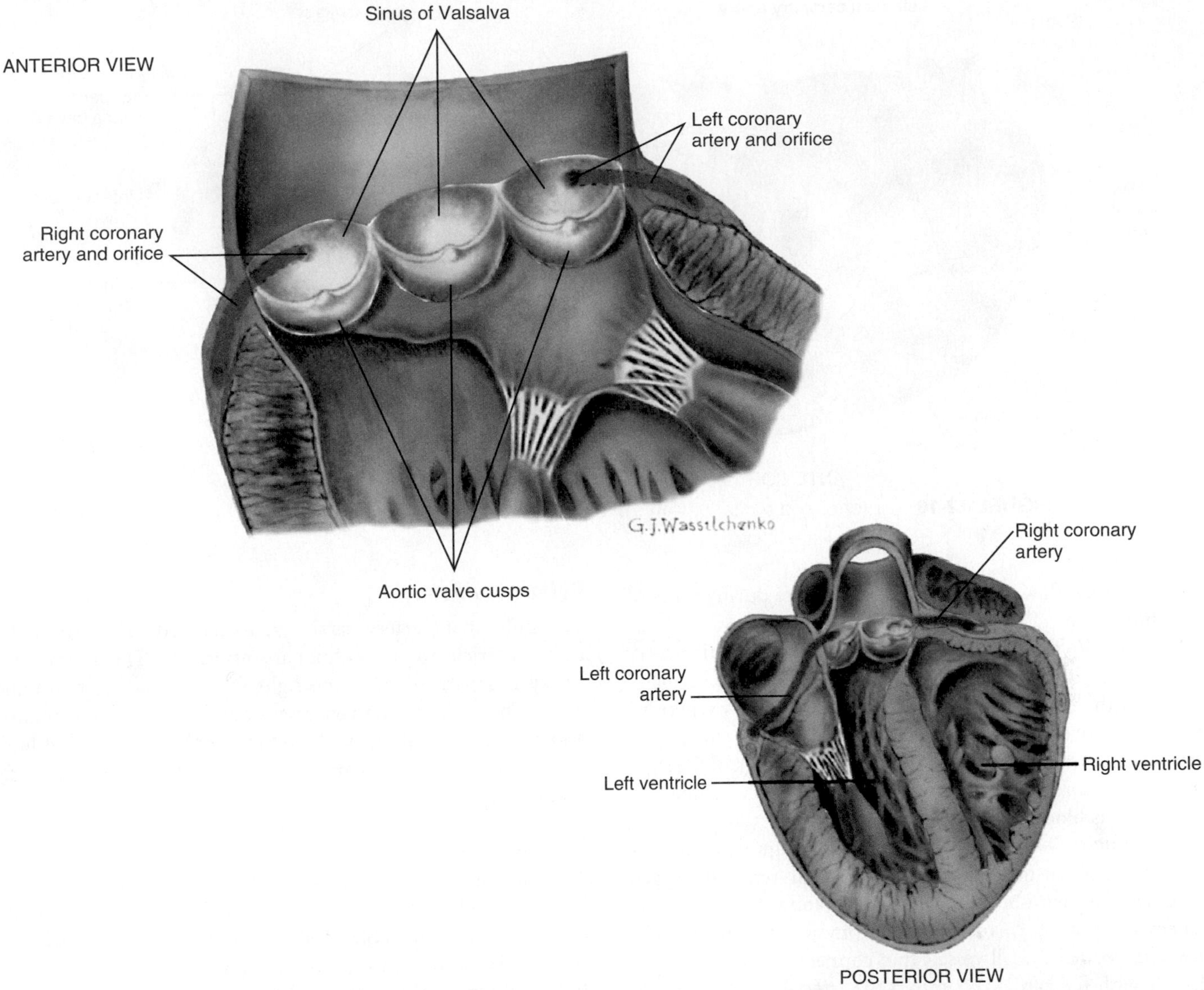

ANTERIOR VIEW

Sinus of Valsalva

Left coronary
artery and orifice

Right coronary
artery and orifice

G.J.Wassilchenko

Aortic valve cusps

Right coronary
artery

Left coronary
artery

Left ventricle

Right ventricle

POSTERIOR VIEW

FIGURE 12-8 Proximity of the right and left coronary arteries to the aortic valve and the sinus of Valsalva.

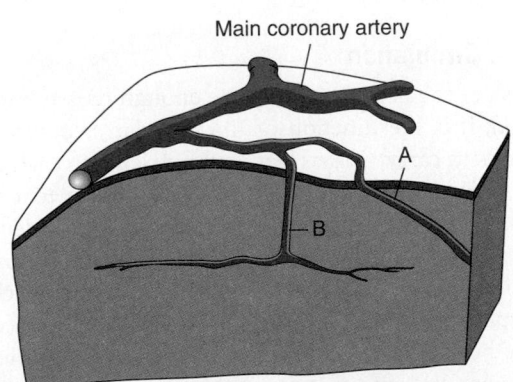

Main coronary artery

A

B

FIGURE 12-9 Intramyocardial Distribution of Coronary Arteries. *A,* Epicardial arteries arise at acute angles from main coronary vessels to supply the epicardial surface of the heart. *B,* Smaller vessels branch at oblique angles from main coronary vessels that penetrate deeper into the myocardium and endocardium (intramural arteries). (Redrawn from Quaal S. *Comprehensive Intraaortic Balloon Pumping.* 2nd ed. St. Louis, MO: Mosby; 1993.)

The coronary arteries are end-arteries, that is, they supply a discrete area of the myocardium and have limited collateral circulation. End-arteries are also susceptible to obstruction by atherosclerotic plaque or thrombus that can result in loss of blood flow to the myocardial muscle normally supplied by that artery. This can be fatal, depending on the location of the obstruction. Blockage of coronary arterial blood flow, especially in the left main coronary artery, usually results in death from massive infarction of the left ventricle. If the blocked artery supplies a smaller section of myocardium, the result may be an MI but not death.

Several clinical situations merit a brief discussion here. During ventricular contraction, no blood flows to the cardiac tissues because of the contracted state of the cardiac muscle and the resulting occlusion of arteries within the musculature. Coronary artery circulation is highest during early diastole, after the aortic valve has closed. During an episode of tachycardia, diastolic time is greatly diminished; hence coronary perfusion time is lessened. This offers an explanation for compromised

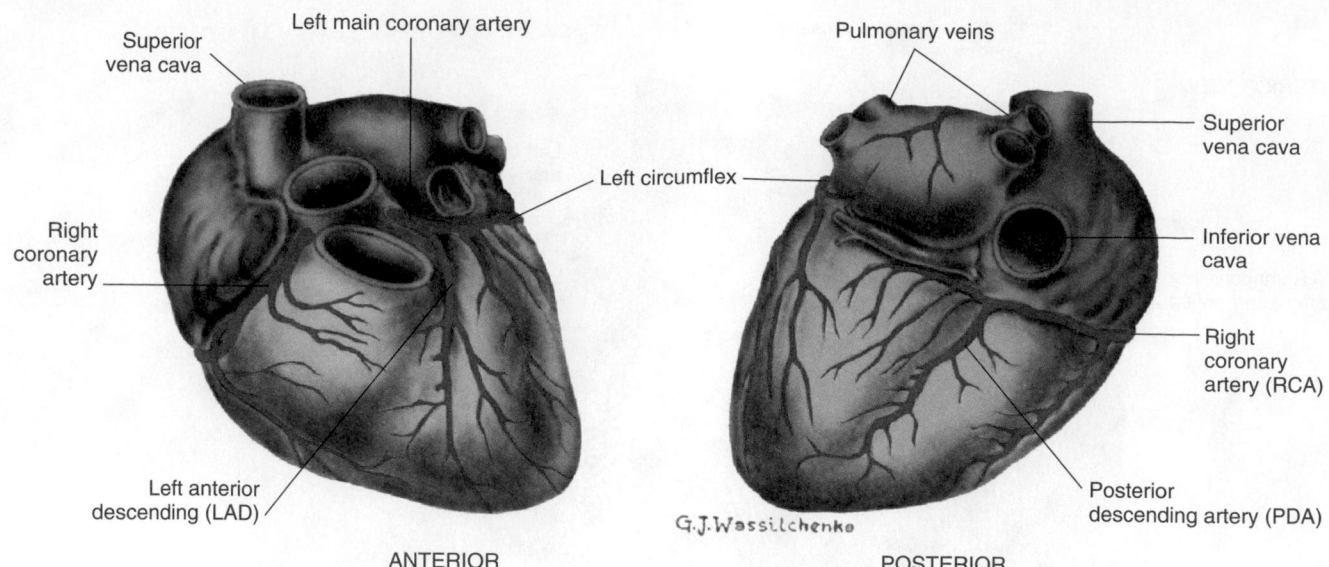

FIGURE 12-10 Anterior and posterior views of the coronary artery circulation and major vessels.

coronary blood flow and fall in blood pressure during times of rapid heart rate.

Coronary Veins. The cardiac (coronary) veins, which carry deoxygenated blood, are adjacent to the paths of the coronary arteries, with one significant difference. The coronary veins ultimately join together to become the *coronary sinus* (the largest cardiac vein), which primarily empties into the back of the right atrium. The coronary venous blood then mixes with the systemic venous blood in the right atrium.[22]

Physiologic Cardiac Shunts. A shunt occurs when deoxygenated blood (usually venous blood with reduced oxygen content) mixes with arterial oxygenated blood. In the heart in a specific situation, this is a normal physiologic process. The *thebesian veins* are small vessels that connect the capillary beds directly with the cardiac chambers via irregular endothelium-lined sinuses within the myocardium. The thebesian veins add a small quantity of deoxygenated blood to the oxygenated blood in the left ventricle.

An example of an abnormal, or pathologic, intracardiac shunt is an opening in the ventricular septum, between the left and right sides of the heart. In the ventricle, this septal opening, called a *ventricular septal defect* (VSD), allows mixing of blood from both ventricles. The clinical impact depends on the size of the intracardiac shunt. A VSD is a congenital opening between the ventricles; a ventricular septal rupture (VSR) can occur as a complication of a large anterior-wall MI, as shown in Figure 15-15.

Major Cardiac Vessels
Aorta
The aorta is the largest artery in the body. It carries oxygenated blood from the left ventricle to the rest of the body. The aorta is separated from the left ventricle by the aortic valve. Just above the aortic valve are two small openings that represent the origins of the right and left coronary carterial systems (see Fig. 12-8). These opening are known by several names, including the *coronary ostia* and the *sinus of Valsalva*.

Pulmonary Artery
The pulmonary artery carries deoxygenated blood from the right ventricle to the pulmonary arterioles. The pulmonary artery is separated from the right ventricle by the pulmonic valve. The main pulmonary artery divides into a right branch and a left branch, directing blood to the right and the left lung vasculature. The pulmonary artery is the only artery in the body that carries deoxygenated blood.

Pulmonary Veins
The four pulmonary veins return oxygenated blood from the lungs to the left atrium. These are the only veins in the body that carry oxygenated blood. The veins drain into the back wall of the left atrium (see Fig. 12-10). No valves inhibit the flow of blood into the left atrium. Blood flow is accomplished by simple hydrostatic pressure gradients. The pressure must be lower in the left atrium than in the pulmonary circulation for flow to occur in a forward direction.

Systemic Circulation
If the task of the heart is to generate enough pressure to pump the blood, it is the function of the vascular structures to act as conduits to carry vital oxygen and nutrients to each cell and also to carry away waste products. The ability to exchange those nutrients and waste products at the cellular level is of primary importance. The vascular system acts not only as a conducting system for blood but also as a control mechanism for the pressure in the heart and vessels. It is the complex interplay between the heart and blood vessels that maintains adequate pressure and velocity within this system for optimal functioning.

Arterial System. Arteries are constructed of three layers (Fig. 12-11): 1) The *adventitia*, the outermost layer, is composed largely of a connective tissue coat to provide strength and shape to the vessel; 2) the *media*, or muscular middle layer, is made up of smooth muscle and elastic tissue. The muscular layer changes the lumen diameter when necessary; and 3) the

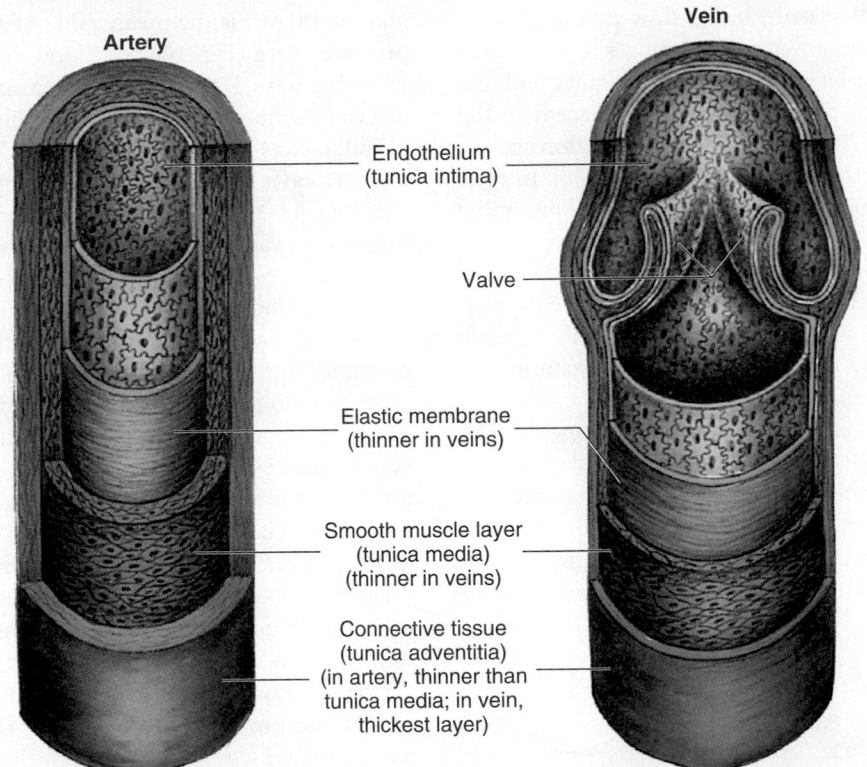

FIGURE 12-11 Cross-section of an artery and vein showing the three layers: tunica intima, tunica media, and tunica adventitia. Note the difference in wall thickness between the artery and the vein and the lack of valves within the artery. (From Thompson JM, et al. *Mosby's Clinical Nursing.* 5th ed. St. Louis, MO: Mosby; 2002.)

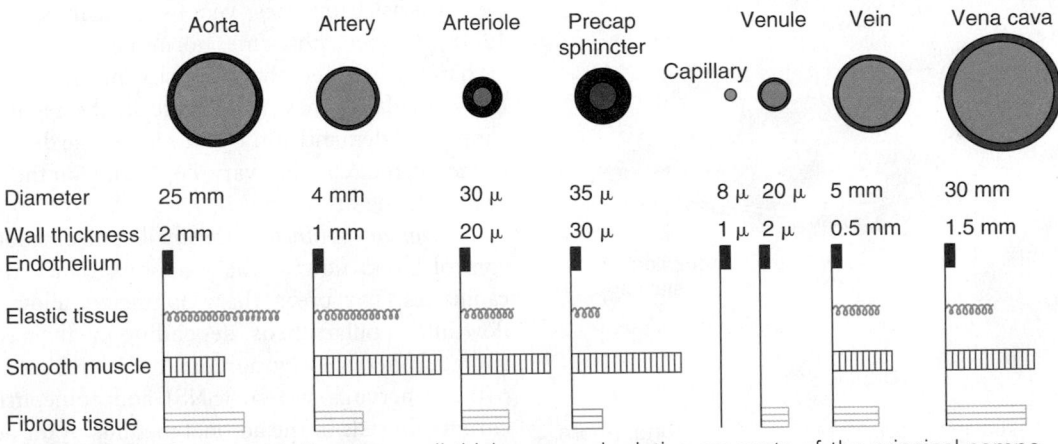

FIGURE 12-12 Internal diameter, wall thickness, and relative amounts of the principal components of the vessel circulatory system. Cross-sections of the vessels are not drawn to scale because of the huge range from aorta to vena cava to capillaries. (From Berne RM, Levy MN. *Cardiovascular Physiology.* 8th ed. St. Louis, MO: Mosby; 2001.)

innermost layer, or *intima*, consists of a thin lining of endothelium and a small amount of elastic tissue. The smooth endothelial lining decreases resistance to blood flow and minimizes opportunity for platelet aggregation.

The intimal and the adventitial layers remain relatively constant in the vascular system, whereas the elastin and smooth muscle in the media vary in proportion, depending on the size and type of the vessel. The aorta contains the greatest amount of elastic tissue. This is necessary because of the sudden shifts in pressure created by the left ventricle. The arterioles, or smaller

arteries, and precapillary sphincters have more smooth muscle than do the larger arteries and aorta because they function to change the luminal diameter when regulating blood pressure and blood flow to tissues (Fig. 12-12).

Blood Flow and Blood Pressure. The pulsatile nature of arterial flow is caused by intermittent cardiac ejection and the stretch of the ascending aorta. The pressure wave initiated by left ventricular ejection (Fig. 12-13) travels considerably faster than does blood itself. When an examiner palpates a pulse, it is the propagation of the pressure wave that is perceived.

In the normal arterial system, blood flow is described as laminar, or streamlined, because the fluid moves in one direction. However, differences exist in the linear velocities within a blood vessel. The layer of blood immediately adjacent to the vessel wall moves relatively slowly because of the friction created as it comes in contact with the motionless vessel wall. In contrast, the more central blood in the lumen travels more rapidly (Fig. 12-14).

Clinical implications include conditions in which the vessel wall has an abnormality such as a small clot or plaque deposit. This disruption in the streamlined flow can set up eddy currents that may predispose the area to platelet aggregation and atherosclerosis.

Blood pressure measurement has several components. The *systolic blood pressure* (SBP) represents the ventricular volume ejection and the response of the arterial system to that ejection. The *diastolic blood pressure* (DBP) value indicates the ventricular resting state of the arterial system. The *pulse pressure* is the difference between the SBP and the DBP. The *mean arterial pressure* (MAP) is the mean value of the area under the blood pressure curve (Fig. 12-15). Blood pressure may be measured in several ways. Direct measurement is accomplished by means of a catheter inserted into an artery. Blood pressure is measured in millimeters of mercury (mm Hg). The most common indirect method is by means of a stethoscope and sphygmomanometer (Fig. 12-16). Figure 12-17 graphically summarizes blood pressures in various portions of the systemic circulatory system.

Vascular resistance is a reflection of arteriolar tone. The large amount of smooth muscle in the arterioles allows for relaxation or contraction of these vessels, which causes changes in the resistance and redistribution of blood flow. Resistance is the opposition to flow caused by the blood vessels. Most changes in resistance are caused by alterations in the tone of the arterial vessel walls, especially in the arterioles. The purpose of this mechanism is to maintain a constant blood pressure in the arterial system. The clinician can never assume that blood flow and blood pressure are identical. For example, poor blood flow to the tissues because of vasoconstricted peripheral arterioles causes the blood to back up and increases the blood pressure. A higher blood pressure is a compensatory mechanism but does not necessarily mean that tissue perfusion is adequate.

It is also possible to calculate the resistance within the systemic vascular system, described by the phrase *systemic vascular resistance* (SVR). When it occurs in the pulmonary circulation, it is termed *pulmonary vascular resistance* (PVR). These derived values are based on calculations from other hemodynamic parameters, as described in Chapter 14 and Appendix B.

Microcirculation. The *microcirculation* consists of arterioles, arterial capillaries, venous capillaries, and venules (Fig. 12-18). Oxygen, nutrients, hormones, and waste products are exchanged between the bloodstream and adjacent cells. The microcirculation has a vital role in the regulation of oxygen supply and demand at the tissue level. The density and anatomy of the microcirculation vary, depending on the metabolic needs of each tissue or organ.

Precapillary sphincters are small cuffs of smooth muscle that control blood flow at the junction of the arterioles and the capillaries. The precapillary sphincters allow selective blood flow into capillary beds, depending on their contractile state, and are innervated by norepinephrine released from the sympathetic nervous system (SNS) and epinephrine released by chromaffin cells in the adrenal medulla of the adrenal glands.[23]

As blood reaches the capillary level, the pulsatile nature of arterial flow is dampened (see Fig. 12-17). Even though the

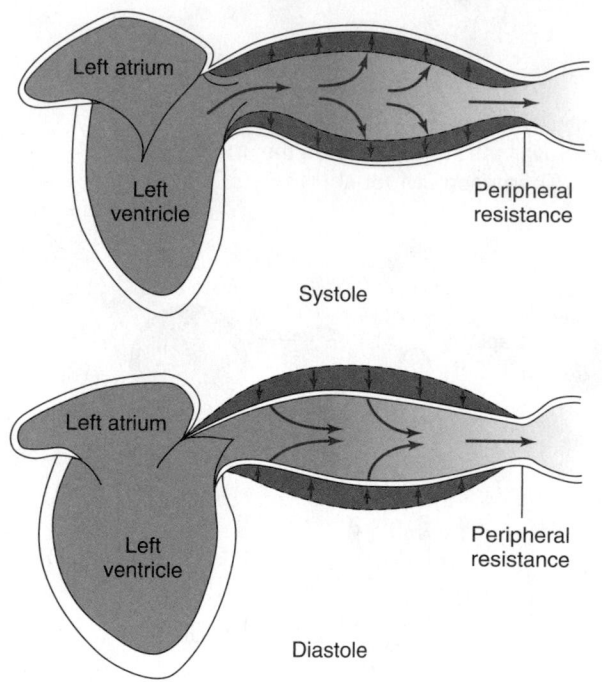

FIGURE 12-13 Elastic and recoil properties of the aorta. (From Berne RM, Levy MN. *Cardiovascular Physiology*. 8th ed. St. Louis, MO: Mosby; 2001.)

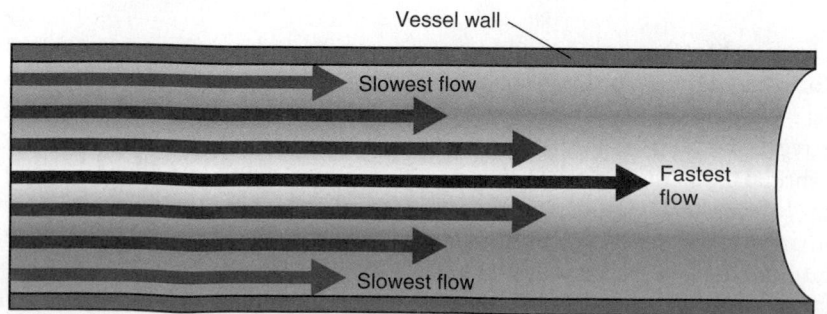

FIGURE 12-14 Laminar flow in an artery.

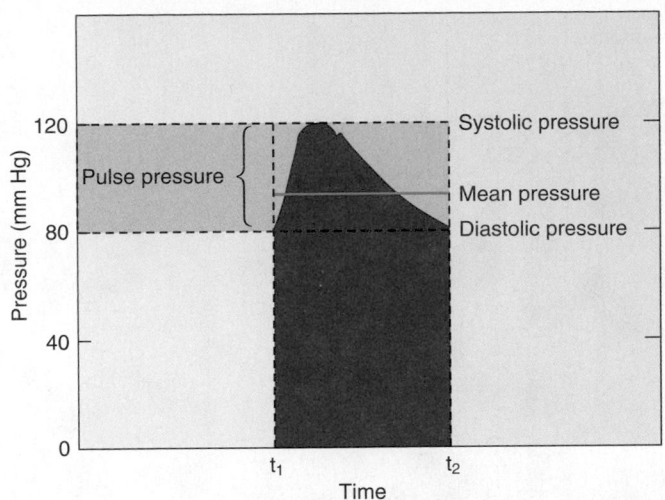

FIGURE 12-15 Arterial systolic, diastolic, pulse, and mean pressures. (From Berne RM, Levy MN. *Cardiovascular Physiology.* 8th ed. St. Louis, MO: Mosby; 2001.)

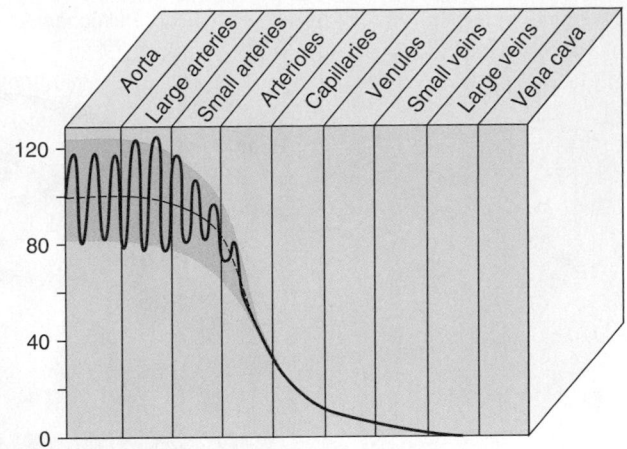

FIGURE 12-17 Blood pressures in various portions of the systemic circulatory system.

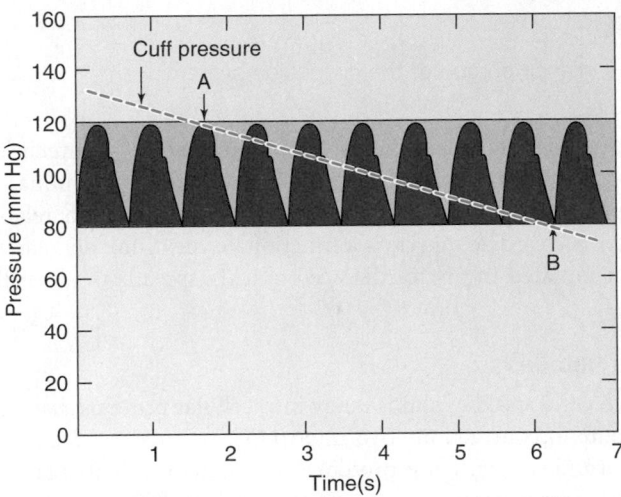

FIGURE 12-16 Principles of blood pressure measurement with a sphygmomanometer. The oblique line represents pressure in the inflatable bag in the cuff. At cuff pressures greater than the systolic pressure (*to the left of* A), no blood progresses beyond the cuff, and no sounds can be detected below the cuff with the stethoscope. At cuff pressures between the systolic and diastolic levels (*between* A *and* B), spurts of blood traverse the arteries under the cuff and produce Korotkoff sounds. At cuff pressures lower than the diastolic pressure (to *the right of* B), arterial flow past the region of the cuff is continuous, and no sounds are audible. (From Berne RM, Levy MN. *Cardiovascular Physiology.* 8th ed. St. Louis, MO: Mosby; 2001.)

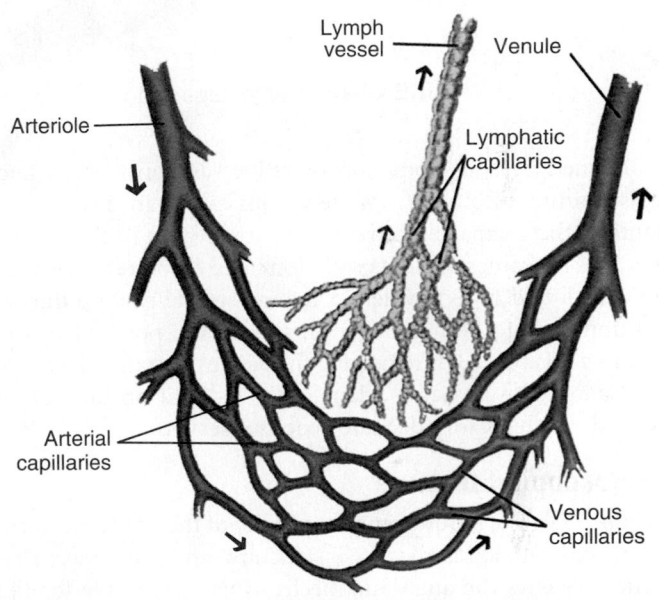

FIGURE 12-18 Microcirculation. Note the branching nature and large cross-sectional area of the capillary bed. (From Thompson JM, et al. *Mosby's Clinical Nursing.* 5th ed. St. Louis, MO: Mosby; 2002.)

Venous System

As blood leaves the capillary system, it passes through the venules and into the veins. Venules and veins contain elastic tissue, smooth muscle, and fibrous tissue (see Fig. 12-12). The veins, however, contain a greater percentage of smooth muscle and fibrous tissue to accommodate the large venous volume and demand for reserve capacity. The majority of circulating blood is contained in the venous system. Veins are referred to as *capacitance vessels* (Fig. 12-19). Approximately 75% of the total blood volume is found in the veins. This enables the body to tap into a large reserve during times of need. For example, when a person changes from a supine position to a sitting position, approximately 7 to 10 mL blood per kilogram of body weight pools in the legs. Potentially, cardiac output could decrease by 20%. However, normal arterial pressure and blood flow are

diameter of a capillary is less than that of an arteriole, the pressure and flow velocity in the capillary bed is low as a result of the large cross-sectional area of the branching capillary bed (see Fig. 12-18). The capillary consists of a single cell layer of endothelium and is devoid of muscle or elastin (see Fig. 12-12). This arrangement allows solutes to diffuse in and out of the capillaries unimpeded by mechanical barriers. The capillaries normally retain large structures such as red blood cells but are highly permeable to smaller solutes such as electrolytes.

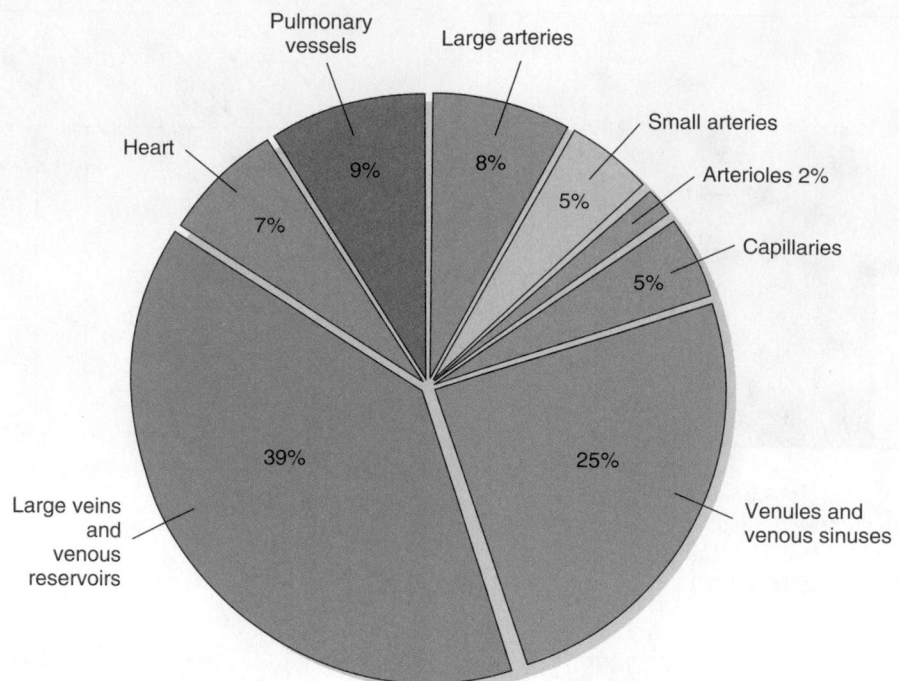

FIGURE 12-19 Percentage of the total blood volume in each portion of the circulation system.

maintained by a combination of reflex vasoconstriction and redistribution of blood from the venous capacitance vessels. In humans, these capacitance reservoirs are greatest in the spleen, liver, and intestines. Patients with decreased blood reserves, who are dehydrated or hypovolemic, require special caution during position changes, especially from the supine position to the standing position. Before helping the patient to stand, the nurse must allow him or her to "dangle" the legs (sit on the side of the bed) to check for adequate venous reserves.

Microscopic Structure

To appreciate the unique pumping ability of the heart, the nurse must understand cardiac cell structure and function. This section reviews the anatomic mechanisms responsible for the contractile process in cardiac muscle cells.

Cardiac Fibers

Cardiac muscle fibers are typically found in a latticework arrangement. The fiber cells (myofibrils) divide, rejoin, and then separate again, but they retain distinct cellular walls and possess a single nucleus. Individual cardiac muscle cells are known as *myocytes*. The myocytes are connected by specialized junctional complexes called *intercalated disks* that assist in the propagation of depolarization. Myocardial muscle cells differ greatly from skeletal muscle, where the cells are fused together to form a continuous fiber with many nuclei.

In general, cardiac myofibrils run on a longitudinal axis, and the fibers appear striped, or striated. When viewed under an electron microscope, these striations are seen to be the contractile proteins (Fig. 12-20). The areas separating each myocardial cell from its neighbor, called *intercalated disks*, are continuous with the *sarcolemma*, or cell membrane. The point at which a longitudinal branch of one cell meets the branch of another is called a *tight junction* (or *gap junction*), which is contained

within the intercalated disks. These junctions offer much less impedance to electrical flow than does the sarcolemma, so depolarization occurs from one cell to another with relative ease. The cardiac muscle is a functional syncytium: depolarization initiated in any cardiac cell quickly spreads to all of the heart.

Cardiac Cells

Each cardiac cell contains many intracellular proteins that contribute to contraction. Two important contractile proteins are *actin* and *myosin*. These proteins abound in the cell in organized longitudinal arrangements. Under electron microscopy, the myosin filaments appear thick, whereas the actin filaments, which are almost twice as prevalent, appear thin. The actin filaments are connected to a *Z-disk* on one end, leaving the other end free to interact with the myosin cross-bridges. In the resting muscle cell, actin and myosin partially overlap. Myosin has three distinct regions: 1) the head, 2) the hinge, and 3) the tail. The ends of the myosin filament that overlap with actin have tiny projections named *myosin heads*, which contain a binding site for actin (Fig. 12-21). For contraction to occur, myosin heads must interact with actin to form cross-bridges (see Fig. 12-21).

The sarcomere is the functional unit of cardiac contraction and is defined as the region between two Z-disks.[24] In the normal resting state, the sarcomere is about 2 to 2.2 mm long (Fig. 12-22). Myosin filaments are situated in the middle of the sarcomere and are attached to the Z-disk of the sarcomere by the protein *titan*.[25, 26] Each sarcomere consists of a central *A-band* (thick filaments) and two halves of the *I-band* (thin filaments), as shown in Figure 12-22C. The I-bands from two adjacent sarcomeres meet at the Z-disk. The central portion of the A-band is the *M-band*, which does not contain actin. Figure 12-22, *C*, shows the position of titin, the thin filaments and the

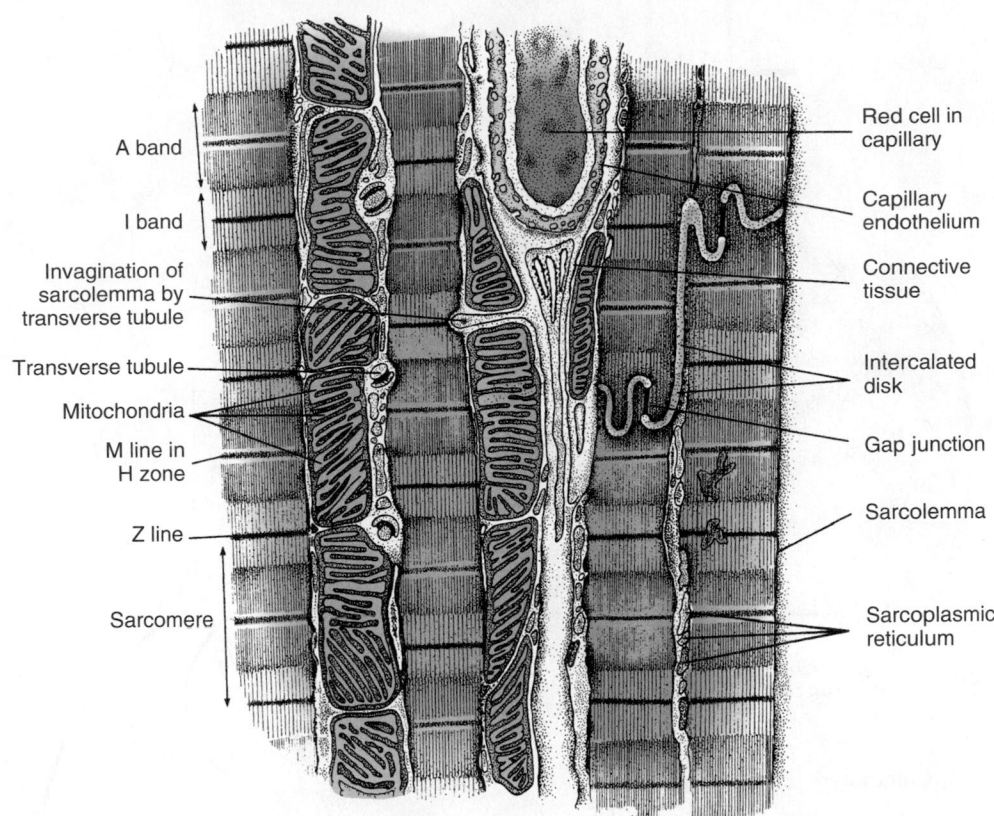

A band

I band

Invagination of
sarcolemma by
transverse tubule

Transverse tubule

Mitochondria

M line in
H zone

Z line

Sarcomere

Red cell in
capillary

Capillary
endothelium

Connective
tissue

Intercalated
disk

Gap junction

Sarcolemma

Sarcoplasmic
reticulum

FIGURE 12-20   Diagram of an electron micrograph of cardiac muscle showing large numbers of mitochondria, intercalated disks with tight junctions, transverse tubules, and longitudinal tubules (also known as the *sarcoplasmic reticulum*) (approximately × 30,000). (From Berne RM, Levy MN. *Cardiovascular Physiology*. 8th ed. St. Louis, MO: Mosby; 2001.)

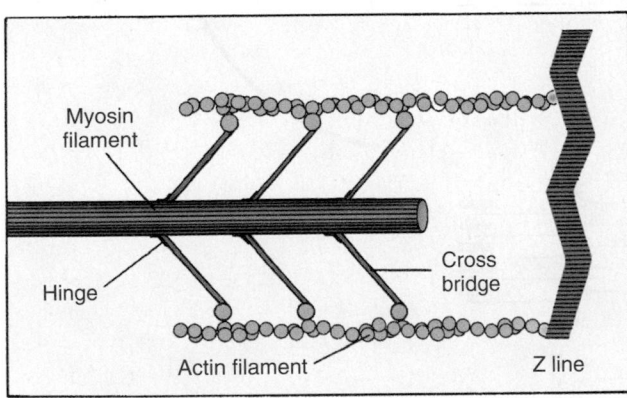
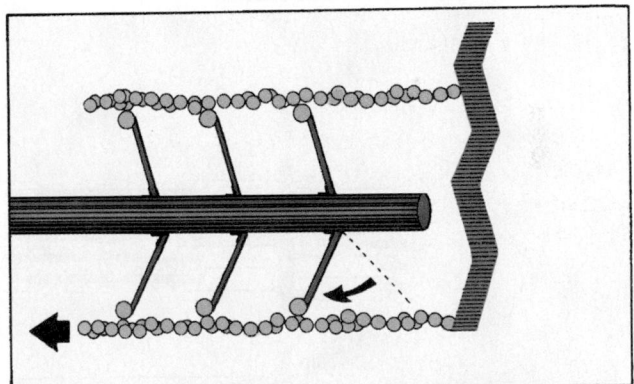

Myosin
filament

Hinge

Cross
bridge

Actin filament

Z line

FIGURE 12-21   Actin and myosin filaments and cross-bridges responsible for cell contraction.

thick filaments in the sarcomere. The thin filament is composed of the helical chains of the actin globular proteins that coil around a long filament of tropomyosin, and three regulatory *troponin* proteins: 1) Tn-T, 2) Tn-C, and 3) Tn-I. The troponin complex is attached to actin at regularly spaced intervals.

Another extremely important intracellular structure necessary for successful contraction is the *sarcoplasmic reticulum*. Calcium ions are stored in the in the sarcoplasmic reticulum and released for use after depolarization (see Fig. 12-22A). Deep invaginations into the sarcomere are called *transverse tubules*, or *T-tubules*.[27] T-tubules are essentially an extension of the cell membrane (sarcolemma); they conduct depolarization

to structures deep within the cytoplasm such as the sarcoplasmic reticulum.[27] T-tubules connect to sarcomeres at the Z-disk, as shown in Figure 12-22B. The Z-disk is composed of interconnecting proteins such as *alpha-actinin* that link actin to the Z-disk. Cardiac cells abound with mitochondria, which contain respiratory enzymes necessary for oxidative phosphorylation (see Fig. 12-20). This enables these cells to keep up with the tremendous energy requirements of repetitive contraction. When cardiac cells are damaged by trauma or ischemia, myocardial cells release protein biomarkers such as troponin, which, when measured by laboratory analysis, can help determine the extent of injury (see Figure 15-12).

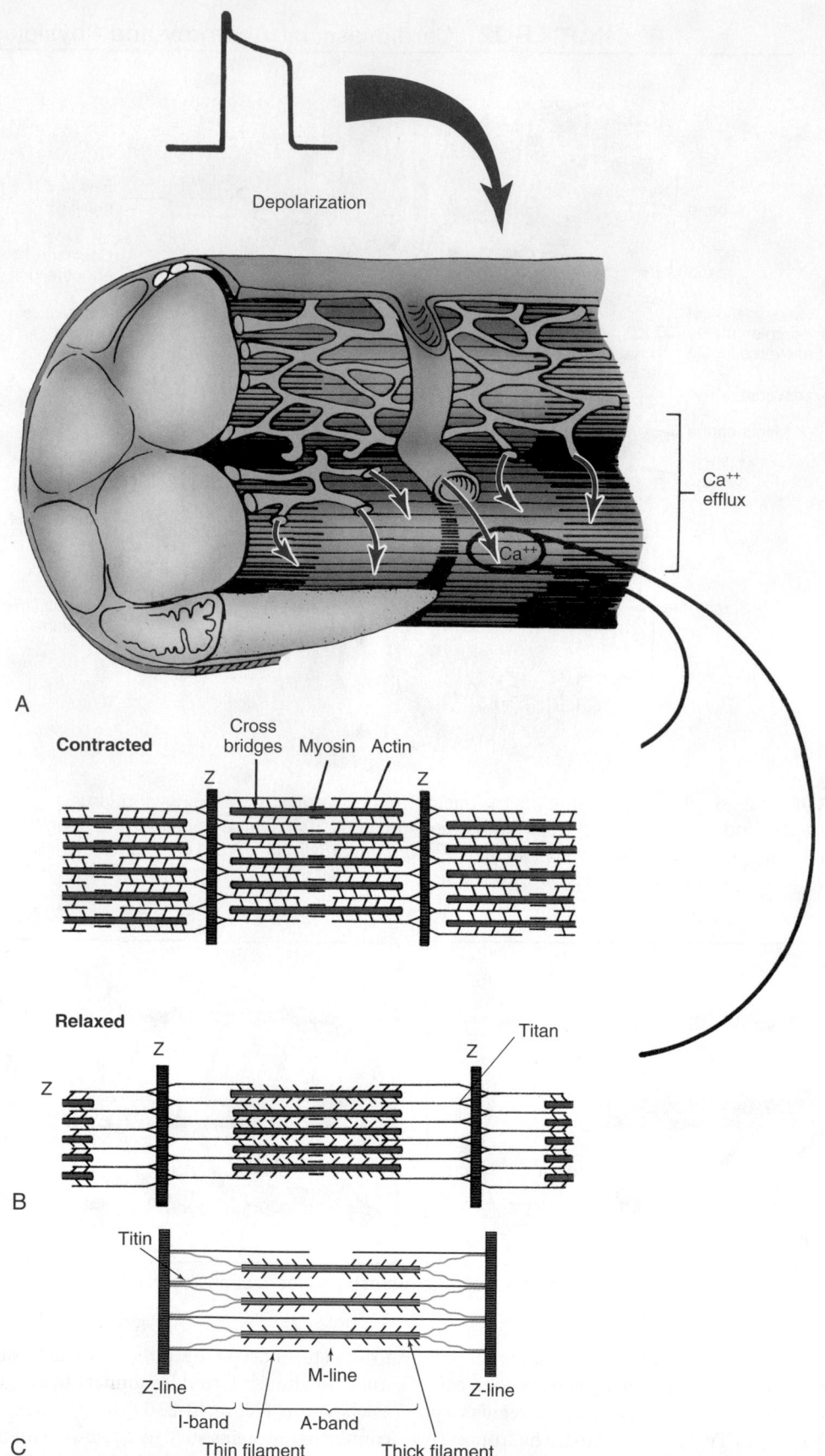

Depolarization

Ca++ efflux

Ca++

A

Contracted

Cross bridges Myosin Actin

Z Z

Relaxed

Z Z Titan

Z

B

Titin

Z-line M-line Z-line

I-band A-band

Thin filament Thick filament

C

FIGURE 12-22 *A,* Depolarization of a myocardial cell causes the release of calcium from the sarcoplasmic reticulum and the transverse tubules. *B,* Calcium release allows for the cross-bridges on myosin filaments to attach to actin filaments to effect cell contraction. *C,* The sarcomere lies between two Z-lines. The sarcomere is composed of a central A-band, which contains thick filaments, and two halves of the I-band, which contain thin filaments. The center of the A-band is the M-line. Titin spans from the Z-line to the M-line. (*A* and *B,* from Quaal S. *Comprehensive Intraaortic Balloon Pumping.* 2nd ed. St. Louis, MO: Mosby; 1993; *C,* adapted with permission from Shiels HA, White E. Commentary: the Frank-Starling mechanism in vertebrate cardiac myocytes. *J Exp Biol.* 2008;211:2005.)

TABLE 12-3   TERMS RELATED TO CARDIAC TISSUE FUNCTION

TERM	DEFINITION
Excitability	Ability of a cell or tissue to depolarize in response to a given stimulus
Conductivity	Ability of cardiac cells to transmit a stimulus from cell to cell
Automaticity	Ability of certain cells to spontaneously depolarize ("pacemaker potential")
Rhythmicity	Automaticity generated at a regular rate
Contractility	Ability of the cardiac myofibrils to shorten in length in response to an electrical stimulus (depolarization)
Refractoriness	State of a cell or tissue during repolarization, when the cell or tissue cannot depolarize regardless of the intensity of the stimulus or requires a much greater stimulus than is normally required

TABLE 12-4   APPROXIMATE CONCENTRATIONS OF POTASSIUM, SODIUM, AND CALCIUM IONS IN A RESTING MYOCARDIAL CELL

	EXTRACELLULAR CONCENTRATION (mEq/L)	INTRACELLULAR CONCENTRATION (mEq/L)
Potassium (K^+)	4	135
Sodium (Na^+)	145	10
Calcium (Ca^{2+})	2	0.1

PHYSIOLOGY

The electrical and mechanical properties of cardiac tissue have fascinated scientists for more than 100 years. These properties include excitability, conductivity, automaticity, rhythmicity, contractility, and refractoriness. The following section relates these concepts specifically to cardiac cells (Table 12-3).

Electrical Activity

Transmembrane Potentials

Electrical potentials across cell membranes are present in essentially all the cells of the body. Some cells, such as nerve and muscle cells, are specialized for conduction of electrical impulses along their membranes. This *electrical potential*, or *transmembrane potential*, refers to the relative electrical difference between the interior of a cell and that of the fluid surrounding the cell. *Ionic channels* are pores in cell membranes that allow for passage of specific ions at specific times or in response to specific signals. Transmembrane potentials and ionic channels are extremely important in myocardial cells because they form the basis for electrical impulse conduction and muscular contraction. Knowledge of the normal structure and function of cardiac ion channels is increasingly important as a basis for understanding the genesis of lethal cardiac dysrhythmias and for the development of cardiac medications designed to treat these channelopathies.

Resting Membrane Potential

In a myocardial cell at rest, the normal resting membrane potential (RMP) is approximately −80 to −90 millivolts (mV). This means that the interior of the cell is relatively negative compared with the exterior medium. The relative negativity of the cell interior is created by an uneven distribution of positively and negatively charged ions. When the cell is at rest, more positively charged ions are outside the cell than are inside the cell.

When the cell is at rest, the intracellular potassium ion (K^+) concentration is very high, and the intracellular sodium ion (Na^+) level is low. Conversely, the extracellular K^+ concentration is relatively low compared with a high concentration of Na^+

(Table 12-4). Calcium (Ca^{2+}) has a much higher concentration outside than inside the cell when the cell is at rest. These large differences in individual ion concentrations create chemical gradients. A *chemical gradient* describes the tendency of an ion to move from an area of higher solute concentration to an area of lower concentration. However, an *electrical gradient* is also present, which causes the positively charged ions to move to an area of relative negativity. For example, the chemical gradient of K^+ forces it to move out of the cell because the intracellular K^+ concentration is so much higher than that of the outside medium. However, as a result of the relative negativity inside the cell (−80 to −90 mV), the electrical gradient works to retain the positively charged K^+ ion. An important factor influencing both gradients is *membrane permeability*, or the selectivity of the membrane to ionic movements. Even at rest, some slight movement of ions occurs across the cell membrane. For example, the cell membrane is approximately 50 times more permeable to K^+ than it is to Na^+. Because K^+ movement out of the cell results in greater negativity inside the cell, K^+ is the principal ion responsible for maintaining the negative RMP.

Phases of the Action Potential

In a myocardial cell, when a sudden increase in permeability of the membrane to Na^+ occurs, it is followed by a rapid sequence of events that lasts a fraction of a second. This sequence of events is termed *depolarization*. The graphic representation of depolarization and repolarization is termed the *action potential (AP)* (Fig. 12-23). Ionic currents cause changes in electrical potentials, which are known as *AP phases 0, 1, 2, 3, and 4*. These phases give the AP a characteristic shape (Table 12-5; see Fig. 12-7).

Phase 0. The sodium crossing the cell membrane causes the cell to become depolarized and the interior of the cell to become more positive. At approximately −65 mV, the membrane reaches the threshold, the point at which the inward Na^+ current overcomes the efflux of K^+. This is accomplished by means of the fast Na^+ channels. With the fast Na^+ channels open, the inward rush of Na^+ is extremely rapid and briefly causes the inside of the cell to become slightly more positive than the outside of the cell. This series of events is graphically described as *phase 0* of the AP and is reflected in the overshoot of the AP, during which the charge is 20 to 30 mV.

Phase 1 and Phase 2. When the rapid influx of Na^+ is terminated, a brief period of partial repolarization occurs as the

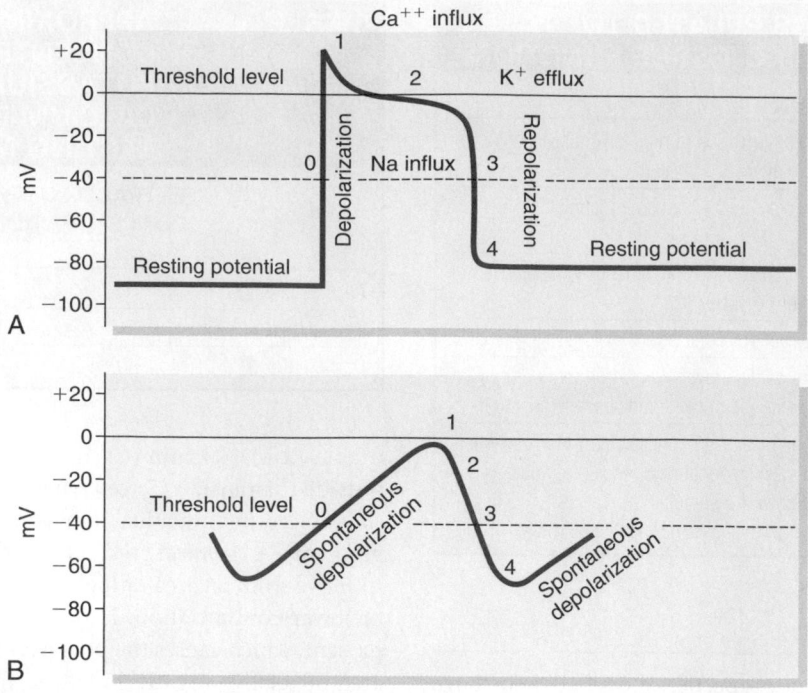

FIGURE 12-23 Cardiac Action Potentials. *A,* Action potential phases 0 to 4 of a non-pacemaker cell. *B,* Action potential of a pacemaker cell. (From Thompson JM, et al. *Mosby's Clinical Nursing.* 5th ed. St. Louis, MO: Mosby; 2002.)

	TABLE 12-5	**PHASES 0 THROUGH 4 OF A CARDIAC CELL ACTION POTENTIAL**	
PHASE	**DESCRIPTION**	**IONIC MOVEMENT**	**MECHANISMS**
0	Upstroke	Na^+ into cell	Fast Na^+ channels open
1	Overshoot	—	Fast Na^+ channels close
2	Plateau	Na^+ and Ca^{2+} into cell, K^+ out	Multiple channels (Ca^{2+}, Na^+, K^+) open to maintain membrane voltage
3	Repolarization	K^+ out of cell	Ca^{2+} and Na^+ channels close; K^+ channel remains open
4	Resting membrane potential	Na^+ out, K^+ in	Na^+–K^+ pump

Ca^{2+}, Calcium; *K^+,* potassium; *Na^+,* sodium.

AP slope returns toward zero (*phase 1* of the AP). The plateau that follows is described as *phase 2*. During this phase, another set of channels, the slow Na^+ and Ca^{2+} channels, open to allow the influx of Ca^{2+} and Na^+. During phase 2, K^+ tends to diffuse out of the cell, balancing the slow inward flux of Na^+ and Ca^{2+} thereby maintaining the plateau of the AP. The Ca^{2+} entering the cell at this phase causes cardiac contraction, which is described later in this chapter. The inward flux of Ca^{2+} during this phase can be influenced by many factors. For example,

calcium channel–blocking medications such as verapamil and diltiazem inhibit the inward Ca^{2+} current into pacemaker tissue, especially the AV node. For this reason, this class of medications is used therapeutically to slow the rate of atrial tachydysrhythmias and protect the ventricle from excessive atrial impulses, as described in the section on cardiac medications in Chapter 16.

Phase 3. The repolarization phase is described as *phase 3*, and it depends on two processes. The first is the inactivation of the slow channels, which prevents further influx of Ca^{2+} and Na^+. The other is the continued efflux of K^+ out of the cell. Both processes cause the intracellular environment to become more negative, thereby re-establishing the RMP. On the AP, phase 3 is seen as a gradual descent during which the interior of the cell becomes more negative relative to the outside.

Phase 4. In *phase 4*, the AP returns to an RMP of −80 to −90 mV. The excess Na^+ that entered the cell during depolarization is removed from the cell in exchange for K^+ by means of the Na^+–K^+ pump. This mechanism returns the intracellular concentrations of Na^+ and K^+ to the levels present before depolarization and is essential for normal ionic balance and preparation for the next depolarization (see Table 12-5).

Fiber Conduction and Excitability. Different parts of the conduction system require different electrical currents and create individual transmembrane APs, as shown in Figure 12-7 earlier in the chapter. Ionic shifts within the endocardium, myocardium, and epicardium are not uniform, although the clinical significance of this finding is not clear. Propagation of an AP along a cardiac fiber occurs as a result of ionic shifts (discussed earlier). As a local section of the cell becomes depolarized, reaches threshold, and completely depolarizes, it affects the adjacent area of the cell and initiates depolarization in that area.

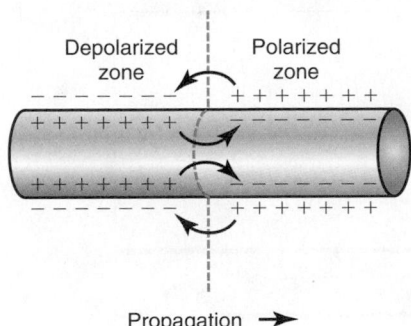

FIGURE 12-24 Schematic representation of the propagation of an action potential along a cell membrane.

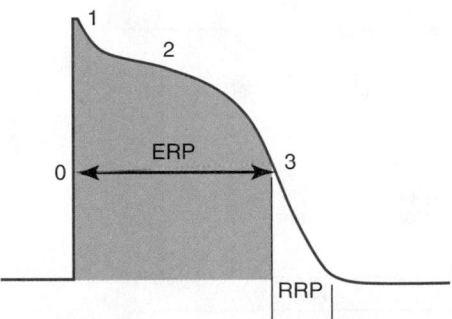

FIGURE 12-25 The two parts of the refractory period. The effective (absolute) refractory period *(ERP)* extends from phase 0 to approximately −50 mV in phase 3. The remainder of the action potential is the relative refractory period *(RRP)*. (From Conover MB. *Understanding Electrocardiography.* 8th ed. St. Louis, MO: Mosby; 2002.)

The AP propagates down the fiber in a wavelike fashion (Fig. 12-24). This is somewhat analogous to a trail of gunpowder. When the gunpowder is lit at one end, a small area ignites, burns, and then ignites the area of gunpowder immediately adjacent to it and on down the line.

The time from the beginning of the AP until the fiber can accept another AP is called the *effective* or *absolute refractory period.* During this period, the cell cannot be depolarized regardless of the amount or intensity of the stimulus. This period lasts from the beginning of depolarization until the interior of the cell has repolarized to approximately −50 mV during phase 3. The absolute refractory period is immediately followed by the *relative refractory period.* At this time, the cell is not fully repolarized but could depolarize with a strong enough stimulus (Fig. 12-25). This period lasts from approximately −50 mV during phase 3 until the cell returns to RMP (phase 4); at that point, the cell is fully repolarized and is again ready to respond to the next stimulus. The concept of relative versus absolute refractory periods is useful for understanding the genesis of ventricular dysrhythmias (see Chapter 14). In brief, a cell cannot be stimulated to depolarize until it has at least partially recovered from the previous impulse. This means that an ectopic impulse cannot be propagated during the absolute refractory period.

Pacemaker Cell versus Non-pacemaker Cell Action Potentials. The AP is representative of the depolarization of non-pacemaker myocardial cells. The AP generated by a Purkinje fiber is similar to that of a ventricular myocardial cell except that phase 2 is usually more prolonged in the Purkinje fiber. Atrial myocardial cells exhibit a shortened plateau (phase 2) compared with ventricular cells. The pacemaker cells of the SA node have an AP that is very different from that of a myocardial cell or a Purkinje cell. In the SA node, the RMP is not as negative, approximately −65 mV. Rather than having an RMP that remains constant, the pacemaker cells slowly depolarize at a steady rate until the threshold is reached (see Fig. 12-23B). The lack of a steady-state RMP is largely the result of a continual Na$^+$ influx through the slow channels. This mechanism explains how the cells can spontaneously depolarize (automaticity). It also provides the basis for understanding alterations in the pacemaker cells. The frequency of pacemaker cell discharge may be altered by changing the rate of depolarization or by raising or lowering the cellular RMP.

Mechanical Activity
Excitation–Contraction Coupling

Electrical activity is the stimulus for mechanical contraction. As the myocardial cell is depolarized during phase 2 of the AP, extracellular Ca^{2+} ions enter the cytoplasm through the cell membrane via special Ca^{2+} channels. The entry of Ca^{2+} ions is the trigger for the release of Ca^{2+} stores from the sarcoplasmic reticulum (calcium-induced calcium release). The cytoplasmic Ca^{2+} then binds with the regulatory Tn-C protein to induce a conformational change in Tn-I; this action induces a conformational change in Tn-T that moves the tropomyosin away from the myosin-binding site on actin. This permits actin to interact with myosin thereby releasing adenosine diphosphate (ADP) and an inorganic phosphate to provide the energy needed for myosin to slide along the actin molecule and initiate contraction. This mechanism is known as *cross-bridge cycling.* The result is myocardial contraction that spreads throughout the myocardium.

Once contraction has occurred, intracellular Ca^{2+} levels are lowered by two processes. Most Ca^{2+} is taken back up into the sarcoplasmic reticulum via a Ca^{2+} and magnesium (Mg^{2+})–dependent, adenosine triphosphate (ATP)–based process. In addition, the Na$^+$–Ca^{2+} exchange system located in the sarcolemma moves Ca^{2+} outside the cell. This decreases the concentration of Ca^{2+} in the cytoplasm, leading to muscular relaxation.

Cardiac Cycle

The term *cardiac cycle* refers to one complete mechanical cycle of the heartbeat, beginning with ventricular contraction and ending with ventricular relaxation.

Atrial Systole

The atria fill by passive filling from the vena cavae (right atrium) and the pulmonary veins (left atrium). During diastole, the mitral and tricuspid valves are open, allowing for passive filling into the ventricles. Following electrical depolarization of the atria (the p-wave), atrial contraction (atrial systole) is initiated, causing additional blood to enter the ventricular chamber. This is also referred to as *atrial kick.* The next action is the closure of the mitral and tricuspid valves.

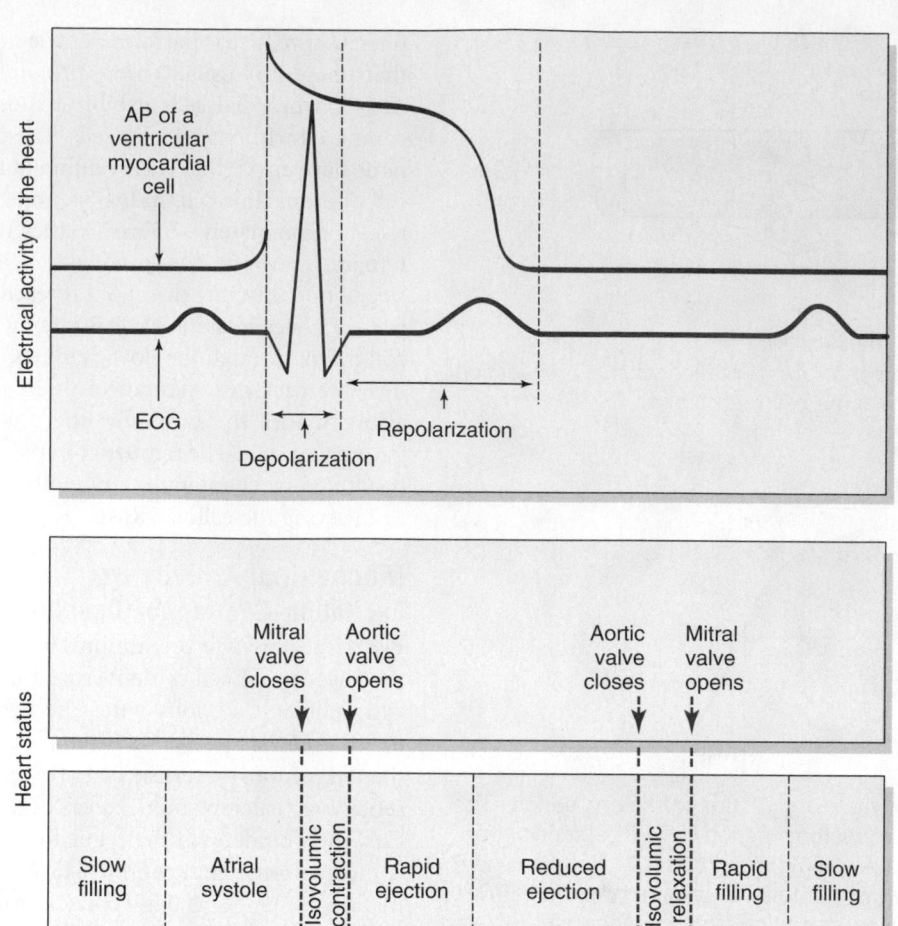

FIGURE 12-26 The Cardiac Cycle.

Isovolumic Contraction

Ventricular depolarization from the QRS electrical stimulus depolarizes the septum and papillary muscles first. The ventricles then begin to tense, starting with the inner endocardium and traversing the myocardium toward the outer epicardium. This increases the pressure within the ventricular chambers. This is known as *isovolumic contraction*, because even though the ventricular muscle is contracting, the volume of blood within the ventricles does not change. In Figure 12-26, this is seen as a rapid rise in left ventricular pressure.

Ventricular Systole

Ventricular systole represents the ventricular ejection portion of the cardiac cycle. As ventricular tension increases, intraventricular pressures exceed the pressure in the aorta and pulmonary arteries, causing the aortic and pulmonic valves to open. The amount of blood ejected from the ventricles with each beat is called the *stroke volume* (SV). In a healthy heart, more than half of the total ventricular blood volume is ejected; the blood that remains in the ventricles is the *residual* or *end-systolic* volume.

The ejection fraction (EF) is the ratio of the SV ejected from the left ventricle per beat to the volume of blood remaining in the left ventricle at the end of diastole (left ventricular end-diastolic volume, or LVEDV). EF is expressed as a percentage, and a normal value is 50% or greater. An EF of less than 35% indicates poor ventricular function (as in cardiomyopathy), poor ventricular filling, obstruction to outflow (as in some valve stenosis conditions), or a combination of these conditions.

Isovolumic Relaxation

The next phase is *isovolumic relaxation*, which occurs between the closure of the semilunar (aortic and pulmonic) valves and the opening of the AV (mitral and tricuspid) valves. All four valves are closed, and the pressure within the ventricular chamber falls to below atrial pressure without any change in intraventricular volume. At this point, the mitral and tricuspid valves open.

Ventricular Diastole

Once the AV valves open, the majority of ventricular filling occurs. The next phase is a reduced ventricular filling period, during which blood flows passively from the periphery and the pulmonary vasculature into the ventricles. The last part of ventricular diastolic filling occurs during atrial contraction, also described as *atrial kick*. This provides approximately 20% of total ventricular filling in normal sinus rhythm. With this, the cycle is complete and ready to begin once again with atrial systole (see Fig. 12-26).

Interplay of the Heart and Vessels: Cardiac Output

Cardiac output (CO) is defined as the volume of blood ejected from the heart in 1 minute. The determinants of CO are heart rate (HR) in beats per minute (beats/min) and stroke volume (SV) in milliliters per beat (mL/beat). The equation is:

$$SV \times HR = CO$$

CO is usually expressed in liters per minute (L/min). Normal CO in the human adult is approximately 4 to 8 L/min; it is approximately 4 to 6 L/min at rest and increases with exercise. CO can be made specific to body size by using the person's height and weight to determine the cardiac index (CI). The CI is equal to CO divided by the individual's body surface area (BSA) calculated from the height and weight. BSA is expressed in square meters (m^2), the normal range is 2.5 to 4.5 L/min/m^2. Changes in SV or HR can change CO. However, all three parameters must be individually assessed as described in the section hemodynamics in Chapter 14.

For example, for a person with an HR of 72 and an SV of 70 mL, the CI would be:

$$72 \text{ (beats/min)} \times 70 \text{ (mL/beat)} = 5.04 \text{ L/min}$$

If the HR were to change to 140 and the SV to 40 mL in this person, the calculation would be:

$$140 \text{ (beats/min)} \times 40 \text{ (mL/beat)} = 5.6 \text{ L/min}$$

Even though CO is higher, clearly the faster HR would not be an improvement in this situation. The decreased SV in the second instance indicates that cardiac decompensation is imminent. SV as a value is influenced by three primary factors: 1) preload, 2) afterload, and 3) contractility (Fig. 12-27).

Preload

The concept of preload was introduced in the early 1900s when Ernest Starling described his findings in an isolated

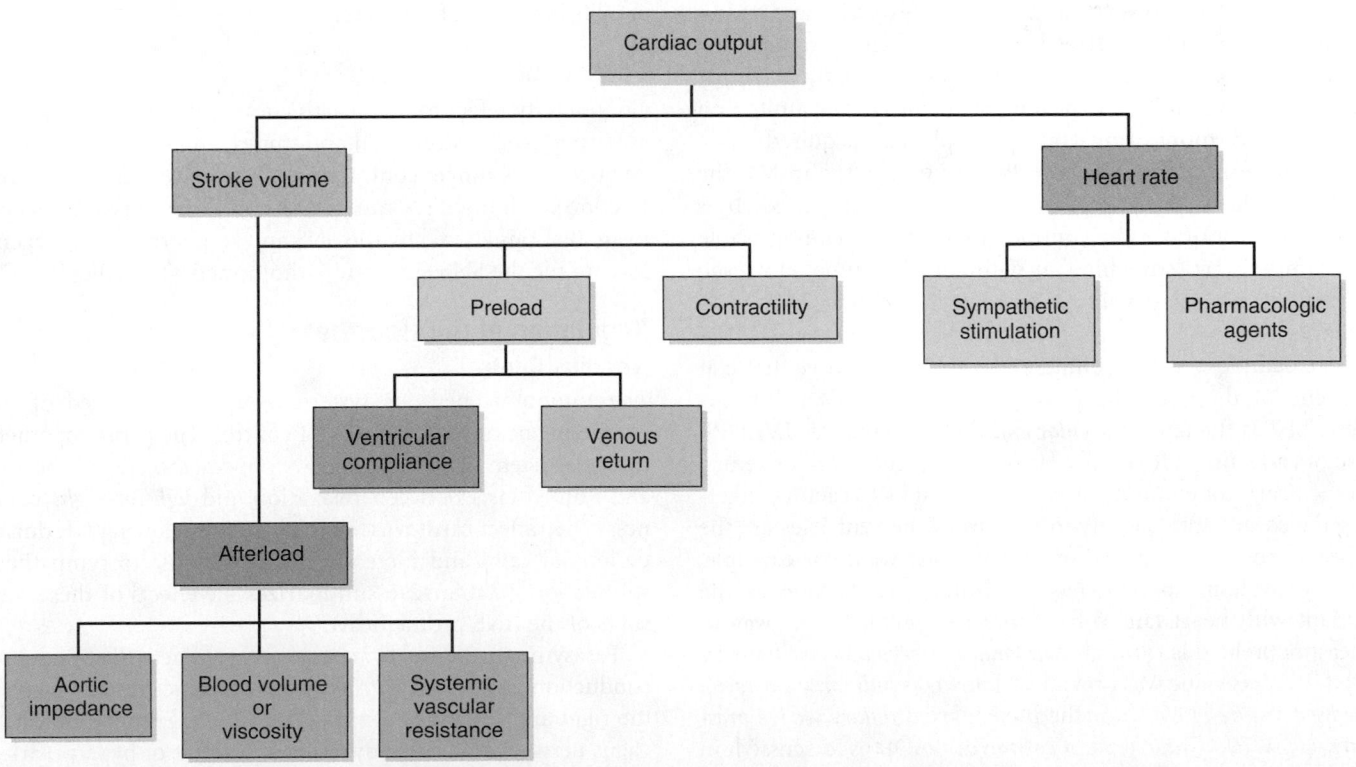

FIGURE 12-27 Determinants of Cardiac Output.

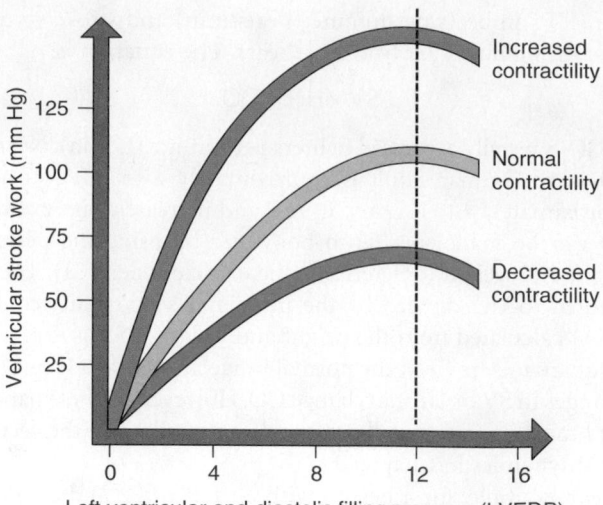

FIGURE 12-28 Starling Curve. As the left ventricular end-diastolic pressure (LVEDP) increases, so does ventricular stroke work or contractility. When left ventricular filling pressure exceeds a maximal point, contractility and cardiac output diminish.

canine heart preparation. Starling found that as he increased the volume infused into a denervated heart, CO increased, until it reached a point at which further infusion caused CO to decrease. This has become known as *Starling's law of the heart*, and it is graphically described as the *Starling curve* (Fig. 12-28). It can best be described on a molecular basis, using as a foundation the discussion of the actin and myosin cross-bridges in the myofibril. As the diastolic volume increases, it stretches the actin and myosin molecules in their resting state. As contraction occurs, contractility increases as a result of the increased stretch. However, if the stretch is excessive and causes actin and myosin to be stretched beyond their cross-bridging limits (>2.2 mm), contractility decreases. This is the basis for Starling's curve. With the advent of intensive care units and sophisticated monitoring, this principle has acquired great significance in clinical practice. For example, after an MI, the ability of the left ventricle to pump may be impaired. It is desirable to optimize the contractility of the remaining viable heart muscle by "stretching" it with added volume. However, if the intravascular volume exceeds the stretch limit, CO diminishes.

Preload, then, is the volume of blood in the left ventricle at the end of diastole. The pressure created by this volume is described as the *left ventricular end-diastolic pressure* (LVEDP). Factors affecting left ventricular preload include venous return to the heart, total blood volume, and atrial kick. Factors affecting the compliance (ability to stretch) of the ventricles are the stiffness and the thickness of the muscular wall. For example, the hypovolemic patient has too little preload, whereas the patient with heart failure has too much preload. One way to measure preload is through *pulmonary artery occlusion pressure (PAOP)*. This value was previously known as *pulmonary arterial wedge pressure (PAWP)* or the *pulmonary capillary wedge pressure (PCWP)*. Clinical application of PAOP is discussed in Chapter 14.

TABLE 12-6	SUMMARY OF THE EFFECTS OF THE PARASYMPATHETIC AND SYMPATHETIC NERVOUS SYSTEMS ON THE HEART		
FUNCTION	**PARASYMPATHETIC**	**SYMPATHETIC**
Automaticity	Decrease	Increase
Contractility	Decrease	Increase
Conduction velocity	Decrease	Increase
Chronotropy (rate)	Decrease	Increase

Afterload

Afterload can be defined as the ventricular wall tension or stress during systolic ejection. It is commonly described by the term *systemic vascular resistance (SVR)* or, less frequently, *peripheral vascular resistance*. An increase in afterload usually means an increase in the work of the heart. Afterload is increased by factors that oppose ejection. Examples of increased afterload include aortic impedance (high diastolic aortic pressure, aortic stenosis), septal hypertrophy (obstruction in the outflow tract), vasoconstriction (increased SVR), and hypertension. Therapeutic management to decrease afterload is aimed at decreasing the work of the heart through the use of vasodilators to decrease the myocardial oxygen demand.

An increase in afterload evokes autoregulation, in which the ventricle adapts to changes in filling pressure without a continued increase in resting fiber length. For example, when the SVR increases abruptly during vasoconstriction, ventricular diastolic pressure rises temporarily until the ventricle reaches a new equilibrium level of pressure.

Contractility

Contractility refers to the heart's contractile force. Also known as *inotropy* (*ino* ["strength"] and *tropy* ["enhancing"]), it can be positive (i.e., stronger contraction) or negative (i.e., weaker contraction). Contractility can be increased by Starling's mechanism. It also is altered by the SNS and by pharmacologic agents that mimic the SNS (i.e., sympathomimetics) (see Fig. 12-27).

Regulation of the Heartbeat
Nervous Control

The autonomic nervous system (ANS) is composed of two competing neurologic systems of control. The parasympathetic nervous system (PNS) and the SNS operate to create a balance and homeostasis between relaxation and *fight-or-flight* readiness. They affect cardiovascular function by slowing HR during periods of calm and increasing it in response to sympathetic stimulation.[23] Table 12-6 summarizes the effects of these divisions of the ANS on the heart.

Parasympathetic fibers are concentrated near the SA and AV conduction tissue and in the atria.[23] Specifically, this involves the right and left vagus nerves (Fig. 12-29). Stimulation of the vagus nerve produces bradycardia as a result of hyperpolarization of phase 4 of the AP, which causes the slope to take longer

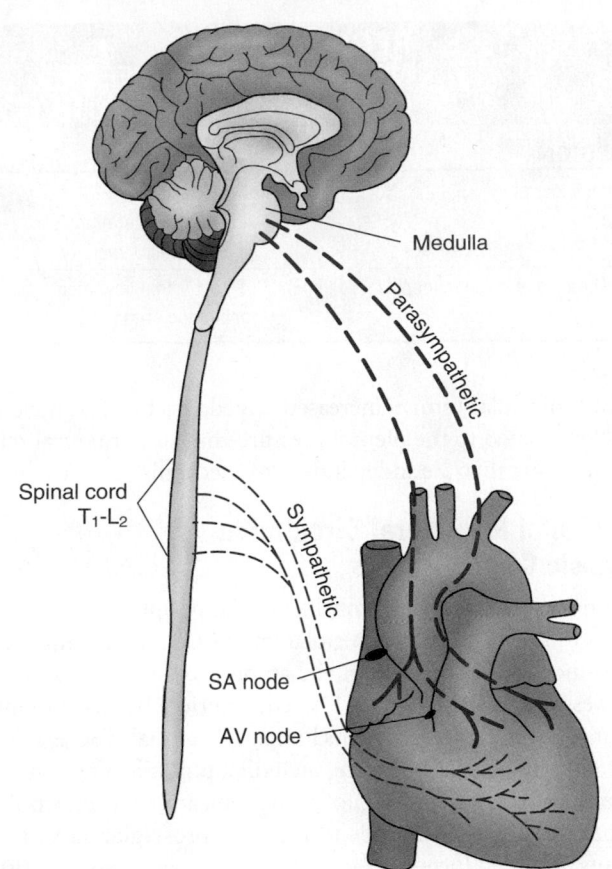

FIGURE 12-29 Autonomic nervous system innervation of nodal tissue and myocardium by parasympathetic vagus nerve fibers and sympathetic chains. (Modified from Quaal S. *Comprehensive Intraaortic Balloon Pumping.* 2nd ed. St. Louis, MO: Mosby; 1993.)

to reach the threshold. Sympathetic tone concomitantly decreases.

Sympathetic nerve fibers are subepicardial and follow the path of the major coronary arteries.[28] When stimulated, sympathetic fibers directly alter ventricular function and increase HR and contractility.

Intrinsic Regulation

Supplementing the nervous control of the heart are several reflexes that serve as feedback mechanisms to the brain. These reflexes work to maintain even blood flow, oxygenation, and perfusion.

Baroreceptors. Baroreceptors, or pressure sensors, are located in the aortic arch and the carotid sinuses.[29] They are more sensitive to wall changes (wall stretch) in these areas than to the absolute pressure. As the receptors sense a change in wall conformation, usually as a result of a change in pressure, the ANS is activated to raise HR (in the case of decreased pressure) or lower it (in response to increased pressure). For example, a decrease in blood pressure alters the baroreceptor input to the vasomotor center in the medulla (brainstem), causing a reflex tachycardia. The baroreflex also initiates changes in venous tone to alter CO according to need. Venoconstriction increases blood return to the heart and augments SV.

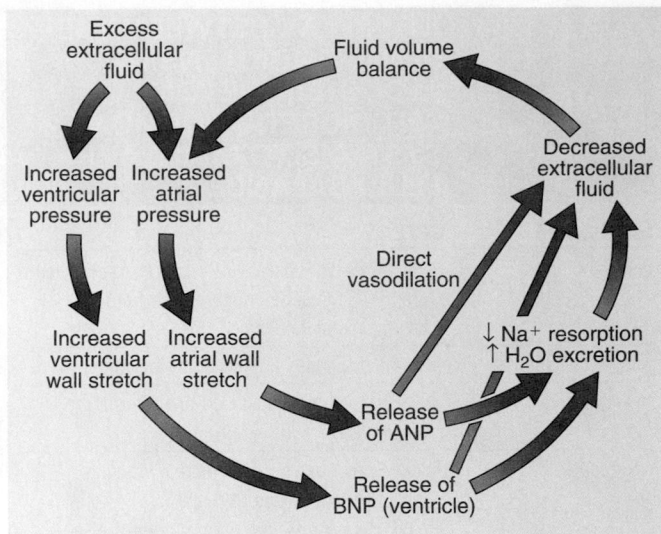

FIGURE 12-30 The release of atrial peptide (ANP) from the atrium and brain natriuretic peptide (BNP) from the ventricle in response to volume overload.

Chemoreceptors. The arterial *chemoreceptors*, or *carotid* and *aortic bodies*, are located in the carotid arteries and at the bifurcation of the aortic arch.[30] They possess a rich capillary blood supply and extensive innervation of the PNS. Their primary function is to maintain homeostasis during hypoxemia.[30] Chemoreceptors signal changes in oxygen tension (Pao_2 <80 mm Hg), or a carbon dioxide tension ($Paco_2$) of greater than 40 mm Hg, but not to changes in acid–base balance (pH). Changes in the pH level are detected by the central chemoreceptors in the brainstem (medulla oblongata). Information about changes in these parameters is communicated to the SNS via the brainstem altering HR. Stimulation of the carotid or aortic chemoreceptors normally causes an increase in respiratory rate and depth.

Right Atrial Receptors. The *Bainbridge reflex* is attributed to receptors in the right and left atria.[31] When the pressure in the right atrium rises sufficiently to stimulate the stretch receptors, it causes a reflex tachycardia. The purpose of this reflex is possibly to protect the right side of the heart from an overload state and to quickly equalize filling pressures of the right and left sides of the heart.

Natriuretic Peptides. Another cardiac control mechanism involves the natriuretic peptide system (Fig. 12-30). The heart secretes two major natriuretic peptides. The atrial myocardium secretes *atrial natriuretic peptide* (ANP) in response to atrial stretch, and the ventricular myocardium secretes *brain natriuretic peptide* (BNP) if stretch of the ventricular chamber occurs. Both peptides cause vasodilatation, increase natriuresis (Na^+ and water loss via the kidneys), and inhibit the SNS and the renin–angiotensin–aldosterone system (RAAS).[32] Clinically, BNP levels are measured to confirm the diagnosis of acute heart failure. A recombinant form of human BNP, nesiritide (Natrecor), is used therapeutically to mimic the clinical effects of BNP and treat symptoms of heart failure.

Renin–Angiotensin–Aldosterone System. The RAAS system is activated by low blood pressure or intravascular volume depletion. The juxtaglomerular cells of the kidney, located

TABLE 12-7	INTERPLAY BETWEEN THE RENIN–ANGIOTENSIN–ALDOSTERONE AND ANTIDIURETIC HORMONE SYSTEMS TO MAINTAIN FLUID BALANCE
HORMONE	**EFFECT***
Renin ↓	Reduction in vascular volume or low arterial blood pressure stimulates renin release from juxtaglomerular cells near the kidney.
Angiotensinogen ↓	Angiotensinogen is produced in the liver.
Angiotensin I ↓	Lungs release ACE to convert angiotensin I to angiotensin II.
Angiotensin II ↓	Angiotensin II activates peripheral vascular receptors to increase SVR and raise arterial blood pressure. Angiotensin II release also stimulates adrenal glands to release aldosterone.
	ADH is released from the posterior pituitary when angiotensin II causes constriction of the renal arterioles and when the hypothalamus detects intracellular dehydration.
Aldosterone	Aldosterone acts on the kidney distal tubules to retain sodium; when salt is retained, so is water.

*Overall effect is to increase intravascular volume and raise blood pressure.
ACE, Angiotensin-converting enzyme; *ADH,* antidiuretic hormone; *SVR,* systemic vascular resistance.

near the afferent arteriole, are activated by low renal blood flow. As shown in Table 12-7, this stimulates release of the hormone renin. Renin converts the protein angiotensinogen to angiotensin I. When angiotensin I passes through the pulmonary vascular bed, it is activated by angiotensin-converting enzyme (ACE) to become angiotensin II. Angiotensin II is a powerful agent with two principal actions: 1) It activates peripheral vascular receptors to vasoconstrict the systemic arterial system and increase blood pressure, and 2) it activates the release of aldosterone from the adrenal glands. Aldosterone works at the distal convoluted tubule in the kidney to retain sodium and, consequently, water. Many medications are used to manipulate the RAAS system to manage symptoms of heart failure (see "Heart Failure" in Chapter 15 and "Cardiac Medications" in Chapter 16).

Respiratory Influences. Other influences involve the respiratory cycle and its effect on HR and SV. Normally, HR varies slightly with the respiratory cycle. The heart usually accelerates on inspiration and decelerates with exhalation (see "Sinus Dysrhythmia" in Chapter 14). Left ventricular SV decreases during normal inspiration. Possible reasons include normal fluctuations in sympathetic and vagal tones during respiration or any of the following alterations: decreased intrathoracic pressure contributing to increased venous return; the Bainbridge reflex; activation of stretch receptors in the lungs; interactions between the respiratory and cardiac centers in the medulla; increased capacity of the pulmonary vessels during lung inflation; decreased left ventricular compliance resulting from increased

TABLE 12-8	REGIONS IN THE MEDULLA THAT AFFECT CARDIOVASCULAR ACTIVITY
REGION	**ACTIVITY**
Dorsal lateral medulla (pressor region)	Vasoconstriction Cardiac acceleration Enhanced contractility
Ventromedial medulla (depressor region)	Direct spinal inhibition Inhibition of the pressor region

right ventricular return; increased impedance to left ventricular outflow related to the pleural pressure changes; or neural reflex mechanisms that are independent of mechanical influences.

Control of Peripheral Circulation
Intrinsic Control

Intrinsic, or local, control of the arterial peripheral circulation is most influential at the arteriolar level. Arterioles are the major resistance vessels because of the amount of smooth muscle in the vessel walls (see Fig. 12-12). The arteriole has the potential for increasing or decreasing its lumen substantially. Several local factors influence this balance, including pharmacologic stimuli from locally released catecholamines, histamine, acetylcholine, serotonin, angiotensin, adenosine, and prostaglandins. These agents can be induced by a variety of mechanisms such as tissue injury, hypoxemia, or hormones. Other factors that influence circulation locally are temperature and carbon dioxide.

Extrinsic Control

Extrinsic control is mediated by two major mechanisms: 1) the ANS and 2) peripheral vascular reflexes.

The ANS exerts dual antagonistic control over most organ systems via sympathetic (constriction) and parasympathetic (dilation) nerve fibers. Stimulation of the vasomotor center in the medulla causes increased mean arterial pressure and HR by enhancing sympathetic outflow and possibly inhibiting parasympathetic outflow. The sympathetic outflow targets resistance arterioles, causing vasoconstriction. Inhibition of these areas produces the opposite effect—vasodilation. Sympathetic fibers causing vasoconstriction supply arteries, arterioles, and veins.

Capacitance vessels (veins) contain up to 75% of the blood volume. Increases in venous tone (venoconstriction) increase the volume of blood returning to the right side of the heart and augment SV. The most richly innervated venous beds are those in splanchnic (spleen) and cutaneous (skin) circulations. The venous and arterial vascular systems are interdependent; they dilate and constrict in unison. One does not act without the other. Table 12-8 summarizes the sympathetic receptors, including location and effects of stimulation.

The control of peripheral circulation is achieved by a combination of intrinsic and extrinsic mechanisms. Additional influences include emotions, temperature, and humoral substances. For example, when red blood cells are exposed to hypoxia at the tissue level, they release the vasodilators nitric oxide and ATP to increase oxygen delivery.

SUMMARY

- Knowledge of normal cardiovascular anatomy and physiology is vital for a complete understanding of the changes that occur in cardiac disease states.
- The major anatomic structures of the heart include the pericardium, myocardium, endocardium, coronary arteries, coronary veins, atria, ventricles, heart valves, and electrical conduction system.

- The electrical conduction system, the mechanical events of the cardiac cycle, the autonomic nervous system, and the preload volume in the veins act synergistically to ensure optimal cardiac output and hemodynamic stability in a state of health.

REFERENCES

1. Anderson RH, Loukas M. The importance of attitudinally appropriate description of cardiac anatomy. *Clin Anat.* 2009;22:47.
2. Dell'Italia LJ. Anatomy and physiology of the right ventricle. *Cardiol Clin.* 2012;30(2):167.
3. Hale SJ, Mirjaili S, Stringer MD. Inconsistencies in surface anatomy: the need for an evidence-based reappraisal. *Clin Anat.* 2010;23:922.
4. Lachman N, Syed FF, Habib A, et al. Correlative anatomy for the electrophysiologist, Part I: the pericardial space, oblique sinus, transverse sinus. *J Cardiovasc Electrophysiol.* 2010;21(12):1421.
5. Loukas M, Walters A, Boon JM, et al. Pericardiocentesis: a clinical anatomy review. *Clin Anat.* 2012;25(7):872.
6. Rabkin SW. Epicardial fat: properties, function and relationship to obesity. *Obes Rev.* 2007;8(3):253.
7. Ouwens DM, Sell H, Greulich S, et al. The role of epicardial and perivascular adipose tissue in the pathophysiology of cardiovascular disease. *J Cell Mol Med.* 2010;14(9):2223.
8. Iacobellis G, Bianco C. Epicardial adipose tissue: emerging physiological, pathophysiological and clinical features. *Cell.* 2011;22(11):450.
9. Anderson RH, Ho SY, Redmann K, et al. The anatomical arrangement of the myocardial cells making up the ventricular mass. *Eur J Cardiothorac Surg.* 2005;28(4):517.
10. Partridge JB, Anderson RH. Left ventricular anatomy: its nomenclature, segmentation, and planes of imaging. *Clin Anat.* 2009;22(1):77.
11. Muresian H. The clinical anatomy of the mitral valve. *Clin Anat.* 2009;22(1):85.
12. Bascelli A, Di Fonso A, Bartoloni G, et al. Functional mitral regurgitation: from normal to pathological anatomy of mitral valve. *Int J Cardiol.* 2012. Epub pre-print.
13. Mordi I, Tzemos N. Bicuspid aortic valve disease: a comprehensive review. *Cardiol Res Pract.* 2012. Epub pre-print.
14. Siu SC, Silversides CK. Bicuspid aortic valve disease. *J Am Coll Cardiol.* 2010;55:2789.
15. Park DS, Fishman GI. The cardiac conduction system. *Circulation.* 2011;123:904.
16. Pejković B, Krajnc I, Anderhuber F, et al. Anatomical aspects of the arterial blood supply to the sinoatrial and atrioventricular nodes of the human heart. *J Int Med Res.* 2008;36(4):691.
17. James TN. The internodal pathways of the human heart. *Prog Cardiovasc Dis.* 2001;43(6):495.
18. Anderson RH, Cook AC. The structure and components of the atrial chambers. *Europace.* 2007;9(suppl 6):vi3.
19. Fedorov VV, Glukhov AV, Chang R. Conduction barriers and pathways of the sinoatrial pacemaker complex: their role in normal rhythm and atrial arrhythmias. *Am J Physiol Heart Circulatory Physiol.* 2012;302(9):H1773.
20. Kurian T, Ambrosi C, Hucker W, et al. Anatomy and electrophysiology of the human AV node. *PACE.* 2010;33(6):754.
21. Loukas M, Groat C, Khangura R, et al. The normal and abnormal anatomy of the coronary arteries. *Clin Anat.* 2009;22:114.
22. Loukas M, Blinsky E, El-Sedfy A, et al. Cardiac veins: a review of the literature. *Clin Anat.* 2009;22:129.
23. Thomas GD. Neural control of the circulation. *Adv Physiol Edu.* 2011;35:28.
24. Gautel M. The sarcomeric cytoskeleton: who picks up the strain? *Curr Opin Cell Biol.* 2011;23:439.
25. LeWinter MM, Granzier H. Cardiac titin : a multifunctional giant. *Circulation.* 2010;121:2137.
26. Pappas CT, Bliss KT, Zieseniss A, et al. The Nebulin family: an actin support group. *Trends Cell Biol.* 2009;21(1):29.
27. Ibrahim M, Gorelik J, Yacoub MH, et al. The structure and function of cardiac t-tubules in health and disease. *Proc Royal Soc Biol Sci.* 2011;278:2714.
28. Zipes DP. Heart-brain interactions in cardiac arrhythmias: role of the autonomic nervous system. *Cleve Clin J Med.* 2008;75(suppl 2):S94.
29. Fadel PJ. Arterial baroreflex control of the peripheral vasculature in humans: rest and exercise. *Med Sci Sports Exerc.* 2008;40(12):2055.
30. Prabhakar NR, Peng YJ. Peripheral chemoreceptors in health and disease. *J Appl Physiol.* 2004;96(1):359.
31. Crystal GJ, Salem RM. The Bainbridge and the "reverse" Bainbridge reflexes: history, physiology, and clinical relevance. *Anesth Analg.* 2012;114(3):520.
32. Maisel A. Circulating natriuretic peptide levels in acute heart failure. *Rev Cardiovasc Med.* 2007;8(suppl 5):S13.

Cardiovascular Clinical Assessment

Mary E. Lough

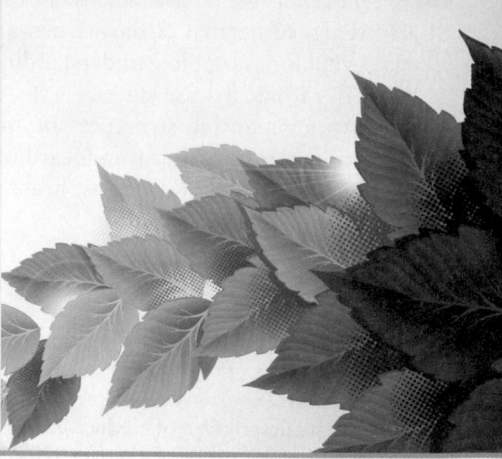

⊖volve WEBSITE

http://evolve.elsevier.com/Urden/criticalcare/

Evolve Features:

- NCLEX Review Questions
- CCRN Review Questions
- PCCN Review Questions
- Mosby's Nursing Skills Procedures
- Animations
- Video Clips
- Glossary

Physical assessment of the patient with cardiovascular disease is a skill that must not be overlooked in the middle of all the technology of the critical care setting.[1] Data collected from a thorough, thoughtful history taking and examination contribute to both the nursing and the medical decisions about therapeutic interventions.

HISTORY

Patient history is important because it provides data that contribute to diagnosis of cardiovascular disease and treatment plan. For a patient in acute distress, the history taking is shortened to just a few questions about the patient's chief complaint, precipitating events, and current medications (Box 13-1). For a patient who is not in obvious distress, the history focuses on the following four areas:

1. Review of the patient's present illness
2. Overview of the patient's general cardiovascular status, including previous cardiac diagnostic studies, interventional procedures, cardiac surgeries, and current medications (i.e., cardiac, noncardiac, and over-the-counter medications)
3. Review of the patient's general health status, including family history of coronary artery disease (CAD), hypertension, diabetes, peripheral arterial disease, or stroke
4. Survey of the patient's lifestyle, including risk factors for CAD

One of the unique challenges in cardiovascular assessment is identifying when "chest pain" is of cardiac origin and when it is not. The following safety information should always be considered:

- If any evidence of CAD or risk of heart disease exists, assume that the chest pain is caused by myocardial ischemia until proven otherwise.
- Questions to elicit the nature of the chest pain cover five basic areas: 1) quality, 2) location, 3) duration of pain, 4) factors that provoke the pain, and 5) factors that relieve the pain. Questions that may help elicit this information are listed in Table 13-1.
- Little correlation may exist between the severity of chest discomfort and the gravity of its cause. This is a result of the subjective nature of pain and the unique presentation of ischemic disease in women, older patients, and individuals with diabetes.
- Subjective descriptors vary greatly among individuals. Not all patients use the word "pain"; some may describe their problem as "pressure," heaviness," discomfort," or "indigestion."
- A correlation is not always present between the location of chest discomfort and its source because of *referred pain*. For example, in patients with gastroesophageal reflux disease (GERD), esophageal spasm can cause visceral substernal chest pain that radiates to the left arm and jaw and may be described by patients as "heartburn."[2]
- Other nonpainful symptoms that may signal cardiac dysfunction are dyspnea, palpitations, cough, fatigue, edema, ischemic leg pain, nocturia, syncope, and cyanosis.

In a meta-analysis of the evaluation of stable, intermittent chest pain, a patient's description of chest pain was found to be the most important predictor of underlying coronary disease.[3] In the evaluation of acute chest pain, the 12-lead

BOX 13-1 DATA COLLECTION

Cardiovascular History

Common Cardiovascular Symptoms
- Chest pains
- Palpitations
- Dyspnea
- Cough, hemoptysis
- Nausea
- Nocturia
- Edema
- Dizziness, syncope, visual changes
- Leg claudication (pain) or paresthesias
- Fatigue

Patient Lifestyle
- Baseline cognitive functioning
- Health habits
  - Use of tea and coffee; over-the-counter medication use; smoking; exercise; sleep; dietary habits
  - Use of illegal recreational drugs (e.g., cocaine)
  - Use of alcohol (occasional, daily)
- Lifestyle pattern and responsibilities
- Working, relaxing, coping, cultural habits
- Social support systems
- Recent life changes within the past 12 months
- Emotional state
- Evidence of psychologic stress, anger, anxiety, depression
- Perception of illness and its meaning for the future

Cardiovascular Risk Factors
- Gender
- Age
- Cultural identity
- Family history of premature CAD (65 years or younger)
- Smoking history
- Hypertension
- Hyperlipidemia
- Sedentary lifestyle
- Diabetes mellitus
- Obesity
- Kidney failure

Medical History

Child
- Murmurs, cyanosis, streptococcal infections, rheumatic fever

Adult
- Diseases and abnormalities
  - Heart failure (right- or left-sided), CAD, heart valve disease, mitral valve prolapse, myocardial infarction, peripheral vascular disease (arterial or venous), diabetes mellitus, hypertension, hyperlipidemia, dysrhythmias, murmurs, endocarditis, visual defects, recent weight changes, psychiatric illnesses, thrombophlebitis, deep vein thrombosis, systemic or pulmonary emboli

- Surgical history
  - *Cardiovascular:* coronary artery bypass grafting, valvular placement, peripheral vascular bypasses or repairs, pacemaker, defibrillator implant (ICD)
  - *Other body systems:* neurologic, gastrointestinal, musculoskeletal, pulmonary, renal, immunologic, hematologic
- Allergies, especially to emergency medications (lidocaine, morphine), radiographic contrast agents, or iodine (shellfish)
- Recent dental work or infection

Family History
- CAD at age 65 years or younger
- Myocardial infarction or early death of unknown origin
- Hypertension
- Stroke
- Diabetes mellitus
- Lipid disorders
- Collagen vascular disease

Current Medication Use
- ACE inhibitors
- Anticoagulants
- Antidysrhythmics
- Antihypertensives
- Antiplatelet agents
- Angiotensin-receptor blockers
- Beta-blockers
- Calcium channel blockers
- Cholesterol-lowering agents
- Digitalis
- Diuretics
- Nitrates
- Hormone replacement therapy
- Oral contraceptives
- Potassium, calcium
- Nonprescription medications or herbal remedies

Cardiac Studies or Interventions Done in the Past
- Cardiac catheterization
- Electrophysiology study
- Cardiac ultrasound (echocardiogram)
- 12-lead electroencephalogram
- Exercise electrocardiography test (stress test)
- Myocardial imaging with radiographic isotopes (e.g., thallium, dipyridamole, dobutamine)
- Thrombolytic therapy
- Percutaneous transluminal coronary angioplasty
- Atherectomy
- Stent placement
- Valvuloplasty

ACE, Angiotensin-converting enzyme; *CAD,* coronary artery disease; *ICD,* implantable cardioverter defibrillator.

TABLE 13-1	CLARIFYING CHEST PAIN SYMPTOMS BY ASKING SPECIFIC QUESTIONS
DETERMINE	**TYPICAL QUESTION**
Location, radiation	Where is it? Does it move or stay in one place?
Quality	What is it like?
Quantity	How severe is it? How frequent? How long does it last?
Chronology	When did it begin? How has it progressed? What are you doing when it occurs? What do you do to get rid of it?
Associated findings	Do you feel any other symptoms at the same time?
Treatment sought and effect	Have you seen a physician in the past for this same problem? What was the treatment?
Personal	What do you think this is from?
Perception	Why do you think it happened now?

electrocardiogram (ECG) was the most useful bedside predictor for a diagnosis of ST-elevation myocardial infarction (STEMI).[3]

PHYSICAL EXAMINATION

A comprehensive physical assessment is fundamental to arriving at an accurate diagnosis. The nurse who has developed the skills of *inspection*, *palpation*, and *auscultation* can be confident when assessing patients with cardiovascular disease. *Percussion*, however, is not employed when assessing the cardiovascular system.

Inspection

Face

The face is observed for the color of the skin (i.e., cyanotic, pale, or jaundiced) and for an apprehensive or painful expression. The patient's skin, lips, tongue, and mucous membranes are inspected for pallor or cyanosis. *Central cyanosis* is a bluish discoloration of the tongue and sublingual area. Multiracial studies indicate that the tongue is the most sensitive site for observation of central cyanosis, which must be recognized and treated as a medical emergency. Pulse oximetry, arterial blood gas analysis, and treatment with 100% oxygen must be instituted immediately.

Thorax

The anterior thorax and posterior thorax are inspected for skeletal deformities that may displace the heart and cause cardiac compromise. The skin on the chest wall and abdomen is inspected for scars, bruises, wounds, and bulges associated with pacemaker or defibrillator implants. Respiratory rate, pattern, and effort are also observed and recorded.

Abdomen

The abdomen is assessed for signs of distention or ascites, which may be associated with right-sided heart failure. Abdominal adiposity is a known risk factor for CAD.

Clubbing of Nail Beds

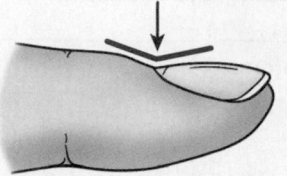

Normal nail shows a slight angle between root of nail bed and finger.

Normal Finger and Nail Bed

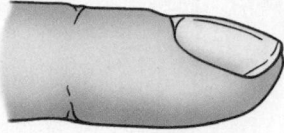

Early clubbing shows loss of angle at root of nail bed. Fingertip is of normal size.

Early Clubbing

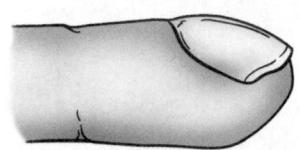

Moderate clubbing shows bulging of angle at root of nail bed. Distal finger/toe is enlarged.

Moderate Clubbing

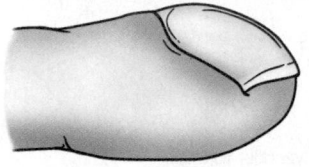

Advanced clubbing shows bulging and widening of nail bed. Distal finger/toe is bulbous.

Advanced Clubbing

FIGURE 13-1 Clubbing of Nail Beds.

Nail Beds and Cyanosis

The nail beds are inspected for signs of discoloration or cyanosis.[4] *Clubbing* in the nail bed is a sign associated with long-standing central cyanotic heart disease or pulmonary disease with hypoxemia.[4,5] "Clubbing" of the nail refers to a nail that has lost the normal angle between the finger and the nail root; the nail becomes wide and convex. The terminal phalanx of the finger also becomes bulbous and swollen.[6] Clubbing is rare and is a sign of severe central cyanosis (Fig. 13-1). *Peripheral cyanosis*, a bluish discoloration of the nail bed, is seen more commonly. Peripheral cyanosis results from a reduction in the quantity of oxygen in the peripheral extremities from arterial disease or decreased cardiac output (CO). Clubbing never occurs as a result of peripheral cyanosis.

Lower Extremities

Legs are inspected for signs of peripheral arterial or venous vascular disease. The visible signs of peripheral arterial vascular disease include pale, shiny legs with sparse hair growth. Recent guidelines indicate that many individuals, especially women, can have peripheral atherosclerosis without obvious signs or symptoms.[7] Venous disease causes edema of the limb, with deep red rubor, brown discoloration, and, frequently, leg ulceration.

TABLE 13-2 INSPECTION AND PALPATION OF EXTREMITIES: COMPARISON OF ARTERIAL AND VENOUS DISEASE

CHARACTERISTIC	ARTERIAL DISEASE	VENOUS DISEASE
Hair loss	Present	Absent
Skin texture	Thin, shiny, dry	Flaking, stasis, dermatitis, mottled
Ulceration	Located at pressure points; painful, pale, dry with little drainage; well-demarcated with eschar or dried; surrounded by fibrous tissue; granulation tissue scant and pale	Usually at the ankle; painless, pink, moist with large amount of drainage; irregular, dry, and scaly; surrounded by dermatitis; granulation tissue healthy
Skin color	Elevational pallor, dependent rubor	Brown patches, rubor, mottled cyanotic color when dependent
Nails	Thick, brittle	Normal
Varicose veins	Absent	Present
Temperature	Cool	Warm
Capillary refill	Greater than 3 seconds	Less than 3 seconds
Edema	None or mild, usually unilateral	Usually present foot to calf, unilateral or bilateral
Pulses	Weak or absent (0 to 1+)	Normal, strong, and symmetric

Modified from Krenzer ME. Peripheral vascular assessment: finding your way through arteries and veins. *AACN Clin Issues.* 1995;6(4):631.

A comparison of typical assessment findings in arterial and venous diseases is presented in Table 13-2.

Posture

Body posture can indicate the amount of effort it takes to breathe. For example, sitting upright to breathe may be necessary for the patient with acute heart failure, and leaning forward may be the least painful position for the patient with pericarditis.

Weight

The weight in proportion to height is assessed to determine whether the patient is obese or cachectic.[8]

Mentation

The patient is observed for signs of confusion or lethargy that may indicate hypotension, low CO, or hypoxemia.

Jugular Veins

The jugular veins of the neck are inspected for a noninvasive estimate of intravascular volume and pressure. The internal jugular veins are observed for *jugular vein distention* (JVD) (Fig. 13-2; Box 13-2). JVD is caused by an elevation in central venous pressure (CVP). This occurs with fluid volume overload, right ventricular dysfunction, pericardial effusion, or any condition that elevates right atrial pressure.[9,10] The right internal jugular vein can be palpated for measurement of CVP in centimeters of water (Fig. 13-3; Box 13-3). Bedside ultrasound is also used to evaluate JVD and estimate CVP.[11]

Abdominojugular Reflux

The abdominojugular reflux sign can assist with the diagnosis of right ventricular failure. This noninvasive test is used in conjunction with measurement of JVD. The procedure for assessing abdominojugular reflux is described in Box 13-4. A positive abdominojugular reflux sign is an increase in the jugular venous pressure (CVP equivalent) of 4 cm or more sustained for at least 15 seconds.[12]

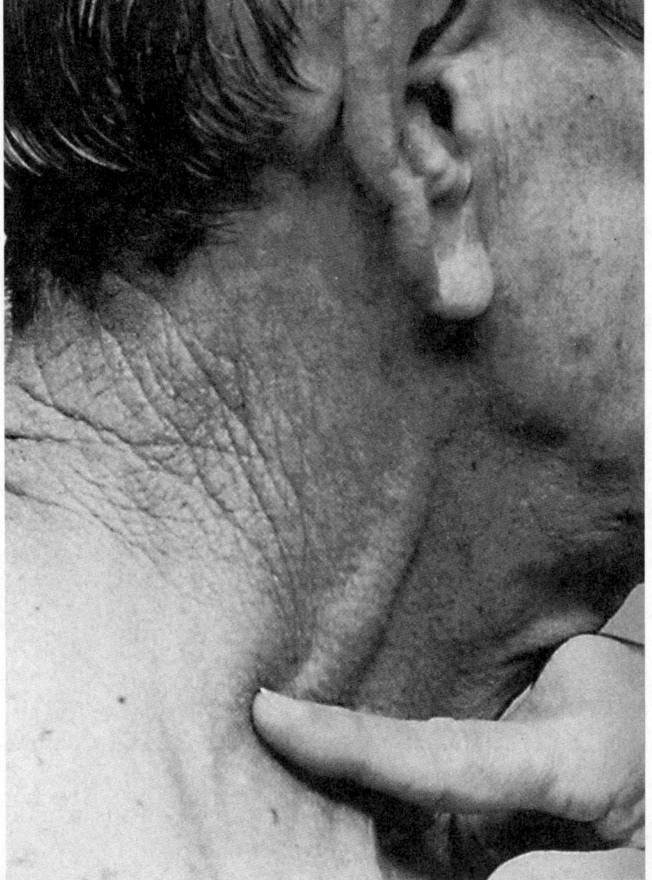

FIGURE 13-2 Assessment of Jugular Vein Distention (JVD). Applying light finger pressure over the sternocleidomastoid muscle, parallel to the clavicle, helps identify the external jugular vein by occluding flow and distending it. The finger pressure is released, and the patient is observed for true distention. If the patient's trunk is elevated to 30 degrees or more, JVD should not be present.

Thoracic Reference Points

The thoracic cage is divided with imaginary vertical lines (sternal, midclavicular, axillary, vertebral, and scapular), and the intercostal spaces are divided by imaginary horizontal lines to serve as reference points in locating or describing cardiac findings (Fig. 13-4). The ribs are numbered from 1 (the first rib below the clavicle) to 12. The intercostal space below each rib is given the same number as the rib that lies above it. The second rib is the easiest to locate because it is attached to the sternum at the angle of Louis. This angle (also called the *sternal angle*) is the bony ridge on the sternum that lies approximately 2 inches below the sternal notch (see Fig. 13-4A). After the second

BOX 13-3 PROCEDURE FOR ASSESSING CENTRAL VENOUS PRESSURE

1. The patient reclines in the bed. The highest point of pulsation in the internal jugular vein is observed during exhalation.
2. The vertical distance between this pulsation (top of the fluid level) and the sternal angle is estimated or measured in centimeters.
3. This number is then added to 5 cm for an estimation of central venous pressure (CVP). The 5 cm is the approximate distance of the sternal angle above the level of the right atrium (see Fig. 13-3).
4. *Documentation:* The degree of elevation of the patient is included in the report (e.g., "CVP estimated at 13 cm, using internal jugular vein pulsation, with the head of the bed elevated 45 degrees").

BOX 13-2 PROCEDURE FOR ASSESSING JUGULAR VEIN DISTENTION

1. Patient reclines at a 30- to 45-degree angle.
2. The examiner stands on the patient's right side and turns the patient's head slightly toward the left.
3. If the jugular vein is not visible, light finger pressure is applied across the sternocleidomastoid muscle just above and parallel to the clavicle. This pressure fills the external jugular vein by obstructing flow (see Fig. 13-2).
4. After the location of the vein has been identified, the pressure is released, and the presence of jugular vein distention (JVD) is assessed.
5. Because inhalation decreases venous pressure, JVD should be assessed at end-exhalation.
6. Any fullness in the vein extending more than 3 cm above the sternal angle is evidence of increased venous pressure. Generally, the higher the sitting angle of the patient when JVD is visualized, the higher is the central venous pressure.
7. *Documentation:* JVD is reported by including the angle of the head of the bed at the time JVD was evaluated (e.g., "Presence of JVD with the head of the bed elevated to 45 degrees").

BOX 13-4 PROCEDURE FOR ASSESSING ABDOMINOJUGULAR REFLUX

1. Ask the patient to relax and breathe normally through an open mouth.
2. Measure the jugular vein distention (JVD) in the patient's right internal jugular vein, following the procedure described in Box 13-2.
3. Apply firm pressure of approximately 20 to 35 mm Hg to the patient's midabdomen for 15 to 30 seconds, and remeasure the JVD during the compression.
4. Measure the right JVD a third time after the compression is released.
5. Ask the patient not to tense or hold the breath during the test. (Doing so increases venous return to the heart and may produce a falsely positive result.)
6. A positive abdominojugular reflux is identified when abdominal compression causes a sustained JVD increase of 4 cm or more. This sign is indicative of right-sided heart failure.
7. A normal abdominojugular reflux is reported if there is no rise in JVD, a transient (<10 seconds) rise in JVD, or a rise in JVD less than or equal to 3 cm sustained throughout compression.

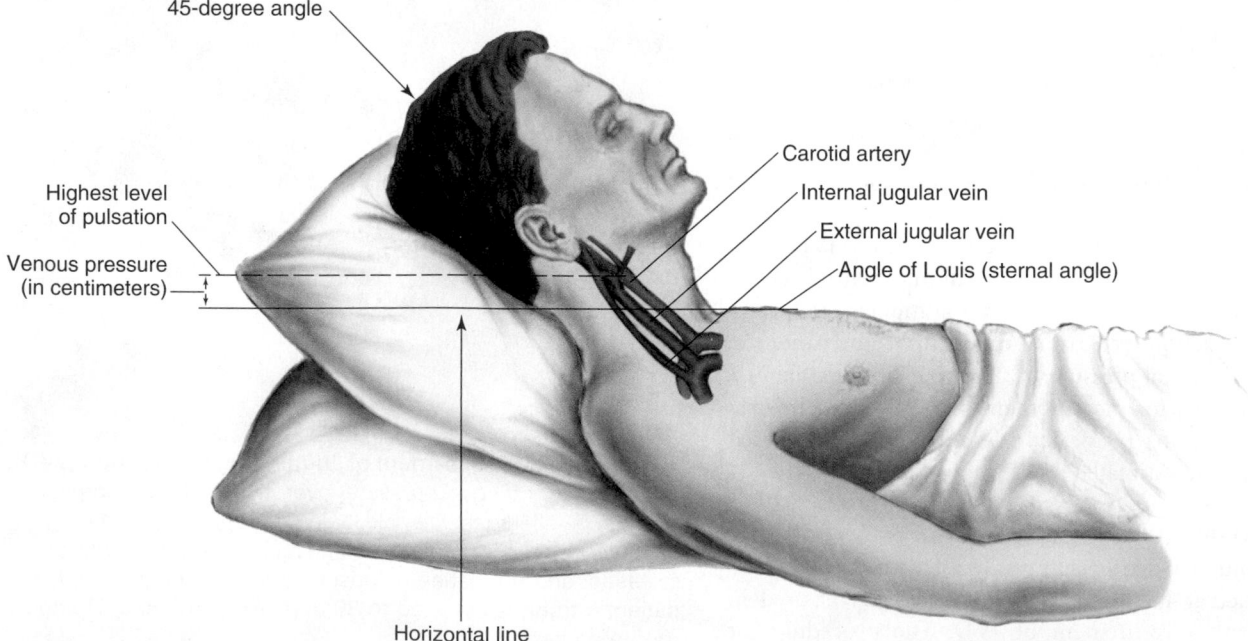

FIGURE 13-3 **Position of Internal and External Jugular Veins.** Pulsation in the internal jugular vein can be used to estimate central venous pressure. (Modified from Thompson JM, et al. *Mosby's Clinical Nursing.* 5th ed. St. Louis, MO: Mosby; 2002.)

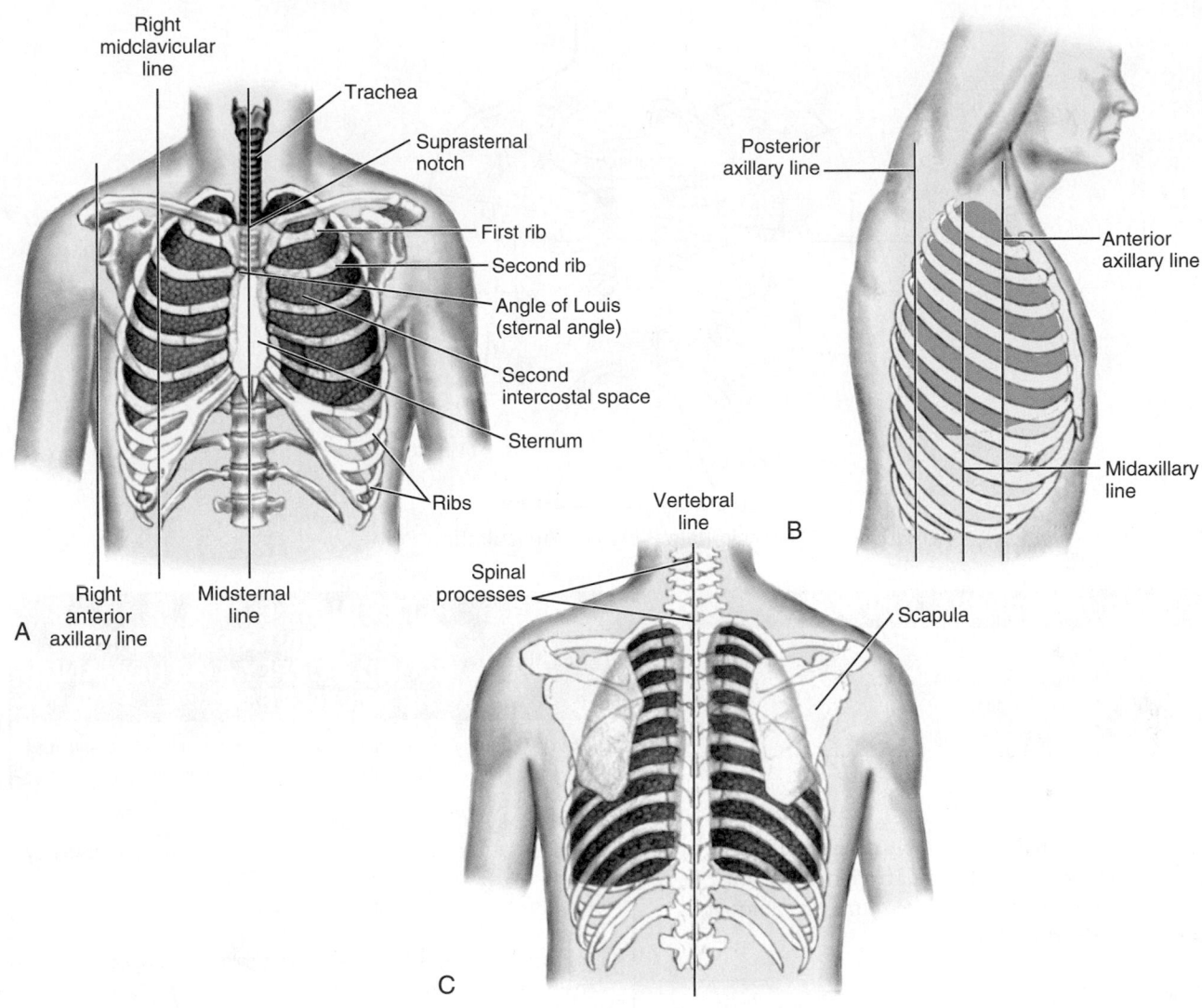

FIGURE 13-4 **Thoracic Landmarks.** *A,* Anterior thorax. *B,* Right lateral thorax. *C,* Posterior thorax.

rib has been located, it can be used as a reference point to count off the other ribs and intercostal spaces.

Apical Impulse

The anterior thorax is inspected for the *apical impulse,* sometimes referred to as the *point of maximal impulse* (PMI). The apical impulse occurs as the left ventricle contracts during systole and rotates forward, causing the left ventricular apex of the heart to hit the chest wall. The apical impulse is a quick, localized, outward movement normally located just lateral to the left midclavicular line at the fifth intercostal space in the adult patient (Fig. 13-5). The apical impulse is the only normal pulsation visualized on the chest wall. In the patient without cardiac disease, PMI may not be noticeable (see Fig. 13-5).

Palpation

Palpation is a technique that uses the sense of touch in the tips of the fingers and the palm of the hand.

Arterial Pulses

Seven pairs of bilateral arterial pulses are palpated. The examination incorporates bilateral assessment of the carotid, brachial, radial, ulnar, popliteal, dorsalis pedis, and posterior tibial arteries. The pulses are palpated separately and compared bilaterally to check for consistency.[13] Pulse volume is graded on a scale of 0 to 3+ (Box 13-5). The abdominal aortic pulse can also be palpated.

Carotid Pulses

The carotid arteries are assessed at the medial midneck region. If blood flow through the carotid arteries is compromised by atherosclerotic plaque, firm palpation could cause total occlusion. The touch is, therefore, light, and the carotid arteries are palpated gently and only one at a time.

Brachial, Ulnar, and Radial Pulses

The brachial pulse is assessed by gently palpating the inner aspect of the slightly bent elbow with the fingers. The radial pulse is palpated in the medial area of the wrist (thumb side).

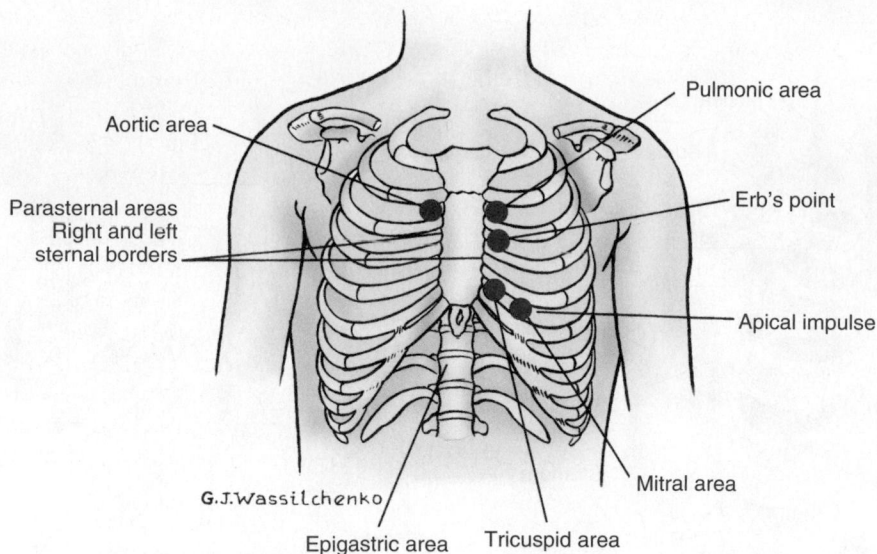

Aortic area

Parasternal areas
Right and left
sternal borders

Pulmonic area

Erb's point

Apical impulse

Mitral area

G.J.Wassilchenko

Epigastric area　Tricuspid area

FIGURE 13-5　Thoracic Palpation and Auscultation Points.

BOX 13-5	PULSE PALPATION SCALE
0	Not palpable
1+	Faintly palpable (weak and thready)
2+	Palpable (normal pulse)
3+	Bounding (hyperdynamic pulse)

The ulnar artery is palpated at the opposite side of the wrist (little finger side). The radial and ulnar arterial pulses must be assessed before an arterial line is inserted; this test, known as the *Allen test*, is described in Box 13-6.

Femoral Pulses

The femoral arteries are palpated by pressing deeply into the groin beneath the inguinal ligament, approximately midway between the anterior superior iliac spine and the symphysis pubis.

Popliteal Pulses

The popliteal pulse is lightly palpated using the fingertips. The patient's leg is very slightly bent, and the clinician's two hands gently cup the patient's knee with the thumbs on top of the kneecap and the fingertips behind the knee.

Dorsalis Pedis and Posterior Tibial Pulses

The pulses of the lower leg and foot are assessed to determine blood flow to the limb and to assess adequacy of CO to the extremities. The dorsalis pedis pulse is located on the upper aspect of the foot. The posterior tibial pulse is located behind the medial malleolus (inner ankle bone) of the lower leg.

Descending Aorta Pulse

When the patient is in the supine position, the abdominal aortic pulsation is located in the epigastric area and can be felt as a forward movement when firm fingertip pressure is applied above the umbilicus. If prominent or diffuse, the pulsation may indicate an abdominal aneurysm.

BOX 13-6	PROCEDURE FOR ASSESSMENT OF ARTERIAL BLOOD SUPPLY TO THE HAND: THE ALLEN TEST

Before a radial artery is punctured or cannulated, the Allen test is performed to assess blood flow to the hand and to ensure that it is adequate.

Allen Test by Visual Inspection
1. If the patient is alert and cooperative, he or she is asked to repeatedly make a tight fist to squeeze the blood out of the hand.
2. The radial artery is compressed with firm thumb pressure by the examiner.
3. The patient is requested to open the hand, palm side up while the radial artery is still occluded.
4. Pressure is released, and the time it takes for the color to return to the hand is noted.

If the ulnar artery is patent, the color will return within 3 seconds. The patient may describe a tingling in the palm as blood flow returns. Delayed color return (a "failed" Allen test) implies that the ulnar artery is inadequate. This means radial artery is the only reliable source of arterial blood flow to the hand and therefore it must not be punctured or cannulated.

Allen Test with Pulse Oximetry
1. If the patient is unable to cooperate to make a fist, an alternative approach is to use a pulse oximeter that displays a pulse waveform.
2. Place the pulse oximeter on the middle finger and establish an adequate pulse amplitude display on the monitor.
3. Simultaneously compress the radial and ulnar arteries until the waveform clearly decreases or vanishes.
4. Release pressure off the ulnar artery only. If the ulnar artery is patent, the pulse amplitude recovers its normal appearance.
5. Repeat the procedure with the radial artery.
6. Arterial catheterization of the radial artery can be accomplished safely only if blood supply to the hand is adequate.

A diminished or absent pulse may indicate low CO, arterial stenosis, or occlusion proximal to the site of the examination. An abnormally strong or bounding pulse suggests the presence of an aneurysm or an occlusion distal to the examination site. If a distal pulse cannot be palpated by using light finger pressure, a Doppler ultrasound stethoscope may enhance diagnostic accuracy. It is important to mark the location of the audible signal with an indelible ink marker pen for future evaluation of pulse quality.

Capillary Refill

Capillary refill assessment is a maneuver that uses the patient's nail beds to evaluate arterial circulation to the extremity and overall perfusion. The nail bed is compressed to produce blanching, after which release of the pressure should result in the return of blood flow and baseline nail color in less than 2 seconds.[14] The severity of arterial insufficiency is directly proportional to the amount of time required to re-establish blood flow and color.

Edema

Edema is fluid accumulation in the extravascular spaces of the body. The dependent tissues within the legs and sacrum are particularly susceptible. Edema may be dependent, unilateral or bilateral, and pitting or nonpitting. The amount of edema is quantified by measuring the circumference of the limb or by pressing the skin of the feet, ankles, and shins against underlying bone. Edema is a symptom associated with several diseases, and further diagnostic evaluation is required to determine the cause. Although no universal scale for pitting edema exists, typical scales use a 0-to-4+ system (Table 13-3).

Auscultation
Blood Pressure Measurement

Blood pressure measurement is an essential component of every complete physical examination. Hypertension is diagnosed as a systolic blood pressure (SBP) of 140 mm Hg or higher, or a diastolic blood pressure (DBP) of 90 mm Hg or above.[15] Prehypertension is defined as SBP in the range of 120 to 139 mm Hg in association with a DBP between 80 to 89 mm Hg.[15] The incidence of hypertension in the United States has increased dramatically as a result of an aging population and an increase in the prevalence of obesity. The risk of hypertension increases with older age. More than 90% of people who have a normal blood pressure at 55 years eventually develop hypertension, according to findings from the Framingham Heart Study.[15]

In the critical care setting, systemic blood pressure can be measured directly or indirectly. Arterial monitoring devices (see Chapter 14) that directly measure arterial pressure by means of an invasive technique, which requires placement of an arterial

catheter, are considered the gold standard. Correct use of a stethoscope and sphygmomanometer or electronic measuring devices can produce indirect blood pressure values that closely reflect direct measurements (within 1 to 3 mm Hg). The following discussion reviews the essential elements of noninvasive blood pressure monitoring.

Noninvasive Blood Pressure Monitoring. The most common peripheral locations for blood pressure monitoring are the bilateral brachial arteries. The pressure is measured in both arms to rule out subclavian arterial stenosis. Normally, the difference in pressure between the arms is less than 10 mm Hg. A finding of more than 15 mm Hg difference between the bilateral arm pressures suggests arterial obstruction on the side with the lower pressure.[16] Asymmetry is documented so that all subsequent measurements can be made on the arm with the higher pressure.

Correct positioning of the extremity being measured is essential. Blood pressure can be measured in any position as long as the arm or the leg is at the level of the heart. Falsely elevated readings are obtained if the arm is at a level lower than the heart, and falsely low pressures are obtained when the arm is at a level higher than the heart.

Orthostatic Hypotension. When a healthy person stands, 10% to 15% of the blood volume is pooled in the legs; this reduces venous return to the right side of the heart, which decreases CO and lowers arterial blood pressure.[17] Transient orthostatic intolerance is part of daily life for many people, but acute orthostatic hypotension is a cause for concern.[18] The fall in blood pressure activates baroreceptors; the subsequent reflex increases in sympathetic outflow and parasympathetic inhibition lead to peripheral vasoconstriction, with increased heart rate and contractility.[17] Postural (orthostatic) hypotension occurs when the SBP or BP drops by 10 to 20 mm Hg, or the diastolic BP drops by 5 mm Hg, after a change from the supine posture to the upright posture. This is usually accompanied by dizziness, lightheadedness, or syncope. If a patient experiences these symptoms, it is important to complete a full set of postural vital signs before increasing the patient's activity level (Box 13-7). Orthostatic hypotension can have many causes.[18] The three most common causes of orthostatic vital sign changes (i.e., drop in blood pressure and rise in heart rate) observed in critical care are as follows:

1. Intravascular volume depletion or fluid loss caused by bleeding, excessive diuresis, or fever
2. Inadequate vascular vasoconstrictor mechanisms to constrict the arterial bed, which can occur in older patients after prolonged immobility or as a result of spinal cord injury
3. Autonomic insufficiency caused by administration of pharmacologic agents such as beta-blockers, angiotensin-converting enzyme (ACE) inhibitors, and calcium-channel blockers

Blood Pressure Cuff Size. Correct size and placement of the inflatable bladder (inside the nondistensible cuff) are crucial to obtaining an accurate blood pressure measurement. The bladder should be long enough to encircle at least 80% of the width of the upper arm (or leg) in adults.[19] Cuffs that are too small can give falsely high readings, and cuffs that are too large can give

TABLE 13-3	PITTING EDEMA SCALE			
		INDENTATION DEPTH		
SCALE	**EDEMA**	**ENGLISH UNITS**	**METRIC UNITS**	**TIME TO BASELINE**
0	None	0	0	
1+	Trace	0-0.25 inch	<6.5 mm	Rapid
2+	Mild	0.25-0.5 inch	6.5-12.5 mm	10-15 sec
3+	Moderate	0.5-1 inch	12.5 mm-2.5 cm	1-2 min
4+	Severe	>1 inch	> 2.5 cm	2-5 min

BOX 13-7 MEASUREMENT OF POSTURAL (ORTHOSTATIC) VITAL SIGNS

Guidelines

1. Record blood pressure (BP) and heart rate (HR) in each position.
2. Do not remove the cuff between measurements.
3. Record all associated signs and symptoms.
4. Clearly document patient position.

Lying	Sitting	Standing
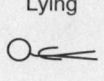	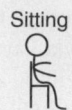	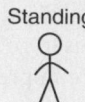

Technique

1. Keep the patient as flat as possible for 10 minutes before the initial assessment.
2. *Patient supine:* Obtain initial BP and HR measurements.
3. *Patient sitting with legs hanging:* Measure immediately and after 2 minutes.
4. *Patient standing:* Measure immediately and after 2 minutes. If BP and HR are stable but orthostasis is suspected, BP and HR can be repeated every 2 minutes. Note that this is rarely practical for the critically ill patient.

Results

Normal Changes

HR increases by 5 to 20 beats/min (transiently).
Systolic BP drops by 10 mm Hg.
Diastolic BP drops by 5 mm Hg.

Positive Orthostasis

Drop in systolic BP by more than 20 mm Hg.
Drop in diastolic BP by more than 10 mm Hg within 3 minutes.

BOX 13-8 OBTAINING ACCURATE BLOOD PRESSURE READINGS

- Compare right and left measurements.
- Position the extremity at the level of the heart.
- Document the position of the patient.
- Ensure proper cuff size.
- Measure readings at eye level at the top of the meniscus.

falsely low readings. Box 13-8 lists the key points to observe when obtaining blood pressure readings.

Korotkoff Sounds. Obtaining systemic blood pressure readings involves auscultation of *Korotkoff sounds*, the sounds created by turbulence of blood flow within a vessel caused by constriction of the blood pressure cuff. The pressure in the cuff is inflated above the normal systolic pressure. As the pressure in the cuff is reduced, Korotkoff sounds change in quality and intensity. These sounds are divided into five stages. The SBP is the highest point at which initial tapping occurs. DBP is equated with the complete disappearance of Korotkoff sounds. Often, a muffling of diastolic sounds occurs before these sounds completely disappear. This has caused debate about which diastolic value to record. Because complete disappearance of Korotkoff sounds corresponds more closely to intra-arterial catheter measurement, it is the value that should be recorded.

Auscultatory Gap. In older patients with systolic hypertension, the presence of an *auscultatory gap* is not uncommon.[19] It is important to inflate the cuff to greater than the patient's normal systolic pressure to avoid this gap and underestimation of SBP. Use of an initial palpation estimate of the SBP taken before auscultation with a stethoscope is one recommended method to accurately determine the upper SBP.

Automated Blood Pressure Devices. Electronic automated devices are frequently used for measuring blood pressure and have replaced the mercury sphygmomanometer in many places. The mercury used in the sphygmomanometer is a nondegradable environmental pollutant that is difficult to dispose of safely. For this reason, mercury sphygmomanometers have been phased out of use in most hospitals.

In readings from automated devices, the systolic number is accurate, but the diastolic value is often calculated from the SBP and the mean arterial pressure (MAP), and therefore, it may not be accurate. Devices placed on the arm or the leg are considered accurate (as long as the cuff size is correct) for systolic measurement and trending of blood pressure. Considerable controversy exists with regard to automated devices being applied to the wrist or the finger, so this method should not be used to monitor blood pressure in any critically ill patient or one with cardiac disease.

Automatic blood pressure cuff placement should be rotated frequently to avoid excessive irritation to the extremity, especially when the automatic cuff is set to cycle more frequently than every 15 minutes.

Pulse Pressure. Pulse pressure describes the difference between systolic and diastolic values. The normal pulse pressure is 40 mm Hg (i.e., the difference between an SBP of 120 mm Hg and a DBP of 80 mm Hg). In the critically ill patient, a low blood pressure is frequently associated with a narrow pulse pressure. For example, a patient with a blood pressure of 90/72 mm Hg has a pulse pressure of 18 mm Hg. The narrowed pulse pressure is a temporary compensatory mechanism caused by arterial vasoconstriction resulting from volume depletion or heart failure. The narrow pulse pressure ensures that the MAP (78 mm Hg, in this example) remains in a therapeutic range to provide adequate organ perfusion.

In contrast, a hypotensive septic patient who exhibits vasodilation will have a wide pulse pressure and inadequate organ perfusion. If the blood pressure is 90/36 mm Hg, the pulse pressure is 54 mm Hg, and the MAP will be an inadequate 54 mm Hg. In both these examples, the SBP is the same (90 mm Hg); the difference in pulse pressure is a function of intravascular volume and vascular tone.

Pulsus Paradoxus. In normal physiology, the strength of the pulse fluctuates throughout the respiratory cycle. When the "pulse" is measured using the SBP, the pressure is observed to decrease slightly during inspiration and to rise slightly during respiratory exhalation. The normal difference is 2 to 4 mm Hg. In some clinical conditions such as cardiac tamponade, the blood pressure decline is abnormally large during inspiration. In general, an inspiratory decline of SBP greater than 10 mm Hg is considered diagnostic of *pulsus paradoxus*.[20-22] The traditional technique for measuring pulsus paradoxus using a sphygmomanometer and a blood pressure cuff and pulse oximetry is

---

BOX 13-9 PROCEDURE FOR MEASURING PULSUS PARADOXUS

Measurement with a Sphygmomanometer

1. The patient should be lying supine in a comfortable position.
2. The breathing pattern should be of normal depth and rate to avoid excessive respiratory interference.
3. Blood pressure is measured following standard procedures (see Boxes 13-7 and 13-8). The sphygmomanometer cuff is inflated to a pressure greater than the systolic blood pressure (SBP), and Korotkoff sounds are auscultated over the brachial artery while the cuff is deflated at rate of approximately 2 to 3 mm Hg per heartbeat.
4. The peak SBP during expiration (i.e., the pressure at which Korotkoff sounds are heard only during expiration) should be identified and then reconfirmed.
5. The cuff is then deflated slowly to establish the SBP at which Korotkoff sounds become audible during both inspiration and expiration.
6. If the auscultated difference between these two SBP values exceeds 10 mm Hg during quiet respiration, a paradoxical pulse is present.

Measurement by Waveform Analysis

1. A pulse oximetry sensor with a visible pulse waveform can be used as an additional measurement device.
2. In the critical care unit, an arterial waveform from an indwelling arterial catheter (if present) can be used to measure the difference in SBP between expiration and inspiration.

BOX 13-10 CHARACTERISTICS OF THE FIRST AND SECOND HEART SOUNDS

First Heart Sound (S_1)
- High pitched
- Loudest in mitral area (apex)

Split S_1
- Normal split less than 20 milliseconds (ms)
- Split heard best in tricuspid area
- Important to differentiate between split S_1 and S_4
- Occurs immediately before carotid upstroke

Second Heart Sound (S_2)
- High pitched
- Loudest in aortic area (base)

Split S_2
- Normal split less than 30 ms
- Split heard best in pulmonic area
- ↑ Split with inhalation
- ↓ Split with exhalation

↑, Increased; ↓, decreased.

---

described in Box 13-9. If the patient is hypotensive, pulsus paradoxus is more accurately assessed in the critical care unit by monitoring a pulse oximetry waveform or an indwelling arterial catheter waveform.[20-22]

Pulsus Alternans. Pulsus alternans describes a regular pattern of pulse amplitude changes that alternate between stronger and weaker beats. This finding is suggestive of end-stage left ventricular heart failure.

Vascular Bruits. The carotid and femoral arteries are auscultated for bruits. A bruit, a high-pitched "sh-sh" sound, is an extracardiac vascular sound that vacillates in volume with systole and diastole. An abnormal bruit is produced as blood flows through a partially occluded vessel. Auscultation of a bruit can expedite the diagnosis of suspected arterial obstruction.

Normal Heart Sounds

Auscultation of the heart is the most challenging part of the cardiac physical examination, and, in an era of increasing technologic demands, it is daunting to new clinicians. To summarize the advice given by most experts, the examiner must do the following:[23-25]

1. Auscultate systematically across the precordium.
2. Visualize the cardiac anatomy under each point of auscultation, expecting to hear the physiologically associated sounds.
3. Memorize the cardiac cycle to enhance the ability to hear abnormal sounds.
4. Practice, practice, practice.

First and Second Heart Sounds. Normal heart sounds are referred to as the *first heart sound* (S_1) and the *second heart sound* (S_2). S_1 is the sound associated with mitral and tricuspid valve closure and is heard most clearly in the mitral and tricuspid areas. S_2 (aortic and pulmonic closure) can be heard best at the second intercostal space to the right and left of the sternum (see Fig. 13-5). Both sounds are high pitched and heard best with the diaphragm of the stethoscope (Box 13-10). Each sound is loudest in an auscultation area located downstream from the actual valvular component of the sound, as shown in Figure 13-6.

Physiologic Splitting of S_1 and S_2. Each normal heart sound has two components: right and left. Mitral valve closure and tricuspid valve closure are both responsible for S_1, and aortic valve and pulmonic valve closure are responsible for S_2. All the components of the split sounds are high pitched and best heard with the diaphragm of the stethoscope (Fig. 13-7). Normally, sounds emitted from the left side are louder than those from the right because left ventricular contraction occurs milliseconds before that of the right ventricle. Physiologic splitting is accentuated by inspiration and usually disappears on expiration. This splitting is most easily detected on inspiration because there is an increased blood return to the right side of the heart and a decreased amount of blood return to the left side of the heart. As a result, pulmonic valve closure is delayed because of the extra time needed for the increased blood volume to pass through the pulmonic valve, and aortic valve closure is early because of the relatively smaller amount of blood ejected from the left ventricle. The resulting heart sound is a split S_2 (the closure of each valve is audible because there is more time between left and right contractions) (see Fig. 13-7).

Pathologic Splitting of S_1 and S_2. A variety of abnormalities can alter the intensity and timing of split heart sounds. For example, during auscultation in the pulmonic area, a pathologic split is audible with a stethoscope if the pulmonic valve closure occurs after the aortic valve closure. Pathologic splitting of S_1 and S_2 is associated with specific cardiovascular conditions such as pulmonary hypertension, pulmonic stenosis, and right ventricular failure and with electrical conduction disturbances such as right bundle branch block and premature ventricular contractions.

Abnormal Heart Sounds

Third and Fourth Heart Sounds. Abnormal heart sounds are known as the *third heart sound* (S_3) and the *fourth heart sound*

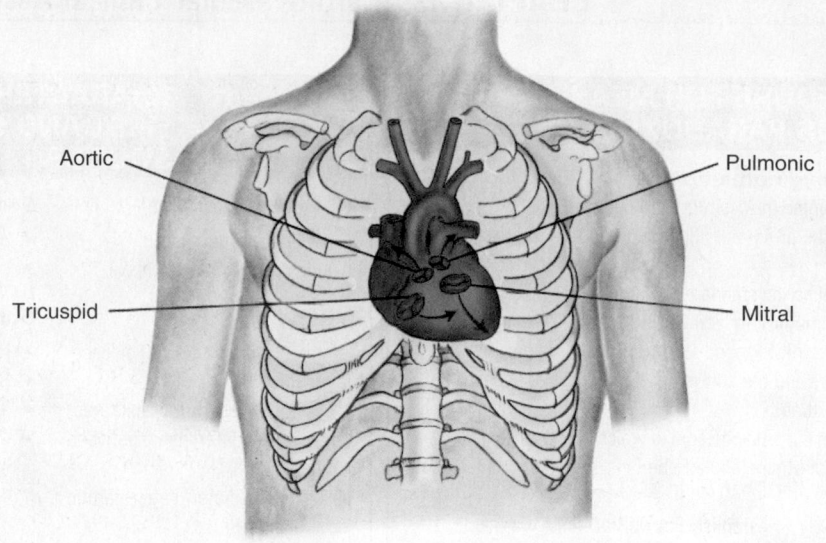

G.J.Wassilchenko

FIGURE 13-6 Transmission of heart sounds to the thorax and their relationship to the anatomic position of the heart valves.

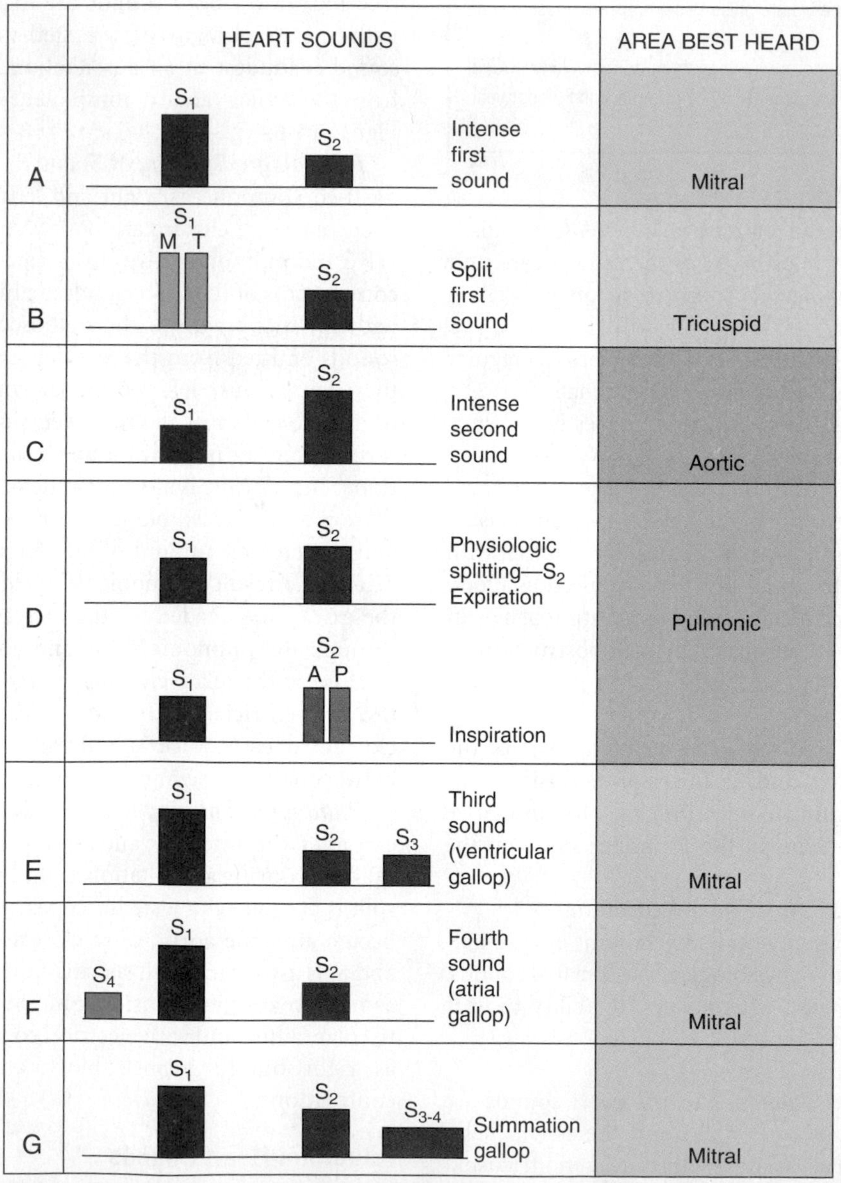

	HEART SOUNDS		AREA BEST HEARD
A	S_1 S_2	Intense first sound	Mitral
B	S_1 M T S_2	Split first sound	Tricuspid
C	S_1 S_2	Intense second sound	Aortic
D	S_1 S_2 — Expiration; S_1 S_2 A P — Inspiration	Physiologic splitting—S_2 Expiration; Inspiration	Pulmonic
E	S_1 S_2 S_3	Third sound (ventricular gallop)	Mitral
F	S_4 S_1 S_2	Fourth sound (atrial gallop)	Mitral
G	S_1 S_2 S_{3-4}	Summation gallop	Mitral

FIGURE 13-7 Characteristics of normal and abnormal heart sounds and the auscultatory area where each is best heard.

(S_4); they are referred to as *gallops* when auscultated during an episode of tachycardia. These low-pitched sounds occur during diastole and are best heard with the bell of the stethoscope positioned lightly over the apical impulse. The characteristics of S_3 and S_4 are detailed in Box 13-11. The presence of S_3 may be normal in children, young adults, and pregnant women because of rapid filling of the ventricle in a young, healthy heart. However, an S_3 in the presence of cardiac symptoms is an indicator of heart failure in a noncompliant ventricle with fluid overload.[26] Not unexpectedly, the development of an S_3 heart sound is strongly associated with elevated levels of brain natriuretic peptide (BNP or proBNP).[26]

Auscultation of an S_4 also leads the examiner to suspect heart failure and decreased ventricular compliance.[27] An S_4, also referred to as an *atrial gallop*, occurs at the end of diastole (just before S_1), when the ventricle is full. It is associated with atrial contraction, also called *atrial kick*.

Heart Murmurs

Heart valve murmurs are prolonged extra sounds that occur during systole or diastole. Murmurs are produced by turbulent flood flow through the chambers of the heart, from forward flow through narrowed or irregular valve openings, or backward regurgitant flow through an incompetent valve.[28] Murmurs occur in both systole and diastole. Most murmurs are caused by structural cardiac changes. The steps to effectively and accurately auscultate for cardiac murmurs are listed in Box 13-12. Murmurs are characterized by specific criteria:

Timing: place in the cardiac cycle (systole/diastole)
Location: where it is auscultated on the chest wall (mitral or aortic area)
Radiation: how far the sound spreads across chest wall
Quality: whether the murmur is blowing, grating, or harsh
Pitch: whether the tone is high or low

BOX 13-11 CHARACTERISTICS OF THE THIRD AND FOURTH HEART SOUNDS

THIRD HEART SOUND (S_3)

Physiologic Causes
- Related to diastolic motion and rapid filling of ventricles in early diastole
- Can be normal in children and young adults (<40 yr)

Pathologic Causes
- Ventricular dysfunction with an increase in end-systolic volume (MI, heart failure, valvular disease, systemic or pulmonary hypertension)
- Hyperdynamic states (anemia, thyrotoxicosis, mitral or tricuspid regurgitation)

Rhythmic Word Association
- Kentucky: S_1, S_2, S_3

Synonyms
- Ventricular gallop
- Protodiastolic gallop

FOURTH HEART SOUND (S_4)

- Related to diastolic motion and ventricular dilation with atrial contraction in late diastole
- May occur with or without cardiac decompensation
- Ventricular hypertrophy with a decrease in ventricular compliance (CAD, systemic hypertension, cardiomyopathy, aortic or pulmonary stenosis, increase in intensity with acute MI or angina)
- Hyperkinetic states (anemia, thyrotoxicosis, arteriovenous fistula)
- Acute valvular regurgitation

Rhythmic Word Association
- "Tennessee": S_4, S_1, S_2

Synonyms
- Atrial gallop
- Presystolic gallop

CAD, Coronary artery disease; *MI*, myocardial infarction.

BOX 13-12 TECHNIQUE OF AUSCULTATION OF HEART SOUNDS AND MURMURS

1. Stethoscope
- Diaphragm
  - Larger surface area
  - Brings out higher frequency and filters out low frequency
  - Use for listening to S_1/S_2 (split S_1/S_2), loud murmurs, pericardial friction rubs
- Bell
  - Smaller surface area
  - Filters out high-frequency sounds and accentuates low-frequency sounds
  - Rest lightly on area (or else it becomes a diaphragm)
2. Location: heart sounds auscultated at APTM
   A: aortic area (second right ICS along sternal border)
   P: pulmonic area (second left ICS along sternal border)
   T: tricuspid area (fourth left ICS along sternal border)
   M: mitral area (fifth ICS at MCL)
3. "Know your bases"
- Base of the heart refers to the right and left second ICS beside the sternum S_2 where the aortic or pulmonic sounds are auscultated

- Apex or left ventricular area refers to the fifth ICS along the MCL
  - Most commonly referred to as the PMI
  - Also referred to as the mitral area
  - S_1 and mitral sounds are loudest here
- Erb's point: second aortic area (third left ICS along sternal border); pericardial friction rubs are heard best here
4. Palpation
- Location
- Palpate carotid pulse (or watch ECG to identify S_1 and S_2)
5. Be quiet and patient!
- Listen for S_1 and S_2 first, ignoring all other sounds
- Inching technique
- After you are sure which is S_1 or S_2, try to determine when the other sound comes in
- Is it systolic or diastolic?
- S_3 and S_4 are best heard with patient in left lateral decubitus position. Note the location (suggests origin of sound)
- Note the timing (S_4 comes just before S_1, and S_3 comes just after S_2)
6. Interpret the sounds based on the clinical condition

ECG, Electrocardiogram; *ICS*, intercostal space; *MCL*, midclavicular line; *PMI*, point of maximal impulse.

BOX 13-13 GRADING OF CARDIAC MURMURS

GRADE	DESCRIPTION
1	Very faint; may be heard only in a quiet environment
2	Quiet but clearly audible
3	Moderately loud
4	Loud; may be associated with a palpable thrill
5	Very loud; thrill easily palpable
6	Very loud; may be heard with stethoscope off the chest Thrill palpable and visible

BOX 13-14 AUSCULTATION OF THE CARDIAC VALVES

Aortic Area
- S_2 loud
- Aortic systolic murmur

Tricuspid Area
- S_1 split
- Right ventricular S_3 and S_4
- Tricuspid valve murmurs
- Murmur of ventricular septal defect

Pulmonic Area
- S_2 loud and split with inhalation
- Pulmonic valve murmurs

Mitral Area
- S_1 loud
- Left ventricular S_3 and S_4
- Mitral valve murmurs

Erb's Point
- S_2 split with inhalation
- Aortic diastolic murmur
- Pericardial friction rub

Intensity: the loudness is graded on a scale of 1 through 6; the higher the number, the louder is the murmur (Box 13-13).

The four most common valvular murmurs auscultated in adults are briefly discussed in the following paragraphs. For more information on valvular anatomy, refer to Chapter 12.

Mitral Stenosis. The term *mitral stenosis* refers to narrowing of the mitral valve orifice. This produces a low-pitched murmur, which varies in intensity and harshness depending on the degree of valvular stenosis. It occurs during diastole, is auscultated at the mitral area (fifth intercostal space, midclavicular line), and does not radiate. As the mitral stenosis progresses, left atrial enlargement occurs, often leading to atrial fibrillation and the development of left atrial thrombi. The increased left atrial pressure also creates pulmonary congestion, breathlessness, moist cough, and symptoms of right-sided heart failure.

Mitral Regurgitation. Mitral regurgitation is described as *acute* or *chronic.* Causes of acute mitral regurgitation include rupture of a papillary muscle after an acute myocardial infarction (MI) and rupture of one or more chordae tendineae. As a result, when the ventricle contracts during systole, a jet of blood is sent in a retrograde manner to the left atrium, causing a sudden increase in left atrial pressure, acute pulmonary edema, and low CO and leading to cardiogenic shock. Chronic mitral regurgitation is most often seen in older adults as the valve structures sag and stretch over time. The murmur of mitral regurgitation is auscultated in the mitral area and occurs during systole. It is high pitched and blowing, although the pitch and intensity vary, depending on the degree of regurgitation. As mitral regurgitation progresses, the murmur radiates more widely.

Aortic Stenosis. The term *aortic stenosis* describes narrowing of the aortic valve orifice. As a result, the left ventricle faces increasing difficulty in ejecting blood to the aorta. The ventricle responds by increasing intraventricular pressure and adding muscle mass (left ventricular hypertrophy), but over time, because of the pressure load and the stenotic aortic valve, the left ventricle will fail and lose contractile force. The decreased blood volume entering the aorta during systole means that the coronary arteries do not fill efficiently, and chest pain is a common symptom of aortic stenosis. This chest pain can be difficult to differentiate from angina caused by CAD, especially in the older adult.[29] Other symptoms include dizziness, syncope, and breathlessness caused by left-sided heart failure. After symptoms occur, the clinical course is poor unless the aortic valve is replaced. Two years after onset of aortic stenosis symptoms, survival is poor without aortic valve replacement.[29] The murmur of aortic stenosis occurs during systole. It is auscultated at the aortic area (second intercostal space, right sternal border). Aortic stenosis produces a low-pitched murmur that does not radiate, although the tone of the murmur varies, depending on the degree of valvular obstruction. Because a strong correlation does not exist among the loudness of the murmur, clinical symptoms, and the severity of the stenosis, it is advisable to perform an ECG to visualize the valve after an aortic stenosis murmur is detected.

Aortic Insufficiency. The term *aortic regurgitation,* also commonly known as *aortic insufficiency,* describes an incompetent aortic valve. It is often described in layperson's terms as a "leaking valve." After the left ventricle has ejected blood into the aorta, the valve normally closes, maintains a tight seal, and prevents blood from moving back into the left ventricle. If the valve cusps do not maintain this seal, the sound of blood flowing back into the left ventricle during diastole is heard as a decrescendo, high-pitched, blowing murmur. This early diastolic murmur is initially audible at the aortic area (second intercostal space, right sternal border), but as the aortic regurgitation progresses, it can be auscultated along the length of the left sternal border. As with all valvular murmurs, the pitch and intensity vary with the degree of regurgitation. Box 13-14 provides expected abnormal findings at each of the key auscultatory areas; Table 13-4 compares the features of the most common valvular murmurs.

Innocent Murmurs

In children, adolescents, and healthy young adults, systolic "high-flow" murmurs are common and are a result of vigorous ventricular contraction. These nonpathologic murmurs are termed *innocent murmurs.* They are always systolic, have a low-to-medium pitch (heard best with the bell of the stethoscope), and are of grade 1 to 2 intensity with a blowing quality. They are often heard best in the tricuspid area and do not radiate (Box 13-15).

Murmurs Associated with Myocardial Infarction

At the bedside, the nurse is often the first person to auscultate a new murmur. The holosystolic or pansystolic murmurs that can occur acutely as a complication of MI are good examples.

TABLE 13-4   CHARACTERISTICS OF SOME MURMURS

DEFECTS	TIMING IN THE CARDIAC CYCLE	PITCH, INTENSITY, QUALITY	LOCATION, RADIATION
Systolic Murmurs			
Mitral regurgitation	S_1 — S_2	High Harsh Blowing	Mitral area May radiate to axilla
Tricuspid regurgitation	S_1 — S_2	High Often faint, but varies Blowing	Tricuspid RLSB, apex, LLSB, epigastric areas Little radiation
Ventricular septal defect	S_1 — S_2	High Loud Blowing	Left sternal border
Aortic stenosis	S_1 — S_2	Chhhh hh Medium Rough, harsh	Aortic area to suprasternal notch, right side of neck, apex
Pulmonary stenosis	S_1 — S_2	Low to medium Loud Harsh, grinding	Pulmonic area No radiation
Diastolic Murmurs			
Mitral stenosis	S_2 — Atrial kick — S_1	Low Quiet to loud with thrill Rough rumble	Mitral area Usually no radiation
Tricuspid stenosis	S_2 — Atrial kick — S_1	Medium Quiet; louder with inspiration Rumble	Tricuspid area or epigastrium Little radiation
Aortic regurgitation	S_2 — S_1	High Faint to medium Blowing	Aortic area to LLSB and aorta Erb's point
Pulmonic regurgitation	S_2 — S_1	Medium Faint Blowing	Pulmonic area No radiation

LLSB, Left lower sternal border; *RLSB*, right lower sternal border.

BOX 13-15   DESCRIPTION OF INNOCENT MURMURS

- Always systolic
- Soft, short (grade 1 or 2, low pitched)
- Modified by change in position
- Normal S_2
- Most common at left sternal border

Papillary Muscle Rupture. The auscultation of a new, high-pitched, holosystolic, blowing murmur at the cardiac apex heralds mitral valve regurgitation resulting from papillary muscle dysfunction. This murmur may be soft (grade 1 or 2) and may occur only during ischemic episodes when the papillary muscle contractility is impaired, but its presence is associated with persistent pain, ventricular failure, and higher mortality. If the murmur is loud (grade 5 or 6), harsh, and radiating in all directions from the apex, the papillary muscle or the chordae tendineae may have ruptured. The clinical auscultation of a new murmur should always be confirmed by transthoracic or transesophageal echocardiography (TEE).[28,30] Papillary muscle rupture is an emergency situation requiring immediate medical and surgical intervention.

Ventricular Septal Rupture. Ventricular septal rupture is a rare emergency situation that can occur after an acute MI. Ventricular septal rupture describes a new opening in the septum between the two ventricles. It creates a harsh, holosystolic murmur that is loudest (by auscultation) along the left sternal border.[31] The clinical picture associated with acute ventricular septal rupture is that of acute ventricular failure and cardiogenic shock. Immediate diagnosis and treatment are necessary to prevent death.

Cardiac Rubs

Pericardial Friction Rub. A *pericardial friction rub* is a sound that can occur within 2 to 7 days after an MI. The friction rub results from pericardial inflammation (*pericarditis*). Classically, a pericardial friction rub is a grating or scratching sound that is both systolic and diastolic, corresponding with cardiac motion within the pericardial sac. It is often associated with chest pain, which can be aggravated by deep inspiration, coughing, swallowing, and changing position. It is important to differentiate pericarditis from acute myocardial ischemia, and the detection of a pericardial friction rub through auscultation can assist in this differentiation, leading to effective diagnosis and treatment.

█ SUMMARY

- An accurate history from the patient, or from a family member or significant other who knows the individual's current state of health, is essential. Signs and symptoms experienced by the patient offer clues as to the underlying causes of the cardiac condition. If the patient exhibits obvious signs of acute distress (shortness of breath, pink-frothy sputum, hypotension, tachycardia, pallor, sweating), or complains of chest pain or pressure, the questions are brief and focused to quickly identify the immediate problem.
- Inspection is used to determine whether the patient is anxious or relaxed. Inspection is also employed to identify serious conditions such as cyanosis, clubbing of fingernails, or significant peripheral edema.
- Palpation of the major pulses is a routine part of the cardiovascular physical examination. Normally, pulses are equal bilaterally. The loss of a pulse on one side may indicate the presence of atherosclerotic arterial vascular disease.
- Auscultation of heart sounds and murmurs is a skill that takes time and practice to master. When performed skillfully, the auscultation can reveal much about cardiac function and blood flow.

REFERENCES

1. Conn RD, O'Keefe JH. Cardiac physical diagnosis in the digital age: an important but increasingly neglected skill (from stethoscopes to microchips). *Am J Cardiol.* 2009;104:590.
2. Ang D, Sifrim D, Tack J. Mechanisms of heartburn. *Nat Clin Pract Gastroenterol Hepatol.* 2008;5(7):383.
3. Chun AA, McGee SR. Bedside diagnosis of coronary artery disease: a systematic review. *Am J Med.* 2004;117(5):334.
4. Tully AS, Trayes KP, Suddiford JS. Evaluation of nail abnormalities. *Am Fam Physician.* 2012;85(8):779.
5. Marrie TJ, Brown N. Clubbing of the digits. *Am J Med.* 2007;120(11):940.
6. Spicknall KE, Zirwas MJ, English JC 3rd. Clubbing: an update on diagnosis, differential diagnosis, pathophysiology, and clinical relevance. *J Am Acad Dermatol.* 2005;52(6):1020.
7. Hirsch AT, et al. A call to action: women and peripheral artery disease: a scientific statement from the American Heart Association. *Circulation.* 2012;125(11):1449.
8. Cornier MA, et al. Assessing adiposity: a scientific statement from the American Heart Association. *Circulation.* 2011;124(18):1996.
9. Jolobe O. Disproportionate elevation of iugular venous pressure in pleural effusion. *Br J Hosp Med.* 2011;72(10):582.
10. Ferrante G, Pugliese F, Di Mario C. Jugular venous pressure: a cardinal sign. *Lancet.* 2010;376(9743):802.
11. Deol GR, Collett N, Ashby A, et al. Ultrasound accurately reflects the jugular venous examination but underestimates central venous pressure. *Chest.* 2011;139:95.
12. Wiese J. The abdominojugular reflux sign. *Am J Med.* 2000;109(1):59.
13. Coats C, Eliott P. The collapsing pulse. *Br J Hosp Med.* 2012;73(5):C78.
14. Lewin J, Maconochie I. Capillary refill time in adults. *Emerg Med J.* 2008;25(6):325.
15. Chobanian AV, Bakris GL, Black HR, et al. Seventh report of the Joint National Committee on Prevention, Detection, Evaluation, and Treatment of High Blood Pressure. *Hypertension.* 2003;42(6):1206.
16. Ochoa VM, Yeghiazarians Y. Subclavian artery stenosis: a review for the vascular medicine practitioner. *Vasc Med.* 2011;16(1):29.
17. Naschitz JE, Rosner I. Orthostatic hypotension: framework of the syndrome. *Postgrad Med J.* 2007;83(983):568.
18. Stewart JM. Mechanisms of sympathetic regulation in orthostatic intolerance. *J Appl Physiol.* 2012.
19. Aronow WS, et al. ACCF/AHA 2011 Expert consensus document on hypertension in the elderly: a report of the American College of Cardiology Foundation Task Force on Clinical Expert Consensus Documents. *Circulation.* 2011;123:2434.
20. Swami A, Spodick DH. Pulsus paradoxus in cardiac tamponade: a pathophysiologic continuum. *Clin Cardiol.* 2003;26(5):215.
21. Stone MK, Bauch TD, Rubal BJ. Respiratory changes in the pulse-oximetry waveform associated with pericardial tamponade. *Clin Cardiol.* 2006;29(9):411.
22. Wu LA, Nishimura RA. Images in clinical medicine. Pulsus paradoxus. *N Engl J Med.* 2003;349(7):666.
23. Treadway K. Heart sounds. *N Engl J Med.* 2006;354(11):1112.
24. Chizner MA. Cardiac auscultation: rediscovering the lost art. *Curr Probl Cardiol.* 2008;33(7):326.
25. Barrett MJ, Lacey CS, Sekara AE, et al. Mastering cardiac murmurs: the power of repetition. *Chest.* 2004;126(2):470.
26. Johnston M, Collins SP, Storrow AB. The third heart sound for diagnosis of acute heart failure. *Curr Heart Fail Rep.* 2007;4(3):164.
27. Gupta S, Michaels AD. Relationship between accurate auscultation of the fourth heart sound and the level of physician experience. *Clin Cardiol.* 2009;32(2):69.
28. Bonow RO, et al. 2008 Focused Update Incorporated into the ACC/AHA 2006 guidelines for the management of patients with valvular heart disease: a report of the American College of Cardiology/American Heart Association Task Force on Practice Guidelines (Writing Committee to Revise the 1998 Guidelines for the Management of Patients With Valvular Heart Disease). *Circulation.* 2008;118:e523.
29. Segal BL. Valvular heart disease, Part 1. Diagnosis and surgical management of aortic valve disease in older adults. *Geriatrics.* 2003;58(9):31.
30. Czarnecki A, Thakrar A, Fang T, et al. Acute severe mitral regurgitation: consideration of papillary muscle architecture. *Cardiovasc Ultrasound.* 2008;6:5.
31. Hanifin C. Cardiac auscultation 101: a basic science approach to heart murmurs. *JAAPA.* 2010;23(4):44-8.

Cardiovascular Diagnostic Procedures

Mary E. Lough, Christine Thompson

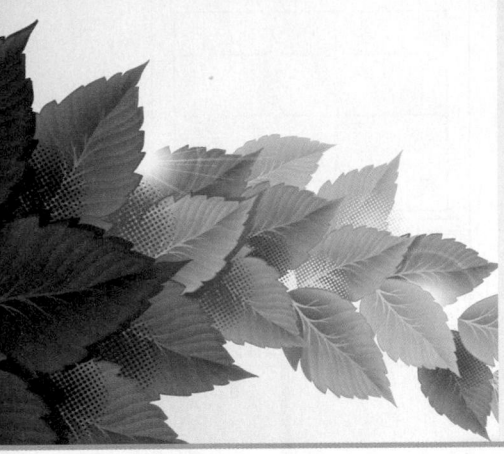

CARDIOVASCULAR ASSESSMENT AND MONITORING

Bedside Hemodynamic Monitoring

Hemodynamic monitoring is at a critical juncture. The technology that launched invasive hemodynamic monitoring is more than 30 years old, and the search to find viable replacement monitoring technologies that are minimal or noninvasive is intense. This has created a new challenge in critical care. Although the use of invasive monitoring is declining, it is still employed for hemodynamically unstable patients. Critical care nurses must be knowledgeable about traditional hemodynamic monitoring methods and be able to apply established physiologic principles in new situations. As the technology evolves, clinicians will apply the same physiologic principles to the new methods to ensure safety and optimal outcomes for each patient. The following discussion of hemodynamic monitoring describes both established and emerging technologies.

Equipment

A traditional hemodynamic monitoring system has four component parts as shown in Figure 14-1 and described in the following list:

1. An invasive catheter and high-pressure tubing connect the patient to the transducer.
2. The transducer receives the physiologic signal from the catheter and tubing and converts it into electrical energy.
3. The flush system maintains patency of the fluid-filled system and catheter.

4. The bedside monitor contains the amplifier with recorder, which increases the volume of the electrical signal and displays it on an oscilloscope and on a digital scale in millimeters of mercury (mm Hg).

Although many different types of invasive catheters can be inserted to monitor hemodynamic pressures, all such catheters are connected to similar equipment (see Fig. 14-1). Even so, there remains variation in the way different hospitals configure their hemodynamic systems. The basic setup consists of the following:

- A bag of 0.9% sodium chloride (normal saline) is used as a flush solution. In some hospitals heparin is added as an anticoagulant. A pressure infusion cuff covers the bag of flush solution and is inflated to 300 mm Hg.
- The system contains intravenous tubing, three-way stopcocks, and an in-line flow device attached for continuous fluid infusion and manual flush. High-pressure tubing must be used to connect the invasive catheter to the transducer to prevent damping (flattening) of the waveform.
- A pressure transducer is used. Modern transducers are disposable, use a silicon chip, and are highly accurate.

Heparin. The use of the anticoagulant heparin added to the normal saline (NS) flush setup to maintain catheter patency remains controversial.[1,2] While many units do add heparin to flush solutions, other critical care units avoid heparin because of concern about development of heparin-induced antibodies that can trigger the autoimmune condition known as heparin-induced thrombocytopenia (HIT).[2] This is sometimes described as a "heparin allergy" and, when present, is associated with a dramatic drop in platelet count and thrombus formation. If

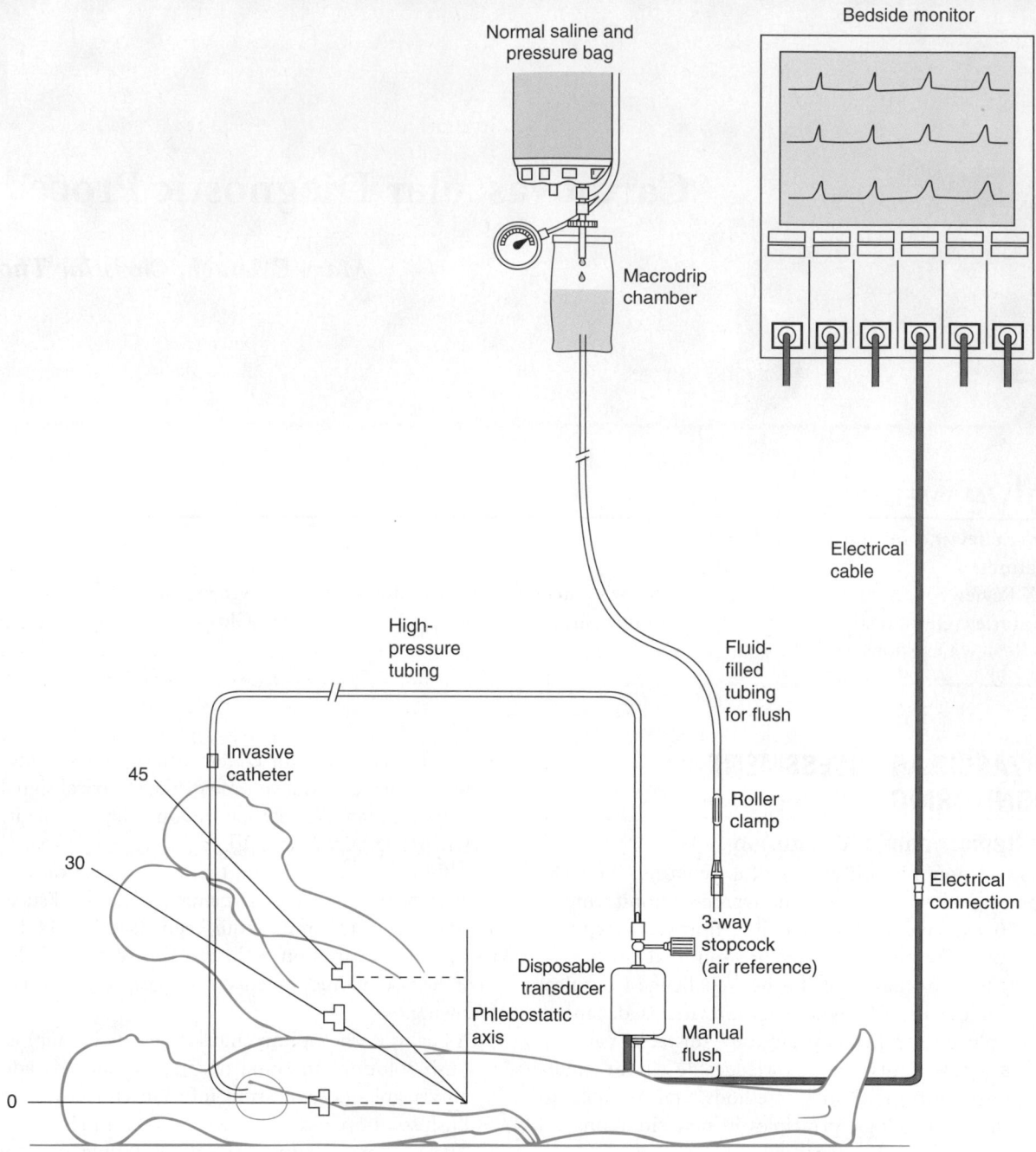

Normal saline and
pressure bag

Bedside monitor

Macrodrip
chamber

Electrical
cable

High-
pressure
tubing

Fluid-
filled
tubing
for flush

Invasive
catheter

45

Roller
clamp

30

Electrical
connection

3-way
stopcock
(air reference)

Disposable
transducer

Phlebostatic
axis

Manual
flush

0

Patient with invasive catheter

FIGURE 14-1   The four parts of a hemodynamic monitoring include an invasive catheter attached to high-pressure tubing to connect to the transducer; a transducer; a flush system, including a manual flush; and a bedside monitor.

heparin is used in the flush infusion, ongoing monitoring of the platelet count is recommended.[3]

Flush solutions, lines, stopcocks, and disposable transducers are changed every 96 hours per current Centers for Disease Control and Prevention (CDC) guidelines.[4] However, there is variation in practice between hospitals; some change the flush solutions every 24 hours. For this reason, it is essential to be familiar with the specific written procedures that concern hemodynamic monitoring equipment in each critical care unit. Dextrose solutions are not recommended as flush solutions in monitoring catheters.[4]

Calibration of Equipment. To ensure accuracy of hemodynamic pressure readings, two baseline measurements are necessary:

1. Calibration of the system to atmospheric pressure, also known as *zeroing the transducer*
2. Determination of the phlebostatic axis for transducer height placement, also called *leveling the transducer*[5]

Zeroing the Transducer. To calibrate the equipment to atmospheric pressure, referred to as zeroing the transducer, the three-way stopcock nearest to the transducer is turned simultaneously to open the transducer to air (atmospheric pressure) and to close it to the patient and the flush system. The monitor is adjusted so that "0" is displayed, which equals atmospheric pressure. Atmospheric pressure is not zero; it is 760 mm Hg at sea level. Using zero to represent current atmospheric pressure provides a convenient baseline for hemodynamic measurement purposes.

Some monitors also require calibration of the upper scale limit while the system remains open to air. At the end of the calibration procedure, the stopcock is returned to the closed position and a closed cap is placed over the open port. At this point, the patient's waveform and hemodynamic pressures are displayed.

Disposable transducers are very accurate, and after they are calibrated to atmospheric pressure, drift from the zero baseline is minimal. Although in theory this means that repeated calibration is unnecessary, clinical protocols in most units require the nurse to calibrate the transducer at the beginning of each shift for quality assurance.

Phlebostatic Axis. The phlebostatic axis is a physical reference point on the chest that is used as a baseline for consistent transducer height placement. To obtain the axis, a theoretic line is drawn from the fourth intercostal space, where it joins the sternum to a midaxillary line on the side of the chest. The midaxillary line is one half of the anteroposterior depth of the lateral chest wall.[5] This point approximates the level of the atria, as shown in Figure 14-1. It is used as the reference mark for central venous pressure (CVP) and pulmonary artery catheter transducers. The level of the transducer "air reference stopcock"

approximates the position of the tip of an invasive hemodynamic monitoring catheter within the chest.

Leveling the Transducer. Leveling the transducer is different from zeroing. This process aligns the transducer with the level of the left atrium. The purpose is to line up the *air–fluid interface* with the left atrium to correct for changes in *hydrostatic pressure* in blood vessels above and below the level of the heart.[5]

A carpenter's level or laser-light level can be used to ensure that the transducer is parallel with the phlebostatic axis reference point. When there is a change in the patient's position, the transducer must be leveled again to ensure accurate hemodynamic pressure measurements are obtained.[5] Errors in measurement can occur if the transducer is placed below the phlebostatic axis because the fluid in the system weighs on the transducer, creating additional hydrostatic pressure, and produces a falsely high reading. For every inch the transducer is below the tip of the catheter, the fluid pressure in the system increases the measurement by 1.87 mm Hg. For example, if the transducer is positioned 6 inches below the tip of the catheter, this falsely elevates the displayed pressure by 11 mm Hg.

If the transducer is placed above this atrial level, gravity and lack of fluid pressure will give an erroneously low reading. For every inch the transducer is positioned above the catheter tip, the measurement is 1.87 mm Hg less than the true value. If several clinicians are taking measurements, the reference point can be marked on the side of the patient's chest to ensure accurate measurements. Box 14-1

◎ BOX 14-1   NIC

Invasive Hemodynamic Monitoring

Definition

Measurement and interpretation of invasive hemodynamic parameters to determine cardiovascular function and regulate therapy as appropriate

Activities

Assist with insertion and removal of invasive hemodynamic lines

Assist with Allen test for evaluation of collateral ulnar circulation before radial artery cannulation, if appropriate

Assist with chest radiograph examination after insertion of pulmonary artery catheter

Monitor heart rate and rhythm

Zero and calibrate equipment every 4 to 12 hours, as appropriate, with transducer at the level of the right atrium

Monitor blood pressure (systolic, diastolic, and mean), central venous/right atrial pressure, pulmonary artery pressure (systolic, diastolic, and mean), and pulmonary capillary/artery wedge pressure

Monitor hemodynamic waveforms for changes in cardiovascular function

Compare hemodynamic parameters with other clinical signs and symptoms

Use closed-system cardiac output setup

Obtain cardiac output by administering cardiac output injectate within 4 seconds, and average three injections that are within less than 1 L of each other

Monitor pulmonary artery and systemic arterial waveforms; if dampening occurs, check tubing for kinks or air bubbles, check connections, aspirate clot from tip of catheter, gently flush system, or assist with repositioning of catheter

Document pulmonary artery and systemic arterial waveforms

Monitor peripheral perfusion distal to catheter insertion site every 4 hours or as appropriate

Monitor for dyspnea, fatigue, tachypnea, and orthopnea

Monitor for forward progression of pulmonary catheter resulting in spontaneous wedge, and notify physician if it occurs

Refrain from inflating balloon more frequently than every 1 to 2 hours, or as appropriate

Monitor for balloon rupture (e.g., assess for resistance when inflating balloon and allow balloon to passively deflate after obtaining pulmonary artery occlusion pressure [PAOP])

Prevent air emboli (e.g., remove air bubbles from tubing; if balloon rupture is suspected, refrain from attempts to reinflate balloon and clamp balloon port)

Maintain sterility of ports

Maintain closed-pressure system to ports, as appropriate

Perform sterile dressing changes and site care, as appropriate

Inspect insertion site for signs of bleeding or infection

Change IV solution and tubing every 24 to 96 hours, based on protocol

Monitor laboratory results to detect possible catheter-induced infection

Administer fluid and/or volume expanders to maintain hemodynamic parameters within specified range

Administer pharmacologic agents to maintain hemodynamic parameters within specified range

Instruct patient and family on therapeutic use of hemodynamic monitoring catheters

Instruct patient on activity restriction while catheters remain in place

Modified from Bulechek GM, et al. *Nursing interventions classification* (NIC). 6th ed. St. Louis: Mosby; 2013.

summarizes other nursing activities associated with hemodynamic monitoring.

Patient Position

Position of the hemodynamically monitored patient would not be an issue if critical care patients only lie flat in the bed. However, lying flat is not always a comfortable position, especially if the patient is alert or if the head of the bed needs to be elevated to decrease the work of breathing.

Head of Bed Backrest Position. Nurse researchers have determined that the CVP, pulmonary artery pressure (PAP), and pulmonary artery occlusion pressure (PAOP)—also called *pulmonary artery wedge pressure* (PAWP)—can be reliably measured at head of bed backrest positions from 0 (flat) to 60 degrees if the patient is lying on his or her back (supine).[5,6] If the patient is normovolemic and hemodynamically stable, raising the head of the bed usually does not affect hemodynamic pressure measurements. If the patient is so hemodynamically unstable or hypovolemic that raising the head of the bed negatively affects intravascular volume distribution, the first priority is to correct the hemodynamic instability and leave the patient in a lower backrest position. In summary, most patients do not need the head of the bed to be lowered to 0 degrees to obtain accurate CVP, PAP, or PAOP readings.

Lateral Position. The landmarks for leveling the transducer are different if the patient is turned to the side. Researchers have evaluated hemodynamic pressure measurement readings with the patients in the 30- and 90-degree lateral positions with the head of the bed flat, and they found the measurements to be reliable.[5] In the 30-degree angle position, the landmark to use for leveling the transducer is one half of the distance from the surface of the bed to the left sternal border.[5] In the 90-degree right-lateral position, the transducer fluid–air interface was positioned at the fourth ICS at the midsternum. In the 90-degree left-lateral position, the transducer was positioned at the left parasternal border (beside the sternum).[5] It is important to know that measurements can be recorded in nonsupine positions, because critically ill patients must be turned to prevent development of pressure ulcers and other complications of immobility.

Intra-arterial Blood Pressure Monitoring
Indications

Intra-arterial blood pressure monitoring is indicated for any major medical or surgical condition that compromises cardiac output (CO), tissue perfusion, or fluid volume status. The system is designed for continuous measurement of three blood pressure parameters: systole, diastole, and mean arterial blood pressure (MAP). The direct arterial access is helpful in the management of patients with acute respiratory failure who require frequent arterial blood gas measurements.

Catheters

The size of the catheter used is proportionate to the diameter of the cannulated artery. In small arteries—such as the radial and dorsalis pedis—a 20-gauge, 3.8-cm to 5.1-cm, nontapered catheter is used most often. If the larger femoral or axillary arteries are used, a 19- or 20-gauge, 16-cm catheter is used.

The catheter insertion is usually percutaneous, although the technique varies with vessel size. Catheters are most often inserted in the smaller arteries, using a "catheter-over-needle" unit in which the needle is used as a temporary guide for catheter placement. With this method, after the unit has been inserted into the artery, the needle is withdrawn, leaving the supple plastic catheter in place. Insertion of a catheter into a larger artery typically uses the Seldinger technique, which involves the following steps:

1. Entry into the artery using a needle
2. Passage of a supple guidewire through the needle into the artery
3. Removal of the needle
4. Passage of the catheter over the guidewire
5. Removal of the guidewire, leaving the catheter in the artery

Insertion and Allen Test. Several major peripheral arteries are suitable for receiving a catheter and for long-term hemodynamic monitoring. The most frequently used site is the radial artery.[2] The femoral artery is a larger vessel that is also frequently cannulated. Other smaller arterials such as the dorsalis-pedis, axillary, or brachial arteries are avoided if possible, and only used when other arterial access is unavailable.

The major advantage of the radial artery is the supply of collateral circulation to the hand provided by the ulnar artery through the palmar arch in most people. Before radial artery cannulation, collateral circulation must be assessed by using Doppler flow or by the modified Allen test according to institutional protocol.[2,7] In the Allen test the radial and ulnar arteries are compressed simultaneously. The patient is asked to clench and unclench the hand until it blanches. One of the arteries is then released, and the hand should immediately flush from that side. The same procedure is repeated for the remaining artery.

Nursing Management

Intra-arterial blood pressure monitoring is designed for continuous assessment of arterial perfusion to the major organ systems of the body. MAP is the clinical parameter most often used to assess perfusion, because MAP represents perfusion pressure throughout the cardiac cycle. Because one third of the cardiac cycle is spent in systole and two thirds in diastole, the MAP calculation must reflect the greater amount of time spent in diastole.[8] This MAP formula can be calculated by hand or with a calculator, where diastole times 2 plus systole is divided by 3 as shown in the formula below:

$$\frac{(\text{Diastole} \times 2) + (\text{Systole} \times 1)}{3} = \text{MAP}$$

A blood pressure of 120/60 mm Hg produces a MAP of 80 mm Hg. However, the bedside hemodynamic monitor may show a slightly different digital number because bedside monitoring computers calculate the area under the curve of the arterial line tracing[8] (Table 14-1).

Infection. Infection was once believed to be rare in arterial catheters because of the rapid arterial blood flow. New evidence suggests that arterial catheters are associated with the same risk of bloodstream infections as central venous catheters (CVCs).[9] This means that infection prevention measures must be just as meticulous for arterial catheters as for CVCs.[9]

TABLE 14-1 HEMODYNAMIC PRESSURES AND CALCULATED HEMODYNAMIC VALUES

HEMODYNAMIC PRESSURE	DEFINITION AND EXPLANATION	NORMAL RANGE
Mean arterial pressure (MAP)	Average perfusion pressure created by arterial blood pressure during the cardiac cycle. The normal cardiac cycle is one third systole and two thirds diastole. These three components are divided by 3 to obtain the average perfusion pressure for the whole cardiac cycle.	70-100 mm Hg
Central venous pressure (CVP)	Pressure created by volume in the right side of the heart. When the tricuspid valve is open, the CVP reflects filling pressures in the right ventricle. Clinically, the CVP is often used as a guide to overall fluid balance.	2-5 mm Hg 3-8 cm water (H_2O)
Left atrial pressure (LAP)	Pressure created by the volume in the left side of the heart. When the mitral valve is open, the LAP reflects filling pressures in the left ventricle. Clinically, the LAP is used after cardiac surgery to determine how well the left ventricle is ejecting its volume. In general, the higher the LAP, the lower the ejection fraction from the left ventricle.	5-12 mm Hg
Pulmonary artery pressure (PAP) PA systolic (PAS) PA diastolic (PAD) PAP mean (PAP_M)	Pulsatile pressure in the pulmonary artery measured by an indwelling catheter.	PAS 20-30 mm Hg PAD 5-10 mm Hg PAP_M 10-15 mm Hg
Pulmonary artery occlusion pressure (PAOP)*	Pressure created by the volume in the left side of the heart. When the mitral valve is open, the PAOP reflects filling pressures in the pulmonary vasculature, and pressures in the left side of the heart are transmitted back to the catheter "wedged" into a small pulmonary arteriole.	5-12 mm Hg
Cardiac output (CO)	Amount of blood pumped out by a ventricle over 1 minute. Clinically, it can be measured using the thermodilution CO method, which calculates CO in liters per minute (L/min).	4-6 L/min (at rest)
Cardiac index (CI)	CO divided by the body surface area (BSA), with tailoring of CO to individual body size. A BSA conversion chart is necessary to calculate CI, which is considered more accurate than CO because it is individualized to height and weight. CI is measured in liters per minute per square meter of BSA (L/min/m²).	2.2-4.0 L/min/m²
Stroke volume (SV)	Amount of blood ejected by the ventricle with each heartbeat, expressed in milliliters (mL). Hemodynamic monitoring systems calculate SV by dividing cardiac output (CO in L/min) by the heart rate (HR) and then multiplying the answer by 1000 to change liters to milliliters (mL).	60-70 mL
Stroke volume index (SI)	SV indexed to the BSA.	40-50 mL/m²
Systemic vascular resistance (SVR)	Mean pressure difference across the systemic vascular bed divided by blood flow. Clinically, SVR represents the resistance against which the left ventricle must pump to eject its volume. This resistance is created by the systemic arteries and arterioles. As SVR increases, CO falls. SVR is measured in Wood units or dyn·sec·cm⁻⁵. If the number of Wood units is multiplied by 80, the value is converted to dyn·sec·cm⁻⁵.	10-18 Wood units or 800-1400 dyn·sec·cm⁻⁵
Systemic vascular resistance index (SVRI)	SVR indexed to BSA.	2000-2400 dyn·sec·cm⁻⁵
Pulmonary vascular resistance (PVR)	Mean pressure difference across pulmonary vascular bed divided by blood flow. Clinically, PVR represents the resistance against which the right ventricle must pump to eject its volume. This resistance is created by the pulmonary arteries and arterioles. As PVR increases, the output from the right ventricle decreases. PVR is measured in Wood units or dyn·sec·cm⁻⁵. PVR is normally one sixth of SVR.	1.2-3.0 Wood units or 100-250 dyn·sec·cm⁻⁵
Pulmonary vascular resistance index (PVRI)	PVR indexed to BSA.	225-315 dyn·sec·cm⁻⁵/m²
Left cardiac work index (LCWI)	Amount of work the left ventricle does *each minute* when ejecting blood. The hemodynamic formula represents pressure generated (MAP) multiplied by volume pumped (CO). A conversion factor is used to change mm Hg to kilogram-meter (kg-m). LCWI is always represented as an indexed volume (BSA chart). LCWI increases or decreases because of changes in pressure (MAP) or volume pumped (CO).	3.4–4.2 kg-m/m²
Left ventricular stroke work index (LVSWI)	Amount of work the left ventricle performs with *each heartbeat*. The hemodynamic formula represents pressure generated (MAP) multiplied by volume pumped (SV). A conversion factor is used to change mL/mm Hg to gram-meter (g-m). LVSWI is always represented as an indexed volume. LVSWI increases or decreases because of changes in the pressure (MAP) or volume pumped (SV).	50-62 g-m/m²

Continued

TABLE 14-1	HEMODYNAMIC PRESSURES AND CALCULATED HEMODYNAMIC VALUES—cont'd	
HEMODYNAMIC PRESSURE	**DEFINITION AND EXPLANATION**	**NORMAL RANGE**
Right cardiac work index (RCWI)	Amount of work the right ventricle performs *each minute* when ejecting blood. The hemodynamic formula represents pressure generated (PAP mean) multiplied by volume pumped (CO). A conversion factor is used to change mm Hg to kilogram-meter (kg-m). RCWI is always represented as an indexed value (BSA chart). Similar to LCWI, the RCWI increases or decreases because of changes in the pressure (PAP mean) or volume pumped (CO).	0.54-0.66 kg-m/m^2
Right ventricular stroke work index (RVSWI)	Amount of work the right ventricle does *each heartbeat*. The hemodynamic formula represents pressure generated (PAP mean) multiplied by volume pumped (SV). A conversion factor is used to change mm Hg to gram-meter (g-m). RVSWI is always represented as an indexed value (BSA chart). Similar to LVSWI, the RVSWI increases or decreases because of changes in the pressure (PAP mean) or volume pumped (SV).	7.9-9.7 g-m/m^2

*Pulmonary artery occlusion pressure (PAOP) was formerly called *pulmonary capillary wedge pressure* (PCW or PCWP) or *pulmonary arterial wedge pressure* (PAWP).

Perfusion Pressure. A MAP greater than 60 mm Hg is necessary to perfuse the coronary arteries. A higher MAP may be required to perfuse the brain and the kidneys. A MAP between 70 and 90 mm Hg is ideal for the cardiac patient to decrease left ventricular (LV) workload. After a carotid endarterectomy or neurosurgery, a MAP of 90 to 110 mm Hg may be more appropriate to increase cerebral perfusion pressure. Systolic and diastolic pressures are monitored in conjunction with the MAP as a further guide to the accuracy of perfusion. If CO decreases, the body compensates by constricting peripheral vessels to maintain the blood pressure. In this situation, the MAP may remain constant but the pulse pressure (difference between systolic and diastolic pressures) narrows. The following examples explain this point:

Mr. A: BP, 90/70 mm Hg; MAP, 76 mm Hg

Mr. B: BP, 150/40 mm Hg; MAP, 76 mm Hg

Both patients have a perfusion pressure of 76 mm Hg, but they are clinically very different. Mr. A is peripherally vasoconstricted, as is demonstrated by the narrow pulse pressure (90/70 mm Hg). His skin is cool to touch, and he has weak peripheral pulses. Mr. B has a wide pulse pressure (150/40 mm Hg), warm skin, and normally palpable peripheral pulses. Nursing assessment of the patient with an arterial line includes comparison of clinical findings with arterial line readings, including perfusion pressure and MAP.

Pulse Pressure. A clinical example of hemodynamic nursing assessment can be seen in patient JW 1 day after coronary artery bypass grafting (CABG). JW recently has been weaned from dopamine (Intropin) and sodium nitroprusside (Nipride) and received an IV diuretic, 20 mg of furosemide (Lasix). He has voided 800 mL of urine via the urinary catheter during the past 2 hours. JW's MAP remains at 80 mm Hg, but his pulse pressure has narrowed by 30 mm Hg from 120/60 to 100/70 mm Hg. His heart rate (HR) has increased from 90 to 110 beats per minute. This clinical situation is not uncommon after furosemide administration, but the narrowed pulse pressure and increased HR may indicate hypovolemia. The nurse caring for

JW will monitor the trend of the MAP. If the MAP begins to decrease and JW shows signs of a low CO, his physician will be notified. In most nonemergency situations, following the trend of the arterial pressure is more valuable than an isolated measurement.

Cuff Blood Pressure. If the arterial line becomes unreliable or dislodged, a cuff pressure can be used as a reserve system.[10] In the normotensive, normovolemic patient, little difference exists between the arm cuff blood pressure and the intravascular catheter pressure, and differences of 5 to 10 mm Hg do not generally alter clinical management. The situation is different if the patient has a low CO or is in shock. The concern is that the cuff pressure may be unreliable because of peripheral vasoconstriction, and an arterial line is generally required. It is usual practice to compare a cuff pressure after the arterial line is inserted. A recent study in hypotensive patients found that a MAP calculated from the arm cuff blood pressure was comparable to the intravascular arterial MAP.[11] However, blood pressure cuffs placed on the thigh or ankle were less accurate in hypotensive patients.[11]

Arterial Pressure Waveform Interpretation

As the aortic valve opens, blood is ejected from the left ventricle and is recorded as an increase of pressure in the arterial system. The highest point recorded is called *systole*. After peak ejection (systole), the force decreases, and the pressure drops. A notch (dicrotic notch) may be visible on the downstroke of this arterial waveform, representing closure of the aortic valve. The *dicrotic notch* signifies the beginning of diastole. The remainder of the downstroke represents diastolic runoff of blood flow into the arterial tree. The lowest point recorded is called *diastole*. A normal arterial pressure tracing is shown in Figure 14-2. Notice that electrical stimulation (QRS) is always first and that the arterial pressure tracing follows the initiating QRS.

Decreased Arterial Perfusion. Specific problems with heart rhythm can translate into poor arterial perfusion if CO decreases. Poor perfusion may be seen as a single, nonperfused beat after a premature ventricular contraction (PVC) (Fig. 14-3) or as multiple, nonperfused beats (Fig. 14-4). In ventricular bigeminy, every second beat is poorly perfused (Fig. 14-5). A

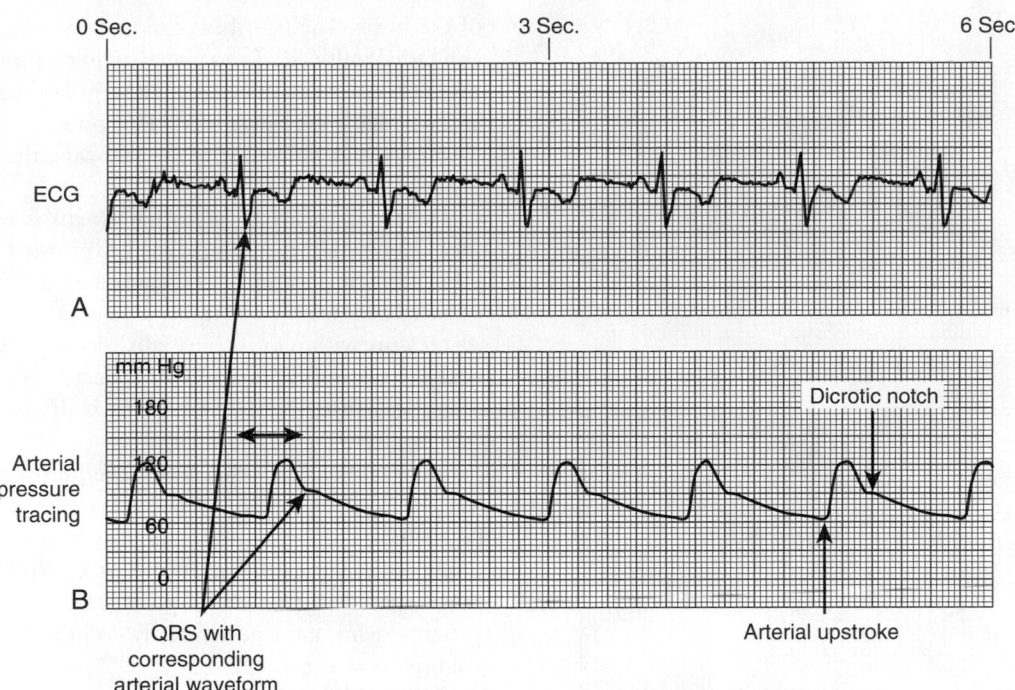

FIGURE 14-2 Simultaneous ECG *(A)* and normal arterial pressure *(B)* tracings.

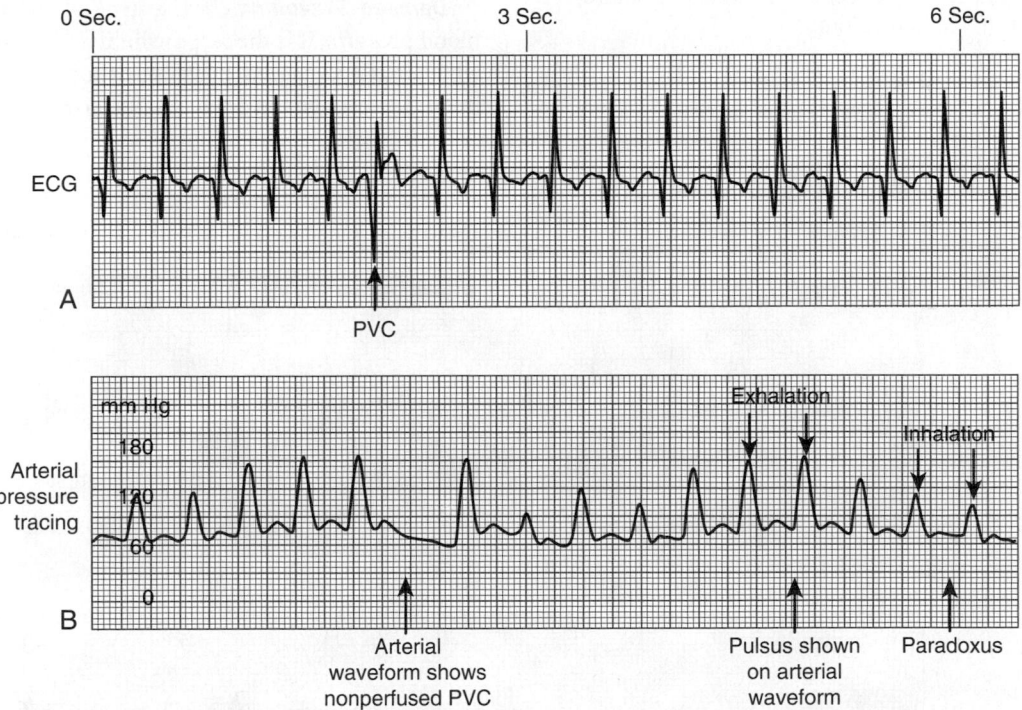

FIGURE 14-3 Simultaneous ECG *(A)* and arterial pressure *(B)* tracings show a normal arterial waveform with a nonperfused premature ventricular contraction (PVC). The arterial waveform also shows evidence of pulsus paradoxus in a patient who is mechanically ventilated.

disorganized atrial baseline resulting from atrial fibrillation creates a variable arterial pulse because of the differences in stroke volume (SV) between each beat (Fig. 14-6). All of these examples illustrate that when two beats are close together, the left ventricle does not have time to fill adequately, and the second beat is inadequately perfused or is not perfused at all.

Pulse Deficit. A pulse deficit occurs when the apical HR and the peripheral pulse are not equal. In the critical care unit, this can be seen on the bedside monitor. Normally, there is one arterial upstroke for each QRS, and if there are more QRS complexes than arterial upstrokes, a pulse deficit is present, as shown in Figures 14-3 and 14-6. To identify a pulse deficit in an unmonitored patient, a stethoscope is placed over the apex

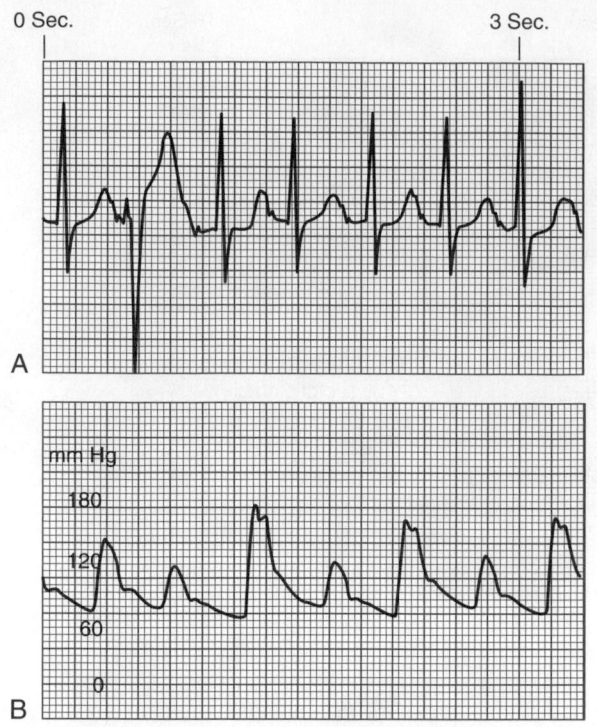

FIGURE 14-4 Simultaneous ECG *(A)* and arterial pressure *(B)* tracings show pulsus alternans. A nonperfused premature ventricular contraction (PVC) is also present.

of the heart. The heartbeat can be heard, but it cannot be felt as a radial pulse. To determine whether a pulse deficit is significant, it is necessary to evaluate the clinical impact on the patient and whether any change in MAP or pulse pressure has occurred. Generally, the more nonperfused beats, the more serious the problem.

Pulsus Paradoxus. Pulsus paradoxus is a decrease of more than 10 mm Hg in the arterial waveform that occurs during inhalation (inspiration). It is caused by a fall in CO as a result of increased negative intrathoracic pressure during inhalation. As pressure within the thorax falls, blood pools in the large veins of the lungs and thorax, and SV is decreased. The procedure for identification of pulsus paradoxus is discussed in Chapter 13 (see Box 13-9).

In certain clinical conditions, the pulsus paradoxus is obvious and can be clearly seen on an arterial waveform. It can be used as a clinical diagnostic test in a patient with cardiac tamponade, pericardial effusion, or constrictive pericarditis.[12] Pulsus paradoxus commonly occurs in hypovolemic surgical patients who are mechanically ventilated with large tidal volumes (see Fig. 14-3).

Pulsus Alternans. In pulsus alternans, every other arterial pulsation is weak. This sometimes occurs in individuals with advanced LV heart failure.

Damped Waveform. If the arterial monitor shows a low blood pressure, it is the responsibility of the nurse to determine whether it is a patient problem or a problem with the equipment, as described in Table 14-2. A low arterial blood pressure

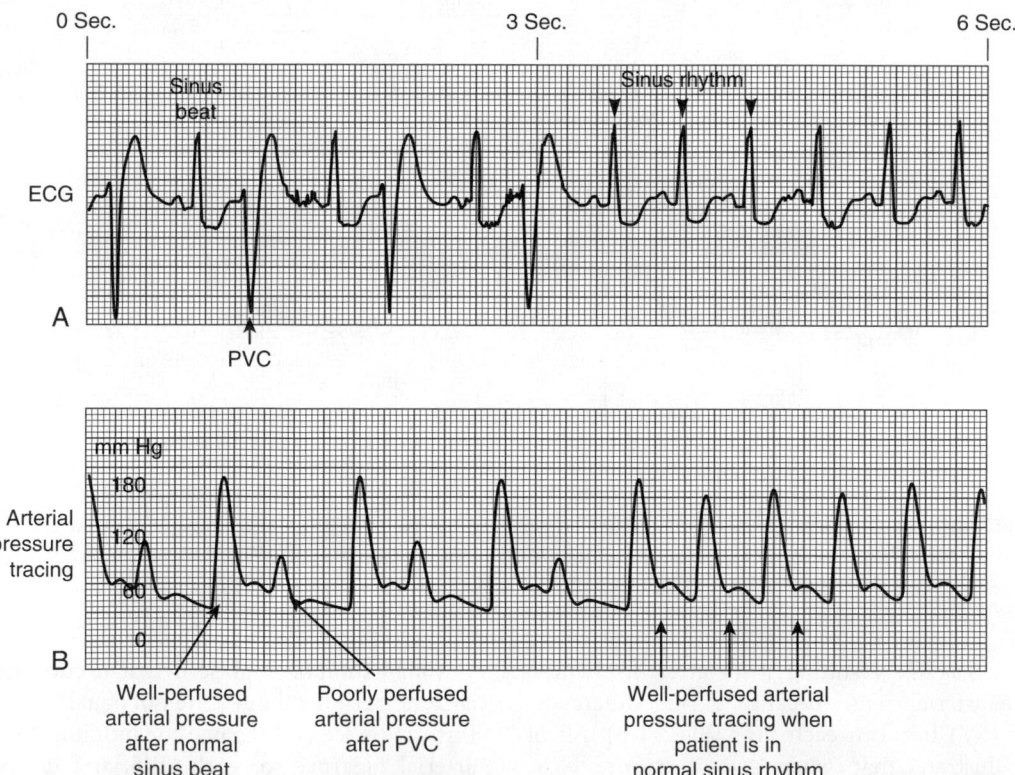

FIGURE 14-5 Simultaneous ECG *(A)* and arterial pressure *(B)* tracings show ventricular bigeminy. Every other ventricular beat is poorly perfused on the arterial pressure waveform. *B* depicts a well-perfused arterial pressure tracing as the patient converts to normal sinus rhythm.

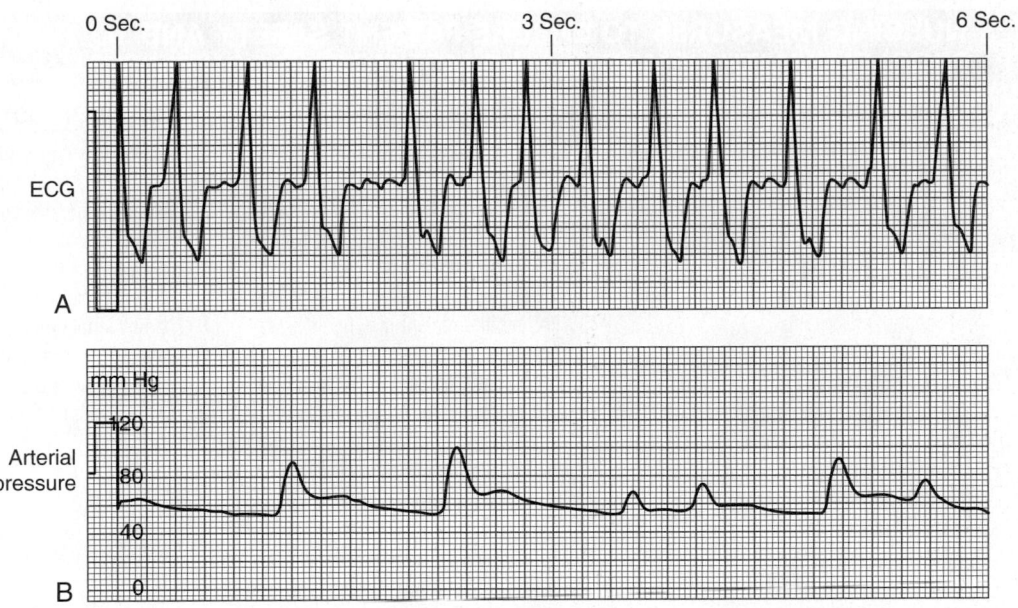

FIGURE 14-6 Simultaneous ECG *(A)* and arterial pressure *(B)* tracings show atrial fibrillation, which results in irregular atrial pulsations. They create differences in beat-to-beat ventricular upstroke volume, resulting in diminished or absent ventricular output, as seen on the arterial waveform.

TABLE 14-2	NURSING MEASURES TO ENSURE PATIENT SAFETY AND TO TROUBLESHOOT PROBLEMS WITH HEMODYNAMIC MONITORING EQUIPMENT		
PROBLEM	**PREVENTION**	**RATIONALE**	**TROUBLESHOOTING**
Overdamping of waveform	Provide continuous infusion of solution containing heparin through an in-line flush device (1 unit of heparin for each 1 mL of flush solution).	Ensure that recorded pressures and waveform are accurate because a damped waveform gives inaccurate readings.	Before insertion, completely flush the line and/or catheter. In a line attached to a patient, back flush through the system to clear bubbles from tubing or transducer.
Underdamping ("overshoot" or "fling")	Use short lengths of noncompliant tubing. Use fast-flush square wave test to demonstrate optimal system damping. Verify arterial waveform accuracy with the cuff blood pressure.	If the monitoring system is underdamped, the systolic and diastolic values will be overestimated by the waveform and the digital values. False high systolic values may lead to clinical decisions based on erroneous data.	Perform the fast-flush square wave test to verify optimal damping of the monitoring system.
Clot formation at end of the catheter	Provide continuous infusion of solution containing heparin through an in-line flush device (1 unit of heparin for each 1 mL of flush solution).	Any foreign object placed in the body can cause local activation of the patient's coagulation system as a normal defense mechanism. The clots that are formed may be dangerous if they break off and travel to other parts of the body.	If a clot in the catheter is suspected because of a damped waveform or resistance to forward flush of the system, gently aspirate the line using a small syringe inserted into the proximal stopcock. Flush the line again after the clot is removed, and inspect the waveform. It should return to a normal pattern.
Hemorrhage	Use Luer-Lock (screw) connections in line setup. Close and cap stopcocks when not in use. Ensure that the catheter is sutured or securely taped in position.	A loose connection or open stopcock creates a low-pressure sump effect, causing blood to back into the line and into the open air. If a catheter is accidentally removed, the vessel can bleed profusely, especially with an arterial line or if the patient has abnormal coagulation factors (resulting from heparin in the line) or has hypertension.	After a blood leak is recognized, tighten all connections, flush the line, and estimate blood loss. If the catheter has been inadvertently removed, put pressure on the cannulation site. When bleeding has stopped, apply a sterile dressing, estimate blood loss, and inform the physician. If the patient is restless, an armboard may protect lines inserted in the arm.

Continued

TABLE 14-2 **NURSING MEASURES TO ENSURE PATIENT SAFETY AND TO TROUBLESHOOT PROBLEMS WITH HEMODYNAMIC MONITORING EQUIPMENT—cont'd**

PROBLEM	PREVENTION	RATIONALE	TROUBLESHOOTING
Air emboli	Ensure that all air bubbles are purged from a new line setup before attachment to an indwelling catheter. Ensure that the drip chamber from the bag of flush solution is more than one half full before using the in-line, fast-flush system. Some sources recommend removing all air from the bag of flush solution before assembling the system.	Air can be introduced at several times, including when central venous pressure (CVP) tubing comes apart, when a new line setup is attached, or when a new CVP or pulmonary artery (PA) line is inserted. During insertion of a CVP or PA line, the patient may be asked to hold his or her breath at specific times to prevent drawing air into the chest during inhalation. The in-line, fast-flush devices are designed to permit clearing of blood from the line after withdrawal of blood samples. If the chamber of the intravenous tubing is too low or empty, the rapid flow of fluid will create turbulence and cause flushing of air bubbles into the system and into the bloodstream.	Because it is impossible to get the air back after it has been introduced into the bloodstream, prevention is the best cure. If air bubbles occur, they must be vented through the in-line stopcocks and the drip chamber must be filled. The left atrial pressure (LAP) line setup is the only system that includes an air filter specifically to prevent air emboli.
Normal waveform with *low* digital pressure	Ensure that the system is calibrated to atmospheric pressure. Ensure that the transducer is placed at the level of the phlebostatic axis.	To provide a 0 baseline relative to atmospheric pressure. If the transducer has been placed *higher* than the phlebostatic level, gravity and the lack of hydrostatic pressure will produce a false *low* reading.	Recalibrate the equipment if transducer drift has occurred. Reposition the transducer at the level of the phlebostatic axis. Misplacement can occur if the patient moves from the bed to the chair or if the bed is placed in a Trendelenburg position.
Normal wave form with *high* digital pressure	Ensure that the system is calibrated to atmospheric pressure. Ensure that the transducer is placed at the level of the phlebostatic axis.	To provide a 0 baseline relative to atmospheric pressure. If the transducer has been placed *lower* than the phlebostatic level, the weight of hydrostatic pressure on the transducer will produce a false *high* reading.	Recalibrate the equipment if transducer drift has occurred. Reposition the transducer at the level of the phlebostatic axis. This situation can occur if the head of the bed was raised and the transducer was not repositioned. Some centers require attachment of the transducer to the patient's chest to avoid this problem.
Loss of waveform	Always have the hemodynamic waveform monitored so that changes or loss can be quickly noted.	The catheter may be kinked, or a stopcock may be turned off.	Check the line setup to ensure that all stopcocks are turned in the correct position and that the tubing is not kinked. Sometimes, the catheter migrates against a vessel wall, and having the patient change position restores the waveform.

waveform is shown in Figure 14-7. In this case, the digital readout correlated well with the patient's cuff pressure, confirming that the patient was hypotensive. This arterial waveform is more rounded, without a dicrotic notch, compared with the normal waveform in Figure 14-2. A damped (flattened) arterial waveform is shown in Figure 14-8. In this case, the patient's cuff pressure was significantly higher than the digital readout, representing a problem with equipment. A damped waveform occurs when communication from the artery to the transducer is interrupted and produces false values on the monitor and oscilloscope. Damping is caused by a fibrin "sleeve" that partially occludes the tip of the catheter, by kinks in the catheter

or tubing, or by air bubbles in the system. Troubleshooting techniques (see Table 14-2) are used to find the origin of the problem and to remove the cause of damping.

Underdamped Waveform. Another cause of arterial waveform distortion is *underdamping,* also called *overshoot* or *fling.* Underdamping is recognized by a narrow, upward systolic peak that produces a falsely high systolic reading compared with the patient's cuff blood pressure, as shown in Figure 14-9. The overshoot is caused by an increase in dynamic response or increased oscillations within the system.

Fast-Flush Square Waveform Test. The monitoring system's dynamic response can be verified for accuracy at the bedside by

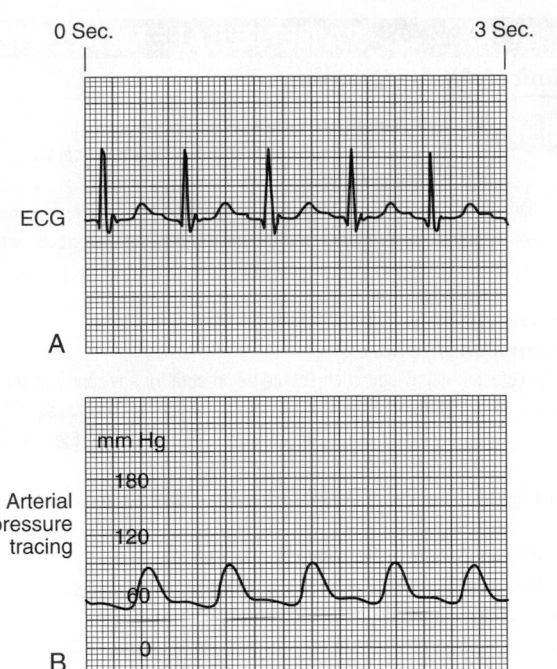

FIGURE 14-7 Simultaneous ECG *(A)* and arterial pressure *(B)* tracings show a low arterial pressure waveform.

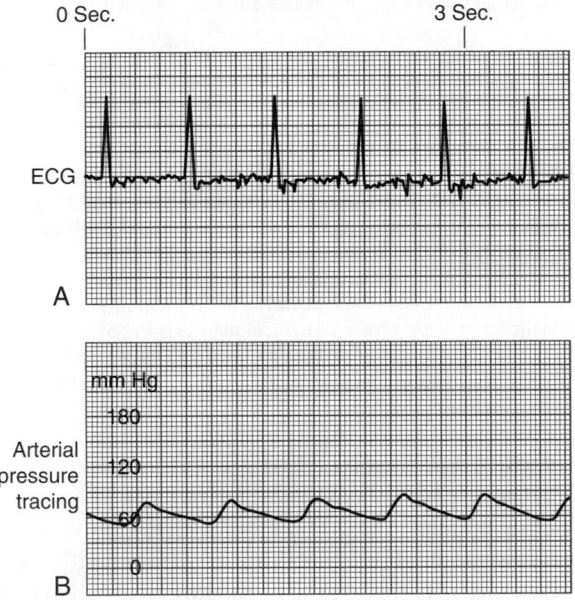

FIGURE 14-8 Simultaneous ECG *(A)* and arterial pressure *(B)* tracings show a damped arterial pressure waveform.

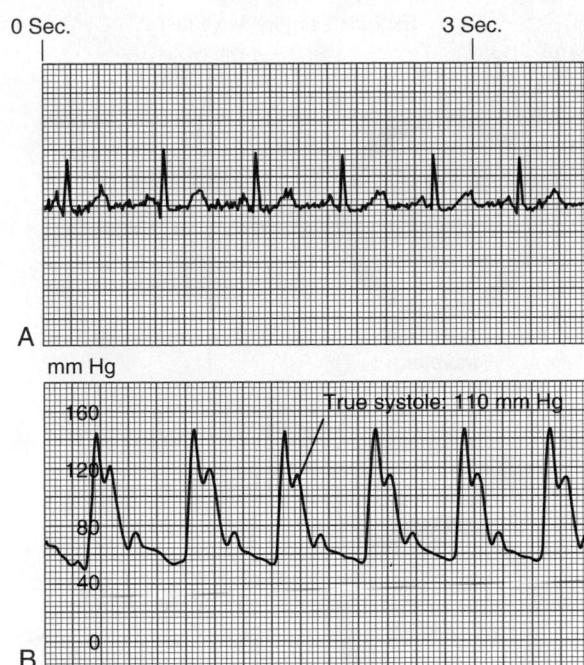

FIGURE 14-9 Simultaneous ECG *(A)* and arterial pressure *(B)* tracings show the overshoot, or fling, caused by a heightened dynamic response in the monitoring system. The monitor recorded an arterial line blood pressure of 141/51 mm Hg. The patient's true blood pressure with a cuff was 110/54 mm Hg. The 110 mm Hg cuff systolic pressure is consistent with the arterial line tracing without "overshoot."

the *fast-flush square waveform test*, also called the *dynamic frequency response test*.[5] The nurse performs this test to ensure that the patient pressures and waveform shown on the bedside monitor are accurate.[5] The test makes use of the manual flush system on the transducer. Normally, the flush device allows only 3 mL of fluid/hr. With the normal waveform displayed, the manual fast-flush procedure is used to generate a rapid increase in pressure, which is displayed on the monitor oscilloscope. As shown in Figure 14-10, the normal dynamic response waveform shows a square pattern with one or two oscillations before the return of the arterial waveform. If the system is overdamped, a sloped (rather than square) pattern is seen. If the system is underdamped, additional oscillations—or vibrations—are seen on the fast-flush square wave test. This test can be performed with any hemodynamic monitoring system. If air bubbles, clots, or kinks are in the system, the waveform becomes damped, or flattened, and this is reflected in the square waveform result.

This is an easy test to perform, and it should be incorporated into nursing care procedures at the bedside when the hemodynamic system is first set up, at least once per shift, after opening the system for any reason, and when there is concern about the accuracy of the waveform.[5] If the pressure waveform is distorted or the digital display is inaccurate, the troubleshooting methods described in Table 14-2 can be implemented. The nurse caring for the patient with an arterial line must be able to assess whether a low MAP or narrowed perfusion pressure represents decreased arterial perfusion or equipment malfunction. Assessment of the arterial waveform on the oscilloscope, in combination with clinical assessment, and use of the square waveform test will yield the answer.

Alarms. All critically ill patients must have the hemodynamic monitoring alarms on and adjusted to sound an audible alarm if the patient should experience a change in blood pressure, HR, respiratory rate, or other significant monitored variable. The key issues concerning monitor alarms are presented in Box 14-2.

Central Venous Pressure Monitoring
Indications

CVP monitoring is indicated whenever a patient has significant alteration in fluid volume (see Table 14-1). The CVP can be

Expected square wave test

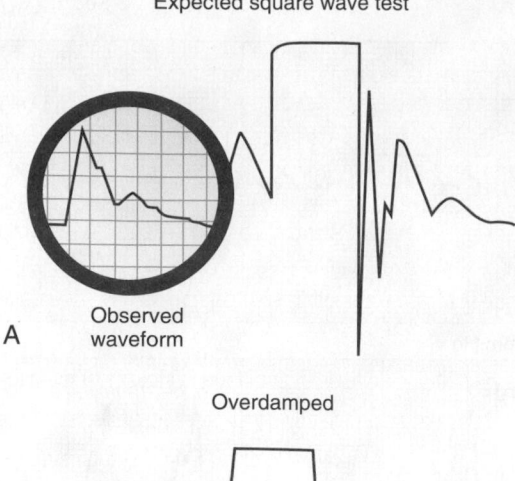

A Observed waveform

Overdamped

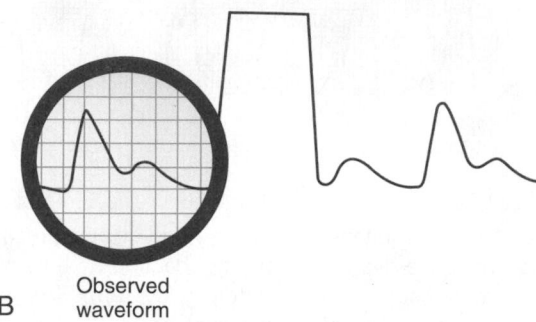

B Observed waveform

Underdamped

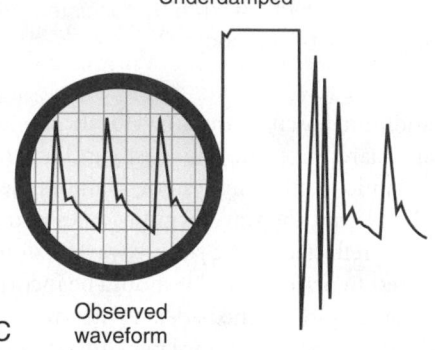

C Observed waveform

FIGURE 14-10 Square Wave Test. *A*, Expected square wave test result. *B*, Overdamped. *C*, Underdamped. (From Darovic GO. *Hemodynamic Monitoring: Invasive and Noninvasive Clinical Application*. 3rd ed. Philadelphia: WB Saunders; 2002.)

used as a guide in fluid volume replacement in hypovolemia and to assess the impact of diuresis after diuretic administration in the case of fluid overload. When a major intravenous line is required for volume replacement, a CVC is a good choice because large volumes of fluid can easily be delivered.

Central Venous Catheters

A range of CVC options are available as single-, double-, triple-, and quad-lumen infusion catheters, depending on the specific needs of the patient. CVCs are made from a variety of materials ranging from polyurethane to silicone; most are soft and flexible. Catheters that are antimicrobial-impregnated or heparin-coated have a lower rate of bloodstream infections.[4]

Insertion. The large veins of the upper thorax—subclavian (SC) and internal jugular (IJ)—are most commonly used for percutaneous CVC line insertion.[4] The femoral vein in the groin

is used when the thoracic veins are not accessible. All three major sites have advantages and disadvantages.

Internal Jugular Vein. The IJ vein is the most frequently used access site for CVC insertion. Compared with the other thoracic veins, it is the easiest to canalize. If the IJ vein is not available, the external jugular (EJ) vein may be accessed, although blood flow is significantly higher in the IJ vein, making it the preferred site. Another advantage of the IJ vein is that the risk of creating an iatrogenic pneumothorax is small. Disadvantages to the IJ vein are patient discomfort from the indwelling catheter when moving the head or neck and contamination of the IJ vein site from oral or tracheal secretions, especially if the patient is intubated or has a tracheostomy. This may be the reason why catheter-related infections are higher in the IJ than the SC position for indwelling catheters left in place for more than 4 days.[13,14]

Subclavian Vein. If the anticipated CVC dwelling time is prolonged more than 5 days, the SC site is preferred. The SC position has the lowest infection rate and produces the least patient discomfort from the catheter. The disadvantages are that the SC vein is more difficult to access and carries a higher risk of iatrogenic pneumothorax or hemothorax, although the risk varies greatly, depending on the experience and skill of the physician inserting the catheter.

Femoral Vein. The femoral vein is considered the easiest cannulation site because there are no curves in the insertion route. The large diameter of the femoral vein carries a high blood flow that is advantageous for specialized procedures such as continuous renal replacement therapy (CRRT) or plasmapheresis. Because there is a higher rate of nosocomial infection with femoral catheters, this site is not recommended.[4] If a femoral venous access has been used, the CVC should be changed to either the SC or IJ location as soon as the patient is hemodynamically stable.[4]

During insertion of a catheter in the SC or IJ vein, the patient may be placed in a Trendelenburg position. Placing the head in a dependent position causes the IJ veins in the neck to become more prominent, facilitating line placement. To minimize the risk of air embolus during the procedure, the patient may be asked to "take a deep breath and hold it" any time the needle or catheter is open to air. The tip of the catheter is designed to remain in the vena cava and should not migrate into the right atrium. Because many patients are awake and alert when a CVC is inserted, a brief explanation about the procedure can minimize patient anxiety and result in cooperation during the insertion. This cooperation is important, because CVC insertion is a sterile procedure and because the supine or Trendelenburg position may not be comfortable for many patients. The electrocardiogram (ECG) should be monitored during CVC insertion because of the associated risk of dysrhythmias.

All central catheters are designed for placement by percutaneous injection after skin preparation and administration of a local anesthetic. Visualization of the vessel with a bedside ultrasound before insertion is recommended to reduce the number of CVC placement attempts.[4] A prepackaged CVC kit typically is used for the procedure. The standard CVC kit contains sterile towels, chlorhexidine and alcohol for skin preparation, a needle introducer, a syringe, guidewire, and a catheter. The Seldinger technique, in which the vein is located by using a "seeking" needle and syringe, is the preferred method of placement. A guidewire is passed through the needle, the needle is removed, and the catheter is passed over the guidewire. After the tip of the catheter is correctly placed in the vena cava, the guidewire is removed. A sterile intravenous tubing and solution is attached, and the catheter is sutured in place. Following upper thoracic CVC placement, a chest radiograph is obtained to verify placement and the absence of an iatrogenic hemothorax or pneumothorax, especially if the SC vein was accessed.

Central Venous Catheter Complications

The CVC is an essential tool in care of the critically ill patient, but it is associated with some risks, and it is the responsibility of all clinicians to be informed about these hazards and to follow hospital procedures to avoid iatrogenic complications. CVC complications include air embolus, catheter-associated thrombus formation, and infection.

Air Embolus. The risk of air embolus, although uncommon, is always present for the patient with a central venous line in place. Air can enter during insertion[15] through a disconnected or broken catheter by means of an open stopcock, or air can enter along the path of a removed CVC.[16,17] This is more likely if the patient is in an upright position, because air can be pulled into the venous system with the increase in negative intrathoracic pressure during inhalation. If a large volume of air is infused rapidly, it may become trapped in the right ventricular outflow tract, stopping blood flow from the right side of the heart to the lungs. Based on animal studies, this volume is approximately 4 mL/kg.[18] If the air embolus is large, the patient will experience respiratory distress and cardiovascular collapse. An auscultatory clinical sign specifically associated with a large venous air embolism is the *mill wheel murmur*.[15,16,19] A mill wheel murmur is a loud, churning sound heard over the middle chest, caused by the obstruction to right ventricular outflow. Treatment involves immediately occluding the external site where air is entering, administering 100% oxygen, and placing the patient on the left side with the head downward (left lateral Trendelenburg position).[19] This position displaces the air from the right ventricular outflow tract to the apex of the heart, where the air may be aspirated by catheter intervention or gradually absorbed by the bloodstream as the patient remains in the left lateral Trendelenburg position. Precautions to prevent an air embolism in a CVP line include using only screw (Luer-Lock) connections, avoiding long loops of intravenous tubing, and using closed-top screw caps on the three-way stopcock.

Thrombus Formation. Clot formation (thrombus) at the CVC site is unfortunately common. Thrombus formation is not uniform; it may involve development of a *fibrin sleeve* around the catheter,[20] or the thrombus may be attached directly to the vessel wall. Other factors that promote clot formation include rupture of vascular endothelium, interruption of laminar blood flow, and physical presence of the catheter, all of which activate the coagulation cascade. The risk of thrombus formation is higher if insertion was difficult or there were multiple needlesticks. Gradual thrombus formation may lead to "sudden" CVC occlusion. Usually, the CVC becomes more difficult to withdraw blood from, or the CVP waveform becomes intermittently damped over a period of hours or even 1 to 2 days and is reported as "needing frequent flushes" to remain patent. This situation is caused by the continued lengthening of a fibrin sleeve that extends along the catheter length from the insertion site past the catheter tip.[20] Some catheters are heparin coated to reduce the risk of thrombus formation, although the risk of HIT does not make this a benign option. Sometimes, CVC complications are additive; for example, the risk of catheter-related infection is increased in the presence of thrombi, where the thrombus likely serves as a culture medium for bacterial growth. Because of concerns over the development of HIT many hospitals use a saline-only flush to maintain CVC patency.[21,22]

Infection. Infection related to the use of CVCs is a major problem. The incidence of infection strongly correlates with the length of time the CVC has been inserted, longer insertion times leading to a higher infection rate.[4,23] CVC-related infection is identified at the catheter insertion site or as a bloodstream infection (septicemia). Systemic manifestations of infection can be present without inflammation at the catheter site. No decrease in bloodstream infections was found when catheters were routinely changed and this practice is no longer recommended.[4] When a CVC is infected it must be removed and a new catheter inserted in a different site. If a catheter infection is suspected, the CVC should not be changed over a guidewire because of the risk of transferring the infection.[4] Most infections are transmitted from the skin, and infection prevention begins prior to insertion of the CVC. Insertion guidelines state that the physician must use effective hand-washing procedures, clean the insertion site with 2% chlorhexidine gluconate in 70% isopropyl, use sterile technique during catheter insertion, and maintain maximal sterile barrier precautions.[4] In many hospitals the nurse is authorized to stop the procedure if these insertion infection control guidelines are not followed. A daily review to determine whether the catheter is still required is recommended to ensure CVCs are removed promptly when no longer needed (Box 14-3).[4]

All clinicians must use good hand-washing technique and follow aseptic procedures during site care and any time the CVC system is entered to withdraw blood, give medications, or change tubing.[4] Site dressings impregnated with chlorhexidine are recommended to lower CVC infection rates.[4]

Nursing Management

In the critically ill patient, the CVC is used to monitor the CVP and waveform. The CVP catheter is used to measure the filling pressures of the right side of the heart. During diastole, when the tricuspid valve is open and blood is flowing from the right atrium to the right ventricle, the CVP accurately reflects right ventricular end-diastolic pressure (RVEDP). The normal CVP is 2 to 5 mm Hg (3 to 8 cm H_2O).

Central Venous Pressure—Volume Assessment. The time-honored practice of using the CVP value to assess central volume status has now been challenged.[24] A landmark systematic review of the literature revealed a weak relationship between the CVP measurement and blood volume.[24] Nor was a low CVP value always reliable in predicting who would respond to a fluid challenge.[24] In patients with a CVP between 0 and 5 mm Hg, up to 25% do not respond to a fluid challenge as expected.[25] Overall only about half of critically ill patients respond as expected to a fluid challenge.[24] In this situation the clinician must look at other indices of poor tissue perfusion such as an elevated lactate level, low base deficit, or decreased urine output.[25]

Passive Leg Raise. Another method to assess fluid responsiveness is to passively raise and support the patient's legs, to allow the venous blood from the lower extremities to rapidly flow into the vena cava and return to the right heart. If this maneuver increases the CVP by at least 2 mm Hg, this suggests that the patient will have a positive response to an IV fluid bolus.[26]

Water Versus Mercury Central Venous Pressure. CVP values are measured in millimeters of mercury (mm Hg) if

---

⚡ BOX 14-3 PATIENT SAFETY ALERT

Prevention of Central Venous Catheter-Related Bloodstream Infections

1. Education, Training, and Staffing
   a. Nurses and other health care providers should receive education about indications for central venous catheter (CVC) use, maintenance, and infection prevention.
   b. Only trained personnel should insert and maintain CVCs.
   c. Adequate staffing levels in critical care units are associated with fewer catheter-related bloodstream infections (CRBSI).
2. Selection of Catheters and Sites
   a. Use subclavian site rather than jugular or femoral insertion sites to minimize infection risk.
   b. Use ultrasound guidance to place CVCs.
   c. Remove any catheter that is no longer essential.
   d. If a CVC was placed in a medical emergency when aseptic technique was not assured, replace CVC within 48 hours.
3. Hand Hygiene and Aseptic Technique
   a. Perform hand hygiene procedures by washing hands with soap and water or alcohol-based hand rubs (ABHR) before and after palpating the CVC site, dressing the site or any other intervention.
   b. New sterile gloves must be worn by the professional inserting the CVC.
   c. New sterile gloves must be donned before touching a new catheter for CVC exchange over guidewire.
   d. Wear clean or sterile gloves when changing the catheter dressing.
4. Maximal Sterile Barrier Precautions
   a. For insertion, use maximal sterile barrier precautions including cap, mask, sterile gown, sterile gloves, and a full-body drape.
5. Skin Preparation
   a. Prepare clean skin with greater than 0.5% chlorhexidine preparation with alcohol before CVC insertion.

b. Antiseptics should be allowed to dry according to the manufacturer's recommendation before CVC insertion.
6. Catheter Site Dressing Regimens
   a. Transparent, semipermeable polyurethane dressings permit continuous visualization of the CVC insertion site.
   b. Replace transparent dressings on CVC sites at least every 7 days.
   c. Monitor the site when changing the dressing or by palpation through an intact dressing.
   d. Replace catheter site dressing whenever the dressing becomes damp, loose, or soiled.
   e. Do not use topical antibiotic ointment or creams on insertion sites (except for dialysis catheters) because of increased fungal infection risk.
   f. Use a chlorhexidine-impregnated sponge dressing at CVC site if CRBSI rate is not decreasing by other means (no recommendation for other types of chlorhexidine dressings).
7. Patient Cleansing
   a. Use 2% chlorhexidine wash for daily skin cleaning to reduce CRBSI.
8. Catheter Securement Device
   a. Use a sutureless catheter securement device to reduce catheter movement, which may reduce infection risk.
9. Antimicrobial Strategies
   a. Use an antimicrobial impregnated CVC when catheters are expected to remain in place for longer than 5 days.
   b. Do not administer systemic antimicrobial prophylaxis to prevent CRBSI.
   c. Do not routinely use anticoagulant therapy to prevent CRBSI.
10. No Routine CVC Replacement
    a. Do not routinely replace CVCs.
    b. Do not replace CVCs on the basis of fever alone.

O'Grady P, et al. Guidelines for the prevention of intravascular catheter-related infections. *Am J Infect Control.* 2011;39(4):S1-S34.

bedside hardwire monitoring is used. If a patient is admitted from a medical–surgical unit with a water manometer CVP and clinicians want to know the relationship between the two values, it involves a straightforward calculation based on the following standard relationship: 1 mm Hg (mercury pressure) is equivalent to 1.36 cm H_2O (water pressure). Although the numeric value in cm H_2O will be higher, the values are clinically equivalent for the specific patient. To convert water manometer pressure to mercury pressure, the water-pressure value is divided by 1.36 ($H_2O \div 1.36$). To convert mercury pressure to water pressure, the mercury value is multiplied by 1.36 (mm Hg $\times$ 1.36).

Removal. Removal of the CVC usually is a nursing responsibility. Complications are infrequent, and the ones to anticipate are bleeding and air embolus. Recommended techniques to avoid air embolus during CVC removal include removing the catheter when the patient is supine in bed (not in a chair) and placing the patient flat or in reverse Trendelenburg position if the patient's clinical condition permits this maneuver. Patients with heart failure, pulmonary disease, and neurologic conditions with raised intracranial pressure (ICP) should not be placed flat. If the patient is alert and able to cooperate, he or she is asked to take a deep breath to raise intrathoracic pressure during removal. After removal, to decrease the risk of air entering by a "track," an occlusive dressing is applied to the site. If bleeding at the site occurs after removal, firm pressure is applied. If a patient has prolonged coagulation times, fresh-frozen plasma or platelets may be prescribed before CVC removal.

Patient Position. To achieve accurate CVP measurements, the phlebostatic axis is used as a reference point on the body, and the transducer or water manometer zero must be level with this point. If the phlebostatic axis is used and the transducer or water manometer is correctly aligned, any head of bed position of up to 60 degrees may be used for accurate CVP readings for most patients.[5] Elevating the head of the bed is especially helpful for the patient with respiratory or cardiac problems who cannot tolerate a flat position.

Central Venous Pressure Waveform Interpretation. The normal right atrial (CVP) waveform has three positive deflections—*a*, *c*, and *v* waves—that correspond to specific atrial events in the cardiac cycle (Fig. 14-11). The *a* wave reflects atrial contraction and follows the P wave seen on the ECG. The downslope of this wave is called the *x* descent and represents atrial relaxation. The *c* wave reflects the bulging of the closed tricuspid valve into the right atrium during ventricular contraction; this wave is small and not always visible but corresponds to the QRS-T interval on the ECG. The *v* wave represents atrial filling and increased pressure against the closed tricuspid valve in early diastole. The downslope of the *v* wave is named the *y* descent and represents the fall in pressure as the tricuspid valve opens and blood flows from the right atrium to the right ventricle.

Cannon Waves. Dysrhythmias can change the pattern of the CVP waveform. In a junctional rhythm or after a PVC, the atria are depolarized after the ventricles if retrograde conduction to the atria occurs. This may be seen as a retrograde P wave on the ECG and as a large combined *ac* or *cannon wave* on the CVP waveform (Fig. 14-12). These cannon waves can be easily detected as large pulses in the jugular veins. Other pathologic conditions, such as advanced right ventricular failure or tricuspid valve insufficiency, allow regurgitant backflow of blood

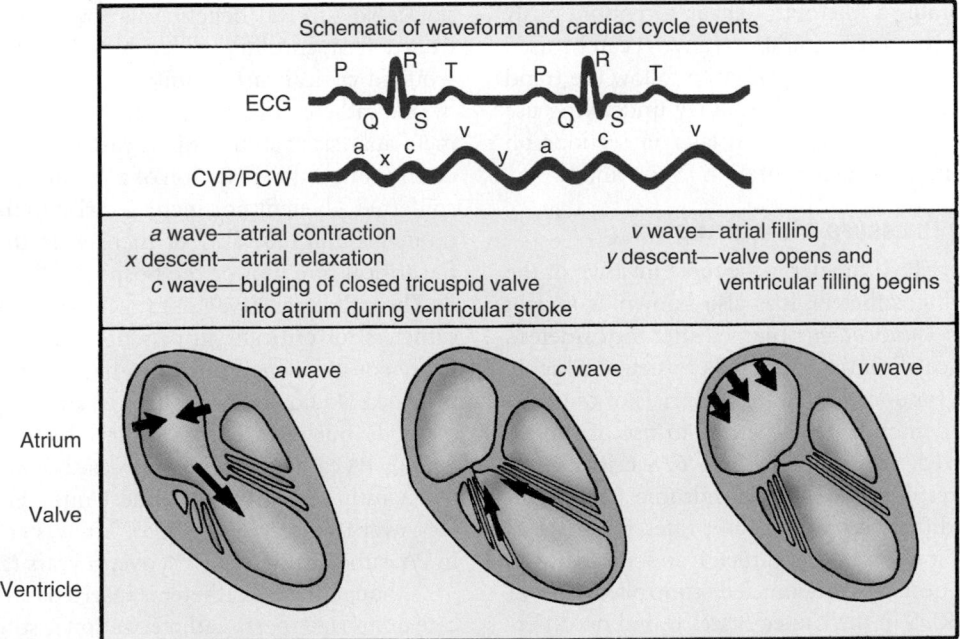

FIGURE 14-11 Cardiac events that produce the CVP waveform with *a*, *c*, and *v* waves. The *a* wave represents atrial contraction. The *x* descent represents atrial relaxation. The *c* wave represents the bulging of the closed tricuspid valve into the right atrium during ventricular systole. The *v* wave represents atrial filling. The *y* descent represents opening of the tricuspid valve and filling of the ventricle.

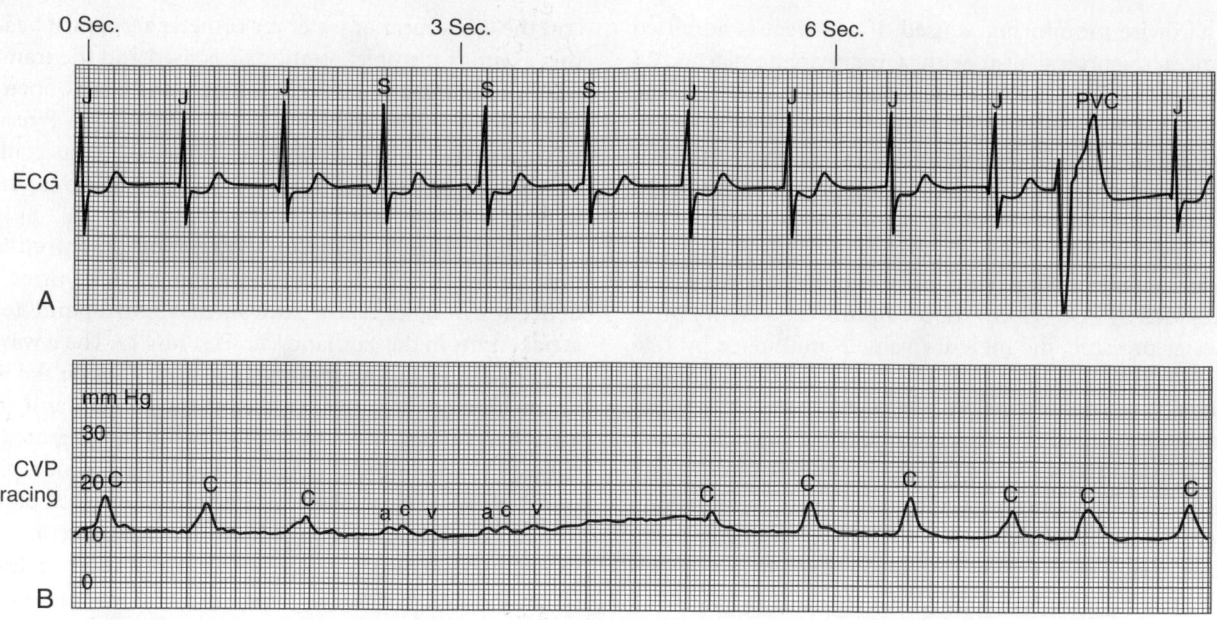

FIGURE 14-12 Simultaneous electrocardiographic *(A)* and central venous pressure (CVP) *(B)* tracings. The CVP waveform shows large cannon waves *(c* waves) corresponding to the junctional beats or premature ventricular contractions *(bottom strip).* As the patient converts to sinus rhythm, the CVP waveform has a normal configuration. *ac,* Normal right atrial pressure tracing; *c,* cannon waves on CVP tracing; *J,* junctional rhythm followed by cannon waves on CVP waveform; *PVC,* premature ventricular contraction followed by cannon wave on CVP; *S,* sinus rhythm followed by normal CVP tracing with *a, c,* and *v* waves.

from the right ventricle to the right atrium during ventricular contraction, producing large *v* waves on the right atrial waveform. In atrial fibrillation, the CVP waveform has no recognizable pattern because of the disorganization of the atria.

Specialized Central Venous Catheters

A CVC that incorporates a fiberoptic sensor to continuously measure central venous oxygen saturation (Scvo₂) can be used as a traditional CVC and additionally used to follow the trend of venous oxygen saturation.[27] The physiology underlying use of this fiberoptic technology is discussed later in sections on monitoring mixed venous oxygen saturation (Svo₂) and Scvo₂.

Pulmonary Artery Pressure Monitoring

The pulmonary artery (PA) catheter is the most invasive of the critical care monitoring catheters. It is also known as a *right heart catheter* or *Swan-Ganz catheter* (named after the catheter's inventors). The practice of routinely using PA catheters is highly controversial. Several randomized, controlled trials of critically ill patients have not demonstrated a benefit to use of the PA catheter. A randomized, controlled trial of 676 critical care patients with acute respiratory distress syndrome (ARDS) in France reported no difference in mortality rates for patients when treatment was guided by PA catheter and for patients without this information.[28] A randomized, controlled trial of 1000 patients with ARDS in the United States found no difference in mortality rates for patients when treatment was guided by a PA catheter and those for whom diagnostic information was obtained from a CVP.[29]

The impact of PA catheterization on mortality rates for patients with acute heart failure has also been examined. A randomized, controlled trial of 433 patients with acute heart failure in the United States reported no difference in mortality based on whether fluid volume management was guided by PA catheter insertion or not.[30] Similar results were reported from a British multicenter trial enrolling more than 1000 critical care patients; there were no differences in mortality or in length of stay.[31] No survival benefit was found in a randomized, controlled trial enrolling older high-risk surgical patients who required critical care monitoring when treatment was guided by PA catheter diagnostics or not.[32] Systematic reviews and meta-analysis of studies of PA catheter use have reached similar conclusions—that insertion of a PA catheter is neutral, it neither conferred a benefit nor increased risk to the patient. There was no increase in mortality or increase in the number of days in the critical care unit or the hospital.[33,34]

These findings have raised concerns about routine use of PA catheters for critically ill patients. The PA catheter is invasive. It previously seemed intuitive that the diagnostic information provided would confer a survival advantage over less invasive methods, but research has shown this is not the case. Consequently PA catheter use has decreased dramatically. The number of PA catheters inserted in the United States has declined by 65% over 10 years (1993-2004).[35] In western Canada the decline in PA catheter use was 50% over 5 years (2002-2006).[36]

Although the PA catheter is inserted less frequently in critical care units, right heart catheterization is still used as a diagnostic tool in the cardiac catheterization laboratory. In many critical care units, the PA catheter is reserved for patients who are refractory to conventional treatment,[37] and in many settings, it has been replaced by less invasive technologies such as echocardiography, as discussed later in this chapter.

Indications

The thermodilution PA catheter is reserved for the most hemodynamically unstable patients, for the diagnosis and evaluation of heart disease,[38] and shock states. The PA catheter is used to evaluate patient response to treatment, as described in Table 14-3. The PA catheter can simultaneously assess PA systolic and diastolic pressures, PA mean pressure, and PAOP (wedge pressure). The PA catheter is used to measure CO, determine mixed venous oxygen saturation, and calculate additional hemodynamic parameters.

Cardiac Output Determinants

CO is the product of HR multiplied by stroke volume (SV). SV is the volume of blood ejected by the heart during each beat (reported in milliliters).

$$HR \times SV = CO$$

The normal adult SV is 60 to 70 mL. The clinical factors that contribute to the heart's SV are preload, afterload, and contractility (Fig. 14-13). These three factors may be monitored using the PA catheter. Another contributor to CO is HR, which is usually recorded from the ECG leads.

Oxygen Supply and Demand

When the peripheral tissues need more oxygen (e.g., during exercise or fever), the normal, healthy heart can augment HR and SV and greatly increase CO. In the critically ill patient, when the tissues require more oxygen, these normal mechanisms are often nonfunctional, and it is the critical care nurse who assesses the need for and then optimizes hemodynamic function. The following discussion is intended to provide a basic understanding of the clinical factors that determine CO and the role of the critical care nurse in caring for the patient with an alteration in any of these factors.

Preload. Clinicians commonly describe the hemodynamic numbers related to preload as *filling pressures*. These values refer to the pressures resulting from the volumes in the atria and ventricles. These pressure numbers include pulmonary artery

---

TABLE 14-3 PULMONARY ARTERY CATHETERS: SELECTED INDICATIONS FOR USE AND RESPONSE TO TREATMENT

DIAGNOSTIC INDICATIONS*	POSSIBLE CAUSE	ASSOCIATED CLINICAL FINDINGS	HEMODYNAMIC PROFILE†	TREATMENT AND EXPECTED RESPONSE
Hypovolemic shock	Trauma Surgery Bleeding Burns Excessive diuresis	Cardiovascular: sinus tachycardia, ↓ BP (SBP <90 mm Hg), weak peripheral pulses Pulmonary: lungs clear Renal: ↓ urinary output Skin: normal skin temperature, no edema Neurologic: variable	Low CO Low CI (2.2 L/min/m²) High SVR (>1600 dyn·sec·cm⁻⁵) Low PAP Low PAOP	Treatment: Fluid challenge Expected hemodynamic response: ↓ HR ↑ BP ↑ PAP ↑ PAOP ↑ CVP ↑ CO/CI ↓ SVR
Septic shock	Sepsis	Cardiovascular: sinus tachycardia, ↓ BP (SBP <90 mm Hg), bounding peripheral pulses Pulmonary: lungs may be clear or congested, depending on the origin of the sepsis Renal: ↓ urinary output Skin: warm and flushed Neurologic: variable	High CO (>8 L/min) High CI Low SVR (<600 dyn·sec·cm⁻⁵) Low PAP Low PAOP Low CVP	Treatment: IV fluid to maintain hemodynamic function Fluid challenge Peripheral vasoconstricting agent (alpha) to ↑ SVR Antibiotics and laboratory cultures to find site of infection Consider rhAPC Expected hemodynamic response: ↓ HR ↑ BP ↑ PAP ↑ PAOP ↑ CVP ↑ CO and CI ↑ SVR SvO_2 = 70%

*Patients undergoing major vascular or cardiac surgery may also have a pulmonary catheter in situ to follow the trend of the cardiac output and cardiac index, SVR systemic vascular resistance and PVR pulmonary vascular resistance, and fluid status during the first 24 hours after surgery.
†See Table 14-1 for definitions and Appendix B for normal values of hemodynamic parameters listed in this table.

Continued

TABLE 14-3	PULMONARY ARTERY CATHETERS: SELECTED INDICATIONS FOR USE AND RESPONSE TO TREATMENT—cont'd			
DIAGNOSTIC INDICATIONS*	**POSSIBLE CAUSE**	**ASSOCIATED CLINICAL FINDINGS**	**HEMODYNAMIC PROFILE†**	**TREATMENT AND EXPECTED RESPONSE**
Multisystem failure shock	Multiple organ dysfunction syndrome (MODS)	Cardiovascular: normal sinus rhythm or sinus tachycardia, ↓ BP, weak peripheral pulses Pulmonary: lungs may be clear or congested, depending on the site of sepsis; acidosis based on arterial blood gas values, may require mechanical ventilation Renal: ↓ urinary output, may have ↑ BUN and ↑ creatinine levels Skin: cool and mottled Neurologic: variable, depending on fluid status and medications used in treatment	Low CO Low CI (<2.2 L/min/m²) High SVR (>1600 dyn·sec·cm⁻⁵) High or low PAP High or low PAOP High or low CVP	Treatment: Vasodilators to ↓ SVR, Antibiotics Support of body system as necessary (e.g., mechanical ventilation, hemodialysis) Expected hemodynamic response: ↓ HR ↑ BP Normalized PAP, PAOP, CVP ↓ SVR ↓ PVR ↑ CO and CI
Cardiogenic shock	LV pump failure caused by acute myocardial infarction or severe mitral or aortic valve disease	Cardiovascular: sinus tachycardia, possibly dysrhythmias, systolic BP <90 mm Hg, S₃ or S₄, weak peripheral pulses Pulmonary: lungs may have crackles or pulmonary edema Renal: ↓ urinary output Skin: cool, pale, and moist	Low CO Low CI (<2.2 L/min/m²) High SVR (>1600 dyn·sec·cm⁻⁵) High PAP High PAOP (>15 mm Hg) High CVP Low SVI Low left CWI Low left VSWI	Treatment: Inotropic medications to ↑ LV contractility Vasodilators or IABP to ↓ SVR Diuretics to ↓ preload Optimization of HR and control of dysrhythmias Expected hemodynamic response: ↓ HR ↑ BP ↓ PAP ↓ PAOP ↓ CVP ↓ SVR ↑ CO and CI ↑ SVI ↑ Left CWI ↑ Left VSWI
Acute respiratory distress syndrome (ARDS) or noncardiogenic pulmonary edema	Trauma Sepsis Shock Inhaled toxins (smoke, chemicals, 100% oxygen) Aspiration of gastric contents Metabolic disorders	Neurologic: may have ↓ mentation caused by low BP and CO Cardiovascular: sinus tachycardia, high or low BP, normal peripheral pulses Pulmonary: poor oxygenation and pulmonary edema, ↑ respiratory rate, or need for mechanical ventilation Renal: ↑ or ↓ urinary output Skin: normal temperature Neurologic: anxiety or confusion associated with respiratory distress and poor oxygenation	Normal CO Normal CI Normal SVR Normal PAOP High PAP High PVR (>250 dyn·sec·cm⁻⁵) Low right CWI Low right VSWI	Treatment: Eliminate cause of ARDS Support pulmonary function as necessary Expected hemodynamic response: ↓ HR Normal BP ↓ PAP ↓ PVR ↑ Right CWI ↑ Right VSWI Normal CO and CI Normal SVR

BP, Blood pressure; *BUN*, blood urea nitrogen; *CI*, cardiac index; *CO*, cardiac output; *CVP*, central venous pressure; *CWI*, cardiac work index; *HR*, heart rate; *IABP*, intra-aortic balloon pump; *IV*, intravenous; *PAOP*, pulmonary artery occlusion pressure; *PAP*, pulmonary artery pressure; *PVR*, pulmonary vascular resistance; *rhAPC*, recombinant human activated protein C; *SBP*, systolic blood pressure; *SVI*, stroke volume index; *SVO₂*, mixed venous oxygen saturation; *SVR*, systemic vascular resistance; *VSWI*, ventricular stroke work index; ↓, decrease or decreased; ↑, increase or increased.

diastolic pressure (PADP) and PAOP (or wedge pressure), which measure preload in the left side of the heart, and CVP, which measures preload in the right side of the heart.

Preload is the *volume* in the ventricle at end-diastole. Because diastole is the filling stage of the cardiac cycle, the volume in the ventricle at end-diastole represents the presystolic volume available for ejection for that cardiac cycle. LV volume can be measured directly during cardiac catheterization but it is not generally measured in the critical care unit. The principle is that the presence of blood within the ventricle creates pressures that can be measured by the PA catheter and transducer and can be displayed on the bedside monitor.

Measurement of Preload. When the PA catheter is correctly positioned with the tip in one of the large branches of the PA,

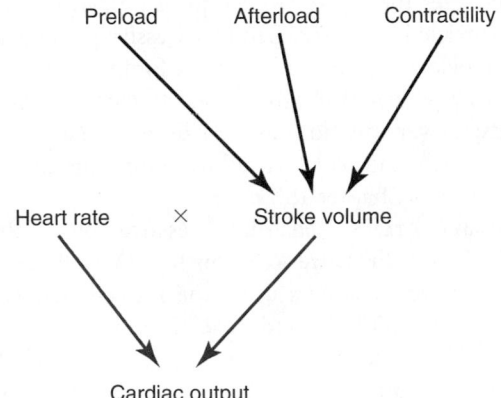

FIGURE 14-13 Preload, afterload, and contractility contribute to the heart's stroke volume. Stroke volume × Heart rate = Cardiac output.

the only valve between the PA catheter tip and the left ventricle is the mitral valve. During diastole, when the mitral valve is open, no obstruction exists between the tip of the PA catheter and the left ventricle (Fig. 14-14). The LV preload volume creates left ventricular end-diastolic pressure (LVEDP). This is measured clinically by the PAOP or "wedge" pressure. The PAOP and PADP are the values most often referred to in this chapter, because they are the values used in clinical practice. Normal left atrial pressure (LAP) or PAOP is 5 to 12 mm Hg.

Frank-Starling Law of the Heart. Clinically the PAOP has significance because a change in LV volume (preload) is reflected by a change in the measured PAOP (wedge pressure). Change in preload relies on the *Frank-Starling law of the heart*. This concept states that the force of ventricular ejection is directly related to two elements:

1. Volume in the ventricle at end-diastole (preload)
2. Amount of myocardial stretch placed on the ventricle as a result

If the volume in the left ventricle is low, CO is also suboptimal. If intravenous fluids (volume) are infused, CO increases as LV volume and myocardial fiber stretch increase. This is true up to a point. Past this point, more fluid volume overdistends the ventricle and stretches the myocardial fibers so much that CO decreases. This scenario is seen clinically in the setting of acute heart failure with pulmonary edema. The increased volume in the overdistended left ventricle raises pressure in the left ventricle, left atrium, and pulmonary veins (that drain into the left atrium), and it ultimately raises pulmonary capillary pressures measured as an increased wedge pressure (PAOP). The impact of preload on CO is represented in Figures 14-15 and 14-16, using the Frank-Starling curve as a model.

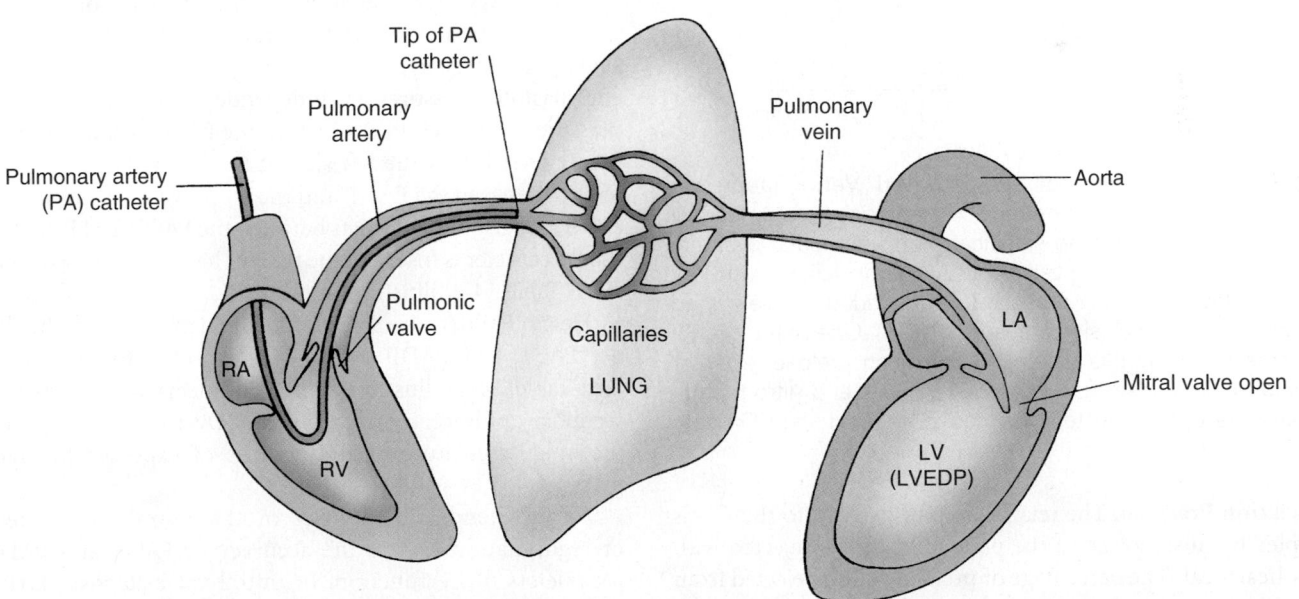

FIGURE 14-14 Relationship of the pulmonary artery occlusion pressure (PAOP) (i.e., wedge pressure) to the left ventricular end-diastolic pressure (LVEDP) (i.e., preload). In most clinical situations, the PAOP accurately reflects the LVEDP. During diastole, when the mitral valve is open, there are no other valves or other obstructions between the tip of the catheter and the left ventricle (LV). The pressure exerted by the volume in the LV is reflected through the left atrium (LA), through the pulmonary veins, and to the pulmonary capillaries. *PA,* Pulmonary artery; *RA,* right atrium; *RV,* right ventricle.

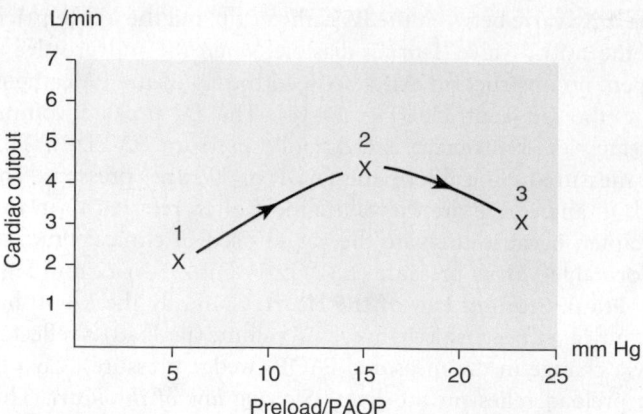

FIGURE 14-15 Impact of Preload on Cardiac Output (CO). *1,* Poor cardiac output with low preload as a result of hypovolemia. *2,* Hypovolemia is corrected after the administration of 2 L of intravenous fluid. The preload volume in the ventricle is increased, and pulmonary artery occlusion pressure (PAOP) has risen. Because of the increased fiber stretch from the increase in preload, CO also has risen. *3,* After the infusion of an additional 2 L of intravenous solution, the myocardial fibers are overdistended, preload (PAOP) has increased, and CO has fallen as the volume in the left ventricle rises.

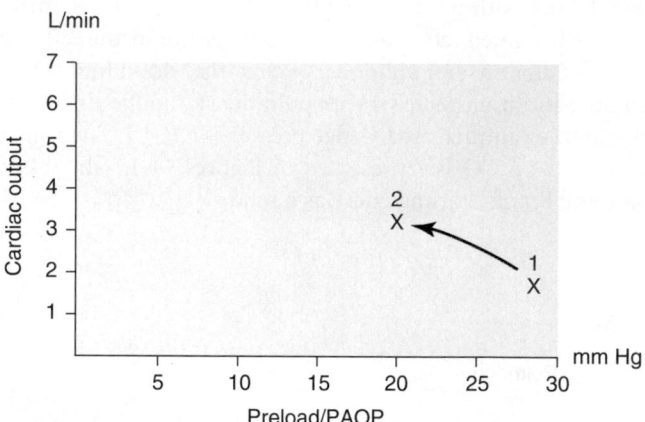

FIGURE 14-16 Impact of Preload and Venodilation on Cardiac Output (CO). *1,* After an acute anterior wall myocardial infarction that has created significant left ventricular dysfunction, this patient has left ventricle (LV) pump failure with low CO and elevated filling pressures identified by an elevated pulmonary artery occlusion pressure (PAOP). One of the clinical problems faced by this patient is too much preload. *2,* After administration of diuretics to reduce volume and nitroglycerin to dilate the venous system, preload is reduced and CO rises.

Ejection Fraction. The relationship of preload to the CO is complex because not all of the preload volume is ejected with every heartbeat. The percentage of preload volume ejected from the left ventricle per beat is measured during cardiac catheterization and is described as the ejection fraction (EF). A normal EF in a healthy heart is 70%. In clinical practice, most cardiologists will accept an EF value of greater than 50% as normal. The volume ejected from the left ventricle with each beat is known as the SV, which can be calculated at the bedside by dividing the CO by the HR per minute (SV = CO ÷ HR).

Cardiac Dysfunction. A significant relationship exists between LVEDP and cardiac muscle dysfunction. As a general rule, the higher the pressure inside the left ventricle, the greater the degree of cardiac dysfunction. The pressure rises at end-diastole (end of filling) because the compromised ventricle cannot eject all of the preload blood volume. For example, in a patient with heart failure, the preload volume may be 100 mL. However, the SV ejected may be only 30 mL. The EF in this patient is 30% (normal EF is greater than 50%). The remaining preload volume (70 mL in this example) significantly elevates LV pressures. When the mitral valve opens at the beginning of diastole, the pressure in the left atrium needs to be slightly higher than pressures in the left ventricle to allow filling. The 70 mL remaining in the ventricle produces high LV diastolic pressures. This elevates the left atrial filling pressure and consequently elevates the PAOP (wedge pressure). In this example, the left ventricle is overstretched by excessive preload, and CO therefore is below normal. A plan of care for this patient includes decreasing LV preload through 1) restriction of intravenous and oral fluids; 2) venodilation; and 3) diuresis. The myocardial dysfunction will lead to heart failure symptoms that are discussed further in Chapter 15.

Pulmonary Artery Diastolic Pressure and Pulmonary Artery Occlusion Pressure Relationship. LVEDP can be estimated by indirect measures using the PA catheter. The most accurate is the PAOP method. The second method involves measuring PADP during diastole when the normal PADP is equal to or 1 to 3 mm Hg higher than the mean PAOP and LVEDP. It is physiologically impossible for the PAOP to be higher than the PADP. The clinician must recalibrate and troubleshoot the monitoring system if this appears to occur (see Table 14-2).

Pulmonary Hypertension. Specific clinical conditions can alter the normal PADP/PAOP relationship.[39] In ARDS with acute pulmonary hypertension, the pulmonary arterial systolic and diastolic pressures are independently raised above the LV pressures. In this clinical situation the PADP will not accurately reflect function of the left side of the heart. The numeric difference between the PADP and the PAOP value is called a *gradient.* If a large gradient exists between the PAOP and PADP when the PA catheter is inserted, the patient has pulmonary hypertension (Table 14-4, illustration C).

Heart Failure. In failure of the left side of the heart, the PAOP and PADP are elevated and approximately equal (see Table 14-4, illustration B). The heart failure may cause secondary pulmonary hypertension. Over time, the damage to the lung vasculature occurs because of exposure to high LV pressure.

Mitral Stenosis. Pathology of the mitral valve—stenosis or regurgitation—alters the accuracy of PAOP and PADP as parameters of LV function. In mitral valve stenosis, LAP and PAOP are increased and cause pulmonary congestion; however, these elevated values do not reflect the LVEDP because a stenotic mitral valve decreases normal blood flow from the left atrium to the left ventricle, decreasing LV preload and consequently lowering LVEDP. A nonstenotic mitral valve is essential for accurate readings because a narrowed mitral valve increases LAP, PAOP, and PADP in the presence of a normal LVEDP.

TABLE 14-4   CLINICAL INTERPRETATION OF PULMONARY ARTERY WAVEFORMS

PA PRESSURE	CLINICAL INTERPRETATION	WAVEFORM INTERPRETATION*
Pulmonary artery systolic (PAS) pressure	PAS pressure reflects the systolic pressure in the pulmonary vasculature. Waveform **A** is a normal waveform. The elevated values in pulmonary hypertension may be caused by idiopathic sources, some congenital heart defects, or lung disease.	
Pulmonary artery diastolic (PAD) pressure	In the patient with healthy lung vasculature, PAD pressure reflects left ventricular end-diastolic pressure (LVEDP), as shown in waveform **B**. Even if the patient experiences heart failure, the pulmonary artery occlusion pressure (PAOP) and PAD increase together.	
	In the presence of acute respiratory distress syndrome or pulmonary hypertension, PAD pressure is not an accurate reflection of PAOP, as shown in waveform **C**.	
Mean pulmonary artery pressure (PAP mean or PAP$_M$)	PAP mean pressure is used in the calculation of pulmonary vascular resistance (PVR) and pulmonary vascular resistance index (PVRI), as described in Table 14-1. High mean pressures can reflect cardiac or pulmonary disease. Low mean pressures reflect hypovolemia. Waveform **D** shows PAP mean placement.	
Pulmonary artery occlusion pressure (PAOP) or pulmonary artery wedge pressure (PAWP)	In the healthy patient, PAOP reflects blood in the left ventricle at end-diastole (LVEDP). The normal PAOP waveform is a left atrial waveform, as shown in waveform **E**.	
	If a patient has mitral valve regurgitation, the *v* waves are larger than normal, increasing PAOP and possibly not reflecting true LVEDP, as shown in waveform **F**. PAOP is elevated in many cardiac disease states in which LV function is compromised. PAOP is low in hypovolemic states.	

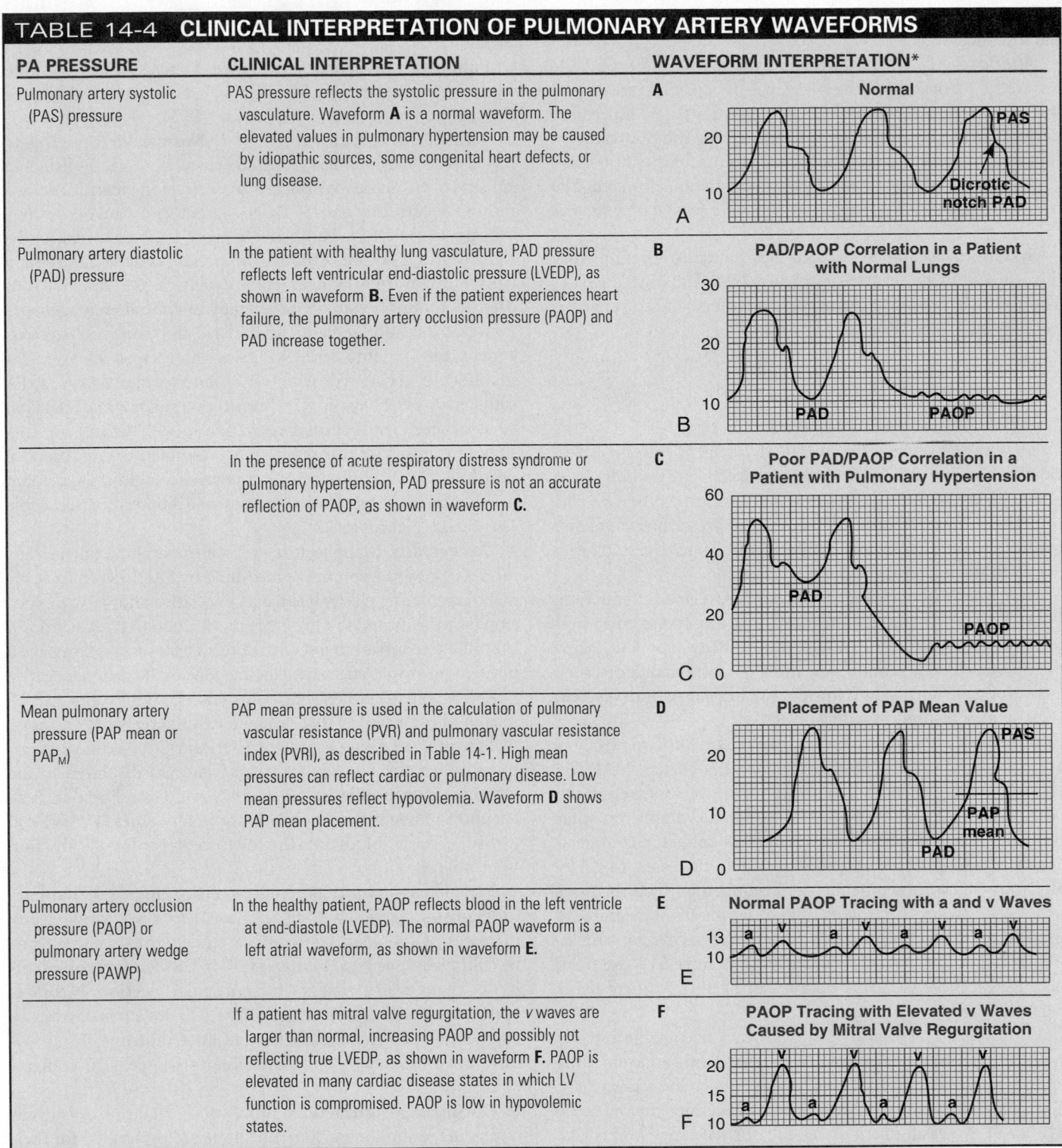

*Pressures on the *y* axis are given in millimeters of mercury (mm Hg).

Mitral Regurgitation. In patients with mitral regurgitation (MR), the mean PAOP reading is artificially elevated because of abnormal backflow of blood from the left ventricle to the left atrium during systole. This PAOP reading is distinguished by very large *v* waves on the PAOP (wedge) tracing and may not reflect the true LVEDP (see Table 14-4, illustration F).

The *v* waves can be dramatically large in some patients. The size of the *v* wave is related to the amount of MR and to the compliance of the left atrium.[40] If the MR is chronic and the left atrium is compliant and can stretch, the *v* waves may be small. In the setting of acute MR after infarction of a papillary muscle, the noncompliant or stiff atrium contributes to the development of large *v* waves. Reading the PAOP tracing in the presence of MR is difficult. If the *v* waves are large (acute MR), they cannot be used to estimate LV preload. If the *v* wave is small (chronic MR), the mean PAOP or LAP can still estimate

LV preload (LVEDP). Echocardiography also is used to confirm the presence of MR.[41]

Afterload. *Afterload* is defined as the pressure the ventricle generates to overcome the resistance to ejection created by the arteries and arterioles. It is a calculated measurement derived from information obtained from the PA catheter. As a response to increased afterload, ventricular wall tension rises. After a decrease in afterload, wall tension is lowered. The technical name for afterload is *systemic vascular resistance* (SVR).

Systemic Vascular Resistance. Resistance to ejection from the left side of the heart is estimated by calculating the SVR. The formula, normally calculated by the bedside computer, is as follows:

$$SVR = \frac{MAP - CVP}{CO} \times 80$$

The normal value is 800 to 1200 dyn·sec·cm^{-5}. To index this value to the patient's body surface area, the cardiac index (CI) is placed in the formula in the same position as the CO. The critical care nurse frequently manipulates prescribed vasoactive medications to therapeutically alter SVR. In general, the lower the SVR, the higher the CO.

Systemic Vascular Resistance and Afterload Reduction. Pharmacologic manipulation of SVR to improve cardiac performance is commonly used with the critically ill patient. When the SVR is elevated, continuous infusions of vasodilators, such as sodium nitroprusside (Nipride), or high-dose nitroglycerin (NTG), may be used to reduce SVR.

If the SVR is extremely low (e.g., less than 500 dyn·sec·cm^{-5}), as may occur in sepsis, the CO will be elevated, and MAP will be low. In this situation, volume and vasopressors are infused to increase MAP and the SVR. After adequate volume resuscitation, the Surviving Sepsis Campaign guidelines recommend centrally administered dopamine, which increases MAP by affecting CO, or norepinephrine (Levophed), which increases MAP by vasoconstriction of the peripheral vasculature to increase SVR.[42] Frequent assessment of the peripheral circulation is required when medications that increase SVR are used, because excessive vasoconstriction can negatively affect tissue perfusion.

One case can serve as an example. Mr. T had a large anterior wall MI 2 days ago. As a result, he has symptoms of acute heart failure, an elevated SVR of 1840 dyn·sec·cm^{-5}, and a low CO of 2.8 L/min. In a heart with decreased contractility after an acute MI, an SVR measurement above the normal range lowers CO. To optimize Mr. T's cardiac function, systemic vasodilators (afterload-reducing medications) are infused to lower the SVR into the normal range. After the administration of sodium nitroprusside (1 to 4 mcg/kg/min), Mr. T's SVR decreased to 970 dyn·sec·cm^{-5}, and his CO increased to 4.1 L/min. In this situation, decreasing the SVR greatly increased the amount of blood ejected from the left ventricle.

For a person with a normal heart without cardiac dysfunction, an elevated SVR may have minimal impact on CO. In summary, the importance of SVR on CO is related to the functional quality of the myocardium. Whether the heart muscle is globally damaged (cardiomyopathy) or regionally damaged (MI), small changes in SVR can produce significant changes in CO.

Pulmonary Vascular Resistance. Resistance to ejection from the right side of the heart is estimated by calculating the pulmonary vascular resistance (PVR). The PVR value is normally one sixth of the SVR. Normal PVR is 100 to 250 dyn·sec·cm^{-5}. The formula to calculate PVR is listed in Appendix B. Acute pulmonary hypertension, identified as a mean PA pressure greater than 25 mm Hg, can occur as a sequela of ARDS.[43] The acute rise in PVR may cause the right ventricle to fail, although LV pressures generally remain within the normal range. Traditionally, a PA catheter was used to monitor vasodilator therapy and fluid management. However, because research trials have not shown a survival benefit for patients with ARDS who received invasive PA monitoring compared with CVP monitoring, today, a PA catheter is rarely used.[28,29] Chronic pulmonary hypertension is associated with chronic elevation of PVR, and in that situation infusions of pulmonary vasodilators are used to decrease PVR.[44] A discussion of pharmacologic management of pulmonary hypertension occurs in Chapter 15; see Table 15-12 and Figure 15-22.

Contractility. Many factors have an impact on contractility, including preload volume as measured by PAOP, SVR, myocardial oxygenation, electrolyte balance, positive and negative inotropic medications, and the amount of functional myocardium available to contribute to contraction. These factors can have a positive inotropic effect, enhancing contractility, or a negative inotropic effect, decreasing contractility. Significant factors related to contractility that can be measured by the PA catheter include preload filling pressures, SVR, and CO. Additional contractility numbers can be calculated and are displayed in the hemodynamic profile on the bedside monitor. These include left and right ventricular stroke work index values (LVSWI and RVSWI). These values estimate the force of cardiac contraction (see Table 14-1).

Preload has an impact on contractility by means of Starling's mechanism. As volume in the ventricle rises, contractility increases. If the ventricle is overdistended with volume, contractility falls (see Figs. 14-15 and 14-16). SVR alters contractility by changes in resistance to ventricular ejection. If SVR is high, contractility is decreased. If SVR is low, contractility is augmented. Hypoxemia acts as a negative inotrope. The myocardium must have oxygen available to the cells to contract efficiently.

Optimizing Contractility. Intravenous medications such as dopamine, dobutamine, and milrinone are prescribed for their positive inotropic effect. The nurse considers the impact of these pharmacologic agents on contractility when following the trend of the patient's hemodynamic profile. No single hemodynamic number reflects contractility. However, if LV contractility is increased in response to treatment, this effect is frequently reflected by changes in PAOP (wedge pressure) and by an increase in CO and LVSWI.

Pulmonary Artery Catheters

The traditional PA catheter, invented by Swan and Ganz, has four lumens for measurement of right atrial pressure (RAP) or

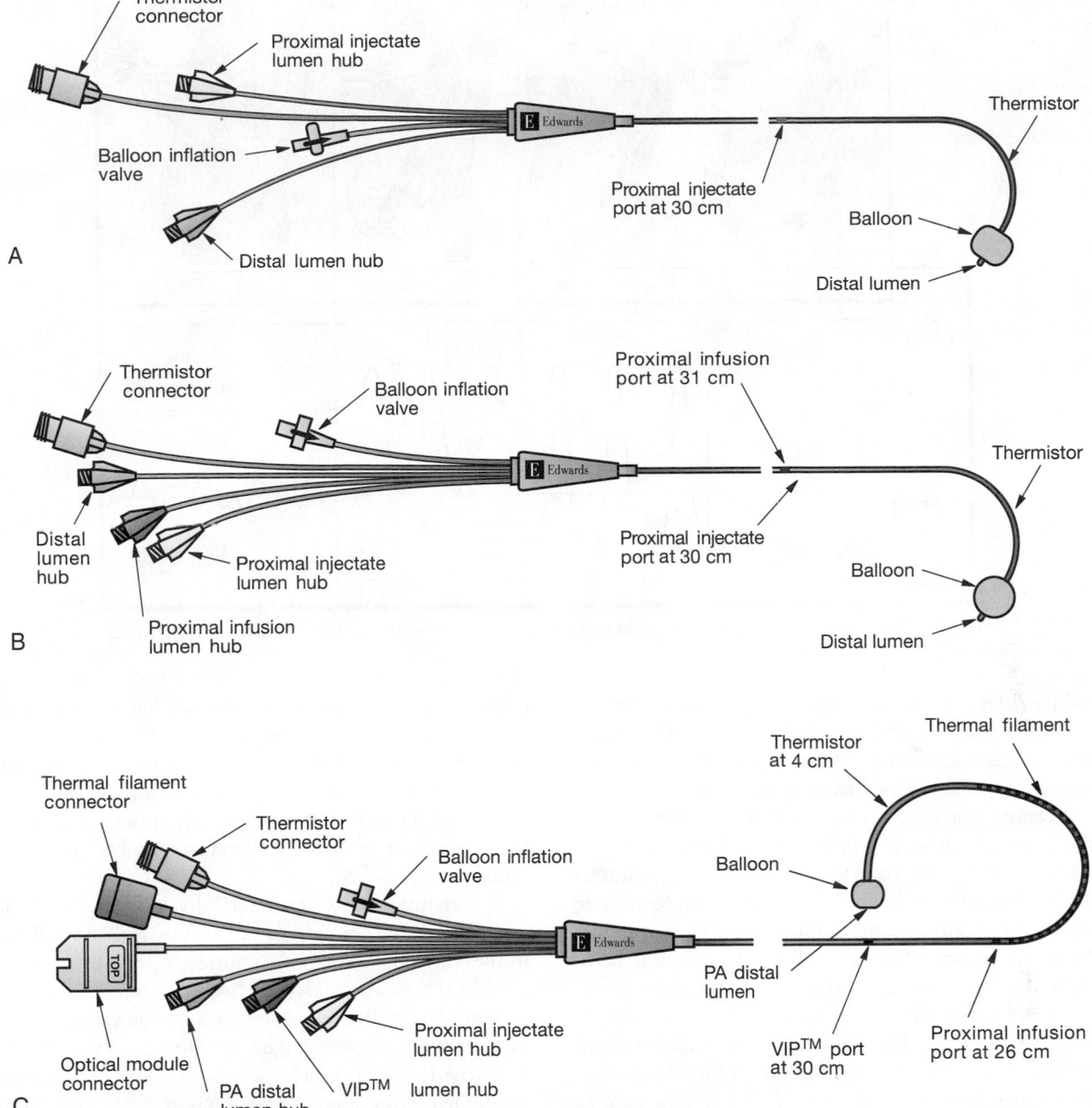

FIGURE 14-17   Types of Pulmonary Artery Catheters. *A,* Four-lumen catheter. *B,* Five-lumen catheter that includes an additional venous infusion port (VIP) into the right atrium. *C,* Seven-lumen catheter that includes a VIP port and two additional lumens, as well as a thermal filament, for continuous cardiac output (CCO) and internal fiber-optic strands for continuous mixed venous oxygen saturation (SvO$_2$) monitoring (i.e., optical module connector). An additional option is to combine the use of the CCO filament and the thermistor response time to calculate continuous right ventricular end-diastolic volume (RECEDV) and right ventricular ejection fraction (RVEF). (Copyright 2001 Edwards Lifesciences LLC. All rights reserved. Reprinted with permission of Edwards Lifesciences, Swan-Ganz is a trademark of Edwards Lifesciences Corporation, registered in the U.S. Patent and Trademark Office.)

CVP, PA pressures, PAOP, and CO (Fig. 14-17A). Multifunction catheters may have additional lumens, which can be used for intravenous infusion (Fig. 14-17B) and to measure continuous SvO$_2$, right ventricular volume, and continuous CO (Fig. 14-17C). Other PA catheters include transvenous pacing electrodes to pace the heart if needed.

The PA flow directed catheter is 110 cm long. The most commonly used size is 7.5 or 8.0 Fr, although 5.0 and 7.0 Fr sizes are available. Each of the four lumens exits into the heart or PA at a different point, graduated along the catheter length (see Fig. 14-17A).

Right Atrial Lumen. The proximal lumen is situated in the right atrium and is used for intravenous infusion, CVP measurement, withdrawal of venous blood samples, and injection of fluid for CO determinations. This port is often described as the *right atrial port,* also called the *CVP port.*

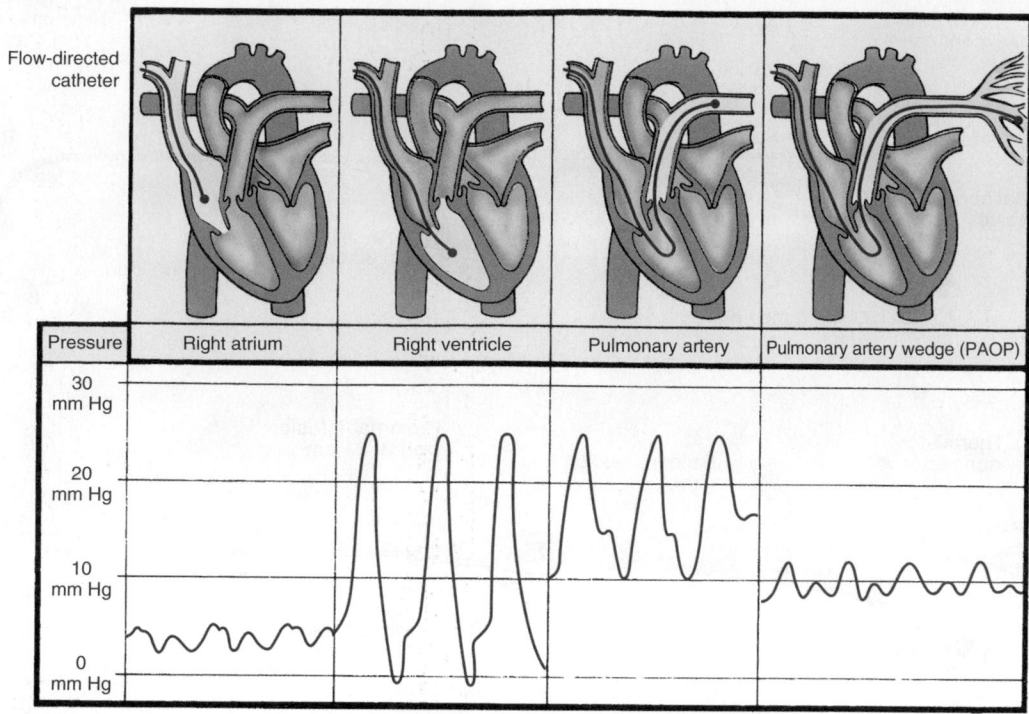

FIGURE 14-18 Pulmonary Artery (PA) Catheter Insertion with Corresponding Waveforms.

Pulmonary Artery Lumen. The distal PA lumen is located at the tip of the PA catheter and is situated in the PA. It is used to record PAPs and can be used for withdrawal of blood samples to measure mixed venous blood gases (e.g., Svo_2).

Balloon Lumen. The third lumen opens into a balloon at the end of the catheter that can be inflated with 0.8 mL (7 Fr) to 1.5 mL (7.5 Fr) of air. The balloon is inflated during catheter insertion after the catheter reaches the right atrium to assist in forward flow of the catheter and to minimize right ventricular ectopy from the catheter tip. The balloon is also inflated to obtain the PAOP measurements when the PA catheter is correctly positioned in the PA.

Thermistor Lumen. The fourth lumen is a thermistor (temperature sensor) used to measure changes in blood temperature. It is located 4 cm from the catheter tip and is used to measure thermodilution CO. The connector end of the lumen is attached directly to the CO computer.

Additional Features. If continuous Svo_2 is measured, the catheter has an additional fiberoptic lumen that exits at the tip of the catheter (see Fig. 14-17C). If cardiac pacing is used, two PA catheter methods are available. One type of catheter has three atrial (A) and two ventricular (V) pacing electrodes attached to the catheter so that when it is properly positioned, the patient can be connected to a pacemaker and be AV paced. The other catheter method uses a specific transvenous pacing wire that is passed through an additional catheter lumen and exits into the right ventricle if ventricular pacing is required. A right ventricular volumetric PA catheter is available that measures SV in the right ventricle.

Insertion

If a PA catheter is to be inserted into a patient who is awake, some brief explanations about the procedure are helpful to ensure that the patient understands what is going to happen. The initial insertion techniques used for placement of a PA catheter are similar to those described for CVC insertion. Because the PA catheter is positioned within the heart chambers and PA on the right side of the heart, catheter passage is monitored using fluoroscopy or waveform analysis on the bedside monitor (Fig. 14-18).

Before inserting the catheter into the vein, the physician—using sterile technique—tests the balloon for inflation and flushes the catheter with NS solution to remove any air. The PA catheter is then attached to the bedside hemodynamic line setup and monitor so that the waveforms can be visualized while the catheter is advanced through the right side of the heart (see Fig. 14-18). A larger introducer sheath (8.5 Fr)—which has the tip positioned in the vena cava and has an additional intravenous side-port lumen—is often used to cannulate the vein first. This introducer sheath is known by several different names in clinical practice, including *sheath, cordis, introducer,* or *side port.* This introducer sheath remains in place, and the supple PA catheter is threaded through it into the vena cava and into the right side of the heart.

Pulmonary Artery Waveform Interpretation

Each chamber of the heart has a distinctive waveform with recognizable characteristics. It is the responsibility of the critical care nurse to recognize each waveform displayed on the bedside monitor when the catheter enters the corresponding chamber during insertion and during routine monitoring.

Right Atrial Waveform. As the PA catheter is advanced into the right atrium during insertion, a right atrial waveform must be visible on the monitor, with recognizable *a, c,* and *v* waves (see Fig. 14-18). The normal mean pressure in the right atrium is 2 to 5 mm Hg. Before passage through the tricuspid valve, the balloon at the tip of the catheter is inflated for two reasons. First, it cushions the pointed tip of the PA catheter so that if the tip comes into contact with the right ventricular wall, it will cause less myocardial irritability and, consequently, fewer ventricular dysrhythmias. Second, inflation of the balloon assists the catheter to float with the flow of blood from the right ventricle into the PA. It is because of these features and the balloon that PA catheters are described as *flow-directional catheters.*

Right Ventricular Waveform. The right ventricular waveform is distinctly pulsatile, with distinct systolic and diastolic pressures. Normal right ventricular pressures are 20 to 30 mm Hg systolic and 0 to 5 mm Hg diastolic. Even with the balloon inflated, it is not uncommon for ventricular ectopy to occur during passage through the right ventricle. All patients who have a PA catheter inserted must have simultaneous ECG monitoring, with defibrillator and emergency resuscitation equipment nearby.

Pulmonary Artery Waveform. As the catheter enters the PA, the waveform again changes. The diastolic pressure rises. Normal PA pressures range from 20 to 30 mm Hg systolic over 10 mm Hg diastolic. A dicrotic notch, visible on the downslope of the waveform, represents closure of the pulmonic valve.

Pulmonary Artery Occlusion Waveform (Wedge). While the balloon remains inflated, the catheter is advanced into the wedge position. This maneuver produces the PAOP. The waveform decreases in size and is nonpulsatile, reflecting a normal left atrial tracing with *a* and *v* wave deflections. This is known as a *wedge tracing,* because the balloon is "wedged" into a small pulmonary vessel, but it is technically described as the PAOP (see Fig. 14-18). The balloon occludes the pulmonary vessel so that the PA catheter tip and lumen are exposed only to left atrial pressure (LAP) and are protected from the pulsatile influence of the right ventricle and PA. When the balloon is deflated, the catheter should spontaneously float back into the PA. When the balloon is reinflated, the wedge tracing should be visible. The normal PAOP ranges from 5 to 12 mm Hg.

After insertion, the introducer is sutured to the skin, the catheter, which lies within the introducer, is secured with tape or with a specialized catheter securement device. A chest radiograph is taken to verify placement. If the catheter is advanced too far into the pulmonary bed, the patient is at risk for pulmonary infarction. If the PA catheter is not sufficiently advanced into the PA, it will not be useful for PAOP readings. However, in many critical care units, if the patient's PADP and PAOP values approximate (within 0 to 3 mm Hg), the PADP is reliably used to follow the trend of LV filling pressure (preload). This prevents possible trauma from frequent balloon inflation; in such a situation, the PA catheter is consciously pulled back into a nonwedging position in the PA.

After insertion of the catheter, the chest radiograph or fluoroscopy is used to verify the PA catheter position to make sure that it is not looped or knotted in the right ventricle and to rule out pneumothorax or hemorrhagic complications. A thin plastic sleeve is placed on the outside of the catheter when it is inserted to maintain sterility of the part of the PA catheter that exits from the patient. If the PA catheter is not in the desired position or if it migrates out of position, it can be repositioned. Use of this external sleeve on PA catheters has been associated with lower rates of bloodstream infection.[4]

Medical Management

Controversy exists in the medical community over the use of PA catheters and rates of use have declined in response to lack of benefit demonstrated in clinical trials. Medical goals of hemodynamic monitoring include assessment of adequacy of perfusion in stable patients, early detection of decreased perfusion, titration of therapy to meet specific therapeutic outcomes, and differentiation of different organ system dysfunctions. Practice guidelines are available for physicians who routinely work with PA catheters.[45]

Nursing Management

The more knowledgeable the critical care nurse can become about use of the PA catheter, the more accurate and effective the nursing management interventions will be.[5] Factors that affect PA measurement are the head-of-bed backrest position and lateral body position relative to transducer height placement, respiratory variation, and use of positive end-expiratory pressure (PEEP).

Patient Position. The patient does not need to be flat for accurate pressure readings to be obtained. In the supine position, when the transducer is placed at the level of the phlebostatic axis, a head-of-bed position from flat up to 60 degrees is appropriate for most patients.[5] It is important to know that PADP and PAOP measurements in the lateral position may be significantly different from those taken when the patient is lying supine. If there is concern about the validity of pressure readings in a particular patient, it is more reliable to take measurements with the patient on his or her back, with the head of bed elevated from flat to 60 degrees as tolerated. After a patient changes position, a stabilization period of 5 to 15 minutes is recommended before taking pressure readings.[5] The stabilization period is usually longer if the patient has LV dysfunction or is hemodynamically unstable.

Respiratory Variation. All PADP and PAOP (wedge) tracings are subject to respiratory interference, especially when the patient is on a positive-pressure, volume-cycled ventilator.[5] During the positive-pressure inhalation phase, the increase in intrathoracic pressure may "push up" the PA tracing, producing an artificially high reading (Fig. 14-19A). During inhalation with spontaneous breaths, negative intrathoracic pressure "pulls down" the waveform, producing an erroneously low measurement (see Fig. 14-19B). To minimize the impact of respiratory variation, the PADP is read at end-expiration, which is the most stable point in the respiratory cycle when intrapleural pressures are close to zero. If the digital number fluctuates with respiration, a printed readout on paper can be obtained to verify true PADP. In some clinical settings, ECG signals or airway pressure and flow are recorded simultaneously with the PADP/PAOP tracing to identify end-expiration.[5]

Positive End-Expiratory Pressure. Some clinical diagnoses, such as ARDS, require the use of high levels of PEEP set with the ventilator to treat refractory hypoxemia. If a PEEP of greater than 10 cm H_2O is used, PAOP (wedge) and PAPs will be artificially elevated, and CO may be negatively affected. Because of

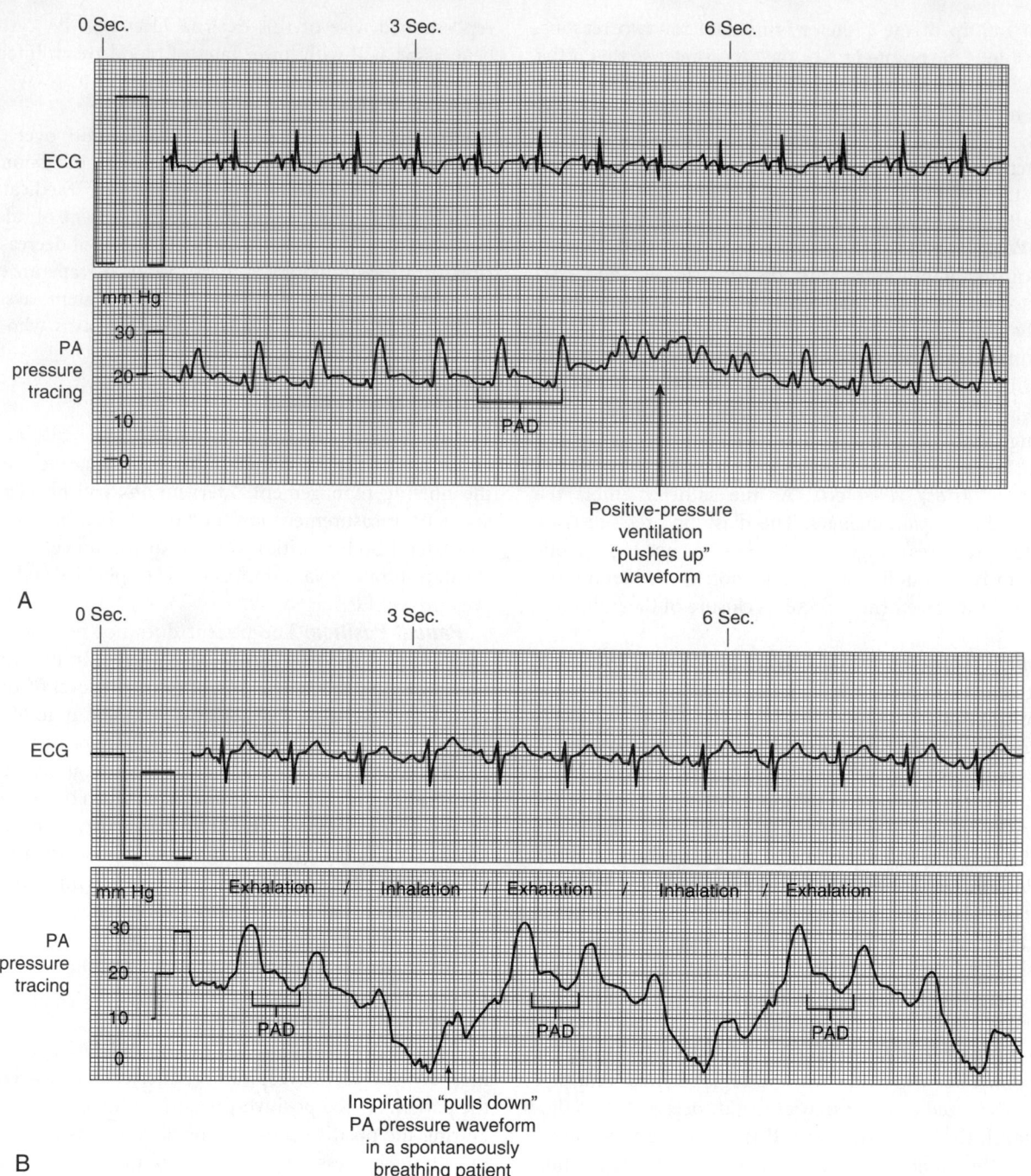

FIGURE 14-19 Pulmonary artery (PA) waveforms that demonstrate the impact of ventilation on PA pressure readings. For accuracy, PA pressures are read at the end of exhalation. *A,* In positive-pressure ventilation, the increase in intrathoracic pressure during inhalation "pushes up" the PA pressure waveform, creating a falsely high reading. *B,* In spontaneous breathing, the decrease in intrathoracic pressure during normal inhalation "pulls down" the PA waveform, creating a falsely low reading.

this impact of PEEP, in the past, patients in some critical care units were taken off the ventilator to record PAP measurements. It has since been shown that this practice closes alveoli, decreases the patient's oxygenation level, and may result in persistent hypoxemia.

Because patients remain on PEEP for treatment, they remain on it during measurement of PAPs. In this situation, the trend of PA readings is more important than one individual measurement. The most important factor is not one individual measurement or the absolute number obtained; it is instead the trend of the measurements being used as a basis for clinical interventions to support and improve cardiopulmonary function in the critically ill.

Avoiding Complications. Potential cardiac complications include ventricular dysrhythmias, endocarditis, valvular damage, cardiac rupture, and cardiac tamponade. Potential pulmonary complications include rupture of a PA, PA thrombosis, embolism or hemorrhage, and infarction of a segment of lung.

The PA catheter tracing is continuously monitored to ensure that the catheter does not migrate forward into a spontaneous wedge or PAOP position. A segment of lung can suffer infarction if the wedged catheter occludes an arteriole for a prolonged period. If the catheter is spontaneously wedged the catheter must be gently pulled back out of the wedge position to prevent pulmonary infarction.

Infection is always a risk with a PA catheter. The risks are similar to those discussed in the section on CVCs (see Box 14-3).

Pulmonary Artery Catheter Removal. PA catheters can be safely removed from the patient by critical care nurses competent in this procedure.[5,46] Removal is not usually associated with major complications. Sometimes there are PVCs as the catheter is pulled through the right ventricle.[5]

Cardiac Output Measurement

The PA catheter measures CO using an intermittent (bolus) or a continuous CO method.

Thermodilution Cardiac Output Bolus Method. The bolus thermodilution method is performed at the bedside and results in CO calculated in liters per minute. Three CO values that are within a 10% mean range are obtained at one time and are averaged to calculate CO. A known amount (5 mL) of iced or, more typically, 10 mL of room-temperature NS solution is injected into the proximal lumen of the PA catheter. The injectate exits into the right atrium and travels with the flow of blood past the thermistor (temperature sensor) located at the distal end of the catheter in the PA. The injectate can be delivered by hand injection using individual syringes of saline. Frequently, a closed in-line system attached to a 500-mL bag of NS is used as a reservoir to deliver the individual injections.

Sometimes, the right atrial (proximal) port is clotted and not usable. If another right atrial port is available, it can be substituted. However, if a usable port is not available, to ensure accurate CO data, a new PA catheter is inserted.

Cardiac Output Curve. The thermodilution CO method uses the indicator-dilution method, in which a known temperature is the indicator. It is based on the principle that the change in temperature over time is inversely proportional to blood flow. Blood flow can be diagrammatically represented as a CO curve on which temperature is plotted against time (Fig. 14-20A). Most hemodynamic monitors display this CO curve, which must then be interpreted to determine whether the CO injection is valid. The normal curve has a smooth upstroke, with a

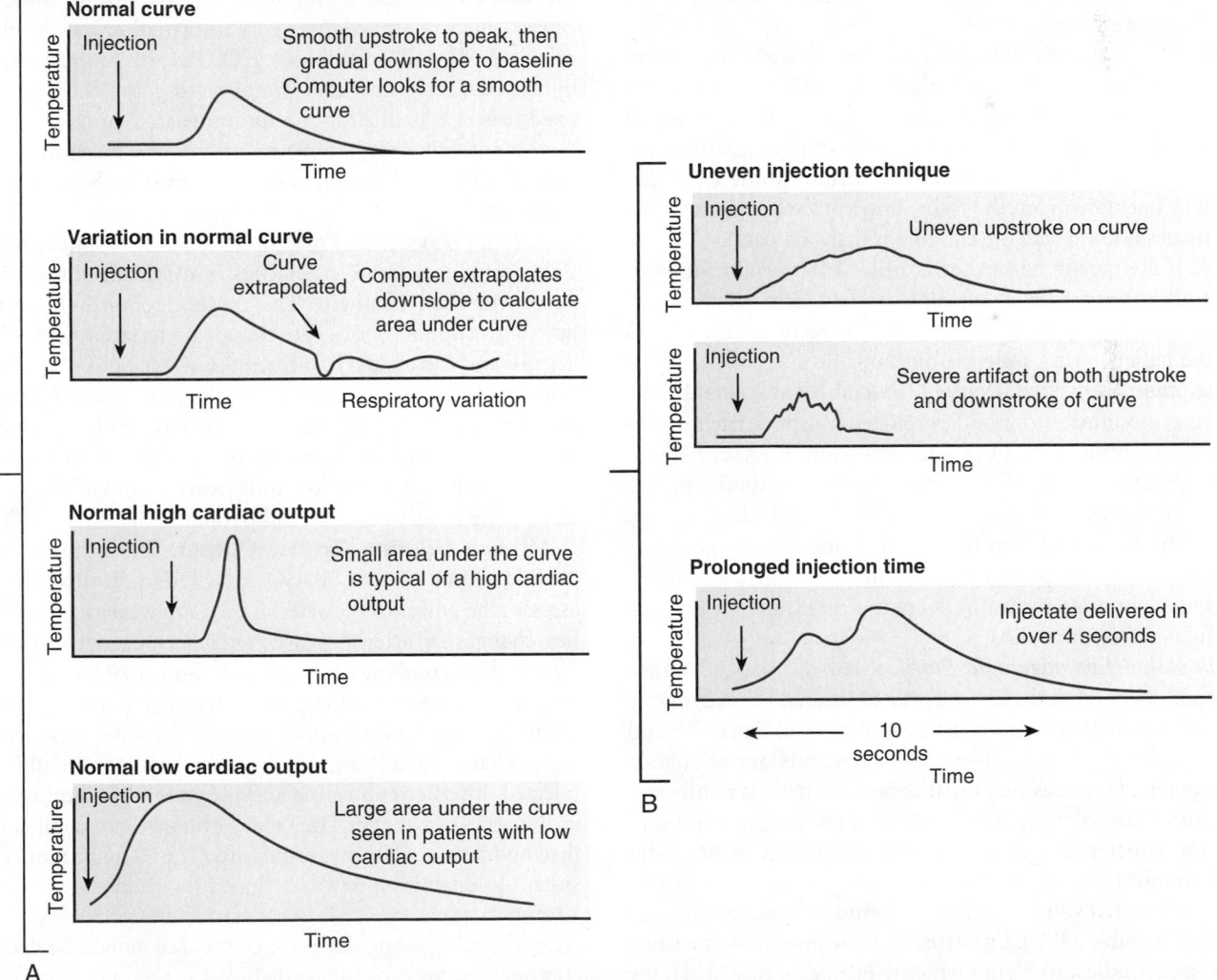

FIGURE 14-20 *A,* Variations in the normal cardiac thermodilution bolus output curve. *B,* Abnormal cardiac output (CO) curves produce an erroneous CO value.

rounded peak and a gradually tapering down-slope. If the curve has an uneven pattern, it may indicate faulty injection technique, and the CO measurement must be repeated. Patient movement or coughing also alters the CO measurement (see Fig. 14-20B).

Injectate Temperature. If the CO is within the normal range, it is equally accurate whether iced or room temperature injectate is used. However, if the COs are extremely high or very low, iced injectate may be more accurate. To ensure accurate readings, the difference between injectate temperature and body temperature must be at least 10° C, and the injectate must be delivered within 4 seconds, with minimal handling of the syringe to prevent warming of the solution. This is particularly important if iced injectate is used. With all delivery systems, the injectate is delivered at the same point in the respiratory cycle, usually end-exhalation.

Patient Position and Cardiac Output. In the normovolemic, stable patient, reliable CO measurements can be obtained in a supine position (patient lying on his or her back) with the head of the bed elevated up to 60 degrees.[5] If the patient is hypovolemic or unstable, leaving the head of the bed in a flat position or only slightly elevated is the most clinically appropriate choice. CO measurements performed when the patient is turned to the side are not considered as accurate as those performed with the patient in the supine position.

Clinical Conditions That Alter Cardiac Output. Two clinical conditions produce errors in the thermodilution CO measurement: tricuspid valve regurgitation and ventricular septal rupture. If the patient has tricuspid valve regurgitation, the expected flow of blood from the right atrium to the PA is disrupted by backflow from the right ventricle to the right atrium. This creates a lower CO measurement than the patient's actual output. If the person has an intracardiac left-to-right shunt, as occurs after ventricular septal rupture, the thermodilution CO measures the large pulmonary volume and records a higher CO than the patient's true systemic output.

Continuous Invasive Cardiac Output Measurement. The bolus thermodilution method is reliable but performed intermittently. Continuous CO monitoring using a PA catheter is also frequently used in clinical practice. One method employs a thermal filament on the PA catheter to emit small energy signals (the indicator) into the bloodstream. These signals are then detected by the thermistor near the tip of the PA catheter. The equivalent of an indicator curve is created, and a CO value is calculated from this data.

Calculated Hemodynamic Profiles. For the patient with a thermodilution PA catheter in place, additional hemodynamic information can be calculated using routine vital signs, CO, and body surface area (BSA). These measurements are calculated using specific formulas that are indexed to a patient's body size using the DuBois body area surface chart or the computer program associated with the current generation of hemodynamic monitors.

The calculated values used in the hemodynamic profiles are described in Table 14-1. Clinical use of these profiles is described in two case studies. In Hemodynamic Profile 1 (Box 14-4), the example is a step-by-step interpretation of the hemodynamic profile to familiarize the reader with use of calculated values. In

Hemodynamic Profile 2 (Box 14-5), the example uses only values indexed to body weight and illustrates the impact of treatment on these values over time.

Noninvasive and Minimally Invasive Measurement of Cardiac Output

As a result of the perceived risks associated with use of the PA catheter, combined with studies that have not shown improved outcomes with routine monitoring, there is tremendous interest in finding less invasive methods of CO measurement. Noninvasive methods include echocardiography or bioimpedance. Minimally invasive techniques can involve vascular catheters or esophageal probes as described in Table 14-5. All have been compared with the PA catheter thermodilution CO method.

Thoracic Electrical Bioimpedance. Thoracic electrical bioimpedance is a noninvasive method of continuous CO measurement. Impedance cardiography works by emitting a low-voltage, high-frequency, alternating electrical current through the thorax by means of four skin electrodes. Two are placed at the base of the neck under the ear and two are placed at the side of the chest in the midaxillary line at the midxyphoid level.[47] The sensing electrodes detect changes in electrical impedance within the thorax. Because blood flow through the thoracic aorta causes shifts in impedance, this information can be used to calculate SV and continuous CO. Use of thoracic electrical bioimpedance in the in-hospital setting is uncommon. One cited reason is that, although bioimpedance provides information about CO, it does not provide other clinical information such as cardiac filling pressures that may be helpful to guide treatment.[48]

Arterial Waveform - Pulse Contour Cardiac Output Methods. Pulse contour waveform analysis is minimally invasive compared with the PA catheter. This method requires the patient to have a functional venous catheter and arterial catheter in place. The SV and CO are derived from the arterial waveform or *pulse contour*. A significant advantage of the pulse contour waveform method is that the patient does not have to be intubated or sedated to tolerate the monitoring system. Three commercial systems that use pulse contour waveform technology have undergone trials in critically ill patients.

Lithium Dilution Cardiac Output. The lithium dilution cardiac output system (LiDCO, LiDCO Ltd., United Kingdom) assesses the power of the arterial pressure waveform and identifies changes in arterial power to reflect changes in SV. The *LiDCO Plus* combines two systems: an initial calibration and ongoing assessment of the pulse waveform guided by a proprietary algorithm. To obtain an accurate baseline measure of SV and CO for calibration, a subtherapeutic dose of lithium is injected into the venous line and measured by a lithium sensor in the arterial catheter. The values obtained are comparable to thermodilution CO measurements.[49-51] Recalibration of the system to establish a new baseline is required about every 4 to 8 hours.[52]

A second system, the *LiDCO rapid*, a noncalibrated pulse contour system, is also available. In general, noncalibrated systems are reported to have lower levels of CO accuracy when compared with bolus thermodilution CO.[53]

BOX 14-4 HEMODYNAMIC PROFILE 1

Admission

Mr. SR has a medical history of cardiomyopathy and chronic obstructive pulmonary disease (COPD). He is admitted to a coronary care unit because of an exacerbation of his biventricular heart failure. He has been complaining about anginal pain and shortness of breath. His nursing diagnoses are Decreased Cardiac Output and Impaired Gas Exchange.

Height	163 cm	PAD	27 mm Hg	PVR	322 dyn·sec·cm^{-5}
Weight	79 kg	PAP$_M$	36 mm Hg	PVRI	612 dyn·sec·cm^{-5}/m^2
Body surface area (BSA)	1.9 m^2	PAOP	26 mm Hg	LCW	2.1 kg-m
		CVP	24 mm Hg	LCWI	1.1 kg-m/m^2
HR	104 beats/min	CO	2.48 L/min	LVSW	2.4 g-m
ABP		CI	1.31 L/min/m^2	LVSWI	10.7 g-m/m^2
Systolic	88 mm Hg	SV	23.8 mL	RCW	1.21 kg-m
Diastolic	51 mm Hg	SI	12.5 mL/m^2	RCWI	0.64 kg-m/m^2
MAP	63 mm Hg	SVR	1257 dyn·sec·cm^{-5}	RVSW	11.7 g-m
PAS	55 mm Hg	SVRI	2388 dyn·sec·cm^{-5}/m^2	RVSWI	6.2 g-m/m^2

Analysis of the Hemodynamic Profile*

PROFILE	ANALYSIS
HR (heart rate)	HR of 104 beats/min is above normal limits (normal, 60-100 beats/min).
ABP (arterial blood pressure)	Narrow pulse pressure of 88/51 mm Hg with a low mean arterial pressure (MAP) of 63 mm Hg (normal MAP, 65-90 mm Hg).
PAP (pulmonary artery pressure)	Pulmonary artery pressures are elevated (55/27 mm Hg), consistent with diagnosis of cardiomyopathy, failure of left side of heart, and COPD (normal PAP, 25/10 mm Hg).
PAOP (pulmonary artery occlusion pressure)	Elevated PAOP (26 mm Hg), consistent with diagnosis of cardiomyopathy and failure of left side of heart (normal PAOP, 5-12 mm Hg).
CVP (central venous pressure)	Elevated CVP (24 mm Hg), consistent with diagnosis of cardiomyopathy, failure of right side of heart, and COPD (normal CVP, 4-6 mm Hg).
CO (cardiac output) and CI (cardiac index)	Poor CO and CI (CO, 2.48 L/min; CI, 1.31 L/min/m^2). Both values are below normal (normal CO, 4-6 L/min; normal CI, 2.2-4 L/min/m^2).
SV (stroke volume) and SI (stroke volume index)	SV and SI are low (SV, 23.8 mL; SI, 12.5 mL/m^2). These results would be anticipated from the low CO (normal SV, 60-70 mL; normal SI, 40-50 mL/min/m^2).
SVR (systemic vascular resistance) and SVRI (systemic vascular resistance index)	SVR and SVRI are at the upper normal range (SVR, 1257 dyn·sec·cm^{-5}; SVRI, 2388 dyn·sec·cm^{-5}/m^2). These values are not contributing to the low CO at this time (normal SVR, 800-1400 dyn·sec·cm^{-5}; normal SVRI, 2000-2400 dyn·sec·cm^{-5}/m^2).
PVR (pulmonary vascular resistance) and PVRI (pulmonary vascular resistance index)	PVR and PVRI are elevated (PVR, 322 dyn·sec·cm^{-5}; PVRI 612 dyn·sec·cm^{-5}/m^2). High PVR may be contributing to the low CO (normal PVR, 100-250 dyn·sec·cm^{-5}; normal PVRI, 225-315 dyn·sec·cm^{-5}/m^2).
LCWI (left cardiac work index) and LVSWI (left ventricular stroke work index)	Both LCWI and LVSWI are below normal (LCWI, 1.1 kg-m/m^2; LVSWI, 10.7 g-m/m^2), indicating that left ventricular myocardial damage may be present. This is consistent with Mr. SR's diagnosis of cardiomyopathy (normal LCWI, 3.4-4.2 kg-m/m^2; normal LVSWI, 50-62 g-m/m^2).
RCWI (right cardiac work index) and RVSWI (right ventricular stroke work index)	RCWI is normal, but RVSWI is below normal (RCWI, 0.64 kg-m/m^2; RVSWI, 6.2 g-m/m^2), indicating that right ventricular myocardial damage may be present. This is consistent with Mr. SR's diagnosis of cardiomyopathy and history of COPD (normal RCWI, 0.54-0.66 kg-m/m^2, normal RVSWI, 7.9-9.7, g-m/m^2).
Nursing impression	The hemodynamic data confirm the nursing clinical diagnosis of poor CO. The goal is to improve CO within the limits of Mr. SR's myocardial dysfunction and COPD. As CO improves and PA pressures decrease, the patient will have less pulmonary congestion, which will improve alveolar gas exchange.

*Formulas and normal values for the hemodynamics values are given in Table 14-1 and in Appendix B.

Pulse Index Contour Cardiac Output. The pulse index contour cardiac output system (PiCCO$_2$) (Pulsion Medical Systems, Germany) obtains CO by two methods, the *transpulmonary CO* (baseline) and a continuous CO measurement obtained by analyzing the systolic component of the arterial waveform.[54,55] Three calibrations using cold saline are required at initial setup (venous injections with arterial sensor). The venous injection can be delivered from jugular or femoral venous access. The transit time is longer from the femoral artery, which causes a systematic overestimate of the CO, but once recognized, this can be accounted for by following the trend of measurements.[56] The manufacturer recommends recalibration every 8 hours, although researchers reported that recalibration is required every 4 to 6 hours or even hourly to maintain accurate CO readings.[57-59]

The PiCCO system also monitors other clinically relevant variables that offer additional information to guide management in critical illness. The *extravascular lung water* (EVLW) index measures the volume of lung water in lung tissue and is a marker of pulmonary edema.[55] Lung water content increases in conditions such as heart failure, pneumonia, and sepsis and higher lung water content is associated with higher mortality. Knowledge of EVLW may influence whether to administer diuretics or volume.

BOX 14-5 HEMODYNAMIC PROFILE 2

1. Admission

Mrs. JL has been admitted to the critical care unit with pulmonary edema. She has a history of anterior wall myocardial infarction and severe chronic obstructive pulmonary disease (COPD).

Height	159 cm	MAP	106 mm Hg	SI	9.9 mL/m^2
Weight	45.8 kg	PAS	53 mm Hg	SVRI	5351 dyn·sec·cm^{-5}/m^2
Body surface area (BSA)	1.40 m^2	PAD	27 mm Hg	PVRI	1046 dyn·sec·cm^{-5}/m^2
		PAP$_M$	44 mm Hg	LCWI	1.9 kg-m/m^2
HR	131 beats/min	PAOP	27 mm Hg	LVSWI	14.3 g-m/m^2
ABP		CVP	19 mm Hg	RCW	0.78 kg-m/m^2
Systolic	160 mm Hg	CO	1.82 L/min	RCWI	5.9 g-m/m^2
Diastolic	80 mm Hg	CI	1.3 L/min/m^2		

Analysis of the Hemodynamic Profile*

In the above hemodynamic profile, notice the fast HR; high MAP; high PA and CVP filling pressures; low CI, SI, LVSWI, and RVSWI; and high SVRI and PVRI. These values are consistent with a diagnosis of failure of the left side of the heart, causing pulmonary edema, which may lead to cardiogenic shock. Treatment is focused on increasing the CI by lowering SVRI and PVRI and using IV sodium nitroprusside and intravenous (IV) nitroglycerin in continuous infusion.

2. Three Hours Later

Height	159 cm	MAP	83 mm Hg	SI	16.5 mL/m^2
Weight	45.8 kg	PAS	41 mm Hg	SVRI	3088 dyn·sec·cm^{-5}/m^2
Body surface area (BSA)	1.40 m^2	PAD	26 mm Hg	PVRI	300 dyn·sec·cm^{-5}/m^2
		PAP$_M$	33 mm Hg	LCWI	2.1 kg-m/m^2
HR	113 beats/min	PAOP	26 mm Hg	LVSWI	18.6 g-m/m^2
ABP		CVP	11 mm Hg	RCWI	0.84 kg-m/m^2
Systolic	104 mm Hg	CO	2.61 L/min	RVSWI	7.4 g-m/m^2
Diastolic	69 mm Hg	CI	1.86 L/min/m^2		

Analysis of Hemodynamic Profile 2

Results 3 hours after sodium nitroprusside administration showed improving hemodynamics, demonstrated as normal MAP and lower intracardiac filling pressures (PA and CVP). However, CI and SI remain low; and SVRI is above normal. Mrs. JL remains in severe left ventricular failure because of her low CI.

3. The Next Day

Height	159 cm	MAP	77 mm Hg	SI	22.5 mL/m^2
Weight	45.8 kg	PAS	31 mm Hg	SVRI	2423 dyn·sec·cm^{-5}/m^2
Body surface area (BSA)	1.40 m^2	PAD	15 mm Hg	PVRI	273 dyn·sec·cm^{-5}/m^2
		PAP$_M$	23 mm Hg	LCWI	2.4 kg-m/m^2
HR	104 beats/min	PAOP	15 mm Hg	LVSWI	22.9 g-m/m^2
ABP		CVP	4 mm Hg	RCWI	0.74 kg-m/m^2
Systolic	111 mm Hg	CO	3.28 L/min	RVSWI	7.1 g-m/m^2
Diastolic	60 mm Hg	CI	2.34 L/min/m^2		

Analysis of Hemodynamic Profile 3

The next day, Mrs. JL's hemodynamics have improved with continued use of sodium nitroprusside and nitroglycerin. The CI value is in the low-normal range, and SVRI and PVRI values are in the high-normal range. LVSWI remains low, reflecting the patient's compromised left ventricle from a prior anterior wall myocardial infarction.

*See Box 14-4 for explanation of abbreviations and Table 14-1 and Appendix B for an explanation of hemodynamic values.

Pulse contour analysis enables the use of *stroke volume variation* (SVV) to assess volume status. SVV measures the difference between the highest and lowest SV over the previous 30 seconds. The caveat is that the patient must be mechanically ventilated and not over-breathing the ventilator. This limits SVV usefulness to anesthesia, deep sedation, or pharmacologic paralysis.[55]

Pulse Contour Cardiac Output Method. The Vigileo Monitor (Edwards Lifesciences, Irvine, CA) uses pulse contour waveform technology but does not require calibration. A specialized sensor (FloTrac sensor) added to the conventional arterial line setup assesses arterial pressure at a frequency of 100 Hz to characterize the arterial pulse waveform. This information is combined with patient variables (age, sex, weight) in a proprietary algorithm to estimate SV and CO.[57,60] The validation studies show conflicting results; some researchers reported that the system was not able to maintain accurate CO readings, and others found it tracked hemodynamic changes accurately in response to vasopressors.[57,60]

All of the pulse contour systems use different proprietary methods for the estimation of aortic impedance. For this reason, even though the mean CO values may be similar, the different methods trend CO values differently over time in response to volume and inotropic interventions.[50,61]

Esophageal Doppler Cardiac Output. The esophagus is used as the monitoring site for patients who are deeply sedated or are under general anesthesia in the operating room. The esophageal Doppler is considered less invasive than a PA

TABLE 14-5 CARDIAC OUTPUT MEASUREMENT

DEVICE NAME	PROBE PLACEMENT	METHOD	CARDIAC OUTPUT CALCULATION	CLINICAL ISSUES
Noninvasive Methods				
Bioimpedance	External electrodes placed on the neck and chest	Thoracic electric bioimpedance	1. A small alternating current is applied across the chest by skin electrodes. 2. Pulsatile changes in thoracic blood volume result in changes in electrical impedance. The rate of change of impedance during systole is measured and used to calculate CO.	Noninvasive. Less accurate with low body temperature.
Minimally Invasive Methods				
Pulse Contour Waveform Methods				
LiDCO (LiDCO Ltd., Cambridge, United Kingdom)	Requires a venous access catheter (central or peripheral) and an arterial catheter with a lithium-monitoring sensor attached	Pulse contour waveform analysis method (calibrated)	Independent calibration with a lithium dilution technique is initially required: 1. A small, subtherapeutic dose of isotonic lithium chloride is injected through the venous catheter. 2. The lithium is detected at the arterial sensor (femoral artery), where a fixed flow pump ensures constant flow. 3. A concentration-time curve is produced for lithium before recirculation. 4. CO is calculated based on the lithium dose given and the measurement of area under the curve.	Easy to set up, uses conventional venous and arterial catheters; can measure extravascular lung water for patients in pulmonary edema. CO measurement is affected by artifact on arterial waveform and by irregular and damped arterial waveforms; can be used in conscious and in unresponsive patients. Requires calibration at least every 8 hours to maintain accuracy; cannot be used in patients on lithium therapy because this interferes with the calibration.
PiCCO (Pulsion Medical Systems, Munich, Germany)	Requires a central venous access catheter and uses a specialized arterial thermistor-tipped catheter in the femoral artery	Pulse contour waveform analysis method that uses transpulmonary thermodilution	1. A set volume of cold saline is injected through the central venous catheter. The arterial thermistor-tipped catheter detects the blood temperature change. 2. Continuous CO measurements are achieved by analyzing the systolic component of the arterial waveform.	CO measurement is affected by artifact on arterial waveform and irregular arterial waveforms. Three calibrations are required initially, and frequent recalibration is required to maintain accuracy.
Vigileo (Edward Lifesciences, Irvine, Calif.)	Requires a functional arterial catheter	Pulse contour waveform analysis method (does not require calibration)	1. Calculates CO by use of the arterial pressure waveform analysis in conjunction with patient data (age, sex, height, weight). 2. Uses an internal proprietary algorithm based on the principle that pulse pressure (difference between systolic and diastolic pressure) is proportional to stroke volume (SV) and inversely proportional to aortic compliance. 3. Aortic pressure is sampled at 100 Hz and is updated every 20 seconds.	Does not require external calibration but requires zeroing of the transducer. Lack of calibration procedures is controversial.

Continued

TABLE 14-5 CARDIAC OUTPUT MEASUREMENT—cont'd

DEVICE NAME	PROBE PLACEMENT	METHOD	CARDIAC OUTPUT CALCULATION	CLINICAL ISSUES
Esophageal Probe Methods				
Esophageal Doppler	Ultrasound probe placed in the lower esophagus	SV is calculated by measurement of the aortic blood velocity in the descending thoracic aorta (by continuous wave Doppler) plus calculation of the cross-sectional area of the aorta; these values are used to calculate the CO.	1. Measurement of the aorta cross-sectional area, measured using M-mode ultrasound, and multiplying this value by blood velocity to calculate flow or CO. 2. The value of total CO is derived from a nomogram using aortic blood velocity, height, weight, and age.	Useful in the operating room or with deeply sedated patients. Probe is stiff, and placement is not well tolerated by conscious patients.
Transesophageal echocardiography (TEE)	Ultrasound probe placed in the esophagus	Probe placement allows imaging of the LV outflow tract. SV is measured by Doppler.	1. The left ventricular (LV) outflow tract area is measured; this value is squared and multiplied by the velocity time interval of blood flow and heart rate (HR). 2. LV SV can be measured, as can HR to use the SV × HR = CO formula.	Useful in the operating room or with deeply sedated patients. Probe is stiff, and placement is not well tolerated by conscious patients. Requires skill to accurately position probe to visualize the LV outflow tract.
Partial CO_2 Rebreathing Method				
$NICO_2$ (Philips, Respironics)	Addition of a partial CO_2 rebreathing circuit to ventilator	Partial CO_2 rebreathing method	CO measurement is based on changes in respiratory CO_2 concentration obtained from a short period of rebreathing. CO_2 elimination is calculated by sensors that measure flow, airway pressure, and CO_2 concentration. These variables are used in the Fick partial rebreathing formula to calculate CO.	Can be used only in intubated and ventilated patients. Specialized additional tubing setup on ventilator. Cannot be used in patients who cannot tolerate hypercapnia (elevated CO_2). CO measurement is altered by intrapulmonary shunt.

CO, Cardiac output; *CO_2*, carbon dioxide; *HR*, heart rate; *LV*, left ventricle; *SV*, stroke volume.

catheter. Insertion of the esophageal Doppler is similar to insertion of a gastric tube, although the probe is relatively inflexible and stiff.[62] The probe is inserted 35 to 40 cm from the teeth. The tip of the probe rests near T5-T6 on the vertebral column, where the esophagus typically is parallel with the descending aorta.[62] There are at least three types of esophageal Doppler monitors available, with proprietary differences in the methods of CO measurement.[63] When the probe is correctly placed, this method has a high degree of accuracy for CO measurement.[63] Accurate CO values depend on correct placement and on the skill of the operator.[64]

Partial Carbon Dioxide Rebreathing Cardiac Output. A different technology involves partial carbon dioxide (CO_2) rebreathing and uses a modified Fick principle for CO applied to CO_2. This noninvasive cardiac output (NICO) system (Novametrix Medical Systems Inc., Wallingford, CT, USA), involves the addition of an extra circuit (tubing loop) to the ventilator tubing, and it can be used only with intubated, mechanically ventilated patients. A sensor that uses infrared light absorption measures CO_2, and a second sensor measures airflow in the circuit tubing to collect data during a breathing cycle. CO_2 production is calculated as the product of minute ventilation and CO_2 concentration. Arterial CO_2 content is

derived from end-tidal CO_2 and the CO_2 dissociation curve. The differences in these values are then used to calculate the CO.[65] The validation studies have produced inconsistent results for the accuracy of the derived CO; this might have resulted from intrapulmonary shunt in the critically ill. This system also requires frequent calibration.

These emerging technologies are likely to improve over time. The impetus for improvement is the push toward less invasive methods to replace the PA catheter. The different technologies have very different advantages and disadvantages, and more innovations are certainly on the horizon.

Continuous Monitoring of Venous Oxygen Saturation

Indications

Continuous monitoring of venous oxygen saturation is indicated for the critically ill patient who has the potential to develop an imbalance between oxygen supply and metabolic tissue demand. This includes patients in severe sepsis or shock, those after high-risk cardiac surgery, and patients with ARDS.[66]

Continuous venous oxygen monitoring permits a calculation of the balance achieved between arterial oxygen supply (Sao_2) and oxygen demand at the tissue level by sampling desaturated venous blood from the PA catheter distal tip. This sample is called *mixed venous oxygen saturation* (Svo₂) because it is a mixture of all of the venous blood drained from many body tissues. The same fiberoptic technology has been used in combination with a fiberoptic triple-lumen CVC. In this situation, the venous blood is sampled from the superior vena cava (SVC), just above the right atrium, and the Scvo₂ is measured.

Under normal conditions, the cardiopulmonary system achieves a balance between oxygen supply and demand. Four factors contribute to this balance:

1. Cardiac output (CO)
2. Hemoglobin (Hgb)
3. Arterial oxygen saturation (Sao₂)
4. Tissue oxygen metabolism (Vo₂)

Three of these factors (CO, Hgb, and Sao₂) contribute to the supply of oxygen to the tissues. Tissue metabolism (Vo₂) determines oxygen consumption or the quantity of oxygen extracted at tissue level that creates the demand for oxygen. The relationships of these factors are illustrated in Figure 14-21.

In addition to measurement of venous oxygen saturation, it is possible to calculate the quantity of oxygen (in mL/min) that is provided to the tissues by the cardiopulmonary system and to assess the amount of oxygen consumed by the body tissues. These calculations rely on principles of oxygen

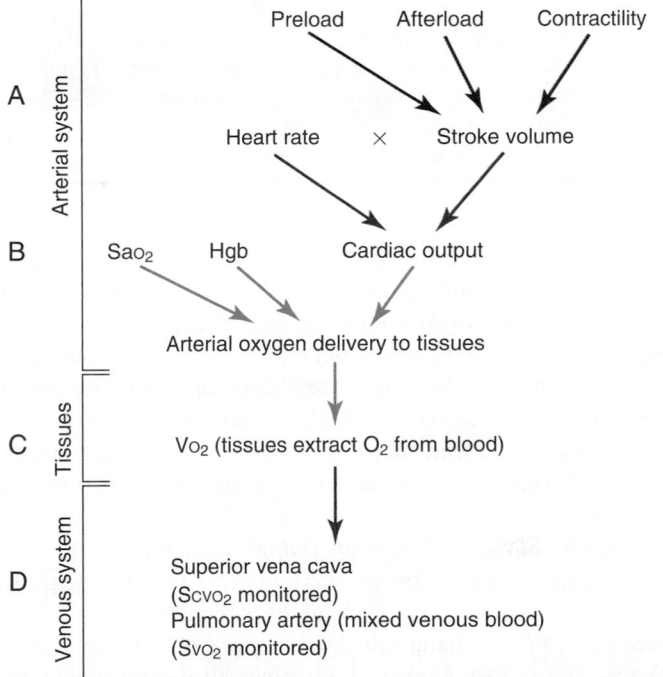

FIGURE 14-21 Several factors contribute to the mixed venous oxygen saturation (Svo₂) value. *A,* Cardiac output (CO) is determined by heart rate (Scvo₂ central venous oxygen saturation HR) × stroke volume (SV). *B,* The oxygen saturation (Sao₂), hemoglobin (Hgb) level, and CO contribute to arterial oxygen delivery at the tissue level. *C,* Tissues extract and use the oxygen carried in the blood. This process of cellular oxygen consumption is Vo₂. *D,* Blood returns to the superior vena cava (recorded as Scvo₂) and then to the pulmonary artery, where the mixed venous blood is recorded as Svo₂.

transport physiology and are the basis for calculation of Svo₂. These formulas are explained in greater detail in Table 14-6 and are listed in Appendix B.

Catheters

The type of catheter used to measure venous oxygen saturation is defined by where the fiberoptic tip is located, either at the tip of a CVC or on the distal tip of a PA catheter.

Svo₂ Catheter. The pulmonary arterial Svo₂ catheter has the traditional four lumens plus a lumen containing two or three optical fibers. The fiberoptics are attached to an optical module that is connected to a small bedside computer. The optical module transmits a narrow band of light down one optical fiber. This light is reflected off the hemoglobin in the blood and returns to the optical module through the receiving fiberoptic. The Svo₂ signal is recorded on a continuous display.

Scvo₂ Catheter. The central venous Scvo₂ technology is incorporated into a multilumen CVC. The fiberoptic catheter tip is positioned in a central vein, such as the SVC. The technology used to measure the venous saturation is identical in both types of catheters, and the same continuous display module is used for both catheters.

The Scvo₂ catheter has been successfully used to guide hemodynamic fluid resuscitation in septic patients.[27] The relationship between the values obtained from the traditional PA (Svo₂) catheter and the central venous (Scvo₂) catheter are very similar, although the Scvo₂ values are slightly higher. The trend of parallel measurements (up or down as patient condition changes) is in the same direction most cases.

Svo₂ or Scvo₂ Calibration. The catheter is calibrated before insertion into the patient through a standardized color reference system, which is part of the catheter package. Insertion technique and sites are identical to those used for placement of conventional PA or CVC catheters. Waveform analysis or venous saturation measurement, or both, can be used for accurate placement. After the catheter is inserted, recalibration is unnecessary unless the catheter becomes disconnected from the optical module.

To recalibrate the fiberoptic module to verify accuracy when the catheter is already inserted in a patient, a mixed venous blood sample (Svo₂) or central venous sample (Scvo₂) must be withdrawn from the appropriate catheter tip and sent to the laboratory for oxygen saturation analysis. In many critical care units, this is a standard daily procedure to ensure that readings used to guide patient care remain accurate.[67]

Nursing Management

Svo₂ monitoring provides a continuous assessment of the balance of oxygen supply and demand for an individual patient. Nursing assessment includes evaluation of the Svo₂ or Scvo₂ value and evaluation of the four factors (Sao₂, CO, Hgb, and Vo₂) that maintain the oxygen supply–demand balance.

Normal Svo₂ Values. Normal Svo₂ is approximately 75% in the healthy individual (range, 60% to 80%). In critically ill patients, an Svo₂ value between 60% and 80% is evidence of adequate balance between oxygen supply and demand.

Normal Scvo₂ Values. The normal values for the Scvo₂ catheter are slightly higher, because the reading is taken before

TABLE 14-6　CALCULATIONS OF OXYGEN TRANSPORT PHYSIOLOGY

NAME	FORMULA	NORMAL VALUE	EXPLANATION
Arterial oxygen saturation (SaO_2)	$\dfrac{HgbO_2}{Hgb + HgbO_2} \times 100$	>96%	SaO_2 is determined by the amount of oxygen bound to hemoglobin (Hgb), termed oxyhemoglobin ($HgbO_2$). $HgbO_2$ is divided by the total hemoglobin ($Hgb + HgbO_2$). Normally, 96% of oxygen is bound to hemoglobin.
Blood oxygen content CaO_2 (arterial) CvO_2 (venous)	(O_2 dissolved) + (O_2 saturation) ($P_{O_2} \times 0.003$) + ($1.34 \times Hgb \times S_{O_2}$)	19-20 mL/dL 12-15 mL/dL	Blood oxygen (O_2) content is the amount of oxygen dissolved in 100 mL (1 dL) of blood. It can be calculated for arterial blood (CaO_2) and for venous blood (CvO_2). Measured in units of mL/dL, it is the combination of dissolved O_2 (PaO_2) and O_2 saturation (SaO_2).
Blood oxygen transport (i.e., oxygen delivery)	$CO \times CaO_2 \times 10$ (arterial) $CO \times CvC_2 \times 10$ (venous)	1000 mL/min 750 mL/min	Oxygen transport represents the amount (mL) of oxygen transported to or from the tissues each minute (mL/min). Arterial O_2 transport is a measure of the O_2 delivered to the tissues. Venous O_2 transport reflects the venous return to the right side of the heart. Oxygen transport is calculated by multiplying the cardiac output (CO) by the oxygen content (CaO_2 or CvO_2) and by the number 10. The difference between normal arterial and normal venous O_2 return represents oxygen consumption by the tissues.
Tissue oxygen consumption (VO_2)	Arterial O_2 transport minus venous O_2 transport ($CO \times CaO_2 \times 10$) − ($CO \times CVO_2 \times 10$)	250 mL/min	Oxygen consumption is the amount of oxygen consumed by the tissues in 1 minute. To calculate VO_2, the arterial oxygen transport and venous oxygen transport values (calculated in mL/min) must be known. The difference is VO_2.
Arterial-venous oxygen difference (a-v O_2 difference)	Arterial O_2 content minus venous O_2 content $CaO_2 - CVO_2$	3.0-5.5 mL/dL	The a-v O_2 difference is the difference between the arterial oxygen content (CaO_2) and the venous oxygen content (CvO_2). Because CaO_2 and CVO_2 are measured in mL/dL, the a-v O_2 difference is also measured in mL/dL.
Mixed venous oxygen saturation (SvO_2)	Arterial O_2 transport minus tissue O_2 consumption equals venous O_2 return ($CO \times CaO_2 \times 10$) − VO_2	60%-80%	SvO_2 is the venous oxygen return that is bound (saturated) to hemoglobin. Saturation is measured as a percentage (%). The SvO_2 value is a function of the amount of oxygen delivered to the tissues minus the amount of oxygen consumed by the tissues (VO_2) and is measured in mL/min. The higher the amount (mL) of oxygen in the venous return, the greater the hemoglobin saturation.

the blood enters the right heart chambers, where the *cardiac sinus* (vein) delivers venous blood drained from the myocardium into the right atrium. The heavily desaturated myocardial blood decreases the oxygen saturation slightly. For this reason, SvO_2 values are always slightly lower than $ScvO_2$ readings in the same patient.[68]

One clinical rule of thumb is to subtract 30 from the SaO_2, and the resulting value should represent an acceptable SvO_2. For example,

SaO_2 is 100% − 30% = 70% SvO_2

SaO_2 is 95% − 30% = 65% SvO_2

If the SvO_2 or $ScvO_2$ value changes by more than 10% and this change is maintained for more than 10 minutes, the clinician must determine which of the four factors is affecting SvO_2.

SvO_2 or $ScvO_2$ and Arterial Oxygen Saturation. A change in SvO_2 or $ScvO_2$ may be caused by a change in arterial oxygen saturation (SaO_2). If the SaO_2 is increased because supplemental oxygen is being administered, the SvO_2 also will increase. If the oxygen supply is disrupted and SaO_2 is decreased, SvO_2 will decrease. The SvO_2 can be decreased by any action or disease that reduces oxygen supply, including ARDS, endotracheal suctioning, removing a patient from the ventilator, or removing

supplementary oxygen. Figure 14-22 demonstrates a drop in SvO_2 during suctioning in a patient with ARDS. Transient decreases in SvO_2 or $ScvO_2$ related to a nursing action such as endotracheal suctioning are not usually a cause for concern. Some patients may be slow to resaturate up to the presuction level of SvO_2 or $ScvO_2$. In this case, an appropriate nursing intervention is to wait until the venous oxygen saturation has again returned to baseline before initiating other nursing activities.

SvO_2 or $ScvO_2$ and Cardiac Output. A change in SvO_2 or $ScvO_2$ may be caused by an alteration in CO. Four hemodynamic factors affect CO: preload, SVR, contractility, and HR (see Fig. 14-21). Changes in one or more of these individual factors affects CO. Figure 14-23 shows an improvement in a patient's SvO_2 concentration from 70% to 80% after volume administration that increased preload (point A). Later, this patient's CO fell abruptly during a short run of ventricular tachycardia (VT) (point B). Any major loss of HR causes a decrease in CO. Alterations in contractility, preload, and afterload (SVR) also have the potential to alter CO.

Because CO is an important component of the continuous SvO_2 value, researchers investigated whether SvO_2 could be substituted for thermodilution CO as a monitoring tool. Studies of

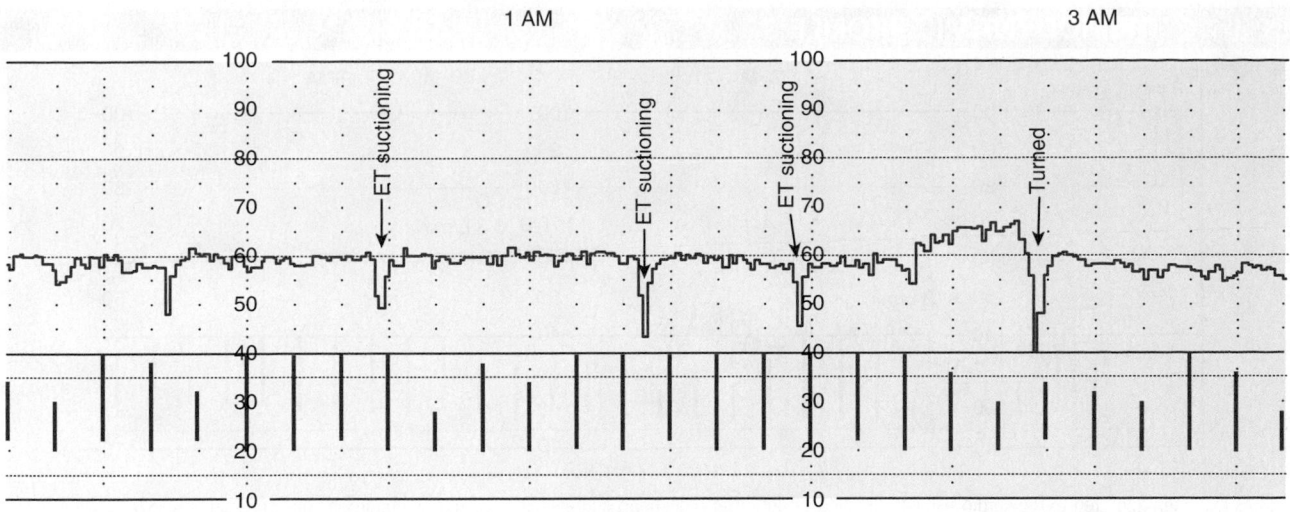

FIGURE 14-22 The SvO₂ value decreases during endotracheal (ET) suctioning. The ET suction decreases the oxygen saturation (SaO₂) level. The baseline SvO₂ value is low (60%) because the patient has acute respiratory distress syndrome (ARDS) and is hypoxemic.

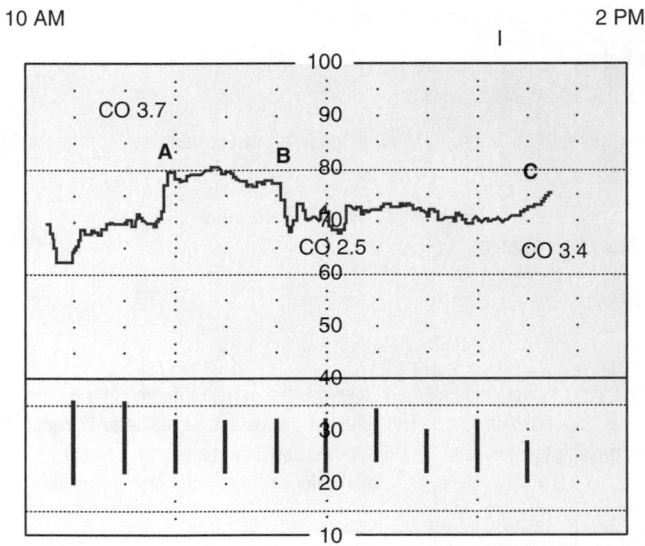

FIGURE 14-23 Impact of Changes in Cardiac Output (CO) on SvO₂ Values. *Point A:* Just before point A, SvO₂ readings are low because CO and pulmonary artery pressures were low as a result of excessive diuresis. Infusion of 500 mL of colloid solution and 1000 mL of lactated Ringer's solution crystalloid increased the SvO₂ level and improved the CO, which rose to 3.7 L/min. *Point B:* A short run of ventricular tachycardia caused the CO to fall abruptly to 2.5 L/min and decreased the SvO₂ value. *Point C:* The beginning of an upward trend in SvO₂ is related to administration of fluids and to improvement in CO and in filling pressures. CO is now 3.4 L/min. The graph represents a 4-hour printout; the space between each dotted line represents 20 minutes.

adult patients after cardiac surgery and acute MI indicate that a sustained change in the SvO₂ value does not automatically mean there has been a change in CO. No consistent or reliable correlation was found between SvO₂ and CO. Instead, a change in SvO₂ indicates a need to check a CO at the bedside to determine the cause of the change in venous oxygen saturation. The SvO₂ measurement is very sensitive and serves as an early warning for changes in patient condition, whether or not the change is the result of an alteration in CO. Monitoring SvO₂ is an additional level of hemodynamic monitoring but does not replace thermodilution CO.

This principle is clearly illustrated in the SvO₂ Hemodynamic Profile 3 (Box 14-6), in which an increase in SvO₂ is not associated with a significant rise in CO. The rationale and explanation for this finding is also discussed in the section on assessment of oxygen consumption.

SvO₂ or ScvO₂ and Hemoglobin. Hemoglobin is the transport mechanism for oxygen in the blood. If the hemoglobin level falls as a result of bleeding or red cell destruction, the body maintains oxygen transport by increasing CO and using oxygen reserves in the venous blood return. The body can compensate efficiently for anemia. In the healthy person, the hemoglobin concentration must be extremely low before SvO₂ decreases. However, in an anemic patient with a compromised cardiovascular system who cannot adequately increase CO, SvO₂ or ScvO₂ declines as venous oxygen reserves are depleted by the body.

SvO₂ or ScvO₂ and Oxygen Consumption. Oxygen consumption Vo₂ describes the amount of oxygen the body tissues consume for normal function in 1 minute. If the body's metabolic demands increase because of exercise or increased metabolic rate, the body increases CO to augment oxygen supply and uses reserve oxygen in the venous system. Normal oxygen delivery to the tissues is 1000 mL (1 L) of oxygen per minute. At rest, a person may consume one fourth of the available oxygen, or 250 mL of oxygen per minute. This leaves a venous oxygen reserve of 750 mL of oxygen per minute (see Table 14-6). For the normal individual, the combination of increased CO and use of considerable venous oxygen reserve provides adequate compensation for increased metabolic needs. However, for the critically ill patient with cardiac or respiratory dysfunction, an increase in activity leading to increased oxygen consumption may overwhelm the cardiopulmonary system and oxygen reserves.

BOX 14-6   HEMODYNAMIC PROFILE 3

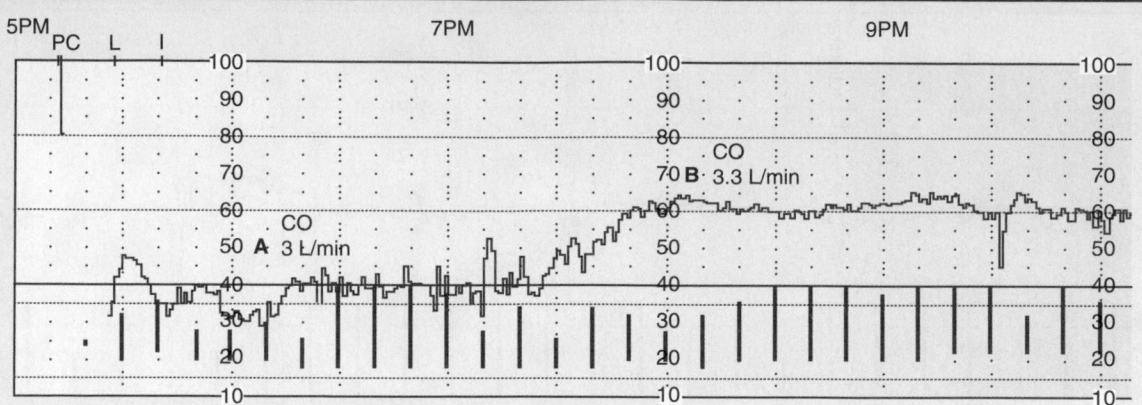

Mr. EH has just been admitted to the cardiovascular critical care unit after open heart surgery. At *point A* in the figure, he has an extremely low SvO$_2$ value of 40%. An SvO$_2$ value below 40% indicates that the oxygen supply is not adequate to meet the demands of the body tissues, resulting in metabolic acidosis. To determine the reason for the low SvO$_2$ level, values must be known for the hemoglobin (Hgb) level, the arterial oxygen saturation (SaO$_2$), the cardiac output (CO), and the tissue oxygen consumption (VO$_2$). EH's Hgb value is 11.6 g/dL (normal male Hgb, 13.5-18.0 g/dL), which is acceptable after major surgery; the SaO$_2$ is 99.6% (normal, 97%), which is high because this patient started receiving mechanical ventilation with 70% oxygen immediately after surgery; and the CO is low at 3.15 L/min (normal, 4-6 L/min). EH is receiving dopamine (5 mcg/kg/min) for his low CO. He is shivering and cold because his body temperature is only 35.2° C after the surgery. Using the values of Hgb of 11.6 g/dL, SaO$_2$ of 99.6%, and CO of 3.15 L/min, it is possible to calculate the tissue oxygen consumption (VO$_2$) for EH.

Arterial Supply	Venous Return
CO (PaO$_2$ × 0.003) + (1.34 × Hgb × SaO$_2$) 10 − CO (PvO$_2$ × 0.0031) + (1.34 × Hgb × S$\bar{v}$O$_2$) 10 = $\dot{V}$O$_2$	

To calculate arterial oxygen supply, the oxygen in the venous return, VO$_2$, and the difference between the arterial (a) and venous (v) oxygen content (a-v O$_2$ difference), insert EH's values **(in boldface)** into the previous formula.

Arterial Supply	Venous Return	$\dot{V}$O$_2$	a-v O$_2$ Difference
3.15 (354 × 0.003) + (1.34 × **11.6** × **0.99**) 10 −	**3.15 (20** × 0.003) + (1.34 × **11.6** × **0.38**) 10		
3.15 (1.0 + 15.3) 10	**3.15** (0.06 + 5.90) 10		
3.15 (16.3) 10	**3.15** (5.90) 10		
505 mL/min (see illustration at top)	183 mL/min		= 322 mL/min 10.4 mL/dL

At *point A* in the preceding illustration, the arterial oxygen supply to the tissues is 505 mL/min (normal, 1000 mL/min), whereas the oxygen returned in the venous blood is only 183 mL/min (normal, 750 mL/min). EH's VO$_2$ is elevated at 322 mL/min (normal, 250 mL/min). The clinical goals for this patient would be to 1) increase the CO; and 2) use sedation or muscle relaxants to decrease oxygen consumption by controlling the shivering. The difference between the oxygen content in the arterial (a) and the venous (v) blood (a-v O$_2$ difference) is very large at 10.4 mL/dL (normal, 3.5-5.0 mL/dL). These calculated values confirm the nursing diagnosis of Ineffective Tissue Perfusion with a decreased CO.

Two hours later, at *point B* (see illustration), EH's SvO$_2$ has improved to a low-normal value of 60%. Additional inotropic medications have been administered. At this time the Hgb is 10.8 g/dL, SaO$_2$ is 99.6%, and CO remains low at 3.3 L/min. The improvement in SvO$_2$ has not been caused by a dramatic increase in CO. When EH's oxygen consumption is calculated at *point B*, it becomes evident that the decrease in physical activity after sedation with morphine to reduce shivering has improved the SvO$_2$. EH's values are emphasized in bold.

Arterial Supply	Venous Return
CO (PaO$_2$ × 0.003) + (1.34 × Hgb × SaO$_2$) 10 − CO (PvO$_2$ × 0.003) + (1.34 × Hgb × S$\bar{v}$O$_2$) 10 = $\dot{V}$O$_2$	

Arterial Supply	Venous Return	$\dot{V}$O$_2$	a-v O$_2$ Difference
3.3 (266 × 0.003) + (1.34 × **10.8** × **0.99**) 10 −	**3.3 (28** × 0.003) + (1.34 × **10.8** × **0.60**) 10		
3.3 (0.82 + 14.32) 10	**3.3** (0.86 + 8.6) 10		
3.3 (15.1) 1	**3.3** (9.4) 10		
498 mL/min	300 mL/min		= 198 mL/min 5.7 mL/dL

At *point B* in the illustration, EH's arterial oxygen supply is still low at 498 mL/min, and the oxygen in his mixed venous blood return remains low at 300 mL/min. VO$_2$ is now lower than normal (typical after sedation) at 198 mL/min. At this time, the a-v O$_2$ difference is almost within the normal limits at 5.7 mL/dL. These findings are confirmed by the low-normal SvO$_2$ value of 60% at *point B*. This case study illustrates the point that tissue oxygen consumption (O$_2$ demand) can be as important as cardiac output (CO) and oxygenation (O$_2$ supply) in determining SvO$_2$ in the patient with a compromised cardiovascular system.

See Table 14-6 for an explanation of abbreviations and Box 14-4 and Appendix B for explanation of hemodynamic values.

TABLE 14-7 ALTERATIONS IN OXYGEN CONSUMPTION

CONDITION OR ACTIVITY	% INCREASE OVER RESTING V_{O_2}	% DECREASE UNDER RESTING V_{O_2}
Clinical Conditions That Increase V_{O_2}		
Fever	10% (for each 1° C above normal)	
Skeletal injuries	10%-30%	
Work of breathing	40%	
Severe infection	60%	
Shivering	50%-100%	
Burns	100%	
Routine postoperative procedures	7%	
Nasal intubation	25%-40%	
Endotracheal tube suctioning	27%	
Chest trauma	60%	
Multiple organ dysfunction syndrome	20%-80%	
Sepsis	50%-100%	
Head injury, with patient sedated	89%	
Head injury, with patient not sedated	138%	
Critical illness in emergency department	60%	
Nursing Activities That Increase V_{O_2}		
Dressing change	10%	
Electrocardiogram	16%	
Agitation	18%	
Physical examination	20%	
Visitor	22%	
Bath	23%	
Chest radiograph examination	25%	
Position change	31%	
Chest physiotherapy	35%	
Weighing on sling scale	36%	
Conditions That Decrease V_{O_2}		
Anesthesia		25%
Anesthesia in burned patients		50%

Modified from White KM, et al. The physiologic basis for continuous mixed venous oxygen saturation monitoring. *Heart Lung.* 1990; 19(5 Pt 2):548.

V_{O_2}, Oxygen consumption.

In the critically ill patient, nursing procedures can increase V_{O_2} by 10% to 36% (Table 14-7). The critical care nurse can observe the effect of increased V_{O_2} during routine nursing care and under conditions that increase metabolic rate. Activities such as turning, giving a backrub, or getting a patient out of bed are often accompanied by a sudden, temporary decrease in the patient's continuous Svo_2 or $Scvo_2$ reading. After the physical activity is finished, most patients resaturate up to their preactivity venous saturation level within a few minutes. In critically ill patients, it may take up to 5 minutes for resaturation (increase in Svo_2 or $Scvo_2$) to occur. In this situation, the appropriate nursing action is to observe the patient clinically in conjunction with monitoring Svo_2 or $Scvo_2$ and to postpone additional maneuvers until the venous saturation has returned to baseline.

Many clinical conditions that dramatically increase V_{O_2} consumption are often seen in critical care units. Conditions such as sepsis, multiple organ dysfunction syndrome (MODS), burns, head injury, and shivering can more than double the normal oxygen tissue requirements (see Table 14-7). Such dramatic increases in V_{O_2} translate into a low Svo_2 or $Scvo_2$ value, even if the CO is normal. This situation is demonstrated in Hemodynamic Profile 3, in which intense shivering resulted in increased tissue oxygen consumption and a low initial Svo_2 value (point A); after sedation, the Svo_2 value increased due to the normalization of tissue oxygen requirements (point B).

Normal Svo_2 or $Scvo_2$. If Svo_2 or $Scvo_2$ is within the normal range of 60% to 80% and the patient is not clinically compromised, the nurse can assume that oxygen supply and demand are balanced for that individual. The situation becomes out of balance when a decrease in oxygen delivery (Sao_2) occurs because of changes in CO or hemoglobin concentration, or an increase in oxygen demand (increased V_{O_2}) occurs.

Low Svo_2 or $Scvo_2$. If Svo_2 or $Scvo_2$ falls below 60% and is sustained, the clinician must assume that oxygen supply is not equal to demand (Table 14-8). It is helpful to assess the cause of decreased Svo_2 or $Scvo_2$ in a logical sequence that reflects knowledge of the meaning of the venous saturation value. The following is one such assessment sequence:

1. Clinically assess the patient.
2. Assess whether the decreased Svo_2 or $Scvo_2$ is caused by low oxygen supply. Verify the effectiveness of the ventilator or oxygen mask, or check Sao_2 from arterial blood gas values.
3. Assess cardiac function by performing a CO measurement.
4. Assess the hemoglobin value by checking recent laboratory results or by withdrawing a blood sample for laboratory analysis.
5. Assess whether the decreased Svo_2 or $Scvo_2$ is the result of a recent patient movement or nursing action that may have temporarily increased V_{O_2}.

The concept of target values is helpful when designing protocols for hemodynamic monitoring. Target values for venous oximetry are an Svo_2 of 70% or above and a $Scvo_2$ of 65% or above. The concept is that patients with values below these targets are at greater risk for organ hypoperfusion and increased mortality. This was seen in a study of intraoperative and postoperative surgical patients, in whom an $Scvo_2$ below 65% was associated with increased mortality.[69,70] Based on studies of patients with sepsis, the Surviving Sepsis Campaign guidelines recommend that $Scvo_2$ be maintained above 70% for septic patients.[42] This represents a clinically useful target to aim for, even as research is ongoing to find the optimal $Scvo_2$ value to predict survival.

If Svo_2 or $Scvo_2$ falls below 40%, and is maintained at this low value, the imbalance of oxygen supply and demand will not be adequate to meet tissue needs at the cellular level. At some

TABLE 14-8 MEASUREMENTS OF MIXED VENOUS OXYGEN SATURATION

Svo$_2$ MEASUREMENT	PHYSIOLOGIC BASIS FOR CHANGES IN Svo$_2$/Scvo$_2$	CLINICAL DIAGNOSIS AND RATIONALE
High Svo$_2$ (80%-95%)	Increased oxygen supply Decreased oxygen demand	Patient receiving more oxygen than required by clinical condition Anesthesia, which causes sedation and decreased muscle movement Hypothermia, which lowers metabolic demand (e.g., during cardiopulmonary bypass) Sepsis caused by decreased ability of tissues to use oxygen at a cellular level False high-positive result because the pulmonary artery catheter is wedged in a pulmonary arteriole (Svo$_2$ only)

Normal Svo$_2$/Scvo$_2$ (60%-80%)
Low Svo$_2$/Scvo$_2$ (<60%)
	Normal oxygen supply and metabolic demand
	Decreased oxygen supply caused by:
	  Low hemoglobin (Hgb)
	  Low arterial saturation (Sao$_2$)
	  Low CO
	  Increased oxygen consumption (Vo$_2$)
		Balanced oxygen supply and demand
		Anemia or bleeding with compromised cardiopulmonary system
		Hypoxemia resulting from decreased oxygen supply or lung disease
		Cardiogenic shock caused by LV pump failure
		Metabolic demand exceeds oxygen supply in conditions that increase muscle movement and increase metabolic rate, including physiologic states such as shivering, seizures, and hyperthermia and nursing interventions such as being weighed on a bed scale and turning

SCVO$_2$, Central venous oxygen saturation; *SVO$_2$*, mixed venous oxygen saturation.

point, the cells change from an aerobic to anaerobic mode of metabolism, which results in the production of lactic acid and is representative of a shock state in which cellular injury or cell death may result. At this point, every attempt must be made to determine the cause of the low Svo$_2$ or Scvo$_2$ and to correct the oxygen supply–demand imbalance. To avoid the risk of lactic acidosis, it is helpful to watch the trend of the Svo$_2$ or Scvo$_2$ and to intervene early with a goal of returning the venous oxygen saturation to 70%.[42]

High Svo$_2$. In certain clinical conditions, Svo$_2$ or Scvo$_2$ may increase to an above-normal level (greater than 80%). This occurs during times of low oxygen demand (decreased Vo$_2$), such as during anesthesia or hypothermia. In some cases of septic shock, the tissue cells cannot use the oxygen supplied to them, and the oxygen is not extracted from the blood at the tissue level. In this situation, the venous oxygen reserve remains elevated, and the Svo$_2$ or Scvo$_2$ value is higher than normal (see Table 14-8). If the Svo$_2$ PA catheter drifts into a wedged position, the Svo$_2$ increases because the fiberoptic tip of the catheter comes into contact with newly oxygenated blood.

Electrocardiography

Electrocardiography is a complex and vitally useful subject. Detailed evaluation of an ECG can provide a wealth of cardiac diagnostic information and often provides the basis upon which other, definitive diagnostic tests are selected. The following sections discuss the many clinical factors that the critical care nurse considers when using ECG monitoring, specific dysrhythmias commonly encountered in clinical practice, and the skills needed for 12-lead ECG analysis. The intent is to provide a sound basis for understanding the value of the many clinical applications of electrocardiography.

Basic Principles of Electrocardiography

The ECG records electrical changes in heart muscle caused by an action potential. It does not record the mechanical contraction, which usually follows electrical depolarization

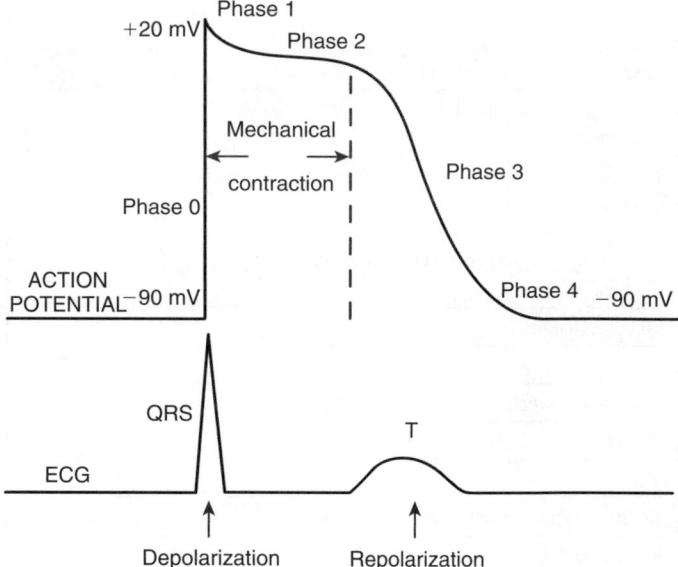

FIGURE 14-24 Correlation of the action potential of a ventricular myocardial cell with the electrical events recorded on the surface ECG. Notice that the ECG pattern is "silent" during phase 2 of the action potential. Mechanical contraction is occurring, but no significant electrical activity is present.

immediately. A brief discussion of the cardiac action potential will explain the concept that electrical changes occurring during electrical stimulation of the myocardial cell produce the deflections seen on the ECG tracing (Fig. 14-24).

Phase 0. During phase 0 (depolarization), the electrical potential changes rapidly from a baseline of −90 mV to +20 mV and stabilizes at about 0 mV. Because this is a significant electrical change, it appears as a wave on the ECG as the QRS.

Phases 1 and 2. During phases 1 and 2, an electrical plateau is created, and during this plateau, mechanical contraction occurs. Because there is no significant electrical change, no waveform appears on the ECG (the recorded tracing is isoelectric with baseline).

Phase 3. During phase 3 (repolarization), the electrical potential again changes, this time a little more slowly, from 0 mV back to −90 mV. This is another major electrical event and is reflected on the ECG as a T wave.

Phase 4. During phase 4 (resting period), the chemical balance is restored by the sodium pump, but because positively charged ions are exchanged on a one-for-one basis, no electrical activity is generated, and no visible change occurs on the ECG tracing. For more information on the cardiac action potential, see "Phases of the Action Potential" in Chapter 12.

Electrocardiographic Leads. All electrocardiographs use a system of one or more leads. The basic 3-lead system consists of three bipolar electrodes that are applied to the chest wall and labeled right arm (RA), left arm (LA), and left leg (LL). The term *bipolar* means that each created ECG lead has a positive and a negative pole. A third electrode acts as a ground. The function of the ground electrode is to prevent the display of background electrical interference on the ECG tracing. Electrodes do not transmit any electricity to the patient; rather, they sense and record intrinsic cardiac electrical activity from the body's surface.

The positive electrode on the skin acts as a camera. If the wave of depolarization travels toward the positive electrode, an upward stroke, or *positive deflection*, is written on the ECG paper (Fig. 14-25A). If the wave of depolarization travels away from the positive electrode, a downward line, or *negative deflection*, is recorded on the ECG (see Fig. 14-25B). When depolarization moves perpendicularly to the positive electrode, a biphasic complex occurs. Sometimes, the complex may even appear almost flat, or isoelectric, if the electrical forces traveling in opposite directions are equal and have the effect of canceling each other (see Fig. 14-25C). The size of the muscle mass being depolarized also has an effect, with the larger muscle mass (usually the left ventricle) having a greater influence on the tracing.

The wave of ventricular depolarization in the healthy heart travels from right to left and from head to toe. The appearance of the waveforms in different ECG leads depend on the location of the positive electrode.

12-Lead Electrocardiogram. The standard 12-lead ECG provides a picture of electrical activity in the heart using 10 different electrode positions to create 12 unique views of electrical activity occurring within the heart.[71-73] A standard 12-lead ECG contains six limb lead images and six chest (precordial) lead images, and the correct placement of these leads is vitally important to avoid misdiagnosis.[74] If a 12-lead ECG is being obtained, the limb electrodes are typically placed on the muscle of the limb avoiding bone, and the patient is asked to remain still. In the critical care unit, the electrodes are typically placed on the torso, near the origin of the limb, avoiding the clavicular bone (LA and RA) and the pelvic bone (LL and RL), as shown in Figure 14-26A. This arrangement is used because patients wear the electrodes for hours or days, and limb movement would distort the electrical baseline. Practically, this means that ECG waveforms on the bedside monitor will not be identical to those obtained by standard 12-lead ECG, for which the limb electrodes are placed directly on corresponding extremities.[71]

Standard Limb Leads. The limb lead tracings are obtained by placing electrodes on all four extremities: left arm (LA), right arm (RA), left leg (LL), and right leg (RL). Leads I, II, and III are *bipolar* limb leads that use limb lead electrodes paired as the positive and negative poles (see Fig. 14-26A). The electrodes are placed in a static position on the body, and the polarity is switched to achieve the desired view. This is done manually on the critical care bedside monitor or automatically by the electrocardiographic machine when a 12-lead ECG is obtained:

Lead I—positive electrode at LA and negative electrode at RA
Lead II—positive electrode at LL and negative electrode at RA
Lead III—positive electrode at LL and negative electrode at LA

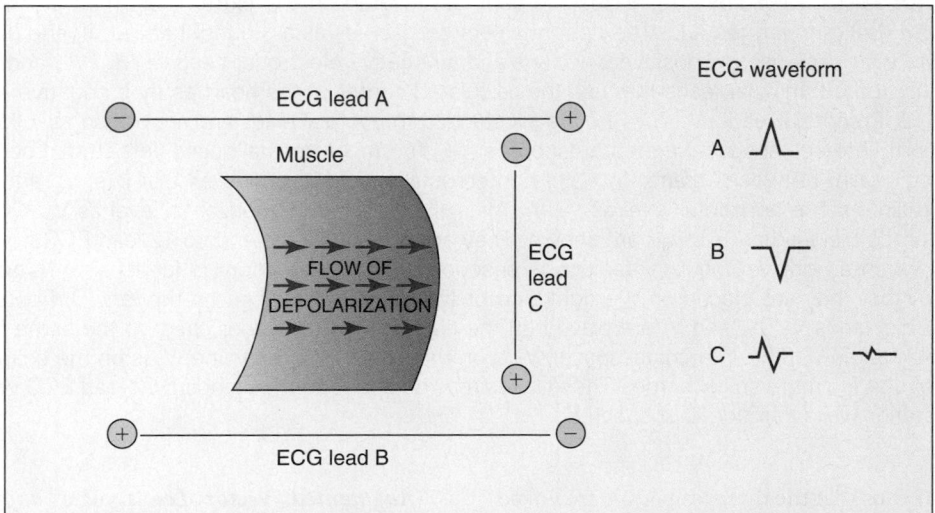

FIGURE 14-25 Effect of lead position on the ECG tracing. *A,* Flow of depolarization toward the positive electrode results in a positive deflection on the ECG. *B,* Flow of depolarization away from the positive electrode results in a negative deflection on the ECG. *C,* Flow of depolarization perpendicular to the positive electrode results in a biphasic or nearly isoelectric deflection on the ECG. This basic principle applies to the P wave and the QRS complex.

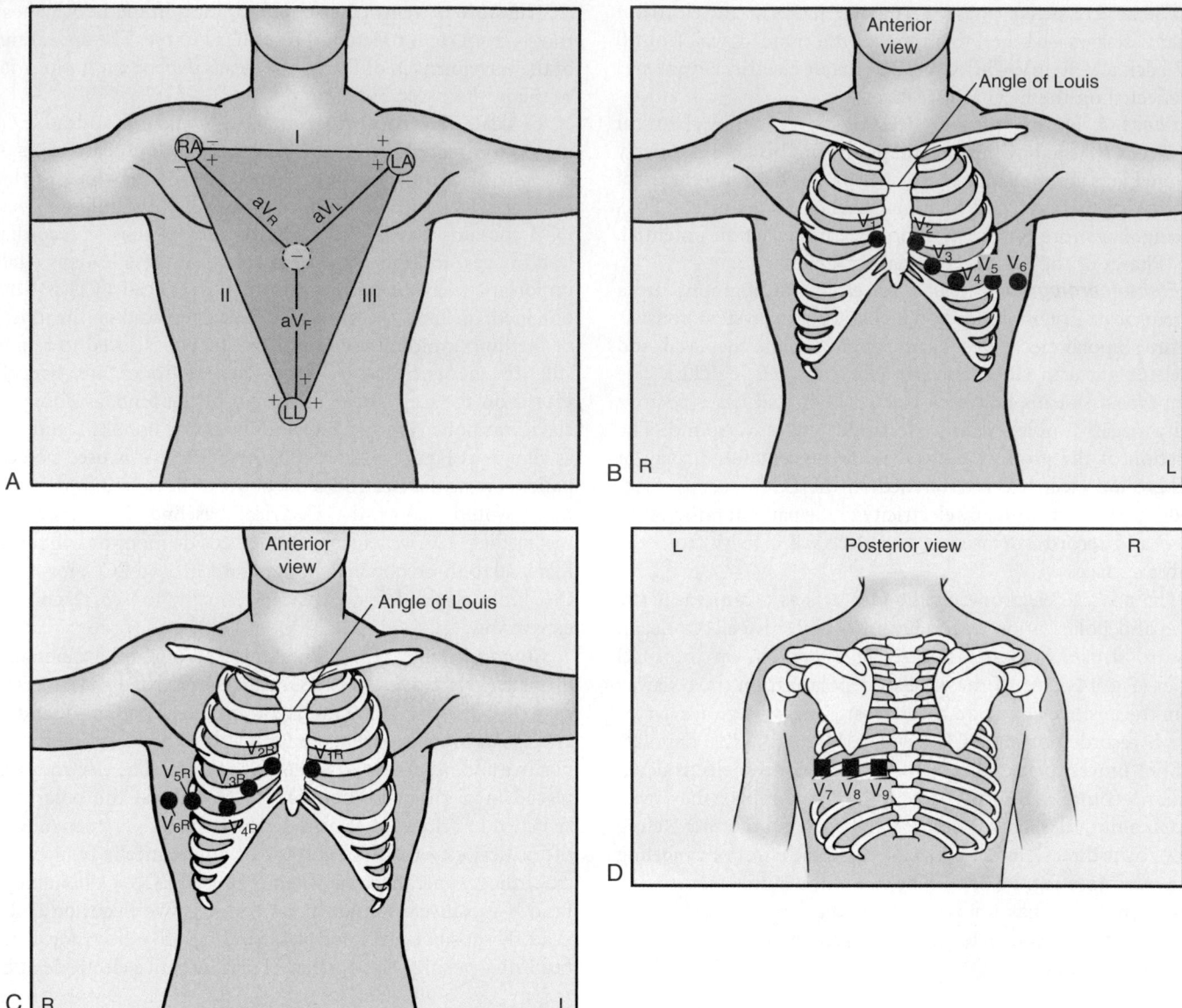

FIGURE 14-26 *A*, Standard limb leads. Leads are located on the extremities: right arm (RA), left arm (LA), and left leg (LL). The right leg electrode serves as a ground. Leads I, II, and III are bipolar, with each using a positive electrode and a negative electrode. Leads aVR, aVL, and aVF are augmented unipolar leads that use the calculated center of the heart as their negative electrode. *B*, Precordial leads. V_1 to V_6 are the six standard precordial leads and are placed as follows: V_1, fourth intercostal space, right sternal border; V_2, fourth intercostal space, left sternal border; V_3, equidistant between V_2 and V_4; V_4, fifth intercostal space, left midclavicular line; V_5, anterior axillary line, same horizontal level as V_4; V_6, midaxillary line, same horizontal level as V_4. *C*, The right precordial leads V_1R to V_6R are shown. They are not part of a standard 12-lead ECG but are used when a right ventricular infarction is suspected. Their placement is identical to V_3 to V_6, except that they are placed on the right side of the chest rather than on the left. *D*, Posterior precordial leads V_7, V_8, and V_9 are placed on the patient's left posterior chest at the same horizontal level as V_4 (fifth intercostal space). V_7 is on the posterior axillary line, V_8 is on the scapular line, and V_9 is on the spinal border. These leads may be added to the standard 12-lead ECG when a posterior wall infarction is suspected.

This configuration means that the three limb leads are linked in a circuit. The information obtained from the three limb leads is used to create a *central reference potential* that reflects the average potential of the RA, LA, and LL electrodes.[71] The central reference potential shown at the center of the electrode triangle in Figure 14-26A is used to calculate the augmented vector leads.

Augmented Vector Leads. The *augmented vector leads*, labeled aVR, aVL, and aVF, are created from the derived electrode pairs previously described. These augmented leads have only one positive electrode (see Fig. 14-26A), with the calculated central reference potential (center of triangle) acting as a negative electrode. Under these circumstances, the ECG tracing obtained is ordinarily very small, so the machine enhances, or *augments*, it by adding enough voltage to render the waveform amplitudes roughly equivalent to the other lead views. The term *vector* refers to directional force. The augmented vector leads are used in the interpretation of myocardial injury and infarction. The limb leads and the augmented vector leads are derived from the four limb electrodes. They constitute the *frontal plane axis* of the 12-lead ECG.[71,75]

Precordial Leads. The six precordial, or left chest, leads are labeled as V leads and are distributed in an arc around the left side of the chest. They are positioned to detect electrical forces traveling from right to left or from front to back. Each of the V leads is independent from the other precordial electrodes and provides a unique view of the cardiac electrical system (see Fig. 14-26B). The six electrodes are placed on the chest in the following locations[71]:

V_1—fourth intercostal space at the right sternal border
V_2—fourth intercostal space at the left sternal border
V_3—midway between V_2 and V_4
V_4—fifth intercostal space in the midclavicular line
V_5—in the horizontal plane of V_4 at the anterior axillary line or, if the anterior axillary line is ambiguous, midway between V_4 and V_6
V_6—in the horizontal plane of V_4 at the midaxillary line

Right Ventricular Precordial Leads. At times, additional leads are helpful in evaluating the extent of myocardium involved in an acute MI. The right ventricle and the posterior wall of the heart are areas that are not clearly seen on a standard 12-lead ECG. The right ventricle can be visualized more fully by adding right-sided chest leads (see Fig. 14-26C). Labeled V_1R, V_2R, V_3R, V_4R, V_5R, and V_6R, they are added to the standard 12-lead ECG when right ventricular infarction is suspected. Right ventricular infarction is commonly accompanied by inferior and posterior wall infarction.[74] The use of the six right ventricular leads expands the diagnostic accuracy of the 12-lead ECG and is sometimes called an *18-lead ECG*.

Posterior Wall Leads. The posterior wall of the heart can be assessed using posterior chest leads (see Fig. 14-26D). These leads are labeled V_7, V_8, and V_9. Although posterior lead placement can be somewhat technically challenging, the information obtained may influence decisions regarding clinical management. The use of the posterior leads expands the diagnostic accuracy of the 12-lead ECG and can be described as a *15-lead ECG*.

Baseline Distortion. The tracing must have a flat baseline, which is that portion of the tracing between the various waveforms. Two forms of artifact can distort the baseline: 60-cycle interference and muscular movement. Sixty cycle-per-second (Hertz) interference (Fig. 14-27A) results from leakage of ambient electrical current in the immediate environment and appears as a generalized thickening of the baseline. It can usually be resolved by ensuring that all electrical equipment at the bedside is electrically grounded. Moving the offending device away from the patient may help, or occasionally it may be necessary to unplug one piece of equipment at a time until the offending device is found. Muscular movement (see Fig. 14-27B) is displayed as a coarse, erratic disturbance of the baseline. In most cases, asking the patient to lie quietly while the

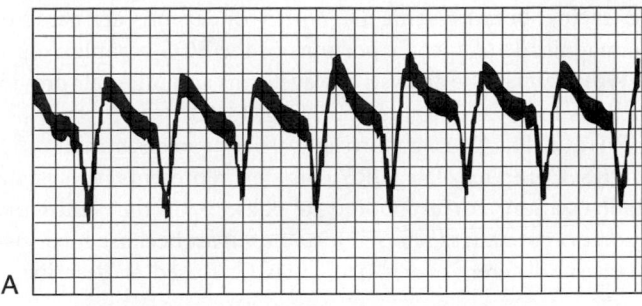

A

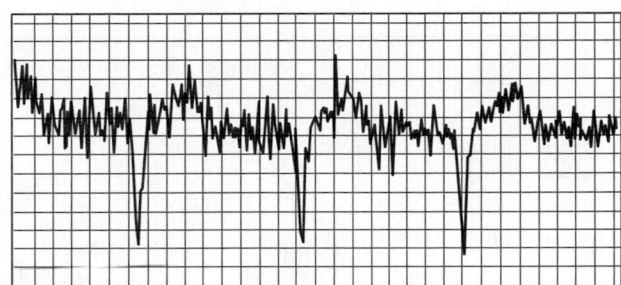

B

FIGURE 14-27 *A*, Artifact from 60-cycle interference. *B*, Artifact caused by muscular movement.

ECG is being run is sufficient. If movement is caused by shivering or seizure activity, it is best to wait until the activity subsides before obtaining the 12-lead ECG. When baseline tremor is caused by Parkinson's disease or another neuromuscular disorder, resolution may not be possible. Electrical artifact has an adverse effect on the accurate interpretation of the tracing and may mimic lethal ventricular dysrhythmias.[76]

Electrocardiographic Analysis

Specialized Electrocardiographic Paper. ECG paper records the speed and magnitude of electrical impulses on a grid composed of small and large boxes (Fig. 14-28). Every large box contains 25 small (1 mm²) boxes within it. At a standard paper speed of 25 mm/sec, looking at the ECG paper from left to right, one small box (1 mm wide) is equivalent to 0.04 second, and one large box (5 mm wide) represents 0.20 second. These ECG boxes represent the time it takes for the electrical impulse to travel through a particular part of the heart and are stated in seconds rather than in millimeters or number of boxes. The vertical scale represents the magnitude, or force, of the electrical signal. The vertical scale is standardized to a specific calibration.

Calibration. At standard calibration, one small box equals 0.1 mm, and one large box equals 0.5 mm. It is important to look for the standardization mark, which is usually located at the beginning of the tracing (Fig. 14-29A). The mark indicates that in response to a standard electrical signal of 1 mV, the calibration signal rises vertically the equivalent of two large boxes to make a calibration mark. ECGs are sometimes run at different calibrations. If at standard calibration some complexes are so tall they run off the paper, the ECG recording is repeated at one-half standard (see Fig. 14-29B), and the calibration mark rises only one large box. If all of the complexes on a standard tracing are very small, it may be repeated at double standard, with the calibration mark going up four large boxes (see Fig. 14-29C). In any case, the calibration must be clearly marked on the tracing, because some diagnostic conclusions are based on the magnitude of specific portions of the ECG complex.

Waveforms. The analysis of waveforms and intervals provide the basis for ECG interpretation (Fig. 14-30).

P Wave. The P wave represents atrial depolarization.

QRS Complex. The QRS complex represents ventricular depolarization, corresponding to phase 0 of the ventricular action potential. It is referred to as a *complex* because it consists of several different waves. The letter Q is used to describe an

initial negative deflection; only if the first deflection from the baseline is negative will it be labeled a Q wave. The letter *R* applies to any positive deflection from baseline. If there are two positive deflections in one QRS complex, the second is labeled R′ ("R prime") and is commonly seen in lead V_1 in patients with right bundle branch block (RBBB). The letter *S* refers to any subsequent negative deflections. Any combination of these deflections can occur and is collectively called the *QRS complex* (Fig. 14-31). The QRS duration is normally less than 0.10 second (2.5 small boxes).

T Wave. The T wave represents ventricular repolarization, corresponding to phase 3 of the ventricular action potential. The onset of the QRS to approximately the midpoint or peak of the T wave represents an absolute refractory period, during which the heart muscle cannot respond to another stimulus no matter how strong that stimulus may be (Fig. 14-32). From the midpoint to the end of the T wave, the heart muscle is in the relative refractory period. The heart muscle has not yet fully recovered, but it can be depolarized again if a strong enough stimulus is received. This can be a particularly dangerous time for ventricular ectopy to occur, especially if any portion of the myocardium is ischemic, because the ischemic muscle takes even longer to fully repolarize. This sets the stage for the disorganized, self-perpetuating depolarizations of various sections of the myocardium known as *ventricular fibrillation* (VF).

Intervals Between Waveforms. The intervals between waveforms are evaluated (see Fig. 14-30).

PR Interval. The PR interval is measured from the beginning of the P wave to the beginning of the QRS complex. Normally, the PR interval is 0.12 to 0.20 second long and represents the time between sinus node discharge and the beginning of ventricular depolarization. Because most of this period results from delay of the impulse in the AV node, the PR interval is an indicator of AV nodal function.

In the electrophysiology laboratory and in some critical care units, these time values are described in milliseconds. There are 1000 milliseconds (msec) in 1 second. Thus, the normal PR interval value can also be written as 120 to 200 msec.

ST Segment. The ST segment is the portion of the wave that extends from the end of the QRS to the beginning of the T wave. Its duration is not measured. Instead, its shape and location are evaluated.[73] The ST segment is normally flat and at the same

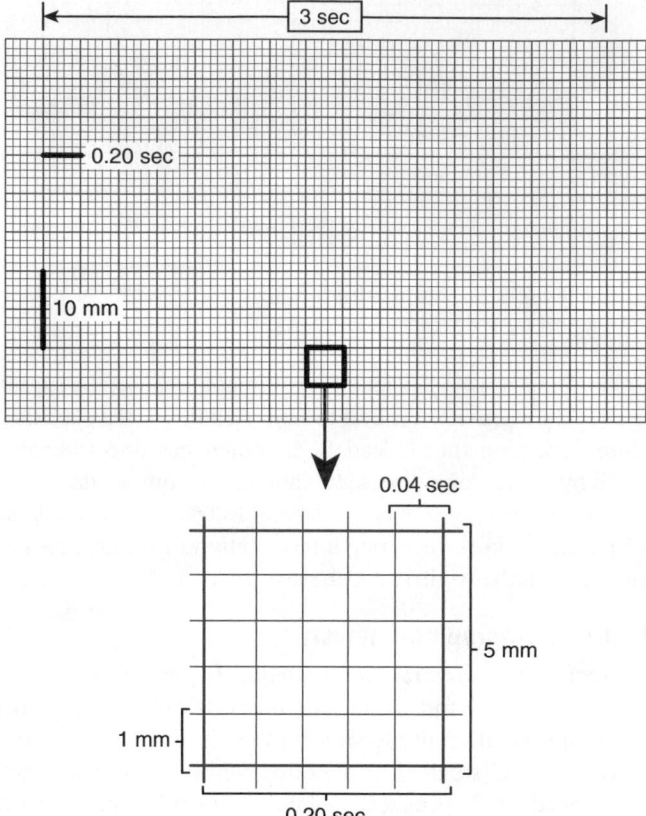

FIGURE 14-28 ECG graph paper. The horizontal axis represents time, and the vertical axis represents the magnitude of voltage. Horizontally, each small box is 0.04 second, and each large box is 0.20 second. Vertically, each large box is 5 mm. Markings are present every 3 seconds at the top of the paper for ease in calculating heart rate.

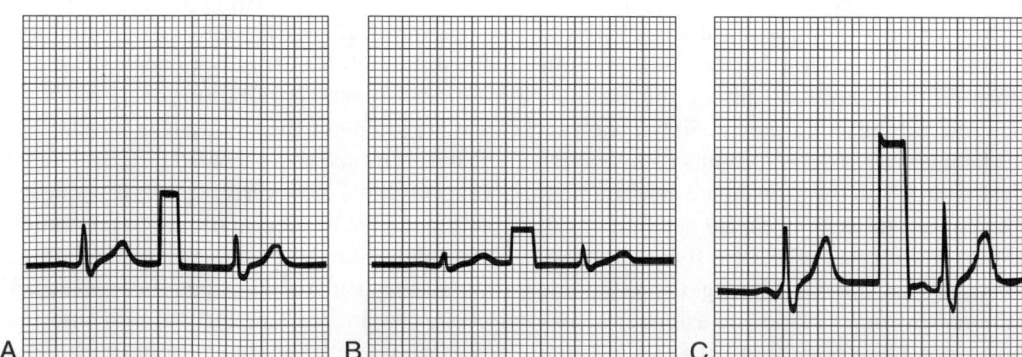

FIGURE 14-29 *A,* The machine is calibrated so that the normal standardization mark is 10 mm tall. *B,* Half standardization is used when QRS complexes are too tall to fit on the paper. *C,* Twice normal standardization is used when QRS complexes are too small to be adequately analyzed.

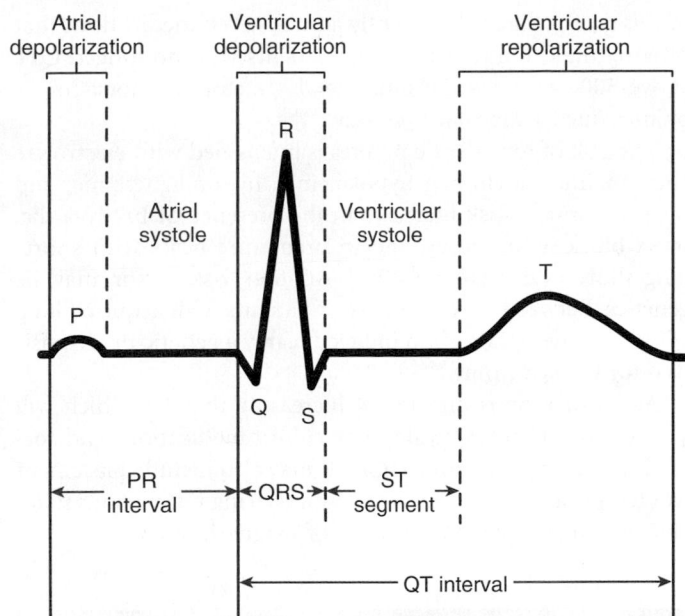

FIGURE 14-30 Normal ECG Waveforms, Intervals, and Correlation with Events of the Cardiac Cycle. The *P wave* represents atrial depolarization, followed immediately by atrial systole. The *QRS* represents ventricular depolarization, followed immediately by ventricular systole. The *ST segment* corresponds to phase 2 of the action potential, during which time the heart muscle is completely depolarized and contraction normally occurs. The *T wave* represents ventricular repolarization. The *PR interval*, measured from the beginning of the P wave to the beginning of the QRS, corresponds to atrial depolarization and impulse delay in the atrioventricular (AV) node. The *QT interval*, measured from the beginning of the QRS complex to the end of the T wave, represents the time from initial depolarization of the ventricles to the end of ventricular repolarization.

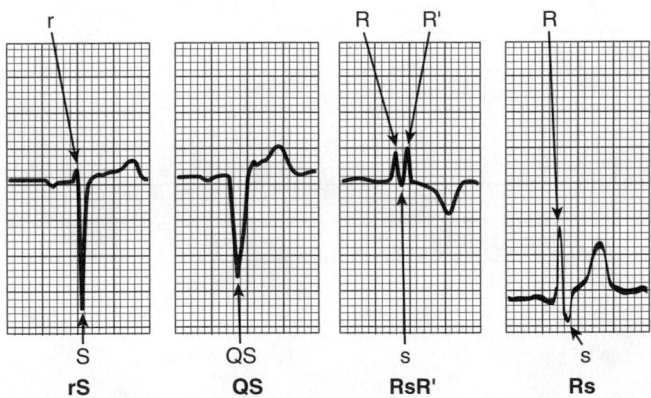

FIGURE 14-31 Examples of QRS Complexes. Small deflections are labeled with lowercase letters, and uppercase letters are used for larger deflections. A second upward deflection is labeled R'.

level as the isoelectric baseline. Any change from baseline is expressed in millimeters and may indicate myocardial ischemia (one small box equals 1 mm). ST segment elevation of 1-2 mm is associated with acute myocardial injury, preinfarction, and pericarditis. ST segment depression (decrease from baseline more of 1-2 mm) is associated with myocardial ischemia.[77] The

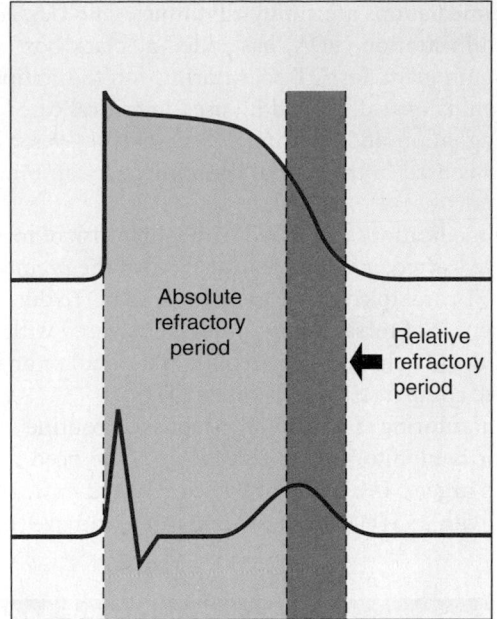

FIGURE 14-32 Absolute and relative refractory periods are correlated with the cardiac muscle's action potential and with an ECG tracing.

ST segment must be monitored carefully in high-risk patients (described later).

QT Interval. The QT interval is measured from the beginning of the QRS complex to the end of the T wave and indicates the total time interval from the onset of depolarization to the completion of repolarization. There is no established bedside monitoring lead recommended for measuring the QT interval.[72] On the 12-lead ECG, the QT interval is usually the longest in precordial leads V_3 and V_4.[72] The important point is that each clinician measures the QT interval using the same ECG lead.[72] At normal HRs, the QT interval is less than one half of the R-R interval when measured from one QRS complex to the next. However, the length of a QT interval depends on HR and must be adjusted according to the HR to be evaluated in a clinically meaningful way.

Because the QT interval shortens at faster HRs and lengthens with slower HRs, it is often written as a "corrected" value (QTc), meaning the QT value was mathematically corrected as if the HR were 60 beats/min. This allows comparison of QTc across a range of HRs. The corrected QT interval (QTc) is calculated by dividing the measured QT interval (in seconds) by the square root of the RR cycle length (see Fig. 14-3).[72] The upper limit of normal for the QTc is 0.48 second (480 msec) in women and less than 0.47 second (470 msec) in men.[72] A QTc of 440 msec is described as borderline.[73] A prolonged QT interval is significant because it can predispose the patient to the development of polymorphic VT, known also as *torsades de pointes*. A long QT interval can be congenital, as a result of genetic inheritance, or it can be acquired from an electrolyte imbalance or medications.[78,79]

Many antidysrhythmic medications can prolong the QT interval, notably class Ia antidysrhythmics (quinidine, procainamide, disopyramide) and class III antidysrhythmics (amiodarone, droneradone, ibutilide, dofetilide, sotalol). Not all high-risk mediations are antidysrhythmics. The U.S. Food and Drug Administration (FDA) has added a "black box" warning and a requirement for QT monitoring for the antipsychotic medication haloperidol (Haldol), used in critical care for treatment of agitation and delirium.[80] See Table 14-9 for a list of medications used in the critical care unit that can prolong the QT interval.

When medications associated with a high risk of torsades de pointes are started, it is important to record the premedication baseline QTc and to continue to monitor the QTc during treatment. The risk of torsades de pointes is increased with prolongation of the QTc beyond 0.5 second (500 msec) or an increase of 60 msec compared to the baseline QTc.[78]

QTc monitoring is not yet an established routine in critical care,[81] nor is monitoring for risk factors. The need to change practice is urgent. In a study of 900 cardiac patients, 18% were admitted with a QTc longer than 500 msec, and over one third of this group were subsequently administered medications that prolong the QT interval.[82] Many patients with prolonged QTc above 500 msec acquire multiple risk factors for torsades de pointes during their hospital stay.[79,80,82]

The risk of torsades de pointes is intensified with electrolyte abnormalities, including hypokalemia, hypomagnesemia, and hypocalcemia.[78] Risk increases in the presence of bradycardia, heart block with pauses, and in premature beats with short-long-short cycles (Box 14-7).[78] Another risk factor may be genetics. Between 10% and 15% of patients with acquired long QT syndrome (medication induced) carry a genetic predisposition for the syndrome.[78]

Acute therapy is directed at increasing the HR, which will shorten the QT interval, stopping culprit medications and correcting electrolyte abnormalities. It may also include placement of a temporary pacemaker and administering intravenous magnesium, especially if serum levels of magnesium are low.

TABLE 14-9   MEDICATIONS THAT MAY CAUSE TORSADES DE POINTES

GENERIC NAME	BRAND NAME	CLINICAL USE	COMMENTS
Arsenic trioxide	Trisenox®	Anticancer for leukemia	
Azithromycin	Zithromax®	Antibiotic	
Bepridil	Vascor®	Antianginal	Females>Males
Chloroquine	Aralen®	Antimalarial	
Chlorpromazine	Thorazine®	Antipsychotic; antiemetic	
Citalopram	Celexa®	Antidepressant	
Clarithromycin	Biaxin®	Antibiotic	
Disopyramide	Norpace®	Antidysrhythmic	Females>Males
Dofetilide	Tikosyn®	Antidysrhythmic	Females>Males
Droperidol	Inapsine®	Sedative; antinausea	
Erythromycin	E.E.S.® Erythrocin®	Antibiotic; increase GI motility	Females>Males
Flecainide	Tambocor®	Antidysrhythmic	
Halofantrine	Halfan®	Antimalarial	Females>Males
Haloperidol	Haldol®	Antipsychotic	TdP risk with IV or excess dosage
Ibutilide	Corvert®	Antidysrhythmic	Females>Males
Mesoridazine	Serenti®	Antipsychotic	
Methadone	Dolophine®	Opiate agonist for pain control	Females>Males
Methadone	Methadose®	Opiate agonist for pain control	Females>Males
Moxifloxacin	Avelox®	Antibiotic	
Pentamidine	NebuPent® Pentam®	Anti-infective for pneumocystis pneumonia	Females>Males
Pimozide	Orap®	Antipsychotic; Tourette's tics	Females>Males
Procainamide	Pronestyl® Procan®	Antidysrhythmic	
Quinidine	Quinaglute® Cardioquin®	Antidysrhythmic	Females>Males
Sotalol	Betapace®	Antidysrhythmic	Females>Males
Thioridazine	Mellaril®	Antipsychotic	
Vandetanib	Caprelsa®	Anticancer for thyroid cancer	

Modified from the *Arizona Center for Education and Research on Therapeutics (CERT)*. http://www.qtdrugs.org. Accessed August 27, 2012. Table only includes medications with a documented risk of torsades de pointes, in the United States. Low-risk medications are not included.

BOX 14-7 RISK FACTORS FOR TORSADES DE POINTES

Prolonged QTc
QTc _500 msec

Medications
Use of QT-prolonging medications
Rapid IV infusion of QT-prolonging medications
Diuretics

Structural Heart Conditions
Heart failure
Myocardial infarction

Metabolic Conditions
Hypokalemia
Hypomagnesemia
Hypocalcemia
Liver failure with decreased medication metabolism

Bradycardia
Sinus bradycardia
Complete heart block
Incomplete heart block with pauses
Premature complexes leading to short-long-short cycles

Genetic Predisposition
Occult (latent) congenital LQTS23,64
Genetic polymorphisms (reduced repolarization reserve)

Age and Sex
Advanced age
Female sex

Torsades de pointes risk increases with a higher number of risk factors, some of which may be clinically silent and difficult to detect.

From Drew BJ, Ackerman MJ, Funk M, et al. Prevention of torsade de pointes in hospital settings: a scientific statement from the American Heart Association and the American College of Cardiology Foundation. *Circulation.* 2010;121(8):1047.

Ventricular Axis. Electrical impulses spread through cardiac muscle tissue in many directions at once when the ventricular muscle is depolarized. Using the 12-lead ECG, all of these individual forces can be averaged to describe the overall direction that current is traveling, which is called the *mean vector*. This mean vector represents the general direction of the wavefront of depolarization within the heart. The mean vector can be plotted on a circular graph known as the *hexaxial reference system* (Fig. 14-33), and a degree value can be assigned to it. This degree represents the overall ventricular axis.[75]

Parameters for ventricular axis in degrees are −30° to +90°.[75] Right-axis deviation is present if the heart's electrical axis falls between +90° and +180°. Right-axis deviation can be further delineated as moderate right-axis deviation when it is between +90° and +120°, and marked right-axis deviation when it is between +120° and +180°.[75]

Left-axis deviation is present if the axis falls between −30° and −90°. Moderate left-axis deviation describes an axis between −30° and −45°. Marked left-axis deviation describes an axis between −45° and −90°.[75]

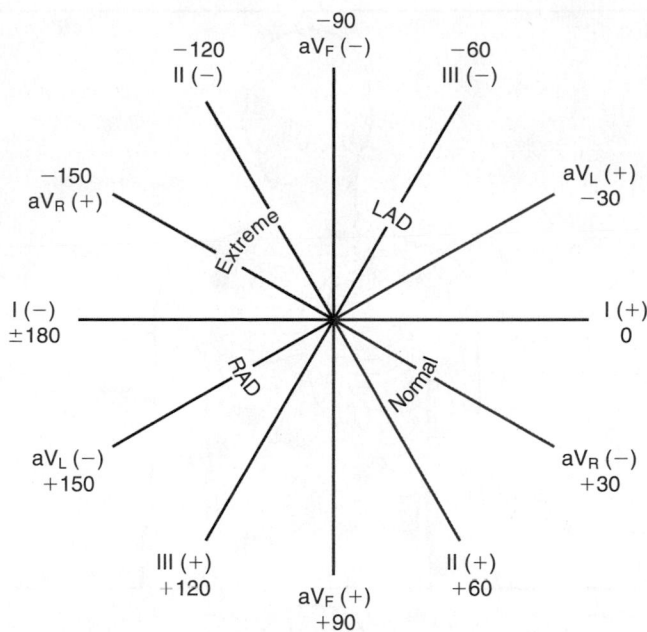

FIGURE 14-33 Hexaxial Reference System. *LAD*, Left-axis deviation; *RAD*, right-axis deviation.

Figure 14-33 shows how these points are located on the hexaxial reference system. If the axis plots in the upper left portion of the circle, also known as the *extreme quadrant* or *northwest quadrant*, it is called an *indeterminate axis*. This axis occurs rarely but can be seen when the wave of depolarization starts at the bottom of the ventricle—near the point of maximal impulse (PMI) or apex of the ventricle—and spreads upward toward the atria. Clinically, this can be seen in beats of ventricular origin, such as PVCs and some pacemaker-initiated beats.

Calculating the Ventricular Axis. The ventricular axis is calculated using the six limb leads (leads I, II, III, and aVR, aVL, aVF) in the three steps outlined below (see ECG example in Fig. 14-34).

Step 1. Find the limb lead with the smallest QRS complex or the one that is the most *equiphasic* (equal portions above and below the baseline). In Figure 14-35, lead aVF is the smallest.

Step 2. Using the hexaxial reference system (see Fig. 14-33), locate the lead that is perpendicular to the one that had the smallest complex. For example, perpendicular to lead aVF is lead I, so the mean vector lies parallel with lead I.

Step 3. The third step is to determine whether the QRS complex is positive or negative in the lead parallel to the mean vector (in this case, lead I). If the QRS is positive, the mean vector is directed *toward* the positive electrode. If the QRS is negative, the mean vector is directed *away* from the positive electrode. In Figure 14-35, the QRS deflection in lead I is upright or positive. The positive pole of lead I is at the right midpoint of the hexaxial reference system and corresponds to a numeric degree of zero, which is within the normal range (see Figure 14-33) (Box 14-8).

Cardiac Monitor Lead Analysis

During continuous cardiac monitoring, adhesive, pregelled electrodes are used to obtain an ECG tracing that is similar to

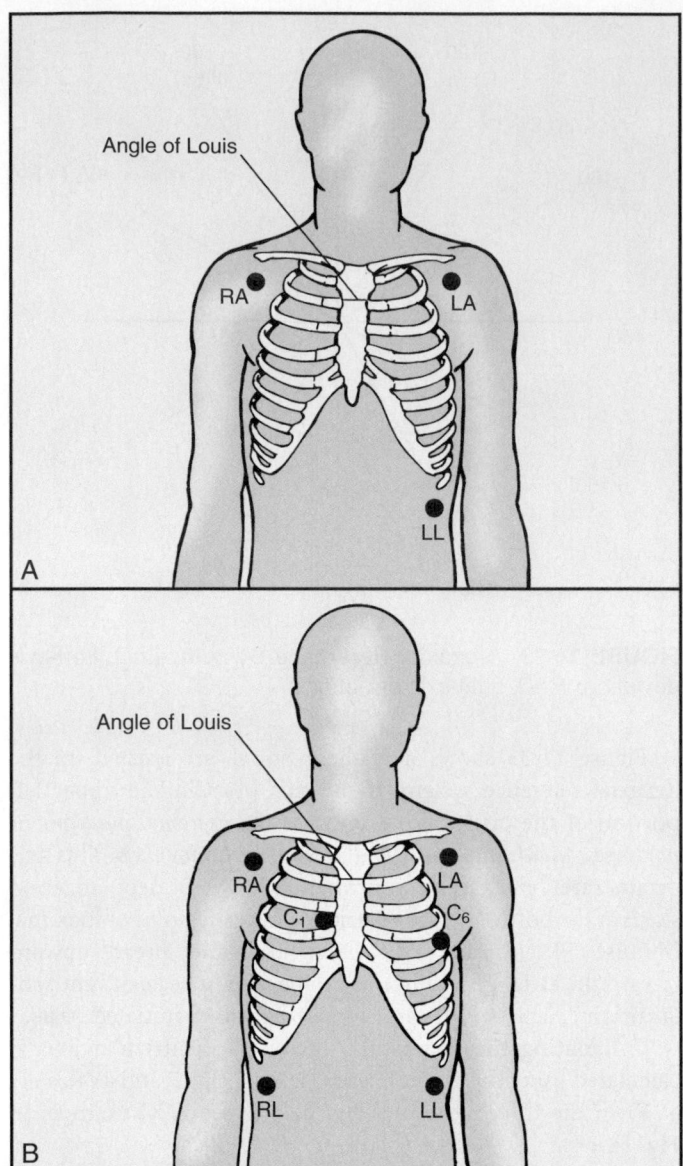

FIGURE 14-34 *A,* Three electrodes and lead-wire cables allow monitoring of three of the limb leads (I, II, and III) and can be rearranged to monitor MCL₁ and MCL₆. *B,* In the multilead monitoring system, five electrodes and lead-wire cables allow monitoring of any of the six standard limb leads (I, II, III, aVR, aVL, or aVF) and any one precordial lead (V₁ or V₆). C₁ indicates the proper position of the chest electrode for monitoring lead V₁, and C₆ indicates the proper position of the chest electrode for monitoring V₆. Color-coded cable attachments allow quick identification and accurate electrode placement.

one or more leads of a 12-lead ECG. At minimum, this requires three electrodes. One of the electrodes acts as a positive pole, one as a negative pole, and one as a ground. In most critical care units, five electrodes are used. Five electrode systems allow the clinician to monitor two leads simultaneously and permit selection of several different leads at any time through a lead selector switch on the monitor. Typical placement of the five electrodes in a multilead system is right arm (RA), left arm (LA), left leg (LL), and right leg (RL), with one chest lead that usually is placed in the V₁ position, as illustrated in Figure 14-34.

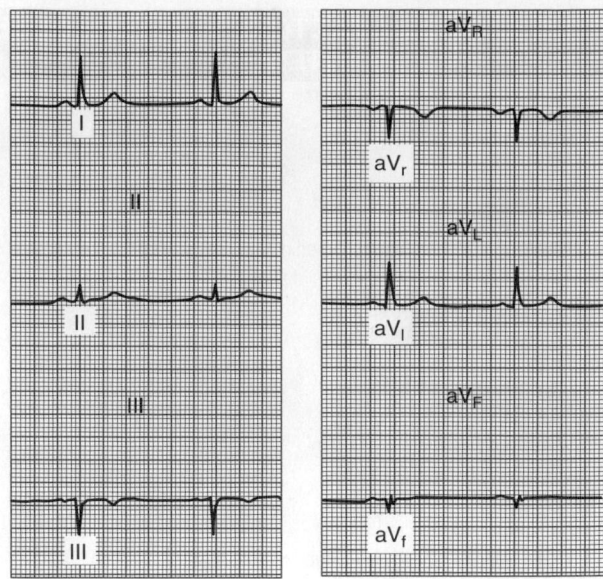

FIGURE 14-35 Limb leads of a normal ECG illustrate a normal axis of 0 degrees.

BOX 14-8 STEPS IN DETERMINING THE AXIS

1. Find the most isoelectric limb lead.
2. Using the hexaxial reference system, find the lead that is perpendicular to the one identified in step 1.
3. Determine whether the QRS is positive or negative in the perpendicular lead.
4. Look at the corresponding positive or negative pole of the perpendicular lead on the hexaxial reference system.
5. The degree listed on the hexaxial reference system is the axis.

The selection of an ECG monitoring lead is not a decision to be made casually or according to habit. The monitoring lead should be chosen in consideration of the patient's clinical condition and recent clinical history.[72] If the patient has experienced ST segment elevation associated with acute coronary syndrome, percutaneous catheter intervention (PCI), or recent cardiac surgery, the leads that exhibited ST segment elevation should used to guide selection of the optimal ECG monitoring leads.[72] Verify correct electrode placement and appropriate lead selection at the beginning of each shift.

Lead II. On a standard 12-lead ECG, lead II is formed by a positive electrode attached to the left leg, a negative electrode attached to the right arm, and a ground electrode on the right leg. It is not practical to connect electrodes to the arms and legs during continuous monitoring, so the electrodes are placed on the torso near the origin of the limbs (see Fig. 14-34). In the critical care unit, most patients have at least five electrodes placed, and the lead is selected by choosing a lead selector button on the monitor. If the monitored heart has a normal electrical axis, lead II displays a waveform that is predominantly upright, with a positive P wave and positive QRS waveform (see Fig. 14-36B). P waves are usually easy to identify in lead II, and it is recommended for monitoring of atrial dysrhythmias. However, it is difficult to identify RBBB and left bundle branch

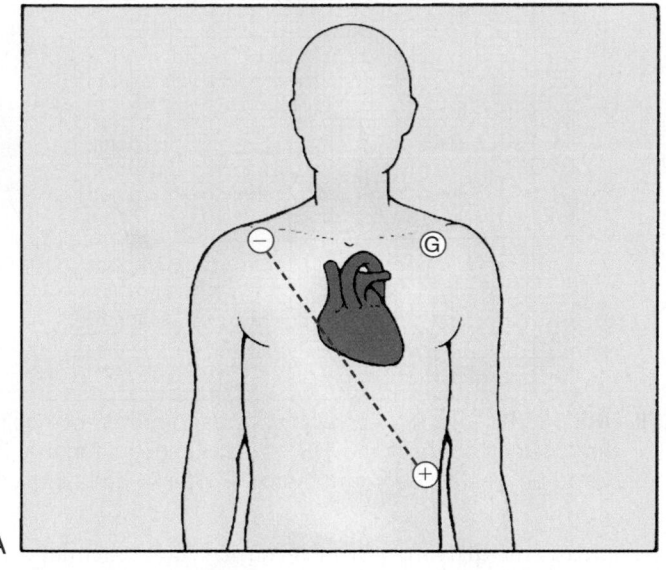

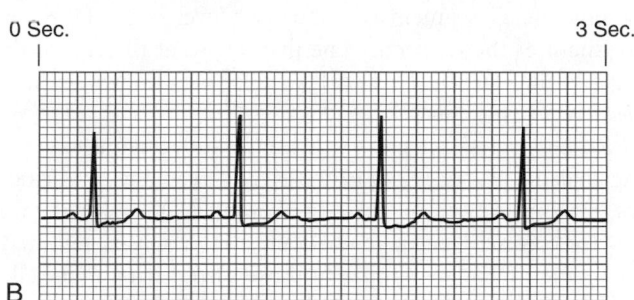

FIGURE 14-36 Monitoring lead II. *A*, Electrode placement. The negative electrode is placed below the right shoulder; the positive electrode is placed on the lower left torso (preferably below the rib cage); and the ground electrode is placed on the left shoulder. *B*, Typical ECG tracing in lead II.

block (LBBB) in this lead, because this is a vertical lead that does not clearly display horizontal interventricular conduction changes. Lead II is also nondiagnostic in differentiating VT from supraventricular tachycardia (SVT) with aberrant conduction. More information on differentiating VT from wide-complex SVT is provided later in this chapter.

Lead V₁. The V_1 electrode is placed at the fourth intercostal space to the right of the sternal border. Most of the electrical activity of the heart is directed toward the left ventricle and away from the V_1 electrode. For this reason, the normal QRS complex in lead V_1 is mostly negative (Fig. 14-37B). Any abnormal electrical activity directed toward the right ventricle, such as in RBBB, results in an upright QRS complex, often in an RSR′ pattern.

V_1 is the optimal lead to select if the critical care nurse needs to analyze ventricular ectopy. V_1 provides information to facilitate differentiation between RBBB versus LBBB pattern, or distinguish between VT and SVT with aberrant conduction; determine whether PVCs originate in the right or left ventricle, and clarify when ST segment changes are caused by the RBBB and when they are the result of ischemia. Lead V_1 is excellent for this purpose. More information on the criteria used to identify these rhythms using the V_1 lead is provided later in this chapter.

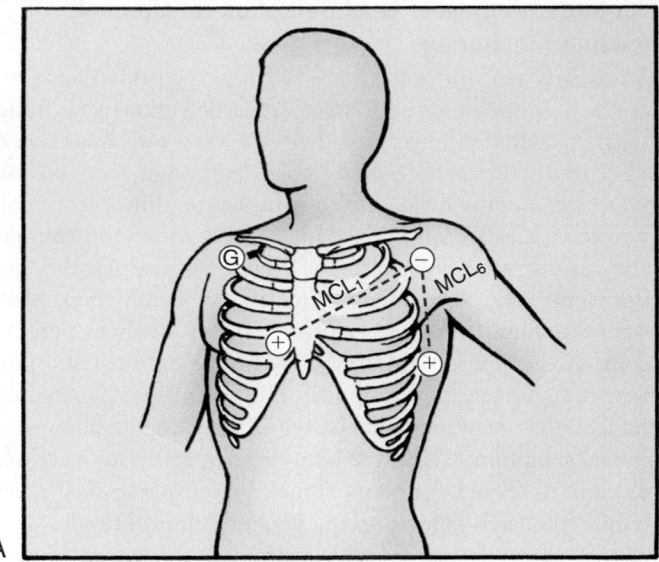

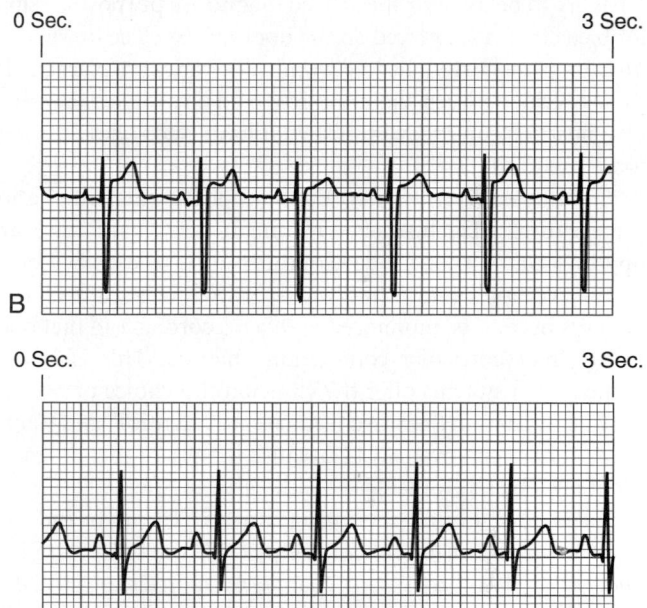

FIGURE 14-37 *A*, Monitoring lead placement for MCL_1 and MCL_6. *B*, Typical ECG tracing for MCL_1. *C*, Typical ECG tracing for MCL_6.

MCL₁. MCL_1 means "modified chest lead using V_1". It is similar to a V_1 lead on a 5-lead or 12-lead ECG. The tracings are similar but not identical. In MCL_1 the negative electrode is placed on the right shoulder and the positive electrode is placed at the fourth intercostal space, just to the right of the sternum (see Fig. 14-37A). This electrode must be placed accurately. MCL_1 is an uncommon lead choice today. It is used only if monitoring with a 3-lead system (such as on a transport monitor, when a "true" V_1 is not available), which is a rare situation within any critical care unit. The normal QRS complex in lead MCL_1 has a mostly negative deflection (see Fig. 14-37B). In contrast, the normal QRS complex in lead MCL_6 has a mostly positive deflection because of the position of the MCL_6 lead placement on the left lateral midaxillary chest wall (see Fig. 14-37C).

Electrocardiographic Lead Selection for Optimal Bedside Monitoring

In the early years of critical care nursing, the primary goals of cardiac monitoring were HR surveillance, detection of "warning" ventricular dysrhythmias (mostly PVCs), and early detection of lethal dysrhythmias (VF or asystole). Although these are still goals of ECG monitoring in the critical care unit, several more complex issues are now concerns. Not all wide QRS-complex tachycardias are ventricular in origin; sometimes they are supraventricular with aberrant ventricular conduction. Many patients are undergoing reperfusion therapy involving percutaneous coronary intervention (PCI), stenting, or fibrinolysis, and these patients require continuous monitoring for ST segment changes that may represent ischemia even in the absence of clinical symptoms. The nurse admitting a patient to the critical care unit or telemetry unit must make a well-planned choice of monitoring leads tailored to the patient's clinical needs. Accuracy of electrode placement is extremely important if these leads are to be used for specialized diagnostic purposes.[77] Upper limb electrodes are placed on the upper chest close to where the limb joins the torso. The lower limb electrodes are placed below the rib cage between the umbilicus and the midaxillary line.[73] Diagnostic accuracy is diminished if limb electrodes are moved too close to the heart.

Continuous Dysrhythmia Monitoring. Patients with serious cardiac diseases such as acute MI, heart failure, and cardiomyopathy are at risk for the development of bundle branch blocks (BBBs), complex ectopy, and wide-complex tachycardias. These patients need to be monitored with a precordial lead that documents interventricular conduction changes. This is lead V_1. Some 5-lead systems offer the clinician the choice of MCL_1 or V_1. The tracings in these two leads are not identical, and V_1 must always be chosen over MCL_1 because it has a higher diagnostic accuracy. The six frontal plane (limb and augmented lead) tracings also offer several monitoring choices that can be individualized to the clinical needs of the patient. Leads I and aVF are selected to detect a sudden change in ventricular axis. If ST segment monitoring is required, the lead is selected according to the area of ischemia. If the ischemic area is not known, leads V_3 and III are recommended to detect ST segment ischemia.[77] In inferior wall injury, leads II, III, and aVF are chosen; if lateral ischemia is present, lead I or aVL may be selected.

Continuous ST Segment Monitoring. A key responsibility of the critical care nurse is monitoring for ECG changes that signify myocardial ischemia.[77] At the bedside, this takes the form of continuous ST segment monitoring using the traditional bedside monitor and ECG electrodes. Increasingly, bedside monitoring systems incorporate ST segment analysis software to detect myocardial ischemia or injury. ST segment changes may be accompanied by classic symptoms such as chest pain, or they may be "silent," without any clinical symptoms except ST segment depression or elevation seen on the ECG monitor.[83]

The best way to choose a lead for monitoring the ST segment to detect ischemia is to look at the patient's 12-lead ECG during an episode of ischemia, if available. The standard 12-lead ECG obtained in an acute coronary syndrome before treatment or during a PCI will reveal the leads that best demonstrate

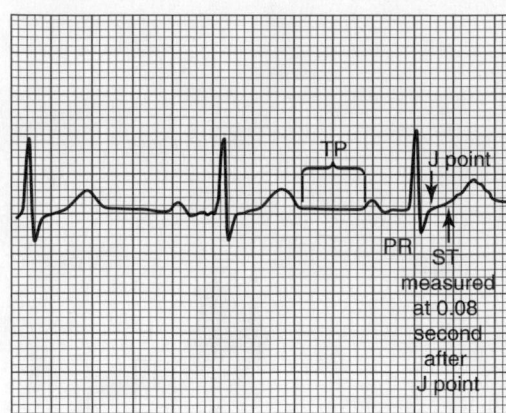

FIGURE 14-38 The TP interval is used as the reference point for the isoelectric line if the HR is slow enough for the TP interval to be clearly seen. If not, the PR interval can be used.

ischemia in that patient.[72,77] Under normal (nonischemic) conditions, the ST segment is at the same level as the TP segment (segment of the isoelectric line that begins at the end of the T wave to the start of the next P wave),[84] also known as the *isoelectric line* (Fig. 14-38).

Patients at risk for silent ischemia include anyone experiencing an acute coronary syndrome even if treated with fibrinolytics, nitrates, or anticoagulation therapy.[83] PCI patients are at risk for coronary artery repeat occlusion or spasm, reflected by ST segment changes similar to those seen during PCI balloon inflation. Any patient admitted to the critical care unit with a history of prior MI, angina, diabetes, or kidney failure is a candidate for ST segment monitoring.[72]

ST segment deviation can have nonischemic causes and can create a false-positive alarm. Common culprits include hyperkalemia, pericarditis, hypokalemia, hypomagnesemia, hypothermia, ventricular aneurysm, hypothyroidism, pulmonary infarction, and medications such as quinidine and digitalis. Patients with subarachnoid hemorrhage (SAH) often demonstrate ST segment changes caused by excessive release of norepinephrine from the myocardial sympathetic nerves. The degree of myocardial necrosis and ST segment elevation depends on the severity of neurologic injury.[85]

ST segment deviation is measured as the number of millimeters of ST segment vertical displacement from the isoelectric line or from the patient's baseline. Because ST segments may slope or arc, the measurement position is typically selected 60 msec to the right of the J point[77] (Fig. 14-39). The J point is chosen to avoid monitoring the upstroke of the T wave. On the bedside monitor, ST segment elevation is displayed as a positive number, whereas ST segment depression is indicated as a negative number (see Fig. 14-39). To be clinically significant, the J point of the ST segment must be displaced up or down from the isoelectric baseline by at least 1 mm or 2 mm (one or two small boxes on ECG paper), depending on the specific ECG lead being monitored.[86] Specific values for recognition of abnormal J-point thresholds in different ECG leads are listed in Box 14-9.

When setting ST segment alarm parameters, the patient's condition is always considered. The alarm may be set at 1 mm above and below the baseline ST segment level in patients at

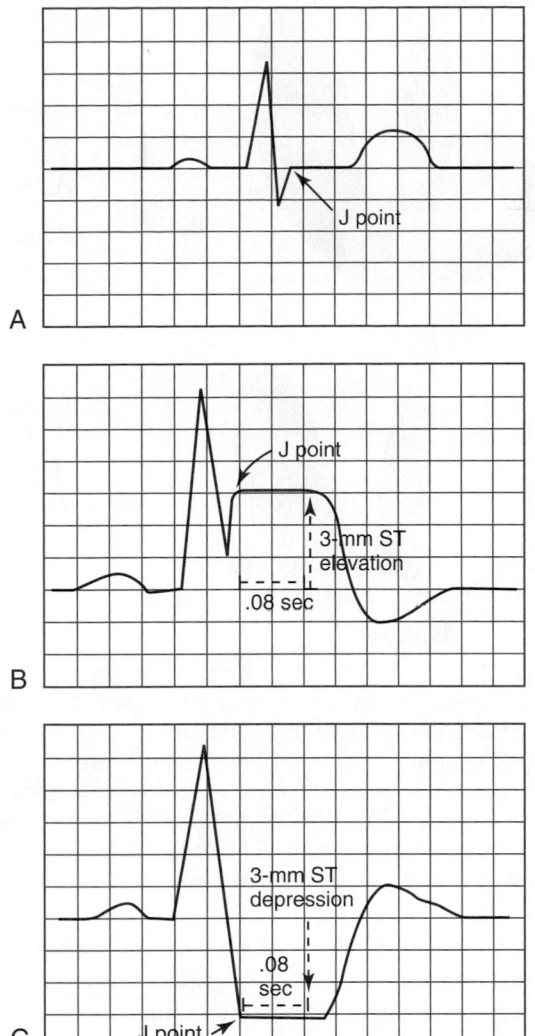

FIGURE 14-39 *A,* Normal position of the J point. *B,* A 3-mm ST segment elevation. *C,* A 3-mm ST segment depression. ST segment changes are measured 60 to 80 msec (0.06 to 0.08 sec) after the J point.

high risk for ischemia. In stable, low-risk patients, the suggested setting is 2 mm above or below the isoelectric line.[72] The rationale for selection of wider ST segment alarm parameters in more stable patients is that this may reduce the number of false ST segment alarms.[72] This is important because stable patients tend to be more active, and when patients change position, it can alter the isoelectric baseline. If there are too many false ST segment alarms, clinicians may be tempted to turn off or not pay attention to the alarm system. Poor electrode contact with the skin also is responsible for false ST segment change alarms, emphasizing the need for correct skin preparation before electrode placement.[72]

Some specific ECG patterns do not lend themselves to ST segment monitoring, particularly rhythms that are associated with a wide QRS and distortion of the ST segment. This includes LBBB and RBBB, paced rhythms, and idioventricular rhythms. Other rhythms that make ST segment monitoring problematic include erratic atrial fibrillation or atrial flutter that obscures the isoelectric baseline.[72] Agitated and restless patients make continuous ST segment monitoring almost impossible.

Atrial Hypertrophy

Atrial chamber enlargement can be suspected from the 12-lead ECG because muscle size influences the ECG tracing. Atrial abnormalities may be identified by the size and shape of the P waves and are usually most obvious in lead II. Traditionally, wide, m-shaped P waves, classically seen in *left atrial hypertrophy* were called *P mitrale,* because left atrial hypertrophy is often caused by mitral stenosis (Fig. 14-40A). Tall, peaked P waves seen with *right atrial hypertrophy* were referred to as *P pulmonale,* because this condition is often the result of chronic pulmonary disease (see Fig. 14-40B). Current ECG guidelines emphasize that P-wave abnormalities can be caused by many conditions and can occur without atrial enlargement. For this reason the ECG is not considered definitive in the identification of atrial hypertrophy.[87] The less specific term atrial abnormality is suggested for P-wave abnormalities when the underlying pathology is unknown.[87]

Ventricular Hypertrophy

Ventricular hypertrophy describes an increase in the size and muscle mass of one or both ventricles. Because a larger muscle is being depolarized, a greater amount of electrical activity is recorded on the ECG during depolarization. In ventricular hypertrophy, the increased muscle mass results in increased QRS voltages particularly in the precordial leads. Upright QRS complexes become taller, and negative QRS complexes become

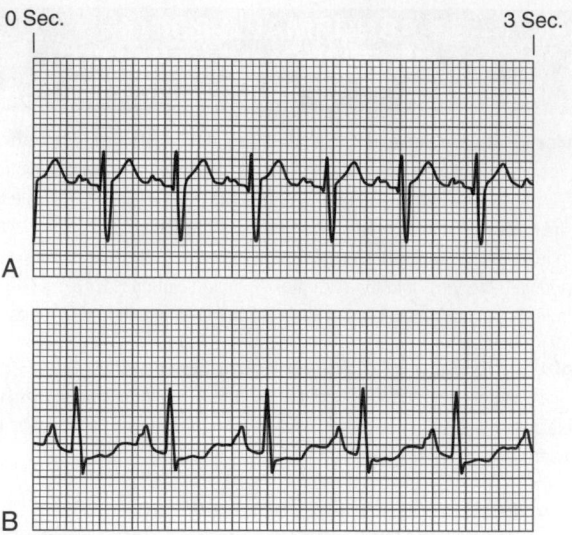

0 Sec.   3 Sec.

A

B

FIGURE 14-40 Atrial Hypertrophy. *A,* In left atrial hypertrophy, the P wave is broad and notched and is sometimes called *P mitrale,* because it is often associated with mitral valve disease. *B,* In right atrial hypertrophy, the P wave is tall and peaked and is sometimes called *P pulmonale,* because it is often associated with pulmonary disease.

even more negative. Often, the QRS becomes slightly wider, because it takes longer to depolarize a larger muscle. The QRS axis often shifts toward the enlarged ventricle, because a greater portion of the total electrical activity of the heart occurs there. Although the 12-lead ECG can suggest hypertrophy, the echocardiogram is the most reliable diagnostic device, because it can visualize ventricular wall thickness and motion.

Ischemia and Infarction

Ischemia occurs when the delivery of oxygen to the tissues is insufficient to meet metabolic demand. Cardiac ischemia in an unstable form occurs because of a sudden decrease in supply, such as when the artery is blocked by a thrombus or when coronary artery spasm occurs.[88,89] Stable angina can occur when a stenotic coronary artery is unable to adapt to a sudden increase in demand created by exercise. Ischemia is by nature a transient process. The balance of supply versus demand is restored, and the cardiac muscle tissue recovers. Conversely, when the imbalance in myocardial oxygen demand/delivery becomes so great that the tissues can no longer survive, myocardial cells infarct and become necrotic. Many nursing and medical interventions are directed toward saving as much ischemic tissue as possible.

Infarction refers to the death and disintegration of muscle cells and their eventual replacement by fibrotic scar tissue. After infarction has occurred, the process cannot be reversed. Thus, careful ECG monitoring and swift intervention to restore myocardial perfusion before infarction can take place is critically important.

Electrocardiographic Changes Indicating Ischemia and Infarction. Ischemia and infarction cause changes in the way cardiac muscle cells respond to electrical stimuli. These changes can usually be seen in a 12-lead ECG tracing.

ST segment elevation is seen when the positive electrode lies directly over an area of transmural (full-wall thickness) injury

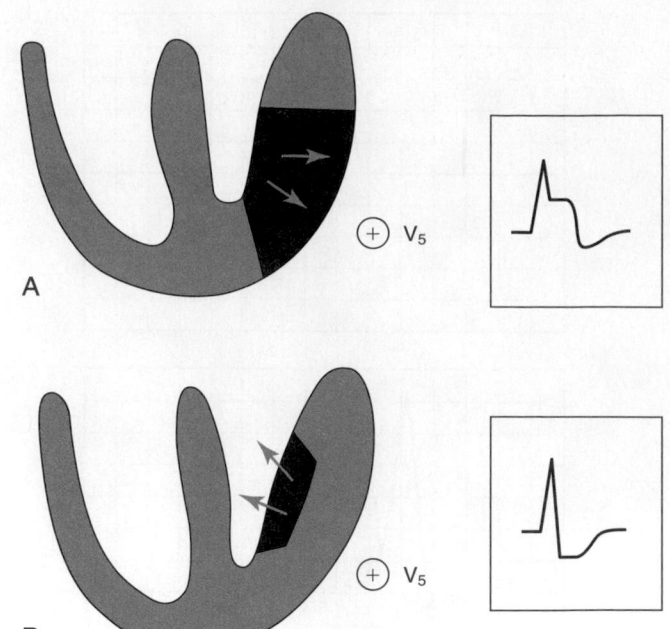

A   (+) V₅

B   (+) V₅

FIGURE 14-41 *A,* Acute transmural ischemia. The electrical forces *(arrows)* responsible for the ST segment are directed outward through the entire thickness of the heart muscle wall, causing ST segment elevation in leads directly over the ischemic area. *B,* Acute subendocardial ischemia. The electrical forces responsible for the ST segment are deviated toward the inner layer of the heart, resulting in ST depression in leads directly over that area of the heart muscle wall.

(Fig. 14-41A). The ST segment changes on the surface ECG are caused by differences in voltage gradients between ischemic and healthy myocardium, referred to as "injury currents."[86] This represents a preinfarction state, and interventions to unblock the occluded coronary artery must be initiated to prevent death of myocardium. ST segment elevation is a precursor to an ST elevation myocardial infarction (STEMI).[89]

Not every myocardial infarction is heralded by ST segment elevation. When the patient has an MI without ST segment elevation, it is described as a non–ST elevation myocardial infarction (NSTEMI), and the diagnosis can be considerably more challenging without the signature ST segment changes seen on the ECG.[88]

ST segment depression occurs when the reduction of blood flow is limited to the endocardium and some normal muscle tissue remains between the ischemic area and the positive electrode (see Fig. 14-41B). ST segment depression is seen because the positive electrode is separated from the ischemic area by normal tissue. T waves most commonly flatten or become inverted.

Infarction involves necrosis (death) of muscle cells with eventual formation of scar tissue. These cells can no longer be depolarized when an impulse reaches them. If the infarction involves the epicardial (outer) layer of the heart muscle or the entire thickness of the heart wall (transmural lesion), the QRS complex changes. Abnormal Q waves typically develop in the leads overlying the affected area. Occasionally, the entire QRS complex becomes smaller without development of Q waves.

TABLE 14-10	ELECTROCARDIOGRAPHIC CHANGES DURING MYOCARDIAL INFARCTION		
LOCATION OF INFARCTION	**ARTERY INVOLVED**	**LEADS INVOLVED**	**ECG CHANGES***
Anterior wall	LAD	V_{3-4}	Q waves, ST ↑,T ↓
Inferior wall	RCA or LCx	II, III, aVF	Q waves, ST ↑,T ↓
Ventricular septum	LAD	V_{1-2}	Q waves, ST ↑,T ↓
Lateral wall	LCx	V_{5-6}, I, aVL	Q waves, ST ↑,T ↓
Posterior wall	RCA or LCx	V_{1-3} (ant*); V_{7-9} (post†)	Tall, upright R; ST ↓; Upright T with ST ↑ V_{7-9}
Right ventricle	Proximal RCA	V_4R (right‡)	ST ↑

*See Figure 14-7B for ECG lead placement.
†See Figure 14-7D for ECG lead placement.
‡See Figure 14-7C for ECG lead placement.
ant, Anterior; *ECG*, electrocardiographic; *LCx*, left circumflex artery; *LAD*, left anterior descending artery; *post*, posterior; *Q waves*, pathologic Q waves; *RCA*, right coronary artery; *right*, right precordium; ↑, elevated; ↓ depressed.

Non–Q-wave Infarction. Not every acute MI results in a pathologic Q wave on the 12-lead ECG. When the typical ECG changes are not present, the diagnosis depends on symptomatic clinical presentation, specific cardiac biomarkers (e.g., cTnI, cTnT, CK-MB), and non-ECG diagnostic tests such as cardiac catheterization. NSTEMI infarctions are less likely to result in a non–Q-wave infarction.

Infarct Location by 12-Lead Electrocardiogram. The location of the infarction can be roughly determined by noting the specific leads in which the ST segment and T-wave changes are seen on the 12-lead ECG. Table 14-10 summarizes the anticipated 12-lead ECG changes.

Right ventricular infarction and posterior wall infarction are particularly difficult to identify on a standard 12-lead ECG, because none of the standard leads directly views these areas. A right ventricular infarction may be suspected and investigated in the setting of an acute inferior wall MI. To avoid missing this diagnosis, right-sided precordial leads (see Fig. 14-26B) can be placed, and a 12-lead ECG obtained for any patient with a suspected inferior right ventricular wall MI.[74] Early identification of right ventricular infarct is important because it requires special management and carries a greater in-hospital mortality risk.[90] Nitrates and other vasodilatory agents commonly administered in acute MI can cause profound hypotension with negative effect on preload and CO.

A posterior wall MI may be suspected in a patient with an acute inferior wall MI when there is ST segment depression in leads V_1, V_2, and V_3 on the standard 12-lead ECG. Tall, upright R waves may also be present. Posterior wall involvement can be verified by adding posterior precordial leads V_7, V_8, and V_9 (see Fig. 14-26D).

Infarct Electrocardiographic Progression. When blood flow in a coronary artery is suddenly occluded, the entire area of heart muscle normally perfused by that artery becomes ischemic. Collateral arterioles usually exist, which overlap and

TABLE 14-11	TIMING OF ELECTROCARDIOGRAPHIC CHANGES
TIME FRAME	**CHANGE**
Immediate	ST segment elevation in leads over the area of infarction
Within a few hours	Giant, upright T waves
Several hours	ST segment normalizes; T waves invert symmetrically
Several hours to days	Q waves or reduced R waves; voltage may remain low permanently

supply the perimeter of this area and may prevent necrosis of some of the affected tissue. At the center of the ischemic area, collateral blood flow is minimal or does not exist at all. Within a few hours, this tissue begins to die. On the ECG tracing, this process is illustrated as follows: within minutes of the onset of infarction, ST segment elevation occurs in the leads directly overlying the affected heart wall. This ST segment elevation persists for a period of hours to 1 day, gradually becoming less severe. Within the first few hours, T waves may become tall and symmetric. They are known as hyperacute T waves, and they indicate acute ischemia. Meanwhile, usually within 4 to 24 hours from the onset of the infarction, abnormal Q waves begin to develop in the affected leads, and T waves begin to invert. Sometimes, instead of Q waves developing, the R waves become smaller. This still indicates necrosis of muscle tissue. The ST segments become isoelectric again in a few days, and the T wave becomes symmetric and deeply inverted in the affected leads. Occasionally, these T-wave changes never resolve. However, the T waves usually return to normal within several months. The Q waves may persist for the remainder of the patient's life, or they may get smaller over time and, in some individuals, disappear altogether. Table 14-11 summarizes the timing of these changes.

Intraventricular Conduction Defects

Intraventricular conduction defects are the result of an abnormal pathway of conduction through the ventricles. Normally, conduction spreads rapidly from the AV node to the bundle of His and from there, down the right and left bundle branches. The right bundle branch is long and thin and terminates in a mass of Purkinje fibers, which spread the wave of depolarization into surrounding right ventricular muscle. After only a short distance, the left bundle branch divides into the left anterior fascicle, the left posterior fascicle, and the left septal fibers (Fig. 14-42). Each of these fascicles causes depolarization of separate areas of the left ventricle. If any part of the conduction system fails, the muscle cells in that area will still depolarize, but not as quickly. Depolarization must then spread from cell to cell, a slower process than activation through specialized conduction pathways.

On the ECG, intraventricular conduction defects cause a widening of the QRS because of the slower spread of depolarization. The affected muscle tissue begins the slower cell-to-cell depolarization just as the other areas in the ventricle are almost

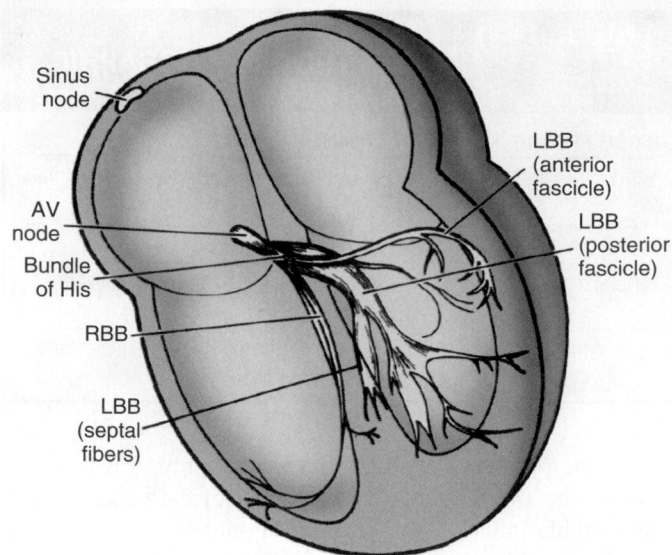

FIGURE 14-42 Cardiac Conduction System. *AV*, Atrioventricular; *LBB*, left bundle branch; *RBB*, right bundle branch. (Modified from Conover MB. *Understanding Electrocardiography*. 8th ed. St. Louis: Mosby; 2002.)

finished. This later depolarization is then tacked onto the end of the normal QRS, making it prolonged and altering its shape.

Any part of the conduction system can be affected. The term *bundle branch block* refers to complete interruption of conduction through the right bundle or the entire left bundle branch.

Right and Left Bundle Branch Blocks. The chest leads are the most useful in identifying complete RBBB and LBBB. V_1 and V_6 are the best leads from which to identify forces traveling in a horizontal direction, because they are located on the right and left sides of the heart, respectively. Figure 14-43A shows the normal sequence of ventricular activation and the usual shape of the QRS complex in V_1 and V_6.

Right Bundle Branch Block. In complete RBBB the QRS complex is wider than 0.12 second (120 msec) (see Fig. 14-43B). This is because the right ventricle is not activated through the normal rapid conduction system. Instead, it must be activated slowly, from one cell to the next. Electrical forces that are not counterbalanced by opposing forces on the left travel toward the right at the end of the ventricular activation. The septum is depolarized first in a normal manner from left to right. Next, the wave of depolarization spreads through the left ventricle and is recorded in lead V_1 as a tiny negative deflection. The final portion of the QRS complex is wide and upright, indicating final electrical forces traveling toward the right. This represents right ventricular depolarization that occurs after LV depolarization is almost complete. In V_1, this QRS complex represents a classic pattern that is labeled rsR' in V_1.[75] The ST segment representing repolarization is also abnormal and makes recognition of ST segment changes related to ischemia difficult to detect by ECG monitoring.

In lead V_6, the positive electrode is on the left side of the chest, and the waveforms are reversed. The final forces of the QRS complex are negative because they are traveling toward the right and away from the positive electrode of V_6. The final negative deflection in V_6 is smaller than the final upright

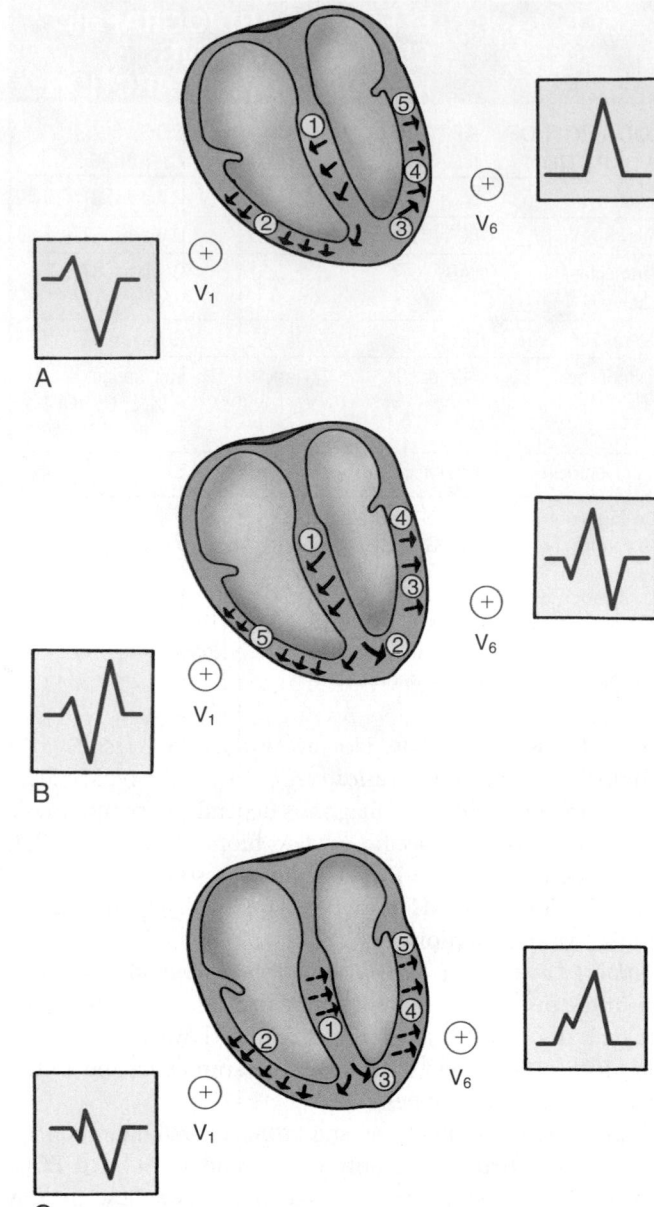

FIGURE 14-43 *A*, Sequence of ventricular depolarization and resulting QRS complex, as seen in leads V_1 and V_6. *B*, Sequence of ventricular depolarization for a right bundle branch block and resulting QRS complex, as seen in leads V_1 and V_6. *C*, Sequence of ventricular depolarization for a left bundle branch block and resulting QRS complex, as seen in leads V_1 and V_6.

deflection in lead V_1, because the positive electrode in V_6 is at a greater distance from the right ventricle.

Left Bundle Branch Block. In complete LBBB (see Fig. 14-43C), the conduction through the left ventricle must spread from cell to cell, which results in a prolonged QRS duration, longer than 0.12 second (120 msec).[75] Because a portion of the common left bundle normally initiates depolarization of the septum, the septum is depolarized in an abnormal direction, from right to left. In lead V_1, this is recorded as an initial negative deflection. Next, the right ventricle is depolarized, which is identified as a small upright notch in the QRS complex as the forces travel briefly toward the positive electrode of V_1.

BOX 14-10	CAUSES OF LEFT-AXIS DEVIATION

- Normal variation
- Mechanical shifts: exhalation; high diaphragm caused by pregnancy, ascites, or abdominal tumor
- Left anterior hemiblock
- Left ventricular hypertrophy
- Wolff-Parkinson-White syndrome
- Hyperkalemia
- Cardiomyopathy

BOX 14-11	CAUSES OF RIGHT-AXIS DEVIATION

- Normal variation
- Mechanical shifts: inhalation, emphysema
- Left posterior hemiblock
- Right ventricular hypertrophy
- Lateral wall myocardial infarction
- Right bundle branch block
- Dextrocardia

Sometimes, this notch is absent. The sequence of events has not changed, but the left ventricle is already beginning to be depolarized cell to cell and may offset the rightward forces of right ventricular depolarization. The final forces travel toward the left as the left ventricle is being depolarized. The left ventricle is a very large muscle mass, and these final electrical forces are large and wide. In lead V_1, the final deflection is a deep, negative deflection (S wave), whereas in lead V_6, these final forces inscribe a tall, upright deflection (R wave).

Presence of an LBBB makes diagnosis of an acute anterior wall MI extremely difficult because the change in repolarization masks ST segment elevation. Perhaps related to this difficulty in interpreting injury, patients with acute coronary syndrome in the presence of LBBB have double the mortality risk in-hospital compared with ACS patients without LBBB.[91]

BBBs may be recognized at the bedside if the patient is being monitored with leads V_1 and V_6, respectively. However, definitive diagnosis of BBB should be made via a 12-lead ECG.[92] A BBB exists when the P wave is followed by a QRS complex that is wider than 0.12 second (120 msec) with other features of the block.[75] The presence of the P wave indicates that the complex did not originate from the ventricles. One quick method to determine which bundle branch is blocked is to look at the last part of the QRS just before it returns to the baseline in leads V_1 and V_6. If upright in V_1 and negative in V_6, an RBBB exists. If negative in V_1 and upright in V_6, an LBBB is present.

Hemiblocks. Hemiblocks involve conduction failure of only part of the left bundle branch. In left anterior fascicular block, also called *left anterior hemiblock*, LV depolarization begins in the left posterior fascicle and spreads anteriorly through Purkinje fibers distal to the block. The QRS is of normal duration, meaning it is less than 0.12 second. However, the frontal-plane axis changes dramatically and becomes more negative than −30 degrees, indicating left-axis deviation (axis between −45 degrees and −90 degrees)[75] (Boxes 14-10 and 14-11). Anterior hemiblock is a relatively frequent finding in patients with arterial hypertension or cardiomyopathy (see Box 14-11).[93]

Left posterior fascicular block is also a hemiblock and is also known by the term *left posterior hemiblock*. The QRS duration is within normal limits (less than 0.12 second).[75] The block in the posterior fascicle changes the normal conduction pathway, so that the anterior portion of the left ventricle is depolarized first. Conduction then spreads slowly to the right, inferiorly and posteriorly. The axis then swings entirely the other direction and becomes greater than +90 degrees, indicating right-axis deviation (axis between 90 and 180 degrees).[75] Isolated posterior hemiblock is rare, and it is almost always associated with concomitant RBBB.[93]

Bifascicular Block. Blockage of either of the two branches of the LV conduction system plus RBBB constitutes a *bifascicular block.* Any combination of these conduction disturbances can occur and can evolve into complete heart block. Normally, bifascicular block (hemiblock plus RBBB) is well tolerated, and no intervention is necessary. The exception is bifascicular block that develops during an acute MI, in which the evolving infarct may warrant placement of a temporary pacemaker prophylactically in case conduction tissue ischemia progresses to complete heart block.

Dysrhythmia Interpretation

In clinical practice, the terms *dysrhythmia* and *arrhythmia* often are used interchangeably. The question of which word is the more accurate is often discussed. Both terms are correct, and either may be used in practice. In this textbook, dysrhythmia is the more commonly used term. A dysrhythmia is any disturbance in the normal cardiac conduction pathway. Dysrhythmias can be detected on a 12-lead ECG, but they often occur only sporadically. For this reason, patients in a critical care unit are monitored continuously using a single- or dual-lead system, and rhythm strips are recorded each shift and any time the patient's heart rhythm changes. Dysrhythmias occur frequently in cardiac and noncardiac critically ill patients. A systematic approach to assess a rhythm disturbance is an indispensable skill. Steps to accurately interpret a rhythm strip are introduced first, followed by specific criteria to evaluate common dysrhythmias encountered in clinical practice.

Heart Rate Determination. The first thing to assess when evaluating a rhythm strip is the ventricular rate. Regardless of the dysrhythmia involved, the ventricular rate holds the key to whether the patient can tolerate the dysrhythmia (i.e., maintain adequate blood pressure, CO, and mentation). If the ventricular rate is consistently greater than 200 or less than 30, emergency measures must be started to correct the rate. A detailed analysis of the underlying rhythm disturbance can proceed later, when the immediate crisis is over. The three methods for calculating rate (Fig. 14-44A) follow:

1. Number of R-R intervals in 6 seconds times 10 (ECG paper is usually marked at the top in 3-second increments, making a 6-second interval easy to identify)
2. Number of large boxes between QRS complexes divided into 300

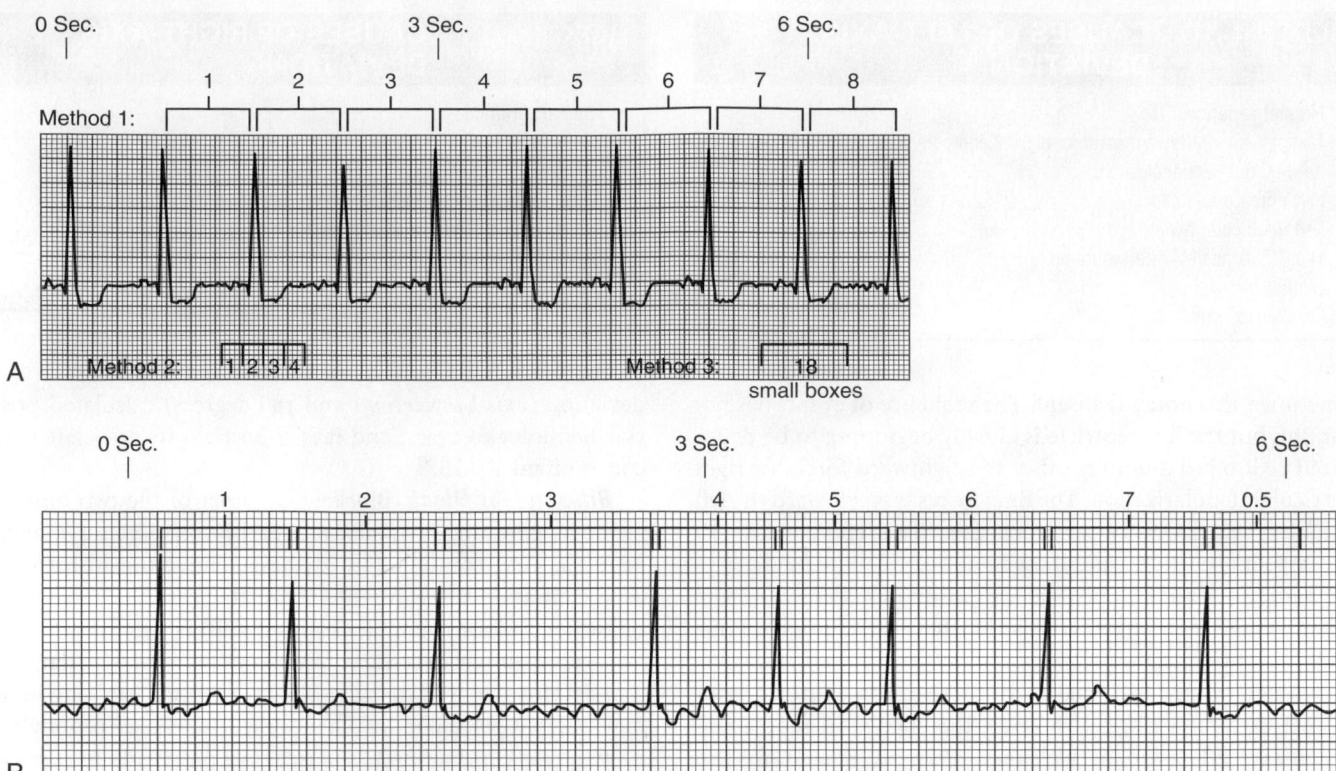

FIGURE 14-44 *A,* Calculation of the HR if the rhythm is regular. Method 1: number of R-R intervals in 6 seconds multiplied by 10 (e.g., 8 × 10 = 80/min). Method 2: number of large boxes between QRS complexes divided into 300 (e.g., 300 ÷ 4 = 75/min). Method 3: number of small boxes between QRS complexes divided into 1500 (e.g., 1500 ÷ 18 = 84/min). *B,* Rate calculation if the rhythm is irregular. Only method 1 can be used (e.g., 7.5 intervals × 10 = 75/min).

3. Number of small boxes between QRS complexes divided into 1500

In the healthy heart, the atrial rate and the ventricular rate are the same. However, in many dysrhythmias, the atrial and ventricular rates are different, and both must be calculated. To find the atrial rate, the PP interval, instead of the R-R interval, is used in one of the three methods listed for determining rate.

The choice of method for calculating the HR depends on the regularity of the rhythm. If the rhythm is irregular, the first method (R-R intervals in 6 seconds × 10) is the only method that can be used (see Fig. 14-44B). If the rhythm is regular, it is more accurate to use the second or third method. The second method can be easier to use when two consecutive R waves fall exactly on dark lines, and it provides a rapid estimate of rate. The third method is recommended when both R waves do not fall exactly on dark lines.

Rhythm Determination. The term *rhythm* refers to the regularity with which the P waves or R waves occur. Calipers assist in determining rhythm. One point of the calipers is placed on the beginning of one R wave, and the other point is placed on the next R wave. Leaving the calipers "set" at this interval, each succeeding R-R interval is checked to be sure it is the same width as the first one measured.

In describing the rhythm, three terms are used. If the rhythm is *regular,* the R-R intervals are the same ±10%. For example, if there are 20 small boxes in an R-R interval, an R wave could be

off by two small boxes, but the rhythm would still be considered regular. If the rhythm is *regularly irregular,* the R-R intervals are not the same, but some sort of pattern is involved, which could be grouping, rhythmic speeding up and slowing down, or any other consistent pattern (Fig. 14-45A). If the rhythm is *irregularly irregular,* the R-R intervals are not the same, and no pattern can be found (see Fig. 14-46B).

P-Wave Evaluation. The P wave is analyzed by answering the following questions. First, is the P wave present or absent? Second, is it related to the QRS? It is hoped that one P wave will be in front of every QRS. Sometimes, two, three, or four P waves may be in front of every QRS. If this pattern is consistent, the P wave and QRS are still related, although not on a 1:1 basis.

PR-Interval Evaluation. The duration of the PR interval, which normally is 0.12 to 0.20 second (120 to 200 msec), is measured first. This is measured from the start of a visible P wave to the beginning of the next QRS (Fig. 14-46). All PR intervals on the strip are verified to be sure they have the same duration as the original interval.

QRS Complex Evaluation. The entire ECG strip must be evaluated to ascertain that the QRS complexes are consistently the same shape and width. The normal QRS duration is 0.06 to 0.10 second (60 to 110 msec). Any QRS longer than 0.10 second is considered abnormal.[75] If more than one QRS shape is on the strip, each QRS must be measured. The QRS is measured from where it leaves the baseline to where it returns to the baseline (see Fig. 14-46).

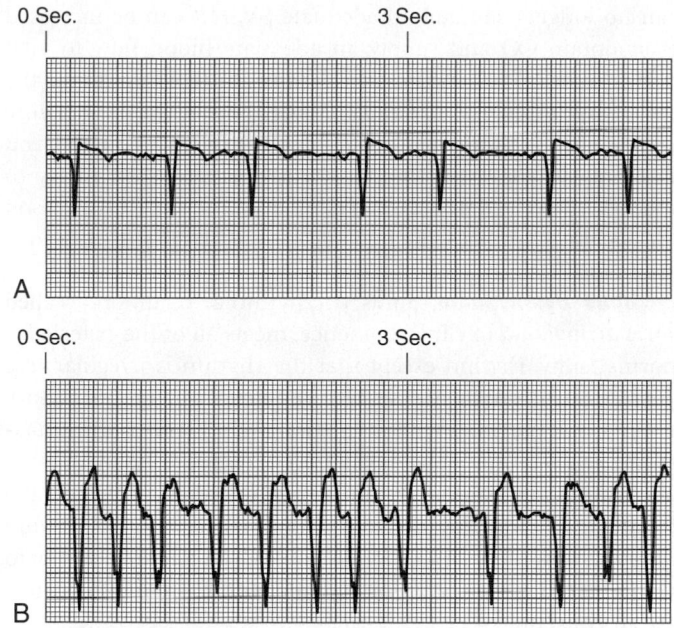

FIGURE 14-45 *A,* Regularly irregular rhythm is irregular but has a consistent pattern in that every other beat is premature. *B,* Irregularly irregular rhythm is irregular with no consistent pattern.

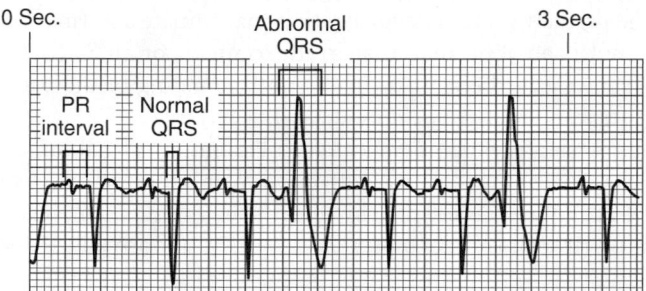

FIGURE 14-46 PR interval measurement, from the beginning of the P wave to the beginning of the QRS complex. The PR interval on this tracing is 0.20 second; the QRS duration illustrates normal and abnormal intervals. The narrow QRS complexes measure 0.08 second, which is normal. The wide QRS complexes measure 0.20 second and are caused by ventricular ectopy.

QT Evaluation. The length of the QT varies with the HR. The QT interval is shorter when the HR is faster. A QT interval corrected for HR (QTc) that is longer than 0.50 second (500 msec) is of concern, as discussed earlier under "QT Interval."

Sinus Rhythms

The cardiac cycle begins when an impulse originates in the sinus node. As the wave of depolarization spreads through the atria, a P wave is inscribed on the ECG. The impulse is delayed briefly in the AV node, which corresponds to the PR interval on the ECG. After leaving the AV node, the wave of depolarization spreads rapidly through the bundle of His and the bundle branches and causes ventricular depolarization, which is recorded as a QRS complex by the ECG. Contraction immediately follows depolarization. Contraction is terminated by repolarization, which is demonstrated as a T wave on the ECG.

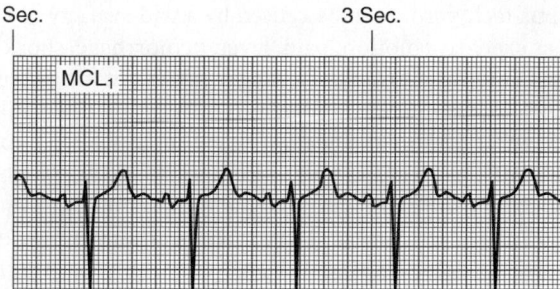

FIGURE 14-47 Normal Sinus Rhythm. The rate is 70, and the rhythm is regular. One P wave is present before each QRS complex. The PR interval is 0.18 second and does not vary throughout the strip. The QRS duration is 0.08 second. All evaluation criteria are within normal limits.

Normal Sinus Rhythm. If all of the events described for sinus rhythms occur in their normal sequence with normal rates and intervals, the patient is in normal sinus rhythm. The following are the criteria for normal sinus rhythm:

Rate. The intrinsic rate of the sinus node is 60 to 100 beats/min. *Intrinsic rate* is the normal rate at which a pacemaker site in the heart depolarizes automatically with no outside influences, such as medications, fever, or exercise. In normal sinus rhythm, the rate must be whatever is normal for the sinus node (60 to 100 beats/min).

Rhythm. The rhythm must be regular ±10%.

P wave. P waves must be present, and only one must precede every QRS complex.

PR interval. The PR interval represents delay in the AV node. In normal sinus rhythm, the PR interval is 0.12 to 0.20 second.

QRS. Size and shape do not matter in this complex, because it depends on lead placement and gain adjustments on the monitor. However, all QRS complexes must look alike. If conduction through the ventricles is normal, the QRS duration is 0.06 to 0.10 second. Figure 14-47 is an example of normal sinus rhythm in V_1.

Sinus Bradycardia. Sinus bradycardia meets all of the criteria for normal sinus rhythm except that the rate is less than 60 beats/min (Table 14-12). It is normally seen in well-trained athletes at rest or in many other individuals during sleep. Other conditions in which sinus bradycardia occurs include vagal stimulation, increased intracranial pressure, medication therapy with digoxin or beta-blockers, and ischemia of the sinus node caused by an acute MI. Sinus bradycardia usually is not treated unless the patient displays symptoms of hypoperfusion, such as hypotension, dizziness, chest pain, or changes in level of consciousness.

Sinus Tachycardia. Sinus tachycardia meets all the criteria for normal sinus rhythm except that the rate is greater than 100 beats/min (see Table 14-12). Rates may be as high as 180 to 200 beats/min in healthy young adults during strenuous exercise. However, in the critical care setting, bed rest is prescribed for most patients. It is wise to be skeptical of any "sinus tachycardia" with a rate greater than 150 and to search for a triggering focus other than the sinus node. For example, atrial flutter waves may be difficult to see at first glance because of baseline distortion caused by the high ventricular rate (Fig. 14-48).

Sinus tachycardia can be caused by a wide variety of factors, such as exercise, emotion, pain, fever, hemorrhage, shock, heart failure, and thyrotoxicosis.[94] Illegal stimulant drugs such as cocaine, "ecstasy," and amphetamines can raise the resting HR significantly.[94] Many medications used in critical care can also cause sinus tachycardia; common culprits are aminophylline, dopamine, hydralazine, atropine, and catecholamines such as epinephrine. Tachycardia is detrimental to anyone with ischemic heart disease because it decreases the time for ventricular filling, decreases SV, and compromises CO. Tachycardia increases heart work and myocardial oxygen demand while decreasing oxygen supply by decreasing coronary artery filling time.

If the cause of the tachycardia can be determined, such as fever or pain, the cause is treated rather than trying to lower the HR directly. Several medications are available to decrease the HR if needed. Calcium channel blockers and beta-blockers are widely used for this purpose. However, a word of caution is warranted. CO is determined by HR and SV. If an injured heart can no longer maintain an adequate SV, HR can be increased to maintain CO and supply an adequate blood flow to vital body tissues. If a medication is administered to force the sinus node to slow, severe and relatively immediate heart failure can result. The sinus node is controlled by many neural and humoral influences in the body, and the rate is set to try to meet the perceived demands; a close examination of the reason for the tachycardia is mandatory before treatment decisions are made.[95]

Sinus Dysrhythmia. Sinus dysrhythmia, commonly called *sinus arrhythmia* in clinical practice, meets all of the criteria for normal sinus rhythm except that the rhythm is irregular (see Table 14-12). This irregularity coincides with the respiratory pattern; HR increases with inhalation and decreases with exhalation (Fig. 14-49). Sinus dysrhythmia often occurs in children and young adults, and the incidence decreases with age. No treatment is required. To avoid being misled by other rhythm disturbances, the examiner must look at all P waves closely to verify that they are all the same shape and that the PR intervals are all constant.

Atrial Dysrhythmias

Atrial dysrhythmias originate from an ectopic focus in the atria, somewhere other than the sinus node. The ectopic impulse occurs prematurely, before the normal sinus impulse occurs. The premature atrial depolarization may initiate a normal QRS complex, an abnormal or aberrant complex, or an SVT. Huge advances have been made in the understanding of the pathogenesis and management of atrial dysrhythmias.

Premature Atrial Contractions. Premature atrial contractions (PACs) are isolated early beats from an ectopic focus in the atria. The underlying rhythm is usually sinus. The regular sinus rhythm is interrupted by an early, abnormally shaped

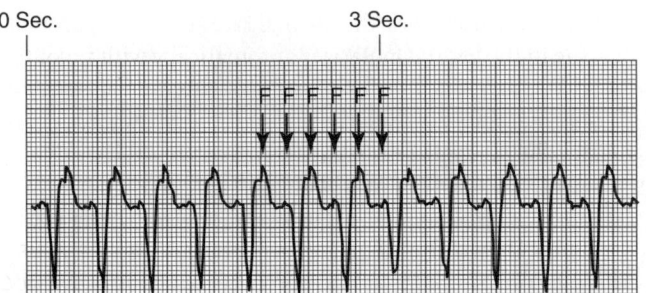

FIGURE 14-48 Although the tracing may be confused with sinus tachycardia, it is atrial flutter with 2:1 conduction. Notice how difficult it is to see the extra flutter waves (F) that are hidden in the QRS complexes.

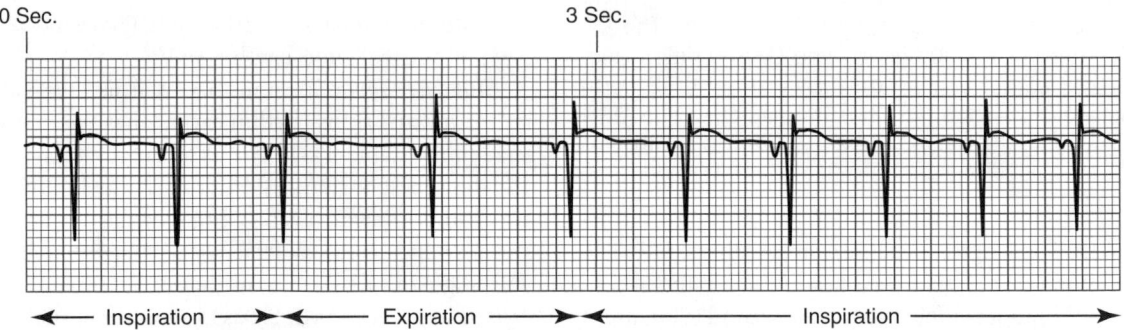

FIGURE 14-49 Sinus Dysrhythmia. Notice the increased heart rate (HR) during inspiration and decreased HR during expiration.

TABLE 14-12	SINUS RHYTHMS			
PARAMETERS	**NORMAL SINUS RHYTHM**	**SINUS BRADYCARDIA**	**SINUS TACHYCARDIA**	**SINUS DYSRHYTHMIA**
Rate	60-100/min	<60/min	>100/min	Variable
Rhythm	Regular	Regular	Regular	Irregular; respiratory variation
P wave	Present, with one per QRS	Present, with one per QRS	Present, with one per QRS	Present, with one per QRS
PR interval	0.12-0.20 sec and constant	0.12-0.20 sec and constant	0.12-0.20 sec and constant	0.12-0.20 sec and constant
QRS	0.06-0.10 sec	0.06-0.10 sec	0.06-0.10 sec	0.06-0.10 sec

atrial P wave. The early atrial wave usually looks different from the sinus P wave and may be inverted. The PR interval may be longer, shorter, or the same as the PR interval of a sinus impulse. The QRS that follows the ectopic atrial P wave can vary in shape depending on the degree of refractoriness of the AV node.

Normal, narrow QRS. If the atrial impulse arrives in the AV node after the AV node is fully repolarized, the impulse is conducted to the ventricles as a normal QRS. If the ventricles are also fully repolarized, conduction through the bundle branches is expected and a normal QRS is recorded on the ECG (Fig. 14-50A).

Wide QRS. Occasionally, the early ectopic P wave can be conducted through the AV node, but part of the conduction pathway through the ventricular bundle branches is blocked. Because the right bundle branch normally has the longest refractory period, it is usually the right bundle branch that is still blocked when the early impulse arrives. This produces a QRS that is wider than 0.12 second (120

msec) or wider than three small boxes on the ECG paper, with a shape consistent with RBBB (see Fig. 14-50B). Conduction through the ventricles that is different from normal is referred to as *aberrant.* Consequently, these early, abnormally conducted PACs are described as *aberrantly conducted PACs.*

Pause with no QRS. Sometimes, the ectopic P wave arrives so early that the AV node is still in its absolute refractory period. In this case, the wave of depolarization does not move past the AV node and no QRS follows. All that is seen on the ECG is an early, abnormal P wave followed by a pause until the next sinus P wave occurs (see Fig. 14-50C). This is called a *nonconducted PAC.* Usually, these P waves are so early that they are superimposed on the T wave of the previous beat, making them difficult to find. The pause that follows is still clearly seen. Whenever an unexpected pause occurs in a rhythm, the T wave preceding the pause must be examined very carefully and compared with other T waves on the same strip to locate distortions that may reveal a hidden early P wave.

PACs can occur in individuals with normal hearts. PACs are accentuated by emotional upheaval, nicotine, caffeine, and digitalis. Mitral valve prolapse is associated with an increased frequency of atrial dysrhythmias. Heart failure can cause PACs because of increased pressure within the atria. As atrial pressure begins to rise, the atrial walls are stretched, causing irritability of atrial cells and the occurrence of PACs.

Supraventricular Tachycardia. The term *supraventricular tachycardia* (SVT) is used clinically to describe a varied group of dysrhythmias that originate above the AV node. SVT is not a specific term; it includes sinus tachycardia, atrial tachycardia, multifocal atrial tachycardia, atrial flutter, atrial fibrillation, and junctional tachycardia. Each of these entities has a distinct pathophysiology, specific therapy, and expected outcome. SVT may also be described as a *narrow-complex tachycardia,* defined as a QRS that is less than 0.12 second (120 milliseconds).[94] After the specific dysrhythmia is identified, it usually is referred to by a specific name, such as atrial fibrillation with a rapid ventricular response. The term SVT is used to describe a rapid, sustained atrial or junctional tachycardia when the exact mechanism is unknown. Women are affected by episodic SVT at about twice the rate of men.[94]

In an acute situation, a rapid dysrhythmia may be difficult to identify precisely. SVT can cause hemodynamic instability. It is important to differentiate VT from SVT; the focus then can be directed toward rate control until the acute situation is resolved and hemodynamic stability is restored. At that point, a more careful analysis is needed to determine the specific dysrhythmia responsible for the SVT. The differentiation of wide-complex SVT from VT requires specific knowledge of the relevant ECG criteria (discussed later).

SVT is not always benign. About 15% of people with SVT experience syncope (lose consciousness). Medications are used to limit the SVT rate and prevent "blackouts" or syncope.[94] SVT that is persistent for weeks or months may lead to a tachycardia-mediated cardiomyopathy.[94] A baseline 12-lead ECG is helpful, and when possible, a 12-lead ECG should be obtained during the palpitations.[94]

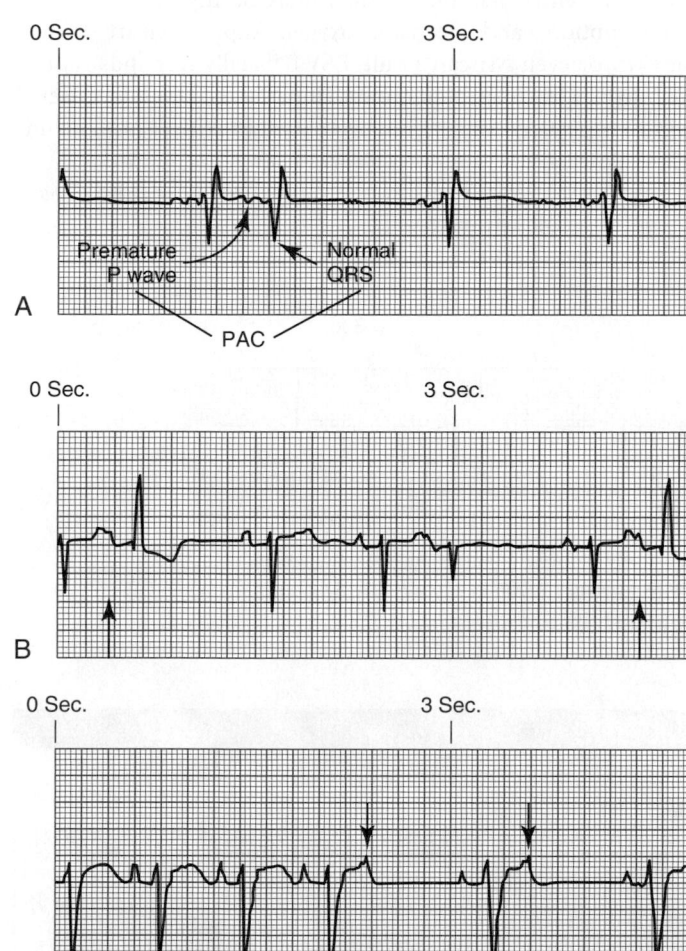

FIGURE 14-50 Premature Atrial Contractions (PACs). *A,* Normally conducted PAC. The early P wave is indicated by the *arrow,* and the QRS that follows has a normal shape and duration. *B,* Nonconducted (blocked) PACs. The early P waves are indicated by *arrows.* Notice how they distort the T waves, making them appear peaked compared with the normal T waves seen after the third and fourth QRS complexes. *C,* Right bundle branch block aberration after a PAC.

Supraventricular Tachycardia with Aberrant Conduction. If the QRS in SVT is wider than 0.12 second, it is important to differentiate between SVT with aberrant conduction and VT (discussed later). SVT with aberrant conduction includes SVT with a BBB and SVT that uses an anomalous congenital additional fiber (accessory pathway), such as Wolff-Parkinson-White syndrome.[94] Patients with SVT with aberrant conduction are frequently misdiagnosed, and evaluation by a specialist is highly recommended.[94]

Paroxysmal Supraventricular Tachycardia. *Paroxysmal* means starting and stopping abruptly. *Paroxysmal supraventricular tachycardia* (PSVT) refers to the sudden interruption of sinus rhythm by an atrial ectopic focus that fires repetitively at a rate of 150 to 250 beats/min and eventually stops as suddenly as it began (Fig. 14-51).

The rhythm of PSVT is perfectly regular because the re-entry loop has a specific length; each circuit through the loop requires exactly the same amount of time to complete. Re-entry within the atria itself or involving the AV node is the mechanism responsible for most SVTs, including PSVT. Other common underlying mechanisms include abnormal automaticity and triggered activity. P waves are present and abnormally shaped, although they may be difficult to identify because they often blend in with the previous T wave because of the rapid rate. It is most helpful if the beginning of the PSVT run is captured and recorded on ECG paper, because the early, abnormal P wave is often easiest to identify in front of the first beat of the run.

The PR interval should be the same for each cycle in the run, but it will probably be different from the PR interval of the patient's own normal sinus rhythm. As with PACs, the QRS complex is usually normal, because after the impulse passes through the AV node, conduction through the ventricles follows the usual pathway (Table 14-13). However, in PSVT (as discussed for SVT), aberrant conduction, often in the form of LBBB or RBBB, can occur with a wide QRS complex (greater than 0.12 second); this creates difficulty in differentiating relatively benign PSVT from its more serious counterpart, VT.

Sometimes, because of refractoriness in the AV node, not all of the ectopic P waves are conducted to the ventricles. Usually, at least every other P wave conducts a QRS, described as a 2:1 ratio, but occasionally, the conduction relation may drop to three P waves for every QRS (3:1 ratio).

PSVT has essentially the same causal factors as PACs. PSVT has greater clinical significance, because it may be sustained for long periods and because it occurs at such a rapid rate. As stressed in the discussion of sinus tachycardia, rapid rates decrease ventricular filling time, increase myocardial oxygen consumption, and decrease oxygen supply. Heart failure, angina, or even MI can result. PSVT usually responds rapidly to medical management, which initially includes the use of vagal maneuvers. Vagal maneuvers used in critical care include the following[94]:

Valsalva maneuver. The patient is asked to "bear down," as if going to the bathroom.

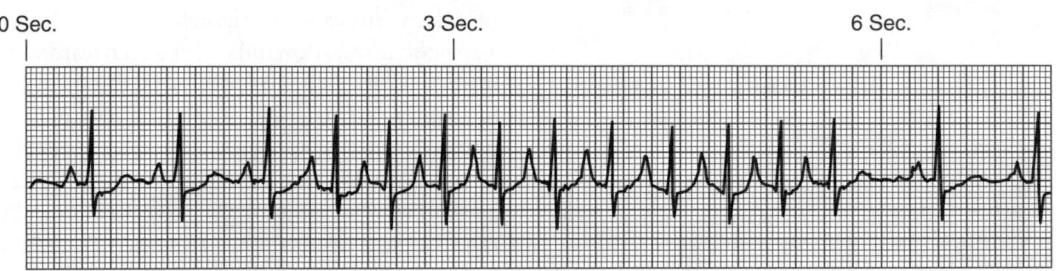

FIGURE 14-51   Paroxysmal Supraventricular Tachycardia (PSVT). Notice that the atrial rate during tachycardia is 158 beats/min. The run starts and stops abruptly.

TABLE 14-13   ATRIAL DYSRHYTHMIAS

PARAMETER	PAROXYSMAL SUPRAVENTRICULAR TACHYCARDIA	MULTIFOCAL ATRIAL TACHYCARDIA	ATRIAL FLUTTER	ATRIAL FIBRILLATION
Rate				
Atrial	150-250/min	100-160/min	250-350/min	>350/min (unable to count it)
Ventricular	Same or less	Same	250-350/min, one half or less	100-180/min (uncontrolled); <100/min (controlled)
Rhythm	Regular	Irregular	Atrial: regular; ventricular: may or may not be regular	Irregularly irregular
P wave	Present; abnormally shaped	Present; three or more different shapes	F waves	Fibrillatory baseline
PR interval	May be normal or prolonged	Variable	Conduction ratio: flutter waves per QRS	Absent
QRS	0.06-0.10 sec	0.06-0.10 sec	0.06-0.10 sec	0.06-0.10 sec

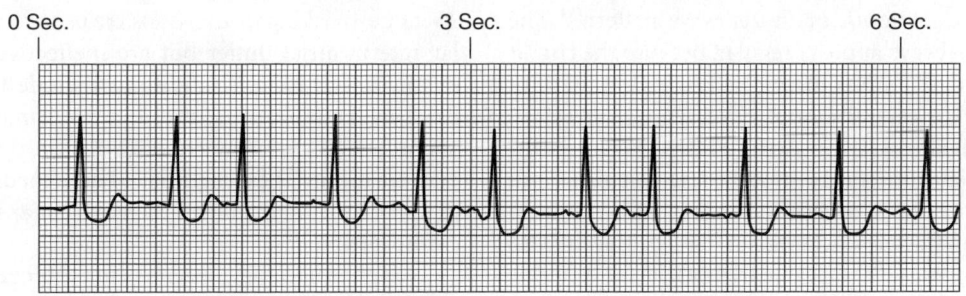

FIGURE 14-52 Multifocal Atrial Tachycardia (MAT). Notice that there are several differently shaped P waves and that the PR intervals vary.

Carotid sinus massage. It is performed on only one side of the neck over the carotid artery by a physician on a patient with a monitored ECG and avoided on older patients who may have atherosclerotic disease of the carotid arteries.

If vagal maneuvers are unsuccessful at terminating the PSVT, the next step usually is the use of intravenous medications if the patient is hemodynamically stable.[94] The intravenous medication of choice to briefly block conduction through the AV node is adenosine (Adenocard). In PSVT, adenosine alone is often sufficient to restore normal sinus rhythm, but if not, it will unmask the ectopic P waves and confirm or provide strong clues to diagnose the SVT.[94] The usual dose is 6 mg given intravenously by rapid push, followed by an NS bolus. If this does not create a temporary AV block or restore sinus rhythm, a 12-mg intravenous dose is administered. Potential dysrhythmic side effects of adenosine include a 1% to 15% chance of initiating atrial fibrillation. Adenosine is contraindicated in patients with severe asthma.[94]

Other intravenous medications that may be used to slow the rate in PSVT are amiodarone (Cordarone), a class III antidysrhythmic with a rapid onset and a short half-life.[94] Alternatively, diltiazem, a class IV calcium channel blocker in the nondihydropyridine group, can be administered. The action of these medications is to slow conduction through the AV node.[94] If intravenous medications do not convert the PSVT or sustained SVT or if the patient becomes hemodynamically unstable, the next step is electrical cardioversion.[94]

Multifocal Atrial Tachycardia. Multifocal atrial tachycardia (MAT), sometimes referred to as *chaotic atrial tachycardia*, occurs when there are numerous irritable atrial foci that intermittently fire and generate an impulse (Fig. 14-52). The atrial rate is greater than 100 beats/min but usually does not exceed 160 beats/min. The distinguishing feature on the ECG is that there are at least three different P-wave shapes, indicating at least three different irritable foci that can generate three different atrial rates.[94] MAT is always irregular and is frequently misdiagnosed and confused with atrial fibrillation.[94] MAT is most commonly seen in older patients with chronic obstructive pulmonary disease (COPD). COPD causes chronic pulmonary hypertension, which causes chronically elevated right atrial and right ventricular pressures. The abnormally high right atrial pressure causes stretching of the right atrial muscle cells and chronic irritability. Because the underlying cause cannot be resolved, this dysrhythmia is refractory to any treatment. There is no role for electrical cardioversion, antidysrhythmic

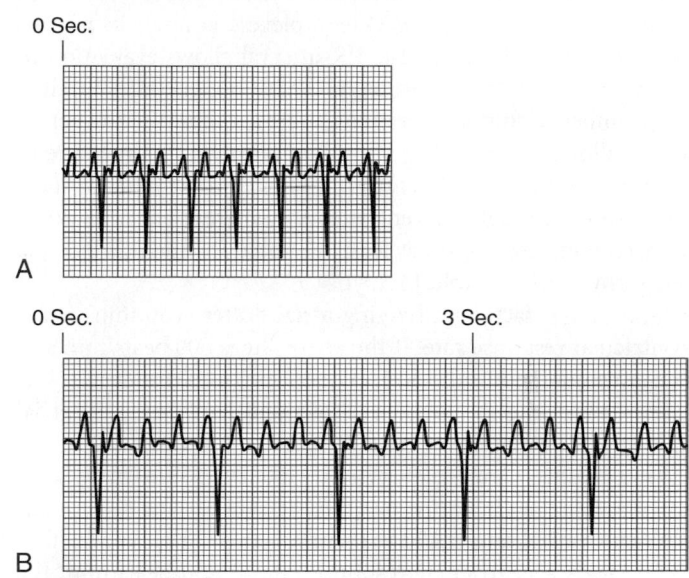

FIGURE 14-53 *A,* Initial strip shows atrial flutter with 2:1 conduction through the atrioventricular (AV) node. *B,* During carotid sinus massage, the AV conduction rate is decreased, more clearly revealing the flutter waves.

medications, or catheter ablation. Therapy is directed at limiting the effect of the COPD and correcting any electrolyte abnormalities.[94]

Atrial Flutter. Atrial flutter is recognized on the ECG by the *sawtooth* atrial pattern. These sawtooth-shaped atrial wavelets are not P waves; they are more appropriately called F waves (atrial flutter waves), as shown in Figure 14-53. Fortunately, the AV node does not allow conduction of all these impulses to the ventricles.

Pathogenesis of Atrial Flutter. Atrial flutter can be started by any isolated atrial impulse, but to be maintained, the atrial flutter requires a *re-entry circular pathway* around macroscopic structures in the atria. Typically, these structures are in the right atrium and involve the vena cava and the tricuspid valve in an area known as the *cavotricuspid isthmus.* The *re-entry loop* typically circles counterclockwise around the tricuspid valve[94] and can circle the inferior vena cava (IVC) or the IVC and the tricuspid valve. To maintain a viable, self-perpetuating re-entry pathway, the loop must avoid the sinoatrial node and be large enough to always meet tissue that is ready to be depolarized (accept a new electrical stimulus). The atrial re-entry rate in atrial flutter is typically between 250 and 350 beats/min, producing the classic sawtooth or flutter wave pattern.[94] The atrial flutter wavelet always appears regular, because the circuit is always the same length and requires exactly the same amount of time to complete the re-entry loop.

Atrial and Ventricular Rates in Atrial Flutter. When evaluating the rate of atrial flutter, it is important to calculate both atrial and ventricular rates. The ventricular rhythm is regular if the same number of flutter waves occurs between each QRS complex—in other words, if the degree of block at the AV node remains constant. Sometimes, the refractoriness in the AV node changes from beat to beat, resulting in an irregular ventricular response. When describing atrial flutter, the term *PR interval* no longer applies; instead, a conduction ratio, such as 3:1 or 4:1 (ratio of atrial waves to QRS complexes) is used. In normal sinus rhythm, measuring the PR interval allows evaluation of the speed of conduction through the AV node; in atrial flutter, the number of flutter waves that bombard the AV node before one is allowed to pass through to the ventricles is a measure of AV nodal conduction. After the impulse has passed the AV node, conduction through the ventricles is unaltered. The QRS duration remains normal or at least the same as it was in normal sinus rhythm (see Table 14-13).

The major factor underlying atrial flutter symptoms is the ventricular response rate. If the atrial rate is 300 beats/min and the AV conduction ratio is 4:1, the ventricular response rate is 75 beats/min and should be well tolerated. However, if the atrial rate is 300 beats/min but the AV conduction ratio is 2:1, the corresponding ventricular rate of 150 beats/min may cause angina, acute heart failure, or other signs of cardiac decompensation. An atrial rate of 250 beats/min with a 1:1 AV conduction ratio yields a ventricular response rate of 250 beats/min; the patient will be extremely symptomatic, and emergency measures are needed to decrease the ventricular rate.

Sometimes, it is difficult to identify the flutter waves, especially if the conduction ratio is 2:1. Vagal maneuvers or adenosine can be useful diagnostic tools to allow better visualization of the flutter waves (see Fig. 14-53A). Vagal maneuvers or intravenous adenosine cannot terminate atrial flutter but do create a temporary AV block to permit visualization of the atrial waveform and thereby facilitate accurate diagnosis, as seen in Figure 14-53B.

Atrial Flutter Management. Pharmacologic cardioversion using ibutilide (Corvert) is effective at converting hemodynamically stable atrial flutter to sinus rhythm in 38% to 76% of patients.[94] The reasons for the variance in conversion in clinical studies is unknown, but it was not related to the length of time the patients had been in atrial flutter. For patients who responded to the ibutilide, the average conversion time after infusion was 30 minutes. One of the complications of ibutilide is polymorphic tachycardia—also known as *torsades de pointes*—but in studies of patients with atrial flutter, the rate of torsades de pointes was less than 3%.[94]

Antidysrhythmic medications are prescribed in two ways to treat atrial flutter: to convert the rhythm to normal sinus rhythm (NSR) and to slow conduction through the AV node. The most effective conversion agent is ibutilide (discussed previously); other, less effective medications include flecainide, propafenone, sotalol, procainamide, and amiodarone.[94] Other

AV node-blocking medications are used to control the ventricular rate in atrial flutter but are ineffective at terminating the dysrhythmia. These medications include the calcium channel blockers, beta-blockers, and digoxin. Amiodarone shares both properties. It can slow conduction through the AV node and convert the atrial dysrhythmia. These medications are effective as a mechanism to control the ventricular rate before electrical cardioversion.[94]

Nonpharmacologic interventions to convert atrial flutter to sinus rhythm are the most effective; they include electrical cardioversion and atrial overdrive pacing. The conversion rate with DC cardioversion is between 95% and 100%.[94] If atrial flutter has been present for more than 48 hours, up to one third of patients will have thrombi in the atria, and anticoagulation is mandated before pharmacologic or electrical cardioversion. The risk of systemic emboli after cardioversion ranges from 2% to 7%.[94] Overdrive atrial pacing is often favored to convert atrial flutter after cardiac surgery. Epicardial wires that are placed at the time of surgery are connected to an external pacemaker. The overall success rate of atrial overdrive pacing is 83% (range, 55% to 100%).[94]

For about 60% of patients, sudden onset of atrial flutter is associated with an acute disease process such as acute MI or exacerbation of pulmonary disease, or it follows cardiac or pulmonary surgery. In this scenario, after the acute disease is managed, the atrial flutter usually responds quickly to standard therapy, and long-term medication management is not required. If at any time the patient with atrial flutter becomes hemodynamically unstable, electrical cardioversion is the recommended emergency intervention.[94]

For patients with atrial flutter unrelated to an acute disease process, permanent termination of the atrial flutter circuit can be achieved by *radiofrequency ablation* (RFA).[96] RFA is a catheter procedure used to create a line of conduction block across one of more sections of the re-entry pathway. The most frequent location for RFA is a narrow band of tissue between the IVC and the tricuspid annulus known as the *cavotricuspid isthmus*.[94] Chapter 16 contains additional information on antidysrhythmic medications for the treatment of atrial dysrhythmias.

Atrial Fibrillation. Atrial fibrillation is the most frequently encountered dysrhythmia in the developed world (Fig. 14-54). It affects an estimated 2.3 million individuals in the United States and 4.5 million people in the European Union. In the

0 Sec.   3 Sec.

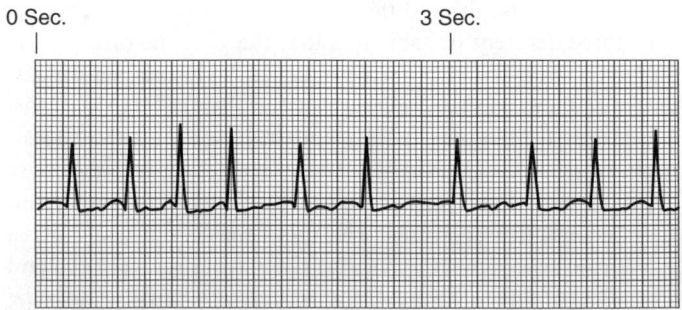

FIGURE 14-54   Atrial Fibrillation. Notice the irregularly irregular ventricular rhythm.

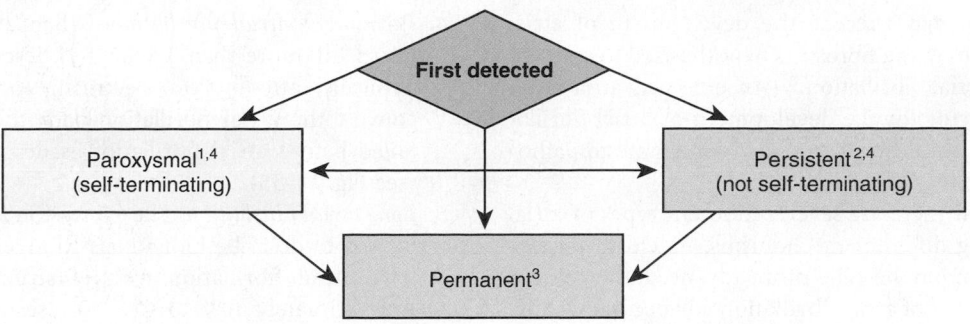

[^1]Episodes that generally last less than or equal to 7 days (most less than 24 h);
[^2]usually more than 6 days;
[^3]cardioversion failed or not attempted; and
[^4]both paroxysmal and persistent AF may be recurrent.

FIGURE 14-55 Patterns of new-onset atrial fibrillation. (From Fuster V, et al. ACC/AHA/ESC 2006 guidelines for the management of patients with atrial fibrillation: a report of the American College of Cardiology/American Heart Association Task Force on Practice Guidelines and the European Society of Cardiology Committee for Practice Guidelines [Writing Committee to revise the 2001 guidelines for the management of patients with atrial fibrillation]: developed in collaboration with the European Heart Rhythm Association and the Heart Rhythm Society. *Circulation.* 2006;114[7]:e257.)

United States, the estimated annual cost to treat atrial fibrillation is about $3,000 per patient per year.[97] When first detected, atrial fibrillation may be described as *paroxysmal* (self-terminating) or *persistent* (not self-terminating); when all attempts at conversion to sinus rhythm have failed, it is described as *permanent* (Fig. 14-55).

Atrial fibrillation may be classified under the broad category of SVT, because the HR is rapid and many patients have symptoms of hypotension and breathlessness during paroxysmal atrial fibrillation when uncontrolled by medication. Nonsinus uncoordinated atrial electrical activation leads to a rapid deterioration in atrial mechanical function. The ECG tracing in atrial fibrillation is notable for an uneven atrial baseline that lacks clearly defined P waves and instead shows rapid oscillations or fibrillatory wavelets that vary in size, shape, and frequency.[97] The atrial fibrillatory waves are particularly easy to identify in the inferior ECG leads II, III, and AVF.

The ventricular response to atrial fibrillation is influenced by several factors: the efficiency of the AV node; autonomic nervous system activity—the level of sympathetic and parasympathetic (vagus nerve) tone; presence of medications that increase or slow conduction through the AV node-bundle branch conduction system; and various underlying heart conditions such as heart failure.[97] Atrial fibrillation displays irregular R-to-R intervals (different timing intervals between the QRS complexes) that do not show any logical pattern. The ability of the AV node and bundle branches to conduct or block the fibrillatory atrial impulses is key to the appearance of the QRS on the surface ECG. In atrial fibrillation, the QRS-complex shape is usually narrow and normal in appearance as long as the pathway through the ventricles is intact after the impulse leaves the AV node. The AV node acts as a filter to protect the ventricles from the hundreds of atrial impulses that occur each minute, although the AV node does not receive all of these atrial impulses. When the atrial muscle tissue immediately surrounding the AV node is in a refractory state, impulses generated in other areas of the atria cannot reach the AV node, which helps to explain the wide variation in R-R intervals during atrial fibrillation (see Table 14-13).

Pathogenesis of Atrial Fibrillation. The pathogenesis of atrial fibrillation has traditionally been ascribed to random electrical foci firing in the atria. Research using high-density atrial mapping, high-speed video recordings, and ECG analysis has uncovered distinct spatial organization within the atria.[97] Atrial fibrillation involves several re-entry circuits within the atria, and in some cases, they originate at specific anatomic sites. The four pulmonary veins that drain into the left atrium are a trigger site for early atrial foci to initiate and propagate re-entry circuits to maintain atrial fibrillation.[97] The earliest atrial ectopic foci have been electrically mapped 2 to 4 cm within the pulmonary veins. The affected pulmonary veins contain thin myocardial sleeves that project into the pulmonary veins from the left atrium. This ectopic tissue resembles discontinuous fingerlike projections about 5 mm thick that extend as far as 4.5 cm into one or more pulmonary veins. The tissue ultimately becomes part of the venous wall. The spread of atrial fibrillation to the rest of the atria is thought to occur through multiple re-entry *wavelets* that are maintained in perpetual motion by a "mother rotor," or dominant re-entry circuit, which functions at a higher frequency, drives the atrial fibrillation, and originates from the ectopic pulmonary vein tissue.

When a single focus can be identified, it is possible to encircle that area and isolate that site using radiofrequency ablation (RFA). There are several different RFA designs used to isolate foci that originate in the four pulmonary veins: encircling all four veins together or isolating individual pulmonary veins or in pairs.[98] This catheter procedure is successfully used in many cardiac electrophysiology centers. Sometimes cryothermy or laser energy may be used for the ablation as an alternative to radiofrequency energy.

The atria demonstrate other pathologic changes in atrial fibrillation, typically atrial fibrosis and loss of atrial muscle mass. Atrial fibrosis may precede the development of atrial fibrillation, and the ongoing fibrosis is hypothesized to contribute to persistent atrial fibrillation.[97] An enlarged atria is an independent risk factor for the development of atrial fibrillation.[99] Additionally, atrial fibrillation can contribute to pathologic atrial enlargement.[99]

It is probable that there are several different types of atrial fibrillation involving different mechanisms. As electrophysiologic mapping techniques become more advanced, the mystery surrounding the origins of atrial fibrillation will become clearer. Although atrial fibrillation may look disorganized on the ECG baseline tracing, an electrical pattern exists within the atria. Knowledge of this pattern will ultimately lead to treatments that can help cure or control atrial fibrillation.

Types of Atrial Fibrillation. Atrial fibrillation is described by several additional labels that are associated with different clinical outcomes:

1. *Paroxysmal atrial fibrillation.* Atrial fibrillation that starts and stops abruptly is called *paroxysmal atrial fibrillation*, and it is often described as self-limiting (see Fig. 14-55).[97,100] The patient can often feel the palpitations and may describe it in different ways, such as "like a bird fluttering in my chest." Sometimes, when the HR is really fast, it is not possible to identify the rhythm as atrial fibrillation and it may initially be labeled as an SVT. It is always helpful to catch the start or ending point of any SVT on an ECG rhythm strip so that the initial stimulus can be identified. A printed rhythm strip also permits a more precise analysis of the dysrhythmia after the patient's clinical condition has been stabilized. In the critical care unit, it is important to document occurrence of paroxysmal atrial fibrillation by placing an ECG rhythm strip in the medical record and noting any associated clinical symptoms. The goal of treatment is to convert the atrial fibrillation back to a sinus rhythm as soon as possible. Electrical or pharmacologic cardioversion is most effective when the atrial fibrillation has been present for less than 24 hours.[97]

2. *Recurrent atrial fibrillation.* When a patient has two or more episodes of paroxysmal atrial fibrillation, it is described as *recurrent.* There is often a period during which patients may go in and out of atrial fibrillation, before the electrical atrial remodeling is complete and atrial fibrillation becomes the dominant and persistent rhythm.[97]

3. *Persistent atrial fibrillation.* When atrial fibrillation is sustained beyond 7 days or there are multiple bouts of paroxysmal atrial fibrillation, it is called *persistent* (see Fig. 14-55).[97] Research studies and clinical experience demonstrate that the longer a person remains in atrial fibrillation, the greater the degree of atrial electrical remodeling, and the more difficult it becomes to convert the atria back to sinus rhythm.[99] Even after electrical cardioversion, when the surface ECG may show sinus rhythm, the mechanical function of the atria may take days or weeks to return to normal contractile function.[99] Following cardioversion the patient remains at risk for a thromboembolic event from dislodged thrombi, and also from the formation of new atrial thrombi if atrial contractile function is not restored.[99]

4. *Permanent atrial fibrillation.* When atrial fibrillation has lasted for more than 1 year it is described as *permanent.* Typically, attempts to electrically or pharmacologically convert the atrial fibrillation back to sinus rhythm have failed before atrial fibrillation is described as permanent (see Fig. 14-55).[97]

5. *Lone atrial fibrillation.* The expression *lone atrial fibrillation* is used to describe individuals younger than 60 years who have atrial fibrillation without structural heart disease. Approximately 30% to 45% of cases of paroxysmal atrial fibrillation, and 20% to 25% of cases of persistent atrial fibrillation, occur in younger patients without demonstrable underlying heart disease.[97]

6. *Atrial fibrillation associated with underlying structural heart disease.* Some cardiac conditions are associated with atrial fibrillation, particularly hypertension, especially with associated LV hypertrophy, heart failure, valvular heart disease, acute MI, myocarditis, and pericarditis.[97,101] In developed countries, rheumatic heart disease, which was prevalent at the beginning of the 20th century, now plays a minor role. When the atrial tissue of patients in persistent atrial fibrillation is examined histologically (tissue analysis), the atria show structural abnormalities beyond the changes known to be caused by the underlying heart condition. These changes are called *electrical atrial remodeling.* The longer the person remains in atrial fibrillation, the less likely is a return to sinus rhythm.[99]

7. *Atrial fibrillation associated with other conditions.* Noncardiac conditions associated with an increased incidence of atrial fibrillation are diabetes, pulmonary embolism, pneumonia, and thyrotoxicosis. After the acute condition is treated, the atrial fibrillation should resolve and not recur. Hyperthyroidism is a correctable cause of atrial fibrillation that can be effectively reversed in most cases by correcting the thyrotoxic condition. If not recognized and treated, excess thyroid hormone makes rate control difficult, increases risk of a thromboembolic event, and causes higher rates of morbidity and mortality.

8. *Silent atrial fibrillation.* In silent atrial fibrillation, the patient is asymptomatic or minimally symptomatic and is unaware of the dysrhythmia. In a recent multicenter study of patients with a new implanted pacemaker where the intracardiac rhythm was monitored, 10% had silent or subclinical atrial fibrillation in the first 3 months.[102] The presence of silent atrial fibrillation is of concern because atrial fibrillation causes a deterioration in atrial mechanical function, formation of atrial emboli, and increased risk of stroke, and it is harder to convert to sinus rhythm the longer it is present.

9. *Cardiac surgery postoperative atrial fibrillation.* Atrial fibrillation occurs in approximately one third of patients after CABG.[99,103] If the CABG is combined with mitral or aortic value replacement, the incidence of atrial fibrillation rises further. Most atrial fibrillation develops on the second to third postoperative day and affects patients with or without a history of atrial fibrillation.[104] Postoperative atrial fibrillation after cardiac surgery is associated with significant hemodynamic instability, increased length of hospital stay,

decreased long-term survival, and increase in the risk of embolic stroke. Beta-blockers are recommended as prophylaxis to reduce the incidence of atrial fibrillation after cardiac surgery.[103]

10. *Atrial electrogram after cardiac surgery.* Atrial and ventricular epicardial temporary pacemaker wires are frequently inserted during cardiac surgery in case postoperative pacing support is required during the postoperative course. The atrial pacing wire or wires are placed on the right ventricle and exit the chest to the lower right side of the sternum. If the atrial pacing lead is connected to an ECG monitoring lead, the atrial tracing is clearly visible and much larger than normal because the recording comes directly from the right atrium. The atrial electrogram (AEG) procedure is not frequently performed but is useful when it is not possible to differentiate whether a patient in SVT has P waves, flutter waves, or atrial fibrillation on the standard surface ECG.[104,105]

Atrial Fibrillation Risk Factors. As more research has focused on the cause of atrial fibrillation, a clearer picture of incidence and risk factors has emerged. Atrial fibrillation is present in 0.4% to 1% in the general population, but the incidence rises to more than 8% among those older than 80 years.[97]

The median age of patients with atrial fibrillation is about 75 years.[97] Atrial fibrillation is the most common cardiac dysrhythmia in the United States and responsible for about one third of dysrhythmia-related hospital admissions.[97] The risk of developing atrial fibrillation is higher for people with a history of hypertension, heart failure, obesity, or MI.[97]

Atrial Fibrillation Management. There continues to be debate about the most effective treatment approach for atrial fibrillation, as shown in the algorithm to treat new-onset atrial fibrillation (Fig. 14-56). In the past, the gold standard goal has been to convert the patient out of the atrial fibrillation back to sinus rhythm. However, for many older patients, remaining out of atrial fibrillation is an unattainable goal. The major therapeutic focus is achieving *rhythm* versus *rate* control. All patients with atrial fibrillation require anticoagulation to prevent thrombotic embolism and stroke, unless individual patient risks outweigh the benefit of therapy.[106]

Rhythm Control. For the hospitalized patient with *new-onset* atrial fibrillation with unstable hemodynamics, the primary focus is generally on rhythm control (conversion to sinus rhythm) using antidysrhythmic medications or electrical cardioversion. Emergency medications used to convert atrial fibrillation to sinus rhythm, also known as a chemical

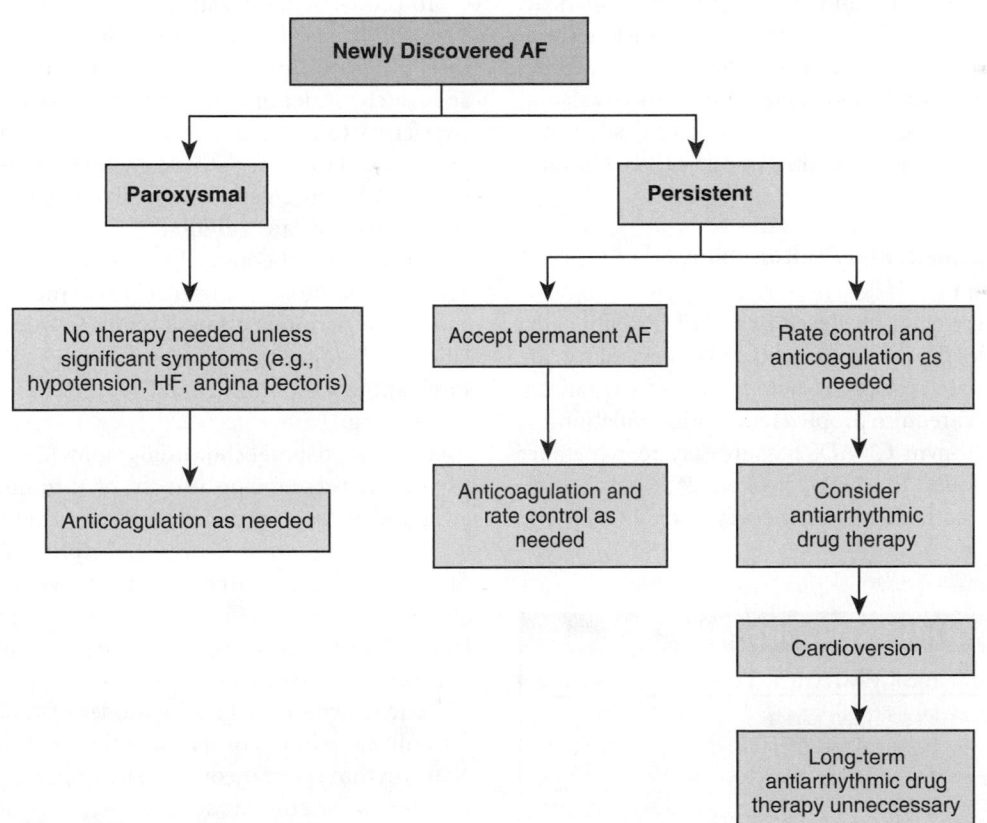

FIGURE 14-56 Management of new-onset atrial fibrillation. (From Fuster V, et al. ACC/AHA/ESC 2006 guidelines for the management of patients with atrial fibrillation: a report of the American College of Cardiology/American Heart Association Task Force on Practice Guidelines and the European Society of Cardiology Committee for Practice Guidelines [Writing Committee to revise the 2001 guidelines for the management of patients with atrial fibrillation]: developed in collaboration with the European Heart Rhythm Association and the Heart Rhythm Society. *Circulation.* 2006;114[7]:e257.)

cardioversion, include amiodarone and ibutilide. Antidysrhythmic medications used long-term to maintain sinus rhythm include amiodarone, dronedarone disopyramide, flecainide, propafenone, quinidine, sotalol, and dofetilide. The selection of the optimal medication is dependent on whether the patient has underlying structural heart disease or not.[106,107] Currently amiodarone is the most commonly prescribed medication for treatment of atrial fibrillation.[106] Even with medication therapy, recurrence of atrial fibrillation is likely. Electrical cardioversion may be successful in converting the atria to sinus rhythm if attempted within a few days or weeks of the onset of atrial fibrillation. Success is less likely if the atrial fibrillation has existed for a long time.[97]

Rate Control. The most frequently prescribed medications used to control the ventricular rate in atrial fibrillation include calcium channel blockers, beta-blockers, and digoxin. These medications work to slow conduction through the AV node. They have no impact on the fibrillating atria. In the past, it was assumed that rate control was an inferior strategy, because the patient stayed in atrial fibrillation, lost "atrial kick," and was presumed to have an increased risk of embolic stroke. Two multicenter trials have altered that perception: the *Atrial Fibrillation Follow-up: Investigation of Rhythm Management* (AFFIRM) and the *RAte Control vs. Electrical Cardioversion for Persistent Atrial Fibrillation* (RACE). These two trials found similar morbidity, mortality, and quality of life in patients treated with rhythm conversion or rate control. For long-term management of permanent atrial fibrillation, rate control is the recommended approach, and therapeutic anticoagulation to prevent embolic stroke is mandatory.[108] Antidysrhythmic medications used to manage atrial fibrillation are listed in Table 16-17 in Chapter 16.

Stroke Risk Assessment and Antithrombotic Therapy in Atrial Fibrillation

Atrial fibrillation, because of the development of thrombi in the atria, greatly increases the risk of embolic stroke. Several scoring mechanisms have been developed to help predict which patients with atrial fibrillation require prophylactic anticoagulation.

CHADS2. The acronym CHADS2 is an easy to remember risk-assessment tool used to predict stroke risk in atrial fibrillation and to guide antithrombotic therapy (Box 14-12). The letters stand for cardiac failure, hypertension, age, diabetes, stroke (double points).[101] The score ranges from 0 to 6. For a score of 0, no treatment or aspirin is recommended; for a score of 1, aspirin or warfarin is recommended; for a score between 2 and 6, anticoagulation with warfarin is recommended.[101] There are newer oral anticoagulants: *dabigatran*, a thrombin-inhibitor, and *rivaroxaban* factor Xa inhibitor, which can be prescribed for atrial fibrillation in patients with higher CHAD2 scores.[109]

CHA2DS2-VASc. Other scoring systems, such as the CHA2DS2-VASc have expanded the risk factor profile to include acute heart failure, hypertension, age 75 years or older (double points), diabetes, stroke (double points), vascular disease, age 65-74, and sex (female).[101]

Electrical and chemical (medication-induced) forms of cardioversion entail the threat of precipitating emboli into the systemic circulation. During atrial fibrillation, the atria do not contract effectively, and blood may pool and promote clots that attach to the atrial walls (mural thrombi).[99] If cardioversion is successful and normal sinus rhythm is restored, the atria again contract forcibly and, if thrombus formation has occurred, may send clots traveling through the pulmonary or systemic circulation. The atrial fibrillation antithrombotic recommendations subsequently described apply equally to patients with atrial flutter.[108]

To prevent embolic stroke, it is important to pay attention to the *48-hour rule*. Patients who have been in atrial fibrillation for 48 hours or longer (how long may not be known) must be adequately anticoagulated with an oral vitamin K antagonist (warfarin) to achieve a target international normalized ratio (INR) of 2.0 to 3.0 for at least 3 weeks before elective cardioversion.[108] After successful cardioversion, patients should be anticoagulated for an additional 4 weeks.[108] Advancements in antithrombotic therapies have resulted in several newer oral agents in addition to warfarin. These medications are available specifically for prevention of stroke in nonvalvular atrial fibrillation[100,108]: dabigatran,[110] rivaroxaban,[111] and apixaban.[112] These three antithrombotics do not require routine anticoagulation monitoring.

Transesophageal echocardiography (TEE) is helpful in identifying the presence or absence of thrombi in the fibrillating atria and is recommended as a screening tool before elective cardioversion.[108] It is especially helpful for patients in atrial fibrillation for less than 48 hours who, in the absence of atrial thrombi, may undergo cardioversion without anticoagulation.[108] TEE is described in more detail under "Transesophageal Echocardiography."

Patients who experience episodes of rapid atrial fibrillation for only a few hours or days at a time and then convert back to sinus rhythm spontaneously (paroxysmal atrial fibrillation) are also at risk for embolic stroke.

Nonpharmacologic Procedures to Treat Atrial Fibrillation. Several catheter interventions to treat atrial fibrillation are being explored, including atrial pacing, cardiac surgery, and catheter isolation of the pulmonary veins.

The Cox-Maze III procedure (typically called the MAZE procedure) is an open heart surgical operation. The surgery is suitable for only a tiny fraction of the individuals who have

---

BOX 14-12   CHADS2 SCORE

LETTER	RISK FACTOR	SCORE
C	Chronic heart failure	1
H	Hypertension	1
A	Age > 75 years	1
D	Diabetes mellitus	1
S	Stroke or TIA	2

The CHADS$_2$ score is used to predict the risk of having a stroke in atrial fibrillation. A higher score is associated with a higher risk of embolic stroke. CHADS$_2$ minimum score = 0; CHADS$_2$ maximum score = 6.
A score of 0 – no treatment or aspirin
A score of 1 – aspirin or warfarin
A score of 2 to 6 – warfarin

atrial fibrillation, usually those who have *lone atrial fibrillation* without other structural heart disease. It is designed to permanently cure atrial fibrillation by "cut and sew" insertion of strategic scar lines into the atria. The success rate, measured as freedom from atrial fibrillation, is 75% to 95% up to 15 years after surgery.[101] The surgical MAZE procedure is now rarely performed. It has been replaced by interventions that use less-invasive catheter-based radiofrequency energy sources to create lines of conduction block (scar) around the pulmonary veins.[98] Alternative catheter-based energy sources include cryoablation and high-intensity focused ultrasound.[101]

The goal of radiofrequency ablation (RFA) is to reduce clinical symptoms associated with atrial fibrillation. Based on the results of published studies, 57% of patients have reduced symptoms postablation even without antidysrhythmic medications.[113] When multiple ablation procedures are performed, the success rate increases to 71% without antidysrhythmic medications, and to 77% with antidysrhythmics.[113] Atrial pacing does not reduce the incidence of atrial fibrillation.[102]

Junctional Dysrhythmias

Only certain areas of the AV node have the property of automaticity. The entire area around the AV node is collectively called the *junction;* impulses generated there are called *junctional.* After an ectopic impulse arises in the junction, it spreads in two directions at once. One wave of depolarization spreads upward into the atria and depolarizes them, causing the recording of a P wave on the ECG. This is called *retrograde (backward) conduction,* and the P wave is inverted when viewed in lead II. At the same time, another wave of depolarization spreads downward into the ventricles through the normal conduction pathway, producing a normal QRS complex. This is called *antegrade (forward) conduction.*

Depending on timing, the P wave 1) may be seen in front of the QRS, with a short PR interval of less than 0.12 second; 2) may be obscured entirely by the QRS; or 3) may immediately follow the QRS.

Premature Junctional Contraction. If only a single ectopic impulse originates in the junction, it is simply called a *premature junctional contraction.* On the ECG, the rhythm is regular from the sinus node, except for one early QRS complex of normal shape and duration. The P wave can be entirely absent. If a P wave can be found, it very closely precedes or follows the QRS. In lead II, the P wave appears inverted (having a negative deflection), because the atria are being depolarized from the AV node upward, which is the opposite direction from the wave of depolarization that occurs when triggered by the sinus node. If the P wave appears before the QRS, the PR interval is less than 0.12 second. Premature junctional contractions have virtually the same clinical significance as do PACs. However, if the patient is receiving digoxin, digitalis toxicity may be suspected. Although digoxin slows conduction through the AV node, it also increases automaticity in the junction.

Junctional Escape Rhythm. Sometimes, the junction becomes the dominant pacemaker of the heart (Table 14-14). Normally, the intrinsic rate of the junction is 40 to 60 beats/min. The intrinsic rate of the sinus node is 60 to 100 beats/min. Under normal conditions, the junction never has a chance to escape and depolarize the heart because it is overridden by the sinus node. However, if the sinus node fails, the junctional impulses can depolarize completely and pace the heart. This is called a *junctional escape rhythm,* and it is a protective mechanism to prevent asystole in the event of sinus node failure. Generally, a junctional escape rhythm (Fig. 14-57) is well tolerated hemodynamically, although efforts must be directed toward restoring sinus rhythm. Sometimes, a pacemaker is

TABLE 14-14 JUNCTIONAL RHYTHMS

PARAMETER	JUNCTIONAL ESCAPE RHYTHM	ACCELERATED JUNCTIONAL RHYTHM	JUNCTIONAL TACHYCARDIA
Rate	40-60/min	60-100/min	>100/min
Rhythm	Regular	Regular	Regular
P waves	May be present or absent; inverted in lead II	May be present or absent; inverted in lead II	May be present or absent; inverted in lead II
PR interval	<0.12 sec	<0.12 sec	<0.12 sec
QRS	0.06-0.10 sec	0.06-0.10 sec	0.06-0.10 sec

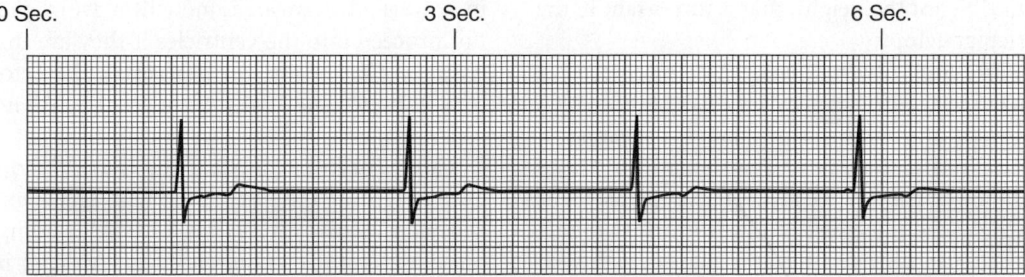

0 Sec.　　　　　3 Sec.　　　　　6 Sec.

FIGURE 14-57 Junctional Escape Rhythm. The ventricular rate is 38. P waves are absent, and the QRS has a normal width.

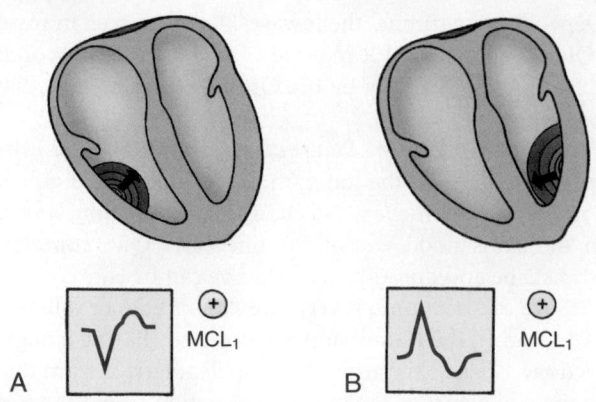

FIGURE 14-58   *A,* Right ventricular premature ventricular contraction (PVC). The spread of depolarization is from right to left, away from the positive electrode in lead V₁ (MCL₁), resulting in a wide, negative QRS complex. *B,* Left ventricular PVC. The spread of depolarization is from left to right, toward the positive electrode in lead V₁ (MCL₁). The QRS complex is wide and upright.

inserted as a protective measure because of concern that the AV junction may also fail.

Junctional Tachycardia and Accelerated Junctional Rhythm. A junctional rhythm can also occur at a faster rate (see Table 14-14). As with sinus rhythm, the term *tachycardia* is reserved for rates greater than 100 beats/min; junctional tachycardia is a junctional rhythm, usually regular, at a rate greater than 100 beats/min. When the junctional rate is greater than 60 beats/min and less than 100 beats/min it is described as an *accelerated junctional rhythm.*[114] Accelerated junctional rhythm is usually well tolerated by the patient, mainly because the HR is within a reasonable range. Junctional tachycardia may not be tolerated as well, depending on the rate and the patient's underlying cardiac reserve. Digitalis toxicity may be suspected if the patient is taking digoxin, because it enhances automaticity of the AV node. For digitalis toxicity, the optimal strategy is to measure the digoxin serum level and withhold digoxin until the dysrhythmia resolves. When digitalis toxicity is life threatening, administer the antidote *Digoxin Immune Fab.*[115]

Ventricular Dysrhythmias

Ventricular dysrhythmias result from an ectopic focus in any portion of the ventricular myocardium. The usual conduction pathway through the ventricles is not used, and the wave of depolarization must spread from cell to cell. As a result, the QRS complex is prolonged and is always greater than 0.12 second. It is the width of the QRS, not the height, that is important in the diagnosis of ventricular ectopy.

Premature Ventricular Contractions. A single ectopic impulse originating in the ventricles is called a PVC. Some PVCs are very small in height but remain wider than 0.12 second. If in doubt, a different lead is evaluated. The shape of the QRS depends on the location of the ectopic focus. If the ectopic focus is in the right ventricle, the impulse spreads from right to left, and the QRS resembles an LBBB pattern, because the left ventricle is the last to be depolarized. In V₁, this is a wide, negative QRS (Fig. 14-58A). If the ectopic focus is in the LV free wall,

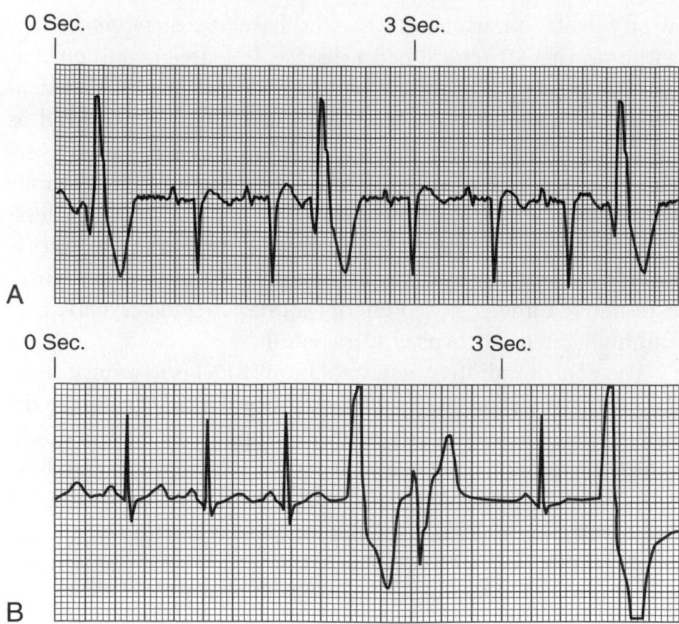

FIGURE 14-59   *A,* Unifocal premature ventricular contractions (PVCs). *B,* Multifocal PVCs.

the wave of depolarization spreads from left to right (see Fig. 14-58B).

Because the ectopic focus may be any cell in the ventricle, the QRS can manifest in an unlimited number of shapes or patterns. If all of the ventricular ectopic beats look the same in a particular lead, they are called *unifocal,* which means that they probably all result from the same irritable focus (Fig. 14-59A). Conversely, if the ventricular ectopics are of various shapes in the same lead, they are called *multifocal* (see Fig. 14-59B). Multifocal ventricular ectopics are more serious than unifocal ventricular ectopics, because they indicate a greater area of irritable myocardial tissue and are more likely to deteriorate into VT or fibrillation. In general, ventricular dysrhythmias have more serious implications than do atrial or junctional dysrhythmias and occur only rarely in healthy individuals.

A PVC originates in a ventricular cell that has become abnormally permeable to sodium, usually as a result of damage of one kind or another. Because of this new permeability to sodium, the cell reaches depolarization threshold before an impulse is received from the sinus node. After the depolarization threshold is reached, the cell automatically depolarizes, initiating total ventricular depolarization. Ordinarily, the ventricular impulse does not conduct back through the AV node; the sinus node is not disturbed and continues to depolarize the atria, resulting in a normal P wave. Conduction from the sinus node will not proceed into the ventricles if they are in a refractory state. Assuming there is no further ventricular ectopy, the next sinus beat conducts normally through the AV node and into the ventricles.

Compensatory Pause. If the interval from the last normal QRS preceding the PVC to the next one is exactly equal to two complete cardiac cycles (Fig. 14-60A), a compensatory pause is present. Because this does not usually occur in PACs or premature junctional contractions, when present, it is somewhat diagnostic of ventricular ectopy. If the normal sinus P wave that

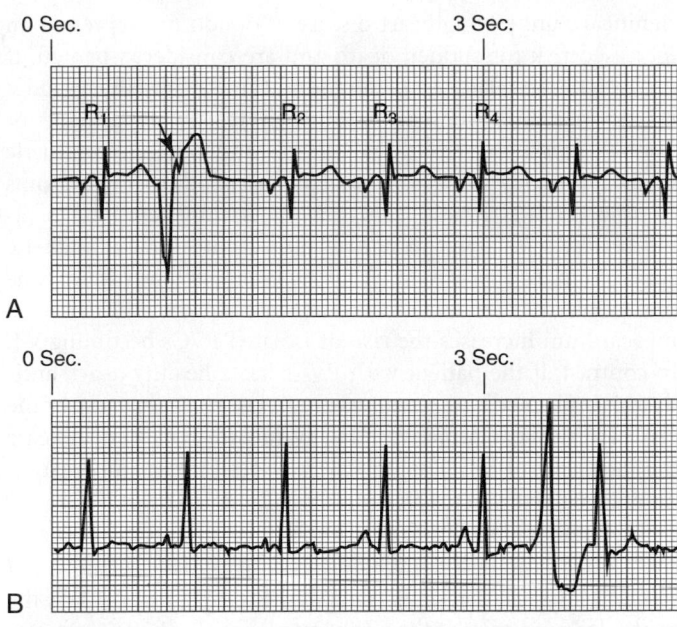

A

B

FIGURE 14-60 *A,* Premature ventricular contraction (PVC) with a fully compensatory pause. The interval between the two sinus beats that surround the PVC (R_1 and R_2) is exactly two times the normal interval between sinus beats (R_3 and R_4). The fully compensatory pause occurs because the sinus node continues to pace despite the PVC. Notice the sinus P wave *(arrow)* hidden in the ST segment of the PVC. This P wave did not conduct through to the ventricles because they had just been depolarized and were still in the absolute refractory period. *B,* Interpolated PVC. The PVC falls between two normal QRS complexes without disturbing the rhythm. Notice that the R-R interval between sinus beats remains the same.

occurs immediately after the PVC finds the ventricles sufficiently recovered to accept another impulse, a normal QRS results and the PVC is sandwiched between two normal beats (see Fig. 14-60B). This PVC is referred to as *interpolated,* meaning *between.* Interpolated PVCs usually occur when the PVC is very early or the normal sinus rate is relatively slow.

Occasionally, the ventricular impulse spreads backward across the AV node to depolarize the atria. When this occurs, the sinus node is reset and no full compensatory pause occurs.

Describing Ventricular Ectopy. PVCs can develop concurrently with any supraventricular dysrhythmia. It is not sufficient to describe a patient's rhythm as "frequent PVCs" or even "frequent unifocal PVCs." The underlying rhythm must always be described first, such as "sinus bradycardia with frequent unifocal PVCs" or "atrial fibrillation with occasional multifocal PVCs." Timing of PVCs can also be described. When a PVC follows each normally conducted beat, *ventricular bigeminy* is present (Fig. 14-61). If a PVC follows every two normal beats, it is called *ventricular trigeminy.*

In individuals with underlying heart disease, PVCs or episodes of self-terminating VT are potentially malignant. Nonsustained VT is defined as three or more consecutive premature ventricular beats at a rate faster than 110 beats/min lasting less than 30 seconds.

Premature Ventricular Contraction Timing. The timing of PVCs can be important, especially if myocardial ischemia is

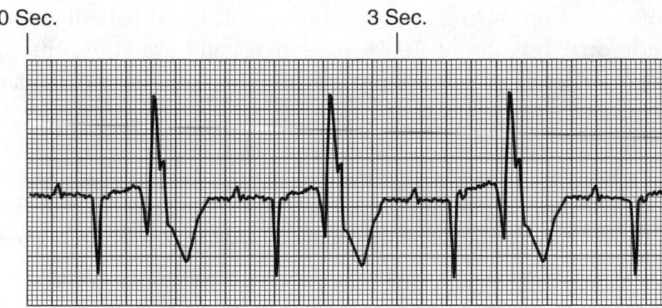

FIGURE 14-61 Ventricular Bigeminy.

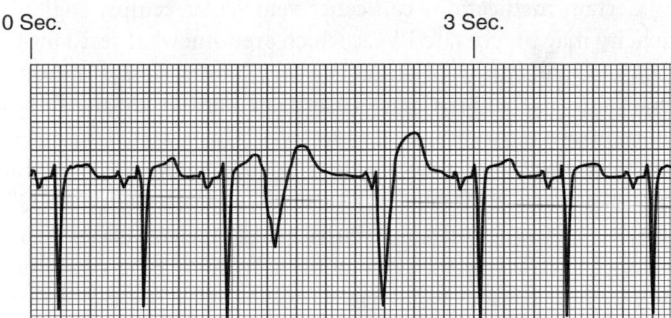

FIGURE 14-62 R-on-T Phenomenon.

present. The relative refractory period, represented on the ECG by the last half of the T wave, is a particularly vulnerable time for ectopy to occur because repolarization is not complete. Repolarization is even more delayed in ischemic tissue, so that various portions of the ventricular muscle are not repolarized simultaneously. If a PVC occurs at this critical point when only a part of the muscle is repolarized, individual segments of muscle can depolarize separately from each other, resulting in VF. This is called the *R-on-T phenomenon* (Fig. 14-62).

Two consecutive PVCs are described as a *couplet,* and three consecutive PVCs are called a *triplet* or a *three-beat run of ventricular tachycardia.* More than three consecutive PVCs are considered VT, but it is still useful to state how many beats of VT occurred if the run was short, lasting fewer than 20 beats.

Causes of Premature Ventricular Contractions. PVCs can result from many causes. They have been known to occur, although rarely, in healthy individuals with no evidence of heart disease. The critical care nurse has an important role in identifying factors that may be causing or at least contributing to PVCs. Acute ischemia is the most dangerous cause of ventricular ectopy. Ischemia causes cell membrane permeability to change, giving rise to early depolarization and the initiation of ectopic impulses. Ventricular ectopy that occurs during an acute ischemic event may require treatment with intravenous amiodarone or other antidysrhythmic medications.

Metabolic abnormalities are common causes of PVCs. Hypokalemia, hypoxemia, and acidosis predispose the cell membrane to instability and may cause ventricular ectopy. Treatment is directed toward identifying the metabolic disturbance and correcting it. Arterial blood gas values and serum potassium and magnesium levels are obtained if no recent results are available. The ability of oxygen and potassium values to change very rapidly in a critically ill patient must not be underestimated. If

PVCs develop during suctioning of an intubated patient, a few additional breaths of 100% oxygen usually are sufficient to restore adequate oxygenation and to eliminate the ventricular ectopy.

Any form of heart disease can lead to ventricular ectopy. Patients with cardiomyopathy or ventricular aneurysms can have chronic, severe ventricular ectopy, which may prove to be refractory to antidysrhythmic agents. Invasive procedures, such as insertion of a PA catheter or cardiac catheterization, can cause PVCs by mechanically irritating the ventricular muscle. In these situations, the ectopy usually resolves with removal or advancement of the catheter.

Certain medications can cause ventricular ectopy. Digitalis toxicity may precipitate PVCs, which are somewhat resistant to conventional antidysrhythmic therapy. Some class I antidysrhythmic medications can cause more serious dysrhythmias than those they were intended to treat. This is called a *prodysrhythmic effect* (also described as a *proarrhythmic effect*), and it can sometimes be fatal. Class 1a medications prolong the QT interval by lengthening the ventricular refractory period. This is a therapeutic effect, but when the QT prolongation becomes excessive, a characteristic form of polymorphic VT called *torsades de pointes* develops (Fig. 14-63). In this dysrhythmia, the VT is very rapid, and the QRS complexes appear to twist in a spiral pattern around the baseline. Clinically, torsades de pointes is poorly tolerated because of the extremely rapid rate. If not terminated, death will ensue. Sometimes, the torsades de pointes stops spontaneously, although the patient may experience a syncopal episode or seizure at the time of the dysrhythmia. Risk factors for development of torsades de pointes are listed in Box 14-7 earlier in the chapter.

Premature Ventricular Contraction Management. Not all ventricular ectopy requires treatment. In individuals without significant underlying heart disease, PVCs do not represent an increased risk for sudden death and are considered benign. If the patient complains of palpitations, therapy initially includes reassurance and elimination of such factors as caffeine or alcohol ingestion, emotional stress, and sympathomimetic medications that increase ventricular irritability. If symptoms continue, mild tranquilizers can be administered or beta-blockers can be given to reduce the response to sympathetic stimulation. Antidysrhythmic medications such as amiodarone or beta-blockers are used during an acute MI when the damaged myocardium increases the risk of isolated PVCs becoming VT. In contrast, if the patient with PVCs has a healthy heart, antidysrhythmic medications are used as a last resort because of the risk of prodysrhythmia, specifically medications that increase the incidence of VT. Chapter 16 provides further information on antidysrhythmic medications, see Table 16-16.

Idioventricular Rhythms. Sometimes an ectopic focus in the ventricle can become the dominant pacemaker of the heart (Table 14-15). If the sinus node and the AV junction fail, the ventricles depolarize at their own intrinsic rate of 20 to 40 times per minute. This is called an *idioventricular rhythm* and is naturally protective mechanism. Rather than trying to abolish the ventricular beats, the aim of treatment is to increase the effective HR and re-establish dominance of a higher pacing site such as the sinus node or the AV junction. Usually, a temporary pacemaker is used to increase the HR until the underlying problems that caused failure of the other pacing sites can be resolved.

An *accelerated idioventricular rhythm* (AIVR) occurs when a ventricular focus assumes control of the heart at a rate greater than its intrinsic rate of 40 beats/min but less than 100 beats/min (Fig. 14-64). Although relatively benign in and of itself, this rhythm must be closely observed for any increase in rate, and the patient must be observed for hemodynamic deterioration.

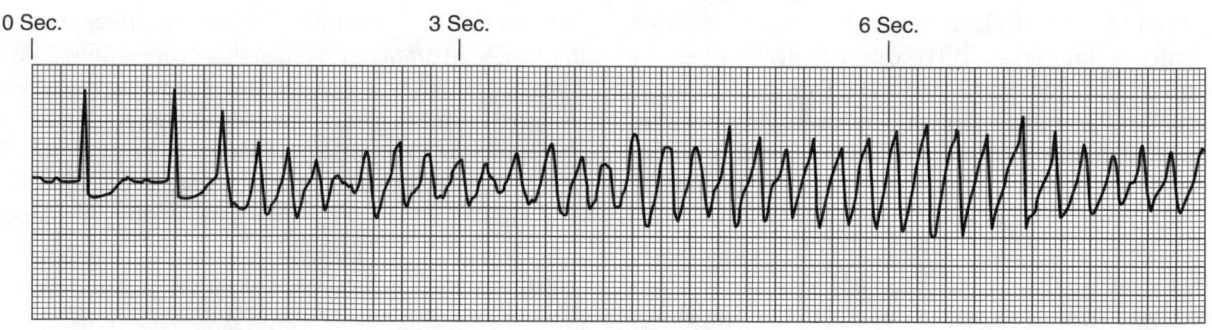

FIGURE 14-63 Torsades de Pointes.

TABLE 14-15 VENTRICULAR RHYTHMS

PARAMETER	IDIOVENTRICULAR RHYTHM	ACCELERATED IDIOVENTRICULAR RHYTHM	VENTRICULAR TACHYCARDIA	VENTRICULAR FIBRILLATION
Rate	20-40/min	40-100/min	>100/min	None
Rhythm	Usually regular	Usually regular	Usually regular	Irregular
P waves	Absent or retrograde	Absent or retrograde	Absent or retrograde	None
PR interval	None	None	None	None
QRS	>0.12 sec	>0.12 sec	>0.12 sec	Fibrillatory waves

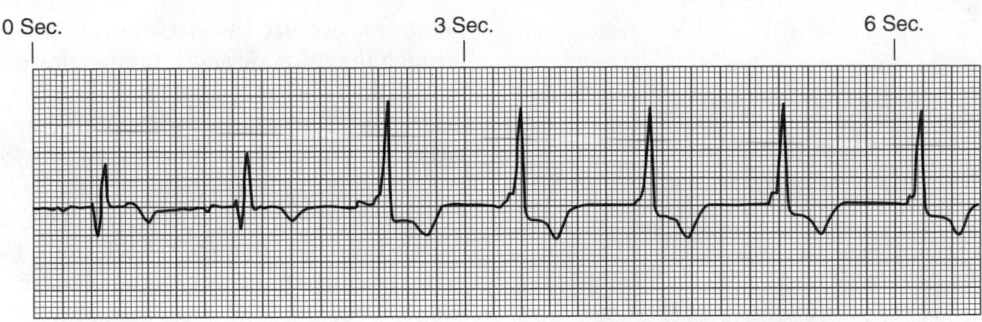

FIGURE 14-64 Accelerated Idioventricular Rhythm (AIVR). The QRS duration is 0.14 second, and the ventricular rate is 65.

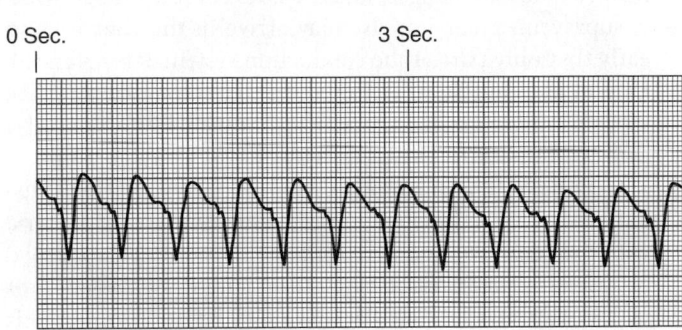

FIGURE 14-65 Ventricular Tachycardia.

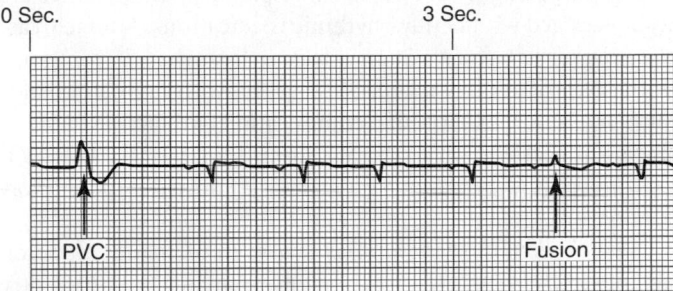

FIGURE 14-66 Ventricular Fusion Beat *(arrows)*. The QRS duration is only 0.08 second, and the shape represents the normal QRS and the previous PVC.

Usually, AIVR is not treated pharmacologically if well tolerated with a stable blood pressure, although a transvenous temporary pacemaker should be inserted electively as a precaution against sudden hemodynamic deterioration. Intravenous lidocaine must never be administered to a patient with an idioventricular rhythm, because it suppresses the ventricular pacemaker and converts the rhythm to asystole.

Ventricular Tachycardia. Ventricular tachycardia (VT) is caused by a ventricular pacing site firing at a rate of 100 times or more per minute, usually maintained by a re-entry mechanism within the ventricular tissue (Fig. 14-65). The complexes are wide, and the rhythm may be slightly irregular, often accelerating as the tachycardia continues (see Table 14-15). In most cases, the sinus node is not affected and it continues to depolarize the atria on schedule. P waves can sometimes be seen on the ECG tracing. They are not related to the QRS and may even appear to conduct a normal impulse to the ventricles if their timing is just right.

If the sinus impulse and the ventricular ectopic impulse meet in the middle of the ventricles, a fusion beat results. Fusion beats are narrower than ventricular beats and look like a cross between the patient's sinus QRS and the ventricular ectopic QRS (Fig. 14-66). When present, P waves and fusion beats are helpful in verifying the diagnosis of VT as opposed to SVT. Differentiation between VT and SVT was discussed earlier.

Most VT occurs in the presence of structural cardiac disease, such as myocardial ischemia, congenital heart disease, valvular dysfunction, and cardiomyopathy. Other triggers include drug toxicities, electrolyte disturbances, and as an adverse reaction to certain antidysrhythmic medications (prodysrhythmia).

VT is a life-threatening dysrhythmia and must be treated quickly. The rapid ventricular rate decreases blood pressure and

the patient may lose consciousness. The loss of the synchronized timing of atrial contraction, which normally adds volume to the ventricles just before contraction and enhances the force of contraction, is lost, greatly reducing CO. If not terminated quickly, VT is likely to degenerate into VF and death.

How VT is clinically managed depends on whether the patient is stable or unstable, as well as whether a pulse and adequate blood pressure are present. Pulseless VT is a life-threatening condition. The patient will lose consciousness and will need immediate cardiopulmonary resuscitation and defibrillation as described in the American Heart Association (AHA) protocols for advanced cardiac life support (ACLS).

Patients with stable or wide-complex "slow VT" who have an HR below 150 beats/min, palpable pulse, and stable blood pressure may be treated pharmacologically with the IV antidysrhythmics amiodarone, procainamide, or sotalol (beta-blocker with Class III antidysrhythmic properties) as described in the ACLS protocols.

After the acute episode is over, patients who have already experienced sustained VT or cardiac arrest continue to be at risk for sudden cardiac death. An extensive clinical evaluation of these patients is warranted, including cardiac catheterization and electrophysiologic testing with programmed ventricular stimulation. Therapy is aimed at preventing a recurrence of sustained VT or VF. It may include treating the underlying cause, administering antidysrhythmic medications, performing ablation of the re-entrant pathway within the ventricle, or inserting an implantable cardioverter defibrillator (ICD).

ICDs can be programmed to deliver several bursts of overdrive pacing to terminate stable VT before cardioversion. This has the advantage of being more comfortable for the patient, since it prevents the discomfort of an internal shock if the

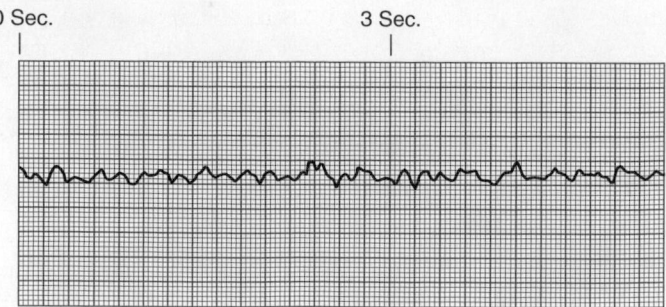

0 Sec.   3 Sec.

FIGURE 14-67   Ventricular Fibrillation.

overdrive pacing is successful. Most patients with an ICD are also managed with antidysrhythmic medications. Antitachycardia (overdrive) pacing is an effective treatment if combined with defibrillation backup. It is risky without defibrillator support, since one of the complications of antitachycardia pacing is acceleration of the VT toward a faster, pulseless VT, polymorphic VT, or even VF. Chapter 16 provides more information on implantable cardioverter defibrillators.

Ventricular Fibrillation. VF is the result of chaotic electrical activity in the ventricles from repetitive, small areas of re-entry or a series of rapid discharges from various foci within the ventricular myocardium. This causes the ventricles to be unable to contract completely and effectively. The ventricles merely quiver, and no forward flow of blood occurs. Without forward flow, no palpable pulse or audible apical heart tones are present. Clinically, VF is indistinguishable from asystole (absence of electrical activity). On the ECG, VF appears as a continuous, undulating pattern without clear P, QRS, or T waves (Fig. 14-67). When VF occurs in the setting of an acute ischemic event and is accompanied by a significant amount of myocardial damage, the survival rate is poor. Resuscitation is often unsuccessful; recurrence rates are high for those who are resuscitated. VF is seen on the ECG as large, erratic undulations of the baseline (coarse VF) or as a mild tremor (fine VF). In VF, the patient does not have a pulse, no blood is being pumped forward, and defibrillation is the only definitive therapy. Coarse VF is more likely to be successfully defibrillated. Antidysrhythmic medications such as intravenous amiodarone are administered if initial attempts at defibrillation fail. As with any cardiac arrest situation, supportive measures such as cardiopulmonary resuscitation (CPR), intubation, and correction of metabolic abnormalities are performed concurrently with definitive therapy.

Differential Diagnosis of a Wide QRS-Complex Tachycardia. Wide-complex tachycardias are typically caused by one of four mechanisms[116]:
1. VT
2. SVT with aberrancy due to conduction slowing in the bundle branch system
3. SVT with antegrade conduction over an accessory pathway
4. Ventricular paced rhythm

The challenge is to recognize the atypical wide-complex tachycardia. Tachycardias that are triggered by an ectopic atrial or junctional focus have a *supraventricular* origin, meaning that they come from an irritable site above the ventricles.[117] Typical SVT has a narrow QRS complex (less than 0.12 second

duration), because the electrical impulse enters the ventricle through the AV node and continues down the normal conduction pathway by means of the bundle branches through the ventricles. VT always has a wide QRS complex (longer than 0.12 second), because the impulse begins somewhere within the ventricles and must spread slowly—cell to cell—without the benefit of the usual conduction system. It is easy to distinguish between typical SVT and VT by QRS width alone. Unfortunately, not all SVTs result in a narrow QRS complex. An SVT presents with a wide QRS complex in three situations:
1. The patient may already have an RBBB or LBBB, resulting in a wide QRS even during sinus rhythm. Understandably, if the patient develops an atrial or junctional tachycardia, the BBB remains unchanged, and the QRS complex is still wide.
2. A supraventricular impulse may arrive in the ventricles so early that only part of the conduction system is repolarized. One of the bundle branches is still refractory, causing the wave of depolarization to spread abnormally (aberrantly) through the ventricles and resulting in a wide QRS complex.
3. Occasionally, an anatomic variant occurs in which the patient has a small strip of muscle tissue connecting the atria with the ventricles and bypassing the AV node. This is called an *accessory pathway*, or *bypass tract*, the most common of which occurs in Wolff-Parkinson-White syndrome. This does not pose a hemodynamic problem in normal sinus rhythm, although it sometimes causes subtle ECG changes that allow it to be detected. However, when rapid atrial dysrhythmias occur, they can be conducted directly to a portion of the ventricular myocardium without normal AV delay. Depolarization through the ventricles then proceeds from cell to cell rather than through the normal and efficient pathway of the conduction system, resulting in a wide QRS-complex tachycardia that closely resembles VT.

Significance of Ventricular Tachycardia and Supraventricular Tachycardia. Standard treatment for VT includes administration of intravenous amiodarone. In contrast, SVT is treated with a variety of medications that work by blocking the AV node conduction pathway—diltiazem, verapamil, amiodarone, or digoxin. A problem occurs if the SVT has occurred as a result of the presence of an accessory pathway and the narrow-complex tachycardia is treated with verapamil or other medications that block the AV node but do not block the Wolff-Parkinson-White accessory pathway. This can result in an extremely fast wide-complex tachycardia through the accessory pathway with acute, severe hypotension or loss of consciousness requiring immediate cardioversion. For this reason, it is important to be sure of the cause of the tachycardia in individuals who are relatively hemodynamically stable before treatment is initiated.

Regardless of the site of origin, a rapid wide QRS-complex tachycardia may not be well tolerated, largely because of the fast HR that prevents adequate ventricular filling during diastole, as well as increasing myocardial oxygen demand while decreasing time available for coronary artery filling. Hemodynamic deterioration is evidenced by syncope, severe hypotension, or ischemic symptoms. In this case, emergency external cardioversion must be performed regardless of whether the tachycardia is of ventricular or supraventricular origin. Correct diagnosis of a wide QRS-complex tachycardia may have an impact on the long-term management of a patient as well. If atrial flutter or fibrillation is determined to be the underlying mechanism, long-term treatment probably includes amiodarone or a beta-blocker to reduce the HR response when these dysrhythmias occur. If VT is determined to be the underlying mechanism in a patient without a history of ventricular dysrhythmias, a careful search for the cause (e.g., hypoxemia, electrolyte imbalance, excess sympathetic stimulation, ischemia) is warranted. Depending on the clinical situation, the patient may require long-term antidysrhythmic therapy. If there is a history of VT or sudden cardiac death and the patient is already on antidysrhythmic therapy, a recurrent episode of VT indicates that the current treatment regimen is not effective and the therapy needs to be changed.

Clinical Differentiation of Ventricular Tachycardia from Supraventricular Tachycardia. Contrary to popular belief, hemodynamic stability or instability does not help to differentiate between VT and SVT with a wide QRS complex. In theory, an SVT is better tolerated, especially if atrial contraction is still occurring before each ventricular contraction (AV synchrony). However, clinically this is often variable. VT may be well tolerated, especially if the rate is less than 150 beats/min. Some patients can be in sustained VT for hours without significant hemodynamic compromise. Conversely, because AV synchrony is lost in atrial fibrillation or atrial flutter, and the ventricular response rate may be very rapid, ventricular filling and CO can be severely compromised.

Careful physical examination can be of value in determining the source of the tachycardia. The jugular venous pulse can be assessed for the presence of cannon *a* waves. When the atria contract at the same time as ventricular systole, the AV valves are closed and the blood in the atria is forced to regurgitate into the venous system. This is seen as a very large pulsation in the jugular vein. If it occurs sporadically (not with every beat), it is a sign of AV dissociation, or independent beating of the atria and ventricles. Heart sounds provide another diagnostic clue. Variation of the intensity of the first heart sound (S_1) from beat to beat favors VT, because this is also indicative of AV dissociation.

The most reliable means of diagnosing a wide QRS-complex tachycardia is through careful analysis of the ECG. HR and rhythm are evaluated first, although they are not the only diagnostic indicators. The QRS width is measured in more than one lead, because the lead with the widest QRS complex is the most reliable indicator of true QRS duration. It is assumed that some portion of the QRS complex is isoelectric in leads where the QRS appears to be narrow. QRS widths of less than 0.14 second favor SVT with aberrant conduction, whereas widths of greater than 0.14 second (140 msec) in an RBBB pattern or of greater than 0.16 second (160 msec) in an LBBB pattern favors VT.[117]

The tracing is examined closely for the presence of P waves. If P waves can be identified and they do not correlate on a 1:1 basis with the QRS complexes, AV dissociation exists and strongly suggests VT. Although P waves may be found in any lead, they are in general most readily visible in leads V_1 or II. When the sinus node remains in control of the atria and a ventricular ectopic focus is in control of the ventricles, it is likely that at some point the timing will be coordinated and, by chance, the sinus impulse will conduct through the AV node and begin to depolarize the ventricles just as the ventricular ectopic focus fires. The resulting QRS complex is a *fusion beat* (see Fig. 14-66), which resembles a blend of the patient's normal QRS and the wide QRS complex of the ventricular dysrhythmia. The presence of fusion beats also strongly suggests VT.

Another helpful diagnostic criterion for VT is a QRS axis in the northwest quadrant of −90 degrees to −180 degrees (Fig. 14-68). An axis in this quadrant means that the wave of

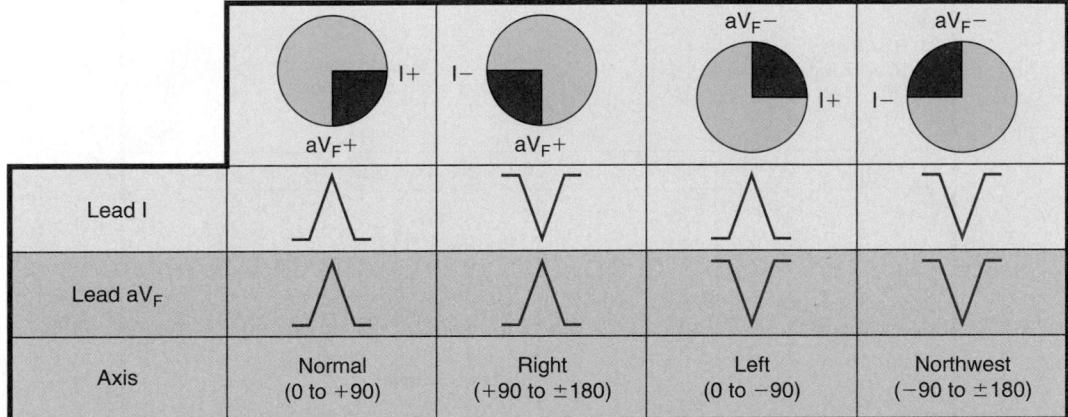

FIGURE 14-68 Determination of QRS axis quadrant by noting predominant QRS polarity in leads I and aVF. *Normal axis:* If QRS during tachycardia is primarily positive in both I and aVF, the axis falls within the normal quadrant from 0 to 90 degrees. *Right-axis deviation:* If the QRS complex is primarily negative in I and positive in aVF, right-axis deviation is present. *Left-axis deviation:* If the QRS complex is predominantly positive in I and negative in aVF, left-axis deviation is present. *Indeterminate axis:* If QRS is primarily negative in both I and aVF, a markedly abnormal "indeterminate," or "northwest," axis is present that is diagnostic of ventricular tachycardia. (From Drew B. Bedside electrocardiographic monitoring: state of the art for the 1990s. *Heart Lung.* 1991;20[6]:610.)

depolarization is directed upward and to the right, exactly the opposite of normal ventricular depolarization. Even when ventricular conduction is abnormal, as in BBBs, ventricular depolarization begins at the level of the AV junction and spreads downward toward the apex, although conduction disturbances direct the current flow more to the right or left than normal. Although not all VT rhythms have an axis in the extreme or northwest quadrant, when this axis is present, it confirms the diagnosis of VT. Figure 14-69 shows how this abnormal axis can be identified from a 5-lead ECG bedside monitor by observing the shape of the QRS in leads I and aVF.

The shape of the QRS complex in the right precordial lead V_1 or MCL_1 and the left precordial lead V_6 or MCL_6 can be diagnostic of VT or SVT with aberrant conduction. Figure

14-69 summarizes these QRS patterns. If the QRS complex is entirely positive from V_1 through V_6 or entirely negative, the diagnosis is VT. This phenomenon is known as *precordial concordance.*

Nursing Management. Proper electrode placement and appropriate lead selection have already been discussed but cannot be overemphasized. In addition to correct lead placement and selection, every effort must be made to record the wide QRS-complex tachycardia on a standard 12-lead ECG. Certainly, emergency treatment must not be delayed if the patient is hemodynamically unstable, but documenting the dysrhythmia by recording a "stat" 12-lead ECG must be given a high priority if time permits. VT and SVT are often nonsustained, and waiting for a physician's order or the arrival of a

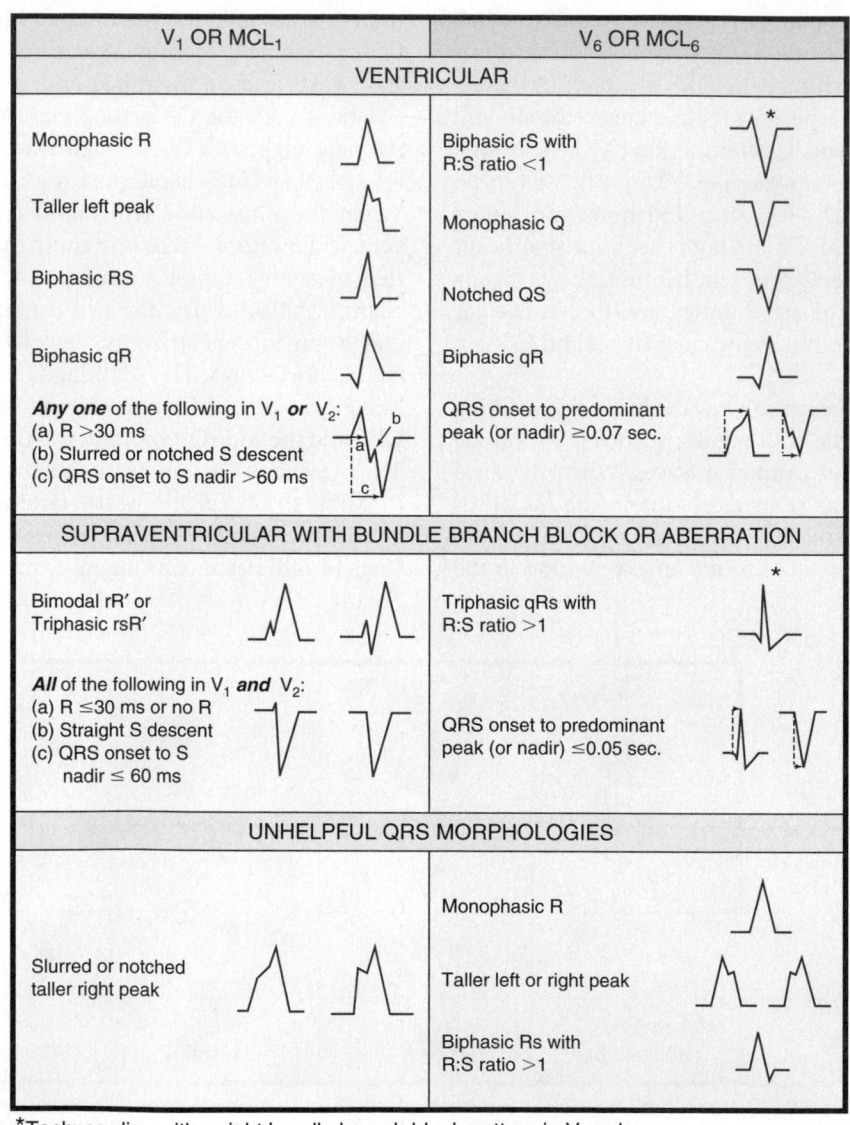

*Tachycardias with a right bundle branch block pattern in V_1 only

FIGURE 14-69 Summary of morphologic clues in V_1 or MCL_1 (*left column*) and in V_6 or MCL_6 (*right column*) that are valuable in distinguishing supraventricular tachycardia with bundle branch block or aberration from ventricular tachycardia. If wide-complex tachycardia with taller right peak pattern (i.e., unhelpful morphology) develops in a patient monitored with a single MCL_1 lead, the nurse changes leads to determine whether the wide complex falls into one of the diagnostic patterns in V_6 (MCL_6). (From Drew B. Bedside electrocardiographic monitoring: state of the art for the 1990s. *Heart Lung.* 1991;20[6]:610.)

TABLE 14-16 ATRIOVENTRICULAR BLOCK

PARAMETER	FIRST DEGREE	SECOND-DEGREE MOBITZ I (WENCKEBACH)	SECOND-DEGREE MOBITZ II	THIRD-DEGREE (COMPLETE)
PR interval	>0.20 sec and constant	Increases with each consecutively conducted P wave	Constant	Varies randomly
P waves	1 P wave for each QRS	Intermittently not conducted, yielding more P waves than QRS complexes	Intermittently not conducted, yielding more P waves than QRS complexes	P waves independent and not related to QRS complexes
QRS	0.06-0.10 sec	0.06-0.10 sec	May be normal, but usually coexists with BBB (>0.12 sec)	0.06-0.10 sec if junctional escape pacemaker activates the ventricles >0.12 sec if ventricular escape pacemaker activates the ventricles

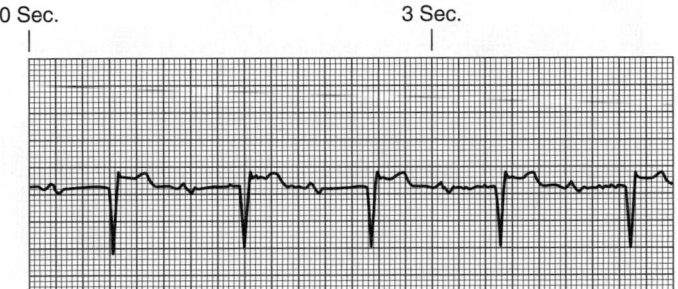

0 Sec.   3 Sec.

FIGURE 14-70 First-Degree Atrioventricular (AV) Block. The PR interval is prolonged to 0.44 second.

technician to perform the test could result in failure to document the atrioventricular conduction disturbance.

Normally, the sinoatrial node triggers electrical depolarization in the heart. From there, the impulse travels through the right atrium to the AV node. The left atrium is depolarized by a conduction fiber known as *Bachman's bundle* that connects the right and left atria. The electrical impulse is briefly delayed in the AV node to allow the atria to contract and the mitral and tricuspid valves to close before the impulse is conducted to the bundle of His, the bundle branches, and the Purkinje fibers.

On the ECG, the ability of the AV node to conduct is evaluated by measuring the PR interval and the relationship of P waves to QRS complexes (Table 14-16). The normal PR interval, measured from the beginning of the P wave to the beginning of the QRS complex, ranges from 0.12 to 0.20 second.

First-Degree Atrioventricular Block. When all atrial impulses are conducted to the ventricles but the PR interval is greater than 0.20 second, a condition known as *first-degree AV block* exists (Fig. 14-70). First-degree AV block can be chronic or acute, and it may be caused by a multitude of conditions. Long-standing first-degree block may occur related to fibrosis and sclerosis of the conduction system, lack of blood supply to the conduction system due to coronary artery disease (CAD), valvular heart disease, myocarditis, and various cardiomyopathies. First-degree heart block that develops acutely is of much greater concern. Causes include drug toxicity related to digoxin, beta-blockers, or amiodarone administration; acute myocardial ischemia or infarction, hyperkalemia, edema after valvular heart surgery, and increased vagal tone. First-degree AV block

represents slowed conduction through the AV node. If the associated QRS is narrow it is likely that the only conduction abnormality is in the AV node. However, if the associated QRS complex is widened, it is likely that there is also damage to the bundle branches as a result of sclerosis, ischemia, or infarction.

Second-Degree Atrioventricular Block. Second-degree AV block can be broadly defined as a condition in which some atrial impulses are conducted to the ventricles, but others are "blocked" at the AV node. This description of intermittent AV conduction covers two patterns with markedly different clinical significance: second-degree AV block is divided into Mobitz type I (also known as *Wenckebach block)* and Mobitz type II.

Mobitz Type I. In Mobitz type I block, the AV conduction times progressively lengthen until a P wave is not conducted. This typically occurs in a pattern of *grouped beats* and is observed on the ECG by a gradually lengthening PR interval, until ultimately the final P wave in the group fails to conduct. In Mobitz type I, the QRS complex is generally of normal width and appearance. Several criteria must be present for Mobitz I (Wenckebach) to be diagnosed:

1. The sinus node is functional and generates impulses that conduct to the AV node at a constant rate. On the ECG the measured P-to-P interval is regular.

2. As each successive atrial impulse arrives earlier into the *relative refractory period* of the impaired AV node, more time is needed to conduct the impulse. On the ECG, this is seen as an incremental increase in the length of each PR interval. The R-to-R interval usually becomes shorter with each beat.

3. The PR interval is shortest in the first beat.
   a. The initial PR interval is often, but not always, of normal length. If first-degree block coexists, the initial PR interval will be prolonged, but this initial PR interval will still have the shortest measured interval of the group.
   b. The initial PR interval is shorter because the AV node has experienced a "rest" or longer recovery time due to the final nonconducted P wave in the group, as subsequently described.

4. The final P wave of the group is not conducted. The atrial impulse arrives during the AV node's absolute refractory period and is not conducted. This is seen on the ECG by a P wave that is *not* followed by a QRS complex (Fig. 14-71).

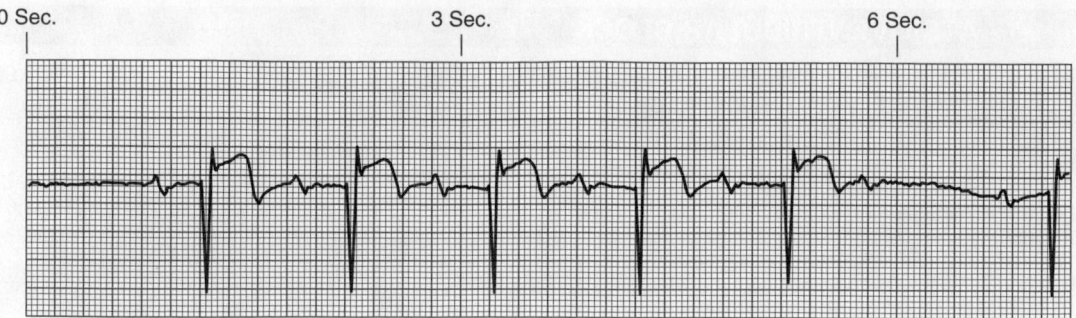

FIGURE 14-71 Mobitz type I (Wenckebach) Second-Degree Atrioventricular (AV) Block. Notice that the PR intervals gradually increase from 0.36 to 0.46 second until a P wave is not conducted to the ventricles.

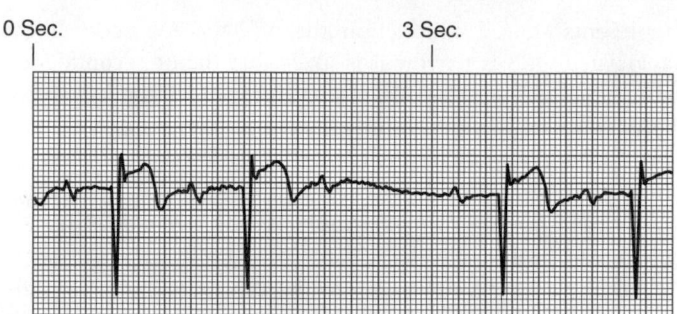

FIGURE 14-72 Mobitz Type II Second-Degree Atrioventricular (AV) Block. Notice that the PR intervals remain constant.

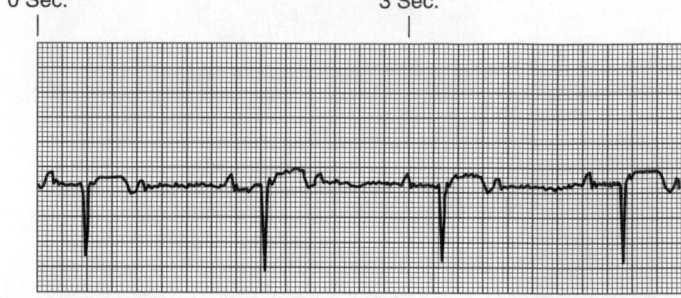

FIGURE 14-73 A 2:1 Atrioventricular (AV) Block. Because no two consecutive P waves are conducted, it is not possible to determine with certainty whether this is a Mobitz I or Mobitz II second-degree AV block.

Mobitz I block has a specific, repeating pattern that catches the eye. The expected groups are 3:2, 4:3, or 5:4. For example, if four P waves are conducted to the ventricles and the fifth one is not, a 5:4 conduction ratio is present (five P waves to four QRS complexes). The nonconducted P ends a *group*. After the pause, the cycle repeats itself. The PR interval typically lengthens the most with the second beat of the cycle.

Mobitz type I does not generally cause significant hemodynamic compromise as long as the ventricular HR is maintained. However, in the presence of ischemia and infarction it may progress to a more severe level of block. If Mobitz type I occurs in the setting of an acute inferior wall infarction, close observation and, occasionally, placement of a temporary pacemaker as a precautionary measure are warranted.

Mobitz Type II. Mobitz type II block is always anatomically located below the AV node in the bundle of His in the bundle branches or even in the Purkinje fibers. This results in an all-or-nothing situation with respect to AV conduction. Sinus P waves are or are not conducted. When conduction does occur, all PR intervals are the same. Because of the anatomic location of the block, on the surface ECG the PR interval is constant and the QRS complexes are wide (Fig. 14-72).

Mobitz II block is more ominous clinically than Mobitz I and may progress to complete AV block. If the block involves the Purkinje fibers, an escape rhythm may not develop. For this reason, it is important to prepare for *transcutaneous cardiac pacing* (TCP) by bringing the TCP device (often combined with a defibrillator) to the bedside as a precaution. TCP refers to

external pacing from outside the chest wall. When pacing is required, two large pacing electrodes are placed on the chest. There is always a diagram on the machine showing where to place the pads on the chest. Consider the possibility that the patient will need a temporary transvenous pacemaker inserted and possibly require a permanent pacemaker before hospital discharge.

2:1 Conduction. Occasionally, only every other P wave is conducted through the AV node (Fig. 14-73). This pattern may indicate Mobitz type I or Mobitz type II, because consecutive conduction of P waves—which reveal a lengthening or constant PR—does not occur. In Mobitz I, the conduction ratios may have decreased from 4:3 to 3:2 to 2:1, but the site and type of block have not changed. The change in conduction ratio may be caused by an increase in atrial rate, or it may change spontaneously.

In 2:1 conduction, it is impossible to be certain whether the block is Mobitz type I or type II from the surface ECG. If it occurs along with other Mobitz I ratios, it is probably still Mobitz I. If it is an isolated occurrence with no other strips for comparison, the QRS width and the PR interval offer valuable clues to the site of the block. In Mobitz I, the QRS is usually normal and the PR interval is usually prolonged. In Mobitz II, the QRS is usually wide and the PR interval is usually normal. During an acute inferior MI, Mobitz type I AV block with 2:1 conduction is much more common than is type II.

Third-Degree Atrioventricular Block. Third-degree, or complete, AV block is a condition in which no atrial impulses

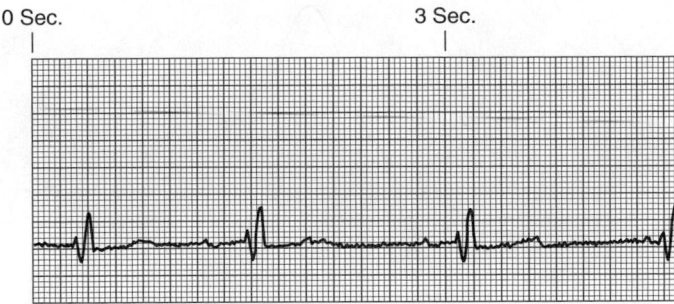

FIGURE 14-74 Third-Degree (Complete) Heart Block.

can conduct from the atria to the ventricles. This is also described by the terms *complete heart block* or *AV dissociation* to indicate that the atria and the ventricles are controlled by different pacemakers. The block can be located at the level of the AV node or below the node within the bundle of His or the bundle branches.[118] It can be caused by infarction, digitalis toxicity, or age-related degeneration of the conduction system in older patients. It is hoped that a junctional focus or ventricular focus will depolarize spontaneously at its intrinsic rate of 20 to 40 beats/min and that ventricular contraction will continue. If not, asystole occurs; there is no pulse, and death will result if pacemaker support is not immediate.

On the ECG, P waves are present and usually occur at regular intervals. If a junctional focus is pacing the heart, normal QRS complexes are present but occur at a rate and timing interval totally independent of the P waves. The PR intervals vary widely, because the P wave and QRS are not related to each other. If a ventricular focus is pacing the heart, the QRS complex is wide and unrelated to the P waves (Fig. 14-74).

Management of Atrioventricular Block. Clinically, the consequences of AV block range from benign to life threatening. First-degree AV block is seldom of immediate concern but bears close observation for progression of the conduction disturbance. Second-degree Mobitz I (Wenckebach) is usually benign as long as the patient is not bradycardic. If hemodynamic compromise is present or deemed likely, a temporary pacemaker can be inserted prophylactically. Second-degree Mobitz II is more serious and often precedes complete AV block. Use of a temporary pacemaker is recommended, but its insertion can be elective if the patient remains hemodynamically stable. Complete heart block causes AV dissociation and is associated with a low CO that requires use of a pacemaker. In complete heart block, the patient may exhibit cannon waves as the dissociated atria contact against closed AV valves and create a "wave" on the atrial pressure waveform. An example of this phenomenon is shown in Figure 14-12. If the patient is hemodynamically unstable, external TCP can be used to maintain an adequate ventricular rate until a transvenous or permanent pacemaker can be inserted.

LABORATORY ASSESSMENT

Laboratory assessment of cardiovascular status is obtained through studies of blood serum. Accurate interpretation of

these laboratory studies, along with the clinical picture, enables the critical care team to diagnose, treat, and assess the response to therapeutic interventions.

Laboratory studies of blood serum are performed to assess the following:
1. Electrolyte levels that can alter cardiac muscle contraction
2. Cardiac biomarkers that reflect myocardial cellular integrity or infarction
3. Hematologic status to evaluate risk of anemia and infection
4. Coagulation times
5. Serum lipid levels
6. Status of other organ systems that can secondarily affect cardiac function

Electrolytes
Potassium
During depolarization and repolarization of nerve and muscle fiber, potassium and sodium exchange occurs intracellularly and extracellularly. The potassium gradient across the cell membrane determines conduction velocity and helps confine pacing activity to the sinus node. Excess or deficiency of potassium can alter myocardial muscle function. Normal serum potassium levels are 3.5 to 4.5 mEq/L.

Hyperkalemia. Elevated serum potassium, called *hyperkalemia*, can be caused by a variety of conditions that include excess potassium administration, extensive skeletal muscle destruction (rhabdomyolysis), tumor lysis syndrome, and kidney failure. Some medications may induce hyperkalemia including potassium-sparing diuretics, angiotensin-converting enzyme (ACE) inhibitors and angiotensin receptor blockers (ARB).[119] Hyperkalemia can elicit significant changes in the ECG because it decreases AV conduction velocity, slows ventricular depolarization, and accelerates repolarization.[120] As the serum levels of potassium rise, tall, narrow peaked T waves are usually, although not uniquely, associated with early hyperkalemia and are followed by prolongation of the PR interval, loss of the P wave, widening of the QRS complex, heart block, and asystole (Fig. 14-75A).[120] Severely elevated serum potassium (greater than 8 mEq/L) causes a wide QRS tachycardia, as shown in the 12-lead ECG in Figure 14-75B. If not corrected, severe hyperkalemia can lead to VF or cardiac standstill. It is important to know that evidence of hyperkalemia is not always visible on the ECG.[121] Furthermore, that research has shown that ECG waveform changes are not a sensitive indicator of elevated potassium levels.[121] When hyperkalemia is suspected, it is safer to draw serial serum potassium levels than to rely on the ECG waveform alone.[121]

This life-threatening condition can be acutely managed with IV insulin to drive the potassium inside the cell and temporarily out of the plasma. Glucose is usually administered at the same time to avoid hypoglycemia as a secondary complication. Potassium is permanently removed from the bloodstream by cation-exchange resin products, such as Kayexalate, placed into the gastrointestinal tract or removed directly from the blood by hemodialysis.[122] Coexisting low serum sodium, calcium, or pH levels potentiate the cardiac effects of hyperkalemia.

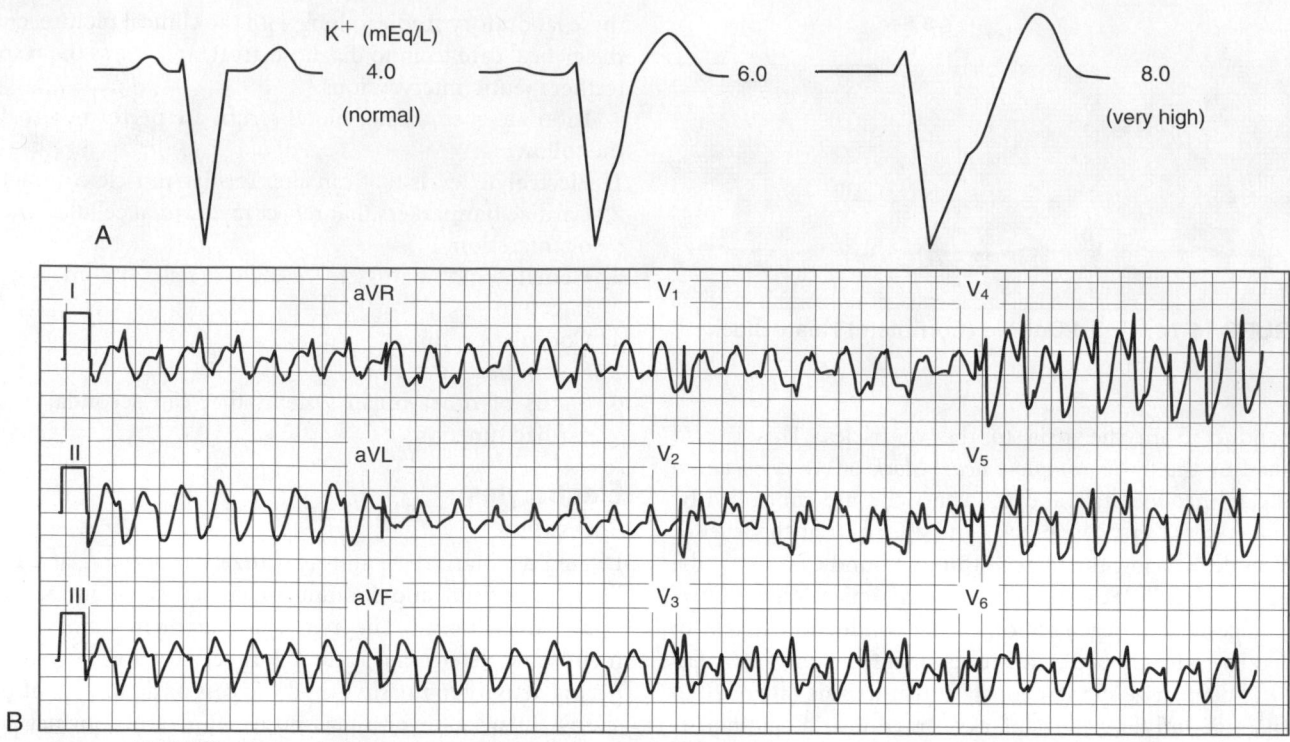

FIGURE 14-75 Effects of Hyperkalemia on the ECG. *A,* Stages in hyperkalemia from normal potassium levels to plasma levels of 8 mEq/L. At approximately 6 mEq/L, the P wave flattens, the QRS broadens, and the ST segment disappears, with the S wave flowing into the tall, tented T wave. *B,* A 12-lead ECG of a patient with a serum potassium level of 9.1 mEq/L.

Hypokalemia. A low serum potassium (K^+) level, called *hypokalemia* (less than 3.5 mEq/L), is commonly caused by gastrointestinal losses, diuretic therapy with insufficient replacement, or chronic steroid therapy. Hypokalemia is also reflected by changes on the ECG (Fig. 14-76). The earliest ECG change is often PVCs, which can deteriorate into VT or VF without appropriate potassium replacement.

Hypokalemia impairs myocardial conduction and prolongs ventricular repolarization. This can be seen by a prominent U wave (a positive deflection after the T wave on the ECG).[122] The U wave is not totally unique to hypokalemia, but its presence is a signal for the clinician to check the serum potassium level.[122] In the critical care unit, where patients are receiving diuretics or have nasogastric tubes to suction, the serum potassium level is checked frequently by the critical care nurse and replaced intravenously to normal levels to prevent dysrhythmias. Great care must be taken when replacing potassium intravenously to ensure it is diluted sufficiently and administered slowly to prevent accidental overdose. Potassium is a high-alert medication, and additional safety procedures are recommended for replacement of this electrolyte (Box 14-13). Table 14-17 provides the electrolyte values that affect cardiac contractility.

Calcium

Calcium (Ca^{2+}) is an important cation in the body. Calcium metabolism is controlled by many factors, including normal parathyroid hormone (PTH) function, calcitonin, and vitamin D acting on target organs such as the kidney, bone, and gastrointestinal tract. Calcium is an important mediator of many cardiovascular functions because of its effect on vascular tone, myocardial contractility, and cardiac excitability.

Serum calcium values are recorded in three possible ways, depending on the hospital laboratory: milliequivalents per liter (mEq/L), milligrams per deciliter (mg/dL), or millimoles per liter (mmol/L).

In the bloodstream, about 50% of calcium is biologically active and is known as *ionized calcium.*[123] The remaining nonactive calcium is bound to protein (primarily albumin) and inorganic ions such as sulfate and phosphate.[123] The normal values for total and ionized serum calcium levels are listed in Table 14-17. The normal serum concentration of ionized calcium is maintained within very narrow limits; changes in ionized calcium level are responsible for the clinical effects of hypercalcemia and hypocalcemia. The only accurate way to determine the level of ionized calcium—described as physiologically active, unbound, or free—is to measure the ionized serum value with a laboratory assay.[123] The mathematically calculated values that extrapolate from total calcium and serum albumin levels have been shown to be inaccurate.[123]

Hypercalcemia. Hypercalcemia is defined as increased amounts of ionized calcium (greater than 4.8 mg/dL or 1.30 mmol/L) or increased amounts of total serum calcium (greater than 10.5 mg/dL or 2.60 mmol/L). Serum calcium levels are increased by bone tumors; primary hyperparathyroidism

Hypokalemia

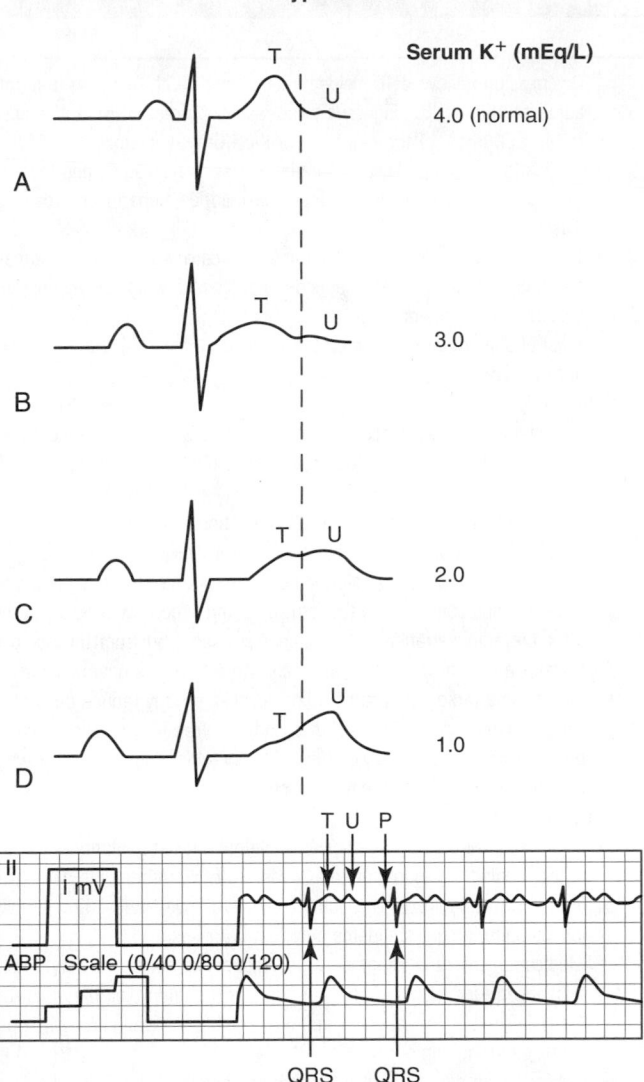

FIGURE 14-76 Effects of Hypokalemia on the ECG. *A*, At a normal serum concentration of 3.5 to 4.5 mEq/L, the amplitude of the T wave is appreciably greater than that of the U wave. *B*, By the time the serum potassium level has dropped to 3 mEq/L, the amplitudes of the T and U waves are approaching each other. *C* and *D*, With a further drop in the level of potassium, the U wave begins to tower over and fuse with the T wave. *E*, ECG tracing from a patient with a serum potassium of 2.6 mEq/L shows a prominent U wave.

caused by elevated PTH levels; excessive intake of supplemental calcium and vitamin D, usually in oral antacids; hypomagnesemia; and as a complication of kidney failure from decreased renal excretion of calcium. Hypercalcemia affects many organs, causes smooth muscle relaxation, and can lead to neurologic changes such as lethargy, confusion, and even coma. Elevated serum calcium has the cardiovascular effect of strengthening contractility and shortening ventricular repolarization, demonstrated on the ECG by a shortened QTc interval.[122] Rhythm disturbances may include bradycardia; first-, second-, and third-degree heart block; and BBB. Hypercalcemia can potentiate the effects of digitalis, precipitate digitalis toxicity, and cause hypertension.[123]

Management of hypercalcemia involves promotion of renal excretion of calcium by diuretics and high-volume intravenous NS at 200 to 300 mL/hr if tolerated by the heart, lungs, and kidneys. Patients who cannot tolerate this clinical regimen should be hemodialyzed using a low-calcium dialysate.

Hypocalcemia. *Hypocalcemia* is defined as an ionized calcium level below normal (less than 4 mg/dL or less than 1.05 mmol/L) or a low total serum calcium level. Hypocalcemia (measured by ionized calcium) is a common finding and is reported to occur in 15% to 20% of critically ill patients, depending on the admitting diagnosis.[124] The more severe the patient's illness, the greater the risk of developing hypocalcemia. Transfusions of blood from the blood bank lower serum calcium levels because the citrate used as an anticoagulant in banked blood binds to the calcium.[123] This is called *citrate chelation.* If citrate is used during hemodialysis or plasmapheresis, it will have the same calcium-binding (chelating) effect. Phosphate also binds to calcium and can lower the serum calcium level. Metabolic alkalosis often coexists with hypocalcemia. The cardiovascular effects of hypocalcemia include decreased myocardial contractility, decreased CO, and hypotension. Rhythm disturbances with severe hypocalcemia are variable, ranging from bradycardia to VT and asystole. When the ionized calcium is low, the ECG may show a prolonged QTc interval[122] (Fig. 14-77). This predisposes a patient to the life-threatening ventricular dysrhythmia called *torsades de pointes.*

Management of hypocalcemia, especially when the ionized calcium is low, involves infusion of intravenous calcium chloride or IV calcium gluconate.[123]

- Calcium chloride provides 27 mg of elemental calcium/mL (272 mg in 10 mL).
- Calcium gluconate provides 9 mg of elemental calcium/mL (90 mg in 10 mL).

Magnesium

Magnesium (Mg^{2+}) is essential for many enzyme, protein, lipid, and carbohydrate functions in the body and is critical for the production and use of energy. The body stores most magnesium in bone (53%), muscle (27%), and soft tissues (19%); only a tiny proportion resides within the bloodstream—red blood cells contain 0.5%, and serum contains 0.3%.[125] As with other electrolytes, the ionized portion of the serum magnesium is the biologically active component that is available for biochemical processes. Serum magnesium is 67% ionized, 19% protein bound, and 14% complexed.[125] The serum magnesium is what is normally measured in a routine blood test. Serum magnesium can be reported in units of mEq/L, mg/dL, or mmol/L, depending on the laboratory running the analysis. The normal serum range is from 1.5 to 2 mEq/L, 1.8 to 2.4 mg/dL, or 0.7 to 1.1 mmol/L. These represent the same serum level of magnesium despite different measurement guidelines used in the report. It is important to anticipate that normal reference values will vary between hospital laboratories.

Hypermagnesemia. The incidence of hypermagnesemia is rare in comparison with hypomagnesemia. It results from kidney failure, tumor lysis syndrome, or iatrogenic overtreatment.

⚡ BOX 14-13 PATIENT SAFETY ALERT

Medication Administration

QSEN 1. Accurate Patient Identification
- Use at least two patient identifiers (not the patient's room number) when taking blood samples or administering medications or blood products. Examples include the patient name or date of birth.

2. Effective Communication Among Caregivers
- An organizational method to decrease the number of medication errors is the use of *computerized physician order entry* (CPOE), as advocated by the Leapfrog group (http://www.leapfroggroup.org).
- Hospitals should have a process for taking verbal or telephone orders that requires a verification "read back" of the complete order by the person receiving the order.
- The Institute of Safe Medication Practices (ISMP) maintains a list of medications with similar-sounding names as name confusion can lead to medication errors. The list is available on the ISMP website at http://www.ismp.org/Tools/confuseddrugnames.pdf. Medication errors can be reported to the Medication Errors Reporting Program (MERP).
- Standardize the abbreviations, acronyms, and symbols used throughout the organization, including a list of abbreviations, acronyms, and symbols not to use.
- Examples of problematic abbreviations include "U" for units and "μg" for micrograms. When handwritten, a capital U can be mistaken for a zero (0); in numerous case reports, an insulin dosage written in U was interpreted as 0. Using the abbreviation "μg" instead of "mcg" for micrograms is also problematic; when handwritten, the Greek letter μ can look like an "m." The error-prone abbreviation is available on the ISMP website at: http://www.ismp.org/Tools/errorproneabbreviations.pdf.
- Use of trailing zeros (e.g., 2.0 versus 2) and use a leading decimal point without a leading zero (e.g., .2 instead of 0.2) are dangerous prescription-writing practices. Misinterpretation has caused 10-fold dosing errors.

3. High-Alert Medication Safety
- Remove concentrated electrolytes (including but not limited to potassium chloride, potassium phosphate, and hypertonic sodium chloride) from patient care units.
- Standardize and limit the number of medication concentrations available in the organization.
- In the first 2 years after enacting a *sentinel event reporting mechanism*, the most common category was medication errors, and the most frequently implicated medication was potassium chloride (KCl). The Joint Commission reviewed 10 incidents of patient death resulting from mis-administration of KCl. Eight were the result of direct infusion of concentrated KCl. In six of the eight cases, the KCl was mistaken for another medication, primarily because of similarities in packaging and labeling. Most often, KCl was mistaken for sodium chloride, heparin, or furosemide (Lasix).
- The Joint Commission suggests that health care organizations *not* make concentrated KCl available outside the pharmacy unless appropriate, specific safeguards are in place.
- A list of a list of high-alert medications is available on the ISMP website at http://www.ismp.org.

4. Infusion Pump Safety
- Ensure free-flow protection on all general-use and patient-controlled analgesia (PCA) intravenous (IV) infusion pumps used in the organization.
- Infusion pumps that do not provide protection from the free flow of IV fluid or medication into the patient are hazardous.
- *Free flow* occurs when IV solution flows freely under the force of gravity without being controlled by the infusion pump. Free flow typically occurs after the administration set is temporarily removed from the pump to transfer a patient to another area, change a patient's gown, or place a patient on a radiography table. Clinicians can greatly reduce this risk by using administration sets with set-based anti–free-flow mechanisms that prevent gravity free flow by closing off the IV tubing to prohibit flow when the administration set is removed from the pump.

5. Hospital Safety
- Each year The Joint Commission develops Hospital National Patient Safety Goals that incorporate medication safety requirements. This information is available on The Joint Commission website at http://www.jointcommission.org/standards_information/npsgs.aspx.
- Medication safety is an important component of hospital safety. Hospitals are graded on the safety of their environment for patients. The "safety score" for each hospital is publicly available at http://www.leapfroggroup.org.

More information can be accessed on the websites of the following three safety organizations:

http://www.jointcommission.org
http://www.usp.org
http://www.leapfroggroup.org

TABLE 14-17 CHEMISTRY VALUES THAT AFFECT CARDIAC CONTRACTILITY AND CONDUCTION

ELECTROLYTE	NORMAL RANGES*		
	mEq/L	mg/dL	mmol/L
Potassium (K$^+$)	3.5-4.5		3.50-4.50
Ionized calcium (Ca)		4.0-5.0	1.00-1.30
Total calcium (Ca^{2+})		8.5-10.5	2.00-2.60
Magnesium (Mg^{2+})	1.5-2.0	1.8-2.4	0.70-1.10

*Laboratory values may be reported as mEq/L, mg/dL, or mmol/L. Each measurement parameter used produces a different value. Some electrolytes are reported with more than one reference value. Different clinical laboratories use different reference values, and the cited reference values may vary slightly between hospital laboratories.

Hypomagnesemia. A total serum magnesium concentration below 1.5 mEq/L defines *hypomagnesemia*. It is commonly associated with other electrolyte imbalances, most notably alterations in potassium, calcium, and phosphorus. Low serum magnesium levels can result from many causes. Hypomagnesemia is caused by insufficient intake in the diet or in total parenteral nutrition (TPN) and is associated with chronic alcohol abuse. In the critical care unit, aggressive diuresis with loop diuretics will lower serum levels.[125] Diarrhea can be a significant cause of magnesium loss because lower gastrointestinal fluids contain up to 15 mEq/L magnesium; vomiting or gastric suction causes less depletion because the upper gastrointestinal fluids contain about 1 mEq/L). Another cause of magnesium depletion is rapid administration of citrated blood products, which causes the citrate to bind to the magnesium, a condition known as *citrate chelation*. In patients with chronic hypomagnesemia, the serum levels are replenished from the bone stores.

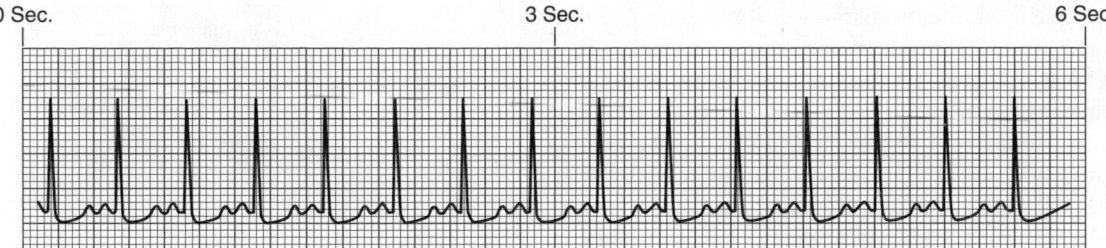

FIGURE 14-77 Abnormal QT Prolongation in a Hypocalcemic Patient. The patient is a 50-year-old woman admitted to the critical care unit with a diagnosis of alcoholic liver disease and malnourishment. Total calcium concentration is 5.1 mg/dL, and the albumin level is 1.3 mg/dL. The QT interval (0.55 second) is markedly prolonged for the heart rate (HR) (100 beats/min). The QT interval varies with the HR and can be corrected (QT_c) as if the HR were 60 beats/min using the formula $\sqrt{QT/RR} = QT_c$. The QT_c should be 0.44 second or less. The QT_c in the ECG tracing shown is 0.55 second. Hypocalcemia lengthens ventricular repolarization. A quick method for assessing the QT interval is to remember that it is usually less than half of the R-R interval. If it is more than one half of the R-R interval, it is prolonged. (From Yucha CB, Toto KH. Calcium and phosphorus derangements. *Crit Care Nurs Clin North Am.* 1994;6[4]:747.)

Hypomagnesemia can also occur in patients who take proton pump inhibitor (PPI) medications to reduce production of gastric acid. This condition improves when the PPIs are stopped.[126]

Hypomagnesemia can cause hypertension and vasospasm, including coronary artery spasm. Some studies have linked magnesium depletion to sudden cardiac death, to an increased incidence of acute MI, and to the occurrence of ventricular dysrhythmias.[125]

In hypomagnesemia, the ECG changes are similar to those seen with hypokalemia and hypocalcemia: prolonged PR and QTc intervals, presence of U waves, T-wave flattening, and a widened QRS complex. Cardiac dysrhythmias may be supraventricular or ventricular and include the polymorphic ventricular rhythm torsades de pointes. In cardiac arrest with pulseless VT with torsades de pointes, IV magnesium 1 to 2 grams diluted in 10 mL D5W may be administered over 15 minutes.[127] It is important to evaluate kidney function when administering magnesium to avoid precipitating hypermagnesium states.

Cardiac Biomarker Studies
Cardiac Biomarkers in Acute Coronary Syndrome
Cardiac biomarkers are proteins that are released from damaged myocardial cells.[128] When myocardial cells are damaged, they release detectable proteins into the bloodstream so that a rise in biomarkers can be correlated with heart muscle injury. The biomarkers that are routinely measured include cardiac *troponin I* (cTnI), cardiac *troponin T* (cTnT), and *CK-MB*. Table 14-18 summarizes the cardiac biomarkers related to myocardial injury and infarction. Unfortunately, in many hospitals, the laboratory turnaround time for results of quantitative cardiac biomarkers is between 60 and 90 minutes, which limits the usefulness of the biomarkers in an emergency. If point-of-care testing at the bedside is used, the results are available more quickly and may be more helpful in the clinical decision-making process.

TABLE 14-18	SERUM BIOMARKERS AFTER ACUTE MYOCARDIAL INFARCTION		
SERUM BIOMARKER	**TIME TO INITIAL ELEVATION (HOURS)***	**PEAK ELEVATION† (HOURS)***	**RETURN TO BASELINE (DAYS)***
Cardiac troponin I (cTnI)	3-12	24	5-10
Cardiac troponin			
T (cTnT)	3-12	12-48	5-14
CK-MB‡	3-12	24	2-3

*Time periods represent average reported values.
†Does not include patients who have had reperfusion therapy.
‡The creatine kinase (CK) enzyme consists of two subunits, the brain type (B) and the muscle type (M).

Creatine Kinase-MB. The creatine kinase (CK) muscle/brain (MB) biomarker (CK-MB) is released as a result of myocardial damage, and serum levels rise 4 to 8 hours after MI, peak at 15 to 24 hours, and remain elevated for 2 to 3 days (see Table 14-18). Serial samples are drawn routinely at 6- or 8-hour intervals, and three samples are usually sufficient to support or rule out the diagnosis of MI. CK-MB is never an isolated test; it is always performed in conjunction with cardiac troponin levels.

Troponin T and Troponin I. The *troponins* are biomarkers for myocardial damage. cTnI and cTnT are more sensitive markers of myocardial injury and infarction than CK-MB. As a result, more patients with myocardial damage are now being detected. Several different methods of laboratory assay are available, which means that normal serum levels will vary between different clinical settings, although cardiac serum cTnI and cTnT levels will be low in the absence of myocardial muscle damage.

The initial elevation of cTnI, cTnT, and CK-MB occurs 3 to 6 hours after the acute myocardial damage. This means that if an individual comes to the emergency department as soon as chest pain is experienced, the biomarkers will not have risen. For this reason, it is clinical practice to diagnose an acute MI by 12-lead ECG and clinical symptoms without waiting for elevation of cardiac biomarkers.

Because cTnI is found only in cardiac muscle, it is a highly specific biomarker for myocardial damage, considerably more specific than CK-MB. As a consequence, patients with a positive cTnI result and a negative CK-MB result usually rule in an acute MI. A negative cTnI result that remains negative many hours after an episode of chest pain is a strong indicator that the patient is not experiencing an acute MI. Even with a negative cTnI result, symptoms of chest pain still indicate that the patient should have a comprehensive cardiac evaluation to determine if there is underlying CAD present that may later lead to complications.

A new development is the advent of high-sensitivity troponin I monitoring (hsTnI).[129] The advantage to using a more sensitive biomarker test is that more patients with acute coronary syndrome (ACS) will be identified, although this will not eliminate the requirement for astute clinical assessment due to the many other conditions associated with elevated troponin levels.[128]

Cardiac Biomarkers and Reperfusion. Management of STEMI includes opening the coronary artery obstructed by a thrombus and reperfusing the injured area as rapidly as possible. Individuals who have recent onset of chest pain (within 12 hours) are candidates for reperfusion therapies, including fibrinolytic agents ("clot busters"), cardiac catheterization with PCIs such as balloon angioplasty, atherectomy, or stent placement. If successful, these interventions may totally abort the MI or limit the amount of cardiac muscle damage, resulting in an early rise and fall of the cardiac biomarkers as illustrated in Figure 15-13 in Chapter 15. After reperfusion, the serum troponin levels rise dramatically and peak early. Cardiac biomarker samples are drawn at admission, before administration of fibrinolytic therapy or PCI, and then at 6-hour or 8-hour intervals for 18 to 24 hours to detect any biomarker rise and assess the return of effective myocardial reperfusion.

Natriuretic Peptide Biomarkers in Heart Failure

Natriuretic peptides are biomarkers that provide additional information with which to accurately evaluate the breathless patient.[130] It can be difficult to identify whether a dyspneic patient has a primary pulmonary problem or is exhibiting symptoms of acute heart failure with pulmonary edema. Cardiac natriuretic peptides are used to help make the correct diagnosis. In decompensated heart failure, the myocytes in the ventricle release B-type natriuretic peptide (BNP) from the ventricles. Three laboratory assays are commercially available to measure BNP: a point-of-care test, a laboratory test for BNP, and a different laboratory test to measure the N-Terminal fragment of pro-BNP (NTpro-BNP). BNP has a half-life of about 20 minutes, whereas NTpro-BNP has a longer half-life of 1 to 2 hours.[131] The choice of test is generally dependent on what is available in the hospital.

The greater the ventricular wall stress, the higher the BNP level rises. The BNP value is combined with the physical examination, the 12-lead ECG, and a chest radiograph to increase the

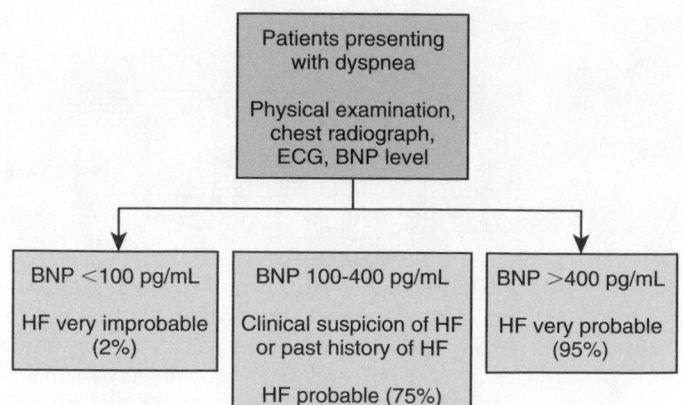

FIGURE 14-78 The B-type natriuretic peptide (BNP) algorithm in the diagnosis of heart failure.

accuracy of heart failure diagnosis (Fig. 14-78).[131] A symptomatic patient with a BNP level below 100 pg/mL or an NTproBNP below 300 pg/mL, is unlikely to be in heart failure, with only a 10% likelihood.[130] Conversely, a patient with a BNP level above 400 pg/dL is almost definitely in heart failure.[130] BNP is an excellent test to rule out acute heart failure.[130] The challenge lies in interpreting the results of patients with a BNP level between 100 and 400 pg/mL, sometimes described as the *gray zone*.[130,131] This highlights the importance of using a spectrum of clinical and diagnostic tests. As the symptoms of heart failure are successfully treated, the BNP level usually decreases toward the normal range.

There are some caveats to the use of natriuretic peptides as biomarkers, principally because they are not unique to the heart. Natriuretic peptides are also released from the endothelium and from the kidney, and this can alter the measured BNP levels. Filtration by the kidney is one of the mechanisms by which BNP is cleared from the bloodstream. BNP levels are higher in patients with kidney failure, especially if the glomerular filtration rate (GFR) is below 60 mL/min/1.7 m². [130,131] BNP levels can also be elevated in high-CO septic shock, possibly because of endothelial natriuretic peptide release or myocardial damage.

BNP levels are lower than expected in obese patients with heart failure, possibly because natriuretic peptide receptors in adipose tissue degrade BNP more rapidly.[131] Conditions such as mitral stenosis that cause pulmonary edema but protect the left ventricle are associated with lower BNP levels than expected from the clinical picture. Even with these caveats, the BNP remains an extremely useful addition for the diagnosis of heart failure.

Hematologic Studies

Hematologic laboratory studies that are routinely ordered for the management of patients with altered cardiovascular status are red blood cell (RBC) or erythrocyte level, hemoglobin level, hematocrit level, and white blood cell (WBC) or leukocyte level.

Red Blood Cells

The normal amount of RBCs in a person varies with age, gender, environmental temperature, altitude, and exercise. Men produce

4.5 to 6 million RBCs/mm³, whereas the normal level for women is 4 to 5.5 million/mm³. *Anemia* is the clinical condition that occurs when not enough red blood cells are available to carry oxygen to the tissues. *Polycythemia* is the condition that occurs when excess RBCs are produced.

Hemoglobin

Hemoglobin levels normally range from 14 to 18 g/dL in men and from 12 to 16 g/dL in women.

Hematocrit

The hematocrit is the volume percentage of RBCs in whole blood. The value is 40% to 54% for men and 38% to 48% for women.

White Blood Cells

Most inflammatory processes that produce necrotic tissue within the heart muscle, such as rheumatic fever, endocarditis, and MI, increase the WBC level. WBCs are also known as leukocytes, and a WBC test may be called a serum leukocyte count. The normal WBC level for both genders is 5000 to 10,000 cells/mm³. The WBC level also increases in response to infection.

Platelets

The normal platelet count is 150,000 to 400,000 cells/mm³. Less commonly, the normal platelet count range will be written as 150 to 400 × 10⁹/L. Normally, the platelet count is the only laboratory value that is reported. Unfortunately, there is no routine test available for critical care patients that can evaluate platelet functionality. Platelets are important because they are the first cells to be activated when the coagulation system is stimulated. Many medications inhibit platelet function and make the platelets "slippery" so that they do not clump together to activate the clotting process. Sometimes, the antiplatelet action of a medication is its intended role, such as with aspirin used to prevent acute coronary syndrome, and it can be an unintended side effect. A low platelet count is called *thrombocytopenia*.

Blood Coagulation Studies

Coagulation studies are ordered to determine blood-clotting effectiveness. Anticoagulants—most notably heparin, direct thrombin inhibitors, warfarin, and platelet inhibitory agents—are administered daily in critical care units for many clinical reasons. It is essential to understand the laboratory tests that are used to monitor the effectiveness of therapeutic anticoagulation.

Prothrombin Time. Most coagulation study results are reported as the length of time in seconds it takes for blood to form a clot in the laboratory test tube. The *prothrombin time* (PT) is no longer directly used to determine the therapeutic dosage of warfarin (Coumadin) necessary to achieve anticoagulation. The PT is not standardized between laboratories so the result of this test is always reported as a standardized *international normalized ratio* (INR).

International Normalized Ratio. The INR was developed by the World Health Organization (WHO) in 1982 to standardize PT results among clinical laboratories worldwide. Table 14-19 shows target INR ranges for different cardiovascular conditions

TABLE 14-19 NORMAL AND THERAPEUTIC COAGULATION VALUES

TEST	CLINICAL CONDITION	NORMAL VALUE	THERAPEUTIC ANTICOAGULANT TARGET VALUE
INR	Normal coagulation	<1.0	
INR	Atrial fibrillation		2.0-3.0
INR	Treatment of DVT/PE		2.0-3.0
INR	Mechanical heart valves		2.0-3.0
aPTT	Normal coagulation	28-38 sec	1.5-2.5 × normal
PTT	Normal coagulation	60-90 sec	1.5-2.0 × normal
ACT*	Normal coagulation	0-120 sec	150-300 sec

*ACT is normal, but therapeutic values may vary with type of activator used.
ACT, Activated coagulation time; *aPPT*, activated partial thromboplastin time; *DVT*, deep vein thrombosis; *INR*, international normalized ratio; *PE*, pulmonary embolism; *PTT*, partial thromboplastin time.

that require anticoagulation. A target INR of 2.5 (range 2.0 to 3.0) is desirable.[132,133]

When a patient is first started on warfarin, it is important to know that it can take 72 hours or more to achieve a therapeutic level of anticoagulation. This is because the half-life of prothrombin is between 36 and 42 hours.[134] This delay in anticoagulation effectiveness also occurs if a patient is being converted from heparin-based anticoagulation—monitored by *activated partial thromboplastin* time (aPTT)—to warfarin-based anticoagulation (monitored by INR). To ensure a safe transition, a period of 48 to 72 hours is required in order to obtain a therapeutic INR value before the heparin is discontinued.

Activated Partial Thromboplastin Time. The aPTT is used to measure the effectiveness of intravenous or subcutaneous ultrafractionated heparin (UFH) therapy. Coagulation monitoring is required with UHF, although not with subcutaneous low–molecular-weight heparin (LMWH), because of lower levels of plasma protein binding. In cases of over-anticoagulation with heparin, the antidote is protamine sulfate.

Anti-Factor Xa Test of Heparin Activity. Some critical care units monitor heparin activity directly using the anti-Factor Xa assay. This is the only test available to monitor the anticoagulant effects of LMWH and the newer antithrombotic medications.[135]

Activated Coagulation Time. An additional test of heparin effect is the *activated coagulation time* (ACT), also known as the *activated clotting time*. The ACT is a *point of care test* that is performed outside of the laboratory setting in areas such as the cardiac catheterization laboratory, the operating room, or critical care units. Normal and therapeutic values for these coagulation studies are shown in Table 14-19.

Serum Lipid Studies

Four primary blood lipid levels are important in evaluating an individual's risk of developing or having progression of CAD:

total cholesterol; low-density lipoprotein cholesterol (LDL-C); triglycerides; and high-density lipoprotein cholesterol (HDLC). When levels of cholesterol low-density lipoproteins (LDLs) and triglycerides are elevated or the level of high-density lipoproteins (HDLs) is low, the patient is considered at risk for developing or having progression of CAD and is offered intensive interventions in diet therapy, exercise prescription, and medication therapy.[136,137] The following lipid biomarkers are frequently ordered together as a "lipid panel."

Total Cholesterol

Cholesterol is a fatlike substance (lipid) that is present in cell membranes, is produced by the liver, and is a precursor of bile acids and steroid hormones. The cholesterol level in the blood is determined partly by genetics and partly by acquired factors such as diet, calorie balance, and level of physical activity. Cholesterol in excess amounts (greater than 200 mg/dL) in the serum forces the progression of atherosclerosis (atherogenesis). Table 14-20 lists the desirable lipid levels to lower the risk of CAD and to reduce morbidity and mortality in patients with established CAD.

Low-Density Lipoproteins

About 60% to 70% of the total serum cholesterol is carried in the bloodstream, complexed as LDL-C. The LDL-C and total serum cholesterol levels are directly correlated with risk for CAD, and high levels of each are significant predictors of future acute MI in persons with established coronary artery atherosclerosis. LDL-C is the major atherogenic lipoprotein and is the primary target for cholesterol-lowering efforts.[136] Guidelines recommend maintaining an LDL-C level below 130 mg/dL for the patient with no history of atherosclerotic disease. A patient with known CAD but who is not high risk should aim for an LDL-C level below 100 mg/dL. The recommended target LDL-C level for high-risk patients with CAD has been lowered to 70 mg/dL.[137]

TABLE 14-20	DESIRABLE LIPID LEVELS
LIPID	**DESIRABLE LEVEL**
Total cholesterol	<200 mg/dL
	<130 mg/dL without CAD
LDL-C	<100 mg/dL with CAD but not considered high risk
	<70 mg/dL with CAD and considered at high risk for future coronary events
Triglycerides	<100 mg/dL
HDL-C	>40 mg/dL (male)
	>50 mg/dL (female)

Data from the Executive Summary of the Third Report of the National Cholesterol Education Program (NCEP) Expert Panel on Detection, Evaluation, and Treatment of High Blood Cholesterol in Adults (Adult Treatment Panel III). *JAMA.* 2001;285(19):2486; Grundy SM, et al. Implications of recent clinical trials for the National Cholesterol Education Program (NCEP) Adult Treatment Panel III (ATP III) Guidelines. *Circulation.* 2004;110:227.
CAD, Coronary artery disease; *HDL-C*, high-density lipoprotein cholesterol; *LDL-C*, low-density lipoprotein cholesterol.

Very-Low-Density Lipoproteins and Triglycerides

The very-low-density lipoproteins (VLDLs) contain 10% to 15% of the total serum cholesterol along with most of the triglycerides in fasting serum.

High-Density Lipoproteins

HDLs are particles that carry 20% to 30% of the total serum cholesterol. A low HDL-C level (below 35 mg/dL) is another independent, significant risk factor for CAD. Several studies also support the finding that HDL-C helps protect against atherogenesis, and a level greater than 50 mg/dL may act as a shield against the risk of CAD. Low HDL-C levels are often associated with elevated triglyceride levels.[138]

Triglycerides

Triglycerides are another form of lipid in the bloodstream that is normally included in the lipid assessment panel. The normal fasting level is less than 100 mg/dl.[138] Elevated triglyceride levels are associated with diabetes mellitus and an increased risk of atherosclerotic disease.

DIAGNOSTIC PROCEDURES

Cardiac Catheterization and Coronary Arteriography

Cardiac catheterization and coronary arteriography are routine diagnostic procedures for patients with known or suspected heart disease. Clinical indications for cardiac catheterization include myocardial ischemia, unstable angina, evolving MI, heart failure with a history that suggests CAD or valvular heart disease, and congenital heart disease. Cardiac catheterization is used to confirm physical findings and to provide a baseline for medical or surgical therapy.[139]

Left-Heart Cardiac Catheterization

During catheterization of the left side of the heart, hemodynamic pressure measurements are taken in the aortic root, the left ventricle, and the left atrium.[140] Radiopaque contrast (dye) is used to visualize the left ventricle (ventriculogram). This information is also used to calculate the LV EF. The coronary arteries are visualized and contrast dye is injected directly into each arterial system. The general term for vessel imaging is *angiogram* (veins and arteries), but the more specific term used to describe the visualization of the coronary arteries is *arteriogram*.

Right-Heart Cardiac Catheterization

Catheterization of the right side of the heart is performed using a thermodilution PA catheter. Information obtained includes hemodynamic pressure measurements in the right atrium, the right ventricle, the PA, and the pulmonary artery occlusion wedge position, as well as the measurement of CO, calculated hemodynamic values, and oxygen saturations and an angiogram of the right-heart chambers using radiopaque contrast.

Procedure

Before the catheterization, the patient meets with the cardiologist to discuss the purpose, benefit, and risks of the study. For many patients, cardiac catheterization is the first major invasive procedure after a diagnosis of possible heart disease. The patient is often very anxious and has many questions. It is important that nursing and medical staff fully answer patients' questions about the catheterization experience.

The morning of the procedure the patient fasts except for ingesting prescribed cardiac medications. Light premedication is given before the patient goes to the catheterization laboratory. If there is a history of allergy, an antihistamine or corticosteroid may be administered to prevent an anaphylactic reaction to the radiopaque contrast. Throughout the cardiac catheterization, the patient remains awake and alert. He or she is positioned on a hard table with a C-shaped camera arm overhead or to the side. This arm can be positioned to view the heart from several different angles.

Prevention of Contrast-Induced Nephropathy. In patients with an elevated serum creatinine, sodium bicarbonate or NS will be administered to protect the kidneys from the damaging effects of the contrast medium.[141] N-acetylcysteine has not been shown to be effective.[141] Up to 10% of acute kidney injury in the hospital occurs as a result of procedures that use IV contrast.[142]

Cardiac catheterization catheters, available in a variety of designs and sizes, are placed in the femoral vein and artery after the patient receives a local anesthetic. The choice of catheters is based on the cardiologist's experience and the diagnostic study required. The femoral artery is used to catheterize the left side of the heart, including the coronary arteries. The femoral vein is frequently used as the access vessel to pass catheters to the right side of the heart. During the study, the patient receives heparin systemically to reduce the risk of emboli. Many patients also receive nitroglycerin to control chest pain, particularly when the coronary arteries are full of contrast material during the coronary arteriographic procedure. At this time, the patient may also experience bradycardia or hypotension. To move the contrast dye more quickly and minimize the vagal effect on HR and blood pressure, the patient may be asked to cough. If bradycardia persists, atropine or, occasionally, a transvenous pacemaker may be used. If hypotension continues, IV fluids are administered as a bolus. At the end of the study, the femoral catheters are removed from the vessels. After the catheterization, when the patient is stable, the cardiologist meets with the patient and family to discuss the findings and plan of care.

Nursing Management

Femoral Artery Site Care. After the diagnostic catheters (and the sheaths through which they are inserted) are removed from the femoral artery and vein, pressure is applied to the femoral vessels until bleeding has stopped. After catheterization, the patient remains flat for up to 6 hours (varies by institutional protocol and catheter size) to allow the femoral arterial puncture site to form a stable clot. Most bleeding occurs within the first 2 to 3 hours after the procedure. During this time, the groin site is checked frequently for evidence of bleeding or hematoma. Three methods may be used to control bleeding at the femoral arterial puncture site after catheter or sheath removal. The most basic method is manual pressure, in which a clinician holds pressure directly on the vein or artery until bleeding stops. The second method uses external mechanical compression over the site (C-clamp or FemoStop). The third method is for the cardiologist to use an *arteriotomy closure device* at the end of the catheterization procedure. One closure device is designed to suture the artery closed as the sheath is removed; another option is placement of a collagen plug into the track of the sheath insertion site. All of these methods are effective. After routine diagnostic cardiac catheterization procedures, there is no difference in the rate of femoral arterial site complications for the different methods. The patient is asked to lie still and not to bend at the hip. It usually takes about 40 minutes for a stable clot to form, but it can take longer in some patients, including those with a large body surface area.

Sometimes, when the patient needs to void urine, the movement can dislodge the clot. If the patient cannot void in the supine position, a urinary catheter is usually inserted for women and a condom catheter is used for men.

Peripheral Pulses. The peripheral pulses located distal to the arterial access site are monitored closely by the critical care nurse. If the femoral artery has been used, dorsal pedal and posterior tibial pulses are assessed. If an alternative access site such as the radial artery is used, the radial pulse is assessed. Pulses are assessed every 15 minutes for the first hour after the catheterization and every 30 minutes to 1 hour thereafter. The limb corresponding to the catheterization site is assessed for changes in color, temperature, pain, or paresthesia to detect early evidence of acute arterial occlusion.

Rehydration. The patient is encouraged to drink large amounts of clear liquids, and the intravenous fluid rate is increased to 100 mL/hr. Fluid is given for rehydration because the radiopaque contrast acts as an osmotic diuretic. This is also used to prevent *contrast-induced nephropathy* or damage to the kidney from the contrast dye used to visualize the heart structures. Patients who have elevated blood urea nitrogen (BUN) or creatinine levels before catheterization are at risk for acute kidney failure from the dye. For these patients, the quantity of contrast material is consciously limited, and fluid boluses are given to preserve kidney function.

Angina. The patient is assessed for chest pain after the procedure. Usually, sublingual nitroglycerin is sufficient to relieve the pain, discomfort, or pressure. Not all patients describe their angina as "pain," and many other descriptors such as "pressure" may be used. Patients are encouraged to use the 0-to-10 pain scale to quantify the angina. A 12-lead ECG must be obtained immediately to identify the coronary arteries involved, and the cardiologist is notified. If the chest pain persists, this may indicate that a clot has formed in a coronary artery, and the patient may need to return to the cardiac catheterization laboratory for an interventional cardiology procedure. More information about PCI is provided in the section "Catheter Interventions for Coronary Artery Disease" in Chapter 16.

Dysrhythmias. Dysrhythmias are always a concern after an invasive cardiovascular diagnostic procedure. They result from the underlying cardiac disease and the low potassium levels that can occur after excessive diuresis.

Patient Education

Because of the invasive nature of cardiac catheterization, many patients express considerable anxiety. Relevant information concerns the sensory details of the procedure, such as lying flat and immobile on a hard table for many hours and sometimes experiencing a feeling of warmth when the dye is injected. Pain is uncommon because opiate analgesics and sedative medications are always provided. Information about possible outcomes—positive and negative—and possible complications must be provided to the patient. Postcatheterization requirements such as lying still and drinking large quantities of fluids are explained. The basic information can be provided using written and audiovisual material, but it is vital to individualize the content and answer any specific concerns or questions. Patients are also asked to report any other unusual symptoms, such as chest pain or nausea.

Electrophysiology Study
Indications

The electrophysiology study (EPS) is an invasive diagnostic tool used to record intracardiac electrical activity. A person may have an EPS performed because of a history of a syncopal episode (loss of consciousness); rapid, wide-complex tachycardia, or other cardiac electrical problems not diagnosed by the noninvasive diagnostic studies such as the 12-lead ECG, treadmill stress test, signal-averaged ECG, or Holter monitoring. The EPS is performed in a specially equipped cardiac catheterization laboratory.

Before the electrophysiology study, written and verbal education is provided to the patient and family to increase their sense of security and to decrease stress and anxiety. All antidysrhythmic medications are discontinued several days before the study so that any ventricular dysrhythmias may be readily induced during the EPS. Anticoagulants, especially warfarin, are also stopped before EPS. Premedication is administered before the study to induce a relaxed state, and during the procedure, the patient is conscious but receives sedative agents (e.g. midazolam or propofol) at regular intervals. The patient fasts 6 hours prior to the EPS and during the procedure lies supine on a hard table with a C-shaped or U-shaped camera arm to the side or directly overhead to verify the position of the EPS catheters in the heart.

Electrophysiology equipment for stimulation of dysrhythmias and monitoring is usually positioned nearby. A peripheral intravenous access line and surface ECG leads are placed, and electrophysiology catheters are inserted into the femoral vein and advanced to the right side of the heart under fluoroscopy. These catheters, similar to pacing catheters, are placed at specific anatomic sites within the heart to record the earliest electrical activity. The catheter placements are demonstrated in Figure 14-79, with catheter tip positions shown at the following locations:

1. High right atrium (HRA) near to the sinoatrial (SA) node
2. AV node
3. Coronary sinus (CS) behind the left atrial/ventricular border
4. Bundle of His (HB) near the tricuspid valve
5. Right ventricle (RV) near the apex

During EPS, *programmed electrical stimulation* is used to trigger the dysrhythmia. This technique delivers pulses of two to four early paced beats by means of a specific catheter to the selected area of myocardium. During the EPS, the

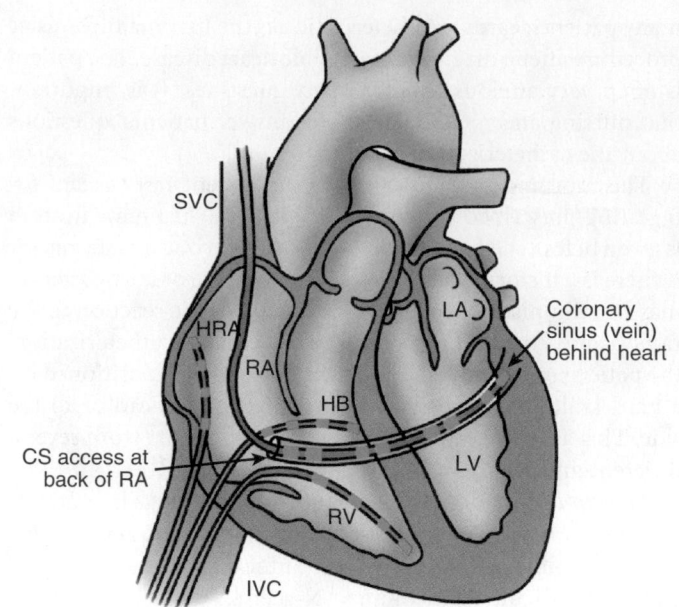

Placement of catheters in the heart in an electrophysiology study.

CS indicates coronary sinus: HB, His bundle; HRA, high right atrium; IVC, inferior vena cava; RV, right ventricle; SVC, superior vena cava.

FIGURE 14-79 Catheter placement within the heart during an electrophysiology study (EPS). *LA*, Left atrium; *LV*, left ventricle; *RA*, right atrium.

electrophysiologist looks for a site of early electrical activation that stimulates the myocardium before the sinoatrial node. The goal of EPS is to discover the origin of dysrhythmias that cannot be evaluated from the surface ECG alone.

Atrial Measurements. Typical measurements during EPS include sinus node recovery time (SNRT) and sinoatrial conduction time (SACT) plus atrial pacing to measure the atrial and AV node refractory periods. Coronary sinus pacing is used to induce left atrial tachydysrhythmias. Atrial pacing usually is performed after the ventricular study to reduce the risk of putting the patient into atrial fibrillation or flutter because of retrograde conduction up the bundle of His and AV node.

Ventricular Measurements. Programmed electrical stimulation is used to induce the ventricular dysrhythmia, especially in patients who have experienced sustained or nonsustained VT, or survived a sudden cardiac death episode. To measure the retrograde V-to-A interval and stimulate the myocardium, the right ventricular catheter is selected to rapidly pace the right ventricle; the catheter then is moved to the right ventricular outflow tract (near the pulmonary valve), and the pacing stimulation is repeated. This protocol produces VT in the majority of patients with a known history of VT or VF.

After the dysrhythmia is induced and diagnosed, it can be converted to normal sinus rhythm by 10 to 15 paced beats delivered at a rate faster than the VT or by cardioversion and defibrillation plus intravenous antidysrhythmic medications. At the end of the study, all of the electrophysiology catheters are removed before the patient returns to the nursing unit.

Implantable Cardioverter Defibrillators. When an electrophysiology follow-up study is required for a patient with an

ICD, the device can substitute for the EP catheters. The ICD has sensing leads, pace termination, backup bradycardia pacing, and cardioversion and defibrillation capabilities. The EPS can be performed by the external ICD programmer in the EPS laboratory. The ICD generator and leads perform programmed electrical stimulation in a manner similar to a full EPS. Chapter 16 provides more information on the therapeutic uses of ICDs.

Chest Radiography
Basic Principles and Technique

Chest radiography is the oldest noninvasive method for visualizing images of the heart, and it remains a frequently used and valuable diagnostic tool. Information about cardiac anatomy and physiology can be obtained with ease and safety at a relatively low cost. In the critical care unit, the nurse may be the first person to view the chest radiograph of an acutely ill patient. Critical care nurses also have an important role in ensuring the quality of the film through proper positioning and instruction of the patient. For these reasons, it is crucial to understand the basics of chest radiography techniques and interpretation as they apply to the cardiovascular and pulmonary systems.

Tissue Densities. As x-rays travel through the chest from the emitting tube to the film plate, they are absorbed to various degrees by the tissues through which they pass (Table 14-21). Very dense tissue, such as bone, absorbs almost all the x-rays, leaving the film unexposed, or white. The heart, the aorta, and the pulmonary vessels and the blood they contain are moderately dense structures, appearing as gray areas on the radiographic film. These vascular structures are surrounded by air-filled lung that allows the greatest penetration of x-rays, resulting in fully exposed (black) areas on the film. Thoracic structures can be studied best by examining their borders. Two structures with the same density, when located next to each other, have no visible border. If a structure is located next to a contrasting density (e.g., vascular structures next to an air-filled lung), even subtle changes in size and shape can be seen.

Standard Views. In most institutions, a standard radiographic examination of the heart and lungs consists of posterior–anterior (PA) and left lateral films. The standard film is taken in the radiology department with the patient in an upright position; the film exposed during a deep, sustained inhalation; and the x-ray tube aimed horizontally 6 feet from the film. This is referred to as a *PA film* because the beam traverses the patient from posterior to anterior.

Portable Chest Radiography. Because most patients in critical care units are too ill to go to the radiology department, chest radiographs are routinely obtained by using portable radiographic machines, with the patient sitting upright or lying supine, depending on the patient's clinical condition and the judgment of the nurse. The film plate is placed behind the patient's back and an anteroposterior (AP) projection is used, in which the x-ray beam enters from the front of the chest.[143] For the supine film, with the patient lying flat on the bed, the x-ray tube can be only approximately 36 inches from the patient's chest because of ceiling height and radiographic equipment construction. This results in a lower quality film from a diagnostic standpoint, because the images of the heart and great vessels are magnified and not as sharply defined. Whenever possible, the upright (AP) film is preferred to the supine (flat) one, because it provides a more accurate image, it shows more of the lung since the diaphragm is lower, and the thoracic structures appear sharper and less magnified.

Nursing Interventions to Produce an Optimal Chest Radiograph. The critical care nurse can have a big impact on the quality of the radiographic film. Several key elements must be considered:

- The radiograph is taken when the patient has taken a deep breath (inspiration). During exhalation, the lungs are less full of air, which can make the lung tissue appear cloudy as if there is additional lung water. The heart also appears larger during exhalation. This could lead to an erroneous diagnosis of heart failure. Alert patients are encouraged to take in a deep breath and hold it while the exposure is obtained. For patients receiving mechanical ventilatory support, the exposure must be timed to coincide with maximal inhalation.
- It is important to remove extrinsic tubing and other movable objects from the patient's thorax to permit optimal visualization of the chest. Hands or arms should not be across the chest while the radiograph is obtained.
- The patient should sit upright in bed if the clinical condition permits this position. Upright radiograph views have a sharper focus because the distance from the patient to the x-ray tube is closer to the standard 72 inches (6 feet).
- The nurse should ensure that the patient is straight in the bed rather than turned or twisted; this permits clearer visualization of the major thoracic structures.

Indications

There is considerable debate over the optimal frequency of the routine chest radiograph in the critical care unit. The American College of Radiology (ACR) expert panel made these recommendations for portable radiographic machines used in the critical care unit:

1. Daily chest radiographs are recommended for patients with acute cardiopulmonary problems and those receiving mechanical ventilation.
2. Patients who require cardiac monitoring but are otherwise stable need only an admission radiograph.
3. A chest radiograph is obtained when a new thoracic device is placed or there is a specific question about the patient's cardiopulmonary status that the radiograph could address.

TABLE 14-21	INTRATHORACIC STRUCTURE RADIOGRAPHIC DENSITIES	
METAL OR BONE (WHITE)	**FLUID (GRAY)**	**AIR (BLACK)**
Ribs, clavicle, sternum, spine	Blood	Lung
Calcium deposits	Heart	
Surgical wires or clips	Veins	
Prosthetic valves	Arteries	
Pacemaker wires	Edema	

Chest Radiograph Analysis: Lines and Tubes

Evaluation of a chest film is a systematic process. All thoracic invasive tubes and lines must be located and identified. Major thoracic structures, including the lungs, pleural space, mediastinum, diaphragm, and vascular structures, are assessed and compared with previous films, if available. Variations from previous films can alert the clinician to possible complications and provide information about the patient's hemodynamic status.

Central Venous Catheter. CVCs are seen on the chest film as moderately radiopaque tubes extending centrally from an SC, IJ, or femoral vein insertion site. The ideal location of the catheter tip is within the SVC so that it is close, but not inside, the right atrium. CVC misplacement during insertion ranges from 1% to 15% of cases.[143] The expertise of the clinician inserting the catheter and variations in patient anatomy are some of the reasons for the wide range of complications. The risk of pneumothorax is 5.6%.[143] A chest radiograph is required after CVC insertion using the IJ or SC vein.

Pulmonary Artery Catheter. A chest radiograph is required after insertion of a PA catheter, also known as a Swan-Ganz catheter. The primary clinical reason for the chest radiograph is to determine the position of the tip of the PA catheter. To wedge correctly, the noninflated catheter tip must lie within 2 cm of the hilar point of the lung and not extend beyond the proximal interlobar arteries.[143] The most serious potential complication is rupture of the PA. This complication is rare but has a mortality rate of more than 70% when it does occur.[143]

Endotracheal Tube. A chest radiograph is always requested after endotracheal intubation, because physical examination is not sufficiently sensitive to determine endotracheal tube (ETT) malposition. Although clinical physical assessment can recognize a misplaced ETT in 2% to 5% of cases, suboptimal positioning is identified in 20% to 25% of cases by chest radiographs.[143]

Enteric Tube. Malposition of enteral feeding tubes occurs in 1% of cases and occurs more frequently with small-bore feeding tubes.[143] Because the consequences of delivering enteral nutrition into a nonenteric space are so severe for the patient, a chest radiograph is required after placement and before beginning tube feeds.[144]

Chest Tube. Chest tubes contain a radiopaque line that makes them clearly visible on the chest radiograph. Chest tubes are located within the pleural or mediastinal space. Pulmonary chest tubes are placed to treat pneumothorax or hemothorax. Most pneumothoraces in the critical care unit are iatrogenic (e.g., ventilator barotrauma) or traumatic (e.g., complication of CVC placement), or they occur after cardiothoracic surgery.[145] One or two mediastinal drainage tubes are commonly inserted during cardiac surgery. One may be positioned superiorly to drain the anterior mediastinum, and the other is directed inferiorly to drain the left posterolateral pericardial space.

Intra-aortic Balloon Catheter. An intra-aortic balloon pump (IABP) provides mechanical support for the failing heart. The catheter that is evaluated on the chest radiograph is a 26- to 28-mm inflatable balloon that surrounds a catheter inserted into the descending aorta, usually percutaneously through the femoral artery. A chest radiograph must be obtained immediately after insertion to evaluate the position of the IABP catheter.[145] The distal tip of the IABP catheter contains a small radiopaque marker that is helpful in determining its position on the chest film. The tip of the IABP catheter must lie below the origin of the left SC artery in the descending thoracic aorta (just below the aortic arch). Even when inserted properly, there is a risk of aortic dissection.[146] Aortic dissection is a life-threatening complication. It can be seen on the chest radiograph as a loss of sharpness of the borders of the descending thoracic aorta.

Pacemaker or Implantable Defibrillator. A *pacemaker* and ICD are cardiovascular devices that can be visualized on a chest film. There is considerable variety in the range of pacing electrodes that are encountered in critical care patients. If the pacemaker is permanently implanted, the entire system is seen on the chest film. If it is only a temporary pacemaker, the pulse generator is external to the body and is not seen on the chest radiograph. The pacing electrodes are radiopaque and look like white wires extending transvenously into the right side of the heart. Pacing wires sutured on the epicardium during cardiac surgery are visible on the right atrium and/or right ventricle. Patients with a history of heart failure may have an additional pacing wire inserted into the coronary sinus (vein) to pace the left ventricle in addition to a right ventricular wire (biventricular pacing). Table 14-22 summarizes the most common cardiovascular devices and their correct position as seen on the chest radiograph.

Chest Radiograph Analysis: Cardiac and Pulmonary Factors

A wealth of physiologic data can be gleaned from a chest radiograph. To be valid, this information must be interpreted in the context of a thorough physical examination and clinical knowledge of the patient's condition.

Cardiac Heart Size. Comparison of the cardiothoracic (CT) ratio (Fig. 14-80) can be used to assess heart size. The normal heart size is less than one half of the diameter of the chest viewed on the radiograph. Patients with chronic heart failure often have cardiomegaly (enlarged heart), which can dramatically occupy much of the thoracic diameter on the film.

TABLE 14-22 CARDIOVASCULAR DEVICES

DEVICE	FUNCTION	POSITION
Pulmonary artery catheter	Measures pulmonary artery occlusion pressure and right-heart pressures	Tip in right or left pulmonary artery
Central venous catheter	Central venous pressure measurement, venous access	Superior vena cava
Left atrium catheter	Left atrial pressure	Left atrium
Mediastinal chest tubes	Mediastinal fluid evacuation	Anterior mediastinum, posterior pericardium
Pacemaker leads	Cardiac pacing	Over right-heart
Intra-aortic balloon catheter	Assists left ventricular function	Tip just below top of aortic arch

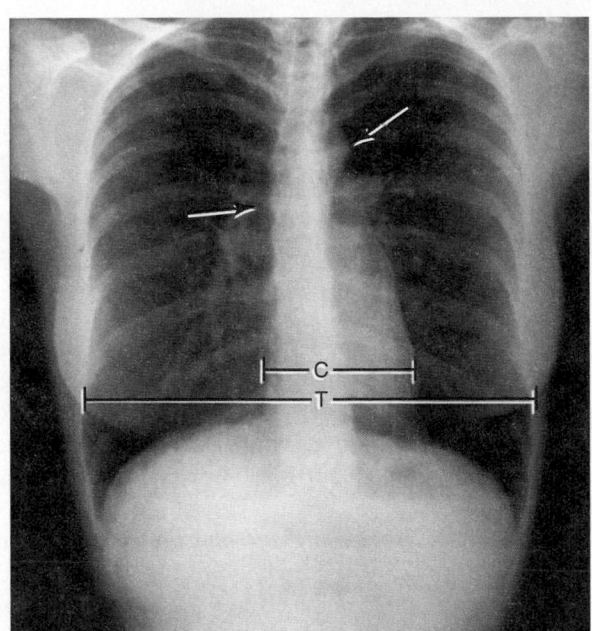

FIGURE 14-80 Determining the cardiothoracic ratio is a technique for estimating heart size on a posteroanterior chest radiograph. Normally, the cardiac diameter is 50% or less of the thoracic diameter when measured during full inhalation. The width of the vascular pedicle *(arrows)* is a more accurate indicator of systemic blood volume. *C,* Maximal cardiac diameter; *T,* maximal thoracic diameter measured to the inside of the ribs.

Pulmonary Edema. Pulmonary edema is a common finding in the critically ill. The "wet lungs" appear on the chest radiograph as white, dense, cloudy areas and may accentuate pulmonary vascular markings. Pulmonary edema shows up very clearly on the chest radiograph, although in the absence of a clinical history the radiograph is not sufficient to determine if the pulmonary edema is from a cardiac or a pulmonary cause.[143] If the pulmonary edema is caused by heart failure, sometimes described as *hydrostatic pulmonary edema*, the fluid may be in a "bat-wing" distribution, with the white areas concentrated in the hilar region (origin of the major pulmonary vessels). However, as the heart failure progresses, the quantity of fluid in the alveolar spaces increases, and the white, fluffy appearance is seen throughout the lung.

If the pulmonary edema is caused by ARDS, also known as *noncardiogenic pulmonary edema*, the distribution of fluid is randomly distributed. It may be described as diffuse bilateral infiltrates.[145]

Pneumonia. Hospital-acquired pneumonia (HAP) is a serious iatrogenic complication that may be detected on a chest radiograph. For the mechanically ventilated patient, the risk is increased because the normal oropharyngeal defenses are bypassed by intubation. This leaves the patient vulnerable for development of *ventilator-associated pneumonia* (VAP), a complication with a reported incidence of between 12% to 29% of cases and a mortality of up to 50%.[143] On the chest radiograph, any appearance of a new or progressive opacity (dense, white area) is a cause for concern and should be clinically investigated. More comprehensive information on pneumonia is provided in Chapter 20.

Pneumothorax. Pneumothorax, or air within the pleural cavity, is diagnosed by chest radiography. Normally, the pleura are not visible because they are adjacent to the chest wall. As the pneumothorax increases in size, the nurse can see the edge of the pleura as the trapped air separates it from the chest wall. The "pneumo" (air) appears black within the pleura. There are no lung markings in the pleural area, and the collapsed lung appears increasingly dense (gray or white). The biggest risk is development of a *tension pneumothorax* that will shift the mediastinal structures. This is also visible on a chest radiograph.

Digital Radiography

Digital radiography systems have been widely implemented in hospitals. In a digital radiograph, the image is divided into discrete elements (pixels) that are assigned a specific value and stored for later display on a computer screen. Pixel sizes vary; the smaller the pixels, the better the resolution. Digital systems have many advantages. No film development is necessary, so the image can be displayed rapidly on a computer screen in the clinical area. The image can be expanded or compressed. This system also lends itself to computer-assisted diagnosis, which involves computer analysis of the image to detect and quantify pathologic findings. If a baseline film has been digitally recorded, the baseline film can be "subtracted" from the current film, highlighting any areas of change, such as increased heart size or new pulmonary infiltrates.

Ambulatory Electrocardiographic Tests

Before coming to the critical care unit, a patient might have had other ECG tests to determine the degree of cardiovascular disease. *Ambulatory electrocardiography* is a technique that records the ECG of patients while they perform their usual activities. It is designed to document abnormal cardiac rhythms that occur at random or that are induced by specific circumstances such as emotional stress or physical activity. Clinical indications include palpitations, dizziness, syncope, and pacemaker evaluation. Two types of recording systems are available: *continuous* and *intermittent*. Many intermittent systems have a short memory loop that permits capture of recent antecedent ECG rhythms that may have precipitated the symptoms of concern.

Continuous Electrocardiographic Recording Systems

Holter monitors are the most widely used continuous recording systems. The patient wears skin electrodes and carries a small box that contains a digital or analog recorder. The monitor is carried by a shoulder strap or clipped to a belt or pocket for 24 hours and then is returned to the hospital or clinic for reading. This is a totally noninvasive procedure with no adverse effects. All Holter monitors record at least two leads to minimize inaccurate interpretation caused by artifact.

Electrocardiographic Monitoring Leads. Usually, five electrodes are placed. Two of them are positive electrodes, corresponding approximately to the V_1 and V_5 positions on a standard 12-lead ECG. Two negative electrodes and one ground also are placed. Occasionally, additional electrodes are used to improve diagnostic capabilities. For example, a separate lead can be used to detect pacemaker spikes if the patient is being monitored for pacemaker dysfunction. The skin electrodes are disposable, pre-gelled, and self-adhering. They should be kept dry—not because of any electrical danger but to prevent their falling off before the recording is completed.

Patient Education. If clear directions are provided to the patient, it will make a big difference to the quality of the final recording. The ambulatory monitor saves all of the ECG tracings for 24 hours. The final recording can display the time that an event occurred. Most also have an event marker, which the patient can press to indicate the onset of symptoms or another event that may be important. The patient is asked to keep a diary of activities, symptoms, and any medications that are taken.

Continuous recording systems are the most thorough form of ambulatory electrocardiography because they record every heartbeat for 24 hours. They do not require the active participation of the patient (although a detailed patient log is helpful) and therefore do not miss asymptomatic ECG changes or dysrhythmias that may be accompanied by a loss of consciousness. When dysrhythmias occur that correlate with symptoms or symptoms occur in the absence of dysrhythmias, one of the primary goals of Holter monitoring has been achieved. Unfortunately, most patients do not have typical symptoms daily. If no significant dysrhythmias or symptoms occur during the 24-hour monitoring period, the test is unhelpful. The only activities that are restricted while wearing a Holter monitor are those that would get the chest electrodes or monitor wet, eliminating swimming and taking a shower or tub bath. Sponge baths are permitted as long as the chest electrodes are avoided.

More recently, newer ECG recording devices have become available that are applied to the skin as a "patch," turned on in the clinic setting and worn continuously. The patient's ECG may be recorded for up to 30 days, after which time the patch device is submitted to the clinic for evaluation of the recorded tracings.

Intermittent Electrocardiographic Recording Systems

A portable monitor that does not record the ECG continuously can also be used to diagnose dysrhythmias. These may also be described as *event monitors*. The patient wears electrodes, but the device is not constantly recording. The patient is instructed to press a button when experiencing symptoms to initiate the recording manually in real time. The big advantage of the intermittent recording system is the ability to leave the recorder in place up to 96 hours, as well as the ability to trigger recording when the symptoms occur.

External Loop Recorders. The external loop recorder records continuously but only keeps the most recent 4 minutes of ECG activity on the memory loop. The memory loop in the device means the patient can press a button and intermittently record a specific event such as heart palpitations during or after the event has occurred. At a later time, the recorder is returned to the hospital or clinic for interpretation of the ECG. The recorder is small and can be clipped to a belt and worn for up to a month.

Implantable Electrocardiographic Recording Systems. For patients whose symptoms are not diagnosed with the traditional methods or who require longer periods of follow-up to diagnose syncope or intermittent dysrhythmias, a small, continuous *implantable loop recorder* may be inserted under the skin of the upper chest. The recorder is about 2 inches by 1 inch by 1 inch. Insertion takes about 20 minutes under local anesthetic. It is especially useful if prior short-term ambulatory ECG recordings have failed to reveal an underlying problem. The inserted loop recorder continuously monitors the ECG rhythm for up to 14 months. After a syncopal episode (loss of consciousness), the patient or a family member places a small, handheld activator on the chest wall over the loop recorder to capture the most recent ECG data. The stored ECG is subsequently analyzed to determine whether the syncopal episode was caused by a dysrhythmia. At this point, after a diagnosis is made, the implantable loop recorder can be safely removed.

Transtelephonic Electrocardiographic Systems. Transtelephonic monitors are intermittent monitoring systems that are not attached to the patient all the time. These monitors consist of a small box, about 4 inches by 2 inches, with four metal electrodes on the bottom. The box is issued to the patient for a specific time, often 1 month, and the patient carries the box at all times. Whenever symptoms are experienced, the patient places the recording box in the center of the chest and places the four metal electrodes in firm contact with the skin.

An alternative method is to use two arm bracelets containing metal electrodes rather than direct chest placement. A button is depressed to activate the recording, which lasts 1 to 2 minutes. The recording is stored until it is convenient for the patient to make a telephone call to send in the recording to a central analysis facility. At that time, the patient's telephone is placed over a transmitter on the box, and the recording is transmitted to the analysis facility, where it is printed out and analyzed as a readable ECG tracing.

Internet Remote Monitoring. The transtelephonic system has been used for many years to remotely follow the function of ICDs or pacemakers. Newer technology options mean that patients who have recent-model ICDs or permanent pacemakers implanted can have their device monitored by an Internet-based, remote monitoring service. The patient dials a prearranged phone number to send the information to a protected site. The information is then downloaded by the dysrhythmia nurse or electrophysiologist to a secure Internet web page in the clinical setting. The clinician can view all the programmable details plus any dysrhythmic events or malfunction of the ICD or the pacemaker. The quantity and quality of information transmitted is superior to that transmitted with older transtelephonic systems. The patient does not need to have a computer available because the information is transmitted using a small portable monitor and any standard telephone line.

Patient Education. A well-informed patient can greatly enhance the quality of the recording. Many patients' symptoms do not occur every day and may be missed during a random 24-hour recording. Often, symptoms tend to occur in association with specific activities. The patient is encouraged to be as active as possible. Keeping an accurate diary of activities is important, because it allows correlation of an identified dysrhythmia with a specific event.

Stress Tests: Exercise with Electrocardiographic Monitoring

Exercise stress testing is a noninvasive test. It consists of an ECG tracing during a period of *physiologic stress* on the heart muscle and its blood supply to uncover and diagnose ischemia, which is not apparent at rest.[147] Physiologic stress is created by asking the patient to walk on a treadmill or to ride a stationary bicycle.

Physiology of Exercise on the Cardiovascular System. Exercise places unique demands on the cardiovascular system. Systemic oxygen consumption increases markedly, requiring the heart to increase CO to meet these demands. Myocardial contractility increases, resulting in greater SV and systolic blood pressure. HR is increased as a result of circulating catecholamines. Normally, as HR and SV rise, CO is increased dramatically, and the tissue needs for oxygen are met. This enhanced myocardial performance is not without a penalty. Even at rest, the heart muscle extracts 70% of the oxygen available in the circulating blood. When the myocardial demand for oxygen increases during exercise, coronary blood flow must increase to maintain an adequate oxygen supply. In people with CAD, coronary blood flow cannot increase sufficiently to meet the high metabolic needs of the myocardium during exercise, and ischemia results.

Stress Test Protocols. Exercise is performed using a treadmill on which the speed and slope can be varied or using a stationary bicycle. A number of protocols have been developed using a treadmill. Two popular ones are the *Bruce protocol*, in which the grade and speed are varied every 3 minutes, and the *Balke protocol*, in which speed remains constant and grade is gradually increased every minute. Regardless of the protocol used, the ECG is monitored continuously. Blood pressure is also measured and recorded every minute.

Heart Rate Criteria in Treadmill Stress Test. The treadmill test is stopped when a target level, based on the patient's maximal stress test HR, is reached. The maximal predicted HR is estimated using the formula:

$$220 - \text{Patient's age}$$

Increasing the HR to 85% to 90% of the predicted maximum is preferred, and in most patients, this level of exercise is sufficient to unmask any significant CAD. The diagnostic value of the test is based on the maximal HR achieved, *not* on the length of time that the patient remains on the treadmill. A well-trained athlete may be able to stay on the treadmill for 15 minutes, whereas an older or sedentary person may tolerate it for only 3 to 5 minutes; however, if 85% of the predicted maximal HR is achieved, both tests are equally diagnostic. A person who is taking beta-blockers may not be able to reach his or her age-adjusted targeted HR because of the bradycardic effect of this class of medications.

The exercise test workload is described as a metabolic equivalent (MET) of oxygen consumption. The definition of 1 MET is 3.5 mL of oxygen per kilogram per minute at rest for a 70 kg, 40-year-old man. The stress test result may be described as "poor exercise tolerance" (less than 5 MET), or "good exercise tolerance" (10 to 11 MET). To put these numbers into a clinical perspective, patients with heart disease who achieved less than 5 MET during an exercise test were four times more likely to die, compared with patients who achieved 10 MET or more.[91]

Clinical Reasons to Stop the Treadmill Test. The test may be aborted before maximal HR is reached if symptoms occur. Reasons to halt the test include the development of moderate to severe angina (chest pain), signs of pallor or poor perfusion, and the patient asking to stop the test. Other signs that can alert the nurse to stop the test include ST segment elevation equal to or greater than 1.0 mm (one small box); ST depression equal to or greater than 2.0 mm (2 small boxes); cardiac dysrhythmias or a marked shift in ventricular axis; and increased symptoms, such as breathlessness or fatigue and a fall in blood pressure of 10 mm Hg or more from baseline.[148] Blood pressure is expected to rise during exercise, but a systolic blood pressure greater than 250 mm Hg or a diastolic blood pressure greater than 115 mm Hg is considered high enough to stop the test.[148]

Treadmill Tests after Myocardial Infarction. A low-level stress test is sometimes performed before discharge from the hospital on patients who have had an acute MI. In this case, the HR is raised to only 120 or 130 beats per minute. ST segment depression or elevation that occurs during the predischarge low-level stress test is a reliable indicator of additional myocardium at risk. However, exercise-induced angina or abnormal blood pressure responses to exercise often do not appear during a low-level stress test, so a "normal" predischarge stress test must be followed later by a test closer to maximal level.

Nursing Management. During the exercise test, the patient is encouraged to continue as long as possible. However, the test is stopped if the patient requests because of symptoms such as fatigue, shortness of breath, leg cramps, significant ECG changes, blood pressure changes, or development of angina. After the exercise test is completed, the patient is assisted into a supine position. The ECG, the pulse rate, and blood pressure are monitored for at least 10 more minutes to detect dysrhythmias or signs of ischemia. The patient is instructed to rest for the next 30 to 60 minutes after release from the exercise laboratory. Hot showers should be avoided for 3 to 4 hours to prevent development of orthostatic hypotension. It is essential that nurses who monitor patients during this test are experienced and knowledgeable about all aspects of stress testing and emergency protocols. Emergency medications and a defibrillator must be available in the test area.

Patient Education. Many patients are anxious about undergoing exercise testing, and the anxiety is often multifactorial. Patients without known heart disease may be afraid that they will "fail" the test, find they have heart disease, and perhaps need open heart surgery. If the patient generally follows a sedentary lifestyle, anxiety may be caused by the fear of "collapsing" on the treadmill or spending several days recovering from exhaustion. Some are afraid that they will be forced to go beyond their endurance. Often, low-level exercise testing is performed before discharge on patients who have been hospitalized for an acute MI. These patients may be afraid that the strain on their heart is too great or that they will die during the test. Effective patient education can do much to allay these fears. In addition to describing the procedure itself, the nurse instructs the patient to fast for 3 hours before the test, refrain from smoking for at least 2 hours before the test, and wear comfortable shoes and loose-fitting clothes. Reassurance that the heart will be monitored closely during the test is also important.

Signal-Averaged Electrocardiogram

The *signal-averaged electrocardiogram* (SAECG) is used to identify late potentials within the QRS complex. These low-amplitude waveforms cannot be detected on a standard surface ECG but can be recorded as an SAECG. Late potentials indicate slow conduction within the ventricular myocardium that can be a substrate for ventricular dysrhythmias and put the individual at risk for sudden cardiac death.[149]

SAECG is a noninvasive test. The patient lies in a supine position and is asked to keep muscle movement to a minimum. Cardiac electrode leads are applied to the anterior and posterior chest walls, and the leads are connected to a signal-averaged ECG computer. This computer produces a high-resolution, high-magnification ECG signal. This "noise-free" ECG is then analyzed for QRS duration and for the presence, duration, and measurement of late myopotentials. After computer analysis, the SAECG is described as negative (normal) or positive (abnormal). A positive SAECG in combination with other specific indicators is a predictor of increased risk for sudden cardiac death.

Many patients with a positive SAECG (abnormal) produce a normal SAECG when placed on antidysrhythmic medications. The SAECG is not analyzed in isolation. It is used in conjunction with other cardiac diagnostic tests, including the EPS. It is a helpful adjunct to the EPS but does not replace it.

Echocardiography

Echocardiography uses *waves of ultrasound* to obtain and display images of cardiac structures. Normal human hearing occurs at a sound frequency of 20 to 20,000 cycles per second (Hz). Ultrasound uses sound frequencies greater than 20,000 Hz. When used to image cardiac structures, the best results are achieved using 1.5 to 10 MHz. Usually, 2.25 MHz is used with adults to allow optimal depth penetration, whereas 3 to 5 MHz is used in pediatric patients to provide a clearer image of the smaller structures.

Ultrasound is reflected best at interfaces between tissues that have different densities. In the heart these are the blood, cardiac valves, myocardium, and pericardium. Because all these structures differ in density, their borders can be seen on the echocardiogram.

Echocardiography is used to detect structural heart abnormalities such as mitral valve stenosis and regurgitation, prolapse of mitral valve leaflets, aortic stenosis and insufficiency, hypertrophic cardiomyopathy, atrial septal defect, thoracic aortic dissection, cardiac tamponade, and pericardial effusion. Echocardiography is quickly becoming a first-line hemodynamic assessment tool in the critical care unit.

Transthoracic Echocardiography

When transthoracic echocardiography (TTE) is performed, the patient is in a supine, a left lateral, or a semirecumbent position. The position used depends on the patient's clinical condition and on which structures are to be examined. A transducer is placed on the skin, with lubricant between the transducer and the skin to improve contact and reduce artifact. The active element in the transducer is a piezoelectric crystal. *Piezoelectric* refers to the ability to transform electrical energy into mechanical energy (in this case, sound energy). The transducer emits ultrasound waves and receives a signal from the reflected sound waves. Periods of sound transmission alternate with periods of sound reception.

Ultrasonic waves do not travel through air very well, and they cannot penetrate very dense structures, such as bone. In adults, the transducer is usually placed in the third or fourth intercostal space to the left of the sternum, because at that point the pericardium is in direct contact with the chest wall and the ultrasonic waves are not obstructed by air or bone. Other positions are sometimes used if the standard location does not provide adequate visualization of the cardiac structures. In the critical care unit, the echocardiograph machine is usually brought to the bedside. The lighting in the room can be dimmed to improve the visual clarity of the images displayed on the screen.

The nursing care consists of monitoring the patient during the procedure, which is usually performed by an echocardiography technician. TTE is completely noninvasive; the nurse explains this and the purpose of the test to the patient and family. The procedure is not uncomfortable, but it may be tiresome for certain patients because of the length of the procedure, which is usually 30 to 60 minutes.

Motion-Mode Echocardiography

In motion-mode (M-mode) TTE, a thin beam of ultrasound is directed through the heart (Fig. 14-81A). Each interface is represented by a dot, and when recorded over time (like an ECG tracing), each dot becomes a line on an oscilloscope. A strip-chart recording can be made of this tracing as the heart beats. Heart motion is recorded over time, and a typical M-mode echo is shown in Figure 14-81B. M-mode echocardiograms are particularly useful in detecting small pericardial effusions and cardiac tamponade.

Two-Dimensional and Three-Dimensional Echocardiograms

The two-dimensional (2-D) echocardiogram uses crystals in the transducer to create a cross-sectional imaging plane. Sections of the heart are then viewed from a number of different angles (Fig. 14-82). The picture is displayed on an oscilloscope, and digital photographs are taken to serve as a permanent record. The 2-D echocardiogram images a whole "slice" of the heart at once and is used for direct measurement of LV volumes and wall mass. The 2-D slice also permits visualization of the cardiac structures in relation to each other and readily identifies valvular dysfunction and wall-motion abnormalities after MI.

A more recent innovation is the three-dimensional (3-D) echocardiogram. It produces a more realistic image of structures such as the mitral valve.[150]

Phonocardiogram

Phonocardiography is combined with echocardiography to evaluate valvular dysfunction. *Phono* (sound), *cardio* (heart), and *gram* (recording) provide a graphic display of the sounds that occur in the heart and great vessels. The transducer is

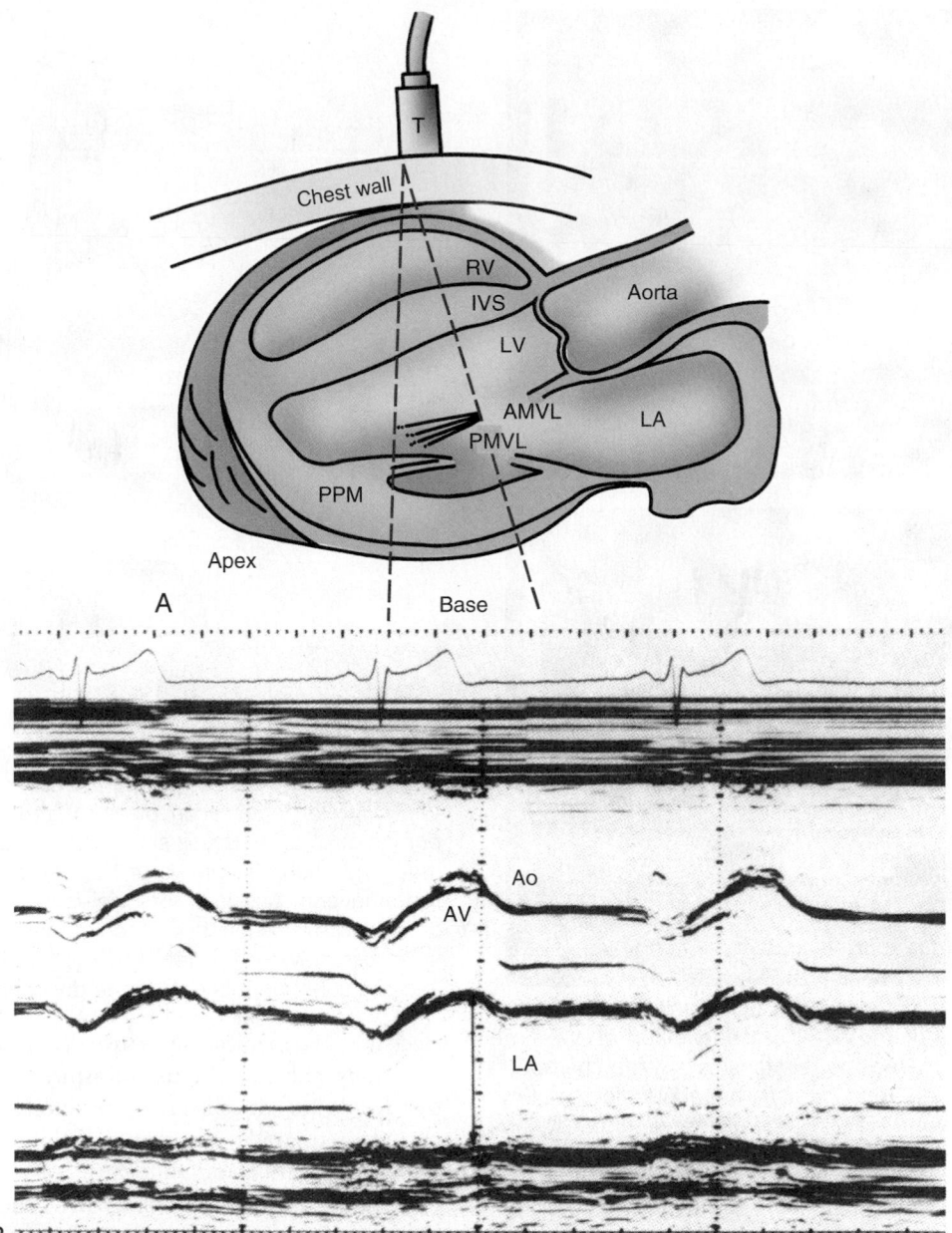

FIGURE 14-81 *A,* Schematic representation of cardiac structures traversed by two echobeams. *B,* Normal, M-mode echocardiogram at the level of the aorta, aortic valve leaflets, and left atrium. *AMVL,* Anterior mitral valve leaflet; *Ao,* aorta; *AV,* aortic valve; *IVS,* interventricular septum; *LA,* left atrium; *LV,* left ventricle; *PMVL,* posterior mitral valve leaflet; *PPM,* posterior papillary muscle; *RV,* right ventricle; *T,* transducer. (B from Kinney M, et al. *Andreoli's Comprehensive Cardiac Care.* 8th ed. St. Louis: Mosby; 1995.)

placed on the chest wall to record heart sounds that correspond to auscultation with a traditional stethoscope. Chapter 13 provides more information on heart sounds.

Color-Flow Doppler Echocardiography

Doppler echocardiography provides a special kind of echocardiogram that assesses blood flow. It uses a pulsed or continuous wave of ultrasound that records frequency shifts of reflected sound waves, showing velocity and direction of blood flow relative to the transducer. Doppler signals are usually displayed in color. Known as *color-flow mapping* or *imaging,* this technique analyzes Doppler signals from multiple intracardiac sites

simultaneously. The Doppler tracing for each site is displayed in a color-coded format superimposed on a real-time 2-D echocardiographic image. Flow toward the transducer is displayed in one color, whereas flow away from the transducer is displayed in a contrasting color. The brightness of the color varies to signify different flow velocities.

Doppler echocardiography is especially useful in individuals with valvular heart disease. The blood flow associated with regurgitation and stenosis can be detected, and estimates can be made of the severity of the disease. Doppler can accurately estimate right ventricular systolic pressure. When several valves are involved, the Doppler technique can clarify the extent of

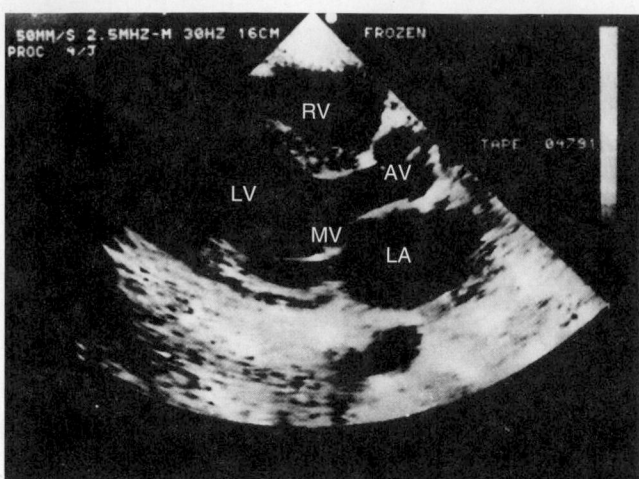

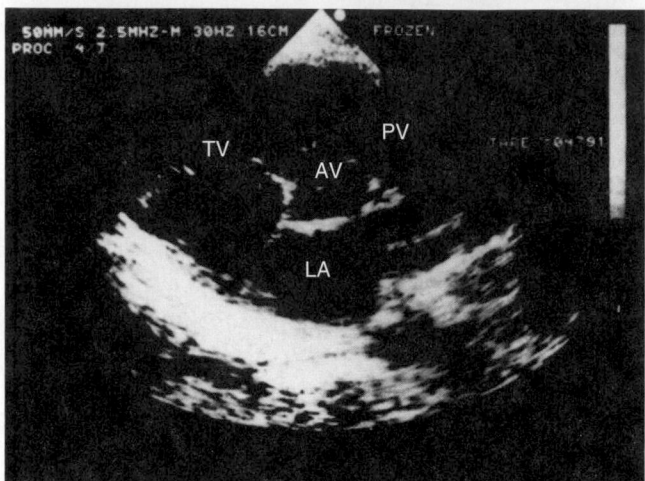

FIGURE 14-82 Two-Dimensional Echocardiogram. Notice that several sections of the heart can be viewed at one time and that it is easier to see the relationships of the chambers. *LA,* Left atrium; *LV,* left ventricle; *MV,* mitral valve; *PV,* pulmonary vein; *RV,* right ventricle; *TV,* tricuspid valve. (From Kinney M, et al. *Andreoli's Comprehensive Cardiac Care.* 8th ed. St. Louis: Mosby; 1995.)

damage to the individual valves. Other uses for Doppler echocardiography include evaluation of congenital shunts, measurement of volume flow and CO, and assessment of new structural abnormalities after acute MI. By measuring flow velocity in the right ventricular outflow tract, mean PAP can be estimated.

Transesophageal Echocardiography

Transesophageal echocardiography (TEE) is a technique in which the transducer (single-plane, biplane, or multiplane device) is mounted on a flexible shaft similar to an endoscope and advanced into the esophagus, from where cardiac structures can be clearly visualized. The multiplane transducer has a single array of crystals that can be rotated in a 180-degree arc, requiring less manipulation of the probe within the esophagus. Because of the close anatomic relationship between the heart and the esophagus, TEE produces high-quality images of intracardiac structures and the thoracic aorta without the interference of the chest wall, bone, or air-filled lung.

The insertion procedure is similar to an upper gastrointestinal endoscopy. The patient is asked to fast for a minimum of 6 hours before the TEE to prevent nausea and vomiting. For an

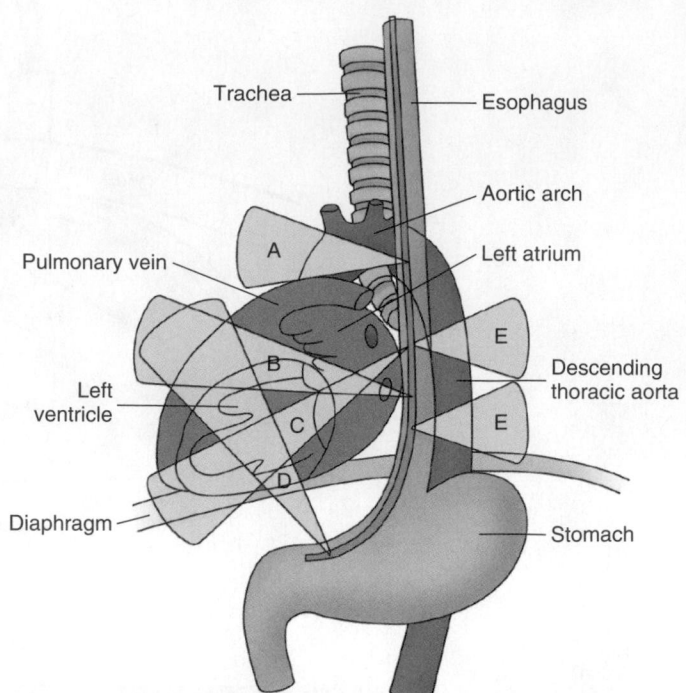

FIGURE 14-83 Diagram of common scan planes during a transesophageal echocardiogram (TEE) with a two-dimensional view. *A,* Horizontal scan plane of the aortic arch and distal portion of aorta. *B,* Basal, short-axis (transverse), long-axis (sagittal), and short-axis views of both atria. *C,* Four-chamber and left atrioventricular long-axis views. A sagittal scan plane can image a cross section of the left ventricle. *D,* Transgastric, short-axis view of the left and right ventricles. *E,* Transverse and sagittal scan sections of the descending aorta.

elective TEE, medication is usually given to inhibit salivary secretions, reducing the risk of aspiration. Analgesic and sedative agents are administered to reduce fear and anxiety and to provide retrograde amnesia. Routine antibiotic prophylaxis against bacteremia and endocarditis is not necessary, although it is considered for high-risk patients such as those with prosthetic valves, previous endocarditis, or very poor dentition. The pharyngeal region is anesthetized with 2% viscous lidocaine and 10% lidocaine spray to lessen the gag reflex and prevent retching and laryngospasm. The patient is usually placed in the left lateral decubitus position, although the supine position can be used in the critical care setting if necessary. A soft bite block is inserted between the teeth to prevent damage to the echoscope. As the echoscope is inserted, the patient is asked to swallow. The echoscope is advanced to 25 cm from the mouth, and imaging is begun (Fig. 14-83). TEE is also used intraoperatively during cardiac surgery for monitoring valve repair and replacement. The images obtained by TEE are superior to transthoracic views in a variety of ways. The entire thoracic aorta can be visualized clearly. Both atrial chambers are clearly seen with TEE, and the left atrial appendage is particularly well visualized, making TEE the procedure of choice for detection of left atrial thrombus. Diagnosis and quantification of atrial septal defects is possible with this method, and the addition of Doppler capabilities allows assessment of atrial shunting. TEE is useful in evaluating patients with valvular disorders, including infective endocarditis to visualize vegetations on the valve leaflets.

Manipulation of the TEE probe within the esophagus can cause a vasovagal response, producing bradycardia and hypotension. The most serious risk of the procedure is esophageal bleeding. Individuals with liver cirrhosis or esophageal varices and patients on a heparin drip are also at risk for esophageal bleeding. During TEE the patient's vital signs are closely monitored with ECG, blood pressure, and clinical observation. If esophageal entry is difficult, it cannot be forced. Emergency resuscitation equipment must be present in case of a severe vasovagal episode (e.g., bradycardia, hypotension). Suction equipment must be at the bedside in the event that the patient vomits or has difficulty handling oral secretions.

Stress Echocardiography

Stress echocardiography is often used in the outpatient setting to identify stable angina. It provides a very accurate picture of the ischemic impact of CAD on the myocardium.[151] Stress echocardiography can diagnose regional (ischemia) and global (cardiomyopathy) abnormalities.[151] It may also be used after MI to evaluate the impact of necrosis on viable wall tissue. Physiologic stress from increased exercise creates an imbalance between myocardial oxygen supply and demand. This causes ischemia and eventually results in wall-motion abnormalities, which are detectable with an echocardiogram. Stress can be applied to the heart by physical and pharmacologic means.[151] One of two methods of physical exertion usually is employed: the patient can exercise on a treadmill or a stationary bicycle. The protocols used for physical echocardiographic stress testing are very similar to those used in the ECG stress test setting previously described (Table 14-23).

Dobutamine Stress Test. When patients are unable to exercise to exercise to raise their heart rates sufficiently to evaluate myocardial response, pharmacologic agents may be used. Dobutamine, a β-1 agonist is most frequently used and will discussed here. It should be noted, however, that alternate agents may be selected to provoke accelerated heart rates for the study, including the vasodilators adenosine and dipyridamole as well as regadenoson (an Adenosine A2A receptor agonist). Choice of agent is based on the patient's concomitant disease states and clinical status.

Pharmacologic stress is most frequently incited with a dobutamine infusion beginning at 5 mcg/kg/min and increasing as needed to 40 or 50 mcg/kg/min to achieve 85% of maximal HR.[151] Dobutamine causes myocardial ischemia through a dramatic increase in myocardial oxygen demand by an increase in HR, contractility, and systemic blood pressure. Potential side effects include hypotension, hypertension, dysrhythmias, nausea, headache, anxiety, and tremor. Atropine is

TABLE 14-23 STRESS TESTING METHODS

TEST PARAMETERS	STRESS ELECTROCARDIOGRAPHY	STRESS ECHOCARDIOGRAPHY	STRESS RADIONUCLIDE IMAGING
Exercise stress test	3-, 5-, or 12-lead ECG leads are attached to the chest and limbs to monitor the ECG *during* the exercise protocol.	The patient exercises according to protocol. Echocardiogram is recorded immediately *after* exercise.	The radiopharmaceutical (thallium 201 or technetium 99m) is injected before exercise. The patient exercises according to the protocol. The heart is scanned *after* exercise to view uptake of the radiotracer.
Pharmacologic stress test	Patient is at rest. IV medications stimulate heart rate (HR) and contractility: Dosage starts with dobutamine at 5 mcg/kg/min and is increased as needed to increase the HR. ECG pattern is monitored during the medication infusions. Other medications include adenosine, regadenoson, and dipyridamole.	Patient is at rest. IV medications stimulate HR and contractility: Dosage starts with dobutamine at 5 mcg/kg/min and is increased as needed to increase the HR. Echocardiogram is recorded during and after the medication infusions. Other medications include adenosine, regadenoson, and dipyridamole.	Patient is at rest. IV medications simulate exercise: Dosage starts with dobutamine 5 mcg/kg/min and is increased as needed to increase the HR. Radionuclide image is scanned during and after pharmacologic stress. Other medications include adenosine, regadenoson, and dipyridamole.
Clinical indications	Used to rule out CAD. Not as helpful if patient has a distorted ECG pattern at baseline due to LBBB, RBBB or internal ventricular pacemaker because ST segment changes are obscured.	Useful for patients with LBBB, RBBB, and implanted pacemaker, because the wall motion is visualized directly.	Helpful for patients with LBBB, RBBB, and implanted pacemaker It is useful before CABG to determine if bypass graft will supply blood to an ischemic area. There is no benefit in grafting an artery to an infarcted area.
Clinical outcome of a positive test result	Chest pain develops. ST segment ECG pattern changes.	Chest pain develops. Wall-motion abnormalities are visualized.	Areas of the heart that do not take up radiotracer are called *cold spots*. A cold spot is ischemic or infarcted tissue. A follow-up scan later the same day (or the next day with some radiotracers) shows whether the cold spot has filled in; if yes, the area is ischemic; if it remains cold, the area is infarcted.

CABG, Coronary artery bypass graft; *CAD*, coronary artery disease; *ECG*, electrocardiographic; *IV*, intravenous; *LBBB*, left bundle branch block; *RBBB*, right bundle branch block.

also administered if the dobutamine infusion alone does not cause an adequate increase in HR. Because of the potential risks of dobutamine stress echocardiography, it is recommended that qualified physicians be engaged in at least 100 studies a year to maintain competence.

Intravascular Ultrasound

Intravascular ultrasound (IVUS) is used as an adjunct diagnostic technique during coronary angiography or during a coronary PCI. A miniature, flexible ultrasound catheter that incorporates a high-frequency transducer (20 to 40 MHz) provides high-resolution images of the coronary arterial wall. This technology is not an alternative to angiography but is used as a complementary diagnostic technique. IVUS permits an anatomic view of the interior of the coronary artery. The cardiologist can visualize the exact location of atherosclerotic plaque or see if a coronary stent has deployed (expanded) correctly against the vessel wall.

Intracardiac Ultrasound

The use of intracardiac ultrasound is increasing. Flexible ultrasound catheters can be directed into the atria and ventricles. Diagnostic uses include direct visualization of intracardiac structures, replacement for TEE during interventional or selected surgical procedures, and views of the atrial or ventricular septum during a repair procedure.

Hand-Carried Ultrasound Devices

Portable ultrasound, or point-of-care ultrasound, is used in many critical care units and emergency departments. Portable ultrasound is designed to increase the accuracy of the bedside physical examination.

Magnetic Resonance Imaging

Magnetic resonance imaging (MRI) is a noninvasive imaging technique that can obtain specific biochemical information from body tissue without the use of ionizing radiation. The procedure does not present any known hazard to living cells. In many respects, the image created is superior to radiography and ultrasonography, because bone does not interfere with MRI.

Indications

Cardiac MRI can provide information about tissue integrity, cardiac wall-motion abnormalities, aneurysms, EF, CO, patency of proximal coronary arteries, and flow rates through coronary artery bypass grafts. MRI is useful in diagnosing complications of MI, such as pericarditis or pericardial effusion, valvular dysfunction, ventricular septal rupture, aneurysm, and intracardiac thrombus.[152]

Blood that is actively flowing does not emit a magnetic resonance signal; it provides a natural dark contrast material in the lumen of proximal coronary arteries. As a result, abnormalities of lumen size such as narrowing—which may provide evidence of obstruction—can be visualized.

How Magnetic Resonance Imaging Works

The physics behind MRI scanning is complex, but the basic concept is simple. Certain atoms within molecules act as tiny bar magnets with north and south poles. The nuclei spin around this axis like a spinning top. Under normal conditions, these small atomic magnets are arranged at random. If a patient is placed within a strong magnetic field, many of the nuclei line up in the same direction as the magnetic force. When a radio-frequency wave is sent, some of the nuclei absorb this energy, causing them to fall out of alignment and wobble like a gyroscope that is winding down. This wobbling out of alignment is called *resonance.* The process of returning to alignment with the magnetic field after the radiofrequency signal is turned off is called *relaxation.* These energy changes can be detected and recorded by the scanner.

Each type of atom has its own unique resonance and relaxation pattern. The easiest one to record is the hydrogen ion, although other atoms such as phosphorus, sodium, and carbon are being studied. Because there are two hydrogen ions per molecule of water, MRI is especially sensitive to changes in tissue water content. Myocardial ischemic injury results in predictable increases in regional myocardial water content, allowing differentiation between normal and ischemic tissue. Infarction leading to myocardial scarring results in tissue with a decreased water content, which can be identified on a magnetic resonance scan as an area of decreased signal intensity.

MRI works well for structures that have little or no motion, such as the brain. Cardiac applications have been limited because of the constant motion of the heart. In an attempt to overcome this limitation, various gating or slicing techniques have been used to time the images at exact phases of the cardiac cycle. The gating can be timed from the R wave of the ECG or from the arterial pulse tracing. Either method is satisfactory as long as the patient is in normal sinus rhythm. With any irregularity of the rhythm, the gating technique becomes much less helpful.

Metal Objects

MRI is a safe procedure. The main hazard is related to the presence of metal substances in the environment. Because the magnetism used is approximately 40,000 times stronger than the magnetic field of the earth, metal objects such as intravenous line poles, infusion pumps, or oxygen tanks can become projectiles if they come close enough to the magnet's pull. No metal objects are permitted in the area of the MRI scanner. The patient must be asked about the presence of any metallic implants (pacemaker) or other metal (residual bullet or shrapnel) that may be moved by the magnetic force during the scan. Aneurysm clips are composed of ferromagnetic materials and can experience significant torque when exposed to the magnetic field. Another consideration is that exposure to the strong magnetic field may cause a cardiac pacemaker or ICD to turn off or switch modes.

Challenges with Magnetic Resonance Imaging

MRI has significant limitations that affect patients in the critical care setting. One of the challenges is that patients must leave the unit and be transported to the nuclear medicine laboratory for MRI. Standard ventilators, monitoring equipment, and infusion pumps cannot be used because these machines contain metal parts. Special ventilators with nonmagnetic accessories are available, as well as nonmetal ECG, pulse oximetry sensors, and infusion pumps.

The narrow size of the magnet bore (tube or tunnel) requires the patient to lie flat and motionless for long periods. The close quarters inside the magnet bore tend to provoke claustrophobia in anyone already predisposed to it, and sedation may be required. The patient who is claustrophobic needs considerable reassurance and education before lying supine and motionless inside the MRI tube. A recent innovation is the use of open MRI scanners. The MRI tube is open at both ends so that the patient's head is not enclosed while the body is scanned.

Cardiac Radionuclide Imaging Studies

Several types of radionuclide imaging tests are available. As with diagnostic ECG and echocardiography, many of the radionuclide tests can be performed at rest and during exercise.[153]

Purpose of Radionuclide Scans

The purpose of a radionuclide scan is to determine whether there is a perfusion defect in cardiac muscle. A scan is indicated for the person with chest pain and known or suspected CAD. The radionuclide scan is especially helpful for the person who has a coexisting LBBB or a permanent pacemaker where the QRS shape is distorted. Both situations make interpretation of acute angina challenging to interpret accurately on the 12-lead ECG. This has opened a window of opportunity for radionuclide imaging, in which the myocardial ability to receive blood flow is visualized directly.[154]

A radionuclide scan adds to the information that has been gained from a cardiac catheterization study and a 12-lead ECG. Coronary artery anatomy and patency is important because regional myocardial blood supply is always from a specific coronary artery and any blockage of an artery can lead to a discrete myocardial perfusion defect, meaning that the blood supply to this area is decreased (ischemic) or absent (infarcted). Although coronary arteriography defines the anatomy of the coronary arteries, it does not show whether the arteries perfuse the cardiac muscle.

Radionuclide Isotopes

The radioisotopes used in cardiac diagnostic imaging are very different from those used in oncology for tumor ablation. Diagnostic isotopes have a short half-life (minutes to hours) and are used in very small amounts to minimize radioactivity risk. Patients do not need to be isolated, and no specific precautions are required for blood, urine, stool, or other body fluids.

Thallium 201. Thallium 201 (^{201}Tl) is a low-energy radioactive isotope. It is an analogue of potassium and acts like potassium when injected into the bloodstream. Because thallium is similar to potassium, it is absorbed from the bloodstream by cardiac muscle cells as part of the sodium–potassium adenosine triphosphatase (ATPase) pump. Thallium uptake depends on two factors: the patency of the coronary arteries and the amount of healthy myocardium with a functional sodium–potassium ATPase pump. Areas of infarcted myocardium (dead tissue) do not take up thallium. After thallium has been injected, a specialized scintillation camera and associated computer system are used to scan the myocardium.

Technetium 99m. Technetium 99m (^{99m}Tc) is also used frequently. It is often attached to other trace substances for diagnostic imaging (^{99m}Tc-sestamibi or ^{99m}Tc-tetrofosmin).[154] These substances are often described as *radiopharmaceuticals*.[154] ^{99m}Tc tracers are highly suited to imaging myocardium during ACS because the tracers do not redistribute over time (they remain in myocardium), allowing a second scan to be performed many hours later if needed.[154] In clinical practice, this is seldom practical, and use of radiopharmaceuticals in emergency situations is rare outside of research studies.[154] These tests are used when the patient's hemodynamic and cardiac condition is stable.

Stress Test Radionuclide Scan

This test takes place in a specialized nuclear medicine department. The walls of the testing space are normally lined with lead to prevent any radioactivity dispersal to other areas. A patent intravenous line is required. A radioisotope flow agent (^{201}Tl or ^{99m}Tc) is injected into the bloodstream before exercise to permit identification of perfused versus nonperfused (cold) areas. After the physical activity, a specialized perfusion-scanning camera is used to scan the heart. As with the other cardiac stress tests, the options to increase the HR and myocardial blood flow are physical exercise by the patient or infusion of a medication to achieve the same effect (see Table 14-23).

Exercise Radionuclide Scan Procedure. Before the *exercise radionuclide scan*, the procedure is fully explained to the patient, including a description of the equipment (ECG monitoring equipment, cardiovascular exercise treadmill or stationary bicycle, and an Anger gamma scintillation camera). The patient is usually fasting, because the scan involves vigorous exercise. Vasodilating medications that may alter the uptake of the radioisotope (nitrates, theophylline, and related medications) are held (not taken by the patient) before any baseline study. Other medications that will not affect the outcome of the study can be taken as usual. A patent intravenous line is inserted before the test. In the laboratory, the patient is asked to exercise vigorously for 1 minute or more or until angina or fatigue develops. At this point, the isotope is injected into the bloodstream. After the injection, the patient is asked to exercise vigorously for another minute to stress the heart and circulate the radioisotope. As soon as possible after exercise (within 10 minutes), the patient is asked to lie on the examination table for the first perfusion scan by the scintillation camera. The camera examines the heart from three angles—anterior, left anterior oblique, and left lateral oblique—to increase accuracy. On the camera screen, the heart image looks like a circle with a hole (doughnut shape). The myocardium appears, but the fluid-filled center does not.

Pharmacologic Radionuclide Scan Procedure. A patient who cannot tolerate a radionuclide-exercise stress test can undergo a pharmacologic radionuclide test at rest. The test can be performed with ^{201}Tl or ^{99m}Tc. In the absence of physical exercise, a dobutamine infusion is used to increase coronary artery and myocardial blood flow.[154] Maximal contractility is achieved with dobutamine at about 10 mcg/kg/min for normal hearts. The goal is to drive the HR to the 85% maximal HR predicted for that individual; if needed, atropine is added to achieve the desired HR. After the first scan, the patient is removed from the scanner and the HR is allowed to return to baseline. After about 5 to 10 minutes, the patient is asked to return to the scanner to ensure the LV wall motion has also returned to baseline.

Radionuclide Test Results. If no perfusion defect is seen, the test is complete for that patient. If a perfusion defect (dark area) is observed in the myocardium, the patient is asked to return for a repeat scan 2 to 4 hours later or the next day, depending on the radioisotope tracer that was used. If a perfusion defect is present 4 hours later, the area is infarcted. This is sometimes described as a *cold spot* or as a *fixed lesion*. If the perfusion defect has taken up the radioisotope since the first test (redistribution), the area is ischemic. An ischemic defect is amenable to reperfusion therapy such as CABG or a catheter-based procedure to open a coronary artery.

Computed Tomography Angiography

Computed tomography (CT) is employed to calculate the Coronary Artery Calcium Score (CACS).[139,155,156] The quantity of calcium in atherosclerotic plaque is measured using electron beam or multidetector CT, then the calcium score is calculated. A score below 100 is considered low risk, while a score above 300 indicates high risk of a future coronary event.[157] Clinically, the CACS is considered along with other risk factor information to evaluate individual risk from atherosclerotic coronary disease.[156]

▌SUMMARY

Hemodynamic Monitoring

- Hemodynamic monitoring is one of the major reasons patients are admitted to the critical care unit.
- Hemodynamic monitoring of CO is in transition from invasive (PA Catheter) to minimally invasive systems (LiDCO, PiCCO, FloTrac) or noninvasive (echocardiography/Doppler) methods.
- Continuous monitoring of venous oxygen saturation (Svo_2 and $Scvo_2$) is indicated for the critically ill patient who has the potential to develop an imbalance between oxygen supply and metabolic tissue demand.

ECG Monitoring

- Accurate ECG lead placement and interpretation of ECG rhythms in the context of a clinical diagnosis yields relevant information that contributes to optimal patient outcomes. This includes recognition of ischemia and infarction on a 12-lead ECG and knowledge of atrial dysrhythmias, ventricular dysrhythmias, and heart blocks.

Cardiac Laboratory Assessment

- Laboratory studies required in cardiac care include electrolyte levels (potassium, sodium, calcium), cardiac biomarkers (Troponin and CK-MB), hematologic status (Hgb, Hct, WBC, platelets), coagulation times (INR, aPTT), serum lipid levels (LDL-C, HDL-C, triglycerides), and laboratory values associated with the status of other organ systems that can secondarily affect cardiac function.

Cardiac Diagnostic Studies

- Specialized diagnostic studies include cardiac catheterization to assess the ventricular chambers and pressures, angiography to assess the coronary arteries, and electrophysiology study to assess the heart's electrical system.
- Interpretation of the chest radiograph is used to noninvasively locate catheters, tubes, and implantable devices and to detect complications such as pulmonary edema, pneumonia, and pneumothorax.
- Echocardiography is frequently used in the critical care unit for rapid assessment of change in cardiac function; use has increased as this technology has become smaller and more portable.
- Ambulatory ECG tests include Holter monitoring, treadmill stress tests, signal-averaged ECG, MRI, and CT.

REFERENCES

1. Mitchell MD, et al. Heparin flushing and other interventions to maintain patency of central venous catheters: a systematic review. *J Adv Nurs.* 2009;65(10):2007.
2. Brzezinski M, Luisetti T, London MJ. Radial artery cannulation: a comprehensive review of recent anatomic and physiologic investigations. *Anesthesia Analg.* 2009;109(6):1763.
3. Warkentin TE, et al. Treatment and prevention of heparin-induced thrombocytopenia: American College of Chest Physicians Evidence-Based Clinical Practice Guidelines. 8th ed. *Chest.* 2008;133(6 Suppl):340S.
4. O'Grady NP, et al. Guidelines for the prevention of intravascular catheter-related infections. *Am J Infection Control.* 2011;39(4 Suppl 1):S1.
5. *American Association of Critical-Care Nurses.* AACN practice alert: pulmonary artery pressure monitoring. http://www.aacn. org/wd/practice/docs/pap-measurement.pdf. 2009. Accessed August 2012.
6. Rauen CA, Makic MB, Bridges E. Evidence-based practice habits: transforming research into bedside practice. *Crit Care Nurse.* 2009;29(2):46; quiz 60-61.
7. Kohonen M, et al. Is the Allen test reliable enough? *Eur J Cardiothorac Surg.* 2007;32(6):902.
8. Shapiro DS, Loiacono LA. Mean arterial pressure: therapeutic goals and pharmacologic support. *Crit Care Clin.* 2010;26(2):285, table of contents.
9. Lucet JC, et al. Infectious risk associated with arterial catheters compared with central venous catheters. *Crit Care Med.* 2010;38(4):1030.
10. Chatterjee A, et al. Results of a survey of blood pressure monitoring by intensivists in critically ill patients: a preliminary study. *Crit Care Med.* 2010;38(12):2335.

11. Lakhal K, et al. Noninvasive monitoring of blood pressure in the critically ill: reliability according to the cuff site (arm, thigh, or ankle). *Crit Care Med.* 2012;40(4):1207.

12. Feihl F, Broccard AF. Interactions between respiration and systemic hemodynamics. Part II: practical implications in critical care. *Intensive Care Med.* 2009;35(2):198.

13. Polderman KH, Girbes AJ. Central venous catheter use. Part 1: mechanical complications. *Intensive Care Med.* 2002;28(1):1.

14. Polderman KH, Girbes AR. Central venous catheter use. Part 2: infectious complications. *Intensive Care Med.* 2002;28(1):18.

15. Maddukuri P, et al. Echocardiographic diagnosis of air embolism associated with central venous catheter placement: case report and review of the literature. *Echocardiography.* 2006;23(4):315.

16. Deceuninck O, et al. Images in cardiovascular medicine. Massive air embolism after central venous catheter removal. *Circulation.* 2007;116(19):e516.

17. Clark DK, Plaizier E. Devastating cerebral air embolism after central line removal. *J Neurosci Nurs.* 2011;43(4):193; quiz 197.

18. Wang AZ, et al. The differences between venous air embolism and fat embolism in routine intraoperative monitoring methods, transesophageal echocardiography, and fatal volume in pigs. *J Trauma.* 2008.

19. Collyer TC, Yates DR, Bellamy MC. Severe air embolism resulting from a perforated cap on a high-flow three-way stopcock connected to a central venous catheter. *Eur J Anaesthesiol.* 2007;24(5):474.

20. Sinno MC, Alam M. Echocardiographically detected fibrinous sheaths associated with central venous catheters. *Echocardiography.* 2012;29(3):E56.

21. Sona C, Prentice D, Schallom L. National survey of central venous catheter flushing in the intensive care unit. *Crit Care Nurse.* 2012;32(1):e12.

22. Schallom ME, et al. Heparin or 0.9% sodium chloride to maintain central venous catheter patency: a randomized trial. *Crit Care Med.* 2012;40(6):1820.

23. Timsit JF, et al. A multicentre analysis of catheter-related infection based on a hierarchical model. *Intensive Care Med.* 2012, Epub in press.

24. Marik PE, Baram M, Vahid B. Does central venous pressure predict fluid responsiveness? A systematic review of the literature and the tale of seven mares. *Chest.* 2008;134(1):172.

25. Kupchik N, Bridges E. Critical analysis, critical care: central venous pressure monitoring: what's the evidence? *Am J Nurs.* 2012;112(1):58.

26. Lakhal K, et al. Central venous pressure measurements improve the accuracy of leg raising-induced change in pulse pressure to predict fluid responsiveness. *Intensive Care Med.* 2010;36(6):940.

27. Christensen M. Mixed venous oxygen saturation monitoring revisited: Thoughts for critical care nursing practice. *Austral Crit Care.* 2012;25(2):78.

28. Richard C, et al. Early use of the pulmonary artery catheter and outcomes in patients with shock and acute respiratory distress syndrome: a randomized controlled trial. *JAMA.* 2003;290(20):2713.

29. Wheeler AP, et al. Pulmonary-artery versus central venous catheter to guide treatment of acute lung injury. *N Engl J Med.* 2006;354(21):2213.

30. Binanay C, et al. Evaluation study of congestive heart failure and pulmonary artery catheterization effectiveness: the ESCAPE trial. *JAMA.* 2005;294(13):1625.

31. Harvey SE, et al. Post hoc insights from PAC-Man—the U.K. pulmonary artery catheter trial. *Crit Care Med.* 2008;36(6):1714.

32. Sandham JD, et al. A randomized, controlled trial of the use of pulmonary-artery catheters in high-risk surgical patients. *N Engl J Med.* 2003;348(1):5.

33. Harvey S, et al. Pulmonary artery catheters for adult patients in intensive care. *Cochrane Database Syst Rev.* 2006;3:CD003408.

34. Shah MR, et al. Impact of the pulmonary artery catheter in critically ill patients: meta-analysis of randomized clinical trials. *JAMA.* 2005;294(13):1664.

35. Wiener RS, Welch HG. Trends in the use of the pulmonary artery catheter in the United States, 1993-2004. *JAMA.* 2007;298(4):423.

36. Koo KK, et al. Pulmonary artery catheters: evolving rates and reasons for use. *Crit Care Med.* 2011;39(7):1613.

37. Richard C, Monnet X, Teboul JL. Pulmonary artery catheter monitoring in 2011. *Curr Opin Crit Care.* 2011;17(3):296.

38. Kahwash R, Leier CV, Miller L. Role of the pulmonary artery catheter in diagnosis and management of heart failure. *Cardiol Clin.* 2011;29(2):281.

39. Opitz CF, et al. Pulmonary hypertension: Hemodynamic evaluation. Updated Recommendations of the Cologne Consensus Conference 2011. *Internat J Cardiol.* 2011; 154(Suppl 1):S13.

40. Bunker N, DiNardo JA. Large left atrial "v" waves after mitral valve replacement. *J Cardiothorac Vasc Anesthesia.* 2009;23(1):69.

41. Ahuja K, et al. Posterior Papillary Muscle Rupture Complicating an ST-segment Myocardial Infarction. *J Emerg Med.* 2011. Epub in press.

42. Dellinger RP, et al. Surviving Sepsis Campaign: international guidelines for management of severe sepsis and septic shock: 2008. *Crit Care Med.* 2008;36(1):296.

43. Price LC, et al. Pathophysiology of pulmonary hypertension in acute lung injury. *Am J Physiol Lung Cell Mol Physiol.* 2012;302(9):L803.

44. Price LC, et al. Pulmonary vascular and right ventricular dysfunction in adult critical care: current and emerging options for management: a systematic literature review. *Crit Care.* 2010;14(5):R169.

45. Practice guidelines for pulmonary artery catheterization: an updated report by the American Society of Anesthesiologists Task Force on Pulmonary Artery Catheterization. *Anesthesiology.* 2003;99(4):988.

46. Oztekin DS, et al. Comparison of complications and procedural activities of pulmonary artery catheter removal by critical care nurses versus medical doctors. *Nurs Crit Care.* 2008;13(2):105.

47. Malfatto G, et al. Transthoracic impedance accurately estimates pulmonary wedge pressure in patients with decompensated chronic heart failure. *Congest Heart Fail.* 2012;18(1):25.

48. Kamath SA, et al. Correlation of impedance cardiography with invasive hemodynamic measurements in patients with advanced heart failure: the BioImpedance CardioGraphy (BIG) substudy of the Evaluation Study of Congestive Heart Failure and Pulmonary Artery Catheterization Effectiveness (ESCAPE) Trial. *Am Heart J.* 2009;158(2):217.

49. Cecconi M, et al. A prospective study of the accuracy and precision of continuous cardiac output monitoring devices as compared to intermittent thermodilution. *Minerva Anestiol.* 2010;76(12):1010.

50. Hadian M, et al. Cross-comparison of cardiac output trending accuracy of LiDCO, PiCCO, FloTrac and pulmonary artery catheters. *Crit Care.* 2010;14(6):R212.

51. Mora B, et al. Validation of cardiac output measurement with the LiDCO pulse contour system in patients with impaired left

ventricular function after cardiac surgery. *Anaesthesia.* 2011;66(8):675.

52. Sundar S, Panzica P. LiDCO systems. *Internat Anesthesiol Clin.* 2010;48(1):87.

53. Broch O, et al. Uncalibrated pulse power analysis fails to reliably measure cardiac output in patients undergoing coronary artery bypass surgery. *Crit Care.* 2011;15(1):R76.

54. Litton E, Morgan M. The PiCCO monitor: a review. *Anaesthes Intensive Care.* 2012;40(3):393.

55. Oren-Grinberg A. The PiCCO Monitor. *Internat Anesthesiol Clin.* 2010;48(1):57.

56. Schmidt S, et al. Effect of the venous catheter site on transpulmonary thermodilution measurement variables. *Crit Care Med.* 2007;35(3):783.

57. Morgan P, Al-Subaie N, Rhodes A. Minimally invasive cardiac output monitoring. *Curr Opin Crit Care.* 2008;14(3):322.

58. Hofer CK, Ganter MT, Zollinger A. What technique should I use to measure cardiac output? *Curr Opin Crit Care.* 2007;13(3):308.

59. Hamzaoui O, et al. Effects of changes in vascular tone on the agreement between pulse contour and transpulmonary thermodilution cardiac output measurements within an up to 6-hour calibration-free period. *Crit Care Med.* 2008;36(2):434.

60. Button D, et al. Clinical evaluation of the FloTrac/Vigileo system and two established continuous cardiac output monitoring devices in patients undergoing cardiac surgery. *Br J Anaesth.* 2007;99(3):329.

61. Monnet X, et al. Arterial pressure-based cardiac output in septic patients: different accuracy of pulse contour and uncalibrated pressure waveform devices. *Crit Care.* 2010;14(3):R109.

62. Turner MA. Doppler-based hemodynamic monitoring: a minimally invasive alternative. *AACN Clin Issues.* 2003;14(2):220.

63. Schober P, Loer SA, Schwarte LA. Perioperative hemodynamic monitoring with transesophageal Doppler technology. *Anesth Analg.* 2009;109(2):340.

64. Robert JM, et al. Residents and ICU nurses get reliable static and dynamic haemodynamic assessments with aortic oesophageal Doppler. *Acta Anaesthesiol Scand.* 2012;56(4):441.

65. Young BP, Low LL. Noninvasive monitoring cardiac output using partial CO(2) rebreathing. *Crit Care Clin.* 2010;26(2):383.

66. Walley KR. Use of central venous oxygen saturation to guide therapy. *Am J Resp Crit Care Med.* 2011;184(5):514.

67. Jesurum J. Protocols for Practice -SVO2 Monitoring. *Crit Care Nurse.* 2004;24(4):73.

68. Marx G, Reinhart K. Venous oximetry. *Curr Opin Crit Care.* 2006;12(3):263.

69. Collaborative Study Group on Perioperative ScvO$_2$ Monitoring. Multicentre study on peri- and postoperative central venous oxygen saturation in high-risk surgical patients. *Crit Care.* 2006;10(6):R158.

70. Maddirala S, Khan A. Optimizing hemodynamic support in septic shock using central and mixed venous oxygen saturation. *Crit Care Clin.* 2010;26(2):323.

71. Kligfield P, et al. Recommendations for the standardization and interpretation of the electrocardiogram: part I: the electrocardiogram and its technology: a scientific statement from the American Heart Association Electrocardiography and Arrhythmias Committee, Council on Clinical Cardiology; the American College of Cardiology Foundation; and the Heart Rhythm Society: endorsed by the International Society for Computerized Electrocardiology. *Circulation.* 2007;115(10):1306.

72. Drew BJ, et al. Practice standards for electrocardiographic monitoring in hospital settings: an American Heart Association scientific statement from the Councils on Cardiovascular Nursing, Clinical Cardiology, and Cardiovascular Disease in the Young: endorsed by the International Society of Computerized Electrocardiology and the American Association of Critical-Care Nurses. *Circulation.* 2004;110(17):2721.

73. Drew BJ, Funk M. Practice standards for ECG monitoring in hospital settings: executive summary and guide for implementation. *Crit Care Nurs Clin North Am.* 2006; 18(2):157, ix.

74. Drew BJ. Pulling it all together: case studies on ECG monitoring. *AACN Adv Crit Care.* 2007;18(3):305.

75. Surawicz B, et al. AHA/ACCF/HRS recommendations for the standardization and interpretation of the electrocardiogram: part III: intraventricular conduction disturbances: a scientific statement from the American Heart Association Electrocardiography and Arrhythmias Committee, Council on Clinical Cardiology; the American College of Cardiology Foundation; and the Heart Rhythm Society: endorsed by the International Society for Computerized Electrocardiology. *Circulation.* 2009;119(10):e235.

76. Baranchuk A, et al. Electrocardiography pitfalls and artifacts: the 10 commandments. *Crit Care Nurs.* 2009;29(1):67.

77. American Association of Critical-Care Nurses. AACN practice alert: ST segment monitoring. http://www.aacn.org/WD/Practice/Docs/PracticeAlerts/ST_Segment_Monitoring_05-2009.pdf. 2009. Accessed August 2012.

78. Drew BJ, et al. Prevention of torsade de pointes in hospital settings: a scientific statement from the American Heart Association and the American College of Cardiology Foundation. *Circulation.* 2010;121(8):1047.

79. Pickham D, et al. High prevalence of corrected QT interval prolongation in acutely ill patients is associated with mortality: results of the QT in Practice (QTIP) Study. *Crit Care Med.* 2012;40(2):394.

80. Muzyk AJ, et al. Examination of baseline risk factors for QTc interval prolongation in patients prescribed intravenous haloperidol. *Drug Safety.* 2012;35(7):547.

81. Funk M, et al. Unnecessary arrhythmia monitoring and underutilization of ischemia and QT interval monitoring in current clinical practice: baseline results of the Practical Use of the Latest Standards for Electrocardiography trial. *J Electrocardiol.* 2010;43(6):542.

82. Tisdale JE, et al. Prevalence of QT interval prolongation in patients admitted to cardiac care units and frequency of subsequent administration of QT interval-prolonging drugs: a prospective, observational study in a large urban academic medical center in the US. *Drug Safety.* 2012;35(6):459.

83. Conti CR, Bavry AA, Petersen JW. Silent ischemia: clinical relevance. *J Am Coll Cardiol.* 2012;59(5):435.

84. Rautaharju PM, et al. AHA/ACCF/HRS recommendations for the standardization and interpretation of the electrocardiogram: part IV: the ST segment, T and U waves, and the QT interval: a scientific statement from the American Heart Association Electrocardiography and Arrhythmias Committee, Council on Clinical Cardiology; the American College of Cardiology Foundation; and the Heart Rhythm Society: endorsed by the International Society for Computerized Electrocardiology. *Circulation.* 2009;119(10):e241.

85. Behrouz R, Sullebarger JT, Malek AR. Cardiac manifestations of subarachnoid hemorrhage. *Expert Rev Cardiovasc Ther.* 2011;9(3):303.

86. Wagner GS, et al. AHA/ACCF/HRS recommendations for the standardization and interpretation of the electrocardiogram: part VI: acute ischemia/infarction: a scientific statement from the American Heart Association Electrocardiography and Arrhythmias Committee, Council on Clinical Cardiology; the American College of Cardiology Foundation; and the Heart Rhythm Society: endorsed by the International Society for Computerized Electrocardiology. *Circulation.* 2009;119(10):e262.

87. Hancock EW, et al. AHA/ACCF/HRS recommendations for the standardization and interpretation of the electrocardiogram: part V: electrocardiogram changes associated with cardiac chamber hypertrophy: a scientific statement from the American Heart Association Electrocardiography and Arrhythmias Committee, Council on Clinical Cardiology; the American College of Cardiology Foundation; and the Heart Rhythm Society: endorsed by the International Society for Computerized Electrocardiology. *Circulation.* 2009;119(10):e251.

88. Jneid H, et al. 2012 ACCF/AHA Focused Update of the Guideline for the Management of Patients With Unstable Angina/Non-ST-Elevation Myocardial Infarction (Updating the 2007 Guideline and Replacing the 2011 Focused Update): A Report of the American College of Cardiology Foundation/American Heart Association Task Force on Practice Guidelines. *Circulation.* 2012.

89. Kushner FG, et al. 2009 Focused Updates: ACC/AHA Guidelines for the Management of Patients With ST-Elevation Myocardial Infarction (updating the 2004 Guideline and 2007 Focused Update) and ACC/AHA/SCAI Guidelines on Percutaneous Coronary Intervention (updating the 2005 Guideline and 2007 Focused Update): a report of the American College of Cardiology Foundation/American Heart Association Task Force on Practice Guidelines. *Circulation.* 2009;120(22):2271.

90. Goldstein JA. Acute right ventricular infarction. *Cardiol Clin.* 2012;30(2):219.

91. Morrow DA. Cardiovascular risk prediction in patients with stable and unstable coronary heart disease. *Circulation.* 2010;121(24):2681.

92. Haataja P, et al. Prevalence of ventricular conduction blocks in the resting electrocardiogram in a general population: The Health 2000 Survey. *Internat J Cardiol.* 2012.

93. Elizari MV, Acunzo RS, Ferreiro M. Hemiblocks revisited. *Circulation.* 2007;115(9):1154.

94. Blomstrom-Lundqvist C, et al. ACC/AHA/ESC guidelines for the management of patients with supraventricular arrhythmias–executive summary. a report of the American college of cardiology/American heart association task force on practice guidelines and the European society of cardiology committee for practice guidelines (writing committee to develop guidelines for the management of patients with supraventricular arrhythmias) developed in collaboration with NASPE-Heart Rhythm Society. *J Am Coll Cardiol.* 2003;42(8):1493.

95. Magder SA. The ups and downs of heart rate. *Crit Care Med.* 2012;40(1):239.

96. Calkins H, et al. HRS/EHRA/ECAS expert consensus statement on catheter and surgical ablation of atrial fibrillation: recommendations for personnel, policy, procedures and follow-up. A report of the Heart Rhythm Society (HRS) Task Force on Catheter and Surgical Ablation of Atrial Fibrillation developed in partnership with the European Heart Rhythm Association (EHRA) and the European Cardiac Arrhythmia Society (ECAS); in collaboration with the American College of

Cardiology (ACC), American Heart Association (AHA), and the Society of Thoracic Surgeons (STS). Endorsed and approved by the governing bodies of the American College of Cardiology, the American Heart Association, the European Cardiac Arrhythmia Society, the European Heart Rhythm Association, the Society of Thoracic Surgeons, and the Heart Rhythm Society. *Europace.* 2007;9(6):335.

97. Fuster V, et al. ACC/AHA/ESC 2006 Guidelines for the Management of Patients with Atrial Fibrillation: a report of the American College of Cardiology/American Heart Association Task Force on Practice Guidelines and the European Society of Cardiology Committee for Practice Guidelines (Writing Committee to Revise the 2001 Guidelines for the Management of Patients With Atrial Fibrillation): developed in collaboration with the European Heart Rhythm Association and the Heart Rhythm Society. *Circulation.* 2006;114(7):e257.

98. Calkins H, et al. 2012 HRS/EHRA/ECAS expert consensus statement on catheter and surgical ablation of atrial fibrillation: recommendations for patient selection, procedural techniques, patient management and follow-up, definitions, endpoints, and research trial design: a report of the Heart Rhythm Society (HRS) Task Force on Catheter and Surgical Ablation of Atrial Fibrillation. Developed in partnership with the European Heart Rhythm Association (EHRA), a registered branch of the European Society of Cardiology (ESC) and the European Cardiac Arrhythmia Society (ECAS); and in collaboration with the American College of Cardiology (ACC), American Heart Association (AHA), the Asia Pacific Heart Rhythm Society (APHRS), and the Society of Thoracic Surgeons (STS). Endorsed by the governing bodies of the American College of Cardiology Foundation, the American Heart Association, the European Cardiac Arrhythmia Society, the European Heart Rhythm Association, the Society of Thoracic Surgeons, the Asia Pacific Heart Rhythm Society, and the Heart Rhythm Society. *Heart Rhythm.* 2012;9(4):632 e621.

99. Schotten U, et al. Pathophysiological mechanisms of atrial fibrillation: a translational appraisal. *Physiol Rev.* 2011;91(1):262.

100. Wann LS, et al. 2011 ACCF/AHA/HRS focused update on the management of patients with atrial fibrillation (updating the 2006 guideline): a report of the American College of Cardiology Foundation/American Heart Association Task Force on Practice Guidelines. *Circulation.* 2011;123(1):104.

101. Camm AJ, et al. Guidelines for the management of atrial fibrillation: the Task Force for the Management of Atrial Fibrillation of the European Society of Cardiology (ESC). *Eur Heart J.* 2010;31(19):2369.

102. Healey JS, et al. Subclinical atrial fibrillation and the risk of stroke. *New Engl J Med.* 2012;366(2):120.

103. Hillis LD, et al. 2011 ACCF/AHA Guideline for Coronary Artery Bypass Graft Surgery: a report of the American College of Cardiology Foundation/American Heart Association Task Force on Practice Guidelines. *Circulation.* 2011;124(23): e652.

104. Kern LS, McRae ME, Funk M. ECG monitoring after cardiac surgery: postoperative atrial fibrillation and the atrial electrogram. *AACN Adv Crit Care.* 2007;18(3):294.

105. Miller JN, Drew BJ. Atrial electrograms after cardiac surgery: survey of clinical practice. *Am J Crit Care.* 2007;16(4):350.

106. Zimetbaum P. Antiarrhythmic drug therapy for atrial fibrillation. *Circulation.* 2012;125(2):381.

107. Chenoweth J, Diercks DB. Management of atrial fibrillation in the acute setting. *Curr Opin Crit Care.* 2012;18(4):333.

108. You JJ, et al. Antithrombotic therapy for atrial fibrillation: Antithrombotic Therapy and Prevention of Thrombosis, 9th ed: American College of Chest Physicians Evidence-Based Clinical Practice Guidelines. *Chest.* 2012;141(2 Suppl):e531S.

109. Schneeweiss S, et al. Comparative efficacy and safety of new oral anticoagulants in patients with atrial fibrillation. *Circ Cardiovasc Qual Outcomes.* 2012;5(4):480.

110. Connolly SJ, et al. Dabigatran versus warfarin in patients with atrial fibrillation. *New Engl J Med.* 2009;361(12):1139.

111. Patel MR, et al. Rivaroxaban versus warfarin in nonvalvular atrial fibrillation. *New Eng J Med.* 2011;365(10):883.

112. Granger CB, et al. Apixaban versus warfarin in patients with atrial fibrillation. *New Engl J Med.* 2011;365(11):981.

113. Calkins H. Catheter ablation to maintain sinus rhythm. *Circulation.* 2012;125(11):1439.

114. Pelter MM, Carey MG. P wave alterations. *Am J Crit Care.* 2007;16(2):187.

115. Yang EH, Shah S, Criley JM. Digitalis toxicity: a fading but crucial complication to recognize. *Am J Med.* 2012;125(4):337.

116. Goldberger ZD, Rho RW, Page RL. Approach to the diagnosis and initial management of the stable adult patient with a wide complex tachycardia. *Am J Cardiol.* 2008;101(10):1456.

117. Alzand BS, Crijns HJ. Diagnostic criteria of broad QRS complex tachycardia: decades of evolution. *Europace.* 2011;13(4):465.

118. Pelter MM, Carey MG. Conduction system disease. *Am J Crit Care.* 2010;19(4):383.

119. Raebel MA. Hyperkalemia associated with use of angiotensin-converting enzyme inhibitors and angiotensin receptor blockers. *Cardiovasc Ther.* 2012;30(3):e156.

120. Freeman K, et al. Effects of presentation and electrocardiogram on time to treatment of hyperkalemia. *Acad Emerg Med.* 2008;15(3):239.

121. Montague BT, Ouellette JR, Buller GK. Retrospective review of the frequency of ECG changes in hyperkalemia. *Clin J Am Soc Nephrol.* 2008;3:324.

122. El-Sherif N, Turitto G. Electrolyte disorders and arrhythmogenesis. *Cardiol J.* 2011;18(3):233.

123. Kelly A, Levine MA. Hypocalcemia in the critically ill patient. *J Intensive Care Med.* 2011, Epub ahead of print.

124. Buckley MS, LeBlanc JM, Cawley MJ. Electrolyte disturbances associated with commonly prescribed medications in the intensive care unit. *Crit Care Med.* 2010;38(Suppl):S253.

125. Noronha JL, Matuschak GM. Magnesium in critical illness: metabolism, assessment, and treatment. *Intensive Care Med.* 2002;28(6):667.

126. Cundy T, Mackay J. Proton pump inhibitors and severe hypomagnesaemia. *Curr Opin Gastroenterol.* 2011;27(2):180.

127. Neumar RW, et al. Part 8: adult advanced cardiovascular life support: 2010 American Heart Association Guidelines for Cardiopulmonary Resuscitation and Emergency Cardiovascular Care. *Circulation.* 2010;122(18 Suppl 3):S729.

128. Patil H, Vaidya O, Bogart D. A review of causes and systemic approach to cardiac troponin elevation. *Clin Cardiol.* 2011;34(12):723.

129. Keller T. Serial changes in highly sensitive troponin I assay and early diagnosis of myocardial infarction. *JAMA.* 2011;306(24):2684.

130. Maisel AS, Daniels LB. Breathing not properly 10 years later: what we have learned and what we still need to learn. *J Am Coll Cardiol.* 2012;60(4):277.

131. Maisel A. Circulating natriuretic peptide levels in acute heart failure. *Rev Cardiovasc Med.* 2007;8(Suppl 5):S13.

132. Holbrook A, et al. Evidence-based management of anticoagulant therapy: Antithrombotic Therapy and Prevention of Thrombosis, 9th ed: American College of Chest Physicians Evidence-Based Clinical Practice Guidelines. *Chest.* 2012;141(2 Suppl):e152S.

133. Whitlock RP, et al. Antithrombotic and thrombolytic therapy for valvular disease: Antithrombotic Therapy and Prevention of Thrombosis, 9th ed: American College of Chest Physicians Evidence-Based Clinical Practice Guidelines. *Chest.* 2012;141(2 Suppl):e576S.

134. Douketis JD, et al. Perioperative management of antithrombotic therapy: Antithrombotic Therapy and Prevention of Thrombosis, 9th ed: American College of Chest Physicians Evidence-Based Clinical Practice Guidelines. *Chest.* 2012;141(2 Suppl):e326S.

135. Gehrie E, Laposata M. Test of the month: the chromogenic antifactor Xa assay. *Am J Hematol.* 2011. Epub ahead of print.

136. Grundy SM, et al. Implications of recent clinical trials for the National Cholesterol Education Program Adult Treatment Panel III guidelines. *Circulation.* 2004;110(2):227.

137. Smith S, et al. AHA/ACCF Secondary Prevention and Risk Reduction Therapy for Patients With Coronary and Other Atherosclerotic Vascular Disease: 2011 Update. A Guideline From the American Heart Association and American College of Cardiology Foundation. *Circulation.* 2011;124:2458.

138. Miller M, et al. Triglycerides and cardiovascular disease: a scientific statement from the American Heart Association. *Circulation.* 2011;123:2292.

139. Patel MR, et al. ACCF/SCAI/AATS/AHA/ASE/ASNC/HFSA/HRS/SCCM/SCCT/SCMR/STS 2012 appropriate use criteria for diagnostic catheterization: a report of the American College of Cardiology Foundation Appropriate Use Criteria Task Force, Society for Cardiovascular Angiography and Interventions, American Association for Thoracic Surgery, American Heart Association, American Society of Echocardiography, American Society of Nuclear Cardiology, Heart Failure Society of America, Heart Rhythm Society, Society of Critical Care Medicine, Society of Cardiovascular Computed Tomography, Society for Cardiovascular Magnetic Resonance, and Society of Thoracic Surgeons. *J Am Coll Cardiol.* 2012;59(22):1995.

140. Nishimura RA, Carabello BA. Hemodynamics in the cardiac catheterization laboratory of the 21st century. *Circulation.* 2012;125(17):2138.

141. Stacul F, et al. Contrast induced nephropathy: updated ESUR Contrast Media Safety Committee guidelines. *Eur Radiol.* 2011;21(12):2527.

142. Isaac S. Contrast-induced nephropathy: nursing implications. *Crit Care Nurse.* 2012;32(3):41.

143. Trotman-Dickenson B. Radiology in the intensive care unit (Part I). *J Intensive Care Med.* 2003;18(4):198.

144. Godoy MCB, et al. Chest radiography in the ICU: part 1, evaluation of airway, enteric, and pleural tubes. *AJR.* 2012;198:563.

145. Trotman-Dickenson B. Radiology in the intensive care unit (part 2). *J Intensive Care Med.* 2003;18(5):239.

146. Godoy MCB, et al. Chest Radiography in the ICU: Part 2, Evaluation of Cardiovascular Lines and Other Devices. *AJR.* 2012;198:572.

147. Miller TD. Stress testing: the case for the standard treadmill test. *Curr Opin Cardiol.* 2011;26(5):363.

148. Gibbons RJ, et al. ACC/AHA 2002 guideline update for exercise testing: summary article: a report of the American College of Cardiology/American Heart Association Task Force on Practice

Guidelines (Committee to Update the 1997 Exercise Testing Guidelines). *Circulation.* 2002;106(14):1883.

149. Marcus FI, Zareba W, Sherrill D. Evaluation of the normal values for signal-averaged electrocardiogram. *J Cardiovasc Electrophysiol.* 2007;18(2):231.

150. Little SH. Three-dimensional echocardiography to quantify mitral valve regurgitation. *Curr Opin Cardiol.* 2012;27(5):477.

151. Douglas PS, et al. ACCF/ASE/AHA/ASNC/HFSA/HRS/SCAI/SCCM/SCCT/SCMR 2011 Appropriate Use Criteria for Echocardiography. A Report of the American College of Cardiology Foundation Appropriate Use Criteria Task Force, American Society of Echocardiography, American Heart Association, American Society of Nuclear Cardiology, Heart Failure Society of America, Heart Rhythm Society, Society for Cardiovascular Angiography and Interventions, Society of Critical Care Medicine, Society of Cardiovascular Computed Tomography, and Society for Cardiovascular Magnetic Resonance Endorsed by the American College of Chest Physicians. *J Am Coll Cardiol.* 2011;57(9):1126.

152. Sommer G, Bremerich J, Lund G. Magnetic resonance imaging in valvular heart disease: clinical application and current role for patient management. *J Magn Reson Imag.* 2012;35:1241.

153. Badheka AO, Hendel RC. Radionuclide cardiac stress testing. *Curr Opin Cardiol.* 2011;26(5):370.

154. Hendel RC, et al. ACCF/ASNC/ACR/AHA/ASE/SCCT/SCMR/SNM 2009 appropriate use criteria for cardiac radionuclide imaging: a report of the American College of Cardiology Foundation Appropriate Use Criteria Task Force, the American Society of Nuclear Cardiology, the American College of Radiology, the American Heart Association, the American Society of Echocardiography, the Society of Cardiovascular Computed Tomography, the Society for Cardiovascular Magnetic Resonance, and the Society of Nuclear Medicine. *Circulation.* 2009;119(22):e561.

155. Mark DB, et al. ACCF/ACR/AHA/NASCI/SAIP/SCAI/SCCT 2010 Expert Consensus Document on Coronary Computed Tomographic Angiography. A Report of the American College of Cardiology Foundation Task Force on Expert Consensus Documents. *Circulation.* 2010;121:2509.

156. Greenland P, et al. ACCF/AHA 2007 Clinical expert consensus document on coronary artery calcium scoring by computed tomography in global cardiovascular risk assessment and in evaluation of patients with chest pain. *Circulation.* 2007;115:402.

157. Grayburn PA. Interpreting the coronary artery calcum score. *N Engl J Med.* 2012;366(4):294.

Cardiovascular Disorders

Elizabeth Scruth, Annette Haynes

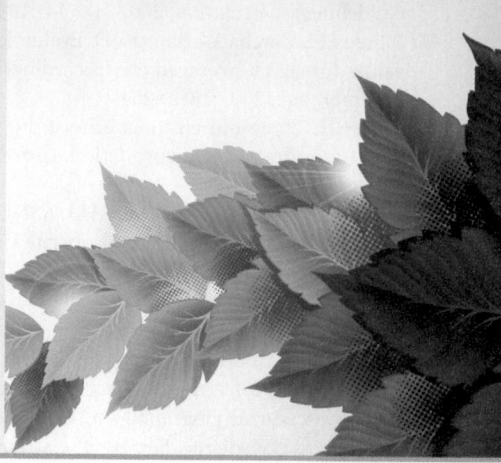

evolve WEBSITE

http://evolve.elsevier.com/Urden/criticalcare/

Evolve Features:

- NCLEX Review Questions
- CCRN Review Questions
- PCCN Review Questions
- Mosby's Nursing Skills Procedures
- Animations
- Video Clips
- Glossary

Cardiovascular disease remains the leading cause of mortality in the United States. In 2008, the overall rate of death attributable to cardiovascular disease (CVD) was 244.8 per 100 000.[1] From 1998 to 2008, the rate of death attributable to CVD declined by 30%.[1] In the United States, a person has a cardiac event approximately every 25 seconds, and every minute someone dies from a cardiac event.[1] CVD causes 1 in 3 deaths in the United States, and 1 in 9 death certificates mentioned heart failure; 1 in 3 people had some form of CVD.[1]

In 2009, 4.2 million cardiovascular operations and procedures were performed on men and 3.3 million on women. Between 2010 and 2030, it is expected that the total medical costs of CVD will triple from 273 billion to 818 billion dollars.[1] The critical care nurse is in a unique position to assist with educating the public on a daily basis about CVD and the risk factors that are modifiable with changes in habits or lifestyles. An understanding of the pathology of CVD processes and clinical management allows the critical care nurse to accurately anticipate and plan interventions. This chapter focuses on cardiac disorders commonly seen in the critical care environment.

CORONARY ARTERY DISEASE

Description and Etiology

The biggest contributor to cardiovascular system–related morbidity and mortality is *coronary artery disease* (CAD). *Atherosclerosis* is a progressive disease that affects arteries throughout the body. In the heart, atherosclerotic changes are clinically known as CAD. This disease process is also known by the term

coronary heart disease (CHD) because other heart structures ultimately become involved in the disease process. The atherosclerotic vascular changes that lead to CAD may begin in childhood. Research and epidemiologic data collected during the past 50 years have demonstrated a strong association between preventable and nonpreventable risk factors and the development of CAD.[1,2] These risk factors are further delineated as *nonmodifiable* and *modifiable coronary risk factors* (Box 15-1).

Risk Factors for Coronary Artery Disease
Age, Gender, and Race

The severe effects of CAD occur as a person ages. In general, CAD symptoms are seen in persons age 45 years and older.[1] Traditionally, CAD has been regarded a primarily male disease. Research is, however, showing that it affects women as well.[1-3] Men typically develop external manifestations of the disease about 5 to 10 years earlier compared with women. The prevalence of cardiovascular disease is higher among women starting at age 75 years.[1-3] CAD rates for postmenopausal women are two to three times higher than those for premenopausal women of the same age.[1] Primary cardiovascular risk factors are different in men and women, with women having higher rates of diabetes and hypertension compared with men.[1]

Family History

A positive family history is one in which a close blood relative has had a myocardial infarction (MI) or stroke before age 60 years. This family history suggests a genetic or lifestyle predisposition to the development of CAD. Individuals with a family history had a 50% greater risk of having an acute MI as

BOX 15-1 CORONARY ARTERY DISEASE RISK FACTORS

Nonmodifiable Risk Factors
- Age
- Gender
- Family history
- Race

Modifiable Risk Factors
- Elevated serum lipids
- Hypertension
- Cigarette smoking
- Prediabetes or diabetes mellitus
- Diet high in saturated fat, cholesterol, and calories
- Elevated homocysteine level
- Metabolic syndrome
- Obesity
- Physical inactivity
- Postmenopause (modification is controversial)

TABLE 15-1 LIPID GUIDELINES AND RISK FOR CORONARY ARTERY DISEASE

ATP III Classification of Total, Low-Density Lipoprotein (LDL), and High-Density Lipoprotein (HDL) Cholesterol and Triglycerides (mg/dL)*

Total Cholesterol	
<200	
200-239	Borderline-high
>240	High
LDL Cholesterol	
<100	Optimal
100-129	Near or above optimal
130-159	Borderline high
160-189	High
>190	Very high
HDL Cholesterol	
<40	Low
>60	High
Triglycerides	
<150	Normal
150-199	Borderline high
200-499	High
>500	Very high

*Values outside the target range increase the risk for coronary artery disease.
HDL, High-density lipoprotein; *LDL*, low-density lipoprotein; *VLDL*, very-low–density lipoprotein.

demonstrated in the INTERHEART study, a large study that looked at risk factors of patients in 52 countries who experienced an MI.[4]

Hyperlipidemia

Hyperlipidemia is a leading factor responsible for severe atherosclerosis and the development of CAD. Millions of adults above age 20 years have total serum cholesterol levels above 240 milligrams per deciliter (mg/dL). Assessing total serum cholesterol and triglyceride levels is essential to the assessment of cardiovascular risk in patients.[1] A lipid panel blood test will measure the following values:

- High-density lipoprotein (HDL) cholesterol
- Low-density lipoprotein (LDL) cholesterol
- Very-low–density lipoprotein (VLDL) cholesterol
- Triglycerides

Treatment of hyperlipidemia has advanced beyond the concept of lowering total cholesterol to treatment of specific lipoprotein abnormalities.[1,3,5] The target levels for specific serum lipids are listed in Table 15-1.

Total Cholesterol. The total cholesterol is the sum of the HDL, LDL, and VLDL cholesterol in the bloodstream. It is used as a starting point for lipid testing. A total cholesterol level higher than 200 mg/dL is an indication to investigate the lipid profile and other risk factors for CAD.[5]

High-Density Lipoprotein Cholesterol. HDL cholesterol is frequently described as the "good cholesterol" because higher serum levels exert a protective effect against acute atherosclerotic events. All the reasons are not completely understood, but one recognized physiologic effect is the ability of HDL to promote the efflux of cholesterol from cells. This process may minimize the accumulation of foam cells in the arterial wall and decrease the risk of developing atherosclerosis.[6] High HDL cholesterol levels confer anti-inflammatory and antioxidant benefits on the arterial wall.[6] In contrast, a low HDL cholesterol level is an independent risk factor for the development of CAD and other atherosclerotic conditions. HDL cholesterol is generally higher in women, and levels can be raised by physical exercise and by stopping smoking. In patients with low HDL cholesterol levels, when lifestyle changes are ineffective, the HDL level can be raised by medications such as extended-release nicotinic acid (niacin) and fibrates.

An HDL cholesterol level below 40 mg/dL in adult males and below 50 mg/dL in adult females is considered low and is a risk factor for heart disease (HD) and stroke.

Low-Density Lipoprotein Cholesterol. LDL cholesterol is usually described as the "bad cholesterol" because high levels are associated with an increased risk of acute coronary syndrome (ACS), stroke, and peripheral arterial disease (PAD). High LDL levels initiate the atherosclerotic process by infiltrating the vessel wall and binding to the matrix of cells beneath the endothelium.[6] LDL cholesterol also exerts an inflammatory effect on the arterial vessel wall.[6] A high LDL cholesterol level is initially managed by nonpharmacologic lifestyle changes, such as weight loss, smoking cessation, low-fat diet, physical exercise, and attainment of a normal body size as measured by the body mass index (BMI). If lifestyle changes are insufficient to reduce the LDL cholesterol level in the bloodstream, the medication category of choice is a *statin*. Numerous research studies have conclusively demonstrated that lowering the LDL cholesterol with statins for primary or secondary prevention is highly effective in lowering mortality from CAD.[1,3] Therapy should be tailored to treat the individual cardiovascular risk profile. The target LDL cholesterol is determined according to the individual's risk profile as described in Table 15-1.

Triglycerides. Triglycerides are serum lipids that constitute an additional atherogenic risk factor. A fasting triglyceride level above 150 mg/dL in adults is considered elevated and is a risk factor for heart disease and stroke. Recent guidelines suggest that triglyceride levels below 100 mg/dL may be optimal.[7] The mean level of triglycerides for American adults ≥20 years of age is 137.6 mg/dL.[1]

Lipoprotein(a). LDL cholesterol can be further analyzed by the category of lipid particles that make up the total LDL value. Researchers have investigated the function of several lipid particles to determine their role in the development of premature atherosclerotic CAD. One particle that has been extensively studied is *lipoprotein(a)*, which is abbreviated Lp(a) and described verbally as "LP little a." Lp(a) is manufactured in the liver and circulates in the bloodstream bound to a large glycoprotein called *apolipoprotein(a)*, abbreviated as apo(a).[8] The Lp(a)–apo(a) lipid particle concentration is elevated in the presence of inflammation, and it stimulates atheroma and clot formation in inflamed arteries.[8] This effect is thought to occur because the apo(a) is structurally similar to plasminogen, a protein essential for clot formation.

Lp(a) levels are 90% genetically determined. Elevated Lp(a) plasma levels constitute the most frequently encountered genetic lipid disorder in families with premature CAD.[8] Testing for Lp(a) is reserved for high-risk patient populations, such as those with a strong family history of premature atherosclerotic disease and for patients with premature CAD who do not exhibit the expected cardiac risk factors. Reduction of Lp(a) levels to below 30 mg/dL is the therapeutic goal. This usually is achieved by ingesting high doses (1500 to 2000 mg/day) of extended-release nicotinic acid (niacin). The Lp(a) level is not reduced by statins, medications that traditionally lower LDL levels, or by physical exercise, a low-fat diet, weight loss, or tight control of blood glucose levels.[8] Lifestyle changes are recommended, and research is ongoing, but a cure has not yet been found.

High-Fat Diet

A diet rich in saturated fats leads to elevated cholesterol levels in the blood. The first line of treatment to lower elevated serum cholesterol is a low-fat, high-fiber diet and increased physical exercise.[9,10] If these measures are not effective, lipid-lowering medications are indicated. This approach sounds simple, but less than one half of the people who qualify for lipid reduction therapy are taking their medications; only one third of treated patients reach their LDL target.

Obesity

Obesity is a disease of modern times. A body mass index (BMI) of greater than 30 kilograms per meter squared (kg/m^2) is considered obese. Global estimates are more than 1 billion overweight adults, and at least 300 million of these people are obese. Obesity is often associated with a sedentary lifestyle accompanied by the calories consumed and portion sizes. A high risk of

---

BOX 15-2 HOW TO CALCULATE AND INTERPRET BODY MASS INDEX

Use a Calculator to Determine the Body Mass Index (BMI)

Metric Units: Divide body weight in kilograms by height in meters; divide the result by height in meters:

$BMI = (Weight_{kg}/Height_m) \div Height_m$

Example: A person weighs 100 kg and is 1.90 m tall:

$BMI = 100/1.90 \div 1.90 = 27.7$

How to Interpret the BMI Result

BMI (kg/m^2)	WEIGHT STATUS
<18.5	Underweight
18.5–24.9	Normal weight
25–29.5	Overweight
>30	Obese

---

coronary heart disease is among the well-established adverse health effects associated with excess weight. Hypertension, hypercholesterolemia, and diabetes are among the clinical conditions that are important mediators of this association.[1-3] Currently, one third of the adult population in the United States is obese.[1] The BMI is a mathematic formula used to assess body weight relative to height. BMI is used to evaluate the threat of excess weight as a risk factor for CAD and permits comparisons of people of different gender, age, height, and body type.[1] BMI is calculated as the weight in kilograms divided by the square of the height in meters (kg/m^2). The BMI calculation in metric units is shown in Box 15-2. A normal BMI is between 18.5 and 25 kg/m^2. A BMI between 25 and 30 kg/m^2 indicates that the person is overweight. A BMI greater than 30 kg/m^2 is the definition of obesity.[1]

The distribution pattern of body fat is a CAD risk factor. The higher the weight carried in the abdominal area, indicated by a large waist, the greater is the risk of CAD. Excess abdominal adiposity (apple body shape) indicates additional fat around the abdominal organs compared with individuals who have a smaller waist and larger hips (pear body shape). A waist size greater than 40 inches in men and 35 inches in women increases their risk for CAD. Physical exercise assists with weight reduction, lowers the risk for CAD, and decreases the risk of developing type 2 diabetes.

Physical Activity

Regular vigorous physical activity using large muscle groups promotes physiologic adaptation to aerobic exercise, which can prevent the development of CAD and reduce symptoms in patients with established cardiovascular disease.[11] Exercise also reduces the incidence of many other diseases, including type 2 diabetes, osteoporosis, obesity, depression, and cancers of the colon and breast.[11] Many research trials have demonstrated the positive effects of physical activity on the other major cardiac risk factors.[11] Exercise alters the lipid profile by decreasing LDL cholesterol and triglyceride levels and increasing HDL cholesterol levels.[11] Exercise reduces insulin resistance at the cellular level, lowering the risk for developing type 2 diabetes, especially if combined with a weight-loss program.[11] Epidemiologic studies indicate that participating in physical athletics in one's youth does not confer protection in later years. A sedentary lifestyle has negative effects, regardless of age, gender, BMI, smoking status, presence or absence of hypertension, or abnormal lipoprotein profile. Lifelong physical activity is necessary to prevent atherosclerotic CAD and stroke.

Hypertension

Hypertension is often described as the "silent killer" because 30% of those affected are unaware they have seriously elevated blood pressure.[1] In the United States, 1 person in 3 has hypertension. Normal blood pressure is described as a systolic blood pressure (SBP) below 120 mm Hg and a diastolic blood pressure (DBP) below 80 mm Hg. *Hypertension* is defined as an SBP greater than 140 mm Hg or DBP greater than 90 mm Hg. *Controlled hypertension* is a term that describes maintaining blood pressure within the normal range with the use of antihypertensive medications.[1] It is essential that patients understand that sustained elevation of blood pressure leads inexorably to atherosclerosis, heart failure, kidney failure, stroke, and heart attack.[12] Hypertension is so widespread in industrialized societies that even a normotensive person at age 55 years has a 90% lifetime risk of developing hypertension. This implies that even normotensive persons should adopt interventions to maintain a normal blood pressure.[1]

Hypertension is a cardiac risk factor because high SBP damages the arterial endothelium, leading to vascular inflammation that encourages the formation of plaque. Hypertension is a complex, multifactorial disease process, which is divided into stages for the purposes of treatment, as shown in Table 15-2.

Prehypertension is an SBP of 120 to 139 mm Hg or DBP above 85 mm Hg.[1,11,12] *Hypertension* is diagnosed when the blood pressure is above 140/90 mm Hg. Hypertension affects another one in three adults in the United States. After the blood pressure is above 140/80 mm Hg, hypertension is described as stage 1 or stage 2 (see Table 15-2).

Projections show that by 2030, an additional 27 million people could have hypertension.[1] The current guidelines recommend the goal of treatment for the person with hypertension without other risk factors is to achieve a blood pressure below 140/80 mm Hg. For the person with hypertension who already has diabetes or kidney disease, the target blood pressure is below 130/80 mm Hg. A normal blood pressure is below 120/80 mm Hg.[11,12]

Lifestyle interventions that can normalize blood pressure include physical exercise, a low-salt diet, limiting alcohol intake, and achieving normal body weight. Most patients are started on a diuretic, and if this is insufficient, they may be placed on an angiotensin-converting enzyme inhibitor (ACEI), angiotensin receptor blocker (ARB), beta-blocker, or calcium channel blocker. Most patients require at least two medications, one each from different medication classifications, to normalize their blood pressure.[12] Hypertensive emergencies with acute organ damage are discussed in the last section of this chapter.

Cigarette Smoking

The greater the number of cigarettes smoked per day, the greater is the risk of developing CAD, acute MI, and stroke.[1] Cigarette smoking unfavorably alters serum lipid levels, decreases HDL cholesterol level, and increases LDL cholesterol and triglyceride levels. Smoking increases the risk of CHD at all levels, including less than five cigarettes per day.[1] Smokers are two to four times more likely to develop CAD compared with nonsmokers.[1] Passive, secondhand smoke exposure also increases cardiovascular risk for nonsmoking adults.[1,13] Nonsmokers who are exposed to secondhand smoke at home or at work increase their risk of developing coronary heart disease by 30%.[1] Current cigarette smoking is a powerful predictor for the development of unstable angina, and myocardial infarction.[1,14,15]

Within 1 year of giving up cigarettes, an ex-smoker's risk of developing CAD decreases significantly. Nicotine is addictive, and giving up smoking is difficult. People need tremendous support to be able to "kick the habit." The good news is that many do quit, and smoking in the United States continues to decline.[1] Chapter 20 provides patient education guidelines on how to stop smoking.

Diabetes Mellitus

Individuals with diabetes mellitus (types 1 and 2) have a higher incidence of CHD compared with the general population. Elevated blood glucose level is a known risk factor for development of vascular inflammation associated with atherosclerosis. For decades, the diagnosis of diabetes was based on plasma glucose criteria. In 2009, the American Diabetes Association recommended the use of the hemoglobin (Hgb) A_{1C} test to diagnose diabetes, with at threshold of 6.5% or greater, which was adopted as standard practice in 2010.[16] The criteria for the diagnosis of diabetes is: A_{1C} 6.5% or greater, a fasting blood glucose 126 mg/dL or greater, or 2-hour plasma glucose 200 mg/dL or greater during an oral glucose tolerance test.[16] Or, in a patient with classic symptoms of hyperglycemia a random plasma glucose above 200 mg/dL signifies diabetes.[16]

A fasting blood glucose concentration between 100 to 125 mg/dL or an A_{1C} of 5.7% to 6.4% represents an increased risk for diabetes (Table 15-3). The upper limit for a normal fasting plasma glucose level is 125 mg/dL.[16,17] Patients with diabetes have an increased risk of developing CAD and have worse clinical outcomes after ACS events.[16,17] In a multinational study of patients who were seen at hospitals with symptoms of ACS,

TABLE 15-2	BLOOD PRESSURE GUIDELINES AND RISK FOR CORONARY ARTERY DISEASE	
CATEGORY	**SYSTOLIC BP* (mm Hg)**	**DIASTOLIC BP* (mm Hg)**
Normal (optimal)*	<120	<80
Prehypertension	120-139	80-89
Stage 1 hypertension	140-159	90-99
Stage 2 hypertension	≥160	≥100

*Values greater than normal increase the risk for CAD and heart failure.
BP, Blood pressure; *CAD,* coronary artery disease.

TABLE 15-3	FASTING BLOOD GLUCOSE AND RISK FOR CORONARY ARTERY DISEASE
BLOOD GLUCOSE LEVEL	**FASTING PLASMA GLUCOSE LEVEL* (mg/dL)**
Normal	70-100
Prediabetes	100-125
Diabetes	126 or higher

*Values greater than normal increase the risk for CAD and kidney failure.
CAD, Coronary artery disease.

almost 1 in 4 had a known history of diabetes.[18] More detailed information on type 2 diabetes and the use of insulin and oral medications to control blood glucose levels and combat insulin resistance is included in Chapters 32 and 33.

Chronic Kidney Disease

Chronic kidney disease is considered a risk equivalent for CAD.[1-3,19] This means that patients with chronic kidney disease have as much risk of experiencing a coronary event as if they already had CAD.[1-3,20] The risk of death for the patient with acute MI rises as the serum creatinine level increases.[20]

Metabolic Syndrome

Metabolic syndrome refers to the clustering of risk factors associated with CVD and type 2 diabetes.[1] About one third of people in the United States have metabolic syndrome. The following are risk factors[1,21]:

- Fasting plasma glucose above 100 mg/dL or taking medications to lower elevated blood glucose.
- HDL cholesterol below 40 mg/dL in men and below 50 mg/dL in women, or taking medications to raise HDL levels.
- Triglycerides above 150 mg/dL or taking medications to lower elevated triglycerides.
- Waist circumference above 40 inches (102 cm) in men, or above 35 inches (88 cm) in women.
- Blood pressure (BP) above 130 mm Hg systolic or above 85 mm Hg diastolic, or taking antihypertensive medications.

Women and Heart Disease

Substantial progress has been made in the awareness, treatment, and prevention of CVD in women.[22] In 2007, CVD still caused approximately one death per minute among women in the United States.[22] After age 65 years, a higher percentage of women than men have hypertension. Average body weight continues to increase, with nearly 2 out of every 3 women in the United States above age 20 years now being overweight or obese.[22] The average age for the first acute MI in men is 65.8 years, and in women, it is 70.4 years.[1] The incidence of CVD is two to three times higher among postmenopausal women than among women who are premenopausal.[1] In the past, it seemed logical to prescribe *hormone replacement therapy* (HRT) to treat the

symptoms of menopause.[22] Current 2011 guidelines do not recommend the use of hormone therapy for primary or secondary prevention of CVD.[22] Data from the Framingham Heart Study indicate the lifetime risk for cardiovascular disease is more than one in two for women at age 40 years, and in the 2007 update of *Guidelines for the Prevention of CVD in Women*, a new algorithm for risk classification in women was adopted that stratified women's risk into 3 categories:

- *At high risk:* documented CAD or CVD risk equivalents, such as the presence of documented CVD, diabetes mellitus, end stage or chronic kidney disease, or 10-year predicted risk for CHD>20%
- *At risk:* given the presence of subclinical vascular disease or poor exercise tolerance on treadmill testing
- *At optimal risk:* in the setting of a Framingham risk score less than 10%, absence of major CVD risk factors, and engagement in a healthy lifestyle.[1,22]

In 2011, these guidelines added an acknowledgement of several 10-year risk equations for the prediction of 10-year global CVD risk, such as the updated Framingham CVD risk profile and the Reynolds risk score for women.[22]

The American Heart Association (AHA) defined a new concept of ideal cardiovascular health in women as follows:

- Absence of clinical CVD and the presence of all ideal levels of total cholesterol (<200 mg/dL)
- Blood pressure (<120/80 mm Hg)
- Fasting blood glucose (<100 mg/dL)
- Adherence to healthy behaviors
- Lean body mass index (<25 kg/m^2)
- Participation in physical activity at recommended levels
- Cessation of smoking
- Pursuit of eating pattern as suggested by *Dietary Approaches to Stop Hypertension* (DASH diet)[23]

Cardiovascular disease kills more than 500,000 women annually in the United States. Mortality rates for women after an acute MI are higher than for men: 38% compared with 25%. Risk factors associated with acute MI more strongly in women than in men include hypertension, diabetes mellitus, alcohol intake, and physical inactivity.[22,23] Many reasons contribute to higher mortality from acute MI in women, and these include waiting longer to seek medical care, having smaller coronary arteries, being older when symptoms occur, and experiencing very different symptoms from those of men of the same age.[24,25,26]

Vascular Inflammation

The link between vascular inflammation and atherosclerotic disease is well established[27,28] (see the section "Pathophysiology of Coronary Artery Disease"). Research to identify prognostic and sensitive inflammatory markers is ongoing.

C-Reactive Protein

The inflammatory marker most frequently cited is *C-reactive protein* (CRP). It is measured as high-sensitivity CRP (hs-CRP).[27-29] CRP is associated with an increased risk of development of other cardiovascular risk factors including diabetes, hypertension, and weight gain.[28-30] The higher the hs-CRP value, the greater is the risk of a coronary event, especially if all

TABLE 15-4 C-REACTIVE PROTEIN AND RISK FOR CORONARY ARTERY DISEASE

CATEGORY	HS-CRP LEVEL* (mg/L)
Low risk (normal)	<1
Moderate risk	1-3
High risk	>3

*Values above 1 mg/dL increase the risk for CAD, but test results are not valid in the presence of infection or other inflammatory condition. Normal values may vary slightly between clinical laboratories; however, values below 1 mg/dL are usually considered normal. A test result greater than 10 mg/L suggests a noncoronary source of inflammation or infection.
CAD, Coronary artery disease; C-reactive, cross-reactive; hs-CRP, high-sensitivity C-reactive protein.
Based on data from Pearson TA, et al. Markers of inflammation and cardiovascular disease, application to clinical and public health practice: a statement for healthcare professionals from the Centers for Disease Control and Prevention and the American Heart Association. Circulation. 2003;107(3):499.

other potential causes of systemic inflammation such as infection can be ruled out. Value ranges for hs-CRP are shown in Table 15-4. If other systemic inflammatory conditions such as bronchitis or urinary tract infection are present, the hs-CRP test loses all predictive value.[28,29] CRP and other inflammatory markers are used to estimate the probability of future acute coronary events.[29,30] During ACS events, there is widespread activation of neutrophils in the cardiac circulation (measured from the coronary sinus), which suggests that inflammation is not limited to one unstable plaque.[31]

Coronary Artery Disease Risk Equivalents

Certain medical conditions are risk equivalents of CAD. A risk equivalent means the person has the same risk of having an acute MI as if he or she had coronary heart disease already. Two noncardiac medical conditions considered risk equivalents for CAD: diabetes mellitus and chronic kidney disease.[30] PAD and cerebral vascular disease are atherosclerotic conditions that are also considered CAD risk equivalents.[30]

Multifactorial Risk

CAD has multifactorial causation; the greater the number of risk factors, the greater the risk of developing CAD.[1,3,30,32] The best time for an individual to make lifestyle changes is before the symptoms of CAD occur. Patients with two or more risk factors or with one or more of the CAD risk-equivalent diseases have the greatest potential to benefit from risk factor reduction and lifestyle change.[30] The major risk factors for developing CAD have been extensively documented in large epidemiologic studies: smoking, family history, adverse lipid profile, and elevated blood pressure.

Primary versus Secondary Prevention of Coronary Artery Disease

If a person has symptoms of CAD or has previously had an ACS event, the goal of any lifestyle change or medication is called secondary prevention, or preventing another heart attack.[11] If an individual matches the risk profile described previously but does not have symptoms of CAD or has not had an acute MI, the treatment plan is described as primary prevention. The constellation of cardiac risk factors is well established and can predict development of CAD for most populations in the developed world.[30]

Pathophysiology of Coronary Artery Disease

CAD is a progressive atherosclerotic disorder of the coronary arteries that results in narrowing or complete occlusion. Atherosclerosis affects the medium-sized arteries that perfuse the heart and other major organs. Normal arterial walls are composed of three layers: 1) the intima (inner lining), 2) the media (middle muscular layer), and 3) the adventitia (outer coat).

Development of Atherosclerosis

Atherosclerosis is a chronic inflammatory disorder that is characterized by an accumulation of macrophages and T lymphocytes in the arterial intimal wall. A high LDL cholesterol concentration is one of the triggers of vascular inflammation. The inflammation injures the wall, allowing the LDL cholesterol to move into the vessel wall below the endothelial surface.[6] Blood monocytes adhere to endothelial cells and migrate into the vessel wall. Within the artery wall, some monocytes differentiate into macrophages that unite with and then internalize LDL cholesterol. The foam cells that result are the marker cells of atherosclerosis.[6]

Elevated LDL cholesterol levels promote low-level endothelial inflammation, which allows lipoproteins to infiltrate the intimal vessel wall. After it has infiltrated under the endothelium, LDL cholesterol tends to stay within the vessel wall rather than return to the circulation. This contrasts with the actions of HDL cholesterol, which enters the vessel wall, helps efflux cholesterol from cells, and then returns to the circulation.[6] The actions of HDL cholesterol may help minimize the number of foam cells in the artery wall.[6]

Atherosclerotic Plaque Rupture

When a mature atherosclerotic plaque develops, it is not uniform in composition. It has a lipid liquid center filled with procoagulant factors. A connective tissue fibrous cap covers the top of the fluid lipid center.[29,31] The abrupt rupture of this cap allows procoagulant lipids to flood into the vessel lumen and rapidly form a coronary thrombosis, as shown in Table 15-5. As the enlarging clot blocks blood flow through the coronary artery, a "heart attack" will occur unless adequate collateral circulation from other coronary vessels occurs. Symptoms and suggested cardiac interventions at appropriate stages in development of CAD are listed in Table 15-5.

Plaques that are likely to rupture are saturated with macrophages and other inflammatory cells. These vulnerable plaques are usually not obstructive and are situated at bends or branch points in the arterial tree.[3] It is not known what factors cause the fibrous cap to rupture or erode. As deep fissures in the cap expose the procoagulant factors to the blood plasma, an unstoppable cycle is put into motion. When platelets in the bloodstream are exposed to collagen, necrotic debris, von Willebrand

TABLE 15-5   TIMELINE OF ATHEROGENESIS DEVELOPMENT DEPICTED BY LONGITUDINAL SECTION OF AN ARTERY

ATHEROGENESIS OR THROMBOGENESIS	ASSOCIATED SYMPTOMS	CARDIAC INTERVENTION
A. Normal artery, normal vessel wall B. Lipids in bloodstream C. Extracellular lipid accumulates in the intima of the artery (atheroma)	No symptoms No symptoms No symptoms	Primary prevention of CAD recommended: consume a low-fat diet, take regular physical exercise, avoid smoking, and achieve normal BMI
D. Lipid accumulation evolves to become a fatty-fibrous (atherosclerotic) lesion; some lesions contain a lipid interior covered by a fibrous cap	Chest pain with exercise that is relieved by rest or NTG (stable angina) or possibly no symptoms until the lesion fills more than 75% of the vessel lumen	PCI if stable angina is present and CAD is diagnosed by cardiac catheterization
E. Rupture of the cap allows lipid in the center to be released into the bloodstream, stimulating clot formation (thrombogenesis)	Chest pain not relieved by rest or NTG (ACS—unstable angina)	Call 911 for immediate transport to a hospital, preferably one with experience treating ACS
F. Fresh clot blocks the vessel; spasm of the artery may occur near the thrombus	Chest pain unrelieved by rest or NTG—severity, location of angina, and associated symptoms vary greatly among individuals (ACS—acute MI)	Emergency intervention to open the artery: fibrinolytic or catheter-based procedure (PCI)
G. Vessel is open, but the atherosclerotic lesion remains	No symptoms	Secondary prevention of CAD to prevent repeat MI; beta-blockers to prevent arrhythmias; ACE-1 medications to prevent ventricular remodeling and heart failure; elective PCI

Illustration modified from Antman EM, et al. ACC/AHA guidelines for the management of patients with ST-elevation myocardial infarction—executive summary. *Circulation.* 2004;110:588.

ACE-I, Angiotensin-converting enzyme inhibitor; *ACS*, acute coronary syndrome; *BMI*, body mass index; *CAD*, coronary artery disease; *MI*, myocardial infarction; *NTG*, nitroglycerin; *PCI*, percutaneous coronary intervention.

factor, and thromboxane, a clot is formed and can occlude the coronary artery. Highly fibrotic plaques do not rupture. The type of atherosclerotic plaque that is prone to rupture has a weak fibrous cap and a large amount of liquid cholesterol within the core (see Table 15-5).

Plaque Regression

A reduction in blood cholesterol decreases atherosclerotic plaque size by decreasing the amount of liquid cholesterol within the plaque core.[9] Lowering cholesterol levels does not change the dimensions of the fibrous or calcified portions of the plaque. However, lower cholesterol levels reduce vascular inflammation and make vulnerable plaque less likely to rupture.

Acute Coronary Syndrome

The term *acute coronary syndrome* (ACS) is used to describe the array of clinical presentations of CAD that range from unstable angina to acute MI (see Table 15-5).[1,2,3,6] An acute MI is generally described by patients as a "heart attack." The following section discusses stable manifestations of CAD (stable angina) and acute manifestations described as an ACS (unstable angina and acute MI). Figure 15-1 is a concept map of ACS.

Angina

Angina pectoris, or chest pain, caused by myocardial ischemia is not a separate disease, but rather a symptom of CAD. It is caused by a blockage or spasm of a coronary artery, leading to diminished myocardial blood supply. The lack of oxygen causes myocardial ischemia, which is felt as chest discomfort, pressure, or pain. Angina may occur anywhere in the chest, neck, arms, or back, but the most commonly described location is pain or pressure behind the sternum. The pain often radiates to the left arm but can also radiate down both arms and to the back, the shoulder, the jaw, or the neck (Fig. 15-2). Angina symptoms are not the same for all individuals, many patients may describe pressure or discomfort rather than pain, and

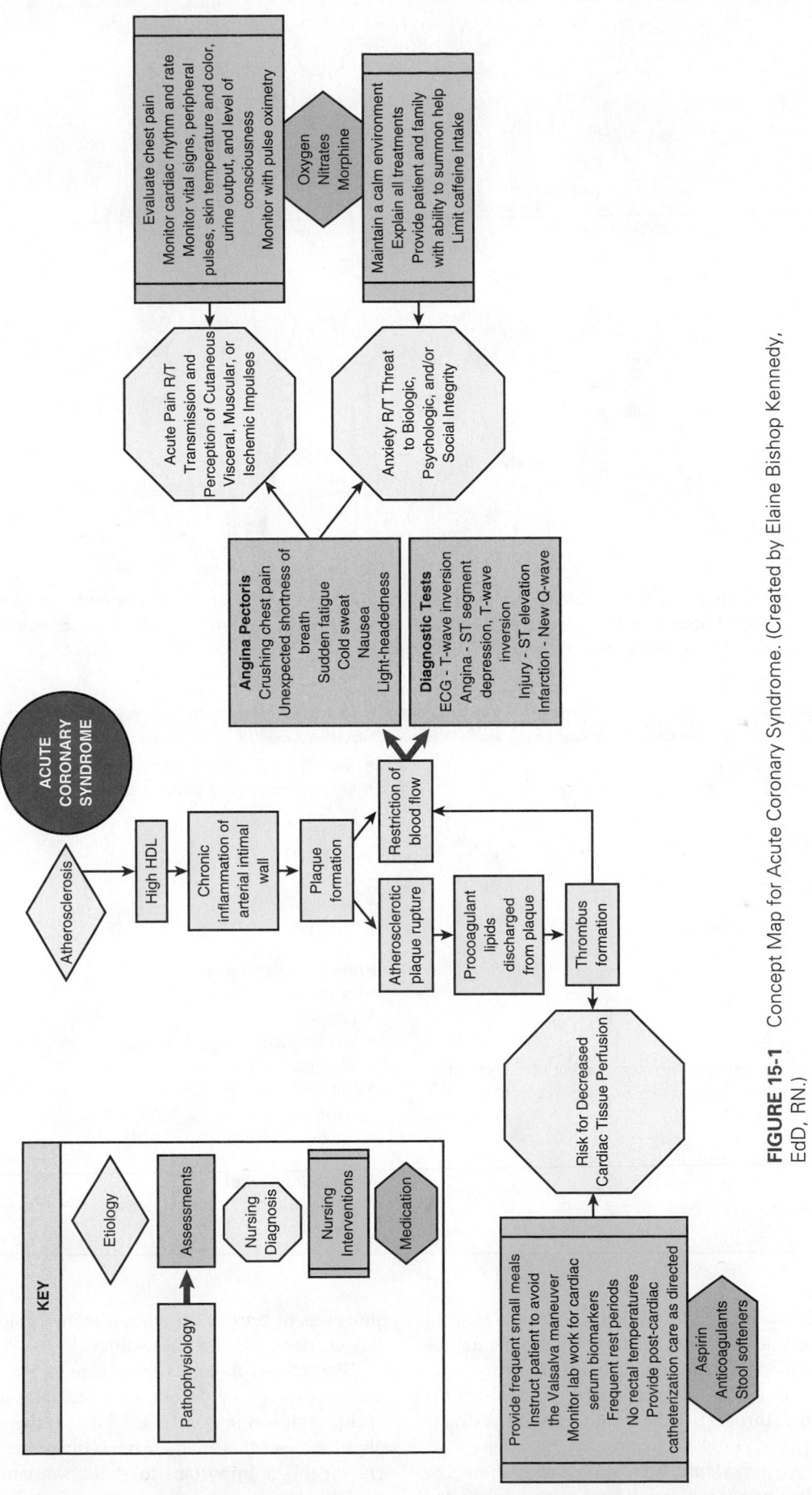

FIGURE 15-1 Concept Map for Acute Coronary Syndrome. (Created by Elaine Bishop Kennedy, EdD, RN.)

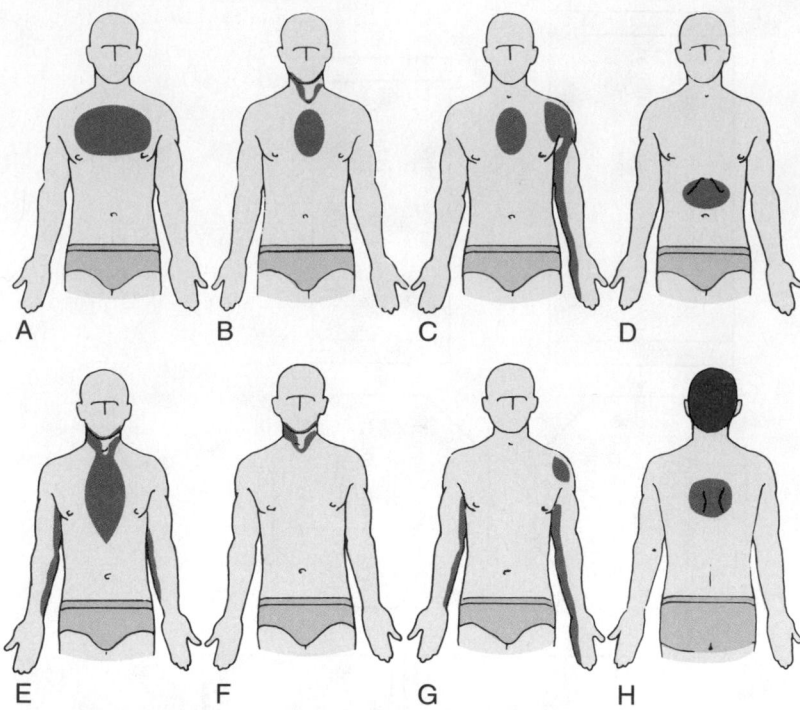

FIGURE 15-2   Common Sites for Anginal Pain. *A,* Upper part of chest; *B,* beneath sternum, radiating to neck and jaw; *C,* beneath sternum, radiating down left arm; *D,* epigastric; *E,* epigastric, radiating to neck, jaw, and arms; *F,* neck and jaw; *G,* left shoulder; *H,* intrascapular.

BOX 15-3   CHARACTERISTICS OF ANGINA PECTORIS

Location
- Beneath sternum, radiating to neck and jaw
- Upper chest
- Beneath sternum, radiating down left arm
- Epigastric
- Epigastric, radiating to neck, jaw, and arms
- Neck and jaw
- Left shoulder, inner aspect of both arms
- Intrascapular

Duration
- Less than 5 minutes
- Less than 5 minutes (stable)
- Longer than 5 minutes or worsening symptoms without relief from rest or sublingual nitroglycerin indicates preinfarction symptoms (unstable)

Quality
- Sensation of pressure or heavy weight on the chest
- Feeling of tightness, like a vise
- Visceral quality (deep, heavy, squeezing, aching)
- Burning sensation

- Shortness of breath, with feeling of suffocation
- Most severe pain ever experienced

Radiation
- Medial aspect of left arm
- Jaw
- Left shoulder
- Right arm

Precipitating Factors
- Exertion or exercise
- Cold weather
- Exercising after a large, heavy meal
- Walking against the wind
- Emotional upset
- Fright, anger
- Coitus

Medication Relief
- Usually within 45 seconds to 5 minutes after sublingual nitroglycerin administration

---

presenting symptoms can be highly individualized, as described in Box 15-3. Patients and families must be taught that angina does not always present in the dramatic heart attack scenario, as often portrayed on television and in movies, in which the person clutches the throat or chest and exhibits extreme distress.[2]

Angina Symptom Equivalents. Men and women should be made aware of angina symptom equivalents such as unexpected

shortness of breath, breaking out in a cold sweat, or sudden fatigue, nausea, or lightheadedness.[15]

Women and Angina. Many women experience a variety of different symptoms before an acute MI and during the acute event, as shown in Box 15-4.[32,33] The recognition and publicity about the fact that many women do not experience "crushing chest pain" is important to avoid women's symptoms being trivialized by clinicians.[37] It is important that women are made

BOX 15-4 CARDIOVASCULAR SYMPTOMS EXPERIENCED BY WOMEN BEFORE ACUTE MYOCARDIAL INFARCTION

SYMPTOMS 1 MONTH BEFORE ACUTE MI	SYMPTOMS DURING ACUTE MI
• Unusual fatigue (71%)	• Shortness of breath (58%)
• Sleep disturbance (48%)	• Weakness (55%)
• Shortness of breath (42%)	• Unusual fatigue (43%)
• Indigestion (39%)	• Cold sweat (39%)
• Anxiety (36%)	• Dizziness (39%)
• Heart racing (27%)	• Nausea (36%)
• Arms weak or heavy (25%)	• Arm heaviness or weakness (35%)
• Changes in thinking or memory (24%)	• Ache in arms (32%)
• Vision change (23%)	• Heat or flushing (32%)
• Loss of appetite (22%)	• Indigestion (31%)
• Hands or arms tingling (22%)	• Pain centered high in chest (31%)
• Difficulty breathing at night (19%)	• Heart racing (23%)

From McSweeney JC, et al: Women's early warning symptoms of acute myocardial infarction. *Circulation.* 2003;108(21):2619.
MI, Myocardial infarction.

aware of *angina symptom equivalents* such as unexplained shortness of breath, breaking out in a cold sweat, or sudden fatigue, nausea, or lightheadedness.[2] More women die every year in the United States of ACS compared with men, a fact that is largely unknown by health care providers.[33,34]

Stable Angina. *Stable angina* is predictable and caused by similar precipitating factors each time; typically, it is exercise induced. Patients become used to the pattern of this type of angina and may describe it as "my usual chest pain." Pain control should be achieved within 5 minutes of rest and by taking sublingual nitroglycerin. Ischemia and chest pain occur when myocardial demand from exertion exceeds the fixed blood oxygen supply. Additional information on CAD and stable angina is provided in Box 15-5.

Unstable Angina. *Unstable angina* is defined as a change in a previously established stable pattern of angina. It is part of the continuum of ACS. Unstable angina usually is more intense than stable angina, may awaken the person from sleep, or may necessitate more than nitrates for pain relief. A change in the level or frequency of symptoms requires immediate medical evaluation. Severe angina that persists for more than 5 minutes, worsens in intensity, and is not relieved by one nitroglycerin tablet is a medical emergency, and the patient or a family member must call 911 immediately.[3] The 911 (Emergency Medical Services [EMS]) system is available to 90% of the population of the United States.[3,35] Family and friends are discouraged from driving a person experiencing unstable angina to the hospital and instead are urged to call 911. Patients should be instructed never to drive themselves but to contact the EMS by calling 911.

Unstable angina is an indication of atherosclerotic plaque instability. It can signal atherosclerotic plaque rupture and thrombus formation that can lead to MI. The patient who comes to the emergency department with recent-onset unstable angina but who has nonspecific or nonelevated ST-segment

changes on the 12-lead electrocardiogram (ECG) may be admitted to the critical care unit to rule out MI. If the symptoms are typical of an MI, it is important to treat the patient according to the latest published guidelines because not all patients who experience an MI have ST-segment elevation on the 12-lead ECG.[2,14,15]

Variant Angina. *Variant angina,* or Prinzmetal angina, is caused by a dynamic obstruction from intense vasoconstriction of a coronary artery.[36] Spasm can occur with or without atherosclerotic lesions. Variant angina commonly occurs when the individual is at rest, and it is often cyclic, occurring at the same time every day. Smoking, alcohol use, and illegal stimulant drug (cocaine) use may precipitate spasm. A definitive diagnosis of variant angina is made during a cardiac catheterization study. Signs of spasm include ST-segment elevation and chest pain. Coronary artery spasm can occur with or without CAD. The prognosis is excellent when no significant coronary artery stenosis exists. Coronary artery spasm is treated with nitroglycerin or calcium channel blockers to vasodilate the coronary arteries.

Silent Ischemia. *Silent ischemia* describes a situation in which objective evidence of ischemia is observed on an ECG monitor but the person does not complain of anginal symptoms. Silent ischemia can occur in many clinical situations, as described in Box 15-6. One third of patients who are having a heart attack do not report chest pain as a symptom.[2] Patients with diabetes are at particular risk for silent ischemia. Many patients who have had type 2 diabetes for more than 10 years have developed *autonomic neuropathy,* which decreases their ability to experience chest pain. Patients with diabetes may misinterpret angina-equivalent symptoms such as nausea, vomiting, and diaphoresis as signaling a disruption in glucose control rather than a sign of myocardial ischemia.

Medical Management

Accurate assessment of chest pain symptoms is essential if unstable angina is to be recognized and treated effectively. Factors to consider when assessing chest pain are listed in Box 15-7. An important reason to ask questions about the chest pain is to differentiate between stable and unstable angina. The change from stable to unstable angina is potentially life threatening for the patient. If the ST segments are elevated or a newly documented left bundle branch block (LBBB) is seen on the 12-lead ECG, the patient should be treated for acute MI.[2] However, if these classic ECG signs are missing and the chest pain continues, the current pharmacologic treatment of choice is aspirin (if the patient cannot tolerate aspirin, then a thienopyridine such as clopidogrel can be given). Patients with definite unstable angina or non–ST elevation myocardial infarction (UA or NSTEMI) should receive dual antiplatelet therapy on admission if an invasive strategy is imminent. A glycoprotein (GP) IIb/IIIa inhibitor is administered unless bivalirudin is chosen; and a loading dose of clopidogrel is given at least 6 hours prior to the procedure. Patients undergoing noninvasive treatment should receive aspirin and a thienopyridine (clopidogrel, prasugrel or ticagrelor) for 1 month and ideally up to 1 year. If symptoms persist, a diagnostic angiography is performed. A stress test should be performed on patients who are

BOX 15-5 EVIDENCE-BASED PRACTICE

Coronary Artery Disease and Stable Angina

QSEN Strong evidence exists that the following lifestyle interventions help to prevent CAD:

- Diet
  - Diet low in salt and high in fiber, fruit, vegetables, and grains.
  - All dietary fat less than 30% of total calories; saturated fat less than 7%.
  - Limit glucose in diet (simple sugars).
  - Limit calories if overweight.
  - Omega-3 fatty acids included in diet.
- Exercise
  - Start by walking more often and increase physical exercise from there. Refer to cardiac rehabilitation program.
- Obesity
  - Achieve healthy body weight.
- Addiction
  - Stop cigarette smoking. Avoid exposure to environmental (secondhand) tobacco smoke at home and at work.
  - Limit alcohol intake.

Strong evidence exists that the following diagnostic procedures help the patient with angina:

- When a patient presents with chest pain, quickly obtaining a detailed history of symptoms, focused physical examination, and risk factor assessment can help determine whether the probability of CAD is low, intermediate, or high.
- Initial laboratory tests include hemoglobin, fasting blood glucose, lipid panel, cardiac enzymes.
- Obtain a baseline 12-lead ECG at rest, even if chest pain is not present.
- Obtain a 12-lead ECG during an episode of chest pain.
- Obtain a chest radiograph if symptoms of heart failure are present.
- Obtain an exercise 12-lead ECG if the condition is stable and symptoms suggest CAD or if the condition is stable with complete LBBB or RBBB that makes the ECG difficult to interpret for ischemia.
- Obtain cardiac echocardiography for patients with a systolic murmur suggestive of aortic stenosis.
- Use cardiac echocardiography to determine extent of left ventricular (LV) hypertrophy or dysfunction.
- Stress cardiac echocardiography is recommended for patients with greater than 1 mm of ST-segment depression at rest (stress may be by physical exercise or by pharmacologic stimulation).
- Coronary angiography (typically as part of a cardiac catheterization procedure) is recommended for patients at high risk for adverse coronary events.

Initial Pharmacologic and Lifestyle Treatment Recommendations

- The goal of treatment is to eliminate chest pain.
- The 10 most important elements of CAD and stable angina management can be remembered using the A to E mnemonic:

  A—Aspirin and antianginal medications: Prescribe daily, low-dose (75 to 325 mg) aspirin; oral nitrates; and sublingual nitroglycerin for episodes of angina.

  B—Beta-blockers and blood pressure: Use ACEI and beta-blockers to decrease blood pressure to less than 140/90 mm Hg if no other CAD risk factors are present and to less than 130/80 mm Hg if diabetes or kidney disease are present.

  C—Cholesterol and cigarettes: Obtain a fasting lipid profile. Recommend diet or lipid reduction medication therapy (statin) to lower LDL-C to less than 100 mg/dL (<70 mg/dL if achievable), increase HDL-C to more than 40 mg/dL for men or more than 50 mg/dL for women, and reduce triglycerides to less than 150 mg/dL.

  Recommend adding plant stanols or sterols (2 g/day) or viscous fiber (>10 g/day), or both, to the diet to further lower LDL-C; add dietary omega-3 fatty acids in the form of fish or capsule (1 g/day). Always ask about tobacco use; strongly recommend smoking cessation; encourage nicotine replacement therapy (nicotine patches or gum) as needed.

  D—Diet and diabetes: Prescribe a low-fat, calorie-appropriate diet and provide nutritional consultation as needed to achieve a fasting blood glucose level of 70 to 100 mg/dL and HbA$_{1c}$ of less than 6.5%.

  E—Education and exercise: Provide education about risk factor modification and the CAD disease process; recommend daily exercise for 30 to 60 minutes (ideal) or at least seven times each week (minimum of 5 days per week). A BMI between 18.5 and 24.9 kg/m^2 and waist less than 40 inches for men or less than 35 inches for women should be recommended. Treat depression, if present. HRT is not recommended as a treatment for symptoms of coronary heart disease. Influenza vaccination is recommended.

Interventional and Surgical Recommendations for Stable High-Risk Patients

Patients are risk stratified according to their symptoms and the results of cardiac diagnostic tests.

- Percutaneous catheter interventions (PCI)
  - PCI is more frequently performed than open heart surgery for relief of anginal symptoms.
- Coronary artery bypass surgery (CABG)
  - For patients with left main occlusion or multivessel disease
  - For patients with two-vessel disease who have significant proximal LAD stenosis and an LV ejection fraction less than 50%

References

Anderson JL, et al. 2011 ACCF/AHA Focused Update Incorporated Into the ACC/AHA 2007 Guidelines for the Management of Patients With Unstable Angina/Non-ST-Elevation Myocardial Infarction: a Report of the American College of Cardiology Foundation/American Heart Association Task Force on Practice Guidelines, *Circulation*. 2011;123:e426.

Fihn SD, et al. 2012 ACCF/AHA/ACP/AATS/PCNA/SCAI/STS Guideline for the Diagnosis and Management of Patients With Stable Ischemic Heart Disease: A Report of the American College of Cardiology Foundation/American Heart Association Task Force on Practice Guidelines, and the American College of Physicians, American Association for Thoracic Surgery, Preventive Cardiovascular Nurses Association, Society for Cardiovascular Angiography and Interventions, and Society of Thoracic Surgeons. *Circulation*. 2012; 126(25):e354-e471.

Mosca L, et al. Effectiveness-based guidelines for the prevention of cardiovascular disease prevention in women-2011 update: a guideline from The American Heart Association. *Circulation*. 2011;123:1243.

Wright SR, et al. 2011 ACC/AHA Focused Update of the guidelines for the management of patients with unstable angina/non-ST elevation myocardial infarction: a report from the American College of Cardiology/American Heart Association Task Force on Practice Guidelines developed in collaboration with the American College of Emergency Physicians, Society for Cardiovascular Angiography and Interventions, and Society for Thoracic Surgeons. *J Am Coll Cardiol*. 2011;57:1920.

ACEI, Angiotensin-converting enzyme inhibitors; *BMI*, body mass index; *CAD*, coronary artery disease; *ECG*, electrocardiogram; *HbA$_{1c}$*, glycosylated hemoglobin; *HDL-C*, high-density lipoprotein cholesterol; *HRT*, hormone replacement therapy; *LAD*, left anterior descending coronary artery; *LBBB*, left bundle branch block; *LDL-C*, low-density lipoprotein cholesterol; *LV*, left ventricle; *RBBB*, right bundle branch block.

BOX 15-6 CLINICAL CHARACTERISTICS OF SILENT ISCHEMIA

- Objective electrocardiographic (ECG) evidence of myocardial ischemia without any chest pain or symptoms
- No anginal symptoms after a previous myocardial infarction (MI), but objective ECG evidence of myocardial ischemia continues
- Symptoms of angina with some episodes of ischemia and no symptoms with other ischemic events; patient may or may not have had a previous MI

BOX 15-7 FACTORS TO CONSIDER WHEN ASSESSING CHEST PAIN

- Onset: Was it sudden or gradual?
- Duration: Did pain last seconds or minutes? How soon after onset did the patient call for help?
- Precipitating factors: Was the patient up and moving around?
- Location: Was pain substernal? Was it located in same area as previous pain?
- Radiation: Did pain radiate to the jaw, neck, arm, or shoulder?
- Quality: Was pain similar to previous anginal pain? less painful or more painful?
- Intensity: On a scale of 1 to 10, where would the patient rate the pain?
- Relieving factors: What made the pain better—changing position, nitroglycerin, oxygen, the presence of the nurse?
- Aggravating factors: Did things such as the environment, telephone calls, or waiting for help worsen the pain?
- Associated symptoms: Was the pain accompanied by nausea, vomiting, diaphoresis, or dyspnea?
- Emotional response: Was there an emotional response that intensified the pain—anxiety, fear, anger?

◎ BOX 15-8 NURSING DIAGNOSES

Coronary Artery Disease and Angina

- Acute Pain, related to transmission and perception of cutaneous, visceral, muscular, or ischemic impulses, p. 1123
- Risk for Decreased Cardiac Tissue Perfusion, p. 1155
- Activity Intolerance, related to cardiopulmonary dysfunction, p. 1119
- Powerlessness, related to lack of control over current situation, p. 1152
- Anxiety, related to threat to biologic, psychologic, or social integrity, p. 1125
- Deficient Knowledge, related to lack of previous exposure to information, p. 1134 (see Box 15-10, Patient Education for Coronary Artery Disease and Angina)

---

not undergoing invasive therapy for their UA/NSTEMI and if negative the GP IIb/IIIa inhibitor can be discontinued and unfractionated heparin (UFH) administered for 48 hours.

Nursing Management

Nursing management of the patient with CAD and angina incorporates a variety of nursing diagnoses (Box 15-8). Nursing interventions focus on early identification of myocardial ischemia, control of chest pain, recognition of complications, maintenance of a calm environment, and patient and family education.

Recognizing Myocardial Ischemia

Complaints of chest discomfort (angina) must be evaluated quickly because angina is an indicator of myocardial ischemia (see Box 15-7). The patient is asked to rate the intensity of the chest discomfort on a scale of 0 to 10. Pain levels must be assessed with sensitivity to differences in cultural manifestations of pain. The term *chest pain* is not to be used exclusively because some patients describe their angina as "pressure" or "heaviness." It is important to document the characteristics of the pain and the patient's heart rate and rhythm, BP, respirations, temperature, skin color, peripheral pulses, urine output, mentation, and overall tissue perfusion. A 12-lead ECG is used to identify the area of ischemic myocardium. The major concern is that the chest pain may represent preinfarction angina, and early identification is essential so that the patient can be immediately treated. Treatment may include transfer to the cardiac catheterization laboratory for a coronary arteriogram and opening of a blocked artery. If the hospital does not have a cardiac catheterization laboratory, GP IIb/IIIa receptor blockers may be infused to prevent the evolution of the acute MI before transfer.[2,14,15]

Relieving Chest Pain MONA

In the critical care unit, control of angina is achieved by a combination of supplemental oxygen, nitrates, analgesia, and surveillance of the angina and of the effects of pharmacologic therapy.

- *Oxygen:* All patients with acute ischemic pain are administered supplemental oxygen to increase myocardial oxygenation. Pulse oximetry is used to guide therapy and maintain oxygen saturation above 90% unless patient has a history of chronic obstructive pulmonary disease (COPD) and is a carbon dioxide (CO_2) retainer.
- *Nitrates:* A combination of intravenous and sublingual nitroglycerin is used to vasodilate the coronary arteries and decrease pain. After nitrate administration, the critical care nurse closely observes the patient for relief of chest pain, for return of the ST segment to baseline, and for the potential development of unwanted side effects such as hypotension and headache. Administration of a nitrate is avoided if the SBP is below 90 mm Hg. Medication interactions with nitrates are another potential cause for concern. The phosphodiesterase inhibitor medication *sildenafil* is prescribed for several conditions including pulmonary hypertension (Revatio) and erectile dysfunction (Viagra). Sildenafil and nitrates in combination may contribute to a precipitous fall in blood pressure.[3]
- *Analgesia:* Morphine (2 to 4 mg given intravenously) is the analgesic opiate of choice for preinfarction angina. It relieves pain and decreases fear and anxiety. After administration, the critical care nurse assesses the patient for pain relief and the development of unwanted side effects such as hypotension and respiratory depression.[2,15]
- *Aspirin:* Chewing an oral non–enteric-coated aspirin (162 to 325 mg) at the beginning of chest pain has been shown to reduce mortality. The nonenteric formulation is preferred because it increases absorption in the mouth when chewed, not swallowed.[2,15]

Maintaining a Calm Environment

Patients admitted to a critical care unit with unstable angina experience extreme anxiety and fear of death. The critical care nurse is faced with the challenge of ensuring that the elements of a calm environment that can alleviate the patient's fear and anxiety are maintained, while being ready at all times to respond to an acute emergency such as a cardiac arrest or to assist with emergency intubation or insertion of hemodynamic monitoring catheters. Additional aspects of acute cardiac care are listed in Box 15-9.

Patient Education

In the critical care unit, the patient's ability to retain educational information is severely affected by stress and pain. Patient education topics that should be discussed when the clinical condition has stabilized are listed in Box 15-10. It is essential to teach avoidance of the Valsalva maneuver, which is defined as forced expiration against a closed glottis. This can be explained to the patient as "bearing down" during defecation or breath holding when repositioning in bed. The Valsalva maneuver causes an increase in intrathoracic pressure, which decreases venous return to the right side of the heart and can be associated with low blood pressure and symptomatic bradycardia.

After the anginal pain is controlled, longer-term education of the patient and the family can begin. Points to cover include: 1) risk factor modification, 2) signs and symptoms of angina, 3) when to call the physician, 4) medications, and 5) dealing with emotions and stress. However, because the acute hospital length of stay for uncomplicated angina is usually less than 3 days, referral to a cardiac rehabilitation program for a controlled exercise program and risk factor modification after discharge may be the most helpful teaching intervention a critical care nurse can provide. Clinical practice guidelines for the management of CAD and stable angina are listed in Box 15-5 earlier in the chapter.

◎ BOX 15-9   NIC

Cardiac Care: Acute

Definition

Limitation of complications for a patient recently experiencing an episode of an imbalance between myocardial oxygen supply and demand resulting in impaired cardiac function

Activities

- Evaluate chest pain (e.g., intensity, location, radiation, duration, and precipitating and alleviating factors).
- Instruct the patient on the importance of immediately reporting any chest discomfort.
- Provide immediate and continuous means to summon nurse, and let the patient and family know calls will be answered immediately.
- Monitor electrocardiogram (ECG) for ST changes, as appropriate.
- Perform a comprehensive appraisal of cardiac status, including peripheral circulation.
- Monitor cardiac rhythm and rate.
- Auscultate heart sounds.
- Recognize the frustration and fright caused by inability to communicate and exposure to strange machinery and environment.
- Auscultate lungs for crackles or other adventitious sounds.
- Monitor the effectiveness of oxygen therapy, if appropriate.
- Monitor determinants of oxygen delivery (e.g., PaO_2 and hemoglobin levels and cardiac output), if appropriate.
- Monitor neurological status.
- Monitor intake and output, urine output, and daily weight, as appropriate.
- Select best ECG lead for continuous monitoring, as appropriate.
- Obtain 12-lead ECG, as appropriate.
- Draw serum, CK, LDH, and AST levels, as appropriate.
- Monitor kidney function (e.g., BUN and Serum Creatine [Cr] levels), as appropriate.
- Monitor liver function tests, if appropriate.
- Monitor lab values for electrolytes that may increase the risk of dysrhythmias (e.g., serum potassium and magnesium), as appropriate.
- Obtain chest radiograph, as appropriate.

- Monitor trends in blood pressure and hemodynamic parameters, if available (e.g., central venous pressure and pulmonary artery occlusion pressure [PAOP]).
- Provide small, frequent meals
- Provide appropriate cardiac diet (i.e., limit intake of caffeine, sodium, cholesterol, and food high in fat)
- Refrain from giving oral stimulants
- Substitute artificial salt, if appropriate
- Limit environmental stimuli
- Maintain an environment conducive to rest and healing
- Avoid causing intense emotional situations.
- Identify the patient's methods of handling stress.
- Promote effective techniques for reducing stress.
- Perform relaxation therapy, if appropriate.
- Refrain from arguing.
- Discourage decision making when the patient is under severe stress.
- Avoid overheating or chilling the patient.
- Refrain from inserting a rectal tube.
- Refrain from taking rectal temperatures.
- Refrain from doing a rectal or vaginal examination.
- Delay bathing, if appropriate.
- Instruct the patient to avoid activities that result in the Valsalva maneuver (e.g., straining during bowel movement).
- Administer medications that will prevent episodes of the Valsalva maneuver (e.g., stool softeners, antiemetics), as appropriate.
- Prevent peripheral thrombus formation (i.e., turn every 2 hours and administer low-dose anticoagulants).
- Administer medications to relieve or prevent pain and ischemia, as needed.
- Monitor effectiveness of medication.
- Instruct the patient and family on the aims of care and how progress will be measured.
- Ensure that all staff are aware of these goals and are working together to provide consistent care.
- Offer spiritual support to the patient and family (i.e., contact a member of the clergy), as appropriate.

Modified from Bulechek GM, et al. *Nursing interventions classification (NIC)*, 6th ed. St. Louis, Mosby; 2013.
AST, Aspartate amino transferase; *BUN*, blood urea nitrogen; *CK*, creatine kinase; *LDH*, lactate dehydrogenase; *PaO₂*, partial pressure of oxygen dissolved in arterial blood.

Coronary Artery Disease and Angina

- Angina: Describe signs and symptoms such as pain, pressure, and heaviness in chest, arms, or jaw.
- Preinfarction or unstable angina: Any chest pain that is not relieved by a sublingual nitroglycerin (NTG) tablet taken 5 minutes apart times 3 doses provides a reason to call 911 (emergency services).
- Use of the 0 to 10 pain scale: Notify critical care nurse or emergency personnel of any changes in pain intensity.
- Use of sublingual NTG for angina: Pain intensity should decrease on the pain scale after NTG administration. At home, NTG must be kept in a dark, air-tight container, or it loses its potency. To ensure potency, the NTG supply must be replaced about every 6 months. Active NTG has a slight burning sensation when placed under the tongue.
- Avoid Valsalva maneuver.
- Risk factor modification tailored to the patient's individual risk factor profile:
  - Decrease fat intake to 30% of total calories a day.
  - Stop smoking.
  - Reduce salt intake.
  - Control hypertension.
  - Treat diabetes and control blood glucose levels (if patient has diabetes).
  - Increase physical activity; achieve ideal body weight.
- Reference to a cardiac rehabilitation program.
- Medication teaching about indications and side effects.
- Follow-up care after discharge.
- Symptoms to report to a health care professional.
- Discussion of how to handle emotional stress and anger.

MYOCARDIAL INFARCTION

Description and Etiology

Myocardial infarction (MI) is the term used to describe irreversible myocardial necrosis (cell death) that results from an abrupt decrease or total cessation of coronary blood flow to a specific area of the myocardium. In the hospital, this is often referred to as an *acute MI*, indicating the sudden onset and the life-threatening nature of the event. Increasingly, an acute MI is described in relation to whether ST-segment elevation is seen on the diagnostic 12-lead ECG. It may be labeled an *acute NSTEMI.*[15] or an *acute STEMI.*[2]

Three mechanisms can block the coronary artery and are responsible for the acute reduction in oxygen delivery to the myocardium:

1. Plaque rupture
2. New coronary artery thrombosis
3. Coronary artery spasm close to the ruptured plaque

Myocardial tissue can best be salvaged within the first 2 hours (120 minutes) after the onset of anginal symptoms, as illustrated in Figure 15-3. The earlier the myocardium is revascularized, the better are the chances of survival.[2,15] Unfortunately, many persons do not seek treatment until the acute phase has passed or delay seeking treatment because of denial of symptoms.

Pathophysiology

Ischemia

The outer region of the infarcted myocardial area is the *zone of ischemia*, or penumbra, as illustrated in Figure 15-4. It is composed of viable cells. Priority interventions are targeted to save this viable muscle. Repolarization in this zone is temporarily

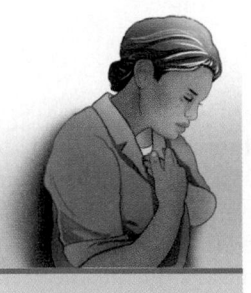
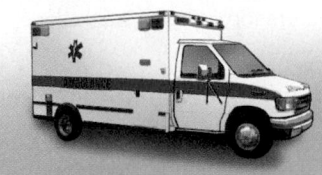

EMS on Scene

- EMS arrival on scene as FMC
- Prehospital 12-lead ECG by EMS to diagnose STEMI

- EMS transport directly to a PCI-Capable hospital with FMC-to-PCI device goal of ≤90 minutes
- Activate hospital PCI team when en route to hospital

- Onset of symptoms
- Call 911

Non-PCI Capable Hospital

- Immediate interhospital transport to a PCI-Capable hospital for patients with STEMI
- Goal is FMC-to-PCI device time of ≤120 minutes.
- When unavoidable time delays will make the FMC-to-PCI device time longer than 120 minutes, fibrinolysis should be selected as the method of reperfusion for patients without contraindications.
- IV fibrinolysis should start within 30 minutes of arrival.

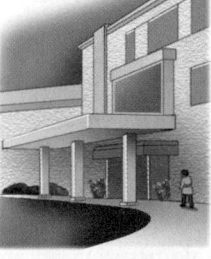

PCI-Capable Hospital

- When a patient is initially seen at a PCI-Capable hospital, the goal is a door-to-PCI device time of under 90 minutes.

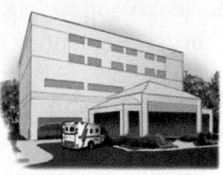

Goal is Total Ischemic Time ≤ 120 Minutes

FIGURE 15-3 Evaluation of prehospital chest pain and acute coronary syndrome and treatment options.[2] *ECG,* Electrocardiogram; *EMS,* emergency medical services; *FMC,* first medical contact; *PCI,* percutaneous coronary intervention; *STEMI,* ST elevation myocardial infarction.

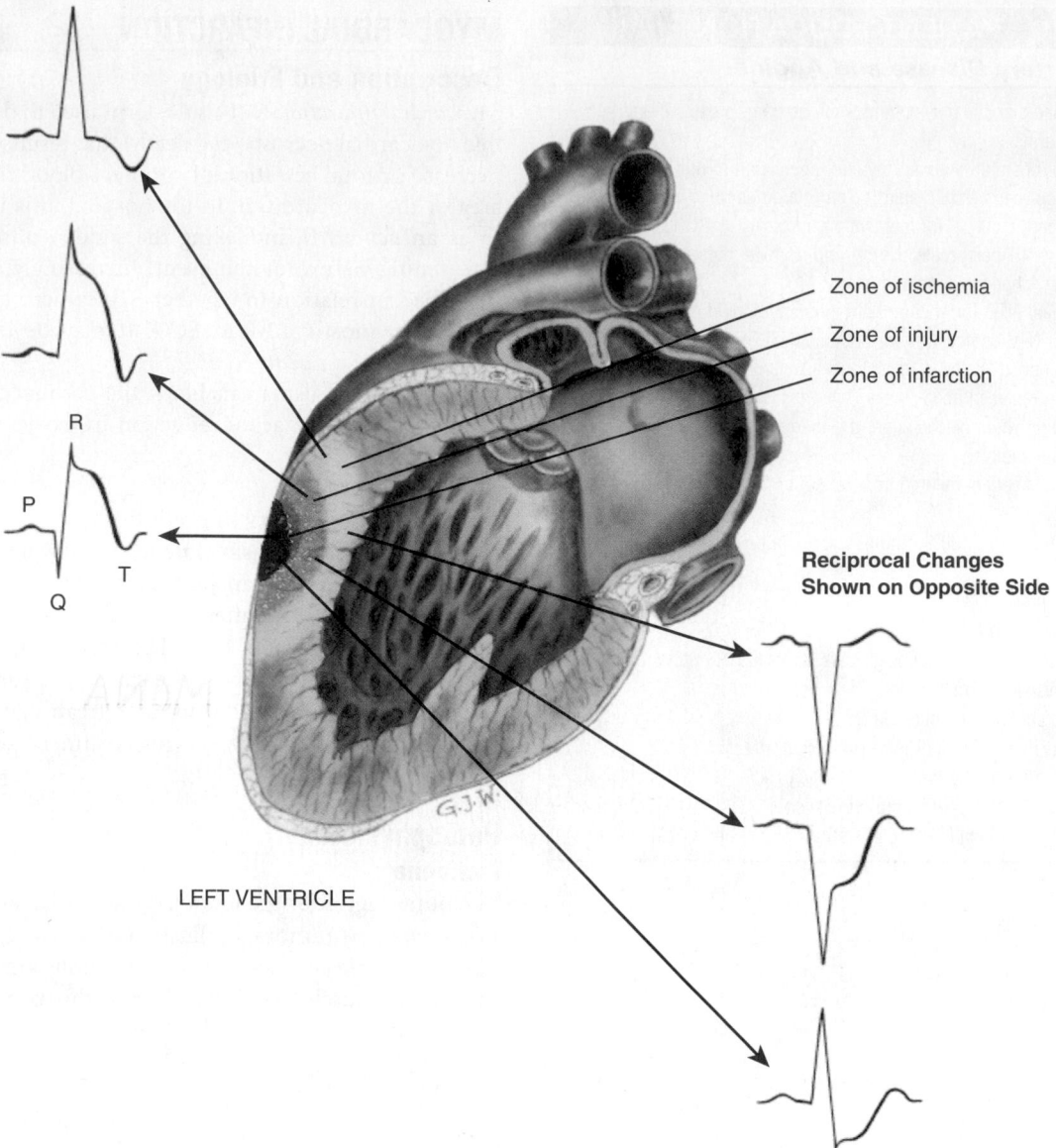

FIGURE 15-4 Zone of ischemia, zone of injury, and zone of infarction are shown through electrocardiograph waveforms and reciprocal waveforms corresponding to each zone.

impaired but eventually will be restored to normal. Repolarization of the cells in this area manifests as T-wave inversion (Fig. 15-5B).

Injury

The infarcted zone is surrounded by injured but still potentially viable tissue in an area known as the *zone of injury* (see Fig. 15-4). Cells in this area do not fully repolarize because of the deficient blood supply. This is recorded on the ECG as elevation of the ST segment (see Fig. 15-5C).

Infarction

The area of dead muscle (necrosis) in the myocardium is known as the *zone of infarction* (see Fig. 15-4). On the ECG, evidence of this zone is seen as new pathologic Q waves, which reflect a lack of depolarization from the cardiac surface involved in the MI (see Fig. 15-5D). As healing takes place, the cells in this area are replaced by scar tissue.

Q-Wave Myocardial Infarction

MIs are classified according to the location on the myocardial surface and the muscle layers affected. Not all infarctions cause necrosis in all layers, as shown in Figure 15-6. A transmural MI involves all three cardiac layers—the *endocardium*, the *myocardium*, and the *epicardium*. A transmural (full-thickness) MI usually provokes significant ECG changes (see Fig. 15-5). This is also described as a *Q-wave MI*. Not every acute MI produces a recognizable series of Q waves on the 12-lead ECG. Some patients who had a demonstrated Q wave on a 12-lead ECG as a result of an acute MI lose the Q wave months or years later. The reasons for this are unknown, but it may represent the development of collateral circulation.

12-Lead Electrocardiographic Changes

The ECG changes produced by an MI demonstrate alteration in myocardial depolarization (QRS complex) and repolarization (ST segment). The changes in repolarization are seen by

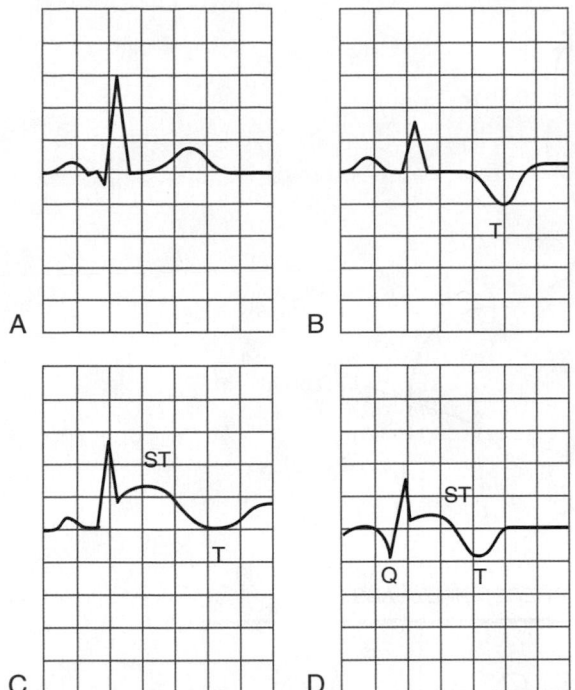

FIGURE 15-5 Electrocardiograph (ECG) Changes Indicative of Ischemia, Injury, and Infarction (Necrosis) of the Myocardium. *A,* Normal ECG. *B,* Ischemia indicated by inversion of the T wave. *C,* Ischemia and current of injury indicated by T-wave inversion and ST-segment elevation. The ST segment may be elevated above or depressed below the baseline, depending on whether the tracing is from a lead facing toward or away from the infarcted area and depending on whether epicardial or endocardial injury occurs. Epicardial injury causes ST-segment elevation in leads facing the epicardium. *D,* Ischemia, injury, and myocardial necrosis. The Q wave indicates necrosis of the myocardium.

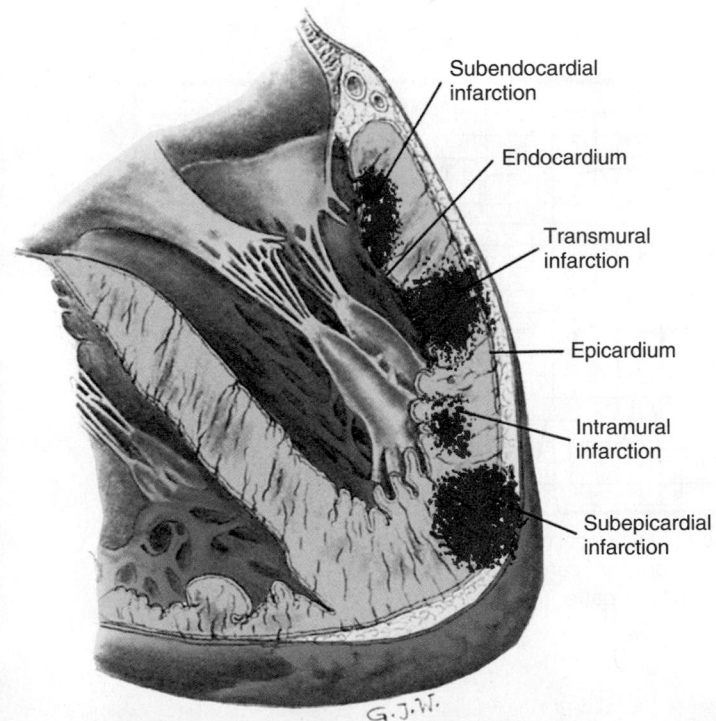

FIGURE 15-6 Location of infarctions in myocardium.

TABLE 15-6	**CORRELATIONS AMONG VENTRICULAR SURFACES, ELECTROCARDIOGRAPHIC LEADS, AND CORONARY ARTERIES**

SURFACE OF LEFT VENTRICLE	ELECTROCARDIOGRAPHIC LEADS	USUALLY INVOLVED
Inferior	II, III, aVF	Right coronary artery
Lateral	V_5-V_6, I, aVL	Left circumflex
Anterior	V_2-V_4	Left anterior descending
Anterior lateral	V_1-V_6, I, aVL	Left main coronary artery
Septal	V_1-V_2	Left anterior descending
Posterior	V_1-V_2	Left circumflex or right coronary artery (reciprocal changes)
	V_7-V_9 (direct)	

I lateral	aVR	V_1 septal	V_4 anterior
II inferior	aVL lateral	V_2 septal	V_5 lateral
III inferior	aVF inferior	V_3 anterior	V_6 lateral

the presence of new Q waves. These new, pathologic Q waves are deeper and wider than tiny Q waves found on the normal 12-lead ECG.[2,32]

Myocardial Infarction Location

The location of infarction is determined by correlating the ECG leads with Q waves and the ST-segment and T-wave abnormalities (Table 15-6). The ECG manifestations that are used to diagnose an MI and pinpoint the area of damaged ventricle include inverted T waves, ST-segment elevation, and pathologic Q waves in specific lead groupings, as described subsequently.

Anterior Wall Infarction. Anterior wall infarction results from occlusion of the proximal left anterior descending artery (see Table 15-6). ST-segment elevation is expected in leads V_1 through V_4 on the 12-lead ECG, as shown in Figure 15-7. If the left main coronary artery is occluded, the ECG manifestations will involve almost all of the precordial leads V_1 through V_6 and leads I and aVL (see Table 15-6). These specific groups of ECG changes that help locate the part of the heart that is infarcting are called *indicative changes.* A large anterior wall MI may be associated with left ventricular pump failure, cardiogenic shock, or death.[13,20]

Left Lateral Wall Infarction. Left lateral wall infarction occurs as a result of occlusion of the circumflex coronary artery. On a 12-lead ECG, new Q waves and ST-segment T-wave changes are seen in leads I, aVL, V_5, and V_6 (Fig. 15-8). In reality, few patients present with only lateral wall ECG changes, and some anterior wall leads (V_3 and V_4) may show evidence of injury or infarction.

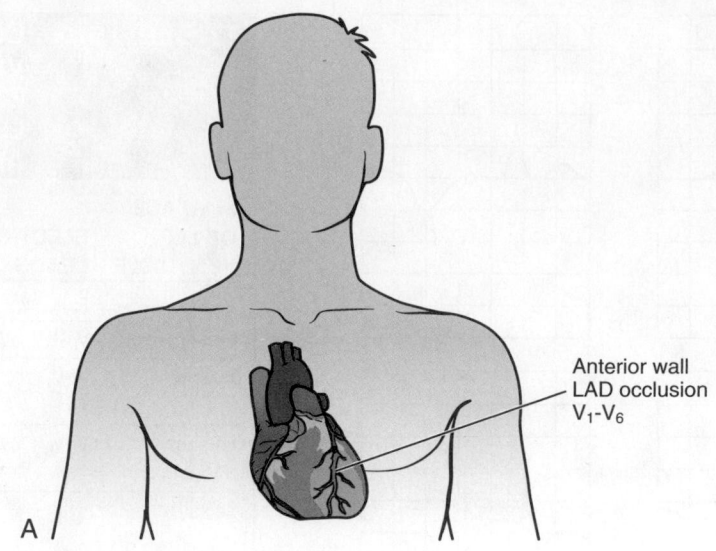

Lead I	AV$_R$	V$_1$	V$_4$
Lead II	AV$_L$	V$_2$	V$_5$
Lead III	AV$_F$	V$_3$	V$_6$

Example of an Acute Anterior Wall MI

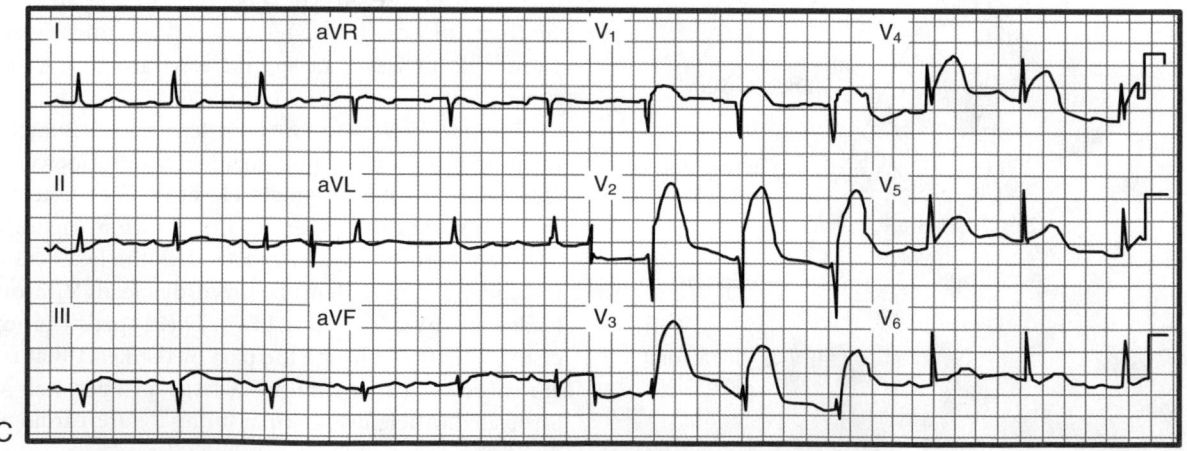

FIGURE 15-7   **Changes Seen on a 12-Lead Electrocardiogram (ECG) with an Anterior Wall Myocardial Infarction (MI).** *A,* Infarction location on the cardiac wall; *B,* ECG leads with expected ST-segment elevation; *C,* a 12-lead ECG from a patient experiencing left anterior wall MI. *LAD,* Left anterior descending artery.

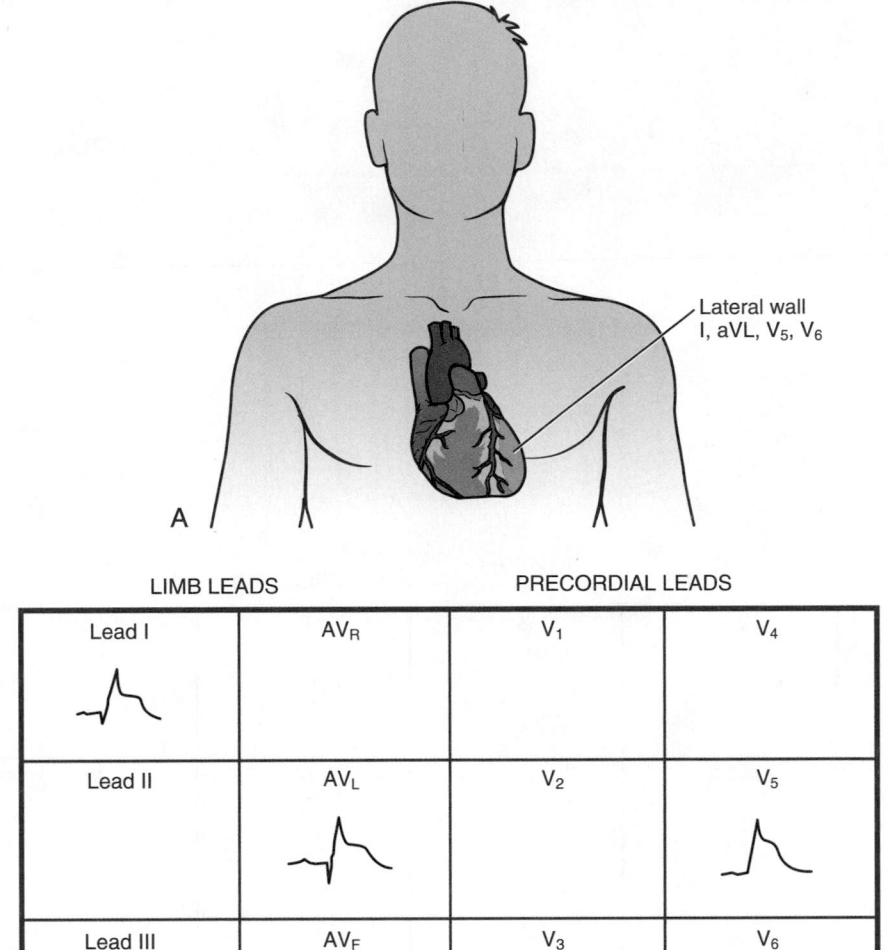

FIGURE 15-8 Changes Seen on a 12-Lead Electrocardiogram (ECG) with a Lateral Wall ST Segment Elevation Myocardial Infarction (STEMI). *A,* Infarction location on the cardiac wall; *B,* ECG leads with expected ST-segment elevation.

Inferior Wall Infarction. Inferior wall infarction occurs with occlusion of the right coronary artery. This infarction manifests by ECG changes in leads II, III, and aV_F (Fig. 15-9). Conduction disturbances are expected with an inferior wall MI and are related to the anatomy of the coronary arterial supply. Because the right coronary artery perfuses the sinoatrial (SA) node in slightly more than half of the population and supplies the proximal bundle of His and the atrioventricular (AV) node in more than 90% of individuals, heart block and other conduction disturbances should be anticipated.

Right Ventricular Infarction. Infarction of the right ventricle occurs when a blockage occurs in a proximal section of the right coronary artery. This places all of the right ventricle and the inferior wall at risk. Right ventricular ischemia can be demonstrated in up to one half of inferior wall STEMIs, although only 10% to 15% show the hemodynamic abnormalities associated with classic infarction of the right ventricle. If massive infarction occurs, the patient can suffer cardiogenic shock,

which carries a mortality rate of more than 50% in this population.[36-38]

The ECG leads on the 12-lead ECG also correlate with the coronary arteries. Leads can also be placed on the right side of the chest to assist in the diagnosis of right ventricular infarction and posteriorly to show a posterior infarction. To detect a right ventricular infarction, specific ECG lead placement is used. Electrodes are placed over the right precordium (chest) in a mirror image of the conventional left-sided leads. It is important to write R on the 12-lead ECG (e.g., V_1R-V_6R) in front of the recorded right ventricular chest leads to ensure that the lead location is clear. The limb leads are not affected. Figure 14-26C in Chapter 14 shows the correct position of the right-sided precordial leads used to diagnose an acute right ventricular MI.[36,37,38] The ECG voltage is much lower in the V_1R-V_6R leads, and when detected, ST-segment elevation is usually seen in V_4R^2 (Fig. 15-10). The right ventricle has a very thin wall, which means that ST-segment elevation is detected

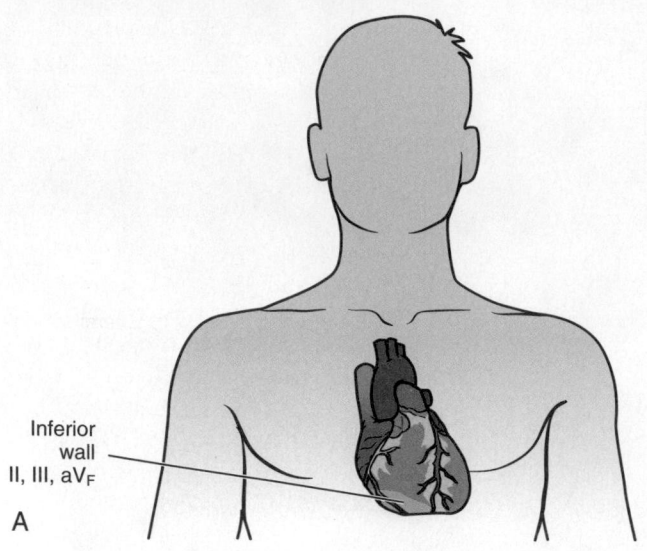

A

Inferior
wall
II, III, aV_F

LIMB LEADS   PRECORDIAL LEADS

Lead I	aV_R	V_1	V_4
Lead II	aV_L	V_2	V_5
Lead III	aV_F	V_3	V_6

B

Example of an Acute Inferior Wall MI

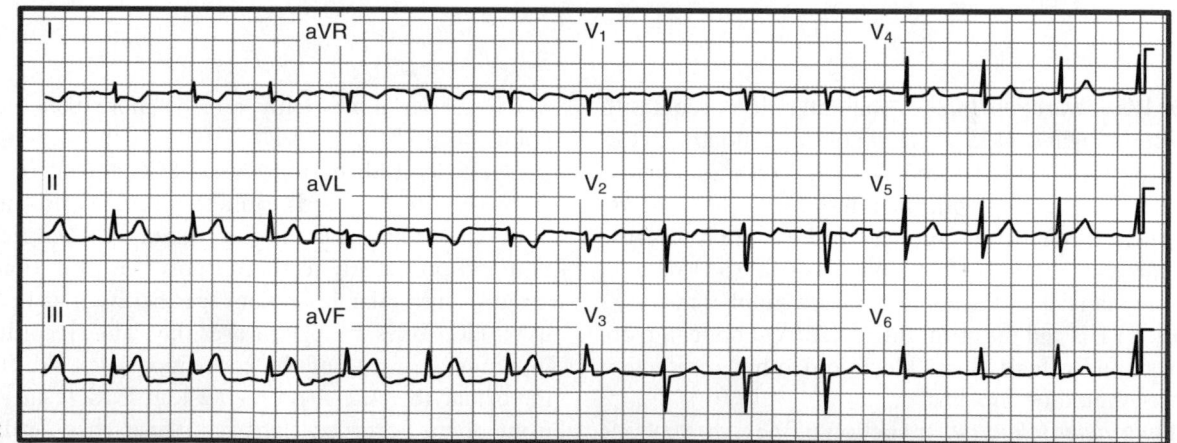

C

FIGURE 15-9   Changes Seen on a 12-Lead Electrocardiogram (ECG) with an Inferior Wall Myocardial Infarction (MI). *A,* Infarction location on cardiac wall. *B,* ECG leads with expected ST-segment elevation. *C,* A 12-lead ECG from a patient experiencing inferior wall MI.

only in the right ventricular leads during the acute phase of the infarction.

Posterior Wall Infarction. Infarction in the posterior wall can occur because of a blockage in the right coronary artery or in the circumflex artery. This occurs because both arteries supply this section of the heart, although the right coronary artery is generally the dominant vessel. A posterior wall MI is difficult to detect but may be identified by specific leads placed in the left scapular area or by very tall R waves in leads V_1 and V_2 (Fig. 15-11). Figure 14-26D in Chapter 14 shows the correct placement of the left posterior leads used to diagnose an acute posterior MI.

Non–ST-Segment Elevation Myocardial Infarction

The 12-lead ECG is a highly useful diagnostic tool. For many years, it was considered the gold standard when diagnosing an acute MI. However, the ST segment is not elevated in every acute MI. One reason for the lack of ST-segment elevation may be that the infarction and subsequent necrosis are not full-thickness lesions. Because some of the muscle in the area can still be depolarized, ST-segment elevation may not occur. This type of MI is also less likely to develop Q waves on a subsequent 12-lead ECG after the acute phase has passed. This situation is diagnostically known as an NSTEMI.[14,15] This condition has previously been described by several names, including non-transmural MI, non–Q-wave MI, and subendocardial MI. Because patients who sustain an NSTEMI do have CAD, it is important that they be treated aggressively to minimize the size of the infarcted area. Without the visual clue of the ST-segment elevation on the 12-lead ECG, the patients cannot receive immediate intravenous fibrinolytic agents, but they can be appropriately managed in an interventional catheterization laboratory and receive GP IIb/IIIa inhibitor therapy, as illustrated in the timeline in Figure 15-3. The 12-lead ECG plays a

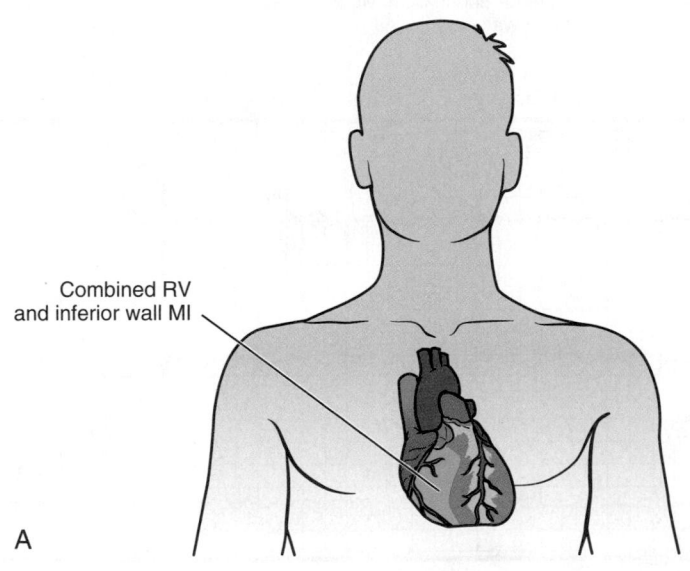

FIGURE 15-10 Changes Seen on a 12-Lead Electrocardiogram (ECG) with an Inferior Right Ventricular ST Segment Elevation Myocardial Infarction (RV STEMI). *A,* Picture of an RV wall MI. *B,* Acute inferior wall MI, with the right coronary artery (RCA) occluded.

Continued

Example of an Acute Inferior Wall and RV Wall MI. Shows ST elevation in leads II, III, AVF, and reciprocal changes (ST depression) in anterior and lateral leads.

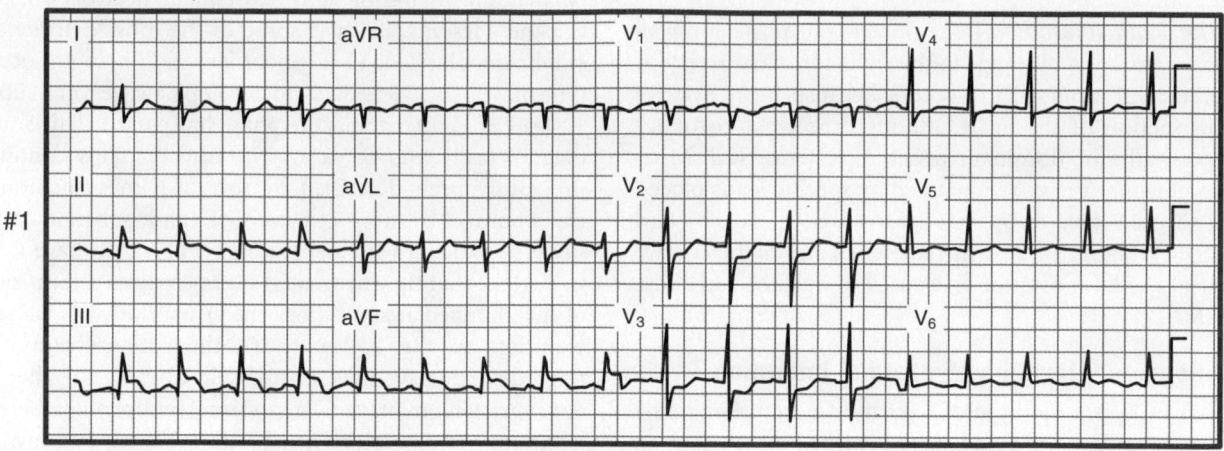

Reciprocal changes seen in V₁, V₂, V₃, V₄, I, and aVL, which provides a clue as to the extent of the MI.
Angiographic changes associated with an occlusion of the RCA.
These findings can range from:
 - Proximal occlusion (near origin of RCA) that will produce inferior MI, posterior MI, and RV MI
 - Middle RCA occlusion that will produce posterior and inferior MI
C - Distal RCA occlusion that will produce inferior wall MI

Example of an Acute RV MI in right precordial leads.

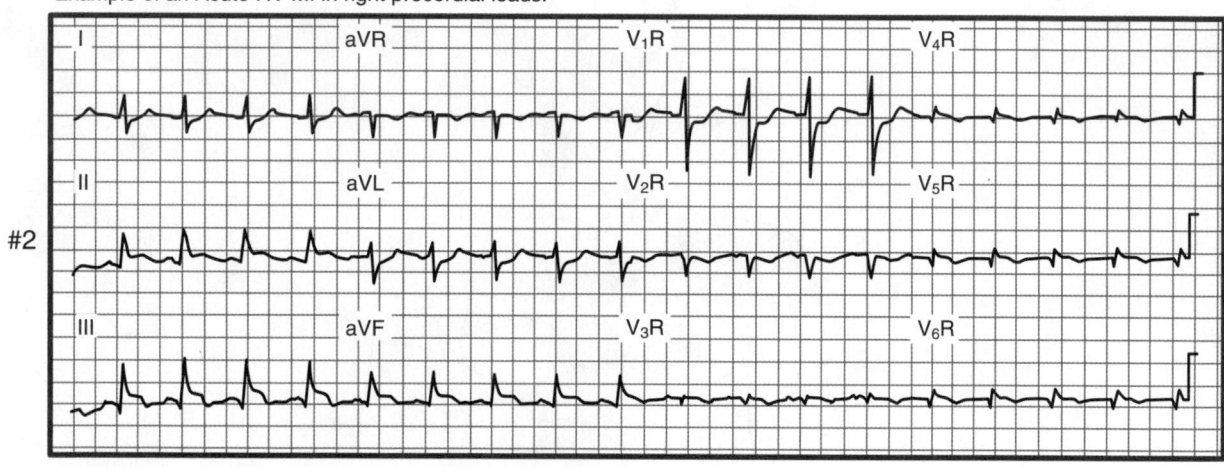

ECG shows ST elevation in right precordial leads (V₃R to V₆R), indicating RV wall injury/infarct.
 Note limb leads are identical in both ECGs.

D **These two 12-lead ECGs are from the same patient with RV MI.**
FIGURE 15-10, cont'd. *C,* Example of an acute inferior RV wall MI with conventional 12-lead ECG. *D,* Example of an acute RV wall MI with a right-sided 12-lead ECG. Both 12-lead ECGs are taken from the same patient.

vital role in identifying the treatment plan for an ACS. Visualizing ST-segment elevation is helpful when present. Patients without ST elevation may still be at risk for becoming unstable and should be monitored (Fig. 15-12). In this case, the definitive diagnosis may be made in the cardiac catheterization laboratory or by elevation of specific cardiac biomarkers.

Cardiac Biomarkers During Myocardial Infarction

In the presence of damage and necrosis of myocardium cardiac biomarkers are released. These biomarkers are also called *cardiac enzymes.* To confirm the diagnosis of acute MI, the serum biomarkers creatine kinase–muscle/brain (CK-MB) and

troponin I or troponin T are measured. Although CK is still used the troponins are valuable because the turn-around time is faster. If the coronary artery is opened by fibrinolytic therapy or a percutaneous catheter intervention (PCI), the biomarkers exhibit a more rapid rise and dramatic fall (Fig. 15-13). Information on biomarkers is also shown in Table 14-18 in Chapter 14.

Complications of Acute Myocardial Infarction

Many patients experience complications occurring early or late in the postinfarction course. These complications may result from electrical dysfunction or from a cardiac contractility

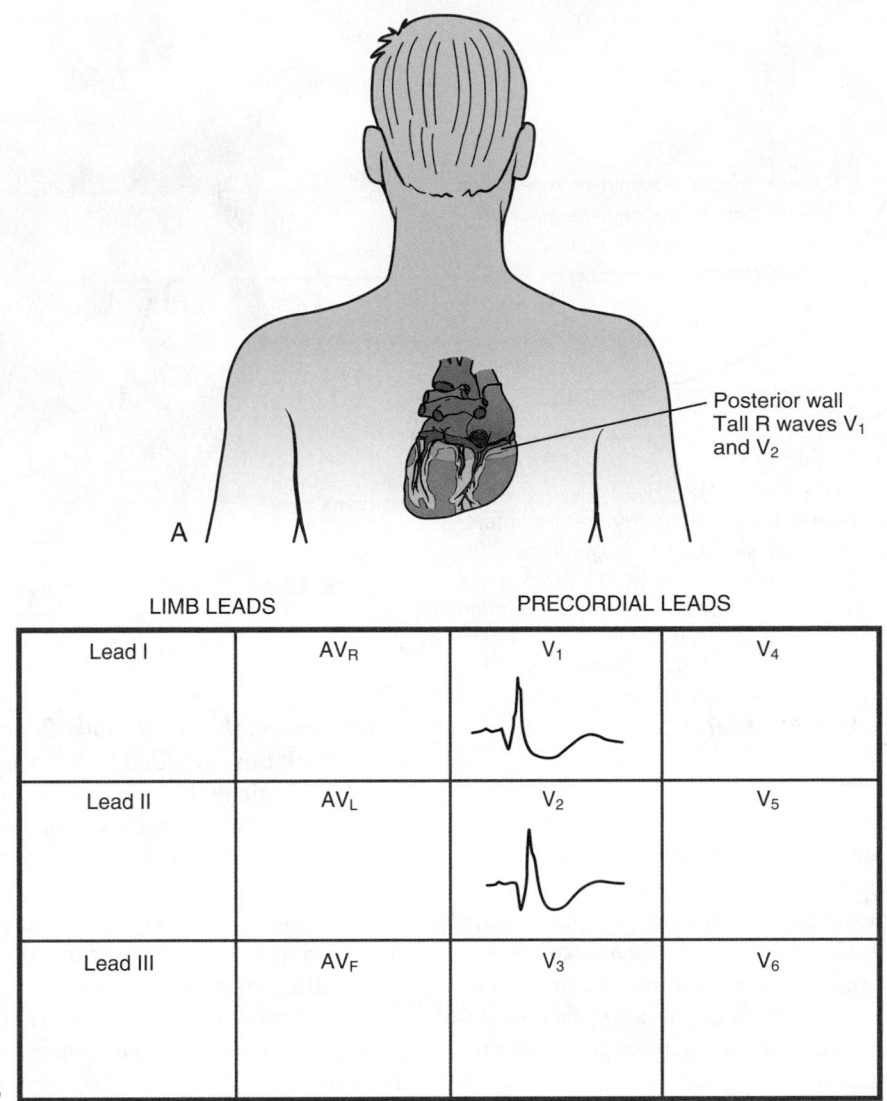

FIGURE 15-11 Changes Seen on a 12-Lead Electrocardiogram (ECG) with ST Segment Elevation Myocardial Infarction (STEMI). *A,* Infarction location on the cardiac wall. *B,* ECG leads with expected ST-segment elevation in the posterior wall STEMI.

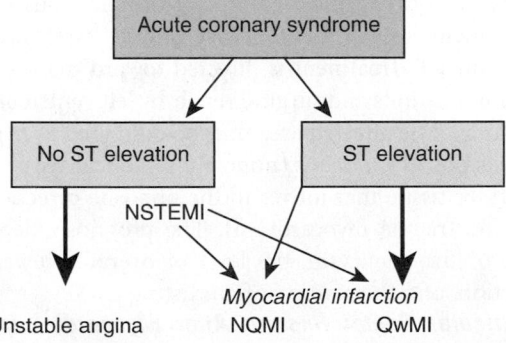

FIGURE 15-12 Acute coronary syndrome. (Modified from Braunwald E, et al. ACC/AHA guideline update for the management of patients with unstable angina and non-ST-segment elevation myocardial infarction—2002: summary article. *Circulation.* 2002;106[14]:1893.)

problem. Electrical dysfunctions include bradycardia, bundle branch blocks, and various degrees of heart block. Pumping complications can cause heart failure, pulmonary edema, and cardiogenic shock. The presence of a new murmur in a patient with an acute MI warrants special attention, as it may indicate rupture of the papillary muscle. The murmur can be indicative of severe damage and impending complications such as heart failure and pulmonary edema.

Sinus Bradycardia. Sinus bradycardia (heart rate less than 60 beats per minute [beats/min]) occurs frequently in patients who sustain an acute MI. It is more prevalent with an inferior wall infarction in the first hour after STEMI. Symptomatic bradycardia with hypotension and low cardiac output is treated with atropine (0.5 to 1.0 mg by intravenous push), repeated every 3 to 5 minutes to a maximum dose of 0.03 mg/kg (e.g., 2 mg for a person who weighs 70 kg) per the *Advanced Cardiac Life Support (ACLS) Guidelines.*

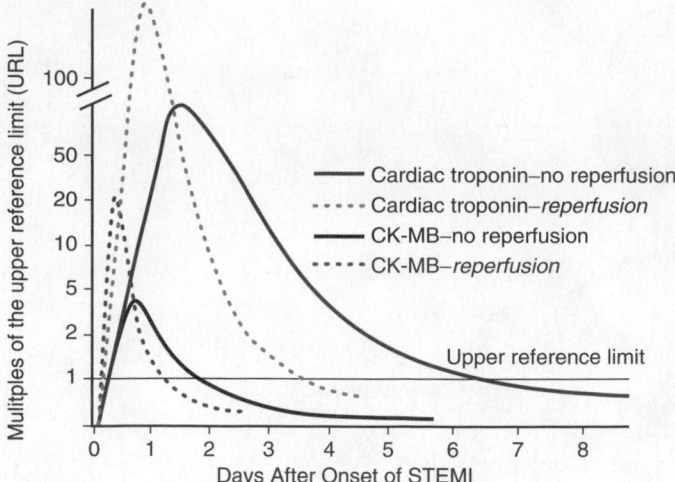

FIGURE 15-13 Cardiac biomarkers during myocardial infarction (MI). (From Antman EM, et al. ACC/AHA guidelines for the management of patients with ST-elevation myocardial infarction—executive summary: a report of the American College of Cardiology/American Heart Association Task Force on Practice Guidelines [Writing Committee to Revise the 1999 Guidelines for the Management of Patients with Acute Myocardial Infarction]. *Circulation.* 2004;110[9]:e82.)

Sinus Tachycardia. Sinus tachycardia (heart rate more than 100 beats/min) most often occurs with an anterior wall MI. Anterior infarctions impair left ventricular pumping ability, thereby reducing the ejection fraction and the stroke volume. In an attempt to maintain cardiac output, the heart rate increases. Sinus tachycardia is corrected by treating the underlying cause, as it greatly increases myocardial oxygen consumption, leading to further ischemia.

Atrial Dysrhythmias. Premature atrial contractions (PACs) occur frequently in patients who sustain an acute MI. Atrial fibrillation (AF) is also common and may occur spontaneously or may be preceded by PACs. With the onset of AF, the loss of organized atrial contraction decreases cardiac output by up to 20%. Patients with new-onset or preexisting AF have higher morbidity rates than patients without AF during an ACS event. ACS patients with new-onset AF experience a greater number of in-hospital adverse events such as reinfarction, shock, pulmonary edema, bleeding, and stroke. Management of AF includes both rate control and rhythm control.[39]

Ventricular Dysrhythmias. Premature ventricular contractions (PVCs) are seen in almost all patients within the first few hours after an MI. They are initially controlled by administering oxygen to reduce myocardial hypoxia and by correcting acid–base or electrolyte imbalances. In the setting of an acute MI, PVCs are pharmacologically treated if they have the following characteristics: frequent (>6/min), closely coupled (R-on-T phenomenon), multiform shapes, and occurrence in bursts of three or more, increasing the risk of sustained ventricular tachycardia (VT). Ventricular fibrillation (VF) is a life-threatening dysrhythmia associated with high mortality in acute MI. Beta-blockers are prescribed after an acute MI to decrease mortality from ventricular dysrhythmias.

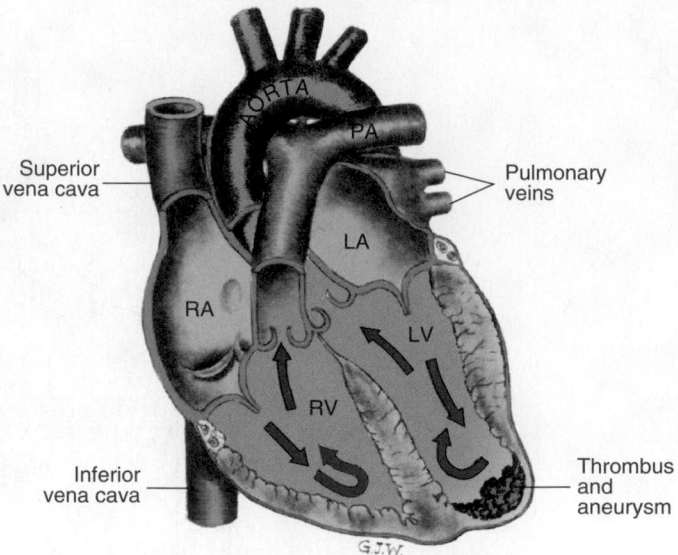

FIGURE 15-14 Ventricular aneurysm after acute myocardial infarction. *LA,* Left atrium; *LV,* left ventricle; *PA,* pulmonary artery; *RA,* right atrium; *RV,* right ventricle.

Atrioventricular Heart Block During Myocardial Infarction. Heart block can occur in 6% to 14% of patients with STEMI, and those patients have increased mortality rates. In STEMI, AV block most often occurs after an inferior wall infarction. Because the right coronary artery supplies the AV node in 90% of the population, right coronary artery occlusion leads to ischemia and infarction of the AV node cells. The development of sudden heart block has become much less common because most patients receive fibrinolysis or undergo PCI to open the occluded vessel. In most cases, transcutaneous pacing is the primary intervention; transvenous pacemakers are used less frequently.

Ventricular Aneurysm After Myocardial Infarction. A ventricular aneurysm (Fig. 15-14) is a noncontractile, thinned left ventricular wall that results from an acute transmural infarction. It most often occurs in the setting of an acute left anterior descending artery occlusion with a wide area of infarcted myocardium. The most effective prevention is early reperfusion of the myocardium, accomplished by opening the thrombosed coronary artery. The most common complications of a ventricular aneurysm are acute heart failure, systemic emboli, angina, and VT. Treatment is directed toward management of these complications and surgical repair by left ventricular aneurysmectomy. The affected area may be described as *hypokinetic* (contracts poorly), *akinetic* (noncontractile scar tissue), or *dyskinetic* (scar tissue that moves in the opposite direction to the normal contractile myocardium). The prognosis depends on the size of the aneurysm, the level of overall left ventricular dysfunction, and the severity of coexisting CAD.

Ventricular Septal Rupture After Myocardial Infarction. Postinfarction rupture of the ventricular septal wall is a rare but potentially lethal complication of an acute anterior wall MI (Fig. 15-15). *Ventricular septal rupture,* also known as *acquired ventricular septal defect* (VSD), is an abnormal communication between the right and left ventricle. This complication occurs in less than 1% of all MIs, and the incidence has declined

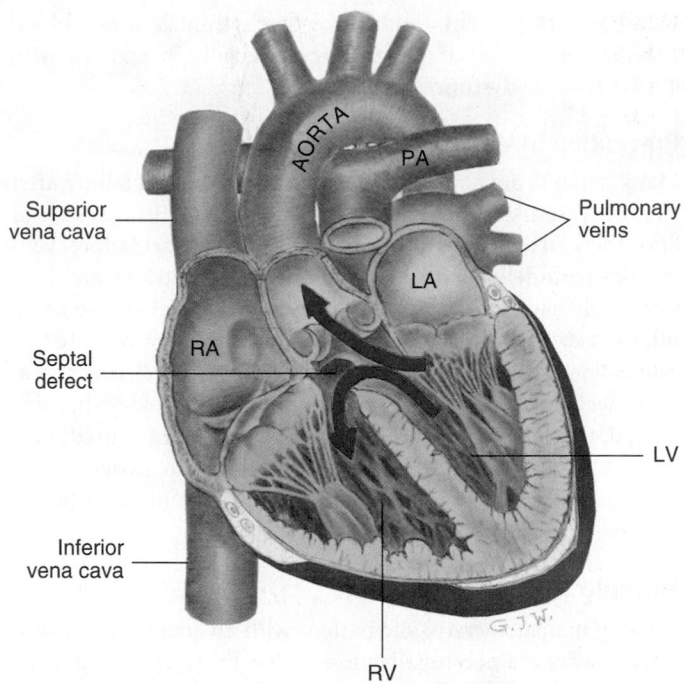

FIGURE 15-15 Ventricular septal rupture after acute myocardial infarction. *LA,* Left atrium; *LV,* left ventricle; *PA,* pulmonary artery; *RA,* right atrium; *RV,* right ventricle.

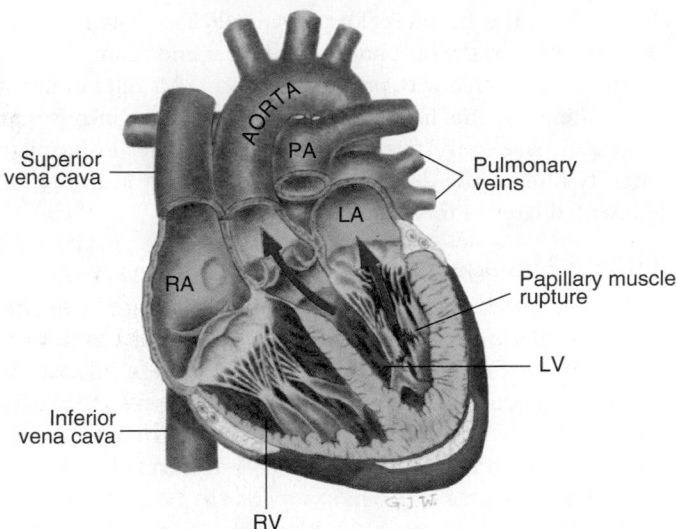

FIGURE 15-16 Papillary muscle rupture after acute myocardial infarction. *LA,* Left atrium; *LV,* left ventricle; *PA,* pulmonary artery; *RA,* right atrium; *RV,* right ventricle.

because most STEMI patients have the blocked coronary artery opened through PCI or fibrinolysis within a short time frame after diagnosis. Nevertheless, rupture of the ventricular septum carries an extremely high mortality rate. Mortality rates between 35% and 73% are typical.[40,41] Most patients with septal rupture also have signs and symptoms of cardiogenic shock. Ventricular septal rupture manifests as severe chest pain, syncope, hypotension, and sudden hemodynamic deterioration caused by shunting of blood from the high-pressure left ventricle into the low-pressure right ventricle through the new septal opening. A holosystolic murmur (often accompanied by a thrill) can be auscultated and is best heard along the left sternal border. Rupture of the septum is a medical and surgical emergency. The patient's condition is stabilized with vasodilators and an intra-aortic balloon pump (IABP) to decrease afterload. The goal of afterload reduction in this patient population is to decrease the amount of blood being shunted to the right side of the heart and consequently to increase the flow of blood to the systemic circulation. If the septal rupture is very small, and the patient's condition is sufficiently stable to wait for scar tissue to form before surgical repair, survival improves. Unfortunately, when the septal opening is large, the massive left to right shunt across the septum makes the chances of survival dismal with or without surgery.[41,42]

Papillary Muscle Rupture After Myocardial Infarction. Papillary muscle rupture can occur when the infarct involves the area around one of the papillary muscles that support the mitral valve. Infarction of the papillary muscles results in ineffective mitral valve closure, and blood is forced back into the low-pressure left atrium during ventricular systole. The rupture may be partial or complete. Complete rupture is catastrophic and precipitates severe acute mitral regurgitation, cardiogenic shock, and high risk of death.

Partial rupture (Fig. 15-16) also results in mitral regurgitation, but the condition can be stabilized with aggressive medical management using the IABP and vasodilators. Urgent surgical intervention is required to replace the mitral valve.[2,43]

Cardiac Wall Rupture After Myocardial Infarction. The incidence of cardiac wall rupture has two peak times. The first occurs within the first 24 hours and the second between the third and fifth postinfarction day when leukocyte scavenger cells are removing necrotic debris, thinning the myocardial wall. The onset is sudden and usually catastrophic, bleeding into the pericardial sac results in cardiac tamponade, cardiogenic shock, pulseless electrical activity (PEA), and death. Survival is rare. If rupture occurs in the hospital, emergency pericardiocentesis is required to relieve the tamponade until a surgical repair can be attempted. The best prevention is early reperfusion of the myocardium.

Pericarditis After Myocardial Infarction. Pericarditis is inflammation of the pericardial sac. It can occur during or after an acute MI. The damaged epicardium becomes rough and inflamed and irritates the pericardium lying adjacent to it, precipitating pericarditis. Pain is the most common symptom of pericarditis, and a pericardial friction rub is the most common initial sign. The friction rub is best auscultated with a stethoscope at the sternal border and is described as a grating, scraping, or leathery scratching. Pericarditis frequently produces a pericardial effusion.[44] After the effusion occurs, the friction rub may disappear. On the 12-lead ECG, pericarditis may manifest as elevation of the ST segment in all of the typically upright leads.[45] Pericarditis is treated with nonsteroidal anti-inflammatory medications (NSAIDs), aspirin, and rest. Pericarditis that occurs as a late complication of acute MI is known as *Dressler's syndrome.*[46]

Heart Failure and Acute Myocardial Infarction. Many patients with acute STEMI also have acute heart failure on admission to the hospital. These patients have often waited longer to come to the hospital and are older and more likely to be female. Compared with patients with acute MI but not heart failure, these patients have a higher risk of adverse in-hospital events and have longer lengths of stay and higher in-hospital mortality rates. More detailed information about heart failure is presented later in this chapter.

Medical Management

Quality outcomes research shows that compliance with the guidelines developed by the American College of Cardiology and the American Heart Association (ACC/AHA) decreases in-hospital mortality after acute MI.[47,48] When the AHA/ACC guidelines for treatment of STEMI or NSTEMI are followed, patients admitted to hospitals have 8.3% in-hospital mortality rate, compared with a 15.3% mortality rate in patients managed at hospitals where the most recent guidelines are not fully utilized.[48,49] The guidelines are research based and are designed to improve the outcome of patients admitted to the hospital with an acute MI. Clinical guidelines address the issues of interventions to open the coronary artery, anticoagulation, prevention of dysrhythmias, intensive glucose control, and prevention of ventricular remodeling after STEMI. To facilitate rapid coronary artery revascularization in STEMI, local hospitals are encouraged to develop a coordinated patient transfer strategy between PCI-capable and non-PCI—capable hospitals, as illustrated in Figure 15-3.[2]

Recanalization of the Coronary Artery

The essential immediate interventions are fibrinolytic therapy or PCI to open the occluded artery for the patient with an acute STEMI.[2] All clinical guidelines emphasize the need for patients with symptoms of ACS to be rapidly triaged and treated.[2]

Anticoagulation

In the acute phase after STEMI, heparin is administered in combination with fibrinolytic therapy to recanalize (open) the coronary artery.[2] For patients who will receive fibrinolytic therapy, an initial heparin bolus of 60 units/kg (maximum 5000 units) is given intravenously, followed by a continuous heparin drip at 12 units/kg/hr (maximum 1000 units/hr) to maintain an activated partial thromboplastin time (aPTT) between 50 and 70 seconds (1.5 to 2.0 times) control for 48 hours or until revascularization.[2]

It is also prudent to administer intravenous UFH or subcutaneous low molecular weight heparin (LMWH) if the person is at risk for thrombus development. For patients with known heparin-induced thrombocytopenia (HIT), as an alternative to LMWH or UFH, a third class of antithrombotic medications is available—direct antithrombotic agents (e.g., hirudin, bivalirudin, argatroban). Patients at risk for thrombotic emboli include those with an anterior wall infarction, AF, previous embolus, cardiomyopathy, or cardiogenic shock.

Dysrhythmia Prevention

The antidysrhythmic with the best safety record after STEMI is amiodarone. Beta-blockers are another class of antidysrhythmics that are recommended for all patients after STEMI.

Beta-blockers prevent ventricular dysrhythmias, lower blood pressure, and prevent reinfarction, especially in patients with left ventricular dysfunction.[2]

Prevention of Ventricular Remodeling

Many patients are at risk for development of heart failure after STEMI. Vasodilating medications (ACEIs or ARBs) can stop or limit the ventricular remodeling that leads to heart failure. Ventricular remodeling is progressive changes in the size, architecture, and shape of the myocardium and occurs because of an injury such as an MI. Ventricular remodeling is modulated by catecholamines and activation of neurohormonal compensatory mechanisms. The heart chamber walls ultimately become dilated, thinned, and poorly contractile. An ACEI is used, or if it is not tolerated, an ARB is indicated for all patients after STEMI.[2] Information about the clinical effects of heart failure is provided later in this chapter.

Nursing Management

Nursing management of the patient with an acute MI incorporates a variety of nursing diagnoses (Box 15-11). Nursing interventions focus on achieving a balance between myocardial oxygen supply and demand, preventing complications, and providing patient and family education.

Balance of Myocardial Oxygen Supply and Demand

In the acute period, if severe heart muscle damage has occurred, myocardial oxygen supply is increased by the administration of supplemental oxygen to prevent tissue hypoxia. This imbalance manifests as many clinical signs (Box 15-12). Cardiac medications play an increasingly important role in balancing supply and demand, and it is the critical care nurse who administers and monitors the effectiveness of these agents. For the patient with a low cardiac output, positive inotropic medications such as dobutamine, dopamine, or both may be administered. Milrinone, a phosphodiesterase inhibitor, which increases contractility by improving sarcolemma calcium uptake and causes

---

◎ BOX 15-11   NURSING DIAGNOSES

Myocardial Infarction

- Acute Pain, related to transmission and perception of cutaneous, visceral, muscular, or ischemic impulses, p. 1123
- Decreased Cardiac Output, related to alterations in preload, p. 1128
- Decreased Cardiac Output, related to alterations in afterload, p. 1128
- Decreased Cardiac Output, related to alterations in contractility, p. 1128
- Decreased Cardiac Output, related to alterations in heart rate or rhythm, p. 1128
- Activity Intolerance, related to cardiopulmonary dysfunction, p. 1119
- Risk for Decreased Cardiac Tissue Perfusion, p. 1155
- Disturbed Sleep Pattern, related to fragmented sleep, p. 1137
- Anxiety, related to threat to biologic, psychologic, or social integrity, p. 1125
- Ineffective Coping, related to situational crisis and personal vulnerability, p. 1150
- Powerlessness, related to lack of control over current situation or disease progression, p. 1152
- Deficient Knowledge, related to lack of previous exposure to information, p. 1134 (see Box 15-13, Patient Education for Myocardial Infarction)

BOX 15-12 CLINICAL MANIFESTATIONS OF ACUTE MYOCARDIAL INFARCTION

- Tachycardia with or without ectopy
- Bradycardia
- Normotension or hypotension
- Tachypnea
- Diminished heart sounds, especially S_1
- If left ventricular dysfunction present, may have S_3, S_4, or both
- Systolic murmur
- Pulmonary crackles
- Pulmonary edema
- Air hunger
- Orthopnea
- Frothy sputum
- Decreased cardiac output
- Decreased urine output
- Decreased peripheral pulses
- Slow capillary refill
- Restlessness
- Confusion
- Anxiety
- Agitation
- Denial
- Anger

BOX 15-13 PATIENT EDUCATION

Myocardial Infarction

- Pathophysiology of coronary artery disease, angina, and acute myocardial infarction
- Angina: Describe signs and symptoms, such as pain, pressure, or heaviness in chest, arms, or jaw
- Use of the 0 to 10 pain scale: Notify critical care nurse or emergency personnel of any changes in chest pain intensity
- Avoid Valsalva maneuver
- Risk factor modification tailored to the patient's individual risk factor profile:
  - Decrease daily fat intake to less than 30% of total calories.
  - Reduce total serum cholesterol to less than 200 mg/dL.
  - Reduce low-density lipoprotein (LDL) cholesterol to less than 70 mg/dL.
  - Stop smoking.
  - Reduce salt intake.
  - Control hypertension.
  - Control diabetes (if patient has diabetes).
  - Increase physical activity.
  - Achieve ideal body weight, if overweight.
- Reference to cardiac rehabilitation program
- Medication teaching about indications and side effects
- Follow-up care after discharge
- Symptoms to report to a health care professional
- Discussion of how to handle emotional stress and anger

positive inotropic effects in the myocardium, may be prescribed. In contrast to dobutamine and dopamine, milrinone does not complete for receptor sites in patients taking beta-blockers. These inotropic agents are used to increase cardiac contractility in the healthy areas of the heart (increasing oxygen supply) while avoiding damage to the recently infarcted areas. Myocardial oxygen supply can be further enhanced by the use of coronary artery vasodilators. Nitroglycerin is often administered for the first 48 hours to increase vasodilation and prevent myocardial ischemia. Research evidence supports the administration of early beta-blockade therapy to decrease myocardial workload and to prevent dysrhythmias. However, if the patient is in cardiogenic shock, beta-blockers are withheld until the cardiac output has improved.[2] Other interventions to decrease cardiac work and myocardial oxygen consumption include bed rest with bedside commode privileges when the patient is clinically stable.

Prevention of Complications

A thorough grasp of the range of potential complications that can occur after STEMI is essential. Cardiac monitoring for early detection of ventricular dysrhythmias is ongoing. Assessment for signs of continued ischemic pain is important because angina is a warning sign of the myocardium being at risk. In response to angina, a 12-lead ECG is obtained to determine if an extension of the infarct exists, and nitroglycerin is administered, and the physician is notified immediately so that interventions may be initiated to limit the size of the MI. Heart failure is a serious complication after STEMI. When the patient's blood pressure is stable, treatment with an ACEI is initiated. These vasodilators are used to prevent left ventricular remodeling and dilation that occurs in many patients after an acute MI. Hypotension is a potential complication of ACEIs, especially with the first dose. It is an important nursing responsibility to monitor blood pressure and patient symptoms after taking this medication. Surveillance to detect obvious and subtle signs of bleeding is also a priority because so many acute MI patients receive antiplatelet, anticoagulant, and fibrinolytic medications.[2,47-49]

In the first 24 hours after a myocardial infarction, diet is progressed as tolerated. Preventing hospital-acquired pneumonia and deep vein thrombosis (DVT) is facilitated by early mobilization and raising the head of the bed 30 degrees or more. An upright position facilitates decrease in venous return, lowering of preload, and decrease in the workload of the myocardium. The patient is taught to avoid increasing intra-abdominal pressure (Valsalva maneuver). Stool softeners may be given to the patient to lessen the risk of constipation from analgesics and bed rest and to decrease the risk of straining. Providing a calming and quiet environment that focuses on the well-being of the patient assists in the recovery phase.

Depression After Myocardial Infarction

Depression is a phenomenon that occurs across a wide spectrum of human experience. Depression is a risk factor for development of coronary artery disease and impedes recovery following acute MI.[50] Key symptoms of depression mentioned frequently by cardiac patients are fatigue, change in appetite, and sleep disturbance.

Patient Education

After the acute phase of an MI, patient and family education becomes a priority. The education focuses on key elements: 1) risk factor reduction, 2) manifestations of angina, 3) when to call a physician or emergency services, 4) medications, and 5) resumption of physical and sexual activities (Box 15-13). It is recommended that a referral is made to a cardiac rehabilitation program to reinforce education that was commenced during hospitalization.[2] Clinical practice guidelines for multidisciplinary care of the patient with an acute MI are listed in Box 15-14.

BOX 15-14 EVIDENCE-BASED PRACTICE

Acute Coronary Syndrome and Acute Myocardial Infarction (Non-STEMI and STEMI)

QSEN **Prevention of Acute Coronary Syndrome**

The term *ACS* is used to define the life-threatening consequences of CAD, notably unstable angina, non-STEMI, and STEMI:

- *Unstable angina* is a term that denotes chest pain that is not relieved by SL nitroglycerin or rest within 5 minutes.
- Non-STEMI is an acute MI *without* ST-segment elevation on the 12-lead ECG.
- STEMI is an acute MI *with* ST-segment elevation on the 12-lead ECG. All of the recommendations are class I, meaning that there is strong research evidence to support these recommendations.

Recommendations That Decrease the Risk of Developing Non-STEMI and STEMI

- Primary care providers should evaluate CAD risk factors for all patients every 3 to 5 years using a validated risk assessment scoring tool.
- The 10-year risk of ACS and acute MI should be assessed for all patients who have more than two major risk factors through the use of evidence based risk assessment tools.
- An intensive risk factor modification program is recommended for patients with established CAD or high-risk equivalents such as diabetes or chronic kidney disease.

Recommendations about Emergency ACS Symptoms

- A patient who has previously diagnosed CAD should take one SL nitroglycerin dose, and the patient (if alone) or a friend or relative should call 911 if chest pain or discomfort is unrelieved or worsening in 5 minutes.
- The same recommendation applies to a patient without known CAD. If pain is unrelieved with rest or worsening at 5 minutes, the patient (if alone) or a friend or relative should call 911.
- Patients with chest discomfort should be transported to the hospital by ambulance rather than be driven by a friend or relative.
- Family members should be advised to take a CPR course before an ACS emergency occurs. This will teach CPR skills, demonstrate use of an AED, and educate participants about the "chain of survival" concept.

Recommendations for Prehospital EMS-Paramedic First Responders

- First responders such as EMS-paramedics can provide early defibrillation and ACLS for patients in cardiac arrest.
- EMS personnel should administer 162 to 325 mg of nonenteric aspirin (chewed, not swallowed) to patients with chest pain and suspected STEMI.
- A prehospital fibrinolysis protocol is reasonable for patients with STEMI if there are physicians in the ambulance or if there is a well-organized EMS service with full-time paramedics plus 12-lead ECG transmission capability and online medical direction.
- Patients older than 75 years and those with cardiogenic shock should be transported to a hospital with the ability to provide fibrinolytics, emergency PCI, or emergency CABG.
- Patients with STEMI who have a contraindication to fibrinolytic therapy should be brought to a hospital capable of emergency PCI or CABG. At the scene, the door-to-departure time should be *less than 30 minutes*. PCI should be initiated *within 90 minutes* after initial medical contact.

Recommendations for Initial Emergency Clinical Management

- Hospitals should establish multidisciplinary teams to facilitate rapid triage of patients who present to the ED with chest pain.

- Use of written protocols is recommended to standardize care. An immediate cardiology consultation is advised if the patient's symptoms fall outside the written protocol.

STEMI

- *Fibrinolytics for STEMI:* Time from coming into contact with the health care system (paramedics or ED) to receiving fibrinolytics should be *less than 30 minutes*. A brief, focused neurologic examination to determine prior stroke or presence of cognitive defects is necessary before administration of fibrinolytics.
- *PCI for STEMI:* Time from coming into contact with the health care system (paramedics or ED) to balloon inflation PCI should be *less than 90 minutes*.

Non-STEMI

- If the level of risk for the patient with non-STEMI is not immediately apparent, a "chest pain unit" within the ED permits close surveillance by competent clinicians without immediate hospital admission.
- Glycoprotein IIb/IIIa inhibitors for non-STEMI, in addition to aspirin and heparin, are indicated if cardiac catheterization or PCI is planned.
- PCI may be indicated for non-STEMI.

Recommendations for Initial Emergency Physical Assessment

Vital Signs

- HR, BP, RR, temperature SpO$_2$, ECG monitor to detect presence of dysrhythmias.

Physical Assessment

- Assess for warm or cool skin, color, capillary refill, peripheral pulses.
- Auscultate heart for cardiac murmur or new S$_3$ or S$_4$.
- Auscultate lungs for air entry plus crackles and wheezes.
- Observe for breathlessness and frothy pink sputum (pulmonary edema).
- Ask patient, family, significant others for relevant history.

Recommendations for Emergency Diagnostics

12-Lead ECG

- The 12-lead ECG should be shown to the ED physician within 10 minutes after the patient's arrival in the ED for all patients with chest discomfort or angina-equivalent symptoms.
- If the first ECG is normal but the patient continues to have symptoms of chest pain or discomfort, the 12-lead ECG should be repeated at 5- to 10-minute intervals, *or* continuous 12-lead ECG monitoring can be used.
- In patients with inferior wall infarction, RV infarction must be suspected and right-sided ECG leads recorded. V4R is the diagnostic lead of choice to diagnose ST-segment elevation in the RV.

Laboratory Studies

- Laboratory tests should be performed as part of the general management of STEMI but should not delay the administration of reperfusion therapy.

Cardiac Biomarkers

- Measurement of cardiac-specific troponins is recommended for patients with coexistent skeletal muscle injury. Clinicians are advised not to wait for results of the biomarker assay before initiating reperfusion therapy. Point-of-care (handheld) biomarker assay results can be used for rapid determination of treatment, but subsequent biomarker assays should be done by quantitative laboratory analysis.

BOX 15-14 EVIDENCE-BASED PRACTICE

Acute Coronary Syndrome and Acute Myocardial Infarction (Non-STEMI and STEMI)—cont'd

Imaging Studies
- *Portable chest radiograph:* Obtaining the chest radiograph must not delay reperfusion therapy unless a major complication such as aortic dissection is suspected.
- *Portable echocardiography (TTE or TEE) or MRI:* A scan should be obtained to distinguish aortic dissection from STEMI, for patients in whom the symptoms are not clear.

Recommendations for Care
Prevent Hypoxia
- Supplemental oxygen administered to maintain oxygen saturation greater than 90%.

Coronary Vasodilation
- Nitroglycerin (0.04 mg SL every 5 minutes for three doses) is administered. If chest pain or discomfort is ongoing, start peripheral IV. Administer IV nitroglycerin for relief of chest pain, control of hypertension, or relief of pulmonary congestion.

Pain Control
- Morphine sulfate (2 to 4 mg IV) is administered; can increase to 2- to 8-mg IV increments at 5- to 15-minute intervals for STEMI pain control.

NSAIDs
- Discontinue NSAIDs (except for aspirin), both nonselective and COX-2 selective agents, at time of presentation with STEMI because of increased risk of mortality, reinfarction, hypertension, heart failure, and myocardial rupture associated with NSAID use.

Aspirin
- Aspirin 162 mg to be chewed by patient for rapid buccal absorption.

Beta-Blockers
- Oral beta-blocker therapy is administered to patients with STEMI who do not have contraindications to beta-blockade, irrespective of fibrinolytic or primary PCI reperfusion.
- Contraindications for beta-blockade with STEMI include signs of heart failure, low cardiac output, cardiogenic shock risk, heart block or prolonged PR interval (>0.24 second), and active asthma or reactive airway disease.
- While considering the options for reperfusion, beta-blockers are given if the patient has tachycardia or hypertension; otherwise, they are started as soon as possible after STEMI.

Angiotensin-Converting Enzymes Inhibitors
- Oral ACE inhibitors are indicated within the first 24 hours after STEMI unless contraindicated.

Recommendations for Emergency Interventions for STEMI
Fibrinolytic Medications
- Fibrinolytic medications are administered to STEMI patients (if PCI is not available) with ST-segment elevation greater than 0.1 mV (1 mm or one small box) in two contiguous precordial (chest) leads *or* two adjacent limb leads, new LBBB or presumed new LBBB, and onset of symptoms less than 12 hours earlier.
- Before administration of fibrinolytic therapy, rule out neurologic contraindications.
- Rule out facial trauma, uncontrolled hypertension, or ischemic stroke within the last 3 months.
- If contraindications to fibrinolysis are present, PCI is the preferred method of reperfusion.

PCI
- Emergency diagnostic coronary angiography should be performed to identify blocked coronary artery before PCI.
- Emergency PCI is recommended over fibrinolytic therapy if symptom onset was longer than 3 hours ago.
- Emergency PCI can be performed within 12 hours after symptom onset for patients with new LBBB or presumed new LBBB.
- Emergency PCI balloon inflation should be done within 90 minutes after arrival at the hospital.

Cardiac Surgery
Emergency CABG surgery is undertaken for specific indications in STEMI:
- Failed PCI with persistent pain or hemodynamic instability
- Recurrent ischemia refractory to medical therapy in patients with suitable anatomy who are not candidates for PCI
- Post-MI VSR or papillary muscle rupture, both of which frequently lead to cardiogenic shock
- Cardiogenic shock less than 36 hours after MI, in patients younger than 75 years with ST-segment elevation, or in patients with new LBBB who have multivessel or left main disease
- Recurrent ventricular dysrhythmias in patients with 50% or greater left main coronary artery lesion or triple-vessel disease or both

Recommendations for Secondary Prevention of Complications
Medications
- ACE inhibitors, to prevent ventricular remodeling
- Beta-blockers, to prevent ventricular dysrhythmias
- Diuretics, if heart failure has developed
- Antihyperlipidemics, if total cholesterol, LDL-C, or triglycerides are elevated

Recommendations for Management of Complications after STEMI *Cardiogenic Shock*
- IABP for patients with hypotension (BP of 90 mm Hg or SBP of 30 mm Hg below baseline)

Ventricular Arrhythmias
- VF or pulseless VT is managed by standard ACLS criteria
- Patients with hemodynamically significant VT more than 2 days after STEMI who have ongoing ventricular dysrhythmias are considered for implantation of an ICD
- Patients with an EF between 30% and 40% at 1 month after STEMI should undergo an EPS, if they are inducible to VT/VF, an ICD is recommended to reduce risk of SCD
- Patients with an EF of less than 30% at 1 month after STEMI are at high risk for SCD

AV block
- Transvenous pacemaker (emergency) or permanent pacemaker (later elective) is inserted for symptomatic second- or third-degree AV block.
- All patients after STEMI who require permanent pacing should also be evaluated for ICD indications.

Provide Relevant Education
Medications
- Written and verbal instructions about medication dosages, administration, and side effects

Continued

Acute Coronary Syndrome and Acute Myocardial Infarction (Non-STEMI and STEMI)—cont'd

Emergency Information

- Give patient and family information about calling 911 if pain/angina-equivalent symptoms persist or are worse after 5 minutes.
- Family members of high-risk patients are advised to take a CPR class and learn about AED.

Risk Factors

- Smoking cessation, hypertension control, weight control, normal blood glucose; low-fat diet; normal lipid panel
- Increase physical activity, no new HRT for women

Cardiac Rehabilitation

- Participation in a cardiac rehabilitation program will help the patient continue the process of risk factor and lifestyle modification.

References

Anderson JL, et al. 2011 ACCF/AHA Focused Update Incorporated Into the ACC/AHA 2007 Guidelines for the Management of Patients With Unstable Angina/Non-ST-Elevation Myocardial Infarction: a Report of the American College of Cardiology Foundation/American Heart Association Task Force on Practice Guidelines. *Circulation*. 2011;123:e426.

O'Gara PT, et al. 2013 ACCF/AHA Guideline for the Management of ST-Elevation Myocardial Infarction: a Report of the American College of Cardiology Foundation/American Heart Association Task Force on Practice Guidelines. *Circulation*. 2013;127(4):e362.

Wright SR, et al. 2011 ACC/AHA Focused Update of the guidelines for the management of patients with unstable angina/non ST elevation myocardial infarction: a report of the American College of Cardiology/American Heart Association Task Force on Practice Guidelines developed in collaboration with the American College of Emergency Physicians, Society for Cardiovascular Angiography and Interventions, and Society for Thoracic Surgeons. *J Am Coll Cardiol*. 2011;57:1920.

ACE, Angiotensin-converting enzyme; *ACLS*, advanced cardiac life support; *ACS*, acute coronary syndrome; *AED*, automated external defibrillator; *AV*, atrioventricular; *BP*, blood pressure, *CABG*, coronary artery bypass graft surgery; *CAD*, coronary artery disease; *COX-2*, cyclooxygenase 2; *CPR*, cardiopulmonary resuscitation; *ECG*, electrocardiogram; *ED*, emergency department; *EF*, ejection fraction; *EMS*, emergency medical services; *EPS*, electrophysiology study; *HR*, heart rate; *HRT*, hormone replacement therapy; *IABP*, intra-aortic balloon pump; *ICD*, implantable cardioverter defibrillator; *IV*, intravenous; *LBBB*, left bundle branch block; *LDL*, low-density lipoprotein cholesterol; *MI*, myocardial infarction; *MRI*, magnetic resonance imaging; *non-STEMI*, non-ST-segment elevation myocardial infarction; *NSAIDs*, nonsteroidal anti-inflammatory drugs; *PCI*, percutaneous coronary intervention; *RR*, respiratory rate; *RV*, right ventricle; *Sao₂*, arterial oxygen saturation; *SCD*, sudden cardiac death; *SL*, sublingual; *Spo₂*, oxygen saturation from external pulse-oximeter; *STEMI*, ST-segment elevation myocardial infarction; *TEE*, transesophageal echocardiogram; *TTE*, transthoracic echocardiogram; *VF*, ventricular fibrillation; *VSR*, ventricular septal rupture; *VT*, ventricular tachycardia.

SUDDEN CARDIAC DEATH

Description

Of those who die suddenly each year of coronary heart disease, 50% of men and 64% of women have no previous symptoms of the disease. Between 70% and 89% of sudden cardiac deaths (SCDs) occur in men, and the annual incidence is three to four times higher in men than in women; however, this disparity decreases with advancing age. People who have had an MI with symptoms that last less than 1 hour or occur in a hospital emergency department have a sudden death rate four to six times higher than that of the general population. SCD represents about 5% of the total annual mortality rate for all causes.[51,52,53]

When the onset of symptoms is rapid, the most likely mechanism of death is VT, which degenerates into VF. Despite aggressive cardiopulmonary resuscitation (CPR) initiated outside the hospital, few who sustain an out-of-hospital cardiac arrest survive to hospital discharge. Strategies that have been shown to improve resuscitation survival involve huge communitywide programs to teach laypersons CPR and how to use an automated external defibrillator (AED). These programs assist with survival to hospital discharge.[1]

Etiology

Most SCD incidents occur in patients with pre-existing ventricular dysfunction resulting from cardiac disease. Specific SCD risk factors include extensive coronary atherosclerosis with or without a history of an acute MI; dilated or hypertrophic cardiomyopathy; valvular heart disease; autonomic nervous system abnormalities; electrical system abnormalities such as AV block, Wolff-Parkinson-White (WPW) syndrome, prolonged QT syndrome, or Brugada syndrome; and taking medications that prolong the QT interval.[54-56] An ejection fraction less than 30% and a history of ventricular dysrhythmias are powerful predictors of SCD. Other risk factors are listed in Box 15-15. Unfortunately, many individuals are unaware of their risk or have not considered other risk factors.

Medical Management

Depending on the length of time the patient was unconscious as a result of the cardiac arrest, cognitive defects may be present because of the lack of cerebral blood flow and resultant hypoxia. The cardiac arrest may also have damaged the myocardium and other tissues. Therapy is tailored to the needs of the patient. For comatose patients at high risk for hypoxic brain injury after cardiac arrest, therapeutic hypothermia is initiated to preserve brain function. In the Framingham study, women experienced SCD at half the rate of men and are on the average 6 to 10 years older than men when they experience the event.[52-59] Prevention focuses on identification and treatment of high-risk cardiac patients (see sections "Implantable Cardioverter Defibrillator" and "Antidysrhythmic Medications" in Chapter 16).

HEART FAILURE

Description and Etiology

The number of patients with heart failure is increasing in the United States. Almost 6 million adults (those above the age of 18 years) in the United States have heart failure. It is estimated that by 2030, an additional 3 million more people will be

BOX 15-15 CAUSES OF SUDDEN CARDIAC DEATH

Acquired SCD Risk

Most SCD patients are older adults and have a history of CAD, MI, and subsequent heart failure.

- Heart failure
  - Ejection fraction <30%
  - Heart structure is abnormal (systolic or diastolic ventricular dysfunction)
  - CAD and a history of MI that has produced scar tissue is the most common cause of VT/VF leading to SCD
- Cardiomyopathy (dilated or ischemic)
  - Patients who are inducible for VT/VF in EPS are at highest risk
  - Risk is decreased by implantation of an ICD and antidysrhythmic medication therapy

Genetic SCD Risk

Genetic cardiovascular disease accounts for 40% of SCD in young adults.

- Brugada syndrome
  - ECG signs: coved-type ST-segment elevation (>2 mm) in right precordial leads, although ECG variations also occur
  - Heart structure appears normal
  - High risk of VT or VF in otherwise young healthy adults
  - VT/VF often occurs at night, at rest
  - Represents 4% of all SCD; average age, 41 years
  - Represents up to 20% of genetic SCD patients
  - Hereditary: autosomal-dominant genetic transmission

- Five times more common in males
- Patients who are inducible in EPS are at increased risk
- Risk reduced by implantation of an ICD
- Wolff-Parkinson-White syndrome
  - Congenital accessory conduction pathway connects the atria and ventricles
  - Accessory pathway is *in addition* to the normal conduction system
  - Accessory pathway allows very rapid transmission of impulses leading to "pre-excitation" of the ventricle that can degenerate into VT/VF, especially if atrial dysrhythmias are present
  - WPW syndrome is usually identified when patient is a teenager or young adult
  - WPW syndrome is often recognized during exercise by palpitations or breathlessness
  - It can be cured in many cases by radiofrequency ablation of the accessory pathway
- Hypertrophic cardiomyopathy
  - Risk of VT/VF with exercise exists.
  - The HOCM form can be cured in many cases by alcohol ablation of the enlarged ventricular septum.
  - For other HCM patients, the risk is reduced by implantation of an ICD.
- Long QT syndrome
  - Risk of VT/VF with exercise exists.
  - The risk is reduced by implantation of an ICD.

CAD, Coronary artery disease; *CV*, cardiovascular; *ECG*, electrocardiogram; *EPS*, electrophysiology study; *HCM*, hypertrophic cardiomyopathy; *HOCM*, hypertrophic obstructive cardiomyopathy; *ICD*, implantable cardioverter defibrillator; *MI*, myocardial infarction; *SCD*, sudden cardiac death; *VF*, ventricular fibrillation; *VT*, ventricular tachycardia; *WPW*, Wolff-Parkinson-White.

diagnosed with heart failure.[1] Figure 15-17 is a concept map of heart failure.

Pathophysiology

Heart failure is a response to cardiac dysfunction, a condition in which the heart cannot pump blood at a volume required to meet the body's needs. Any condition that impairs the ability of the ventricles to fill or eject blood can cause heart failure. CAD with resultant necrotic damage to the left ventricle is the underlying cause of heart failure in most patients. Other major conditions that lead to heart failure include valvular dysfunction, infection (myocarditis or endocarditis), cardiomyopathy, and uncontrolled hypertension.[60] Hypertension is the precursor of heart failure in men and women.[1,60]

Assessment and Diagnosis

Heart failure is typically classified on the basis of the New York Heart Association (NYHA) criteria. Patients are assigned into four groups, I through IV, according to the severity of symptoms and degree of patient activity eliciting symptoms (Table 15-7). Research-based clinical guidelines suggest adding a second level of classification that emphasizes the progressive nature of heart failure through stages identified by increasing distress and intensified clinical interventions (Table 15-8).[60] Heart failure can manifest in many different ways, depending on how far ventricular remodeling and dysfunction have advanced. Heart failure may be discovered because of a known clinical syndrome such as acute MI or because of decreased exercise tolerance, fluid retention, or admission to the critical care unit for an unrelated condition.[60] For patients with fluid retention, the most reliable clinical sign of fluid volume overload is jugular venous distention.[60] The procedure used to estimate jugular venous distention is described in Figure 13-2 in Chapter 13.

The first step in the diagnosis is to determine the underlying structural abnormality creating the ventricular dysfunction and symptoms. Various imaging tests are available to visualize cardiac anatomy, and laboratory tests are used to evaluate the impact of hormonal or electrolyte imbalance. The results of these tests permit the cardiology team to design a treatment plan to control symptoms and possibly correct the underlying cause. All patients do not have the same type of heart failure.

Left Ventricular Failure

Failure of the left ventricle is defined as a disturbance of the contractile function of the left ventricle, resulting in a low cardiac output state. This leads to vasoconstriction of the arterial bed that raises systemic vascular resistance (SVR), a condition also described as "high afterload," and creates congestion and edema in the pulmonary circulation and alveoli. Patients presenting with left ventricular failure have one of the following: 1) decreased exercise tolerance, 2) fluid retention, or 3) discovery during examination of noncardiac problems.[60] Clinical manifestations of left ventricular failure include decreased peripheral perfusion with weak or diminished pulses; cool, pale extremities; and, in later stages, peripheral cyanosis (Table 15-9). Over time, with progression of the disease state, the fluid accumulation behind the dysfunctional left ventricle elevates pulmonary pressures, contributes to pulmonary congestion and

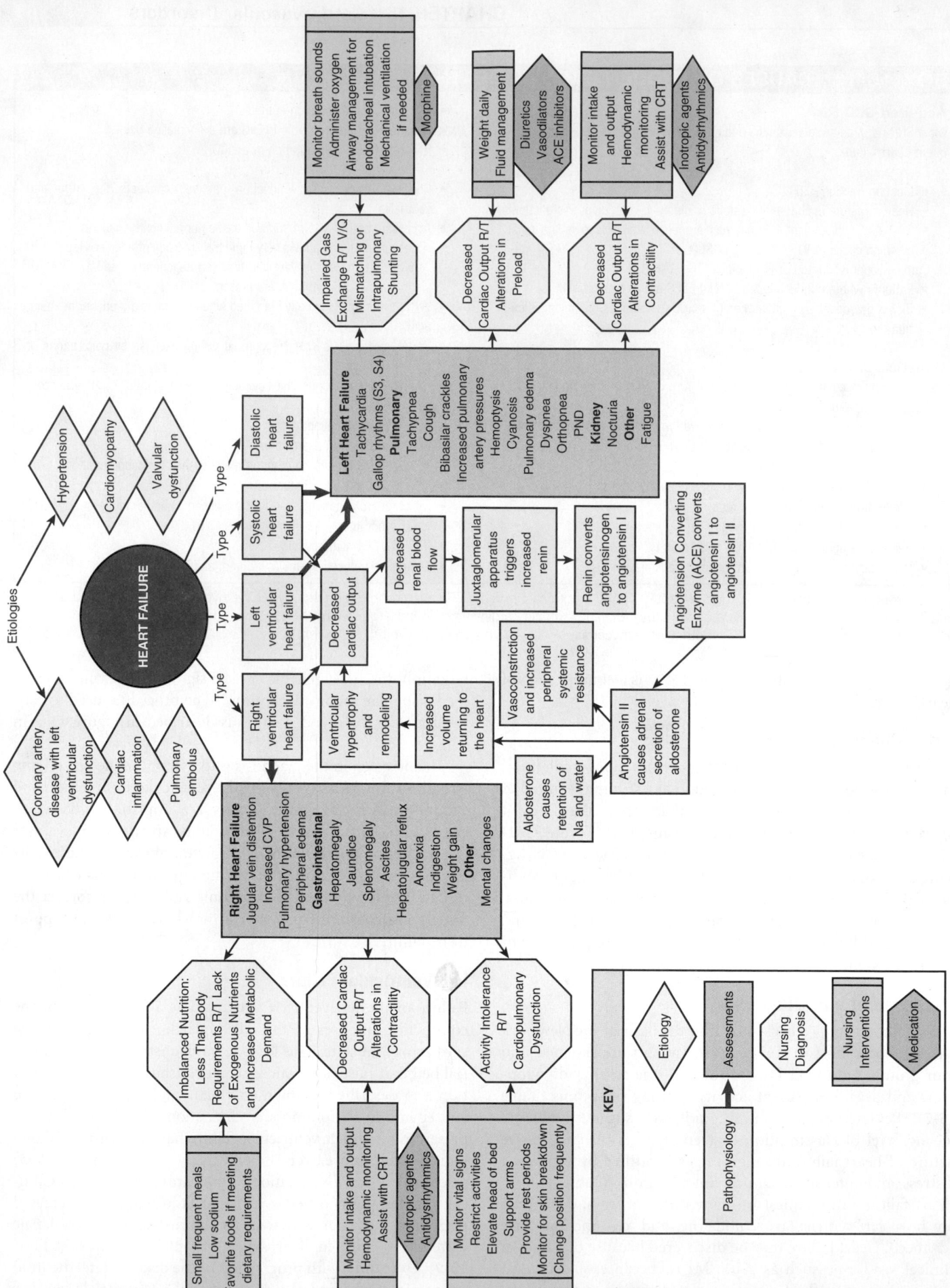

FIGURE 15-17 Concept map for heart failure. (Created by Elaine Bishop Kennedy, EdD, RN.)

edema, and produces dysfunction of the right ventricle, resulting in failure of the right side of the heart.

Right Ventricular Failure

Failure of the right side of the heart is defined as ineffective right ventricular contractile function. Pure failure of the right ventricle may result from an acute condition such as a pulmonary embolus or a right ventricular infarction, but it is most commonly caused by failure of the left side of the heart. The common manifestations of right ventricular failure are jugular venous distention, elevated central venous pressure (CVP), weakness, peripheral or sacral edema, hepatomegaly (enlarged liver), jaundice, and liver tenderness. Gastrointestinal symp-

toms include poor appetite, anorexia, nausea, and an uncomfortable feeling of fullness (see Table 15-9).

Systolic Heart Failure

The term *systolic dysfunction* describes an abnormality of the heart muscle that markedly decreases contractility during systole (ejection) and lessens the quantity of blood that can be pumped out of the heart. Patients with a diagnosis of systolic heart failure (SHF) have signs and symptoms of heart failure combined with a below-normal ejection fraction. Left ventricular systolic dysfunction is the classic picture that most clinicians consider when thinking about heart failure. In addition to the signs and symptoms of left heart failure (described earlier), the patient has a low ejection fraction. How low the ejection fraction has to be to qualify as SHF is still being debated, but the value usually is below 50%;[65] some clinicians cite numbers below 45% or 40%.[67,68] Symptoms of SHF include dyspnea, exercise intolerance, and fluid volume overload.

CAD and its sequelae represent the underlying cause in two thirds of patients with systolic heart failure.[60] The remaining patients with systolic dysfunction have *nonischemic cardiomyopathy* (described as *dilated cardiomyopathy*),[62] which results from an identifiable cause such as hypertension, thyroid disease, cardiac valvular disease, alcohol use, or myocarditis.[60] If the cause is unknown, systolic dysfunction is described as *idiopathic dilated cardiomyopathy*. SHF increases with age. Clinical findings that are required to make a diagnosis of SHF include the following:

TABLE 15-7 NEW YORK HEART ASSOCIATION FUNCTIONAL CLASSIFICATION OF HEART FAILURE

CLASS	DEFINITION
I	Normal daily activity does not initiate symptoms.
II	Normal daily activities initiate onset of symptoms, but symptoms subside with rest.
III	Minimal activity initiates symptoms; patients are usually symptom free at rest.
IV	Any type of activity initiates symptoms, and symptoms are present at rest.

TABLE 15-8 PROGRESSION OF HEART FAILURE

STAGE	STRUCTURAL HEART DISORDER	SYMPTOMS	MANAGEMENT
A	No, but at risk because of hypertension CAD Diabetes mellitus	None	Preventive treatment of known risk factors Hypertension Lipid disorders Cigarette smoking Diabetes mellitus Discourage alcohol and illicit drug use
B	Yes, but without symptoms Previous MI Family history of CM Asymptomatic valvular disease or CM	None	Treat all risk factors If indicated, use the following: • ACE inhibitors • Beta-blockers
C	Yes, with prior or current symptoms	Shortness of breath Fatigue Reduced exercise tolerance	Treat all risk factors and HF symptoms: • Diuretics • ACE inhibitors • Beta-blockers • Digitalis • Dietary salt restriction
D	Yes, with refractory HF symptoms despite maximal specialized interventions (pharmacologic, medical, nursing) Recurrently hospitalized for HF symptoms	Marked symptoms at rest despite maximal medical therapy	Refractory HF requires interventions from previous stages (A—C), plus the following: • Continuous IV inotropic support • Mechanical assist devices • Heart transplantation • Hospice care

Modified from Hunt SA, et al. ACC/AHA 2005 guideline update for the diagnosis and management of chronic heart failure in the adult: a report of the American College of Cardiology/American Heart Association Task Force on Practice Guidelines. *Circulation.* 2005;112(12):e154.
ACE, Angiotensin-converting enzyme; *CAD,* coronary artery disease; *CM,* cardiomyopathy; *HF,* heart failure; *IV,* intravenous; *MI,* myocardial infarction.

TABLE 15-9 CLINICAL MANIFESTATIONS OF RIGHT- AND LEFT-SIDED HEART FAILURE

LEFT VENTRICULAR FAILURE		RIGHT VENTRICULAR FAILURE	
SIGNS	SYMPTOMS	SIGNS	SYMPTOMS
Tachypnea	Fatigue	Peripheral edema	Weakness
Tachycardia	Dyspnea	Hepatomegaly	Anorexia
Cough	Orthopnea	Splenomegaly	Indigestion
Bibasilar crackles	Paroxysmal nocturnal dyspnea	Hepatojugular reflux	Weight gain
Gallop rhythms (S₃ and S₄)	Nocturia	Ascites	Mental changes
Increased pulmonary artery pressures		Jugular venous distention	
Hemoptysis		Increased central venous pressure	
Cyanosis		Pulmonary hypertension	
Pulmonary edema			

- Signs and symptoms of heart failure
- Left ventricular systolic dysfunction with an ejection fraction below normal

In systolic heart failure, the ventricular chambers change their shape, a detrimental development known as *ventricular remodeling.* The negative impact on the cardiac cells is different from the dysfunction and loss of myocytes from myocardial ischemia and infarction.

Significant hemodynamic changes occur as systolic dysfunction progresses. In systolic heart failure, the left ventricular end-diastolic volume (LVEDV) is high, which raises the left ventricular end-diastolic pressure (LVEDP) compared with a normal heart. The increase in intracardiac volume and pressure causes a rise in left atrial and pulmonary venous pressures. This means that all blood flowing into the heart through the pulmonary vascular bed is exposed to increased hydrostatic pressure, which is necessary to fill the congested heart. The increase in pulmonary vascular pressure causes transudation of fluid from the pulmonary capillaries into the alveolar interstitium, and this fluid is ultimately forced through the walls of the alveoli, causing pulmonary edema. The pulmonary complications of heart failure are described in greater detail later. The elevated left heart pressures eventually raise pressures in the right side of the heart and lead to secondary right heart failure.

Diastolic Heart Failure

The term *diastolic dysfunction* describes an abnormality of the heart muscle that makes it unable to relax, stretch, or fill during diastole. Diastolic heart failure (DHF) is caused by left ventricular dysfunction.[63] DHF is treated differently from SHF.

Studies have shown that patients with DHF have a preserved ejection fraction defined as 45% or greater. Principal causes are similar to SHF (described earlier): CAD, myocardial ischemia, AF, uncontrolled hypertension in 75% of cases, and left ventricular hypertrophy in about 40%.[64] Some conditions that are known to markedly alter diastolic function include hypertrophic cardiomyopathy, restrictive cardiomyopathy, and infiltrative diseases such as amyloidosis and neoplastic infiltrate.[60,64] The incidence of DHF is highest among patients older than 75 years, and the condition disproportionately affects older women. It is postulated that the process of aging impacts diastolic function negatively, imposing stiffness and fibrosis on the cardiac muscle and cardiovascular vessels.

Clinical findings that are required to make a diagnosis of DHF include the following:[60,61,63]
- Signs and symptoms of heart failure
- Normal or only mildly abnormal left ventricular systolic dysfunction
- Abnormal left ventricular relaxation, filling, diastolic distensibility, or diastolic stiffness

Normally, diastole is the filling stage of the cardiac cycle when the ventricle relaxes completely. The abnormal hemodynamics of DHF can be elicited by diagnostic tests such as cardiac catheterization and a stress echocardiogram (see Stress Echocardiography in Chapter 14). An ejection fraction above the range of 40% to 50% is considered normal for this population.

In DHF, the LVEDP is high, whereas the LVEDV is paradoxically low compared with normal hearts.[63] Another diagnostic clue is that many patients with DHF have normal intracardiac pressures at rest, but during exercise, the LVEDP and pulmonary vascular pressures rise rapidly.[63] This occurs because the noncompliant, stiff ventricle cannot increase stroke volume during exercise; cardiac output remains low, even though physical demand is high. Patients with DHF often experience a sudden rise in blood pressure and sinus tachycardia during exercise; they are exercise intolerant and experience fatigue, dyspnea, pulmonary venous congestion, and even pulmonary edema.[60,64,65]

Systolic Diastolic Heart Failure versus Diastolic Heart Failure

It turns out to be impossible to accurately determine whether a patient has SHF or DHF from clinical assessment alone.[63] Both types of heart failure produce similar signs and symptoms. The level of symptoms and quality of life vary between individuals and between men and women, even when the ejection fraction and presumed cardiac dysfunction are the same.[66] This may occur because most symptoms come from the neurohormonal compensatory mechanisms (described later) rather than the cardiac output. An elevated B-type natriuretic peptide (BNP) level (>100 picogram per milliliter [pg/mL]) is very useful to diagnose heart failure in patients with fluid overload and shortness of breath.[66] The BNP value tends to be higher in patients with a diagnosis of SHF compared with those with DHF, although the difference is not reliable enough to be used to differentiate the two types of heart failure in clinical practice.[67] The more severe the heart failure, the higher is the BNP level. The primary use of the BNP test is to determine whether the patient has heart failure.

The definitive diagnosis of the type of heart failure is often made using Doppler echocardiography. A two-dimensional echocardiogram coupled with Doppler flow studies to determine whether abnormalities of the myocardium, heart valves, or pericardium are present and which chambers are involved is the single-most powerful diagnostic test in the evaluation of patients with heart failure. Calculation of the ejection fraction can be determined using Doppler echocardiography or during a cardiac catheterization. These diagnostic tests also show that some patients exhibit combined SHF and DHF.[60,63]

It is not possible to distinguish whether a patient has SHF or DHF simply by looking at the medications they are prescribed. The same medications are used to treat the two types of heart failure, although the underlying rationales may be different.[61] For example, beta-blockers are used in DHF to slow the heart rate, to prolong diastole to give more time for ventricular filling, and to modify the ventricular response to exercise, especially for patients who have a preserved ejection fraction.[61] When beta-blockers are prescribed for treatment of SHF, the intent is to preserve long-term inotropic (contractile) function and prevent ventricular remodeling.[61] Diuretics are used to treat both types of heart failure, although a smaller dosage is generally needed in DHF.[61] ACEIs and ARBs are also used to treat both types of heart failure. The medications used to treat heart failure are further discussed in Chapter 16 (see Table 16-21).

Acute Heart Failure versus Chronic Heart Failure

Acute or chronic heart failure is determined by the rapid progression of the syndrome, the presence and activation of compensatory mechanisms, and the presence or absence of fluid accumulation in the interstitial space (see Table 15-8). In clinical practice guidelines, the terms *acute* and *chronic* have replaced the older name of *congestive heart failure* (CHF) because not all heart failure involves pulmonary congestion. However, the description of a patient by CHF remains commonly employed in clinical practice.

Acute heart failure has a sudden onset, with no compensatory mechanisms. The patient may experience acute pulmonary edema, low cardiac output, or even cardiogenic shock. Patients with chronic heart failure are hypervolemic, have sodium and water retention, and have structural heart chamber changes such as dilation or hypertrophy.[60]

Chronic heart failure is an ongoing process, with symptoms that may be made tolerable by medication, diet, and a reduced activity level. The deterioration into acute heart failure can be precipitated by the onset of dysrhythmias, acute ischemia, sudden illness, or cessation of medications. This may necessitate admission to a critical care unit. Hypertension is the primary precursor of heart failure in women, whereas coronary heart disease, specifically MI, is the primary cause of heart failure in men.[60]

Neurohormonal Compensatory Mechanisms in Heart Failure

When the heart begins to fail and the cardiac output is no longer sufficient to meet the metabolic needs of tissues, the body activates several major compensatory mechanisms: the sympathetic nervous system, the renin-angiotensin-aldosterone system (RAAS), and, if hypertension is present, the development of ventricular hypertrophy (see Table 15-8). This process ultimately reshapes the ventricle in a process described as *ventricular remodeling*. These pathophysiologic processes and the pharmacologic measures taken to limit ventricular remodeling are described in this section.

The sympathetic nervous system compensates for low cardiac output by increasing heart rate and blood pressure. As a result, levels of circulating catecholamines are increased, resulting in peripheral vasoconstriction. In addition to raising blood pressure and heart rate, catecholamines cause shunting of blood from nonvital organs such as the skin to vital organs such as the heart and brain. This mechanism, although initially helpful, may become a negative factor if elevation of heart rate increases myocardial oxygen demand while shortening the amount of time for diastolic filling and coronary artery perfusion.

Activation of renin-angiotensin-aldosterone system (RAAS) in heart failure promotes fluid retention.[56,68] The RAAS is activated by low cardiac output that causes the hormone renin to be secreted by the kidneys. A physiologic chain of events is then set in motion that leads to volume overload. The renin acts on angiotensinogen in the bloodstream and converts it to angiotensin I; when angiotensin passes through the lung tissues, it is activated by angiotensin-converting enzyme (ACE), an enzyme that converts the angiotensin I to angiotensin II, a powerful vasoconstrictor that increases SVR, raises blood pressure, and increases the workload of the left ventricle; the increased SVR further lowers cardiac output. The mineralocorticoid hormone aldosterone is released from the adrenal glands and stimulates sodium retention by means of the distal tubules of the kidney. In response to the low cardiac output, the renal arterioles constrict, decrease glomerular filtration, and increase reabsorption of sodium from the proximal and distal tubules. To break the RAAS cycle of fluid retention in heart failure, two types of medications are prescribed to interrupt the steps. To inhibit the conversion of angiotensin I to angiotensin II, an ACEI is prescribed (see Table 16-21 (Medications used for Heart Failure) in Chapter 16). These agents prevent arterial vasoconstriction, decrease blood pressure and SVR, and decrease the amount of ventricular remodeling that often occurs with heart failure. A medication that inhibits angiotensin II directly may be prescribed instead. The medications in this category are ARBs.[68] Aldactone (spirolactone) is a medication from a different category that is also prescribed to break the RAAS cycle. Aldactone is a mineralocorticoid receptor antagonist that inhibits (blocks) the retention of sodium from the distal tubules of the kidney.[56,68] Figure 15-18 depicts the mechanism of action by which these medications act on the RAAS.

Ventricular hypertrophy is the final compensatory mechanism. It is also strongly associated with pre-existing hypertension. Because myocardial hypertrophy increases the force of contraction, hypertrophy helps the ventricle overcome an increase in afterload. When this mechanism is no longer efficient for the ventricle, it will remodel by dilation.

Ventricular remodeling occurs as a result of the previously described mechanisms. The shape of the ventricle is changed,

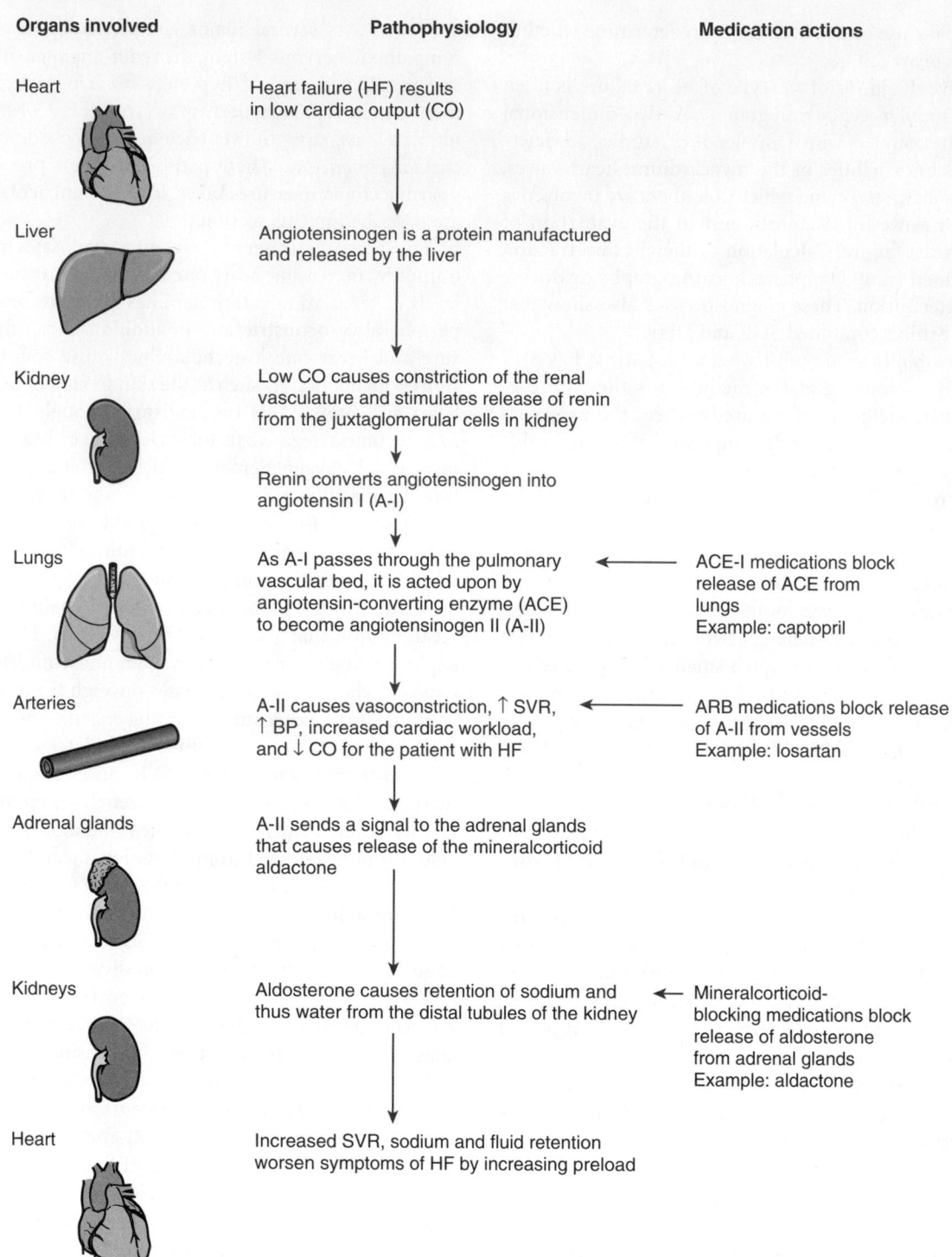

Organs involved	Pathophysiology	Medication actions
Heart	Heart failure (HF) results in low cardiac output (CO)	
Liver	Angiotensinogen is a protein manufactured and released by the liver	
Kidney	Low CO causes constriction of the renal vasculature and stimulates release of renin from the juxtaglomerular cells in kidney	
	Renin converts angiotensinogen into angiotensin I (A-I)	
Lungs	As A-I passes through the pulmonary vascular bed, it is acted upon by angiotensin-converting enzyme (ACE) to become angiotensinogen II (A-II)	← ACE-I medications block release of ACE from lungs Example: captopril
Arteries	A-II causes vasoconstriction, ↑ SVR, ↑ BP, increased cardiac workload, and ↓ CO for the patient with HF	← ARB medications block release of A-II from vessels Example: losartan
Adrenal glands	A-II sends a signal to the adrenal glands that causes release of the mineralcorticoid aldactone	
Kidneys	Aldosterone causes retention of sodium and thus water from the distal tubules of the kidney	← Mineralcorticoid-blocking medications block release of aldosterone from adrenal glands Example: aldactone
Heart	Increased SVR, sodium and fluid retention worsen symptoms of HF by increasing preload	

FIGURE 15-18 Renin-angiotensin-aldosterone system (RAAS), its role in heart failure, and medication actions.

or is remodeled, to resemble a round bowl. A dilated ventricle has poor contractility and is enlarged without hypertrophy. Research trial evidence indicates that synergistic use of medications from different categories—ACEI or ARB, aldactone, as well as beta-blockade—can halt or reduce the progression of heart failure remodeling.[69,70,71]

Pulmonary Complications of Heart Failure

The clinical manifestations of acute heart failure result from tissue hypoperfusion and organ congestion and are progressive.

The severity of clinical manifestations progresses as heart failure worsens. Initially, manifestations appear only with exertion, but eventually, they also occur at rest.[60]

Shortness of Breath in Heart Failure

The patient experiences the feeling of shortness of breath first with exertion, but as heart failure worsens, symptoms are also present at rest. A diagnostic blood test is available to assist clinicians in differentiating whether a patient's shortness of breath is caused by cardiac failure or by pulmonary complications.

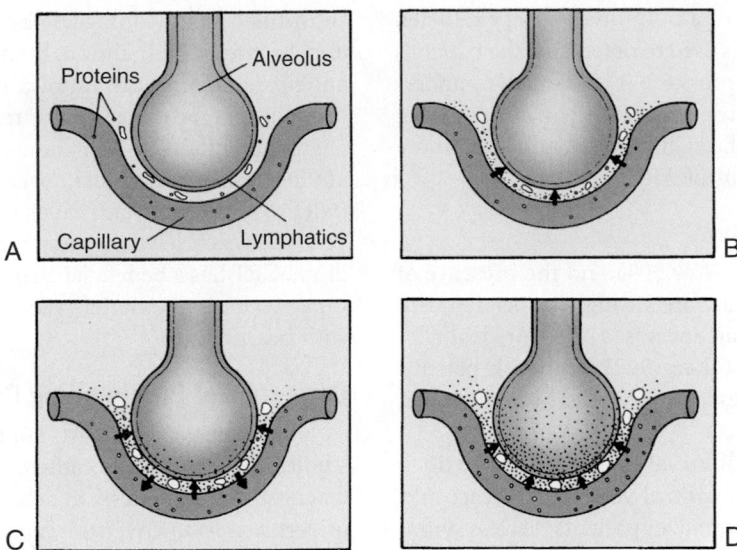

FIGURE 15-19   As pulmonary edema progresses, it inhibits oxygen and carbon dioxide exchange at the alveolar capillary interface. *A,* Normal relationship; *B,* increased pulmonary capillary hydrostatic pressure causes fluid to move from the vascular space into the pulmonary interstitial space; *C,* lymphatic flow increases in an attempt to pull fluid back into the vascular or lymphatic space; *D,* failure of lymphatic flow and worsening of left-sided heart failure results in further movement of fluid into the interstitial space and the alveoli.

BNP, a cardiac neurohormone released by the ventricles in response to volume expansion and pressure overload, is elevated in DHF and SHF. Heart failure increases left ventricular wall tension because of the excess preload in the ventricles. When the BNP blood level is greater than 100 pg/mL, the dyspnea is most likely related to cardiac failure rather than pulmonary failure.[72,73] The more severe the heart failure, the higher is the BNP value.[73] If the patient has concomitant kidney disease, the BNP clinical diagnostic point to diagnose heart failure rises to greater than 200 pg/mL.[74,75] Breathlessness in heart failure is described by the following terms:

- *Dyspnea:* the patient's sensation of shortness of breath, which from pulmonary vascular congestion and decreased lung compliance
- *Orthopnea:* difficulty breathing when lying flat because of an increase in venous return that occurs in the supine position
- *Paroxysmal nocturnal dyspnea:* a severe form of orthopnea in which the patient awakens from sleep gasping for air
- *Cardiac asthma:* dyspnea with wheezing, a nonproductive cough, and pulmonary crackles that progress to the gurgling sounds of pulmonary edema

Pulmonary Edema in Heart Failure

Pulmonary edema, or protein-laden fluid in the alveoli, inhibits gas exchange by impairing the diffusion pathway between the alveolus and the capillary. It is caused by increased left atrial and ventricular pressures and results in an excessive accumulation of serous or serosanguineous fluid in the interstitial spaces and alveoli of the lungs. The formation of pulmonary edema has two stages. The first stage is not as severe and is characterized by interstitial edema, engorgement of the perivascular and peribronchial spaces, and increased lymphatic flow (Fig. 15-19B). The later stage is characterized by alveolar edema resulting from fluid moving into the alveoli from the interstitium (see Fig. 15-19C). Eventually, blood plasma moves into the alveoli faster than the lymphatic system can clear it, interfering with diffusion of oxygen, depressing the arterial partial pressure of oxygen (Pao_2), and leading to tissue hypoxia (see Fig. 15-19D).

Patients experiencing heart failure and pulmonary edema are extremely breathless and anxious and have a sensation of suffocation. They expectorate pink, frothy sputum and feel as if they are drowning. They may sit bolt upright, gasp for breath, or thrash about. The respiratory rate is elevated, and accessory muscles of ventilation are used, with nasal flaring and bulging neck muscles. Respirations are characterized by loud inspiratory and expiratory gurgling sounds. Diaphoresis is profuse, and the skin is cold, ashen, and sometimes cyanotic. This reflects low cardiac output, increased sympathetic stimulation, peripheral vasoconstriction, and desaturation of arterial blood.

Arterial Blood Gases in Pulmonary Edema. Arterial blood gas values are variable. In the early stage of pulmonary edema, respiratory alkalosis may be present because of hyperventilation, which eliminates CO_2. As the pulmonary edema progresses and gas exchange becomes impaired, acidosis (pH <7.35) and hypoxemia ensue. A chest radiograph usually confirms an enlarged cardiac silhouette, pulmonary venous congestion, and interstitial edema.

Cardiogenic Pulmonary Edema versus Noncardiogenic Pulmonary Edema. In the critical care unit, when a patient develops pulmonary edema, it is often a challenge to determine whether the cause is cardiac, known as *cardiogenic pulmonary edema,* or the origin is pulmonary or systemic in origin. The latter is referred to as *noncardiogenic pulmonary edema* or, more commonly, *acute respiratory distress syndrome* (ARDS). Options to determine the cause of the pulmonary edema include use of the serum BNP level[67] or insertion of a pulmonary artery catheter. The pulmonary artery catheter is used to determine the patient's "pulmonary arterial occlusion" pressure. It is essential to understand the different causes because the treatment of each form of pulmonary edema is specific. Chapter 20 provides more information on the management of ARDS.

Dysrhythmias and Heart Failure

A ventricular ejection fraction below 30% and the presence of NYHA class III or IV heart failure are strongly associated with ventricular dysrhythmias and an increased risk for death.[76,77] Because sustained VT or VF initiates SCD, high-risk patients with severe heart failure are prescribed antidysrhythmic medications and have an ICD inserted.[76,77]

Many patients with heart failure also have AF. Digoxin is frequently prescribed for AF to control ventricular heart rate. Digoxin does not prolong life but makes patients feel less symptomatic. Digoxin may also work synergistically with specific beta-blockers (e.g., carvedilol) and make the symptoms more tolerable for patients with severe heart failure.[76,77]

Medical Management

The goals of the medical management of heart failure are to relieve symptoms, enhance cardiac performance, and correct known precipitating causes.

Relief of Symptoms and Enhancement of Cardiac Performance

In the acute phase of advanced heart failure, the patient may have a pulmonary artery catheter in place so that left ventricular function can be monitored closely. Control of symptoms involves management of fluid overload and improvement of cardiac output by decreasing SVR and increasing contractility. Diuretics are administered to decrease preload and to eliminate excess fluid from the body.[69] If pulmonary edema develops, additional diuretics are used. Morphine is given to facilitate peripheral dilation and decrease anxiety. Afterload is decreased by vasodilators such as sodium nitroprusside (Nipride) and nitroglycerin. Sodium nitroprusside is a balanced vasodilator medication that relaxes arterial resistance and venous capacitance vessels. By reducing both preload and afterload, it can relieve congestion and also improve cardiac output, particularly in patients with increased SVR. It is useful in favorably redistributing total LV stroke volume in patients with either mitral or aortic insufficiency such that regurgitant flow is reduced while forward flow is increased.[78] Nitrates are used to decrease preload and vasodilate the coronary arteries if CAD is an underlying cause of the acute heart failure. For some patients, an IABP is temporarily required.[79] Contractility is initially increased by continuous infusion of positive inotropic medications (dopamine) or by combination inodilators such as dobutamine or milrinone.

After the acute exacerbation is resolved, the patient is transitioned to oral agents as the intravenous medications are weaned off. Before the transition out of the critical care unit, the patient with heart failure will receive ACEIs to inhibit left ventricular chamber remodeling and slow left ventricular dilation.[60,68,70] If the patient does not tolerate ACEIs, ARBs may be substituted.[69] Low dosage beta-blockers such as carvedilol may also be prescribed, although strict surveillance is required to anticipate and avoid untoward negative inotropic effects.[77] Digoxin may be added to the regimen, especially if the person has concomitant AF.[80] Nonpharmacologic interventions that are increasingly used include *cardiac resynchronization therapy* (CRT).[81] CRT is biventricular pacing, where the right and left ventricles each have a pacing lead in contact with the myocardium. CRT has a beneficial effect on clinical symptoms, exercise capacity, and systolic left ventricular performance in patients with heart failure.[81,82,83]

Correction of Precipitating Causes

After symptoms of heart failure are controlled, diagnostic studies such as cardiac catheterization, echocardiography, and diagnostic imaging tests to determine myocardial perfusion are undertaken to uncover the cause of the heart failure and tailor long-term management to treat the cause. Some structural problems such as valvular disease may be amenable to surgical correction.

Palliative Care for End-Stage Heart Failure

In 2004, a consensus statement on palliative and supportive care in advanced heart failure was published.[84] Heart failure is a progressive disease, and patients will not recover.[60,84] At a point in the trajectory of heart failure, many patients with NYHA class IV heart failure will become candidates for palliative care.[84] The primary aim of palliative care is symptom management and the relief of suffering. Fundamental to all symptom management strategies for heart failure is the optimization of medications, according to current guidelines.[60,84] The most common symptoms of advanced heart failure are dyspnea, pain, and fatigue.[84]

Nursing Management

Nursing management of the patient with heart failure incorporates a variety of nursing diagnoses (Box 15-16). Nursing management interventions are designed to achieve optimal cardiopulmonary function, promote comfort and emotional support, monitor the effectiveness of pharmacologic therapy, ensure nutritional intake is sufficient, and provide patient and family education.

⊚ **BOX 15-16   NURSING DIAGNOSES**

Acute Heart Failure

- Impaired Gas Exchange, related to ventilation/perfusion mismatching or intrapulmonary shunting, p. 1144
- Decreased Cardiac Output, related to alterations in preload, p. 1128
- Decreased Cardiac Output, related to alterations in contractility, p. 1128
- Decreased Cardiac Output, related to alterations in heart rate or rhythm, p. 1128
- Activity Intolerance, related to cardiopulmonary dysfunction, p. 1119
- Anxiety, related to threat to biologic, psychologic, or social integrity, p. 1125
- Ineffective Coping, related to situational crisis and personal vulnerability, p. 1150
- Deficient Knowledge, related to lack of previous exposure to information, p. 1134 (see Box 15-17, Patient Education for Acute Heart Failure)

Optimizing Cardiopulmonary Function

The patient's ECG is evaluated for dysrhythmias that may be present as a result of medication toxicity or electrolyte imbalance. Patients with heart failure are prone to digoxin toxicity because of decreased renal perfusion and electrolyte imbalances. Breath sounds are auscultated frequently to determine the adequacy of respiratory effort and to assess for onset or worsening of pulmonary congestion. Oxygen is administered through a nasal cannula to relieve dyspnea. Diuretics or vasodilators are used to decrease excessive preload and afterload.[60,69] If the patient is not hypotensive, morphine may be administered to decrease hyperventilation and anxiety. If the patient's ventilatory status worsens, the nurse must be prepared for endotracheal intubation and mechanical ventilation. Obtaining daily weights is important until the weight stabilizes at a "dry" weight. Generally, the daily weight is used in fluid management and a weekly weight is optimally used for tracking body weight (e.g., muscle, fat).

Promoting Comfort and Emotional Support

During periods of breathlessness, activity must be restricted. Bed rest usually is prescribed for the patient, who is positioned with the head of the bed elevated to allow for maximal lung expansion. The arms can be supported on pillows so that no undue stress is placed on the shoulder muscles. The legs may be placed in a dependent position to encourage venous pooling, thereby decreasing venous return. Rest periods must be carefully planned and adhered to and independence within the patient's activity prescription fostered. Vital signs are recorded before an activity is begun and after it is completed. Signs of activity intolerance such as dyspnea, fatigue, sustained increase in pulse, and onset of dysrhythmias are documented and reported to the physician. Activity is gradually increased according to the patient's tolerance. Skin breakdown is a risk because of the combination of bed rest, inadequate nutrition, peripheral edema, and decreased perfusion to the skin and subcutaneous tissue. Frequent position changes and mobilization can help to provide comfort and prevent this complication.

Monitoring the Effects of Pharmacologic Therapy

Patients experiencing acute heart failure require aggressive pharmacologic therapy.[78,80,85] The critical care nurse must know the action, side effects, therapeutic levels, and toxic effects of the diuretics and venodilators used to decrease preload, the positive inotropic agents used to increase ventricular contractility, the vasodilators used to decrease afterload, and any antidysrhythmics used to control heart rate and prevent dysrhythmias. The patient's hemodynamic response to these agents is closely monitored. Fluid intake and output balances are tabulated daily or even hourly in the critical care unit.

Nutritional Intake

Patients experiencing heart failure often have decreased appetite and nausea, so small, frequent meals may be more appropriate than the standard three large meals. Food must be as tasty as possible; favorite foods and foods from home may be incorporated into the diet as long as the foods are compatible with nutritional restrictions such as low levels of sodium to decrease

---

BOX 15-17   PATIENT EDUCATION

Acute Heart Failure

- Heart failure: pathophysiology of heart failure
- Fluid balance: low-salt diet to reduce fluid retention; intake and output measurement; signs of fluid overload, such as peripheral edema
- Daily weight: increase or loss of 1 to 2 pounds in a few days is a sign of fluid gain or loss, not true weight gain or loss
- Breathlessness: increasing shortness of breath, wheezing, and sleeping upright on pillows or in a recliner are symptoms that must be monitored and reported to a health care professional
- Activity: activity conservation with rest periods as heart failure progresses
- Medications: as medications are complex, information must be given in writing and orally
  - Preload: purpose of diuretics, increased urine output, and control of fluid volume
  - Afterload: purpose of vasodilators or angiotensin-converting enzyme (ACE) inhibitors in decreasing the workload of the heart
  - Heart rate: purpose of digoxin is to control atrial fibrillation, a frequent dysrhythmia in heart failure
  - Contractility: with the exception of digoxin, no oral contractility medications are approved by the U.S. Food and Drug Administration (FDA)
  - Anticoagulation: patients with distended atria and enlarged ventricles or with atrial fibrillation may be prescribed an anticoagulant such as warfarin (Coumadin); risks of bleeding, importance of correct dosages, prothrombin times, international normalized ratio (INR), and nutritional-pharmacologic interactions are emphasized
- Follow-up care
- Symptoms to report to a health care professional

---

the risk of fluid retention. Each patient must be assessed for nutritional imbalance individually. Not all patients with heart failure have the same nutritional needs.

Patient Education

The nurse assesses the patient's and family's understanding of the pathophysiology and individual risk factor profile for heart failure.[84] Primary topics of education include 1) the importance of a daily weight, 2) fluid restrictions, and 3) written information about the multiple medications used to control the symptoms of heart failure (Box 15-17).[60] Many patients with a diagnosis of heart failure also require education about lifestyle changes such as smoking cessation, weight loss, energy conservation, and how to incorporate exercise and sodium restriction into their daily lives.[70,86,87] Achieving the optimal outcomes for the patient with heart failure require contributions from a team of educated health care clinicians.[70,85,86,87,88] Collaborative multidisciplinary goals, developed from clinical practice guidelines for the management of the patient with symptoms of heart failure, are listed in Box 15-18.

CARDIOMYOPATHY

Description and Etiology

Cardiomyopathy is a disease of the heart muscle: *cardio* (heart), *myo-* (muscle), and *-pathy* (pathology). Cardiomyopathies are classified on the basis of structural abnormalities and, if known, genotype. Cardiomyopathies are categorized as *extrinsic*, being caused by external factors such as hypertension, ischemia,

BOX 15-18   EVIDENCE-BASED PRACTICE

Heart Failure

 A collaborative heart failure management team provides an integrated approach to care to achieve clinical stability for the patient.

1. Ensure systematic assessment and management.
   - To achieve an absence of "congestion" and to stabilize patient's condition at the best "stage" possible when in hospital (see Tables 15-7 and 15-8)
   - To maintain the same stability once discharged home and to avoid hospital readmission
2. Counsel and educate patient and family after discharge from hospital. Patients and families should understand the following:
   - Heart failure disease process
   - Heart failure medications, dosages, medication schedule, medication side effects
   - Fluid balance related to salt-restriction diet (2 g/day of sodium), daily weight, diuretic regimen
   - When to call health care provider
   - Risk of additional complications: sudden cardiac death, progressive heart failure, need for other cardiac procedures (pacemaker, ICD, PCI) or cardiac

surgery (bypass graft, valve replacement); mechanical assist device or heart transplantation, as needed by some patients
   - Purpose of "advance directive" for health care decisions
3. Promote patient compliance with treatment regimen.
   - Patient needs support from concerned companions and health care professionals.
   - Patient should remain physically active and involved with life.
4. Facilitate hospital discharge; implement outpatient models of health care delivery.
   - Close communication between inpatient and outpatient health care providers is essential.

Reference

Jessup M, et al. 2009 focused update: ACCF/AHA Guidelines for the Diagnosis and Management of Heart Failure in Adults: a report of the American College of Cardiology Foundation/American Heart Association Task Force on Practice Guidelines: developed in collaboration with the International Society for Heart and Lung Transplantation. *Circulation.* 2009;119(14):1977-2016.

ICD, Implantable cardioverter-defibrillator; *PCI,* percutaneous coronary intervention.

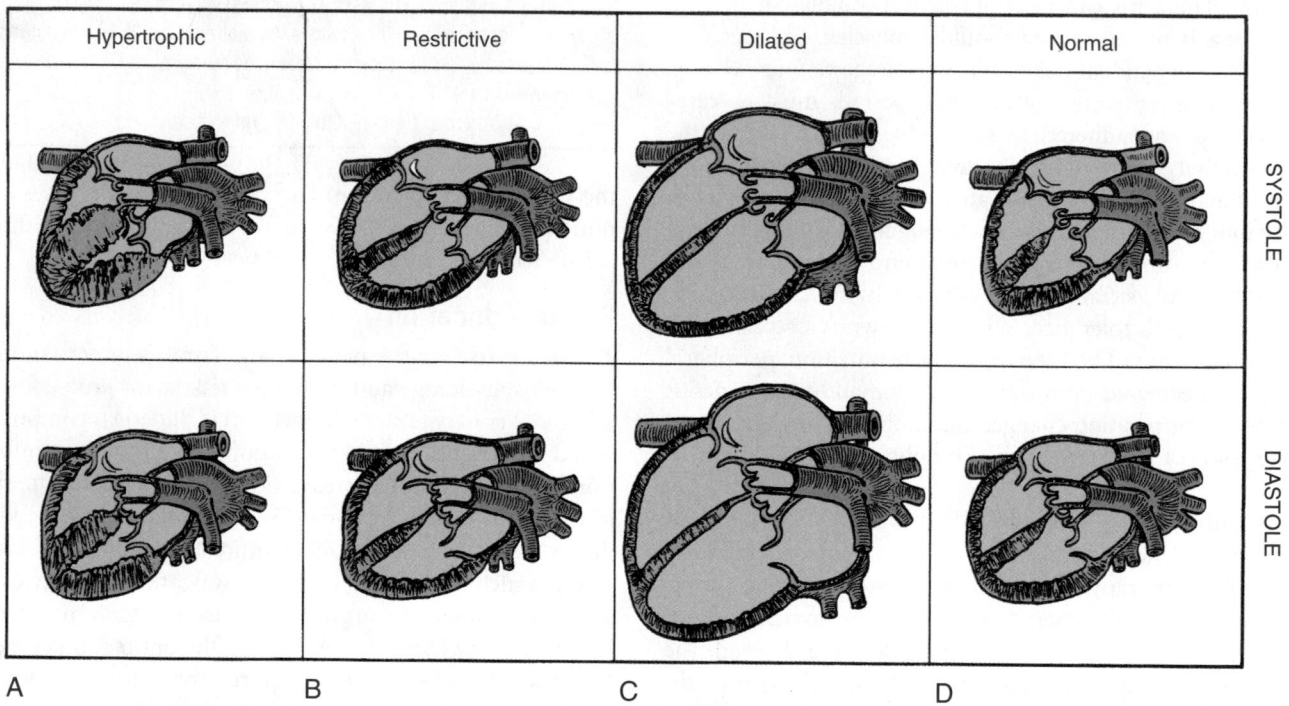

FIGURE 15-20   Types of cardiomyopathies and differences in ventricular diameter during systole and diastole compared with a normal heart. *A,* Hypertrophic; *B,* restrictive; *C,* dilated; *D,* normal.

inflammation, valvular dysfunction or as *intrinsic*, which correspond to myocardial diseases without identifiable external causes.[89,90] The two main forms of primary cardiomyopathies are the hypertrophic and dilated cardiomyopathies. Most of hypertrophic cardiomyopathy and 20% to 50% of dilated cardiomyopathy are familial, showing a genetic disposition.[90] The cardiomyopathic categories are hypertrophic, restrictive, and dilated, as illustrated in Figure 15-20.

Hypertrophic Obstructive Cardiomyopathy

Hypertrophic cardiomyopathy (HCM) is a genetically inherited disease that affects the myocardial sarcomere.[90,91] As HCM progresses, the left ventricle becomes stiff, noncompliant, and hypertrophied, sometimes in an asymmetric fashion.[89] HCM occurs in two forms. A well-known, but less frequent manifestation is a stiff, noncompliant myocardial muscle, with left ventricular hypertrophy and hypertrophy of the upper ventricular septum. This left ventricular septal hypertrophy obstructs outflow through the aortic valve, especially during exercise (see Fig. 15-20A). It also pulls the papillary muscle out of alignment, causing mitral regurgitation. Other patients with HCM have generalized left ventricular hypertrophy, but the septum is not more enlarged than the rest of the myocardium[89] HCM causes significant diastolic dysfunction because the muscle-bound, stiff, noncompliant heart muscle does not allow adequate filling during diastole.

Two advances in diagnostic medicine have propelled understanding of the differences between these two forms of HCM. *Two-dimensional transthoracic echocardiography* (TTE) is often useful as the first diagnostic test to identify HCM.[89] TTE enables visualization of septal anatomy, septal movement, and ventricular wall thickness and motion. The second advance is *diagnostic genetics*. Genetic testing for HCM usually is performed at a center with expertise in this area.[89] HCM is inherited as an autosomal dominant trait, and the clinical expression is caused by mutations in any of one of 10 genes. Each different gene encodes different protein components of the myocardial sarcomere.[89] Genetic analysis is an area of ongoing research that will undoubtedly help clarify other aspects of this cardiomyopathy within the next decade.

Symptoms are similar to those seen with heart failure, with the addition of myocardial ischemia, supraventricular tachycardia (SVT), VT, syncope, and stroke.[89,90,91] Symptoms usually are more intense with physical exercise, especially in the obstructive form of HCM, in which the aortic outflow tract is obstructed by the enlarged left ventricular septum. Because a known association exists between HCM and SCD, limitation of physical activity may be recommended. Causes of SCD are thought to stem from ventricular dysrhythmias and AF.[89] The atrial dysrhythmias are related to increased age and atrial enlargement. Pharmacologic management includes beta-blockers to decrease left ventricular workload, medications to control and prevent atrial and ventricular dysrhythmias, anticoagulation if AF or left ventricular thrombi are present, and medications to manage heart failure. Interventional procedures include insertion of an ICD to decrease the risk of SCD, and percutaneous alcohol ablation of the intraventricular septum to decrease the size of the septal wall.[89,90]

Dilated Cardiomyopathy

Dilated cardiomyopathy (DCM) is characterized by gross dilation of both ventricles without muscle hypertrophy (see Fig. 15-20C). Several distinct causes of dilated cardiomyopathy exist. DCMs have both primary and secondary causes and are the most common cause of heart failure. DCM results from valvular, ischemic, toxins, metabolic, infectious and systemic causes.[90]

Ischemic Dilated Cardiomyopathy. Ischemic DCM results from repeated myocardial injury or infarction resulting in reduction of ejection fraction. It is the most common cause of DCM in the United States. The patient has signs and symptoms of SHF and a low ejection fraction.[62,90] Treatment consists of the use of ACE inhibitors in symptomatic and asymptomatic patients and beta-blockers and digoxin in symptomatic patients.

Idiopathic Dilated Cardiomyopathy. When the cause of DCM is unknown, it is called *idiopathic DCM*. In some cases, the occurrence is linked to genetic inheritance. Scientific advances in molecular genetics permit detailed studies of families with a high incidence of DCM. It is thought that 10% to 50% of *familial idiopathic DCM* cases reflect genetic transmission.[91-93] In affected families, various genetic mutations occur in the gene that codes for the sarcomere contractile protein in the heart. The heritable trait can be expressed as an autosomal dominant or recessive inheritance pattern.[91-92] Preliminary research indicates that the genetic picture is highly individual for different family groups, even if the clinical picture appears similar.[91-93]

Other Causes of Dilated Cardiomyopathy. Many other nonischemic, nongenetic causes of DCM exist. Injury can be caused by valvular heart dysfunction that has placed extreme pressure or volume on the chambers, and viral or bacterial infections such as myocarditis can lead to inflammatory changes that permanently remodel the heart.[93] Other noncardiac causes include infiltration by systemic collagens as in amyloidosis or sarcoidosis.[94,95]

In DCM, the myocardial muscle fibers contract poorly, resulting in global left ventricular dysfunction, low cardiac output, atrial and ventricular dysrhythmias, blood pooling that leads to ventricular thrombi and embolic episodes, refractory heart failure, and premature death. The goals of the medical management of DCM are similar to those for systolic heart failure: improvement of pump function, removal of excess fluid, control of heart failure symptoms, anticipation and management of complications, and prevention of SCD.

Restrictive Cardiomyopathy

Restrictive cardiomyopathy (RCM) is the least commonly encountered cardiomyopathy in the developed countries (see Fig. 15-20B). As with the other cardiomyopathies, this form can be idiopathic or can have a known cause.[94] RCMs involve abnormalities of diastolic function with preserved systolic function.[50,93] DHF, low cardiac output, dyspnea, orthopnea, and liver engorgement are the most common clinical manifestations of RCM. An elevated jugular venous pressure, S_4 and late S_3 may be present. Both ventricles are typically small with decreased volumes and large atria. The atrial septum and cardiac valves may be thickened, and pericardial effusion may also be present.[50] Medical management is aimed at improving symptoms and preventing tachycardia. Diuretics reduce pulmonary pressure and fluid volume relieving of dyspnea. Nitrates can also provide relief. Patients are advised to reduce sodium intake, weigh daily, and restrict water intake. ACE inhibitors and ARBs improve stroke volume and reduce myocardial oxygen demand.[50]

Nursing Management

Nursing management of the patient with cardiomyopathy incorporates a variety of nursing diagnoses related to the symptoms of heart failure. These nursing diagnoses are reviewed in Box 15-19. Nursing interventions are individualized according to the type of cardiomyopathy and are focused on achievement of a stable fluid balance, monitoring the effects of pharmacologic therapy, safely increasing mobility, and providing patient

⊚ BOX 15-19 NURSING DIAGNOSES
Cardiomyopathy

- Decreased Cardiac Output, related to alterations in preload, p. 1128
- Decreased Cardiac Output, related to alterations in afterload, p. 1128
- Decreased Cardiac Output, related to alterations in contractility, p. 1128
- Decreased Cardiac Output, related to alterations in heart rate or rhythm, p. 1128
- Impaired Gas Exchange, related to ventilation/perfusion mismatching or intrapulmonary shunting, p. 1144
- Activity Intolerance, related to cardiopulmonary dysfunction, p. 1119
- Anxiety, related to threat to biologic, psychologic, or social integrity, p. 1125
- Powerlessness, related to lack of control over current situation or disease progression, p. 1152
- Deficient Knowledge, related to lack of previous exposure to information, p. 1134 (see Box 15-20, Patient Education for Cardiomyopathy)

BOX 15-20 PATIENT EDUCATION
Cardiomyopathy

Cardiomyopathy produces symptoms of heart failure; patient education covers many of the same issues discussed for heart failure.

- Cardiomyopathy: explain pathophysiology of cardiomyopathy and heart failure
- Fluid balance: low-salt diet to reduce fluid retention; intake and output measurement; signs of fluid overload, such as peripheral edema
- Daily weight: increase or loss of 1 to 2 pounds in a few days is a sign of fluid gain or loss, not true weight gain or loss
- Breathlessness: increasing shortness of breath, wheezing, and sleeping upright on pillows are symptoms that must be monitored and reported to a health care professional
- Activity: activity conservation with rest periods as heart failure progresses
- Medications: as medications are complex, information must be given in writing and orally
  - Preload: purpose of diuretics, increased urine output, and control of fluid volume
  - Afterload: purpose of vasodilators or angiotensin-converting enzyme (ACE) inhibitors in decreasing the workload of the heart
  - Heart rate: purpose of digoxin is to control atrial fibrillation, a frequent dysrhythmia in heart failure; purpose of amiodarone is to control ventricular and atrial dysrhythmias, which are common in heart failure
  - Contractility: with the exception of digoxin, no oral contractility medications are approved by the U.S. Food and Drug Administration (FDA)
  - Decrease sympathetic response: purpose of carvedilol (beta-blocker) is to lower cardiac response to adrenergic stimulation
  - Anticoagulation: patients with distended atria, enlarged ventricles, or atrial fibrillation may be prescribed anticoagulants (Coumadin) or aspirin, or both; risk of bleeding, importance of correct dosages, prothrombin times, international normalized ratio (INR), and nutritional-pharmacologic interactions are emphasized
- Follow-up care
- Symptoms to report to a health care professional

and family education. As with heart failure, a collaborative team of compassionate, knowledgeable professionals is required to provide effective care and education for these challenging patients.[50]

Patient Education

Education is tailored to the type of cardiomyopathy and to any associated conditions (Box 15-20).

PULMONARY HYPERTENSION

Description and Etiology

Pulmonary hypertension (PH) is a progressive, ultimately fatal disease of the pulmonary vasculature. PH results from progressive narrowing of the small pulmonary vessels resulting in increase in pulmonary vascular resistance. Pulmonary arterial hypertension (PAH) is the largest subdivision of this complex disease.[96] PAH is a disease of the small pulmonary arteries that is characterized by vascular proliferation and remodeling.[97] If untreated, PH progresses to right ventricular failure and death.[97] It is discussed with cardiovascular diseases that affect the arteries because it affects arterial vessels. PH may arise as an isolated condition or be associated with other diseases.

World Health Organization Classification of Pulmonary Hypertension

The World Health Organization (WHO) classification of PH was most recently updated in 2008 at the Fourth World Symposium of Pulmonary Hypertension. This updated model groups disorders according to similarities in pathophysiology and treatment (Table 15-10).[98] Some of the causes of PH likely to be seen in a critical care unit are discussed in the following sections. Whatever the cause, the presence of PH significantly increases morbidity and mortality of any underlying cardiac or pulmonary disease. PH is a serious and frequently life-threatening condition that needs aggressive treatment.[97]

Functional Classification of Pulmonary Hypertension

A functional classification describes a grouping of physical symptoms that limit a patient's activity as a result of their disease condition. The AHA has used a functional classification for heart failure symptoms for many years (see Table 15-7). The NYHA heart failure classification was used for PAH symptoms, until 2003, when a disease-specific functional classification was developed (Table 15-11). The premise is the same as the NYHA classification, with the understanding that a higher number means that the patient is more symptomatic, has greater limitation of activity, and risks higher mortality. The functional classification level strongly predicts mortality and is used to guide PAH therapy.[99,100]

Idiopathic Pulmonary Arterial Hypertension

If the cause of the PH is unknown, it is called idiopathic pulmonary hypertension (IPAH) and is classified as WHO group I (see Table 15-10). IPAH is characterized by the following features (Fig. 15-21):
- Intimal endothelial cell proliferation and medial thickening due to vascular smooth muscle cell proliferation
- Muscularization of precapillary arterioles
- Angioproliferative plexiform lesions of the endothelial cells develop from proliferation and fibrosis of the endothelium and increase obstruction

IPAH is rare, with an incidence of approximately three to six cases per million people per year. It has a female-to-male ratio of almost 3:1 and the mean age at diagnosis is 37 years.[96,101] PH has an insidious onset, and diagnosis is difficult because of the nonspecific nature of the symptoms (e.g., dyspnea, fatigue).

TABLE 15-10 WHO CLASSIFICATION OF PULMONARY HYPERTENSION

Group 1	Pulmonary arterial hypertension (PAH) Idiopathic PAH Heritable BMPR2, ALK1, endoglin (with or without hereditary hemorrhagic telangiectasia) Associated PAH (APAH) induced by medications, unknown drugs and toxins Connective tissue diseases HIV infection Portal hypertension Congenital heart disease Schistosomiasis Chronic hemolytic anemia Persistent pulmonary hypertension of the newborn
Group 1′	Pulmonary veno-occlusive disease (PVOD), pulmonary capillary hemangiomatosis (PCH), or both
Group 2	Pulmonary hypertension from left heart disease Systolic dysfunction Diastolic dysfunction Valvular disease
Group 3	Pulmonary hypertension from lung diseases, hypoxia, or both Chronic obstructive pulmonary disease Interstitial lung disease Other pulmonary diseases with mixed restrictive and obstructive pattern Sleep-disordered breathing Alveolar hypoventilation disorders Chronic exposure to high altitude Developmental abnormalities
Group 4	Chronic thromboembolic pulmonary hypertension
Group 5	PH with unclear mechanisms, multifactorial mechanisms, or both Hematological disorders: myeloproliferative disorders, splenectomy Systemic disorders: sarcoidosis, pulmonary Langerhans cell histiocytosis, lymphangioleiomyomatosis, neurofibromatosis, vasculitis Metabolic disorders: glycogen storage disease, Gaucher disease, thyroid disorders Other: tumoral obstruction, fibrosing mediastinitis, chronic kidney failure on dialysis

From Simmoneau G, et al. Updated clinical classification of pulmonary hypertension. *JACC Cardiovasc Intervent.* 2009;54(1):S43.
ALK-1, Activin receptor-like kinase 1 gene; *APAH,* associated pulmonary arterial hypertension; *BMPR2,* bone morphogenetic protein receptor, type 2; *HIV,* human immunodeficiency virus; *PAH,* pulmonary arterial hypertension; *WHO,* World Health Organization.

Frequently, by the time a firm diagnosis is made, the patient is highly symptomatic with anginal chest pain, near-syncope or syncope, and right ventricular heart failure.[112] Without treatment, PAH patients had estimated median survival rates at 1, 3, and 5 years of 68%, 48%, and 34%, respectively. Treatment increases survival by 20% to 30%.[96,102,103]

Heritable Pulmonary Arterial Hypertension

Heritable PAH, previously known as *familial pulmonary arterial hypertension* (FPAH), is a condition with genetic mutations classified in WHO group I (see Table 15-10). Several genes

TABLE 15-11 FUNCTIONAL CLASSIFICATION OF PULMONARY HYPERTENSION: WHO CLASSIFICATION

CLASS	SYMPTOMS
Class I	Patients with pulmonary hypertension but without resulting limitation of physical activity; ordinary physical activity does not cause undue dyspnea of fatigue, chest pain or near syncope
Class II	Patients with pulmonary hypertension resulting in slight limitation of physical activity; they are comfortable at rest; ordinary physical activity causes undue dyspnea or fatigue, chest pain or near syncope
Class III	Patients with pulmonary hypertension resulting in marked limitation of physical activity; they are comfortable at rest; less than ordinary activity causes undue dyspnea or fatigue, chest pain or near syncope
Class IV	Patients with pulmonary hypertension with inability to carry out any physical activity without symptoms; these patients manifest signs of right heart failure. Dyspnea and/or fatigue may even be present at rest. Discomfort is increased by any physical activity

From Barst RJ, et al. Diagnosis and differential assessment of pulmonary arterial hypertension. *J Am Coll Cardiol.* 2004;43:40S.

associated with heritable PAH have been confirmed, including *BMPR2* (bone morphogenic protein receptor II), actin receptor-like kinase 1 (*ALK1*), and endoglin (with or without hereditary hemorrhagic telangiectasia). *BMPR2* is the associated genetic abnormality in 70% of these cases.[98,104] Transmission of the *BMPR2* mutation leads to alteration of apoptosis that favors cellular proliferation.[104] In families with this gene, the children of patients have a 50% risk of inheriting the gene. However, not everyone who inherits the gene will exhibit the signs and symptoms of the disease, the reasons for which are not understood.[97] In this subgrouping, the pathogenesis of PH is thought to be caused by multiple genetic and environmental stimuli. This has led to the development of a "multiple-hit hypothesis." This hypothesis predicts that modifier genes and environmental stimuli influence primary gene abnormalities such as the *BMPR2* mutation to develop into clinically evident PAH.[111]

Medications, illegal drugs, and toxin-induced PAH include agents with identified risk of inducing PAH. The first identified group included aminorex and fenfluramine derivatives used for weight loss. Since these agents were removed from market other agents, including toxic rapeseed oil, St. John's Wort, and anti-obesity agents containing phenylpropanolamine, have been identified as increasing the risk for developing IPAH.[97,98] Amphetamine use is a likely risk for developing PH, with meth-amphetamine demonstrating a strong relationship to IPAH.[98] The risk of developing PAH increases with exposure to toxic drug or environmental stimuli.

Associated with Pulmonary Arterial Hypertension

Associated pulmonary arterial hypertension (APAH) may be related to other risk factors or conditions. This is classified as a

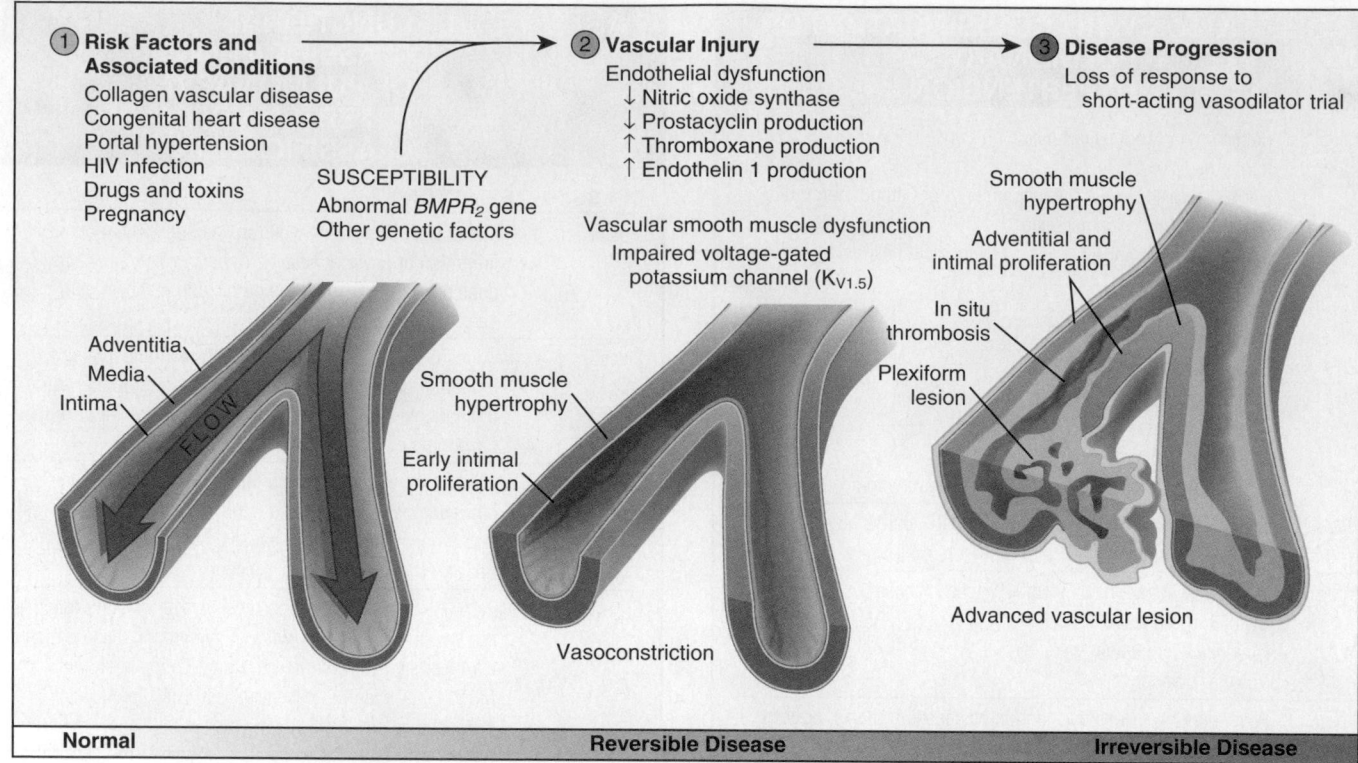

FIGURE 15-21 Pathogenesis of pulmonary arterial hypertension.

WHO group I disease (see Table 15-10). APAH includes a number of conditions associated with lesions in the small pulmonary muscular arterioles, for example, collagen vascular disease, human immunodeficiency virus (HIV) infection, portal hypertension, congenital systemic to pulmonary shunts, schistosomiasis, and chronic hemolytic anemia.

Pulmonary Veno-occlusive Disease and Pulmonary Capillary Hemangiomatosis

Pulmonary veno-occlusive disease (PVOD), pulmonary capillary hemangiomatosis (PCH), or both are included in IPAH because of pathologic similarities. These conditions are relocated from previous classification groups and renamed *Group1'* because they have similar pathologic changes. Similar clinical presentation, risk factors, and familial association suggest that this subgrouping represents different components of a single disease spectrum.[97,98,104]

Pulmonary Hypertension Due to Left Heart Disease

PH that results from left heart disease is classified as a WHO group II condition (see Table 15-10). This is the most common form of PH with systolic dysfunction, diastolic dysfunction, and valvular disease composing distinct etiologies.[98,104] Pulmonary venous hypertension (PVH) causes PH by a different mechanism from those of other forms of PH. It occurs as a result of elevated pressures in the left side of the heart that subsequently raise the pulmonary venous pressure. Patients with PVH have a history of CAD, acute MI, valvular disease, heart failure, or DCM. Pulmonary hypertension develops initially as a passive process of back-pressure that produces upstream elevation in the pulmonary venous and ultimately pulmonary arterial pressure (PAP). Prolonged pressure elevation leads to an increase in pulmonary arteriolar resistance and persistent vascular changes.[98]

Pulmonary Hypertension Associated with Lung Disease or Hypoxemia

Chronic lung disease is often associated with hypoxemia and may entrain PH. In this group, which is classified as WHO group III (see Table 15-10), PH is caused by alveolar hypoxia secondary to lung disease, impaired control of breathing, or chronic exposure to high altitude.[98] All patients with PH feel short of breath with exercise, but patients with COPD or interstitial lung disease (cystic fibrosis, pulmonary fibrosis, and emphysema) are breathless even at rest. All patients with obstructive pulmonary disease have worse survival rates when pulmonary hypertension progresses.[113] Pulmonary function tests and sleep apnea studies are performed as part of the diagnostic workup for patients with PAH and lung disease.[102,104]

Chronic Thromboembolic Pulmonary Hypertension

PAH that results from chronic thromboembolic conditions such as chronic thromboembolic pulmonary hypertension (CTEPH) is classified as WHO group IV (see Table 15-10). PAH can happen acutely in response to a large pulmonary embolus that blocks flow to the pulmonary vascular bed. PAH can also occur after multiple microembolic thrombi that obstruct the smaller pulmonary arteries. CTEPH carries up to 4% incidence after acute pulmonary emboli.[97] If the risk of pulmonary emboli is recognized in the patient with hypercoagulability, this condition is potentially preventable. The guidelines recommend that when PH is diagnosed, a *ventilation/perfusion scan* (V/Q scan) be performed to determine the presence or absence of pulmonary emboli.[98,104] Treatment in a center of excellence with experience in pulmonary thromboendarterectomy is highly recommended for this condition as skill in the procedure and required support systems are essential.[97,98]

Pulmonary Hypertension with Unclear and Multifactorial Mechanisms

Group V in the WHO classification (see Table 15-10) covers miscellaneous conditions, including hematologic disorders (myleoproliferative disorders, splenectomy) systemic disorders (sarcoidosis, neurofibromatosis, vasculitis), metabolic disorders (glycogen storage, Gaucher disease, thyroid disorders) and other (tumoral obstruction, fibrosing mediastinitis, chronic kidney failure).

Pathophysiology

The pulmonary vascular bed is normally a high-flow, low-pressure, low-resistance system that easily adjusts to changes in cardiac output, oxygen demand, and exercise.[96] In the presence of PH, these characteristics are lost. Progressive and sustained elevation of pulmonary pressures with increased pulmonary vascular resistance leads to increased pressure on the right ventricle, increased right ventricular workload, right ventricular hypertrophy, heart failure, and death.

The three major components in the pathogenesis of chronic PH are: 1) endothelial dysfunction and vasoconstriction, 2) vascular remodeling, and 3) thrombosis. A fourth component is the development of plexiform lesions that irreversibly obliterate the pulmonary arterioles (see Fig. 15-21).[99] Impaired endothelial cell function results in vasoconstriction caused by decreased endothelial cell-derived nitric oxide (NO), decreased prostacyclin, and an increase in the vasoconstrictor endothelin. This results in thrombi within the pulmonary arterioles from increased thrombosis and diminished thrombolysis. Overproduction of substances that cause vasoconstriction, such as thromboxane and endothelin, or a decrease in endothelial factors that cause vasodilatation, specifically endothelial prostacyclin and NO, or a combination of these factors, may be the catalyst.[104]

Assessment and Diagnosis

The diagnosis of PH is difficult. Pulmonary hypertension is often a diagnosis of exclusion when all other diagnostic theories are exhausted. The clinical symptoms of PH are nonspecific in the early stages of the disease and reflect the inability of the pulmonary vascular bed to accommodate increased cardiac output with exercise. These factors support findings that presence of symptoms often last more than 2 years before diagnosis.[105,106]

Physical Assessment

The severity of PH clinical symptoms are classified using the WHO pulmonary hypertension functional classes I to IV (see Table 15-10). Revised PH treatment algorithm. This is similar to the NYHA classification for heart failure.[96] Physical examination clues that reveal right ventricular failure include elevated jugular venous pressure (JVP), a palpable right ventricular heave, hepatomegaly, ascites, and peripheral edema. Auscultation of heart sounds may reveals a prominent pulmonic component to the second heart sound, and a holosystolic blowing murmur from tricuspid regurgitation. Pulmonary edema suggests left ventricular dysfunction or a noncardiac cause such as ARDS.[100]

The patient's signs and symptoms early in PAH include fatigue and shortness of breath caused by impaired oxygen transport and reduced cardiac output. Later symptoms include syncope from systemic hypotension as a result of low cardiac output and angina from the under-filled right and left ventricles. Patients may have intestinal edema, which can cause constipation, abdominal pain, malabsorption, and anorexia.[99]

Diagnostic tests that can assist with PAH diagnosis include the 12-lead ECG, the echocardiogram, and a right-sided cardiac catheterization. The most helpful noninvasive test is the echocardiogram. Echocardiography can estimate right atrial pressure and PAP, and it can determine the degree of right ventricular dysfunction.[100] Signs of significant disease include right ventricular dilation and hypertrophy; septal bowing into the left ventricle, creating a D-shaped left ventricle; right ventricular hypokinesis; tricuspid regurgitation; right atrial enlargement; and a dilated inferior vena cava.

The 12-lead electrocardiogram (ECG) is a noninvasive test that may show right axis deviation and right ventricular hypertrophy resulting from PAH. The 12-lead ECG is an adjunct test that can indicate strain on the right ventricle, but used alone, it cannot diagnose PH.

The most helpful invasive diagnostic test is right-sided cardiac catheterization because it can provide verifiable numbers. To diagnose PAH, the mean PAP must be greater than 25 mm Hg at rest.[102] Precise analysis of mixed venous oxygen saturation (SVO_2) during insertion and passage of the pulmonary artery catheter through the cardiac chamber can allow diagnosis of intracardiac shunts. A pulmonary artery occlusion pressure (PAOP) less than 15 mm Hg rules out left ventricular heart disease.[100,102] Information on diagnostic use of the pulmonary artery catheter and (SVO_2) is included in the section on "Hemodynamics" in Chapter 14.

The ability of the pulmonary vessels to vasodilate in response to administration of a pulmonary arterial vasodilator, called a *positive vasoreactivity test*, is an important component of the cardiac catheterization study when used to diagnose PAH. Vasoactive medications such as inhaled NO (iNO), intravenous adenosine, or intravenous epoprostenol (prostacyclin) are used. The ability of the pulmonary vasculature to dilate determines how helpful pharmacologic pulmonary arterial vasodilators are likely to be. A positive response includes a reduction in mean PAP of at least 10 mm Hg to achieve a mean PAP below 40 mm Hg with an increased or unchanged cardiac output. Only about 10% to 20% of patients with PH have a positive response to vasodilators.[99,104]

If the diagnostic tests are performed when PH is advanced, the PAP may almost equal the systemic aortic pressure, and the pulmonary arterioles may not vasodilate in response to vasodilator medications. In this scenario, the enlarged right ventricle puts pressure on the intraventricular septum and compresses the left ventricle. The smaller, compressed left ventricle greatly reduces left ventricular stroke volume and cardiac output.[97,99]

Formal assessment of exercise tolerance is important for evaluation and ongoing treatment of PAH. The *6-minute walk distance* (6MWD) and a variety of treadmill exercise tests are used for this evaluation. In the 6MWD, the patient walks as far as possible for 6 minutes. The distance walked in 6 minutes has a strong association with mortality among patients with IPAH.[96,102] Evaluation of serial 6MWD tests can monitor the severity, response to treatment, or progression of the disease.[104]

Medical Management

Medical management focuses on early diagnosis, use of appropriate pharmacologic therapies, and prevention of complications. Goals of therapy include alleviation of symptoms, improvements in quality of life, and survival. Improvements are measured by changes in functional class and exercise

tolerance.[97] Clinical practice guidelines for this complex and progressive disease recommend referral to a medical center specializing in the management of PH.[104]

Medications

Table 15-12 presents pulmonary hypertension medications. Most patients are maintained on multiple medications that include oral endothelin receptor antagonists, phosphodiesterase-5 (PDE-5) inhibitors, pulmonary vasodilators, prostacyclin derivatives, calcium channel blockers (early stage only), anticoagulants, diuretics, and oxygen. Figure 15-22 provides an example of how these medications can be combined as part of the treatment regimen.[102,105]

Calcium channel blockers improve survival of PH patients who demonstrate a significantly positive vasoreactivity test result during the right-sided cardiac catheterization (responders).[105,107] Long-acting calcium channel blockers include nifedipine, diltiazem, and amlodipine.[107] Most patients with PH are

TABLE 15-12 PHARMACOLOGIC MANAGEMENT

Pulmonary Hypertension Medications

MEDICATION	DOSAGE	ACTION	SPECIAL CONSIDERATIONS
Endothelin Receptor Antagonist (ERA)		Blocks vasoconstriction and smooth muscle proliferation	
Bosentan (Tracleer)	62.5-125 mg PO bid		Monitor LFTs
Ambrisentan (Letairis)	5-10 mg PO daily		Monitor LFTs
Phosphodiesterase-5 (PDE-5) Inhibitors		Pulmonary vasodilation and decreases smooth muscle proliferation	Concomitant use with nitrates can result in irreversible hypotension
Sildenafil (Revatio)	20 mg PO tid IV bolus 10mg tid		
Tadalafil (Adcirca)	40 mg PO daily		
Pulmonary Vasodilator			
Inhaled nitric oxide (iNO)		Dilates pulmonary vasculature	Abrupt withdrawal results in rebound pulmonary hypertension; NO production leads to methemoglobinemia
Prostacylin Derivatives		Dilates pulmonary and peripheral vessels; antiproliferative, antiplatelet	Rebound pulmonary hypertension if abruptly discontinued or dose decreased
Epoprostenol (Flolan) (Veletri)	Start at 2-4 ng/kg/min continuous IV Ranges 20-40 ng/kg/day		Flolan needs to be refrigerated or covered with icebags for short half-life; Veletri is stable at room temperature
Treprostinil (Remodulin) (Tyvaso oral inhalation)	20-80 ng/kg/mg continuous infusion SC/IV 3 inhal (18 mcg) 4-9 times/day		Pain at injection site
Iloprost	2.5-5 mcg (6-9 inhalations) nebulized/qid		Hemoptysis
Anticoagulant			Maintain INR with oral vitamin K antagonist therapy
Calcium Channel Blocker		Vasodilator	Can cause hypotension, *only* useful in positive vasoreactor patients
Nifedipine	120-240 mg/day		
Diltiazem	240-720 mg/day		
Amlodipine	Up to 20 mg/day		
Diuretics		Decrease volume overload	Monitor electrolytes and kidney function closely

INR, International normalized ratio; *IV,* intravenous; *LFT,* liver function test; *NO,* nitric oxide; *PO,* by mouth; *SC,* subcutaneous.

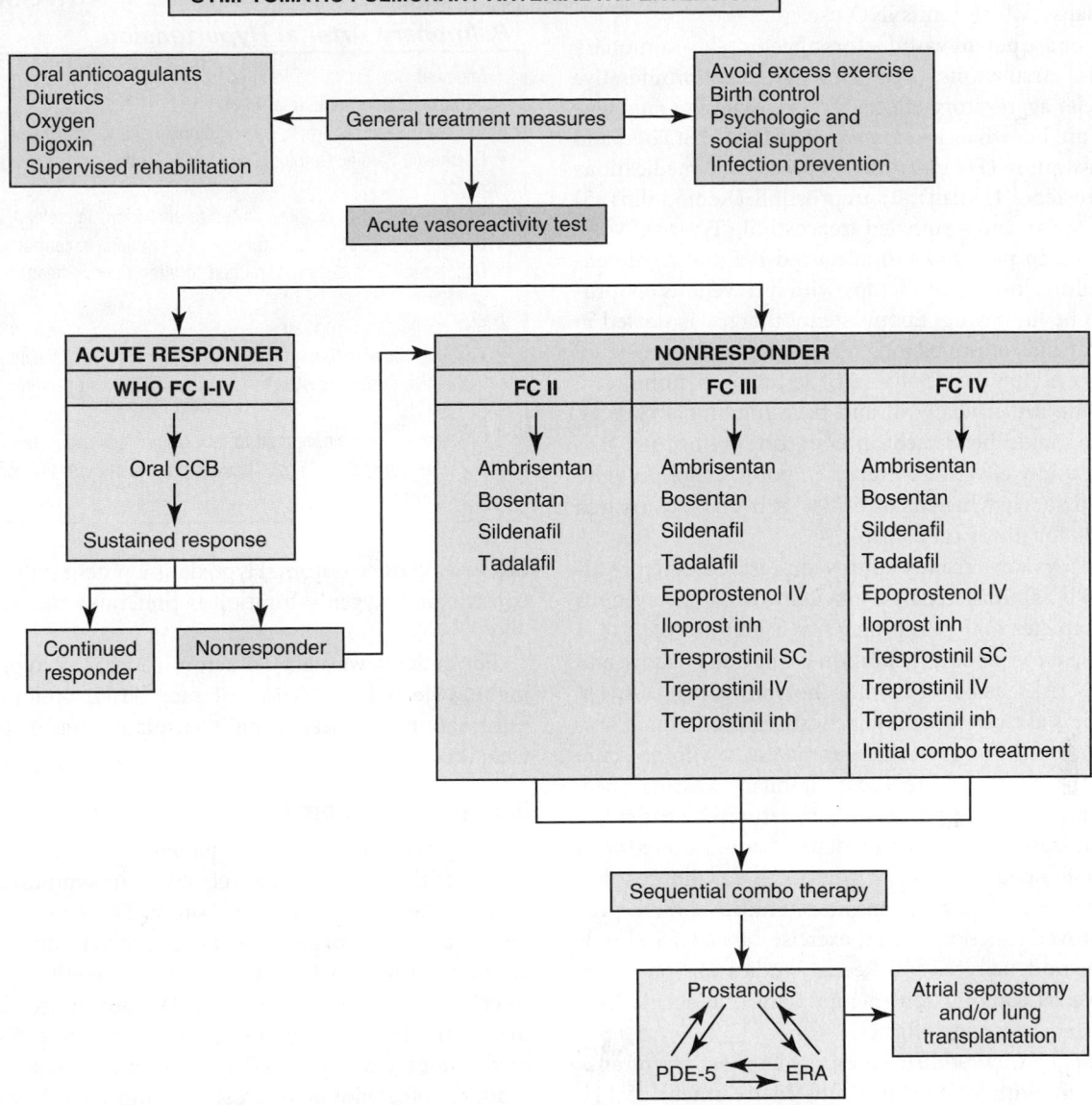

SYMPTOMATIC PULMONARY ARTERIAL HYPERTENSION

FIGURE 15-22 Combination medication therapy used to treat pulmonary arterial hypertension (PAH). (Based on Badesch DB, et al. Diagnosis and assessment of pulmonary arterial hypertension. *JACC.* 2009;54[1]:S55.)

nonresponders and are more effectively managed with one of the newer medications developed specifically to treat PH (described later).[102,105]

Endothelin receptor antagonists are used for treating PH. Endothelin 1 is a potent vasoconstrictor and smooth muscle mitogen capable of inducing smooth muscle cell hypertrophy. Two types of endothelin receptors are: 1) endothelin A, which causes vasoconstriction and smooth muscle proliferation and 2) endothelin B, which causes vasodilatation and is involved in clearance of endothelin. Bosentan is an oral endothelin receptor antagonist.[102,105] Bosentan (Tracleer) is approved for WHO classes III and IV. In IPAH and scleroderma-related disorders, it improves symptoms, functional class, hemodynamics, and exercise capacity measured by 6MWD.[118,125] Ambrisentan (Letairis) is useful in treating IPAH and PH resulting from connective tissue and congenital heart disease. It improves

symptoms, time to clinical worsening, exercise capacity, and functional class.[98,107,108]

PDE-5 inhibitors are designed to inhibit the degradation of cyclic guanosine monophosphate (cGMP). These medications promote pulmonary vasodilatation and decrease vascular smooth muscle cell proliferation. Sildenafil (Revatio) and tadalafil (Adcirca) are potent inhibitors of PDE-5; they are used to treat erectile dysfunction and are an effective treatment option for PAH.[105] Started as monotherapy, sildenafil is also used as part of a multi-medication treatment regimen.[102,107]

NO is a potent *vasodilator* that dilates the pulmonary vasculature in ventilated lung units. It improves oxygenation and reduces PAP.[100,105] Inhaled NO (iNO) is useful in critically ill mechanically ventilated patients, especially in combination with dobutamine or milrinone. Abrupt withdrawal of iNO can lead to methemoglobinemia, nitrogen dioxide (NO_2)

production, and rebound pulmonary hypertension with hemodynamic collapse, which limits iNO use.

Prostacyclins are potent vasodilators affecting the pulmonary and systemic circulations, and they have antiproliferative and antiplatelet aggregatory effects.[102,107] Prostacyclin analogue medications are known as *prostanoids*. The four U.S. Food and Drug Administration (FDA)–approved prostanoid medications are 1) epoprostenol (Flolan), 2) treprostinil (Remodulin), 3) iloprost (Ventavis), and 4) inhaled treprostinil (Tyvaso).[99,107,109]

- *Epoprostenol*: In patients with advanced PH and right ventricular failure, long-term therapy with intravenous epoprostenol can be life saving. Epoprostenol therapy is started in the hospital and continued long term at home. Epoprostenol has a short elimination half-life of less than 5 minutes.[107] Patients who are critically ill and have functional class IV symptoms should be started on epoprostenol because it is the most rapidly effective therapy.[102] Epoprostenol provides a sustained survival benefit of 62.8% at 3 years, compared with 35.4% for historical controls.[97,99]
- *Treprostinil*: A more recently approved prostanoid, treprostinil sodium is administered by a subcutaneous or intravenous infusion catheter and pump and has a half-life of 3 to 4 hours. Subcutaneous administration is safe and effective and avoids the risks associated with the indwelling catheter. However, it is associated with injection-site pain, which may not be tolerated. These prostacyclin analogues do not cure the PH, but all vasodilate the pulmonary vascular bed, control symptoms, and prolong life in responsive patients.
- *Iloprost*: Iloprost is an inhaled prostanoid administered with an ultrasonic nebulizer 6 to 12 times each day. Iloprost has a serum half-life of 20 to 25 minutes. Studies show it provides improved functional class, exercise capacity, and pulmonary hemodynamics.[102,105] Recent studies on long-term use and use as combination therapy with oral agents have demonstrated safety and efficacy.
- *Tyvaso (inhaled treprostinil)*: Tyvaso is the most recent analogue studied with successful results in treatment of PH. Tyvaso improved 6MWD when used in combination therapy with bosentan or sildenafil therapy.[109] Tyvaso is an inhaled prostanoids administered with a handheld nebulizer four times daily.

Anticoagulation is an essential component of pharmacologic management. Risk factors for venous thromboembolism such as heart failure, right ventricular dysfunction, low stroke volume and decreased arterial pulse pressure, a sedentary lifestyle, and a thrombophilic predisposition are found in PH. Warfarin (Coumadin) improves survival in patients with IPAH and APAH. The usual target international normalized ratio (INR) of 2 to 3 is reduced to 1.5 to 2.5 when used with prostacyclin analogues.[99,107]

Diuretics are used to prevent right ventricular volume overload, edema, ascites, and malabsorption associated with bowel edema. Serum electrolytes and kidney function are closely monitored.[104]

Supplemental oxygen (O_2) use is a key component of therapy for chronic PH.[102] Chronic hypoxemia from impaired cardiac output results in mixed venous desaturation. Hypoxemia can also be related to right to left shunting through patent foramen ovale or heart defects.[104] Oxygen inhalation decreases PAP and

---

◉ BOX 15-21 NURSING DIAGNOSES

Pulmonary Arterial Hypertension

- Impaired Gas Exchange, related to ventilation/perfusion mismatching or intrapulmonary shunting, p. 1144
- Activity Intolerance, related to cardiopulmonary dysfunction, p. 1119
- Decreased Cardiac Output, related to alterations in afterload (pulmonary), p. 1128
- Decreased Cardiac Output, related to alterations in preload, p. 1128
- Decreased Cardiac Output, related to alterations in contractility, p. 1128
- Decreased Cardiac Output, related to alterations in heart rate or rhythm, p. 1128
- Risk for Infection, p. 1160
- Anxiety, related to threat to biologic, psychologic, or social integrity, p. 1125
- Ineffective Coping, related to situational crisis and personal vulnerability, p. 1150
- Deficient Knowledge, related to lack of previous exposure to information, p. 1134 (see Box 15-22, Patient Education for Pulmonary Arterial Hypertension)

---

improves cardiac output. Hypoxia is a potent pulmonary vasoconstrictor. Oxygen saturation is preferably maintained above 90%.[100]

For patients who are refractory to pharmacologic management, a heart-lung transplant may be an option.[102] Detailed information on heart-lung transplantation is provided in Chapter 37.

Nursing Management

Nursing management of the patient with PH incorporates a variety of nursing diagnoses related to the symptoms of breathlessness and right-sided heart failure. These nursing diagnoses are reviewed in Box 15-21. Nursing interventions are individualized according to how advanced the symptoms of PH are. Interventions focus on lowering PAP, administration of pharmacologic therapy, monitoring of the effects and safety of all medications, treating pain that can occur at the site of injection (with epoprostenol or treprostinil), and providing patient and family education.

Patient Education

If the cause for PH is known the patient should receive education prior to discharge. All patients should be provided with a written medication list with the name and purpose of all their medications. Specific education topics can include 1) the use and care of a handheld nebulizer, tunneled intravenous catheter, or subcutaneous pump for administration; 2) infection control; and 3) sterile preparation of the prostacyclin analogue medication.[110,111] The name of the health care professional to contact for questions related to the PH is also important (Box 15-22). A collaborative team of empathetic, educated professionals is essential to provide effective care for these challenging patients (Box 15-23).

ENDOCARDITIS

Description and Etiology

Endocarditis is an inflammation on the endothelial surface of the heart, specifically thrombotic-fibrin vegetations on the

---

BOX 15-22 PATIENT EDUCATION

Pulmonary Arterial Hypertension

- Pathophysiology of pulmonary arterial hypertension and disease process
- Symptoms: dyspnea at rest or, more commonly, with exertion
- Activity conservation with scheduled rest periods
- Medications: purpose, side effects, special considerations
  - Epoprostenol (Flolan): intravenous (IV) by pump, half-life of 2 to 3 minutes
  - Treprostinil (Remodulin): IV or subcutaneous (SC) by pump, half-life of 3 hours
  - Ventavis and Veletri inhalation
  - Bosentan (Tracleer): oral
  - Sildenafil (Viagra): oral concomitant use with nitrates contraindicated as may result in profound hypotension
- Pain management at insertion site of IV or SC catheter
- Use of handheld nebulizer for inhaled Iloprost or Tyvaso
- Anticoagulation: purpose of international normalized ratio (INR); monitoring of skin, gums, urine, and stool for signs of bleeding; precautions to prevent bleeding when on anticoagulation (e.g., soft toothbrush, electric razor when shaving, avoid contact sports)
- Follow-up care after discharge
- Symptoms to report to a health care professional

---

cardiac valves. This irritation can be related to infectious or noninfectious sources sources.[112]Although most commonly associated with valve leaflets, chordae, chamber walls, paraprosthetic tissue, implanted shunts, conduits, and fistulas may also be affected.[113] The older term of bacterial endocarditis has been replaced by *infectious endocarditis* (IE) because nonbacterial organisms can be the infective source of the endothelial inflammation. The incidence of IE has not declined over the past 30 years, with 15,000 cases reported each year and a mortality rate of almost 40%.[114] IE is the fourth most common cause of life-threatening infectious syndromes (after urosepsis, pneumonia, and intra-abdominal sepsis). The risk of acquiring IE is higher among patients with congenital heart disease, valvular heart disease, and prosthetic heart valves. Approximately 75% of patients have a pre-existing structural abnormality of involved cardiac valve. Increasing incidence of invasive health care interventions such as implantable pacemakers and ICDs, body piercings, intravenous drug abuse (IVDA), and an increase in the number of older patients with degenerative valve disease increase the numbers at risk for IE.[112,114] Involvement of right heart valves is highly suspicious for IVDA.[112] Among intravenous drug abusers, the incidence of IE is 60 times that of age-matched controls.[115]

Development of IE depends on the following events:[116]
- Presence of a nonbacterial thrombotic lesion on a cardiac valve or endothelium
- Bacteremia (bacteria in bloodstream)
- Bacteria attaching to the nonbacterial thrombotic lesion
- Proliferation of bacteria on and within the lesion that may develop into a vegetation

Research suggests the source of the organism is less likely than previously thought to be related to a specific invasive procedure such as a urogenital procedure or dental work. Instead, IE results from the confluence of multiple daily bacteremic events in the presence of a susceptible cardiac lesion.[116]

Pathophysiology

IE results from a bacterial or fungal organism in the bloodstream that successfully colonizes the cardiac endothelium. It is fatal if not treated. Bacterial organisms, typically streptococci, staphylococci, and enterococci, are the most common pathogens. An increase in multidrug-resistant organisms has led to increased numbers of patients, more serious complications, and higher mortality rates.[116,117] Sites where endocarditis vegetations occur correlate with aberrant intracardiac flow caused by valvular damage or septal defects. After the vegetations have colonized, bacteria multiply at a rapid rate inside a protective platelet-fibrin casing that sequesters the infection.[114]

Assessment and Diagnosis

Diagnosis must be made as soon as possible to initiate treatment and identify patients at high risk for complications. Diagnosis is guided by classic manifestations of bacteremia or fungemia, evidence of active valvulitis, peripheral emboli, and immunologic vascular phenomena.

Modified Duke Criteria

The 2008 AHA scientific statement on IE supports use of the modified Duke criteria for diagnosis, early identification, and treatment of IE. This system stratifies patients with suspected IE into three categories: 1) definite cases, 2) possible cases, and 3) rejected cases (Table 15-13). A definite diagnosis of IE requires 2 major criteria, 1 major and 3 minor criteria, or 5 minor criteria. A possible diagnosis of IE requires 1 major criteria and 1 minor criteria or 3 minor criteria.[116-118]

Blood Cultures

Initial symptoms include fever, sometimes accompanied by rigor (shivering), fatigue, malaise, with up to 50% of patients complaining of myalgias and joint pain.[112] Blood cultures are drawn during periods of elevated temperature to detect the infective organism. At least 10 mL of venous blood should be placed in each of the blood culture containers to ensure that the organism will be detected.[115] Culture-negative endocarditis occurs in up to one third of cases and usually is related to prior antibiotic use or infection by a "fastidious" organism, which does not proliferate under conventional laboratory culture conditions.[113] White blood cell (WBC) counts are typically elevated, and the symptoms are identified in the Duke criteria (see Table 15-13).

Chest Radiograph

Cough and pleuritic chest pain are present in 40% to 60% of cases. The first noninvasive test is often a chest radiograph to detect nodular infiltrates, cardiomegaly, and enlarged pulmonary vessels.

Echocardiogram

The other essential noninvasive test is an echocardiogram of the heart valves to visualize vegetations. Transthoracic echocardiography (TTE) may be initially performed, but transesophageal echocardiography (TEE) is even more valuable because of the clarity of the heart valve images. TEE is more sensitive in detection of vegetations and abscesses.[117] Color-flow

BOX 15-23 EVIDENCE-BASED PRACTICE

Pulmonary Arterial Hypertension

QSEN Recommendations for Early Detection and Screening for Pulmonary Arterial Hypertension

- Relatives of patients with heritable pulmonary arterial hypertension (HPAH) are recommended to undergo prenatal genetic testing before any pregnancy.
- Pregnancy is not recommended for female patients with PH.
- If PH is suspected, a 12-lead ECG is required as an early screening test to rule out other possible cardiac anomalies. The ECG is not diagnostic for PH.
- If PH is suspected, a chest radiograph can reveal features supportive of a PH diagnosis.
- If PH is suspected, Doppler echocardiography is recommended to noninvasively evaluate RV systolic pressures and to assess for anatomic abnormalities such as RA or RV enlargement, LV involvement, and intracardiac shunting.

Recommendations for Diagnostic Tests to Further Evaluate Pulmonary Arterial Hypertension

- In patients with unexplained PH, testing for connective tissue disease and HIV infection is recommended.
- In patients with probable connective tissue PH, a V/Q scan is recommended to identify perfusion blocks and severity of disease progression.
- Pulmonary function tests are recommended to rule out other causes of lung disease.
- Lung biopsy is not recommended. It carries a high risk and low diagnostic yield.
- Right-sided heart catheterization is recommended, as is acute vasoreactivity testing using a short-acting agent such as IV epoprostenol, IV adenosine, or inhaled NO.
- Serial assessments of functional class and endurance on a 6-minute walk are recommended.

Recommendations for General Management of Pulmonary Arterial Hypertension

- Anticoagulation with warfarin (Coumadin) should be considered.
- Diuretics should be administered, as indicated.

- Supplemental oxygen should be used as necessary to maintain oxygen saturations higher than 90% at all times.
- Referral to a center that specializes in treatment of PAH is strongly recommended.

Recommendations for Medications to Treat Pulmonary Arterial Hypertension

- CCB is recommended for patients with positive vasoreactivity testing.
- All patients should be considered for long-term therapy with a combination of the following medications (see Fig. 15-22):
  - Endothelin-receptor antagonists
    - Bosentan (oral)
    - Ambrisentan (oral)
  - Phosphodiesterase inhibitors
    - Sildenafil
    - Tadalafil
  - Prostanoids
    - Epoprostenol (IV)
    - Treprostinil (SC, IV, inhaled)
    - Iloprost (inhaled)
- Patients with PAH in functional class IV are candidates for long-term treatment with IV epoprostenol.

References

Badesch DB, et al. Diagnosis and assessment of pulmonary arterial hypertension. *JACC Cardiovasc Intervent.* 2009;54(1):S55.

McLaughlin V, et al. ACCF/AHA 2009 Expert consensus document on pulmonary hypertension. *JACC Cardiovasc Intervent.* 2009;53(17):1573.

CCB, Calcium channel blocker; *ECG,* electrocardiogram; *HIV,* human immunodeficiency virus; *IV,* intravenous; *LV,* left ventricle; *mPAP,* mean pulmonary artery pressure; *NO,* nitrous oxide; *PAH,* pulmonary arterial hypertension; *RA,* right atrium; *RV,* right ventricle; *SC,* subcutaneous; *V/Q,* ventilation-perfusion.

mapping is especially useful to visualize the severity a valvular regurgitation.[118]

Complications

Heart failure is the most frequent complication of IE and the most frequent cause of death. Embolic complications are the second most common complication occurring in 22% to 50% of IE cases: 65% of the emboli occur in the central nervous system (CNS) and can cause a stroke. Pulmonary embolism (PE) occurs in 66% to 75% of IVDA cases that involve vegetations on the tricuspid valve. Other organs affected by emboli include liver, spleen, kidney, abdominal mesenteric artery, and peripheral vessels. Septic emboli may be visible on the fingers and toes. Rate of emboli formation rapidly declines with appropriate intravenous antimicrobial administration.[117] Risk of death increases with the development of emboli and decreased arterial perfusion to vital organs. Clinical manifestations of endocarditis that may be discovered on physical examination are listed in Box 15-24.

Medical Management

Treatment requires prolonged intravenous therapy with adequate doses of antimicrobial agents tailored to the specific IE microbe and patient circumstances. The antibiotic management of native valve endocarditis (NVE) is frequently different from treatment of prosthetic valve endocarditis (PVE) or IVDA endocarditis. Antibiotic treatment is prolonged, administered in high doses intravenously and may involve combination therapy.[117] Best outcomes are achieved if therapy is initiated before hemodynamic compromise.[115]

In many cases, antimicrobial medications are not sufficient to cure the IE. Cardiac surgery to excise the damaged native or prosthetic valve is required for persistent vegetation, valve dysfunction, perivalvular extension, and aggressive fungal or antibiotic resistant bacteria. Usually, valve surgery is delayed until the patient is stable.[115] An increasing number of patients with uncomplicated IE are being discharged earlier than in the past and are continuing the intravenous antimicrobial therapy at

TABLE 15-13 MODIFIED DUKE CRITERIA

MAJOR CRITERIA*	MINOR CRITERIA*
Blood culture positive for IE	Predisposition: persons with a heart condition or an injectable drug user
Evidence of endocardial involvement	Fever: temperature >38°C Vascular phenomena: major arterial emboli, septic pulmonary infarcts, mycotic aneurysm, intracranial hemorrhage, conjunctival hemorrhages and Janeway lesions Immunologic phenomena: glomerulonephritis, Osler nodes, Roth spots, and rheumatoid factor Microbial evidence: positive blood culture that does not meet any major criterion or serologic evidence of active infection with organism consistent with IE

*A *definite* diagnosis of infective endocarditis (IE) requires two major criteria, or one major and three minor criteria, or five minor criteria. A *possible* diagnosis of IE requires one major criteria and one minor criteria or three minor criteria.
Based on data from Baddour LM, et al. Infective endocarditis: diagnosis, antimicrobial therapy, and management of complications. A statement for healthcare professionals from the Committee on Rheumatic Fever, Endocarditis, and Kawasaki Disease, Council on Cardiovascular Disease in the Young, and the Councils on Clinical Cardiology, Stroke, and Cardiovascular Surgery and Anesthesia, American Heart Association: endorsed by the Infectious Diseases Society of America. *Circulation.* 2005;111(23):e394; Wilson W, et al. Prevention of infective endocarditis: guidelines from the American Heart Association. A guideline from the American Heart Association Rheumatic Fever, Endocarditis, and Kawasaki Disease Committee, Council on Cardiovascular Disease in the Young, and the Council on Clinical Cardiology, Council on Cardiovascular Surgery and Anesthesia, and the Quality of Care and Outcomes Research Interdisciplinary Working Group. *Circulation.* 2007;116(15):1736.

BOX 15-24 CLINICAL MANIFESTATIONS OF ENDOCARDITIS

- Fever
- Splenomegaly
- Hematuria
- Petechiae
- Cardiac murmurs
- Easy fatigability
- Osler nodes (small, raised, tender areas most commonly found in pads of fingers and toes)
- Splinter hemorrhages in nail beds
- Roth spots (round or oval spots consisting of coagulated fibrin; seen in the retina and lead to hemorrhage)

home by means of a surgically or peripherally implanted long-term central venous catheter.[117]

Nursing Management

Nursing management of the patient with IE incorporates a variety of nursing diagnoses (Box 15-25). Nursing interventions focus on timely antimicrobial administration to resolve the infection, prevent complications, provide pain medication, and individualize patient education.

BOX 15-25 NURSING DIAGNOSES

Endocarditis

- Decreased Cardiac Output, related to alterations in preload, p. 1128
- Decreased Cardiac Output, related to alterations in afterload, p. 1128
- Decreased Cardiac Output, related to alterations in contractility, p. 1128
- Decreased Cardiac Output, related to alterations in heart rate or rhythm, p. 1128
- Activity Intolerance, related to cardiopulmonary dysfunction, p. 1119
- Acute Pain, related to transmission and perception of cutaneous, visceral, muscular, or ischemic impulses, p. 1123
- Risk for Infection, related to invasive procedures, p. 1160
- Anxiety, related to threat to biologic, psychologic, or social integrity, p. 1125
- Deficient Knowledge, related to lack of previous exposure to information, p. 1134 (see Box 15-26, Patient Education for Endocarditis)

BOX 15-26 PATIENT EDUCATION

Endocarditis

- Pathophysiology of endocarditis
- Medications: importance of long-term intravenous antibiotics for eradication
- Temperature: daily temperature monitoring
- Infection control: prophylactic antibiotics related to dental work or other invasive procedures after current medical crisis is controlled
- Activity tolerance: increase activity as tolerated and rest periods, as needed
- Heart failure: if symptoms of heart failure are present, education is given on fluid and sodium restriction, fluid balance, diuretic management, daily weight, and controlling breathlessness
- Follow-up care after discharge
- Symptoms to report to a health care professional

Resolving the Infection

IE requires a long course of intravenous antibiotics, usually for 4 to 6 weeks. This is begun in the hospital and continued at home with an indwelling central catheter after the patient is in stable condition.[117] Nursing assessment includes monitoring for signs of worsening infection such as persistent temperature elevation, malaise, weakness, easy fatigability, and night sweats, or new emboli on hands or feet (Box 15-26).

Preventing Complications

Between 20% and 60% of patients with IE experience complications.[114] The nursing assessment is attuned to the early detection of changes such as shortness of breath or chest pain with hemoptysis. As valvular dysfunction accelerates, acute heart failure develops. Cardiac assessment includes auscultation of heart sounds to detect the presence of or change in a cardiac murmur. This can be caused by worsening heart failure or by pulmonary emboli. Changes in level of consciousness, visual changes, or complaints of headache should always be reported immediately because of the risk of emboli. Evaluation of liver and kidney function is essential to monitor the health of those organs because of the risk of emboli. With the complex and prolonged antibiotic therapy required for treating IE, adverse medication reactions constitute another important consideration.

BOX 15-27 EVIDENCE-BASED PRACTICE

Infective Endocarditis and Infective Endocarditis Prophylaxis

QSEN **Diagnosis of Infective Endocarditis**

The Modified Duke Criteria are recommended to guide diagnosis (see Table 15-13). Endocarditis prophylaxis is recommended for patients with the following:

- Prosthetic heart valve with a history of infective endocarditis
- Valve repair
- Complex cyanotic congenital heart disease
- Congenital valve malformation such as bicuspid aortic valve
- HCM with latent or resting obstruction
- MVP with valvular regurgitation and/or thickened valve leaflets

Special considerations apply for patients with prosthetic valve and IE:

- Patients with a risk for IE who have unexplained fever for more than 48 hours should have at least two sets of blood cultures obtained from different sites.
- Surgical valve replacement is indicated for patients with IE of a prosthetic valve who present in heart failure.

Antimicrobial Therapy

Four features mark the antimicrobial therapy administered for IE:

1. It is prolonged.
2. It is bactericidal.
3. It is intravenous.
4. It is high dosage.

At least two sets of blood cultures are obtained every 24 to 48 hours until the infection is cleared from the bloodstream. IV antimicrobial therapy is continued after hospital discharge in the home setting.

Complications from Infective Endocarditis

- Emboli from infected heart valves occur in 22% to 50% of IE cases and 65% of embolic events involve the CNS. The rate of embolic events drops significantly during and after 2 to 3 weeks of appropriate antimicrobial therapy.
- Acute heart failure has the greatest impact on overall prognosis.

Complications from Antibiotics

- Toxicity from the high doses of antibiotics may impair kidney function or vestibular function (balance).
- Diarrhea and colitis can be caused by a reaction to the antibiotic therapy or by overgrowth by *Clostridium difficile*.

Indications for Surgery

- Removal of infected device
- Increase in size of valve vegetation despite appropriate antimicrobial therapy
- Mitral or aortic regurgitation with acute heart failure unresponsive to medical therapy
- One or more embolic events during the first 2 weeks of antimicrobial therapy

References

Nishimura RA, et al. ACC/AHA 2008 guideline update on valvular heart disease: focused update on infective endocarditis. *Circulation.* 2008;118:887.

Wilson W, et al. Prevention of infective endocarditis: guidelines from the American Heart Association: a guideline from the American Heart Association Rheumatic Fever, Endocarditis, and Kawasaki Disease Committee, Council on Cardiovascular Disease in the Young, and the Council on Clinical Cardiology, Council on Cardiovascular Surgery and Anesthesia, and the Quality of Care and Outcomes Research Interdisciplinary Working Group. *Circulation.* 2007;116(15):1736.

HCM, Hypertrophic cardiomyopathy; *IE,* infective endocarditis; *MVP,* mitral valve prolapse.

Patient Education

The person with IE needs to know the manifestations of infection, how to take an oral temperature, and what medical procedures increase risk of a recurrence of IE. A written list of all medications must be supplied (see Box 15-26). It is essential to reinforce to patients the necessity to provide a comprehensive endocarditis history to their other health care providers such as the dentist or the podiatrist.[117,118] The known IVDA has a unique set of challenges to overcome.[119] Multidisciplinary support for the patient to meet the challenge of opiate withdrawal and psychologic dependence is essential to prevent a relapse.[135] Many clinicians participate in the care of a patient with IE (Box 15-27).

VALVULAR HEART DISEASE

Description and Etiology

The term *valvular heart disease* describes structural and functional abnormalities of single or multiple cardiac valves. The result is an alteration in blood flow across the valve. The two types of valvular lesions are *stenotic* and *regurgitant.* These are described with reference to the specific cardiac valves involved.

Admission of patients with valvular disease to the critical care unit is generally related to surgical replacement or an exacerbation of heart failure. In the past, in the United States, most valvular lesions were rheumatic in origin, and damage was a direct result of group A beta-hemolytic streptococcal pharyngitis. As a result of aggressive treatment of "strep throat," this has become a rare problem. Valve lesions are now more commonly related to congenital disorders and older patients. These patients are more likely to present with symptoms of heart failure and degenerative valve changes.[120-123] These changes may be described as myxomatous leaflet degeneration or annular calcification.[118,120]

Pathophysiology

Mitral Valve Stenosis

The term *mitral valve stenosis* describes a progressive narrowing of the mitral valve orifice. Primary cause is rheumatic carditis with rare occurrences related to congenital malformations. Mitral stenosis occurs in twice as many women as men.[120] Symptoms occur when the normal valve size is reduced to 2 cm^2 or less. Symptoms occur at rest when the valve area is reduced below 1 cm^2.[120] Narrowing is caused by aging valve tissue or by acute rheumatic valvulitis (Table 15-14A). The diffuse valve leaflets fibrose and fuse, reducing mobility and thickening the chordae tendineae. As a result, the mitral valve can no longer open or close passively in response to left atrial and ventricular pressure changes. Blood flow across the valve is impeded. Mitral stenosis increases the risk of developing AF because of the high pressures in the left atrium that will stimulate left atrial remodeling and enlargement. Development of AF will significantly increase symptoms and may increase the need for surgical replacement of the valve.

Mitral Valve Regurgitation

Mitral valve regurgitation may result from rheumatic disease, aging of the valve, endocarditis, collagen vascular disease, or papillary muscle dysfunction[120] (see Table 15-14B). In mitral regurgitation, the valve annulus, leaflets, chordae tendineae, and papillary muscles may all be dysfunctional, or the dysfunction may be isolated to just one component of the valve. Mitral valve regurgitation results in retrograde flow of blood into the left atrium with each ventricular contraction. It is always described as chronic or acute because of the very different impact on the left-sided chambers.

In chronic mitral valve regurgitation, the left atrium has dilated to accommodate the additional regurgitant volume, whereas the left ventricle has hypertrophied (increased muscle) to maintain an adequate stroke volume and cardiac output. In

---

TABLE 15-14 VALVULAR DYSFUNCTION

	PATHOPHYSIOLOGY	CLINICAL MANIFESTATIONS	PHYSICAL SIGNS
A. Mitral valve stenosis ┊ **indicates stenosis** A ↓	**Mitral Valve Stenosis** Left atrium must generate more pressure to propel blood beyond the lesion Rise in left atrial pressure and volume reflected retrograde into pulmonary vessels Right ventricular hypertrophy Right ventricular failure	Dyspnea on exertion Fatigue and weakness Pronounced respiratory symptoms (e.g., orthopnea, paroxysmal nocturnal dyspnea) Mild hemoptysis with bronchial capillary rupture Susceptibility to pulmonary infections	Chest radiograph: pulmonary congestion, redistribution of blood flow to upper lobes ECG: Atrial fibrillation and other atrial dysrhythmias Auscultation: diastolic murmur, accentuated S_1, opening snap Catheterization: elevated pressure gradient across valve; increased left atrial pressure, pulmonary artery occlusion pressure, and pulmonary artery pressure; low cardiac output
B. Mitral valve regurgitation 🌳 **indicates backward flow from a valve that is leaking or regurgitant** B	**Mitral Valve Regurgitation** LV dilation and hypertrophy Left atrial dilation and hypertrophy	Weakness and fatigue Exertional dyspnea Palpitations Severe symptoms precipitated by LV failure, with consequent low output and pulmonary congestion	Chest radiograph: left atrial and LV enlargement, variable pulmonary congestion ECG: P mitrale, LV hypertrophy, atrial fibrillation Auscultation: murmur throughout systole Catheterization: opacification of left atrium during LV injection, *v* waves, increased left atrial and LV pressures Variable elevations of pulmonary pressures
C. Aortic valve stenosis ┊ **indicates stenosis** C	**Aortic Valve Stenosis** LV hypertrophy Progressive failure of ventricular emptying Pulmonary congestion Failure of right side of heart, with systemic venous congestion Sudden cardiac death	Exertional dyspnea Exercise intolerance Syncope Angina Heart failure (LV failure)	Chest radiograph: poststenotic aortic dilation, calcification ECG: LV hypertrophy Auscultation: systolic ejection murmur Catheterization: significant pressure gradient, increased LV end-diastolic pressure

Continued

TABLE 15-14   VALVULAR DYSFUNCTION—cont'd

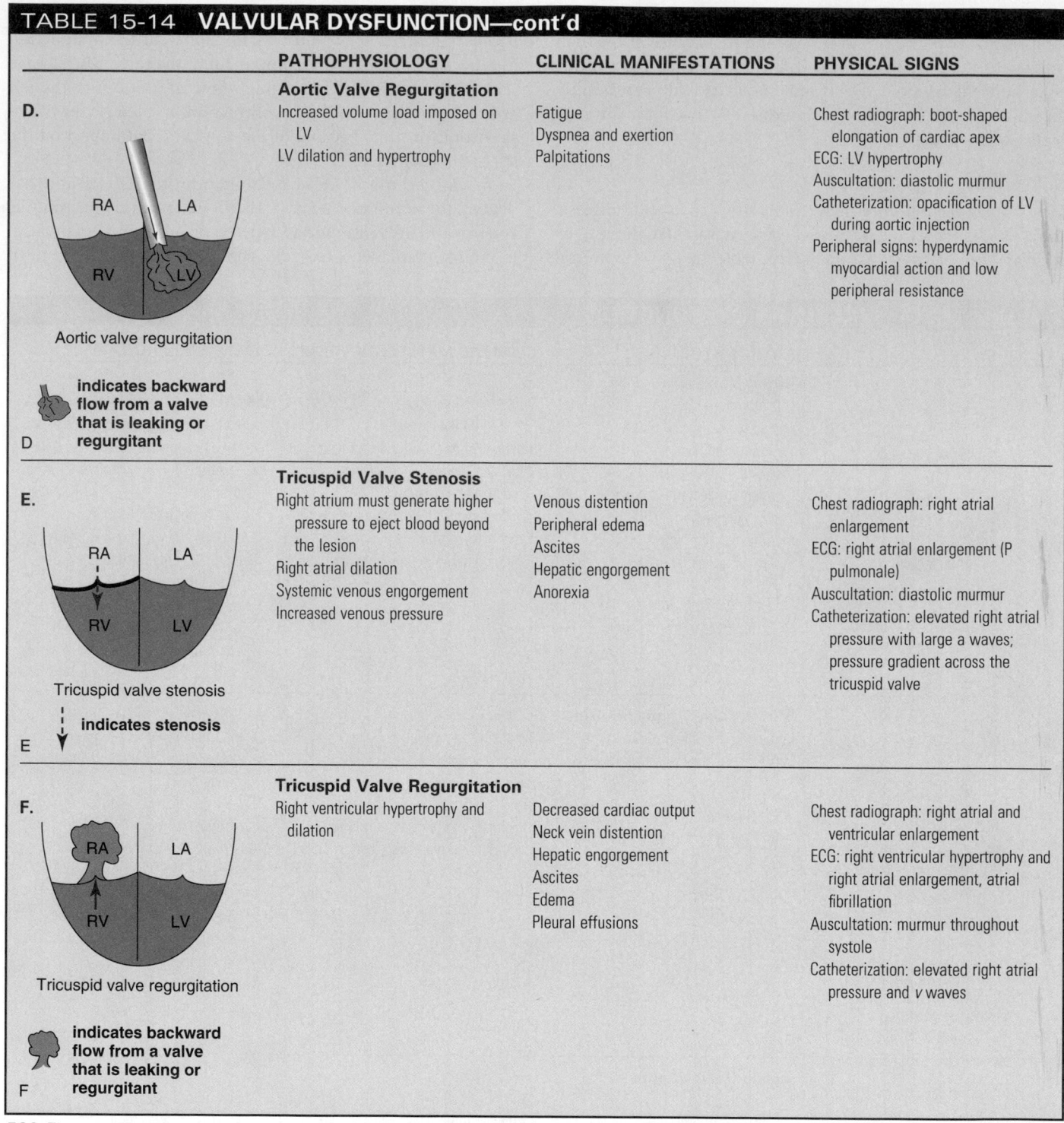

	PATHOPHYSIOLOGY	CLINICAL MANIFESTATIONS	PHYSICAL SIGNS
D. Aortic valve regurgitation ◆ indicates backward flow from a valve that is leaking or regurgitant	**Aortic Valve Regurgitation** Increased volume load imposed on LV LV dilation and hypertrophy	Fatigue Dyspnea and exertion Palpitations	Chest radiograph: boot-shaped elongation of cardiac apex ECG: LV hypertrophy Auscultation: diastolic murmur Catheterization: opacification of LV during aortic injection Peripheral signs: hyperdynamic myocardial action and low peripheral resistance
E. Tricuspid valve stenosis ┊ indicates stenosis	**Tricuspid Valve Stenosis** Right atrium must generate higher pressure to eject blood beyond the lesion Right atrial dilation Systemic venous engorgement Increased venous pressure	Venous distention Peripheral edema Ascites Hepatic engorgement Anorexia	Chest radiograph: right atrial enlargement ECG: right atrial enlargement (P pulmonale) Auscultation: diastolic murmur Catheterization: elevated right atrial pressure with large a waves; pressure gradient across the tricuspid valve
F. Tricuspid valve regurgitation ◆ indicates backward flow from a valve that is leaking or regurgitant	**Tricuspid Valve Regurgitation** Right ventricular hypertrophy and dilation	Decreased cardiac output Neck vein distention Hepatic engorgement Ascites Edema Pleural effusions	Chest radiograph: right atrial and ventricular enlargement ECG: right ventricular hypertrophy and right atrial enlargement, atrial fibrillation Auscultation: murmur throughout systole Catheterization: elevated right atrial pressure and v waves

ECG, Electrocardiogram; *LV*, left ventricular; *P mitrale*, m-shaped P waves that occur in left atrial hypertrophy and are often caused by mitral stenosis; *P pulmonale*, tall, peaked P waves that occur in right atrial hypertrophy and are often caused by chronic pulmonary disease.

contrast, acute mitral valve regurgitation is precipitated by chordae tendineae or papillary muscle rupture resulting from an acute MI or IE.[120] This is a medical emergency. The left atrium cannot accommodate the sudden increase in volume and pressure, and use of an IABP, inotropic and afterload-reducing pharmacological support are often required to increase forward output and to reduce pulmonary congestion.[139] After the patient's condition has stabilized, surgical replacement or repair of the incompetent valve is performed.[120]

Aortic Valve Stenosis

The term *aortic valve stenosis* describes a narrowing of the aortic valve area. It can result from aging, rheumatic valvulitis, or deterioration of a congenital bicuspid valve[120,122] (see Table 15-14C). The pathologic hallmarks are inflammation, fibrous valvular thickening, and tissue calcification resembling bone formation.[124] When the aortic valvular opening is reduced to less than 1.5 cm^2, the condition is classified as mild. Cardiac catheterization or Doppler echocardiography can identify a gradient of less than 25 mm Hg across the valve.[120] The *gradient* represents the difference in systolic pressure between the left ventricle and the aorta. A significant pressure difference is a diagnostic hallmark of valvular stenosis. If the valve orifice has narrowed to 1 cm^2 or less, the gradient will be greater than 40 mm Hg, and the diagnosis will be upgraded to severe aortic valve stenosis.[120] The impedance of left ventricular ejection into the aorta results in increased left ventricular systolic pressure, left ventricular hypertrophy, and eventually left ventricular dilation. When symptoms such as angina, dyspnea, syncope, and other indicators of heart failure develop, it is critical to intervene to prevent further damage to the left ventricle. Aortic valve replacement is usually indicated. Congenitally abnormal valves may require replacement by the forth to sixth decades, and the degenerative changes are often tolerated until about 72 years of age.[122]

Aortic Valve Regurgitation

Aortic regurgitation, also known as *aortic insufficiency*, can occur as a result of rheumatic fever, systemic hypertension, Marfan syndrome, syphilis, rheumatoid arthritis, aging valve tissue, or discrete subaortic stenosis (see Table 15-14D). Aortic valve incompetence results in a reflux of blood back into the left ventricle during ventricular diastole. To accommodate this extra volume, the left ventricle initially dilates and then hypertrophies in an attempt to empty more completely and to meet the needs of the peripheral circulation. Aortic valve replacement is recommended for symptomatic patients with well-preserved or moderate left ventricular dysfunction.[120]

Tricuspid Valve Stenosis

Tricuspid valve stenosis is rarely an isolated lesion (see Table 15-14E). It often occurs in conjunction with mitral or aortic disease. Its origin most often is rheumatic fever or a complication of IVDA and resultant endocarditis.[120] Tricuspid valve stenosis increases the pressure work of the usually low-pressure right atrium, resulting in right atrial hypertrophy. The right atrium dilates in an attempt to accommodate the residual right atrial volume and the incoming venous return. As a result, systemic venous congestion occurs—the consequences of which include jugular venous congestion, liver failure, hepatomegaly, ascites, and peripheral edema.

Tricuspid Valve Regurgitation

Tricuspid valve regurgitation usually results from advanced failure of the left side of the heart that eventually affects the right side of the heart, severe pulmonary hypertension, or as a complication of IE. Other causes include carcinoid, rheumatoid arthritis, radiation therapy, trauma, and Marfan syndrome[120] (see Table 15-14F).

Pulmonic Valve Disease

Pulmonary valve disease is not a common disorder in adults. It is most often related to congenital anomalies and produces failure of the right side of the heart.[125] Acquired cases are most often related to carcinoid or rheumatic fever pathologies. Initial symptoms present as dyspnea and can progress to severe heart failure symptomatology. Balloon

valvuloplasty has proven successful for treatment of these patients.[125]

Mixed Valvular Lesions

Many persons have *mixed valvular lesions* as an element of stenosis and regurgitation. Mixed lesions can accentuate the severity of a condition. For example, when combined, aortic stenosis and aortic regurgitation increase left ventricular volume and pressure and thereby multiply the degree of left ventricular work.

Medical Management

Management of valvular disorders includes pharmacologic therapy to control symptoms of heart failure and then cardiac surgical repair or replacement of the affected valve.[120,124] When surgery is not feasible, balloon dilation is a rare option selected for individuals too ill to undergo a major cardiac surgical procedure.[126] Percutaneous valve devices including stent valves and mitral clips are being evaluated as a less invasive alternative.[127-129]

Nursing Management

Nursing management of the patient with valvular disease incorporates a variety of nursing diagnoses (Box 15-28). Nursing management interventions focus on achievement of adequate cardiac output, maintenance of fluid balance, and patient and family education.

Cardiac Output

Low cardiac output is a common finding in patients with valvular heart disease. It can occur because of decreased forward flow through a stenotic valve, bidirectional flow across an incompetent valve, or associated heart failure. Vital signs and the effect of positive inotropic and afterload-reducing agents are assessed and documented. If the patient has hemodynamic catheters inserted, cardiac output and hemodynamic parameters are measured and evaluated. Patient care activities are carefully planned to provide adequate rest periods to prevent fatigue.

Fluid Balance

Fluid status is evaluated by auscultation of breath sounds for crackles, heart sounds for presence of an S_3, daily weights to trend a "sudden weight gain," and presence of peripheral edema. The appearance of pulmonary crackles or an S_3 heart sound confirms volume overload. The jugular vein is assessed for signs

---

◎ BOX 15-28 NURSING DIAGNOSES

Valvular Heart Disease

- Decreased Cardiac Output, related to alterations in preload, p. 1128
- Decreased Cardiac Output, related to alterations in afterload, p. 1128
- Decreased Cardiac Output, related to alterations in contractility, p. 1128
- Decreased Cardiac Output, related to alterations in heart rate or rhythm, p. 1128
- Activity Intolerance, related to cardiopulmonary dysfunction, p. 1119
- Deficient Knowledge, related to lack of previous exposure to information, p. 1134 (see Box 15-29, Patient Education for Valvular Heart Disease)

of increased distention. Diuretics and vasodilators are administered to counteract excess fluid retention. The patient is weighed daily, and fluid intake and output are monitored and recorded.

Patient Education

Education for the patient with acute or chronic heart failure caused by valvular dysfunction includes: 1) information related to diet, 2) fluid restrictions, 3) the actions and side effects of heart failure medications, 4) the need for prophylactic antibiotics before undergoing any invasive procedures, and 5) when to call the health care provider to report a negative change in cardiac symptoms (Box 15-29).

Many patients also require information about valvular heart surgery. Achieving the optimal outcomes for the patient with valve disease requires contributions from a team of educated health care clinicians. Collaborative multidisciplinary priorities are listed in Box 15-30. The heart valve replacement section in Chapter 16 provides more information on surgical management.

ATHEROSCLEROTIC DISEASES OF THE AORTA

Description

Two aortic conditions are described—aortic aneurysm and aortic dissection. Both disease states are the result of progressive atherosclerotic disease and systemic arterial hypertension.

BOX 15-29 PATIENT EDUCATION

Valvular Heart Disease

- Pathophysiology of valvular disease
- Infection control: prophylactic antibiotics related to dental work or other invasive procedures
- Heart failure: if symptoms of heart failure are present, education is provided on fluid and sodium restriction, fluid balance, diuretic management, daily weight, and controlling breathlessness
- Surgery: if open-heart surgery was performed, information about postsurgical recovery is provided
- Medications: medications may be complex, and information must be given in writing and orally
- Preload: purpose of diuretics, increased urine output, and control of fluid volume
- Afterload: purpose of vasodilators or angiotensin-converting enzyme (ACE) inhibitors in decreasing the workload of the heart
- Heart rate: purpose of digoxin is to control the rate in atrial fibrillation, a frequent dysrhythmia in heart failure
- Contractility: with the exception of digoxin, no oral contractility medications are approved by the U.S. Food and Drug Administration (FDA)
- Anticoagulation: patients with distended atria, enlarged ventricles, atrial fibrillation, or mechanical valves may be prescribed anticoagulants (Coumadin); risks of bleeding, importance of correct dosages, prothrombin times, international normalized ratio (INR), and nutritional-pharmacologic interactions are emphasized
- Follow-up care after discharge
- Symptoms to report to a health care professional

BOX 15-30 EVIDENCE-BASED PRACTICE

Valvular Heart Disease

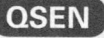 Class I recommendations with strong evidence are provided.

Recommendations for Detection and Surveillance of Valvular Disease by Echocardiography
- Echocardiography is noninvasive and is used for all initial diagnosis and serial follow-up evaluations.

Recommendations for Aortic Stenosis
- Echocardiography is the primary diagnostic tool.
- Coronary arteriography is used before AVR if CAD is suspected.
- AVR recommended for symptomatic patients with severe AS; AVR can be combined with CABG surgery when CAD is present.

Recommendations for Aortic Regurgitation
- Echocardiography is the primary diagnostic tool.
- Cardiac catheterization is used if noninvasive tests are inconclusive.
- AVR is indicated for symptomatic patients with severe AR irrespective of LV systolic function.
- AVR is indicated for nonsymptomatic patients with severe AR with LV systolic dysfunction (ejection fraction <0.5 [50%]); AVR can be combined with CABG surgery if CAD is present.

Recommendations for Mitral Stenosis
- Echocardiography is the primary diagnostic tool.

- Anticoagulation is indicated in patients with MS and atrial fibrillation (paroxysmal, persistent, or permanent) and for patients with MS in sinus rhythm with a prior embolic event or left atrial thrombus.
- Cardiac catheterization if noninvasive tests are inconclusive.
- Mitral valve repair (preferable), or mitral valve replacement is indicated for symptomatic (NYHA functional class III or IV) moderate or severe MS if percutaneous mitral balloon valvuloplasty is contraindicated.

Recommendations for Mitral Regurgitation
- Echocardiography is the primary diagnostic tool.
- Cardiac catheterization if noninvasive tests are inconclusive or if additional hemodynamic measurements are required.
- Mitral valve repair is the operation of choice over valve replacement in most patients with chronic MR.

See Box 15-27 for recommendations related to management of patients with valve disease and prosthetic valves.

References

Bonow RO, et al. ACC/AHA 2006 guidelines for the management of patients with valvular heart disease: executive summary. *Circulation.* 2006;114: 450-527.

Nishimura RA, et al. ACC/AHA 2008 guideline update on valvular heart disease: focused update on infective endocarditis: a report of the American College of Cardiology/American Heart Association Task Force on Practice Guidelines. *Circulation.* 2008;11(8):887-895.

AR, Aortic regurgitation; *AS,* aortic stenosis; *AVR,* aortic valve replacement; *CABG,* coronary artery bypass graft; *CAD,* coronary artery disease; *IE,* infective endocarditis; *LV,* left ventricular; *MR,* mitral regurgitation; *MS,* mitral stenosis; *NYHA,* New York Heart Association.

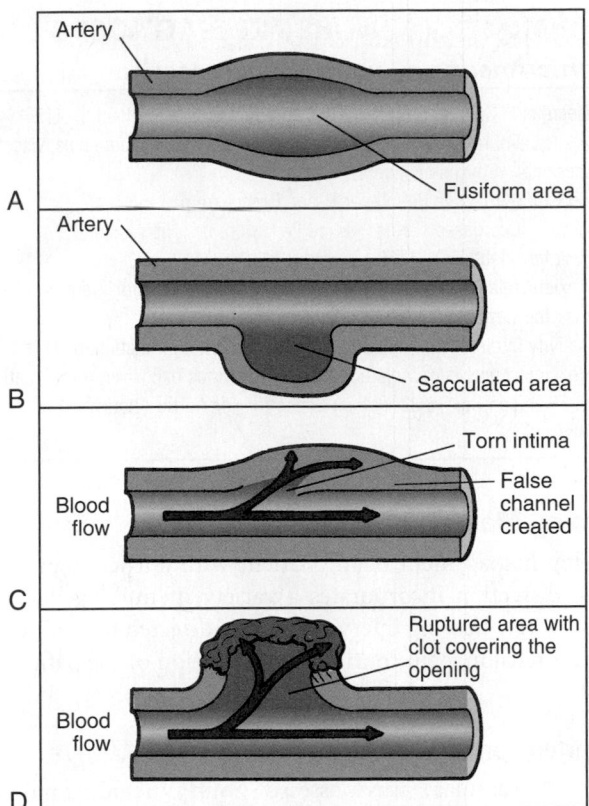

FIGURE 15-23 Four Types of Vascular Injury. *A,* In the fusiform aneurysm, an entire segment of an artery is dilated, taking on a spindle or bulbous shape. Fusiform aneurysms occur most often in the abdominal aorta and result from atherosclerosis; *B,* a sacculated aneurysm involves only one side of an artery and usually is located in the ascending aorta; *C,* dissection occurs because of a tear in the intima, resulting in the shunting of blood between the intima and media of a vessel; *D,* pseudoaneurysm can result from arterial trauma, such as that caused by an arterial introducer sheath or intra-aortic balloon catheter, when the arterial opening does not heal normally and is covered by a clot that may rupture at any time.

Aortic Aneurysm

An *aortic aneurysm* is a localized dilation of the arterial wall that results in an alteration in vessel shape and blood flow, and two types of vascular aneurysms exist (Fig. 15-23A and B). Aortic aneurysm is diagnosed most commonly in older adults. Abdominal aortic aneurysm is four times more common compared with thoracic aneurysm.

Aortic Dissection

An *aortic dissection* occurs when a column of blood separates the vascular layers. This creates a false lumen, which communicates with the true lumen through a tear in the intima (see Fig. 15-23C).

Etiology

Of the patients with an aortic aneurysm, 90% have a history of systemic hypertension. Other causes of aortic aneurysm include the following: atherosclerotic changes in the thoracic and abdominal aorta, blunt trauma, Marfan syndrome, pregnancy, and injury or dissection.

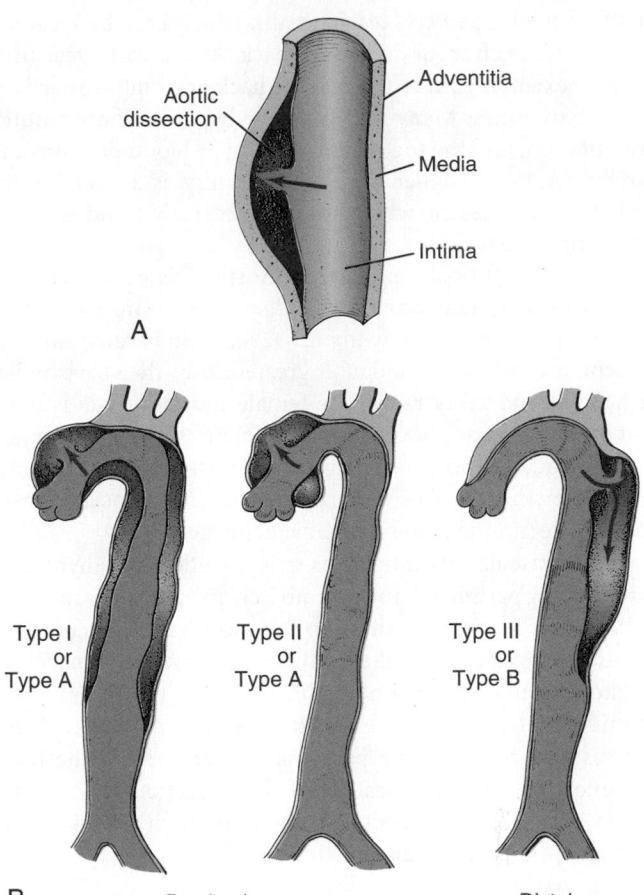

FIGURE 15-24 Aortic Dissection. *A,* Separation of vascular layers. *B,* Classification of aortic dissection. (Modified from Price SA, Wilson LM. *Pathophysiology: Clinical Concepts of Disease Processes.* 5th ed. St. Louis: Mosby; 1997.)

Assessment and Diagnosis

An aortic aneurysm does not always produce symptoms. It may be detected during routine abdominal examination as a palpable, pulsatile mass located in the umbilical region of the abdomen to the left of the midline. A thoracic aneurysm may be identified on a routine chest radiograph. An aortic dissection is usually identified emergently by the onset of acute pain.

Aortic Aneurysm

An aneurysm less than 4 cm in diameter can be managed on an outpatient basis with frequent blood pressure monitoring and ultrasound testing to document any changes in the size of the aneurysm. Management includes weight loss, smoking cessation, and hypertension control, as appropriate. An aortic aneurysm larger than 5 cm in diameter requires evaluation for surgical repair or placement of an aortic stent to eliminate the risk of rupture (see Chapter 16).

Aortic Dissection

Aortic dissections are classified according to the site of the tear. Two classification systems are used in clinical practice. These use the letters A and B or the numerals I, II, or III, as shown in Figure 15-24. The classic clinical presentation is the sudden onset of intense, severe, tearing pain, which may be localized initially in the chest, abdomen, or back. As the aortic tear (dissection) extends, pain radiates to the back or distally toward the lower extremities. Many patients have hypertension on initial presentation, and the focus is on control of blood pressure and early operation. Higher surgical mortality is found among patients who present with shock, hypotension, and signs of poor organ perfusion.[130]

The International Registry of Aortic Dissection (IRAD) records indicate that acute aortic dissection is more common in men (72%) than in women (32%), but because women present at an older age and after greater delay, they have higher in-hospital mortality rates. The female mortality rate is twice that of an age-matched population of men.[131] Risk of aneurysm rupture and likelihood of poor outcome after rupture is greater with women.[130-132] Morbidity and mortality associated with aortic dissection increase with advancing age.[130,131]

Cardiovascular warning signs may include severe hypertension, fleeting peripheral pulses, limb ischemia, or a new murmur indicative of aortic regurgitation. The most frequent acute neurologic changes include altered mental status and coma.[133] An ascending aortic dissection produces pain in the central chest or midscapular region of the back. A descending aortic dissection usually manifests by pain that radiates down the back, abdomen, or legs. The location of the dissection may be estimated according to the site of pain, although this does not eliminate the need for diagnostic procedures.

The two most helpful initial diagnostic tests are TTE and computed tomography (CT) because both permit rapid visualization of the thoracic structures. The chest radiograph is helpful only if the mediastinum is already widened. Diagnostic findings that identify high-risk patients include a widened mediastinum or an excessively dilated aorta. The definitive invasive diagnostic procedure is an aortogram (aortic angiogram with radiopaque contrast).

Medical Management

Medical management of an aortic aneurysm depends on what symptoms are seen and on hemodynamics. If the patient is stable, management is focused on controlling hypertension and educating the patient about the need for corrective surgery before the aneurysm is more than 5 cm wide. If the patient is seen with an acute aortic dissection, management involves immediate control of hypertension with intravenous medications and control of pain with opiates.[134,135] Progression of the dissection is evaluated by the patient's report of worsening or new pain. If the patient presents with hypotension or in cardiogenic shock, blood pressure support measures to maintain tissue perfusion are initiated. In such cases, emergency surgery may be performed. Surgery is usually required for dissections that involve the ascending aorta to prevent death from cardiac tamponade. This includes type A or type I and type II dissections (see Fig. 15-24). The surgical procedure includes resection of the affected area, followed by graft placement and restoration of blood flow to major branches of the aorta. Replacement of the aortic valve is performed if the dissection involves the valve. Dissections that involve the descending aorta (type B or type III) do not always require surgery.

BOX 15-31 NURSING DIAGNOSES
Aortic Aneurysm and Aortic Dissection

- Decreased Cardiac Output, related to alterations in preload, p. 1128
- Acute Pain, related to transmission and perception of cutaneous, visceral, muscular, or ischemic impulses, p. 1123
- Risk for Ineffective Peripheral Tissue Perfusion, p. 1158
- Risk for Decreased Cardiac Tissue Perfusion, p. 1155
- Risk for Infection, p. 1160
- Anxiety, related to threat to biologic, psychologic, or social integrity, p. 1125
- Risk for Ineffective Renal Perfusion, p. 1159
- Activity Intolerance, related to cardiopulmonary dysfunction, p. 1119
- Deficient Knowledge, related to lack of previous exposure to information, p. 1134 (see Box 15-32, Patient Education for Aortic Aneurysm and Aortic Dissection)

Nursing Management

Nursing management of the patient with aortic aneurysm or aortic dissection incorporates a variety of nursing diagnoses (Box 15-31). Nursing interventions are directed toward control of hypertension, pain control, and education of the patient and family.

Hypertension Management

The cardiovascular status is assessed hourly, including monitoring blood pressure in both arms, checking peripheral pulses bilaterally, auscultating for an aortic murmur, and monitoring the ECG for ischemic changes or dysrhythmias. Patients usually require an arterial line and receive potent antihypertensive medications such as labetalol, which combines beta-blocking activity to reduce cardiac output and lower blood pressure and peripheral alpha-blocking activity to vasodilate the arteries and decrease blood pressure.

Pain Control

Acute pain is a classic sign of aortic dissection. Opiates and sedatives are administered to control pain, decrease anxiety, and increase comfort. Because these medications can mask the pain of further dissection, they are administered judiciously. The patient's neurovascular status is assessed hourly. Documentation includes the presence and distribution of pain, pallor, paresthesia, paralysis, and movement of the limb.

Patient Education

In the acute period, education is limited to an explanation of the critical care environment and the importance of blood pressure control. If additional procedures such as aortography, CT, or surgery are to be performed, the critical care nurse assists with these explanations (Box 15-32). Recommendations for prevention and treatment of atherosclerotic aortic aneurysm and dissection are listed in Box 15-33.

PERIPHERAL ARTERIAL DISEASE

Description

Peripheral vascular disease (PVD) is divided into peripheral arterial disease (PAD) and peripheral venous disease. Venous disease is a chronic condition that is managed on an outpatient

BOX 15-32 PATIENT EDUCATION

Aortic Aneurysm and Aortic Dissection

- Pathophysiology of atherosclerotic aortic disease: aortic aneurysm or aortic dissection
- Hypertension control: hypertension increases the risk of aneurysm rupture or aortic dissection
- Pain control: use of 0 to 10 pain scale; information about availability of pain medications for acute pain
- Preprocedure teaching for aortic angiogram, computed tomography scan, or transesophageal echocardiogram
- Preoperative teaching for aortic surgical repair
- Risk factor modification: after the acute episode, if the cause of the aortic aneurysm or aortic dissection is atherosclerosis, an individual risk factor profile is developed for each patient; strategies to discuss include the following: decrease daily fat intake to less than 30% of total calories, achieve total blood cholesterol level of less than 200 mg/dL, stop smoking, reduce salt intake, control hypertension, treat diabetes if patient has diabetes, increase physical activity, achieve and maintain ideal body weight
- Symptoms to report to a health care professional: pain, signs and symptoms of infection
- Follow-up care after discharge

basis and does not require admission to a critical care unit. In contrast, PAD may require critical care admission for an acute thrombotic occlusion or after a vascular surgical procedure. PAD can occur in any peripheral artery. It is especially painful in the arteries that supply the lower extremities. The following descriptions relate to PAD.

Etiology

Atherosclerosis is a common cause of chronic arterial occlusion in older adults. PAD affects less than 4% of people younger than 40 years but has an impact on almost 22% of those older than 70 years.[136,137] Risk factors are the same for PAD and CAD. Most patients diagnosed with PAD have at least one risk factor that predisposes them to development of CAD.[136,137] Diabetes, smoking, hypertension, hyperlipidemia, and male gender increase the risk of peripheral arterial occlusion.[136,137,139] As with CAD, the presence of kidney disease increases the incidence of concomitant PAD.[136]

Pathophysiology

The most commonly affected vessels in the lower extremities are the superficial femoral artery and the popliteal artery in the legs, followed by the distal aorta and iliac arteries.

Assessment and Diagnosis

Ankle-Brachial Index

The ankle-brachial index (ABI) is a noninvasive test used to estimate the severity of arterial disease in the leg by comparing it with the measured arterial pressure in the arm. The SBP is measured on the arm and on the leg (just above the ankle). A cuff is used to occlude the pressure, and the SBP is measured at the posterior tibial pulse and the dorsalis pedis pulse locations.[136,137,140] The SBP can be palpated with the fingers or auscultated using a handheld 5- to 7-megahertz (MHz) Doppler device. To calculate the ABI, the arm SBP is divided into the

ankle SBP number.[136,137,140] A normal ABI value is between 0.9 and 1.0, signifying that the peripheral arteries are normal. Patients with an ABI value between 0.71 and 0.9 have mild PAD; those with an ABI between 0.41 to 0.7 have moderate PAD; and an ABI less than 0.4 indicates severe PAD.[136] Generally, as the ABI value decreases, symptoms of peripheral ischemia increase.

Intermittent Claudication

Arterial occlusion obstructs blood flow to the distal extremity. The lack of blood flow produces ischemic muscle pain known as *intermittent claudication*. This cramping, aching pain while walking is often the first symptom of PAD. The pain is relieved by rest and may remain stable in occurrence and intensity for many years. Symptoms do not occur until more than 75% of the vessel lumen is occluded.

As with other atherosclerotic conditions, PAD is typically asymptomatic until the disease process is well advanced. Clinicians who rely on history of leg pain alone severely underestimate PAD in the early stages. Only about 10% of population with PAD has classic symptoms of intermittent claudication (leg pain associated with PAD). Up to 50% of patients with PAD are asymptomatic, and the remaining 40% have a variety of leg symptoms different from classic claudication.[137] The ABI can be used as a screening tool to detect the presence of PAD before symptoms occur.[136,137] Prevention measures can then be discussed with the patient.

Rest Pain

As PAD progresses, patients may develop pain at rest. Pain at rest threatens the viability of the limb and requires immediate catheter or surgical intervention to relieve the blockage and restore circulation to the extremity.

Acute Occlusion

The symptoms of acute occlusion from thrombosis are sudden onset of severe pain, loss of pulses, collapse of superficial veins, coldness, pallor, and impaired motor and sensory function. As with rest pain, acute occlusion requires immediate intervention to open the artery.

Atrophic Tissue Changes

Skin changes associated with PAD include thickening of the nails and drying of the skin. Hair loss is common on the lower leg, feet, and toes. Pallor and a temperature gradient may be present as a line of demarcation between areas that have adequate arterial perfusion and areas that are poorly perfused. Wasting of muscle or soft tissue may be seen. As the atherosclerotic arterial disease progresses, skin ulcerations and gangrene can occur.

Medical Management

Medical therapy is geared toward controlling or eliminating risk factors, providing effective foot care, and suggesting alterations in lifestyle to promote rest and pain relief. Pharmacologic management may include the use of anticoagulants, vasodilators, or antiplatelet agents. If these therapies do not produce positive results, the patient may be a candidate for percutaneous

BOX 15-33 EVIDENCE-BASED PRACTICE

Aortic Aneurysm and Aortic Dissection

QSEN **Recommendations for Prevention of Atherosclerotic Aortic Aneurysm and Dissection**

- Hypertension is a major risk factor. There are no specific recommendations related to BP control and aortic disease. Reduction of BP to less than 130/80 mm Hg is consistent with recommendations for other atherosclerotic diseases (coronary and cerebrovascular).
- Cigarette smoking is a major risk factor for aortic disease. Smoking cessation is essential.
- Routine use of statins has been found to decrease the aneurysm rupture rate and may be effective in decreasing AAA growth rate.
- Aortic dissection also occurs as a complication of blunt chest trauma from high-speed motor vehicular trauma.

Recommendations for Treatment of Aortic Dissection

- Admission to the critical care unit for monitoring of heart rate and BP.
- Reduction of systolic BP using IV beta-blockers (Esmolol) or beta-blocker plus alpha-blocker combination (Labetalol). Beta-blockers are recommended because they reduce the force of blood ejected from the ventricle against the weakened aortic wall.
- If further systolic BP reduction is necessary, IV vasodilators (sodium nitroprusside) are added in addition to beta-blockers.
- Intubation and mechanical ventilation are recommended if profound hemodynamic instability exists.
- Pain relief (morphine sulfate) and sedation are recommended.
- Diagnosis of aortic dissection is made by clinical signs and location of the site of the tear and false lumen. CT is the most common diagnostic test in an emergency. MRI is often used for chronic stable dissections. TTE followed by TEE may also be used.
- Treatment recommendations depend on the classification of the dissection:
  - Type A (type I, type II) dissections that involve the aortic arch are repaired surgically to prevent aortic rupture or cardiac tamponade.
  - Type B (type III) dissections are recommended for medical treatment. Surgery or endovascular repair is recommended only in cases of

persistent chest pain, aortic expansion, periaortic hematoma, or mediastinal hematoma.
- Type A aortic dissection is a high-risk diagnosis with an overall hospital mortality rate of 25%. Patients with type A dissections who are admitted to the hospital with hypotension have a higher risk of adverse events.

Recommendations for Treatment of Elective Abdominal Aortic Aneurysm

- Formation of AAA or dissection before the sixth decade of life is uncommon.
- Based on current evidence, a 5.5-cm aneurysm diameter is the best threshold for repair in the "average" male patient. Vascular surgery experts recommend that women have elective repair of aneurysm at 4.5 to 5 cm. Individual anatomy, patient age, and physical size must also be considered.
- Until the results of long-term randomized trials are available, the choice between endoluminal repair (stent) and open abdominal surgery depends on patient and physician preferences.

References

Chaikof EL, et al. The care of patient with an abdominal aortic aneurysm: the Society for Vascular Surgery practice guidelines. *J Vasc Surg.* 2009;50(4):S2-S49.

Feldman M, Shah M, Elefteriades A. Medical management of acute type A aortic dissection. *Ann Thorac Cardiovasc Surg.* 2010;15(5):286.

Grootenboer N, et al. Systematic review and meta-analysis of sex differences in outcome after intervention for abdominal aortic aneurysm. *Br J Surg.* 2010;97(8):1169-1179.

Hiratzka L, et al. 2010 ACCF/AHA/AATS/ ACR/SCA/SCAO/ SIR/STS/SVM Guidelines for the diagnosis and management of patients with thoracic aortic disease. *Circulation.* 2010;121(13):e266.

Moll FL, et al. Management of abdominal aortic aneurysms. Clinical practice guidelines for the European Society of Vascular Surgery. *Eur J Vasc Endovasc Surg.* 2011;41:S1.

AAA, Abdominal aortic aneurysm; *BP,* blood pressure; *CT,* computed tomography; *IV,* intravenous; *MRI,* magnetic resonance imaging; *TTE,* transthoracic echocardiography; *TEE,* transesophageal echocardiography.

transluminal angioplasty (PTA), stent placement, or vascular bypass surgery. PTA or stent placement is effective if the lesion (blockage) is discrete and localized. However, if the arterial disease is diffuse, bypass surgery is usually performed. If gangrene (cell death) is present, limb or partial limb amputation is required.

Nursing Management

Nursing management of the patient with PAD incorporates a variety of nursing diagnoses (Box 15-34). Nurses assess the quality of the peripheral arterial pulses, intervene to maintain skin integrity and control pain, and educate the patient and family about PVD.

Arterial Pulses

Assessments of peripheral pulses, limb color, and temperature are critical in the evaluation of an ischemic limb. Arterial pulses are typically diminished, transiently present (intermittent vessel spasm), or absent distal to the site of occlusion. Patients with

BOX 15-34 NURSING DIAGNOSES

Peripheral Arterial Disease

- Acute Pain, related to transmission and perception of cutaneous, visceral, muscular, or ischemic impulses, p. 1123
- Risk for Ineffective Peripheral Tissue Perfusion, p. 1158
- Activity Intolerance, related to prolonged immobility or deconditioning, p. 1119
- Anxiety, related to threat to biologic, psychologic, or social integrity, p. 1125
- Powerlessness, related to lack of control over current situation or disease progression, p. 1152
- Deficient Knowledge, related to lack of previous exposure to information, p. 1134 (see Box 15-35, Patient Education for Peripheral Arterial Disease)

diabetes have a much higher incidence of PVD (arterial and venous) compared with the general population. Most hospitals use a standard scale to improve documentation of pulses. If the pulse cannot be palpated, Doppler ultrasonography may be used to assess blood flow.

Skin Integrity

Care is taken to protect the limb from injury and development of pressure ulcers. Healing is often impaired because of poor arterial blood flow or diabetes. Feet may be protected from injury by cotton or lamb's wool placed between the toes or by a bed cradle. However, for an acute ischemic limb, removal of the thrombus is the only treatment that can salvage ischemic tissue.

Pain Control

The term for pain during exercise in the presence of PAD is *intermittent claudication*. Leg pain that occurs after exercise, caused by increased muscle oxygen demand, can be effectively managed by stopping the exertion. However, pain at rest (without exercise) is a warning sign of an anoxic limb. The pain of an acute ischemic limb is extreme, and morphine is used for pain control. Ultimately, removal of the arterial obstruction is the only method to eliminate the pain.

Patient Education

Education topics include risk factor modification that emphasizes similar lifestyle changes to those recommended for patients with CAD, including smoking cessation, promoting exercise, maintenance of ideal body weight, inspection of the feet and legs, foot care, avoidance of foot trauma, and medications. Many patients with PAD underestimate their risk of stroke or acute MI and do not understand that the risk factors for PAD are the same for all of the cardiovascular atherosclerotic diseases.[136,137,139] Walking is good exercise for increasing blood flow to the lower extremities and is highly recommended for the person with PAD.[137,141,142]

If a surgically implanted prosthetic bypass graft is in place, teaching must include information about IE precautions. If the patient has diabetes, education about diabetes management is included in the teaching plan. Box 15-35 lists the salient points to include when teaching patients and families about PAD. Symptoms of PAD are listed in Box 15-36.

CAROTID ARTERY DISEASE

Description

The bifurcation of the carotid arteries is a common site of atherosclerotic plaque development (Fig. 15-25). Because these arterioles carry the blood supply to the brain, when they are obstructed, the presenting symptoms are neurologic. Treating carotid artery disease, a readily treatable obstruction, can prevent a stroke. Blood supply to the brain is provided by two separate arterial systems: 1) the vertebral arteries and 2) the internal carotid arteries, whose branches anastomose to form the circle of Willis. Any abrupt interruption in circulation for 4 to 6 minutes can produce permanent brain damage. When circulation to an area is impaired gradually, collateral circulation is often able to develop and maintain an adequate supply of blood to that area of the brain. Abrupt interruption in blood supply leads to an area of brain tissue becoming ischemic and often permanently damaged.

BOX 15-35 PATIENT EDUCATION

Peripheral Arterial Disease

- Pathophysiology of peripheral arterial disease
- Daily inspection and care of feet and legs
- Avoidance of trauma to feet or legs
- Increase walking distance gradually
- Risk factor modification: after the acute episode, if the cause of peripheral arterial disease is atherosclerosis, an individual risk factor profile is developed for each patient; strategies to discuss include the following: decrease daily fat intake to less than 30% of total calories, achieve total blood cholesterol level of less than 200 mg/dL, stop smoking, reduce salt intake, control hypertension, control diabetes if patient has diabetes, increase physical activity, achieve and maintain ideal body weight
- Preprocedure teaching about angiogram, percutaneous angioplasty, or stent placement in the lower extremities
- Risks and benefits of fibrinolytic therapy for acute peripheral arterial occlusion
- Preoperative teaching for revascularization surgery
- Rehabilitation education, if amputation is indicated
- Medications
- Antithrombotic therapy: usually, aspirin to decrease platelet adhesiveness
- Low-density lipoprotein cholesterol (LDL-C) lipid-lowering agents: 3-hydroxy-3-methylglutaryl coenzyme A (HMG CoA) reductase inhibitors
- Antihypertensive agents: antihypertensive medications and how to self-monitor blood pressure
- Symptoms to report to a health care professional: pain (chest or legs), leg or foot trauma
- Follow-up care after discharge

Etiology

The most common cause of carotid artery disease is atherosclerosis.[139,143] Uncommon causes include fibromuscular dysplasia, irradiation, and arteritis. The risk factors for development of atherosclerotic carotid artery disease and stroke are similar to those for CAD and PAD. Patients with any of these conditions must be educated about the other disease processes. The modifiable risk factors include uncontrolled hypertension (SBP >160 mm Hg), AF, smoking, diabetes with uncontrolled blood glucose levels, and hyperlipidemia.[144,145] Women taking HRT after menopause also have an increased risk of stroke.[144] The incidence of carotid stenosis increases with age. Asymptomatic carotid artery stenosis with greater than 50% occlusion is present in 22% to 28% of men and women older than 50 years, and the risk of stroke doubles with each successive decade after age 55 years. The presence of coexisting CAD also increases incidence of stroke, with a relative risk of 1.73 for men and 1.55 for women.[144]

The major mechanisms by which atherosclerosis in the carotid arteries creates ischemic symptoms are embolization and thrombosis. Ulcerated carotid lesions with accumulated platelet and fibrin produce thrombi that travel along with cholesterol deposits to become emboli to the brain. Stenotic areas in the carotid arteries are prone to thrombosis because of sluggish flow across the lesions. Doppler studies can examine the carotid arteries noninvasively. If a stroke is suspected, an emergency CT scan of the head is the appropriate diagnostic test.[139,143]

BOX 15-36   EVIDENCE-BASED PRACTICE

Peripheral Arterial Disease

QSEN   PAD affects 8 million men and women 40 years old or older in the United States. An international multidisciplinary group of clinicians has summarized evidence from clinical trials to begin the process of developing clinical guidelines.

Recommendations to Increase Awareness of PAD and Its Consequences

- Patients who are at highest risk of developing PAD are those who smoke cigarettes, have diabetes, and are older. In screening asymptomatic patients in high-risk groups, 30% to 50% of patients have PAD and do not know it.
- Other PAD risk factors include hypertension, hyperlipidemia, male sex, elevated C-reactive protein levels, elevated plasma fibrinogen levels, elevated blood glucose, prior MI, heart failure, and history of TIA or stroke.
- Patients with symptomatic PAD had a four to five times increased risk of stroke and a 20% to 60% increased risk of MI with a twofold to sixfold increased risk of death from coronary heart disease compared with those without PAD.
- Many patients are not aware of the link between PAD and cardiac and cerebrovascular atherosclerotic disease.

Recommendations to Improve Identification of Patients with Symptomatic PAD

- Because PAD is asymptomatic in the early stages of the disease, the ABI is recommended as a screening tool in high-risk patients. (See text for information on how to measure the ABI.)
- If the diagnosis is not made until the patient complains of intermittent claudication (pain with walking), the disease is already at an advanced stage.

Recommendations to Treat Risk Factors Associated with PAD

- Smokers should stop smoking. This is not easy to do. Physician advice with frequent follow-up and pharmacologic therapy (nicotine replacement and bupropion) demonstrate 1-year success rates of 5%, 16%, and 30%, respectively.
- If the patient is hyperlipidemic, achieve a normal lipid panel: reduce total serum cholesterol to less than 200 mg/dL and LDL-C to less than 70 mg/dL.
- Studies have not specifically examined the effect of controlling hypertension and diabetes on rates of PAD. However, extrapolating from the cardiac literature, researchers recommend reducing BP to less than 130/80 mg Hg and maintaining blood glucose within the normal range (70 to 110 mg/dL; HbA$_{1c}$ ≤ 7%).
- Low-dose aspirin or another platelet-inhibitor medication is recommended.
- Exercise rehabilitation is recommended with promotion of daily walking. The goal is to increase the ability of the patient to walk longer distances without leg pain.

References

Alonso-Coello P, et al. *Antithrombotic therapy in peripheral artery disease: antithrombotic therapy and prevention of thrombosis*, 9th ed. American College of Chest Physicians evidence-based clinical guidelines. *Chest.* 2012;141:e669S-e690S.

Hirsch AT, et al. ACC/AHA 2005 practice guidelines for the management of patients with peripheral arterial disease. *Circulation.* 2006;113:e463.

ABI, Ankle brachial index; *BP,* blood pressure; *C-reactive,* cross-reactive; *HbA$_{1c}$,* glycosylated hemoglobin; *LDL-C,* low-density lipoprotein cholesterol; *PAD,* peripheral arterial disease; *MI,* myocardial infarction; *TIA,* transient ischemic attack.

Carotid artery disease can remain asymptomatic for many years. After emboli are dislodged, the manifestations of carotid artery disease are neurologic and include hemiparesis, dysphasia, dysarthria, global aphasia, diplopia, vertigo, syncope, confusion, and monocular blindness. Neurologic symptoms that resolve completely within a short time are classified as *transient ischemic attacks* (TIAs). Symptoms that do not resolve are described as ischemic strokes.[146] If a patient has recently experienced a TIA, the risk of stroke is increased by more than 10% in the first 22 days, with the risk as high as 17% in the first 90 days.[1,144] Additional information on the neurologic management of the patient experiencing a stroke is provided in Chapter 24.

Medical Management

Medical management is focused on lowering the atherosclerotic risk factors that can be controlled by the patient. This includes regulation of hypertension, smoking cessation, seeking medical attention for treatable cardiac abnormalities such as AF, reducing weight, and reducing the cholesterol level to less than 200 mg/dL. Antithrombotic therapy (warfarin, aspirin, or other antiplatelet therapy) must be prescribed for patients with AF with a comprehensive individualized assessment of the relative risk of embolism versus the risk of bleeding complications.[144,147]

Asymptomatic patients who have carotid stenosis pose a quandary. In these patients, the risk of stroke needs to be weighed against the risks of surgery—specifically, the increased risk of stroke during surgery. Current clinical guidelines suggest that patients with carotid stenosis greater than 60% will benefit from carotid surgical endarterectomy when performed by a surgeon with a history of less than 3% rates of operative morbidity and mortality.[144] The role of stent placement in the carotid artery has also shown similar success with skilled interventionalist.[144,148-153] Patients with carotid artery stenosis need to be informed about the risks involved with any procedure and their risk for future cerebrovascular events, such as stroke.

Nursing Management

Nursing management is focused on assessment of adequate cerebral perfusion represented by vital signs, respiratory pattern, level of consciousness, pupil reaction, pupil size, and possible cranial nerve deficits manifested by difficulty in swallowing, loss of gag reflex, changes in speech, and loss of facial symmetry. The National Institutes of Health (NIH) stroke scale is used to predict patient outcome on initial and ongoing assessment of TIA and stroke-related symptoms.[146] The nurse educates the patient and family about the causes of the current event and provides information on preventing further cerebrovascular

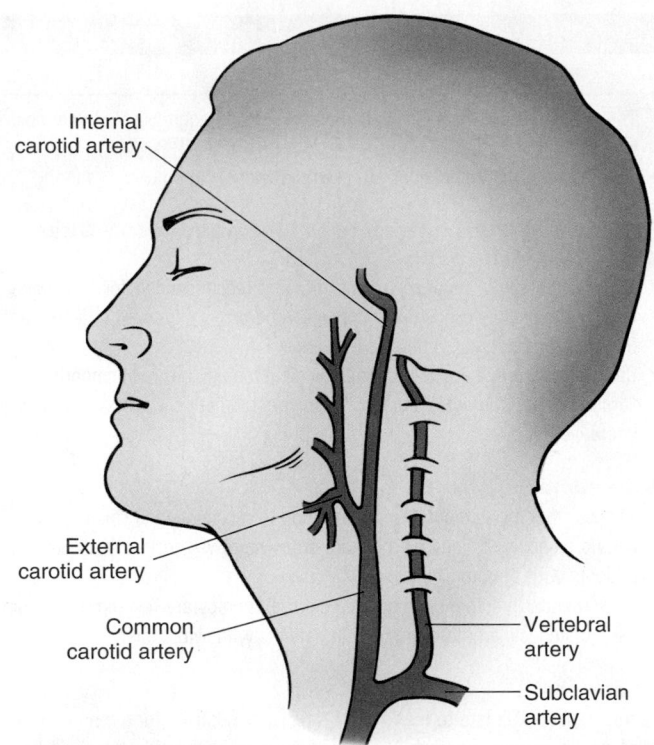

FIGURE 15-25 **Common, Internal, and External Carotid Arteries.** Atherosclerotic plaque develops in the common carotid artery at the bifurcation into the internal and external carotid arteries. Plaque can develop in the common, internal, and external carotid arteries.

⊚ BOX 15-37 NURSING DIAGNOSES

Carotid Artery Disease

- Acute Pain, related to transmission and perception of cutaneous, muscular, or ischemic impulses, p. 1123
- Risk for Ineffective Cerebral Tissue Perfusion, p. 1156
- Anxiety, related to threat to biologic, psychologic, or social integrity, p. 1125
- Deficient Knowledge, related to lack of previous exposure to information, p. 1134 (see Box 15-38, Patient Education for Carotid Artery Disease)

events. Several nursing diagnoses are associated with management of the patient with carotid artery disease (Box 15-37).

Neurologic Assessment

Neurologic assessment of the patient with carotid artery disease is divided into two parts: 1) level of consciousness, mental alertness, and cerebral perfusion and 2) cranial nerve function. A neurologic assessment is performed to make sure that the patient has not suffered a TIA or stroke. Questions to ascertain level of consciousness relate to time and place and reason for hospital admission. Mental alertness is assessed by the ability with which the patient responds to these and other questions. The person is asked to move all four limbs on command. To assess specific cranial nerves, the patient is asked to make a grimace, which should demonstrate bilateral facial symmetry; to stick out the tongue to ensure it is midline; and to swallow and speak, which should be done without difficulty (see "Cranial Nerves" in Chapter 22 and "Rapid Neurologic Examination" in Chapter 23).

BOX 15-38 PATIENT EDUCATION

Carotid Artery Disease

- Pathophysiology of atherosclerotic carotid artery disease
- Pathophysiology of embolic stroke (emboli from carotid artery)
- Warning signs of impending stroke
- Risk factor modification: after the acute episode, if the cause of the carotid artery disease is atherosclerosis, an individual risk factor profile is developed for each patient; strategies to discuss include the following: decrease daily fat intake to less than 30% of total calories, achieve total blood cholesterol level of less than 200 mg/dL, stop smoking, reduce salt intake, control hypertension, control diabetes if patient has diabetes, increase physical activity, achieve and maintain ideal body weight
- Signs and symptoms to report to a health care professional
- Follow-up care after discharge

Patient Education

If a patient is admitted to a critical care unit who has known carotid artery disease and has not had a cerebrovascular event, preventive education is essential. It is important to discuss the mechanism of stroke in carotid artery disease. A stroke is most often caused by an embolic thrombus that has traveled in the bloodstream to a specific area of the brain. The thrombus may have originated in the atria during an episode of AF or in the carotid arteries. In the carotid arteries, a thrombus can develop across the narrowed carotid artery lumen, reducing flow and causing widespread cerebral hypoperfusion. Many patients who have atherosclerotic carotid artery disease also have CAD or PAD and diabetes or hypertension.[139,144] The major areas of patient education are listed in Box 15-38. Recommendations for prevention of carotid artery disease are listed in Box 15-39.

VENOUS THROMBOEMBOLISM

Description

Venous thromboembolism (VTE) comprises two related conditions: 1) DVT and 2) PE. DVT is a clot (thrombus) that forms in a large vein in the leg, pelvis, and, less commonly, the arm. It is often accompanied by inflammation, pain, tenderness, and redness at the site of the thrombus. The concern is that the thrombus may migrate as a VTE through the venous circulation to the pulmonary vascular bed, causing a PE, development of pulmonary hypertension, or death.[154,155]

Etiology

At least 900,000 episodes of VTE leading to hospitalization and 300,000 related deaths occur in the United States annually.[156] Patients in the critical care unit face additional risks from invasive procedures, immobility, and vascular inflammation. Other risk factors for VTE include increasing age, obesity, immobility, trauma, spinal cord injury, active cancer, major surgery, pregnancy, family history, heart failure, and sepsis.[156] VTE incidence is similar for men and women, unless a woman is taking HRT or a contraceptive pill, which increases her risk. Inherited coagulation disorders and hypercoagulability, also called *genetic thrombophilia*, confer a propensity for clotting and increase the DVT risk profile in patients with this genetic inheritance.[157-159]

BOX 15-39   **EVIDENCE-BASED PRACTICE**
Carotid Artery Disease

QSEN   **Recommendations for Prevention of Carotid Artery Disease**

- Smokers should stop smoking and avoid exposure to environmental tobacco smoke (second-hand tobacco smoke). Smoking doubles the risk of stroke.
- Achieve a normal BP, preferably less than 120/80 mm Hg, for individuals at high risk of stroke. Oral antihypertensive medications are prescribed if the target BP is not met with diet and exercise alone. Reduction of BP greatly reduces stroke incidence.
- Achieve and maintain normal weight. The target weight-to-height ratio is a BMI between 18.5 and 24.9 kg/m². A BMI above 25 kg/m² defines obesity. Obese patients are also identified as having a large waist circumference: more than 40 inches for men or more than 35 inches for women.
- Have serum lipids checked, and attain a normal lipid profile. Many patients are prescribed lipid-lowering medications to achieve the following goals:
  - Total cholesterol below 200 mg/dL
  - LDL-C below 70 mg/dL if patient has CV disease risk factors (all patients with carotid arterial disease are likely to fall in this category), diabetes, or kidney disease
  - Triglycerides below 150 mg/dL
- Normal fasting blood glucose level should be between 70 and 110 mg/dL. If the patient has diabetes, the HbA$_{1c}$ should be near normal or below 7%.
- A healthy diet should be instituted. Reduce saturated fat and add fruits and vegetables. Add omega-3 fatty acids as part of the treatment regimen to lower elevated triglycerides.
- Regular exercise is essential. The optimal goal is 30 to 60 minutes daily or at least three times weekly.

Recommended Medications

- Aspirin (50 to 325 orally each day) or other platelet-inhibitor medications are recommended. The combination of aspirin plus extended-release dipyridamole and clopidogrel monotherapy are acceptable options for initial antiplatelet therapy.

- The statin class of medications is recommended to aggressively lower lipid levels.
- Antihypertensive medications are used to lower BP into normal range.

Recommendations Interventions for Carotid Artery Disease
Asymptomatic Patients

- Medical therapy without revascularization is recommended for low-grade carotid stenosis, which is defined as a carotid artery narrowed to less than 60% in asymptomatic patients.
- Carotid endarterectomy and optimal medical therapy are recommended for carotid stenosis greater than 60% in asymptomatic patients with low-operative risk.

Symptomatic Patients

- Medical therapy without revascularization is recommended for low-grade carotid stenosis, defined as a carotid artery narrowed to less than 50% in patients with symptoms.
- Carotid endarterectomy and optimal medical therapy are recommended for carotid stenosis greater than 50% in patients with symptoms.

References

Adams RJ, et al. Update to the AHA/ASA recommendations for the prevention of stroke in patients with stroke and transient ischemic attack. *Stroke*. 2008;39(5):1647.

Goldstein LB, et al. Guidelines for the primary prevention of stroke: a guideline for healthcare professionals from the American Heart Association/ American Stroke Association. *Stroke*. 2011;42(2):517.

Hobson RW, et al. Management of atherosclerotic carotid artery disease: clinical practice guidelines of the Society for Vascular Surgery. *J Vasc Surg*. 2008;48:480.

BMI, Body mass index; *BP*, blood pressure; *CAD*, coronary artery disease; *CV*, cardiovascular; *HbA$_{1c}$*, glycosylated hemoglobin; *LDL-C*, low-density lipoprotein cholesterol.

In the critical care population, the incidence of DVT is 28% to 32% with rates of 60% to 70% in the trauma and stroke populations.[158]

Three major predisposing factors are traditionally described as Virchow's triad: 1) stasis of blood, 2) endothelial injury, and 3) hypercoagulability. Theories on the role of inflammation are adding to the risk profile of thrombosis generation.[158,159] Usually, two of these three conditions must be present for thrombosis to occur. Patients in critical care units generally have one or more risk factors that predispose them to the development of a venous thrombus. The hospitalized patient has more than a 100-fold increased incidence of acute VTE compared with the general public.[157] The incidence of DVT increases with age and markedly increases the patient's risk of fatal PE (see "Pulmonary Embolism" in Chapter 20).

Assessment and Diagnosis

Development of DVT may be insidious. Many patients with DVT are asymptomatic. Pain, if present, is described as an aching or throbbing sensation, which worsens with ambulation. A positive Homans sign, which is pain in the calf on dorsiflexion of the foot, heightens the suspicion of a DVT but is not considered a reliable marker. If DVT is present in the upper extremity, the entire arm swells. Other clinical manifestations include redness with swelling, increased skin temperature, dilation of superficial veins, and mottling and cyanosis caused by stagnant blood flow. In the critical care unit population, symptoms are often masked by intubation, sedation, and altered levels of consciousness.[158]

Venous Ultrasound and D-Dimer

When DVT is suspected, a noninvasive venous ultrasonography typically is used to evaluate vein patency.[160] If the thrombus is large and the vein is easy to visualize, the presence of a DVT can be confirmed by this method alone. However, when the results of the ultrasonography are inconclusive, the addition of the D-dimer blood test increases diagnostic accuracy. The D-dimer test measures the presence of cross-linked fibrin derivatives in the serum. It is a sensitive marker of thrombosis but it lacks specificity. If the normal D-dimer serum value is elevated it signifies the presence of clots, but the thrombi could be located anywhere in the body. Ultrasonography can help localize the location of the DVT. Together, these two tests represent a useful and powerful diagnostic strategy.[159,160] When the

D-dimer value is normal (not elevated), a DVT (or other thrombosis) can safely be ruled out.

Diagnosis of Pulmonary Embolism

If PE is suspected, CT of the thorax may be obtained. Contrast-enhanced CT-arteriography is faster and has greater sensitivity and specificity for detecting emboli in the pulmonary arteries.[160] A V/Q scan is most likely to be diagnostic in the absence of disease, but it is less helpful in critically ill patients. A normal perfusion scan result effectively rules out acute PE.[160]

Current guidelines recommend evaluating the risk factors for each patient on an individual basis. Maintaining a high index of suspicion and using thromboprophylaxis for at-risk patients is essential. If VTE is suspected, using clinical assessment, venous ultrasonography, and the D-dimer assay to confirm or negate the presence of VTE.[154,155]

Medical Management
Prevention of Venous Thromboembolism

Major therapeutic emphasis is placed on prophylaxis for critically ill patients at high risk for VTE.[158] Preventive measures include prophylactic anticoagulation with subcutaneous LMWH or UFH, increasing mobility, and use of sequential compression devices placed on the lower extremities. Normally, the simple action of walking helps return blood to the right side of the heart and prevents venous stasis that may lead to development of venous thrombi. For critically ill patients, immobility is often imposed because of the severity of the illness. After they become stable, most patients are assisted out of bed and helped to walk to restore the circulatory pump.

Management of Diagnosed Venous Thromboembolism

Initially, the patient is confined to bed rest with elevation of the limb, and anticoagulation therapy is initiated. Analgesics are prescribed to reduce discomfort.

Anticoagulation

Anticoagulants are prescribed to reduce further clotting. The risks and benefits of therapeutic anticoagulation are discussed with the patient and family before therapy begins. In the acute phase, the VTE can be treated with intravenous heparin or subcutaneous LMWH. Subsequently, oral warfarin (Coumadin) may be used. Antiplatelet therapy with aspirin or other medications is added to prevent VTE recurrence. Antiplatelet therapy alone does not provide protection against development of VTE.[154,155] Anticoagulation with rivaroxabon (orally active direct Xa inhibitor) is also an option.[154] None of the aforementioned antithrombotics dissolves the existing clot, but these medications can prevent new thrombi from forming. Lytic therapy usually is reserved for massive PE. Patients receiving anticoagulation therapy require careful assessment for bleeding tendencies, including obtaining frequent bleeding studies—aPTT, or INR. Stool and urine are tested for presence of occult blood; gums are inspected for bleeding; and when endotracheal suctioning is required, it is important to be gentle and to assess for presence of blood in the aspirate. After the patient begins to ambulate, custom-fitted below-the-knee elastic stockings are ordered.[155] Complaints or observation of dyspnea or chest pain must be quickly evaluated to assess the risk of PE. Medical

BOX 15-40 NURSING DIAGNOSES
Venous Thromboembolism

- Activity Intolerance, related to prolonged immobility or deconditioning, p. 1119
- Acute Pain, related to transmission and perception of cutaneous, visceral, muscular, or ischemic impulses, p. 1123
- Powerlessness, related to lack of control over current situation or disease progression, p. 1152
- Anxiety, related to threat to biologic, psychologic, or social integrity, p. 1125
- Deficient Knowledge, related to lack of previous exposure to information, p. 1134 (see Box 15-41, Patient Education for Venous Thromboembolism)

management with anticoagulants is adequate for most patients; however, those at risk for PE (patients with cancer, bleeding disorders, or spinal cord injury) may require surgical intervention for protection. Possible procedures include venous embolectomy and insertion of an inferior vena cava filter.[159]

Nursing Management

The focus of nursing management is to prevent the development of DVT. For the patient with DVT, the interventions include rest the affected extremity, prevention of complications that may result from VTE, and monitoring anticoagulant therapy. Several nursing diagnoses are used in the management of the patient with VTE (Box 15-40).

Activity with Deep Vein Thrombosis

For the patient who has developed a DVT, it was previously thought physical activity should be limited to prevent dislodgement of emboli. Recent studies with support from updated treatment guidelines find during the acute phase, once anticoagulation is initiated self-care activities need not be limited, and graduated ambulation is encouraged.[155] Range-of-motion exercises can be performed with any unaffected limb. The patient is instructed to avoid bending at the knees or hips because this impedes venous return. Antiembolism stockings that have been custom fitted can be used. It is not clear when it is safe to resume normal activity such as walking after DVT. Usually, it is resumed after a Doppler study shows no evidence of DVT in the extremity and after symptoms have abated. Prevention strategies again become important because the patient remains at risk for a recurrence. In general, early ambulation after surgery or other procedures and avoidance of bed rest are the most effective prevention strategies.

Risk of Pulmonary Embolism

The patient with a VTE is closely monitored for signs of PE and instructed to report immediately any chest pain, dyspnea, hemoptysis, or tachypnea. Risk factors for VTE are almost identical to those for PE. For patients who must remain immobile because of their clinical condition, external pneumatic compression devices, antiembolism stockings, and low-dose heparin are commonly used.[154,155,159]

Anticoagulation

Anticoagulant therapy is monitored by obtaining daily coagulation values—aPTT if the patient is receiving intravenous heparin and daily INR if the patient is receiving warfarin (Coumadin).[136] Although the American College of Clinical Pharmacology (ACCP) clinical practice guidelines limit routine coagulation monitoring recommendations for LMWH to anti-Xa levels in pregnant women only, this approach may be expanded to all patients in the future.[136] Signs of bleeding are monitored, and symptoms are treated promptly. For the critically ill patient, hemoglobin levels and hematocrit are monitored daily, and stools are assessed for occult blood. Avoidable mechanical trauma is minimized. The alert patient should be instructed to use a soft toothbrush and, if needed, an electric razor.

Patient Education

Patient education emphasizes VTE prevention for all patients who are immobile in the critical care unit for any length of time. This includes explanations about activity prophylaxis such as early ambulation after major surgery, external pneumatic compression boots, and low-dose heparin.

For patients who have a diagnosed DVT, education is focused on identifying symptoms to report, avoidance of trauma to the limb, and elevation of the limb to decrease venous pooling and increase blood flow. If the patient is on anticoagulation medications, the risks and benefits of this therapy are discussed, as well as the risk of VTE and pulmonary embolus. The patient is instructed to report any chest pain, shortness of breath, or respiratory distress (Box 15-41). A collaborative team of clinicians who are aware of current clinical recommendations is essential to provide effective care for all critical care patients at risk for VTE (Box 15-42).

HYPERTENSIVE EMERGENCY

Description

Hypertensive emergency is relatively uncommon. It is seen in less than 1% of patients who have hypertension, but when present, it is life threatening and demands early recognition and management to minimize morbidity and mortality. It was formerly known as *hypertensive crisis* or *malignant hypertension*. With the advent of so many categories of antihypertensive medications, this condition can be effectively managed in the critical care setting. Two forms of acute hypertension are recognized:

- *Hypertensive emergencies* pose a risk of end-organ damage and are life-threatening conditions. The target organ can be the heart (acute MI), the brain (stroke), or the kidney (kidney failure).

DVT, Deep vein thrombosis; *INR*, international normalized ratio; *IV*, intravenous; *LMWH*, low-molecular-weight heparin; *SQ*, subcutaneous; *UFH*, unfractionated heparin; *VTE*, venous thromboembolism.

- *Hypertensive urgencies* are characterized by a serious elevation in blood pressure but do not put the patient at risk for end-organ damage.[161-163]

Etiology

Hypertensive emergency may occur in patients with no history of the condition or can be precipitated by noncompliance with or inadequate medication therapy. In patients with no known history of hypertension, causes of hypertensive emergency include the following:

1. Acute kidney failure
2. Acute CNS events: hypertension frequently accompanies subarachnoid hemorrhage (SAH), intracerebral hemorrhage, or a stroke
3. Acute aortic dissection: hypertension frequently precedes dissection
4. Pregnancy-induced eclampsia: intense arterial vascular constriction, which raises blood pressure and decreases blood supply to the placenta
5. Pheochromocytoma: an adrenal tumor that produces epinephrine and norepinephrine and raises blood pressure as a result of the circulating catecholamines
6. Drug-induced hypertension: illegal drugs, particularly cocaine or amphetamines

TABLE 15-15	HYPERTENSIVE EMERGENCIES
EMERGENCY	**POSSIBLE CAUSES**
Cardiovascular Compromise	
Chest pain	Unstable angina, myocardial infarction, aortic dissection
Acute heart failure	Myocardial infarction, severe hypertension
Hypertension after vascular surgery	Aortic aneurysmectomy, carotid endarterectomy, coronary artery bypass grafting
Central Nervous System Compromise	
Papilledema	Increased intracranial pressure—mass lesion Malignant hypertension—any cause
Headache, agitation, lethargy, confusion	Hypertensive encephalopathy—any cause, subarachnoid hemorrhage, stroke
Coma	Stroke, advanced hypertensive encephalopathy, trauma, tumor
Seizures	Advanced hypertensive encephalopathy, CNS tumor, eclampsia, stroke (less common)
Focal neurologic deficit	Stroke, CNS tumor, hypertensive encephalopathy
Acute kidney failure	Malignant hypertension, vasculitis, scleroderma, glomerulonephritis
Catecholamine excess	Pheochromocytomas, MAOI in combination with certain medications and foods; abrupt withdrawal of antihypertensive medications such as clonidine, guanabenz, or beta-blockers

CNS, Central nervous system; *MAOI,* monoamine oxidase inhibitor.

7. Medication-food interactions: hypertensive response to tyramine-containing foods or beverages (beer or aged cheese) or during treatment with a monoamine oxidase inhibitor (MAOI), which is now rare because most patients are prescribed other antidepressant medications

Pathophysiology

The exact trigger of a hypertensive crisis is often unknown. However, most patients suffer from known hypertension before the event, and the sudden rise in blood pressure is often related to the underlying disease process. Clinical manifestations of hypertensive emergency are listed in Table 15-15.

Assessment and Diagnosis

Hypertensive emergency can manifest as any of the following symptoms, depending on the target organ involved:
1. CNS compromise, identified by headache, blurred vision, change in level of consciousness, or coma
2. Cardiovascular compromise, identified by the chest pain of ACS or aortic dissection
3. Acute kidney failure, identified by a sudden absence of urine output
4. Catecholamine excess

Worsening of symptoms may indicate hypertensive encephalopathy. Diagnostic studies include blood pressure measurement in both arms and placement of an intra-arterial line for close monitoring of blood pressure. A 12-lead ECG reading is taken to evaluate for evidence of acute MI or left ventricular hypertrophy.

Medical Management
Hypertensive Emergencies

Hypertensive emergencies are defined as an acute blood pressure elevation greater than 180/120 mm Hg complicated by impending or progressive target organ dysfunction.[161-163] Hypertensive emergencies with the risk of end-organ damage necessitate admission of the patient to the critical care unit, where intravenous antihypertensive therapy can be administered and blood pressure can be monitored continuously by means of an arterial line. Several intravenous medications in many different medication classes are available for acute reduction of blood pressure. Ideally, the medication should be targeted to the specific condition. Sodium nitroprusside is frequently the first medication used to lower blood pressure in hypertensive emergency. Sodium nitroprusside is useful because of its half-life of seconds. It is not suitable for long-term use because of development of a metabolite that causes cyanide-like toxicity.[163-166] Short-acting beta-blockers that are effective are labetalol and esmolol. Beta-blockers are especially effective if aortic dissection is present. For patients with heart failure, the intravenous ACEI enalaprilat lowers blood pressure. The vasodilator nitroglycerin (NTG) is used for patients with hypertension who have chest pain. For patients with kidney dysfunction, the dopamine receptor antagonist (DA_1) fenoldopam may be used to lower blood pressure and increase blood flow to the kidneys.[163,164,167] Hydralazine is the intravenous agent of choice in eclampsia because it does not cross the placental barrier. The calcium channel blocker nicardipine and the combination alpha-beta blocker labetalol are less likely to decrease cerebral blood flow and have been used in patients with CNS compromise.[1639-165] The alpha-blocker phentolamine is used for patients in pheochromocytoma crisis.[161,164] Sometimes, combinations of the above-mentioned agents are more effective in hypertension control. The intravenous diuretic furosemide (Lasix) is useful in patients with fluid retention.[163,166,167]

Initial goals of therapy in hypertensive emergencies limit reducing mean arterial blood pressure by no more than 20% to 25% over a period of several minutes to several hours.[162,167] Variability depends on the target organ that is affected. When the brain is the target organ, cerebral hypoperfusion can occur if blood pressure is lowered too rapidly. The guidelines for treating stroke do not recommend a rapid reduction of blood pressure. If the blood pressure is excessively high, the aim is to reduce by not more than 20% to 15% in the first 24 hours.[163,165] The blood pressure spontaneously decreases during the first 10 days after a stroke.[167] For the patient with CAD experiencing a hypertensive emergency, the need to maintain adequate DBP to allow for coronary artery filling is paramount.[161,163] If vasodilator therapy drops the diastolic pressure too far—when coronary artery filling occurs—myocardial ischemia may result.[168] The question of how much to decrease the blood pressure in a hypertensive emergency is not simply a matter of reading the number on the monitor from the patient's arterial line; it involves an assessment of the underlying pathology and an

Hypertensive Emergency

- Risk for Ineffective Cerebral Tissue Perfusion, p. 1156
- Risk for Ineffective Peripheral Tissue Perfusion, p. 1158
- Anxiety, related to threat to biologic, psychologic, or social integrity, p. 1125
- Deficient Knowledge, related to lack of previous exposure to information, p. 1134 (see Box 15-44, Patient Education for Hypertensive Emergency)

BOX 15-44 **PATIENT EDUCATION**

Hypertensive Emergency

- Pathophysiology of hypertensive crisis
- Normal and abnormal blood pressure values
- Self-monitoring of blood pressure at home
- Connection between hypertension and other atherosclerotic diseases such as coronary artery disease, peripheral arterial disease (PAD), and cerebrovascular disease
- Warning signs of a "heart attack" or myocardial infarction
- Warning signs of a "brain attack" or stroke
- Warning signs of intermittent claudication or PAD
- Risk factors modification: after the acute episode, if the cause of the carotid artery disease is atherosclerosis, an individual risk factor profile is developed for each patient; strategies to discuss include the following: decrease daily fat intake to less than 30% of total calories, achieve total blood cholesterol level of less than 200 mg/dL, stop smoking, reduce salt intake, control hypertension, control diabetes if patient has diabetes, increase physical activity, achieve and maintain ideal body weight
- Medications: antihypertensive medications, rationale, and side effects
- Signs and symptoms to report to a health care professional
- Follow-up care after discharge

appreciation of the physiologic requirements of the affected target organ. The "Vasodilator Medications" section in Chapter 16 provides more information on specific agents.

Hypertensive Urgencies

Hypertensive urgencies may not necessitate admission to a critical care unit because organ damage is not evident and the patient may be treated with rapid-acting oral antihypertensive agents. Many medication categories are available, including ACEIs, ARBs, calcium channel blockers, and beta-blockers. A loop diuretic (e.g., furosemide) often is prescribed in addition to the antihypertensive agents when the patient has fluid retention.

Nursing Management

The focus of nursing management for the patient with hypertensive crisis is to return the blood pressure to the desired range without introducing other complications as a result of therapy. After the hypertension is controlled, the nurse identifies the factors that resulted in this life-threatening condition. Several nursing diagnoses are associated with hypertensive crisis (Box 15-43).

During the acute phase, the patient is observed closely for clinical manifestations in other organ systems, including the neurologic, cardiac, and renal systems.[167] Neurologic compromise may be manifested by mental confusion, stupor, seizures, coma, or stroke. Cardiac compromise may be exhibited by aortic dissection, myocardial ischemia, or dysrhythmias. Acute kidney failure may not be evident immediately, but urine output, BUN, and serum creatinine values are evaluated over several days to determine whether the kidneys were affected by the hypertensive episode. When short-acting intravenous antihypertensive agents are administered, blood pressure is closely monitored. If potent antihypertensive medications such as sodium nitroprusside or labetalol are being used, an arterial line must be inserted, and the medications must be infused through an infusion pump.[168]

Patient Education

Patient education during the acute phase of a hypertensive emergency is limited to an explanation of the need to control blood pressure and the purpose of the equipment used in the critical care unit. After the hypertensive crisis is resolved, the focus of education is on lifestyle changes to modify risk factors. Hypertension is emphasized as a risk factor for atherosclerotic arterial disease of the heart, brain, and peripheral arterial system. A more complete discussion of hypertension as a cardiovascular risk factor is provided at the beginning of this chapter. The major points to discuss with the patient are listed in Box 15-44. Management of hypertensive emergencies and urgencies are listed in Box 15-45.

Hypertensive Emergencies

QSEN **Definition**
Hypertensive emergency is defined as an acute BP elevation greater than 180/120 mm Hg complicated by impending or progressive target organ dysfunction.

Recommendations
- Early identification of hypertensive emergency in the emergency room and admission to a critical care unit is recommended.
- Patients with hypertensive emergency should have continuous BP monitoring.

- IV medications are used to reduce BP (not necessarily to normal) to prevent or limit target organ damage.
- Initial goal is to reduce BP by no more than 25%. For example, reduce SBP to 160 mm Hg and DBP to 100 to 110 mm Hg in the 2 to 6 hours after admission.
- Decreasing the BP gradually is recommended to avoid cerebral, coronary, or kidney ischemia.
- Medications that cause rapid falls in blood pressure are not recommended in the management of acute hypertensive emergency. For this reason, short-acting nifedipine is *not* endorsed (SL or IV).

BOX 15-45 **EVIDENCE-BASED PRACTICE**

Hypertensive Emergencies—cont'd

- Further gradual reductions in BP can be achieved in the following 24 to 48 hours.

Special Situations: Hypertension and Acute Ischemic Stroke

- For patients admitted with an ischemic stroke, no clinical evidence exists to support rapid reduction in BP.
- For patients with SBP greater than 220 mm Hg or DBP between 120 and 140 mm Hg, BP should be lowered cautiously by 10% to 15% only.
- If the DBP is greater than 140 mm Hg, SNP is recommended to cautiously lower the SBP by about 10%.
- If the SBP is greater than 185 mm Hg or the DBP greater than 110 mm Hg, the use of thrombolytic therapy (tPA) is contraindicated within the first 3 hours after an acute ischemic stroke. The BP must be lowered before the administration of tPA.
- Careful monitoring of the patient for signs of neurologic deterioration related to the lower pressure is mandated in all situations.

Special Situation: Hypertension and Aortic Dissection

- Patients with aortic dissection should have their SBP lowered to less than 100 mm Hg if tolerated.

Ultimate Blood Pressure Target Goal

- The goal of therapy for all patients is a target BP of 140/90 mm Hg or lower before discharge from the hospital. Some patients will require oral medications to achieve this target.
- Target BP is 130/80 mm Hg or lower for patients with known hypertension, kidney failure, diabetes, or cardiovascular disease. Almost all patients with these conditions will require oral medications to achieve their target BP. Many patients require two or more oral medications.

Reference

Chobanian AV, et al. Seventh report of the Joint National Committee on Prevention, Detection, Evaluation, and Treatment of High Blood Pressure. *Hypertension*. 2003;42(6):1206.

BP, Blood pressure; *DBP*, diastolic blood pressure; *IV*, intravenous; *SBP*, systolic blood pressure; *SL*, sublingual; *SNP*, sodium nitroprusside; *tPA*, tissue plasminogen activator.

SUMMARY

- The number of patients with cardiovascular disease in the United States continues to grow.
- Considerable research and clinical progress has clarified the diagnosis and management of many cardiac conditions.
- Atherosclerosis provides a common link among CAD, atherosclerotic aortic disease, PAD, and carotid artery disease. The risk factors and general management strategies for all of these diseases are the same.
- Acute MI, aortic aneurysm, aortic dissection, and embolic stroke represent the acute manifestations of chronic disease progression.
- Heart failure is a consequence of damaged heart muscle that results from MI, cardiomyopathy, valve disease, or hypertension.

Pulmonary Hypertension

- Pulmonary hypertension is a progressive sustained increase in pulmonary pressures with resultant right heart failure and ultimately death.
- Medical management focuses on multidrug therapies and prevention of complications.
- Nursing management includes symptom management, education on multidrug treatments, including IV site care and developing extended support systems.

Endocarditis

- Endocarditis is an infection on the endocardial surface of the heart, heart valves, or both.
- Medical management requires prolonged intravenous antibiotic treatment. Some patients require excision of the involved valve for eradication of infection.
- Nursing management includes monitoring for worsening symptoms and patient education on the need for prolonged medication for treatment, including intravenous site care.

Valvular Heart Disease

- Valvular heart disease is the structural and functional abnormalities of cardiac valves.
- Medical management includes medications to control symptoms and surgical interventions to repair or replace involved valve.
- Nursing management includes medication titration to improve flow through involved valves, monitoring patient symptoms and responses to treatment, and organizing patient care activities to prevent fatigue.

Atherosclerosis of the Aorta

- Aortic disease results from progressive atherosclerosis and hypertension. This includes aneurysmal and local dilatation of the wall and aortic dissection where blood separates the vascular layers.
- Medical management depends on symptoms and hemodynamics. Corrective surgery is aimed at aneurysms more than 5 cm wide. Acute dissection requires immediate control of hypertension and pain, with surgical correction required for dissection of the ascending aorta.
- Nursing management focuses on monitoring for changes in the cardiovascular status, administering medications for significant blood pressure reduction and pain control.

Peripheral Artery Disease

- PAD includes chronic venous disease and acute arterial changes.
- Medical management aims at controlling or eliminating risk factors, pharmacologic management including anticoagulants vasodilators and antiplatelets, and surgical interventions of PTCA, stents, or vascular bypass.
- Nursing care includes assessment of pulses, maintenance of skin integrity, and pain control.

Carotid Artery Disease

- Carotid artery disease results in obstruction of the major arterial supply to the brain.
- Medical management focuses on limiting risks and when obstruction is greater than 60% performing surgical endarterectomy.
- Nursing management includes monitoring neurologic assessment and educating patients and family of stroke symptoms.

Venous Thromboembolism

- VTE includes both DVT and PE with clot formation and obstruction of large vessels.
- Medical management focuses on prevention and treatments with anticoagulation.

- Nursing management is aimed at prevention with activity started as soon as possible for critically ill patients and monitoring the effects of anticoagulation.

Hypertensive Emergency

- Hypertensive emergency is defined as acute blood pressure elevation greater than 180/120 mm Hg and may include symptoms of CNS or cardiovascular compromise, acute kidney failure, or catecholamine excess.
- Medical management is aimed at use of appropriate medications to initially decrease by no more than 20% to 25% over several hours.
- Nursing management is focused on close symptom monitoring with judicious use of blood pressure lowering medications.

REFERENCES

1. Roger VL, et al. American Heart Association. Heart Disease and Stroke Statistics-2012 Update: A Report From the American Heart Association. *Circulation*. 2012;125:e2.
2. O'Gara, et al. 2013 ACCF/AHA Guideline for the Management of ST-Elevation Myocardial Infarction: a Report of the American College of Cardiology Foundation/American Heart Association Task Force on Practice Guidelines. *Circulation*. 2013;127(4):e362.
3. Fihn SD, et al. 2012 ACCF/AHA/ACP/AATS/PCNA/SCAI/STS Guideline for the Diagnosis and Management of Patients With Stable Ischemic Heart Disease: a Report of the American College of Cardiology Foundation/American Heart Association Task Force on Practice Guidelines, and the American College of Physicians, American Association for Thoracic Surgery, Preventive Cardiovascular Nurses Association, Society for Cardiovascular Angiography and Interventions, and Society of Thoracic Surgeons. *Circulation*. 2012;126(25):e354-e471.
4. Yusef S, et al. INTERHEART Study Investigators. Effect of potentially modifiable risk factors associated with myocardial infarction in 52 countries (The INTERHEART Study): case-control study. *Lancet*. 2004;364 (9438):937.
5. Adult Treatment Panel. Third Report of the National Cholesterol Education Program (NCP) Expert Panel on Detection, Evaluation, and Treat of High Blood Cholesterol in Adults (Adult Treatment Panel III) final report. *Circulation*. 2002;106(25):3143.
6. Barter PJ, et al. Antiinflammatory properties of HDL. *Circ Res*. 2004;95(8):764.
7. Miller M, et al. Triglycerides and Cardiovascular Disease: a Scientific Statement From the American Heart Association. *Circulation*. 2011;123:2292.
8. Futterman LG, Lemberg L. Lp(a) lipoprotein: an independent risk factor for coronary heart disease after menopause. *Am J Crit Care*. 2001;10(1):63.
9. Executive summary of the third report of the National Cholesterol Education Program (NCEP) Expert Panel on Detection, Evaluation, and Treatment of High Blood Cholesterol in Adults (Adult Treatment Panel III). *JAMA*. 2001;285(19):2486.
10. Grundy SM, et al. Implications of recent clinical trials for the National Cholesterol Education Program Adult Treatment Panel III guidelines. *Circulation*. 2004;110(2):227.
11. Smith SC, et al. AHA/ACC Secondary Prevention and Risk Reduction Therapy for Patients with Coronary and Other Atherosclerotic Vascular Disease. 2011 Update: A Guideline from the American Heart Association and American College of Cardiology Foundation. *Circulation*. 2011;24:2458.
12. Chobanian AV, et al. Seventh report of the Joint National Committee on Prevention, Detection, Evaluation, and Treatment of High Blood Pressure. *Hypertension*. 2003;42(6):1206.
13. Sargent RP, et al. Reduced incidence of admissions for myocardial infarction associated with public smoking ban: before and after study. *BMJ*. 2004;328(7446):977.
14. Wright SR, et al. 2011 ACC/AHA Focused Update of the guidelines for the management of patients with unstable angina/non-ST-elevation myocardial infarction: a report of the American College of Cardiology/American Heart Association Task Force on Practice Guidelines developed in collaboration with The American College of Emergency Physicians, Society for Cardiovascular Angiography and Interventions, and Society for Thoracic Surgeons. *J Am Coll Cardiol*. 2011;57:1920.
15. Anderson JL, et al. 2011 ACCF/AHA Focused Update Incorporated Into the ACC/AHA 2007 Guidelines for the Management of Patients With Unstable Angina/Non -ST-Elevation Myocardial Infarction: a Report of the American College of Cardiology Foundation/American Heart Association Task Force on Practice Guidelines. *Circulation*. 2011;123:e426.
16. Standards of Medical Care in Diabetes. American Diabetes Association. *Diabetes Care*. 2012;35(Suppl).
17. McGuire DK, et al. Association of diabetes mellitus and glycemic control strategies with clinical outcomes after acute coronary syndromes. *Am Heart J*. 2004;147(2):246.
18. Franklin K, et al. Implications of diabetes in patients with acute coronary syndromes: the Global Registry of Acute Coronary Events. *Arch Intern Med*. 2004;164(13):1457.
19. Smink PA, et al. Albuminuria, Estimated GFR, Traditional Risk Factors, and Incident Cardiovascular Disease: The PREVEND (Prevention of Renal and Vascular Endstage Disease) Study. *Am J Kidney Dis*. 2012;60(5):804.
20. Vassaiwala S, Cannon CR, Foronow GC. Quality of care and outcomes among patients with acute myocardial infarction by level of kidney function at admission: report from the Get With The Guidelines Coronary Artery Disease Program. *Clin Cardiol*. 2012;35(9):541.

21. Gami AS, et al. Metabolic syndrome and risk of incident cardiovascular events and death: a systematic review and meta-analysis of longitudinal studies. *J Am Coll Cardiol.* 2007;49(4):403.

22. Mosa L, et al. Effectiveness–Based Guidelines for the Prevention of Cardiovascular Disease in Women-2011 Update: A Guideline From the American Heart Association. *Circulation.* 2011;123:1243.

23. Llyod-Jones DM, et al. On behalf of the American Heart Association Strategic Planning Task Force and Statistics Committee. Defining and setting national goals for cardiovascular health promotion and disease reduction: the American Heart Association's Strategic Impact Goal through 2020 and beyond. *Circulation.* 2010;121:586.

24. Anderson GL, et al. Effects of conjugated equine estrogen in postmenopausal women with hysterectomy: the Women's Health Initiative randomized controlled trial. *JAMA.* 2004;291(14):1701.

25. Mosca L, et al. Evidence-based guidelines for cardiovascular disease prevention in women: 2007 update. *Circulation.* 2007;115:1481.

26. Lefler LL, Bondy KN. Women's delay in seeking treatment with myocardial infarction: a meta synthesis. *J Cardiovasc Nurs.* 2004;19(4):251.

27. Kavousi M, et al. Evaluation of newer risk markers for coronary heart disease. A cohort study. *Ann Intern Med.* 2012;156:438.

28. Aronow WS. Homocysteine: the association with atherosclerotic vascular disease in older persons. *Geriatrics.* 2003;58(9):22, 27.

29. Pearson TA, et al. Markers of inflammation and cardiovascular disease: application to clinical and public health practice: a statement for healthcare professionals from the Centers for Disease Control and Prevention and the American Heart Association. *Circulation.* 2003;107(3):499.

30. Greeland P, et al. 2010 ACCF/AHA Guideline for Cardiovascular Risk in Asymptomatic Adults. A Report of the American College of Cardiology Foundation/American Heart Association Task Force on Practice Guidelines. Writing Committee Members. *Circulation.* 2010;122:e584.

31. Buffon A, et al. Widespread coronary inflammation in unstable angina. *N Engl J Med.* 2002;347(1):5.

32. Levine GN, et al. 2011 ACC/AHA/SCAI Guideline for Percutaneous Coronary Intervention: executive Summary: A Report of the American College of Cardiology Foundation/ American Heart Association Task Force on Practice Guidelines and the Society for Cardiovascular Angiography and Interventions. *Circulation.* 2011;124:2574.

33. McSweeney JC, et al. Women's early warning symptoms of acute myocardial infarction. *Circulation.* 2003;108(21):2619.

34. Bairey Merz N, et al. Women's ischemic syndrome evaluation: current status and future research directions. Report of the National Heart, Lung and Blood Institute workshop, October 2-4, 2002: executive summary. *Circulation.* 2004;109(6):805.

35. Goldberg RJ, et al. Community trends in the use and characteristics of persons with acute myocardial infarction who are transported by emergency medical services. *Heart Lung.* 2012;41(4):323.

36. Keller KB, Lemberg L. Prinzmetal's angina. *Am J Crit Care.* 2004;13(4):350.

37. Jacobs AK, et al. Cardiogenic shock caused by right ventricular infarction: a report from the SHOCK registry. *J Am Coll Cardiol.* 2003;41(8):1273.

38. Goldstein JA. Acute right ventricular infarction. *Cardiol Clin.* 2012;30(2):219.

39. Wann SL, et al. 2011 ACC/AHA/HRS Focused Update on the Management of Patients with Atrial Fibrillation (Update on Dabigatran). A Report of the American College of Cardiology Foundation/American Heart Association Task Force on Practice Guidelines. *Circulation.* 2011;123:1140.

40. Birnbaum Y, et al. Ventricular septal rupture after acute myocardial infarction. *N Engl J Med.* 2002;347(18):1426.

41. Crenshaw BS, et al. Risk factors, angiographic patterns, and outcomes in patients with ventricular septal defect complicating acute myocardial infarction. GUSTO-I (Global Utilization of Streptokinase and TPA for Occluded Coronary Arteries) Trial Investigators. *Circulation.* 2000;101(1):27.

42. Deja MA, et al. Post infarction ventricular septal defect: can we do better. *Eur J Cardiothorac Surg.* 2000;18(2):194.

43. Meris A, et al. Mechanisms and predictors of mitral regurgitation after high-risk myocardial infarction. *J Am Soc Echocardiogr.* 2012;25(5):535.

44. Seferović PM, et al. Pericardial syndromes: an update after the ESC guidelines 2004. *Heart Fail Rev.* 2012, August 2 ahead of print.

45. Wang K, et al. ST-segment elevation in conditions other than acute myocardial infarction. *N Engl J Med.* 2003;349(22):2128.

46. Paelinck B, Dendale PA. Images in clinical medicine: cardiac tamponade in Dressler's syndrome. *N Engl J Med.* 2003;348(23):1.

47. Wu AH, et al. Hospital outcomes in patients presenting with congestive heart failure complicating acute myocardial infarction: a report from the Second National Registry of Myocardial Infarction (NRMI-2). *J Am Coll Cardiol.* 2002;40(8):1389.

48. Krumholz HM, et al. Patterns of hospital performance in acute myocardial infarction and heart failure 30-day mortality and readmission. *Circ Cardiovasc Quality Outcomes.* 2009;5(2):407.

49. Eagle KA, et al. Adherence to evidence-based therapies after discharge for acute coronary syndromes: an ongoing prospective, observational study. *Am J Med.* 2004;117(2):73.

50. O'Neil A, et al: Depression as a predictor of work resumption following myocardial infarction (MI): a review of recent research evidence. *Health and Quality of Life Outcomes.* 2010;8:95.

51. Balady GJ, et al. Core Components of Cardiac Rehabilitation/ Secondary Prevention Programs: 2007 Update A Scientific Statement From the American Heart Association Exercise, Cardiac Rehabilitation, and Prevention Committee, the Council on Clinical Cardiology; the Councils on Cardiovascular Nursing, Epidemiology and Prevention, and Nutrition, Physical Activity, and Metabolism; and the American Association of Cardiovascular and Pulmonary Rehabilitation. *Circulation.* 2007;115:2675.

52. Fox CS, et al. Temporal trends in coronary heart disease mortality and sudden cardiac death from 1950 to 1999: the Framingham Heart Study. *Circulation.* 2004;110(5):522.

53. Chugh SS, et al. Current burden of sudden cardiac death: multiple source surveillance versus retrospective death-certificate based review in a large U.S. community. *J Am Coll Cardiol.* 2004;44(6):1268.

54. Priori SG, et al. Task Force on Sudden Cardiac Death of the European Society of Cardiology. *Eur Heart J.* 2001;22(16):1374.

55. Antzelevitch C, et al. Brugada syndrome: report of the second consensus conference; endorsed by the Heart Rhythm Society

and the European Heart Rhythm Association. *Circulation*. 2005;111(5):659.

56. Goldberger JJ, et al. American Heart Association/American College of Cardiology Foundation/Heart Rhythm Society scientific statement on noninvasive risk stratification techniques for identifying patients at risk for sudden cardiac death: a scientific statement from the American Heart Association Council on Clinical Cardiology Committee on Electrocardiography and Arrhythmias and Council on Epidemiology and Prevention. *J Am Coll Cardiol*. 2008;52(14):1179.

57. Epstein AE, et al. ACC/AHA/HRS 2008 guideline for device-based therapy of cardiac rhythm abnormalities: a report of the American College of Cardiology/American Heart Association Task Force on Practice Guidelines (Writing Committee to Revise the ACC/AHA/NASPE 2002 Guideline Update for Implantation of Cardiac Pacemakers and Antiarrhythmic Devices) developed in collaboration with American Association of Thoracic Surgery and the Society of Thoracic Surgeons. *J Am Coll Cardiol*. 2008;51(21):1.

58. Steinbeck G. Evolution of implantable cardioverter defibrillator indications: comparison of guidelines in the United States and Europe. *J Cardiovasc Electrophysiol*. 2002;13(suppl 1):S96.

59. Ghani A, et al. Sex based differences in cardiac arrhythmias, ICD utilization and cardiac resynchronization therapy. *Neth Heart*. 2011;19 (1):35.

60. Jessup M, et al. 2009 Focused Update AHA/ ACC Guidelines for the diagnosis and management of chronic heart failure in the adult: a report of the American College of Cardiology/American Heart Association Task Force on Practice Guidelines: Developed in collaboration with the International Society for Heart and Lung Transplantation. *Circulation*. 2009;119:1977.

61. Greenberg B. Acute decompensated heart failure: treatment and challenges. *Circulation*. 2012;76(3):532.

62. Henry LB. Left ventricular systolic dysfunction and ischemic cardiomyopathy. *Crit Care Nurs Q*. 2003;26(1):16.

63. Haney S, Sur D, Zu X. Diastolic heart failure: a review and primary care perspective. *J Am Board Fam Med*. 2005;18(3):189.

64. Bolliger K, Sadar AM. Care and management of the patient with right heart failure secondary to diastolic dysfunction: an advanced practice perspective and case review. *Crit Care Nurs Q*. 2003;26(1):22.

65. Aurigemma GP, Gaasch WH. Clinical practice: diastolic heart failure. *N Engl J Med*. 2004;351(11):1097.

66. Corra-de-Araujo R, et al. Gender differences across racial and ethnic groups in the quality of care for acute myocardial infarction and heart failure associated with comorbidities. *Women's Health Issues*. 2006;16:44.

67. Maisel AS, et al. Bedside B-type natriuretic peptide in the emergency diagnosis of heart failure with reduced or preserved ejection fraction. Results from the Breathing Not Properly (BNP) multinational study. *J Am Coll Cardiol*. 2003;41(11):2010.

68. Butler J, et al. Update on aldosterone antagonists use in heart failure with reduced left ventricular ejection fraction. Heart Failure Society of America Guidelines Committee. *J Card Fail*. 2012;18:265.

69. Patten RD, Soman P. Prevention and reversal of LV remodeling with neurohormonal inhibitors. *Curr Treat Options Cardiovasc Med*. 2004;6(4):313.

70. Mullens W, et al. Importance of venous congestion, for worsening renal function in advanced decompensated heart failure. *J Am Coll Cardiol*. 2009;53:589.

71. Dimopoulos K, et al. Meta-analyses of mortality and morbidity effects of an angiotensin receptor blocker in patients with chronic heart failure already receiving an ACE inhibitor (alone or with a beta-blocker). *Int J Cardiol*. 2004;93(2-3):105.

72. McCullough PA, Sandberg KR. B-type natriuretic peptide and renal disease. *Heart Fail Rev*. 2003;8(4):355.

73. Maisel AS, et al. Impact of age, race, and sex on the ability of B-type natriuretic peptide to aid in the emergency diagnosis of heart failure: results from the Breathing Not Properly (BNP) multinational study. *Am Heart J*. 2004;147(6):1078.

74. Maisel A, et al. State of the art: using natriuretic peptide levels in clinical practice. *Europ J Heart Fail*. 2008;10:824.

75. Kociol RD, et al. Admission, discharge, or change in B-type natriuretic peptide and long-term outcomes: data from Organized Program to Initiate Lifesaving Treatment in Hospitalized Patients with Heart Failure (OPTIMIZE- HF) linked to Medicare claims. *Circ Heart Fail*. 2011;4:628.

76. Buxton AE, et al. Relation of ejection fraction and inducible ventricular tachycardia to mode of death in patients with coronary artery disease: an analysis of patients enrolled in the multicenter unsustained tachycardia trial. *Circulation*. 2002;106(19):2466.

77. Gattis WA, et al. Predischarge initiation of Carvedilol in patients hospitalized for decompensated heart failure: results of the Initiation Management Predischarge: Process for Assessment of Carvedilol Therapy in Heart Failure (IMPACT HF) trial. *J Am Coll Cardiol*. 2004;43:1434.

78. Greenberg B. Acute decompensated heart failure: treatment and challenges. *Circulation J*. 2012;76(3):532.

79. Chen EW, et al. Relation between hospital intra-aortic balloon counterpulsation volume and mortality in acute myocardial infarction complicated by cardiogenic shock. *Circulation*. 2003;108(8):951.

80. Yancy CW. Vasodilator therapy for decompensated heart failure. *J Am Coll Cardiol*. 2008;52:208.

81. Sing PJ, Gras D. Biventricular pacing: current trends and future strategies. *Eur Heart J*. 2012;33:305.

82. Arshad A, et al. Cardiac Resynchronization therapy is more effective in women than in men: the MADIT-CRT (Multicenter Automatic Defibrillator Implantation Trial with Cardiac Resynchronization Therapy) trial. *J Am Coll Cardiol*. 2011;57:813.

83. Linde C, Ellenbogen K, McAllister FA. Cardiac resynchronization therapy (CRT): clinical trials, guidelines, and target populations. *Heart Rhythm*. 2012;8(Suppl):S3.

84. Goodlin SJ, et al. Consensus statement: palliative and supportive care in advanced heart failure. *J Card Fail*. 2004;10(3):200.

85. Prasad R, Pugh PJ. Drug and device therapy for patients with chronic heart failure. *Expert Rev Cardiovascular Ther*. 2012;10(3):313.

86. Evangalista LS, et al. Health literacy and the patient with heart failure: implications for patient care and research. A consensus statement of the Heart Failure Society of America. *J Card Fail*. 2010;16:9.

87. Gary SF, et al. ACCF/AHA/ACP/HFSA/ISHLT 2010 Clinical Competence Statement on Management of Patients with Advanced Heart Failure and Cardiac Transplant. *Circulation*. 2010;122:644.

88. Sneed NV, Paul SC. Readiness for behavioral changes in patients with heart failure. *Am J Crit Care.* 2003;12(5):444.

89. Gersh BJ, et al. 2011 AHA/ACC Guideline for the Diagnosis and Treatment of Hypertrophic Cardiomyopathy. A report of the American College of Cardiology Foundation/American Heart Association Task Force on Practice Guidelines. *Circulation.* 2011;124:e783.

90. Friedrich FW, Carrier L. Genetics of hypertrophic and dilated cardiomopathy. *Current Pharm Biotechn.* 2012;13(13):2467.

91. Kamisago M, et al. Mutations in sarcomere protein genes as a cause of dilated cardiomyopathy. *N Engl J Med.* 2000;343(23):1688.

92. Li D, et al. Novel cardiac troponin T mutation as a cause of familial dilated cardiomyopathy. *Circulation.* 2001;104(18):2188.

93. Murphy RT, et al. Novel mutation in cardiac troponin I in recessive idiopathic dilated cardiomyopathy. *Lancet.* 2004;363(9406):371.

94. Ammash NM, et al. Clinical profile and outcome of idiopathic restrictive cardiomyopathy. *Circulation.* 2000;101(21):2490.

95. McNamara DM, et al. Clinical and demographic predictors of outcomes in recent onset dilated cardiomyopathy: results of the IMAC (Intervention in Myocarditis and Acute Cardiomyopathy)-2 study. *J Am Coll Cardiol.* 2008;58:1112 e8.

96. Gupta V. Inhalation therapy for pulmonary hypertension. *Critical reviews in therapeutic drug carrier systems.* 2010;27.

97. McLaughlin VM, et al. ACCF/AHA 2009 Expert consensus document on pulmonary hypertension. *JACC.* 2009;53(17):1573.

98. Simmoneau G, et al. Updated clinical classification of pulmonary hypertension. *JACC.* 2009;54(1):S43.

99. Rubenfire M, et al. Pulmonary hypertension in the critical care setting: classification, pathophysiology, diagnosis, and management. *Crit Care Clin.* 2007;23(4):801.

100. Zamanian RT, et al. Management strategies for patients with pulmonary hypertension in the intensive care unit. *Crit Care Med.* 2007;35(9):2037.

101. Shah SJ. Pulmonary hypertension. *JAMA.* 2012;308(13):1366.

102. Badesch DB, et al. Diagnosis and Assessment of pulmonary arterial hypertension. *JACC.* 2009;54(1):S55.

103. Keogh. Survival after the initiation of combination therapy in patients with pulmonary arterial hypertension: an Australian collaborative report. *Intern Med J.* 2011;41(3):235.

104. Galiè N, et al. Guidelines for the diagnosis and treatment of pulmonary hypertension. *Eur Heart J.* 2009;30(20):2493.

105. Barst RJ, et al. Updated evidence-based treatment algorithm in pulmonary arterial hypertension. *JACC.* 2009;54(1):S78.

106. Brown LM, et al. Delay in recognition of pulmonary arterial hypertension: factors identified from the REVEAL registry. *Chest.* 2011;140(1):19.

107. Anderson JR, Nawarskas JJ. Pharmacotherapeutic management of pulmonary arterial hypertension. *Cardiol Rev.* 2010;18(3):148.

108. Iheagwara NL, Thomas TF. Pharmacologic treatment of pulmonary hypertension. *US Pharm.* 2010;35(8):HS11.

109. McLaughlin VV, et al. Addition of inhaled treprostinil to oral therapy for pulmonary arterial hypertension. *JACC.* 2010;55(18):1915.

110. Doran AK, et al. Guidelines for the prevention of central venous catheter-related blood stream infections with prostanoid therapy for pulmonary arterial hypertension. *Int J Clin Pract Suppl.* 2008;160:5.

111. Widlitz AC, McDevitt S, Ward GR, Krichman A. Practical aspects of continuous intravenous treprostinil therapy. *CCN.* 2007;27(2):41.

112. Luttenberger K, DiNapoli M. Subacute bacterial endocarditis: making the diagnosis. *Nurs Prac.* 2011;36(3):31-38.

113. Lester SJ, Wilansky S. Endocarditis and associated complications. *Crit Care Med.* 2007;35(8 suppl):S384.

114. Bashore M, et al. Update on infective endocarditis. *Curr Probl Cardiol.* 2006;31 (4):274.

115. Horstkotte D, et al. Guidelines on prevention, diagnosis and treatment of infective endocarditis—executive summary: the Task Force on Infective Endocarditis of the European Society of Cardiology. *Eur Heart J.* 2004;25(3):267.

116. Wilson W, et al. Prevention of infective endocarditis: guidelines from the American Heart Association. A guideline from the American Heart Association Rheumatic Fever, Endocarditis, and Kawasaki Disease Committee, Council on Cardiovascular Disease in the Young, and the Council on Clinical Cardiology, Council on Cardiovascular Surgery and Anesthesia, and the Quality of Care and Outcomes Research Interdisciplinary Working Group. *Circulation.* 2007;116(15):1736.

117. Baddour LM, et al. Infective endocarditis: diagnosis, antimicrobial therapy, and management of complications. A statement for healthcare professionals from the Committee on Rheumatic Fever, Endocarditis, and Kawasaki Disease, Council on Cardiovascular Disease in the Young, and the Councils on Clinical Cardiology, Stroke, and Cardiovascular Surgery and Anesthesia, American Heart Association: endorsed by the Infectious Diseases Society of America. *Circulation.* 2005;111(23):e394.

118. Nishimura RA, et al. ACC/AHA 2008 guideline update on valvular heart disease: focused update on infective endocarditis. A report of the American College of Cardiology/American Heart Association Task Force on Practice Guidelines. *Circulation.* 2008;11(8):887.

119. Broyles LM, Korniewicz DM. The opiate-dependent patient with endocarditis: addressing pain and substance abuse withdrawal. *AACN Clin Issues.* 2002;13(3):432.

120. Bonow RO, et al. ACC/AHA 2006 guidelines for the management of patients with valvular heart disease: a report of the American College of Cardiology/American Heart Association Task Force on Practice Guidelines (Writing Committee to Revise the 1988 Guidelines for the Management of Patients with Valvular Heart Disease) developed in collaboration with the Society of Cardiovascular Anesthesiologists; endorsed by the Society for Cardiovascular Angiography and Interventions and the Society of Thoracic Surgeons. *Circulation.* 2006;114(5):e84.

121. Foster E. Mitral regurgitation due to degenerative mitral-valve disease. *N Engl J Med.* 2010;363(2):156.

122. Siu SC, Silverside CK. Bicuspid aortic valve. *JACC.* 2010;55(2):2789.

123. Carbello BA. The current therapy for mitral regurgitation. *JACC.* 2008;52(5):319.

124. Akat K, et al. Aortic valve calcification: basic science to clinical practice. *Heart.* 2009;95(8):616.

125. Fitzgerald KP. The pulmonary valve. *Cardiol Clin.* 2011;29(2):223.

126. Rosengart TK, et al. Percutaneous and minimally invasive valve procedures: a scientific statement from the American Heart

Association Council on Cardiovascular Surgery and Anesthesia, Council on Clinical Cardiology, Function Genomics and Translation Biology Interdisciplinary Working Group, and Quality of Care and Outcomes Research Interdisciplinary Working Group. *Circulation*. 2008;117(13):1750.

127. Jilaihawi H, Hussaini A, Kar S. Mitraclip: a novel percutaneous approach to mitral valve repair. *Biomed Biotech*. 2011;12(8):633.

128. Makkar RR, et al. Transcatheter aortic-valve replacement for inoperable severe aortic stenosis. *N Engl J Med*. 2012;336(18):1696.

129. Bonow RO, et al. ACC/AHA 2006 guidelines for the management of patients with valvular heart disease: executive summary. *Circulation*. 2006;114:450.

130. Moll FL, et al. Management of abdominal aortic aneurysms. Clinical practice guidelines for the European Society of Vascular Surgery. *Eur J Vasc Endovasc Surg*. 2011;41:S1.

131. Grootenboer N, et al. Systematic review and meta-analysis of sex differences in outcome after intervention for abdominal aortic aneurysm. *Br J Surg*. 2010;97(8):1169.

132. Norman PE, Powell JT. Abdominal aortic aneurysm: the prognosis in women is worse than in men. *Circulation*. 2007;115(22):2865.

133. Hiratzka L, et al. 2010 ACCF/AHA/AATS/ ACR/SCA/SCAO/ SIR/STS/SVM Guidelines for the diagnosis and management of patients with thoracic aortic disease. *Circulation*. 2010;121(13):e266.

134. Feldman M, Shah M, Elefteriades A. Medical management of acute Type A aortic dissection. *Ann Thorac Cardiovasc Surg*. 2010;15(5):286.

135. Chaikof EL, et al. The care of patient with an abdominal aortic aneurysm: The Society for Vascular Surgery practice guidelines. *J Vasc Surg*. 2009;50(4):S2.

136. Hirsch AT, et al. ACC/AHA 2005 practice guidelines for the management of patients with peripheral arterial disease (lower extremity, renal, mesenteric, and abdominal aortic): a collaborative report from the American Association for Vascular Surgery/Society for Vascular Surgery, Society for Cardiovascular Angiography and Interventions, Society for Vascular Medicine and Biology, Society of Interventional Radiology, and the ACC/AHA Task Force on Practice Guidelines (Writing Committee to Develop Guidelines for the Management of Patients with Peripheral Arterial Disease). Endorsed by the American Association of Cardiovascular and Pulmonary Rehabilitation; National Heart, Lung, and Blood Institute; Society for Vascular Nursing; TransAtlantic Inter-Society Consensus; and Vascular Disease Foundation. *Circulation*. 2006;113(11):e463.

137. Olin JW, et al. ACCF/AHA/ACR/ACAI/SIR/SVM/SVN/SVS 2010 performance measures for adults with peripheral artery disease. *Vasc Med*. 2010;15(6):481.

138. Argacha JF, et al. Acute effects of passive smoking on peripheral vascular function. *Hypertension*. 2008;51(6):1506.

139. Tendara M, et al. ESC guidelines on the diagnosis and treatment of peripheral artery disease. *Eur Heart J*. 2011;32:2851.

140. McDermott MM, et al. The ankle-brachial index is associated with the magnitude of impaired walking endurance among men and women with peripheral arterial disease. *Vasc Med*. 2010;15(4):251.

141. Garg PK, et al. Physical activity during daily life and mortality in patients with peripheral arterial disease. *Circulation*. 2006;114(3):242.

142. Murphy TP, et al. Supervised exercise versus primary stenting for claudication resulting from aortoiliac peripheral artery disease. Outcomes from the Claudication: Exercise versus endoluminal revascularization (CLEVER) study. *Circulation*. 2011;125(1):130.

143. Meschia JF, et al. Diagnosis and invasive management of carotid atherosclerotic stenosis. *Mayo Clin Proc*. 2007;82(7):851.

144. Goldstein LB, et al. Guidelines for the primary prevention of stroke: a guideline for healthcare professionals from the American Heart Association/ American Stroke Association. *Stroke*. 2011;42(2):517.

145. Alonso-Coello P, et al. Antithrombotic therapy in peripheral artery disease: Antithrombotic therapy and prevention of thrombosis, 9th ed: American College of Chest Physicians evidence-based clinical guidelines. *Chest*. 2012;141(2 Suppl):e669S.

146. Alexandrov AW. Methodologic challenges in the design and conduct of hyperacute stroke research. *AACN Adv Crit Care*. 2008;19(2):186.

147. Kiernan TJ, Yan BP, Jaff MR. Antiplatelet therapy for the primary and secondary prevention of cerebrovascular events in patients with extracranial carotid artery disease. *J Vasc Surg*. 2009;50(2):431.

148 Gurm HS, et al. Long-term results of carotid stenting versus endarterectomy in high-risk patients. *N Engl J Med*. 2008;358(15):1572.

149. Mas JL, et al. Endarterectomy versus stenting in patients with symptomatic severe carotid stenosis. *N Engl J Med*. 2006;355(16):1660.

150. Mantese VA, et al. The carotid revascularization endarterectomy versus stenting trial (CREST) stenting versus carotid endarterectomy for carotid disease. *Stroke*. 2010;41:S31.

151. Adams RJ, et al. Update to the AHA/ASA recommendations for the prevention of stroke in patients with stroke and transient ischemic attack. *Stroke*. 2008;39 (5):1647.

152. Hopkins LN, et al. Carotid artery revascularization in high surgical risk patients with the NexStent and the Filterwire EX/EZ: 1-year results in the CABERNET trial. *Catheter Cardiovasc Interv*. 2008;71(7):950.

153. Iyer SS, et al. Carotid artery revascularization in high-surgical-risk patients using the Carotid WALLSTENT and FilterWire EX/EZ: 1-year outcomes in the BEACH Pivotal Group. *JACC*. 2008;51(4):427.

154. Geerts WH, et al. Prevention of venous thromboembolism: American College of Chest Physicians Evidence-Based Clinical Practice Guidelines (8th edition). *Chest*. 2008;133(6 suppl):381S.

155. Kearon C, et al. Antithrombotic therapy for VTE diseases, Antithrombotic therapy and prevention of thrombosis, 9th ed: American College of Chest Physicians evidence-based clinical practice guidelines. *Chest*. 2012;141(2 Suppl):e419S.

156. Wakefield TW, et al. Mechanisms of venous thrombosis and resolution. *Arterioscler Thromb Vasc Biol*. 2008;28(3):387.

157. Heit JA. The epidemiology of venous thromboembolism in the community. *Arterioscler Thromb Vasc Biol*. 2008;28(3):370.

158. Chan CM, Shorr AF. Venous thromboembolic disease in the intensive care unit. *Semin Resp Crit Care Med*. 2010;30(1):39.

159. Tapson VF. Acute pulmonary embolism. *N Engl J Med*. 2008;358(10):1037.

160. Moll S. A clinical perspective of venous thromboembolism. *Arterioscler Thromb Vasc Biol*. 2008;28(3):373.

161. Elliott WJ. Clinical features in the management of selected hypertensive emergencies. *Prog Cardiovasc Dis*. 2006;48(5):316.

162. Varon J. Treatment of acute severe hypertension: current and newer agents. *Drugs*. 2008;68(3):283.

163. Papadopoulos D, et al. Hypertension Crisis. *Blood Press*. 2010;19:328.

164. Feldstein C. Management of hypertensive crises. *Am J Ther*. 2007;14(2):135.

165. Marik PE, Varon J. Hypertensive crises: challenges and management. *Chest*. 2007;131(6):1949.

166. Van den Born BJH, et al. Dutch guidelines for management of hypertensive crisis- 2010 revisions. *Netherlands J Medicine*. 2011;69(5):248.

167. Slama M, Modeliar SS. Hypertension in the intensive care unit. *Curr Opin Cardiol*. 2006;21(4):279.

168. Chobanian AV, et al. Seventh report of the Joint National Committee on Prevention, Detection, Evaluation, and Treatment of High Blood Pressure. *Hypertension*. 2003;42(6):1206.

16

Cardiovascular Therapeutic Management

Joni Dirks, Julie Waters

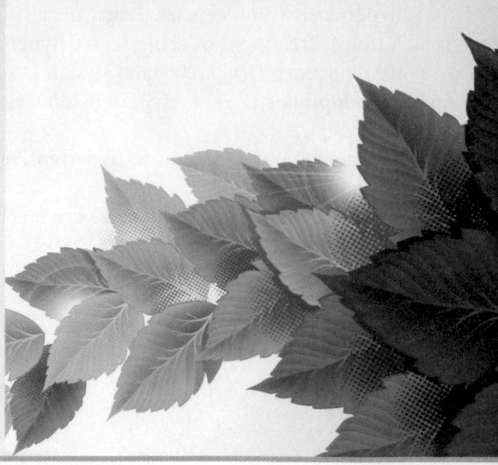

PACEMAKERS

Pacemakers are electronic devices that can be used to initiate the heartbeat when the heart's intrinsic electrical system cannot effectively generate a rate adequate to support cardiac output. Pacemakers may be used temporarily, either supportively or prophylactically, until the condition responsible for the rate or conduction disturbance resolves. They also may be used on a permanent basis if the patient's condition persists despite adequate therapy. The use of permanent pacemakers as a form of device-based therapy has expanded significantly in the last decade.[1]

This section emphasizes temporary pacemakers, because the critical care nurse is responsible for preventing, assessing, and managing pacemaker malfunctions when these devices are used in the clinical setting. A brief discussion of permanent pacemakers is provided, and similarities between implanted and temporary pacemakers are presented where appropriate.

Indications for Temporary Pacing

The clinical indications for instituting temporary pacemaker therapy are similar regardless of the cause of the rhythm disturbance that necessitates the placement of a pacemaker (Box 16-1). The causes range from ischemia and electrolyte imbalances to sequelae related to acute myocardial infarction (MI) or cardiac surgery.

Therapeutic Indications

Dysrhythmias that are unresponsive to medications and result in compromised hemodynamic status are a definite indication for pacemaker therapy. The goal of therapy in the case of bradydysrhythmia is to increase the ventricular rate and thereby enhance cardiac output. Alternately, overdrive pacing can be used to decrease the rate of a rapid supraventricular or ventricular rhythm. This rapid pacing of the heart (i.e., overdrive pacing) functions to prevent the breakthrough ectopy that can result from a slow rate or to interrupt an ectopic focus and allow the natural pacemaker to regain control. Temporary pacing may be used in the treatment of symptomatic bradycardia or progressive heart block that occurs as a result of myocardial ischemia, medication overdose, or illegal drug toxicity. After cardiac surgery, temporary pacing may be used to improve a transiently depressed, rate-dependent cardiac output. Conduction disturbances that occur after valvular surgery can be managed effectively with temporary pacing.

Diagnostic Indications

Several diagnostic uses for temporary pacing have evolved. Electrophysiology studies (EPS) are performed in cardiac catheterization laboratories equipped with specialized pacing equipment. During an EPS, catheters with pacing electrodes are used to diagnose the patient's potential for dysrhythmias.[2] These electrodes are used to induce dysrhythmias in patients with recurrent symptomatic tachydysrhythmias. This allows the physician to closely evaluate the particular dysrhythmia and determine appropriate therapy. For those patients whose tachydysrhythmia is found to be refractory to conventional antidysrhythmic therapy, radiofrequency (RF) current catheter ablation of the responsible tissue can be done safely and effectively in the electrophysiology laboratory. After a mapping procedure has localized the site of dysrhythmia formation, short bursts of RF current are delivered through the catheter, destroying the offending tissue with heat. Ablation has been shown to be an effective treatment for patients with symptomatic supraventricular tachycardias that result from atrioventricular (AV) node re-entry or accessory pathways, such as Wolff-Parkinson-White syndrome.[3,4] Catheter ablation may also be used as a therapeutic strategy for selected patients with atrial fibrillation.[5]

Intracardiac electrograms—recordings of cardiac electrical activity obtained from pacing electrodes—may provide useful diagnostic information. The atrial electrogram (AEG) is an amplified recording of atrial activity that can be obtained through the use of an atrial pacing electrode or an esophageal pill electrode and a standard electrocardiogram (ECG) machine. It may be used after cardiac surgery to facilitate the diagnosis of supraventricular dysrhythmias in patients with temporary atrial epicardial wires already in place.[6]

The Pacemaker System

A pacemaker system is a simple electrical circuit consisting of a pulse generator and a pacing lead (an insulated electrical wire) with one, two, or three electrodes.

Pacing Pulse Generator

The pulse generator is designed to generate an electrical current that travels through the pacing lead and exits through an electrode (exposed portion of the wire) that is in direct contact with the heart. This electrical current initiates a myocardial depolarization. The current then seeks to return by one of several pathways to the pulse generator to complete the circuit.

The power source for a temporary external pulse generator is a standard 9-volt alkaline battery inserted into the generator. Implanted permanent pacemaker batteries are usually long-lived lithium cells.

Pacing Lead Systems

The pacing lead used for temporary pacing may be bipolar or unipolar. In a bipolar system, two electrodes (positive and negative) are located within the heart, whereas in a unipolar system, only one electrode (negative) is in direct contact with the myocardium. In both systems, the current flows from the negative terminal of the pulse generator, down the pacing lead to the negative electrode, and into the heart. The current is then picked up by the positive electrode (ground) and flows back up the lead to the positive terminal of the pulse generator.

The bipolar lead used in transvenous pacing has two electrodes on one catheter (Fig. 16-1). The distal, or negative, electrode is at the tip of the pacing lead and is in direct contact with the heart, usually inside the right atrium or ventricle. Approximately 1 cm from the negative electrode is a positive electrode. The negative electrode is attached to the negative terminal, and the positive electrode is attached to the positive terminal of the pulse generator, either directly or by means of a bridging cable (see Fig. 16-1B).

An epicardial lead system is often used for temporary pacing after cardiac surgery. The bipolar epicardial lead system has two separate insulated wires (one negative and one positive electrode) that are loosely secured with sutures to the cardiac chamber to be paced. Both leads are in contact with the myocardial tissue, so either wire may be used as the negative, or pacing, electrode. The remaining wire is then used as the positive, or ground, electrode.

A unipolar pacing system (epicardial or transvenous) has only one electrode (the negative electrode) making contact with the heart. For a permanent pacemaker, the positive electrode can be created by the metallic casing of the subcutaneously implanted pulse generator (Fig. 16-2), or as is the case with a unipolar epicardial lead system, the positive electrode can be formed by a piece of surgical steel wire sewn into the subcutaneous tissue of the chest or the metal portion of a surface ECG electrode.

Because the unipolar pacing system has a wide sensing area as a result of the relatively long distance between the negative and positive electrodes, it has better sensing capabilities than does a bipolar system. However, this feature makes the unipolar system more susceptible to sensing extraneous signals, such as the electrical artifacts created by normal muscle movements (i.e., myopotentials) or by external electromagnetic interference (EMI), which may result in inappropriate inhibition of the pacing stimulus. This problem is of more concern in permanent pacing systems, in which the "can" of the pacemaker generator may be used as a part of the pacing circuit. Because the can is located near a large muscle mass, upper body movement can result in the inappropriate sensing of myopotentials.[7]

Pacing Routes

Several routes are available for temporary cardiac pacing (Box 16-2). Permanent pacing usually is accomplished transvenously, although when a thoracotomy is otherwise indicated, as in cardiac surgery, the physician may elect to insert permanent epicardial pacing wires.

Transcutaneous cardiac pacing involves the use of two large skin electrodes, one placed anteriorly and the other posteriorly on the chest, connected to an external pulse generator. It is a rapid, noninvasive procedure that nurses can perform in the emergency setting and is recommended in the advanced cardiac life support (ACLS) algorithm for the treatment of symptomatic bradycardia that does not respond to atropine.[8] Improved technology related to stimulus delivery and the development of large electrode pads that help disperse the energy have helped reduce the pain associated with cutaneous nerve and muscle stimulation. Discomfort may still be an issue for some patients, particularly when higher energy levels are required to achieve capture. This route is typically used as a short-term therapy

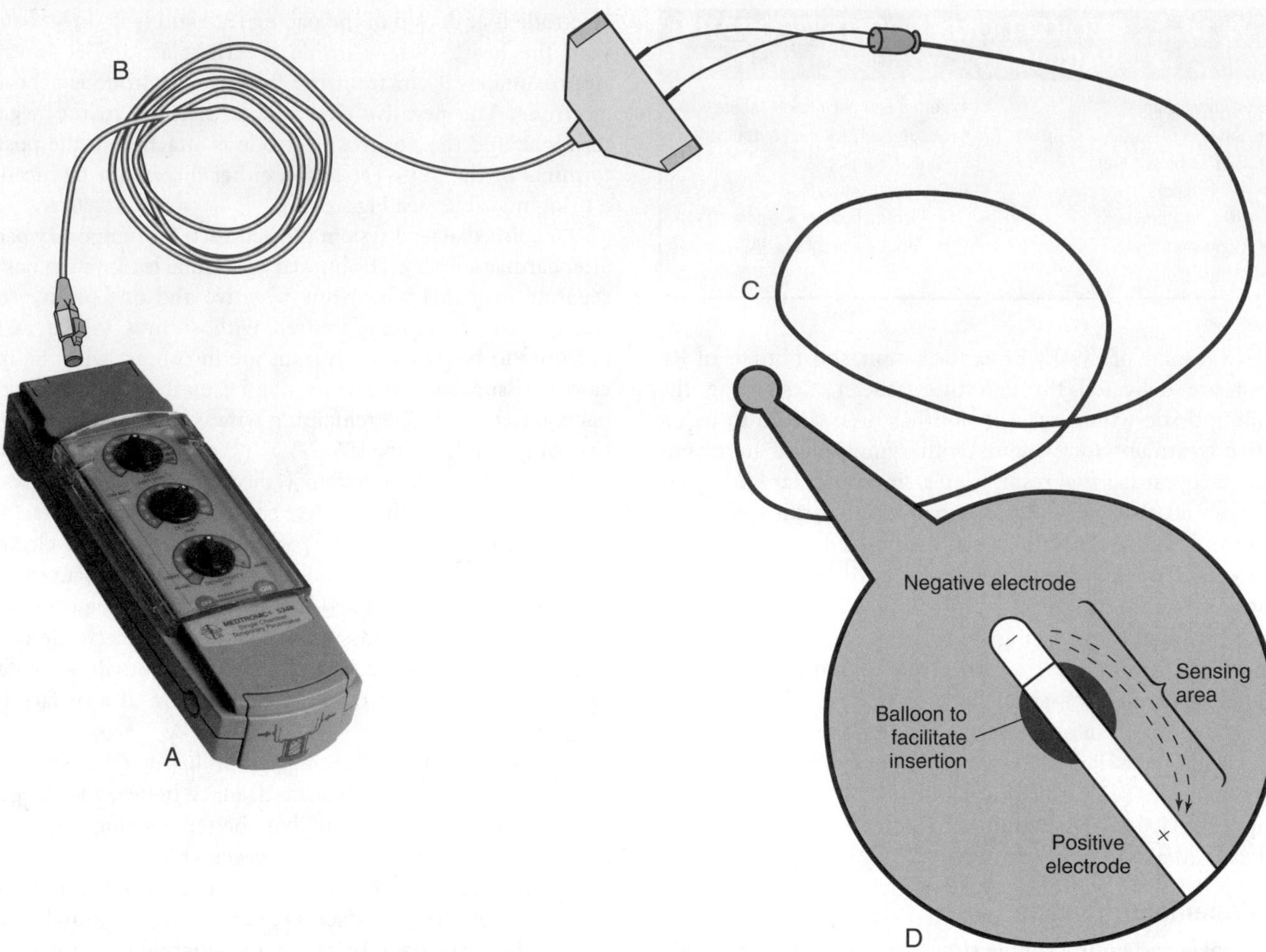

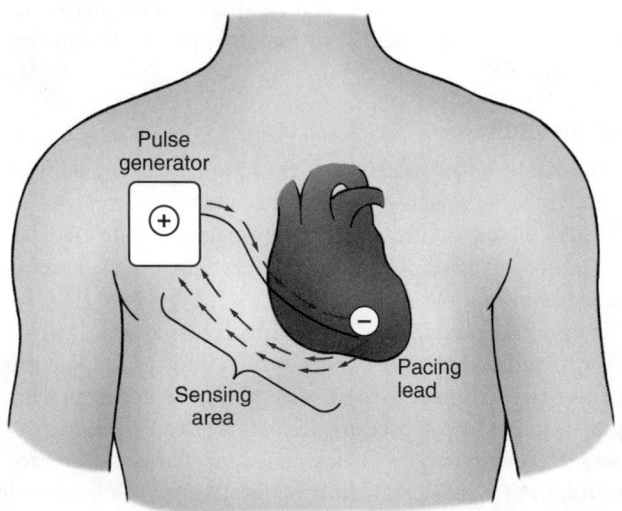

B

C

Negative electrode

Sensing area

Balloon to facilitate insertion

Positive electrode

A

D

FIGURE 16-1 The components of a temporary bipolar transvenous catheter. *A,* Single-chamber temporary (external) pulse generator. *B,* Bridging cable. *C,* Pacing lead. *D,* Enlarged view of the pacing lead tip. (*A,* Reproduced with permission of Medtronic, Inc.)

Pulse generator

⊕

Sensing area

Pacing lead

⊖

FIGURE 16-2 The components of a permanent unipolar transvenous pacing system.

BOX 16-2 ROUTES FOR TEMPORARY PACING

Transcutaneous
Emergency pacing is achieved by depolarizing the heart through the chest by means of two large skin electrodes.

Epicardial
Pacing electrodes are sewn to the epicardium during cardiac surgery.

Transvenous (Endocardial)
The pacing electrode is advanced through a vein into the right atrium or right ventricle, or both.

until the situation resolves or another route of pacing can be established.

The insertion of temporary epicardial pacing wires has become a routine procedure during most cardiac surgical cases. Ventricular and, in many cases, atrial pacing wires are loosely sewn to the epicardium. The terminal pins of these wires are pulled through the skin before the chest is closed. If both chambers have pacing wires attached, the atrial wires exit subcostally to the right of the sternum and the ventricular wires exit in the same region but to the left of the sternum. These wires can be

TABLE 16-1 NASPE/BPEG GENERIC CODE

POSITION I: CHAMBERS PACED	POSITION II: CHAMBERS SENSED	POSITION III: RESPONSE TO SENSING	POSITION IV: RATE MODULATION	POSITION V: MULTISITE PACING
0 = None	0 = None	0 = None	0 = None	0 = None
A = Atrium	A = Atrium	T = Triggered	R = Rate Modulation	A = Atrium
V = Ventricle	V = Ventricle	I = Inhibited		V = Ventricle
D = Dual (A + V)	D = Dual (A + V)	D = Dual (T + I)		D = Dual (A + V)

Modified from Bernstein AD, et al. The Revised NASPE/BPEG generic pacemaker code for antibradycardia, adaptive-rate and multisite pacing. *PACE.* 2002;25:260.
BPEG, British Pacing and Electrophysiology Group; *NASPE,* North American Society of Pacing and Electrophysiology.

BOX 16-3 PACEMAKER TERMINOLOGY

Fixed-Rate (Asynchronous)
Delivers a pacing stimulus at a set (fixed) rate regardless of the occurrence of spontaneous myocardial depolarization; occurs in nonsensing modes

Demand (Synchronous)
Delivers a pacing stimulus only when the heart's intrinsic pacemaker fails to function at a predetermined rate; the pacing stimulus is either inhibited or triggered by the sensing of intrinsic activity

Atrioventricular Sequential (Dual-Chamber)
Delivers a pacing stimulus to both atrium and ventricle in physiologic sequence with sufficient atrioventricular delay to permit adequate ventricular filling

---

TABLE 16-2 EXAMPLES OF TEMPORARY PACING MODES

PACING MODE	DESCRIPTION
Asynchronous	
AOO	Atrial pacing, no sensing
VOO	Ventricular pacing, no sensing
DOO	Atrial and ventricular pacing, no sensing
Synchronous	
AAI	Atrial pacing, atrial sensing, inhibited response to sensed P waves
VVI	Ventricular pacing, ventricular sensing, inhibited response to sensed QRS complexes
DVI	Atrial and ventricular pacing, ventricular sensing; both atrial and ventricular pacing are inhibited if a spontaneous ventricular depolarization is sensed
DDD	Both chambers are paced and sensed; inhibited response of the pacing stimuli to sensed events in their respective chambers; triggered response to sensed atrial activity to allow for rate-responsive ventricular pacing

---

removed several days after surgery by gentle traction at the skin surface with minimal risk of bleeding.[9]

Temporary transvenous endocardial pacing is accomplished by advancing a pacing electrode wire through a vein, often the subclavian or internal jugular vein, and into the right atrium or right ventricle (RV). Insertion can be facilitated through direct visualization with fluoroscopy or by the use of the standard ECG. In some cases, the pacing wire is inserted through a special pulmonary artery catheter by means of a port that exits in the right atrium or RV.

Five-Letter Pacemaker Codes

In the 1960s, pacemaker terminology was limited to *fixed-rate* and *demand* pacing; *AV sequential* pacing was introduced in the early 1970s. Although these terms are still useful for understanding pacemaker function (Box 16-3), the continued expansion of functional capabilities of pulse generators has made it necessary to develop a more precise classification system. In 1974, the Inter-Society Commission for Heart Disease (ICHD) adopted a three-letter code for describing the various pacing modalities available. The code has since undergone several revisions, including the addition of two more letters representing programming characteristics and multisite pacing functions, to accommodate the development of newer devices that are rate responsive or that pace from more than one site within the atria and the ventricles. Table 16-1 describes the current five-letter code.[10] The original three-letter code remains adequate to describe temporary pacemaker function.

The original code is based on three categories, each represented by a letter. The first letter refers to the cardiac chamber that is paced. The second letter designates which chamber is sensed, and the third letter indicates the pacemaker's response to the sensed event. These three letters are used to describe the mode of pacing. For example, a VVI pacemaker paces the ventricle when the pacemaker fails to sense an intrinsic ventricular depolarization, but sensing of a spontaneous ventricular depolarization inhibits ventricular pacing. A VOO pacemaker paces the ventricle at a fixed rate and has no sensing capabilities. In DDD pacing, atrial and ventricular leads are used for pacing and sensing. In response to sensed activity, the pacemaker inhibits the pacing stimulus; a sensed P wave in the atrium inhibits the atrial spike, and a sensed R wave in the ventricle inhibits the ventricular pacing spike. A sensed P wave may also be used to trigger a ventricular pacing stimulus if normal conduction through the AV node is impaired. Table 16-2 provides a description of temporary pacing modes.

Physiologic pacing has traditionally been used to describe modes in which the normal physiologic, or sequential, relationship between atrial and ventricular stimulation and contraction is maintained. AV synchrony increases the volume in the ventricle before contraction and helps to improve cardiac output.

This may be achieved with atrial pacing in patients who have an intact conduction system or by dual chamber pacing when atrial-to-ventricular conduction is impaired (i.e., during heart block). More recently, physiologic pacing has evolved to include the maintenance of ventricular synchrony as well. Strategies to achieve this include minimizing the use of ventricular pacing and simultaneous pacing of both right and left ventricles.[1]

Pacemaker Settings

The controls on all external temporary pulse generators are similar. Their functions must be thoroughly understood so that pacing can be initiated quickly in an emergency situation and troubleshooting can be facilitated if problems with the pacemaker arise.

The *rate control* (Fig. 16-3) regulates the number of impulses that can be delivered to the heart per minute. The rate setting depends on the physiologic needs of the patient, but it usually is maintained between 60 and 80 beats/min. Pacing rates for overdrive suppression of tachydysrhythmias may greatly exceed these values. Some generators have special controls for overdrive pacing that allow for rates of up to 800 stimuli per minute. If the pacemaker is operating in a dual-chamber mode, the ventricular rate control also regulates the atrial rate.

The *output dial* regulates the amount of electrical current, measured in milliamperes (mA), that is delivered to the heart to initiate depolarization. The point at which depolarization occurs, called *threshold*, is indicated by a myocardial response to the pacing stimulus (i.e., capture). Threshold can be determined by gradually decreasing the output setting until 1:1 capture is lost. The output setting is then slowly increased until 1:1 capture is re-established; this threshold to pace is less than 1 mA with a properly positioned pacing electrode. The output is set two to three times higher than threshold, because thresholds tend to fluctuate over time. Box 16-4 details the procedure for measuring pacing thresholds. Separate output controls for atrium and ventricle are used with a dual-chamber pulse generator.

The *sensitivity control* regulates the ability of the pacemaker to detect the heart's intrinsic electrical activity. Sensitivity is measured in millivolts (mV) and determines the size of the intracardiac signal that the generator will recognize. If the sensitivity is adjusted to its most sensitive setting—a setting of 0.5 to 1 mV—the pacemaker can respond even to low-amplitude electrical signals coming from the heart. Turning the sensitivity to its least sensitive setting (i.e., adjusting the dial to a setting of 20 mV or to the area labeled *async*) results in inability of the pacemaker to sense any intrinsic electrical activity and causes the pacemaker to function at a fixed rate. A sense indicator (often a light) on the pulse generator signals each time intrinsic cardiac electrical activity is sensed. A pulse generator may be designed to sense atrial activity or ventricular activity, or both. Box 16-5 describes the procedure for measuring sensitivity. The sensitivity is set at half of the value of the sensitivity threshold to ensure that all appropriate intrinsic cardiac signals are sensed.

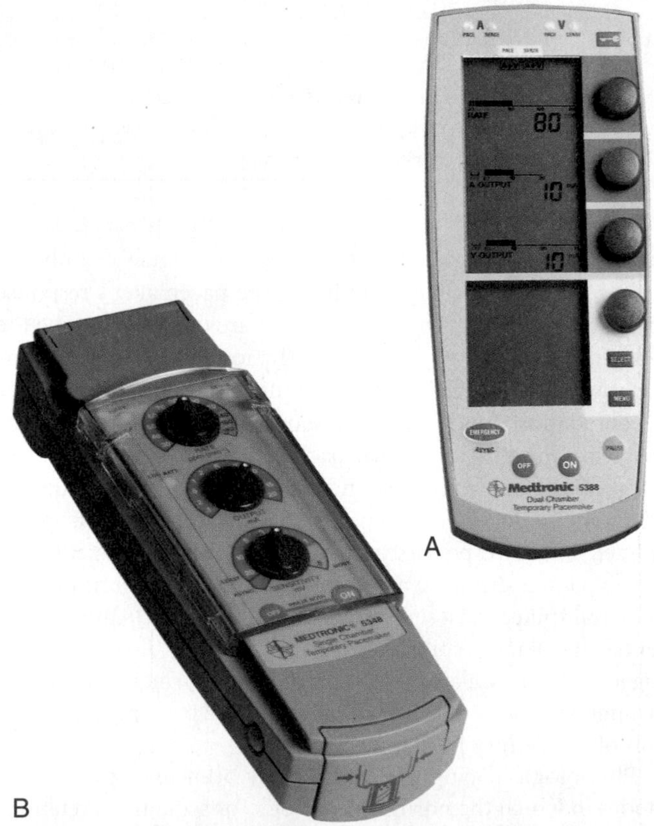

FIGURE 16-3 Temporary pulse generators (external). *A,* Dual-chamber pulse generator. *B,* Single-chamber pulse generator. (Reproduced with permission of Medtronic, Inc.)

BOX 16-4 DETERMINING THE TEMPORARY PACEMAKER PACING THRESHOLD

1. Adjust the pacemaker rate setting so that patient is 100% paced. It may be necessary to increase the pacing rate to achieve this setting.
2. Gradually decrease the output (milliampere, mA) setting until 1:1 capture is lost. The pacing threshold is the point at which capture is lost.
3. Slowly increase the output setting until 1:1 capture is re-established. With a properly positioned pacing electrode, the pacing threshold should be less than 1 mA.
4. Set the output setting two to three times higher than measured threshold, because thresholds tend to fluctuate over time.
5. If a dual-chamber pulse generator is being used, evaluate pacing thresholds for the atrial and ventricular leads separately.

BOX 16-5 DETERMINING THE TEMPORARY PACEMAKER SENSITIVITY THRESHOLD

- Set the sensitivity control to its most sensitive setting.
- Adjust the pulse generator rate to 10 beats/min less than the patient's intrinsic rate (the flash indicator should flash regularly).
- Reduce the generator output to the minimal value to eliminate the risk of competing with the intrinsic rhythm.
- Gradually increase the sensitivity value until the sense indicator stops flashing and the pace indicator starts flashing.
- Decrease sensitivity until the sense indicator begins to flash again; this is the sensitivity threshold.
- Adjust the sensitivity setting on the generator to half of the threshold value; restore the generator output and rate to their original values.

For example, if the measured sensitivity threshold is 3.0 mV, the generator is set at 1.5 mV. The pacemaker's sensing ability can be quickly evaluated by observing for a change in pacing rhythm in response to spontaneous depolarizations.

The *AV interval control* (available only on dual-chamber generators) regulates the time interval between the atrial and ventricular pacing stimuli. This interval is analogous to the PR interval that occurs in the intrinsic ECG. Proper adjustment of this interval to between 150 and 250 milliseconds (msec) preserves AV synchrony and permits maximal ventricular stroke volume and enhanced cardiac output.

Temporary dual chamber pacemakers have other settings that are required in the DDD mode (see Fig. 16-3B). The *lower rate*, or *base rate*, determines the rate at which the generator will pace when intrinsic activity falls below the set rate of the pacemaker. The *upper rate* determines the fastest ventricular rate the pacemaker will deliver in response to sensed atrial activity. This setting is needed to protect the patient's heart from being paced in response to rapid atrial dysrhythmias. The *pulse width*, which can be adjusted from 0.05 to 2 msec, controls the length of time that the pacing stimulus is delivered to the heart. There also is an *atrial refractory period*, programmable from 150 to 500 msec, which regulates the length of time, after a sensed or paced ventricular event, during which the pacemaker cannot respond to another atrial stimulus. An emergency button is also available on most models to allow for rapid initiation of asynchronous (DOO) pacing during an emergency.

On all temporary pacemakers, an on/off switch is provided with a safety feature that prevents the accidental termination of pacing. On new generators, there is also a locking feature to prevent unintended changes to the prescribed settings.

Pacing Artifacts

All patients with temporary pacemakers require continuous ECG monitoring. The pacing artifact is the spike that is seen on the ECG tracing as the pacing stimulus is delivered to the heart. A *P wave* is visible after the pacing artifact if the atrium is being paced (Fig. 16-4A). Similarly, a *QRS complex* follows a ventricular pacing artifact (see Fig. 16-4B). With dual-chamber pacing, a pacing artifact precedes both the P wave and the QRS complex (see Fig. 16-4C).

Not all paced beats look alike. For example, the artifact (spike) produced by a unipolar pacing electrode is larger than that produced by a bipolar lead (Fig. 16-5). The QRS complex of paced beats appears different, depending on the location of the pacing electrode. If the pacing electrode is positioned in the RV, a left bundle branch block (LBBB) pattern is displayed on the ECG. A right bundle branch block (RBBB) pattern is visible if the pacing stimulus originates from the left ventricle (LV).

Pacemaker Malfunctions

Most pacemaker malfunctions can be categorized as abnormalities of pacing or of sensing. Problems with pacing can involve failure of the pacemaker to deliver the pacing stimulus, a pacing

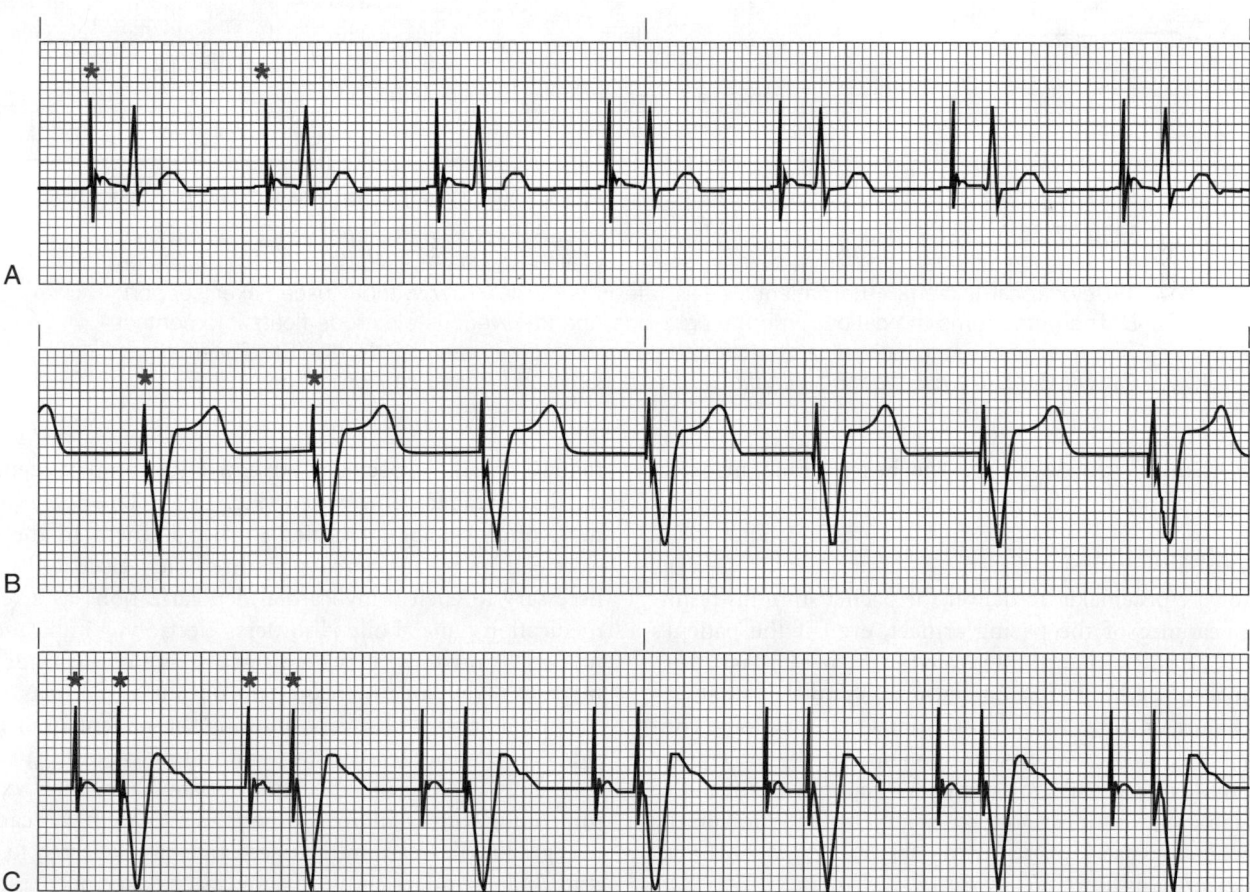

FIGURE 16-4 Pacing examples. *A*, Atrial pacing. *B*, Ventricular pacing. *C*, Dual-chamber pacing. Each asterisk represents a pacemaker impulse.

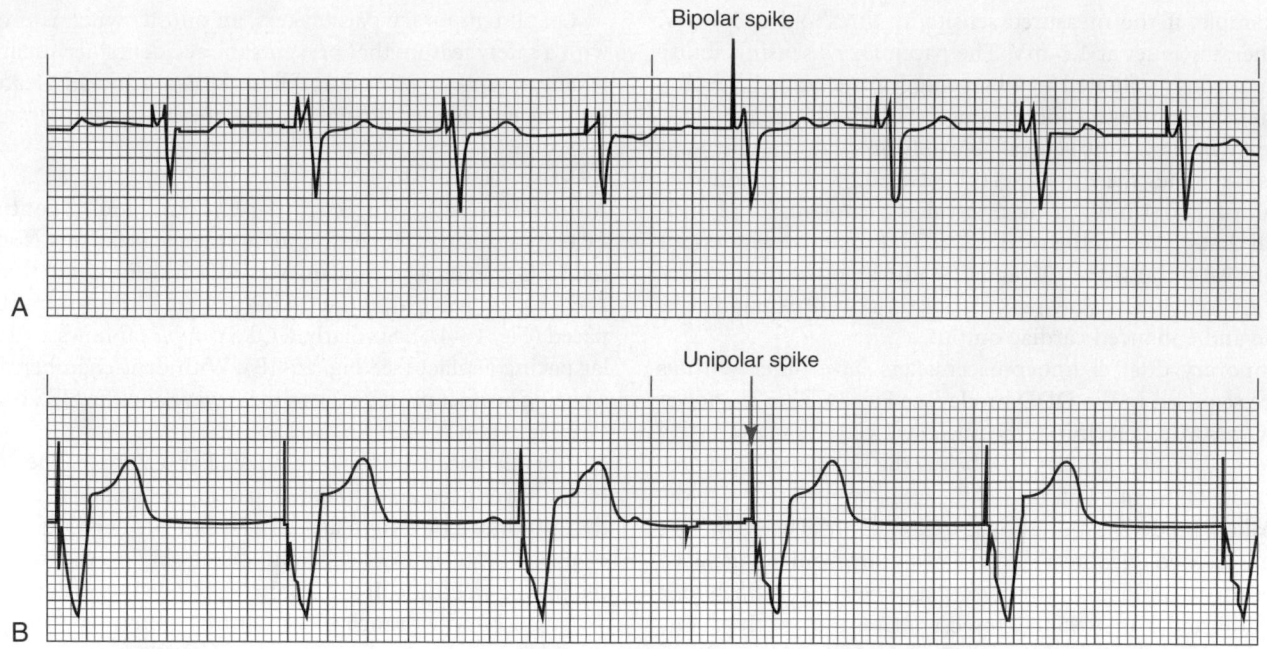

Bipolar spike

Unipolar spike

A

B

FIGURE 16-5   Bipolar and unipolar pacing. *A,* Bipolar pacing artifact. *B,* Unipolar pacing artifact. (Modified from Conover MB. *Understanding Electrocardiography.* 8th ed. St. Louis: Mosby; 2003.)

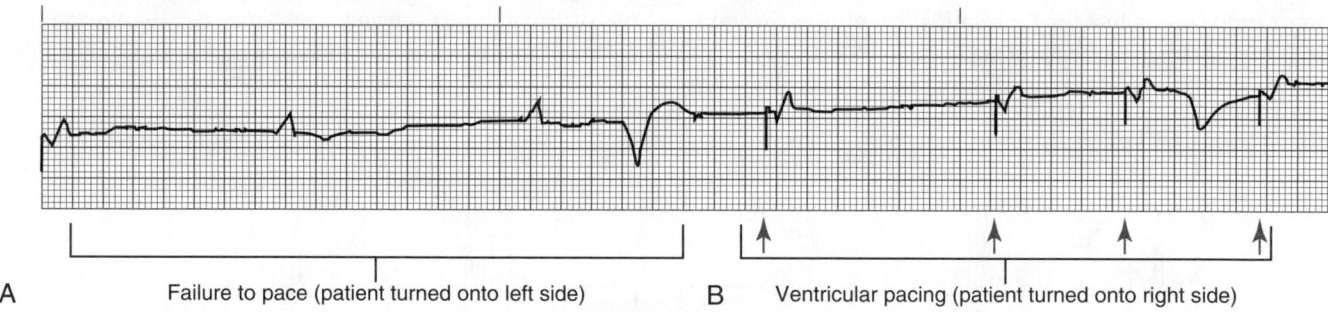

A   Failure to pace (patient turned onto left side)   B   Ventricular pacing (patient turned onto right side)

FIGURE 16-6   Pacemaker malfunction: failure to pace. *A,* Patient with a transvenous pacemaker is turned onto the left side. Immediately, there is a failure to pace (i.e., loss of pacer artifacts on the electrocardiogram). The patient's heart rate is extremely low without pacemaker support. *B,* The nurse turns the patient onto the right side, the transvenous electrode floats into contact with the right ventricular wall, and pacing is resumed. (From Kesten KS, Norton CK. *Pacemakers: Patient Care, Troubleshooting, Rhythm Analysis.* Baltimore: Resource Applications; 1985.)

stimulus that fails to depolarize the heart, or an incorrect number of pacing stimuli per minute.

Pacing Abnormalities

Failure of the pacemaker to deliver the pacing stimulus results in disappearance of the pacing artifact, even if the patient's intrinsic rate is less than the set rate on the pacer (Fig. 16-6). This can occur intermittently or continuously and can be attributed to failure of the pulse generator or its battery, a loose connection between the various components of the pacemaker system, broken lead wires, or stimulus inhibition as a result of EMI. Tightening connections, replacing the batteries or the pulse generator itself, or removing the source of EMI may restore pacemaker function.

If the pacing stimulus fires but fails to initiate a myocardial depolarization, a pacing artifact will be present but will not be

followed by the expected P wave or QRS complex, depending on the chamber being paced (Fig. 16-7). This *loss of capture* most often can be attributed to displacement of the pacing electrode or to an increase in threshold (electrical stimulus necessary to elicit a myocardial depolarization) as a result of medications, metabolic disorders, electrolyte imbalances, or fibrosis or myocardial ischemia at the site of electrode placement. In many cases, increasing the output (mA) elicits capture. For transvenous leads, repositioning the patient onto the left side may improve lead contact and restore capture.

Pacing can occur at inappropriate rates. For example, impending battery failure in a permanent pacemaker can result in a gradual decrease in the paced rate, also referred to as *rate drift.* Inappropriate stimuli from a pacemaker may result in a pacemaker-mediated tachycardia. This usually is caused by sensing of inappropriate signals in a dual-chamber pacemaker

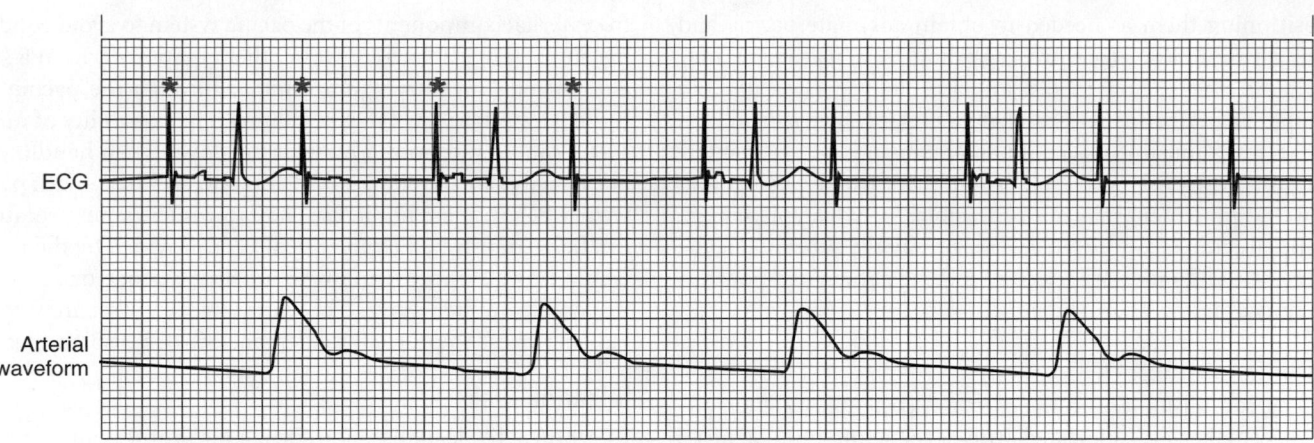

FIGURE 16-7 Pacemaker malfunction: failure to capture. Atrial pacing and capture occur after pacer spikes 1, 3, 5, and 7. The remaining pacer spikes fail to capture the tissue, resulting in loss of the P wave, no conduction to the ventricles, and no arterial waveform. Each asterisk represents a pacemaker impulse.

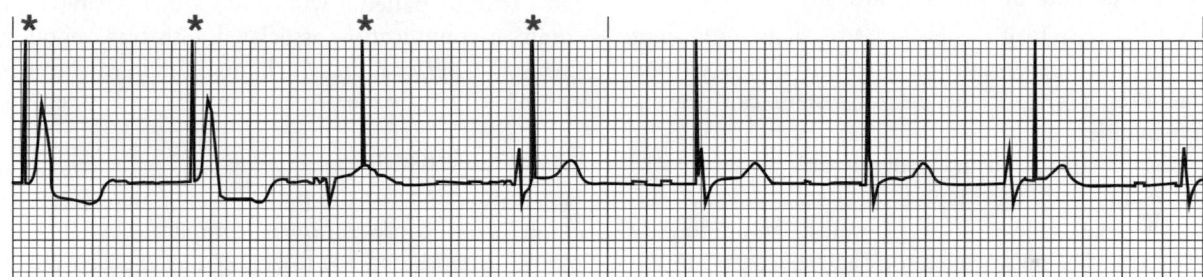

FIGURE 16-8 Pacemaker malfunction: undersensing. After the first two paced beats, a series of intrinsic beats occur; the pacemaker unit fails to sense these intrinsic QRS complexes. These spikes do not capture the ventricle because they occur during the refractory period of the cardiac cycle. Each *asterisk* represents a pacemaker impulse.

that is in a trigger mode, such as DDD. The tachycardia can be terminated by placing a magnet over the generator to transiently suspend sensing.[11]

Sensing Abnormalities

Sensing abnormalities include both undersensing and oversensing.

Undersensing. Undersensing is the inability of the pacemaker to sense spontaneous myocardial depolarizations. Undersensing results in competition between paced complexes and the heart's intrinsic rhythm. This malfunction is manifested on the ECG by pacing artifacts that occur after or are unrelated to spontaneous complexes (Fig. 16-8). Undersensing can result in the delivery of pacing stimuli into a relative refractory period of the cardiac depolarization cycle (see Fig. 12-25 in Chapter 12). A ventricular pacing stimulus delivered into the downslope of the T wave (R-on-T phenomenon) is a real danger with this type of pacer aberration, because it may precipitate a lethal dysrhythmia. The nurse must act quickly to determine the cause and initiate appropriate interventions. Often, the cause can be attributed to inadequate wave amplitude (height of the P or R wave). If this is the case, the situation can be promptly remedied by increasing the sensitivity by moving the sensitivity dial toward its lowest setting. Other possible causes include

inappropriate (asynchronous) mode selection, lead displacement or fracture, loose cable connections, and pulse generator failure.

Oversensing. Oversensing occurs as a result of inappropriate sensing of extraneous electrical signals that leads to unnecessary triggering or inhibition of stimulus output, depending on the pacer mode. The source of these electrical signals can range from tall peaked T waves to EMI in the critical care environment. Because most temporary pulse generators are programmed in demand modes, oversensing results in unexplained pauses in the ECG tracing as the extraneous signals are sensed and inhibit pacing. Often, moving the sensitivity dial toward 20 mV (less sensitive) stops the pauses. With permanent pacemakers, a magnet may be placed over the generator to restore pacing in an asynchronous mode until appropriate changes in the generator settings can be programmed.

Medical Management

The physician determines the pacing route based on the patient's clinical situation. Transcutaneous pacing typically is used in emergent situations until a transvenous lead can be secured. If the patient is undergoing heart surgery, epicardial leads may be electively placed at the end of the operation. The physician places the transvenous or epicardial pacing lead or leads, repositioning them as needed to obtain adequate pacing and sensing thresholds. Decisions regarding lead placement may later limit the pacing modes available to the clinician. For example, to perform dual-chamber pacing, both atrial and ventricular leads must be placed. In an emergency, however, interventions are focused on establishing ventricular pacing, and atrial lead placement may not be feasible. After lead placement, the initial settings for output and sensitivity are determined, the pacing rate and mode are selected, and the patient's response to pacing is evaluated.

Nursing Management

Nursing responsibilities in the care of a patient with a temporary pacemaker are associated with several nursing diagnoses and can be combined into four primary areas: assessment and prevention of pacemaker malfunction, protection against microshock, surveillance for complications such as infection, and patient education.

Prevention of Pacemaker Malfunction

Continuous ECG monitoring is essential to facilitate prompt recognition of and appropriate intervention for pacemaker malfunction. Proper care of the pacing system can prevent pacing abnormalities.

The temporary pacing lead and bridging cable must be properly secured to the body with tape to prevent accidental displacement of the electrode, which can result in failure to pace or sense. The external pulse generator can be secured to the patient's waist with a strap or placed in a telemetry bag for the mobile patient. If the patient is on a regimen of bed rest, the pulse generator can be suspended with twill tape from an IV pole mounted overhead on the ceiling. This prevents tension on the lead while the patient is moved (given adequate length of bridging cable) and alleviates the possibility of accidental dropping of the pulse generator.

The nurse inspects for loose connections between the leads and pulse generator on a regular basis. Replacement batteries and pulse generators must always be available on the unit. Although the battery has an anticipated life span of 1 month, it probably is sound practice to change the battery if the pacemaker has been operating continually for several days. Newer generators provide a low-battery signal 24 hours before complete loss of battery function occurs to prevent inadvertent interruptions in pacing. The pulse generator must always be labeled with the date on which the battery was replaced.

It is important to be aware of all sources of EMI within the critical care environment that may interfere with the pacemaker's function. Sources of EMI in the clinical area include electrocautery, defibrillation current, radiation therapy, magnetic resonance imaging devices, and transcutaneous electrical nerve stimulation (TENS) units.[12] In most cases, if EMI is suspected of precipitating pacemaker malfunction, conversion to the asynchronous mode (fixed rate) can maintain pacing until the cause of the EMI is removed.

Microshock Protection

Because the pacing electrode provides a direct, low-resistance path to the heart, the nurse takes special care while handling the external components of the pacing system to avoid conducting stray electrical current from other equipment. Even a small amount of stray current transmitted through the pacing lead could precipitate a lethal dysrhythmia. The possibility of microshock can be minimized by wearing gloves when handling the pacing wires and by proper insulation of terminal pins of pacing wires when they are not in use (Box 16-6). The latter precaution can be accomplished by the use of caps provided by the manufacturer or by improvising with a plastic syringe or section of disposable rubber glove. The wires are taped securely to the patient's chest to prevent accidental electrode displacement.

Infection Risk

Infection at the lead insertion site is a rare but serious complication associated with temporary pacemakers. The site is carefully inspected for purulent drainage, erythema, and edema, and the patient is observed for signs of systemic infection. Site care is performed according to the institution's policies and procedures. Although most infections remain localized, endocarditis can occur in patients with endocardial pacing leads. A less common complication associated with transvenous pacing is myocardial perforation, which can result in rhythmic hiccoughs or cardiac tamponade.

Patient Education

Patient teaching for the person with a temporary pacemaker emphasizes the prevention of complications (Box 16-7). The patient is instructed not to handle any exposed portion of the lead wire and to notify the nurse if the dressing over the insertion site becomes soiled, wet, or dislodged. The patient also is advised not to use any electrical devices brought in from home that could interfere with pacemaker functioning. Patients with temporary transvenous pacemakers need to be taught to

---

⚡ **BOX 16-6** **PATIENT SAFETY ALERT**

Prevention of Microshock

QSEN
- Wear gloves when handling pacing wires
- Secure all connections between pulse generator, pacing cable, and leads
- Insulate lead tips with nonconducting materials when not attached to generator (manufacturer's cap, finger cot, plastic syringe)
- Keep dressings and pacing equipment dry
- Make sure all electrical equipment is properly grounded
- Use battery-operated shavers

BOX 16-7 **PATIENT EDUCATION**

Temporary Pacemaker

- Description of pacemaker therapy
- Care of the pacemaker system
  Minimize handling of leads or cables
  Notify nurse if dressing becomes wet or loose
- Activity restrictions (minimize upper-extremity movement with transvenous leads)
- Electrical safety precautions (no electric razors)
- Symptoms to report (dizziness)

TABLE 16-3 PERMANENT PACEMAKER RATE-RESPONSE PACING MODES

PULSE GENERATOR	DESCRIPTION
AAIR	AAI features plus rate-responsive pacing; used for patients with a symptomatic bradycardia who have a paceable atrium and intact atrioventricular conduction
VVIR	VVI features plus rate-responsive pacing; used for patients with an atrium that is unpaceable as a result of chronic atrial fibrillation or other atrial dysrhythmia
DDDR	DDD features plus rate-responsive pacing; used for patients with a symptomatic bradycardia in which the atrium is paceable but atrioventricular conduction is, or may become, unreliable

restrict movement of the affected extremity to prevent lead displacement.

Permanent Pacemakers

Almost 400,000 permanent pacemakers are implanted annually in the United States, and critical care nurses are likely to encounter these devices in their clinical practice.[13] These pacemakers were originally designed to provide an adequate ventricular rate in patients with symptomatic bradycardia. Today, the goal of pacemaker therapy is to simulate, as much as possible, normal physiologic cardiac depolarization and conduction. Sophisticated generators permit rate-responsive pacing, effecting responses to sensed atrial activity (DDD) or to a variety of physiologic sensors (body motion or minute ventilation). For patients who do not have a functional sinus node that can increase their heart rate, rate-responsive pacemakers may improve exercise capacity and quality of life.[14] Table 16-3 describes the types of rate-responsive pacing generators in clinical use. The concept of physiologic pacing continues to evolve, because studies have indicated that pacing initiated from the RV apex—even in a dual-chamber mode—may promote heart failure in patients with permanent pacemakers.[1] This has prompted further research to identify alternative sites for pacing and modes that can maximize intrinsic AV conduction and minimize ventricular pacing.[15]

The patient who undergoes implantation of a permanent pacemaker is usually in the hospital for less than 24 hours. Longer lengths of stay are expected for patients with serious complications such as MI or cardiogenic shock. Technologic advances in the computer industry have had a major impact on permanent pacemakers. Microprocessors have allowed for the development of increasingly smaller generators despite the incorporation of more complex features. Today's generators are smaller, more energy-efficient, and more reliable than previous models. The most recent enhancement has been the release of a pacemaker that is compatible with magnetic resonance imaging (MRI).[16] An example of a modern pacemaker is shown in Figure 16-9. A rapidly expanding role for permanent pacemakers has been the use of these devices as a type of nonpharmacologic therapy for treatment of conditions such as heart failure and atrial fibrillation.

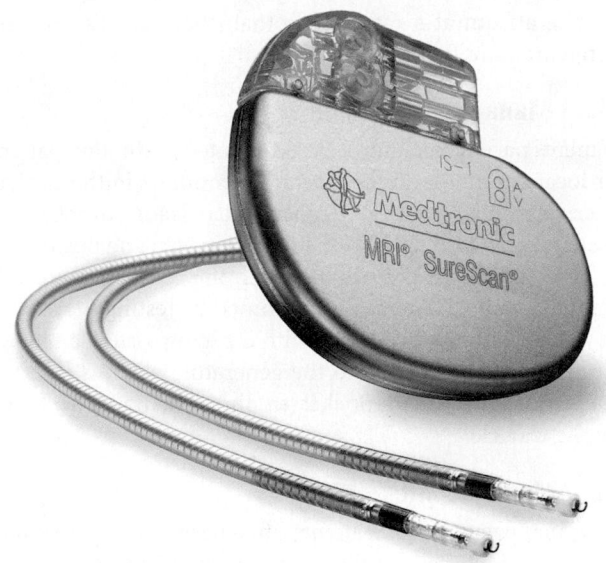

FIGURE 16-9 A permanent pacemaker (Medtronic Revo MRI™ SureScan®). (Reproduced with permission of Medtronic, Inc.)

Cardiac Resynchronization Therapy

About one third of patients with severe heart failure have ventricular conduction delays (prolonged QRS duration or bundle branch block). These conduction delays have been shown to create a lack of synchrony between the contractions of the LV and RV. The hemodynamic consequences of this dyssynchrony include impaired ventricular filling with decreased ejection fraction, cardiac output, and mean arterial pressure.[17] Cardiac resynchronization therapy (CRT) uses atrial pacing plus stimulation of both the LV and RV (biventricular pacing), in an attempt to optimize atrial and ventricular mechanical activity. The CRT device uses three pacing leads, one each in the right atrium and the RV and a specially designed transvenous lead that is inserted through the coronary sinus to pace the LV.[18] Because many patients with heart failure are also at risk for sudden cardiac death, biventricular pacing is available on some implantable cardioverter defibrillators (ICDs). A number of clinical trials have shown that CRT improves symptoms, functional status, and mortality in patients with moderate to advanced heart failure.[18] New research indicates that CRT may also be beneficial in preventing the progression of heart failure in less symptomatic patients.[19]

Atrial Fibrillation Suppression

There is a growing incidence of atrial fibrillation, and atrial pacing has been proposed as a possible preventive therapy for this dysrhythmia in selected patients. Atrial pacing in patients with bradycardia has been shown to lower the recurrence of atrial fibrillation, especially compared with ventricular pacing. Atrial-based modes that promote intrinsic conduction and minimize episodes of ventricular pacing are most effective.[1] Most pacemakers can be programmed to *mode switch* to a non–P-wave tracking mode if rapid atrial rates are sensed.[20] Strategies for patients with paroxysmal atrial fibrillation, which include pacing both atriums (bi-atrial pacing) and transiently pacing the atrium at a rate higher than the patient's intrinsic sinus rate, require further study.[1]

Medical Management

Permanent pacemakers may be implanted with the patient under local anesthesia in the operating room or in the cardiac catheterization laboratory. Transvenous leads usually are inserted through the cephalic or subclavian vein and positioned in the right atrium or RV, or both, with fluoroscopic guidance. Satisfactory lead placement is determined by testing the stimulation and sensitivity thresholds with a pacing system analyzer. The leads are then attached to the generator, which is inserted into a surgically created pocket in the subcutaneous tissue below the clavicle.

Nursing Management

Nursing management for patients after permanent pacemaker implantation includes monitoring for complications related to insertion and for pacemaker malfunction. Postoperative complications are rare but include cardiac perforation and tamponade, pneumothorax, hematoma, lead displacement, and infection.[20,21]

Identification of permanent pacemaker malfunction is the same as that described previously for temporary pacemakers. To evaluate pacemaker function, the nurse must know at least the pacemaker's programmed mode of pacing and the lower rate setting. With permanent pacemakers, settings are adjusted noninvasively through a specialized programmer that uses pulsed magnetic fields or an RF signal. If a pacemaker problem is suspected, ECG strips are obtained, and the physician is notified so that the pacemaker settings can be reprogrammed as needed. If the patient experiences symptoms of decreased cardiac output, he or she may require support with temporary transcutaneous pacing until the problem is corrected.

Critical care nurses also may be involved in monitoring patients with permanent pacemakers after discharge. Some units are equipped with transtelephonic monitoring equipment that allows patients to transmit information over the telephone from a monitoring device in their home. Transmission of the patient's ECG can provide information to confirm proper pacemaker function (capture and sensing) and to determine battery status (rate). Newer technology that uses an Internet-based remote monitoring system for pacemaker follow-up offers significant advantages and may soon replace standard transtelephonic ECG evaluation.[22]

The foregoing discussion provides an introduction to the basic concepts of pacemaker therapy. However, the nurse who cares for patients with permanent or temporary pacemakers must be familiar with ever more sophisticated modes of pacemaker function. Only by keeping pace with current technology can the nurse accurately interpret pacer function and thereby safely and effectively care for patients with pacemakers.

IMPLANTABLE CARDIOVERTER DEFIBRILLATORS

An implantable cardioverter defibrillator (ICD) is an electronic device that is used in the treatment of tachydysrhythmias. The ICD is capable of identifying and terminating life-threatening ventricular dysrhythmias. Initially, an ICD was recommended only for patients who had survived an episode of cardiac arrest caused by ventricular fibrillation (VF) or ventricular tachycardia (VT). As clinical trials found improved survival with ICD therapy when compared to treatment with antidysrhythmic medications, ICD use was expanded to include primary prevention of sudden cardiac death.[23] Current heart failure guidelines recommend ICD implantation in high-risk patients (i.e., those with a left ventricular ejection fraction less than 35%) even without evidence of VT or VF on an EPS.[24] This expanded use of ICDs has resulted in over 100,000 implants per year in the United States.[13]

The ICD System

The ICD system consists of leads and a generator and is similar to a pacemaker but with some key differences. The leads contain not only electrodes for sensing and pacing, but also integrated defibrillator coils capable of delivering a shock. The generator is larger, to accommodate a more powerful battery and a high-voltage capacitor, along with the microprocessor.[25] It is surgically placed in the subcutaneous tissue of the pectoral region in the upper chest (Fig. 16-10). The early model generators could defibrillate or cardiovert only lethal dysrhythmias. The current generation of devices delivers a tiered therapy, with options for programmable antitachycardia pacing, bradycardia backup pacing, low-energy cardioversion, and high-energy defibrillation. With tiered therapy, antitachycardia pacing is used as the first line of treatment in some cases of VT. If the VT can be pace-terminated successfully, the patient will not receive a shock from the generator and may not even realize that the ICD terminated the dysrhythmia. If programmed bursts of pacing do not terminate the VT, the ICD will cardiovert the rhythm. If the dysrhythmia deteriorates into VF, the ICD is programmed to defibrillate at a higher energy. If the dysrhythmia terminates spontaneously, the device will not discharge. Occasionally, the electrical rhythm may deteriorate to asystole or a slow idioventricular rhythm; in such cases, the bradycardia backup pacing function is activated.

Product development for ICDs has resulted in dual-chamber devices with leads in both atria and ventricles. The introduction of atrial leads allows for dual-chamber pacing to optimize hemodynamic performance and atrial sensing to more accurately discriminate between atrial and ventricular tachycardias and to decrease the incidence of inappropriate shocks. ICDs may also incorporate triple-lead systems (leads in one atrium and both ventricles) to allow for CRT and defibrillation in one device. Other developments in ICD technology include improved diagnostic and telemetry functions, such as the ability to provide real-time electrograms obtained from the ICD electrodes or the ability to perform remote device interrogation by telephone or Internet.[25]

Insertion of ICD

The ICD has progressed in both programmable functions and insertion technique. Initially, all ICDs were implanted surgically during open heart surgery or via thoracotomy, with electrode patches attached directly to the heart. Today's smaller

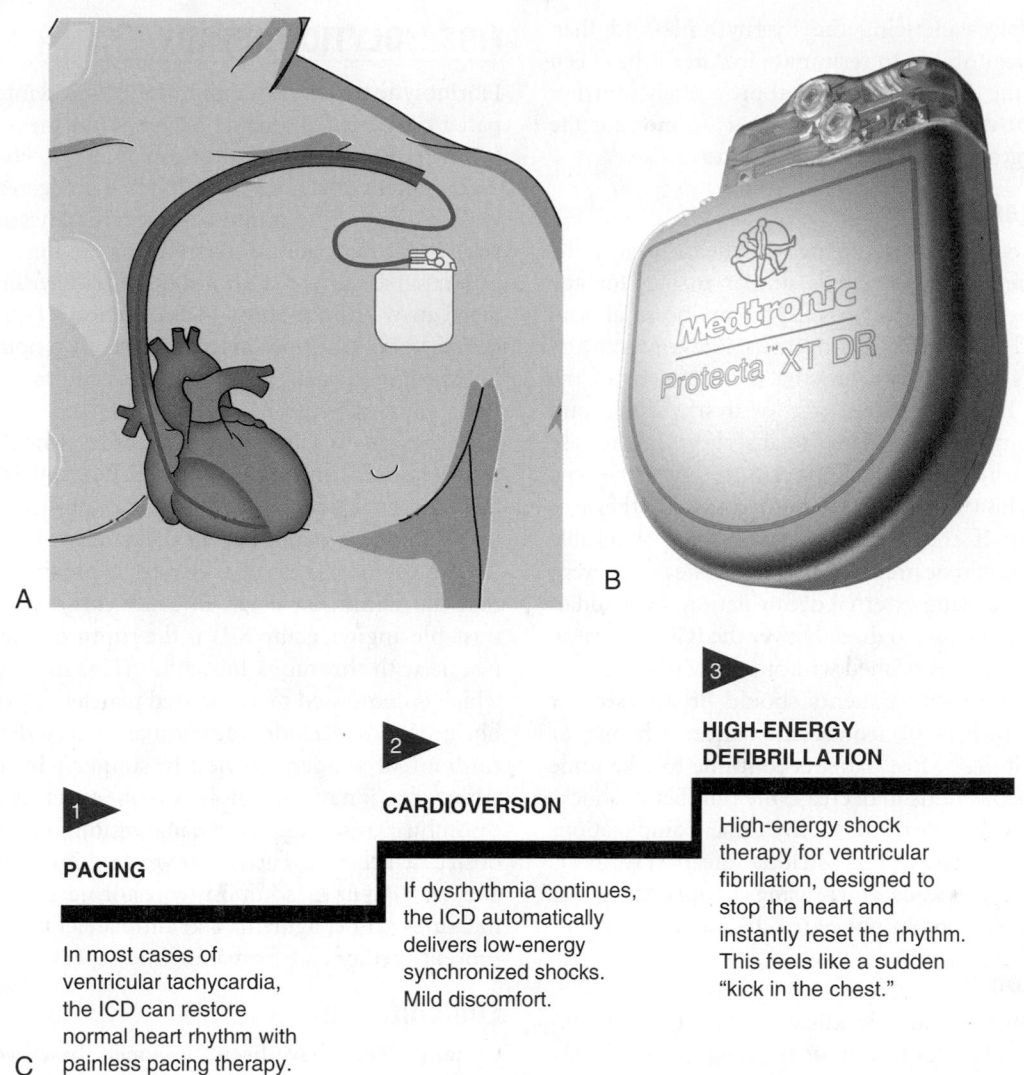

A

B

3
HIGH-ENERGY DEFIBRILLATION

2
CARDIOVERSION

1
PACING

In most cases of ventricular tachycardia, the ICD can restore normal heart rhythm with painless pacing therapy.

If dysrhythmia continues, the ICD automatically delivers low-energy synchronized shocks. Mild discomfort.

High-energy shock therapy for ventricular fibrillation, designed to stop the heart and instantly reset the rhythm. This feels like a sudden "kick in the chest."

C

FIGURE 16-10 Placement of an implantable cardioverter defibrillator (ICD) with a transvenous lead system. *A,* The generator is placed in a subcutaneous "pocket" in the pectoral region. The pacing, cardioversion, and defibrillation functions are all contained in a lead (or leads) inserted into the right atrium and ventricle. *B,* An example of a dual-chamber ICD (Medtronic Gem II DR) with tiered therapy and pacing capabilities. *C,* Tiered therapy is designed to use increasing levels of intensity to terminate ventricular dysrhythmias. (*B,* Reproduced with permission of Medtronic, Inc.)

generators, combined with the use of transvenous leads, obviate the need for major surgery. Transvenous electrode leads are inserted into the subclavian vein and advanced into the right side of the heart, where contact with the endocardium is achieved. To improve defibrillation efficacy, an additional subcutaneous patch may be placed with some models. The endocardial leads are connected to the generator by tunneling through the subcutaneous tissue, and thoracotomy is avoided. Procedural complications are infrequent but may include hematoma, pneumothorax, or lead dislodgement.[26]

Medical Management

Medical management in the ICD patient begins before implantation with a thorough evaluation of the patient's dysrhythmia and underlying cardiac function. A number of noninvasive studies are available to help identify patients at risk for sudden cardiac death, including signal-averaged ECG,

echocardiography, baroreceptor sensitivity testing, and heart rate variability studies. Typically, patients identified as being at risk for sudden cardiac death undergo an EPS to determine the origin of the dysrhythmia and the effect of antidysrhythmic agents in suppressing or altering the rate of the dysrhythmia. Further assessment of cardiac status is made to determine whether additional interventions (e.g., revascularization, cardiac resynchronization therapy) are indicated to improve cardiac function. This part of the workup may include cardiac catheterization, stress testing, and echocardiography. Based on the evaluation, decisions are made regarding the implantation approach (e.g., thoracotomy at the time of surgery, nonthoracotomy) and the type of therapy required (e.g., antitachycardia pacing, cardioversion, defibrillation).

An electrophysiologist performs the initial programming of the device at the time of implantation. During implantation, defibrillation threshold testing is performed to test device integrity. This involves inducing the dysrhythmia and then evaluating the device's ability to terminate it. After it has been determined that the ICD functions appropriately, further follow-up is conducted on an outpatient basis to monitor the number of discharges and the battery life of the device.

Nursing Management

If the ICD system was implanted during open heart surgery, the postoperative nursing management is similar to that for any patient undergoing cardiac surgery. If an endocardial lead system is implanted, the nursing management is less intense and the hospital stay is shorter. The nursing management of the patient with an ICD includes assessing for dysrhythmias and monitoring for complications related to insertion. In the case of a ventricular dysrhythmia, it is important to know the type of ICD implanted, how the device functions, and whether it is activated (i.e., on). If the patient experiences a shockable rhythm, the nurse should be prepared to defibrillate in the event that the device fails. During external defibrillation, the paddles or patches should not be placed directly over the ICD generator, as long as this can be accomplished without delay of defibrillation.[27] For recurring shocks, patients should be assessed for underlying causes, such as electrolyte imbalance, ischemia, or worsening heart failure.[25] Most patients continue to take some antidysrhythmic medications to decrease the number of shocks required and to slow the rate of the tachycardia. Complications associated with the permanent ICD include infection from the implanted system, broken leads, and sensing of supraventricular tachydysrhythmias resulting in unneeded discharges.

Patient Education

To facilitate a positive psychologic adjustment to the ICD, education of the patient and family about the device is vital (Box 16-8). Preoperative teaching for the ICD patient includes information about how the device works and what to expect during the implantation procedure. After implantation, education is focused on aspects of living with an ICD. Patients need information pertaining to scheduled device follow-up and instructions about what to do if they experience a shock. Many institutions have successfully used family support groups for this patient population. Finally, since the ICD is an adjunctive treatment rather than a for cure heart failure, patients need to understand the importance of continued risk-factor modification and prescribed medications.

BOX 16-8 PATIENT EDUCATION

Implantable Cardioverter Defibrillator

- Pathophysiology of the underlying disease process, including sudden cardiac death, ventricular dysrhythmias, and heart disease
- Information regarding how the implantable cardioverter defibrillator is programmed to function
- Actions to take if a shock occurs
- Importance of continuing antidysrhythmic and heart failure medications
- Activity limitations related to driving and avoiding strong magnetic fields
- Signs and symptoms of device failure
- Follow-up schedule with health care professional
- Cardiopulmonary resuscitation (CPR) training for family members

---

FIBRINOLYTIC THERAPY

Fibrinolytic therapy is an important clinical intervention for the patient experiencing acute ST-elevation myocardial infarction (STEMI). Before the introduction of fibrinolytic agents, medical management of acute MI was focused on decreasing myocardial oxygen demands to minimize myocardial necrosis and preserve ventricular function. Today, efforts to limit the size of the infarction are directed toward timely reperfusion of the jeopardized myocardium through restoration of blood flow in the culprit vessel (the open artery theory). Two options are available for opening the artery—fibrinolytics and mechanical intervention. Although mechanical catheter-based intervention has been proven to yield better outcomes when performed in a timely fashion, only one-third of U.S. hospitals are estimated to have this capability.[28] For this reason, fibrinolytic therapy continues to play a major role in the treatment of acute MI.

The use of fibrinolytic therapy is predicated on the theory that the significant event in acute coronary syndromes (e.g., unstable angina, acute MI) is the rupture of an atherosclerotic plaque with thrombus formation (Fig. 16-11). The thrombus, which is composed of aggregated platelets bound together with fibrin strands, occludes the coronary artery, depriving the myocardium of oxygen previously supplied by that artery. The administration of a fibrinolytic agent results in lysis of the acute thrombus, resulting in recanalization, or opening, of the obstructed coronary artery and restoration of blood flow to the affected tissue. In addition to restoring perfusion, adjunctive measures (anticoagulants and antiplatelet therapy) are taken to prevent further clot formation and repeat occlusion.

Eligibility Criteria

Certain criteria have been developed, based on research findings, to determine the patient population that would most likely benefit from the administration of fibrinolytic therapy. Patients with recent onset of chest pain (less than 12 hours' duration) and persistent ST elevation (greater than 0.1 mV in two or more contiguous leads) are considered candidates for fibrinolytic therapy.[29] Patients who present with bundle branch blocks that may obscure ST-segment analysis and a history suggesting an acute MI are also considered candidates for therapy (see "Myocardial Infarction" in Chapter 15). The goal of therapy is to administer fibrinolytic therapy within 30 minutes after presentation ("door to needle"), because early reperfusion yields the greatest benefit.[30]

Exclusion criteria are usually based on the increased risk of bleeding incurred from the use of fibrinolytics. Patients who have stable clots that might be disrupted by fibrinolytic therapy (recent surgery, facial or head trauma,) usually are not considered candidates for fibrinolytic therapy. Other common criteria for the use of fibrinolytic therapy are presented in Box 16-9.

Currently, fibrinolytic therapy is not indicated for patients with unstable angina or non–ST-elevation myocardial infarction (NSTEMIs).[31] It is believed that these conditions result from plaque rupture with the formation of an only partially occlusive thrombus. Fibrinolysis breaks up the clot and releases thrombin, and this can paradoxically increase the material necessary for further thrombosis.[32] Instead, these patients are

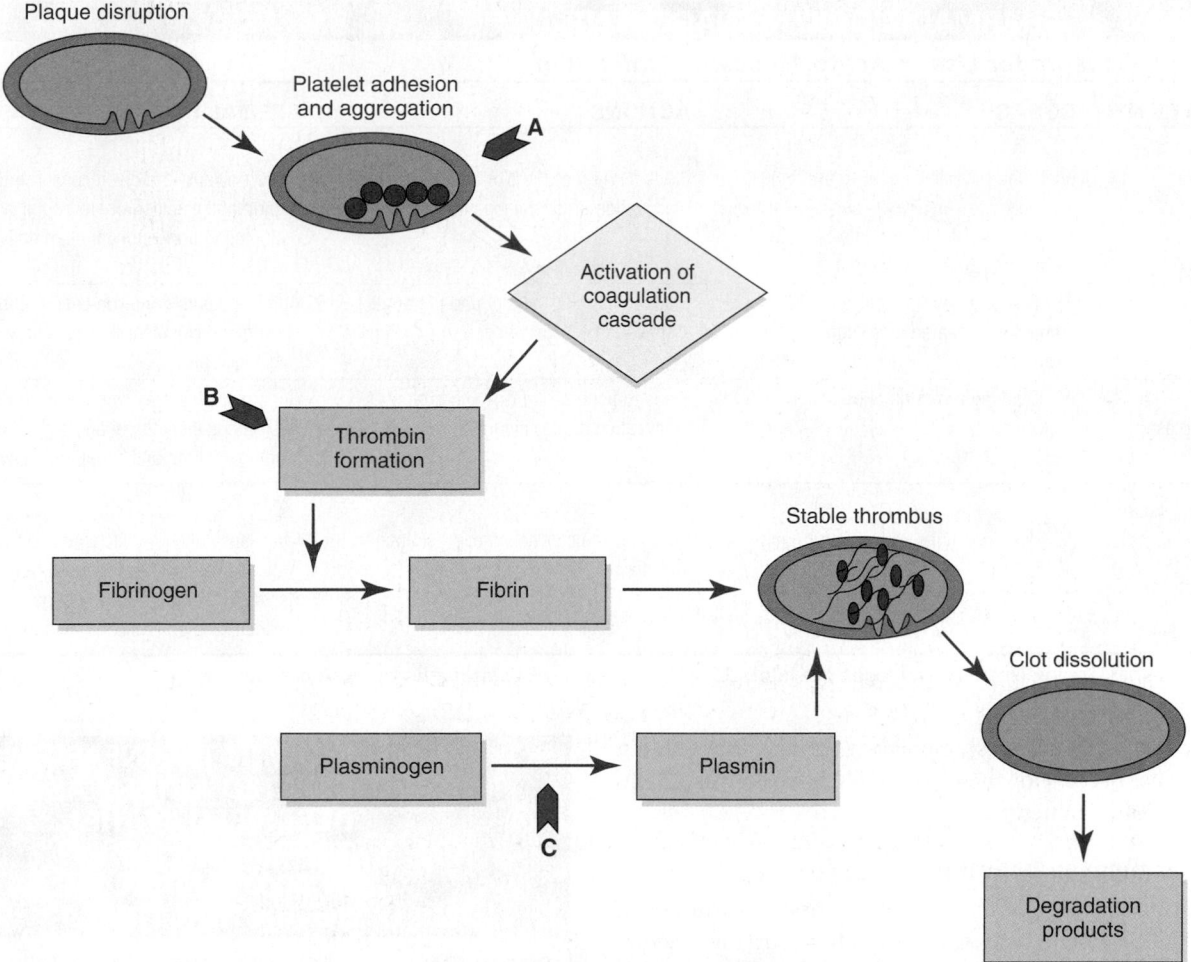

FIGURE 16-11 Thrombus formation and site of action of medications used in the treatment of acute myocardial infarction. *A*, Site of action of antiplatelet agents such as aspirin, thienopyridines, and glycoprotein IIb/IIIa inhibitors. *B*, Heparin bonds with antithrombin III and thrombin to create an inactive complex. *C*, Fibrinolytic agents convert plasminogen to plasmin, an enzyme responsible for degradation of fibrin clots.

BOX 16-9 **FIBRINOLYTIC THERAPY SELECTION CRITERIA**

- No more than 12 hours from onset of chest pain and preferably within 30 minutes of STEMI diagnosis
- ST-segment elevation on electrocardiogram or new-onset left bundle branch block
- Ischemic chest pain unresponsive to sublingual nitroglycerin
- No conditions that might cause a predisposition to hemorrhage

---

treated with antiplatelet agents (e.g., aspirin, clopidogrel, glycoprotein IIb/IIIa inhibitors) and antithrombin medications (e.g., heparin).

Fibrinolytic Agents

Four fibrinolytic agents are currently available for intravenous treatment of acute STEMI. All of these agents stimulate lysis of the clot by converting inactive plasminogen to plasmin, an enzyme responsible for degradation of fibrin (see Fig. 16-11). The first generation fibrinolytic agents (e.g., streptokinase, urokinase) had their primary effect on circulating plasminogen. Newer fibrinolytic agents (e.g., alteplase, reteplase, tenecteplase)

have a greater effect on clot plasminogen than on circulating plasminogen and are therefore considered clot selective. A comparison of currently approved fibrinolytic agents is provided in Table 16-4. Because patients with an area of plaque disruption are still at risk for clot formation and reocclusion, fibrinolytic therapy is used in conjunction with anticoagulants and antiplatelet agents. Current guidelines recommend that anticoagulant therapy be administered for a minimum of 48 hours after reperfusion. Unfractionated heparin (UFH) has been used traditionally, but low–molecular-weight heparin (LMWH) and fondaparinux are also acceptable options.[33] Antiplatelet therapy with clopidogrel is recommended for 14 days, and aspirin should be continued indefinitely.[30]

Streptokinase

Streptokinase (SK) is a fibrinolytic agent derived from beta-hemolytic streptococci, which, when combined with plasminogen, catalyzes the conversion of plasminogen to plasmin, the enzyme responsible for clot dissolution in the body. Because SK is a bacterial protein, it can produce a variety of allergic reactions, including anaphylaxis. In addition the fibrinolytic action of SK is systemic (non-clot specific) and prolonged

TABLE 16-4 PHARMACOLOGIC MANAGEMENT
Fibrinolytic Agents for Use in Acute Myocardial Infarction

MEDICATION	DOSAGE	ACTIONS	SPECIAL CONSIDERATIONS
Clot-Specific			
tPA (alteplase)	IV: 100 mg over 90 min with the first 15 mg given as a bolus over 2 minutes (dose is adjusted based on weight for patients ≤67 kg)	Binds to fibrin at the clot and promotes activation of plasminogen to plasmin	Anticoagulants are given concurrently. Aspirin and clopidogrel are begun with administration and continued daily.
rPA (reteplase)	IV: 10 units given as a bolus over 2 minutes, repeated in 30 min	Binds to fibrin at the clot and promotes activation of plasminogen to plasmin	Anticoagulants are given concurrently. Aspirin and clopidogrel are begun with administration and continued daily.
TNKase (tenecteplase)	IV: 30-50 mg based on body weight, given as a single bolus	Binds to fibrin at the clot and promotes activation of plasminogen to plasmin	Anticoagulants are given concurrently. Aspirin and clopidogrel are begun with administration and continued daily.
Non–Clot-Specific			
SK (streptokinase)	IV: 1.5 million units given over 60 min	Catalyzes the conversion of plasminogen to plasmin, which causes lysis of fibrin; has systemic lytic effects	May cause allergic reactions and hypotension. Anticoagulants are given concurrently. Aspirin and clopidogrel are begun with administration and continued daily.

IV, Intravenous; *rPA*, recombinant plasminogen activator; *SQ*, subcutaneous; *tPA*, tissue plasminogen activator.

(half-life of 20 to 25 minutes), increasing the risk for bleeding complications. Because of these issues, SK is no longer widely used in the United States.

Tissue Plasminogen Activator

Marketed under the trade name Activase, tissue plasminogen activator (tPA), or alteplase, is a naturally occurring enzyme (i.e., nonantigenic) that is clot specific and has a very short half-life (3 to 4 minutes). It converts plasminogen to plasmin after binding to the fibrin-containing clot. This clot-specific action results in an increased concentration and activity of plasmin at the site of the clot, where it is needed. Several different intravenous dosing regimens have been proposed and tested in the clinical setting, but accelerated-dose tPA is considered most effective means of establishing early patency of the occluded vessel.[34]

Recombinant Plasminogen Activator

Recombinant plasminogen activator (rPA), or reteplase, is a variant of the natural human enzyme tPA. Reteplase is less fibrin selective and has a longer half-life than tPA, making it suitable for bolus administration rather than as a continuous infusion. This new-generation plasminogen activator is given as a double bolus and then followed with adjunctive therapies. Unlike tPA, reteplase does not require weight-based dosing. Studies have shown that reteplase is as effective as tPA in the treatment of acute MI and is easier to administer.[34]

Tenecteplase

Tenecteplase (TNKase) is the newest of the fibrinolytic agents. It is a genetically engineered variant of alteplase with slower plasma clearance and better fibrin specificity. Studies have shown that TNKase is as effective as alteplase, with similar rates of bleeding complications between the two agents.[35] TNKase requires only a single bolus injection, which may help facilitate

BOX 16-10 FLOW IN THE INFARCT-RELATED ARTERY AS DESCRIBED IN THE THROMBOLYSIS IN MYOCARDIAL INFARCTION TRIAL

PERFUSION GRADES	FLOW IN THE INFARCT-RELATED ARTERY
TIMI 3	Normal or brisk flow through the coronary artery
TIMI 2	Partial flow, slower than in normal vessels
TIMI 1	Sluggish flow with incomplete distal filling
TIMI 0	No flow beyond the point of occlusion

Modified from The TIMI Study Group. The thrombolysis in myocardial infarction (TIMI) trial: phase I findings. *N Engl J Med.* 1985;312:932. *TIMI*, Thrombolysis in Myocardial Infarction Trial.

more rapid treatment both in and out of the hospital. Although the need for weight-based dosing is a potential disadvantage of this medication, TNKase is currently the most widely used fibrinolytic agent in the United States.[34]

Outcomes of Fibrinolytic Therapy

The benefit of fibrinolytic therapy correlates with the degree of restoration of normal blood flow in the infarct-related artery. Coronary artery patency is defined by angiographic perfusion grades developed by the Thrombolysis in Myocardial Infarction (TIMI) study group in 1985 (Box 16-10).[36] Achievement of TIMI grade 3 flow is associated with the best long-term survival. Studies also indicate that rapid restoration of normal blood flow, within 90 minutes after treatment, results in improved LV function and reduced mortality. The three fibrin-specific fibrinolytics have been shown to achieve TIMI 3 flow in 60% of patients at 90 minutes.[29] The area of fibrinolytic therapy continues to evolve, and medication dose ranges and regimens are subject to change when research findings are updated. Whereas fibrinolytic agents target the fibrin portion of the clot, other treatment strategies are focusing on the platelet portion of the clot (see Fig. 16-11). Oral antiplatelet agents (aspirin or clopidogrel) are administered in conjunction with fibrinolytics. The effectiveness of combining intravenous antiplatelet agents (glycoprotein IIb/IIIa receptor antagonists) with a lower dose of a fibrinolytic has been evaluated in clinical trials. Combination therapy provided reperfusion rates equivalent to those obtained with a fibrinolytic alone, but was associated with an increased risk of bleeding.[34] There was speculation that a planned strategy for administering fibrinolytics or glycoprotein IIb/IIIa receptor antagonists, or both, to patients who must be transported to another facility for percutaneous intervention would improve outcomes. Although promising in theory, this facilitated "upstream" approach to revascularization may increase the risk for bleeding complications in some patients.[37]

Evidence of Reperfusion

Several phenomena may be observed after the reperfusion of an artery that has been completely occluded by a thrombus (Box 16-11). While recognition of these noninvasive markers of recanalization is important for assessing the patient's response to fibrinolytic therapy, they are less reliable than angiography in determining whether reperfusion has been successful.

Pain and Reperfusion Dysrhythmias

One possible sign of reperfusion is the abrupt cessation of chest pain as blood flow is restored to the ischemic myocardium. Another potential indicator of reperfusion is the appearance of various "reperfusion dysrhythmias." A variety of dysrhythmias can occur—premature ventricular contractions (PVCs), bradycardias, heart block, VT—but accelerated idioventricular rhythms have shown the best correlation with reperfusion.[35] Reperfusion dysrhythmias are usually self-limiting or nonsustained, and aggressive antidysrhythmic therapy is not required. However, vigilant monitoring of the patient's ECG is essential, because a stable condition can deteriorate rapidly and the dysrhythmias may necessitate emergency treatment.

ST Segment

Another noninvasive marker of recanalization is rapid return to baseline of the elevated ST segments, which indicates restoration of blood flow to previously ischemic myocardial tissue. A monitoring lead should be chosen that clearly demonstrates ST elevation before initiation of therapy[38] (see "Continuous ST-Segment Monitoring" in Chapter 14). The inability to achieve 50% resolution of the ST elevation within 60 minutes of administering the medication is generally considered criteria for failure of fibrinolytic therapy.[35]

Cardiac Biomarkers

Serial measurement of serum biomarkers may serve as further evidence of successful reperfusion following fibrinolytics. Cardiac specific creatine kinase and troponin rise rapidly and then decrease markedly after reperfusion of the ischemic myocardium. This phenomenon is called *washout*, because it is thought to result from the rapid readmission of substances released by damaged myocardial cells into the circulation after restoration of blood flow (see "Cardiac Biomarkers" in Chapter 14).

Residual Coronary Artery Stenosis

Fibrinolytic therapy has been determined to be a successful strategy for reopening occluded coronary arteries in the setting of acute MI. It limits infarct size, salvaging myocardium and significantly reducing morbidity and mortality associated with cardiogenic shock and VF. However, residual coronary artery stenosis resulting from the atherosclerotic process remains, even after successful fibrinolysis. Subsequent prevention of reocclusion is critical to preserving myocardial function and preventing the risk of late complications. Fibrinolytic therapy is therefore recognized as an emergency procedure to restore patency until more definitive therapy can be initiated to effectively reduce the degree of stenosis (an interventional catheter procedure) or to bypass the offending occlusion (coronary artery bypass grafting [CABG]).

Nursing Management

Nursing management of the patient undergoing fibrinolytic therapy begins with identifying potential candidates. In many institutions, checklists are used to facilitate the rapid identification of patients who are candidates for fibrinolytics. The nurse prepares the patient for fibrinolytic therapy by starting intravenous lines and obtaining baseline laboratory values and vital signs. Throughout the administration of the fibrinolytic agent, assessment of the patient continues for clinical indicators of reperfusion and complications related to therapy. Several nursing diagnoses are linked to management of the patient receiving fibrinolytic therapy (Box 16-12).

The most common complication related to thrombolysis is bleeding, from the fibrinolytic therapy itself and also because the patients routinely receive anticoagulation therapy to minimize the possibility of rethrombosis. The nurse must continually monitor for clinical manifestations of bleeding (Box 16-13). Mild gingival bleeding and oozing around venipuncture sites is common and not a cause of concern. Should serious bleeding

---

BOX 16-11 NONINVASIVE EVIDENCE OF REPERFUSION

- Cessation of chest pain
- Reperfusion dysrhythmias, primarily ventricular
- Return of elevated ST segments to baseline
- Early and marked peaking of creatine kinase and troponins

◎ BOX 16-12 NURSING DIAGNOSES

Fibrinolytic Therapy

- Risk for Decreased Cardiac Tissue Perfusion, p. 1155
- Acute Pain related to transmission and perception of cutaneous, visceral, muscular, or ischemic impulses, p. 1123
- Anxiety related to threat of biologic, psychological, or social integrity, p. 1125
- Deficient Fluid Volume related to absolute loss, p. 1132
- Deficient Knowledge related to lack of previous exposure to information, p. 1134 (see Box 16-14, Patient Education for Fibrinolytic Therapy)

BOX 16-13 SIGNS OF INADEQUATE HEMOSTASIS RELATED TO FIBRINOLYTIC THERAPY

- Bleeding or hematoma at puncture sites
- Hematuria, hematemesis, hemoptysis, melena, epistaxis
- Bruising or petechiae (pinpoint hemorrhages)
- Flank ecchymoses with complaints of low back pain (suggestive of retroperitoneal bleeding)
- Gingival bleeding
- Change in neurologic status (intracranial bleeding)
- Deterioration in vital signs, decreased hematocrit values (internal bleeding)

BOX 16-14 PATIENT EDUCATION

Fibrinolytic Therapy

- Pathophysiology of atherosclerosis
- Risk-factor management
- Description of fibrinolytic agent and how it works
- Measures to minimize bleeding and bruising associated with fibrinolytic therapy
- Recognition and actions to take for recurrent ischemic symptoms
- Information regarding prescribed medications (antiplatelet agents, anticoagulants)

occur, such as intracranial or internal bleeding, all fibrinolytic and antithrombotic therapies are discontinued and volume expanders or coagulation factors, or both, are administered.

In addition to accurate assessment of the patient for evidence of bleeding, nursing management includes preventive measures to minimize the potential for bleeding. For example, patient handling is limited, injections are avoided if at all possible, and additional pressure is provided to ensure hemostasis at venipuncture and arterial puncture sites. Intravenous lines are placed before lytic therapy is administered, and a heparin lock may be used for obtaining laboratory specimens during treatment.

Patient Education

Education for the patient receiving fibrinolytic therapy includes information regarding the actions of fibrinolytic agents, with emphasis on precautions to minimize bleeding (Box 16-14). For example, the patient is cautioned against vigorous tooth brushing and told to refrain from using straight-edge razors. Information is provided regarding ongoing risk-factor management in the prevention of atherosclerotic CAD.

CATHETER INTERVENTIONS FOR CORONARY ARTERY DISEASE

During the past 3 decades, the use of catheter procedures to open coronary arteries blocked or narrowed by CAD has expanded dramatically. These procedures are collectively referred to as *percutaneous coronary intervention* (PCI). Today, PCI includes balloon angioplasty, atherectomy, and stent implantation. Advances in device technology, along with more effective anticoagulant and antiplatelet regimens, have reduced complication rates and improved procedural outcomes.[39]

Patients undergoing scheduled PCI based interventions generally remain in the hospital overnight and then go home. In the setting of emergency PCI, associated with an MI the hospital stay lasts a few days depending on the cardiovascular work-up that is required.

Percutaneous transluminal coronary angioplasty (PTCA), frequently abbreviated to *balloon angioplasty* or simply *angioplasty*, was introduced in 1977 as an alternative to coronary surgical revascularization. PTCA avoided many of the risks associated with cardiac surgery (general anesthesia, sternotomy, extracorporeal circulation, and mechanical ventilation), but its success was hampered by complications related to the procedure (acute closure) and restenosis or renarrowing of the vessel after the procedure. Research in this area has continued, and a growing number of interventional devices have been developed to address the limitations of conventional angioplasty.

Indications for Catheter-Based Interventions

Indications for catheter-based interventions have been considerably broadened since the initial application of balloon angioplasty. Whereas only patients with single-vessel CAD were once considered for PTCA, patients with multivessel disease, even those who have previously undergone saphenous vein grafting, internal mammary artery (IMA) grafting, or fibrinolytic therapy for acute MI, may now be candidates for catheter intervention. Previously seen as a rescue procedure to reduce a severe stenosis that persisted after fibrinolytic therapy, PCI has become preferred as the initial method of treatment for acute MI (primary PCI).[33]

Earlier restrictions regarding the characteristics and location of the atherosclerotic lesion have also changed with operator experience and improved technology. Distal, moderately calcified, and bifurcation stenoses are considered suitable for PCI. Left main coronary artery lesions, although considered high risk, can be successfully treated under certain conditions. It is now possible to traverse and dilate a totally occluded vessel.[40] Lesion morphology related to shape, size, location, and amount of calcification has been more clearly defined through clinical experience and is used to guide the selection of specific catheter-based interventions (see "Coronary Artery Disease" in Chapter 15).

Surgical Backup

Initially, most institutions required that patients preparing to undergo PCI be candidates for CABG. Complications such as intimal dissection with abrupt closure of the vessel could arise during the procedure, requiring the patient to undergo emergency CABG. Today, most dissections are effectively treated with stent placement, with less than 1% of patients requiring emergency bypass surgery. Nevertheless, the availability of cardiac surgical services on site is still recommended. There is currently an exception made for institutions that offer PCI only for treatment of acute STEMI. In this setting, an organized plan for emergent transfer to a surgical center may be used in lieu of on-site surgical access.[41] The emphasis on surgical backup may lessen in the future, as recent studies showed equivalent outcomes for elective PCI performed in hospitals with and without on-site surgery.[42,43]

CABG = Coronary Artery Bypass Grafting

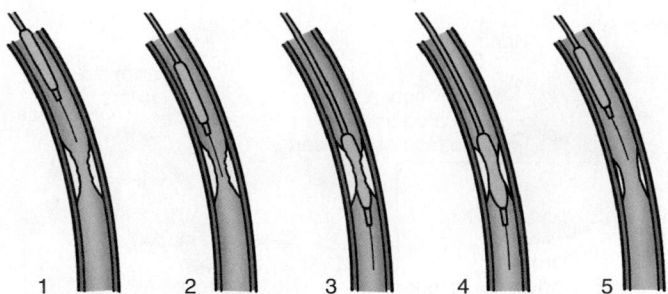

FIGURE 16-12 Percutaneous transluminal coronary angioplasty (PTCA) is used to open a stenotic vessel occluded by atherosclerosis.

Percutaneous Transluminal Coronary Angioplasty

Percutaneous transluminal coronary angioplasty (PTCA) involves the use of a balloon-tipped catheter that, when advanced through an atherosclerotic lesion (atheroma), can be inflated intermittently for the purpose of dilating the stenotic area and improving blood flow through it (Fig. 16-12). The high inflation pressure of the balloon stretches the vessel wall, fractures the plaque, and enlarges the vessel lumen. After balloon deflation, the vessel exhibits some degree of elastic recoil, resulting in a residual stenosis of approximately 30%. A successful angioplasty procedure is one in which the stenosis is reduced to less than 50% of the vessel lumen diameter.[44]

Although PTCA has relatively high success rates in initially opening occluded vessels, this technique by itself has major limitations, including the risk of acute vessel closure and a high frequency of restenosis. In the early application of angioplasty, acute closure occurred in up to 8% of patients as a result of dissection of the vessel wall and associated thrombus formation or vessel spasm. Restenosis occurred in more than one third of patients who underwent PTCA within the first 6 months and was diagnosed when patients experienced a recurrence of anginal symptoms.[39] Studies showed that restenosis was influenced by the final lumen diameter achieved by the procedure, the severity of elastic recoil of the vessel walls in response to the balloon inflation, and the amount of intimal hyperplasia that occurred as the vessel healed over the treated area. Patient characteristics such as a history of diabetes or unstable angina were also found to increase the risk of restenosis.[45]

In the current era of PCI, design enhancements have led to low-profile catheters that are able to traverse tortuous anatomy and noncompliant balloons that prevent overdistention of the vessel.[44] Another modification has been the cutting balloon—a device that produces incisions in the plaque before the balloon is dilated. Even with these improvements PTCA is rarely used alone as an intervention, except to treat lesions in very small coronary arteries.[44] Nevertheless, balloon angioplasty remains an essential adjunctive technique in PCI for dilating vessels and for deploying intracoronary stents.

Atherectomy

Atherectomy is the excision and removal of the atherosclerotic plaque by cutting, shaving, or grinding. Two specialized coronary catheters are used in coronary intervention: directional coronary atherectomy (DCA) and rotational ablation (Rotablator). Initially, it was thought that removing (rather than compressing) the atherosclerotic plaque would decrease the rate of restenosis. Despite significant improvements in initial procedural success, atherectomy failed to significantly reduce the rate of restenosis. Atherectomy is useful for removing plaque in calcified or fibrotic lesions, which helps increase wall compliance and facilitate angioplasty and stent placement. In the current era, atherectomy devices are used in less than 5% of PCI procedures.[44]

Directional Coronary Atherectomy

The DCA catheter consists of a rotating, cup-shaped blade within a windowed cylindrical chamber on one side and a low-inflation balloon on the other. The catheter is positioned within the lesion, and the balloon is inflated, forcing the atheromatous plaque into the chamber window. The cutting blade is then used to shave the protruding plaque, which is collected within the chamber. The ability to turn the catheter in various directions within the vessel led to the name of the device. A DCA catheter is pictured in Figure 16-13A. Because DCA extracts pieces of atheroma that can be studied microscopically (rather like a biopsy specimen), it has contributed significantly to our understanding of atherosclerosis and restenosis.

Rotablator

The Rotablator device has a high-speed, rotating, diamond-coated bur that drills through the plaque, creating tiny particles (see Fig. 16-13B). The particulate matter is carried through the bloodstream and disposed of by the reticuloendothelial system. This is the most frequently used device to debulk heavily calcified lesions that cannot be dilated by angioplasty or prevent delivery of a coronary stent. Rotational atherectomy may also be used for chronic total occlusion and for calcified bifurcation lesions.[44]

Coronary Stents

A major development in the field of interventional cardiology has been the coronary stent prosthesis. A stent is a metal structure that is introduced into the coronary artery over a guidewire and expanded into the vessel wall at the site of the lesion. Bare metal stents were first used to treat acute or threatened vessel closure after failed PTCA. The stent acted as a scaffold to tack dissection flaps against the vessel wall and provided mechanical support to minimize elastic recoil. Subsequent studies confirmed the clinical benefits of stents, which led to elective coronary stenting as a primary procedure. Stent implantation was initially limited to large vessels (greater than 3 mm) with proximal, discrete lesions. Improvements in stent design and operator technique allow for their deployment in smaller vessels with diffuse disease, vessels with lesions at bifurcations, and vessels with thrombus. Multiple stents may be implanted sequentially within a vessel to fully cover the area of the lesion. Stents are currently the predominant form of PCI and are used in more than 90% of all interventional procedures.[44]

Numerous stents are available. They are composed of various types of metal (stainless steel, titanium, cobalt chromium) and come in a variety of configurations (e.g., mesh, coil). Most stents are balloon expandable (Fig. 16-14).

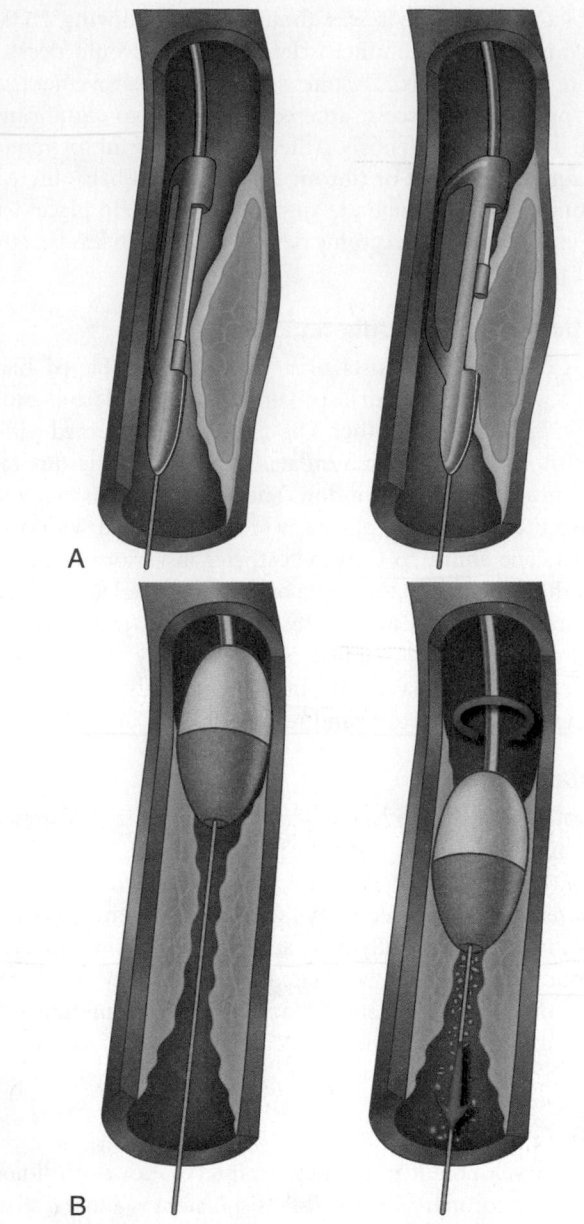

FIGURE 16-13 Atherectomy devices. *A*, Directional coronary atherectomy catheter. *B*, Rotational atherectomy catheter.

Stent Thrombosis

Early use of stents was hampered by a high incidence of sub-acute stent thrombosis. This thrombosis tended to occur during the first 2 to 14 days after stent placement, and resulted in MI in the majority of cases.[39] Later it was found that stent throm-bosis was in part due to inadequate stent expansion within the vessel—which could be remedied by applying high-pressure balloon inflations within the stent during deployment. In addi-tion, antiplatelet therapy was found to be more important than anticoagulation in preventing stent thrombosis.[39] Because platelet activation is a complex process involving multiple path-ways, combination therapy with two or more agents has proven most effective.[46] The current standard of care for PCI typically includes dual antiplatelet therapy with aspirin and a thienopyri-dine. These oral agents are administered before the procedure and continued at discharge.[47] Clopidogrel, a second-generation thienopyridine, has been studied extensively but may be

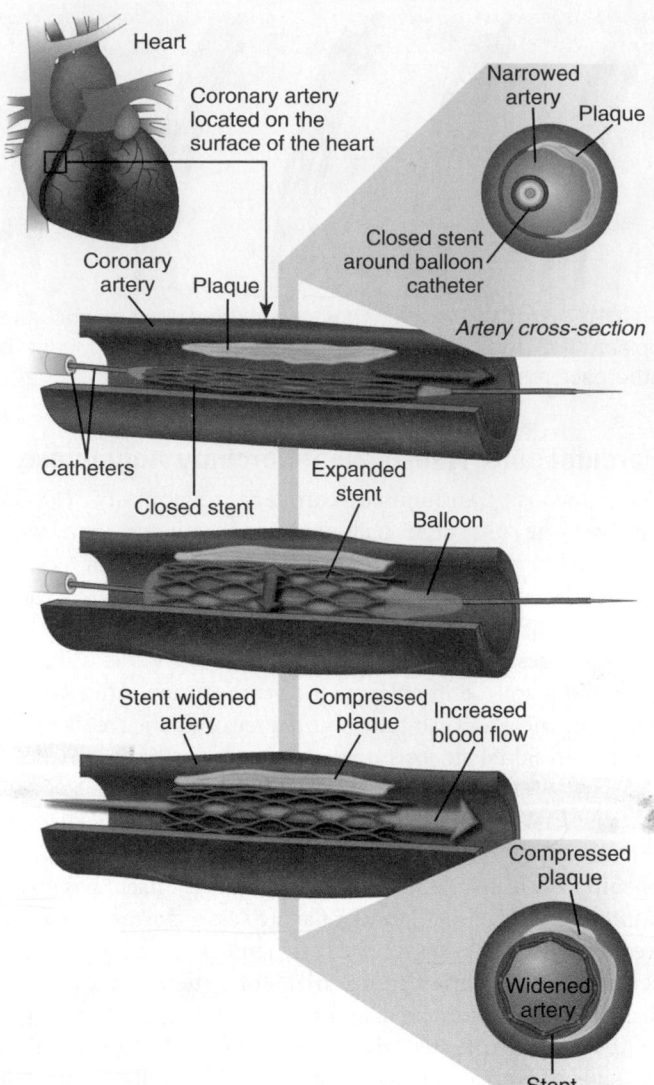

FIGURE 16-14 The intracoronary stent is a balloon-expandable stent.

ineffective in up to 26% of patients.[39] Prasugrel is a newer third-generation thienopyridine that offers a faster onset of action, higher levels of platelet inhibition, and lower incidence of resis-tance.[48] Recently the FDA approved a novel antiplatelet agent, ticagrelor. Advantages of this agent in comparison to clopido-grel and prasugrel are its short half-life and reversible anti-platelet effect. Disadvantages include the need for twice-daily dosing and higher cost.[48a] A description of oral antiplatelet agents is provided in Table 16-5.

More potent intravenous antiplatelet agents—glycoprotein IIb/IIIa inhibitors—may also be used during PCI procedures, especially in high-risk patients.[47] These medications act on the glycoprotein IIb/IIIa receptors on the platelet membrane to inhibit the final phase of platelet aggregation and prevent plate-lets from binding with fibrinogen. Abciximab (ReoPro) was the first of the glycoprotein IIb/IIIa inhibitors to be approved by the U.S. Food and Drug Administration (FDA) as an adjunct to PTCA for the prevention of abrupt closure of arteries in high-risk patients. Later, two additional agents, eptifibatide (Integri-lin) and tirofiban (Aggrastat), were approved. A description of intravenous antiplatelet agents is provided in Table 16-6.

TABLE 16-5 PHARMACOLOGIC MANAGEMENT

Oral Antiplatelet Agents

MEDICATION	DOSAGE	ACTION	SPECIAL CONSIDERATIONS
Aspirin	81-325 mg	Inhibits synthesis of thromboxane A_2 resulting in irreversible inhibition of platelet activation	Lower doses are recommended when given with other antithrombotics
Clopidogrel (Plavix)	300-600 mg loading dose 75-150 mg maintenance	Irreversibly inhibits the ADP $P2Y_{12}$ platelet receptor to block platelet activation	Onset of action 2-4 hr Should be held 5-7 days before elective surgery to decrease risk of bleeding Some patients may have a genetic resistance to clopidogrel, resulting in inadequate platelet inhibition
Prasugrel (Effient)	60 mg loading dose 10 mg daily maintenance	Irreversibly inhibits the ADP $P2Y_{12}$ platelet receptor to block platelet activation	Onset of action 15-30 minutes Should be held 5-7 days before elective surgery to decrease risk of bleeding Contraindicated in patients with prior TIA or stroke; not recommended in patients >75 years of age
Ticagrelor (Brilinta)	180 mg loading dose 90 mg twice daily maintenance	Reversibly inhibits the ADP $P2Y_{12}$ platelet receptor to block platelet activation	Onset of action 30 minutes Should be held 5 days before elective surgery to decrease risk of bleeding Contraindicated in patients with a history of ICH or severe hepatic impairment Maintenance aspirin dose above 100 mg reduces effectiveness

ADP, Adenosine diphosphate; *ICH*, intracranial hemorrhage; *TIA*, transient ischemic attack.

TABLE 16-6 PHARMACOLOGIC MANAGEMENT

Intravenous Antiplatelet Agents

MEDICATION	DOSAGE	ACTION	SPECIAL CONSIDERATIONS
Abciximab (ReoPro)	ACS: 0.25 mg/kg IVP, then 10 mcg/min until PCI (continue infusion for a minimum of 18 hrs to a maximum of 26 hrs) PCI: 0.25 mg/kg IVP, then 0.125 mcg/kg/min × 12 hrs	Inhibits the GP IIb/IIIa receptors responsible for platelet aggregation	Used concomitantly with aspirin and anticoagulants May affect platelet function for up to 48 hrs after infusion
Eptifibatide (Integrilin)	ACS: 180 mcg/kg IV bolus, followed by continuous infusion of 2 mcg/kg/min up to 72 hrs PCI: 180 mcg/kg IV bolus immediately before PCI (repeat after 10 minutes) followed by continuous infusion of 2 mcg/kg/min for 12-24 hrs	Reversibly binds to the glycoprotein GP IIb/IIIa platelet receptor and inhibits platelet aggregation	Concomitant aspirin and anticoagulants may be administered Platelet function returns to baseline within 6-8 hrs Contraindicated in patients with significant kidney dysfunction
Tirofiban (Aggrastat)	ACS: 0.4 mcg/kg/min for 30 min, then continued at 0.1 mcg/kg/min for 48-108 hrs PCI: 25 mcg/kg bolus followed by an infusion of 0.15 mcg/kg/min for up to 18 hrs	Reversibly binds to the glycoprotein GP IIb/IIIa platelet receptor and inhibits platelet aggregation	Administered in combination with heparin for patients undergoing PCI Platelet function returns to baseline within 4-8 hrs Dosage should be reduced in patients with kidney dysfunction

ACS, Acute coronary syndrome; *IV*, intravenous; *IVP*, intravenous push; *PCI*, percutaneous coronary intervention.

In-Stent Restenosis

Bare metal stents have been shown to decrease the incidence of restenosis when compared with balloon angioplasty, most likely as a result of achieving the largest possible lumen diameter at the time of the intervention.[44] Stents have not, however, proved to be a cure for restenosis as was once hoped. Restenosis within the stent is caused by intimal hyperplasia and can occur in a diffuse pattern throughout the stent, as discrete lesions within the body of the stent, or at the stent margins. The incidence of in-stent restenosis requiring intervention is approximately 20%

within the first 6 months after implantation of a bare metal stent.[45] Factors that increase the risk of in-stent restenosis are listed in Box 16-15.

Drug-Eluting Stents

In an effort to minimize restenosis, drug-eluting stents (DES) were developed. These stents have polymer coatings impregnated with medications that are released slowly into the endothelium at the site of stent placement to inhibit cellular proliferation. DES coated with sirolimus (an

Drug eluting stents

immunosuppressive medication used to prevent organ transplant rejection) and paclitaxel (an anticancer agent) have been approved by the FDA.[45] In initial trials, DES were found to decrease the 6-month restenosis rate to less than 10%, and they soon became the predominant stent, implanted in 90% of patients. Later trials demonstrated similar efficacy between bare metal stents and DES in long-term outcomes (stent thrombosis, MI, or death) and raised concerns regarding the possibility of late stent thrombosis (greater than 1 year) in DES.[39] As a result, DES usage has decreased somewhat to around 75% of patients.[45] Because a DES delays endothelialization, dual antiplatelet therapy must be continued for a longer period to prevent stent thrombosis. A DES is also considerably more expensive than a bare metal stent. A comparison of bare metal stents and DES is provided in Table 16-7.

Future Research

Current DES are coated with permanent polymers that remain after the medication is released. These polymers are thought to cause inflammation and may lead to impaired endothelialization.[45] Stent research is now focused on polymers that would dissolve once the stent-medication was released, leaving a bare metal stent in the vessel. Another area of research is a biodegradable stent that would provide an initial scaffolding to hold the vessel open, and then dissolve leaving only the healed vessel. Both of these options could potentially reduce the need for long-term antiplatelet therapy.[39]

Procedure

PCI is performed in the cardiac catheterization laboratory under fluoroscopy. Patients typically receive antiplatelet therapy (a thienopyridine and aspirin) before beginning the procedure. An introducer catheter, or sheath, is inserted percutaneously into the femoral artery. Alternatively, access to the arterial system can be obtained through the radial or brachial artery. In some cases, a venous sheath is inserted and used to perform a right-heart catheterization or to insert a pacing catheter, or both. A catheter with pacing capabilities may be indicated if dilation of the right coronary artery or circumflex artery is anticipated, because the blood supply to the conduction system of the heart may be interrupted, requiring emergency pacing. The patient is systemically anticoagulated to prevent clots from forming on or in any of the catheters. Unfractionated heparin has been used traditionally, initiated with a weight-based bolus and then titrated to achieve a target activated clotting time. Other anticoagulants may be selected based on physician preference or if the patient cannot tolerate heparin. Several of these newer agents have been shown to decrease the risk of bleeding complications when compared to UFH.[49] Options for anticoagulant agents are described in Table 16-8. A special guiding catheter, designed to engage the coronary ostia, is inserted through the arterial sheath and advanced in a retrograde manner through the aorta. Nitroglycerin or calcium channel blockers may be given at this time to prevent coronary artery spasm and to maximize coronary vasodilation during the procedure. A guidewire is then advanced down the coronary artery and negotiated across the occluding atheroma. The balloon catheter is advanced over this guidewire and positioned across the lesion. The balloon is inflated and deflated repetitively until evidence of dilation is demonstrated on an angiogram (Fig. 16-15). For lesions that do not respond well to angioplasty, additional plaque removal may be done with an atherectomy device.

In most procedures, vessel dilation is followed by deployment of an intracoronary stent. A stent is positioned at the target site, the stent is expanded, and the catheter is removed, leaving the stent in place. Intravascular ultrasound is used by some clinicians to evaluate the vessel lumen diameter after stent deployment to ensure optimal expansion.[41] Information obtained by ultrasonography provides a better estimate of residual plaque than that provided by angiography, because contrast material may surround the lattice-work of the stent, giving the appearance of a large lumen even when the stent is not fully open. The patient is transferred to the coronary care or angioplasty unit after the procedure for care and observation. Heparin or other anticoagulants are usually discontinued immediately after the procedure, to facilitate early sheath removal. Sheaths are removed when the activated clotting time (ACT) returns to normal in heparinized patients, or sooner if other anticoagulants or a vascular closure device is used. If glycoprotein IIb/IIIa inhibitors were initiated during the

Percutaneous coronary intervention

BOX 16-15 RISK FACTORS FOR IN-STENT RESTENOSIS

Patient Factors
- Diabetes mellitus
- Acute or chronic kidney failure

Anatomic Factors
- Longer lesions (>20 mm)
- Small vessel diameter (<3 mm)
- Complex, branched lesions

TABLE 16-7 COMPARISON OF BARE METAL AND DRUG-ELUTING STENTS

CHARACTERISTICS	BARE METAL STENT	DRUG-ELUTING STENT
Restenosis rate (at 6 months)	15%-20%	5%-10%
Cost	$	$$$
Duration of dual antiplatelet therapy	Minimum of 1 month for non-ACS patients, at least 12 months for stents implanted for ACS	Minimum of 12 months for either non-ACS or ACS patients, and longer if tolerated
Recommended lesion features	Short lesions <20 mm Large vessel diameter >3 mm	Longer lesions >20 mm Small vessel diameter <3.5 mm

ACS, Acute coronary syndrome.

TABLE 16-8 PHARMACOLOGIC MANAGEMENT

Anticoagulants

MEDICATION	DOSAGE	ACTION	SPECIAL CONSIDERATIONS
Unfractionated Heparin			
Heparin sodium	Initial bolus 60 units/kg (max dose 4000 units), followed by 12 units/kg/hr infusion	Enhances activity of antithrombin III, a natural anticoagulant to prevent clot formation	Effectiveness of treatment may be monitored by aPTT or ACT Response is variable because of binding with plasma proteins Effects may be reversed with protamine sulfate Risk of developing HIT Should not be given to patients already receiving therapeutic SQ enoxaparin
Low Molecular Weight Heparin			
Enoxaparin (Lovenox)	30 mg IV bolus, followed by 1 mg/kg SC every 12 hrs For patients already on SC dosing, an additional bolus of 0.3 mg/kg is given if last dose was >8 hrs prior to PCI	Enhances activity of antithrombin III	More predictable response than heparin, because enoxaparin is not largely bound to protein No need for aPTT or ACT monitoring Lower risk of HIT than with UFH Administer within 30 minutes of initiation of fibrinolytic therapy
Direct Thrombin Inhibitors			
Bivalirudin (Angiomax)	0.75 mg/kg IV bolus, followed by infusion at 1.75 mg/kg/hr during PCI If infusion continued >4 hrs, rate is decreased to 0.2 mg/kg/hr	Directly inhibits thrombin	May be administered alone or in combination with glycoprotein IIb/IIIa inhibitors Produces a dose-dependent increase in aPTT and ACT Coagulation times return to baseline within one hour after stopping infusion Dose should be reduced for patients with kidney dysfunction No reversal agent is available May be used instead of UFH for patients with HIT
Argatroban (Argatroban)	Loading dose of 100 mcg/kg IV bolus over 1 minute, followed by infusion of 1 mcg/kg/min (low-dose) or 3 mcg/kg/min (high-dose)	Directly inhibits thrombin	May be used instead of UFH for patients with HIT ACT is monitored during PCI, while aPTT is used during prolonged infusion Abrupt discontinuation may lead to a rebound hypercoagulable state
Factor Xa Inhibitor			
Fondaparinux (Arixtra)	2.5 mg IV, followed by 2.5 mg SC once daily	Selective inhibitor of factor Xa	May be used in conjunction with fibrinolytics For PCI, must be administered with another anticoagulant (i.e., UFH) to prevent catheter thrombosis Long half-life (>17 hrs) Contraindicated in patients with kidney failure

ACT, Activated clotting time; *aPTT*, activated partial thromboplastin time; *HIT*, heparin-induced thrombocytopenia; *MI*, myocardial infarction; *PCI*, percutaneous coronary intervention; *SC*, subcutaneous.

procedure, they may be continued for 12 to 24 hours, depending on the agent used. Dual antiplatelet therapy with aspirin and a thienopyridine (clopidogrel, prasugrel or ticagrelor) is routinely prescribed at discharge. Recommendations for thienopyridine administration vary based on the type of stent used (see Table 16-7), whereas aspirin is continued indefinitely.

Acute Complications

The incidence of serious cardiac complications after PCI, including coronary spasm, coronary artery dissection, and acute coronary thrombosis, has decreased significantly with improvements in technology. Stents have proved efficacious in the repair of coronary dissections, decreasing the need for emergency bypass surgery. Acute thrombosis has decreased with the established use of dual antiplatelet agents. Bleeding and hematoma formation at the site of vascular cannulation, compromised blood flow to the involved extremity, and retroperitoneal bleeding with femoral access occur infrequently, but are associated with increased morbidity and lengthened hospitalization.[50] Other complications that can occur in the period immediately after PCI include contrast-induced kidney failure, dysrhythmias, and vasovagal response (hypotension, bradycardia, and diaphoresis) during manipulation or removal of introducer sheaths.

Late Complications

Restenosis after PCI continues to be a problem, although rates are much lower with DES than with angioplasty alone. Patients at greatest risk are those with complex lesions, multivessel disease, or diabetes.[45] Treatment options for in-stent restenosis

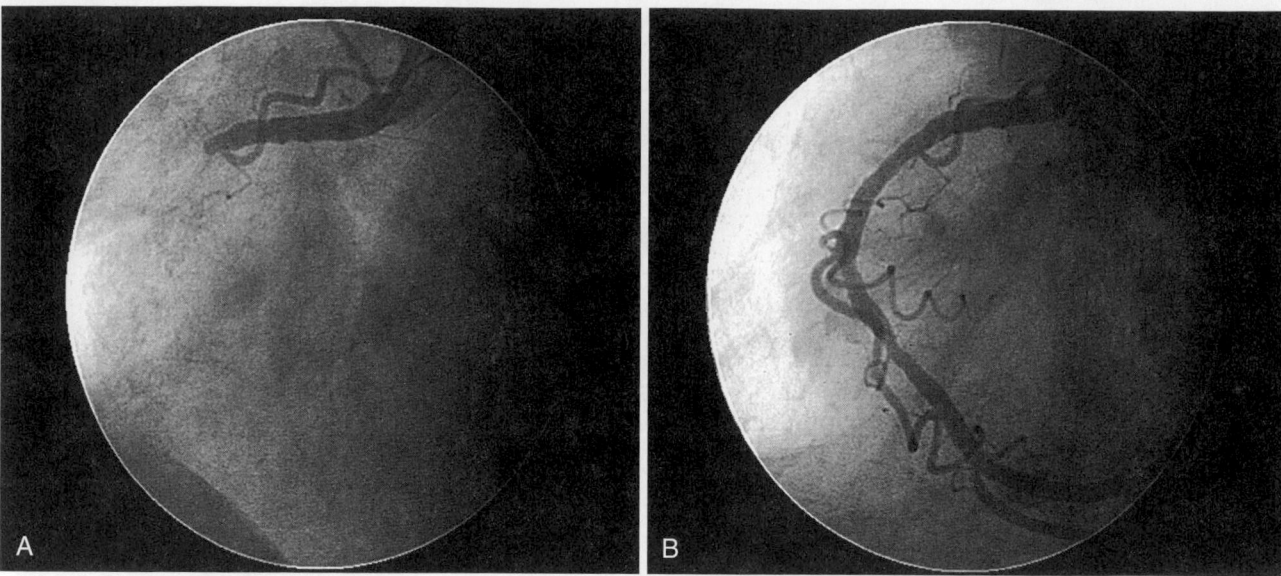

FIGURE 16-15 *A,* Coronary arteriogram of an acute proximal total occlusion of the right coronary artery (RCA). The patient had sudden onset of chest pain at home and was emergently admitted to the cardiac catheterization laboratory. *B,* The same vessel as in A after successful coronary atherectomy and intracoronary fibrinolytic therapy to open the occluded artery. Symptoms of chest pain resolved after the procedure.

◎ BOX 16-16 NURSING DIAGNOSES

Percutaneous Transluminal Coronary Angioplasty, Coronary Atherectomy, and Stenting

- Risk for Decreased Cardiac Tissue Perfusion, p. 1155
- Risk for Ineffective Peripheral Tissue Perfusion, p. 1158
- Activity Intolerance related to prolonged immobility or deconditioning, p. 1119
- Acute Pain related to transmission and perception of cutaneous, visceral, muscular, or ischemic impulse, p. 1123
- Anxiety related to threat to biologic, psychological, or social integrity, p. 1125
- Deficient Knowledge related to lack of previous exposure to information, p. 1134 (see Box 16-18, Patient Education for Percutaneous Transluminal Coronary Angioplasty, Coronary Atherectomy, and Stenting)

---

include balloon dilation, debulking with an atherectomy device, implantation of another DES or brachytherapy—the localized delivery of intracoronary radiation through specialized catheters. Because healing within the stent is delayed, late thrombosis may occur in patients with DES. Late thrombosis, although rare, is associated with a 45% mortality rate. Premature discontinuation of antiplatelet therapy is the strongest predictor of late stent thrombosis, especially with DES.[45]

Nursing Management

Nursing management and nursing diagnoses after PCI focus on accurate assessment of the patient's condition and prompt intervention (Box 16-16). The nurse at the bedside is in a unique position to continuously monitor for clinical manifestations of potential problems and to take quick and appropriate action to minimize the deleterious effects of complications related to the interventional catheter procedure.

Angina

It is essential that the nurse observe the patient for recurrent angina or ST elevation, which are clinical indicators of myocardial ischemia. Monitoring leads should be selected that will reflect ischemia in the vessels that were treated during the intervention. Angina during interventional cardiology procedures is an expected occurrence at the time of balloon inflation or manipulation within the coronary artery. Intraprocedural angina is caused by the temporary interruption of blood flow through the involved artery, which should subside with deflation or removal of the balloon or nitroglycerin administration, or both. Angina after a coronary interventional procedure may be caused by transient coronary vasospasm, or it may signal a more serious complication—acute thrombosis. In any case, the nurse must act quickly to assess for manifestations of myocardial ischemia and initiate clinical interventions as indicated. The physician usually orders intravenous nitroglycerin to be titrated to alleviate chest pain. Continued angina despite maximal vasodilator therapy usually rules out transient coronary vasospasm as the source of ischemic pain, and a return to the cardiac catheterization laboratory must be considered.

Prevention of Contrast Induced Acute Kidney Injury

Patients undergoing PCI are exposed to significant amounts of contrast dye, with its associated nephrotoxicity. Protective strategies may be implemented before the procedure, especially for patients with evidence of baseline kidney impairment. This may include preprocedural hydration and infusion of sodium bicarbonate.[51] While an early study indicated that administration of *N*-acetylcysteine (Mucomyst) might be beneficial, current guidelines do not recommend it for prevention of contrast-induced acute kidney injury.[41] After PCI, hydration is important to maintain adequate flow through the kidneys. Intravenous fluids are administered, and patients are encouraged to take oral fluids as tolerated.

Vascular Site Care

While the sheath is in place or after its removal, bleeding or hematoma at the insertion site may occur due to the effects of anticoagulation. The nurse observes the patient for bleeding or swelling at the puncture site and for changes in vital signs (hypotension, tachycardia) that could indicate hemorrhage. If a femoral approach was used, the nurse also assesses the patient for back pain, which can indicate retroperitoneal bleeding from the internal arterial puncture site.

Peripheral ischemia can also occur secondary to cannulation of the vessel, so nursing care includes frequent assessment of the adequacy of circulation to the involved extremity (Box 16-17). The patient is instructed to keep the limb straight and minimize movement. Additional activity restrictions vary depending on the size and location of the sheath, type of anticoagulation prescribed, methods used to achieve hemostasis, and institutional protocols. For femoral access, the head of the bed is not elevated more than 30 degrees while the sheath is in place (to prevent dislodgment) and for a period of time after its removal (to prevent bleeding). For brachial or radial access, a splint may be used to prevent flexion of the arm or wrist. After sheath removal, direct pressure is applied to the puncture site for 15 to 30 minutes until hemostasis is achieved. If direct pressure is inadequate or the patient is at higher risk for bleeding, a C-clamp or other compression device may be used to apply continuous pressure for 1 to 2 hours to ensure adequate hemostasis. Patients usually are allowed to resume ambulation 2 to 6 hours after the procedure, or sooner if a vascular closure device is employed.[52]

In the last decade, a number of products have been introduced to facilitate adequate hemostasis at the femoral access site after sheath removal. Active closure devices utilize mechanical sutures, collagen plugs, or metal clips to close the vessel when the sheath is removed. Advantages of these devices include a reduced time to hemostasis (under 5 minutes) regardless of the patient's level of anticoagulation, earlier ambulation, and increased patient comfort.[50] The Perclose closure device contains needles and sutures that are used to suture the artery closed after the interventional procedure (Fig. 16-16). AngioSeal is a vascular hemostatic device that uses a collagen plug to seal the arterial puncture site. Gentle pressure is maintained over the puncture site for approximately 5 minutes, until hemostasis is achieved. The StarClose vascular closure device consists of a tiny circumferential nitinol (nickel and titanium) clip that is applied to surface of the vessel to close the femoral artery at the end of the procedure.

Reports of complications and increased cost have limited the use of active closure devices.[50,53] To avoid these complications, a number of products have been developed to enhance manual compression and shorten the time required to achieve hemostasis. Some of these devices rely on the delivery of prothrombotic materials by a patch, whereas others increase local pressure over the puncture site. These devices do not offer immediate closure, but may decrease the time to ambulation.[50] A comparison of vascular closure systems is provided in Table 16-9.

Patient Education

In most cases, patients undergoing elective angioplasty, atherectomy, or stent procedures are hospitalized for approximately 24 hours. All patients require education about their medication regimen and about risk-factor modification (Box 16-18). Because of the abbreviated hospital stay, the nurse often has time to do little more than identify the offending risk factors and initiate basic instruction. Patients are referred to local cardiac rehabilitation centers for more extensive teaching and follow-up to facilitate understanding and compliance with risk-factor modification.

Another point of instruction that must be addressed is the patient's knowledge deficit related to discharge medications. Patients are sent home on a regimen of antiplatelet medications and medications for secondary prevention, such as lipid-lowering agents and blood pressure medications. A nitrate such as isosorbide may be prescribed to promote vasodilation, or, if the patient has demonstrated evidence of a vasospastic component to the disease, calcium channel blockers may be used. It is essential that the patient clearly understands the rationale for therapy and the potential side effects of each medication. Patients also need to understand the importance of not discontinuing their antiplatelet therapy; deaths have been reported when patients discontinued this therapy before elective procedures.[46] It is important that patients be provided with written information and a number to call if problems occur.

Percutaneous Valve Repair
Balloon Valvuloplasty

Percutaneous catheter technology has also been adapted to allow for nonsurgical interventions for stenotic cardiac valves. Current guidelines recommend balloon aortic valvuloplasty for adults only as a bridge to surgery for patients with unstable hemodynamics and who are at a high risk for AVR or in patients with aortic stenosis who are not surgical candidates.[54] Balloon aortic valvuloplasty has a limited role in adults, because restenosis and clinical deterioration occur within 6 to 12 months in most patients, and there has been no significant difference in long-term survival shown between it and medical therapy alone.[55,56]

Balloon valvuloplasty is performed in the cardiac catheterization laboratory by placing a balloon across the stenotic valve and inflating it to reduce stenosis.[57] Regurgitant flow can result, particularly after mitral valvuloplasty, and may result in the need for emergent valve replacement if severe. The risks of balloon valvuloplasty are similar to those inherent in most catheterization procedures and include cardiac perforation, thromboembolic events, dysrhythmias, and vascular complications

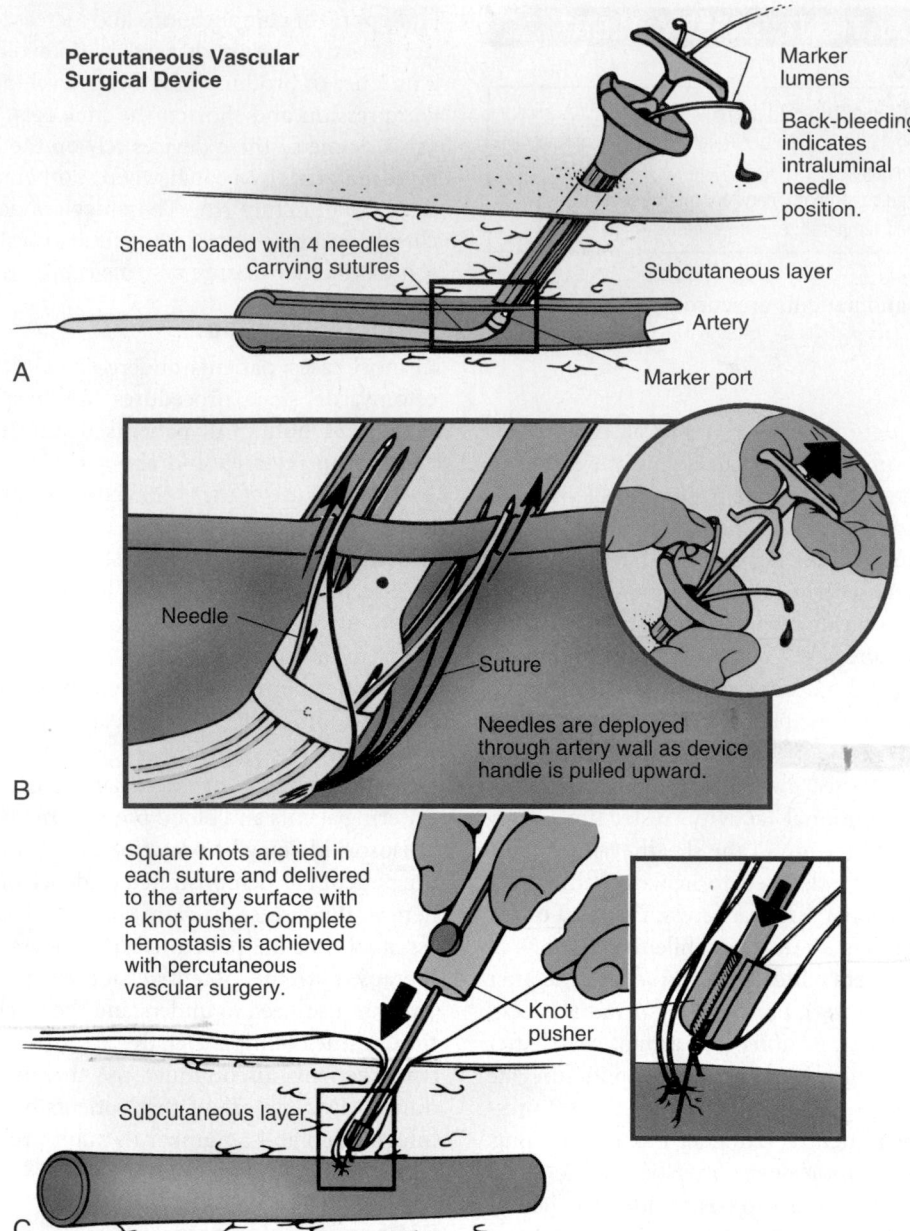

Percutaneous Vascular Surgical Device

Marker lumens

Back-bleeding indicates intraluminal needle position.

Sheath loaded with 4 needles carrying sutures

Subcutaneous layer

Artery

Marker port

A

Needle

Suture

Needles are deployed through artery wall as device handle is pulled upward.

B

Square knots are tied in each suture and delivered to the artery surface with a knot pusher. Complete hemostasis is achieved with percutaneous vascular surgery.

Knot pusher

Subcutaneous layer

C

FIGURE 16-16 Example of a percutaneous vascular surgical device used to close the femoral artery after catheter interventions for coronary artery disease. *A,* Insertion of the device into the femoral artery. *B,* After the interventional procedure, the device is removed by pulling upward to allow the needles in the device to close the artery. *C,* The sutured artery is secured with a knot pusher. (Courtesy Perclose, Inc., Redwood City, Calif.)

caused by the sheath. Postprocedural nursing management is similar to that for other percutaneous cardiac catheter procedures.

Transcatheter Aortic Valve Replacement

Transcatheter aortic valve replacement (TAVR) is a transformational therapy for patients who have severe aortic stenosis but who are extremely high-risk surgical candidates or who are inoperable by virtue of associated comorbidities.[55] TAVR can be done with spinal or general anesthesia in a cardiac catheterization lab or in a hybrid operating room. Transcatheter aortic valves are bioprosthetic valves that are loaded onto a stent or frame, which are then expanded to anchor the valve in the aortic

annulus with no sutures required.[57] Different approaches are used to deploy the device, but once it is in place, contrast medium is used to ensure correct positioning of the catheter valve across the aortic annulus.[57]

While TAVR has been shown to have excellent clinical outcomes in high-risk patients, complications are fairly common due to the complexity of the procedure and the morbidity of the patients. Vascular complications are the most frequent adverse outcome of TAVR, especially with the transfemoral approach due to the large-caliber sheaths and severe atherosclerosis of the arteries.[55] The incidence of early ischemic stroke (within the first 30 days) and need for permanent pacemakers postoperatively continues to be of major concern.[58,59,60] Factors

TABLE 16-9 VASCULAR CLOSURE DEVICES

TECHNOLOGY AND EXAMPLES	DESCRIPTION	COMMENTS
Patch Chito-Seal Clo-Sur P.A.D. D-Stat Syvek Patch	Patches that contain materials to promote clotting are applied directly to the puncture site, along with manual compression.	Less expensive than active closure devices No foreign material is left in the patient
Suture Perclose A-T ProGlide	Sutures deployed through the sheath are used to close the arteriotomy site.	Allows for immediate reaccess through the site if needed (see Fig. 16-16) Device failure may require surgical repair
Plug or Sealant Angio-Seal Duett Mynx	Placement of a procoagulant sealant such as collagen or thrombin is used to close the artery. Angio-Seal also includes an intravascular suture to anchor the collagen plug in place. The Mynx system uses a balloon catheter to inject sealant into the puncture site tract.	Reaccess must be done 1 cm above the previous arterial access site to avoid dislodging the sealant Extrusion of the sealant into the vessel may compromise the arterial lumen Components are absorbed within 30-90 days, depending on the sealant used
Clip or Staple EVS-Angiolink StarClose	Circumferential staples or clips are deployed at the site of the arteriotomy to close the vessel.	Extravascular clip does not compromise the artery lumen

BOX 16-18 PATIENT EDUCATION

Percutaneous Transluminal Coronary Angioplasty, Coronary Atherectomy, and Stenting

- Pathophysiology of atherosclerosis
- Risk-factor modification (diet, exercise, smoking cessation, weight loss)
- Information about prescribed medications (e.g., antiplatelet agents, antihypertensives, nitrates, calcium channel blockers, lipid-lowering medications)
- Symptoms to report to the health care professional (chest pain, shortness of breath, bleeding or drainage from the access site)
- Follow-up appointments

affecting regurgitation through the valve include the ratio of the valve size to the annulus size, positioning of the valve, and calcification of the native valve, all of which may contribute to mild or severe paravalvular aortic regurgitation.[61] Postoperative assessment includes monitoring hemodynamics and fluid balance, observing for signs of stroke and kidney injury along with identifying rhythm disturbances that may require back-up pacing or medical interventions. Multiple comorbid diseases have usually made patients candidates for TAVR and thus nursing care must focus on preventing complications associated with these conditions.[57]

CARDIAC SURGERY

Nursing management of the patient undergoing cardiac surgery is demanding but exciting work that requires the talents of an experienced team of critical care nurses. The following discussion introduces basic cardiac surgical techniques and principles of cardiopulmonary bypass and highlights the key points about postoperative care of the adult patient who requires valve replacement or coronary artery revascularization.

Coronary Artery Bypass Surgery (Graft)

Since its introduction almost 50 years ago, CABG has proved to be safe and effective in relieving angina symptoms and improving survival in most patients. Although there has been a great deal of evolution involving less invasive techniques, improved pharmacologic therapy, and education regarding lifestyle modifications, CABG surgery continues to demonstrate an important role in the treatment of coronary artery disease. Information on "Coronary Artery Disease" is presented in Chapter 15 and "Catheter Interventions for Coronary Artery Disease" are discussed earlier in this chapter.

Almost three decades ago, the combined results of three major randomized trials established the survival benefit of CABG compared to medical therapy in certain patients with stable angina. Early studies demonstrated CABG was more effective than medical therapy for improving survival in patients with left main or 3-vessel CAD and at relieving anginal symptoms.[62] Medical therapy is recommended if the ischemia is prevented by antianginal medications that are well tolerated by the patient.[62] Surgical revascularization has been shown to be more efficacious than PCI in patients with multivessel or left main coronary disease.[63,64] Bypass surgery may allow for more complete revascularization, because it can be used on vessels that are not amenable to treatment with a percutaneous approach, such as those with total occlusions or excessive tortuosity. However, as medical therapy and surgical procedures continue to evolve, updated studies and evaluations are required to guide optimal treatment.

Myocardial revascularization involves the use of a conduit, or channel, designed to bypass an occluded coronary artery.

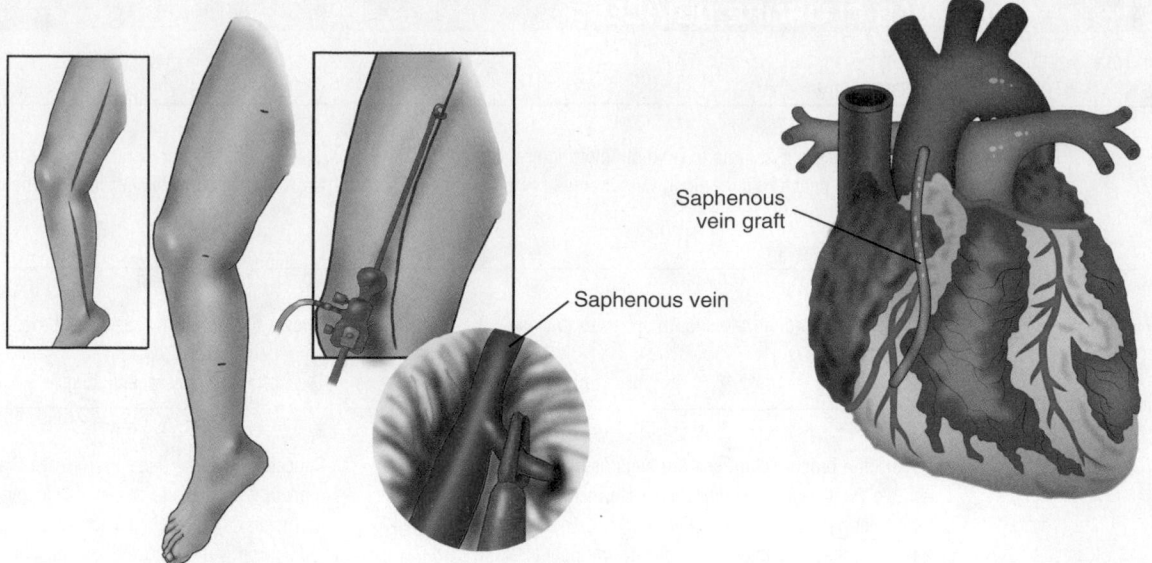

FIGURE 16-17 Saphenous Vein Graft. (Leg illustration from Moser D, Riegel B. *Cardiac Nursing: A Companion to Braunwald's Heart Disease.* Philadelphia: Saunders; 2007.)

Surgeons must evaluate which conduits will provide the best graft patency and long-term outcomes for their patients. The long saphenous vein graft (SVG) is the most frequently utilized conduit for CABG surgery. Saphenous vein grafting involves the anastomosis of an excised portion of the saphenous vein proximal to the aorta and distal to the coronary artery below the obstruction (Fig. 16-17). Harvesting technique plays a crucial role in the long-term patency of the saphenous vein and can be accomplished via an open surgical incision or, more commonly now, via an endoscopic approach. Endoscopic vein harvesting has been associated with decreased length of stay and increased patient satisfaction but has also been linked to a possible risk of early graft failure and so requires further research.[65] Vein grafts have traditionally had a high rate of arteriosclerosis, which has limited their long-term patency. Recent studies suggest that SVGs can achieve 5-year patency rates of over 80%, through improved harvesting techniques along with management strategies such as the use of statins, antiplatelet agents, and smoking cessation.[66,67]

Traditionally, arterial conduits have demonstrated improved patency rates over venous conduits due to their ability to resist atherosclerotic development. Recommendations have been made for complete arterial revascularization in healthy patients less than 60 years of age and may also be reasonable when the target vessels in the right coronary system have a critical stenosis.[62] The IMA, which usually remains attached to its origin at the subclavian artery, is swung down and anastomosed distal to the coronary artery (Fig. 16-18). Either the right IMA or the left IMA may be used as a conduit. The IMA is currently recommended as the conduit of choice for CABG, with a standard practice of attaching the LIMA to the artery that supplies the largest myocardial territory (most often the left anterior descending [LAD] artery).[68] Of note, emergency CABG may preclude the use of the IMA because of the extra time required to mobilize the artery and the inability to effect cardioplegia through this conduit. The IMA has continued to demonstrate

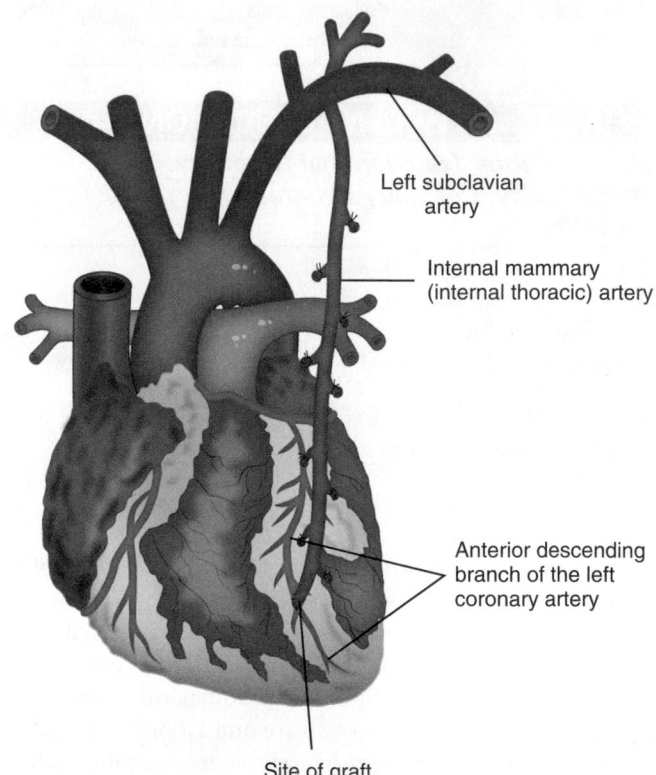

FIGURE 16-18 Internal mammary artery graft.

excellent long-term patency with estimated rates of 85% to 92% at 15 years.[68]

The potential benefit of long-term patency associated with arterial conduits has revived interest in the use of radial artery grafts. First introduced as a potential conduit for myocardial revascularization in the 1970s, radial artery grafts were abandoned because of a high incidence of early graft occlusion and vasospasm. Increased patency rates have been attributed to improved harvesting techniques, better appreciation of competitive flow, and the intraoperative use of vasodilators.[69] Even

TABLE 16-10	CONDUITS USED FOR CORONARY ARTERY BYPASS GRAFTS	
TYPE OF GRAFT	**ADVANTAGES**	**DISADVANTAGES**
Saphenous vein	Easily harvested Length allows for multiple grafts No anatomic limitations to graft sites	Long-term patency still to be determined Requires at least two anastomosis sites
Internal mammary artery	Proven patency rates Requires only one anastomosis	Requires extensive dissection Not accessible for emergency bypass Associated with increased chest wall discomfort postoperatively Anatomic limitations to bypassing some areas of the heart
Radial artery	Improved patency rates Easily harvested	Requires adequate collateral flow to the hand through the ulnar artery May be associated with higher rates of vasospasm Requires two anastomosis sites

though the issue of postoperative administration of calcium channel blockers to prevent vasospasm of the artery has been debated, many patients continue to receive them. A comparison of conduits used for myocardial revascularization is provided in Table 16-10.

Valvular Surgery

Valvular disease results in various hemodynamic dysfunctions that can usually be managed medically as long as the patient remains symptom-free. There is reluctance to intervene surgically early in the course of this disease because of the surgical risks and long-term complications associated with prosthetic valve replacement. These consequences, however, must be weighed against the possibility of irreversible deterioration in LV function that may develop during the compensated asymptomatic phase (see "Valvular Heart Disease" in Chapter 15).

Surgical therapy for aortic valve disease consists primarily of aortic valve replacement, although repairs may be done for selected regurgitant valves.[54] Three surgical procedures are available to treat mitral valve disease: commissurotomy, valve repair, and valve replacement. Commissurotomy is performed for mitral stenosis; the fused leaflets are incised, and calcium deposits are debrided to increase valve mobility. Repair of damaged leaflets may be accomplished with pericardial patches. In the setting of mitral regurgitation, valve repair may include reshaping of the leaflets and the use of a ring to reduce the size of the dilated mitral annulus, enhancing leaflet coaptation (annuloplasty). Although it is technically more demanding, valve repair is preferred over replacement to avoid the complications inherent with a prosthetic valve: the risk of thromboembolic events and the need for long-term anticoagulation.[70] If reconstruction of the mitral valve is not possible, it is replaced.

Prosthetic valves are designed with an orifice, through which blood flows, and an occluding structure that opens and closes.

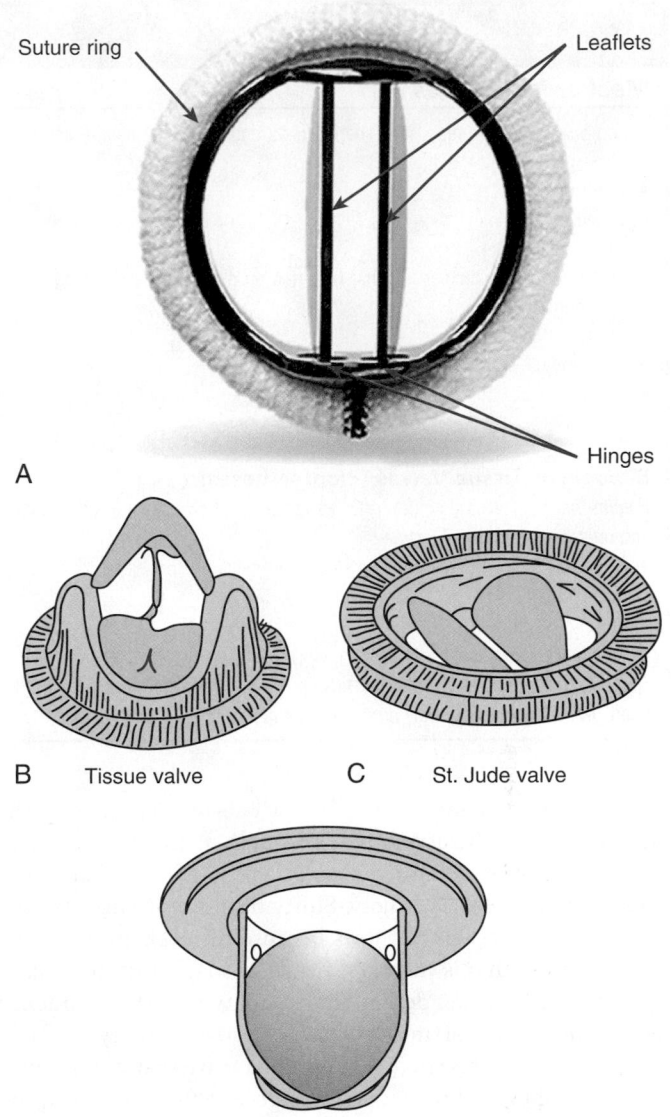

FIGURE 16-19 *A*, Mechanical bileaflet valve. *B*, Prosthetic tissue valve. *C*, Mechanical bileaflet valve (St. Jude). *D*, Starr-Edwards ball-and-cage valve. *A*, *B*, and *C* depict valves currently in use; ball-and-cage valve *(D)* is no longer in clinical use. (*A*, Courtesy St. Jude Medical.)

The two categories of prosthetic valves are mechanical valves and biologic valves, or tissue valves. *Mechanical valves* are made from combinations of metal alloys, pyrolytic carbon, Dacron, and Teflon and have rigid occluding devices (Fig. 16-19). Their construction renders them highly durable, but all patients with mechanical valves require anticoagulation to reduce the incidence of thromboembolism. *Biologic valves* are constructed from animal or human cardiac tissue and have flexible occluding mechanisms. Because of their low thrombogenicity, tissue valves offer the patient freedom from therapeutic anticoagulation. Their durability, however, is limited by their tendency toward early calcification. Box 16-19 provides a description of various valvular prostheses.

BOX 16-19 CLASSIFICATION OF PROSTHETIC CARDIAC VALVES

Mechanical Valves

Tilting-disc: a free-floating, lens-shaped disk mounted on a circular sewing ring
- Medtronic Hall
- Omniscience
- Monostrut

Bi-leaflet: two semicircular leaflets, mounted on a circular sewing ring that opens centrally
- St. Jude Medical
- Duromedics
- CarboMedics
- On-X/ATS

Biologic or Tissue Valves (Bioprostheses)

Porcine heterograft: a porcine aortic valve mounted on a semiflexible stent and preserved in glutaraldehyde
- Hancock
- Carpentier-Edwards
- Toronto Stentless (St. Jude)
- Free Style Stentless (Medtronic)

Homograft: a human heart valve (aortic or pulmonic) harvested from a donated heart and cryopreserved; may or may not be mounted on a support ring

The first mechanical valve had a ball-in-cage design. The Starr-Edwards valve is the only example of this type of valve still in use today. Later valves used a tilting-disc mechanism to occlude blood flow. The Björk-Shiley tilting-disc valve was discontinued in the United States because of mechanical failure, but patients with this valve are still alive today. Most valves used today have a bi-leaflet design, the first of which was introduced by St. Jude Medical in 1977. One of the primary goals in mechanical valve research is to design a valve that can alleviate the causes of thrombosis: surface roughness, turbulent flow, and stagnation in valve pivots. The choice of a valvular prosthesis depends on many factors. Because mechanical valves are more durable, for example, they may be preferred for a young person who is anticipated to have a relatively long life span ahead. Similarly, a bioprosthesis (tissue valve) may be chosen for an older adult patient; the valve has a reduced longevity, but this disadvantage is offset by the older patient's shorter life expectancy.[54] For patients with medical contraindications to anticoagulation and for those whose past compliance with medications has been questionable, a tissue valve may be selected.[71] Technical considerations, such as the size of the annulus (or the anatomic ring in which the valve sits), also can influence the choice of valve; for example, a bioprosthesis may be too big for a small aortic root.

Cardiopulmonary Bypass

CABG surgery can be performed using cardiopulmonary bypass (CPB) "on-pump" or it can be done without it, which is often referred to as "off-pump" CABG (OPCAB). CPB is a mechanical means of circulating and oxygenating a patient's blood while diverting most of the circulation from the heart and lungs during cardiac surgical procedures. The extracorporeal circuit consists of cannulas that drain off venous blood, an oxygenator that oxygenates the blood, and a pump head that propels the arterialized blood back to the ascending aorta—which has been cross-clamped to prevent the back flow of blood into the heart. The patient is systemically heparinized before initiation of bypass to prevent clotting within the bypass circuit. After the patient is taken off the CPB machine, protamine sulfate is given to reverse the effects of the heparin.

In response to findings that the low cardiac output syndrome often seen postoperatively might be a result of intraoperative myocardial ischemia or necrosis, efforts have been directed toward providing additional protection to the myocardium during bypass. Rapidly stopping the heart in diastole by perfusing the coronary arteries with a cold potassium cardioplegic (heart-paralyzing) agent has been the method of choice for intraoperative myocardial protection. Cardioplegia solution is used to achieve cardiac arrest, allowing the surgeon to operate while the heart is stopped. Warm and cold cardioplegia solutions have been evaluated, with no significant difference found to support the use of one solution over another at this point.[72] Regardless of the type of cardioplegic solution used, it must be reinfused at regular intervals during bypass to keep the heart in an arrested state and to minimize myocardial oxygen requirements.

Systemic hypothermia during bypass can reduce tissue oxygen requirements to 50% of normal, which affords the major organs additional protection from ischemic injury. Lowering the body temperature to about 28° C (82.4° F) is accomplished through a heat exchanger incorporated into the pump. The blood is warmed to normal body temperature before bypass is discontinued.

The technique of hemodilution also is used to enhance tissue oxygenation by improving blood flow through the systemic and pulmonary microcirculation during bypass. *Hemodilution* refers to the dilution of the patient's own (autologous) blood with the isotonic crystalloid solution used to prime the pump. Capillary perfusion is enhanced by hemodilution, because the reduced viscosity (stickiness) of the blood decreases both resistance to flow through the capillaries and the possibility of microthrombi formation. At the completion of cardiopulmonary bypass, the large quantities of "pump blood" that remain in the bypass circuit can be collected and used for initial postoperative volume replacement.

Numerous clinical sequelae can result from cardiopulmonary bypass (Table 16-11). Knowledge of these physiologic effects allows the nurse to anticipate problems and intervene effectively in the postoperative period.

Some surgeons may elect to perform OPCAB with the goal of avoiding the potential complications associated with CPB and cross-clamping of the aorta. Several techniques are used to stabilize the operative area during an OPCAB procedure. Immobilization devices that use compression or suction to create an immobile area have been developed to stabilize cardiac wall motion at the site of the anastomosis. Medications that temporarily decrease the heart rate (e.g., esmolol, diltiazem) or cause transient cardiac asystole (e.g., adenosine) may also be used to further limit cardiac motion. Patients still receive heparin but in lower doses than with CPB. Because there is

TABLE 16-11 PHYSIOLOGIC EFFECTS OF CARDIOPULMONARY BYPASS

EFFECTS	CAUSES
Intravascular fluid deficit (hypotension)	Third-spacing Postoperative diuresis Sudden vasodilation (medications, rewarming)
Third-spacing (weight gain, edema)	Decreased plasma protein concentration Increased capillary permeability
Myocardial depression (decreased cardiac output)	Hypothermia Increased systemic vascular resistance Prolonged cardiopulmonary bypass pump run Pre-existing heart disease Inadequate myocardial protection
Coagulopathy (bleeding)	Systemic heparinization Mechanical trauma to platelets Depressed release of clotting factors from liver as a result of hypothermia
Pulmonary dysfunction (decreased lung mechanics and impaired gas exchange)	Decreased surfactant production Pulmonary microemboli Interstitial fluid accumulation in lungs
Hemolysis (hemoglobinuria)	Red blood cells damaged in pump circuit
Hyperglycemia (rise in serum glucose concentration)	Decreased insulin release Stimulation of glycogenolysis
Hypokalemia (low serum potassium concentration)	Intracellular shifts during bypass and postoperative diuresis
Hypomagnesemia (low serum magnesium concentration)	Postoperative diuresis resulting from hemodilution
Neurologic dysfunction (decreased level of consciousness, motor/sensory deficits)	Inadequate cerebral perfusion Microemboli to brain (air, plaque fragments, fat globules)
Hypertension (transient rise in blood pressure)	Catecholamine release and systemic hypothermia causing vasoconstriction

no heat exchanger on the pump, the patient's body temperature may be lower postoperatively, which may potentiate bleeding.[73]

Despite the fact that OPCAB was developed to decrease complications associated with CPB, results have been mixed. The use of OPCAB was shown to reduce the rates of transfusions, reoperation for perioperative bleeding, respiratory complications, and acute kidney injury.[74] However, with conventional CABG there tended to be more complete revascularization, and better graft patency.[75] The perceived neurologic benefits of OPCAB also do not appear to bear out as there have been no differences shown in neuropsychologic outcomes between the groups.[75] OPCAB may be most beneficial in patients with significant comorbid conditions and in those with contraindications to cardiopulmonary bypass.

Postoperative Management

Medical and nursing management of the postoperative cardiac surgery patient are often overlapping. The physician prescribes therapeutic interventions and identifies specific hemodynamic end points that are individualized for each patient. The nurse is then responsible for applying these therapies to maintain the patient's hemodynamic parameters within the desired range. For example, orders may be written to maintain the patient's blood pressure, filling pressures, cardiac output, and systemic vascular resistance (SVR) within a desired range, using a combination of volume, vasodilator, and inotropic infusions. In most institutions, standard protocols are used to facilitate the

◉ BOX 16-20 NURSING DIAGNOSES

Open Heart Surgery

- Decreased Cardiac Output related to alterations in preload, p. 1128
- Decreased Cardiac Output related to alterations in afterload, p. 1128
- Decreased Cardiac Output related to alterations in contractility, p. 1128
- Decreased Cardiac Output related to alterations in heart rate or rhythm, p. 1128
- Impaired Gas Exchange related to ventilation/perfusion mismatching or intrapulmonary shunting, p. 1144
- Ineffective Airway Clearance related to excessive secretions or abnormal viscosity of mucus, p. 1148
- Activity Intolerance related to cardiopulmonary dysfunction, p. 1119
- Deficient Fluid Volume related to absolute loss, p. 1132
- Risk for Infection, p. 1160
- Acute Pain related to transmission and perception of cutaneous, visceral, muscular, or ischemic impulses, p. 1123
- Anxiety related to threat to biologic, psychological, or social integrity, p. 1125
- Disturbed Sleep Pattern related to fragmented sleep, p. 1137
- Deficient Knowledge related to lack of previous exposure to information, p. 1134 (see Box 16-22, Patient Education for Open Heart Surgery)

postoperative nursing diagnoses and management of cardiac surgical patients (Box 16-20).

Cardiovascular Support

Postoperative cardiovascular support often is indicated because of a low output state resulting from pre-existing heart disease, a prolonged cardiopulmonary bypass pump run, inadequate myocardial protection, or some combination of these factors. Cardiac output can be maximized by adjustments in heart rate, preload, afterload, and contractility.

Heart Rate. In the presence of low cardiac output, the heart rate can be appropriately regulated by means of temporary pacing or medication therapy. Temporary atrial and/or ventricular epicardial pacing usually is instituted when the heart rate drops to less than 60 beats/min and the patient is hypotensive, requiring a supportive rate of 80 to 100 beats/min. In the case of tachycardia, intravenous beta-blockers (esmolol) or calcium channel blockers (diltiazem) may be used in the acute postoperative period to slow supraventricular rhythms. Electrolyte disturbances such as hypokalemia, hypomagnesemia, hypocalcemia, and hypercalcemia must be closely monitored and corrected to prevent postoperative dysrhythmias.

Atrial fibrillation occurs in roughly one third of patients after cardiac surgery, with a peak occurrence in the first 2 to 3 days after surgery. This rhythm may induce hemodynamic compromise, prolong hospitalization, and increase the patient's risk of stroke. Prophylactic administration of beta-blockers is recommended to decrease the incidence of atrial fibrillation and its clinical sequelae, or amiodarone as an alternative for those who have contraindications to beta-blockers.[62]

Preload. In most patients, reduced preload is the cause of low postoperative cardiac output. The most common causes of decreased preload are due to hypovolemia from bleeding and fluid shifts caused by the systemic inflammatory response.[76] To enhance preload, volume may be administered in the form of crystalloid, colloid, or packed red cells. Traditionally, preload has been evaluated by intermittent pressure readings obtained from catheters placed in the right atrium or pulmonary artery. A growing body of research suggests that static indices such as central venous pressure (CVP) and pulmonary artery occlusion pressure (PAOP) have a very weak relationship with the patient's intravascular volume and are not helpful in predicting if a patient will be a fluid responder.[77,78] Dynamic measures of preload responsiveness (i.e., pulse pressure variation [PPV] and systolic pressure variation [SPV]) have been shown to more accurately predict an increase in cardiac output in response to a volume challenge in postoperative CABG patients.[79]

Afterload. Many patients who have had cardiac surgery demonstrate postoperative hypertension. Although it is transient, postoperative hypertension can precipitate or exacerbate bleeding from the mediastinal chest tubes. The high SVR (afterload) resulting from the intense vasoconstriction can increase LV workload. Vasodilator therapy with intravenous sodium nitroprusside or nitroglycerin often is used to reduce afterload, control hypertension, and improve cardiac output. Increased afterload may be partially due to the peripheral vasoconstrictive effects of hypothermia, which can be managed with careful rewarming.

A significant percentage of patients experience hypotension after cardiopulmonary bypass due to peripheral vasodilation. This is believed to occur, in part, because of the systemic inflammatory response to cardiopulmonary bypass. Therapy for hypotension after cardiac surgery usually includes volume loading and vasopressors such as phenylephrine to tighten the peripheral vasculature and maintain an adequate mean arterial pressure.

Contractility. If the adjustments in heart rate, preload, and afterload fail to produce significant improvement in cardiac output, contractility can be enhanced with positive inotropic support or intra-aortic balloon pumping (IABP) to augment circulation (discussed later).

Temperature Regulation

Hypothermia can contribute to depressed myocardial contractility, vasoconstriction, and ventricular dysrhythmias in the patient who has had cardiac surgery. Hypothermia may also contribute to postoperative bleeding, because the functioning of clotting factors is depressed during hypothermia. After surgery, patients may be rewarmed with the use of warm blankets or forced-air warming devices. Excessive temperature elevations must be avoided with the goal of maintaining a target body temperature of 36° C to 37° C (96.8° F to 98.6° F).

Control of Bleeding

Postoperative bleeding from the mediastinal chest tubes can be caused by inadequate hemostasis, disruption of suture lines, or coagulopathy associated with cardiopulmonary bypass or hypothermia. Bleeding is more likely to occur with IMA grafts as a result of the extensive chest wall dissection required to free the IMA. If bleeding in excess of 150 mL/hr occurs early in the postoperative period, clotting factors (fresh-frozen plasma, fibrinogen, and platelets), protamine, or desmopressin may be administered. Medications used in the treatment of postoperative bleeding are described in Table 16-12. Thromboelastography (TEG) is now also being used to determine which part of the clotting cycle is deficient in order to help guide the selection of appropriate factors or medications.

TABLE 16-12	MEDICATIONS USED TO TREAT POSTOPERATIVE BLEEDING	
MEDICATION	**DOSE**	**ACTION AND SIDE EFFECTS**
Aminocaproic acid (Amicar)	Loading dose: 4-5 g over 1 hr, followed by continuous infusion of 1 g/hr for 8 hrs or until bleeding is controlled	Inhibits conversion of plasminogen to plasmin to prevent fibrinolysis, helping to stabilize clots
Desmopressin acetate (DDAVP)	0.3 mcg/kg IV over 20-30 min	Improves platelet function by increasing levels of factor VIII. Side effects include facial flushing, tachycardia, headache, and hypotension
Protamine sulfate	25-50 mg IV slowly over 10 min	Neutralizes the anticoagulant effect of heparin. Can cause hypotension, bradycardia, and allergic reactions

Autotransfusion devices, which facilitate the collection and reinfusion of shed mediastinal blood, previously were used in some institutions. Routine autotransfusion of shed mediastinal blood is no longer recommended, because it may further exacerbate bleeding by activating the extrinsic clotting pathway and increase the risk of infection.[80] The use of positive end-expiratory pressure (PEEP) in conjunction with mechanical ventilation may be helpful in controlling excessive bleeding in some cases by increasing the intrathoracic pressure enough to effect tamponade of oozing mediastinal blood vessels.[80] Rewarming the patient reverses the depressed manufacture and release of clotting factors that results from hypothermia. However, persistent mediastinal bleeding—usually in excess of 500 mL in 1 hour or 300 mL/hr for 2 consecutive hours despite normalization of clotting studies—is an indication for re-exploration of the surgical site.

Blood conservation strategies should be used to limit the number of transfusions as the administration of packed red blood cells has been independently associated with increased complications and increased mortality.[62,81] At what point packed red blood cells should be administered is not known—some recommendations support transfusion when the hemoglobin is less than 7g/dL, while others suggest the decision be based upon the individual clinical situation.[80,82]

Chest Tube Patency

Chest tube stripping to maintain patency of the tubes is controversial because of the high negative pressure generated by routine methods of stripping. It is believed to result in tissue damage that can contribute to bleeding. This risk must be carefully weighed against the real danger of cardiac tamponade if blood is not effectively drained from around the heart. Chest tube stripping often is advocated in instances of excessive postoperative bleeding. However, the technique of "milking" the chest tubes is advisable for routine postoperative care, because this technique generates less negative pressure and decreases the risk of bleeding.

Cardiac Tamponade

A potentially lethal complication, cardiac tamponade may occur after surgery if blood accumulates in the mediastinal space, impairing the heart's ability to pump. Signs of tamponade include elevated and equalized filling pressures (e.g., CVP, PADP, PAOP), decreased cardiac output, decreased blood pressure, jugular venous distention, pulsus paradoxus, muffled heart sounds, sudden cessation of chest tube drainage, and a widened cardiac silhouette on radiographs. A bedside echocardiogram may be done to confirm tamponade. Interventions for tamponade may include emergency sternotomy in the critical care unit or a return to the operating room for surgical evacuation of the clot.

Pulmonary Care

Mechanical ventilation is utilized initially to provide adequate alveolar oxygenation and ventilation in the postoperative period. Protocols that facilitate early extubation (less than 6 hours after surgery) have been implemented in most institutions and have been shown to decrease pulmonary complications after cardiac surgery.[83] Early extubation requires a multidisciplinary approach that incorporates anesthesiologists, surgeons, nurses, and respiratory therapists. Potential candidates must be identified before surgery so that the anesthetic regimen supports early extubation.

After surgery, patients are evaluated for hemodynamic stability, adequate control of bleeding, normothermia, and the ability to follow commands. Once these criteria have been met, most institutions have a weaning protocol to follow that often involves a continuous positive airway pressure (CPAP) trial to evaluate the patient's readiness to extubate. Patients who exhibit hemodynamic instability or intraoperative complications or who have underlying pulmonary disease may require longer periods of mechanical ventilation. After extubation, supplemental oxygen is administered, and patients are medicated for incisional pain to facilitate aggressive pulmonary toilet and early mobility, which is essential to helping prevent postoperative complications.[76]

Neurologic Complications

The neurologic dysfunction often seen in patients who have had cardiac surgery has been attributed to decreased cerebral perfusion, cerebral microemboli, hypoxia and the systemic inflammatory response. The dysfunction can range from subtle cognitive changes to signs of acute stroke. Neurologic dysfunction was thought to be primarily caused by CPB, but newer evidence is demonstrating no difference in neuropsychologic outcomes between on-pump and off-pump and indicates that cognitive decline may be influenced more by patient-related factors such as the degree of pre-existing cerebral vascular disease or diabetes.[72,75,84]

The risk of delirium is increased in cardiac surgery patients, especially older adults, and is associated with increased mortality, and reduced quality of life and cognitive function.[85] Nursing staff can play a critical role in the prevention and recognition of delirium. Nonpharmacologic interventions involve reorienting patients, providing visual and hearing aids, early mobilization, sleep promotion, and the judicious use of medications known to potentiate delirium.[86] Treatment of delirium may require the use of medications such as haloperidol (Haldol) or atypical antipsychotics. Liberalization of visitation policies to allow family members a prolonged presence at the bedside is also highly desirable.

Infection

Postoperative fever is fairly common after cardiopulmonary bypass. However, persistent temperature elevation to greater than 101° F (38.3° C) must be investigated. Sternal wound infections and infective endocarditis are the most devastating infectious complications, but leg wound infections, pneumonia, and urinary tract infections also can occur. Infection rates are greater in patients with diabetes, malnutrition, chronic diseases, obesity, and those requiring emergent or prolonged surgery. Using a continuous insulin infusion to maintain blood glucose concentrations less than or equal to 180 mg/dL while avoiding hypoglycemia may reduce the incidence of adverse events, including deep sternal wound infections.[62]

Acute Kidney Injury

Almost one third of patients develop acute kidney injury after cardiac surgery, owing often to a combination of ischemic processes.[87] Kidney dysfunction in the postoperative period requires frequent monitoring of urine output and serum creatinine levels. Because of fluid retention, diuresis is often required to help mobilize fluids from the interstitial to the intravascular space and may be done with the administration of medications or may be allowed to occur naturally. The patient's potassium levels may be depleted with the diuresis, requiring that levels be closely monitored and replaced.

Guidelines for Coronary Artery Bypass Grafting

The American College of Cardiology and the American Heart Association have developed a set of clinical practice guidelines for care of the patient undergoing CABG.[62] These guidelines are designed to support clinical decision making with research evidence (Box 16-21).

BOX 16-21 EVIDENCE-BASED PRACTICE

Coronary Artery Bypass Graft Surgery

QSEN A summary is provided of evidence and evidence-based review recommendations for management of the coronary artery bypass graft (CABG) surgery patient.

Strong Evidence to Support the Following
CABG for Patients
- Emergency CABG for patients with acute MI when primary PCI has failed or cannot be performed, coronary anatomy is suitable for CABG and persistent ischemia and/or hemodynamic instability refractory to nonsurgical therapy is present
- Emergency CABG for patients undergoing surgical repair of postinfarction mechanical complications of MI, those with cardiogenic shock, or those with life-threatening ventricular dysrhythmias in the presence of left main stenosis or 3-vessel CAD
- Undergoing noncoronary cardiac surgery if ≥50% stenosis of left main or ≥70% stenosis of other major coronary arteries
- Significant (≥50%) stenosis of left main
- Significant (≥70%) stenosis in 3 major coronary arteries or in the proximal LAD plus 1 other major coronary artery
- CABG or PCI in patients with 1 or more significant (≥70%) coronary artery stenosis with unacceptable angina despite guideline-directed medical therapy
- Patients undergoing CABG who have at least moderate aortic stenosis should undergo an aortic valve replacement (AVR)
- Patients undergoing CABG who have severe ischemic mitral valve regurgitation not likely to resolve with revascularization should undergo a mitral valve repair or replacement

Anesthetic Considerations
- Anesthetic management should be directed toward early postoperative extubation and accelerated recovery of low- to medium-risk patients

Bypass Graft Conduits
- If possible, the left internal mammary artery (LIMA) should be used to bypass the left anterior descending artery (LAD)

Antiplatelet Therapy
- Aspirin should be administered preoperatively, if not done, initiated within 6 hours postoperatively and continued indefinitely
- In elective cases, clopidogrel and ticagrelor should be discontinued 5 days before surgery and prasugrel for at least 7 days

Management of Hyperlipidemia
- All patients should receive statin therapy unless contraindicated

Blood Glucose Management
- Continuous IV insulin to maintain an early postoperative blood glucose concentration ≤180 mg/dL while avoiding hypoglycemia to reduce adverse events

Dysrhythmia Management
- Beta-blockers should be administered for at least 24 hours before CABG, reinstituted as soon as possible after surgery, and prescribed at discharge unless contraindicated in order to reduce the incidence and clinical sequelae of atrial fibrillation

Angiotensin-Converting Enzyme (ACE) Inhibitors and Angiotensin-Receptor Blockers (ARBs)
- ACE inhibitors and ARBs should be instituted or restarted postoperatively and continued indefinitely for patients with LVEF ≤40%, hypertension, diabetes, or chronic kidney disease

Smoking Cessation
- All smokers should receive educational counseling and be offered smoking cessation therapy during CABG hospitalization

Cardiac Rehabilitation
- Cardiac rehabilitation should be offered to all eligible patients after CABG

Reduction in Risk of Infection
- Preoperative antibiotic administration should be used in all patients to reduce the risk of postoperative infection

Bleeding/Transfusions
- Aggressive attempts at blood conservation are indicated to reduce the need for RBC transfusions

Moderate Evidence to Support the Following
CABG for Patients
- In patients with multivessel CAD with recurrent angina or MI within the first 48 hours of STEMI presentation as an alternative to a more delayed strategy
- CABG or PCI for selected patients ≥75 years of age with ST-segment elevation or left bundle branch block who are suitable for revascularization irrespective of the time interval from MI to the onset of shock
- Emergency CABG after failed PCI to retrieve a foreign body in a crucial anatomic location or for hemodynamic compromise in patients with impairment of the coagulation system and without previous sternotomy
- Significant (≥70%) stenosis in 2 major coronary arteries with extensive myocardial ischemia or target vessels supplying a large area of viable myocardium
- Mild-moderate LV systolic dysfunction (EF 35%-50%) and significant (≥70% stenosis) multivessel CAD or proximal LAD stenosis with viable myocardium present
- Complex 3-vessel CAD (SYNTAX score >22) with or without involvement of the proximal LAD who are good candidates for CABG
- CABG over PCI to improve survival in patients with multivessel CAD and diabetes mellitus, particularly if a LIMA graft can be anastomosed to the LAD

BOX 16-21 EVIDENCE-BASED PRACTICE

Coronary Artery Bypass Graft Surgery—cont'd

- Patients undergoing CABG who have moderate ischemic mitral valve regurgitation not likely to resolve with revascularization should undergo a mitral valve repair or replacement

Hybrid Coronary Revascularization
- The planned combination of LIMA-to-LAD artery grafting and PCI of ≥1 non-LAD coronary arteries is reasonable for 1) limitations to CABG such as heavily calcified proximal aorta or poor target vessels for CABG; 2) lack of suitable graft conduits; 3) unfavorable LAD artery for PCI

Antiplatelet Therapy
- Clopidogrel 75 mg daily is a reasonable alternative in patients who cannot take aspirin

Beta-Blockers
- Preoperative beta-blockers, particularly in patients with an EF >30%, can reduce the risk of in-hospital mortality
- Can reduce the incidence of perioperative myocardial ischemia

Emotional Dysfunction and Psychosocial Considerations
- Cognitive behavior therapy or collaborative care for patients with clinical depression after CABG can be beneficial to reduce objective measures of depression

Carotid Artery Disease
- For patients with a previous transient ischemic attack or stroke and a significant (50%-99%) carotid artery stenosis, consider carotid

revascularization in conjunction with CABG. Sequence and timing (staged or simultaneous) should be determined by the relative magnitude of cerebral and myocardial dysfunction

Infection Prevention
- Leukocyte-filtered blood can be useful to reduce the rate of overall perioperative infection and in-hospital death

Adjuncts to Myocardial Protection
- Insertion of an intra-aortic balloon pump (IABP) is reasonable to reduce the mortality rate in CABG patients who are considered to be at high risk (e.g., LVEF <30% or left main CAD)
- Assessment of cardiac biomarkers in the first 24 hours after CABG may be considered

Dysrhythmia Management
- For patients who cannot take beta-blockers, amiodarone is an alternative to reduce the incidence of postoperative atrial fibrillation
- Digoxin and nondihydropyridine calcium channel blockers can be useful to control the ventricular rate in the setting of atrial fibrillation but are not indicated for prophylaxis

Reference
Hillia LD, et al. 2011 ACCF/AHA guideline for coronary artery bypass graft surgery: executive summary: a report of the American College of Cardiology Foundation/American Heart Association Task Force on Practice Guidelines. *Circulation.* 2011;124(23):2610.

BOX 16-22 PATIENT EDUCATION

Open Heart Surgery

- Pathophysiology of disease (coronary artery or valvular disease)
- Risk-factor modification to prevent coronary artery disease (smoking cessation, regular exercise, weight loss)
- Postoperative incisional care
- Activity limitations (no lifting, pushing, or pulling of anything heavier than 10 pounds for 6 to 8 weeks; no driving for 6 to 8 weeks)
- Recommended exercise progression after surgery
- Recommended diet after surgery
- Information regarding prescribed medications (including prescribed pain medication)
- Anticipated mood changes after surgery
- Follow-up appointment for clinic or primary physician
- Additional information for valve patients
- Symptoms of endocarditis
- Antibiotic prophylaxis before invasive procedures
- Information regarding anticoagulant therapy and follow-up

Patient Education

Patient education includes information related to the surgical procedure, risk-factor management, and prevention of atherosclerosis. Patients who have undergone valve surgery may also require information regarding the need for antibiotic prophylaxis before invasive procedures and specific instructions pertaining to their anticoagulation regimen (Box 16-22).

Technical Advances
Minimally Invasive Cardiac Surgery

Continuously evolving techniques have expanded the options for patients undergoing cardiac surgery, with a general transition from surgical to minimally invasive (mini-thoracotomy and small port) therapies along with percutaneous approaches. In minimally invasive direct coronary artery bypass graft (MIDCABG) surgery, a small left anterior thoracotomy incision is used to directly harvest the left IMA, which is then anastomosed to the LAD. Mitral valve repair procedures also continue to show a steady increase in the rate done with a minimally invasive approach, either robotically assisted or direct.[88]

Development of robotic surgical technology now allows surgeons to view a computer-enhanced image while manipulating instruments through a totally endoscopic port-only approach using robotic arms. Total endoscopic coronary artery bypass can either be done on an arrested heart or on a beating heart. Robotically assisted CABG is demonstrating acceptable safety standards with patients experiencing a rapid return to normal activities.[89] Significant surgeon and team learning curves limit these procedures to dedicated centers and highly specialized cardiac surgeons at this time.

Hybrid coronary revascularization combines catheter-based procedures along with surgical interventions to treat CAD, with the idea of capitalizing on the benefits of each. Most commonly, a LIMA bypass graft to the LAD is done surgically with PCI to one or two additional target vessels.[90] Patients who are hemodynamically unstable or with cardiogenic shock would generally be excluded from this procedure.[90] With the increasing availability of hybrid-operating rooms, there will be more of these approaches done simultaneously instead of the surgical team trying to decide whether to complete the surgery or percutaneous intervention first.

Surgical Treatment of Cardiac Dysrhythmias

The *maze procedure* is a surgical intervention for patients with atrial fibrillation that has not responded to medical therapy. As an open chest procedure, it is usually performed on patients who need open heart surgery for another reason, such as a CABG or valve replacement. A series of scars are made in the atrial tissue to create an electrical maze that disrupts the re-entrant pathways and directs the sinus impulse through the AV node. The procedure also includes surgical isolation of the pulmonary veins, which are thought to be responsible for initiation of atrial fibrillation, and removal of the left and right atrial appendages. The goal of treatment is not only to prevent the recurrence of atrial tachydysrhythmias but to restore sinus rhythm and AV synchrony, if possible. If the sinus node is no longer functioning, a pacemaker may be implanted to restore an AV sequential rhythm. Initially, the scars were created with a "cut and sew" technique, but the development of specialized ablation catheters enabled the creation of lesion lines with other energy sources, such as RF current, microwave energy, or cryoablation, laser, and high-intensity focused ultrasound.[91] The Cox-Maze procedure has become the gold standard for the surgical treatment of atrial fibrillation.[91] Modifications of the procedure have led to less invasive thorascopic versions performed off-pump. Patients require continued monitoring for arrhythmias as atrial fibrillation is common for months afterward while the scar tissue fully matures.

Although future trends in the surgical management of cardiac disease are difficult to predict, the critical care nurse must continue to be prepared to meet the challenge of providing a high level of nursing management at the bedside. A solid knowledge base and keen assessment skills are prerequisites for the accurate anticipation of problems and prompt intervention necessary to stabilize the patient and prevent the occurrence of life-threatening complications.

MECHANICAL CIRCULATORY ASSIST DEVICES

Mechanical circulatory assist devices are used in the treatment of heart failure when conventional pharmacologic therapy has proved ineffective. The primary goals of mechanical assist devices are to decrease myocardial workload and maintain adequate perfusion to vital organs. If the acute heart failure is reversible, a short duration of ventricular assistance is used to allow the myocardium time to recover. If the condition is irreversible, a mechanical assist device may be used as a bridge to heart transplantation for qualified candidates or as a destination therapy for those who have no other surgical options.

Intra-aortic Balloon Pump

Intra-aortic balloon pump (IABP) is the most commonly used temporary mechanical circulatory assist device for supporting failing circulation (Box 16-23). The intra-aortic balloon (IAB)

BOX 16-23　INDICATIONS FOR USE OF THE INTRA-AORTIC BALLOON PUMP

- Failure to wean from cardiopulmonary bypass
- Unstable angina refractory to medications
- Recurrent angina after acute MI
- Hemodynamic support for high-risk PCI and CABG
- Complications of acute MI
  - Cardiogenic shock
  - Papillary muscle dysfunction or rupture with mitral regurgitation
  - Ventricular septal rupture
- Refractory ventricular dysrhythmias
- Septic shock
- Bridge to definitive therapy: cardiac transplantation or ventricular assist device

---

BOX 16-24　PHYSIOLOGICAL EFFECTS OF THE INTRA-AORTIC BALLOON PUMP

Increased
- Coronary blood flow
- Cardiac output
- Urine output
- Improved mentation

Decreased
- Signs of myocardial ischemia: angina, ST-segment changes, ventricular dysrhythmias
- Afterload
- Preload
- Myocardial oxygen demand
- Pulmonary congestion
- Heart rate

---

catheter consists of a single, sausage-shaped polyurethane balloon that is wrapped around the distal end of a vascular catheter and positioned in the descending thoracic aorta just distal to the takeoff of the left subclavian artery. When attached to a bedside pumping console and properly synchronized to the patient's cardiac cycle, the IAB inflates during diastole and deflates just before systole. Its therapeutic effects are based on the hemodynamic principles of diastolic augmentation and afterload reduction (Box 16-24).

Initially, as the balloon is inflated in diastole concurrent with aortic valve closure, the blood in the aortic arch above the level of the balloon is displaced retrograde (backward) toward the aortic root, augmenting diastolic coronary arterial blood flow and increasing myocardial oxygen supply (Fig. 16-20A). The blood volume in the aorta below the level of the balloon is propelled forward toward the peripheral vascular system, which may enhance systemic perfusion. Subsequently, the deflation of the balloon just before the opening of the aortic valve creates a potential space or vacuum in the aorta, toward which blood flows unimpeded during ventricular ejection (see Fig. 16-20B). This decreased resistance to LV ejection, or decreased afterload, facilitates ventricular emptying and reduces myocardial oxygen demands. The overall physiologic effect of IABP therapy is an

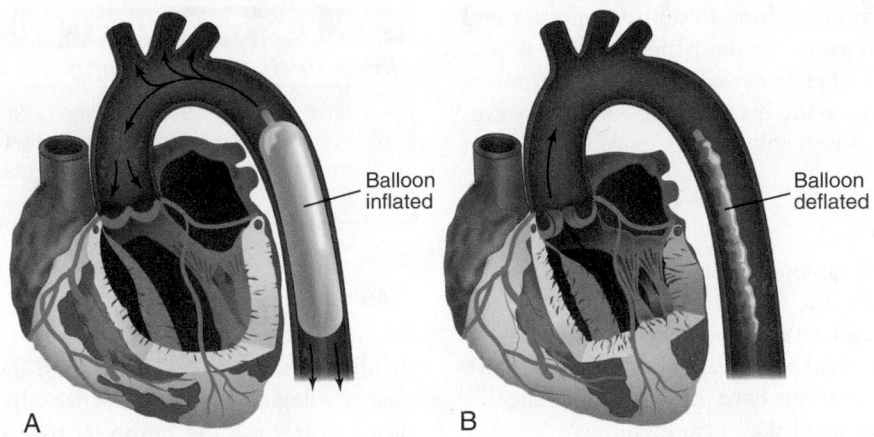

FIGURE 16-20 Mechanisms of action of the intra-aortic balloon pump. *A*, Diastolic balloon inflation augments coronary blood flow. *B*, Systolic balloon deflation decreases afterload.

improvement in the balance between myocardial oxygen supply and demand. Contraindications to IABP include aortic aneurysm, significant aortic valve insufficiency, and severe peripheral vascular disease.[92,93]

Medical Management

The IAB may be inserted in the operating room, the cardiac catheterization laboratory, or the critical care unit. The IAB catheter is usually inserted percutaneously through the femoral artery and advanced to the correct position in the descending thoracic aorta. The physician may insert the balloon through an introducer sheath or perform a sheathless insertion to minimize the degree of vessel occlusion created by the catheter. If percutaneous catheter placement is not feasible, the catheter may be placed through surgical cut-down or by a direct thoracic approach. After insertion, the balloon is attached to the console, filled with the prescribed volume of helium, and pumping is then initiated. If the balloon fails to unwrap completely during filling, the physician may rapidly inflate and deflate the balloon manually, using a syringe.

Nursing Management

The management of the pumping console and its timing functions may be performed by the nurse caring for the patient or delegated to specially trained personnel. There are multiple factors that may affect the efficacy of the IABP, including position of the balloon within the aorta, balloon displacement volume, inflation/deflation timing, signal quality, the patient's cardiac function, and hemodynamic variables, which include circulating blood volume, blood pressure, and vascular resistance.[92,94] Clinicians need to be aware of these factors in order to adequately assess for and ensure optimal IABP performance.

Balloon Catheter Position

The balloon catheter must be maintained in proper position to optimize its effectiveness and minimize complications. The balloon may migrate proximally and occlude the left subclavian artery or the carotids, or it may move distally, compromising renal and mesenteric circulation. Careful assessment of the left radial pulse, level of consciousness, urinary output, and gastrointestinal symptoms is essential. Measures to prevent accidental

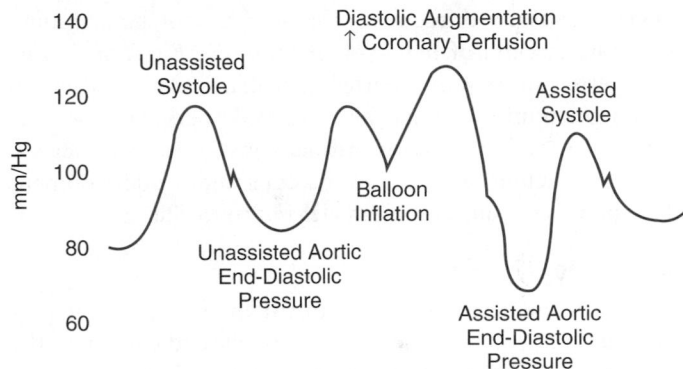

FIGURE 16-21 The timing and effect of balloon counterpulsations. Timing is adjusted by synchronizing balloon inflation with the dicrotic notch on the arterial waveform, resulting in an elevated diastolic pressure. Inflation is maintained throughout diastole to augment coronary perfusion. Deflation occurs just before the next systole, resulting in a reduced systolic pressure and decreased afterload.

displacement of the balloon catheter include ensuring that the IAB is secured to the patient's skin, that the patient observes complete bed rest with the head of the bed elevated no more than 30 degrees, and avoids any flexion of the involved hip.

Timing

The IABP is dependent upon proper timing to ensure optimal hemodynamic benefits.[95] Although systems now adjust the timing automatically, clinicians must still be aware of how to set the timing, understand the method utilized, and evaluate its affects. The ECG and arterial pressure tracings are constantly monitored to verify the timing and effect of balloon counterpulsation (Fig. 16-21). For counterpulsation to occur, the pump must receive a trigger signal to identify the beginning and end of the cardiac cycle. The trigger can be the R wave of the ECG, the upstroke of the arterial pressure waveform, or a pacemaker spike.[93]

Dysrhythmias

Dysrhythmias can adversely affect the timing of balloon inflation and deflation, so rhythm disturbances must be detected and treated promptly. Current IABPs have automatic timing features that use internal algorithms to adjust inflation and deflation in response to changes in the patient's heart rate or rhythm. There are also catheters available that incorporate a fiberoptic sensor to enhance the quality of the arterial waveform, which allows beat-to-beat adjustments to improve timing accuracy.[96]

Vascular Complications

One complication of IABP support is lower extremity ischemia resulting from occlusion of the femoral artery by the catheter itself or by emboli caused by thrombus formation on the balloon (see Box 16-17, Patient Safety for Peripheral Ischemia). Although ischemic complications have decreased with sheathless insertion techniques and the introduction of smaller balloon catheters (7 versus 9.5 Fr), evaluation of peripheral circulation remains an important nursing assessment. The presence and quality of peripheral pulses distal to the catheter insertion site are assessed frequently, along with color, temperature, and capillary refill of the involved extremity. Signs of diminished perfusion must be reported immediately. Anticoagulation (e.g., heparin infusion) may be prescribed to decrease the incidence of thrombosis. Other vascular complications associated with IABP include acute aortic dissection and the development of pseudoaneurysms at the catheter insertion site.

Balloon Perforation

Another potential complication of IABP therapy is balloon perforation. Perforation occurs because of repeated contact of the balloon membrane with calcified plaque in the aorta as the balloon inflates and deflates. The patient is monitored for evidence of a balloon leak, such as a gas leak alarm from the pump console or the presence of blood in the IAB tubing. If a balloon leak is detected, pumping is stopped and the physician is immediately notified so that the balloon can be removed. If the balloon is not promptly removed or pumping is attempted after the perforation, the IAB may become entrapped as the blood hardens within the catheter, creating a mass. If this occurs, the balloon must be surgically removed.

Preventing Further Complications

Log rolling, in which the patient is moved from side to side every 2 hours, is used to maintain skin integrity and to prevent pulmonary atelectasis. Because thrombocytopenia may occur as a result of mechanical destruction of the platelets by the pumping action of the balloon, platelet counts are closely monitored and the patient is observed for evidence of bleeding. Since infection of the insertion site is a potential complication, the dressing is changed in accordance with the hospital policy for other invasive lines.

Psychologic Needs

The psychologic needs of the patient must be considered while on IABP therapy. Sleep deprivation is common and is related in part to the continuous nursing management requirements for the patient and the noise level in the unit, including the sounds made by the balloon pumping device. Anxiety related to fear of nonrecovery and loss of control because of forced immobility is a common occurrence.

Weaning

Weaning from the IABP is considered after hemodynamic stability has been achieved with no—or only minimal—pharmacologic support. One weaning procedure consists of slowly decreasing the pumping frequency from every beat to every fourth beat, as tolerated. Another, less common, weaning method involves a gradual decrease in balloon volume. To prevent thrombus formation on the balloon surface, the IABP must remain at a minimal pumping ratio (or volume) until its removal.

Patient Education

Patient education for the patient with an IAB is presented in Box 16-25. Many of the IABP manufacturers provide helpful educational booklets designed for patients and families.

Ventricular Assist Devices

The ventricular assist device (VAD) is designed to support or replace a failing natural heart with flow assistance. Diversion of varying amounts of systemic blood flow around a failing ventricle by means of a pump reduces cardiac workload while maintaining adequate perfusion to sustain end-organ function. VADs can be used to support a failing RV or LV, or both.[92]

VADs are currently indicated for three types of clinical applications. The first category of patients includes those who, despite aggressive medical therapy, continue to demonstrate persistent heart failure but who have the potential for regaining normal heart function if the heart is given time to rest. This category, called *bridge to recovery*, consists of patients who have acute postsurgical myocardial dysfunction, are in refractory cardiogenic shock after acute MI, or have acute viral myocarditis. The second category, called *bridge to transplantation* (BTT), includes those patients with decompensated chronic heart failure who need circulatory support until heart transplantation can be performed. The third category, called *destination therapy* (DT), is comprised of patients with severe heart failure who are not candidates for heart transplantation and for whom all other medical options have been exhausted. Several VADs have received FDA approval for DT or BTT, with a number of other devices in clinical trials. All consist of a blood pump, cannula, controller, and some type of power source. Some devices displace blood to create pulsatile flow, but most systems now generate continuous flow and are therefore pulseless. Percutaneous VADs allow for rapid, minimally invasive, short-term support for patients in cardiogenic shock until recovery occurs or a long-term device can be placed.[97] There is no single ideal system, so device selection is based on individual VAD capabilities and institutional preference (Table 16-13). The left ventricular assist device (LVAD) is used most commonly because LV failure

TABLE 16-13 VENTRICULAR ASSIST DEVICES

TYPE	INDICATIONS	DESCRIPTION
Temporary		
CentriMag	Short-term univentricular or biventricular support	A continuous-flow pump that produces blood flow from 0-10 L/min Blood flow is produced by the rotation of a magnetically suspended impeller, eliminating contact between components Placed either through an open chest or by percutaneous methods
Impella LP 2.5 and Impella LP 5.0	Short-term left ventricular support	A continuous-flow pump that has a percutaneously inserted catheter, allowing flows of 2.5 L/min or 5 L/min for the version that requires a surgical cut-down for implantation The catheter is placed retrograde across the aortic valve to pull blood from the left ventricle, which is returned to ascending aorta
TandemHeart	Short-term left or right ventricular support	A percutaneously inserted device that provides continuous flow up to 5 L/min LVAD: Inflow is obtained from a catheter positioned in the left atrium (by a transseptal approach), and outflow is through the femoral artery RVAD: inflow is obtained from a catheter positioned in the right atrium and outflow is through the pulmonary artery Device allows for transport to a center for long-term therapy
Long-Term		
HeartWare	Long-term left-ventricular support as bridge to transplantation or destination therapy	A continuous flow rotary pump with centrifugal design that produces nonpulsatile flow Its small size allows for placement above the diaphragm in the pericardial space The pump has no points of mechanical contact, which reduces the damage to red blood cells
HeartMate II	Long-term left ventricular support Approved for bridge to transplantation and destination therapy	An electrically driven rotary pump that produces nonpulsatile flow Smaller size allows for implantation in patients with body surface area <1.5 m² Anticoagulation and antiplatelet therapy are required

LVAD, Left ventricular assist device; *RVAD*, right ventricular assist device.

occurs more often than does RV failure (Fig. 16-23). Use of biventricular support (bi-VAD) may be needed in the acute phase, because RV failure often follows LV failure.[98] Inlet cannulas that divert blood from the heart to the LVAD for LV support are placed in the left atrium or the LV apex, with the outlet cannula attached to the ascending aorta or femoral artery. For the right ventricular assist device (RVAD) the inlet cannula would be placed on the right side with the outlet cannula in the pulmonary artery (Fig. 16-22). Additional options for biventricular failure are the total artificial hearts (TAHs), which can be used for BTT or DT.[99] Flow rates between 1 and 10 L/min are used by the different devices to maintain adequate cardiac output while decreasing ventricular workload.

Nursing Management

Nursing diagnoses and management for a patient with a VAD include monitoring for hemodynamic changes and for complications related to the device. The same interventions to optimize cardiac output by manipulation of heart rate, preload, afterload, and contractility that are used for cardiac surgery patients apply to patients with a VAD. Adequate filling volumes are essential to maintain pump flow. Afterload reduction may be needed to improve output from the unassisted ventricle when univentricular support is used. Complications common to all types of VADs include bleeding, infection, thromboembolism, and device failure, although complication rates vary among the different models.[99] Complications associated specifically with continuous-flow VADs have been arteriovenous malformations and progressive aortic valve insufficiency.[100]

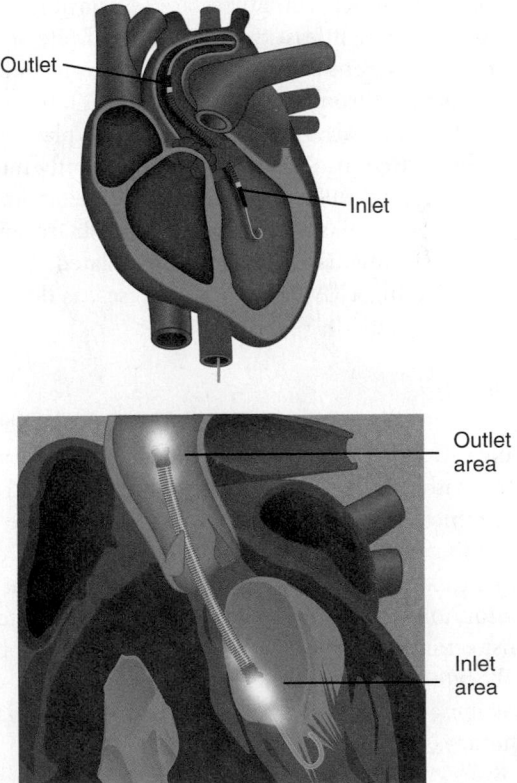

FIGURE 16-22 Diagram of the Impella ventricular assist device. Blood is pulled into the catheter from the left ventricle and returned to the ascending aorta.

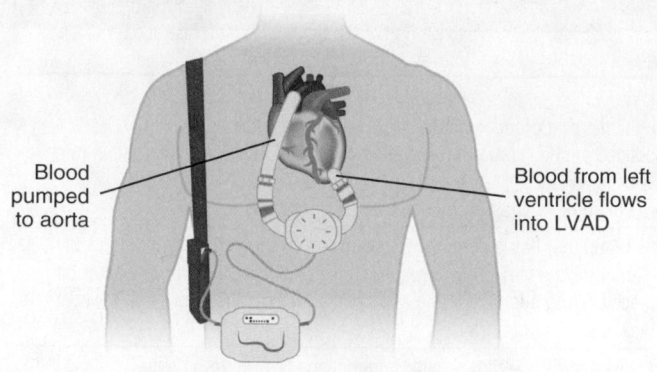

Blood pumped to aorta

Blood from left ventricle flows into LVAD

FIGURE 16-23 Diagram of a left ventricular assist device (LVAD) system.

Device Failure

Although the incidence of device failure continues to decrease, it is a life-threatening event because of the nature of this therapy. VAD designs vary considerably, and troubleshooting methods for device failure are unique to each device. The nurse must be aware of signs of device malfunction as well as patient factors (volume status, dysrhythmias, RV failure) that may affect VAD function.

Anticoagulation

The requirement for anticoagulation varies with the type of VAD, the flow rate, and institutional protocol. If patients are anticoagulated with heparin, nurses are responsible for maintaining clotting times at least twice the normal rate and monitoring for complications of bleeding. Coagulation studies, such as activated partial thromboplastin time (aPTT), prothrombin time (PT), international normalized ratio (INR), platelet counts, and thromboelastogram (TEG) must be frequently monitored during support. Continued bleeding may necessitate withholding the heparin infusion and administering fresh-frozen plasma and platelets. If patients are not anticoagulated, the risk of thrombi obstructing a VAD cannula increases, as does the risk of an embolic event.

Infection

Patients with a VAD are at considerable risk for localized and septicemic infections. Infectious risks are posed by the presence of invasive catheters and the surgically implanted VAD. Infection is prevented by the use of strict aseptic technique with all invasive tubing and dressing changes. Site care varies, depending on institutional protocols and the type of VAD that is used. Nurses monitor patients for infection by measuring temperatures, inspecting insertion sites and incisions, and obtaining daily leukocyte counts. If an infection is suspected, pan-cultures (blood, urine, and sputum) are taken to guide appropriate antibiotic therapy.

Continuous-flow Hemodynamics

Because continuous-flow VADs provide circulatory support throughout the cardiac cycle, patients will have a decreased arterial pulse pressure, which may result in a flat pressure

waveform.[101] For these patients, pulse oximetry is not always reliable and automatic blood pressure monitors may or may not provide a reading, so Dopplers are often required for manual blood pressures.[102] Nurses must often rely on basic assessments such as circulation, mentation, and urine output to determine if the patient is receiving adequate support.

Patient Education

The rapid and acute nature of cardiogenic shock limits the nurse's ability to prepare patients and families for VAD insertion. Despite the critical nature of the illness, nurses explain the reason for the use of the VAD and provide information about the critical care environment and equipment (Box 16-26). The number of VAD patients discharged to home continues to increase. These patients and their families require education related to care of the device and reinforcement on the components of heart failure management.

VASCULAR SURGERY

Vascular surgery may be used as a treatment for arterial occlusive disease or to correct structural abnormalities such as aneurysms. With the evolution in endovascular technology, many patients with vascular disease can now be effectively treated with percutaneous procedures. The choice between an open surgical procedure and an endovascular intervention depends on a number of factors, including the type/location of the vascular lesion, life expectancy, comorbid conditions, and patient preference. Because atherosclerosis is a diffuse disease that affects both the peripheral vessels and the coronary arteries, patients undergoing arterial vascular surgery are at high risk for perioperative cardiac events. The nursing care of patients after vascular surgery focuses not only on observations for surgical complications such as hematoma or reocclusion but also on prompt recognition and appropriate treatment of complications that may arise from the impact of the procedure on preexisting cardiac, pulmonary, or kidney disease.

Carotid Endarterectomy

Carotid endarterectomy (CEA) may be beneficial in both symptomatic and asymptomatic patients with stenoses greater than 50% to 70%.[103] The procedure is performed through a neck incision that allows for visualization of the vessel. The plaque is removed, and the vessel is closed directly or with a patch composed of saphenous vein or a prosthetic material. A Jackson-Pratt drain may be placed at the end of the procedure to minimize hematoma formation. Complications after CEA include perioperative MI, cerebral ischemia or infarction, bleeding, and cranial nerve damage.

Postoperative Nursing Management

Patients require 12 to 24 hours of intensive nursing assessment in the period immediately after CEA. Complications are rare but may be life threatening and require rapid intervention. Serial assessments are performed, and the surgeon is promptly notified of significant changes in the patient's status.

Neurologic Assessment

Frequent neurologic assessments are performed as the patient awakens from anesthesia and then hourly for the first 12 hours. These assessments should include level of consciousness, orientation, pupil response, motor function, and evaluation of cranial nerve function (e.g., swallowing or gag reflexes, hoarseness, tongue movement, facial drooping). Compression, traction, or inadvertent severing can damage nerves that lie in or near the surgical field. The most common injuries are damage to the laryngeal and hypoglossal nerves. Most cranial nerve dysfunction resolves within a short time.[104]

Bleeding

Bleeding is assessed by observation of the dressing for drainage or swelling and measurement of output from the neck drain, if present. If hematoma formation occurs internally, it may impinge on the trachea, so the patient is also monitored for signs of a compromised airway. In addition to monitoring respiratory rate and oxygen saturation, the nurse assesses the patient for tracheal deviation and for symptoms of upper airway obstruction such as stridor or wheezing. A small venous hematoma may respond to manual pressure, but larger arterial hematomas that expand rapidly require emergent return to the operating room for re-exploration and evacuation.

Cardiovascular Monitoring

Continuous ECG monitoring with ST-segment monitoring is used to detect myocardial ischemia after CEA. Bradycardia is common as a result of baroreceptor stimulation during the operative procedure but is usually hemodynamically tolerated as long as the patient's blood pressure is adequate. Manipulation of the carotid bulb during the surgery often results in hemodynamic instability in the immediate postoperative period. An arterial line is usually placed to allow for prompt detection and treatment of hypotension or hypertension. Adequate blood pressure control in the postoperative period is of paramount importance. Hypertension increases the risk of bleeding at the suture line and is typically treated with short-acting vasodilators such as sodium nitroprusside. A relative hypotension compared with the patient's baseline value results in inadequate cerebral perfusion and potential neurologic deficits, so vasopressors such as phenylephrine may be used to maintain an adequate blood pressure.

Carotid Stents

Although CEA has been the gold standard for treatment of patients with significant carotid artery stenosis, carotid stenting is increasingly being used as an alternative in patients considered to be at high surgical risk.[105] This procedure is performed with the use of local anesthesia and percutaneous cannulation similar to that used in coronary stenting. The use of embolic protection devices to trap and remove embolic particles generated during the procedure improves neurologic outcomes.[104] A recent multicenter study demonstrated equivalent outcomes between the two procedures, with fewer minor strokes in the CEA group and a lower risk of MI for carotid artery stenting.[106]

Nursing care of patients following carotid stenting is similar to that provided following CEA. Typically, patients are monitored in a critical care unit overnight to allow for frequent neurologic assessments and treatment of hemodynamic instability.[105] Patients are also monitored for potential complications related to vascular access sheaths.

Abdominal Aortic Aneurysm Repair

An abdominal aortic aneurysm (AAA) is usually repaired when the aneurysm is 5 cm or larger, creating symptoms, or rapidly expanding. This is done to prevent the high mortality associated with abdominal rupture. Repair involves insertion of a prosthetic graft to support the portion of the vessel weakened by the aneurysm. Options for graft placement include either an open surgical procedure or a less invasive endovascular approach.

Surgical Repair

Surgery is performed with the patient under general anesthesia and involves access through a midline abdominal incision or a flank incision (retroperitoneal approach). Clamping of the aorta proximal and distal to the dilated area isolates the aneurysm. The aneurysmal portion of the aorta is replaced with a prosthetic graft, which is then enclosed within the aneurysmal sac.

Postoperative complications include myocardial ischemia or infarction, bleeding, acute kidney injury, and distal embolization.[107] Rarely, colon or spinal cord ischemia may occur because of interruption of blood flow during aortic cross-clamping or embolization. After the surgical procedure, patients are monitored in the critical care unit for 24 to 48 hours, with a total length of hospital stay being 5 to 9 days.

Postoperative Management

Nursing assessment of vital signs along with assessment of peripheral perfusion is performed frequently in the early postoperative period. Continuous ECG monitoring with ST-segment analysis is used to detect myocardial ischemia. An arterial line is placed to allow for prompt detection and treatment of hypotension or hypertension. Hypertension increases the risk of bleeding at the suture lines and is often treated with short-acting vasodilators such as sodium nitroprusside. Hypotension may result in compromised perfusion to organs or the extremities and is treated with volume replacement and vasopressors as needed. Hourly assessment of urine output is performed to evaluate kidney function. If urine output is less than 30 mL/hr, diuretics may be used after correction of hypovolemia. The dressing is assessed for bleeding, and potential signs of internal hemorrhage from the graft site (hypotension, complaints of back pain) are further evaluated with serial hematocrit measurements. Patients without preoperative pulmonary conditions may be rapidly weaned from ventilatory support, with supplemental oxygen given as needed to maintain oxygen saturation in the normal range.

Endovascular Stent Grafts

The endoluminal placement of stent grafts provides a less invasive approach for repair of an AAA. In this procedure, a sutureless vascular graft is implanted into the abdominal aorta through a femoral arteriotomy. The stent isolates the aneurysmal wall from intraluminal blood pressure to prevent further expansion or rupture of the aneurysm.[108] This procedure can be performed with the patient under epidural anesthesia, with minimal blood loss and a shorter length of stay. Initially introduced as an alternative for patients who would otherwise be deemed inoperable due to comorbid conditions, this procedure is now performed in the majority of elective cases.[107] Although the operative mortality and morbidity may be less with endovascular stents, randomized studies have shown no significant difference in long-term survival between open surgical and endovascular interventions in patients with AAA.[109] In addition, follow-up surveillance is essential following stent placement since late complications such as endoleak and device migration can occur, necessitating reintervention.[110]

Peripheral Vascular Procedures

Arteriosclerosis obliterans is a condition in which atherosclerosis produces progressive obstruction of medium-to-larger arteries. These lesions commonly occur at bifurcations of the abdominal aorta and the iliac, femoral, popliteal or tibial, and peroneal arteries. Progression of peripheral arterial disease can lead to critical limb ischemia. This may initially manifest as intermittent claudication, but if left untreated, it can progress to rest pain, ulceration, or even gangrene. Initial treatment focuses on lifestyle modification, such as smoking cessation, exercise therapy, adequate diabetic control, effective treatment of hypertension, and management of dyslipidemia. Pharmacologic interventions such as antiplatelet and antithrombotic agents may be used. If these strategies fail, patients may be considered for revascularization by means of surgical bypass or a percutaneous intervention (angioplasty, atherectomy, or stent placement). Regardless of the type of procedure selected, inflow is always established first—through repair of vascular defects that compromise flow into the femoral vessels. If symptoms persist, this is followed by repair of outflow lesions in vessels in the lower leg.[111]

Because there are a number of endovascular and surgical options available for the treatment of PAD, treatment decisions can be complicated. The risks of the procedure need to be weighed against the anticipated benefits, including long-term patency and options for further treatment if needed. Consensus guidelines have been issued that include treatment recommendations based on lesion morphology, but these continue to evolve with improvements in technology and operator expertise.[112]

Surgical Revascularization

Surgical revascularization utilizes graft material to bypass the diseased portion of the vessel, thus improving distal blood flow. Procedures are usually performed under general anesthesia, although regional anesthesia may be used in some cases. Conduits available for peripheral vascular bypass include vein grafts (reversed saphenous vein, arm vein, or human umbilical vein)

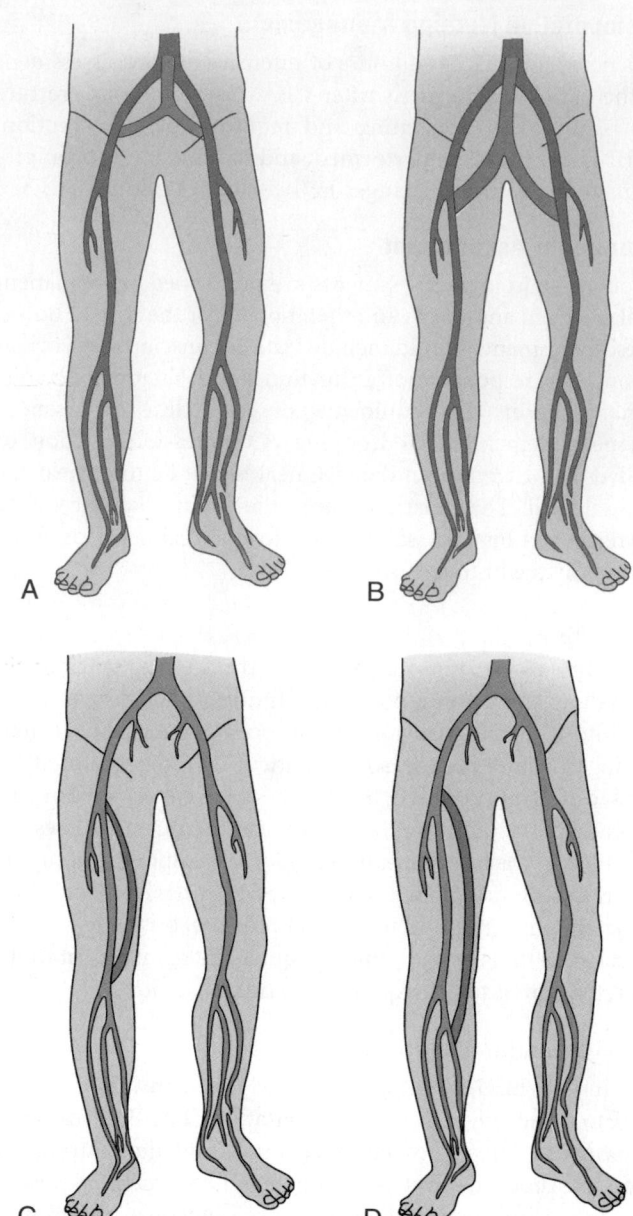

FIGURE 16-24 Peripheral arterial bypass procedures. Inflow procedures: *A,* aortoiliac bypass; *B,* aortobifemoral bypass. Outflow procedures: *C,* femoropopliteal bypass; *D,* femorotibial bypass.

and synthetic grafts made of polytetrafluoroethylene. As in CABG, the type of conduit used has an impact on the patency rate of the graft. While synthetic grafts perform well in larger vessels (higher flow), veins are preferred in smaller vessels because of better patency rates.[113] Types of peripheral vascular procedures are shown in Figure 16-24.

Percutaneous Interventions

Percutaneous interventions used in the coronary arteries—angioplasty, atherectomy, and stenting—can be performed to treat occlusion or narrowing in the peripheral vasculature as well. Similar advances in catheter design and the development of intravascular stents have resulted in a dramatic increase in the number of endovascular procedures performed for PAD. No longer limited to the treatment of short, focal stenoses or for poor surgical candidates, these devices are now routinely used as first-line therapy. Atherectomy is employed more often, since the diameter of peripheral vessels can more easily accommodate the larger catheters required for these procedures. Intravascular stents may be used in combination with percutaneous translu-minal angioplasty (PTA), depending on lesion morphology and location. Mechanical movement of the leg can increase the inci-dence of stent fracture and poor endothelialization, limiting their use in some areas.[114] Complications of interventional vas-cular procedures include hematoma formation at the site of the arteriotomy, formation of a pseudoaneurysm, distal emboliza-tion, and thrombotic occlusion.

Acute occlusion of a peripheral artery may occur as a result of local thrombosis, emboli, trauma, or compression. Left untreated, the resultant ischemia may lead to amputation of the affected limb. Catheter-based interventions that may be used to recanalize acutely occluded arteries include intra-arterial infu-sions of fibrinolytic medications and the use of thrombectomy devices to fragment and remove the clot. If these interventions are unsuccessful, revascularization may be performed.[115] In the setting of limb-threatening ischemia, surgical repairs are more durable and are recommended for patients with an expected lifespan of more than 2 years.[110]

Nursing Management. The primary focus of nursing care in the immediate postprocedural period is assessment of the adequacy of perfusion to the affected limb and identification of complications. Pulse checks are performed frequently, and the physician is notified of any decrease in the strength of the Doppler signal. Adequate blood pressure is essential to maintain perfusion through the repaired vessel or graft. Because distal perfusion is compromised in this patient population, nursing measures to prevent skin breakdown (e.g., sheepskin, frequent repositioning, foot cradles) are implemented. If the repair was performed above the renal arteries, kidney function may be impaired as a result of interruption of renal blood flow during the procedure. Urine output is therefore assessed hourly and supported with fluids and diuretics as needed. Because patients with peripheral vascular disease are at high risk for cardiac events, ST-segment monitoring is performed to detect episodes of myocardial ischemia throughout the perioperative period.

EFFECTS OF CARDIOVASCULAR MEDICATIONS

Multiple medications are used in the treatment of critically ill cardiovascular patients. The critical care nurse is responsible for preparation and administration of these pharmacologic thera-pies and often is required to titrate the dose on the basis of the patient's hemodynamic response. The medications used to treat cardiovascular disease are rapidly changing and expanding as more is learned about the pathophysiology of cardiac disease and as improved formulas are developed by pharmaceutical companies. The critical care nurse who has a general under-standing of the mechanisms of action of the various pharma-cologic classifications can readily apply this knowledge to new medications within the same classification. The following dis-cussion provides a concise review of medications commonly administered to support cardiovascular function in the critical

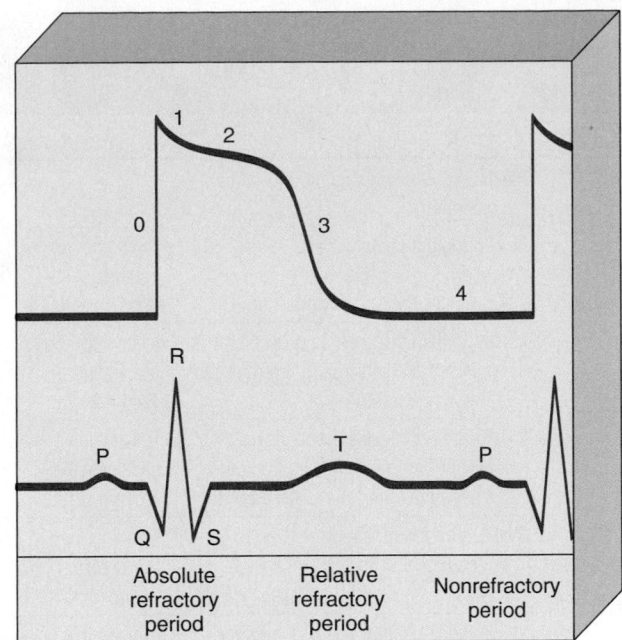

FIGURE 16-25 The phases of the cardiac action potential and their relationship to the heart's refractory periods. *Phase 0,* Depolarization with rapid influx of sodium. *Phase 1,* Rapid repo-larization with rapid efflux of potassium ions and decreased sodium conductance. *Phase 2,* Plateau with slow influx of sodium and calcium ions. *Phase 3,* Repolarization with contin-ued efflux of potassium ions. *Phase 4,* Resting phase with restoration of ionic balance by sodium and potassium pumps.

care setting. The emphasis is on intravenously administered medications that are used for the acute rather than the chronic management of cardiovascular conditions.

Antidysrhythmic Medications

Antidysrhythmic medications comprise a diverse category of pharmacologic agents used to terminate or prevent an array of abnormal cardiac rhythms. These commonly are classified according to their primary effect on the action potential of cardiac cells (Fig. 16-25). The classification scheme shown in Table 16-14 is the most commonly used system. Classification of newer agents is more difficult, because some of these agents have characteristics of more than one class and others have no characteristics of the current system.

Class I

Class I agents are sodium channel blockers that decrease the influx of sodium ions through "fast" channels during phase 0 depolarization. This prolongs the absolute (effective) refractory period, thereby decreasing the risk of premature impulses from ectopic foci. These medications also depress automaticity by slowing the rate of spontaneous depolarization of pacemaker cells during the resting phase (phase 4).

Class I antidysrhythmic medications can be further subdi-vided into three groups according to their potency as sodium channel inhibitors and their effect on phase 3 repolarization. Class IA agents—quinidine, procainamide, and disopyramide—block both the fast sodium channels and phase 3 repolarization,

TABLE 16-14 CLASSIFICATION OF ANTIDYSRHYTHMIC AGENTS

CLASS	ACTION	MEDICATIONS
I	Blocks sodium channels (stabilizes cell membrane)	
IA	Blocks sodium channels and delays repolarization, lengthening the duration of the action potential	Quinidine Procainamide Disopyramide
IB	Blocks sodium channels and accelerates repolarization, shortening the duration of the action potential	Lidocaine Mexiletine Tocainide
IC	Blocks sodium channels and slows conduction through the His-Purkinje system, prolonging the QRS duration	Flecainide Encainide Propafenone
II	Blocks beta-receptors	Esmolol Metoprolol Propranolol
III	Slows repolarization and prolongs the duration of the action potential	Amiodarone Ibutilide Sotalol Dofetilide Dronedarone
IV	Blocks calcium channels	Diltiazem Verapamil

TABLE 16-15 EFFECTS OF ADRENERGIC RECEPTORS

RECEPTOR	LOCATION	RESPONSE TO STIMULATION
Alpha (α)	Vessels of skin, muscles, kidneys, and intestines	Vasoconstriction of peripheral arterioles
Beta$_1$ (β_1)	Cardiac tissue	Increased heart rate Increased conduction Increased contractility
Beta$_2$ (β_2)	Vascular and bronchial smooth muscle	Vasodilation of peripheral arterioles Bronchodilation

For example, bronchospasm can be precipitated by noncardioselective beta-blockers in a patient with chronic obstructive pulmonary disease (COPD) caused by blockade of the effects of Beta$_2$-receptors in the lungs. Beta-blockers also are negative inotropes and must be used cautiously in patients with LV dysfunction. Although numerous beta-blockers are marketed, only esmolol, metoprolol, and propranolol are available as intravenous agents for the treatment of acute dysrhythmias. Of these, esmolol (Brevibloc) offers significant advantages for the critically ill patient because of its short half-life (approximately 9 minutes). It is used in the treatment of supraventricular tachycardias, such as atrial fibrillation and atrial flutter.

Class III

Class III agents include amiodarone, dofetilide, dronedarone, ibutilide, and sotalol. These agents markedly slow the rate of phase 3 repolarization, increasing the effective refractory period and the action potential duration. Although their effects on the action potential are similar, these medications differ greatly in their mechanism of action and their side effects. At this time, sotalol is approved only for oral use. Intravenous amiodarone was originally approved for the treatment of serious ventricular dysrhythmias refractory to other medications. Because of its effectiveness, it is now used for both atrial and ventricular dysrhythmias.[117] Dofetilide (Tikosyn) is a new class III antidysrhythmic agent used for the conversion to and maintenance of normal sinus rhythm in patients with highly symptomatic atrial fibrillation or atrial flutter. Because dofetilide prolongs the refractoriness of both atrial and ventricular tissue, prolongation of the QT interval can occur and is associated with an increased risk of torsades de pointes.[118] Therapy with dofetilide is initiated in a hospital setting under close monitoring. Ibutilide (Covert) is a short-term antidysrhythmic agent used for the rapid conversion of acute atrial fibrillation or atrial flutter to sinus rhythm. Ibutilide is administered as a 10-minute infusion in a carefully monitored clinical setting. The most serious side effect of ibutilide is its potential for inducing life-threatening dysrhythmias, especially torsades de pointes.[119]

Class IV

Class IV agents are calcium channel blockers that inhibit the influx of calcium through slow calcium channels during the plateau phase (phase 2). This effect occurs primarily in tissue

thus prolonging the action potential duration. Clinically, this may result in measurable increases in the QRS duration and lengthening of the QT interval. All class IA agents may depress myocardial contractility, with disopyramide having the most potent negative inotropic effect. Medications in class IB have only a moderate effect on sodium channels and accelerate phase 3 repolarization to shorten the action potential duration; lidocaine, mexiletine, and tocainide belong in this group. Class IC agents are the most potent sodium channel blockers and have little effect on repolarization. Class IC agents increase the PR and QRS intervals. Included in this group are encainide, flecainide, and propafenone. The results of the Cardiac Arrhythmia Suppression Trial (CAST) indicated that treatment with encainide and flecainide may be associated with increased mortality, and the use of these agents in clinical practice has decreased.[116]

Class II

Class II agents are beta-adrenergic blockers (beta-blockers). They inhibit dysrhythmias mediated by the sympathetic nervous system by competing with endogenous catecholamines for available receptor sites. As a result, spontaneous depolarization during the resting phase (phase 4) is depressed, and AV conduction is slowed. Antidysrhythmic medications in this class can be further subdivided into cardioselective agents (those that block only Beta$_1$-receptors) and noncardioselective agents (those that block both Beta$_1$- and Beta$_2$-receptors). Knowledge of the effects of adrenergic-receptor stimulation allows for anticipation of both the therapeutic responses brought about by beta-blockade and the potential adverse effects of these agents (Table 16-15).

in which slow calcium channels predominate, primarily the sinus and AV nodes and the atrial tissue. Verapamil was the first medication in this category available as an intravenous antidysrhythmic. It depresses sinus and AV node conduction and is effective in terminating supraventricular tachycardias caused by AV nodal re-entry. Diltiazem (Cardizem) has become available in intravenous form and is thought to be as effective as verapamil in treating supraventricular dysrhythmias, with fewer hypotensive side effects. Because accessory pathways are not affected by calcium channel blockade, both of these agents must be avoided when treating atrial fibrillation or flutter in patients with Wolff-Parkinson-White syndrome.[8]

Unclassified Antidysrhythmics

Adenosine (Adenocard) is an antidysrhythmic agent that remains unclassified under the current system. Adenosine occurs endogenously in the body as a building block of adenosine triphosphate (ATP). Given in intravenous boluses, adenosine slows conduction through the AV node, causing transient AV block. It is used clinically to convert supraventricular tachycardias and to facilitate differential diagnosis of rapid dysrhythmias. Because of its short half-life, adenosine is administered intravenously as a rapid bolus, followed by a saline flush. The bolus is delivered as centrally as possible, so that the medication reaches the heart before it is metabolized.[8] Side effects are transient, because adenosine is rapidly taken up by the cells and is cleared from the body within 10 seconds.

Magnesium is also unclassified under the present system. Although its action as an antidysrhythmic agent is not entirely understood, clinical studies suggest that it may reduce the incidence of both ventricular and supraventricular dysrhythmias in selected patient populations. It is considered the treatment of choice in patients with torsades de pointes. For acute treatment, 1 to 2 g of magnesium is administered over 1 to 2 minutes. In patients with confirmed hypomagnesemia, this bolus may be followed with a 24-hour infusion.[8]

Side Effects

Antidysrhythmic medications carry the risk of serious side effects, some of which can be life threatening. The major side effects of the intravenous antidysrhythmic agents are listed in Table 16-16. The most severe complication is the potential for a prodysrhythmic effect. This may result in worsening of the underlying dysrhythmia, the occurrence of a new dysrhythmia,

---

TABLE 16-16 PHARMACOLOGIC MANAGEMENT

Selected Antidysrhythmic Agents

MEDICATION	DOSAGE	ACTIONS	SPECIAL CONSIDERATIONS
Adenosine	6 mg IV rapid push; if unsuccessful, repeat with 12 mg over 1-2 sec; follow with IV fluid 10 mL flush (NS or D$_5$W)	Blocks the AV node to terminate SVT, PSVT	Transient; flushing, dyspnea, hypotension
Digoxin	0.5-1 mg loading dose in divided doses; maintenance dose of 0.125-0.375 mg daily	Conversion and/or rate control in SVT, AFib, AF	Bradycardia, heart block Toxicity: CNS and GI symptoms
Diltiazem	Bolus dose of 0.25 mg/kg IV over 2 min, followed by an infusion of 5-15 mg/hr	Conversion and/or rate control in SVT, AFib, AF	Bradycardia, hypotension, AV block
Esmolol	Loading dose of 500 mcg/kg over 1 min, followed by an infusion of 50 mcg/kg/min for 4 min; repeat procedure every 5 min, increasing infusion by 25-50 mcg/kg/min to maximum of 200 mcg/kg/min	Conversion and/or rate control in SVT, AFib, AF Also used to decrease rate of sinus tachycardia	Hypotension, bradycardia, heart failure
Ibutilide	0.010-0.025 mg/kg infused over 10 min (may repeat once) or 1 mg diluted in 50 mL infused over 10 min (may repeat once)	Conversion of AFib, AF	Minimal side effects except for rare polymorphic VT (torsades de pointes)
Propranolol	1-3 mg IV every 5 min, not to exceed 0.1 mg/kg	Conversion and/or rate control in SVT	Bradycardia, heart block, heart failure
Verapamil	5-10 mg IV, may repeat in 15-30 min	Conversion and/or rate control in SVT	Hypotension, bradycardia, heart failure
Lidocaine	1-1.5 mg/kg bolus, followed by continuous infusion of 1-4 mg/min	Treatment of ventricular dysrhythmias (PVCs, VT, VF)	CNS toxicity, nausea, vomiting with repeated doses
Amiodarone	*VT/VF arrest:* 300 mg IV push; may repeat with 150 mg in 3-5 min (maximum dose, 2.2 g/24 hr) *Pulsatile VT, AFib, AF:* 150 mg IV over 10 min, followed by 360 mg over 6 hrs (1 mg/min); maintenance infusion of 0.5 mg/min	Treatment of atrial (AFib, AF, SVT) and ventricular (PVCs, VT, VF) dysrhythmias	Hypotension, abnormal liver function tests
Procainamide	Loading dose of 12-17 mg/kg at a rate of 20 mg/min, followed by infusion of 1-4 mg/min	Treatment of atrial (AF, SVT) and ventricular (PVCs, VT) dysrhythmias	Hypotension, GI effects Widening of QRS and QT lengthening

AF, Atrial flutter; *AFib*, atrial fibrillation; *AV*, atrioventricular; *CNS*, central nervous system; *D$_5$W*, 5% dextrose in water; *GI*, gastrointestinal; *IV*, intravenous; *NS*, normal saline; *PSVT*, paroxysmal supraventricular tachycardia; *PVCs*, premature ventricular contractions; *ST*, sinus tachycardia; *SVT*, supraventricular tachycardia; *VF*, ventricular fibrillation; *VT*, ventricular tachycardia.

or the development of a bradydysrhythmia. For example, torsades de pointes is a prodysrhythmia caused by a number of medications that prolong the QT interval on the ECG. Because the development of a prodysrhythmia is unpredictable, the nurse plays an important role in evaluating ECG changes, monitoring serum medication levels, and assessing patient symptoms. Antidysrhythmic agents may also alter the amount of energy required for defibrillation and pacing. For example, increases in the dose of an antidysrhythmic medication may increase the amount of output (mA) required to depolarize the myocardium.

Treatment of Atrial Fibrillation

More than 2 million people in the United States have atrial fibrillation, and extensive research has been done on the treatment of this disorder. The goals of pharmacologic therapy for atrial fibrillation include re-establishing and maintaining sinus rhythm, decreasing the rapid ventricular response during episodes of atrial fibrillation, and preventing the risk of thromboembolism. Table 16-17 reviews current medications used in the treatment of atrial fibrillation. Results of some clinical trials suggest that rate control is equivalent to restoration of sinus rhythm in terms of mortality, with less incidence of adverse medication effects.[119] In 2010, the FDA approved two new anticoagulant agents for embolism prophylaxis in patients with non-valvular atrial fibrillation. Dabigatrin (Pradaxa) is a direct thrombin inhibitor and Rivaroxaban is a factor Xa inhibitor. These agents have advantages over warfarin in that they have fewer medication interactions and do not require routine monitoring.[120] Concerns have been raised, however, over possible risks of life-threatening hemorrhage because neither of these drugs has an antidote. In addition, a recent meta-analysis found that Dabigatrin use was associated with an increased incidence of myocardial infarction.[121]

Inotropic Medications

Critically ill patients with compromised cardiac function often require the use of medications to enhance myocardial contractility (positive inotropes). Clinically available inotropes include cardiac glycosides, sympathomimetics, and phosphodiesterase

digoxin

TABLE 16-17 MEDICATIONS USED FOR ATRIAL FIBRILLATION

TREATMENT GOAL	CLASSIFICATION AND MEDICATIONS	SPECIAL CONSIDERATIONS
Conversion or maintenance of sinus rhythm	Class IA Quinidine Procainamide (Pronestyl) Disopyramide (Norpace)	Class IA agents prolong QT intervals and may cause torsades de pointes. Rate control should be achieved before initiation of therapy.
	Class IC Flecainide (Tambocor) Propafenone (Rythmol)	Class IC agents are prodysrhythmic in patients with CAD or previous MI and should be avoided in these patients.
	Class III Amiodarone (Cordarone) Dofetilide (Tikosyn) Dronedarone (Multaq) Ibutilide (Corvert) Sotalol (Betapace)	Amiodarone and sotalol also have beta-blocking properties and may help with rate control. Treatment with dofetilide requires careful monitoring for prodysrhythmic effects. Ibutilide is an IV agent and is used for conversion only.
Control of ventricular rate	Beta-blockers Esmolol (Brevibloc) Metoprolol (Lopressor) Propranolol (Inderal)	IV esmolol may be used in acute settings to control ventricular rate. Oral agents are used for maintenance therapy. Beta-blockers provide good rate control during exercise.
	Calcium channel blockers Diltiazem (Cardizem) Verapamil (Isoptin)	Intravenous calcium channel blockers may be used in emergency situations, followed by oral agents for maintenance therapy.
	Digitalis compounds Digoxin (Lanoxin)	Digoxin does not effectively control rate with exercise, so it may be used in combination with other medications.
Prevention of thromboembolism	Anticoagulants Heparin Warfarin (Coumadin) Dabigatran (Pradaxa) Rivaroxaban (Xarelto)	Heparin may be used in emergency situations, before cardioversion. Warfarin is used long term, with monitoring to achieve an INR of 2-3. Dabigatran is an oral direct thrombin inhibitor approved to reduce the risk of thromboembolism in patients with nonvalvular AFib. This medication does not require routine anticoagulant monitoring. Rivaroxaban is a Factor Xa inhibitor approved to reduce the risk of thromboembolism in patients with non-valvular Afib. This medication does not require routine anticoagulant monitoring.
	Antiplatelet agents Aspirin	Aspirin may be used in patients with contraindications to warfarin or in low-risk patients younger than 65 years.

AFib, Atrial fibrillation; *CAD*, coronary artery disease; *INR*, international normalized ratio; *IV*, intravenous; *MI*, myocardial infarction.

TABLE 16-18 PHYSIOLOGIC EFFECTS OF SYMPATHOMIMETIC AGENTS

MEDICATIONS	DOSAGE	RECEPTOR ACTIVATED*				CARDIOVASCULAR EFFECTS		
		ALPHA	BETA$_1$	BETA$_2$	DOPA	CO	HR	SVR
Dobutamine	<5 mcg/kg/min	0	↑↑↑	↑	0	↑↑	↑	↓↓
	5-20 mcg/kg/min	0	↑↑↑	↑↑	0	↑↑↑	↑↑	↓↓
Dopamine	<3 mcg/kg/min	0	↑	↑	↑↑↑	0/↑	0/↑	0
	3-10 mcg/kg/min	↑↑	↑↑↑	↑	↑↑↑	↑↑↑	↑	↑
	11-20 mcg/kg/min	↑↑↑	↑↑↑	↑	↑↑	↑↑	↑↑	↑↑↑
Epinephrine	<2 mcg/min	0	↑	↑↑	0	0/↑	0/↑	↓
	2-8 mcg/min	↑↑	↑↑↑	↑↑	0	↑↑↑	↑↑	↑
	9-20 mcg/min	↑↑↑	↑↑↑	↑↑	0	↑↑	↑↑	↑↑↑
Isoproterenol	1-7 mcg/min	0	↑↑↑	↑↑↑	0	↑↑↑	↑↑↑	↓↓↓
Norepinephrine	<2 mcg/min	↑↑↑	↑↑	0	0	↑	0/↑	↑↑↑↑
	2-16 mcg/min	↑↑↑↑	↑↑	0	0	↓	↑	↑↑↑↑
Phenylephrine	10-100 mcg/min	↑↑↑↑	0	0	0	0	↓	↑↑↑

*See Table 16-14 for actions of receptors.
0, No effect; *↑*, increased (number of arrows indicates degree of effect); *↓*, decreased (number of arrows indicates degree of effect); *CO*, cardiac output; *HR*, heart rate; *SVR*, systemic vascular resistance.

inhibitors. These agents increase myocardial contractility, resulting in improved cardiac output, more complete emptying of the ventricles, and decreased filling pressures.

Cardiac Glycosides

Cardiac glycosides include digitalis and its derivatives. Although these medications have been used for centuries, their slow onset of action and risk of toxicity make them more appropriate for management of chronic heart failure. Because digoxin also causes slowing of the sinus rate and a decrease in AV conduction, it may be administered intravenously in the acute care setting to control supraventricular dysrhythmias.

Sympathomimetic Agents

Sympathomimetic agents stimulate adrenergic receptors, thereby simulating the effects of sympathetic nerve stimulation. Included in this category are naturally occurring catecholamines (epinephrine, dopamine, and norepinephrine) and synthetic catecholamines (dobutamine and isoproterenol). The cardiovascular effects of these medications, which vary according to their selectivity for specific receptor sites, are often dose dependent as well. Table 16-18 describes the cardiovascular effects of sympathomimetic agents at various dosages.

Dopamine (Intropin) is one of the most widely used medications in the critical care setting. It is a chemical precursor of norepinephrine, which, in addition to both alpha- and beta-receptor stimulation, can activate dopaminergic receptors in the renal and mesenteric blood vessels. The actions of dopamine are dose related, although there is some overlap in effect.[122] At low dosages of 1 to 2 mcg/kg/min, dopamine stimulates dopaminergic receptors, causing renal and mesenteric vasodilation. The resultant increase in renal perfusion increases urinary output. However, it is clear that this increase in urine output does not confer protection against the development of acute kidney injury. Moderate dosages result in stimulation of beta$_1$-receptors to increase myocardial contractility and improve cardiac output. At dosages greater than 10 mcg/kg/min, dopamine predominantly stimulates alpha-receptors, resulting in vasoconstriction that often negates both the beta-adrenergic and the dopaminergic effects.

Dobutamine (Dobutrex) is a synthetic catecholamine with predominantly beta$_1$-adrenergic effects. It also produces some beta$_2$ stimulation, resulting in a mild vasodilation. Dobutamine is as effective as dopamine in increasing myocardial contractility and is useful in the treatment of heart failure, especially in hypotensive patients who cannot tolerate vasodilator therapy. The usual dosage range is 2.5 to 20 mcg/kg/min, titrated on the basis of hemodynamic parameters.

Epinephrine (Adrenalin) is produced by the adrenal gland as part of the body's response to stress. This agent has the ability to stimulate both alpha- and beta-receptors, depending on the dose administered (see Table 16-18). At doses of 1 to 2 mg/min, epinephrine binds with beta-receptors to increase heart rate, cardiac conduction, contractility, and vasodilation, thereby increasing cardiac output. As the dosage is increased, alpha-receptors are stimulated, resulting in increased vascular resistance and increased blood pressure. At these doses, epinephrine's impact on cardiac output depends on the heart's ability to pump against the increased afterload. Epinephrine accelerates the sinus rate and may precipitate ventricular dysrhythmias in the ischemic heart. Other side effects include restlessness, angina, and headache.

Norepinephrine (Levophed) is similar to epinephrine in its ability to stimulate beta- and alpha-receptors, but it lacks the beta$_2$ effects of epinephrine. At low infusion rates, beta$_1$-receptors are activated to produce increased contractility, augmenting cardiac output. At higher doses, the inotropic effects are limited by marked vasoconstriction mediated by alpha-receptors. Clinically, norepinephrine is used most often as a vasopressor to elevate blood pressure in shock states.

Isoproterenol (Isuprel) is a pure beta-receptor stimulant with no alpha-adrenergic effects. It produces dramatic increases in heart rate, conduction, and contractility through beta$_1$ stimulation and vasodilation through beta$_2$ stimulation. Isoproterenol also produces vasodilation of the pulmonary arteries and bronchodilation. It greatly increases the automaticity of cardiac cells and frequently precipitates dysrhythmias, such as PVCs and even VT. These effects limit its usefulness in most patients and it is rarely used.

Phosphodiesterase Inhibitors

Phosphodiesterase inhibitors are inotropic agents that also are potent vasodilators (inodilators). Medications in this classification inhibit the enzyme phosphodiesterase, resulting in increased levels of cyclic adenosine monophosphate (AMP) and intracellular calcium. Amrinone (Inocor) and milrinone (Primacor) were the first of these agents approved for use in the United States. Increases in cardiac output occur as a result of increased contractility (inotropic effects) and decreased afterload (vasodilative effects). Amrinone may cause thrombocytopenia, so use of this medication has decreased. Milrinone is associated with a lower rate of thrombocytopenia but can induce atrial and ventricular dysrhythmias (PVCs, VT) in a significant number of patients.[123]

Vasodilator Medications

Vasodilators are pharmacologic agents that improve cardiac performance by various degrees of arterial or venous dilation, or both. The goal of vasodilator therapy may be reduction of preload or of afterload, or both. Afterload reduction is accomplished by vasodilation of arterial vessels. This results in decreased resistance to LV ejection and may improve cardiac output without increasing myocardial oxygen demands. Reduction of preload is accomplished by dilation of venous vessels to increase capacitance. This results in decreased filling pressures for a failing heart. These medications may be classified into four groups on the basis of mechanism of action (Table 16-19).

Direct Smooth Muscle Relaxants

Direct-acting vasodilators include sodium nitroprusside, nitroglycerin, and hydralazine. These medications produce relaxation of vascular smooth muscle through the activation of nitric oxide, which results in decreased peripheral vascular resistance (PVR). Hypotension may occur as a result of peripheral vasodilation, and headaches may be caused by cerebral vasodilation. Compensatory mechanisms can occur in response to the drop in blood pressure. These include baroreceptor activation that causes reflex tachycardia and activation of the renin-angiotensin-aldosterone system (RAAS) (see Fig. 15-18 in Chapter 15), with resultant sodium and water retention.

Sodium nitroprusside (Nipride) is a potent, rapidly acting venous and arterial vasodilator that is particularly suitable for rapid reduction of blood pressure in hypertensive emergencies and perioperatively. It also is effective for afterload reduction in the setting of severe heart failure. Sodium nitroprusside is administered by continuous intravenous infusion, with the dosage titrated to maintain the desired blood pressure and SVR. Prolonged administration can result in thiocyanate toxicity, manifested by nausea, confusion, and tinnitus.[124]

TABLE 16-19 PHARMACOLOGIC MANAGEMENT

Selected Vasodilator Agents

MEDICATION	DOSAGE	ACTION	SPECIAL CONSIDERATIONS
Sodium nitroprusside (Nipride)	0.25-6 mcg/kg/min IV infusion	Potent arterial and moderate venous dilation	May cause hypotension and reflex tachycardia, thiocyanate toxicity with prolonged infusions or kidney dysfunction
Nitroglycerin (Tridil)	5-300 mcg/min IV infusion	Potent venodilator, with arterial effects at higher doses	May cause headache, reflex tachycardia, hypotension
Calcium Channel Blockers			
Clevidipine (Cleviprex)	1-2 mg/hr IV infusion, titrated to 32 mg/hr (500 mg/24 hr)	Potent arterial dilator, with no effect on venous capacitance (preload)	Hypotension, reflex tachycardia, nausea, vomiting, rebound hypertension
Nicardipine (Cardene)	5 mg/hr IV, titrated to 15 mg/hr	Potent arterial dilator, no effect on preload	Hypotension, headache, reflex tachycardia
ACE Inhibitors			
Enalaprilat (Vasotec)	0.625 mg IV over 5 min, then every 6 hr	Moderate dilation of both arteries and veins	Hypotension, elevation of liver enzymes
α-Adrenergic Blockers			
Labetalol (Normodyne)	20-80 mg IV bolus every 10 min, then 1-2 mg/min infusion	Moderate dilation of both arteries and veins	Orthostatic hypotension, bronchospasm, AV block
Phentolamine (Regitine)	1-5 mg IV slowly every 6 hr	Moderate dilation of both arteries and veins	Hypotension, tachycardia

AV, Atrioventricular; *IV*, intravenous; *PO*, by mouth.

Intravenous nitroglycerin (Tridil) causes both arterial and venous vasodilation, but its venous effect is more pronounced. It is used in the critical care setting for the treatment of acute heart failure, because it reduces cardiac filling pressures, relieves pulmonary congestion, and decreases cardiac workload and oxygen consumption. Nitroglycerin dilates the coronary arteries and is a useful adjunct in the treatment of unstable angina and acute MI. The initial dosage is 10 mcg/min, and the infusion is titrated upward to achieve the desired clinical effect: a reduction or elimination of chest pain, decreased PAOP (wedge pressure), or a decrease in blood pressure. The most common side effects of this medication are hypotension, reflex tachycardia, and headache. Nitroglycerin becomes less effective with prolonged infusions, as tolerance develops within 24 to 48 hours.[124]

Hydralazine (Apresoline) is a potent arterial vasodilator. It is not given as a continuous infusion; rather, it is administered in slow intravenous doses of 5 to 10 mg every 4 to 8 hours. Occasionally, hydralazine is given as an intermediate agent during the transition between weaning of a continuous infusion and initiation of oral antihypertensive medications. The major side effect is reflex tachycardia mediated by the sympathetic nervous system. Hydralazine is preferred for treatment of eclampsia or pre-eclampsia, because only minimal amounts cross the placenta.[124]

Calcium Channel Blockers

Calcium channel blockers are a chemically diverse group of medications with differing pharmacologic effects (Table 16-20).

Nifedipine (Procardia), nicardipine (Cardene), and clevidipine (Cleviprex) are dihydropyridines. Medications in this group of calcium channel blockers (with the suffix *-pine*) are used primarily as arterial vasodilators. These agents reduce the influx of calcium in the arterial resistance vessels. Both coronary and peripheral arteries are affected. They are used in the critical care setting to treat hypertension. Nifedipine is available only in an oral form, but in the past it was prescribed sublingually during

hypertensive emergencies. Reports of adverse events associated with sublingual nifedipine prompted the FDA to issue a warning against using this administration route.[125] Nicardipine was the first available intravenous calcium channel blocker, and as such could be more easily titrated to control blood pressure. Because this medication has vasodilatory effects on coronary and cerebral vessels, it has proven beneficial in treating hypertension in patients with coronary artery disease or ischemic stroke. Side effects of nicardipine are related to vasodilation and include hypotension, reflex tachycardia, flushing, headache, and ankle edema.

Clevidipine is a new-short acting calcium channel blocker that allows for even more precise titration of blood pressure in the management of acute hypertension. Advantages of this agent include its short half-life (about 1 minute), rapid onset of action, predictable dose response, and minimal effect on heart rate.[126] Because Clevidipine is mixed in a phospholipid emulsion, it can cause allergic reactions in patients with allergies to soybeans or eggs.[124]

Diltiazem (Cardizem) is from the benzothiazine group of calcium channel blockers. Verapamil (Calan, Isoptin) is part of the phenylalkylamine group. The different classifications account for the differing actions of these calcium channel blockers. These medications dilate coronary arteries but have little effect on the peripheral vasculature. They are used in the treatment of angina, especially that which has a vasospastic component, and as antidysrhythmics in the treatment of supraventricular tachycardias.

Angiotensin-Converting Enzyme Inhibitors

Angiotensin-converting enzyme (ACE) inhibitors produce vasodilation by blocking the conversion of angiotensin I to angiotensin II. Because angiotensin is a potent vasoconstrictor, limiting its production decreases PVR. In contrast to the direct vasodilators and nifedipine, ACE inhibitors do not cause reflex tachycardia or induce sodium and water retention. However, these medications may cause a profound fall in blood pressure,

TABLE 16-20 PHARMACOLOGIC MANAGEMENT

Classification of Calcium Channel Blockers

MEDICATION	DOSAGE	ACTIONS	SPECIAL CONSIDERATIONS
Dihydropyridines			
Nicardipine (Cardene)	5 mg/hr IV, titrated to 15 mg/hr	Short-term control of hypertension	Hypotension, headache, nausea
Nifedipine (Procardia)	10-30 mg PO	Hypertension	Hypotension, headache, reflex tachycardia
Clevidipine (Cleviprex)	1-2 mg/hr IV infusion, titrated to 32 mg/hr	Short-term control of hypertension	Hypotension, reflex tachycardia, nausea, vomiting, rebound hypertension
Benzothiazepines			
Diltiazem (Cardizem)	Bolus dose of 0.25 mg/kg IV over 2 min, followed by an infusion of 5-15 mg/hr	Treatment of SVT, AFib, AF, angina	Bradycardia, hypotension, atrioventricular block
Phenylalkylamines			
Verapamil (Calan, Isoptin)	5-10 mg IV, may repeat in 15-30 min	Treatment of AF, PSVT	Hypotension, bradycardia, heart failure

AF, Atrial flutter; *AFib,* atrial fibrillation; *IV,* intravenous; *PO,* by mouth; *PSVT,* paroxysmal supraventricular tachycardia; *SVT,* supraventricular tachycardia.

especially in patients who are volume-depleted. Blood pressure must be monitored carefully, especially at the initiation of therapy.

ACE inhibitors are used in patients with heart failure to decrease SVR (afterload) and PAOP (preload). Most of these agents are only available in an oral form. Enalaprilat is available in an intravenous form and may be used to decrease afterload in more emergent situations.

B-Type Natriuretic Peptide

Nesiritide (Natrecor) is a vasodilator used in the treatment of acute heart failure. This agent is a recombinant form of human brain natriuretic peptide (BNP), the hormone released by cardiac cells in response to ventricular distention. The primary effects of nesiritide include decreased filling pressures (PAOP, CVP), reduced vascular resistance (SVR, PVR), and increased urine output. Compared with traditional vasodilator therapy for acute heart failure, nesiritide reportedly is as effective as the traditional agents and has fewer side effects (e.g., headache, tachycardia).[127] The recommended dose is an intravenous bolus of 2 mcg/kg, followed by a continuous infusion of 0.01 mcg/kg/min. The primary side effect is hypotension. If this occurs, nesiritide may need to be discontinued for a time and then restarted at a lower dose after the patient has stabilized.[128] Analysis of early clinical studies indicated that this medication may be associated with an increased risk of worsening kidney function (elevated serum creatinine) and short-term mortality compared with traditional treatment of acute decompensated heart failure. More recent studies offered conflicting results, demonstrating a lower mortality and possible kidney protective effects.[127]

Alpha-Adrenergic Blockers

Peripheral adrenergic blockers block alpha-receptors in arteries and veins, resulting in vasodilation. Orthostatic hypotension is a common side effect and may result in syncope. Long-term therapy also may be complicated by fluid and water retention.

Labetalol (Normodyne), a combined peripheral alpha-blocker and cardioselective beta-blocker, is used in the treatment of acute stroke and hypertensive emergencies.[128] Because the blockade of beta$_1$-receptors permits the decrease of blood pressure without the risk of reflexive tachycardia and increased cardiac output, Labetalol also is useful in the treatment of acute aortic dissection.[125]

Phentolamine (Regitine) is a nonselective peripheral alpha-blocker that deceases blood pressure through arterial vasodilation. It is administered by slow IV push, 1 to 5 mg every 6 hours to reduce blood pressure. Phentolamine is used only in very specific circumstances for catecholamine-induced hypertension or illegal-drug related toxicities (e.g., cocaine). Phentolamine is the medication of choice to control blood pressure and sweating caused by *pheochromocytoma*, an epinephrine (adrenalin)-secreting tumor that can arise from the adrenal medulla.[124]

Phentolamine also is used to treat the *extravasation of dopamine* or other vasopressors into peripheral tissues. If this occurs, 5 to 10 mg is diluted in 10 mL normal saline and administered intradermally into the infiltrated area as soon as possible following the extravasation.

Dopamine Receptor Agonists

Fenoldopam (Corlopam) is a unique type of vasodilator, a selective, specific dopamine (D$_1$) receptor agonist.[129] Fenoldopam is a potent vasodilator that affects peripheral, renal, and mesenteric arteries. It is administered by continuous intravenous infusion beginning at 0.1 mcg/kg/min and titrated up to the desired blood pressure effect, with a maximum recommended dose of 0.5 mcg/kg/min. It can be administered as an alternative to sodium nitroprusside or other antihypertensives in the treatment of hypertensive emergencies. Fenoldopam can be used safely in patients with kidney dysfunction.[124]

Vasopressors

Vasopressors are sympathomimetic agents that mediate peripheral vasoconstriction through stimulation of alpha-receptors (see Table 16-15). This results in increased SVR and elevates blood pressure. Some of these medications (epinephrine and norepinephrine) also have the ability to stimulate beta-receptors. Vasopressors are not widely used in the treatment of critically ill cardiac patients, because the dramatic increase in afterload is taxing to a damaged heart. Occasionally, vasopressors may be used to maintain organ perfusion in shock states. For example, phenylephrine (Neo-Synephrine) or norepinephrine (Levophed) may be administered as a continuous intravenous infusion to maintain organ perfusion by increasing SVR in cases of severe sepsis or septic shock.

Vasopressin, also known as antidiuretic hormone (ADH), has become popular in the critical care setting for its vasoconstrictive effects. At higher doses, vasopressin directly stimulates V1 receptors in vascular smooth muscle, resulting in vasoconstriction of capillaries and small arterioles. A one-time dose of 40 units intravenously is recommended in the ACLS guidelines as first-line therapy for VF, pulseless VT asystole, or pulseless electrical activity (PEA).[8] In septic shock vasopressin levels have been reported to be lower than anticipated for a shock state. Vasopressin continuous infusion of 0.03 unit/min may be added to the norepinephrine infusion in refractory shock per sepsis guidelines.[122] Patients must be assessed for side effects such as heart failure caused by the antidiuretic effects, and monitored for increased risk of ischemia in the myocardium, spleen, and periphery. Vasopressin should be infused through a central line to avoid the risk of peripheral extravasation and resultant tissue necrosis. Placement of an arterial line in shock-states to monitor blood pressure and SVR is recommended.

Medication Treatment of Heart Failure

Over 6 million Americans have heart failure, making it a major chronic health issue.[13] The goals of treatment in heart failure include alleviating symptoms, slowing the progression of the disease, and improving survival. Findings from a number of randomly controlled clinical trials have resulted in guidelines for the pharmacologic treatment of heart failure.[17] More information about heart failure is available in Chapter 15. Table 16-21 reviews the medications currently recommended for the treatment of heart failure. Types of medications that have been found to worsen heart failure should be avoided, including most antidysrhythmics, calcium channel blockers, and nonsteroidal anti-inflammatory medications.[17]

TABLE 16-21 MEDICATIONS USED FOR HEART FAILURE

CLASSIFICATION AND MEDICATIONS	MECHANISM OF ACTION	EFFECTS	SPECIAL CONSIDERATIONS
ACE Inhibitors Captopril (Capoten) Enalapril (Vasotec) Lisinopril (Prinivil)	Interferes with the renin-angiotensin-aldosterone system by preventing conversion of angiotensin I to angiotensin II	Decreases afterload Decreases preload Reverses ventricular remodeling	Agents appear equivalent in treatment of heart failure Monitor closely for hypotension when initiating therapy May be contraindicated in patients with elevated creatinine, indicating kidney failure
Angiotensin Receptor Blockers Candesartan (Atacand) Valsartan (Diovan)	Interferes with the renin-angiotensin-aldosterone system by blocking the effect of angiotensin II at the angiotensin II receptor site	Decreases afterload Decreases preload Reverses ventricular remodeling	Used as primary therapy or as an alternative for patients who can't tolerate ACE inhibitors due to side effects such as severe cough Can also be used in combination with an ACE inhibitor for systolic dysfunction; monitor renal function and serum potassium levels
Beta-Blockers Metoprolol Succinate (Toprol XL) Bisoprolol (Zebeta) Carvedilol (Coreg)	Counteracts the SNS response activated in heart failure by blocking receptor sites Metoprolol and bisoprolol are cardioselective beta-blockers, whereas carvedilol blocks alpha- and beta-receptor sites	Slows heart rate Prevents dysrhythmias Decreases blood pressure Reverses ventricular remodeling	Not initiated during decompensated stage of heart failure Use cautiously in patients with reactive airway disease, poorly controlled diabetes, bradydysrhythmias, or heart block Carvedilol dose is increased slowly, while monitoring for symptoms caused by vasodilation, such as dizziness or hypotension
Aldosterone Antagonists Spironolactone (Aldactone) Eplerenone (Inspra)	Counteracts the effects of aldosterone, which include sodium and water retention	Decreases preload Decreases myocardial hypertrophy	May increase serum potassium
Inotropes Digoxin (Lanoxin)	Affects the Na⁺,K⁺-ATPase pump in myocardial cells to increase the strength of contraction	Increases contractility Increases cardiac output Prevents atrial dysrhythmias	Risk of toxicity is increased with hypokalemia

ACE, Angiotensin-converting enzyme; *Na⁺/K⁺-ATPase*, sodium-potassium adenosine triphosphatase; *SNS*, sympathetic nervous system.

BOX 16-27 CASE STUDY

Patient with a Cardiac Problem

Brief Patient History

Mrs. G is a 54-year-old African American woman who has been having intermittent indigestion for the past month. She has a history of hypertension and hyperlipidemia. She was admitted as an in-patient on a medical floor for management of her blood pressure and is scheduled to undergo endoscopy tomorrow. Mrs. G suddenly becomes diaphoretic and complains of nausea and epigastric pain.

Clinical Assessment

The rapid response team is called to evaluate Mrs. G. When the team arrives at her bedside, she continues to complain of pain, which now radiates to her neck and back. She has some slight shortness of breath and is vomiting.

Diagnostic Procedures

The admission electrocardiogram (ECG) shows ST-segment elevation in II, III, and AVF.

Baseline vital signs include the following: blood pressure of 160/90 mm Hg, heart rate of 98 beats/min (sinus rhythm), respiratory rate of 18 breaths/min, temperature of 99° F, and O₂ saturation of 94%.

Medical Diagnosis

Mrs. G is diagnosed with an inferior myocardial infarction.

Questions

1. What major outcomes do you expect to achieve for this patient?
2. What problems or risks must be managed to achieve these outcomes?
3. What interventions must be initiated to monitor, prevent, manage, or eliminate the problems and risks identified?
4. What interventions should be initiated to promote optimal functioning, safety, and well-being of the patient?
5. What possible learning needs do you anticipate for this patient?
6. What cultural and age-related factors may have a bearing on the patient's plan of care?

SUMMARY

Pacemakers

- Pacemakers are electronic devices that can be used to initiate a heartbeat when the heart's intrinsic electrical system cannot generate a rate adequate to support cardiac output.
- The goal of therapy with either temporary or permanent pacemakers is to simulate normal physiologic cardiac depolarization and conduction.
- Nursing responsibilities for patients with pacemakers include assessment and prevention of pacemaker malfunction, protection against microshock, surveillance for complications, and patient education.

Implanted Cardioverter Defibrillators

- An implantable cardioverter defibrillator (ICD) is an electronic device that is used to terminate life-threatening ventricular dysrhythmias, through pacing, cardioversion, or defibrillation.
- Nursing management of the patient with an ICD includes assessing for dysrhythmias, monitoring for complications, and patient education.

Fibrinolytic Therapy

- Fibrinolytic therapy is used to restore blood flow through an occluded coronary artery in patients with an acute ST-elevation myocardial infarction (STEMI).
- Nursing care for patients receiving fibrinolytic agents includes identifying appropriate candidates for therapy, administering the fibrinolytic agent, assessing for evidence of reperfusion, and monitoring for bleeding complications.

Catheter Interventions for Coronary Artery Disease

- Percutaneous coronary intervention (PCI) describes procedures that utilize catheters to open blocked or narrowed coronary arteries and includes balloon angioplasty, atherectomy, and stent implantation.
- Antiplatelet therapy is considered an essential adjunct to PCI to help maintain vessel patency both during and after the procedure.
- Complications associated with PCI include coronary artery spasm, dissection, and thrombosis, contrast-induced kidney injury, and bleeding at the vascular access site.
- Percutaneous valve repair offers an alternative to surgery for high-risk patients.

Cardiac Surgery

- CABG surgery provides myocardial revascularization by using a conduit to bypass an occluded coronary artery.
- Valvular surgery is used to either repair a cardiac valve or replace it with a mechanical or biologic valve.
- Cardiopulmonary bypass (CPB) is an extracorporeal circuit used to circulate and oxygenate a patient's blood during some cardiac surgical procedures.
- Complications associated with cardiopulmonary bypass include intravascular fluid deficits, myocardial depression, coagulopathy, pulmonary dysfunction, hemolysis, hyperglycemia, electrolyte disturbances, neurologic dysfunction, and hypertension.

- Postoperative nursing management for cardiac surgery patients includes optimizing cardiac function (heart rate, preload, afterload, and contractility), temperature regulation, control of bleeding, and monitoring for complications.

Mechanical Circulatory Assist Devices

- Mechanical circulatory assist devices are used in the treatment of heart failure to decrease myocardial workload and maintain adequate perfusion to vital organs.
- Indications for the IABP include failure to wean from CPB, unstable or recurrent angina, complications of an acute MI, hemodynamic support for high-risk interventions, septic shock, and as a bridge to definitive therapy.
- Nursing interventions for IABP patients include monitoring for and preventing complications, assessing for proper timing, evaluating hemodynamic changes, and providing patient education.
- VADs can be used on a temporary basis as a bridge to recovery or transplant or permanently, as destination therapy.
- Nursing management for the patient with a VAD consists of monitoring for hemodynamic changes and complications related to device failure, bleeding, infection, and thromboembolism.

Vascular Surgery

- Vascular surgery may be used as a treatment for arterial occlusive disease or to correct structural abnormalities such as aneurysms.
- Many patients with vascular disease can now be effectively treated with percutaneous procedures (angioplasty, atherectomy, endovascular stents) rather than open surgical repair.
- Nursing care focuses on observing for vascular complications such as hematoma or reocclusion, as well as the prompt recognition and treatment of complications arising from comorbidities such as cardiac, pulmonary, and kidney disease.

Effects of Cardiovascular Medications

- Multiple medications are used in the treatment of critically ill patients, and the nurse is responsible for administration, titration, and monitoring for side effects.
- Antidysrhythmic medications are used to terminate or prevent abnormal cardiac rhythms and are classified according to their primary effect on the action potential of cardiac cells.
- Inotropic agents increase myocardial contractility resulting in improved cardiac output, more complete emptying of the ventricles, and decreased filling pressures.
- Vasodilators have varying effects on arterial and venous dilation and can be used to reduce preload, afterload, or both.
- Vasopressors mediate peripheral vasoconstriction, which results in an increase in SVR and elevates blood pressure.
- Goals of pharmacologic treatment of heart failure include alleviating symptoms, slowing the progression of the disease, and improving survival.

REFERENCES

1. Kalahasty G, Ellenbogen K. The role of pacemakers in the management of patients with atrial fibrillation. *Cardiol Clin.* 2009;27:137.

2. Bosen DM. Beyond ECGs: understanding electrophysiology testing. *Nurs Crit Care.* 2010;5(3):38.

3. Colucci RA, et al. Common types of supraventricular tachycardia: diagnosis and management. *Am Fam Physician.* 2010;82(8):942.

4. Mainigi SK, et al. Usefulness of radiofrequency ablation of supraventricular tachycardia to decrease inappropriate shocks from implantable cardioverter–defibrillators. *Am J Cardiol.* 2012;109:231.

5. Wann LS, et al. 2011 ACCF/AHA/HRS focused update on the management of patients with atrial fibrillation (updating the 2006 guideline): a report of the American College of Cardiology Foundation/American Heart Association Task Force on Practice Guidelines. *Circulation.* 2011;123:104.

6. Preuss T, Wiegand DL. Atrial electrogram. In: Weigand DL. *AACN Procedure Manual for Critical Care.* 6th ed. Philadelphia: Saunders; 2011.

7. Stone ME, et al. Perioperative management of patients with cardiac implantable electronic devices. *Br J Anaesthesia.* 2011;107(suppl 1):i16.

8. Neumar RW, et al. Part 8: adult advanced cardiovascular life support: 2010 American Heart Association Guidelines for Cardiopulmonary Resuscitation and Emergency Cardiovascular Care. *Circulation.* 2010;122(suppl 3):S729.

9. Mishra PK, et al. Temporary epicardial pacing wire removal: is it an innocuous procedure? *Interact Cardiovasc Thorac Surg.* 2010;11:854.

10. Bernstein AD, et al. The revised NASPE/BPEG generic pacemaker code for antibradycardia, adaptive-rate and multi-site pacing. *Pacing Clin Electrophysiol.* 2002;25:260.

11. Crossley GH, et al. HRS/ ASA expert consensus statement on the perioperative management of patients with implantable defibrillators, pacemakers and arrhythmia monitors: facilities and patient management. *Heart Rhythm.* 2011;8:1114.

12. Dyrda K, Khairy P. Implantable rhythm devices and electromagnetic interference: myth or reality? *Expert Rev Cardiovasc Ther.* 2008;6(6):823.

13. Roger VL, et al. Heart disease and stroke statistics—2012 update: a report from the American Heart Association. *Circulation.* 2012;125:e12.

14. Kaszala K, Ellenbogen KA. Device sensing: sensors and algorithms for pacemakers and implantable cardioverter defibrillators. *Circulation.* 2010;122(1):1328.

15. Tops LF, et al. The effects of right ventricular apical pacing on ventricular function and dyssynchrony: implications for therapy. *J Am Coll Cardiol.* 2009;54:764.

16. Mitka M. First MRI-safe pacemaker receives conditional approval from FDA. *JAMA.* 2011;305(10):985.

17. Hunt SH, et al. 2009 focused update incorporated into the ACC/AHA 2005 guidelines for the diagnosis and management of heart failure in adults. *Circulation.* 2009;119(14):e1.

18. Ho JK, Mahajam A. Cardiac resynchronization therapy for treatment of heart failure. *Anesth Analg.* 2010;111:1353.

19. Al-Majed NS, et al. Meta-analysis: cardiac resynchronization therapy for patients with less symptomatic heart failure. *Ann Intern Med.* 2011;154:401.

20. Kaszala K, Huizar JF, Ellenbogen KA. Contemporary pacemakers: what the primary care physician needs to know. *Mayo Clin Proc.* 2008;83(10):1170.

21. Baddour LM, et al. Update on cardiovascular implantable electronic device infections and their management: a scientific statement from the American Heart Association. *Circulation.* 2010;121(3):458.

22. Crossley GH, et al. Clinical benefits of remote versus transtelephonic monitoring of implanted pacemakers. *J Am Coll Cardiol.* 2009;54(22):2012.

23. Thompson BS. Sudden cardiac death and heart failure. *AACN Adv Crit Care.* 2009;20(4):356.

24. Aronow WS. Implantable cardioverter-defibrillators. *Am J Therapeut.* 2010;17:e208.

25. Turakhia MP. Sudden cardiac death and implantable cardioverter-defibrillators. *Am Fam Physician.* 2010;82(11):1357.

26. Curtis JP, et al. Association of physician certification and outcomes among patients receiving an implantable cardioverter-defibrillator. *JAMA.* 2009;301(16):1661.

27. Link MS, et al. Part 6: electrical therapies-automated external defibrillators, defibrillation, cardioversion, and pacing: 2010 American Heart Association Guidelines for Cardiopulmonary Resuscitation and Emergency Cardiovascular Care. *Circulation.* 2010;122(suppl 3):S706.

28. Concannon TW, et al. A percutaneous coronary intervention lab in every hospital? *Circ Cardiovasc Qual Outcomes.* 2012;5:14.

29. O'Connor RE, et al. Part 10: acute coronary syndromes: 2010 American Heart Association Guidelines for Cardiopulmonary Resuscitation and Emergency Cardiovascular Care. *Circulation.* 2010;122(suppl 3):S787.

30. O'Gara PT, et al. 2013 ACCF/AHA Guideline for the Management of ST-Elevation Myocardial Infarction: a report of the American College of Cardiology Foundation/American Heart Association Task Force on Practice Guidelines. *Circulation.* 2013;127(4):e362.

31. Wright RS, et al. 2011 ACCF/AHA focused update of the guidelines for the management of patients with unstable angina/non ST-elevation myocardial infarction. *J Am Coll Cardiol.* 2011;57:1920.

32. Yiadom MY. Emergency department treatment of acute coronary syndromes. *Emerg Med Clin N Am.* 2011;29:699.

33. Loomba RS, Arora R. ST elevation myocardial infarction guidelines today: a systematic review exploring updated ACC/AHA STEMI guidelines and their application. *Am J Therapeut.* 2009;16(5):e7.

34. Kumar A, Cannon CP. Acute coronary syndromes: diagnosis and management, part II. *Mayo Clin Proc.* 2009;84(11):1021.

35. Antman EM, Morrow DA. ST Elevation myocardial infarction management. In: Bonow RO, et al. *Braunwald's Heart Disease.* 9th ed. Philadelphia: Saunders; 2011:1111.

36. The TIMI Study Group. The Thrombolysis In Myocardial Infarction (TIMI) trial: phase I findings. *N Engl J Med.* 1985;312:932.

37. Hanna EB, Hennebry TA, Abu-Fadel MS. Combined reperfusion strategies in ST-segment elevation MI: rationale and current role. *Clev Clinic J Med.* 2010;77(9):629.

38. American Association of Critical Care Nurses. AACN practice alert: ST segment monitoring. http://www.AACN.org, revised 2009. Accessed March 29, 2012.

39. St. Laurent PS. Acute coronary syndromes: new and evolving therapies. *Crit Care Nurs Clin N Am*. 2011;23: 559.

40. Galla JM Whitlow PL. Coronary chronic total occlusion. *Cardiol Clin*. 2010;28:71.

41. Levine GN, et al. 2011 ACCF/AHA/SCAI guideline for percutaneous coronary intervention and executive summary. *Circulation*. 2011;124:2574.

42. Aversano T, Lemmon CC, Liu L. Outcomes of PCI at hospitals with or without on-site cardiac surgery. *N Engl J Med*. 2012;1.

43. Singh M, et al. Percutaneous coronary intervention at centers with and without on-site surgery: a meta-analysis. *JAMA*. 2011;306(22):2487.

44. Pompa JJ, Bhatt DL. Percutaneous coronary intervention. In: Bonow RO, et al. *Braunwald's Heart Disease*. 9th ed. Philadelphia: Saunders. 2011;1270-1300.

45. Garg S, Serruys PW. Coronary stents: current status. *JACC*. 2010;56(10)(suppl):S1.

46. Devabhakthuni S, Seybert AL. Oral antiplatelet therapy for the management of acute coronary syndromes: defining the role of prasugrel. *Crit Care Nurse*. 2011;31(1):51.

47. Kim SJ, Giugliano RP, Jang IK. Adjunctive pharmacologic therapy in percutaneous coronary intervention: Part I antiplatelet therapy. *Coron Artery Dis*. 2011;22:100.

48. Fletcher B, Thalinger KK. Prasugrel as antiplatelet therapy in patients with acute coronary syndromes or undergoing percutaneous coronary intervention. *Crit Care Nurse*. 2010;30(5):45.

48a. Jneid H, et al. 2012 ACCF/AHA Focused update of the guideline for the management of patients with unstable angina/non–ST-elevation myocardial infarction (updating the 2007 guideline and replacing the 2011 focused update): a report of the American College of Cardiology Foundation/American Heart Association Task Force on Practice Guidelines. *Circulation*. 2012;126:875.

49. Kim SJ, Giugliano RP, Jang IK. Adjunctive pharmacologic therapy in percutaneous coronary intervention: part II anticoagulant therapy. *Coron Artery Dis*. 2011;22:113.

50. Dauerman HL, et al. Bleeding avoidance strategies: consensus and controversy. *JACC Cardiovasc Interv*. 2011;58(1):1.

51. Dirkes S. Acute kidney injury: not just acute renal failure anymore? *Crit Care Nurse*. 2011;31(1):37.

52. Shoulders-Odom B. Management of patients after percutaneous coronary interventions. *Crit Care Nurse*. 2008;28(5):26.

53. Biancari F, et al. Meta-analysis of randomized trials on the efficacy of vascular closure devices after diagnostic angiography and angioplasty. *Am Heart J*. 2010;159(4):518.

54. Bonow RO, et al. ACC/AHA guidelines for the management of patients with valvular heart disease: a report of the American College of Cardiology/American Heart Association task force. *J Am Coll Cardiol*. 2006;48(3):e1.

55. Holmes DR, et al. 2012 ACCF/AATS/SCAI/STS Expert Consensus Document on Transcatheter Aortic Valve Replacement. *Ann Thorac Surg*. 2012;93:1340.

56. Rosengart TK, et al. Percutaneous and minimally invasive valve procedures: a scientific statement from the AHA Council on Cardiovascular Surgery and Anesthesia, Council on Clinical Cardiology, Functional Genomics and Translational Biology Interdisciplinary Working Group, and Quality of Care and Outcomes Research Interdisciplinary Working Group. *Circulation*. 2008;117:1750.

57. McRae ME, et al. Transcatheter and transapical aortic valve replacement. *Crit Care Nurs*. 2009;29(1):22.

58. Pruit, G et al. Incidence rate and predictors of permanent pacemaker implantation after transcatheter aortic valve implantation. 2011:885 *EUROPACE: Abstract*.

59. Makkar RR, et al. Transcatheter aortic-valve replacement for inoperable severe aortic stenosis. *N Engl J Med*. Epub ahead of print. March 26, 2012.

60. Kempfert J, et al. Transapical aortic valve implantation: analysis of risk factors and learning experience in 299 patients. *Circulation*. 2011;144(supp1):S124.

61. Kodali SK, et al. Two-year outcomes after Transcatheter or surgical aortic-valve replacement. *N Engl J Med*. Epub ahead of print. March 26, 2012.

62. Hillis LD, et al. 2011 ACCF/AHA Guideline for coronary artery bypass surgery: a report of the American College of Cardiology Foundation/American Heart Association task force on practice guidelines. *Circulation*. 2011;124(23):e652.

63. Weintraub WS, et al. Comparative effectiveness of revascularization strategies. *N Engl J Med*. Epub ahead of print. March 27, 2012.

64. Cohen DJ, et al. Quality of life after PCI with drug-eluting stents or coronary-artery bypass surgery. *N Engl J Med*. 2011;364:1016.

65. Lopes R, et al. Endoscopic versus open vein-graft harvesting in coronary artery bypass surgery. *N Engl J Med*. 2009;361: 235.

66. Hayward P, et al. Comparable patencies of the radial artery and right internal thoracic artery or saphenous vein beyond 5 years: results from the Radial Artery Patency and Clinical Outcomes trial. *J Thorac Cardiovasc Surg*. 2010;139:60.

67. Buxton BF, et al. Choice of conduits for coronary artery bypass grafting: craft or science? *Eur J Cardiothorac Surg*. 2009;35:658.

68. Bello S, et al. Conduits for coronary artery bypass surgery: the quest for the second best. *J Cardiovasc Med*. 2011;12(6): 411.

69. Sabik JF III, Blackstone EH. Coronary artery bypass graft: patency and competitive flow. *J Am Coll Cardiol*. 2008;51:126.

70. Piaschyk M, et al. A journey through heart valve surgery. *Crit Care Nurs*. 2011;23:587.

71. Huang G, Rahimtoola S. Prosthetic heart valve. *Circulation*. 2011;123:2602.

72. South T. Coronary artery bypass surgery. *Crit Care Nurs*. 2011;23:573.

73. Martin CG, Turkelson SL. Nursing Care of the patient undergoing coronary artery bypass grafting. *J Cardiovasc Nurs*. 2006;21(2):109.

74. Lamy A, et al. Off-pump or on-pump coronary-artery bypass grafting at 30 days. *N Engl J Med*. Epub ahead of print. March 26, 2012.

75. Shroyer AL, et al. On-pump versus off-pump coronary-artery bypass surgery. *N Engl J Med*. 2009;361(19):1827.

76. Mullen-Fortino M, et al. Critical care of a patient after CABG surgery. *Nursing 2009 Crit Care*. 2009;4(4):46.

77. Kupchik N, Bridges E. Central venous pressure monitoring: what's the evidence? *Am J Nurs*. 2012;112(2):58.

78. Bridges EJ. Arterial pressure based stroke volume and functional hemodynamic monitoring. *J Cardiovasc Nurs*. 2008;23(2):105.

79. Kramer A, et al. Pulse pressure variation predicts fluid responsiveness following coronary artery bypass surgery. *Chest.* 2004;126(5):1563.

80. Ferraris VA, et al. Perioperative blood transfusion and blood conservation in cardiac surgery: the Society of Thoracic Surgeons and the Society of Cardiovascular Anesthesiologists clinical practice guideline. *Ann Thorac Surg.* 2007;83:s27.

81. Napolitano LM, et al. Clinical practice guideline: red blood cell transfusion in adult trauma and critical care. *J Trauma Injury Infect Crit Care.* 2009;67(6):1439.

82. Collins TA. Packed red blood cell transfusions in critically ill patients. *Crit Care Nurs.* 2011;31(1):25.

83. Camp S, et al. Quality improvement program increases early tracheal extubation rate and decreases pulmonary complications and resource utilization after cardiac surgery. *J Card Surg.* 2009;24(4):414.

84. Selnes OA. Etiology of cognitive changes after CABG surgery: more than just the pump? *Nature.* 2008;5(6):314.

85. Koster S. Consequences of delirium after cardiac operations. *Ann Thorac Surg.* 2012;93:705.

86. Allen J, Alexander E. Prevention, recognition, and management of delirium in the intensive care unit. *AACN Adv Crit Care.* 2012;23(1):5.

87. Karkouti K, et al. Acute kidney injury after cardiac surgery: focus on modifiable risk factors. *Circulation.* 2009;119:495.

88. Ad N, et al. Institutional and national trends in isolated mitral valve surgery over the past decade. *Curr Opin Cardiol.* 2008;23:99.

89. Bonatti J, et al. Robotically assisted totally endoscopic coronary bypass surgery. *Circulation.* 2011;124:236.

90. Bonatti J, et al. Hybrid coronary revascularization: which patients? when? how? *Curr Opin Cardiol.* 2010;25:568.

91. Calkins H, et al. HRS/EHRA/ECAS expert consensus statement on catheter and surgical ablation of atrial fibrillation: recommendations for personnel, policy, procedures and follow-up. *J Heart Rhythm.* 2007;4(6):815.

92. Kale P, Fang JC. Devices in acute heart failure. *Crit Care Med.* 2008;36(1):S121.

93. Trost JC, Hillis D. Intra-aortic balloon counterpulsation. *Am J Cardiol.* 2006;97:1391.

94. Hanlon-Pena PM, Quaal S. Intra-aortic balloon pump timing: review of the evidence supporting current practice. *Am J Crit Care.* 2011;20(4):323.

95. Hanlon-Pena PM, Quaal S. Resource document: evidence supporting current practice in timing assessment. *Am J Crit Care.* 2011;20(4):e99.

96. Sarkar K, Kini AS. Percutaneous left ventricular support devices. *Card Clinic.* 2010;28:169.

97. Basra SS, et al. Current status of percutaneous ventricular assist devices for cardiogenic shock. *Curr Opin Cardiol.* 2011;26:548.

98. Puhlman M. Continuous-flow left ventricular assist device and the right ventricle. *AACN Adv Crit Care.* 2012;23(1):86.

99. Mitter N, Sheinberg R. Update on ventricular assist devices. *Curr Opin Anaesthesiol.* 2010;23:57.

100. Atluri P, et al. The next decade in mechanical assist: advances that will help the patient and the doctor. *Curr Opin Cardiol.* 2011;26:256.

101. Myers T. Temporary ventricular assist devices in the intensive care unit as a bridge to decision. *AACN Adv Crit Care.* 2012; 23(1):55.

102. Christensen D. Physiology of continuous-flow pumps. *AACN Adv Crit Care.* 2012;23(1): 46.

103. Brott TG, et al. ASA/ACCF/AHA/AANN/ACR/ASNR/CNS/ SAIP/SCAI/SIR/SNIS/ SVM/SVS Guideline on the management of patients with extracranial carotid and vertebral artery disease. *J Am Coll Cardiol.* 2011;57:e16.

104. Perkins WJ, Lanzino G, Brott TG. Carotid stenting vs endarterectomy: new results in perspective. *Mayo Clin Proc.* 2010;85(12):1101.

105. Oran NT, Oran I. Carotid angioplasty and stenting in carotid artery stenosis: neuroscience nursing implications. *J Neuroscience Nurs.* 2010;42(1):3.

106. Binning MJ, Khalessi AA, Hopkins LN. Carotid revascularization endarterectomy versus stenting trial (CREST): current and future implications for carotid artery stenting. *Interv Cardiol.* 2010;2(6):779.

107. Chadi SA, et al. Trends in management of abdominal aortic aneurysms. *J Vasc Surg.* 2012;55(4):924.

108. Greenhalgh RM, et al. Endovascular versus open repair of abdominal aortic aneurysm. *N Engl J Med.* 2010; 362(20):1863.

109. Jackson RS, Chang DC, Freischlag JA. Comparison of long-term survival after open vs endovascular repair of intact abdominal aortic aneurysm among Medicare beneficiaries. *JAMA.* 2012;307(15):1621.

110. Rooke TW, et al. 2011 ACCF/AHA Focused update of the guideline for the management of patients with peripheral artery disease (updating the 2005 guideline). *Circulation.* 2011;124:2020.

111. Weinberg MD, et al. Peripheral artery disease. Part 2: medical and endovascular treatment. *Nat Rev Cardiol.* 2011;8:429.

112. Norgren L, et al. Inter-society consensus for the management of peripheral arterial disease (TASC II). *J Vasc Surg.* 2007; 45(Suppl S):S5.

113. Kapadia MR, et al. Modified prosthetic vascular conduits. *Circulation.* 2008;117:1873.

114. Gandhi S Sakhuja R, Slovut DP. Recent advances in percutaneous management of iliofemoral and superficial femoral artery disease. *Cardiol Clin.* 2011;29: 381.

115. Jaffrey Z, et al. Acute limb ischemia. *Am J Med Sci.* 2011;342(3):226.

116. Ganjehei L, et al. Pharmacologic management of arrhythmias. *Texas Heart Institute J.* 2011;38(4):344.

117. Roberts M. Clinical utility and adverse effects of amiodarone therapy. *AACN Adv Crit Care.* 2010;21(4):333.

118. Simmons S. Critical care drugs: dofetilide. *Nursing 2011 Crit Care.* 2011;6(2):8.

119. Gutierrez C, Blanchard DG. Atrial fibrillation: diagnosis and treatment. *Am Fam Physician.* 2011;83(1):61.

120. Furie K, et al. Oral antithrombotic agents for the prevention of stroke in nonvalvular atrial fibrillation: a science advisory for healthcare professionals from the American Heart Association/American Stroke Association. *Stroke.* 2012;43:3442.

121. Uchino K, Hernandez AV. Dabigatran association with higher risk of acute coronary events: meta-analysis of noninferiority randomized controlled trials. *Arch Intern Med.* 2012;172(5):397.

122. Hollenberg SM. Inotrope and vasopressor therapy in septic shock. *Crit Care Nurs Clin N Am.* 2011;23: 127.

123. Coons JC, McGraw M, Murali S. Pharmacotherapy for acute heart failure syndromes. *Am J Health-Syst Pharm.* 2011;68:21.

124. Hays AJ, Wilkerson TD. Management of hypertensive emergencies: a drug therapy perspective for nurses. *AACN Adv Crit Care.* 2010;21(1):5.

125. Rodriguez MA, Kumar SK, DeCaro M. Hypertensive crisis. *Cardiol Rev.* 2010;18:102.

126. Pollack CV, et al. Clevidipine, an intravenous dihydropyridine calcium channel blocker, is safe and effective for the treatment of patients with acute severe hypertension. *Ann Emerg Med.* 2009;53:329.

127. Elkayam U, et al. Vasodilators in the management of acute heart failure. *Crit Care Med.* 2008;36(suppl 1):S95.

128. Falk SA. Anesthetic considerations for the patient undergoing therapy for advanced heart failure. *Curr Opin Anesthesiol.* 2011;24:314.

129. Smithburger PL, et al. Recent advances in the treatment of hypertensive emergencies. *Crit Care Nurse.* 2010;30(5):24.

Pulmonary Anatomy and Physiology

Kathleen M. Stacy

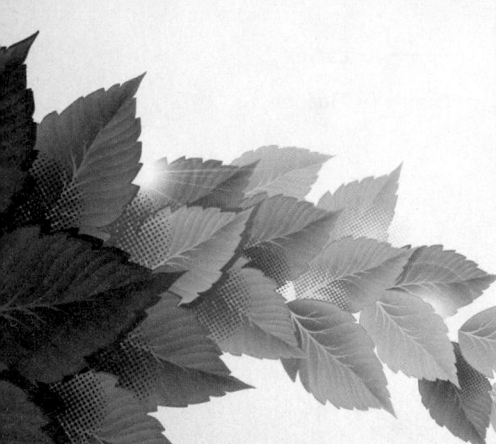

evolve WEBSITE

http://evolve.elsevier.com/Urden/criticalcare/

Evolve features:

- NCLEX Review Questions
- CCRN Review Questions
- PCCN Review Questions
- Mosby's Nursing Skills Procedures
- Animations
- Video Clips
- Glossary

The pulmonary system consists of the thorax, conducting airways, respiratory airways, and pulmonary blood and lymph supply. The primary functions of the pulmonary system are ventilation and respiration. *Ventilation* is the movement of air in and out of the lungs. *Respiration* is the process of gas exchange by means of movement of oxygen from the atmosphere into the bloodstream and movement of carbon dioxide from the bloodstream into the atmosphere. The anatomic structures that constitute the pulmonary system are intimately related to function, and structural abnormalities can readily translate into pulmonary disorders. An applicable knowledge of anatomy and physiology is imperative in caring for the patient with pulmonary dysfunction.

THORAX

The thorax contains the major organs of respiration. It consists of the thoracic cage, lungs, pleura, and muscles of ventilation. Together, these structures form the ventilatory pump, which performs the work of breathing.

Thoracic Cage

The thoracic cage is a cone-shaped structure that is rigid but flexible. It must be somewhat rigid to protect the underlying structures, but it must be flexible to accommodate inhalation and exhalation. The cage consists of 12 thoracic vertebrae, each with a pair of ribs. Posteriorly, each rib is attached to its own vertebra, but anteriorly, attachment varies (Fig. 17-1). The first seven pairs of ribs are attached directly to the sternum. The 8th, 9th, and 10th pairs are attached by cartilage to the ribs above. Because the 11th and 12th ribs have no anterior attachment,

they sometimes are referred to as *floating ribs*. The second rib is attached to the sternum at the angle of Louis, which is the raised ridge that can be felt just below the suprasternal notch.[1]

Lungs

The lungs are cone-shaped organs that have a total volume of approximately 3.5 to 8.5 liters. The superior portion is known as the *apex*, and the inferior portion is known as the *base*. The apical portion of each lung rises a few centimeters above the clavicle (see Fig. 17-1). Each lung is firmly attached to the thoracic cavity at the hilum and at the pulmonary ligament.[2]

Lobes and Segments

The lungs are divided into lobes and segments (Fig. 17-2), with the lobes being separated by pleural membrane-covered fissures. The right lung, which is larger and heavier than the left, is divided into upper, middle, and lower lobes. The left lung is divided into only an upper and a lower lobe.[2] A portion of the left lung, the lingula, corresponds anatomically with the right middle lobe. The horizontal fissure divides the right upper lobe from the right middle lobe. The oblique fissure divides the right upper and middle lobes from the lower lobe and the left upper lobe from the lower lobe. The lobes are divided into 18 segments, each of which has its own bronchus branching immediately off a lobar bronchus. Ten segments are located in the right lung and eight in the left lung.[1]

Mediastinum

The area between the two lungs, the mediastinum, contains the heart, great vessels, lymphatics, and the esophagus. A portion of the mediastinal area contains the root of the lungs, also

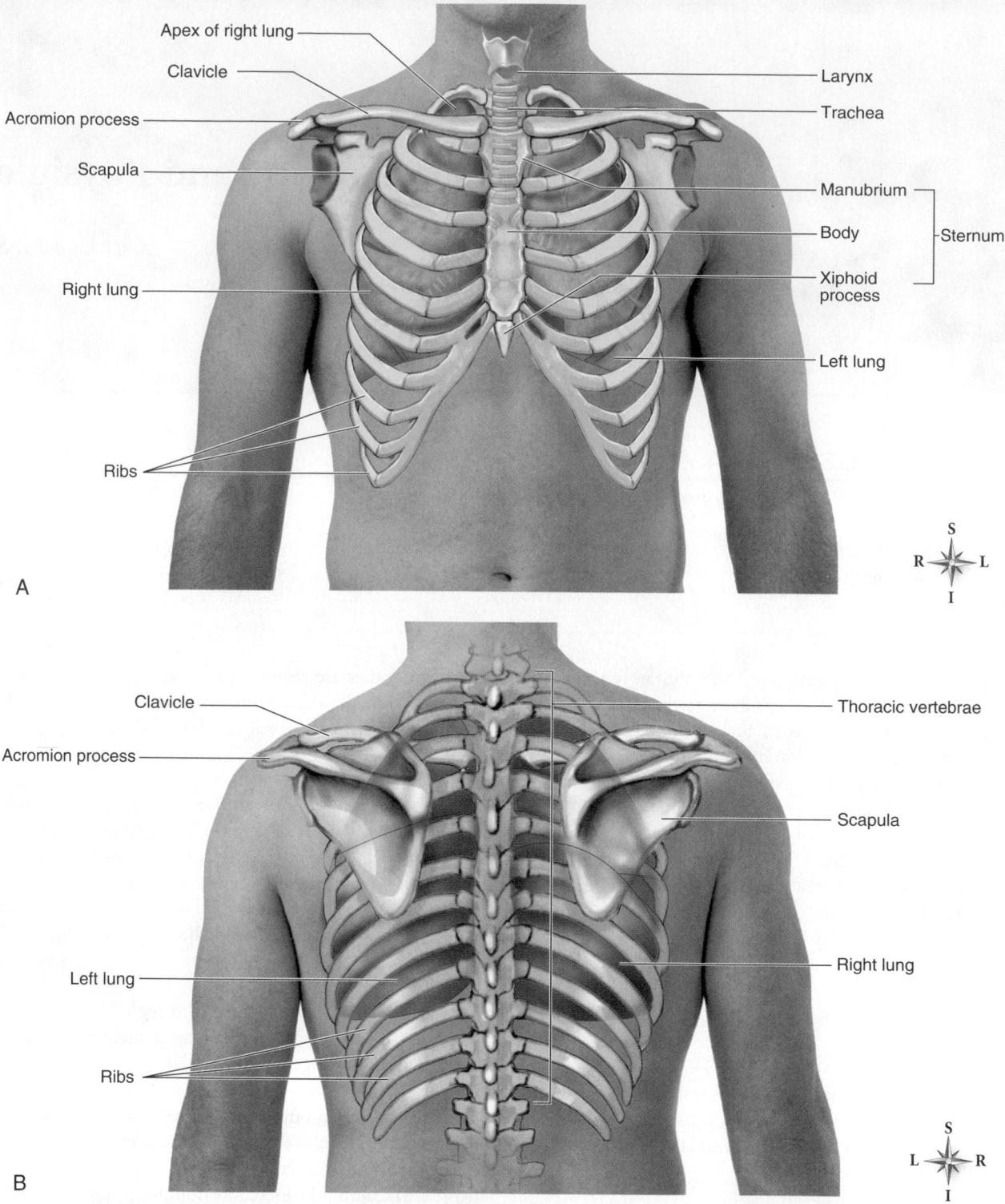

FIGURE 17-1 **Bony Structures of the Chest.** These structures form a protective and expandable cage around the lungs and heart. *A*, Anterior view. *B*, Posterior view. (Adapted from Thompson JM, Wilson SF. *Health assessment for nursing practice*. St. Louis: Mosby; 1996. In Patton KT, Thibodeau GA, eds. *Anatomy and Physiology*. 8th ed. St. Louis: Mosby; 2013.)

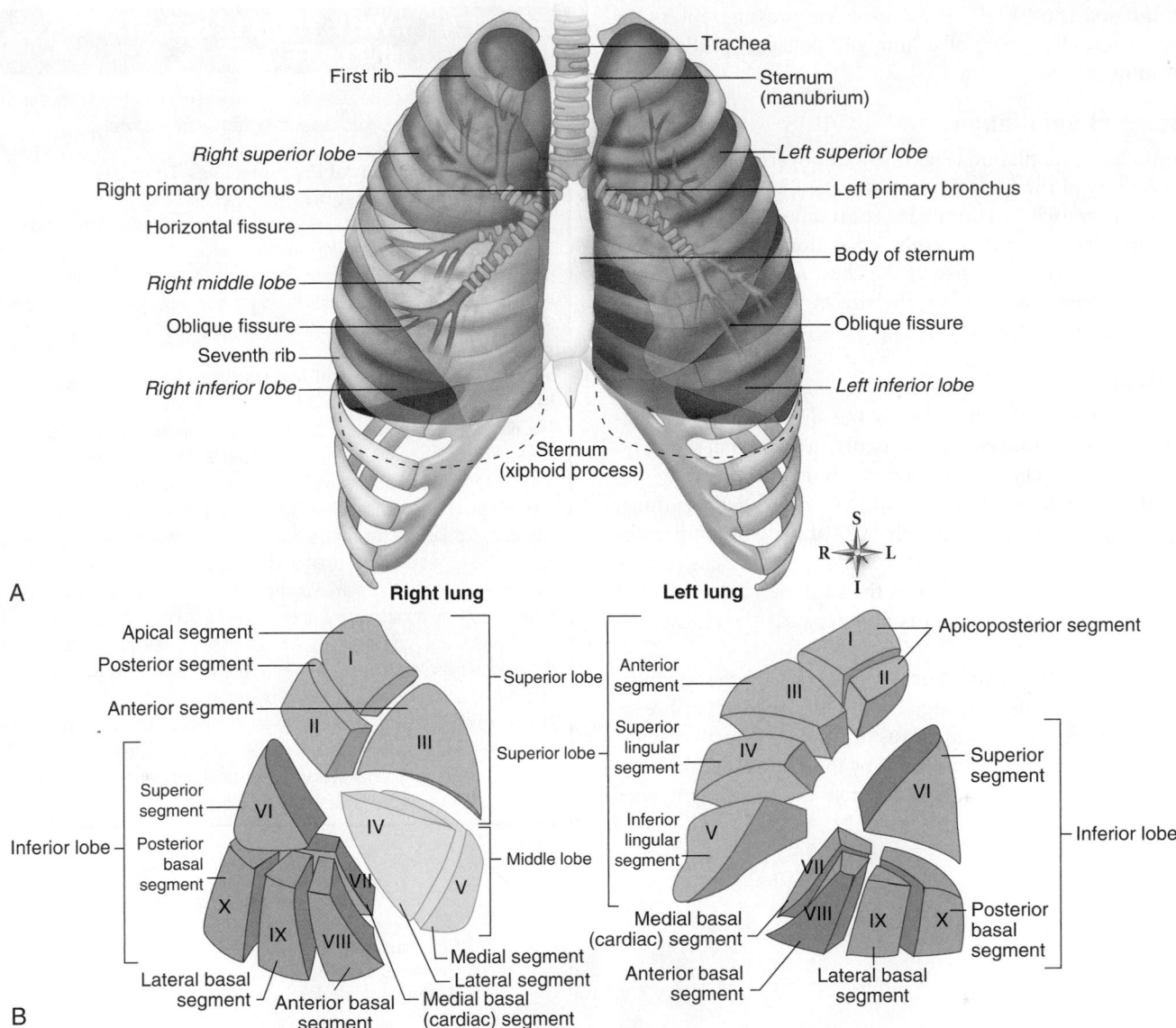

FIGURE 17-2 **Lobes and Segments of the Lungs.** *A,* Anterior view of the lungs, bronchi, and trachea. *B,* Expanded diagram showing the bronchopulmonary segments. (From Patton KT, Thibodeau GA, eds. *Anatomy and Physiology.* 8th ed. St. Louis: Mosby; 2013.)

known as the hilum, in which the visceral and parietal pleural membranes form a sheath around the main stem bronchi, the major blood vessels, and the nerves that enter and exit the lungs.[2]

Pleura

The pleura is a thin membrane that lines the outside of the lungs and the inside of the chest wall. The visceral pleura adheres to the lungs, extending onto the hilar bronchi and into the major fissures. The parietal pleura lines the inner surface of the chest wall and mediastinum.[2] The two pleural surfaces are separated by an airtight space, which contains a thin layer of lubricating fluid. Pleural fluid allows the visceral and parietal pleural membranes to glide against each other during inhalation and exhalation.[1,3] The pleural space has the capacity to hold much more fluid than its normal volume of a few milliliters.[1]

Intrapleural Pressure

The pleural space has a pressure within it called the *intrapleural pressure,* which differs from the intrapulmonary (pressure within the lungs) and atmospheric pressures.[4] Under normal conditions, intrapleural pressure is less than intrapulmonary pressure and less than atmospheric pressure, with a normal range of −4 to −10 cm H_2O during exhalation and inhalation, respectively.[3] A deep inhalation can generate intrapleural pressures of −12 to −18 cm H_2O. This negative intrapleural pressure results from forces within the chest wall that exert pressure to pull the parietal pleura outward and away from the visceral pleura, while the elastic fibers within the lungs exert pressure to pull the visceral pleura inward away from the parietal pleura. The constant pull of the two pleural membranes in opposite directions causes the pressure within the space to be subatmospheric.[4] The negative pressure in the pleural space keeps the lungs inflated (Box 17-1). If atmospheric pressure enters the pleural space, all or part of a lung will collapse, producing a pneumothorax.[1]

Muscles of Ventilation

The muscles of ventilation (Fig. 17-3) are governed by the regulatory activity of the central nervous system, which sends messages to the muscles to stimulate contraction and relaxation. This muscular activity controls inhalation and exhalation. Muscles that increase the size of the chest are called *muscles of inhalation;* those that decrease the size of the chest are called *muscles of exhalation.*[5]

Inhalation

The main muscle of inhalation is the diaphragm. The diaphragm is a dome-shaped, fibromuscular septum that separates the thoracic and abdominal cavities. It is connected to the sternum, ribs, and vertebrae. During normal, quiet breathing, the diaphragm does approximately 80% of the work of breathing. On inhalation, the diaphragm contracts and flattens, pushes down on the viscera, and displaces the abdomen outward. Diaphragmatic contraction also lifts and expands the rib cage to some extent.[1,5,6]

The action of the diaphragm is governed by the medulla, which sends its impulses through the phrenic nerve. The phrenic nerve arises from the cervical plexus through the fourth cervical nerve, with secondary contributions by the third and fifth cervical nerves. For this reason and because the diaphragm does

---

BOX 17-1   WHY THE LUNGS STAY INFLATED

The lungs stay inflated because the pressure surrounding them (intrapleural) is always less than the pressure within them (intrapulmonary).

Why Is the Intrapleural Pressure Less Than the Intrapulmonary Pressure?

The intrapleural pressure is always 1) less then intrapulmonary pressure; 2) less than atmospheric pressure; and 3) considered negative because of the pull of the two pleural membranes in opposite directions. The parietal pleura is pulled outward by forces within the chest wall, whereas the visceral pleural is pulled inward by the force of the elastic fibers within the lungs.

Why Do the Two Pleural Membranes Pull in Opposite Directions?

The parietal pleura, attached to the chest, is pulled outward because the elastic fibers within the intercostal muscles exert outward pressure on the ribs. These fibers are in a relaxed state when the rib cage is fully expanded, such as during a deep inhalation. The visceral pleura is attached to the lungs and is pulled inward because the elastic fibers within the lungs that are responsible for elastic recoil exert pressure to make the lungs smaller. Elastic fibers in the lung are in a relaxed position only when the lung is at its smallest configuration, as occurs with a pneumothorax. Because of the opposite pull of the chest wall and the lung and because the pleural membranes are attached to these structures, there is a constant pull of the two membranes in opposite directions. The subatmospheric pressure that results within the pleural space and the greater-than-atmospheric intrapulmonary pressure within the lungs allows the lungs to remain inflated. Anything that causes the pressure within the pleural space to rise to atmospheric pressure or above will cause the lung to collapse—a pneumothorax.

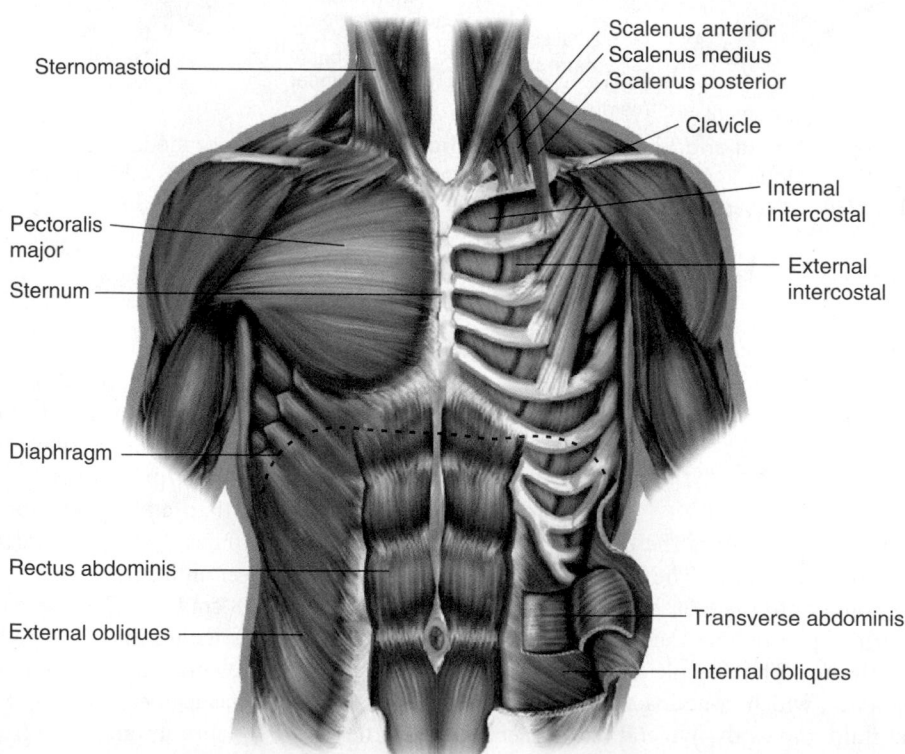

FIGURE 17-3 Muscles of Ventilation. (From Wilkin RL, et al, eds. *Egan's Fundamentals of Respiratory Care.* 8th ed. St. Louis: Mosby; 2003.)

most of the work of inhalation, trauma involving levels C3 to C5 causes ventilatory dysfunction.[5]

Other muscles of inhalation include those that lift the rib cage. The most important of these are the external intercostal muscles, which elevate the ribs and expand the chest cage outward. The scalene, anterior serratus, and sternocleidomastoid muscles also participate to elevate the first two ribs and sternum.[1,5,6]

Exhalation

Exhalation in the healthy lung is a passive event requiring very little energy. Exhalation occurs when the diaphragm relaxes and moves back up toward the lungs. The intrinsic elastic recoil of the lungs assists with exhalation. Because exhalation is a passive act, there are no true muscles of exhalation other than the internal intercostal muscles, which assist the inward movement of the ribs. During exercise, however, exhalation becomes a more active event, requiring some participation of the accessory muscles of ventilation. Several muscles of the abdomen are thought to contribute to active exhalation.[4,5]

Accessory Muscles

The accessory muscles of ventilation usually are considered to be those that enhance chest expansion during exercise but that are not active during normal, quiet breathing. These muscles include the scalene, sternocleidomastoid, and other chest and back muscles, such as the trapezius and the pectoralis major.[1,5,6]

CONDUCTING AIRWAYS

The conducting airways consist of the upper airways, the trachea, and the bronchial tree. The purposes of the conducting airways are to warm and humidify the inhaled air, to act as a protective mechanism that prevents the entrance of foreign matter into the gas exchange areas, and to serve as a passageway for air entering and leaving the gas exchange regions of the lungs.[1-3]

Upper Airways

The upper airways consist of the nasal and oral cavities, the pharynx, and the larynx (see Fig. 17-4). Their main contribution to ventilation is the conditioning of inspired air. *Conditioned*

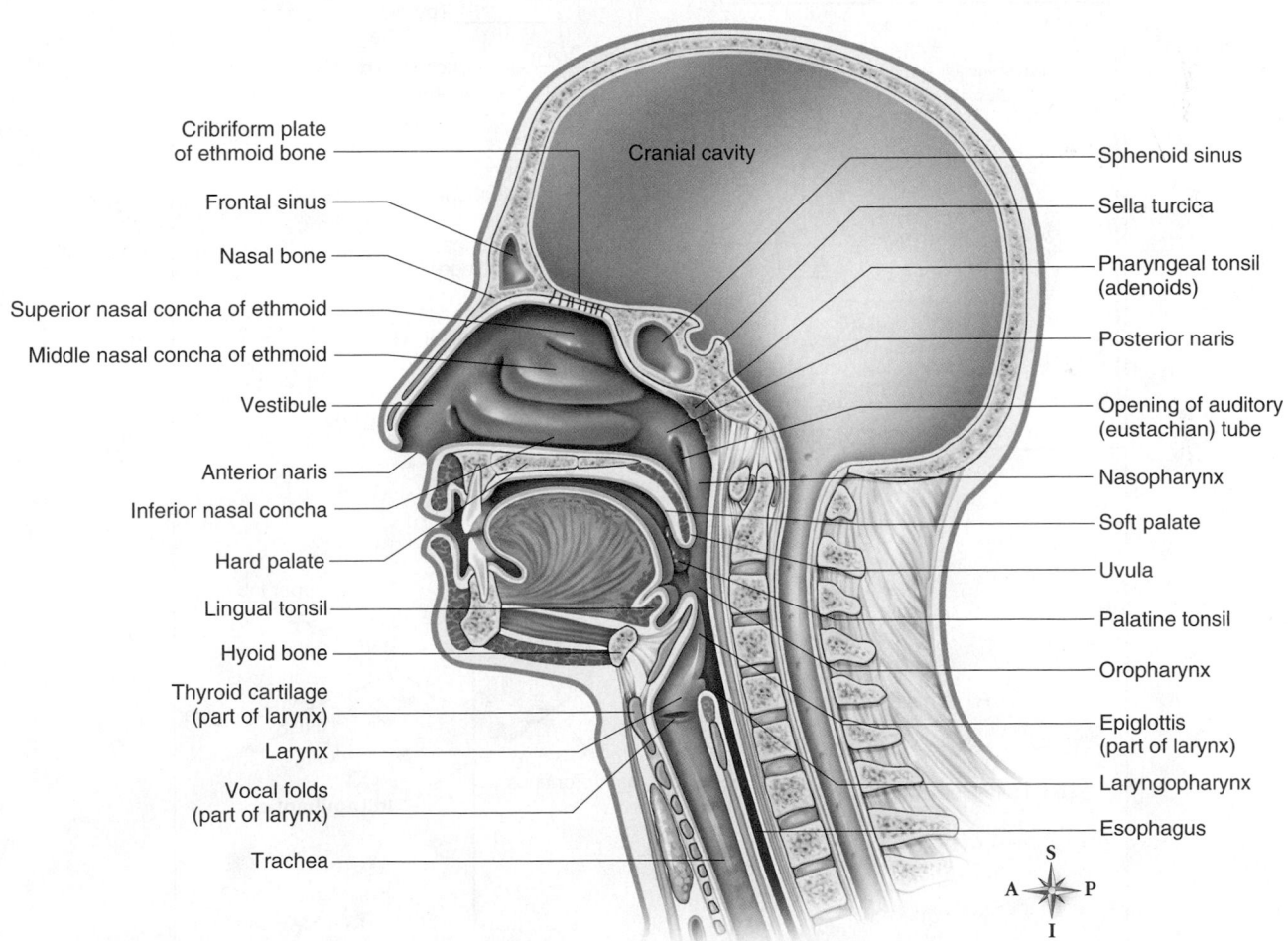

FIGURE 17-4 Upper Respiratory Tract. In this midsagittal section through the upper respiratory tract, the nasal septum has been removed to reveal the turbinates (nasal conchae) of the lateral wall of the nasal cavity. The three divisions of the pharynx (nasopharynx, oropharynx, and laryngopharynx) are also visible. (From Patton KT, Thibodeau GA, eds. *Anatomy and Physiology.* 8th ed. St. Louis: Mosby; 2013.)

air is air that has been warmed, humidified, and cleansed of some irritants. Warming and humidifying, which are essential to prevent irritation of the lower airways, occur mainly within the nose by means of a dense vascular network that lines the nasal passages. The air is cleansed by the coarse hairs that line the nasal passages and filter large inhaled particles.[1,3]

Epiglottis

The epiglottis is located in the upper airways. It protects the lower airways by closing the opening to the trachea during swallowing so that food passes into the esophagus and not the trachea. The epiglottis is a thin, leaf-shaped, elastic cartilage that is located directly posterior to the root of the tongue and attached to the thyroid cartilage (see Fig. 17-4). It opens widely during inhalation, permitting air to pass through the trachea into the lower airways.[1]

Trachea

The trachea is a hollow tube approximately 11 cm (4.5 inches) long and 2.5 cm (1 inch) in diameter (Fig. 17-5). It begins at the cricoid cartilage and ends at the bifurcation (major carina) from which the two main stem bronchi arise. The carina is positioned approximately at the level of the aortic arch, the fifth thoracic vertebra,[7] or just below the level of the angle of Louis.[1] The trachea consists of smooth muscle supported anteriorly by 16 to 20 C-shaped, cartilaginous rings. They prevent tracheal collapse during bronchoconstriction and strong coughing. The posterior wall of the trachea lies contiguous with the anterior wall of the esophagus. Having no cartilaginous support, this wall is composed only of muscle tissue, which is separated from the anterior esophageal wall by loose connective tissue (see Fig. 17-5, inset).[1]

Bronchial Tree

The two main stem bronchi are structurally different (see Fig. 17-5). The left bronchus is slightly narrower than the right, and because of its position above the heart, the left bronchus angles directly toward the left lung at approximately 45 to 55 degrees from the midline. The right bronchus is wider and angles at 20 to 30 degrees from the midline. Because of this angulation and

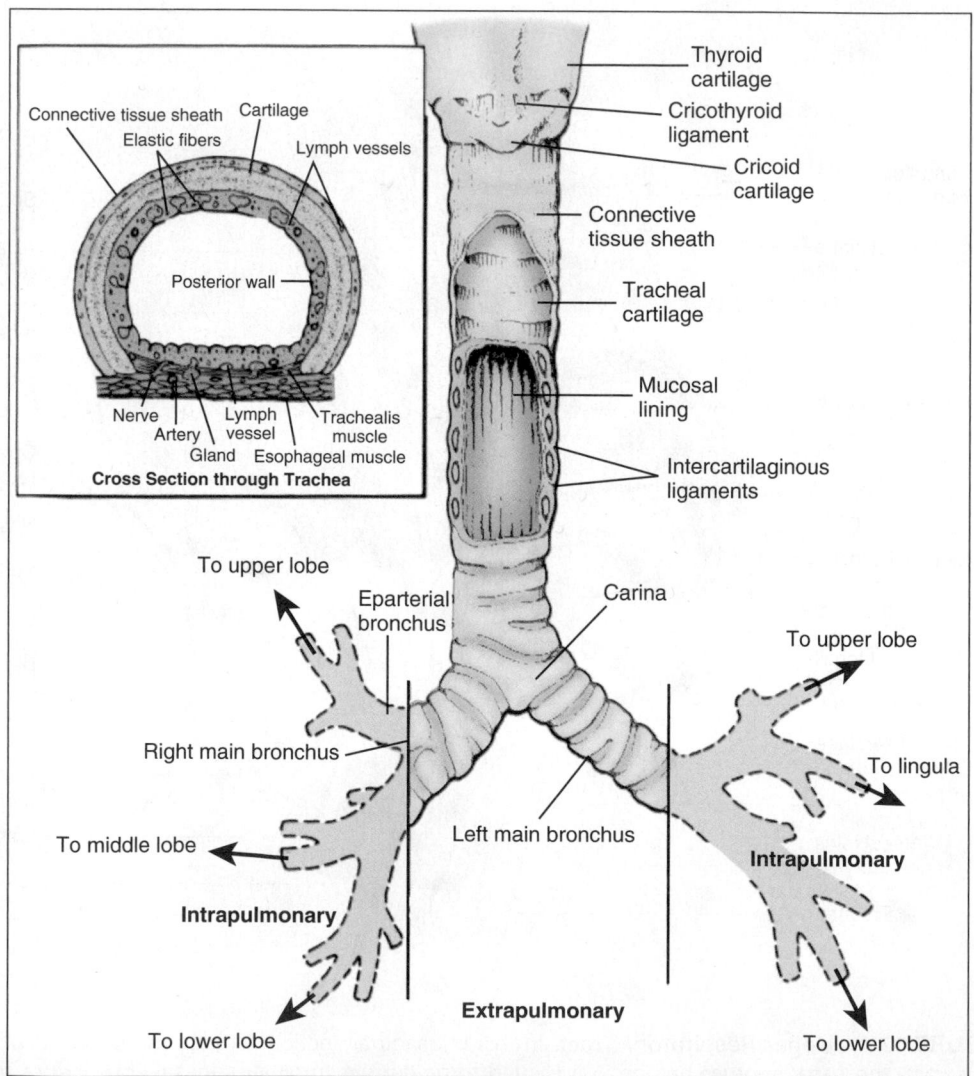

FIGURE 17-5 Anterior view of the trachea and primary bronchi and a cross section *(inset)* through a part of the trachea, including a C-shaped cartilaginous element. (From Martin DE. *Respiratory Anatomy and Physiology.* St. Louis: Mosby; 1988.)

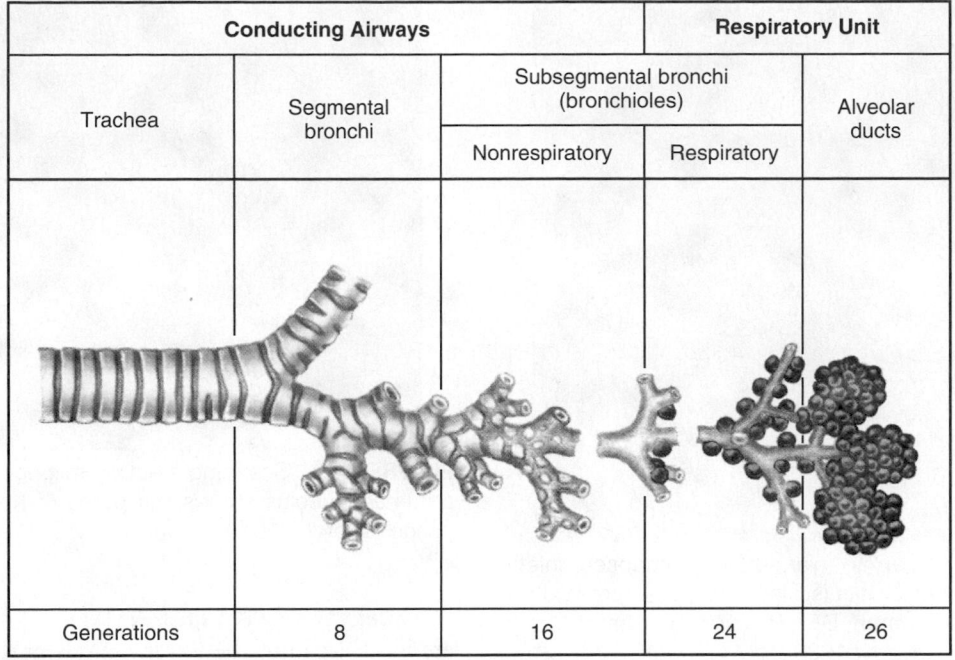

Conducting Airways				Respiratory Unit
Trachea	Segmental bronchi	Subsegmental bronchi (bronchioles)		Alveolar ducts
		Nonrespiratory	Respiratory	
Generations	8	16	24	26

FIGURE 17-6 Conducting and Respiratory Airways. Notice the escalating branching with increasing generations. (From Thompson JM, et al, eds. *Mosby's Clinical Nursing*. 5th ed. St. Louis: Mosby; 2002.)

the forces of gravity, the most common site of aspiration of foreign objects is through the right main stem bronchus into the lower lobe of the right lung.[2,3]

Bronchi

Each branching of the tracheobronchial tree produces a new generation of tubes (Fig. 17-6). The main stem bronchi are the first generation; the next branch, the five lobar bronchi, is the second generation. The third generation includes the 18 segmental bronchi. The fourth through approximately the ninth generations are referred to as the small bronchi, beginning with the subsegmental bronchi. In these bronchi, diameters decrease; however, because the number of bronchi increases with each generation, the total cross-sectional area increases with each generation. This great increase in the cross-sectional area of the lung is significant because it allows easy ventilation despite decreasing airway lumens.[1]

Bronchioles

The final subdivision of the conducting airways is the bronchioles. These tubes have a diameter less than 1 mm and have no connective tissue and cartilage within their walls. Their walls do, however, contain smooth muscle.[2] When smooth muscle constriction occurs, these airways may close completely because of the lack of structural support. The terminal bronchioles form the last branch of the conducting airways, after which the gas exchange areas of the lungs begin. There are more than 32,000 terminal bronchioles total.[1]

Defense System

The main defense system within the airways is the mucociliary escalator, or mucous blanket, a combination of mucus and cilia. The mucus, which floats atop the cilia (Fig. 17-7), traps foreign

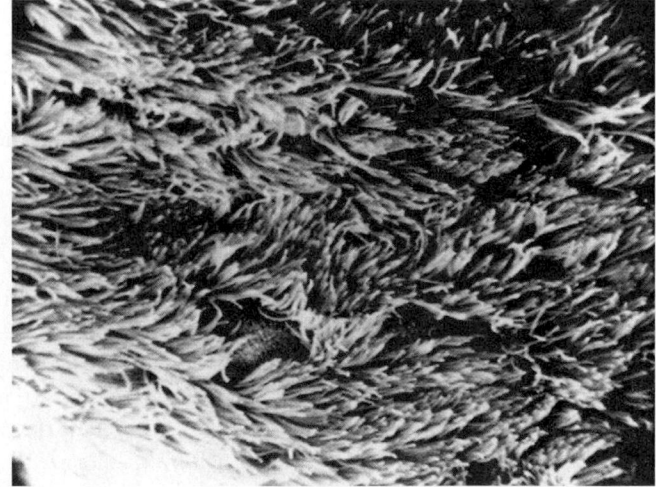

FIGURE 17-7 Scanning electron micrograph of the luminal surface and cilia of a bronchiole from a normal adult male (×2000). (From Ebert RV, Terracio MJ. Observation of the secretion on the surface of the bronchioles with the scanning electron microscope. *Am Rev Respir Dis*. 1975;112:4901.)

particles. Ciliary movement then propels the entire mucous blanket and any trapped particles upward toward the pharynx at an average speed of 1 mm/min in the smaller bronchioles and 12 mm/min in the larger airways and trachea. After the pharynx is reached, the mucus is swallowed or cleared. The submucous glands of the airways produce approximately 100 mL of mucus per day, with all but about 10 mL resorbed through the bronchial lining. The mucociliary escalator is so efficient that almost no particles larger than 3 microns reach the alveoli.[8]

The cough reflex is another protective mechanism in the lungs. Excessive amounts of foreign particles in the trachea and

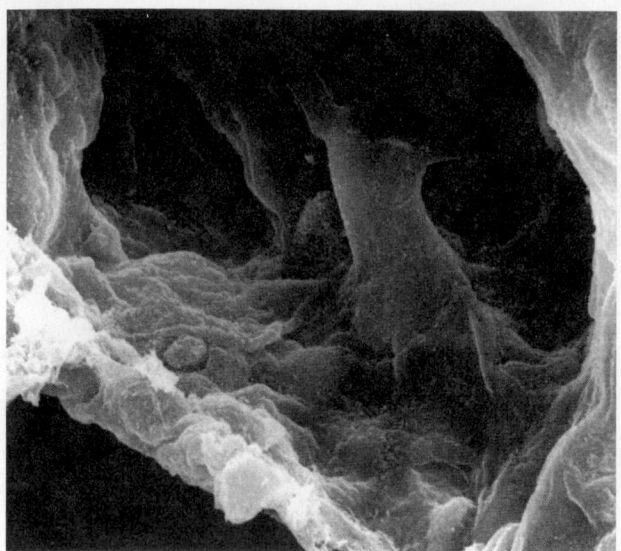

FIGURE 17-8 Detail of an alveolar surface composed chiefly of type I alveolar epithelial cells (scale: 1 cm of picture width = 3.46 microns). (From Martin DE. *Respiratory Anatomy and Physiology*. St. Louis: Mosby; 1988.)

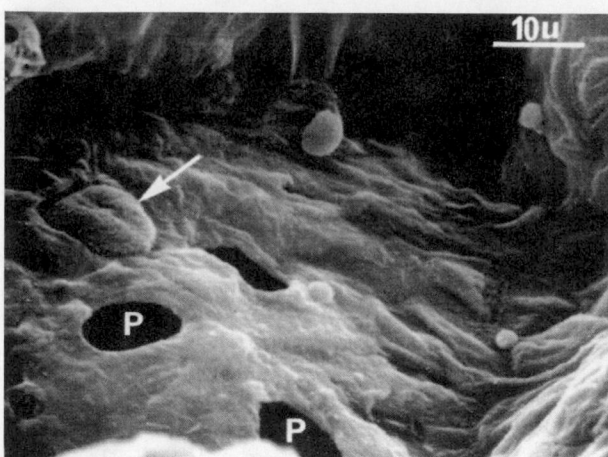

FIGURE 17-9 Scanning electron micrograph of the surface of a human alveolus shows the pores of Kohn *(P)* and a macrophage *(arrow)* (×1500). (Courtesy M.S. Wang, MD.)

bronchi can initiate the cough reflex. Once initiated, the rapid expulsion of air carries away any foreign particles with it.[9]

RESPIRATORY AIRWAYS

The respiratory airways consist of the respiratory bronchioles and the alveoli. The respiratory airways also are known as the *terminal respiratory units*, or the *acini*. Gas exchange takes place in these areas of the lungs.

Respiratory Bronchioles

Each terminal bronchiole gives rise to two respiratory bronchioles, with each branching two to four more times.[2] The respiratory bronchioles form the transition zone of the lungs, acting as conducting airways and gas exchange units. While air is moving through them, alveolar outpouchings on their surfaces allow gas exchange to take place (see Fig. 17-6).[1]

Alveoli

Each respiratory bronchiole gives rise to several alveolar ducts, which terminate in clusters of 10 to 16 alveoli (see Fig. 17-6). Each terminal respiratory unit contains approximately 100 alveolar ducts and 2000 alveoli.[2] The alveolus is the primary site of gas exchange and the end point in the respiratory tract. Approximately 300 million alveoli are in the two lungs. The alveoli are composed of several types of cells, including type I and II alveolar epithelial cells and alveolar macrophages.[1,3]

Type I Alveolar Epithelial Cells

Type I alveolar epithelial cells comprise approximately 90% of the total alveolar surface within the lungs (Fig. 17-8). They are the chief structural cells of the alveolar wall and play a major role in the maintenance of the gas-blood barrier and gas exchange. Type I cells are extremely susceptible to injury and become inflamed when exposed to inhaled toxins.[1]

Collateral Air Passages. A variety of collateral air passages are located within the lower regions of the lungs. Within the walls of the type I cells are the pores of Kohn (Fig. 17-9), which allow collateral movement of air between alveoli. The canals of Lambert are collateral air pathways that exist between the alveoli and the respiratory and terminal bronchioles. They are of particular benefit when a respiratory bronchiole is blocked or collapsed, because they allow gas to pass into alveoli distal to the blockage. Collateral air passages are of significant benefit in any pathologic condition of the lung that results in obstruction of airflow into a portion of the lungs. However, these pores and canals also allow the movement of microorganisms through lung tissue.[1,2]

Type II Alveolar Epithelial Cells

Type II alveolar epithelial cells occur in much greater numbers than type I cells, but because of their minute size, they comprise a smaller portion of the total alveolar wall. After injury to the alveolar wall, type II cells rapidly divide to line the surface; later, they transform into type I cells. The most important function of the type II cells is their ability to produce, store, and secrete pulmonary surfactant (Fig. 17-10).[1,3]

Surfactant. Surfactant is a phospholipid composed of fatty acids bound to lecithin. Like other surfactants, such as detergents and soaps, pulmonary surfactant functions to lower surface tension of the alveoli. Whereas with detergents and soaps this decrease in surface tension cleans clothes, within the lungs, it stabilizes the alveoli, increases lung compliance, and eases the work of breathing. When pulmonary disease disrupts the normal synthesis and storage of surfactant, the lungs become less compliant, and the work of breathing increases. Severe loss of surfactant results in alveolar instability and collapse and impairment of gas exchange.[10]

Defense System

Alveolar macrophages are monocytes that originate in the bone marrow and are released into the bloodstream (Fig. 17-11).[1-3] On entering the pulmonary capillary circulation, they move through the capillary membrane wall into the interstitial space

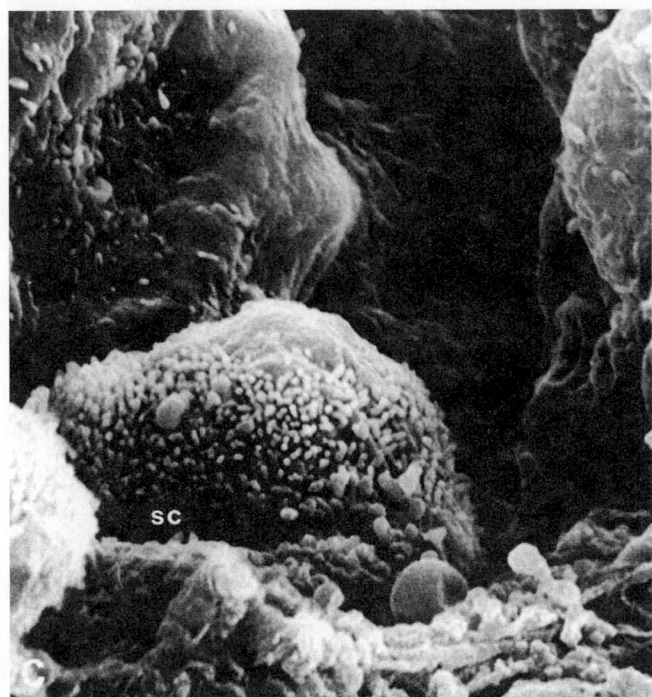

FIGURE 17-10 Type II Alveolar Epithelial Cell. Notice the presence of brush microvilli on all except the bald top of the round luminal surface. Type II cells produce surfactant (scale: 1 cm of picture width = 0.85 micron). (From Martin DE. *Respiratory Anatomy and Physiology*. St. Louis: Mosby; 1988.)

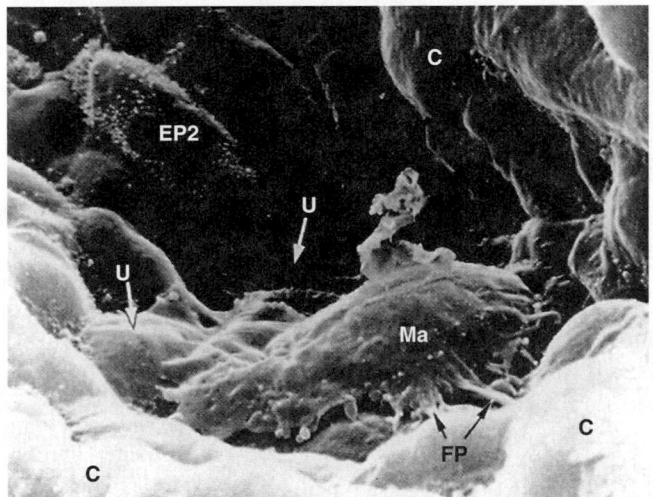

FIGURE 17-11 Scanning electron micrograph of a healthy human lung shows an alveolar macrophage *(Ma)* attached to the epithelium partly by filopodia *(FP)* and forming an undulating membrane *(U)* in the direction of forward movement to the left. Several capillaries *(C)* are evident, and a type II alveolar epithelial cell *(EP2)* can be seen in the background (original magnification ×3700.) (From Gehr P, et al. The normal human lung: ultrastructure and morphometric estimation of diffusion capacity. *Respir Physiol*. 1978;32[2]:121.)

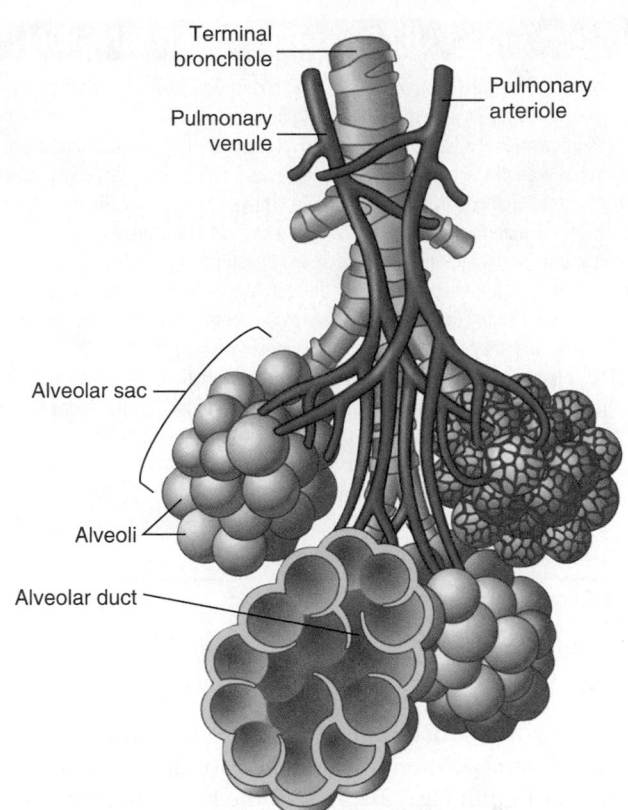

FIGURE 17-12 Terminal Ventilation and Perfusion Units of the Lung. (Modified from Patton KT, Thibodeau GA, eds. *Anatomy and Physiology*. 8th ed. St. Louis: Mosby; 2013.)

hydrogen peroxide, lysozyme, and other substances that kill microorganisms.[2,3]

PULMONARY BLOOD AND LYMPH SUPPLY

Two vascular systems and one lymphatic system make up the pulmonary blood and lymph supply. The pulmonary circulation is the vascular system that forms the gas exchange network surrounding the alveoli. The bronchial circulation is the vascular system that perfuses the tracheobronchial tree.[1]

Pulmonary Circulation

The pulmonary circulatory system begins at the pulmonary artery, which receives venous blood from the right side of the heart. The pulmonary artery then divides into left and right branches and continues to branch until it forms the capillaries that surround the alveoli (Fig. 17-12). After gas exchange takes place, the blood is returned to the left side of the heart through the pulmonary veins.[1,2]

Pulmonary Artery Pressures

The pulmonary circulation is by far the largest vascular bed within the body, and it is the only one that receives the entire cardiac output. Just as the systemic circulation has a systolic and a diastolic blood pressure, so does the pulmonary circulation. However, because of the relative lack of smooth muscle within the vessels of the pulmonary circulation, the pressures are vastly lower than within the systemic circulation.[1,3] Pulmonary artery systolic (PAS) pressure ranges from 15 to 30 mm Hg,

(to the left of Figure 17-12 labels:)
Terminal bronchiole
Pulmonary venule
Pulmonary arteriole
Alveolar sac
Alveoli
Alveolar duct

and through to the alveoli. In the alveoli, the monocytes transform into macrophages and assume a phagocytic role. They move from alveolus to alveolus through the pores of Kohn, keeping the alveoli clean and sterile through phagocytosis and microbial killing activity, which includes the secretion of

BOX 17-2 PULMONARY HYPERTENSION

Pulmonary hypertension is defined as increased pressure (PAS greater than 35 mm Hg and PAM less than 25 mm Hg at rest or less than 30 mm Hg with exertion) within the pulmonary arterial system. It occurs when the cross-sectional area of the pulmonary bed decreases as a result of vasoconstriction or structural changes in the vascular bed. These changes may be a result of a variety of pathophysiologic conditions, including impedance to pulmonary venous drainage (e.g., mitral stenosis); increased pulmonary blood flow (e.g., septal defect); impedance to flow through large pulmonary arteries (e.g., pulmonary embolus) or small pulmonary blood vessels (e.g., collagen vascular diseases); and impedance to flow from hypoxic vasoconstriction.

The pulmonary hypertension resulting from hypoxic vasoconstriction, although caused in part by vasospasm, is largely a result of alterations in the structure of the blood vessels of the pulmonary circulation, which results in an increase in the medial thickness and a reduction in the size of the vascular lumen. Pulmonary hypertension increases the afterload of the right ventricle and, when chronic, can result in right ventricular hypertrophy (cor pulmonale) and failure.

PAM, Pulmonary artery mean pressure; *PAS*, pulmonary artery systolic pressure.

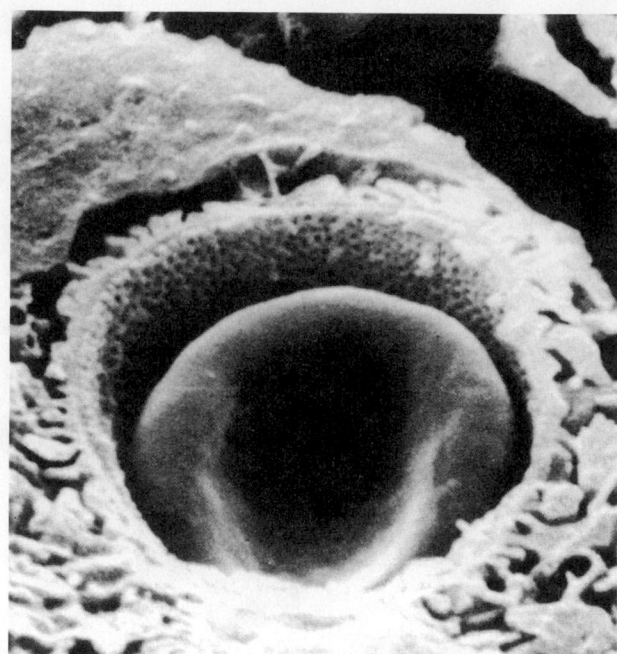

FIGURE 17-13 Scanning Electron Micrograph of a Red Blood Cell in a Capillary. Notice that the diameters of both are similar. In many instances, the red blood cells course through even smaller capillaries, often through capillaries that are one half of the diameter of the red blood cell. This is possible because the cells are pliable, mainly as a result of their biconcave disk shape. (From Martin DE. *Respiratory Anatomy and Physiology.* St. Louis: Mosby; 1988.)

pulmonary artery diastolic (PAD) pressure ranges from 4 to 12 mm Hg, and pulmonary artery mean (PAM) pressure ranges from 9 to 18 mm Hg.[11] Because of the low pulmonary artery pressures, right ventricular wall thickness needs to be only approximately one third of left ventricular wall thickness. However, just as hypertension can occur within the systemic circulation, it also can occur within the pulmonary circulation (Box 17-2).[12]

Alveolar-Capillary Membrane

The vessels of the alveolar-capillary membrane form a network around each alveolus that is so dense it forms an almost continuous sheet of blood covering the alveoli.[2] The interior diameter of each capillary segment is just large enough to allow red blood cells to squeeze by in single file so that their cell membranes touch the capillary walls (Fig. 17-13).[3] In this way, oxygen and carbon dioxide need not pass through significant amounts of plasma when diffusing into and out of the alveoli, making a highly efficient vehicle for gas exchange. Each red blood cell spends approximately three fourths of a second in the alveolar-capillary network and is exposed to the alveolar gas of two or three alveoli.[1] In that short time, hemoglobin is brought from its normal venous blood saturation level of 75% to its arterial saturation of more than 96%.[3] Hemoglobin levels have been shown to reach normal within only a 0.25-second exposure to alveolar gas; under conditions such as in tachycardia, in which the red blood cells spend less time within the pulmonary capillary network, normal oxygenation can still occur.[3]

Membrane Layers

The alveolar-capillary membrane is less than 0.5 micron thick[13] and is composed of several layers of cells: the alveolar epithelium, the alveolar basement membrane, the interstitial space, the capillary basement membrane, and the capillary endothelium (Fig. 17-14). Oxygen and carbon dioxide traverse easily across these layers, which present no barrier to diffusion because the membrane is very thin.[3]

Bronchial Circulation

The bronchial circulation, also known as the *systemic blood supply to the lungs*, is the system that perfuses the tracheobronchial tree, the visceral pleura, interstitial and connective tissue, some arteries and veins, lymph nodes, and the nerves within the thoracic cavity. The bronchial arteries that perfuse structures in the left side of the thorax branch off the aorta, and those that perfuse the right-sided structures branch from the intercostal, subclavian, or internal mammary artery. After perfusing the specific lung structures, most of the venous blood returns to the right side of the heart; however, some venous blood from the bronchial circulation returns directly into the pulmonary veins and the left atrium.[14]

Physiologic Shunting

The left atrium normally contains pure oxygenated blood, with a hemoglobin saturation level of 100%. The mixing of venous blood from the bronchial circulation with the oxygenated blood in the left atrium decreases the saturation of left atrial blood to a range between 96% and 99%. For this reason, while a person is breathing room air, the oxygen saturation of arterial blood is less than 100%. The dumping of venous blood into the left atrium is known as an *anatomic shunt*. The thebesian veins, which drain the right coronary circulation, are also responsible for the addition of venous blood to the left atrium. These two

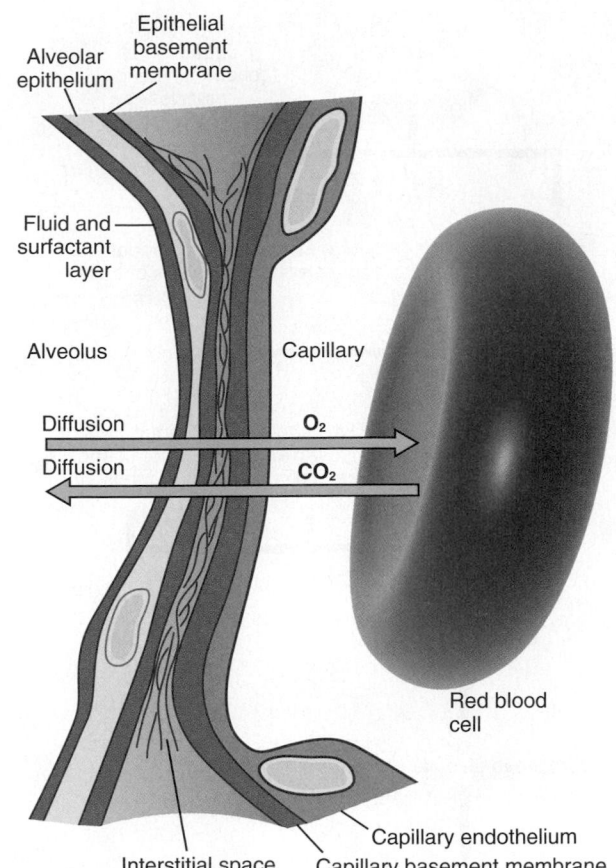

FIGURE 17-14 Layers of the Alveolar-Capillary Membrane. (From Hall JE, ed. *Guyton and Hall Textbook of Medical Physiology.* 12th ed. Philadelphia: Saunders; 2011.)

systems constitute the normal anatomic shunt, which comprises approximately 3% to 5% of the total cardiac output.[15]

Lymphatic Circulation

The lungs are more richly supplied with lymphatic tissue than any other organ, perhaps because of their constant exposure to the external environment. The lymphatic vessels parallel much of the pulmonary vasculature and the tracheobronchial tree to the level of the terminal and respiratory bronchioles. Lymphatic vessels also are located within the connective tissue of lung parenchyma and within the pleural membranes. These vessels eventually drain into the primary lymph nodes located at the hila of the lungs. The lymphatic system in the lungs serves two purposes. As part of the immune system, it is responsible for removing foreign particles and cell debris from the lungs and for producing antibody- and cell-mediated immune responses. It also is responsible for removing fluid from the lungs and for keeping the alveoli clear.[1-3]

VENTILATION

Air moves into and out of the lungs because of the difference between intrapulmonary pressure (pressure inside the lungs) and atmospheric pressure (Fig. 17-15). The movement of air into the lungs is known as *inhalation* see (Fig. 17-15), and the movement of air out of the lungs is known as *exhalation* (Fig. 17-16). At the command of the central nervous system, the muscles of ventilation contract, the thorax and lungs expand, and intrapulmonary pressure falls. When the pressure falls below atmospheric pressure, air enters the lungs, and inhalation occurs. At the end of inhalation, the muscles of ventilation relax, the thorax contracts and the lungs are compressed, and intrapulmonary pressure rises. When the pressure rises above atmospheric pressure, air exits the lungs, and exhalation occurs.[4,16]

Work of Breathing

The work of breathing is the amount of work that must be performed to overcome the elastic and resistive properties of the lungs. The elastic properties are determined by lung recoil, chest wall recoil, and the surface tension of the alveoli. The resistive properties are determined by airway resistance.[1,16,17] Normally, the work of breathing occurs during inhalation, but even exhalation can be a strain when lung recoil, chest wall recoil, or airway resistance is abnormal.[4,16]

During normal, quiet ventilation, only 1% to 2% of basal oxygen consumption is required by the pulmonary system.[17] During heavy exercise, the amount of energy required by the pulmonary system can become progressively greater. The work of breathing can be a factor that limits exercise in the patient with pulmonary disease. Pathologic conditions of the pulmonary system can drastically change the energy requirement for ventilation. Pulmonary diseases that decrease lung compliance (e.g., atelectasis, pulmonary edema), decrease chest wall compliance (e.g., kyphoscoliosis), increase airway resistance (e.g., bronchitis, asthma), or decrease lung recoil (e.g., emphysema) can increase the work of breathing so much that one third or more of the total body energy is used for ventilation (Box 17-3).[4,16]

Pulmonary Volumes and Capacities

Pulmonary ventilation can be described in terms of volumes and capacities (Fig. 17-17). Tidal volume (V_T) is the amount of air inhaled and exhaled with each breath. Inspiratory reserve volume (IRV) is the maximum amount of air that can be inhaled over and above the normal tidal volume. Expiratory reserve volume (ERV) is the maximum amount of air that can be exhaled beyond the normal tidal volume. The residual volume (RV) is the amount of air left in the lungs after a complete exhalation. Inspiratory capacity (IC) is the sum of the tidal volume and the inspiratory reserve. Functional residual capacity (FRC) is the sum of the expiratory reserve volume and the residual volume. Vital capacity (VC) is the sum of the inspiratory reserve volume, the tidal volume, and the expiratory reserve volume. Total lung capacity (TLC) is the sum of all four volumes and represents the maximal amount of air that can be inhaled.[3,16]

Physiologic Dead Space

The portion of total ventilation that participates in gas exchange is known as *alveolar ventilation*. The portion of ventilation that does not is known as *wasted ventilation*. The areas in the lungs that are ventilated but in which no gas exchange occurs are known as *dead space regions*. The conducting airways are referred to as *anatomic dead space* because they are ventilated but not perfused and therefore not able to participate in gas

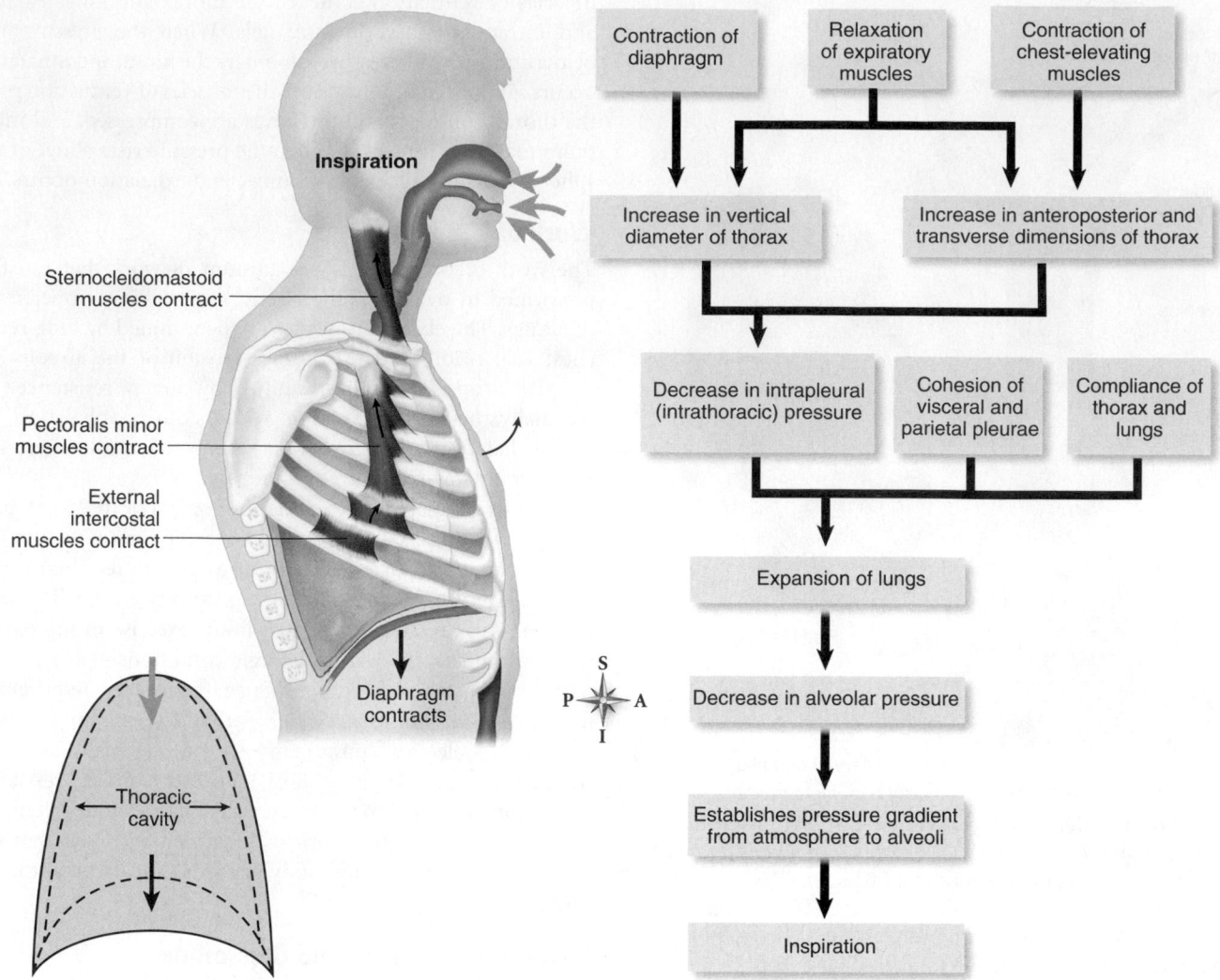

FIGURE 17-15 **The Mechanism of Inspiration.** Note the role of the diaphragm and the chest-elevating muscles (pectoralis minor and external intercostals) in increasing thoracic volume, which decreases pressure in the lungs and thus draws air inward. (From Patton KT, Thibodeau GA, eds. *Anatomy and Physiology.* 8th ed. St. Louis: Mosby; 2013.)

exchange. Some ventilation goes to unperfused alveoli. Without perfusion, gas exchange cannot take place, and the ventilation is wasted. These unperfused alveoli are known as *alveolar dead space.* Anatomic dead space plus alveolar dead space is called *physiologic dead space.*[3,15,16]

Regulation of Ventilation

Regulation of ventilation by the brain is complex and not completely understood. Ventilation is regulated by a triad comprising a controller (located within the central nervous system), a group of effectors (muscles of ventilation), and a variety of sensors that include chemoreceptors (central and peripheral) and mechanoreceptors (located in chest wall and lungs). Efferent nerve fibers convey impulses from the controller to the effectors, whereas afferent nerve fibers carry impulses from some of the sensors to the controller (Fig. 17-18).[18]

Controller

The central nervous system houses what is known as the *controller of ventilation.* The controller is not located in one specific

area; rather, it is in several areas that work together to provide coordinated ventilation. The brainstem regulates automatic ventilation, the cerebral cortex allows voluntary ventilation, and neurons housed in the spinal cord process information from the brain and from the peripheral receptors, allowing them to send final information to the muscles of ventilation.[18]

Brainstem. In the brainstem, the medulla oblongata and the pons are involved in ventilation. Four different groups of neurons are thought to participate in the regulation of inhalation and exhalation. The dorsal respiratory group, located in the medulla, is responsible for the basic rhythm of ventilation. Cells in this area are thought to automatically fire and trigger inhalation. The pneumotaxic center in the pons is responsible for limiting inhalation and triggering exhalation. This response also facilitates control of the rate and pattern of respiration. The ventral respiratory group, located in the medulla, is responsible for inspiration and expiration during periods of increased ventilation. The apneustic center in the lower pons is thought to work with the pneumotaxic center to regulate the depth of inspiration.[18]

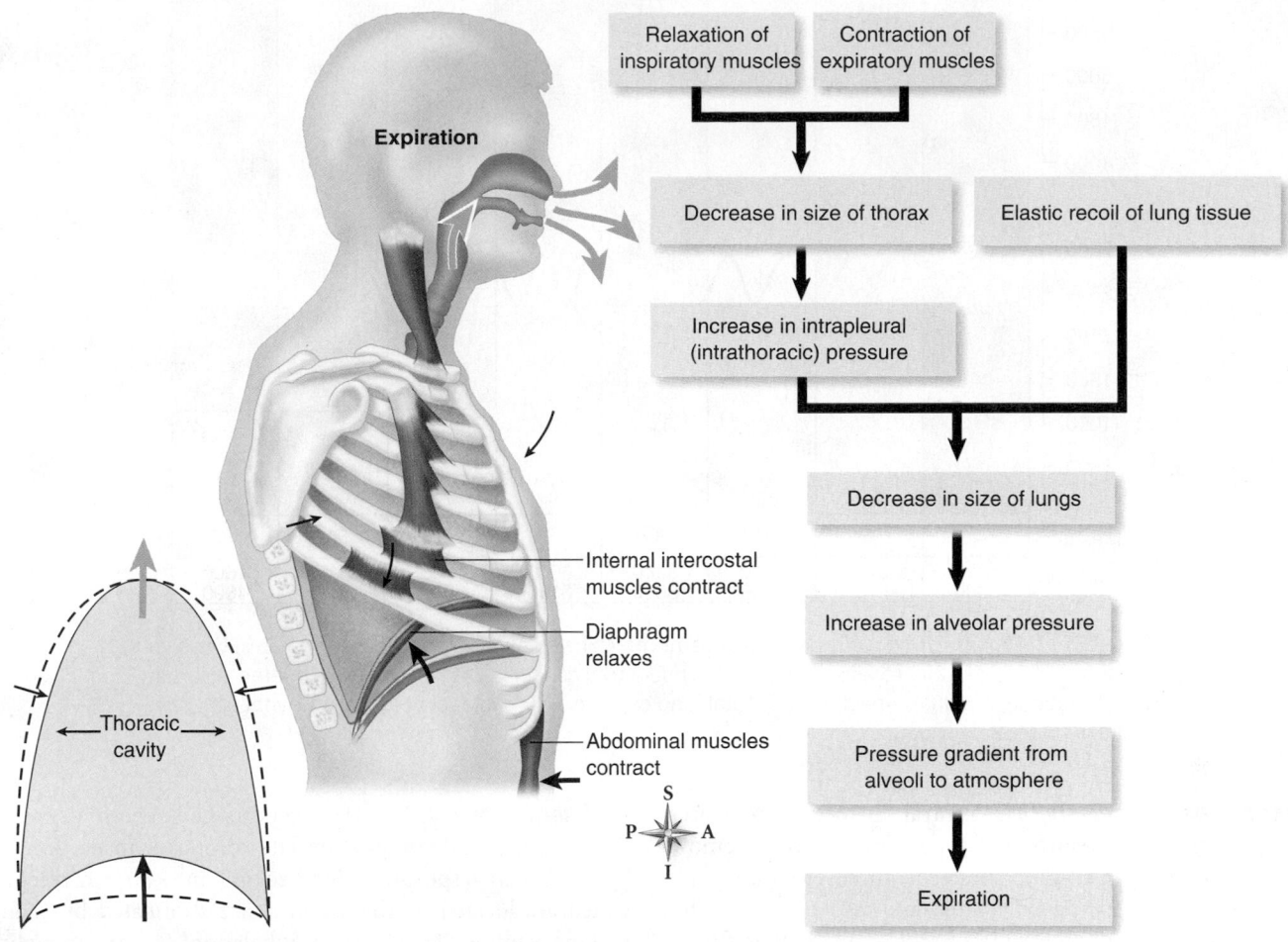

Expiration

Relaxation of inspiratory muscles

Contraction of expiratory muscles

Decrease in size of thorax

Elastic recoil of lung tissue

Increase in intrapleural (intrathoracic) pressure

Decrease in size of lungs

Increase in alveolar pressure

Pressure gradient from alveoli to atmosphere

Expiration

Internal intercostal muscles contract

Diaphragm relaxes

Abdominal muscles contract

Thoracic cavity

FIGURE 17-16 **The Mechanism of Expiration.** Note that relaxation of the diaphragm plus contraction of chest-depressing muscles (internal intercostals) reduces thoracic volume, which increases pressure in the lungs and thus pushes air outward. (From Patton KT, Thibodeau GA, eds. *Anatomy and Physiology.* 8th ed. St. Louis: Mosby; 2013.)

BOX 17-3 HOW LUNG DISEASE CAN ALTER VENTILATION

Normal muscular action of the diaphragm, flexibility of the rib cage, elasticity of the lungs, and airway diameter are instrumental in allowing easy inhalation and exhalation. Any interference with these actions impairs normal ventilation. Pulmonary diseases can be categorized as obstructive or restrictive, depending on how the underlying cause affects normal ventilation.

Restrictive diseases limit lung or chest wall movement and include diffuse interstitial lung fibrosis, atelectasis, kyphoscoliosis, and severe chest wall pain. These conditions can be acute or chronic, and because they restrict lung or chest wall expansion, or both, patients have smaller tidal volumes but an increased ventilatory rate to maintain minute ventilation.

Obstructive diseases impede normal airflow. The classic examples are emphysema, in which airflow is decreased because of a decrease in lung recoil, and asthma, in which airflow is decreased because of diffuse airway narrowing. Emphysema results in lungs that inflate easily but, lacking the normal elastic recoil, do not compress to assist with exhalation. Patients with emphysema may have little difficulty inhaling but struggle to exhale.

Cerebral Cortex. The cerebral cortex functions by allowing voluntary ventilation to override the automatic controls of the medulla and pons. Voluntary ventilatory control is most important during behavioral states such as crying, laughing, singing, and talking. During these states, voluntary control may override the automatic control, which responds chiefly to chemical stimuli and to changes in lung inflation.[3,18]

Effectors

The effectors of ventilation are the muscles of ventilation (see Fig. 17-3). In considering their function in the control of ventilation, the most important issue is that they function in a coordinated fashion. The central nervous system regulates this function.[18]

Sensors

The main sensors for the regulation of ventilation are the central and peripheral chemoreceptors (see Fig. 17-18). These chemoreceptors respond to changes in the chemical composition of the blood or other fluid around them. Other sensors that are found in the lung include the irritant receptors, stretch receptors, and the juxtacapillary (J) receptors.[3,18]

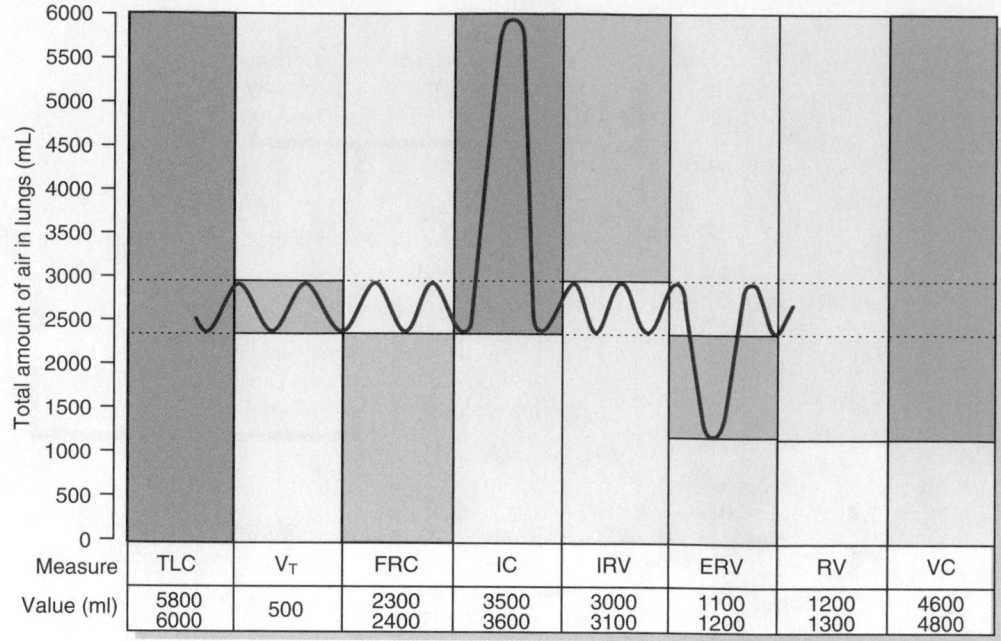

FIGURE 17-17 For lung volume measurements, all values are approximately 25% less in women. *ERV*, Expiratory reserve volume; *IC*, inspiratory capacity; *IRV*, inspiratory reserve volume; *FRC*, functional residual capacity; *TLC*, total lung capacity; *RV*, residual volume; *VC*, vital capacity; V_T, tidal volume.

Central Chemoreceptors. The central chemoreceptors are located near the ventral surface of the medulla in the chemosensitive area (see Fig. 17-18). These chemoreceptors are surrounded by cerebral extracellular fluid and respond primarily to changes in the hydrogen ion concentration of that fluid. Ventilation increases when the hydrogen ion concentration rises and decreases when the hydrogen ion concentration falls. A rise in the partial pressure of carbon dioxide ($Paco_2$) causes the movement of carbon dioxide across the blood-brain barrier into the cerebrospinal fluid, stimulating the movement of hydrogen ions into the brain's extracellular fluid. These hydrogen ions then stimulate the chemoreceptors, and ventilation is increased. The increase in ventilation causes exhalation of excess carbon dioxide, the $Paco_2$ falls, and ventilation returns to normal. Central chemoreceptors are not affected by changes in the partial pressure of oxygen (Pao_2).[18]

Peripheral Chemoreceptors. The peripheral chemoreceptors are located above and below the aortic arch and at the bifurcation of the common carotid arteries (see Fig. 17-18). The most important action of the peripheral chemoreceptors is their response to changes in the Pao_2, because they are the primary receptors that increase ventilation in response to arterial hypoxemia. Immediate hyperventilation, one of the principal compensatory mechanisms in response to hypoxemia, is governed by these chemoreceptors. The peripheral chemoreceptors also respond to changes in $Paco_2$ and hydrogen ion concentration. An increase in either results in an increase in ventilation. Studies indicate that the peripheral chemoreceptors probably are more involved with short-term response to carbon dioxide, whereas the central chemoreceptors are responsible for the long-term response to carbon dioxide.[18]

Other Receptors. Irritant receptors lie between airway epithelial cells, and they stimulate bronchoconstriction and hyperpnea in response to inhaled irritants. Stretch receptors, which are located in the airways, are stimulated by changes in lung volume. They inhibit inhalation and are thought to protect the lung from overinflation (Hering-Breuer reflex). J receptors lie in the alveolar walls close to the capillaries. They are stimulated by engorgement of the pulmonary capillaries and an increase in the interstitial fluid volume. Stimulation of the J receptors is thought to cause rapid, shallow breathing.[19]

RESPIRATION

Respiration refers to the movement of oxygen and carbon dioxide. Gas exchange that takes place at the lung level through the alveolar-capillary membrane is referred to as *external respiration*. The diffusion of gases in and out of the cells at the tissue level is referred to as *internal respiration*.[3]

Diffusion

Oxygen and carbon dioxide move throughout the body by diffusion. Diffusion moves molecules from an area of high concentration to an area of low concentration. The difference in the concentrations of the gases is referred to as the *driving pressure*. The greater the driving pressure of the gas through the membrane, the greater the rate of diffusion.[3] Within the lungs, diffusion occurs because of the difference in the driving pressure between the pulmonary capillaries and the alveoli. Oxygen is in high concentration within the alveoli and exerts a higher driving pressure as compared with the pulmonary capillaries; therefore, oxygen moves by diffusion from the

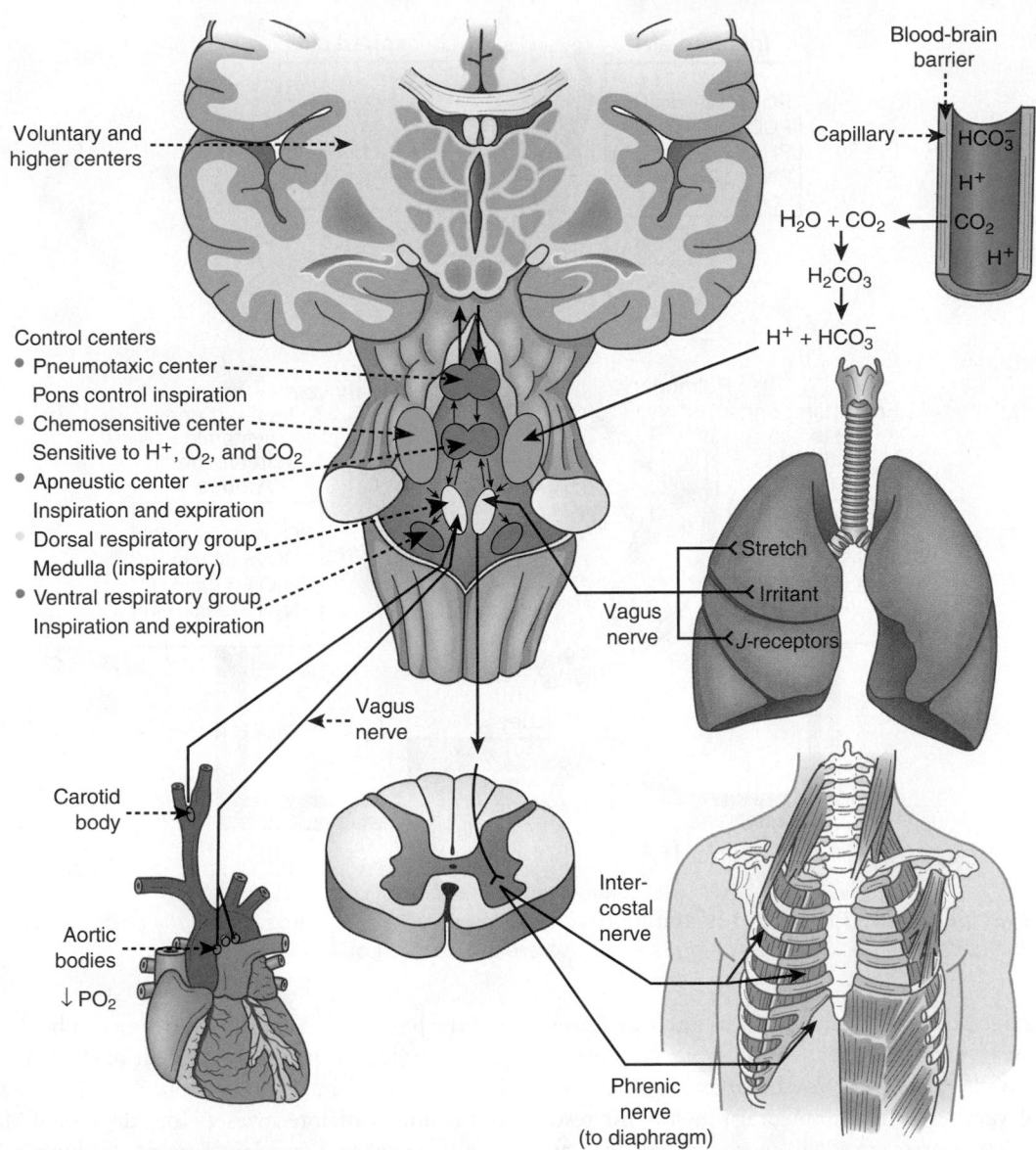

FIGURE 17-18 Respiratory Control System. (From McCance KL, et al, eds. *Pathophysiology: The Biologic Basis for Disease in Adults and Children.* 6th ed. St. Louis: Mosby; 2010.)

alveoli into the pulmonary capillaries. Carbon dioxide is in higher concentration and has a higher driving pressure within the pulmonary capillaries compared with the alveoli; therefore, carbon dioxide diffuses out of the capillaries into the alveoli, where it is exhaled (Fig. 17-19). The driving pressure of oxygen is lower at higher altitudes because the effects of gravity on the gases are lessened,[20] and it is higher when supplemental oxygen is administered.[21]

In addition to the driving pressure of gases, several other factors affect the rate of diffusion. They include the thickness of the alveolar-capillary membrane,[3] the surface area of the membrane,[22] and the diffusion coefficient of the gas.[21] An increase in the thickness of the alveolar-capillary membrane (e.g., pulmonary edema, fibrosis)[3] or a decrease in the surface area of the membrane (e.g., pneumonectomy, lobectomy, pulmonary embolus, emphysema)[22] decreases the rate of diffusion. The diffusion coefficient of each gas is determined by its solubility. The higher the diffusion coefficient, the faster the gas

diffuses. Carbon dioxide has a much higher diffusion coefficient than oxygen, and carbon dioxide diffuses 20 times more rapidly than does oxygen.[21]

VENTILATION/PERFUSION RELATIONSHIPS

Ventilation (V) and perfusion (Q) should be equally matched at the alveolar capillary membrane level for optimal gas exchange to take place, but because of normal regional variations in the distribution of ventilation and perfusion, this is not the case. Normally, alveolar ventilation is approximately 4 L/min, and pulmonary capillary perfusion is approximately 5 L/min. The normal ventilation/perfusion ratio (V/Q) is 4:5, or 0.8.[15,21]

Distribution of Ventilation

The distribution of ventilation throughout the lungs is not even. This is the result of a variety of factors, including the configuration of the thorax and the effects of gravity on

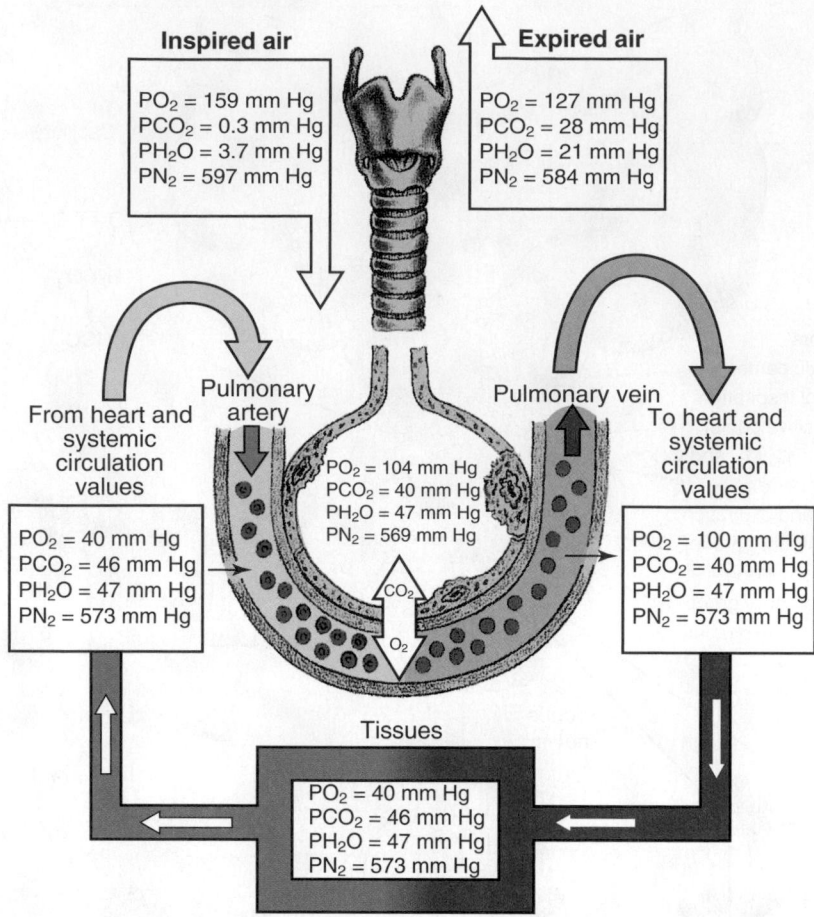

Inspired air
$PO_2 = 159$ mm Hg
$PCO_2 = 0.3$ mm Hg
$PH_2O = 3.7$ mm Hg
$PN_2 = 597$ mm Hg

Expired air
$PO_2 = 127$ mm Hg
$PCO_2 = 28$ mm Hg
$PH_2O = 21$ mm Hg
$PN_2 = 584$ mm Hg

Pulmonary artery

Pulmonary vein

From heart and systemic circulation values
$PO_2 = 40$ mm Hg
$PCO_2 = 46$ mm Hg
$PH_2O = 47$ mm Hg
$PN_2 = 573$ mm Hg

$PO_2 = 104$ mm Hg
$PCO_2 = 40$ mm Hg
$PH_2O = 47$ mm Hg
$PN_2 = 569$ mm Hg

CO_2

O_2

To heart and systemic circulation values
$PO_2 = 100$ mm Hg
$PCO_2 = 40$ mm Hg
$PH_2O = 47$ mm Hg
$PN_2 = 573$ mm Hg

Tissues

$PO_2 = 40$ mm Hg
$PCO_2 = 46$ mm Hg
$PH_2O = 47$ mm Hg
$PN_2 = 573$ mm Hg

FIGURE 17-19 Process of Respiration. (From McCance KL, et al, eds. *Pathophysiology: The Biologic Basis for Disease in Adults and Children.* 6th ed. St. Louis: Mosby; 2010.)

intrapleural pressure. The thorax allows more lung expansion at the base than at the apex, which permits more ventilation to the base and limits ventilation to the apex. Gravity also produces regional variations in intrapleural pressure. At rest, the negative intrapleural pressure at the apex is greater than at the base, and alveoli in the apexes are larger and have more air left in them at the end of expiration. Because the alveoli are larger, they are less compliant and more difficult to inflate. On inhalation, the alveoli at the base expand more because they have less pressure to overcome.[3,15,16] In the upright person, the base of the lung receives about four times more ventilation than the apex.[16] In the supine person, gravity produces the same effects in the dependent zones of the lungs (posterior regions).[3,15,16]

Distribution of Perfusion

The distribution of perfusion through the lungs is related to gravity and intraalveolar pressures. Because of the effects of gravity, the pressure in the capillaries in the lungs is higher in the bases than in the apexes. This promotes preferential blood flow to the gravity-dependent areas of the lungs. Intraalveolar pressures also vary throughout the different regions of the lungs, with the highest pressure in the apexes and the lowest pressure in the bases. In some areas of the lungs, the intraalveolar pressure has the potential of exceeding capillary hydrostatic pressure, resulting in an absence of blood flow to these areas.

On the basis of this concept, the lung can be divided into three zones. Zone 1 is the nondependent portion of the lung, which has the potential of no perfusion. Zone 2 is the middle portion of the lung, which receives various degrees of blood flow. Zone 3 is the gravity-dependent area of the lung, which receives a constant blood flow (Fig. 17-20).[3,15]

Ventilation/Perfusion Mismatch

A variety of factors can affect the matching of ventilation to perfusion in the lungs, and their relationship can be considered as a continuum (Fig. 17-21). At one end of the continuum, the alveolus is receiving ventilation but is not receiving any perfusion and is unable to participate in gas exchange. This situation is referred to as *alveolar dead space*. On the other end of the continuum, the alveolus is receiving perfusion but is not receiving any ventilation and is unable to participate in gas exchange. This situation is referred to as *intrapulmonary shunting*. In this case, the blood is returned to the left side of the heart unoxygenated.[21] Between these two extremes exist an infinite number of ventilation/perfusion mismatches. Situations in which ventilation exceeds perfusion V/Q > 0.8 are considered to be *dead space producing*, whereas situations in which perfusion exceeds ventilation V/Q < 0.8 are considered to be *shunt producing*. Although minor mismatching of ventilation may not significantly affect gas exchange, significant alterations in the relationship result in hypoxemia.[15,21]

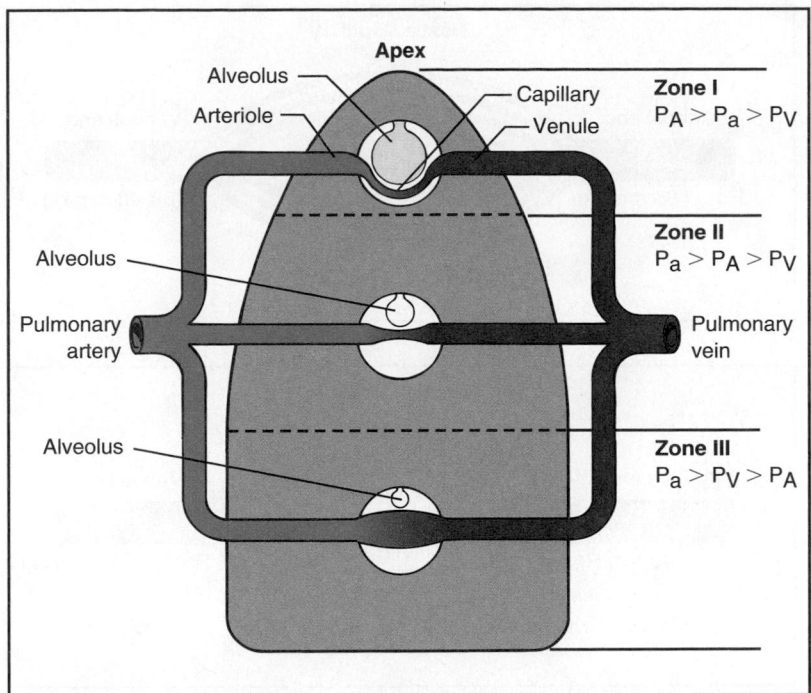

FIGURE 17-20 The Effects of Gravity and Alveolar Pressure on Pulmonary Blood Flow. Notice the three lung zones. In zone I, alveolar pressure (PA) is greater than arterial and venous pressure, and no blood flow occurs. In zone II, arterial pressure (Pa) exceeds alveolar pressure, but alveolar pressure exceeds venous pressure (PV). Blood flow occurs in this zone, but alveolar pressure compresses the venules (venous ends of the capillaries). In zone III, both arterial and venous pressures are greater than alveolar pressure and blood flow fluctuates, depending on the difference between arterial and venous pressures. (From McCance KL, et al, eds. *Pathophysiology: The Biologic Basis for Disease in Adults and Children.* 6th ed. St Louis: Mosby; 2010.)

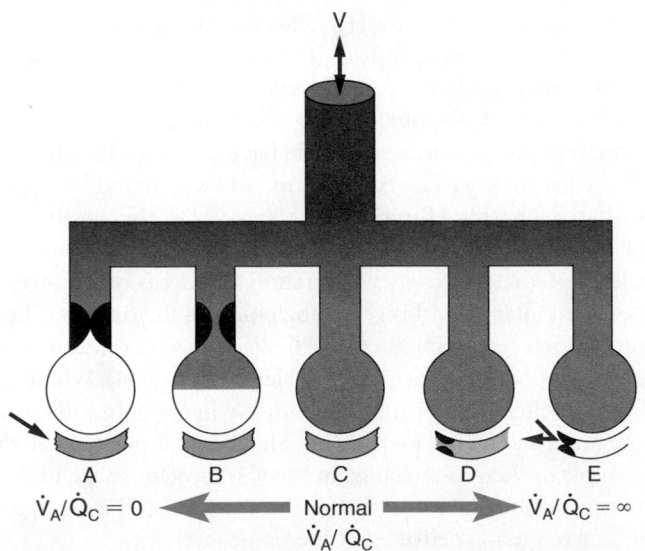

FIGURE 17-21 Continuum of Ventilation/Perfusion (V/Q) Relationships. *A,* Intrapulmonary shunting. *B,* (V/Q) mismatching is a shunt-producing situation. *C,* Normal (V/Q) ratio. *D,* (V/Q) mismatching is a dead space-producing situation. *E,* Alveolar dead space. (From Misasi RS, Keyes JL. Matching and mismatching ventilation and perfusion in the lung. *Crit Care Nurse.* 1996;16[3]:23.)

Hypoxic Vasoconstriction

The distribution of perfusion is affected by the amount of oxygen in the alveoli. Although most blood vessels in the body dilate in response to hypoxia, the pulmonary vessels constrict when the Pao_2 is less than 60 mm Hg. This event, known as *hypoxic vasoconstriction,* usually occurs when a portion of the pulmonary capillaries perfuses unventilated or underventilated alveoli. It is thought to be a compensatory response used to limit the return of unoxygenated blood to the left side of the heart. If the response is prolonged and generalized throughout the lungs, pulmonary hypertension (Box 17-2) will result.[3]

GAS TRANSPORT

Gas transport refers to the movement of oxygen and carbon dioxide to and from the tissue cells. The transportation vehicle is the bloodstream, which is moved by the pumping action of the heart (cardiac output). At the tissue level, oxygen and carbon dioxide move into and out of the cell by diffusion. Oxygen diffuses into the cell because of the pressure gradient that exists between oxygen in the capillary and oxygen in the cell (Fig. 17-22A). Carbon dioxide diffuses into the capillary because of the pressure gradient that exists between carbon dioxide in the cell and carbon dioxide in the capillary (see Fig. 17-22B).[3]

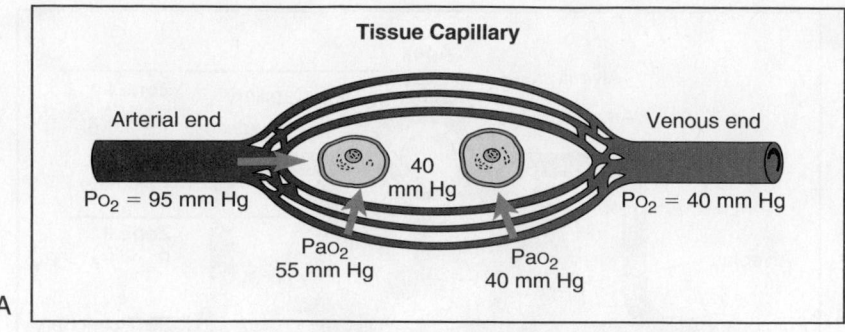

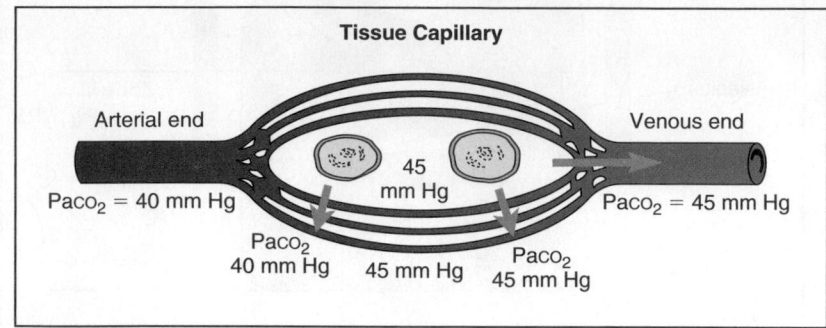

FIGURE 17-22   Internal Respiration. *A*, Diffusion of oxygen from a tissue capillary into a tissue cell. *B*, Diffusion of carbon dioxide from a tissue cell into a tissue capillary.

Oxygen Content

Oxygen is transported to the tissues by the blood in two ways. It is dissolved in plasma (Pao_2) or bound to hemoglobin molecules (oxygen saturation [Sao_2]). Most of the oxygen is transported by hemoglobin, with the portion of oxygen dissolved in plasma equal to approximately 3% of the total oxygen within the blood.[23] The pressure exerted by the oxygen dissolved in plasma is important because this oxygen diffuses across the capillary membrane into the cells first and serves as the vehicle for the unloading of the oxygen from the hemoglobin molecule. As dissolved oxygen leaves the plasma and diffuses into the cells, the molecules of oxygen move off the hemoglobin molecule, dissolve into the plasma, and diffuse into the cells.[20] For this process to begin, a pressure gradient must exist between the oxygen level in the capillary and the oxygen level in the cell.

Oxygen Content Formula

The amount of oxygen in the arterial blood can be calculated using the arterial oxygen content (Cao_2) formula. The amount of oxygen in the venous blood can be calculated using the venous oxygen content (Cvo_2) formula (see Appendix B).[23]

Oxyhemoglobin Dissociation Curve

The relationship between dissolved oxygen and hemoglobin-bound oxygen is plotted as the oxyhemoglobin dissociation curve (Fig. 17-23). The sigmoid shape of the oxyhemoglobin dissociation curve illustrates several essential points about the relationship between the two ways oxygen is carried. The steep lower portion of the curve, at Pao_2 levels of 10 to 60 mm Hg, shows that the peripheral tissues can withdraw large amounts of oxygen from the hemoglobin molecule with only a small

change in Pao_2, preserving the gradient for the continued unloading of hemoglobin.[20,23] The area at Pao_2 levels of 60 to 100 mm Hg is called the *flat upper portion* of the curve. This portion shows that the saturation of hemoglobin remains high even as the Pao_2 declines. For example, in a healthy person, a Pao_2 of 60 mm Hg yields an oxygen saturation level of 89%, whereas a Pao_2 of 100 mm Hg yields an oxygen saturation level of 98%. The great drop in Pao_2 (from 100 to 60 mm Hg) causes only a small drop in oxygen saturation (from 98% to 89%).[21,23]

Shifts in the Oxyhemoglobin Dissociation Curve. Under normal circumstances, hemoglobin has a steady and predictable affinity for oxygen. The combination of oxygen and hemoglobin based on this affinity is responsible for the position of the oxyhemoglobin dissociation curve in which a given Pao_2 yields a predictable oxygen saturation.[20,23] Occasionally, events occur that alter the affinity hemoglobin has for oxygen. These events include changes in pH, $Paco_2$, temperature, and 2,3-diphosphoglycerate (2,3-DPG) levels (Box 17-4). When this affinity is altered, the position of the oxyhemoglobin dissociation curve shifts (see Fig. 17-23). Shifts in the position of the curve mean there is a change in the way oxygen is taken up by the hemoglobin molecule at the alveolar level and a change in the way oxygen is delivered at the tissue level.[21,23]

Shift to the Right. When the curve is shifted to the right (see Fig. 17-23, curve C), there is a lower oxygen saturation level for any given Pao_2; in other words, hemoglobin has less affinity for oxygen. Although the saturation level is lower than expected, a right shift enhances oxygen delivery at the tissue level because hemoglobin unloads more readily. Factors that cause this change in oxygen-hemoglobin affinity and shift the curve to the right include fever, increased $Paco_2$, acidosis, and increased 2,3-DPG levels.[21,23]

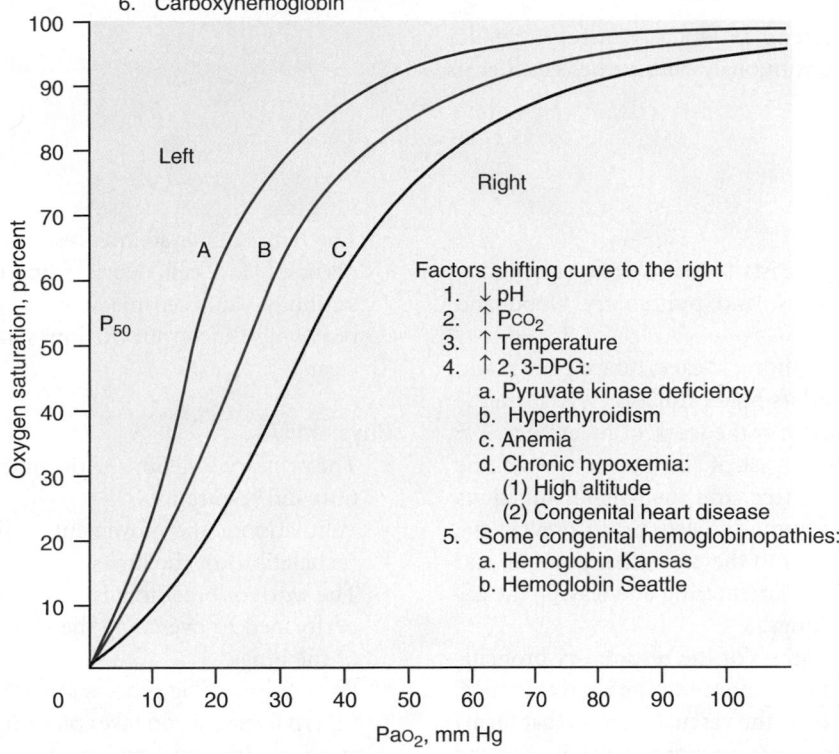

Factors shifting curve to the left
1. ↑ pH
2. ↓ PCO₂
3. ↓ Temperature
4. ↓ 2, 3-DPG:
   a. Hexokinase deficiency
   b. Hypothyroidism
   c. Bank blood
5. Some congenital hemoglobinopathies:
   a. Hemoglobin Ranier
   b. Hemoglobin Hiroshima
   c. Hemoglobin San Francisco
6. Carboxyhemoglobin

Factors shifting curve to the right
1. ↓ pH
2. ↑ PCO₂
3. ↑ Temperature
4. ↑ 2, 3-DPG:
   a. Pyruvate kinase deficiency
   b. Hyperthyroidism
   c. Anemia
   d. Chronic hypoxemia:
      (1) High altitude
      (2) Congenital heart disease
5. Some congenital hemoglobinopathies:
   a. Hemoglobin Kansas
   b. Hemoglobin Seattle

FIGURE 17-23 Oxyhemoglobin Dissociation Curve. *A,* The curve is shifted to the left because of hemoglobin's increased affinity for oxygen. *B,* The standard oxyhemoglobin dissociation curve. *C,* The curve is shifted to the right because of hemoglobin's decreased affinity for oxygen. (Modified from Kinney MR, et al, eds. *AACN's Clinical Reference for Critical Care Nursing.* 4th ed. St. Louis: Mosby; 1998.)

BOX 17-4 WHAT IS 2,3-DPG?

2,3-Diphosphoglycerate (2,3-DPG), an organic phosphate found primarily in red blood cells, has the ability to alter the affinity of hemoglobin for oxygen. When the level of 2,3-DPG increases within the red blood cells, hemoglobin's affinity for oxygen is decreased (a shift in the oxyhemoglobin curve to the right), making more oxygen available to the tissues. Increased synthesis of 2,3,-DPG is an important component of the adaptive responses in healthy persons to an acute need for more tissue oxygen. Tissue hypoxia stimulates production of 2,3-DPG, and increased amounts have been found in patients with anemia, right-to-left shunts, or acute heart failure, and in persons residing at high altitudes.

A decrease in the amount of 2,3-DPG is detrimental to tissue oxygenation because it causes hemoglobin's affinity for oxygen to increase (a shift in the oxyhemoglobin curve to the left). Decreased 2,3-DPG levels occur with hypophosphatemia, septic shock, and the use of banked blood. Blood preserved with acid citrate dextrose loses most of its red cell 2,3-DPG within several days. Blood preserved with citrate phosphate dextrose maintains its 2,3-DPG levels for several weeks. Transfusion of blood with a low level of 2,3-DPG cannot be beneficial for tissue oxygenation until the 2,3-DPG level is restored, which may take 18 to 24 hours.

Shift to the Left. When the curve is shifted to the left (see Fig. 17-23, curve A), the reverse occurs. There is a higher arterial saturation for any given Pao₂ because hemoglobin has an increased affinity for oxygen. Although the saturation level is higher, oxygen delivery to the tissues is impaired because hemoglobin does not unload as easily. Factors that contribute to this effect include hypothermia, alkalemia, decreased Paco₂, and decreased 2,3-DPG levels.[21,23]

Abnormalities of Hemoglobin

Hemoglobin carries approximately 97% of the total amount of oxygen held within the bloodstream. This great carrying capacity depends on hemoglobin that is normal in amount and molecular structure. Most hemoglobin abnormalities affect the oxygen-carrying capability of this molecule. The most common abnormality involving hemoglobin is a decrease in amount. This can be an acute or a chronic situation (anemia). Abnormal hemoglobin structure also can pose problems, such as hemoglobin S, which is responsible for sickle cell anemia. Hemoglobin S has less affinity for oxygen than does normal hemoglobin.

Normal hemoglobin can become abnormal hemoglobin under certain conditions. Methemoglobin and carboxyhemoglobin are two examples. Methemoglobin occurs when the iron atoms within the hemoglobin molecule are oxidized from the ferrous state to the ferric state. Methemoglobin does not carry oxygen. Carboxyhemoglobin occurs when carbon monoxide combines with hemoglobin. Carbon monoxide uses the same binding site as oxygen and has a much greater affinity for hemoglobin.[21]

Carbon Dioxide Content

Carbon dioxide, one of the end products of aerobic cellular metabolism, is produced continuously within the cells. On its way from the cells to the lungs, carbon dioxide is transported within the plasma and the erythrocytes. Carbon dioxide is transported, physically dissolved as the $Paco_2$ (5%), bound to blood proteins (including hemoglobin) in the form of carbaminohemoglobin compounds (5% to 1%), and combined with water to form carbonic acid (8% to 9%), some of which dissociates into hydrogen ions and bicarbonate. In the lungs, these methods of carbon dioxide carriage are reversed as the carbon dioxide leaves the plasma and erythrocytes for exhalation.[21]

SUMMARY

Anatomy

- The pulmonary system consists of the thorax, conducting airways, respiratory airways, and pulmonary blood and lymph supply.
- The thorax consists of the thoracic cage, lungs, pleura, and muscles of ventilation, and its major function is to form the ventilatory pump and perform the work of breathing.
- The conducting airways consist of the upper airways, the trachea, and the bronchial tree, and their major functions are to warm and humidify the inhaled air, to prevent the entrance of foreign matter into the gas exchange areas, and to serve as a passageway for air entering and leaving the gas exchange regions of the lungs.
- The respiratory airways consist of the respiratory bronchioles and the alveoli, and their major function is gas exchange.
- The pulmonary circulation is the vascular system that forms the gas exchange network surrounding the alveoli, and the bronchial circulation is the vascular system that perfuses the tracheobronchial tree.

- The lymphatic system is responsible for removing foreign particles and cell debris from the lungs, for producing antibody- and cell-mediated immune responses, and for removing fluid from the lungs and for keeping the alveoli clear.

Physiology

- The primary functions of the pulmonary system are ventilation and respiration.
- Ventilation is the movement of air in (inhalation) and out (exhalation) of the lungs.
- The work of breathing is the amount of work that must be performed to overcome the elastic and resistive properties of the lungs.
- Respiration is the process of gas exchange.
- External respiration takes place at the lung level through the alveolar-capillary membrane.
- Internal respiration is the diffusion of gases in and out of the cells at the tissue level.

REFERENCES

1. Hicks GH. The respiratory system. In: Kacmarek RM, et al., eds. *Egan's Fundamentals of Respiratory Care.* 10th ed. St Louis: Mosby; 2013.
2. Albertine KH. Anatomy of the lungs. In: Mason RJ, et al, eds. *Murray and Nadel's Textbook of Respiratory Medicine.* 5th ed. Philadelphia: Elsevier; 2010.
3. Brashers VL. Structure and function of the pulmonary system. In: McCance KL, et al, eds. *Pathophysiology: The Biologic Basis for Disease in Adults and Children.* 6th ed. St. Louis: Mosby; 2010.
4. Murali R, Park K, Leslie KO. The pleura in health and disease. *Semin Respir Crit Care Med.* 2010;31:649.
5. Maish MS. The diaphragm. *Surg Clin N Am* 90:955, 2010.
6. Benditt JO, McCool FD. Respiratory system and neuromuscular diseases. In: Mason RJ, et al, eds. *Murray and Nadel's Textbook of Respiratory Medicine.* 5th ed. Philadelphia: Elsevier; 2010.
7. Minnich DJ, Mathisen DJ. Anatomy of the trachea, carina, and bronchi. *Thorac Surg Clin.* 2007;17:571.
8. Antunes MB, Cohen NA. Mucociliary clearance–a critical upper airway host defense mechanism and methods of assessment. *Curr Opin Allergy Clin Immunol.* 2007;7:5.
9. Amin MR, Belafsky PC. Cough and swallowing dysfunction. *Otolaryngol Clin North Am.* 2010;43:35.
10. Enhorning G. Surfactant in airway disease. *Chest.* 2008;133:975.
11. Polanco PM, Pinsky MR. Practical issues of hemodynamic monitoring at the bedside. *Surg Clin N Am.* 2006;86:1431.
12. Gayat E, Mebazaa A. Pulmonary hypertension in critical care. *Curr Opin Crit Care.* 2011;17:439.
13. Wagner PD, et al. Ventilation, blood flow, and gas exchange. In: Mason RJ, et al, eds. *Murray and Nadel's Textbook of Respiratory Medicine.* 5th ed. Philadelphia: Elsevier; 2010.
14. Charana NB, et al. Functional anatomy of bronchial veins. *Pulm Pharmacol Ther.* 2007;20:100.
15. Misasi RS, Keyes JL. Matching and mismatching ventilation and perfusion in the lung. *Crit Care Nurse.* 1996;16(3):23.
16. Chatburn RL, Daoud EG. Ventilation. In: Kacmarek RM, et al, eds. *Egan's Fundamentals of Respiratory Care.* 10th ed. St. Louis: Mosby; 2013.
17. Ayas NT, et al. Respiratory system mechanics and energetics. In: Mason RJ, et al, eds. *Murray and Nadel's Textbook of Respiratory Medicine.* 5th ed. Philadelphia: Elsevier; 2010.
18. Corne S, Bshouty Z. Basic principles of control of breathing. *Respir Care Clin.* 2005;11:147.

19. Eckert DJ, et al. Central sleep apnea pathophysiology and treatment. *Chest.* 2007;131:595.
20. Moore LG, et al. Humans at high altitude: hypoxia and fetal growth. *Respir Physiol Neurobiol.* 2011;178:181.
21. Hirsch CA. Gas exchange and transport. In: Kacmarek RM, et al, eds. *Egan's Fundamentals of Respiratory Care.* 10th ed. St. Louis: Mosby; 2013.
22. Hébert PC, et al. Physiologic aspects of anemia. *Crit Care Clin.* 2004;20:187.
23. Berry BE, Pinard AE. Assessing tissue oxygenation. *Crit Care Nurse.* 2002;22(3):22.

CHAPTER

18

Pulmonary Clinical Assessment

Kathleen M. Stacy

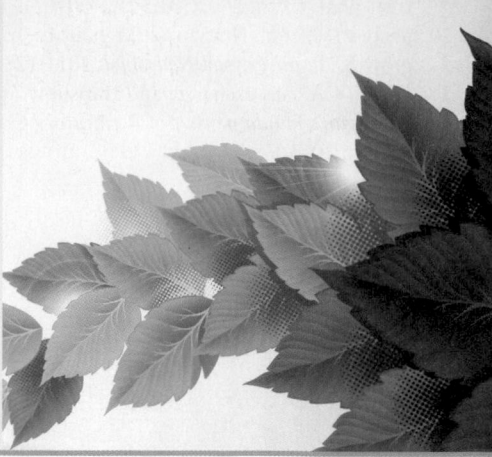

evolve WEBSITE

http://evolve.elsevier.com/Urden/criticalcare/

Evolve features:

- NCLEX Review Questions
- CCRN Review Questions
- PCCN Review Questions
- Mosby's Nursing Skills Procedures
- Animations
- Video Clips
- Glossary

Assessment of the patient with pulmonary dysfunction is a systematic process that incorporates an inquiry into the chronology of the present illness, better known as a *history*, and an investigation of the current physical manifestations, better known as a *physical examination*. The purpose of the assessment is twofold: first, to recognize changes in the patient's pulmonary status that necessitate nursing or medical intervention, and second, to determine the ways in which the patient's pulmonary dysfunction is interfering with his or her self-care activities. After completion, the assessment serves as the foundation for developing the management plan for the patient. The assessment process can be brief or can involve a detailed history and examination, depending on the nature and immediacy of the patient's situation. Whatever the setting, the nurse should develop and practice a sequential pattern of assessment to avoid omitting portions of the examination.

HISTORY

Taking a thorough and accurate history is an essential part of the assessment process. The patient's history provides the foundation and direction for the rest of the assessment. The overall goal of the patient interview is to expose key clinical manifestations that will facilitate the identification of the underlying cause of the illness. This information then assists in the development of an appropriate management plan.

The initial presentation of the patient determines the rapidity and direction of the interview. For a patient in acute distress, the history should be curtailed to just a few questions about the patient's chief complaint and precipitating events. For a patient in no obvious distress, the history should focus on five areas: 1)

review of the patient's present illness; 2) overview of the patient's general respiratory status; 3) examination of the patient's general health status; 4) survey of the patient's family and social background; and 5) description of the patient's current symptoms.[1] Specific items regarding each of these areas are outlined in the Box 18-1.

Symptoms that are common in the pulmonary patient include dyspnea, cough, wheezing, edema, palpitations, fatigue, chest pain, hemoptysis, and sputum abnormalities. Information should be elicited regarding the location, onset and duration, characteristics, setting, aggravating and alleviating factors, associated symptoms, and efforts to treat the symptoms. If the cough is productive, the patient should be asked questions about the color, amount, odor, and consistency of the sputum.[2-5]

PHYSICAL EXAMINATION

Four techniques are used in physical assessment: inspection, palpation, percussion, and auscultation. *Inspection* is the process of looking intently at the patient. *Palpation* is the process of touching the patient to judge the size, shape, texture, and temperature of the body surface or underlying structures. *Percussion* is the process of creating sound waves on the surface of the body to determine abnormal density of any underlying areas. *Auscultation* is the process of concentrated listening with a stethoscope to determine characteristics of body functions.[6,7]

Inspection

Inspection of the patient should focus on three areas: 1) observation of the tongue and sublingual area; 2) assessment of chest

BOX 18-1   DATA COLLECTION

Common Pulmonary Symptoms

Cough
- Onset and duration:
  - Sudden or gradual
  - Episodic or continuous
- Characteristics:
  - Dry or wet
  - Hacking, hoarse, barking, or congested
  - Productive or nonproductive
- Sputum:
  - Present or absent
  - Frequency of production
  - Appearance—color (e.g., clear, mucoid, purulent, blood-tinged, mostly bloody), foul odor, frothy
  - Amount
- Pattern:
  - Paroxysmal
  - Related to time of day, weather, activities, talking, or deep breathing
  - Change over time
- Severity:
  - Causes fatigue
  - Disrupts sleep or conversation
  - Produces chest pain
- Associated symptoms:
  - Shortness of breath
  - Chest pain or tightness with breathing
  - Fever
  - Upper respiratory tract signs (sore throat, congestion, increased mucus production)
  - Noisy respirations or hoarseness
  - Gagging or choking
  - Anxiety, stress, or panic reactions
- Efforts made to treat:
  - Prescription or nonprescription medications
  - Vaporizers
  - Effective or ineffective

Shortness of Breath or Dyspnea on Exertion
- Onset and duration:
  - Sudden or gradual
  - Gagging or choking episode a few days before onset
- Pattern:
  - Related to position—improves when sitting up or with head elevated; number of pillows used to alleviate problems
  - Related to activity—exercise or eating; extent of activity that produces dyspnea
  - Related to other factors—time of day, season, or exposure to something in the environment
  - Harder to inhale or harder to exhale
- Severity:
  - Extent activity is limited
  - Breathing itself causes fatigue
  - Anxiety about getting enough air
- Associated symptoms:
  - Pain or discomfort—exact location in respiratory tree
  - Cough, diaphoresis, swelling of ankles, or cyanosis
- Efforts made to treat:
  - Prescription or nonprescription medications
  - Oxygen
  - Effective or ineffective

Chest Pain
- Onset and duration:
  - Gradual or sudden
  - Associated with trauma, coughing, or lower respiratory tract infection
- Associated symptoms:
  - Shallow breathing
  - Uneven chest expansion
  - Fever
  - Cough
  - Radiation of pain to neck or arms
  - Anxiety about getting enough air
- Efforts made to treat:
  - Heat, splinting, or pain medication
  - Effective or ineffective

Pulmonary Risk Factors
- Tobacco use—current and past:
  - Type of tobacco—cigarettes, cigars, pipes, or smokeless
  - Duration and amount—age started, inhale when smoking, amount used in the past and present
  - Pack years—number of packs per day multiplied by number of years patient has smoked
  - Efforts to quit—previous attempts and current interest
- Work environment:
  - Nature of work
  - Environmental hazards: chemicals, vapors, dust, pulmonary irritants, or allergens
  - Use of protective devices
- Home environment:
  - Location
  - Possible allergens—pets, house plants, plants and trees outside the home, or other environmental hazards
  - Type of heating
  - Use of air conditioning or humidifier
  - Ventilation
  - Stairs to climb

Medical History

Child
- Infectious respiratory diseases:
  - Strep throat
  - Mumps
  - Tonsillitis
- Asthma
- Cystic fibrosis
- Immunizations

Adult
- Previous diagnosis of pulmonary disorders—dates of hospitalization
- Chronic pulmonary disease—date, treatment, and compliance with therapy:
  - Tuberculosis
  - Bronchitis
  - Emphysema
  - Bronchiectasis
  - Asthma
  - Sinus infection

Continued

BOX 18-1   **DATA COLLECTION**

Common Pulmonary Symptoms—cont'd

- Other chronic disorders—cardiovascular, cancer, musculoskeletal, neurologic, immune:
    Obstruction of one or both nares
    Mouth breathing often necessary (especially at night)
    History of nasal discharge
    Compromised immune system function
- Nosebleed
- Sleep apnea:
    Obstructive
    Central
- Previous tests:
    Allergy testing
    Pulmonary function tests
    Tuberculin and fungal skin tests
    Chest radiographs

Surgical
- Thoracic trauma
- Thoracic surgery
- Nasal surgery or injury

Family History
- Tuberculosis
- Cystic fibrosis
- Emphysema
- Allergies
- Asthma
- Atopic dermatitis
- Smoking by household members
- Malignancy

Current Medication Use
- Inhalators
- Steroids
- Antibiotics
- Immunizations
    Pneumococcal (Pneumovax)

---

wall configuration; and 3) evaluation of respiratory effort. If possible, patients should be positioned upright, with their arms resting at their sides.[3] Inspection usually begins during the interview process.[2]

Tongue and Sublingual Area

The tongue and sublingual area should be observed for a blue, gray, or dark purple tint or discoloration indicating the presence of central cyanosis. *Central cyanosis* is a sign of hypoxemia, or inadequate oxygenation of the blood, and it is considered to be a life-threatening condition. It occurs when the amount of reduced hemoglobin (unsaturated hemoglobin) exceeds 5 g/dL. The fingers and toes may also appear discolored, an indication of the presence of peripheral cyanosis.[8]

Chest Wall Configuration

Assessment of chest wall configuration incorporates observations about the size and shape of the patient's chest. Normally, the ratio of anteroposterior diameter to lateral diameter ranges from 1:2 to 5:7 (Fig. 18-1A).[2,4,5] An increase in the anteroposterior diameter is suggestive of chronic obstructive pulmonary disease (COPD).[2,4,5] The shape of the chest should be inspected for any structural deviations. Some of the more frequently seen abnormalities are pectus excavatum, pectus carinatum, barrel chest, and spinal deformities. In *pectus excavatum* (funnel chest), the sternum and lower ribs are displaced posteriorly, creating a funnel or pit-shaped depression in the chest. This causes a decrease in the anteroposterior diameter of the chest and may interfere with respiratory function. In *pectus carinatum* (pigeon breast), the sternum projects forward, causing an increase in the anteroposterior diameter of the chest. The *barrel chest* also results in an increase in anteroposterior diameter of the chest and is characterized by displacement of the sternum forward and the ribs outward (see Fig. 18-1B). Spinal

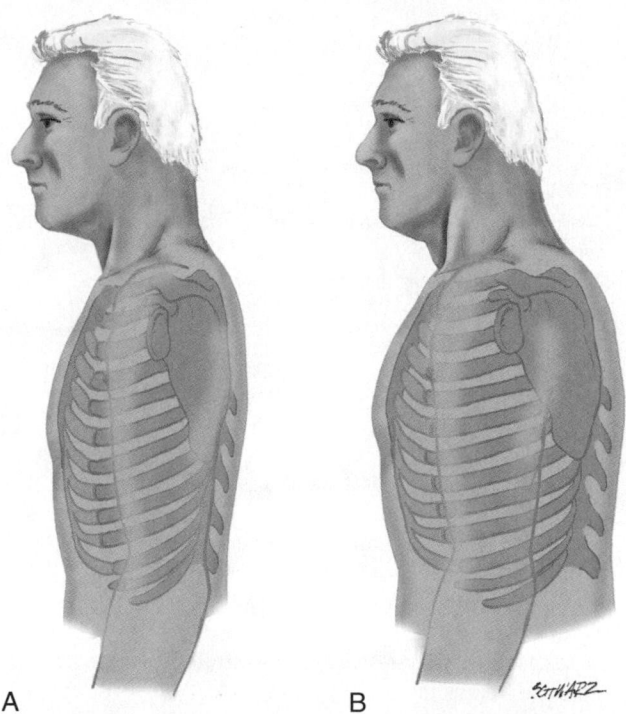

FIGURE 18-1   Chest Wall Configuration. *A*, Normal configuration. *B*, Increased anteroposterior diameter. Notice the contrast in the angle of the slope of the ribs. (From Kacmarek RM, et al, eds. *Egan's Fundamentals of Respiratory Care*. 10th ed. St. Louis: Mosby; 2013.)

deformities such as *kyphosis*, *lordosis*, and *scoliosis* also may be present and can interfere with respiratory function.[9]

Respiratory Effort

Evaluation of respiratory effort incorporates observations on the rate, rhythm, symmetry, and quality of ventilatory

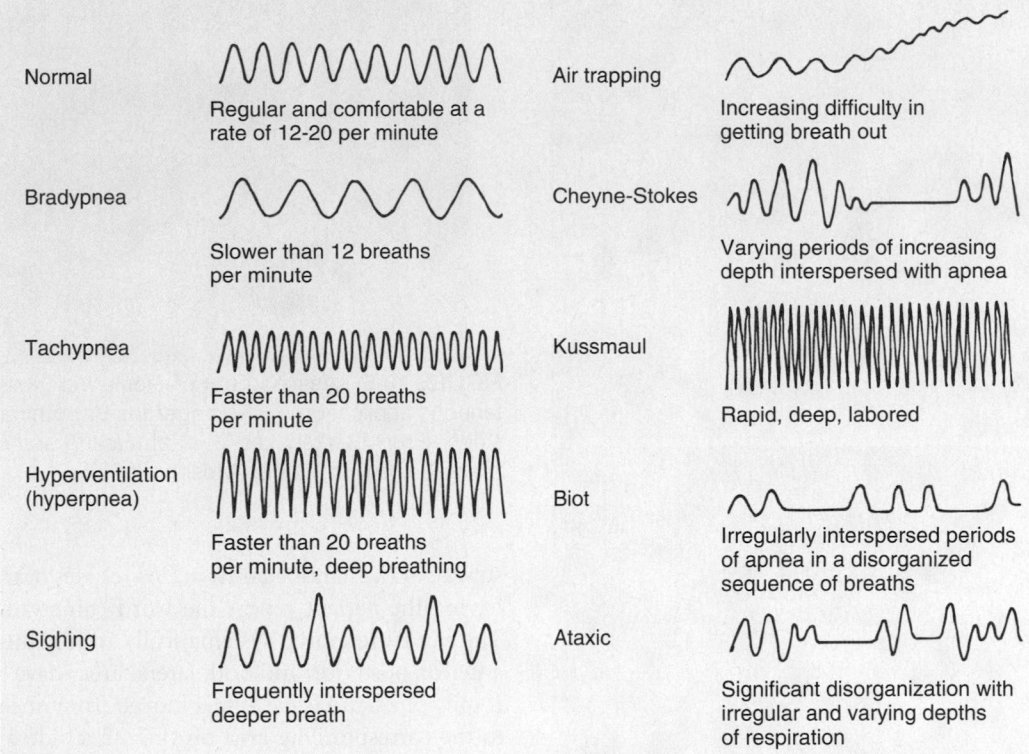

Normal	Regular and comfortable at a rate of 12-20 per minute	Air trapping	Increasing difficulty in getting breath out
Bradypnea	Slower than 12 breaths per minute	Cheyne-Stokes	Varying periods of increasing depth interspersed with apnea
Tachypnea	Faster than 20 breaths per minute	Kussmaul	Rapid, deep, labored
Hyperventilation (hyperpnea)	Faster than 20 breaths per minute, deep breathing	Biot	Irregularly interspersed periods of apnea in a disorganized sequence of breaths
Sighing	Frequently interspersed deeper breath	Ataxic	Significant disorganization with irregular and varying depths of respiration

FIGURE 18-2 **Patterns of Respiration.** (From Seidel HM, et al. *Mosby's Guide to Physical Examination.* 7th ed. St. Louis: Mosby; 2011.)

movements.[2] Normal breathing at rest is effortless and regular and occurs at a rate of 12 to 20 breaths per minute.[3] There are a number of abnormal respiratory patterns (Fig. 18-2). Some of the more commonly seen patterns in patients with pulmonary dysfunction are tachypnea, hyperventilation, and air trapping. *Tachypnea* is manifested by an increase in the rate and decrease in the depth of ventilation. *Hyperventilation* is manifested by an increase in the rate and depth of ventilation. Patients with COPD often experience obstructive breathing, or *air trapping*. As the patient breathes, air becomes trapped in the lungs and ventilations become progressively more shallow until the patient actively and forcefully exhales.[10]

Additional Assessment Areas

Other areas of focus for the careful assessment are patient position, active effort to breathe, use of accessory muscles, presence of intercostal retractions, unequal movement of the chest wall, flaring of nares, and pausing midsentence to take a breath.[2,4,5] The presence of other iatrogenic features, such as chest tubes, central venous lines, artificial airways, and nasogastric tubes, should be identified because they may affect assessment findings.

Palpation

Palpation of the patient should focus on three aspects: 1) confirmation of the position of the trachea; 2) assessment of thoracic expansion; and 3) evaluation of fremitus. The thorax should be assessed for any areas of tenderness, lumps, or bony deformities. The anterior, posterior, and lateral areas of the chest should be evaluated in a systematic fashion.[2]

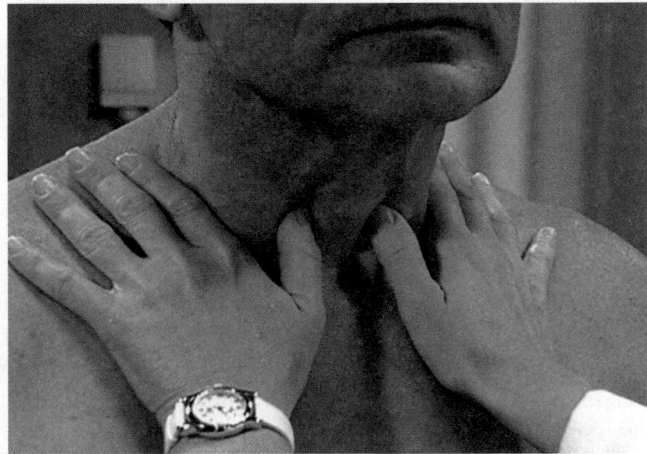

FIGURE 18-3 **Assessment of the Position of the Trachea.** (From Seidel HM, et al. *Mosby's Guide to Physical Examination.* 6th ed. St. Louis: Mosby; 2006.)

Position of the Trachea

Confirmation of the position of the trachea is performed to verify that the trachea is midline. It is assessed by placing the fingers in the suprasternal notch and moving upward (Fig. 18-3).[10] Deviation of the trachea to either side may indicate a pneumothorax, unilateral pneumonia, diffuse pulmonary fibrosis, a large pleural effusion, or severe atelectasis. With atelectasis, the trachea shifts to the same side as the problem, and with pneumothorax, the trachea shifts to the opposite side of the problem.[9]

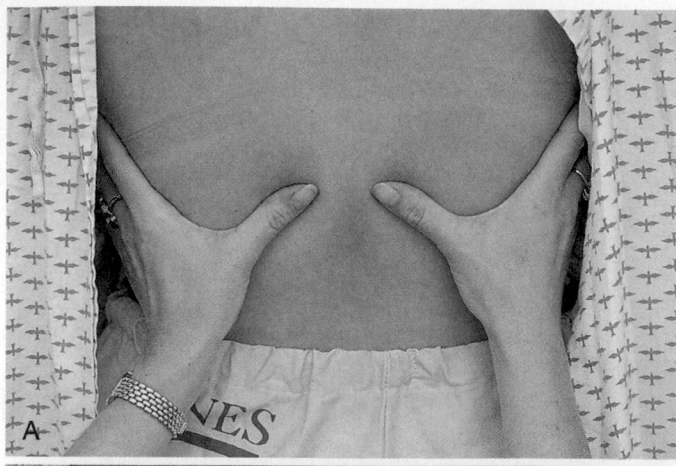

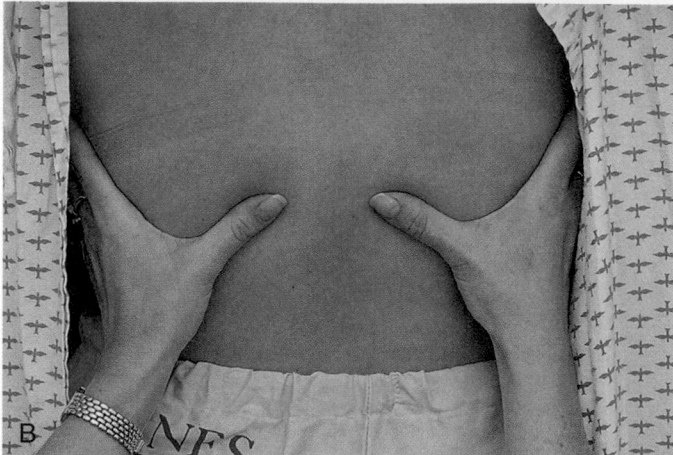

FIGURE 18-4 Assessment of Thoracic Expansion. *A,* Position of hands for palpation of posterior thorax excursion. *B,* As patient inhales, movement of chest excursion separates nurse's thumbs. (From Perry AG, Potter PA. *Clinical Nursing Skills and Techniques.* 7th ed. St. Louis: Mosby; 2010.)

Thoracic Expansion

Assessment of thoracic expansion involves measuring the degree and symmetry of respiratory movement. It is assessed by placing the hands on the anterolateral chest with the thumbs extended along the costal margin, pointing to the xiphoid process, or on the posterolateral chest with the thumbs on either side of the spine at the level of the 10th rib (Fig. 18-4). The patient is instructed to take a few normal breaths and then a few deep breaths. Chest movement is assessed for equality, which signifies symmetry of thoracic expansion.[3,9,10] Asymmetry is an abnormal finding that can occur with pneumothorax, pneumonia, or other disorders that interfere with lung inflation. The degree of chest movement is felt to ascertain the extent of lung expansion. The thumbs should separate 3 to 5 cm during deep inspiration.[5,10] Lung expansion of a hyperinflated chest is less than that of a normal one.[5,10]

Tactile Fremitus

Assessment of tactile fremitus is performed to identify, describe, and localize any areas of increased or decreased afremitus. Fremitus refers to the palpable vibrations felt through the chest wall when the patient speaks. It is assessed by placing the palmar

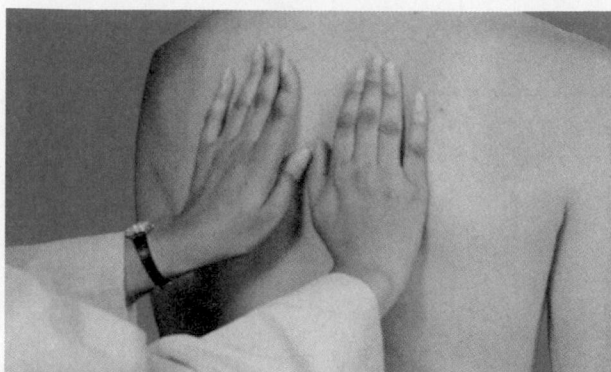

FIGURE 18-5 Assessment of tactile fremitus, showing simultaneous application of the fingertips of both hands to compare sides. (From Barkauskas V, et al. *Health and Physical Assessment.* 3rd ed. St. Louis: Mosby; 2002.)

surface of the hands against opposite sides of the chest wall and having the patient repeat the word "ninety-nine" (Fig. 18-5). The hands are moved systematically around the thorax until the anterior, posterior, and both lateral areas have been assessed.[9,10] If only one hand is used, it is moved from one side of the chest to the corresponding area on the other side of the chest until all areas have been assessed.[10]

Fremitus varies from patient to patient and depends on the pitch and intensity of the voice. Fremitus is described as normal, decreased, or increased. With normal fremitus, vibrations can be felt over the trachea but are barely palpable over the periphery.[2] With decreased fremitus, there is interference with the transmission of vibrations. Examples of disorders that decrease fremitus include pleural effusion, pneumothorax, bronchial obstruction, pleural thickening, and emphysema. With increased fremitus, there is an increase in the transmission of vibrations. Examples of disorders that increase fremitus include pneumonia, lung cancer, and pulmonary fibrosis.[5]

Percussion

Percussion of the patient should focus on two concerns: evaluation of the underlying lung structure and assessment of diaphragmatic excursion. Although the technique is not used often, percussion is a useful method for confirming suspected abnormalities.

Underlying Lung Structure

Evaluation of the underlying lung structure is performed to estimate the amounts of air, liquid, or solid material present. It is performed by placing the middle finger of the nondominant hand on the chest wall. The distal portion, between the last joint and the nail bed, is then struck with the middle finger of the dominant hand. The hands are moved systematically and side to side around the thorax to compare similar areas until the anterior, posterior, and both lateral areas have been assessed (Fig. 18-6). Five tones can be elicited: resonance, hyperresonance, tympany, dullness, and flatness. These tones are distinguished by differences in intensity, pitch, duration, and quality. Table 18-1 describes the different percussion tones and their associated conditions.[3,9]

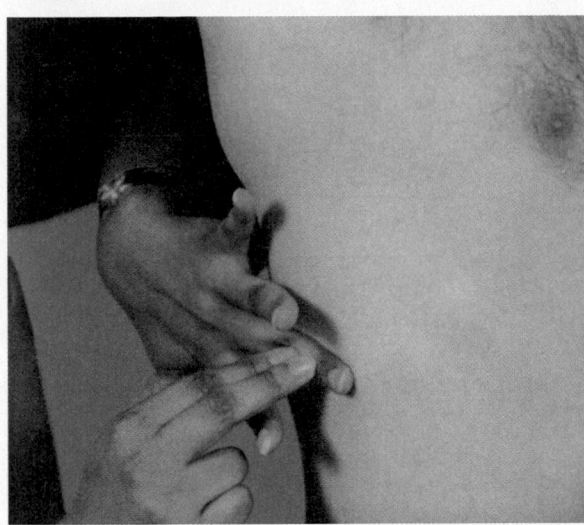

FIGURE 18-6 Assessment of Underlying Lung Structures. (From Barkauskas V, et al. *Health and Physical Assessment*. 3rd ed. St. Louis: Mosby; 2002.)

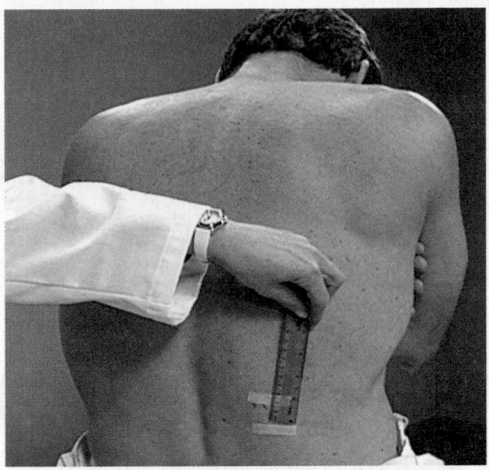

FIGURE 18-7 Measuring Diaphragmatic Excursion. Excursion distance is usually 3 to 5 cm. (From Seidel HM, et al. *Mosby's Guide to Physical Examination*. 7th ed. St. Louis: Mosby; 2011.)

TABLE 18-1	PERCUSSION TONES AND THEIR ASSOCIATED CONDITIONS	
TONE	**DESCRIPTION**	**CONDITION**
Resonance	Intensity: loud Pitch: low Duration: long Quality: hollow	Normal lung Bronchitis
Hyperresonance	Intensity: very loud Pitch: very low Duration: long Quality: booming	Asthma Emphysema Pneumothorax
Tympany	Intensity: loud Pitch: musical Duration: medium Quality: drumlike	Large pneumothorax Emphysematous blebs
Dullness	Intensity: medium Pitch: medium-high Duration: medium Quality: thudlike	Atelectasis Pleural effusion Pulmonary edema Pneumonia Lung mass
Flatness	Intensity: soft Pitch: high Duration: short Quality: extremely dull	Massive atelectasis Pneumonectomy

Diaphragmatic Excursion

Assessment of diaphragmatic excursion is accomplished by measuring the difference in the level of the diaphragm on inspiration and expiration. It is performed by instructing the patient to inhale and hold the breath. The posterior chest is percussed downward, over the intercostal spaces, until the dull sound produced by the diaphragm is heard. The spot is marked. The patient is then instructed to take a few breaths in and out, exhale completely, and then hold his or her breath. The posterior chest is percussed again, and the new area of dullness over the

diaphragm is located and marked. The difference between the two spots is identified and measured (Fig. 18-7). Normal diaphragmatic excursion is 3 to 5 cm.[10] It is decreased in disorders or conditions such as ascites, pregnancy, hepatomegaly, and emphysema. It is increased in pleural effusion or disorders that elevate the diaphragm, such as atelectasis or paralysis.[9]

Auscultation

Auscultation of the patient should focus on three areas: 1) evaluation of normal breath sounds; 2) identification of abnormal breath sounds; and 3) assessment of voice sounds. Auscultation requires a quiet environment, proper positioning of the patient, and a bare chest.[11] Breath sounds are best heard with the patient in the upright position.[5]

Normal Breath Sounds

Evaluation of normal breath sounds is performed to assess air movement through the pulmonary system and to identify the presence of abnormal sounds. It is performed by placing the diaphragm of the stethoscope against the chest wall and instructing the patient to breathe in and out slowly with his or her mouth open.[2] The inspiratory and expiratory phases should be assessed. Auscultation should be done in a systematic sequence: side-to-side, top-to-bottom, posteriorly, laterally, and anteriorly (Fig. 18-8).[5]

Normal breath sounds are different, depending on their location. There are three categories: vesicular, bronchovesicular, and bronchial. Figure 18-9 describes the characteristics of normal breath sounds and their associated conditions.[2,5,11]

Abnormal Breath Sounds

Identification of abnormal breath sounds occurs after the normal breath sounds have been clearly delineated. There are three categories of abnormal breath sounds: absent or diminished breath sounds, displaced bronchial breath sounds, and adventitious breath sounds. Table 18-2 describes the various abnormal pulmonary breath sounds and their associated conditions.[2,5,11]

An *absent* or *diminished breath sound* indicates that there is little or no airflow to a particular portion of the lung (a small

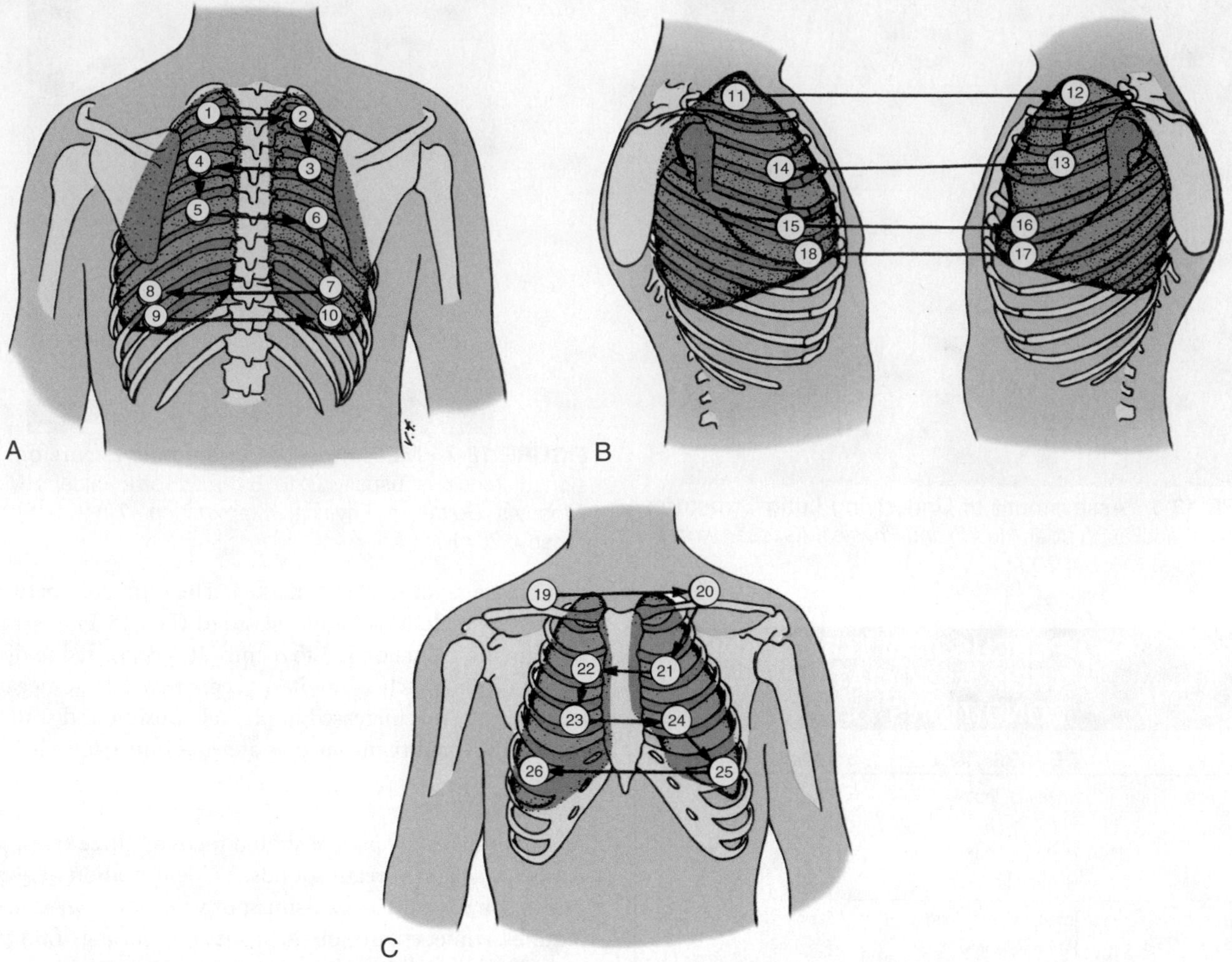

FIGURE 18-8 **Auscultation Sequence.** *A,* Posterior. *B,* Lateral. *C,* Anterior. (From Perry AG, Potter PA. *Clinical Nursing Skills and Techniques.* 7th ed. St. Louis: Mosby; 2010.)

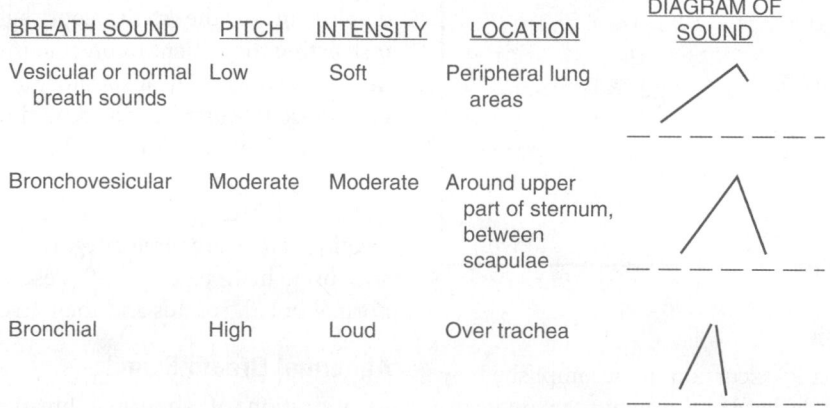

BREATH SOUND	PITCH	INTENSITY	LOCATION	DIAGRAM OF SOUND
Vesicular or normal breath sounds	Low	Soft	Peripheral lung areas	
Bronchovesicular	Moderate	Moderate	Around upper part of sternum, between scapulae	
Bronchial	High	Loud	Over trachea	

FIGURE 18-9 **Characteristics of Normal Breath Sounds.** (From Kacmarek RM, Diamas S. *The Essentials of Respiratory Care.* 4th ed. St. Louis: Elsevier; 2005.)

TABLE 18-2 ABNORMAL BREATH SOUNDS AND THEIR ASSOCIATED CONDITIONS

ABNORMAL SOUND	DESCRIPTION	CONDITION
Absent breath sounds	No airflow to particular portion of lung	Pneumothorax Pneumonectomy Emphysematous blebs Pleural effusion Lung mass Massive atelectasis Complete airway obstruction
Diminished breath sounds	Little airflow to particular portion of lung	Emphysema Pleural effusion Pleurisy Atelectasis Pulmonary fibrosis
Displaced bronchial sounds	Bronchial sounds heard in peripheral lung fields	Atelectasis with secretions Lung mass with exudates Pneumonia Pleural effusion Pulmonary edema
Crackles (rales)	Short, discrete popping or crackling sounds	Pulmonary edema Pneumonia Pulmonary fibrosis Atelectasis Bronchiectasis
Rhonchi	Coarse, rumbling, low-pitched sounds	Pneumonia Asthma Bronchitis Bronchospasm
Wheezes	High-pitched, squeaking, whistling sounds	Asthma Bronchospasm
Pleural friction rub	Creaking, leathery, loud, dry, coarse sounds	Pleural effusion Pleurisy

segment or an entire lung).[11] *Displaced bronchial breath sounds* are normal bronchial sounds heard in the peripheral lung fields instead of over the trachea. This condition is usually indicative of fluid or exudate in the alveoli.[11] *Adventitious breath sounds* are extra or added sounds heard in addition to the other sounds previously discussed. They are classified as crackles, rhonchi, wheezes, and friction rubs.

Crackles, also called *rales*, are short, discrete popping or crackling sounds produced by fluid in the small airways or alveoli or by the snapping open of collapsed airways during inspiration. They can be heard on inspiration and expiration and may clear with coughing.[2,5,11] Crackles can be further classified as fine, medium, or coarse, depending on pitch.[3,5]

Rhonchi are coarse, rumbling, low-pitched sounds produced by airflow over secretions in the larger airways or narrowing of the large airways. They are heard mainly on expiration and sometimes can be cleared with coughing. Rhonchi can be further classified as bubbling, gurgling, or sonorous, depending on the characteristics of the sound.[11]

Wheezes are high-pitched, squeaking, whistling sounds produced by airflow through narrowed small airways. They are heard mainly on expiration but may be heard throughout the ventilatory cycle. Depending on their severity, wheezes can be further classified as mild, moderate, or severe.[11]

A *pleural friction rub* is a creaking, leathery, loud, dry, coarse sound produced by irritated pleural surfaces rubbing together. It is usually heard best in the lower anterolateral chest area during inspiration and expiration. Pleural friction rubs are caused by inflammation of the pleura.[2,5]

Voice Sounds

Assessment of voice sounds is particularly useful in detecting lung consolidation or lung compression. Three abnormal types of voice sounds are bronchophony, whispering pectoriloquy, and egophony.

Bronchophony describes a condition in which the spoken voice is heard on auscultation with higher intensity and clarity than usual. Normally, the spoken word is muffled when heard through the stethoscope. It is assessed by placing the diaphragm of the stethoscope against the posterior side of the patient's chest and instructing the patient to say "ninety-nine." Bronchophony is present when the sound heard is clear, distinct, and loud.

Whispering pectoriloquy describes a condition of unusually clear transmission of the whispered voice on auscultation. Normally, the whispered word is unintelligible when heard through the stethoscope. It is assessed by placing the stethoscope against the posterior side of the patient's chest and instructing the patient to whisper "one, two, three." Whispering pectoriloquy is present when the sound heard is clear and distinct.

Egophony describes a condition in which the voice sounds increase in intensity and develop a nasal bleating quality on auscultation. It is assessed by placing the stethoscope against the posterior side of the patient's chest and instructing the patient to say "e-e-e." Egophony is present when the "e" sound changes to an "a" sound.[2,4,11]

ASSESSMENT FINDINGS OF COMMON DISORDERS

Table 18-3 presents a variety of common pulmonary disorders and their associated assessment findings.

TABLE 18-3 ASSESSMENT FINDINGS FREQUENTLY ASSOCIATED WITH COMMON LUNG CONDITIONS

CONDITION*	BREATH SOUNDS	DESCRIPTION
NORMAL LUNG 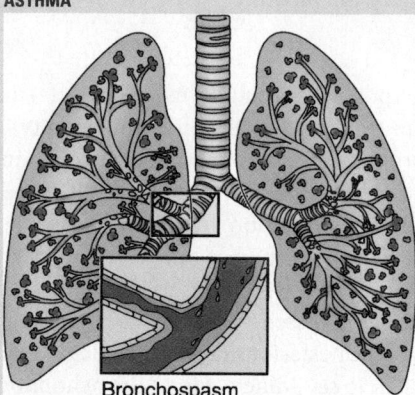	INSPIRATION > EXPIRATION Pitch: Low Intensity: Soft Adventitious sounds: None 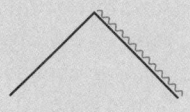	Tracheobronchial tree and alveoli are clear; pleurae are thin and close together; chest wall is mobile.
ASTHMA Bronchospasm	INSPIRATION = EXPIRATION Pitch: moderate Intensity: soft Adventitious sounds: expiratory sibilant wheezes	Asthma is characterized by intermittent episodes of airway obstruction caused by bronchospasm, excessive bronchial secretion, or edema of bronchial mucosa; resultant airway resistance, especially during expiration, produces symptoms of wheezing, dyspnea, and chest tightness.
ATELECTASIS 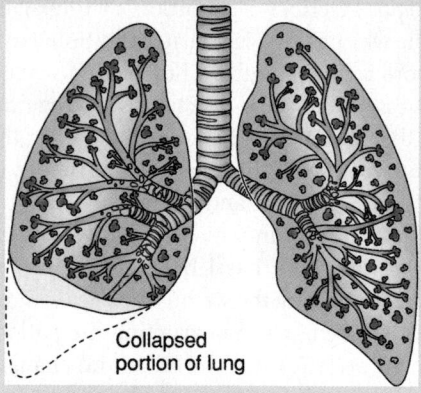 Collapsed portion of lung	INSPIRATION > EXPIRATION *Over empty area:* Pitch: Low or absent Intensity: Soft or absent Adventitious sounds: fine, high-pitched crackles over terminal portion of inspiration if bronchus patent *Over consolidated lung:* Bronchial breath sounds, crackles, and wheezes 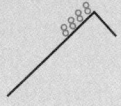	Atelectasis is collapse of alveolar lung tissue, and findings reflect presence of a small, airless lung; this condition is caused by complete obstruction of a draining bronchus by a tumor, thick secretions, or an aspirated foreign body, or by compression of lung.
BRONCHIECTASIS 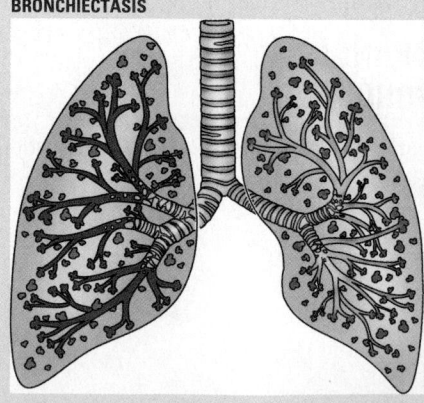	INSPIRATION > EXPIRATION Pitch: Low Intensity: Soft Adventitious sounds: Crackles (sometimes disappear after) 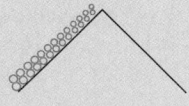	Bronchiectasis is abnormal dilation of bronchi or bronchioles, or both (coughing).

INSPECTION	PALPATION	PERCUSSION	AUSCULTATION
Good, symmetric rib and diaphragmatic movement Anteroposterior diameter < transverse diameter Respirations 12-20 breaths/min and regular	Trachea: Midline Expansion: Adequate, symmetric Tactile fremitus: Moderate and symmetric No lesions or tenderness	Resonant Diaphragmatic excursion: 3-5 cm	Breath sounds: Vesicular Vocal resonance: Muffled Adventitious sounds: None, except for a few transient crackles at bases
Cyanosis Air trapping with audible wheezing Use of accessory muscles of respiration Increased respiratory rate	Tactile fremitus: Decreased	Hyperresonant	Breath sounds: Distant Vocal resonance: Decreased Adventitious sounds: Wheezes
Less chest motion on affected side Affected side retracted, with ribs appearing close together Cough Rapid, shallow breathing	Trachea: Shifted to affected side Expansion: Decreased on affected side Tactile fremitus: Decreased or absent	Dull to flat over collapsed lung Hyperresonant over remainder of affected hemithorax	Breath sounds: Decreased or absent Vocal resonance: Varies in intensity, usually reduced or absent in affected area Adventitious sounds: Fine, high-pitched crackles may be heard over terminal portion of inspiration
If mild, respirations are normal If severe, tachypnea Less expansion of affected side Cough with purulent sputum	Trachea: Midline or deviated toward affected side Expansion: Decreased on affected side Tactile fremitus: Increased	Resonant or dull	Breath sounds: Usually vesicular Vocal resonance: Usually muffled Adventitious sounds: Crackles

Continued

TABLE 18-3 ASSESSMENT FINDINGS FREQUENTLY ASSOCIATED WITH COMMON LUNG CONDITIONS—cont'd

CONDITION*	BREATH SOUNDS	DESCRIPTION
BRONCHITIS, ACUTE 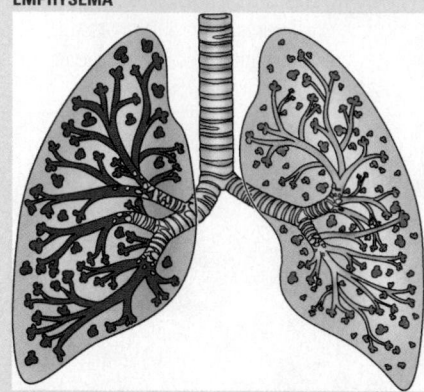	INSPIRATION ≥ EXPIRATION Pitch: Low Intensity: Soft Adventitious sounds: Localized crackles, expiratory sibilant wheezes 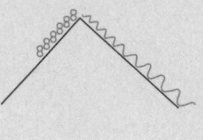	Acute bronchitis is inflammation of bronchial tree characterized by partial bronchial obstruction and secretions or constrictions; it results in abnormally deflated portions of lung.
EMPHYSEMA 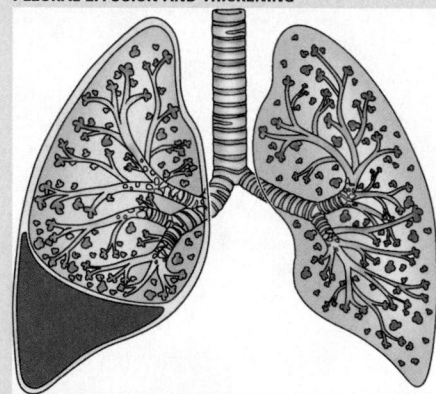	INSPIRATION = EXPIRATION Pitch: Low to very low Intensity: Soft to very soft Adventitious sounds: Occasional rhonchi and/or sibilant wheezes; fine inspiratory crackles 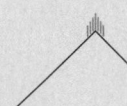	Emphysema is a permanent hyperinflation of lung beyond terminal bronchioles, with destruction of alveolar walls; airway resistance is increased, especially on expiration.
PLEURAL EFFUSION AND THICKENING 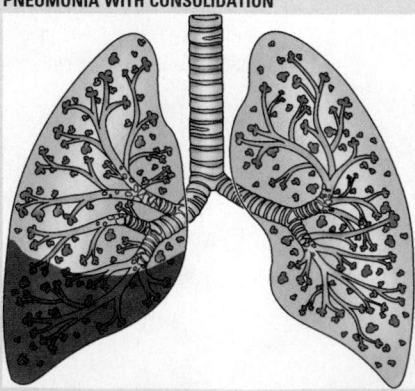	INSPIRATION > EXPIRATION Pitch: Low to absent Intensity: Soft to absent Adventitious sounds: Occasional pleural friction rub 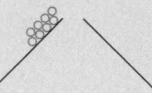	Pleural effusion is a collection of fluid in pleural space; if pleural effusion is prolonged, fibrous tissue may also accumulate in pleural space; clinical picture depends on amount of fluid or fibrosis present and rapidity of development; fluid tends to gravitate to most dependent areas of thorax, and adjacent lung is compressed.
PNEUMONIA WITH CONSOLIDATION	INSPIRATION = EXPIRATION Pitch: High Intensity: Loud Adventitious sounds: Inspiratory crackles in terminal third of inspiration	Pneumonia with consolidation occurs when alveolar air is replaced by fluid or tissue; physical findings depend on amount of parenchymal tissue involved.

INSPECTION	PALPATION	PERCUSSION	AUSCULTATION
If severe, tachypnea and cyanosis Rasping cough with mucoid sputum	Tactile fremitus: Normal to increased	Resonant	Breath sounds: Vesicular Vocal resonance: Moderate Adventitious sounds: Localized crackles, sibilant wheezes
Dyspnea with exertion Barrel chest Tachypnea Use of accessory muscles of respiration	Expansion: Limited Tactile fremitus: Decreased	Resonant to hyperresonant Diaphragmatic excursion: Decreased	Breath sounds: Decreased intensity; often prolonged expiration Vocal resonance: Muffled or decreased Adventitious sounds: Occasional wheezes; often fine crackles in late inspiration
Tachypnea Decreased in definition of intercostal spaces on affected side Dyspnea	Trachea: Deviation toward normal side Expansion: Decreased on affected side Tactile fremitus: Decreased or absent	Dull to flat No diaphragmatic excursion on affected side	Breath sounds: Decreased or absent Vocal resonance: Muffled or absent; if fluid compresses lung, sounds may be bronchial over compression, and bronchophony, egophony, and whisper pectoriloquy may be present Adventitious sounds: Pleural friction rub sometimes present
Tachypnea Guarding and less motion on affected side	Expansion: Limited on affected side Tactile fremitus: Usually increased, but may be weak if a bronchus leading to affected area is plugged	Dull to flat	Breath sounds: Increased in intensity; bronchovesicular or bronchial breath sounds over affected area Vocal resonance: Increased bronchophony, egophony, whisper pectoriloquy present Adventitious sounds: Inspiratory crackles terminal third of inspiration

Continued

TABLE 18-3 ASSESSMENT FINDINGS FREQUENTLY ASSOCIATED WITH COMMON LUNG CONDITIONS—cont'd

CONDITION*	BREATH SOUNDS	DESCRIPTION
PNEUMOTHORAX 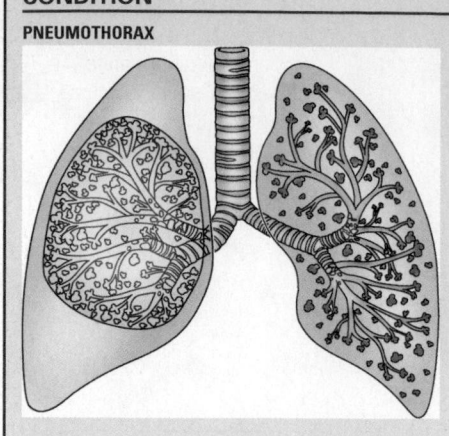	INSPIRATION > EXPIRATION Pitch: Low to absent Intensity: Soft to absent Adventitious sounds: None	Pneumothorax implies air in pleural space: 1. Closed type: Air in pleural space does not communicate with air in lung 2. Open type: Air in pleural space freely communicates with air in lung; air in pleural space is atmospheric 3. Tension type: Air in pleural space communicates with air in lungs only on inspiration; air pressure in pleural space is greater than atmospheric pressure Physical signs depend on degree of lung collapse and presence or absence of pleural effusion.
PULMONARY FIBROSIS, DIFFUSE 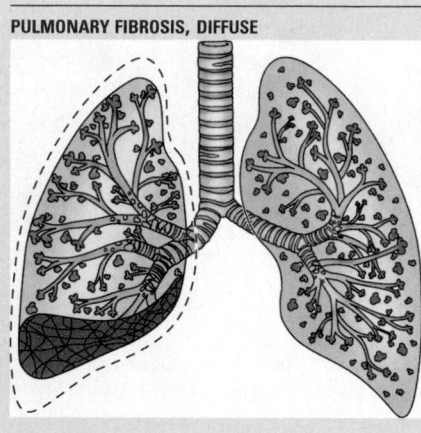	INSPIRATION = EXPIRATION Pitch: Low to absent Intensity: Soft to absent Adventitious sounds: Crackles 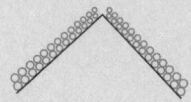	Pulmonary fibrosis is presence of excessive amount of connective tissue in lungs; consequently, lungs are smaller than normal and less compliant, lower lobes are usually affected most.

From Barkauskas V, et al. *Health and Physical Assessment*. 3rd ed. St. Louis: Mosby; 2002.
*Note: Although some disease conditions are bilateral, one diseased lung and one normal lung are illustrated for each condition to provide contrast. When an abnormality is illustrated, the pathologic condition is illustrated on the left side and the normal lung is on the right side of the illustration.

SUMMARY

History
- A review of the patient's current illness and symptoms, including presence or absence of shortness of breath, chest pain, and cough, is an essential part of the patient's medical history.
- As the patient's condition permits, additional information regarding his or her general respiratory status, general health status, and family and social background, including tobacco use, work environment, and home environment, should be obtained.

Clinical Assessment
- Inspection should focus on the tongue and sublingual area, chest wall configuration, and respiratory effort.

- Palpation should focus on position of the trachea, thoracic expansion, and fremitus (normal, decreased, or increased).
- Percussion (when performed) should focus on underlying lung structure and diaphragmatic excursion.
- Auscultation should focus on the presence or absence of normal breath sounds (vesicular, bronchovesicular, and bronchial), abnormal breath sounds (diminished or absent breath sounds, displaced bronchial breath sounds, and adventitious breath sounds), and voice sounds (bronchophony, whispering pectoriloquy, and egophony).
- Adventitious breath sounds are classified as crackles, rhonchi, wheezes, and friction rubs.
- Auscultation is done in a systematic fashion, side-to-side, top-to-bottom, posteriorly, laterally, and anteriorly.

INSPECTION	PALPATION	PERCUSSION	AUSCULTATION
Restricted lung expansion on affected side If large, tachypnea Bulging in intercostal spaces on affected side Cyanosis	Trachea: Deviated toward normal side Expansion: Decreased on affected side Tactile fremitus: Absent	Hyperresonant Decreased diaphragmatic excursion	Breath sounds: Usually decreased or absent; if open pneumothorax, have an amorphous quality Vocal resonance: Decreased or absent Adventitious sounds: None
Dyspnea on exertion Tachypnea Thoracic expansion diminished Cyanosis	Trachea: Deviated to most affected side	Resonant to dull	Breath sounds: Reduced or absent, bronchovesicular or bronchial Vocal resonance: Increased, whisper pectoriloquy may be present Adventitious sounds: Crackles on inspiration

REFERENCES

1. Baid H. The process of conducting a physical assessment: a nursing perspective. *Br J Nurs.* 2006;15:710.
2. Simpson H. Respiratory assessment. *Br J Nurs.* 2006;15:484.
3. Reinke LF. Respiratory assessment. In: Geiger-Bronksy M, Wilson DJ, eds. *Respiratory Nursing: A Core Curriculum.* New York: Springer; 2008.
4. Finesilver C. Pulmonary assessment: what you need to know. *Prog Cardiovasc Nurs.* 2003;18:83.
5. Kallet RH. Bedside assessment of the patient. In: Kacmarek RM, et al, eds. *Egan's Fundamentals of Respiratory Care.* 10th ed. St. Louis: Mosby; 2013.
6. Stiesmeyer JK. A four-step approach to pulmonary assessment. *Am J Nurs.* 1993;93(8):22.
7. Fitzgerald MA. The physical exam. *RN.* 1991;54(11):34.
8. Higginson R, Jones B. Respiratory assessment in critically ill patients: airway and breathing. *Br J Nurs.* 2009;18:456.
9. Schraufnagel DE, Murray JF. History and physical examination. In: Mason RJ, et al, eds. *Murray and Nadel's Textbook of Respiratory Medicine.* 5th ed. Philadelphia: Elsevier; 2010.
10. Seidel HM, et al. *Mosby's Guide to Physical Examination.* 7th ed. St. Louis: Mosby; 2011.
11. Wilkins RL, et al. *Fundamentals of Lung and Heart Sounds.* 3rd ed. St. Louis: Mosby; 2004.

Pulmonary Diagnostic Procedures

Jeanne M. Maiden

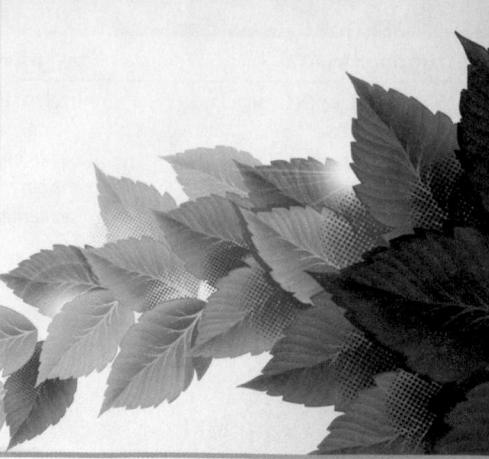

⊖volve WEBSITE

http://evolve.elsevier.com/Urden/criticalcare/

Evolve features:

- NCLEX Review Questions
- CCRN Review Questions
- PCCN Review Questions
- Mosby's Nursing Skills Procedures
- Animations
- Video Clips
- Glossary

To complete the assessment of the critically ill pulmonary patient, a review of the patient's laboratory studies and diagnostic tests is performed. Although many procedures exist for diagnosing pulmonary disease, their application in the critically ill patient is limited. Only studies and tests that are used in the critical care setting are presented here. Bedside monitoring devices are also discussed.

LABORATORY STUDIES

Arterial Blood Gases

Interpretation of arterial blood gas (ABG) levels can be difficult, especially if the nurse is under pressure to do it quickly and accurately. One method that can help ensure accuracy when analyzing ABG levels is to follow the same steps of interpretation each time. A specific method to be used each time that blood gas values must be interpreted is presented here (Box 19-1).

Steps for Interpretation of Blood Gas Levels

Step 1. Look at the Pao_2 level, and answer this question: Does the Pao_2 show hypoxemia? The Pao_2 is a measure of the partial pressure (P) of oxygen dissolved in arterial (a) blood plasma. Sometimes, Pao_2 is shortened to Po_2. It is reported in millimeters of mercury (mm Hg). Pao_2 reflects 3% of total oxygen in the blood.[1]

The normal range of Pao_2 values for persons breathing room air at sea level is 80 to 100 mm Hg. However, the normal range is age dependent for infants and for persons 60 years old or older. The normal level for infants breathing room air is between 50 and 70 mm Hg.[2] The normal level for persons 60 years old or older decreases with age as changes occur in the ventilation/perfusion (V/Q) matching in the aging lung.[1,3] The correct Pao_2 for older persons can be ascertained as follows: 80 mm Hg (the lowest normal value) minus 1 mm Hg for every year of age above 60 years. Using this formula, a 65-year-old individual can have a Pao_2 as low as 75 mm Hg (80 mm Hg − 5 mm Hg = 75 mm Hg) and still be within the normal range. An acceptable range for an 80-year-old person (20 years older than 60 years) is 60 mm Hg (80 mm Hg − 20 mm Hg = 60 mm Hg).

At any age, a Pao_2 lower than 40 mm Hg represents a life-threatening situation that necessitates immediate action.[1] A Pao_2 value less than the predicted lowest value indicates hypoxemia, which means that a lower-than-normal amount of oxygen is dissolved in plasma.[1]

The Pao_2 level should be analyzed before those of other blood gas components. A Pao_2 of less than 40 mm Hg severely compromises tissue oxygenation and calls for the immediate administration of supplemental oxygen or mechanical ventilation, or both. The test results for the Pao_2 level can be analyzed quickly. If the Pao_2 level is more than the lowest value for the patient's age, it is normal.

Step 2. Look at the pH level, and answer this question: Is the pH on the acid or alkaline side of 7.40? The pH is the hydrogen ion (H^+) concentration of plasma. Calculation of pH is accomplished by using the partial pressure of carbon dioxide ($Paco_2$) and the plasma bicarbonate level (HCO_3^-). The formula used is the Henderson-Hasselbalch equation (see Appendix B).[4]

The normal pH of arterial blood is 7.35 to 7.45, and the mean is 7.40. If the pH level is less than 7.40, it is on the acid

<table>
<tr><td colspan="2">

BOX 19-1 STEPS FOR INTERPRETATION OF BLOOD GAS LEVELS

Step 1
Look at the PaO_2 level, and answer this question: Does the PaO_2 level show hypoxemia?

Step 2
Look at the pH level, and answer this question: Is the pH level on the acid or alkaline side of 7.40?

Step 3
Look at the $PaCO_2$ level, and answer this question: Does the $PaCO_2$ level show respiratory acidosis, alkalosis, or normalcy?

Step 4
Look at the HCO_3^- level, and answer this question: Does the HCO_3^- level show metabolic acidosis, alkalosis, or normalcy?

Step 5
Look again at the pH level, and answer this question: Does the pH show a compensated or an uncompensated condition?

</td></tr>
</table>

BOX 19-2 UNCOMPENSATED ARTERIAL BLOOD GAS VALUES

EXAMPLE 1		**EXAMPLE 2**	
PaO_2:	90 mm Hg	PaO_2:	90 mm Hg
pH:	7.25	pH:	7.25
$PaCO_2$:	50 mm Hg	$PaCO_2$:	40 mm Hg
HCO_3^-:	22 mEq/L	HCO_3^-:	17 mEq/L

Interpretation: Uncompensated respiratory acidosis   *Interpretation:* Uncompensated metabolic acidosis

side of the mean. A pH level less than 7.35 is known as *acidemia*, and the overall condition is called *acidosis*. If the pH level is greater than 7.40, it is on the alkaline side of the mean. A pH level greater than 7.45 is known as *alkalemia*, and the overall condition is called *alkalosis*.[1,4,5]

Step 3. *Look at the $PaCO_2$ level, and answer this question: Does the $PaCO_2$ show respiratory acidosis, alkalosis, or normalcy?* The $PaCO_2$ is a measure of the partial pressure of carbon dioxide dissolved in arterial blood plasma, and it is reported in millimeters of mercury (mm Hg). It is the acid–base component that reflects the effectiveness of ventilation in relation to the metabolic rate.[4] In other words, the $PaCO_2$ value indicates whether the patient can ventilate well enough to rid the body of the carbon dioxide produced as a consequence of metabolism.

The normal range for $PaCO_2$ is 35 to 45 mm Hg. This range does not change as a person ages. A $PaCO_2$ value greater than 45 mm Hg defines *respiratory acidosis*, which is caused by alveolar hypoventilation. Hypoventilation can result from chronic obstructive pulmonary disease (COPD), oversedation, head trauma, anesthesia, drug overdose, neuromuscular disease, or hypoventilation with mechanical ventilation.[6]

Ventilatory failure results when the $PaCO_2$ level exceeds 50 mm Hg. Acute ventilatory failure occurs when the $PaCO_2$ level is greater than 50 mm Hg and the pH level is less than 7.30. It is referred to as *acute* because the pH is abnormal, not allowing enough time for the body to compensate by returning the pH to the normal range. Chronic ventilatory failure is defined as a $PaCO_2$ value greater than 50 mm Hg and a pH level greater than 7.30.[1,7]

A $PaCO_2$ value that is less than 35 mm Hg defines *respiratory alkalosis*, which is caused by alveolar hyperventilation. Hyperventilation can result from hypoxia, anxiety, pulmonary embolism, pregnancy, and hyperventilation with mechanical ventilation or as a compensatory mechanism for metabolic acidosis.[4]

Step 4. *Look at the HCO_3^- level, and answer this question: Does the HCO_3^- show metabolic acidosis, alkalosis, or normalcy?* Bicarbonate (HCO_3^-) is the acid–base component that reflects kidney function. The bicarbonate level is reduced or increased in the plasma by renal mechanisms. The normal range is 22 to 26 mEq/L.[4,5]

A bicarbonate level of less than 22 mEq/L defines *metabolic acidosis*, which can result from ketoacidosis, lactic acidosis, renal failure, or diarrhea. The cumulative effect is a gain of acids or a loss of base. A bicarbonate level that is greater than 26 mEq/L defines *metabolic alkalosis*, which can result from fluid loss from the upper gastrointestinal tract (vomiting or nasogastric suction), diuretic therapy, severe hypokalemia, alkali administration, or steroid therapy.[4,5,6]

Step 5. *Look again at the pH level, and answer this question: Does the pH show a compensated or an uncompensated condition?* If the pH level is abnormal (less than 7.35 or greater than 7.45), the $PaCO_2$ value or the HCO_3^- level, or both, will also be abnormal. This is an *uncompensated* condition because the body has not had enough time to return the pH to its normal range.[4,5,6,8] Box 19-2 provides two examples of uncompensated ABGs. If the pH level is within normal limits and the $PaCO_2$ value and the HCO_3^- level are abnormal, the condition is *compensated* because the body has had enough time to restore the pH to within its normal range.[4,5,6,8]

Differentiating the primary disorder from the compensatory response can be difficult. The primary disorder is the abnormality that caused the pH level to shift initially. It is determined according to the pH level; the primary disorder is considered to be the one on whichever side of 7.40 the pH level occurs.[4,8] Box 19-3 provides two examples of compensated ABGs. Partial compensation may be present and is evidenced by abnormal pH, $PaCO_2$, and HCO_3^- levels, indications that the body is attempting to return the pH to its normal range.[4,8]

Table 19-1 summarizes the changes in the acid–base components that accompany various acid–base disorders.[4,5,8] In addition to the parameters previously discussed, other factors must be considered when reviewing a patient's ABGs, including oxygen saturation, oxygen content, base excess and deficit, and anion gap analysis. Table 19-2 summarizes conditions that may potentiate acid–base abnormalities.[4,5,8]

Oxygen Saturation

Oxygen saturation is a measure of the amount of oxygen bound to hemoglobin, compared with hemoglobin's maximal capability for binding oxygen. It can be assessed as a component of the ABG (SaO_2) or can be measured noninvasively using a pulse

BOX 19-3 COMPENSATED ARTERIAL BLOOD GAS VALUES

EXAMPLE 1

Pao$_2$:	90 mm Hg
pH:	7.37
Paco$_2$:	60 mm Hg
HCO$_3$:	38 mEq/L

Interpretation: Compensated respiratory acidosis with metabolic alkalosis. (The acidosis is considered the main disorder and the alkalosis the compensatory response, because the pH is on the acid side of 7.40.)

EXAMPLE 2

Pao$_2$:	90 mm Hg
pH:	7.42
Paco$_2$:	48 mm Hg
HCO$_3$:	35 mEq/L

Interpretation: Compensated metabolic alkalosis with respiratory acidosis. (The alkalosis is considered the main disorder and the acidosis the compensatory response, because the pH is on the alkaline side of 7.40.)

TABLE 19-1 ARTERIAL BLOOD GAS ASSESSMENT

DISORDER	pH	Paco$_2$	HCO$_3^-$
Respiratory Acidosis			
Uncompensated	<7.35	>45 mm Hg	22-26 mEq/L
Partially compensated	<7.35	>45 mm Hg	>26 mEq/L
Compensated	7.35-7.39	>45 mm Hg	>26 mEq/L
Respiratory Alkalosis			
Uncompensated	>7.45	<35 mm Hg	22-26 mEq/L
Partially compensated	>7.45	<35 mm Hg	<22 mEq/L
Compensated	7.41-7.45	<35 mm Hg	<22 mEq/L
Metabolic Acidosis			
Uncompensated	<7.35	35-45 mm Hg	<22 mEq/L
Partially compensated	<7.35	<35 mm Hg	<22 mEq/L
Compensated	7.35-7.39	<35 mm Hg	<22 mEq/L
Metabolic Alkalosis			
Uncompensated	>7.45	35-45 mm Hg	>26 mEq/L
Partially compensated	>7.45	>45 mm Hg	>26 mEq/L
Compensated	7.41-7.45	>45 mm Hg	>26 mEq/L
Combined (or mixed) respiratory and metabolic acidosis	<7.35	>45 mm Hg	<22 mEq/L
Combined (or mixed) respiratory and metabolic alkalosis	>7.45	<35 mm Hg	>26 mEq/L

TABLE 19-2 CAUSES OF ACID-BASE DISORDERS

DISORDERS	POTENTIAL CAUSE

Respiratory Acidosis	Chronic obstructive pulmonary disease
	Acute airway obstruction
	Central nervous system depression
	   Sedatives
	   Anesthetics
	   Opioids
	Trauma
	   Spinal cord
	   Brain
	   Chest wall
	Neuromuscular disease
	   Poliomyelitis
	   Myasthenia gravis
	   Guillain-Barré syndrome
	Hypoventilation with mechanical ventilation

Respiratory Alkalosis	Hypoxia Anxiety Fear Pain Stimulants Pulmonary embolism Hyperventilation with mechanical ventilation
Metabolic Acidosis	Lactic acidosis Ketoacidosis Renal failure (uremia) Rhabdomyolysis Ingestion of acids (methanol, salicylates, ethylene glycol) Diarrhea Renal tubular acidosis Ureterosigmoidoscopy Ileostomy Pancreatic fistula
Metabolic Alkalosis	Steroid therapy Vomiting Gastrointestinal suction Diuretic therapy Hypokalemia Hypovolemia Hypochloremia Sodium bicarbonate intake

oximeter (Spo$_2$).[9,10] Oxygen saturation is reported as a percentage or as a decimal; normal values are greater than 95% when the patient is on room air. Normally, the saturation level cannot reach 100% (on room air) because of physiologic shunting.[1] However, when supplemental oxygen is administered, oxygen saturation may approach 100% so closely that it is reported as 100%.

Proper evaluation of the oxygen saturation level is vital. For example, an Sao$_2$ of 97% means that 97% of the available hemoglobin is bound with oxygen. The word *available* is essential to evaluating the Sao$_2$ level, because the hemoglobin level is not always within normal limits and oxygen can bind only with what is available. A 97% saturation level associated with 10 g/dL of hemoglobin does not deliver as much oxygen to the tissues as does a 97% saturation level associated with 15 g/dL of hemoglobin. Assessing only the Sao$_2$ level and finding it within normal limits does not ensure that the patient's oxygenation status is normal. The hemoglobin level must also be evaluated before a decision on oxygenation status can be made.[1,9,10]

Oxygen Content

Oxygen content (Cao$_2$) is a measure of the total amount of oxygen carried in the blood, including the amount dissolved in plasma (measured by the Pao_2) and the amount bound to the hemoglobin molecule (measured by the Sao_2). Cao_2 is reported in milliliters of oxygen carried per 100 mL of blood. The normal value is 20 mL of oxygen per 100 mL of blood. To calculate the oxygen content, the Pao_2, the Sao_2, and the hemoglobin level are used (see Appendix B). A change in any one of these parameters will affect the Cao_2.[1]

The value of assessing the Cao_2 is best illustrated by the examples in Table 19-3. The ABG parameters that are used most commonly to evaluate oxygenation status (Pao_2 and Sao_2) are both normal. Assessing only the Pao_2 and the Sao_2 would lead to the invalid conclusion that Patient B's oxygenation status is normal. However, consideration of the hemoglobin level and the Cao_2 reveals that the oxygenation of Patient B's blood is significantly abnormal.

Base Excess and Base Deficit

Base excess and base deficit reflect the nonrespiratory contribution to acid–base balance and are reported in milliequivalents per liter (mEq/L) above or below the normal range of −2 mEq/L to +2 mEq/L. A negative base level is reported as a *base deficit*, which correlates with *metabolic acidosis*, whereas a positive base level is reported as a *base excess*, which correlates with *metabolic alkalosis*.[1,4,8]

Classic Shunt Equation and Oxygen Tension Indices

The efficiency of oxygenation can be assessed by measuring the degree of intrapulmonary shunting that occurs in a patient at any one time, using the classic shunt equation and oxygen tension indices. *Intrapulmonary shunting* (QS/QT [the portion of cardiac output not exchanging with alveolar blood divided by the total cardiac output]) refers to venous blood that flows to the lungs without being oxygenated because of nonfunctioning alveoli.[1] Other names for this condition include shunt effect, low V/Q, wasted blood flow, and venous admixture.[1,11,12]

Direct determination of intrapulmonary shunting requires the use of the classic shunt equation (see Appendix B), which is invasive and cumbersome. A shunt greater than 10% is considered abnormal and indicative of a shunt-producing disorder. A shunt greater than 30% is a serious and potentially life-threatening condition, which requires pulmonary intervention.[1,11,12]

Often, intrapulmonary shunting is estimated by using the oxygen tension indices. One advantage to these methods is the ease of performance, although they have been found to be unreliable in critically ill patients.[1,11] An estimate of intrapulmonary shunting can be determined by computing the difference between the alveolar and arterial oxygen concentrations. Normally, alveolar (A) and arterial (a) Po_2 values are approximately equal. When they are not, it indicates that venous blood is passing malfunctioning alveoli and returning unoxygenated to the left side of the heart.[1,11] The most common oxygen tension indices used to estimate intrapulmonary shunting are the Pao_2/Fio_2 ratio, the Pao_2/Pao_2 ratio, and the A-a gradient ($P[A - a]o_2$).

Pao_2/Fio_2 Ratio

The Pao_2/Fio_2 ratio is clinically the easiest formula to calculate because it does not call for the computation of the alveolar Po_2. Normally, the Pao_2/Fio_2 ratio is greater than 286; the lower the value, the worse the lung function.[1,9,11]

Pao_2/Pao_2 Ratio

The Pao_2/Pao_2 ratio (arterial/alveolar O_2 ratio) is normally greater than 60%. The disadvantage to using this formula is that it calls for the computation of the alveolar Po_2 (see Appendix B), but the advantage is that it is unaffected by changes in the Fio_2, as long as the underlying lung condition is stable.[1,11]

Alveolar-Arterial Gradient

The A-a gradient ($P[A - a]o_2$) is normally less than 20 mm Hg on room air for patients younger than 61 years. This estimate of intrapulmonary shunting is the least reliable clinically, but it is used often in clinical decision making. One of the major disadvantages to using this formula is that it is greatly influenced by the amount of oxygen the patient is receiving.[1,11-13]

Serial determinations of the estimates of intrapulmonary shunting provide the practitioner with objective data on which to base clinical decisions.[1,11,12] Table 19-4 shows the change in intrapulmonary shunting in the hypoxemic patient using the previously described oxygen tension indices to estimate severity of shunting.

TABLE 19-3 ASSESSING OXYGENATION STATUS

PATIENT	Pao_2 LEVEL (mm Hg)	Sao_2 LEVEL (%)	Hgb (g/dL)	Cao_2 (mL/dL)
A	100	97	15	19.8
B	100	97	10	13.3

Cao_2, Arterial oxygen content; *Hgb*, hemoglobin; *Pao_2*, arterial partial pressure of oxygen; *Sao_2*, arterial oxygen saturation.

TABLE 19-4 CALCULATION OF INTRAPULMONARY SHUNTING

Fio_2	Pao_2 LEVEL (mm Hg)	Pao_2 LEVEL (mm Hg)	Pao_2/Fio_2	a/A RATIO (%)	A-a GRADIENT (mm Hg)
0.21	40	97	190	41	57
0.50	80	300	160	27	220
1.0	150	610	150	25	460

Modified from Murray JF, Nadel JA, eds. *Textbook of Respiratory Medicine*. Philadelphia: WB Saunders; 1988.

A, Alveolar; *a*, arterial; *Fio_2*, fraction of inspired oxygen; *Pao_2*, arterial partial pressure of oxygen.

Dead Space Equation

The efficiency of ventilation can be measured using the clinical dead space (V_D/V_T) equation (see Appendix B). The formula measures the fraction of tidal volume not participating in gas exchange. A dead space value greater than 0.6 indicates a dead space-producing disorder and is considered abnormal. The major limitations to using this formula are that it requires the measurement of exhaled carbon dioxide to complete and that the work of breathing by patients must remain stable during the collection.[12,14]

Sputum Studies

Careful analysis of sputum specimens is crucial for the rapid identification and treatment of pulmonary infections. The most difficult aspect of sputum examination is proper collection of the specimen. Collection of a good sputum sample requires a conscious, cooperative, and sufficiently hydrated patient.[12] When the patient has difficulty producing sputum, heated, nebulized saline may help to loosen secretions for expectoration.[12] Chest physiotherapy combined with nebulization improves the success rate. Collection of a sputum specimen is best done in the morning, because a greater volume of secretions is present as a result of nighttime pooling. Brushing the teeth and rinsing the oropharyngeal airway is recommended to reduce contamination before collecting a sample.[12,15]

Many critically ill patients cannot cough effectively, and sputum collection by other means is required. These methods include tracheobronchial aspiration, transtracheal aspiration, and the use of a fiberoptic bronchoscopy with a protected brush catheter. Because each method has its own benefits and risks, the patient's clinical condition determines the appropriate technique.[12]

Many critically ill patients have endotracheal or tracheostomy tubes already in place. Collecting sputum specimens from these patients requires special attention to technique (Box 19-4). Deep specimens are obtained to avoid collecting specimens that contain resident upper airway flora that may have migrated down the tube. Colonization of the lower airways with upper airway flora can occur within 48 hours of intubation.[16]

After a sputum specimen is obtained, it is examined for volume, physical properties, mucopurulence, and color. Next, a microscopic examination is done to identify the source of the specimen. If a bacterial infection is suspected, a Gram stain is performed, followed by culture and sensitivity (C&S) assessments.[12,15,16]

DIAGNOSTIC PROCEDURES

Bronchoscopy

Fiberoptic bronchoscopy is a relatively safe procedure done at the bedside, and it is most often used as a diagnostic and therapeutic tool (Fig. 19-2). Diagnostic indications include hemoptysis, infectious pneumonia, difficult intubation, pulmonary injury after chest trauma, acute burn inhalation injury, aspiration lung injuries, and acute upper airway obstruction. Therapeutic indications include the aspiration of foreign bodies, removal of obstructing secretions, atelectasis, difficult intubation, and resection of small, benign growths from the airway.[12,17,18]

Before the bronchoscopy, a complete medical history is obtained, and a thorough examination, including a chest x-ray examination, is performed.[12,17] Preprocedural evaluation of the patient includes clotting studies (prothrombin time [PT], partial thromboplastin time [PTT], and platelet count) and evaluation of the ABG levels.[12,17] Hypoxemic patients need supplemental oxygen during the procedure. The patient must have no oral intake for 6 to 8 hours before the bronchoscopy to reduce the risk of aspiration.[12,17]

Although a topical anesthetic can be used alone, it is usually supplemented by an intravenous sedative or analgesic, or both. A benzodiazepine for sedative effects and a opioid analgesic are

---

BOX 19-4 PROCEDURE FOR COLLECTION OF TRACHEAL OR ENDOTRACHEAL SPUTUM SPECIMEN

1. Clear the endotracheal or tracheostomy tube of all local secretions, avoiding deep airway penetration.
2. Attach a sputum trap to a sterile suction catheter, and advance the catheter into the trachea while trying to avoid contact with the endotracheal tube or tracheostomy tube (Fig. 19-1).
3. After the catheter is fully advanced, apply suction until secretions return to the sputum trap. When enough secretions are collected, discontinue suctioning, and remove the catheter.
4. Do not apply suction while the catheter is being withdrawn, because this can contaminate the sample with sputum from the upper airway. Do not flush the catheter with sterile water, because this dilutes the sample.
5. If the catheter becomes plugged with secretions, place it in a sterile container, and send it to the laboratory. The specimen must be transported immediately or refrigerated if a delay is necessary.

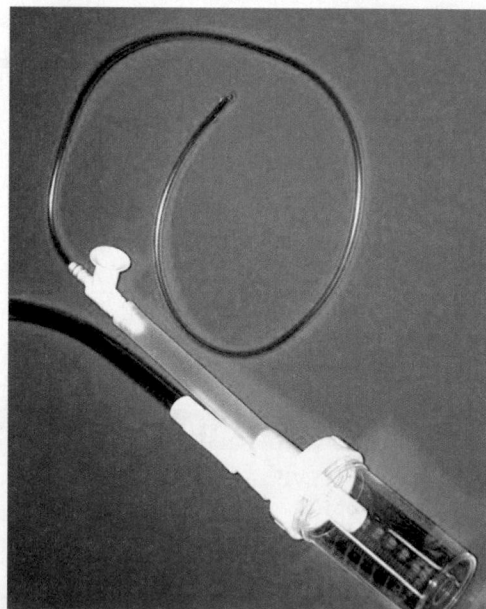

FIGURE 19-1 Specimen Container. (From Kacmarek RM, et al, eds. *Egan's Fundamentals of Respiratory Care.* 10th ed. St. Louis: Mosby; 2013.)

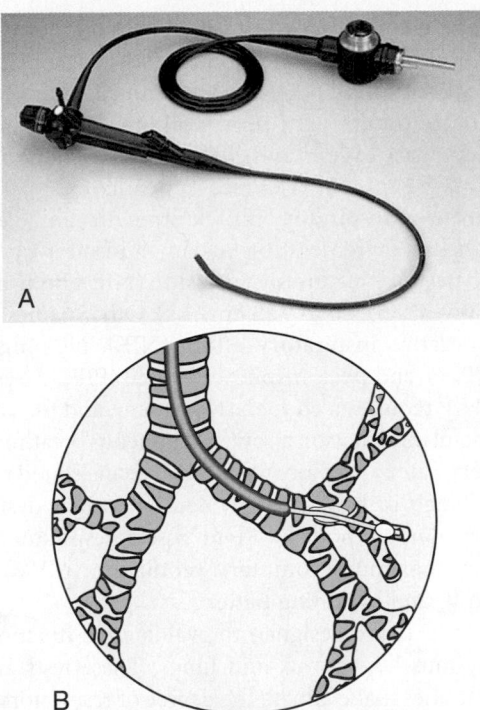

FIGURE 19-2 Fiberoptic Bronchoscope. *A,* The transbronchoscopic balloon-tipped catheter and the flexible fiberoptic bronchoscope. *B,* The catheter is introduced into a small airway and the balloon is inflated with 1.5 to 2 mL of air to occlude the airway. Bronchial alveolar lavage is performed by injecting and withdrawing 30-mL aliquots of sterile saline solution, gently aspirating after each instillation. Specimens are sent to the laboratory for analysis. (From Christensen BL, Kockrow EO, eds. *Adult Health Nursing.* 6th ed. St. Louis: Mosby; 2011.)

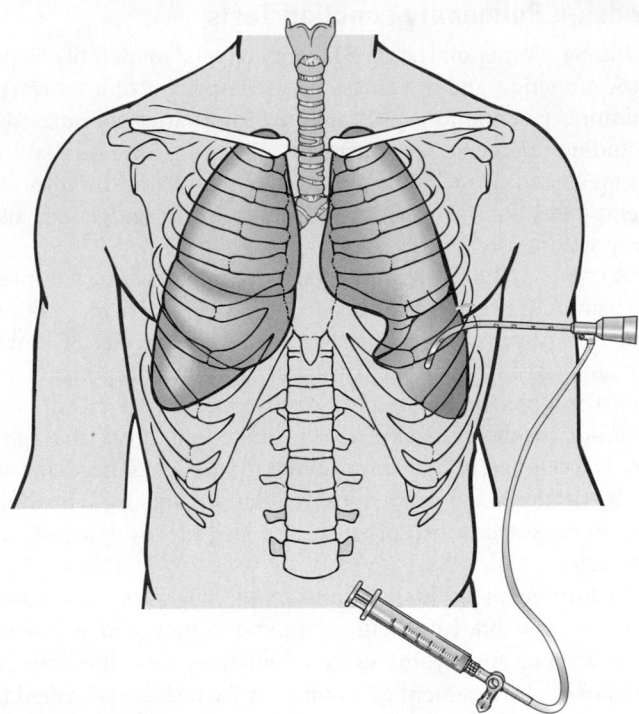

FIGURE 19-3 Thoracentesis. The needle has penetrated the fluid-filled pleural space to remove fluid. (From Christensen BL, Kockrow EO, eds. *Adult Health Nursing.* 6th ed. St. Louis: Mosby; 2011.)

administered intravenously during the procedure.[12,17,18] Preprocedural medications for a diagnostic bronchoscopy may include atropine and intramuscular codeine. Atropine lessens the vasovagal response and reduces the secretions, whereas codeine decreases the cough reflex. When bronchoscopy is performed therapeutically to remove secretions, the patient has decreased cough and gag reflexes, which may impair secretion clearance.[12,17,18] Maintenance of the airway is essential to prevent complications.

Complications of the procedure may be related to the procedure itself, the anesthetic, or an ancillary procedure. Minor complications include laryngospasm, bronchospasm, epistaxis, fever, vomiting, altered pulmonary mechanics, and hemodynamic instability. Major complications include anaphylaxis, infection, hypotension, cardiac dysrhythmias, pneumothorax, hemorrhage, respiratory failure, hypoxemia, and cardiopulmonary arrest.[12,17,18]

Thoracentesis

Thoracentesis is a simple, usually uncomplicated procedure done at the bedside for the removal of fluid or air from the pleural space (Fig. 19-3). It is used most often as a diagnostic measure; it may also be performed therapeutically for the drainage of a pleural effusion or empyema.[19,20] No absolute contraindications to thoracentesis exist, although there are some risks

that may contraindicate the procedure in all but emergency situations. These risk factors include unstable hemodynamics, coagulation defects, mechanical ventilation, the presence of an intraaortic balloon pump, and patients who are uncooperative. In most clinical situations, diagnostic thoracentesis can be delayed until these risk factors are eliminated.[19]

The patient is placed in a sitting position with legs over the side of the bed and with hands and arms supported on a padded overbed table. If the patient's condition precludes sitting, the side-lying position with the back flush with the edge of the bed and the affected side down can be used.[19,20,21] The patient is cautioned not to move or cough during the procedure.[21] During the thoracentesis, the site of the needle insertion is usually determined by previous chest x-ray examination, computed tomography (CT) scan, or chest percussion. A local anesthetic is used to minimize the patient's discomfort during insertion of the thoracentesis needle.[9]

Complications associated with thoracentesis include pain, pneumothorax, and re-expansion pulmonary edema. Pneumothorax can occur as a result of introduction of air into the pleural space, puncture of the lung, or rupture of the visceral pleura.[19,20,21] Re-expansion pulmonary edema can occur when a large amount of effusion fluid (approximately 1000 to 1500 mL) is removed from the pleural space. Removal of the fluid increases the negative intrapleural pressure, which can lead to edema when the lung does not reexpand to fill the space. The patient experiences severe coughing and shortness of breath. The onset of these symptoms is an indication to discontinue the thoracentesis.[21]

Bedside Pulmonary Function Tests

Pulmonary function tests (PFTs) are designed to quantify respiratory function and are an essential component of a thorough pulmonary evaluation. PFTs are used for a variety of purposes, including preoperative assessment, evaluating lung mechanics, diagnosing and tracking pulmonary diseases, and monitoring therapy. Results are individualized according to age, gender, and body size.[22]

A complete PFT consists of four components: lung volumes, mechanics of breathing, diffusion, and ABGs. PFTs may take as long as 2 hours to complete. Because of the severity of illness encountered in the critical care area, all four components are rarely completed. Most often, measurements of pulmonary function in the critically ill are limited to areas that give the practitioner information about the patient's need for or ability to wean from mechanical ventilation. This section covers the areas tested most often at the bedside of critically ill individuals.

Measurement of lung volumes and capacities (Box 19-5) provides valuable information about the origin of a disease process. Four lung volumes and four lung capacities can be measured. Measurement of volumes at the bedside is limited to tidal volume and vital capacity. A vital capacity of 10 to 15 mL/kg usually is a minimally accepted value for weaning, with a respiratory rate of less than 24 breaths/min.[12,22,23]

Assessment of the mechanics of breathing includes measurement of the flow of gas, lung and chest compliance, respiratory muscle strength, and tissue resistance. In the critical care area, dynamic and static compliance are measured at the bedside. *Compliance* is a measure of the distensibility of the lungs (how easily they are inflated). Dynamic compliance is measured during the breathing cycle. A value of 46 to 66 mL/cm H_2O is normal (see Appendix B). Measurement of dynamic compliance does not differentiate among resistance forces. Conditions that increase resistance therefore alter the dynamic compliance value. Dynamic compliance decreases with any decrease in lung compliance or increase in airway resistance, as occurs with

bronchospasm and retained secretions. Static compliance is measured under no-flow conditions so that resistance forces are removed. Static compliance decreases with any decrease in lung compliance, as occurs with pneumothorax, atelectasis, pneumonia, pulmonary edema, and chest wall restrictions. A normal range is 57 to 85 mL/cm H_2O (see Appendix B).[12,22]

Assessment of inspiratory muscle strength can be evaluated through the measurement of maximal inspiratory pressure (MIP) and negative inspiratory pressure (NIP). Both should be more negative than −20 to −25 cm H_2O. Other names for these tests are negative inspiratory effort (NIE), peak inspiratory pressure (PIP), and peak inspiratory force (PIF). Assessing the MIP and NIP requires a cooperative patient, and the values can provide useful information about spontaneous breathing ability. Maximal expiratory pressure (MEP) can be measured to test the ability to cough in patients with neuromuscular dysfunction. Other common methods used to assess respiratory muscle strength are maximum voluntary ventilation (MVV), minute ventilation V_E and breathing pattern.[12,22]

Dynamic PFTs are designed to evaluate the function of the respiratory muscles, thorax, and lungs. These tests are timed breathing studies that evaluate the degree of respiratory impairment and include forced vital capacity (FVC), peak expiratory flow rate (PEFR), forced expiratory volume in 1 second (FEV_1), and forced expiratory volume divided by the forced vital capacity (FEV_1/FVC). Forced expiratory flow ($FEF_{25\%-75\%}$) is the mean rate of airflow over the middle half of the FVC, and it is a good index of airway resistance. When these studies are performed at the bedside, they require the use of spirometry for volume measurement. The tests can be performed with intubated or nonintubated patients. In the intubated patient, the spirometer is attached to the end of the endotracheal tube. In the nonintubated patient, a nose clip is placed on the patient, and the patient is instructed to breathe through a spirometer tube. The patient is seated on the side of the bed if possible.[12,22,23] Table 19-5 provides a description of each of these parameters.

Ventilation/Perfusion Scanning

Ventilation/perfusion (V/Q) scanning is indicated when a serious alteration of the normal V/Q relationship is suspected. V/Q studies are ordered most often to diagnose and follow a suspected pulmonary embolus. V/Q scanning is approximately 90% accurate in determining this diagnosis. Comparing the perfusion scan with the results of a clinical examination may improve this percentage somewhat.[24]

The V/Q scan consists of a ventilation scan and a perfusion scan. The ventilation scan is performed by having the patient inhale a radiolabeled gas and air mixture through a mask. The perfusion scan is performed by intravenously injecting the patient with a radioisotope. Scintillation cameras record the gamma radiation images produced by the isotope as it is breathed or perfused into the lung. When an obstruction of the isotope's flow into an area of the lung occurs, the diminished radioactivity is reflected in the camera image of that zone.[24]

Because the results are less than 100% accurate in predicting pulmonary emboli, most V/Q scans are interpreted in one of four ways. The scan is interpreted as normal when the perfusion scan is normal, and the probability of pulmonary embolism

---

BOX 19-5 LUNG VOLUMES AND CAPACITIES

- *Tidal volume* (V_T): The volume of air exhaled after a normal resting inhalation: V_T × respiratory rate = minute ventilation. Normal value is 500 mL.
- *Inspiratory reserve volume* (IRV): The amount of additional air that can be taken in after a normal inhalation. Normal value is 3000 to 3100 mL.
- *Inspiratory capacity* (IC): The maximal amount of air that can be inhaled after a normal exhalation. Normal value is 3500 to 3600 mL.
- *Expiratory reserve volume* (ERV): The additional amount of air that can be exhaled after a normal resting exhalation. Normal value is 1100 to 1200 mL.
- *Vital capacity* (VC): The maximal amount of air that can be exhaled after a maximal inhalation. Normal value is 4600 to 4800 mL.
- *Residual volume* (RV): The amount of air left in the lung after maximal exhalation. Normal value is 1200 to 1300 mL.
- *Functional residual capacity* (FRC): The amount of air left in the lung after a normal exhalation, equal to the total of the ERV and RV. Normal value is 2300 to 2400 mL.
- *Total lung capacity* (TLC): The maximal volume of air in the lung after a maximal inspiration, which is the total of all lung volumes. Normal value is 5800 to 6000 mL.

TABLE 19-5	BEDSIDE PULMONARY FUNCTION TESTS
TEST	**DESCRIPTION**
Respiratory rate (f)	Number of breaths per minute
Tidal volume (V_T)	Volume of air exhaled after a normal resting inhalation
Minute ventilation V_E	Volume of air expired per minute (tidal volume respiratory rate = minute ventilation)
Maximal voluntary ventilation (MVV)	Maximal amount of air that can be moved into and out of the lungs in 1 minute
Forced vital capacity (FVC)	Maximal amount of air that can be forcefully exhaled from the lungs after maximal inhalation
Maximal inspiratory pressure (MIP)	Maximal negative pressure generated on inhalation
Maximal expiratory pressure (MEP)	Maximal positive pressure generated on exhalation
Peak expiratory flow rate (PEFR)	Maximal flow rate achieved during forced exhalation
Forced expiratory flow at midpoint of vital capacity ($FEF_{25\%-75\%}$)	Measure of the average flow rate during the middle 50% of exhalation
Forced expiratory flow at 1 second (FEV_1)	Volume of air exhaled during the first second of forced exhalation

BOX 19-6	STEPS FOR INTERPRETATION OF A CHEST RADIOGRAPH

Step 1

Look at the different densities (black, gray, and white), and answer this question: *What is air, fluid, tissue, and bone?*

Step 2

Look at the shape or form of each density, and answer this question: *What normal anatomic structure is this?*

Step 3

Look at the right and left sides, and answer this question: *Are the findings the same on both sides, or are there physiologic and pathophysiologic differences?*

Step 4

Look at all the structures (bones, mediastinum, diaphragm, pleural space, and lung tissue), and answer this question: *Are any abnormalities present?*

Step 5

Look for all tubes, wires, and lines, and answer this question: *Are the tubes, wires, and lines in the proper place?*

approaches zero. A low probability interpretation is given when there are small V/Q mismatches, focal V/Q matches with no corresponding radiographic abnormalities, or the perfusion defects are considerably smaller than the radiographic abnormalities. This finding is associated with a 12% chance of pulmonary embolus.[24,25] An intermediate or indeterminate probability is assigned when there are severe diffuse airflow obstructions, perfusion defects corresponding in size and position to radiographic abnormalities, and a single, moderate V/Q mismatch without a corresponding radiographic abnormality. A high probability interpretation is used when the perfusion defects are substantially larger than the radiographic abnormalities or when there is one or more large or two or more moderate V/Q mismatches with no corresponding radiographic abnormalities. This finding is seen infrequently but has a highly predictive value.[24,25,26]

Chest Radiography

Chest radiography is an important diagnostic procedure for any critically ill patient. Chest x-ray examinations aid in the diagnosis of various disorders and complications and assist in the evaluation of treatment.[27]

When interpreting a chest radiograph, a systematic method is used for viewing it (Box 19-6). Areas of the radiographic film that are assessed include bones, mediastinum, diaphragm, pleural space, and lung tissue. Fig. 19-4 provides an example of a normal chest radiograph.

Bones

The clavicles, ribs, thoracic and cervical spine, and scapulas are assessed. The clavicles should be symmetric, and the ribs should

be an equal distance apart. Intervertebral disk spaces should be evident, indicating an adequately exposed inspiratory film.[27] The thoracic and cervical spine should be straight, without signs of curvature. The scapulas usually appear as areas of added density in the upper lung fields. There should be no evidence of fractures, calcification and lesions (increased density), or demineralization (decreased density).[27,28]

Mediastinum

The structures assessed in the mediastinal area are the aortic knob and the trachea. The trachea should be positioned in the midline, with a slight deviation to the right as it approaches the carina.[27] Shifting of the mediastinal structures can occur with atelectasis and removal of all or a portion of a lung (toward the area of involvement), pneumothorax (away from the area of involvement), pleural effusion, and tumors.[27,28]

Diaphragm

The diaphragm should be clearly visible, with sharp costophrenic angles seen where the chest wall and the tapered edges of the diaphragm meet.[27,28] The level of the diaphragm (on deep inspiration) should appear at the 10th or 11th rib,[27,28] with the right side 1 to 2 cm higher than the left side.[27] A gastric air bubble may be found under the left side of the diaphragm.[27,28] An elevated diaphragm may be seen in pregnancy, obesity, conditions that cause air or fluid to accumulate in the peritoneal space, and intestinal obstruction.[27] An elevated hemidiaphragm is associated with several conditions, including phrenic nerve injury, previous chest surgery, subphrenic abscess, trauma, stroke, tumor, pneumonia, and radiation therapy.[27] Flattening of the diaphragm can be a sign of increased air in the lungs, as occurs with chronic COPD or a pleural effusion.[27,28] Obliteration or "blunting" of the costophrenic angle can occur with pleural effusion, atelectasis, or pneumothorax.[27,28]

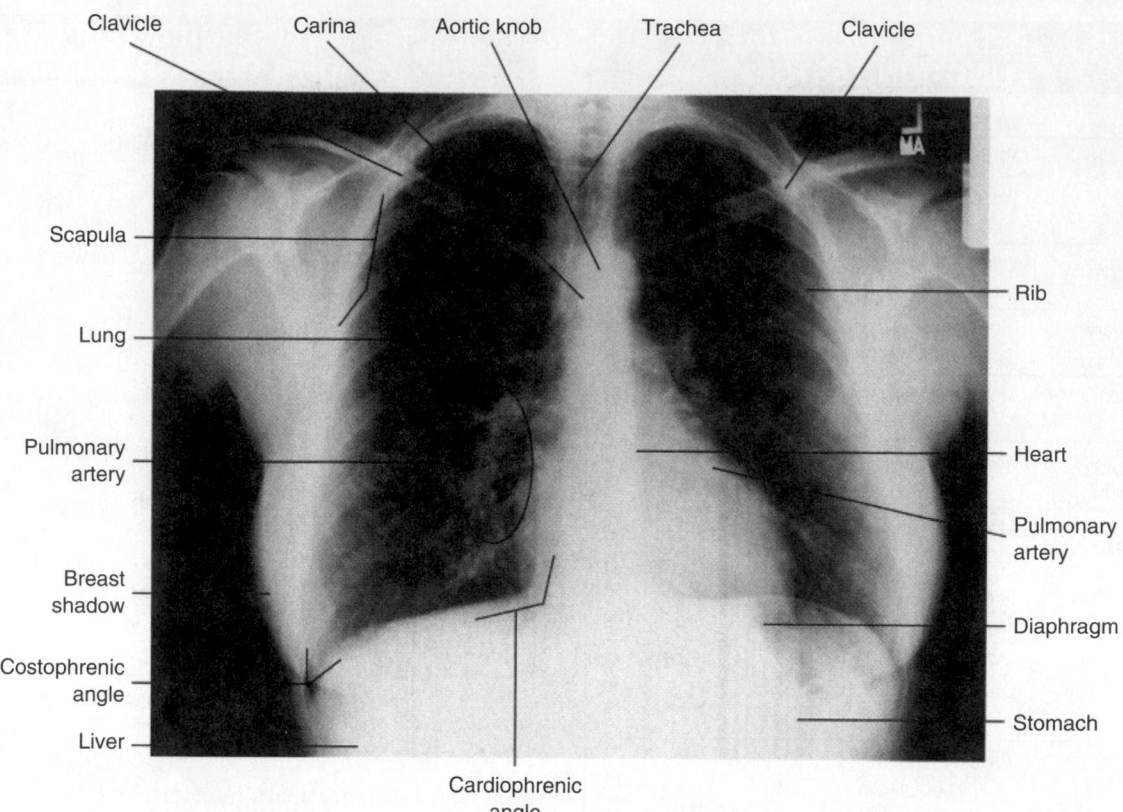

FIGURE 19-4 Location of Structures on a Normal Chest Radiograph. (From Dettenmeir PA. *Radiographic Assessment for Nurses.* St. Louis: Mosby; 1995.)

Pleural Space

Identification of the pleural space on a chest radiograph is an abnormal finding. The pleural space is not visible unless air (pneumothorax) or fluid (pleural effusion) enters it. As fluid accumulates in the pleural space, it surrounds the lung and eventually compresses it. With a pleural effusion, blunting of the costophrenic angle may be evident first, with flattening of the diaphragm and obscuring of the heart borders occurring as the effusion grows.[28] With a pneumothorax, the pleural edges become evident as the examiner looks through and between the images of the ribs on the film. A thin line appears just parallel to the chest wall, indicating where the lung markings have pulled away from the chest wall.[27,28] The collapsed lung manifests as an area of increased density separated by an area of radiolucency (blackness).

Lung Tissue

The lung tissue is viewed for any areas of increased density or increased radiolucency that may indicate an abnormality. Increased density can be the result of accumulation of fluid in the lungs (e.g., water, pus, blood, edema fluid) or collapse of lung tissue (e.g., with atelectasis or pneumothorax). Increased radiolucency is caused by increased air in the lungs, as may occur with COPD.[27,28] In some patients, a fine line may be present on the right side at about the level of the sixth rib in the midlung field. This is a normal finding and represents the horizontal fissure, which separates the right upper lobe from the right middle lobe.[27,28]

Tubes, Wires, and Lines

The chest radiograph is assessed for proper placement of all tubes, wires, and lines. When properly positioned, an endotracheal tube is 2 to 3 cm above the carina, and a nasogastric tube runs the length of the esophagus, with the tip in the stomach.[27] The origin of a central venous catheter is observed as a thin, continuous, radiopaque line at the level of the jaw, progressing toward the superior vena cava in an internal jugular approach, whereas a subclavian approach originates in the clavicular area. A pulmonary artery catheter is viewed running through the right atrium and right ventricle into the pulmonary artery.[27,28] Additional items that may be present include temporary or permanent pacing wires, a permanent pacing generator, an implantable cardioverter defibrillator (ICD), a peripherally inserted central catheter (PICC), chest tubes (pleural or mediastinal), electrocardiographic (ECG) electrodes, and surgical markers and clips.[27,28]

Nursing Management

Nursing management of a patient undergoing a diagnostic procedure involves a variety of interventions, which include preparing the patient psychologically and physically for the procedure, monitoring the patient's responses to the procedure, and assessing the patient after the procedure. Preparing the patient includes teaching the patient about the procedure, answering any questions, and positioning the patient for the procedure. Monitoring the patient's responses to the procedure includes observing the patient for signs of pain, anxiety,

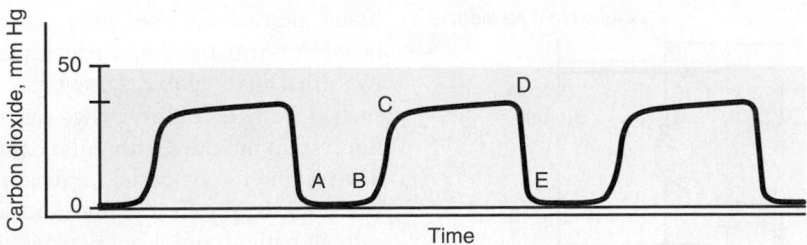

FIGURE 19-5 Normal findings on a capnogram. $A \rightarrow B$ indicates the baseline; $B \rightarrow C$, the expiratory upstroke; $C \rightarrow D$, the alveolar plateau; D, the partial pressure of end-tidal carbon dioxide; and $D \rightarrow E$, the inspiratory downstroke. (From Frakes M. Measuring end-tidal carbon dioxide: clinical applications and usefulness. *Crit Care Nurse.* 2001;21[5]:23.)

or respiratory distress and monitoring vital signs, breath sounds, and oxygen saturation. Assessing the patient after the procedure includes observing for complications of the procedure and medicating the patient for any postprocedural discomfort.

BEDSIDE MONITORING

Capnography

Capnography is the measurement of exhaled carbon dioxide (CO_2) gas; it is also known as *end-tidal CO_2* monitoring. Normally, alveolar and arterial CO_2 concentrations are equal in the presence of normal V/Q relationships. In a patient who is hemodynamically stable, the end-tidal CO_2 (P_{ETCO_2}) can be used to estimate the $Paco_2$, with the P_{ETCO_2} levels 1 to 5 mm Hg less than $Paco_2$ levels. The practitioner must determine first that a normal V/Q relationship exists before correlation of the P_{ETCO_2} and the $Paco_2$ can be assumed.[12-29] Causes of increased P_{ETCO_2} include situations in which CO_2 production is increased, such as hyperthermia, sepsis, and seizures, or in which alveolar ventilation is decreased, such as respiratory depression. Causes of decreased P_{ETCO_2} include situations in which CO_2 production is decreased, such as hypothermia, cardiac arrest, and pulmonary embolism, or in which alveolar ventilation is increased, such as hyperventilation.[12,29]

In the critical care area, continuous capnography is used for assessment and monitoring of the patient's ventilatory status in a variety of situations, including weaning from mechanical ventilation and undergoing procedural sedation. Assessment of changes in physiologic dead space can be carried out with end-tidal CO_2 monitoring, based on the degree of difference between the $Paco_2$ and the P_{ETCO_2}. As the severity of pulmonary impairment increases, so does the disparity between the $Paco_2$ and the P_{ETCO_2}, as indicated by an increased gradient. A gradient of greater than 5 mm Hg can be seen with underperfused alveolar-capillary units (dead space-producing situations) and nonperfused alveolar-capillary units (alveolar dead space). Increased dead space ventilation is a result of decreased pulmonary blood flow or cardiac output and lung disease. This leads to an abnormality in the transfer of CO_2 from the blood to the lung. The result is a P_{ETCO_2} level that is lower than the $Paco_2$ because of the mixing of carbon dioxide between perfused and nonperfused units. The end result is an increased or widened $Paco_2$/P_{ETCO_2} gradient.[12,29]

The noninvasive measurement of P_{ETCO_2} enables assessment of the adequacy of cardiopulmonary resuscitation and endotracheal tube placement. Decreased pulmonary blood flow is associated with lower P_{ETCO_2} values, reflected clinically by decreased cardiac output, as in the case of cardiopulmonary resuscitation.[12,29] During endotracheal intubation, a low P_{ETCO_2} reading indicates that the tube is positioned in the stomach, because the amount of carbon dioxide in the esophagus is expected to be low.[12,29]

There are three forms of capnography: mainstream, sidestream, and proximal diverting. All forms can be used in intubated patients, but side-stream and microstream capnography can also be used in nonintubated patients, broadening the application of end-tidal CO_2 monitoring. Mainstream capnography measures the CO_2 level directly by a sensor in the exhalation port of the ventilator tubing. During exhalation, gas passes over the sensor, and the information is transferred by an electrical cable to the display unit. The display unit produces a waveform, called a *capnogram* (Fig. 19-5), and a numeric recording (P_{ETCO_2}). Disadvantages to this form of capnography include the weight of the sensor on the ventilator tubing and possible obstruction of the sensor by secretions and condensation. In side-stream capnography, the CO_2 gas is continuously aspirated through a side port in the ventilator tubing or nasal cannula and is measured and analyzed by a side unit. Disadvantages to this form of capnography include obstruction of the sampling tube with secretions and slow response time. Proximal diverting capnography is a newer and improved version of side-stream capnography that transports gas a short distance from the airway to a site where the sensor is located thereby reducing the bulkiness at the airway.

Capnography and partial pressure of end-tidal carbon dioxide (P_{ETCO_2}) analysis have many diverse applications in the critical care area, but the practitioner must never assume the P_{ETCO_2} values reflect arterial values of the partial pressure of carbon dioxide ($Paco_2$) without waveform analysis. Any change in the waveform can indicate a change in the patient's pulmonary status and warrants further evaluation. Loss of the waveform may signal loss of effective respirations.[12,29]

Pulse Oximetry

Pulse oximetry is a noninvasive method for monitoring oxygen saturation (Spo_2). It is indicated in any situation in which the patient's oxygenation status requires continuous observation. It

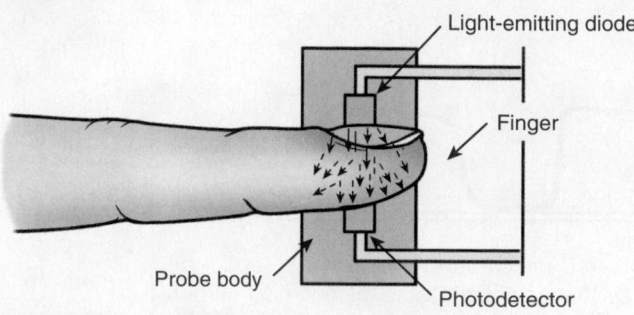

FIGURE 19-6 Pulse Oximeter Finger Probe. (From Wilkins RL, et al, eds. *Egan's Fundamentals of Respiratory Care.* 8th ed. St. Louis: Mosby; 2006.)

consists of a microprocessor and a probe that attaches to the patient's forehead, finger, ear, toe, or nose. The probe consists of two light-emitting diodes and a photodetector (Fig. 19-6). The diodes transmit red and infrared light wavelengths through the pulsating arterial vascular bed to the photodetector on the other side. The percentage of oxygen saturation is determined by the difference in absorbance of the red and infrared light caused by the difference in color between oxygen-bound (bright red) and oxygen-unbound (dark red) hemoglobin. The photodetector converts the light signals into an electric signal that is sent to the microprocessor, which converts it to a digital reading. The pulse oximeter is considered very accurate; readings vary less than 4% to 5% at a saturation level greater than 70%. However, several physiologic and technical factors limit the monitoring system.[9,12]

Physiologic Limitations

Physiologic limitations of pulse oximetry include elevated levels of abnormal hemoglobins, presence of vascular dyes, and poor tissue perfusion. The pulse oximeter cannot differentiate between normal and abnormal hemoglobin. Elevated levels of abnormal hemoglobin falsely elevate the Spo_2. Vascular dyes such as methylene blue, indigo carmine, indocyanine green, and fluorescein interfere with pulse oximetry and can lead to falsely low readings. Poor tissue perfusion to the area with the probe leads to loss of pulsatile flow and signal failure.[9,12] In the critically ill patient, pulse oximetry is reliable only for monitoring the patient's oxygenation status. It is not a reliable method for monitoring the patient's ventilatory status. The ability of a pulse oximeter to detect hypoventilation is accurate only when the patient is breathing room air.[9] Because most critically ill patients require some form of oxygen therapy, pulse oximetry is not a reliable method of detecting hypercapnia and should *not* be used for this purpose.

Technical Limitations

Technical limitations of pulse oximetry include bright lights, excessive motion, and incorrect placement of the probe. Bright lights may interfere with the photodetector and cause inaccurate results. The probe must be covered to limit optical interference. Excessive motion can mimic arterial pulsations and can lead to false readings. Incorrect placement of the probe can lead to inaccurate results, because part of the light can reach the photodetector without having passed through blood (optical shunting).[9,12] Interventions to limit these problems include using the proper probe in the appropriate spot (e.g., not using a finger probe on the ear), applying the probe according to the directions, and ensuring that the area being monitored has adequate perfusion.[9,24]

SUMMARY

Laboratory Studies

- Interpretation of ABG levels involves looking at the Pao_2 (normal range, 80 to 100 mm Hg), the pH (normal range, 7.35 to 7.45), the $Paco_2$ (normal range, 35 to 45 mm Hg), and HCO_3^- (normal range, 22 to 26 mEq/L).
- The efficiency of oxygenation can be assessed by measuring the degree of intrapulmonary shunting using the classic shunt equation and oxygen tension indices (Pao_2/Fio_2 ratio, the Pao_2/Pao_2 ratio, and the A-a gradient).
- Sputum specimens are crucial for the rapid identification and treatment of pulmonary infections.

Diagnostic Procedures

- Fiberoptic bronchoscopy and thoracentesis are often used as diagnostic and therapeutic procedures.
- PFTs are used for preoperative assessment, evaluating lung mechanics, diagnosing and tracking pulmonary diseases, and monitoring therapy.

- V/Q scanning is indicated when a serious alteration of the normal V/Q relationship is suspected, such as with a pulmonary embolus.
- Chest x-ray examination aids in the diagnosis of various pulmonary disorders and assists in the evaluation of treatments.

Bedside Monitoring

- Capnography is a noninvasive method used to monitor a patient's ventilatory status by measurement of exhaled carbon dioxide gas.
- Pulse oximetry is a noninvasive method used to monitor a patient oxygenation status by measurement of oxygen saturation.

REFERENCES

1. Hirsch CA. Gas exchange and transport. In: Kacmarek RM, et al., eds. *Egan's Fundamentals of Respiratory Care.* 10th ed. St. Louis: Mosby; 2013.

2. Goldsmith J, Karotkin E. Appendix. In: Goldsmith J, Karotkin E, eds. *Assisted Ventilation of the Neonate.* 5th ed. St. Louis: Saunders; 2011.

3. Meiner SE. Theories of aging. In: Meiner SE, ed. *Gerontology Nursing.* 4th ed. St. Louis: Mosby; 2011.

4. Beach W. Acid base balance. In: Kacmarek RM, et al., eds. *Egan's Fundamentals of Respiratory Care.* 10th ed. St. Louis: Mosby; 2013.

5. Noble K. The ABC's of arterial blood gases. *J Perianesth Nurs.* 2009;24:401.

6. Ruholl L. Arterial blood gases: analysis and responses. *Medsurg Nurs.* 2006;15:343.

7. Aboussouan, L. Respiratory failure and the need for ventilator support. In: Kacmarek RM, et al., eds. *Egan's Fundamentals of Respiratory Care.* 10th ed. St. Louis: Mosby; 2013.

8. Sood P, et al. Interpretation of arterial blood gas. *Indian J Crit Care Med.* 2010;14(2):57.

9. Siobal MS. Analysis and monitoring of gas exchange. In: Kacmarek RM, et al., eds. *Egan's Fundamentals of Respiratory Care.* 10th ed. St. Louis: Mosby; 2013.

10. Schultz S. Oxygen saturation monitoring with pulse oximetry. In: Wiegand DJHM, ed. *AACN's Procedure Manual for Critical Care.* 6th ed. St. Louis: Elsevier; 2011.

11. Burns S. Shunt calculation. In: Wiegand DJHM, ed. *AACN's Procedure Manual for Critical Care.* 6th ed. St. Louis: Elsevier; 2011.

12. Pierce LNB. *Management of the Mechanically Ventilated Patient.* 2nd ed. St. Louis: Saunders; 2007.

13. Kacmarek RM, Volsko TA. Physiology of ventilatory support. In: Kacmarek RM, et al., eds. *Egan's Fundamentals of Respiratory Care.* 10th ed. St. Louis: Mosby; 2013.

14. Vines DL. Respiratory Monitoring in the intensive care unit. In: Wilkins RL, et al., eds. *Clinical Assessment in Respiratory Care.* 6th ed. St. Louis: Mosby; 2010.

15. Fink J, Arzu A. Humidity and bland aerosol. In: Kacmarek RM, et al., eds. *Egan's Fundamentals of Respiratory Care.* 10th ed. St. Louis: Mosby; 2013.

16. Hirsch CA. Airway clearance therapy. In: Kacmarek RM, et al., eds. *Egan's Fundamentals of Respiratory Care.* 10th ed. St. Louis: Mosby; 2013.

17. Altobelli N. Airway management. In: Kacmarek RM, et al., eds. *Egan's Fundamentals of Respiratory Care.* 10th ed. St. Louis: Mosby; 2013.

18. Murgu S, et al. Flexible bronchoscopy assisted by non invasive positive pressure ventilation. *Crit Care Nurse.* 2011;31(3):70.

19. Kasmani R, et al. Re-expansion pulmonary edema following thoracentesis. *CMAJ.* 2010;182:2000.

20. Josephson T, et al. Amount drained at ultrasound guided thoracentesis and risk of pneumothorax. *Acta Radiol.* 2009;50:42.

21. Strange C. Pleural diseases. In: Kacmarek RM, et al., eds. *Egan's Fundamentals of Respiratory Care.* 10th ed. St. Louis: Mosby; 2013.

22. Douce FH. Pulmonary function testing. In: Kacmarek RM, et al., eds. *Egan's Fundamentals of Respiratory Care,* 10th ed. St. Louis: Mosby; 2013.

23. Siner J, Manthous C. Liberation from mechanical ventilation: what monitoring matters? *Crit Care Clin.* 2007;23:613.

24. Tonelli AR, et al. Pulmonary vascular disease. In: Kacmarek RM, et al., eds. *Egan's Fundamentals of Respiratory Care.* 10th ed. St. Louis: Mosby; 2013.

25 Gandara E, Wells P. Diagnosis: use of clinical probability algorithms, *Clin Chest Med.* 2010;31:629.

26. Magna M, et al. Diagnostic approach to deep vein thrombosis and pulmonary embolism in the critical care setting. *Crit Care Clin.* 2011;27:841.

27. Specht N, Stoller J. Review of thoracic imaging. In: Kacmarek RM, et al., eds. *Egan's Fundamentals of Respiratory Care.* 10th ed. St. Louis: Mosby; 2013.

28. Hagberg C. *Benumof's Airway Management: Principles and Practices.* 2nd ed. Philadelphia: Mosby; 2007.

29. Adams AB. Monitoring the patient in the intensive care unit. In: Kacmarek RM, et al., eds. *Egan's Fundamentals of Respiratory Care.* 10th ed. St. Louis: Mosby; 2013.

Pulmonary Disorders

Kathleen M. Stacy

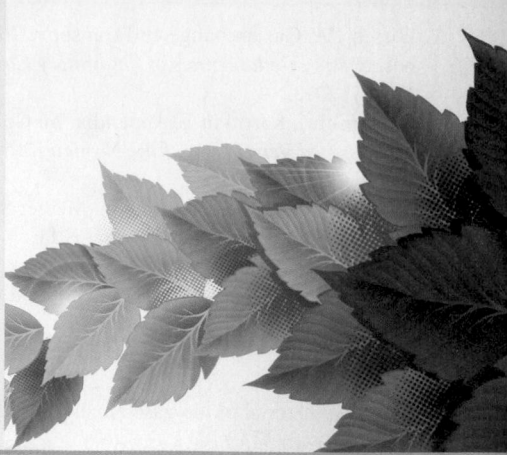

Understanding the pathology of the disease, the areas of assessment on which to focus, and the usual medical management allows the critical care nurse to more accurately anticipate and plan nursing interventions. This chapter focuses on pulmonary disorders commonly seen in the critical care environment.

ACUTE LUNG FAILURE

Description

Acute lung failure (ALF),[1] also known as acute respiratory failure, is a clinical condition in which the pulmonary system fails to maintain adequate gas exchange.[1,2] It is the most common type of organ failure seen in the critical care unit, with approximately 56% of the patients in the critical care unit experiencing it.[1] The mortality rate for patients with ALF is between 30% to 40%, with more than one third of patients not surviving to discharge.[3]

ALF results from a deficiency in the performance of the pulmonary system (Fig. 20-1).[2,4] It usually occurs secondary to another disorder that has altered the normal function of the pulmonary system in such a way as to decrease the ventilatory drive, decrease muscle strength, decrease chest wall elasticity, decrease the lung's capacity for gas exchange, increase airway resistance, or increase metabolic oxygen requirements.[1,5]

ALF can be classified as hypoxemic normocapnic respiratory failure (type I) or hypoxemic hypercapnic respiratory failure (type II), depending on analysis of the patient's arterial blood gases (ABGs). In type I respiratory failure, the patient presents with a low PaO_2 and a normal $PaCO_2$, whereas in type II respiratory failure, PaO_2 is low and $PaCO_2$ is high.[2,4]

Etiology

The etiologies of ALF may be classified as *extrapulmonary* or *intrapulmonary,* depending on the component of the respiratory system that is affected. Extrapulmonary causes include disorders that affect the brain, the spinal cord, the neuromuscular system, the thorax, the pleura, and the upper airways. Intrapulmonary causes include disorders that affect the lower airways and alveoli, the pulmonary circulation, and the alveolar-capillary membrane.[1,6] Table 20-1 lists the different etiologies of ALF and their associated disorders.

Pathophysiology

Hypoxemia is the result of impaired gas exchange and is the hallmark of ALF. Hypercapnia may be present, depending on the underlying cause of the problem. The main causes of hypoxemia are alveolar hypoventilation, ventilation/perfusion (V/Q) mismatching, and intrapulmonary shunting.[1,2,7] Type I respiratory failure usually results from V/Q mismatching and intrapulmonary shunting, whereas type II respiratory failure usually results from alveolar hypoventilation, which may or may not be accompanied by V/Q mismatching and intrapulmonary shunting.[2]

Alveolar Hypoventilation

Alveolar hypoventilation occurs when the amount of oxygen being brought into the alveoli is insufficient to meet the metabolic needs of the body.[6] This can be the result of

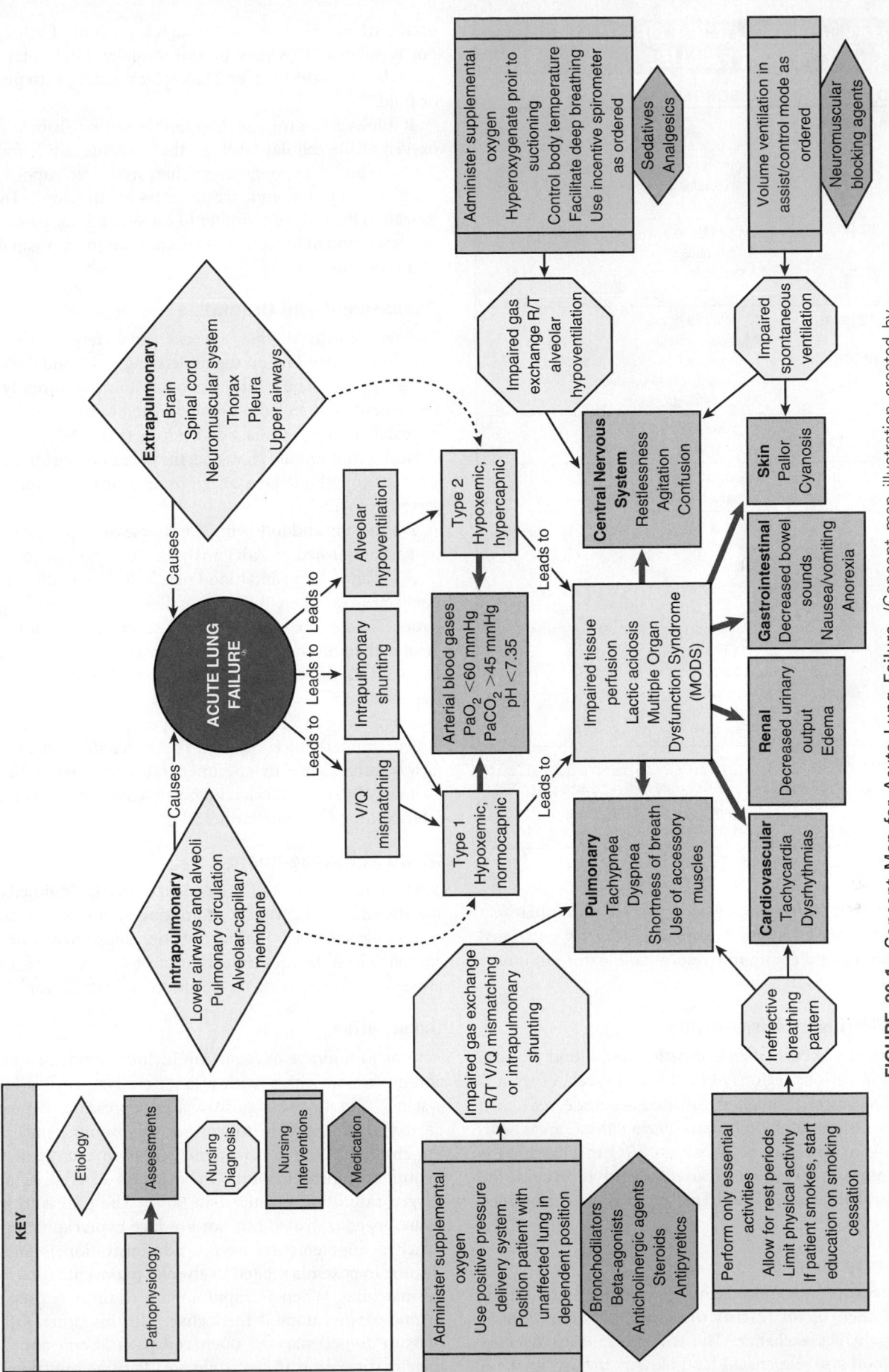

FIGURE 20-1 Concept Map for Acute Lung Failure. (Concept map illustration created by Elaine Bishop Kennedy, EdD, RN.)

TABLE 20-1	ETIOLOGIES OF ACUTE LUNG FAILURE	
AFFECTED AREA	**DISORDERS***
Extrapulmonary	
Brain	Drug overdose
	Central alveolar hypoventilation syndrome
	Brain trauma or lesion
	Postoperative anesthesia depression
Spinal cord	Guillain-Barré syndrome
	Poliomyelitis
	Amyotrophic lateral sclerosis
	Spinal cord trauma or lesion
Neuromuscular system	Myasthenia gravis
	Multiple sclerosis
	Neuromuscular-blocking antibiotics
	Organophosphate poisoning
	Muscular dystrophy
Thorax	Massive obesity
	Chest trauma
Pleura	Pleural effusion
	Pneumothorax
Upper airways	Sleep apnea
	Tracheal obstruction
	Epiglottitis
Intrapulmonary	
Lower airways and alveoli	Chronic obstructive pulmonary disease (COPD)
	Asthma
	Bronchiolitis
	Cystic fibrosis
	Pneumonia
Pulmonary circulation	Pulmonary emboli
Alveolar-capillary membrane	Acute respiratory distress syndrome (ARDS)
	Inhalation of toxic gases
	Near-drowning

*Not an inclusive list.

increasing metabolic oxygen needs or decreasing ventilation.[5] Hypoxemia caused by alveolar hypoventilation is associated with hypercapnia and commonly results from extrapulmonary disorders.[1,2,7]

Ventilation/Perfusion Mismatching

V/Q mismatching occurs when ventilation and blood flow are mismatched in various regions of the lung in excess of what is normal. Blood passes through alveoli that are underventilated for the given amount of perfusion, leaving these areas with a lower-than-normal amount of oxygen. V/Q mismatching is the most common cause of hypoxemia and is usually the result of alveoli that are partially collapsed or partially filled with fluid.[1,2,7]

Intrapulmonary Shunting

The extreme form of V/Q mismatching, intrapulmonary shunting, occurs when blood reaches the arterial system without participating in gas exchange. The mixing of unoxygenated (shunted) blood and oxygenated blood lowers the average level of oxygen present in the blood. Intrapulmonary shunting

occurs when blood passes through a portion of a lung that is not ventilated. This may be the result of 1) alveolar collapse secondary to atelectasis; or 2) alveolar flooding with pus, blood, or fluid.[1,2,7]

If allowed to progress, hypoxemia can result in a deficit of oxygen at the cellular level. As the tissue demands for oxygen continue and the supply diminishes, an oxygen supply/demand imbalance occurs and tissue hypoxia develops. Decreased oxygen to the cells contributes to impaired tissue perfusion and the development of lactic acidosis and multiple organ dysfunction syndrome.[8]

Assessment and Diagnosis

The patient with ALF may experience a variety of clinical manifestations, depending on the underlying cause and the extent of tissue hypoxia. The clinical manifestations commonly seen in the patient with ALF are usually related to the development of hypoxemia, hypercapnia, and acidosis (Fig. 20-2).[9] Because the clinical symptoms are so varied, they are not considered reliable in predicting the degree of hypoxemia or hypercapnia[2] or the severity of ALF.

Diagnosing and following the course of respiratory failure is best accomplished by ABG analysis. ABG analysis confirms the level of $Paco_2$, Pao_2, and blood pH. ALF is generally accepted as being present when the Pao_2 is less than 60 mm Hg. If the patient is also experiencing hypercapnia, the $Paco_2$ will be greater than 45 mm Hg. In patients with chronically elevated $Paco_2$ levels, these criteria must be broadened to include a pH less than 7.35.[9]

A variety of additional tests are performed depending on the patient's underlying condition. These include bronchoscopy for airway surveillance or specimen retrieval, chest radiography, thoracic ultrasound, thoracic computed tomography (CT), and selected lung function studies.[10]

Medical Management

Medical management of the patient with ALF is aimed at treating the underlying cause, promoting adequate gas exchange, correcting acidosis, initiating nutrition support, and preventing complications. Medical interventions to promote gas exchange are aimed at improving oxygenation and ventilation.[1]

Oxygenation

Actions to improve oxygenation include supplemental oxygen administration, either with a low flow system or a high flow system,[11] and the use of positive airway pressure.[12] The purpose of oxygen therapy is to correct hypoxemia, and although the absolute level of hypoxemia varies in each patient, most treatment approaches aim to keep the arterial hemoglobin oxygen saturation greater than 90%.[9] The goal is to keep the tissues' needs satisfied but not produce hypercapnia or oxygen toxicity.[9] Supplemental oxygen administration is effective in treating hypoxemia related to alveolar hypoventilation and V/Q mismatching. When intrapulmonary shunting exists, supplemental oxygen alone is ineffective.[11] In this situation, positive pressure is necessary to open collapsed alveoli and facilitate their participation in gas exchange. Positive pressure is delivered via invasive and noninvasive mechanical ventilation. To

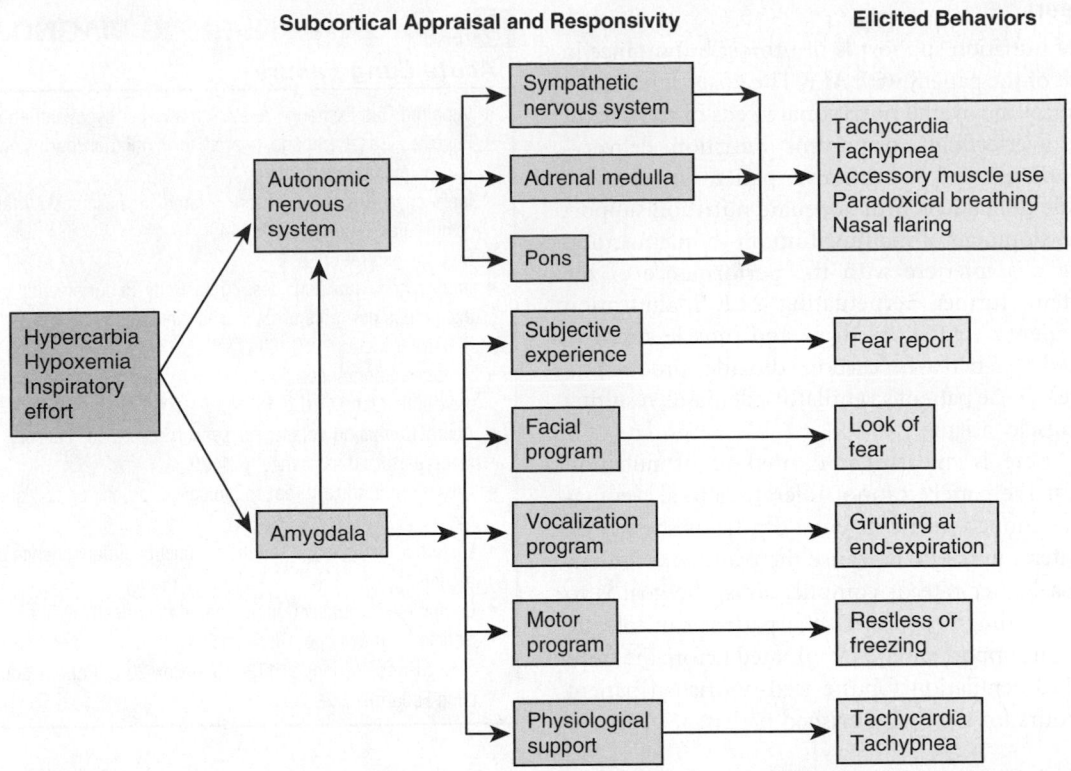

Subcortical Appraisal and Responsivity

Elicited Behaviors

FIGURE 20-2 Model of Respiratory Distress Behaviors Activated from Subcortical Stimulation. (From Campbell ML. Respiratory distress: a model of responses and behaviors to an asphyxial threat for patients who are unable to self-report. *Heart Lung.* 2008;37:53.)

avoid intubation, positive pressure is usually administered initially noninvasively via a mask.[13] For further information on supplemental oxygen therapy and noninvasive ventilation, see Chapter 21.

Ventilation

Interventions to improve ventilation include the use of noninvasive and invasive mechanical ventilation. Depending on the underlying cause and the severity of the ALF, the patient may be treated initially with noninvasive ventilation.[13] However, one study found that those patients with a pH of less than 7.25 at initial presentation had an increased likelihood of the need for invasive mechanical ventilation.[14] The selection of ventilatory mode and settings depends on the patient's underlying condition, severity of respiratory failure, and body size. Initially the patient is started on volume ventilation in the assist/control mode. In the patient with chronic hypercapnia, the settings should be adjusted to keep the ABG values within the parameters expected to be maintained by the patient after extubation.[15] For further information on mechanical ventilation see Chapter 21.

Pharmacology

Medications to facilitate dilation of the airways may also be of benefit in the treatment of the patient with ALF. Bronchodilators, such as beta$_2$-agonists and anticholinergic agents, aid in smooth muscle relaxation and are of particular benefit to patients with airflow limitations. Methylxanthines, such as aminophylline, are no longer recommended because of their negative side effects. Steroids also are often administered to decrease

airway inflammation and enhance the effects of the beta$_2$-agonists. Mucolytics and expectorants are also no longer used since they have been found to be of no benefit in this patient population.[16]

Sedation is necessary in many patients to assist with maintaining adequate ventilation. It can be used to comfort the patient and decrease the work of breathing, particularly if the patient is fighting the ventilator. Analgesics should be administered for pain control.[17,18] In some patients, sedation does not decrease spontaneous respiratory efforts enough to allow adequate ventilation. Neuromuscular paralysis may be necessary to facilitate optimal ventilation. Paralysis also may be necessary to decrease oxygen consumption in the severely compromised patient.[18]

Acidosis

Acidosis may occur in the patient for a number of reasons. Hypoxemia causes impaired tissue perfusion, which leads to the production of lactic acid and the development of metabolic acidosis. Impaired ventilation leads to the accumulation of carbon dioxide and the development of respiratory acidosis. Once the patient is adequately oxygenated and ventilated, the acidosis should correct itself. The use of sodium bicarbonate to correct the acidosis has been shown to be of minimal benefit to the patient and thus is no longer recommended as first-line treatment. Bicarbonate therapy shifts the oxygen-hemoglobin dissociation curve to the left and can worsen tissue hypoxia. Sodium bicarbonate may be used if the acidosis is severe (pH less than 7.1), refractory to therapy, and causing dysrhythmias or hemodynamic instability.[19]

Nutrition Support

The initiation of nutrition support is of utmost importance in the management of the patient with ALF. The goals of nutrition support are to meet the overall nutritional needs of the patient while avoiding overfeeding, to prevent nutrition delivery-related complications, and to improve patient outcomes.[20] Failure to provide the patient with adequate nutrition support results in the development of malnutrition. Both malnutrition and overfeeding can interfere with the performance of the pulmonary system, further perpetuating ALF. Malnutrition decreases the patient's ventilatory drive and muscle strength, whereas overfeeding increases carbon dioxide production, which then increases the patient's ventilatory demand, resulting in respiratory muscle fatigue.[21]

The enteral route is the preferred method of nutrition administration. If the patient cannot tolerate enteral feedings or cannot receive enough nutrients enterally, he or she will be started on parenteral nutrition. Because the parenteral route is associated with a higher rate of complications, the goal is to switch to enteral feedings as soon as the patient can tolerate them.[20,21] Nutrition support should be initiated before the third day of mechanical ventilation for the well-nourished patient and within 24 hours for the malnourished patient.[20,21]

Complications

The patient with ALF may experience a number of complications including ischemic-anoxic encephalopathy,[22] cardiac dysrhythmias,[23] venous thromboembolism (VTE),[24] and gastrointestinal bleeding.[25] Ischemic-anoxic encephalopathy results from hypoxemia, hypercapnia, and acidosis.[22] Dysrhythmias are precipitated by hypoxemia, acidosis, electrolyte imbalances, and the administration of beta$_2$-agonists.[23] Maintaining oxygenation, normalizing electrolytes, and monitoring medication levels will facilitate the prevention and treatment of encephalopathy and dysrhythmias.[22,23] VTE is precipitated by venous stasis resulting from immobility and can be prevented through the use of intermittent pneumatic compression devices and low-dose unfractionated heparin or low–molecular-weight heparin (LMWH).[24] Gastrointestinal bleeding can be prevented through the use of histamine receptor antagonists, cytoprotective agents, or proton pump inhibitors.[25] In addition, the patient is at risk for the complications associated with an artificial airway, mechanical ventilation, enteral and parenteral nutrition, and peripheral arterial cannulation.

Nursing Management

Nursing management of the patient with ALF incorporates a variety of nursing diagnoses (Box 20-1). Nursing care is directed by the specific cause of the respiratory failure, although some common interventions are used. The nurse has a significant role in optimizing oxygenation and ventilation, providing comfort and emotional support, maintaining surveillance for complications, and educating the patient and family.

Optimizing Oxygenation and Ventilation

Nursing interventions to optimize oxygenation and ventilation include positioning, preventing desaturation, and promoting secretion clearance.

Positioning. Positioning of the patient with ALF depends on the type of lung injury and the underlying cause of hypoxemia. For those patients with V/Q mismatching, positioning is used to facilitate better matching of ventilation with perfusion to optimize gas exchange.[26] Because gravity normally facilitates preferential ventilation and perfusion to the dependent areas of the lungs, the best gas exchange would take place in the dependent areas of the lungs.[11] Thus the goal of positioning is to place the least affected area of the patient's lung in the most dependent position. Patients with unilateral lung disease should be positioned with the healthy lung in a dependent position.[26,27] Patients with diffuse lung disease may benefit from being positioned with the right lung down, because it is larger and more vascular than the left lung.[27,28] For those patients with alveolar hypoventilation, the goal of positioning is to facilitate ventilation. These patients benefit from nonrecumbent positions such as sitting or a semierect position.[29] In addition, semirecumbency has been shown to decrease the risk of aspiration and inhibit the development of hospital-associated pneumonia.[30] Frequent repositioning (at least every 2 hours) is beneficial in optimizing the patient's ventilatory pattern and V/Q matching.[31]

Preventing Desaturation. A number of activities can prevent desaturation from occurring. These include performing procedures only as needed, hyperoxygenating the patient before suctioning, providing adequate rest and recovery time between various procedures, and minimizing oxygen consumption. Interventions to minimize oxygen consumption include limiting the patient's physical activity, administering sedation to control anxiety, and providing measures to control fever.[29] The patient should be continuously monitored with a pulse oximeter to warn of signs of desaturation.

Promoting Secretion Clearance. Interventions to promote secretion clearance include providing adequate systemic hydration, humidifying supplemental oxygen, coughing, and suctioning. Postural drainage and chest percussion and vibration have been found to be of little benefit in the critically ill patient[32,33] and thus are not discussed here.

To facilitate deep breathing, the patient's thorax should be maintained in alignment and the head of the bed elevated 30 to 45 degrees. This position best accommodates diaphragmatic descent and intercostal muscle action.

Once the patient is extubated, deep breathing and incentive spirometry should be started as soon as possible. Deep breathing involves having the patient take a deep breath and holding it for approximately 3 seconds or longer. Incentive spirometry involves having the patient take at least 10 deep, effective breaths per hour using an incentive spirometer. These actions help prevent atelectasis and re-expand any collapsed lung tissue. The chest should be auscultated during inflation to ensure that all dependent parts of the lung are well ventilated and to help the patient understand the depth of breath necessary for optimal effect. Coughing should be avoided unless secretions are present because it promotes collapse of the smaller airways.

Educating the Patient and Family

Early in the patient's hospital stay, the patient and family should be taught about ALF, its etiologies, and its treatment. As the patient moves toward discharge, teaching should focus on the interventions necessary for preventing the reoccurrence of the precipitating disorder (Box 20-2). If the patient smokes, he or she should be encouraged to stop smoking and be referred to a smoking cessation program (Box 20-3). In addition, the importance of participating in a pulmonary rehabilitation program should be stressed.

Collaborative management of the patient with ALF is outlined in Box 20-4.

BOX 20-2　PATIENT EDUCATION

Acute Lung Failure

- Pathophysiology of disease
- Specific etiology
- Precipitating factor modification
- Importance of taking medications
- Breathing techniques (e.g., pursed-lip breathing, diaphragmatic breathing)
- Energy conservation techniques
- Measures to prevent pulmonary infections (e.g., proper nutrition, hand washing, immunization against *Streptococcus pneumoniae* and influenza viruses)
- Signs and symptoms of pulmonary infections (e.g., sputum color change, shortness of breath, fever)
- Cough enhancement techniques (e.g., cascade cough, huff cough, end-expiratory cough, augmented cough)

Additional information for the patient can be found at the following websites:

American Lung Association: **http://www.lung.org**

Smokefree.gov: **http://smokefree.gov**

Healthfinder—U.S. Department of Health and Human Services: **http://healthfinder.gov**

WebMD: **http://www.webmd.com**

NHLBI ARDS Network: **http://www.ardsnet.org**

The ARDS Foundation: **http://www.ardsusa.org/facts.htm**

ACUTE RESPIRATORY DISTRESS SYNDROME

Description

Acute respiratory distress syndrome (ARDS) is a systemic process that is considered to be the pulmonary manifestation of multiple organ dysfunction syndrome.[34] It is characterized by noncardiac pulmonary edema and disruption of the alveolar-capillary membrane as a result of injury to either the pulmonary vasculature or the airways.[35]

Many different diagnostic criteria have been used to identify ARDS, which has led to confusion, particularly among researchers. In 2012, in an attempt to address the limitations of the existing definition of ARDS, the ARDS Definition Task Force drafted a new definition (known as the Berlin Definition) of ARDS. This definition eliminated the term "acute lung injury" and proposed three distinct categories (mild, moderate, and severe) of ARDS based on the severity of hypoxemia. The Berlin Definition of ARDS is as follows:

- Timing—within 1 week of known clinical insult or new or worsening respiratory symptoms
- Chest imaging—bilateral opacities not fully explained by effusions, lobar/lung collapse or nodules
- Origin of edema—respiratory failure not fully explained by heart failure or fluid overload; need objective assessment to exclude hydrostatic edema if no risk factor present
- Oxygenation—mild (200 mg Hg less than Pao_2/Fio_2 less than or equal to 300 mm Hg with positive end-respiratory airway pressure [PEEP] or constant positive airway pressure [CPAP] greater than or equal to 5 cm H_2O); Moderate (100 mg Hg less than Pao_2/Fio_2 less than or equal to 200 mm Hg with PEEP greater than or equal to 5 cm H_2O); or Severe (Pao_2/Fio_2 less than or equal to 100 mm Hg with PEEP greater than or equal to 5 cm H_2O).[36]

The mortality rate for ARDS is estimated to be 34% to 58%.[37]

Etiology

A wide variety of clinical conditions is associated with the development of ARDS. These are categorized as *direct* or *indirect*, depending on the primary site of injury (Box 20-5).[35,38] Direct injuries are those in which the lung epithelium sustains a direct insult. Indirect injuries are those in which the insult occurs elsewhere in the body and mediators are transmitted via the bloodstream to the lungs. Sepsis, aspiration of gastric contents, diffuse pneumonia, and trauma were found to be major risk factors for the development of ARDS.[37]

Pathophysiology

The progression of ARDS can be described in three phases: exudative, fibroproliferative, and resolution. ARDS is initiated with stimulation of the inflammatory-immune system as a result of a direct or indirect injury (Fig. 20-3). Inflammatory mediators are released from the site of injury, resulting in the activation and accumulation of the neutrophils, macrophages, and platelets in the pulmonary capillaries. These cellular mediators initiate the release of humoral mediators that cause damage to the alveolar-capillary membrane.[38]

BOX 20-3 EVIDENCE-BASED PRACTICE

Smoking Cessation Guidelines

QSEN The following are the key recommendations of the updated guideline *Treating Tobacco Use and Dependence,* based on the literature review and expert panel opinion:

1. Tobacco dependence is a chronic disease that often requires repeated intervention and multiple attempts to quit. Effective treatments exist, however, that can significantly increase rates of long-term abstinence.
2. It is essential that clinicians and health care delivery systems consistently identify and document tobacco use status and treat every tobacco user seen in a health care setting.
3. Tobacco dependence treatments are effective across a broad range of populations. Clinicians should encourage every patient willing to make a quit attempt to use the counseling treatments and medications recommended in this Guideline.
4. Brief tobacco dependence treatment is effective. Clinicians should offer every patient who uses tobacco at least the brief treatments shown to be effective in this Guideline.
5. Individual, group, and telephone counseling are effective, and their effectiveness increases with treatment intensity. Two components of counseling are especially effective, and clinicians should use these when counseling patients making a quit attempt:
- Practical counseling (problem solving/skills training)
- Social support delivered as part of treatment
6. Numerous effective medications are available for tobacco dependence, and clinicians should encourage their use by all patients attempting to quit smoking—except when medically contraindicated or with specific populations for which there is insufficient evidence of effectiveness (i.e., pregnant women, smokeless tobacco users, light smokers, and adolescents).

- Seven first-line medications (5 nicotine and 2 non-nicotine) reliably increase long-term smoking abstinence rates:
  - Bupropion SR
  - Nicotine gum
  - Nicotine inhaler
  - Nicotine lozenge
  - Nicotine nasal spray
  - Nicotine patch
  - Varenicline
- Clinicians also should consider the use of certain combinations of medications identified as effective in this Guideline.
7. Counseling and medication are effective when used by themselves for treating tobacco dependence. The combination of counseling and medication, however, is more effective than either alone. Thus, clinicians should encourage all individuals making a quit attempt to use both counseling and medication.
8. Telephone quitline counseling is effective with diverse populations and has broad reach. Therefore, clinicians and health care delivery systems should both ensure patient access to quitlines and promote quitline use.
9. If a tobacco user currently is unwilling to make a quit attempt, clinicians should use the motivational treatments shown in this Guideline to be effective in increasing future quit attempts.
10. Tobacco dependence treatments are both clinically effective and highly cost-effective relative to interventions for other clinical disorders. Providing coverage for these treatments increases quit rates. Insurers and purchasers should ensure that all insurance plans include the counseling and medication identified as effective in this Guideline as covered benefits.

From Fiore MC, et al. *Treating Tobacco Use and Dependence: 2008 Update* (Clinical Practice Guideline). Rockville, MD: U.S. Department of Health and Human Services, Public Health Service; 2008. Available from http://www.ncbi.nlm.nih.gov/books/NBK63952/.

BOX 20-4 COLLABORATIVE MANAGEMENT

Acute Lung Failure

- Identify and treat underlying cause.
- Administer oxygen therapy.
- Intubate patient.
- Initiate mechanical ventilation.
- Administer medications:
  - Bronchodilators
  - Steroids
  - Sedatives
  - Analgesics
- Position patient to optimize ventilation/perfusion matching.
- Suction as needed.
- Provide adequate rest and recovery time between various procedures.
- Correct acidosis.
- Initiate nutritional support.
- Maintain surveillance for complications:
  - Encephalopathy
  - Cardiac dysrhythmias
  - Venous thromboembolism
  - Gastrointestinal bleeding
- Provide comfort and emotional support.

BOX 20-5 RISK FACTORS FOR ACUTE RESPIRATORY DISTRESS SYNDROME

Direct Injury

Aspiration
Near-drowning
Toxic inhalation
Pulmonary contusion
Pneumonia
Oxygen toxicity
Transthoracic radiation

Indirect Injury

Sepsis
Nonthoracic trauma
Hypertransfusion
Cardiopulmonary bypass
Severe pancreatitis
Embolism—air, fat, amniotic fluid
Disseminated intravascular coagulation (DIC)
Shock states

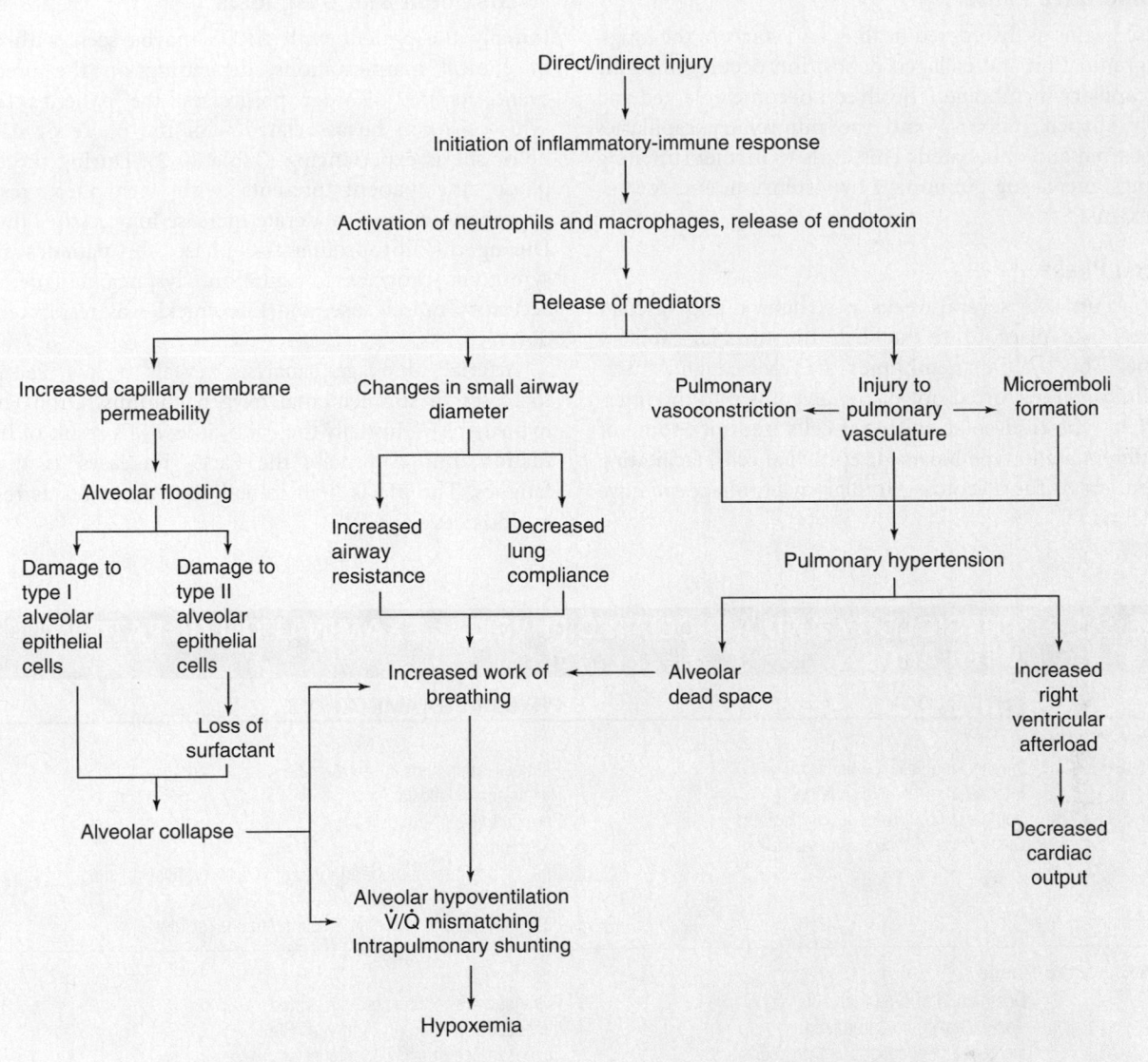

Direct/indirect injury

Initiation of inflammatory-immune response

Activation of neutrophils and macrophages, release of endotoxin

Release of mediators

Increased capillary membrane permeability

Alveolar flooding

Damage to type I alveolar epithelial cells

Damage to type II alveolar epithelial cells

Loss of surfactant

Alveolar collapse

Changes in small airway diameter

Increased airway resistance

Decreased lung compliance

Increased work of breathing

Alveolar hypoventilation
$\dot{V}/\dot{Q}$ mismatching
Intrapulmonary shunting

Hypoxemia

Pulmonary vasoconstriction ← Injury to pulmonary vasculature → Microemboli formation

Pulmonary hypertension

Alveolar dead space

Increased right ventricular afterload

Decreased cardiac output

FIGURE 20-3 Pathophysiology of Acute Respiratory Distress Syndrome.

Exudative Phase

Within the first 72 hours after the initial insult, the exudative phase or acute phase ensues. Once released, the mediators cause injury to the pulmonary capillaries, resulting in increased capillary membrane permeability leading to the leakage of fluid filled with protein, blood cells, fibrin, and activated cellular and humoral mediators into the pulmonary interstitium. Damage to the pulmonary capillaries also causes the development of microthrombi and elevation of pulmonary artery pressures. As fluid enters the pulmonary interstitium, the lymphatics are overwhelmed and unable to drain all the accumulating fluid, resulting in the development of interstitial edema. Fluid is then forced from the interstitial space into the alveoli, resulting in alveolar edema. Pulmonary interstitial edema also causes compression of the alveoli and small airways. Alveolar edema causes swelling of the type I alveolar epithelial cells and flooding of the alveoli. Protein and fibrin in the edema fluid precipitate the formation of hyaline membranes over the alveoli. Eventually, the type II alveolar epithelial cells are also damaged, leading to

impaired surfactant production. Injury to the alveolar epithelial cells and the loss of surfactant lead to further alveolar collapse.[38,39]

Hypoxemia occurs as a result of intrapulmonary shunting and V/Q mismatching secondary to compression, collapse, and flooding of the alveoli and small airways. Increased work of breathing occurs as a result of increased airway resistance, decreased functional residual capacity (FRC), and decreased lung compliance secondary to atelectasis and compression of the small airways. Hypoxemia and the increased work of breathing lead to patient fatigue and the development of alveolar hypoventilation. Pulmonary hypertension occurs as a result of damage to the pulmonary capillaries, microthrombi, and hypoxic vasoconstriction leading to the development of increased alveolar dead space and right ventricular afterload. Hypoxemia worsens as a result of alveolar hypoventilation and increased alveolar dead space. Right ventricular afterload increases and leads to right ventricular dysfunction and a decrease in cardiac output (CO).[38]

Fibroproliferative Phase

This phase begins as disordered healing and starts in the lungs. Cellular granulation and collagen deposition occur within the alveolar-capillary membrane. The alveoli become enlarged and irregularly shaped (fibrotic) and the pulmonary capillaries become scarred and obliterated. This leads to further stiffening of the lungs, increasing pulmonary hypertension, and continued hypoxemia.[38,39]

Resolution Phase

Recovery occurs over several weeks as structural and vascular remodeling take place to re-establish the alveolar-capillary membrane. The hyaline membranes are cleared and intra-alveolar fluid is transported out of the alveolus into the interstitium. The type II alveolar epithelial cells multiply, some of which differentiate to type I alveolar epithelial cells, facilitating the restoration of the alveolus. Alveolar macrophages remove cellular debris.[38,39]

Assessment and Diagnosis

Initially the patient with ARDS maybe seen with a variety of clinical manifestations, depending on the precipitating event. As the disorder progresses, the patient's signs and symptoms can be associated with the phase of ARDS that he or she is experiencing (Table 20-2). During the exudative phase, the patient presents with tachypnea, restlessness, apprehension, and moderate increase in accessory muscle use. During the fibroproliferative phase, the patient's signs and symptoms progress to agitation, dyspnea, fatigue, excessive accessory muscle use, and fine crackles as respiratory failure develops.[40,41]

Arterial blood-gas analysis reveals a low Pao_2, despite increases in supplemental oxygen administration (refractory hypoxemia).[40] Initially the $Paco_2$ is low as a result of hyperventilation, but eventually the $Paco_2$ increases as the patient fatigues. The pH is high initially but decreases as respiratory acidosis develops.[40,41]

TABLE 20-2	PHYSIOLOGY AND ASSOCIATED PHYSICAL EXAMINATION OF PATIENT WITH ARDS	
PHASE	**PHYSIOLOGY**	**PHYSICAL EXAMINATION**
Exudative Phase		
	Parenchymal surface hemorrhage	Restless, apprehensive, tachypneic
	Interstitial or alveolar edema	Respiratory alkalosis
	Compression of terminal bronchioles	Pao_2 normal
	Destruction of type I alveolar cells	CXR: normal
		Chest examination: moderate use of accessory muscles, lungs clear
		Pulmonary artery pressures: elevated
		Pulmonary artery occlusion pressure: normal or low
Fibroproliferative Phase		
	Destruction of type II alveolar cells	Pulmonary artery pressures: elevated
	Gas exchange compromised	Increased workload on right ventricle
	Increased peak inspiratory pressure	Increased use of accessory muscles
	Decreased compliance (static and dynamic)	Fine crackles
		Increasing agitation related to hypoxia
	Refractory hypoxemia:	CXR: interstitial or alveolar infiltrates; elevated diaphragm
	• Intra-alveolar atelectasis	Hyperventilation; hypercarbia
	• Increased shunt fraction	Decreased Svo_2
	• Decreased diffusion	Widening alveolar-arterial gradient
	Decreased functional residual capacity	Increased work of breathing
	Interstitial fibrosis	Worsening hypercarbia and hypoxemia
	Increased dead space ventilation	Lactic acidosis (related to aerobic metabolism)
		Alteration in perfusion:
		• Increased heart rate
		• Decreased blood pressure
		• Change in skin temperature and color
		• Decreased capillary filling
		End-organ dysfunction:
		• Brain: change in mentation, agitation, hallucinations
		• Heart: decreased cardiac output→angina, HF, papillary muscle dysfunction, dysrhythmias, MI
		• Renal: decreased urinary or GFR
		• Skin: mottled, ischemic
		• Liver: elevated SGOT, bilirubin, alkaline phosphatase, PT/PTT; decreased albumin

Modified from Phillips JK. Management of patients with acute respiratory distress syndrome. *Crit Care Nurs Clin North Am.*1999;11(2):233.
ARDS, acute respiratory distress syndrome; *PaO₂,* arterial oxygen pressure; *CXR,* chest radiograph; *SvO₂,* venous oxygen saturation; *HF,* heart failure; *MI,* myocardial infarction; *GFR,* glomerular filtration rate; *SGOT,* serum glutamate oxaloacetate transaminase; *PT,* prothrombin time; *PTT,* partial thromboplastin time.

Initially the chest x-ray film may be normal, because changes in the lungs do not become evident for up to 24 hours. As the pulmonary edema becomes apparent, diffuse, patchy interstitial and alveolar infiltrates appear. This progresses to multifocal consolidation of the lungs, which appears as a "whiteout" on the chest x-ray film.[40]

Medical Management

Medical management of the patient with ARDS involves a multifaceted approach. This strategy includes treating the underlying cause, promoting gas exchange, supporting tissue oxygenation, and preventing complications. Given the severity of hypoxemia, the patient is intubated and mechanically ventilated to facilitate adequate gas exchange.[42]

Ventilation

Traditionally the patient with ARDS was ventilated with a mode of volume ventilation, such as assist/control ventilation (A/CV) or synchronized intermittent mandatory ventilation (SIMV), with tidal volumes adjusted to deliver 10 to 15 mL/kg. Current research now indicates that this approach may have actually led to further lung injury. It is now known that repeated opening and closing of the alveoli cause injury to the lung units (atelectrauma), resulting in inhibited surfactant production, and increased inflammation (biotrauma), resulting in the release of mediators and an increase in pulmonary capillary membrane permeability. In addition, excessive pressure in the alveoli (barotrauma) or excessive volume in the alveoli (volutrauma) leads to excessive alveolar wall stress and damage to the alveolar-capillary membrane, resulting in air escaping into the surrounding spaces.[42] Thus several different approaches have been developed to facilitate the mechanical ventilation of the patient with ARDS.

Low Tidal Volume. Low tidal volume ventilation uses smaller tidal volumes (6 mL/kg) to ventilate the patient, in an attempt to limit the effects of barotrauma and volutrauma. The goal is to provide the maximum tidal volume possible while maintaining end-inspiratory plateau pressure less than 30 cm H_2O. To allow for adequate carbon dioxide elimination, the respiratory rate is increased to 20 to 30 breaths/min.[42,43]

Permissive Hypercapnia. Permissive hypercapnia uses low tidal volume ventilation in conjunction with normal respiratory rates, in an attempt to limit the effects of atelectrauma and biotrauma. Normally, to maintain normocapnia the patient's respiratory rate would have to be increased to compensate for the small tidal volume. In ARDS though, increasing the respiratory rate can lead to worsening alveolar damage. Thus the patient's carbon dioxide level is allowed to rise, and the patient becomes hypercapnic. As a general rule, the patient's $Paco_2$ should not rise faster than 10 mm Hg per hour and overall should not exceed 80 to 100 mg Hg. Because of the negative cardiopulmonary effects of severe acidosis, the arterial pH is generally maintained at 7.20 or greater. To maintain the pH, the patient is given intravenous sodium bicarbonate or the respiratory rate and/or tidal volume are increased. Permissive hypercapnia is contraindicated in patients with increased intracranial pressure, pulmonary hypertension, seizures, and heart failure.[44]

Pressure Control Ventilation. In pressure control ventilation (PCV) mode, each breath is delivered or augmented with a preset amount of inspiratory pressure as opposed to tidal volume, which is used in volume ventilation. Thus the actual tidal volume the patient receives varies from breath to breath. PCV is used to limit and control the amount of pressure in the lungs and decrease the incidence of volutrauma. The goal is to keep the patient's plateau pressure (end-inspiratory static pressure) lower than 30 cm H_2O. A known problem with this mode of ventilation is that as the patient's lungs get stiffer, it becomes harder and harder to maintain an adequate tidal volume and severe hypercapnia can occur.[42,43]

Inverse Ratio Ventilation. Another alternative ventilatory mode that is used in managing the patient with ARDS is inverse ratio ventilation (IRV), either pressure controlled or volume controlled. IRV prolongs the inspiratory (I) time and shortens the expiratory (E) time, thus reversing the normal I : E ratio. The goal of IRV is to maintain a more constant mean airway pressure throughout the ventilatory cycle, which helps keep alveoli open and participating in gas exchange. It also increases FRC and decreases the work of breathing. In addition, as the breath is delivered over a longer period of time, the peak inspiratory pressure in the lungs is decreased. A major disadvantage to IRV is the development of auto–PEEP. As the expiratory phase of ventilation is shortened, air can become trapped in the lower airways, creating unintentional PEEP (or auto-PEEP), which can cause hemodynamic compromise and worsening gas exchange. Patients on IRV usually require heavy sedation with neuromuscular blockade to prevent them from fighting the ventilator.[42,43]

High-Frequency Oscillatory Ventilation. Another alternative ventilatory mode that is used in patients who remain severely hypoxemic despite the treatments previously described is high-frequency oscillatory ventilation (HFOV). The goal of this method of ventilation is similar to that of IRV in that it uses a constant airway pressure to promote alveolar recruitment while avoiding overdistention of the alveoli. HFOV uses a piston pump to deliver very low tidal volumes at very high rates or oscillations (300 to 3000 breaths/min).[45]

Oxygen Therapy

Oxygen is administered at the lowest level possible to support tissue oxygenation. Continued exposure to high levels of oxygen can lead to oxygen toxicity, which perpetuates the entire process. The goal of oxygen therapy is to maintain an arterial hemoglobin oxygen saturation of 90% or greater using the lowest level of oxygen—preferably less than 0.50.[35]

Positive End-Expiratory Pressure. Because the hypoxemia that develops with ARDS is often refractory or unresponsive to oxygen therapy, it is necessary to facilitate oxygenation with PEEP. The purpose of using PEEP in the patient with ARDS is to improve oxygenation while reducing Fio_2 to less toxic levels. PEEP has several positive effects on the lungs, including opening collapsed alveoli, stabilizing flooded alveoli, and increasing FRC. Thus PEEP decreases intrapulmonary shunting and increases compliance. PEEP also has several negative effects including: 1) decreasing CO as a result of decreasing venous return secondary to increased intrathoracic pressure; and 2) barotrauma, as a result of gas escaping into the surrounding spaces secondary to alveolar rupture. The amount of PEEP a patient requires is determined by evaluating both arterial hemoglobin oxygen saturation and CO. In most cases, a PEEP of 10 to 15 cm H_2O is adequate. If PEEP is too high, it can result in overdistention of the alveoli, which can impede pulmonary capillary blood flow, decrease surfactant production, and worsen intrapulmonary shunting. If PEEP is too low, it allows the alveoli to collapse during expiration, which can result in more damage to alveoli.[42]

Extracorporeal and Intracorporeal Gas Exchange. Extracorporeal and intracorporeal gas exchanges are last-resort techniques used in the treatment of severe ARDS when conventional therapy has failed. These methods allow the lungs to rest by facilitating the removal of carbon dioxide and providing oxygen external to the lungs by means of an "artificial lung," or membrane/fiber oxygenator. Extracorporeal membrane oxygenation (ECMO), extracorporeal carbon dioxide removal ($ECCO_2R$), and intravascular oxygenation (IVOX) are three techniques that employ this type of technology. ECMO is similar to cardiopulmonary bypass in that blood is removed from the body and pumped through a membrane oxygenator, where CO_2 is removed and O_2 is added, and then returned to the body. $ECCO_2R$ is a variation of ECMO in which the primary focus is removal of CO_2. IVOX facilitates oxygenation and ventilation with the use of a fiber oxygenator that is implanted in the inferior vena cava. All of these techniques pose serious bleeding problems to the patient, and none has been shown to improve patient outcome.[46,47]

Tissue Perfusion

Adequate tissue perfusion depends on an adequate supply of oxygen being transported to the tissues. An adequate CO and hemoglobin level is critical to oxygen transport. CO depends on heart rate, preload, afterload, and contractility. A variety of fluids and medications are used to manipulate this parameter. Newer approaches to fluid management include maintaining a very low intravascular volume (pulmonary artery occlusion pressure of 5 to 8 mm Hg) with fluid restriction and diuretics, while supporting the CO with vasoactive and inotropic medications. The goal is to decrease the amount of fluid leakage into the lungs.[48]

Nursing Management

Nursing management of the patient with ARDS incorporates a variety of nursing diagnoses (Box 20-6). Nursing interventions include optimizing oxygenation and ventilation, providing comfort and emotional support, and maintaining surveillance for complications.

Optimizing Oxygenation and Ventilation

Nursing interventions to optimize oxygenation and ventilation include positioning, preventing desaturation, and promoting secretion clearance. For further discussion on these interventions, see Nursing Management of Acute Lung Failure earlier in this chapter. One additional nursing intervention that can be used to improve the oxygenation and ventilation of the patient with ARDS is prone positioning.

⊚ BOX 20-6 NURSING DIAGNOSES
Acute Respiratory Distress Syndrome

- Impaired Gas Exchange related to ventilation/perfusion mismatching or intrapulmonary shunting, p. 1144
- Decreased Cardiac Output related to alterations in preload, p. 1128
- Imbalanced Nutrition: Less Than Body Requirements related to lack of exogenous nutrients or increased metabolic demand, p. 1143
- Risk for Aspiration, p. 1154
- Risk for Infection, p. 1160
- Anxiety related to threat to biological, psychological, and/or social integrity, p. 1125
- Disturbed Body Image related to functional dependence on life-sustaining technology, p. 1136
- Compromised Family Coping related to critically ill family member, p. 1127

Prone Positioning. A number of studies have shown that prone positioning the patient with ARDS results in an improvement in oxygenation. Although a number of theories propose how prone positioning improves oxygenation, the discovery that with ARDS there is greater damage to the dependent areas of the lungs probably provides the best explanation. It was originally thought that ARDS was a diffuse homogenous disease that affected all areas of the lungs equally. It is now known that the dependent lung areas are more heavily damaged than the nondependent lung areas. Turning the patient prone improves perfusion to less damaged parts of lungs and improves V/Q matching and decreases intrapulmonary shunting. Prone positioning appears to be more effective when initiated during the early phases of ARDS.[49] For more information on prone positioning see Chapter 21.

Collaborative management of the patient with ARDS is outlined in Box 20-7.

PNEUMONIA

Description

Pneumonia is an acute inflammation of the lung parenchyma that is caused by an infectious agent that can lead to alveolar consolidation. Pneumonia can be classified as community-acquired pneumonia (CAP), hospital-acquired pneumonia (HAP), or health care-associated pneumonia (HCAP).[50] Pneumonia is referred to as community-acquired when it occurs outside of the hospital or within 48 hours of admission to the hospital.[51] Severe CAP requires admission to the critical care unit and accounts for about 22% of all patients with pneumonia. The mortality for this patient group is approximately 18% to 56%, with increasing age as a major risk factor.[52] Pneumonia is referred to as hospital-acquired when it occurs while in the hospital for at least 48 hours.[50] Ventilator-associated pneumonia (VAP) is a subgrouping of HAP that refers to development of pneumonia after the insertion of an artificial airway.[50] VAP is the most common critical care unit-acquired infection.[53] Pneumonia is referred to as health care-associated when it is acquired in health care environments outside of the traditional hospital setting.[54]

BOX 20-7 COLLABORATIVE MANAGEMENT

Acute Respiratory Distress Syndrome (ARDS)

- Administer oxygen therapy.
- Intubate patient.
- Initiate mechanical ventilation:
  - Permissive hypercapnia
  - Pressure control ventilation
  - Inverse ratio ventilation
- Use PEEP.
- Administer medications:
  - Bronchodilators
  - Sedatives
  - Analgesics
  - Neuromuscular blocking agents
- Maximize cardiac output:
  - Preload
  - Afterload
  - Contractility
- Prone patient.
- Suction as needed.
- Provide adequate rest and recovery time between various procedures.
- Initiate nutritional support.
- Maintain surveillance for complications:
  - Encephalopathy
  - Cardiac dysrhythmias
  - Venous thromboembolism
  - Gastrointestinal bleeding
  - Atelectrauma
  - Biotrauma
  - Volutrauma
  - Barotrauma
  - Oxygen toxicity
- Provide comfort and emotional support.

BOX 20-8 RISK FACTORS FOR HOSPITAL-ACQUIRED PNEUMONIA

Host-Related
Advanced age
Altered level of consciousness
Chronic obstructive pulmonary disease
Altered immune system
Severity of illness
Poor nutrition
Hemodynamic compromise
Trauma
Smoking
Dental plaque

Treatment-Related
Mechanical ventilation
Endotracheal intubation
Unintentional extubation
Bronchoscopy
Nasogastric tube
Previous antibiotic therapy
Elevated gastric pH secondary to histamine receptor antagonists, proton pump inhibitors, and enteral feedings
Upper abdominal surgery
Thoracic surgery
Supine position

Infection Control-Related
Poor hand-washing practices

pathogens most frequently associated with VAP are *S. aureus* and *P. aeruginosa*. Risk factors for HAP can be categorized as host-related, treatment-related, and infection control-related (Box 20-8).[55]

Etiology

The spectra of etiologic pathogens of pneumonia vary with the type of pneumonia, as do the risk factors for the disease.

Severe Community-Acquired Pneumonia

Pathogens that can cause severe CAP include *Streptococcus pneumoniae*, *Legionella* species, *Haemophilus influenzae*, *Moraxella catarrhalis*, *Staphylococcus aureus*, *Mycoplasma pneumoniae*, respiratory viruses, *Chlamydia pneumoniae*, and *Pseudomonas aeruginosa*.[51] A number of factors increase the risk for developing CAP, including alcoholism, chronic obstructive pulmonary disease (COPD), and comorbid conditions such as diabetes, malignancy, and coronary artery disease. Impaired swallowing and altered mental status also contribute to the development of CAP, because they result in an increased exposure to the various pathogens due to chronic aspiration of oropharyngeal secretions.[51]

Hospital-Acquired Pneumonia

Pathogens that can cause HAP include *Escherichia coli*, *H. influenzae*, methicillin-sensitive *S. aureus*, *S. pneumoniae*, *P. aeruginosa*, *Acinetobacter baumannii*, methicillin-resistant *S. aureus* (MRSA), *Klebsiella* spp., and *Enterobacter* spp. Two of the

Health Care-Associated Pneumonia

Pathogens that can cause HCAP are similar to those causing both CAP and HAP with *P. aeruginosa* and MRSA being the most common in the United States.[54] Risk factors for HCAP include prior hospitalization (hospitalized for 2 or more days within the last 90 days), receiving hemodialysis, receiving intravenous antibiotic therapy, chemotherapy or wound care within 30 days, residing in a long-term care facility or with family member with multidrug-resistant infection, and an immunocompromised state. These patients are at a higher risk of developing multidrug-resistant organisms.[56]

Pathophysiology

Development of acute pneumonia implies a defect in host defenses, a particularly virulent organism, or an overwhelming inoculation event. Bacterial invasion of the lower respiratory tract can occur by inhalation of aerosolized infectious particles, aspiration of organisms colonizing the oropharynx, migration of organisms from adjacent sites of colonization, direct inoculation of organisms into the lower airway, spread of infection to the lungs from adjacent structures, spread of infection to the lung through the blood, and reactivation of latent infection (usually in the setting of immunosuppression). The most common mechanism appears to be aspiration of oropharyngeal organisms.[57] Table 20-3 lists the precipitating conditions that can facilitate the development of pneumonia.

Figure 20-4 depicts the pathophysiology of HAP. Colonization of the patient's oropharynx with infectious organisms is a major contributor to the development of HAP. Normally the oropharynx has a stable population of resident flora that may be anaerobic or aerobic. When stress occurs, such as with illness, surgery, or infection, pathogenic organisms replace normal resident flora. Previous antibiotic therapy also affects the resident flora population, making replacement by pathologic organisms more likely. The pathogens are then able to invade the sterile lower respiratory tract.[55]

Disruption of the gag and cough reflexes, altered consciousness, abnormal swallowing, and artificial airways all predispose the patient to aspiration and colonization of the lungs and subsequent infection. Histamine$_2$ agonists, antacids, and enteral feedings also contribute to this problem because they raise the pH of the stomach and promote bacterial overgrowth. The nasogastric tube then acts as a wick, facilitating the movement of bacteria from the stomach to the pharynx, where the bacteria can be aspirated.[55]

Infection results in pulmonary inflammation with or without significant exudates. Increased capillary permeability occurs, leading to increased interstitial and alveolar fluid. V/Q mismatching and intrapulmonary shunting occurs, resulting in hypoxemia as lung consolidation progresses. Untreated pneumonia can result in ALF and initiation of the inflammatory-immune response. In addition, the patient may develop a pleural effusion. This is the result of the vascular response to inflammation, whereby capillary permeability is increased and fluid from the pulmonary capillaries diffuses into the pleural space.[58]

Prevention of VAP is discussed under the mechanical ventilation section of Chapter 21.

TABLE 20-3	PRECIPITATING CONDITIONS OF PNEUMONIA
CONDITION	**ETIOLOGIES**
Depressed epiglottal and cough reflexes	Unconsciousness, neurologic disease, endotracheal or tracheal tubes, anesthesia, aging
Decreased cilia activity	Smoke inhalation, smoking history, oxygen toxicity, hypoventilation, intubation, viral infections, aging, COPD
Increased secretion	COPD, viral infections, bronchiectasis, general anesthesia, endotracheal intubation, smoking
Atelectasis	Trauma, foreign body obstruction, tumor, splinting, shallow ventilations, general anesthesia
Decreased lymphatic flow	Heart failure, tumor
Fluid in alveoli	Heart failure, aspiration, trauma
Abnormal phagocytosis and humoral activity	Neutropenia, immunocompetent disorders, patients receiving chemotherapy
Impaired alveolar macrophages	Hypoxemia, metabolic acidosis, cigarette smoking history, hypoxia, alcohol use, viral infections, aging

COPD, Chronic obstructive pulmonary disease.

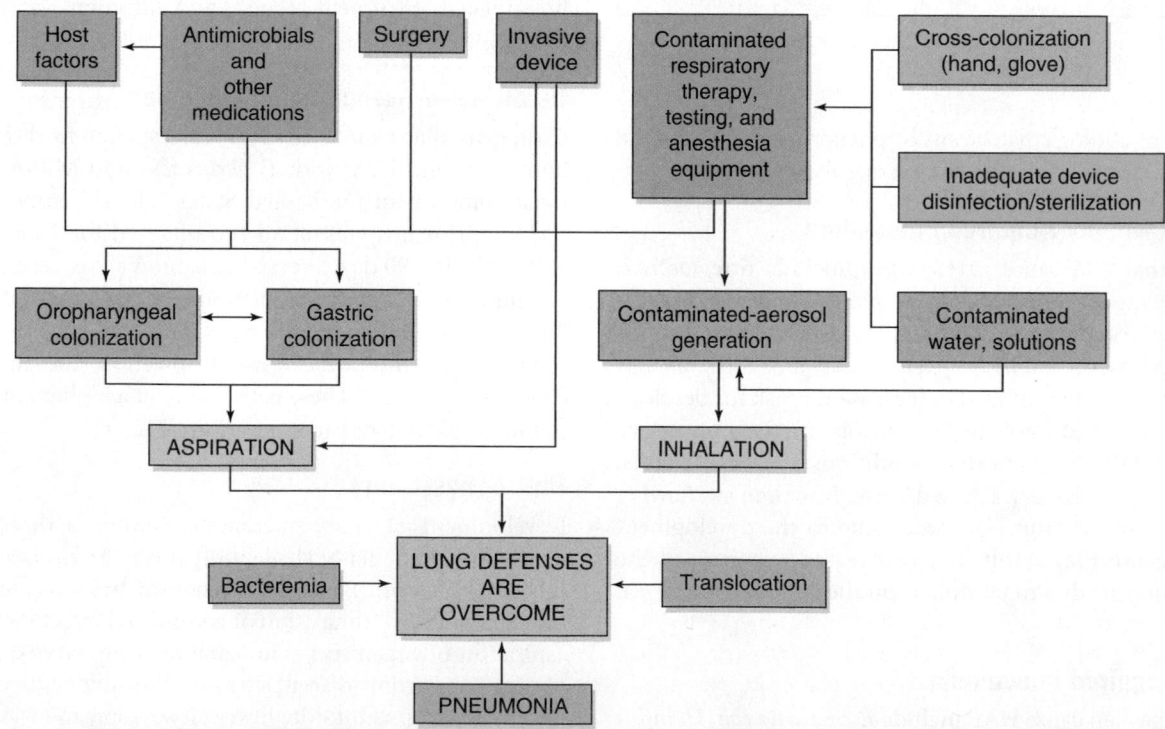

FIGURE 20-4 Pathophysiology of Pneumonia. (From Tablan OC, et al. Guideline for prevention of nosocomial pneumonia. The Hospital Infection Control Practices Advisory Committee, Centers for Disease Control and Prevention. *Am J Infect Control.* 1994;22:247.)

Assessment and Diagnosis

The clinical manifestations of pneumonia will vary with the offending pathogen. The patient may first be seen with a variety of signs and symptoms including dyspnea, fever, and cough (productive or nonproductive). Coarse crackles on auscultation and dullness to percussion may also be present.[53] Patients with severe CAP may manifest confusion and disorientation, tachypnea, hypoxemia, uremia, leukopenia, thrombocytopenia, hypothermia, and hypotension.[57]

Chest radiography is used to evaluate the patient with suspected pneumonia. The diagnosis is established by the presence of a new pulmonary infiltrate. The radiographic pattern of the infiltrates will vary with the organism.[51] A sputum Gram stain and culture are done to facilitate the identification of the infectious pathogen. In 50% of cases, though, a causative agent is not identified.[51] A diagnostic bronchoscopy may be needed, particularly if the diagnosis is unclear or current therapy is not working.[55] In addition, a complete blood count with differential, chemistry panel, blood cultures, and ABGs is obtained.[51]

Medical Management

Medical management of the patient with pneumonia should include antibiotic therapy, oxygen therapy for hypoxemia, mechanical ventilation if ALF develops, fluid management for hydration, nutritional support, and treatment of associated medical problems and complications. For patients having difficulty mobilizing secretions, a therapeutic bronchoscopy may be necessary.[58]

Antibiotic Therapy

Although bacteria-specific antibiotic therapy is the goal, this may not always be possible because of difficulties in identifying the organism and the seriousness of the patient's condition. The time involved obtaining cultures should be balanced against the need to begin some treatment based on the patient's condition. Empiric therapy has become a generally acceptable approach. In this approach, choice of antibiotic treatment is based on the most likely etiologic organism while avoiding toxicity, superinfection, and unnecessary cost. If available, Gram stain results should be used to guide choices of antibiotics. Antibiotics should be chosen that offer broad coverage of the usual pathogens in the hospital or community. Failure to respond to such therapy may indicate that the chosen antibiotic regimen does not appropriately cover all of the etiologic pathogens or that a new source of infection has developed.[51,55]

Currently the Centers for Medicare and Medicaid Services (CMS) and The Joint Commission (TJC) standards for managing patients with CAP require that the first dose of antibiotics be administered within 6 hours of arrival to the hospital. This timeframe is very controversial and has been the subject of much debate. Those in favor of the standard believe that early antibiotic administration leads to improved outcomes while those not in favor of the standard believe it leads to the overuse of antibiotics. More research is needed to clarify the issue.[59]

Independent Lung Ventilation

In patients with unilateral pneumonia or severely asymmetric pneumonia, this alternative mode of mechanical ventilation

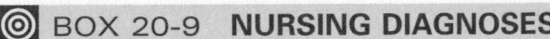
may be necessary to facilitate oxygenation. As the alveoli in the affected lung become flooded with pus, the lung becomes less compliant and difficult to ventilate. This results in a shifting of ventilation to the good lung without a concomitant shift in perfusion and thus an increase in V/Q mismatching. Independent lung ventilation (ILV) allows each lung to be ventilated separately, thus controlling the amount of flow, volume, and pressure each lung receives. A double-lumen endotracheal tube is inserted, and each lumen is usually attached to a separate mechanical ventilator. The ventilator settings are then customized to the needs of each lung to facilitate optimal oxygenation and ventilation.[60]

Nursing Management

Nursing management of the patient with pneumonia incorporates a variety of nursing diagnoses (Box 20-9). Nursing interventions include optimizing oxygenation and ventilation, preventing the spread of infection, providing comfort and emotional support, and maintaining surveillance for complications. The patient's response to the antibiotic therapy should be monitored for adverse effects.

Optimizing Oxygenation and Ventilation

Nursing interventions to optimize oxygenation and ventilation include positioning, preventing desaturation, and promoting secretion clearance. For further discussion on these interventions, see Nursing Management of Acute Lung Failure earlier in this chapter.

Preventing the Spread of Infection

Prevention should be directed at eradicating pathogens from the environment and interrupting the spread of organisms from person to person. Significant progress has been made in removing contaminants from the patient environment through proper disinfection of respiratory equipment and increased use of disposable supplies. Other possible environmental sources of pathogens include suctioning equipment and indwelling lines. These invasive tools must be given proper aseptic care.[55]

Proper hand hygiene is the single most important measure available to prevent the spread of bacteria from person to

---

BOX 20-10 QUALITY IMPROVEMENT

Hand Hygiene Guidelines

QSEN The following are the key recommendations of the Hand Hygiene Task Force, based on the literature review and expert panel opinion:

- Wash hands with soap and water when visibly dirty or contaminated with blood and other body fluids.
- When washing hands with soap and water, wet hands first with water, apply an amount of product recommended by the manufacturer to hands, and rub hands together vigorously for at least 15 seconds, covering all surfaces of the hands and fingers. Rinse hands with water and dry thoroughly with a disposable towel. Use towel to turn off the faucet. Avoid using hot water, because repeated exposure to hot water may increase the risk of dermatitis.
- If hands are not visibly soiled, use an alcohol-based hand rub for routinely decontaminating hands.
- When decontaminating hands with an alcohol-based hand rub, apply product to palm of one hand and rub hands together, covering all surfaces of hands and fingers, until hands are dry (follow the manufacturer's recommendations regarding the volume of product to use).

- Decontaminate hands before and after having direct contact with patients.
- Decontaminate hands before and after donning gloves.
- Wear gloves when contact with blood or other potentially infectious materials, mucous membranes, or non-intact skin could occur.
- Change gloves during patient care if moving from a contaminated body site to a clean body site.
- Remove gloves after caring for a patient. Do not wear the same pair of gloves for the care of more than one patient, and do not wash gloves between uses with different patients.
- Decontaminate hands after contact with inanimate objects (including medical equipment).
- Do not wear artificial fingernails or extenders when having direct contact with patients at high risk (e.g., those in critical care units or operating rooms).
- Keep natural nails tips less than 1/4-inch long.

From Boyce JM, et al, Advisory Committee, and the HICPAC/SHEA/APIC/IDSA Hand Hygiene Task Force. Recommendations of the Healthcare Infection Control Practices Advisory Committee. *MMWR Recomm Rep.* 2002;51(RR16):1.

BOX 20-11 COLLABORATIVE MANAGEMENT

Pneumonia

- Administer oxygen therapy.
- Initiate mechanical ventilation as required.
- Administer medications:
  - Antibiotics
  - Bronchodilators
- Position patient to optimize ventilation/perfusion matching.
- Suction as needed.
- Provide adequate rest and recovery time between various procedures.
- Maintain surveillance for complications:
  - Acute lung failure
- Provide comfort and emotional support.

---

person (Box 20-10). Hand hygiene should occur before and after touching a patient or their surroundings, before performing a procedure, and after exposure to any body fluids.[61] In addition, meticulous oral care, including suctioning of the secretions pooling above the cuff of the artificial airway, is critical to decreasing the bacterial colonization of the oropharynx.[55] Oral care is further discussed in Chapter 21.

Collaborative management of the patient with pneumonia is outlined in Box 20-11.

ASPIRATION PNEUMONITIS

Description

The presence of abnormal substances in the airways and alveoli as a result of aspiration is misleadingly called *aspiration pneumonia.* This term is misleading because the aspiration of toxic substances into the lung may or may not involve an infection. *Aspiration pneumonitis* is a more accurate title, because injury to the lung can result from the chemical, mechanical, and/or bacterial characteristics of the aspirate.[62]

Etiology

A number of factors have been identified that place the patient at risk for aspiration (Table 20-4). Gastric contents and oropharyngeal bacteria (see Pneumonia earlier in this chapter) are the most common aspirates of the critically ill patient.[62-64] The effects of gastric contents on the lungs will vary based on the pH of the liquid. If the pH is less than 2.5, the patient will develop a severe chemical pneumonitis resulting in hypoxemia. If the pH is greater than 2.5, the immediate damage to the lungs will be lessened but the elevated pH may have promoted bacterial overgrowth of the stomach.[62,63] Once the bacteria-laden gastric contents are aspirated into the lungs, overwhelming bacterial pneumonia can develop.[63]

Pathophysiology

The type of lung injury that develops after aspiration is determined by a number of factors, including the quality of the aspirate and the status of the patient's respiratory defense mechanisms.

Acid Liquid

The aspiration of acid (pH less than 2.5) liquid gastric contents results in the development of bronchospasm and atelectasis almost immediately. Over the next 4 hours, tracheal damage, bronchitis, bronchiolitis, alveolar-capillary breakdown, interstitial edema, and alveolar congestion and hemorrhage occur.[64] Severe hypoxemia develops as a result of intrapulmonary shunting and V/Q mismatching. As the disorder progresses, necrotic debris and fibrin fill the alveoli, hyaline membranes form, and hypoxic vasoconstriction occurs, resulting in elevated pulmonary artery pressures.[63,64] The clinical course will follow one of

TABLE 20-4 RISK FACTORS FOR ASPIRATION/ASPIRATION-RELATED PNEUMONIA

RISK FACTOR	RATIONALE
Decreased LOC, either because of CNS problems or use of sedatives	Decreased ability to protect airway from oropharyngeal secretions and regurgitated gastric contents Cough and gag reflexes diminish as LOC diminishes, whether from CNS disorder or sedation Slowed gastric emptying Decreased tone of lower esophageal sphincter
Supine position	Increases probability of gastroesophageal reflux
Presence of a nasogastric tube	Interferes with closure of lower esophageal sphincter Biofilm on tube predisposes to aspiration of pathogenic organisms
Vomiting	Sudden and forceful entry of gastric contents into oropharynx predisposes to aspiration Predisposes to displacement of feeding tube ports into esophagus
Feeding tube ports positioned in esophagus	Infused feedings reflux into oropharynx
Tracheal intubation	Reduction in upper airway defense related to ineffective cough, desensitization of the oropharynx and larynx, disuse atrophy of laryngeal muscles, and esophageal compression by an inflated cuff
Mechanical ventilation	Positive abdominal pressure predisposes to aspiration of gastric contents, probably by increasing gastroesophageal reflux
Accumulation of subglottic secretions above endotracheal cuff	Subglottic secretions can leak around cuff into the lower respiratory tract, especially when cuff is deflated
Inadequate cuff inflation of tracheal devices	Persistent low cuff pressure (e.g., 20 cm H_2O) predisposes to aspiration of oropharyngeal secretions and refluxed gastric contents
Gastric feeding site when gastric emptying significantly impaired	Accumulation of formula and gastrointestinal secretions predisposes to gastroesophageal reflux and aspiration
High GRVs	High GRVs predispose to gastroesophageal reflux and aspiration
Bolus feedings	Volume of infused formula may exceed the tolerance of patients who have poor cough and gag reflexes
Poor oral health	Colonized oropharyngeal secretions may be aspirated into respiratory tract
Advanced age	Older patients tend to have a reduced swallowing ability and are more likely to have neurologic disorders that increase aspiration risks Strong association between advanced age and probability of developing pneumonia once aspiration has occurred
Hyperglycemia	Even mild hyperglycemia can cause delayed gastric emptying by disrupting postprandial antral contractions

From Metheny NA. Strategies to prevent aspiration-related pneumonia in tube-fed patients. *Respir Care Clin N Am.* 2006;12:603.
CNS, central nervous system; *GRVs,* gastric residual volumes; *LOC,* level of consciousness.

three patterns: 1) rapid improvement in 1 week; 2) initial improvement followed by deterioration and development of ARDS or pneumonia; or 3) rapid death from progressive ALF.[64]

Acid Food Particles

The aspiration of acid (pH less than 2.5) nonobstructing food particles can produce the most severe pulmonary reaction because of extensive pulmonary damage. Severe hypoxemia, hypercapnia, and acidosis occur.[63,64]

Nonacid Liquid

The aspiration of nonacid (pH greater than 2.5) liquid gastric contents is similar to acid liquid aspiration initially, but minimal structural damage occurs. Intrapulmonary shunting and V/Q mismatching usually start to reverse within 4 hours, and hypoxemia clears within 24 hours.[63,64]

Nonacid Food Particles

The aspiration of nonacid (pH greater than 2.5) nonobstructing food particles is similar to acid aspiration initially, with significant edema and hemorrhage occurring within 6 hours. After the initial reaction, the response changes to a foreign-body-type reaction with granuloma formation occurring around the food particles within 1 to 5 days.[64] In addition to hypoxemia, hypercapnia and acidosis occur as a result of hypoventilation.[62,63]

Assessment and Diagnosis

Clinically, the patient presents with signs of acute respiratory distress, and gastric contents may be present in the oropharynx. The patient will have shortness of breath, coughing, wheezing, cyanosis, and signs of hypoxemia. Tachypnea, tachycardia, hypotension, fever, and crackles also are present. Copious amounts of sputum are produced as alveolar edema develops.[62,63]

ABGs reflect severe hypoxemia. Chest x-ray film changes appear 12 to 24 hours after the initial aspiration, with no one pattern being diagnostic of the event. Infiltrates will appear in a variety of distribution patterns depending on the position of the patient during aspiration and the volume of the aspirate. If bacterial infection becomes established, leukocytosis and positive sputum cultures occur.[63]

Medical Management

Management of the patient with aspiration lung disorder includes both emergency and follow-up treatment. When

◎ **BOX 20-12   NURSING DIAGNOSES**

Aspiration Pneumonitis

- Impaired Gas Exchange related to ventilation/perfusion mismatching or intrapulmonary shunting, p. 1144
- Ineffective Airway Clearance related to excessive secretions or abnormal viscosity of mucus, p. 1148
- Risk for Aspiration, p. 1154
- Risk for Infection, p. 1160
- Anxiety related to threat to biological, psychological, and/or social integrity, p. 1125
- Ineffective Coping related to situational crisis and personal vulnerability, p. 1150
- Compromised Family Coping related to critically ill family member, p. 1127

aspiration is witnessed, emergency treatment should be instituted to secure the airway and minimize pulmonary damage. The patient's head should be turned to the side and the oral cavity and upper airway should be suctioned immediately to remove the gastric contents.[63,64] Direct visualization by bronchoscopy is indicated to remove large particulate aspirate or to confirm an unwitnessed aspiration event. Bronchoalveolar lavage is not recommended because this practice disseminates the aspirate in lungs and increases damage.[64]

After airway clearance, attention should be given to supporting oxygenation and hemodynamics. Hypoxemia should be corrected with supplemental oxygen or mechanical ventilation with PEEP, if necessary.[63,64] Hemodynamic changes result from fluid shifts into the lungs that can occur after massive aspirations. Monitoring intravascular volume is essential, and judicious amounts of replacement fluids should be instituted to maintain adequate urinary output and vital signs.[63,64]

Empiric antibiotic therapy is usually not indicated following aspiration of gastric contents. However, if VAP is suspected or the aspiration event occurred in the presence of a small bowel obstruction or colonized gastric contents, then antibiotic therapy should be considered.[64] Corticosteroids have not demonstrated to be of any benefit in the treatment of aspiration pneumonitis and thus are not recommended.[63,64]

Nursing Management

Nursing management of the patient with aspiration lung disorder incorporates a variety of nursing diagnoses (Box 20-12). Nursing interventions include optimizing oxygenation and ventilation, preventing further aspiration events, providing comfort and emotional support, and maintaining surveillance for complications.

Optimizing Oxygenation and Ventilation

Nursing interventions to optimize oxygenation and ventilation include positioning, preventing desaturation, and promoting secretion clearance. For further discussion on these interventions, see Nursing Management of Acute Lung Failure earlier in this chapter.

Preventing Aspiration

One of the most important interventions for preventing aspiration is identifying the patient at risk for aspiration (Box 20-13).

BOX 20-13   EVIDENCE-BASED PRACTICE

Aspiration Prevention Guidelines

QSEN   The following are the expected practice guidelines from the updated AACN Practice Alert: *Preventing Aspiration:*

1. Maintain head-of-bed elevation at an angle of 30 to 45 degrees, unless contraindicated. [Level B]
2. Use sedatives as sparingly as feasible. [Level C]
3. For tube-fed patients, assess placement of the feeding tube at 4-hour intervals. [Level C]
4. For patients receiving gastric tube feedings, assess for gastrointestinal intolerance to the feedings at 4-hour intervals. [Level C]
5. For tube-fed patients, avoid bolus feedings in those at high risk for aspiration. [Level E]
6. Consult with physician about obtaining a swallowing assessment before oral feedings are started for recently extubated patients who have experienced prolonged intubation. [Level C]
7. Maintain endotracheal cuff pressures at an appropriate level, and ensure that secretions are cleared from above the cuff before it is deflated. [Level B]

Levels of Evidence:

Level A—Meta-analysis of quantitative studies or metasynthesis of qualitative studies with results that consistently support a specific action, intervention, or treatment

Level B—Well-designed, controlled studies with results that consistently support a specific action, intervention, or treatment

Level C—Qualitative studies, descriptive or correlational studies, integrative reviews, systematic reviews, or randomized controlled trials with inconsistent results

Level D—Peer-reviewed professional and organizational standards with the support of clinical study recommendations

Level E—Multiple case reports, theory-based evidence from expert opinions, or peer-reviewed professional organizational standards without clinical studies to support recommendations

Level M—Manufacturer's recommendations only

Modified from *American Association of Critical-Care Nurses.* AACN practice alert: preventing aspiration. http://www.aacn.org/WD/practice/docs/practicealerts/aacn-aspiration-practice-alert.pdf. 2011. Accessed July 2012.

Actions to prevent aspiration include confirming feeding tube placement, checking for signs and symptoms of feeding intolerance, elevating the head of the bed at least 30 to 45 degrees, feeding the patient via a small-bore feeding tube or gastrostomy tube, avoiding the use of a large-bore nasogastric tube, ensuring proper inflation of artificial airway cuffs, and frequent suctioning of the oropharynx of an intubated patient to prevent secretions from pooling above the cuff of the tube. For patients at risk for aspiration or intolerant of gastric feedings, the feeding tube should be placed in the small bowel.[65]

Collaborative management of the patient with aspiration pneumonitis is outlined in Box 20-14.

PULMONARY EMBOLISM

Description

A pulmonary embolism (PE) occurs when a clot (thrombotic embolus) or other matter (nonthrombotic embolus) lodges in the pulmonary arterial system, disrupting the blood flow to a region of the lungs (Fig. 20-5). The majority of thrombotic emboli arise from the deep leg veins, particularly the iliac, femoral, and popliteal veins.[66] Other sources include the right ventricle, the upper extremities, and the pelvic veins. Nonthrombotic emboli arise from fat, tumors, amniotic fluid, air, and foreign bodies. This section of the chapter focuses on thrombotic emboli.

Etiology

A number of predisposing factors and precipitating conditions put a patient at risk for developing a PE (Box 20-15). Of the three predisposing factors (i.e., hypercoagulability, injury to vascular endothelium, and venous stasis [Virchow's triad]), endothelial injury appears to be the most significant.[66]

Pathophysiology

A massive PE occurs with the blockage of a lobar or larger artery, resulting in occlusion of more than 40% of the pulmonary vascular bed. Blockage of the pulmonary arterial system has both pulmonary and hemodynamic consequences.[67] The effects on the pulmonary system are increased alveolar dead space, bronchoconstriction, and compensatory shunting.[68] The hemodynamic effects include an increase in pulmonary vascular resistance and right ventricular workload.[69,70]

Increased Dead Space

An increase in alveolar dead space occurs because an area of the lung is receiving ventilation without being perfused. The ventilation to this area is known as *wasted ventilation,* because it does not participate in gas exchange. This effect leads to alveolar dead space ventilation and an increase in the work of breathing. To limit the amount of dead space ventilation, localized bronchoconstriction occurs.[70]

Bronchoconstriction

Bronchoconstriction develops as a result of alveolar hypocarbia, hypoxia, and the release of mediators. Alveolar hypocarbia occurs as a consequence of decreased carbon dioxide in the affected area and leads to constriction of the local airways, increased airway resistance, and redistribution of ventilation to perfused areas of the lungs. A variety of mediators are released from the site of the injury, either from the clot or the surrounding lung tissue, which further causes constriction of the airways. Bronchoconstriction promotes the development of atelectasis.[70]

Compensatory Shunting

Compensatory shunting occurs as a result of the unaffected areas of the lungs having to accommodate the entire CO. This creates a situation in which perfusion exceeds ventilation and blood is returned to the left side of the heart without participating in gas exchange. This leads to the development of hypoxemia.[70]

Hemodynamic Consequences

The major hemodynamic consequence of a PE is the development of pulmonary hypertension, which is part of the effect of a mechanical obstruction when more than 50% of the vascular bed is occluded. In addition, the mediators released at the injury site and the development of hypoxia cause pulmonary vasoconstriction, which further exacerbates pulmonary hypertension. As the pulmonary vascular resistance increases, so does the workload of the right ventricle as reflected by a rise in pulmonary artery (PA) pressures. Consequently, right ventricular failure occurs, which can lead to decreases in left ventricular preload, CO, and blood pressure, and shock.[67-70]

Assessment and Diagnosis

The patient with a PE may have any number of presenting signs and symptoms, with the most common being tachycardia and tachypnea. Additional signs and symptoms that may be present include dyspnea, apprehension, increased pulmonic component of the second heart sound (P_1), fever, crackles, pleuritic chest pain, cough, evidence of deep vein thrombosis (DVT), and hemoptysis.[67] Syncope and hemodynamic instability can occur as a result of right ventricular failure.[69]

Initial laboratory studies and diagnostic procedures that may be done are ABG analysis, D-dimer, electrocardiogram (ECG), chest radiography, and echocardiography (ECHO). ABGs may show a low Pao_2, indicating hypoxemia; a low $Paco_2$, indicating hypocarbia; and a high pH, indicating a respiratory alkalosis. The hypocarbia with resulting respiratory alkalosis is caused by tachypnea.[68] An elevated D-dimer will occur with a PE and a number of other disorders. A normal D-dimer will not occur with a PE and thus can be used to rule out a PE as the diagnosis.[67] The most frequent ECG finding seen in the patient with a PE is sinus tachycardia.[66] The classic ECG pattern associated with a PE—S wave in lead I, and Q wave with inverted T wave in lead III—is seen in fewer than 20% of patients.[69] Other ECG findings associated with a PE include right bundle branch block, new-onset atrial fibrillation, T-wave inversion in the anterior or inferior leads, and ST segment changes.[70] Chest x-ray findings vary from normal to abnormal and are of little value in confirming the presence of a PE. Abnormal findings include cardiomegaly, pleural effusion, elevated hemidiaphragm, enlargement of the right descending pulmonary artery (Palla's sign), a wedge-shaped density above the diaphragm (Hampton's hump), and the presence of atelectasis.[68] An ECHO, either transthoracic or transesophageal, is also useful in the identification of a PE, because it can provide visualization of

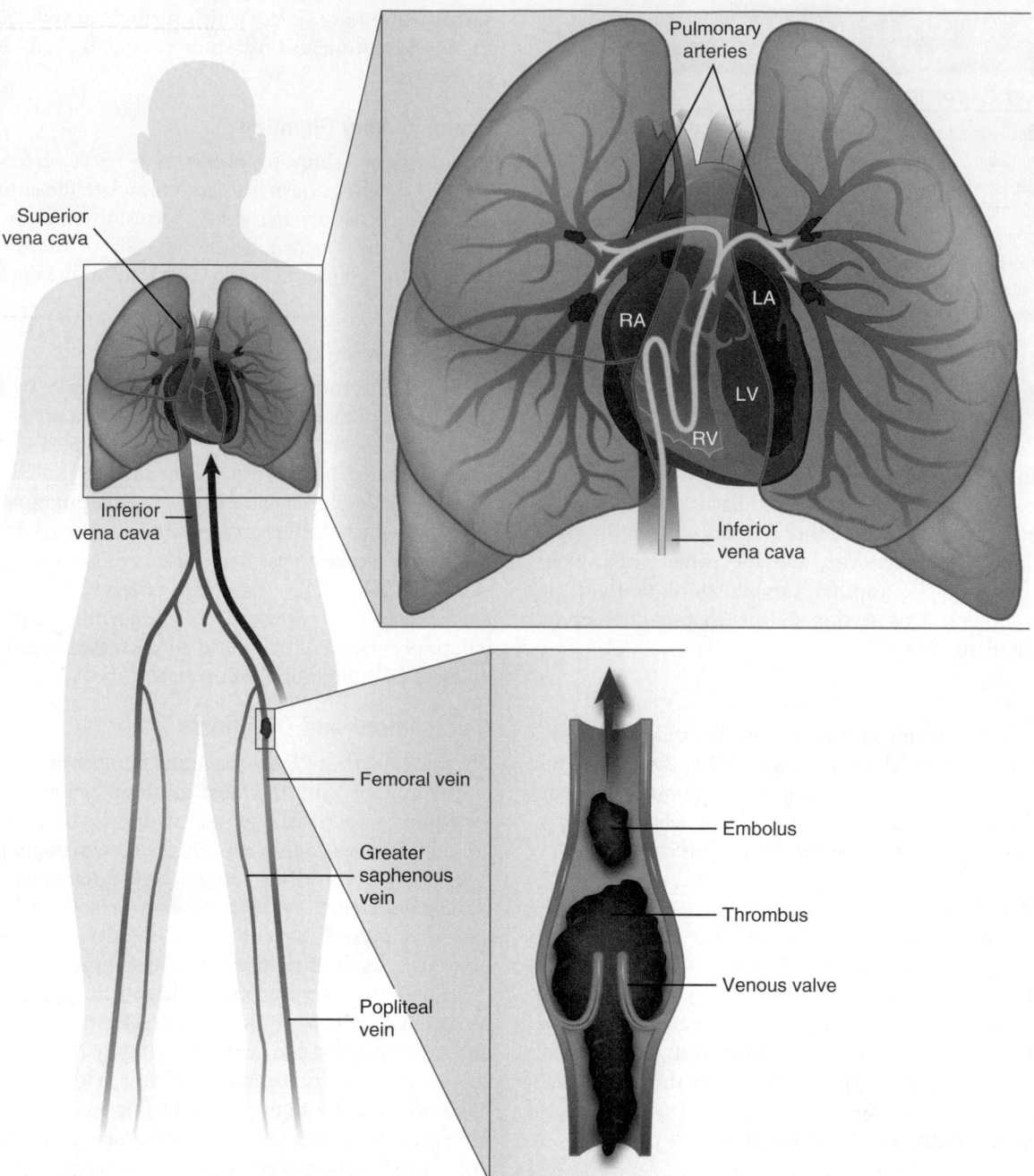

FIGURE 20-5 Pathophysiology of Pulmonary Embolism. Pulmonary embolism usually originates from the deep veins of the legs, most commonly the calf veins. These venous thrombi originate predominantly in venous valve pockets and at other sites of presumed venous stasis (inset, bottom). If a clot propagates to the knee vein or above, or if it originates above the knee, the risk of embolism increases. Thromboemboli travel through the right side of the heart to reach the lungs. *LA,* left atrium; *LV,* left ventricle; *RA,* right atrium; *RV,* right ventricle. (Modified from Tapson VF. Acute pulmonary embolism. *N Engl J Med.* 2008;358:1037.)

any emboli in the central pulmonary arteries. In addition, it can be used for assessing the hemodynamic consequences of the PE on the right side of the heart.[67]

Differentiating a PE from other illnesses can be difficult because many of its clinical manifestations are found in a variety of other disorders.[66] Thus a variety of other tests may be necessary, including a V/Q scintigraphy, pulmonary angiogram, and DVT studies.[67,78,70] Given the advent of more sophisticated CT scanners, the spiral CT is also being used to diagnose a

PE.[68-70] A definitive diagnosis of a PE requires confirmation by a high-probability V/Q scan, an abnormal pulmonary angiogram or CT, or strong clinical suspicion coupled with abnormal findings on lower extremity DVT studies.[68]

Medical Management

Medical management of the patient with a PE involves both prevention and treatment strategies. Prevention strategies include the use of prophylactic anticoagulation with low-dose or

BOX 20-15 RISK FACTORS FOR PULMONARY THROMBOEMBOLISM

Predisposing Factors

Venous stasis
  Atrial fibrillation
  Decreased cardiac output (CO)
  Immobility
Injury to vascular endothelium
  Local vessel injury
  Infection
  Incision
  Atherosclerosis
Hypercoagulability
  Polycythemia

Precipitating Conditions

Previous pulmonary embolus
Cardiovascular disease
  Heart failure
  Right ventricular infarction
  Cardiomyopathy
  Cor pulmonale

Surgery
  Orthopedic
  Vascular
  Abdominal
Cancer
  Ovarian
  Pancreatic
  Stomach
  Extrahepatic bile duct system
Trauma (injury or burns)
  Lower extremities
  Pelvis
  Hips
Gynecologic status
  Pregnancy
  Postpartum
  Birth control pills
  Estrogen replacement therapy

TABLE 20-5 REGIMENS FOR VENOUS THROMBOEMBOLISM PROPHYLAXIS

CONDITION	PROPHYLAXIS
General surgery	Unfractionated heparin 5000 units SC TID or
	Enoxaparin 40 mg SC QD or
	Dalteparin 2500 or 5000 units SC QD
Orthopedic surgery	Warfarin (target INR 2.0 to 3.0) or
	Enoxaparin 30 mg SC BID or
	Enoxaparin 40 mg SC QD or
	Dalteparin 2500 or 5000 units SC QD or
	Fondaparinux 2.5 mg SC QD
Neurosurgery	Unfractionated heparin 5000 units SC BID or
	Enoxaparin 40 mg SC QD and
	Graduated compression stockings/intermittent pneumatic compression
	Consider surveillance lower extremity ultrasonography
Oncological surgery	Enoxaparin 40 mg SC QD
Thoracic surgery	Unfractionated heparin 5000 units SC TID and
	Graduated compression stockings/intermittent pneumatic compression
Medical patients	Unfractionated heparin 5000 units SC TID or
	Enoxaparin 40 mg SC QD or
	Dalteparin 5000 units SC QD or
	Fondaparinux 2.5 mg SC QD or
	Graduated compression stockings/intermittent pneumatic compression for patients with contraindications to anticoagulation
	Consider combination pharmacological and mechanical prophylaxis for very high-risk patients
	Consider surveillance lower extremity ultrasonography for intensive care unit patients

From Piazza G, Goldhaber SZ. Acute pulmonary embolism: part II treatment and prophylaxis. *Circulation.* 2006;114(3):e42.
INR, International normalized ratio; *SC,* subcutaneous; *TID,* 3 times daily; *QD,* daily; *BID,* twice daily.

adjusted-dose heparin, LMWH, or oral anticoagulants (Table 20-5). The use of pneumatic compression has also been demonstrated as effective methods of prophylaxis in low-risk patients.[24]

Treatment strategies include preventing the recurrence of a PE, facilitating clot dissolution, reversing the effects of pulmonary hypertension, promoting gas exchange, and preventing complications. Medical interventions to promote gas exchange include supplemental oxygen administration, intubation, and mechanical ventilation.[67]

Prevention of Recurrence

Interventions to prevent the recurrence of a PE include the administration of unfractionated or LMWH and warfarin (Coumadin).[69] Heparin is administered to prevent further clots from forming and has no effect on the existing clot. The heparin should be adjusted to maintain the activated partial thromboplastin time (aPTT) in the range of 2 to 3 times of upper normal.[69] Warfarin should be started at the same time, and when the international normalized ratio (INR) reaches 3.0, the heparin should be discontinued. The INR should be maintained between 2.0 and 3.0. The patient should remain on warfarin for 3 to 12 months, depending on his or her risk for thromboembolic disease.[69]

Interruption of the inferior vena cava is reserved for patients in whom anticoagulation is contraindicated. The procedure involves placement of a percutaneous venous filter (e.g., Greenfield filter) into the vena cava, usually below the renal arteries. The filter prevents further thrombotic emboli from migrating into the lungs.[71]

Clot Dissolution

The administration of fibrinolytic agents in the treatment of PE has had limited success. Currently, fibrinolytic therapy is reserved for the patient with a massive PE and concomitant hemodynamic instability. Either recombinant tissue-type plasminogen activator (rt-PA) or streptokinase may be used. The therapeutic window for using fibrinolytic therapy is up to 14 days though the most benefit is usually obtained when given within 48 hours.[72]

If the fibrinolytic therapy is contraindicated, a pulmonary embolectomy may be performed to remove the clot. Generally it is performed as an open procedure while the patient is on cardiopulmonary bypass. An emerging alternative to surgical embolectomy is catheter embolectomy. It appears to be particularly useful if surgical embolectomy is not available or is contraindicated. It appears to be most successful when performed within 5 days of the occurrence of the PE.[73]

Reversal of Pulmonary Hypertension

To reverse the hemodynamic effects of pulmonary hypertension, additional measures may be taken. These include the administration of inotropic agents and fluid. Fluids should be administered to increase right ventricular preload, which would stretch the right ventricle and increase contractility, thus

BOX 20-16 EVIDENCE-BASED PRACTICE

Venous Thromboembolism Prevention Guidelines

QSEN The following are the expected practice guidelines from the updated AACN Practice Alert: *Venous Thromboembolism Prevention:*

1. Assess all patients upon admission to the critical care unit for risk factors of venous thromboembolism (VTE) and anticipate orders for VTE prophylaxis based on risk assessment. [Level D]
2. Clinical eligibility and regimens for VTE prophylaxis include:
   - Moderate-risk patients (medically ill and postoperative patients): low-dose unfractionated heparin, LMWH, or fondaparinux [Level B]
   - High-risk patients (major trauma, spinal cord injury, or orthopedic surgery): LMWH, fondaparinux, or oral vitamin K antagonist [Level B]
   - Patients with high risk for bleeding: mechanical prophylaxis including graduated compression stockings and/or intermittent pneumatic compression devices [Level B]
   - Mechanical prophylaxis may also be anticipated in conjunction with anticoagulant-based prophylaxis regimens
3. Review daily—with the physician and during multidisciplinary rounds—each patient's current VTE risk factors including clinical status, necessity for central venous catheter (CVC), current status of VTE prophylaxis, risk for bleeding, and response to treatment. [Level E]
4. Maximize patient mobility whenever possible and take measures to reduce the amount of time the patient is immobile because of the effects of

treatment (e.g., pain, sedation, neuromuscular blockade, mechanical ventilation). [Level E]
5. Ensure that mechanical prophylaxis devices are fitted properly and in use at all times except when being removed for cleaning and/or inspection of skin. [Level E]

Levels of Evidence:

Level A—Meta-analysis of quantitative studies or metasynthesis of qualitative studies with results that consistently support a specific action, intervention, or treatment

Level B—Well-designed, controlled studies with results that consistently support a specific action, intervention, or treatment

Level C—Qualitative studies, descriptive or correlational studies, integrative reviews, systematic reviews, or randomized controlled trials with inconsistent results

Level D—Peer-reviewed professional and organizational standards with the support of clinical study recommendations

Level E—Multiple case reports, theory-based evidence from expert opinions, or peer-reviewed professional organizational standards without clinical studies to support recommendations

Level M—Manufacturer's recommendations only

Modified from American Association of Critical-Care Nurses. *AACN Practice Alert: Venous Thromboembolism Prevention.* http://www.aacn.org/WD/Practice/Docs/PracticeAlerts/VTE%20Prevention%2004-2010%20final.pdf; 2010. Accessed July 2012.

overcoming the elevated pulmonary arterial pressures. Inotropic agents also can be used to increase contractility to facilitate an increase in CO.[69,70]

Nursing Management

Prevention of PE should be a major nursing focus, because the majority of critically ill patients are at risk for this disorder. Nursing actions are aimed at preventing the development of DVT (Box 20-16), which is a major complication of immobility and a leading cause of PE. These measures include the use of pneumatic compression devices, active/passive range-of-motion exercises involving foot extension, adequate hydration, and progressive ambulation.[24]

Nursing management of the patient with a PE incorporates a variety of nursing diagnoses (Box 20-17). Nursing interventions include optimizing oxygenation and ventilation, monitoring for bleeding, providing comfort and emotional support, maintaining surveillance for complications, and educating the patient and family.

Optimizing Oxygenation and Ventilation

Nursing interventions to optimize oxygenation and ventilation include positioning, preventing desaturation, and promoting secretion clearance. For further discussion on these interventions, see Nursing Management of Acute Lung Failure earlier in this chapter.

Monitoring for Bleeding

The patient receiving anticoagulant or fibrinolytic therapy should be observed for signs of bleeding. The patient's gums, skin, urine, stool, and emesis should be screened for signs of

⊚ BOX 20-17 NURSING DIAGNOSES

Pulmonary Embolus

- Impaired Gas Exchange related to ventilation/perfusion mismatching or intrapulmonary shunting, p. 1144
- Acute Pain related to transmission and perception of cutaneous, visceral, muscular, or ischemic impulses, p. 1123
- Risk for Aspiration, p. 1154
- Anxiety related to threat to biological, psychological, and/or social integrity, p. 1125
- Powerlessness related to lack of control over current situation or disease progression, p. 1152
- Compromised Family Coping related to critically ill family member, p. 1127
- Deficient Knowledge: Discharge Regimen related to lack of previous exposure to information, p. 1134 (see Box 20-18, Patient Education for Pulmonary Embolus).

overt or covert bleeding. In addition, monitoring the patient's INR or aPTT is critical to managing the anticoagulation therapy.

Educating the Patient and Family

Early in the patient's hospital stay, the patient and family should be taught about pulmonary embolus, its etiologies, and its treatment (Box 20-18). As the patient moves toward discharge, teaching should focus on the interventions necessary for preventing the reoccurrence of DVT and subsequent emboli, signs and symptoms of DVT and anticoagulant complications, and measures to prevent bleeding. If the patient smokes, he or she should be encouraged to stop smoking and be referred to a smoking cessation program.

BOX 20-18 PATIENT EDUCATION

Pulmonary Embolus

- Pathophysiology of disease
- Specific etiology
- Precipitating factor modification
- Measures to prevent deep vein thrombosis (DVT) (e.g., avoid tight-fitting clothes, crossing legs, and prolonged sitting or standing; elevate legs when sitting; exercise)
- Signs and symptoms of DVT (e.g., redness, swelling, sharp or deep leg pain)
- Importance of taking medications
- Signs and symptoms of anticoagulant complications (e.g., excessive bruising, discoloration of the skin, changes in color of urine or stools)
- Measures to prevent bleeding (e.g., use soft-bristle toothbrush, caution when shaving)

Additional information for the patient can be found at the follow websites:

Vascular Web: **http://www.vascularweb.org/vascularhealth/Pages/pulmonary-embolism.aspx**

Healthfinder—US Department of Health and Human Services: **http://healthfinder.gov**

WebMD: **http://www.webmd.com**

BOX 20-19 COLLABORATIVE MANAGEMENT

Pulmonary Embolus

- Administer oxygen therapy.
- Intubate patient.
- Initiate mechanical ventilation.
- Administer medications:
  - Fibrinolytic therapy
  - Anticoagulants
  - Bronchodilators
  - Inotropic agents
  - Sedatives
  - Analgesics
- Administer fluids.
- Position patient to optimize ventilation/perfusion matching.
- Maintain surveillance for complications:
  - Bleeding
  - Acute respiratory distress syndrome
- Provide comfort and emotional support.

Collaborative management of the patient with a pulmonary embolus is outlined Box 20-19.

STATUS ASTHMATICUS

Description

Asthma is a COPD that is characterized by partially reversible airflow obstruction, airway inflammation, and hyperresponsiveness to a variety of stimuli.[74] Status asthmaticus is a severe asthma attack that fails to respond to conventional therapy with bronchodilators, which may result in ALF.[75,76]

Acute Lung Failure

Etiology

The precipitating cause of the attack is usually an upper respiratory infection, allergen exposure, or a decrease in antiinflammatory medications. Other factors that have been implicated include overreliance on bronchodilators, environmental pollutants, lack of access to health care, failure to identify worsening airflow obstruction, and noncompliance with the health care regimen.[75]

Pathophysiology

An asthma attack is initiated when exposure to an irritant or trigger occurs, resulting in the initiation of the inflammatory-immune response in the airways. Bronchospasm occurs along with increased vascular permeability and increased mucus production. Mucosal edema and thick, tenacious mucus further increase airway responsiveness. The combination of bronchospasm, airway inflammation, and hyperresponsiveness results in narrowing of the airways and airflow obstruction. These changes have significant effects on the pulmonary and cardiovascular systems.[75]

Pulmonary Effects

As the diameter of the airways decreases, airway resistance increases, resulting in increased residual volume, hyperinflation of the lungs, increased work of breathing, and abnormal distribution of ventilation. V/Q mismatching occurs, which results in hypoxemia. Alveolar dead space also increases as hypoxic vasoconstriction occurs, resulting in hypercapnia.[75]

Cardiovascular Effects

Inspiratory muscle force also increases in an attempt to ventilate the hyperinflated lungs. This results in a significant increase in negative intrapleural pressure, leading to an increase in venous return and pooling of blood in the right ventricle. The stretched right ventricle causes the intraventricular septum to shift, thereby impinging on the left ventricle. In addition, the left ventricle has to work harder to pump blood from the markedly negative pressure in the thorax to elevated pressure in systemic circulation. This leads to a decrease in CO and a fall in systolic blood pressure on inspiration (pulsus paradoxus).[75]

Assessment and Diagnosis

Initially the patient may present with a cough, wheezing, and dyspnea. As the attack continues, the patient develops tachypnea, tachycardia, diaphoresis, increased accessory muscle use, and pulsus paradoxus greater than 25 mm Hg. Decreased level of consciousness, inability to speak, significantly diminished or absent breath sounds, and inability to lie supine herald the onset of ALF.[74-76]

Initial ABGs indicate hypocapnia and respiratory alkalosis caused by hyperventilation. As the attack continues and the patient starts to fatigue, hypoxemia and hypercapnia develop.[76] Lactic acidosis also may occur as a result of lactate overproduction by the respiratory muscles. The end result is the development of respiratory and metabolic acidosis.[77]

Deterioration of pulmonary function tests despite aggressive bronchodilator therapy is diagnostic of status asthmaticus and indicates the potential need for intubation. A peak expiratory flow rate (PEFR) less than 40% of predicted or forced expiratory volume in 1 second (FEV$_1$; maximum volume of gas that the patient can exhale in 1 second) less than 20% of predicted indicates severe airflow obstruction, and the need for intubation with mechanical ventilation may be imminent.[78]

Medical Management

Medical management of the patient with status asthmaticus is directed toward supporting oxygenation and ventilation. Bronchodilators, corticosteroids, oxygen therapy, and intubation and mechanical ventilation are the mainstays of therapy.[76]

Bronchodilators

Inhaled beta$_2$-agonists and anticholinergics are the bronchodilators of choice for status asthmaticus. Beta$_2$-agonists promote bronchodilation and can be administered by nebulizer or metered-dose inhaler (MDI). Usually larger and more frequent doses are given, and the medication is titrated to the patient's response. Anticholinergics that inhibit bronchoconstriction are not very effective by themselves, but in conjunction with beta$_2$-agonists, they have a synergistic effect and produce a greater improvement in airflow. The routine use of xanthines is not recommended in the treatment of status asthmaticus because they have been shown to have no therapeutic benefit.[75-78]

A number of studies have focused on the bronchodilator abilities of magnesium. Although it has been demonstrated that magnesium is inferior to beta$_2$-agonists as a bronchodilator, in patients who are refractory to conventional treatment, magnesium may be beneficial. A bolus of 1 to 4 g of intravenous magnesium given over 10 to 40 minutes has been reported to produce desirable effects.[75,76,78]

A number of other studies are evaluating the effects of leukotriene inhibitors such as zafirlukast, montelukast, and zileuton in the treatment of status asthmaticus. Leukotrienes are inflammatory mediators known to cause bronchoconstriction and airway inflammation. Research suggests that these agents may be beneficial as bronchodilators in those patients who are refractory to beta$_2$-agonists.[78]

Systemic Corticosteroids

Intravenous or oral corticosteroids also are used in the treatment of status asthmaticus. Their anti-inflammatory effects limit mucosal edema, decrease mucus production, and potentiate beta$_2$-agonists. It usually takes 6 to 8 hours for the effects of the corticosteroids to become evident.[76] The use of inhaled corticosteroids for the treatment of status asthmaticus remains undecided at this time.[75,76] Initial studies indicate they may be beneficial in certain patient populations.[76]

Oxygen Therapy

Initial treatment of hypoxemia is with supplemental oxygen. High-flow oxygen therapy is administered to keep the patient's Spo$_2$ greater than 92%.[75] Another therapy currently under investigation is the use of heliox. A mixture of helium and oxygen, heliox has a lower density and higher viscosity than an oxygen and air mixture. Heliox is believed to reduce the work of breathing and improve gas exchange because it flows more easily through constricted areas. Studies have shown that it reduces air trapping and carbon dioxide and helps relieve respiratory acidosis.[75]

Intubation and Mechanical Ventilation

Indications for mechanical ventilation include cardiac or respiratory arrest, disorientation, failure to respond to bronchodilator therapy, and exhaustion.[75,77,78] A large endotracheal tube (8 mm) should be used to decrease airway resistance and to facilitate suctioning of secretions. Ventilating the patient with status asthmaticus can be very difficult. High inflation pressures should be avoided because they can result in barotrauma. The use of PEEP should be monitored closely because the patient is prone to developing air trapping. Patient–ventilator asynchrony also can be a major problem. Sedation and neuromuscular paralysis may be necessary to allow for adequate ventilation of the patient.[75,77]

Nursing Management

Nursing management of the patient with status asthmaticus incorporates a variety of nursing diagnoses (Box 20-20). Nursing interventions include optimizing oxygenation and ventilation, providing comfort and emotional support, maintaining surveillance for complications, and educating the patient and family.

Optimizing Oxygenation and Ventilation

Nursing interventions to optimize oxygenation and ventilation include positioning, preventing desaturation, and promoting secretion clearance. For further discussion on these interventions, see Nursing Management of Acute Lung Failure earlier in this chapter.

Educating the Patient and Family

Early in the patient's hospital stay, the patient and family should be taught about asthma, its triggers, and its treatment (Box 20-21). As the patient moves toward discharge, teaching should focus on the interventions necessary for preventing the recurrence of status asthmaticus, early warning signs of worsening airflow obstruction, correct use of an inhaler and a peak flowmeter, measures to prevent pulmonary infections, and signs and symptoms of a pulmonary infection. If the patient smokes, he or she should be encouraged to stop smoking and be referred

---

◎ BOX 20-20   NURSING DIAGNOSES

Status Asthmaticus

- Impaired Gas Exchange related to alveolar hypoventilation, p. 1144
- Impaired Gas Exchange related to ventilation/perfusion mismatching or intrapulmonary shunting, p. 1144
- Ineffective Breathing Pattern related to musculoskeletal fatigue or neuromuscular impairment, p. 1149
- Ineffective Airway Clearance related to excessive secretions or abnormal viscosity of mucus, p. 1148
- Risk for Infection, p. 1160
- Anxiety related to threat to biological, psychological, and/or social integrity, p. 1125
- Disturbed Body Image related to actual change in body structures, function, or appearance, p. 1136
- Compromised Family Coping related to critically ill family member, p. 1127
- Deficient Knowledge: Discharge Regimen related to lack of previous exposure to information, p. 1134 (see Box 20-21, Patient Education for Status Asthmaticus)

BOX 20-21 PATIENT EDUCATION

Status Asthmaticus

- Pathophysiology of disease
- Specific etiology
- Early warning signs of worsening airflow obstruction (20% drop in peak expiratory flow rate [PEFR] below predicted or personal best, increase in cough, shortness of breath, chest tightness, wheezing)
- Treatment of attacks
- Importance of taking prescribed medications and avoidance of over-the-counter asthma medications
- Correct use of an inhaler (with and without spacer device)
- Correct use of a peak flow meter
- Removal or avoidance of environmental triggers (e.g., pollen; dust; mold spores; cat and dog dander; cold, dry air; strong odors; household aerosols; tobacco smoke; air pollution)
- Measures to prevent pulmonary infections (e.g., proper nutrition and hand washing, immunization against *Streptococcus pneumoniae* and influenza viruses)
- Signs and symptoms of pulmonary infection (e.g., sputum color change, shortness of breath, fever)
- Importance of participating in pulmonary rehabilitation program

Additional information for the patient can be found at the follow websites:
- Asthma and Allergy Foundation of America: **http://www.aafa.org**
- American Lung Association: **http://www.lung.org**
- Healthfinder—US Department of Health and Human Services: **http://healthfinder.gov**
- WebMD: **http://www.webmd.com**

BOX 20-22 COLLABORATIVE MANAGEMENT

Status Asthmaticus

- Administer oxygen therapy. Intubate patient.
- Initiate mechanical ventilation.
- Administer medications:
  - Bronchodilators
  - Corticosteroids
  - Sedatives
- Maintain surveillance for complications:
  - Acute lung failure
- Provide comfort and emotional support.

TABLE 20-6 AIR LEAK DISORDERS

TYPE	DESCRIPTION
Pneumothorax *Spontaneous*	
Primary	Disruption of the visceral pleura that allows air from the lung to enter the pleural space; occurs spontaneously in patients *without* underlying lung disease
Secondary	Disruption of the visceral pleura that allows air from the lung to enter the pleural space; occurs spontaneously in patients *with* underlying lung disease
Traumatic	
Open	Laceration in the parietal pleura that allows atmospheric air to enter the pleural space; occurs as a result of penetrating chest trauma
Closed	Laceration in the visceral pleura that allows air from the lung to enter the pleural space; occurs as a result of blunt chest trauma
Iatrogenic	Laceration in the visceral pleura that allows air from the lung to enter the pleural space; occurs as a result of therapeutic or diagnostic procedures, such as central line insertion, thoracentesis, and needle aspiration
Tension	Occurs when air is allowed to enter the pleural space but not to exit it; as pressure increases inside the pleural space, the lung collapses and the mediastinum shifts to the unaffected side; may result from a spontaneous or traumatic pneumothorax
Barotrauma/Volutrauma	
Pulmonary interstitial emphysema	Air in the pulmonary interstitial space
Subcutaneous emphysema	Air in the subcutaneous tissues
Pneumomediastinum	Air in the mediastinal space
Pneumopericardium	Air in the pericardial space
Pneumoperitoneum	Air in the peritoneal space
Pneumoretroperitoneum	Air in the retroperitoneal space

to a smoking cessation program. In addition, the importance of participating in a pulmonary rehabilitation program should be stressed.

Collaborative management of the patient with status asthmaticus is outlined in Box 20-22.

AIR LEAK DISORDERS

Description

Air leak disorders consist of those conditions that result in extra-alveolar air accumulation. These disorders are commonly divided into two categories: pneumothorax[79,80] and barotrauma.[81] A pneumothorax occurs with the accumulation of air or other gas in the pleural space.[79,80] Barotrauma is the result of excessive pressure in the alveoli that can lead to extreme alveolar wall stress and damage to the alveolar-capillary membrane, causing air to escape into the surrounding spaces.[81] The individual air leak disorders are described in Table 20-6.

Etiology

The two main causes of air leak disorders are 1) disruption of the parietal or visceral pleura, which allows air to enter the pleural space[79,80]; and 2) rupture of alveoli, which allows air to enter the interstitial space.[81] Disruption of the parietal pleura occurs as the result of penetrating trauma to the chest wall, which allows atmospheric air to enter the pleural space (traumatic open pneumothorax).[79,80] Disruption of the visceral pleura occurs as the result of entry of air into the pleural space from the lung. This may be caused by blunt chest wall trauma (traumatic closed pneumothorax), diagnostic or therapeutic procedures (traumatic iatrogenic pneumothorax), diseases of the pulmonary system (secondary spontaneous pneumothorax), or ruptured subpleural blebs (primary spontaneous pneumothorax).[79,80] Alveolar rupture occurs as the result of a change in the pressure gradient between the alveoli and the surrounding interstitial space. An increase in alveolar pressure or a decrease in interstitial pressure can lead to overdistention of the alveoli, rupture, and air leakage into the interstitial space. One of the most common causes of barotrauma is mechanical ventilation.[81]

Pathophysiology

The pathologic consequences of pneumothorax and those of barotrauma or volutrauma are different.

Pneumothorax

Regardless of the cause, the entry of air into the pleural space compresses the affected lung. As the lung collapses, the alveoli become underventilated, causing V/Q mismatching and intrapulmonary shunting. If the pneumothorax is large, hypoxemia ensues and ALF quickly develops. Increased pressure within the chest can lead to shifting of the mediastinum, compression of the great vessels, and decreased CO.[79,80]

Barotrauma

After air enters the interstitial space, it travels though the pulmonary interstitium (pulmonary interstitial emphysema), out through the hilum, and into the mediastinum (pneumomediastinum), pleural space (pneumothorax), subcutaneous tissues (subcutaneous emphysema), pericardium (pneumopericardium), peritoneum (pneumoperitoneum), and retroperitoneum (pneumoretroperitoneum).[81] Except for pneumothorax, the resultant disorders are usually fairly benign. Pneumomediastinum has been associated with decreased venous return and upper airway obstruction,[82] and pneumopericardium has been associated with cardiac tamponade.[83]

Assessment and Diagnosis

The clinical manifestations of a pneumothorax depend on the degree of lung collapse. If the pneumothorax is large, decreased respiratory excursion on the affected side may be noticed, along with bulging intercostal muscles. The trachea may deviate away from the affected side. Percussion reveals hyperresonance with decreased or absent breath sounds over the affected area. ABG analysis demonstrates hypoxemia and hypercapnia.[79,80] A chest radiograph confirms the pneumothorax with increased translucency evident on the affected side (Fig. 20-6).[80,84]

The clinical manifestations of barotrauma are much more subtle. Subcutaneous emphysema is manifested by crepitus, usually around the face, neck, and upper chest.[80] Stabbing substernal pain with position changes and with increased ventilation is the most commonly reported symptom of a pneumomediastinum.[82] A clicking or crunching sound synchronous with the heart sounds may be heard over the apex of the heart (Hamman sign).[82] A friction rub may be heard with a pneumopericardium.[83] Barotrauma is also confirmed by radiography. Extra-alveolar air, as evidenced by increased

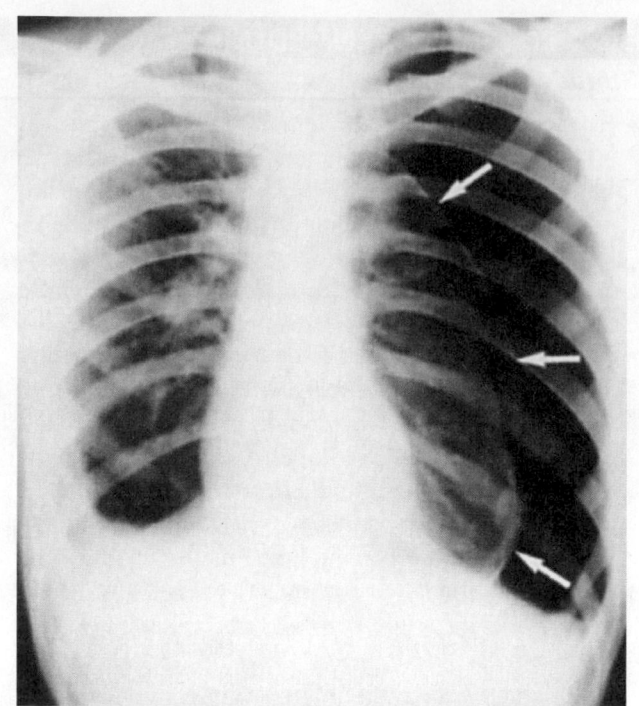

FIGURE 20-6 Left-Sided Tension Pneumothorax. Notice the shift of the heart and mediastinum to the right. (From Des Jardin T, Burton GC. *Clinical Management and Assessment of Respiratory Disease.* 3rd ed. St. Louis: Mosby; 1995.)

translucency, is present in the affected area (e.g., chest, abdomen).[85]

Medical Management

Medical management of air leak disorders varies depending on the severity of the specific disorder. Usually, only a pneumothorax would require treatment, and that would depend on its size. A pneumothorax of less than 15% usually requires no treatment other than supplemental oxygen administration, unless complications occur or underlying lung disease or injury is present.[79,80]

A pneumothorax greater than 15% requires intervention to evacuate the air from the pleural space and facilitate re-expansion of the collapsed lung.[80,86] Interventions include aspiration of the air with a needle and placement of a small-bore (12 to 20 Fr) or large-bore (24 to 40 Fr) chest tube. Chest tubes are inserted into the pleural space to remove fluid or air, reinstate the negative intrapleural pressure, and re-expand a collapsed lung.[80,86] The trend appears to be toward placement of a small-bore tube, as the smaller tubes are more comfortable for the patient and just as effective as large-bore tubes. Patients on mechanical ventilation with a pneumothorax due to barotrauma are best managed with large-bore chest tubes.[87]

Chest tubes are usually inserted in the fourth or fifth intercostal space on the midaxillary line. After the tube is inserted, it is attached to a Heimlich valve or an underwater-seal drainage system. The Heimlich valve is a small one-way valve device that allows air to exit from the pleural space but not enter it (Fig. 20-7). It can be used alone or attached to a drainage bag.[80]

An underwater-seal drainage system is a disposable plastic unit that has three separate chambers: a water-seal chamber, a

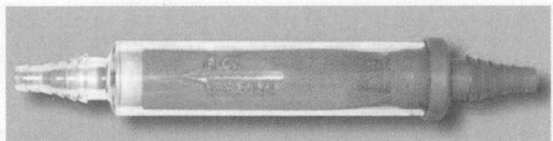

FIGURE 20-7 Heimlich Valve. (Courtesy and © Becton, Dickinson and Company.)

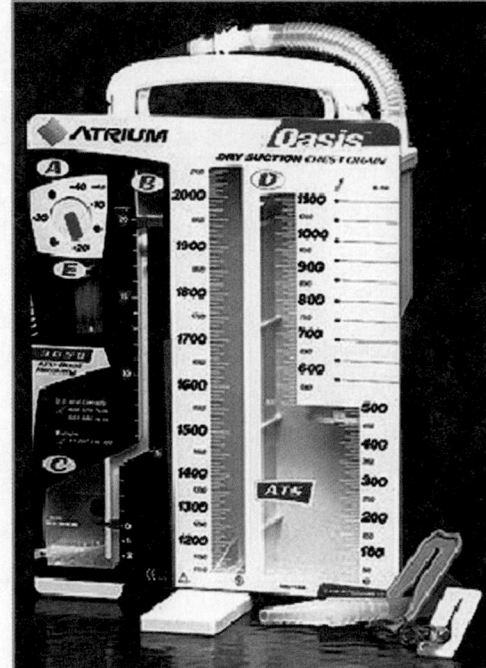

FIGURE 20-8 Underwater-Seal Drainage System. (Courtesy Atrium Medical Corporation, Hudson, NH.)

suction-control chamber, and a drainage-collection chamber (Fig. 20-8). Usually the water-seal chamber is filled to the 2-cm level and the suction-control chamber is adjusted to the desired level of suction. The water-seal chamber acts as a one-way valve, allowing air to escape from the chest but not to enter it. After the chest tubes are placed, the suction-control chamber is attached to an external suction regulator, which is adjusted until the desired level of suction is established (usually 20 cm H_2O). Any fluid draining from the chest will be evident in the collection chamber. Connection points of the drainage tubing are sealed with tape, and an occlusive dressing is applied over the chest tube insertion site. After the tubes are inserted and connected to either device, a chest radiograph should be obtained to confirm re-expansion of the lung.[80,88]

Surgical intervention may be necessary in patients with a persistent air leak or failure of the lung to expand within 3 to 5 days. The preferred procedure is a video-assisted thoracoscopic surgery.[86] Two conditions that require emergency intervention for immediate relief are a tension pneumothorax and a tension pneumopericardium.

Tension Pneumothorax

A tension pneumothorax develops when air enters the pleural space on inhalation and cannot exit on exhalation. As pressure

inside the pleural space increases, it results in collapse of the lung and shifting of the mediastinum and trachea to the unaffected side (see Fig. 20-6). The resultant effect is decreased venous return and compression of the unaffected lung. Clinical signs include diminished breath sounds, hyperresonance to percussion, tachycardia, and hypotension. Treatment comprises administration of supplemental oxygen and insertion of a large-bore needle or catheter into the second intercostal space at the midclavicular line of the affected side. This action relieves the pressure within the chest. The needle should remain in place until the patient is stabilized and a chest tube is inserted.[79,86]

Tension Pneumopericardium

A tension pneumopericardium develops when air enters the pericardial space and has no outlet for exiting. As pressure inside the pericardium increases, it results in compression of the heart and the development of cardiac tamponade. A pericardiocentesis should be performed immediately to relieve the pressure within the pericardial sac.[83]

Nursing Management

Nursing management of the patient with an air leak disorder incorporates a variety of nursing diagnoses (Box 20-23). Nursing interventions should focus on optimizing oxygenation and ventilation, maintaining the chest tube system, providing comfort and emotional support, and maintaining surveillance for complications.

Optimizing Oxygenation and Ventilation

Nursing interventions to optimize oxygenation and ventilation include positioning, preventing desaturation, and promoting secretion clearance. For further discussion on these interventions, see Nursing Management of Acute Lung Failure earlier in this chapter.

Maintaining the Chest Tube System

Maintaining the chest tube system involves careful attention to the suction applied and to maintenance of unobstructed drainage tubes. Kinks and large loops of tubing should be avoided, because they impede drainage and air evacuation, which may prevent timely lung re-expansion or may result in a tension pneumothorax. Retained drainage also becomes an excellent medium for bacterial growth. The water-seal chamber must

Air Leak Disorders

- Administer oxygen therapy
- Intubate patient as needed
- Initiate mechanical ventilation as needed
- Evacuate air from the pleural space
  - Percutaneous catheter attached to Heimlich valve
  - Chest tube to water seal or suction
- Maintain surveillance for complications
  - Acute lung failure
- Maintain the chest drainage system
- Provide comfort and emotional support

Decreased gas exchange
  Ventilation/perfusion mismatching
  Intrapulmonary shunting
  Alveolar hypoventilation
  Anemia
  Acute heart failure
Increased ventilatory workload
  Decreased lung compliance
  Increased airway resistance
  Small endotracheal tube
  Decreased ventilatory sensitivity
  Improper positioning
  Abdominal distention
  Dyspnea
Increased ventilatory demand
  Increased pulmonary dead space
  Increased metabolic demands
  Improper ventilator mode/ settings
  Metabolic acidosis
  Overfeeding

Decreased ventilatory drive
  Respiratory alkalosis
  Metabolic alkalosis
  Hypothyroidism
  Sedatives
Malnutrition
Increased respiratory muscle fatigue
  Increased ventilatory workload
  Increased ventilatory demand
  Malnutrition
  Hypokalemia
  Hypomagnesemia
  Hypophosphatemia
  Hypothyroidism
  Critical illness polyneuropathy
  Inadequate muscle rest

routinely be observed for unexpected bubbling caused by an air leak in the system.[88]

If unexpected bubbling is present, the source must be identified. To determine whether the source is within the system or within the patient, systematic brief clamping of the drainage tube should be performed. The nurse should place a padded clamp on the drainage tubing as close to the occlusive dressing as possible. If the air bubbling stops, the air leak is located between the patient and the clamp. The leak can be within the patient or at the insertion site. The clamp should then be removed and the chest tube site exposed. The tube should be inspected at the site where it enters the chest to ensure that all the eyelets are within the patient. If an eyelet port is outside the chest, it can be a source of an air leak and must be occluded, which may require the attention of the physician. After the insertion site has been eliminated as a leakage source, the chest dressing should be reapplied, completely and securely covering the site. If the air bubbling does not stop when a clamp is placed on the chest tube, the leak must be located between the clamp and the drainage collector. It can be found by releasing the clamp and moving it down the tubing a few inches at a time until the bubbling stops. After the area of the leak is located, it can be taped to re-establish a seal, or the system can be replaced.[88]

A sterile occlusive dressing and a bottle of sterile water should be available at the patient's bedside at all times. If the chest tube system is inadvertently interrupted, the tube should be placed a few centimeters into the bottle of water while the drainage system is re-established. A sterile occlusive dressing is applied to the chest wall if the chest tube is accidentally removed. Immediate implementation of these techniques minimizes or prevents the formation of a pneumothorax and avoids greater complications.

Throughout the duration of chest tube placement, the patient should be assessed periodically for re-expansion of the lung and for complications of chest tube drainage. The nurse should assess the thorax and lungs, paying particular attention to any tracheal deviation, asymmetry of chest movement, presence of subcutaneous emphysema, characteristics of breathing, quality of lung sounds, and presence of tympany or percussion sounds, which are indicative of pneumothorax.

Collaborative management of the patient with an air leak disorder is outlined in Box 20-24.

LONG-TERM MECHANICAL VENTILATOR DEPENDENCE

Description

Long-term mechanical ventilator dependence (LTMVD) is a secondary disorder that occurs when a patient requires assisted ventilation longer than expected given the patient's underlying condition.[89] It is the result of complex medical problems that do not allow the weaning process to take place in a normal and timely manner. A review of the literature reveals a great deal of confusion regarding an exact definition of LTMVD, particularly in regard to an actual time frame. In 2005, the National Association for Medical Direction of Respiratory Care (NAMDRC) Consensus Panel recommended that LTMVD (which they referred to as prolonged mechanical ventilation) be defined as "the need for ≥21 consecutive days of mechanical ventilation for ≥6 hours per day."[90]

Etiology and Pathophysiology

A wide variety of physiologic and psychologic factors contribute to the development of LTMVD. Physiologic factors include those conditions that result in decreased gas exchange, increased ventilatory workload, increased ventilatory demand, decreased ventilatory drive, and increased respiratory muscle fatigue (Box 20-25).[91] Psychologic factors include those conditions that result in loss of breathing pattern control, lack of motivation and confidence, and delirium (Box 20-26).[92] The development of LTMVD also is affected by the severity and duration of the patient's current illness and any underlying chronic health problems.[93]

BOX 20-26 PSYCHOLOGIC FACTORS CONTRIBUTING TO LONG-TERM MECHANICAL VENTILATION DEPENDENCE

Loss of breathing pattern control
  Anxiety
  Fear
  Dyspnea
  Pain
  Ventilator asynchrony
  Lack of confidence in ability to breathe
Lack of motivation and confidence
  Inadequate trust in staff
  Depersonalization
  Hopelessness
  Powerlessness
  Depression
  Inadequate communication
Delirium
  Sensory overload
  Sensory deprivation
  Sleep deprivation
  Pain
  Medications

BOX 20-27 NURSING DIAGNOSES
Long-Term Mechanical Ventilation Dependence

- Impaired Spontaneous Ventilation related to respiratory muscle fatigue or neuromuscular impairment, p. 1145
- Dysfunctional Ventilatory Weaning Response related to physical, psychosocial, or situational factors, p. 1138
- Risk for Aspiration, p. 1154
- Imbalanced Nutrition: Less Than Body Requirements related to lack of exogenous nutrients or increased metabolic demand, p. 1143
- Risk for Infection, p. 1160
- Acute Confusion related to sensory overload, sensory deprivation, and sleep pattern disturbance, p. 1120
- Disturbed Body Image related to functional dependence on life-sustaining technology, p. 1136
- Relocation Stress Syndrome related to transfer out of the intensive care unit, p. 1153
- Powerlessness related to lack of control over current situation or disease progression, p. 1152
- Compromised Family Coping related to critically ill family member, p. 1127

Medical and Nursing Management

The goal of medical and nursing management of the patient with LTMVD is successful weaning. The Third National Study Group on Weaning from Mechanical Ventilation, sponsored by the American Association of Critical-Care Nurses, proposed the Weaning Continuum Model, which divides weaning into three stages: preweaning, weaning process, and weaning outcome.[94] It is within this framework that the management of the long-term ventilator-dependent patient is described. In addition, the common nursing diagnoses for this patient population are listed in Box 20-27.

Preweaning Stage

For the long-term ventilator-dependent patient, the preweaning phase consists of resolving the precipitating event that necessitated ventilatory assistance and preventing the physiologic and psychologic factors that can interfere with weaning. Before any attempts at weaning, the patient should be assessed for weaning readiness, an approach should be determined, and a method should be selected.[92,93]

Weaning Preparedness. The patient should be physiologically and psychologically prepared to initiate the weaning process by addressing those factors that can interfere with weaning. Aggressive medical management to prevent and treat V/Q mismatching, intrapulmonary shunting, anemia, heart failure, decreased lung compliance, increased airway resistance, acid–base disturbances, hypothyroidism, abdominal distention, and electrolyte imbalances should be initiated. In addition, interventions to decrease the work of breathing should be implemented, such as replacing a small endotracheal tube with a larger tube or a tracheostomy, suctioning airway secretions, administering bronchodilators, optimizing the ventilator settings and trigger sensitivity, and positioning the patient in straight alignment with the head of the bed elevated at least 30 degrees. Enteral or parenteral nutrition should be started and the patient's nutritional state optimized. Physical therapy should be initiated for the patient with critical illness polyneuropathy because increased mobility facilitates weaning. A means of communication should be established with the patient. Sedatives can be administered to provide anxiety control, but the avoidance of respiratory depression is critical.[95]

Weaning Readiness. Although a variety of different methods for assessing weaning readiness have been developed, none has proven to be very accurate in predicting weaning success in the patient with LTMVD. One study did indicate that the presence of left ventricular dysfunction, fluid imbalance, and nutritional deficiency increased the duration of mechanical ventilation. Another study suggested that the upward trending of the albumin level may be predictive of weaning success. Because so many variables can affect the patient's ability to wean, any assessment of weaning readiness should incorporate these variables. Cardiac function, gas exchange, pulmonary mechanics, nutritional status, electrolyte and fluid balance, and motivation should all be considered when making the decision to wean. This assessment should be ongoing to reflect the dynamic nature of the process.[96]

Weaning Approach. Although weaning the patient requiring short-term mechanical ventilation is a relatively simple process that can usually be accomplished with a nurse and respiratory therapist, weaning the patient with LTMVD is a much more complex process that usually requires a multidisciplinary team approach. Multidisciplinary weaning teams that use a coordinated and collaborative approach to weaning have demonstrated improved patient outcomes and decreased weaning times. The team should consist of a physician; a nurse; a respiratory therapist; a dietitian; a physical therapist; and a case manager, a clinical outcomes manager, or a clinical nurse specialist. Additional members, if possible, should include an occupational therapist, a speech therapist, a discharge planner, and a social worker. Working together, the team members should develop a comprehensive plan of care for the patient that is efficient, consistent, progressive, and cost effective.[97] Several studies have demonstrated successful weaning through the use of nurse and respiratory therapist-managed protocols.[98]

Collaborative management of the patient requiring long-term mechanical ventilation is outlined in Fig. 20-9.

LONG-TERM DEPENDENCE ON MECHANICAL VENTILATION*

DATE Criteria: —Vent >3 days —Medically stable —Unsuccessful initial weaning attempt	WEANING PHASE	EXTENDING WEANING PHASE	EXTUBATION/ DECANNULATION	POST WEANING PHASE	
				VENTILATOR FACILITY PLACEMENT	TERMINAL WEANING
CONSULTS	Pulmonary Physician/Intensivist Wean Team assessment	Consider psychiatric evaluation Wean Team rounds qweek	SNF Pulmonary Coordinator	Placement Coordinator	Chaplain
DIAGNOSTICS/ MONITORING	As ordered ECG monitoring Continuous Spo₂ monitoring VS with weaning and q2-4h	As ordered ↑↑ VS with weaning and q8-12h	As ordered D/C ECG monitoring Spot check Spo₂ qam VS q8-12h	As ordered D/C ECG monitoring Continuous Spo₂ monitoring VS q8-12h	D/C diagnostics ECG monitoring D/C Spo₂ monitoring D/C routine VS
TREATMENTS	Pressure reduction therapy or lateral rotation therapy	↑	↑	↑	↑
MEDICATIONS	Anxiety management Dyspnea management Pain management Sleep management Stress ulcer prophylaxis DVT prophylaxis Additional medications as ordered Bronchodilators as ordered	↑↑↑↑↑↑↑ Antidepressant therapy	↑↑↑↑↑↑↑	↑↑↑↑↑↑↑↑	Pain control Dyspnea control D/C all other medications
RESPIRATORY	Continue mechanical ventilation Maintain endotracheal tube Initiate/progress weaning trials to extubation or tracheostomy inserted Monitor for weaning intolerance Monitor for airway/cuff problems Monitor secretions/suction prn	↑ Place tracheostomy Progress weaning trials to T-piece ↑↑	D/C mechanical ventilation Extubate or button trach/decannulate IS q1-2h WA; advancing to q4h WA Monitor for respiratory distress ↑↑	Place on home ventilator Tracheostomy Continue/progress weaning trials until transfer Monitor for weaning intolerance ↑↑	D/C mechanical ventilation Tracheostomy D/C weaning trials
ACTIVITY	Maintain HOB 30-45 Provide regular sleep periods Initiate PROM q4h WA Dangle/OOB in chair qd	Sleep 6-8 hours/night OOB in chair 2-3x/d Ambulate with PT/RT assist Bathe patient prior to 2200 ↑	↑↑ D/C PROM Progressive ambulation ↑	↑↑ Continue PROM q4h WA ↑↑	↑ Complete bed rest D/C all activity
PHYSICAL THERAPY	PT evaluation Initiate/progress therapy to qd Strengthening/balance	PT reevaluation Progress therapy to 2x/d (if needed) Transfer/pre-gait training	Progress to 3h/d if going to Rehab ↑↑	↑ Continue PT plan	D/C therapy

*This clinical pathway is a tool to assist health care providers in achieving quality patient outcomes by providing appropriate and timely patient care. It is intended to establish a community standard of care, replace a clinician's medical judgment, establish a protocol for all patients, or exclude alternative therapies.

ADLs, Activities of daily living; *CM,* case manager; *D/C,* discontinue; *DVT,* deep vein thrombosis; *ECG,* electrocardiogram; *HOB,* head of bed; *I&O,* intake and output; *IV,* intravenous; *LCSW,* licensed clinical social worker; *M-F,* Monday through Friday; *OT,* occupational therapy; *OOB,* out of bed; *PEG,* percutaneous endoscopic gastrostomy; *PICC,* peripherally inserted central catheter; *P-M,* Passy-Muir; *PROM,* passive range of motion; *PT,* physical therapy; *RD,* registered dietitian; *RT,* respiratory therapy; *SNF,* skilled nursing facility; *SO,* significant other; *ST,* speech therapy; *UE,* upper extremity; *VS,* vital signs; *WA,* when awake; *WT,* weight.

Continued

LONG-TERM DEPENDENCE ON MECHANICAL VENTILATION*

DATE	WEANING PHASE	EXTENDING WEANING PHASE	EXTUBATION/ DECANNULATION	POST WEANING PHASE — VENTILATOR FACILITY PLACEMENT	TERMINAL WEANING
SPEECH THERAPY		ST evaluation for P-M valve and swallowing Initiate/progress P-M valve to at least 60 min	ST reevaluation for swallowing Initiate swallowing therapy if positive for aspiration	ST reevaluation Continue ST plan	D/C therapy
OCCUPATIONAL THERAPY	OT evaluation Initiate/progress therapy to 3x/wk Initiate self-hygiene/grooming	OT reevaluation Progress therapy to qd (M-F) Hygiene, grooming, and sitting Graded UE strengthening	↑↑ Dress and bathing training Stand for ADLs	↑ Continue OT plan	D/C therapy
NUTRITION	RD evaluation Initiate/progress nutritional support to enteral feedings Monitor I&O qd Weigh patient qwk Insert small-bore feeding tube Maintain IV access	RD reevaluation Continue enteral feedings/start oral feedings if negative for aspiration ↑↑ Place PEG Insert PICC	↑ Progress to total oral feedings if negative for aspiration ↑↑↑ D/C feeding tube and IV access when no longer needed	↑ Continue RD plan ↑ Maintain PEG Maintain PICC	D/C nutritional support D/C I&O D/C weights
SOCIAL SERVICES	LCSW evaluation Identify sources of support and prior level of functioning Support for SO Conduct initial SO conferences	LCSW reevaluation Maintain communication with SO ↑ Conduct follow-up SO conference	↑↑ Conduct SO conferences as needed	↑ Continue LCSW plan Conduct transfer SO conference	↑↑ ↑↑
TEACHING	Orient patient/SO to environment/procedures/equipment Explain weaning plan to patient/SO	↑ ↑	Initiate/complete disease management education Explain discharge plan to patient/SO	Orient patient/SO to environment/procedures/equipment Explain transfer plan to patient/SO	Explain terminal weaning to patient (as appropriate)/SO
DISCHARGE PLANNING	CM evaluation Clarify payor issues Transfer to long-term ventilator unit	CM reevaluation Initiate referral process (as indicated) Initiate transfer summary form Transfer to acute care no earlier than 72h after D/C ventilator	↑ Complete referral process Complete transfer summary form Discharge to SNF/rehab/home (with home care) no earlier than 72h after D/C tracheostomy	↑ Arrange transportation ↑ Transfer/discharge to ventilator facility	
EXPECTED OUTCOMES To be reviewed qwk at WT rounds	• LTMV-WT evaluation completed • Skin remains intact • Anxiety controlled • Rests at regular periods • OOB in chair qd • Participates in PT qd • Participates in OT 3×/wk • Meets needs on enteral nutrition • Initial SO conference done • Transferred to 2 West • Weaned to T-piece/tracheostomy completed <21 days after intubation • Absence of complications	• Skin remains intact • Anxiety controlled • Rest 6 hours at night • OOB in chair 2×/d • Participates in PT 2×/d • Participates in OT qd (M-F) • Uses P-M valve for 60 min • Swallowing evaluated before oral feeding initiated • Meets needs on enteral nutrition • Follow-up SO conference done • Transferred to 4T • Weaned to T-piece • Absence of complications	• Extubated/decannulated without difficulty • Trach buttoned prior to decannulation • Discharged no earlier than 72h after decannulation • Patient education completed • Discharged without delay • Absence of complications	• Transferred/discharged without delay • Absence of complications	• SO conference done • Dyspnea controlled • Life support withdrawn without problems

FIGURE 20-9 Interdisciplinary Plan of Care for Long-Term Mechanical Ventilation Dependence.

B

Weaning Method. A variety of weaning methods are available, but no one method has consistently proven to be superior to the others. These methods include T-tube (T-piece), CPAP, pressure support ventilation (PSV), and SIMV. One recent multicenter study lends evidence to support the use of PSV for weaning over T-tube or SIMV weaning. Often these weaning methods are used in combination with each other, such as SIMV with PSV, CPAP with PSV, or SIMV with CPAP.[91,93]

Weaning Process Stage

For the long-term ventilator patient, the weaning process phase consists of initiating the weaning method selected and minimizing the physiologic and psychologic factors that can interfere with weaning.[91,92] It is imperative that the patient not become exhausted during this phase, because this can result in a setback in the weaning process.[95] During this phase, the patient is assessed for weaning progress and signs of weaning intolerance.[93]

Weaning Initiation. Weaning should be initiated in the morning while the patient is rested. Before starting the weaning process, the patient is provided with an explanation of how the process works, a description of the sensations to expect, and reassurances that he or she will be closely monitored and returned to the original ventilator mode and settings if any difficulty occurs.[93] This information should be reinforced with each weaning attempt. One study showed that family presence during the weaning trial was beneficial and that the trials were longer when the family was present.[99]

T-tube and CPAP weaning are accomplished by removing the patient from the ventilator and then placing the patient on a T-tube or by placing the patient on CPAP mode for a specified duration of time, known as a weaning trial, for a specified number of times per day. When the weaning trial is over, the patient is placed on the assist-control mode or similar mode and allowed to rest to prevent respiratory muscle fatigue. Gradually the duration of time spent weaning is increased, as is the frequency, until the patient is able to breathe spontaneously for 24 hours. If PSV is used in conjunction with CPAP, the PSV is initially set to provide the patient with an assisted tidal volume

of 10 to 12 mL/kg, and this is gradually weaned until a level of 6 to 8 cm H_2O of pressure support is achieved. SIMV and PSV weaning are accomplished by gradually decreasing the number of breaths or the amount of pressure support the patient receives by a specified amount until the patient is able to breathe spontaneously for 24 hours.[93]

Weaning Progress. Weaning progress can be evaluated using various methods. Evaluation of weaning progress when using a weaning method that gradually withdraws ventilatory support, such as SIMV or PSV, can be accomplished by measuring the percentage of the minute ventilation requirement that is provided by the ventilator. If the percentage steadily decreases, weaning is progressing. Evaluation of weaning progress when using a weaning method that removes ventilatory support, such as T-tube or CPAP, can be accomplished by measuring the amount of time the patient remains free from support. If the time steadily increases, weaning is progressing.[93]

Weaning Intolerance. Once the weaning process has begun, the patient should be continuously assessed for signs of intolerance. When present, these signs indicate when to place the patient back on the ventilator or to return the patient to the previous ventilator settings. Commonly used indicators include dyspnea; accessory muscle use; restlessness; anxiety; change in facial expression; changes in heart rate and blood pressure; rapid, shallow breathing; and discomfort.[96] Table 20-7 lists the different weaning intolerance indicators and actions that can be taken to control or prevent them.

Facilitative Therapies. Additional therapies may be needed to facilitate weaning in the patient who is having difficulty making weaning progress. These therapies include ventilatory muscle training and biofeedback. Inspiratory muscle training is used to enhance the strength and endurance of the respiratory muscles. Biofeedback can be used to promote relaxation and assist in the management of dyspnea and anxiety.[93]

Weaning Outcome Stage

Two outcomes are possible for a patient with LTMVD: weaning completed and incomplete weaning.[93]

Weaning Completed. Weaning is deemed successful when a patient is able to breathe spontaneously for 24 hours without

TABLE 20-7   WEANING INTOLERANCE INDICATIONS AND INTERVENTIONS

INDICATOR	ETIOLOGY	INTERVENTION
Pulmonary Signs (Emotional)		
Altered breathing pattern	Inadequate understanding of weaning process	Build trust in staff; consistent care providers
Dyspnea intensity		Encouragement; concrete goals for extubation
Change in facial expression	Inability to control breathing pattern	Involve patient in process and planning daily activities; Efficient communication established
	Environmental factors	Organize care; avoid interruptions during weaning; Adequate sleep; Calm, caring presence of nurse; nonsedating anxiolytics; Measure dyspnea; Fan; music; Biofeedback; relaxation; breathing control; Family involvement; normalizing daily activities

TABLE 20-7 WEANING INTOLERANCE INDICATIONS AND INTERVENTIONS—cont'd

INDICATOR	ETIOLOGY	INTERVENTION
Pulmonary Signs (Physiologic)		
Accessory muscle use	Airway obstruction	Suction/air-mask bag unit ventilation; manually ventilate patient
Prolonged expiration	Secretions/atelectasis	
Asynchronous movements of chest and abdomen	Bronchospasm Patient position/kinked	Bronchodilators Sitting upright in bed or chair or per patient preference
Retractions	ET tube	
Facial expression changes	Increased workload or muscle	
Dyspnea	Fatigue	
Shortened inspiratory time	Caloric intake	Dietary assessment
Increased breathing frequency, decreased V_T	Electrolyte imbalances Inadequate rest Patient/ventilator interactions Increased V_E requirement Infection Overfeeding Respiratory alkalosis Anxiety Pain	Assess electrolytes; give replacements as necessary Rest between weaning trials (i.e., SIMV frequency rate >5) Assess ventilator settings (i.e., flow rate, trigger sensitivity) Muscle training if appropriate Check for infection (treat if indicated) Appropriate caloric intake Baseline ABGs achieved (ventilate according to pH) Coaching to regularize breathing pattern; give nonsedating anxiolytics Judicious use of analgesics
CNS Changes		
Restless/irritable	Hypoxemia/hypercarbia	Increase FiO_2
Decreased responsiveness		Return to mechanical ventilation Discern etiology and treat
CV Deterioration		
Excessive change in BP or HR	Heart failure	Diuretics as ordered
	Increase venous return	Beta-blockers
Dysrhythmias	Ischemia	Increase FiO_2
Angina		Return to mechanical ventilation
Dyspnea		Discern etiology and treat

Modified from Knebel AR. When weaning from mechanical ventilation fails. *Am J Crit Care.* 1992;1(3):19.
ET, endotracheal; *SIMV,* synchronized intermittent mandatory ventilation; V_E, respiratory minute volume; V_T, tidal volume; *ABGs,* arterial blood gases; FiO_2, fraction of inspired oxygen; *CNS,* central nervous system; *CV,* cardiovascular; *BP,* blood pressure; *HR,* heart rate.

ventilatory support. Once this occurs, the patient may be extubated or decannulated at any time, though this is not necessary for weaning to be considered successful.[94]

Incomplete Weaning. Weaning is deemed incomplete when a patient has reached a plateau (5 days at the same ventilatory support level without any changes) in the weaning process despite managing the physiologic and psychologic factors that impede weaning. Thus the patient is unable to breathe spontaneously for 24 hours without full or partial ventilatory support. Once this occurs, the patient should be placed in a subacute ventilator facility or discharged home on a ventilator with home care nursing follow-up.[94]

BOX 20-28 INTERNET RESOURCES

American Association of Critical-Care Nurses: **http://www.aacn.org**
Society for Critical Care Medicine: **http://www.sccm.org**
Respiratory Nursing Society: **http://respiratorynursingsociety.org**
American Association of Respiratory Care: **http://www.aarc.org**
American College of Chest Physicians: **http://www.chestnet.org/accp**
NHLBI ARDS Network: **http://www.ardsnet.org**
American College of Physicians: **http://www.acponline.org**
American Lung Association: **http://www.lung.org**

American Medical Association: **http://www.ama-assn.org**
American Thoracic Society: **http://www.thoracic.org**
Centers for Disease Control and Prevention: **http://www.cdc.gov**
National Institutes for Health: **http://www.nih.gov**
PubMed Health: **http://www.ncbi.nlm.nih.gov/pubmedhealth**
American Society for Parenteral and Enteral Nutrition: **http://www.nutritioncare.org**

SUMMARY

Acute Lung Failure

- ALF is a clinical condition in which the pulmonary system fails to maintain adequate gas exchange; it results from a deficiency in the performance of the pulmonary system.
- Hypoxemia is the hallmark of ALF and is the result of impaired gas exchange due to alveolar hypoventilation, V/Q mismatching, or intrapulmonary shunting.
- Medical management focuses on treatment of the underlying cause, promotion of adequate gas exchange, correction of acidosis, initiation of nutrition support, and prevention of complications (i.e., ischemic-anoxic encephalopathy, cardiac dysrhythmias, VTE, and gastrointestinal bleeding).
- Nursing actions include optimizing oxygenation and ventilation (by positioning, preventing desaturation, and promoting secretion clearance), providing comfort and emotional support, maintaining surveillance for complications, and educating the patient and family.

Acute Respiratory Distress Syndrome

- ARDS is characterized by noncardiac pulmonary edema and disruption of the alveolar-capillary membrane as a result of injury to the pulmonary vasculature or the airways.
- The hallmark of ARDS is refractory hypoxemia.
- Medical management focuses on treatment of the underlying cause, promotion of gas exchange, support of tissue oxygenation, and prevention of complications.
- Nursing actions include optimizing oxygenation and ventilation, providing comfort and emotional support, and maintaining surveillance for complications.

Pneumonia

- Pneumonia is an acute inflammation of the lung parenchyma caused by an infectious agent that can lead to alveolar consolidation and can be classified as community acquired or hospital acquired.
- Medical management focuses on the initiation of antibiotic therapy, administration of oxygen and mechanical ventilation, management of fluids and nutrition support, and treatment of complications.
- Nursing actions include optimizing oxygenation and ventilation, preventing the spread of infection, providing comfort and emotional support, and maintaining surveillance for complications.

Aspiration Pneumonitis

- Aspiration pneumonitis is the presence of abnormal toxic substances in the airways and alveoli, resulting in injury to the lungs.
- Medical management focuses on clearance of the toxic substance from the airways, support of oxygenation, and maintenance of hemodynamics.
- Nursing actions include optimizing oxygenation and ventilation, preventing further aspiration events, providing comfort and emotional support, and maintaining surveillance for complications.

Pulmonary Embolism

- A PE occurs when a clot (thrombotic embolus) or other matter (nonthrombotic embolus) lodges in the pulmonary arterial system, disrupting the blood flow to a region of the lungs.
- Medical management focuses on prevention of the recurrence of PE, initiation of clot dissolution, reversal of the effects of pulmonary hypertension, promotion of gas exchange, and prevention of complications.
- Nursing actions include optimizing oxygenation and ventilation, monitoring for bleeding, providing comfort and emotional support, maintaining surveillance for complications, and educating the patient and family.

Status Asthmaticus

- Status asthmaticus is a severe asthma attack that fails to respond to conventional therapy with bronchodilators; it may result in ALF.
- Medical management focuses on support of oxygenation (by bronchodilators, corticosteroids, and oxygen therapy) and ventilation.
- Nursing actions include optimizing oxygenation and ventilation, providing comfort and emotional support, maintaining surveillance for complications, and educating the patient and family.

Air Leak Disorders

- Air leak disorders consist of those conditions that result in extra-alveolar air accumulation; they are classified into two categories, pneumothorax and barotrauma/volutrauma.
- Two conditions that require emergency intervention for immediate relief are a tension pneumothorax and a tension pneumopericardium.
- Nursing actions include optimizing oxygenation and ventilation, maintaining the chest tube system, providing comfort and emotional support, and maintaining surveillance for complications.

Long-Term Mechanical Ventilation Dependence

- LTMVD is a secondary disorder that occurs when a patient requires assisted ventilation for longer than expected given the patient's underlying condition.
- Weaning can be divided into three stages: preweaning, weaning process, and weaning outcome.
- The preweaning phase consists of resolving the precipitating event that necessitated ventilatory assistance and preventing the physiologic and psychologic factors that can interfere with weaning.
- The weaning process phase consists of initiating the weaning method selected and minimizing the physiologic and psychologic factors that can interfere with weaning.
- Weaning is deemed successful when the patient is able to breathe spontaneously for 24 hours without ventilatory support.

REFERENCES

1. Mac Sweeney R, et al. Acute lung failure. *Semin Respir Crit Care Med.* 2011;32:607.

2. Aboussouan LS. Respiratory failure and the need for ventilatory support. In: Kacmarek RM, et al., eds. *Egan's Fundamentals of Respiratory Care.* 10th ed. St. Louis: Mosby; 2013.

3. Linderman DJ, Janssen WJ. Critical care medicine for the hospitalist. *Med Clin North Am.* 2008;92:467.

4. Balk R, Bone RC. Classification of acute respiratory failure. *Med Clin North Am.* 1983;67:551.

5. Curtis JR, Hudson LD. Emergent assessment and management of acute respiratory failure in COPD. *Clin Chest Med.* 1994;15:481.

6. Raju P, Manthous CA. The pathogenesis of respiratory failure: an overview. *Respir Care Clin N Am.* 2000;6:195.

7. Del Sorbo L, et al. Hypoxemic respiratory failure. In: Mason RJ, et al, eds. *Murray and Nadel's Textbook of Respiratory Medicine.* 5th ed. Philadelphia: Saunders; 2010.

8. Loiacono LA, Shapiro DS. Detection of hypoxia at the cellular level. *Crit Care Clin.* 2010;26:409.

9. Sigillito RJ, DeBlieux PM. Evaluation and initial management of the patient in respiratory distress. *Emerg Med Clin North Am.* 2003;21:239.

10. Dakin J, Griffiths M. The pulmonary physician in critical care 1: pulmonary investigations for acute respiratory failure. *Thorax.* 2002;57:79.

11. Misasi RS, Keyes JL. Matching and mismatching ventilation and perfusion in the lung. *Crit Care Nurse.* 1996;16(3):23.

12. Kernick J, Magarey J. What is the evidence for the use of high flow nasal cannula oxygen in adult patients admitted to critical care units? A systematic review. *Aust Crit Care.* 2010;23:53.

13. Soo Hoo GW. Noninvasive ventilation in adults with acute respiratory distress: a primer for the clinician. *Hosp Pract (Minneap).* 2010;38(1):16.

14. Soo Hoo GW, Hakimian N, Santiago SM. Hypercapnic respiratory failure in COPD patients: response to therapy. *Chest.* 2000;117:169.

15. Ward NS, Dushay KM. Clinical concise review: mechanical ventilation of patients with chronic obstructive pulmonary disease. *Crit Care Med.* 2008;36:1614.

16. Make B, Belfer MH. Primary care perspective on chronic obstructive pulmonary disease management. *Postgrad Med.* 2011;123:145.

17. Sessler CN, Varney K. Patient-focused sedation and analgesia in the ICU. *Chest.* 2008;133:552.

18. Luer J. Sedation and neuromuscular blockade in mechanically ventilated patients. In: Burns SM, ed. *Care of Mechanically Ventilated Patients.* 2nd ed. Sudbury, MD: Jones and Bartlett; 2007.

19. Kraut JA, Madias NE. Metabolic acidosis: pathophysiology, diagnosis and management. *Nat Rev Nephrol.* 2010;6:274.

20. Martindale RG, et al. Guidelines for the provision and assessment of nutrition support therapy in the adult critically ill patient: Society of Critical Care Medicine and American Society for Parenteral and enteral Nutrition: Executive Summary. *Crit Care Med.* 2009;37:1757.

21. Parrish CR, Krenitsky J, Willcutts K. Nutritional support for mechanically ventilated patients. In: Burns SM, ed. *Care of Mechanically Ventilated Patients.* 2nd ed. Sudbury, MD: Jones and Bartlett; 2007.

22. Gunther ML, Moran di A, Ely EW. Pathophysiology of delirium in the intensive care unit. *Crit Care Clin.* 2008;24:45.

23. Frazier SK. Cardiovascular effects of mechanical ventilation and weaning. *Nur Clin North Am.* 2008;43:1.

24. McLeod AG, Geerts W. Venous thromboembolism prophylaxis in critically ill patients. *Crit Care Clin.* 2011;27:765.

25. Ali T, Harty RF. Stress-induced ulcer bleeding in critically ill patients. *Gastroenterol Clin North Am.* 2009;38:245.

26. Wong WP. Use of body positioning in the mechanically ventilated patient with acute respiratory failure: application of Sackett's rules of evidence. *Physiother Theory Pract.* 1999;15:25.

27. Johnson KL, Meyenburg T. Physiological rationale and current evidence for therapeutic positioning of critically ill patients. *AACN Adv Crit Care.* 2009;20:228.

28. Lasater-Erhard M. The effect of patient position on arterial oxygen saturation. *Crit Care Nurse.* 1995;15:31.

29. Cosenza JJ, Norton LC. Secretion clearance: state-of-the-art from a nursing perspective. *Crit Care Nurse.* 1986;6(4):23.

30. Lawrence P, Fulbrook P. The ventilator care bundle and its impact on ventilator-associated pneumonia: a review of the evidence. *Nurs Crit Care.* 2011;16:222.

31. Krishnagopalan S, et al. Body positioning of intensive care patients: clinical practice versus standards. *Crit Care Med.* 2002;30:2588.

32. Stiller K. Physiotherapy in intensive care: towards an evidence-based practice. *Chest.* 2000;118:1801.

33. McCool FD, Rosen M. Nonpharmacologic airway clearance therapies: ACCP evidence-based clinical practice guidelines. *Chest.* 2006;129(suppl 1):250S.

34. Krau SD. Making sense of multiple organ dysfunction syndrome. *Crit Care Nurs Clin North Am.* 2007;19:87.

35. Crouser ED, et al. Acute lung injury, pulmonary edema, and multiple system organ failure. In: Kacmarek RM, et al., eds. *Egan's Fundamentals of Respiratory Care.* 10th ed. St. Louis: Mosby; 2013.

36. The ARDS Definition Task Force. Acute respiratory distress syndrome: the Berlin Definition. *JAMA.* 2012;307:2526.

37. Blank R, Napolitano LM. Epidemiology of ARDS and ALI. *Crit Care Clin.* 2011;27:439.

38. George KJ. A systematic approach to care: adult respiratory distress syndrome. *J Trauma Nurs.* 2008;15(1):19.

39. Tsushima K, et al. Acute lung injury review. *Intern Med.* 2009;48:621.

40. Ragaller M, Richter T. Acute lung injury and acute respiratory distress syndrome. *J Emerg Trauma Shock.* 2010;3:43.

41. Mackay A, Al-Haddad M. Acute lung injury and acute respiratory distress syndrome. *Con Edu Anaesth Crit Care & Pain.* 2009;9:152.

42. Putensen C, et al. Meta-analysis: ventilation strategies and outcomes of the acute respiratory distress syndrome and acute lung injury. *Ann Intern Med.* 2009;151:566.

43. Haas CF. Mechanical ventilation with lung protective strategies: what works? *Crit Care Clin.* 2011;27:469.

44. Yilmaz M, Gajic O. Optimal ventilator settings in acute lung injury and acute respiratory distress syndrome. *Eur J Anaesthesiol.* 2008;25:89.

45. Ali A, Ferguson ND. High-frequency oscillatory ventilation in ALI/ARDS. *Crit Care Clin.* 2011;27:487.

46. Lynch JE, et al. Extracorporeal CO_2 removal in ARDS. *Crit Care Clin.* 2011;27:609.

47. Park PK, et al. Extracorporeal membrane oxygenation in adult acute respiratory distress syndrome. *Crit Care Clin.* 2011;27:627.

48. Liu KD, Matthay MA. Advances in critical care for the nephrologist: acute lung injury/ARDS. *Clin J Am Soc Nephrol.* 2008;3:578.

49. Alsaghir AH, Martin CM. Effect of prone positioning in patients with acute respiratory distress syndrome: a meta-analysis. *Crit Care Med.* 2008;36:603.

50. American Thoracic Society, Infectious Diseases Society of America. Guidelines for the management of adults with hospital-acquired, ventilator-associated, and healthcare-associated pneumonia. *Am J Respir Crit Care Med.* 2005;171:388.

51. Nair GB, Niederman MS. Community-acquired pneumonia: an unfinished battle. *Med Clin N Am.* 2011;95:1143.

52. Sligl WI, et al. Age still matters: prognosticating short- and long-term mortality for critically ill patients with pneumonia. *Crit Care Med.* 2010;38:2126.

53. Shorr AF, et al. Diagnostics and epidemiology in ventilator-associated pneumonia. *Ther Adv Resp Dis.* 2011;5:121.

54. Labelle A, Kollef MH. Healthcare-associated pneumonia: approach to management. *Clin Chest Med.* 2011;32:507.

55. Kieninger AN, Lipsett PA. Hospital-acquired pneumonia: pathophysiology, diagnosis, and treatment. *Surg Clin North Am.* 2009;89:439.

56. Kollef MH, et al. Health care-associated pneumonia (HCAP): a critical appraisal to improve identification, management, and outcomes—proceedings of the HCAP Summit. *Clin Infect Dis.* 2008;46(Suppl 4):S296.

57. Mandell LA, et al. Infectious Diseases Society of America/American Thoracic Society consensus guidelines on the management of community-acquired pneumonia in adults. *Clin Infect Dis.* 2007;44(suppl 2):S27.

58. Miskovich-Riddle L, Keresztes PA. CAP management guidelines. *Nurse Pract.* 2006;31(1):43.

59. Pines JM. Timing of antibiotics for acute, severe infections. *Emerg Med Clin North Am.* 2008;26:245.

60. Anantham D, Jagadesan R, Tiew PE. Clinical review: independent lung ventilation in critical care. *Crit Care.* 2005;9:594.

61. Kendall A, et al. Point-of-care hand hygiene: preventing infection behind the curtain. *Am J Infect Control.* 2012;40(4 Suppl 1):S3.

62. Paintal HS, Kuschner WG. Aspiration syndromes: 10 clinical pearls every physician should know. *Int J Clin Prac.* 2007;61:846.

63. Marik PE. Pulmonary aspiration syndrome. *Curr Opin Pulm Med.* 2011;17:148.

64. Raghavendran K, et al. Aspiration-induced lung injury. *Crit Care Med.* 2011;39:818.

65. Mizock BA. Risk of aspiration in patients on enteral nutrition: frequency, relevance, relation to pneumonia, risk factors, and strategies for risk reduction. *Curr Gastroenterol Rep.* 2007;9:338.

66. Adams AG, Awsare BK. Review for hospitalists: acute pulmonary embolism. *Hosp Pract (Minneap).* 2011;39(4):55.

67. Carlbom DJ, Davidson BL. Pulmonary embolism in the critically ill. *Chest.* 2007;132:313.

68. Dweik RA, Arroliga AC. Pulmonary vascular disease. In: Kacmarek RM, et al., eds. *Egan's Fundamentals of Respiratory Care.* 10th ed. St. Louis: Mosby; 2013.

69. Tapson VF. Acute pulmonary embolism. *N Eng J Med.* 2008;358:1037.

70. Wood KE. Major pulmonary embolism. *Crit Care Clin.* 2011;27:885.

71. Fairfax LM, Sing RF. Vena cava interruption. *Crit Care Clin.* 2011;27:781.

72. Kearon C, et al. Antithrombotic therapy for venous thromboembolic disease: American College of Chest Physicians Evidence-Based Clinical Practice Guidelines (8th Edition). *Chest.* 2008;133(suppl 6):454S.

73. Samoukovic G, et al. The role of pulmonary embolectomy in the treatment of acute pulmonary embolism: a literature review from 1968 to 2008. *Interact Cardiovasc Thorac Surg.* 2010;11:265.

74. Fanta CH. Asthma. *N Engl J Med.* 2009;360:1002.

75. Holgate ST. The mechanisms, diagnosis, and management of severe asthma in adults. *Lancet.* 2006;368:780.

76. Sims JM. An overview of asthma. *Dimens Crit Care Nurs.* 2006;25:264.

77. Cairns CB. Acute asthma exacerbations: phenotypes and management. *Clin Chest Med.* 2006;27:99.

78. Restrepo RD, Peters J. Near-fatal asthma: recognition and management. *Curr Opin Pulm Med.* 2008;14:13.

79. Strange C. Pleural diseases. In: Kacmarek RM, et al., eds. *Egan's Fundamentals of Respiratory Care.* 10th ed. St. Louis: Mosby; 2013.

80. van Berkel V, et al. Pneumothorax, bullous disease, and emphysema. *Surg Clin N Am.* 2010;90:935.

81. Flanders S, Gunn S. Pulmonary issues in acute and critical care: pulmonary embolism and ventilator-induced lung injury. *Crit Care Nurs Clin N Am.* 2011;23:617.

82. Takada K, et al. Management of spontaneous pneumomediastinum based on clinical experience of 25 cases. *Respir Med.* 2008;102:1329.

83. Haan JM, Scalea TM. Tension pneumopericardium: a case report and a review of the literature. *Am Surg.* 2006;72:330.

84. Specht NL, Stoller JK. A review of thoracic imaging. In: Kacmarek RM, et al., eds. *Egan's Fundamentals of Respiratory Care.* 10th ed. St. Louis: Mosby; 2013.

85. Jones R. Recognition of pneumoperitoneum using bedside ultrasound in critically ill patients presenting with acute abdominal pain. *Am J Emerg Med.* 2007;25:838.

86. Yarmus L, Feller-Kopman D. Pneumothorax in the critically ill patient. *Chest.* 2012;141:1098.

87. Light RW. Pleural controversy: optimal chest tube size for drainage. *Respirology.* 2011;16:244.

88. Durai R, et al. Managing a chest tube and drainage system. *AORN.* 2010;91:275.

89. Knebel AR, et al. Weaning from mechanical ventilation: concept development. *Am J Crit Care.* 1994;3:416.

90. MacIntyre NR, et al. Management of patients requiring prolonged mechanical ventilation: report of a NAMDRC Consensus Conference. *Chest.* 2005;128:3937.

91. Caroleo S, et al. Weaning from mechanical ventilation: an open issue. *Minerva Anestesiol.* 2007;73:417.

92. MacIntyre NR. Psychological factors in weaning from mechanical ventilatory support. *Respir Care.* 1995;40:277.

93. Burns SM. Weaning from mechanical ventilation. In: Burns SM, ed. *Care of Mechanically Ventilated Patients.* 2nd ed. Sudbury, MD: Jones and Bartlett; 2007.

94. Knebel AR, et al. Weaning from mechanical ventilatory support: refinement of a model. *Am J Crit Care.* 1998;7:149.

95. El-Khatib MF, Bou-Khalil P. Clinical review: Liberation from mechanical ventilation. *Crit Care.* 2008;12:221.

96. Cox CE, Carson SS. Prolonged mechanical ventilation. In: MacIntyre NR, Branson RD, eds. *Mechanical Ventilation.* 2nd ed. St. Louis: Saunders; 2009.

97. White V, et al. Multidisciplinary team developed and implemented protocols to assist mechanical ventilation weaning: a systematic review of literature. *Worldviews Evid Based Nurs.* 2011;8:51.

98. Girard TD, Ely EW. Protocol-driven ventilator weaning: reviewing the evidence. *Clin Chest Med.* 2008;29:241.

99. Happ MB, et al. Family presence and surveillance during weaning from prolonged mechanical ventilation. *Heart Lung.* 2007;36:47.

Pulmonary Therapeutic Management

Kathleen M. Stacy

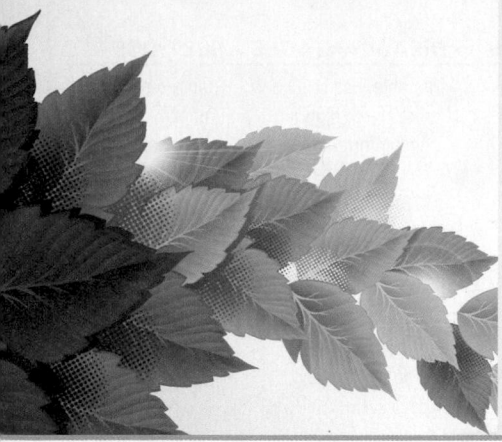

evolve WEBSITE

http://evolve.elsevier.com/Urden/criticalcare/
Evolve features:

- NCLEX Review Questions
- CCRN Review Questions
- PCCN Review Questions
- Mosby's Nursing Skills Procedures
- Animations
- Video Clips
- Glossary

OXYGEN THERAPY

Normal cellular function depends on the delivery of an adequate supply of oxygen to the cells to meet their metabolic needs. The goal of oxygen therapy is to provide a sufficient concentration of inspired oxygen to permit full use of the oxygen-carrying capacity of the arterial blood; this ensures adequate cellular oxygenation, provided the cardiac output and hemoglobin concentration are adequate.[1,2]

Principles of Therapy

Oxygen is an atmospheric gas that must also be considered a medication because—like most other medications—it has detrimental as well as beneficial effects. Oxygen is one of the most commonly used and misused medications. As a medication, it must be administered for good reason and in a proper, safe manner. Oxygen is usually ordered in liters per minute (L/min), as a concentration of oxygen expressed as a percentage (e.g., 40%), or as a fraction of inspired oxygen (Fio_2) such as 0.4.

The primary indication for oxygen therapy is hypoxemia.[3] The amount of oxygen administered depends on the pathophysiologic mechanisms affecting the patient's oxygenation status. In most cases, the amount required should provide an arterial partial pressure of oxygen (Pao_2) of greater than 60 mm Hg or an arterial hemoglobin saturation (Sao_2) of greater than 90% during rest and exercise.[2] The concentration of oxygen given to an individual patient is a clinical judgment based on the many factors that influence oxygen transport such as hemoglobin concentration, cardiac output, and arterial oxygen tension.[1,2]

After oxygen therapy has begun, the patient is continuously assessed for level of oxygenation and the factors affecting it. The patient's oxygenation status is evaluated several times daily until the desired oxygen level has been reached and has stabilized. If the desired response to the amount of oxygen delivered is not achieved, the oxygen supplementation is adjusted, and the patient's condition is re-evaluated. It is important to use this dose-response method so that the lowest possible level of oxygen is administered that will still achieve a satisfactory Pao_2 or Sao_2.[2,3]

Methods of Delivery

Oxygen therapy can be delivered by many different devices (Table 21-1). Common problems with these devices include system leaks and obstructions, device displacement, and skin irritation. These devices are classified as low-flow, reservoir, or high-flow systems.[3]

Low-Flow Systems

A low-flow oxygen delivery system provides supplemental oxygen directly into the patient's airway at a flow of 8 L/min or less. Because this flow is insufficient to meet the patient's inspiratory volume requirements, it results in a variable Fio_2 as the supplemental oxygen is mixed with room air. The patient's ventilatory pattern affects the Fio_2 of a low-flow system: as this pattern changes, differing amounts of room air gas are mixed with the constant flow of oxygen. A nasal cannula is an example of a low-flow device.[3]

Reservoir Systems

A reservoir system incorporates some type of device to collect and store oxygen between breaths. When the patient's inspiratory flow exceeds the oxygen flow of the oxygen delivery system,

TABLE 21-1 OXYGEN THERAPY SYSTEMS

CATEGORY	DEVICE	FLOW	FiO$_2$ RANGE (%)	FiO$_2$ STABILITY	ADVANTAGES	DISADVANTAGES	BEST USE
Low-flow	Nasal cannula	0.25-8 L/min (adults) ≤2 L/min (infants)	22-45	Variable	Use on adults, children, infants; easy to apply; disposable, low cost; well tolerated	Unstable, easily dislodged; high flows uncomfortable; can cause dryness or bleeding; polyps, deviated septum may block flow	Stable patient needing low FiO$_2$; home care patient requiring long-term therapy
	Nasal catheter	0.25-8 L/min	22-45	Variable	Use on adults, children, infants; good stability; disposable, low cost	Difficult to insert; high flows increase back pressure; needs regular changing; polyps, deviated septum may block insertion; may provoke gagging, air swallowing, aspiration	Procedures in which cannula is difficult to use (bronchoscopy); long-term care for infants
	Transtracheal catheter	0.25-4 L/min	22-35	Variable	Lower oxygen usage or cost; eliminates nasal/skin irritation; improved compliance; increased exercise tolerance; increased mobility; enhanced image	High cost; surgical complications; infection; mucus plugging; lost tract	Home care or ambulatory patients who need increased mobility or who do not accept nasal oxygen
Reservoir	Reservoir cannula	0.25-4 L/min	22-35	Variable	Lower oxygen usage/cost; increased mobility; less discomfort because of lower flows	Unattractive, cumbersome; poor compliance; must be regularly replaced; breathing pattern affects performance	Home care or ambulatory patients who need increased mobility
	Simple mask	5-12 L/min	35-50	Variable	Use on adults, children, infants; quick, easy to apply; disposable, inexpensive	Uncomfortable; must be removed for eating; prevents radiant heat loss; blocks vomitus in unconscious patients	Emergencies, short-term therapy requiring moderate FiO$_2$
	Partial rebreathing mask	6-10 L/min (prevent bag collapse on inspiration)	35-60	Variable	Same as simple mask; moderate to high FiO$_2$	Same as simple mask; potential suffocation hazard	Emergencies, short-term therapy requiring moderate to high FiO$_2$
	Nonrebreathing mask	6-10 L/min (prevent bag collapse on inspiration)	55-70	Variable	Same as simple mask; high FiO$_2$	Same as simple mask; potential suffocation hazard	Emergencies, short-term therapy requiring high FiO$_2$
	Nonrebreathing circuit (closed)	3 × V$_E$ (prevent bag collapse on inspiration)	21-100	Fixed	Full range of FiO$_2$	Potential suffocation hazard; requires 50 psi air or oxygen; blender failure common	Patients requiring precise FiO$_2$ at any level (21%–100%)

TABLE 21-1 OXYGEN THERAPY SYSTEMS—cont'd

CATEGORY	DEVICE	FLOW	FiO₂ RANGE (%)	FiO₂ STABILITY	ADVANTAGES	DISADVANTAGES	BEST USE
High-flow	Air-entrainment mask (AEM)	Varies; should provide output flow >60 L/min	24-50	Fixed	Easy to apply; disposable, inexpensive; stable, precise FiO₂	Limited to adult use; uncomfortable, noisy; must be removed for eating; FiO₂ >0.40 not ensured; FiO₂ varies with back-pressure	Unstable patients requiring precise low FiO₂
	Air-entrainment nebulizer	10-15 L/min input; should provide output flow of at least 60 L/min	28-100	Fixed	Provides temperature control and extra humidification	FiO₂ <28% or >0.40 not ensured; FiO₂ varies with back-pressure; high infection risk	Patients with artificial airways requiring low to moderate FiO₂
	Blending system (open)	Should provide output flow of at least 60 L/min	21-100	Fixed	Full range of FiO₂	Requires 50 psi air + oxygen; blender failure or inaccuracy common	Patient with high V_E who need high FiO₂
	High-flow cannula system	Up to 40 L/min (depending on system)	35-90	Variable or fixed depending on system and input flow	Wide range of FiO₂ and relative or absolute humidity; use on adults, children, infants	FiO₂ not ensured depending on input flow and patient breathing pattern; infection risk	Patients of all ages with high or variable V_E who need supplemental oxygen, positive pressure, or humidity

Modified from Heuer AJ. Medical gas therapy. In: Wilkins RL, et al, eds. *Egan's Fundamentals of Respiratory Care*. 10th ed. St. Louis: Mosby; 2013.
FiO₂, Fraction of inspired oxygen; V_E, minute volume.

the patient is able to draw from the reservoir of oxygen to meet his or her inspiratory volume needs. Less mixing of the inspired oxygen occurs with room air than in a low-flow system. A reservoir oxygen delivery system can deliver a higher FiO₂ than a low-flow system. Examples of reservoir systems are simple face masks, partial rebreathing masks, and nonrebreathing masks.[3]

High-Flow Systems

With a high-flow system, the oxygen flows out of the device and into the patient's airways in an amount sufficient to meet all inspiratory volume requirements. This type of system is not affected by the patient's ventilatory pattern. A high-flow system uses either an air-entrainment system or blending system to mix air and oxygen to achieve the desired FiO₂. An air-entrainment mask is an example of a high-flow system that delivers precisely controlled oxygen at the lower FiO₂ range.[3]

One of the newest high-flow systems is the high-flow nasal cannula. With this system, warmed and humidified oxygen is delivered to the patient via a nasal cannula using a blending system. This system has been shown to improve oxygenation and ventilation and decrease the work of breathing in the patient with acute lung failure. It also is more comfortable and better tolerated than similar therapies.[4]

Complications of Oxygen Therapy

Oxygen, like most medications, has adverse effects and complications resulting from its use. The adage, "If a little is good, a lot is better," does not apply to oxygen. The lung is designed to handle a concentration of 21% oxygen, with some adaptability

to higher concentrations, but adverse effects and oxygen toxicity can result if a high concentration is administered for too long.[5]

Oxygen Toxicity

The most detrimental effect of breathing a high concentration of oxygen is the development of oxygen toxicity. It can occur in any patient who breathes oxygen concentrations of greater than 50% for longer than 24 hours. Patients most likely to develop oxygen toxicity are those who require intubation, mechanical ventilation, and high oxygen concentrations for extended periods.[3]

Hyperoxia, or the administration of higher-than-normal oxygen concentrations, produces an overabundance of oxygen free radicals. These radicals are responsible for the initial damage to the alveolar–capillary membrane. Oxygen free radicals are toxic metabolites of oxygen metabolism. Normally, enzymes neutralize the radicals, preventing any damage from occurring. During the administration of high levels of oxygen, the large number of oxygen free radicals produced exhausts the supply of neutralizing enzymes. Damage to the lung parenchyma and vasculature occurs, resulting in the initiation of acute respiratory distress syndrome (ARDS).[2,5]

A number of clinical manifestations are associated with oxygen toxicity. The first symptom is substernal chest pain that is exacerbated by deep breathing. A dry cough and tracheal irritation follow. Eventually, definite pleuritic pain occurs on inhalation, followed by dyspnea. Upper airway changes may include a sensation of nasal stuffiness, sore throat, and eye and ear discomforts. Chest radiographs and pulmonary function tests show no abnormalities until symptoms are severe.

Complete, rapid reversal of these symptoms occurs as soon as normal oxygen concentrations are restored.[5]

Carbon Dioxide Retention

In patients with severe chronic obstructive pulmonary disease (COPD), carbon dioxide (CO_2) retention may occur as a result of administration of oxygen in high concentrations. A number of theories have been proposed for this phenomenon. One states that the normal stimulus to breathe (i.e., increasing CO_2 levels) is muted in patients with COPD and that decreasing oxygen levels become the stimulus to breathe. If hypoxemia is corrected by the administration of oxygen, the stimulus to breathe is abolished; hypoventilation develops, resulting in a further increase in the arterial partial pressure of carbon dioxide ($Paco_2$).[2,3] Another theory is that the administration of oxygen abolishes the compensatory response of hypoxic pulmonary vasoconstriction. This results in an increase in perfusion of underventilated alveoli and the development of dead space, producing ventilation–perfusion mismatch. As alveolar dead space increases, so does the retention of CO_2.[2,3] One further theory states that the rise in CO_2 is related to the ratio of deoxygenated to oxygenated hemoglobin (Haldane effect). Deoxygenated hemoglobin carries more CO_2 compared with oxygenated hemoglobin. Administration of oxygen increases the proportion of oxygenated hemoglobin, which causes increased release of CO_2 at the lung level.[5] Because of the risk of CO_2 accumulation, all patients who are chronically hypercapnic require careful low-flow oxygen administration.[3]

Absorption Atelectasis

Another adverse effect of high concentrations of oxygen is absorption atelectasis. Breathing high concentrations of oxygen washes out the nitrogen that normally fills the alveoli and helps hold them open (residual volume). As oxygen replaces the nitrogen in the alveoli, the alveoli start to shrink and collapse. This occurs because oxygen is absorbed into the bloodstream faster than it can be replaced in the alveoli, particularly in areas of the lungs that are minimally ventilated.[2,3]

Nursing Management

Nursing management of the patient receiving oxygen is outlined in Box 21-1. Key nursing interventions include ensuring the oxygen is being administered as ordered and observing for complications of the therapy. Confirming that the oxygen therapy device is properly positioned and replacing it after removal is important. During meals, an oxygen mask should be changed to a nasal cannula if the patient can tolerate one. The patient receiving oxygen therapy should also be transported with the oxygen. In addition, oxygen saturation should be periodically monitored using a pulse oximeter.

ARTIFICIAL AIRWAYS

Pharyngeal Airways

Pharyngeal airways are used to maintain airway patency by keeping the tongue from obstructing the upper airway. The two types of pharyngeal airways are *oropharyngeal* and *nasopharyngeal airways*. Complications of these airways include

---

◎ BOX 21-1 NIC

Oxygen Therapy

Definition
Administration of oxygen and monitoring of its effectiveness

Activities
- Clear oral, nasal, and tracheal secretions, as appropriate.
- Restrict smoking.
- Maintain airway patency.
- Set up oxygen equipment and administer through a heated, humidified system.
- Administer supplemental oxygen, as ordered.
- Monitor the oxygen liter flow.
- Monitor position of oxygen delivery device.
- Instruct patient about importance of leaving oxygen delivery device on.
- Periodically check oxygen delivery device to ensure that the prescribed concentration is being delivered.
- Monitor the effectiveness of oxygen therapy (e.g., pulse oximetry, arterial blood gases) as appropriate.
- Assure replacement of oxygen mask or cannula whenever the device is removed.
- Monitor patient's ability to tolerate removal of oxygen while eating.
- Change oxygen delivery device from mask to nasal prongs during meals, as tolerated.
- Observe for signs of oxygen-induced hypoventilation.
- Monitor for signs of oxygen toxicity and absorption atelectasis.
- Monitor oxygen equipment to ensure that it is not interfering with the patient's attempts to breathe.
- Monitor patient's anxiety related to need for oxygen therapy.
- Monitor for skin breakdown from friction of oxygen device.
- Provide for oxygen when patient is transported.
- Instruct patient to obtain a supplementary oxygen prescription before air travel or trips to high altitude, as appropriate.
- Consult with other health care personnel about use of supplemental oxygen during activity, sleep, or both.
- Instruct patient and family about use of oxygen at home.
- Arrange for use of oxygen devices that facilitate mobility and teach patient accordingly.
- Convert to alternate oxygen delivery device to promote comfort, as appropriate.

From Bulechek GM, et al. *Nursing Interventions Classification (NIC).* 6th ed. St. Louis: Mosby; 2013.

---

trauma to the oral or nasal cavity, obstruction of the airway, laryngospasm, gagging, and vomiting.[6,7]

Oropharyngeal Airway

An oropharyngeal airway is made of plastic and is available in various sizes. The proper size is selected by holding the airway against the side of the patient's face and ensuring that it extends from the corner of the mouth to the angle of the jaw. If the airway is improperly sized, it will occlude the airway.[6,7] An oral airway is placed by inserting a tongue depressor into the patient's mouth to displace the tongue downward and then passing the airway into the patient's mouth, slipping it over the patient's tongue (Fig. 21-1).[7] When properly placed, the tip of the airway lies above the epiglottis at the base of the tongue. It should be used only in an unconscious patient who has an absent or diminished gag reflex.[6,7]

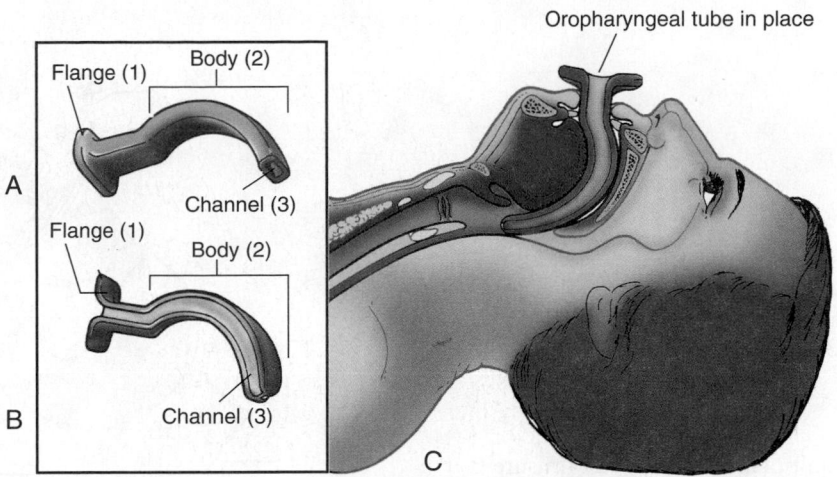

FIGURE 21-1 **Oropharyngeal Airways.** *A,* Guedel airway. *B,* Berman airway. *C,* Airway in place. (From Barnes TA. Emergency cardiovascular life support. In: Kacmarek RM, et al, eds. *Egan's Fundamentals of Respiratory Care.* 10th ed. St. Louis: Mosby; 2013.)

TABLE 21-2	ADVANTAGES OF OROTRACHEAL, NASOTRACHEAL, AND TRACHEOSTOMY TUBES	
OROTRACHEAL TUBES	**NASOTRACHEAL TUBES**	**TRACHEOSTOMY TUBES**
Easier access	Easily secured and stabilized	Easily secured and stabilized
Avoids nasal and sinus complications	Reduces risk of unintentional extubation	Reduces risk of unintentional decannulation
Allows for larger-diameter tube, which facilitates: • Work of breathing • Suctioning • Fiberoptic bronchoscopy	Well tolerated by patient Enables swallowing and oral hygiene Facilitates communication Avoids need for bite block	Well tolerated by patient Enables swallowing, speech, and oral hygiene Avoids upper airway complications Allows for larger-diameter tube, which facilitates: • Work of breathing • Suctioning • Fiberoptic bronchoscopy

Nasopharyngeal Airway

A nasopharyngeal airway is usually made of plastic or rubber and is available in various sizes. The proper size is selected by holding the airway against the side of the patient's face and ensuring that it extends from the tip of the nose to the ear lobe.[6,7] A nasal airway is placed by lubricating the tube and inserting it midline along the floor of the naris into the posterior pharynx.[7] When properly placed, the tip of the airway lies above the epiglottis at the base of the tongue.[6,7]

Endotracheal Tubes

An endotracheal tube (ETT) is the most commonly used artificial airway for providing short-term airway management. Indications for endotracheal intubation include maintenance of airway patency, protection of the airway from aspiration, application of positive-pressure ventilation, facilitation of pulmonary toilet, and use of high oxygen concentrations.[8] An ETT may be placed through the orotracheal or the nasotracheal route.[9,10] In most situations involving emergency placement, the orotracheal route is used because it is simpler and allows the use of a larger-diameter ETT.[10,11] Nasotracheal intubation provides greater patient comfort over time and is preferred in

patients with a jaw fracture.[9,11,12] The advantages of orotracheal and nasotracheal intubation are presented in Table 21-2.

ETTs are available in various sizes, which are based on the inner diameters of the tubes, and have a radiopaque marker that runs the length of the tube. On one end of the tube is a cuff that is inflated with the use of the pilot balloon. Because of the high incidence of cuff-related problems, low-pressure, high-volume cuffs are preferred. On the other end of the tube is a 15-mm adaptor that facilitates connection of the tube to a manual resuscitation bag (MRB), T-tube, or ventilator (Fig. 21-2).[13]

Rapid Sequence Intubation

Rapid sequence intubation (RSI) is a seven-step process that is often used to intubate the critically ill patient. It is considered safer for the patient as it decreases the risk of aspiration.[14]

Step 1—Preparation. Before intubation, the necessary equipment is gathered and organized to facilitate the procedure. Readily available equipment should include a suction system with catheters and tonsil suction, an MRB with a mask connected to 100% oxygen, a laryngoscope handle with assorted blades, a variety of sizes of ETTs, and a stylet. Before the

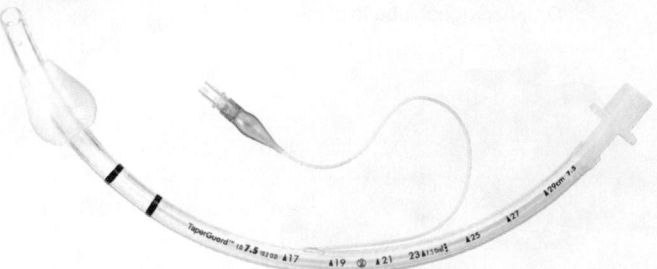

FIGURE 21-2 Endotracheal Tube. (Image used by permission from Nellcor Puritan Bennett LLC, Boulder, CO.)

procedure is initiated, all equipment is inspected to ensure that it is in working order. The patient should be prepared for the procedure, if possible, with an intravenous catheter in place and should be monitored with a pulse oximeter.[14]

Step 2—Preoxygenation. Once everything is ready, the patient is preoxygenated with 100% oxygen for 3 to 5 minutes via a tight-fitting face mask. If the patient is unable to maintain adequate spontaneous ventilations, then assisted ventilations are initiated with an MRB. The goal is to avoid positive pressure ventilation, if possible, as this intervention increases the chances of gastric distention and the risk of aspiration. If an MRB is used, cricoid pressure should be initiated.[14]

Step 3—Pretreatment. While the patient is being preoxygenated, the patient is pretreated with adjunct medications to decrease the physiologic response to intubation. These medications include lidocaine, fentanyl, and atropine. A very low dose of a paralytic agent may be administered to prevent fasciculations. The use of these medications is dependent on the patient's underlying condition. If possible, pretreatment should occur 3 minutes prior to the next step.[14]

Step 4—Paralysis with Induction. Next, a sedative agent and a paralytic agent are administered in "rapid sequence" to achieve induction and paralysis. A variety of sedative agents, including etomidate, midazolam, ketamine, and propofol, are used to facilitate rapid loss of consciousness. Induction dosages for these medications are usually slightly higher than the typical dosages used for sedation. The two most administered neuromuscular blocking agents used to facilitate skeletal muscle relaxation are succinylcholine and rocuronium.[14]

Step 5—Protection and Positioning. The procedure is initiated by positioning the patient with the neck flexed and head slightly extended in the "sniff" position. The oral cavity and pharynx are suctioned, and any dental devices are removed. Next cricoid pressure is applied to protect the airway by preventing vomiting and subsequent aspiration of gastric contents.[14]

Step 6—Placement of the Endotracheal Tube. Next, the ETT is inserted into the trachea (Fig. 21-3), and placement is confirmed.[14] Each intubation attempt is limited to 30 seconds to prevent hypoxemia. After the ETT is inserted, the patient is assessed for bilateral breath sounds and chest movement. Absence of breath sounds is indicative of an esophageal intubation, whereas breath sounds heard over only one side is

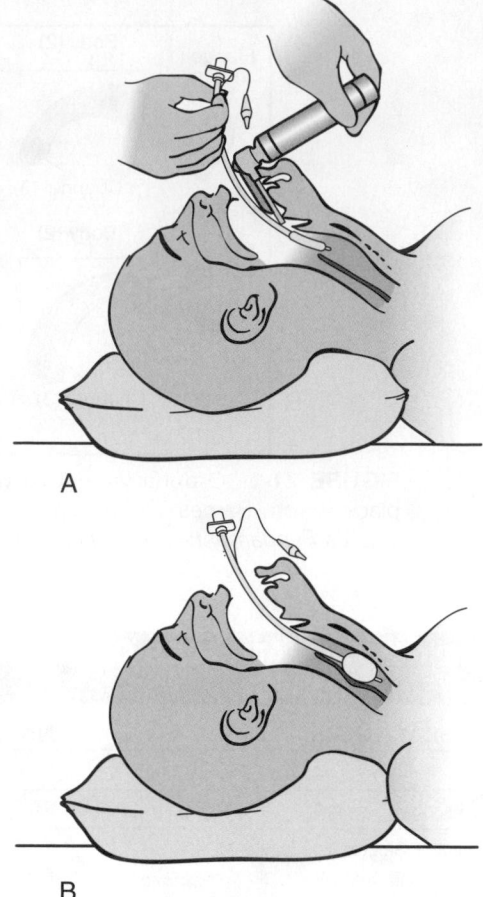

A

B

FIGURE 21-3 Insertion of Tube with Laryngoscope in Place. *A,* Insert the tube with the tip initially against the right buccal mucosa so that a clear view of the vocal cords can be maintained at all times. As it advances, watch the tube pass through the cord. *B,* The tube is correctly placed when the tip is 2 to 3 cm beyond the vocal cords. (From Savage S. Tracheal intubation. In: Pfenninger JL, Fowler GC, eds. *Pfenninger and Fowler's Procedures for Primary Care.* 3rd ed. Philadelphia: Elsevier; 2011.)

indicative of a main stem intubation. A disposable end-tidal CO_2 detector (Fig. 21-4) is used to initially verify correct airway placement, after which the cuff of the tube is inflated and the tube is secured. Finally, a chest radiograph is obtained to confirm placement.[9-11] The tip of the ETT should be approximately 3 to 4 cm above the carina when the patient's head is in the neutral position.[10]

Step 7—Post Intubation Management. After final adjustment of the position is complete, the level of insertion (marked in centimeters on the side of the tube) at the teeth is noted. The ETT is then secured to patient's face using tape or a commercial tube holder (Fig. 21-5). Securing the tube stabilizes it to prevent movement and potential dislodgement.[9,10,15]

Complications

A number of complications can occur during the intubation procedure, including nasal and oral trauma, pharyngeal and hypopharyngeal trauma, vomiting with aspiration, and cardiac

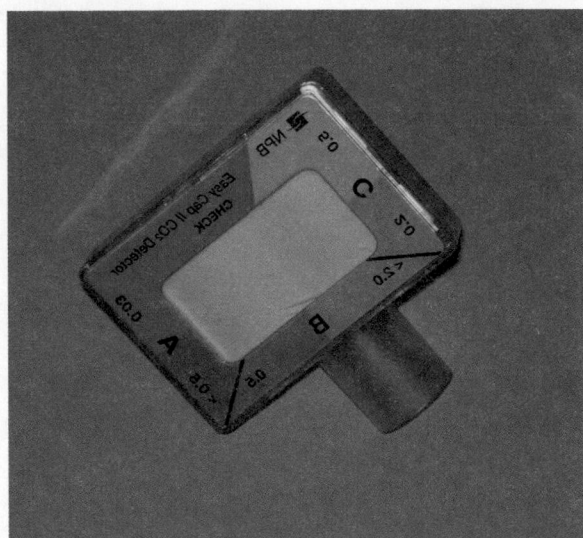

FIGURE 21-4 Disposable colorimetric carbon dioxide detector for confirming tracheal intubation. (From Altobelli N. Airway management. In: Kacmarek RM et al, eds. *Egan's Fundamentals of Respiratory Care*. 10th ed. St. Louis: Mosby; 2013.)

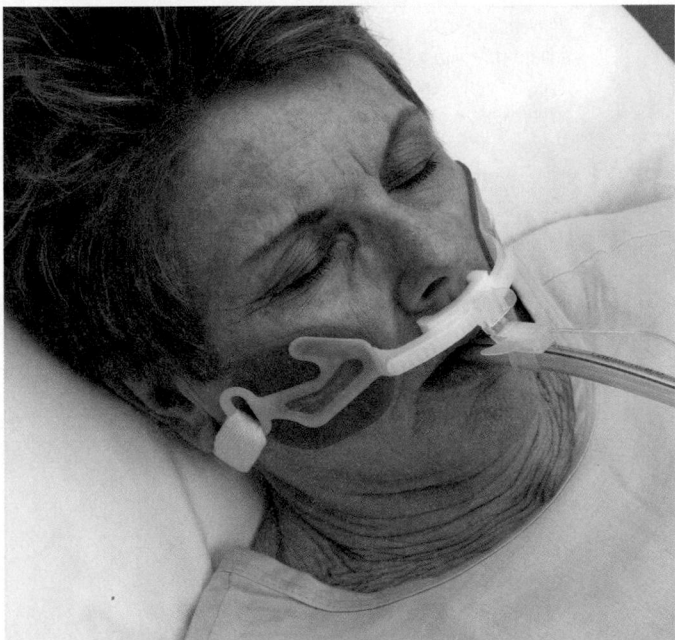

FIGURE 21-5 Commercial tube holder—Anchor Fast oral endotracheal tube fastener. (Courtesy Hollister Incorporated, Libertyville, IL.)

arrest.[15] Tracheal rupture is a rare and often fatal complication that is associated with emergent intubation.[16] Hypoxemia and hypercapnia can also occur, resulting in bradycardia, tachycardia, dysrhythmias, hypertension, and hypotension.[8,12,15]

Several complications can occur while the ETT is in place, including nasal and oral inflammation and ulceration, sinusitis and otitis, laryngeal and tracheal injuries, and tube obstruction and displacement. Other complications can occur days to weeks after the ETT is removed, including laryngeal and tracheal

stenosis and a cricoid abscess (Table 21-3). Delayed complications usually require some form of surgical intervention.[17,18]

Tracheostomy Tubes

A tracheostomy tube is the preferred method of airway maintenance in the patient who requires long-term intubation. Although no ideal time to perform the procedure has been identified, it is commonly accepted that if a patient has been intubated or is anticipated to be intubated for longer than 7 to 10 days, a tracheostomy should be performed.[19] A tracheostomy is also indicated in several other situations such as the presence of an upper airway obstruction due to trauma, tumors, or swelling and the need to facilitate airway clearance due to spinal cord injury, neuromuscular disease, or severe debilitation.[20,21]

A tracheostomy tube provides the best route for long-term airway maintenance because it avoids the oral, nasal, pharyngeal, and laryngeal complications associated with an ETT. The tube is shorter, of wider diameter, and less curved than an ETT; the resistance to air flow is less, and breathing is easier. Additional advantages of a tracheostomy tube include easier secretion removal, increased patient acceptance and comfort, capability of the patient to eat and talk if possible, and easier ventilator weaning.[11,20] See Table 21-2 for a list of the advantages of a tracheostomy tube.

Tracheostomy tubes are made of plastic or metal and may have one or two lumens. Single-lumen tubes consist of the tube; a built-in cuff, which is connected to a pilot balloon for inflation purposes; and an obturator, which is used during tube insertion. The double-lumen tubes consist of the tube with the attached cuff, the obturator, and an inner cannula that can be removed for cleaning and then reinserted or, if disposable, replaced by a new sterile inner cannula. The inner cannula can quickly be removed if it becomes obstructed, making the system safer for patients with significant secretion problems. Single-lumen tubes provide a larger internal diameter for airflow, so airflow resistance is reduced, and the patient can ventilate through the tube with greater ease. Plastic tracheostomy tubes also have a 15-mm adaptor on the end (Fig. 21-6).[20,21]

Tracheostomy Procedure

A tracheostomy tube is inserted by an open procedure or a percutaneous procedure. An open procedure is usually performed in the operating room, whereas a percutaneous procedure can be done at the patient's bedside.[21-23]

Complications

A number of complications can occur during the tracheostomy procedure, including misplacement of the tracheal tube, hemorrhage, laryngeal nerve injury, pneumothorax, pneumomediastinum, and cardiac arrest.[17,21,22] Several complications can occur while the tracheostomy tube is in place, including stomal infection, hemorrhage, tracheomalacia, tracheoesophageal fistula, tracheoinnominate artery fistula, and tube obstruction and displacement.[21,22] A number of complications can occur days to weeks after the tracheostomy tube is removed, including

TABLE 21-3   COMPLICATIONS OF ENDOTRACHEAL TUBES

COMPLICATIONS	CAUSES	PREVENTION AND TREATMENT
Tube obstruction	Patient biting tube Tube kinking during repositioning Cuff herniation Dried secretions, blood, or lubricant Tissue from tumor Trauma Foreign body	*Prevention:* Place bite block. Sedate patient PRN. Suction PRN. Humidify inspired gases. *Treatment:* Replace tube.
Tube displacement	Movement of patient's head Movement of tube by patient's tongue Traction on tube from ventilator tubing Self-extubation	*Prevention:* Secure tube to upper lip. Restrain patient's hands as needed. Sedate patient PRN. Ensure that only 2 inches of tube extend beyond lip. Support ventilator tubing. *Treatment:* Replace tube.
Sinusitis and nasal injury	Obstruction of the paranasal sinus drainage Pressure necrosis of nares	*Prevention:* Avoid nasal intubations. Cushion nares from tube and tape or ties. *Treatment:* Remove all tubes from nasal passages. Administer antibiotics.
Tracheoesophageal fistula	Pressure necrosis of posterior tracheal wall, resulting from overinflated cuff and rigid nasogastric tube	*Prevention:* Inflate cuff with minimal amount of air necessary. Monitor cuff pressures every 8 hours. *Treatment:* Position cuff of tube distal to fistula. Place gastrostomy tube for enteral feedings. Place esophageal tube for secretion clearance proximal to fistula.
Mucosal lesions	Pressure at tube and mucosal interface	*Prevention:* Inflate cuff with minimal amount of air necessary. Monitor cuff pressures every 8 hours. Use appropriate size tube. *Treatment:* May resolve spontaneously. Perform surgical intervention.
Laryngeal or tracheal stenosis	Injury to area from end of tube or cuff, resulting in scar tissue formation and narrowing of airway	*Prevention:* Inflate cuff with minimal amount of air necessary. Monitor cuff pressures every 8 hours. Suction area above cuff frequently. *Treatment:* Perform tracheostomy. Place laryngeal stent. Perform surgical repair.
Cricoid abscess	Mucosal injury with bacterial invasion	*Prevention:* Inflate cuff with minimal amount of air necessary. Monitor cuff pressures every 8 hours. Suction area above cuff frequently. *Treatment:* Perform incision and drainage of area. Administer antibiotics.

PRN, As needed.

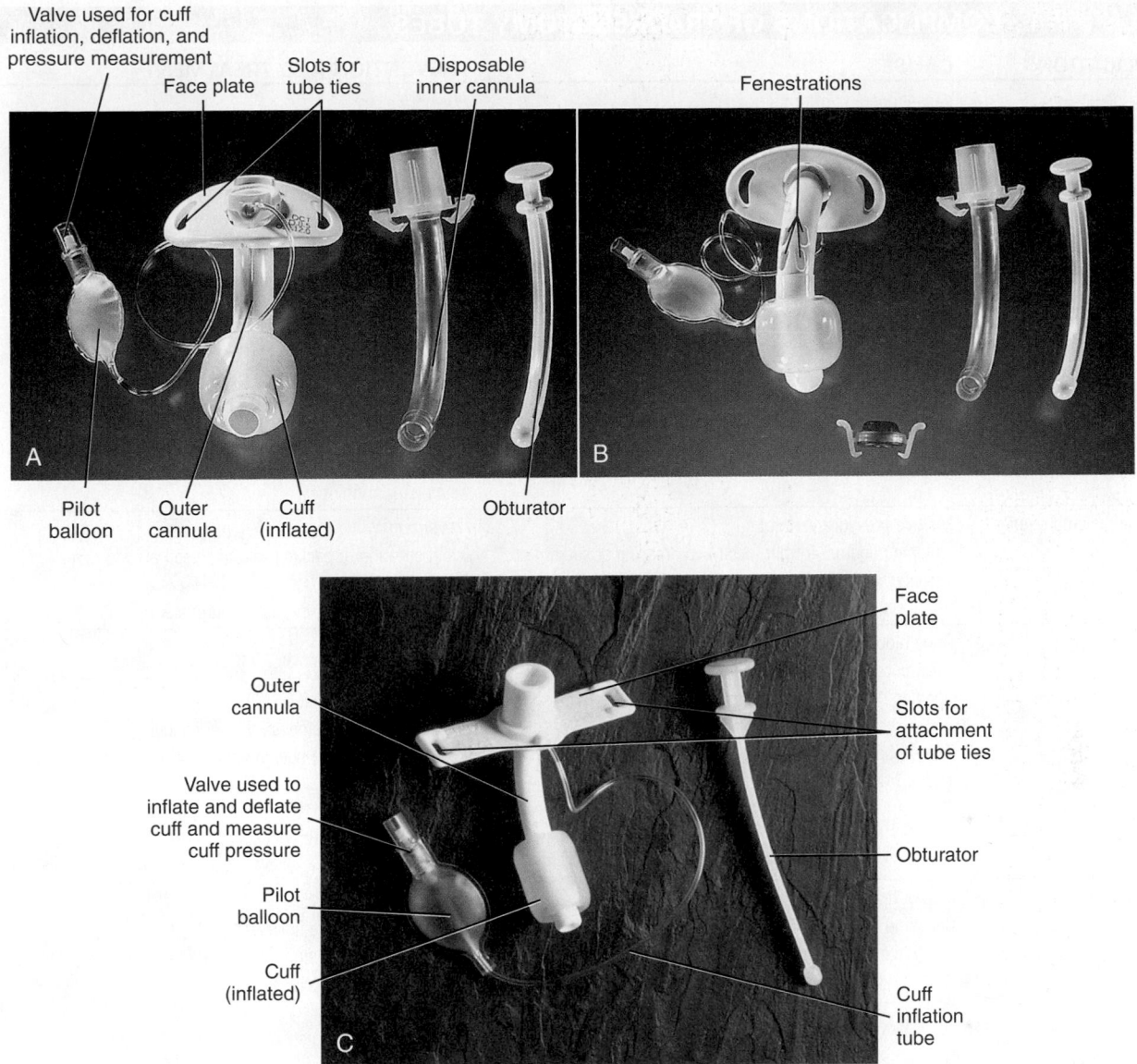

FIGURE 21-6   Tracheostomy Tubes. *A,* Dual-lumen cuffed tracheostomy tube with disposable inner cannula. *B,* Dual-lumen cuffed fenestrated tracheostomy tube. *C,* Single-lumen cannula cuffed tracheostomy tube. (From Rees HC. Care of patients requiring oxygen therapy or tracheostomy. In: Ignatavicius DD, Workman ML, eds. *Medical-Surgical Nursing.* 7th ed. St. Louis: Elsevier; 2013.)

tracheal stenosis and tracheocutaneous fistula (Table 21-4). Delayed complications usually require some form of surgical intervention.[21]

Nursing Management

Nursing management of the patient with an endotracheal or tracheostomy tube requires some additional measures to address the effects associated with tube placement on the respiratory and other body systems (Box 21-2). Nursing interventions for the patient with an artificial airway include providing humidification, managing the cuff, suctioning, establishing a method of communication, and providing oral hygiene. Because the tube bypasses the upper airway system, warming and humidifying of air must be performed by external means. Because the cuff of the tube can cause damage to the walls of the trachea, proper cuff inflation and management are

imperative. In addition, the normal defense mechanisms are impaired and secretions may accumulate; thus, suctioning may be needed to promote secretion clearance. Because the tube does not allow air flow over the vocal cords, developing a method of communication is also very important. Last, observing the patient to ensure proper placement of the tube and patency of the airway is essential.

Patient safety is critically important when caring for a patient with an artificial airway, as loss of the tube can result in loss of the patient's airway. In the event of unintentional extubation or decannulation, the patient's airway should be opened with the head tilt–chin lift maneuver and maintained with an oropharyngeal or nasopharyngeal airway. If the patient is not breathing, he or she should be manually ventilated with a manual resuscitation bag and face mask with 100% oxygen. In the case of a tracheostomy, the stoma should be covered to prevent air

TABLE 21-4 COMPLICATIONS OF TRACHEOSTOMY TUBES

COMPLICATIONS	CAUSES	PREVENTION AND TREATMENT
Hemorrhage	Vessel opening after surgery Vessel erosion caused by tube	*Prevention:* Use appropriate size tube. Treat local infection. Suction gently. Humidify inspired gases. Position tracheal window not lower than third tracheal ring. *Treatment:* Pack lightly. Perform surgical intervention.
Wound infection	Colonization of stoma with hospital flora	*Prevention:* Perform routine stoma care. *Treatment:* Remove tube, if necessary. Perform aggressive wound care and débridement. Administer antibiotics.
Subcutaneous emphysema	Positive-pressure ventilation Coughing against a tight, occlusive dressing or sutured or packed wound	*Prevention:* Avoid suturing or packing wound closed around tube. *Treatment:* Remove any sutures or packing, if present.
Tube obstruction	Dried blood or secretions False passage into soft tissues Opening of cannula positioned against tracheal wall Foreign body Tissue from tumor	*Prevention:* Suction PRN. Humidify inspired gases. Use a tube with a removable inner cannula. Position tube so that opening does not press against tracheal wall. *Treatment:* Remove or replace inner cannula. Replace tube.
Tube displacement	Patient movement Coughing Traction on ventilatory tubing	*Prevention:* Use commercial tube holder. Use tubes with adjustable neck plates for patients with short necks. Support ventilatory tubing. Sedate patient PRN. Restrain patient, as needed. *Treatment:* Cover stoma and manually ventilate patient by mouth. Replace tube.
Tracheal stenosis	Injury to area from end of tube or cuff, resulting in scar tissue formation and narrowing of airway	*Prevention:* Inflate cuff with minimal amount of air necessary. Monitor cuff pressures every 8 hours. *Treatment:* Perform surgical repair.
Tracheoesophageal fistula	Pressure necrosis of posterior tracheal wall, resulting from overinflated cuff and rigid nasogastric tube	*Prevention:* Inflate cuff with minimal amount of air necessary. Monitor cuff pressures every 8 hours. *Treatment:* Perform surgical repair.
Tracheoinnominate artery fistula	Direct pressure from the elbow of the cannula against the innominate artery Placement of tracheal stoma below fourth tracheal ring Downward migration of the tracheal stoma, resulting from traction on tube High-lying innominate artery	*Prevention:* Position tracheal window not lower than third tracheal ring. *Treatment:* Hyperinflate cuff to control bleeding. Remove tube and replace with endotracheal tube, and apply digital pressure through stoma against the sternum. Perform surgical repair.
Tracheocutaneous fistula	Failure of stoma to close after removal of tube	*Treatment:* Perform surgical repair.

PRN, As needed.

BOX 21-2   NIC

Artificial Airway Management

Definition

Maintenance of endotracheal and tracheostomy tubes and prevention of complications associated with their use

Activities

- Perform hand hygiene.
- Use universal precautions.
- Use personal protective equipment (gloves, goggles, and mask), as appropriate.
- Provide an oropharyngeal airway or bite block to prevent biting on the endotracheal tube, as appropriate.
- Provide 100% humidification of inspired air, oxygen, or gas.
- Provide adequate systemic hydration via oral or intravenous fluid administration.
- Inflate endotracheal or tracheostoma cuff using minimal occlusive volume (MOV) technique or minimal leak technique (MLT).
- Maintain inflation of the endotracheal or tracheostoma cuff at 15 to 25 mm Hg during mechanical ventilation and during and after feeding.
- Monitor cuff pressures every 4 to 8 hours during expiration using a three-way stopcock, calibrated syringe, and manometer.
- Check cuff pressure immediately after delivery of any general anesthesia or manipulation of endotracheal tube.
- Institute endotracheal suctioning, as appropriate.
- Suction the oropharynx and secretions from the top of the tube cuff before deflating cuff.
- Change endotracheal tapes or ties every 24 hours, inspect the skin and oral mucosa, and reposition ET to the other side of the mouth.
- Loosen commercial endotracheal tube holders at least once a day, and provide skin care.
- Auscultate for presence of lung sounds bilaterally after insertion and after changing endotracheal or tracheostomy ties.
- Note the centimeter reference marking on endotracheal tube to monitor for possible displacement.
- Assist with chest radiographic examination, as needed, to monitor position of tube.
- Minimize leverage and traction on the artificial airway by suspending ventilator tubing from overhead supports, using flexible catheter mounts and swivels, and supporting tubes during turning, suctioning, and ventilator disconnection and reconnection.
- Monitor for presence of crackles and rhonchi over large airways.
- Monitor secretions: color, amount, and consistency.
- Perform oral care (i.e., use toothbrush, swabs, mouth and lip moisturizer), as needed.
- Monitor for decrease in exhale volume and increase in inspiratory pressure in patients receiving mechanical ventilation.
- Institute measures to prevent spontaneous decannulation (i.e., secure artificial airway with tape or ties, administer sedation and muscle paralyzing agent, use arm restraints), as appropriate.
- Provide additional intubation equipment and Ambu bag in a readily available location.
- Provide trachea care every 4 to 8 hours, as appropriate: clean the inner cannula, clean and dry the area around the stoma, and change tracheostomy ties.
- Inspect skin around tracheal stoma for drainage, redness, irritation and bleeding.
- Inspect and palpate for air under skin every 8 hours.
- Monitor for presence of pain.
- Maintain sterile technique when suctioning and providing tracheostomy care.
- Shield the tracheostomy from water.
- Tape the tracheostomy obturator to head of bed.
- Tape a second tracheostomy (same type and size) and forceps to head of bed.
- Institute chest physiotherapy, as appropriate.
- Ensure that endotracheal or tracheostomy cuff is inflated during feedings, as appropriate.
- Elevate head of the bed 30 degrees or more, or assist patient to a sitting position in a chair during feedings, as appropriate.

From Bulechek GM, et al. *Nursing Interventions Classification (NIC)*, 6th ed. St. Louis: Mosby; 2013.

---

from escaping through it. If the tracheostomy remains open then consideration should be given to ventilating the patient through the stoma instead of the mouth.

One recent study examined patients' perception of endotracheal tube–related discomforts. Forty-six percent of the patients reported remembering having the endotracheal tube while in the critical care unit. The majority of these patients found the discomfort associated with the ETT and the inability to speak very stressful. In addition, some of the patient's continued to have problems with hoarseness, sore throat, and voice changes days to months later.[24]

Humidification

Humidification of air normally is performed by the mucosal layer of the upper respiratory tract. When this area is bypassed, as occurs with ETT and tracheostomy tubes or when supplemental oxygen is used, humidification by external means is necessary. Various humidification devices add water to inhaled gas to prevent drying and irritation of the respiratory tract, to prevent undue loss of body water, and to facilitate secretion

removal.[25,26] The humidification device should provide inspired gas conditioned (heated) to body temperature and saturated with water vapor.[27]

Cuff Management

Because the cuff of the ETT or tracheostomy tube is a major source of the complications associated with artificial airways, proper cuff management is essential. To prevent the complications associated with cuff design, only low-pressure, high-volume cuffed tubes are used in clinical practice.[13,28] Even with these tubes, cuff pressures can be generated that are high enough to lead to tracheal ischemia and injury. Proper cuff inflation techniques and cuff pressure monitoring are critical components of the care of the patient with an artificial airway.[10,28] Figure 21-7 is an example of a one device used to measure cuff pressures.

Cuff Inflation Techniques. Two cuff inflation techniques are used: 1) the minimal leak (ML) technique and 2) the minimal occlusion volume (MOV) technique. The ML technique consists of injecting air into the cuff until no leak is heard and then

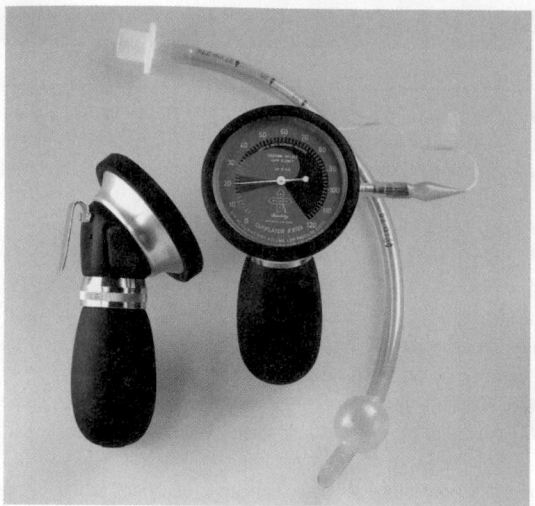

FIGURE 21-7 An aneroid pressure manometer for cuff inflation and measuring cuff pressures. (From Rees HC. Care of patients requiring oxygen therapy or tracheostomy. In: Ignatavicius DD, Workman ML, eds. *Medical-Surgical Nursing*. 7th ed. St. Louis: Elsevier; 2013.)

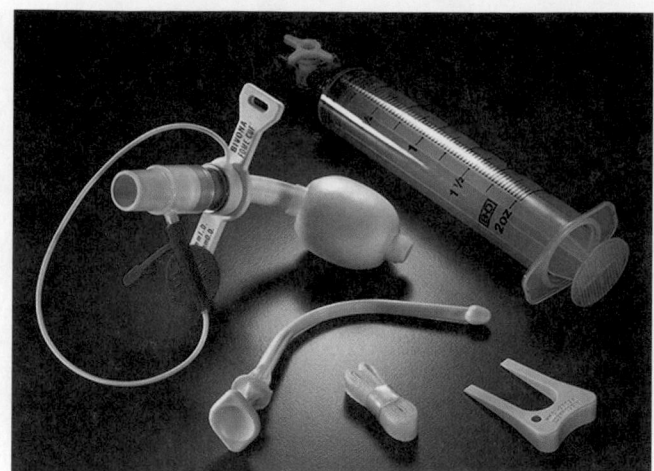

FIGURE 21-8 Foam cuff tracheostomy tube. (Courtesy Smiths Medical, Inc., London, England.)

withdrawing the air until a small leak is heard on inspiration. Problems with this technique include difficulty maintaining positive end-expiratory pressure (PEEP) and aspiration around the cuff. The MOV technique consists of injecting air into the cuff until no leak is heard at peak inspiration. This technique generates higher cuff pressures than does the ML technique. The selection of one technique over the other is determined by individual patient needs. If the patient needs a seal to provide adequate ventilation or is at high risk for aspiration, the MOV technique is used. If these are not concerns, usually the ML technique is used.[10,11,28]

Cuff Pressure Monitoring. Cuff pressures are monitored at least every shift with a cuff pressure manometer. Cuff pressures should be maintained at 20 to 25 mm Hg (24 to 30 cm H_2O) because greater pressures decrease blood flow to the capillaries in the tracheal wall and lesser pressures increase the risk of aspiration. Pressures in excess of 25 mm Hg (30 cm H_2O) should be reported to the physician. Cuffs are not routinely deflated because this increases the risk of aspiration.[10,28]

Foam Cuff Tracheostomy Tubes. One tracheostomy tube on the market has a cuff made of foam that is self-inflating (Fig. 21-8). It is deflated during insertion, after which the pilot port is opened to atmospheric pressure (room air), and the cuff self-inflates. After inflation, the foam cuff conforms to the size and shape of the patient's trachea, thereby reducing the pressure against the tracheal wall. The pilot port can be left open to atmospheric pressure or attached to the mechanical ventilator tubing, allowing the cuff to inflate and deflate with the cycling of the ventilator. Routine maintenance of a foam cuff tracheostomy tube includes aspirating the pilot port every 8 hours to measure cuff volume, to remove any condensation from the cuff area, and to assess the integrity of the cuff. Removal is accomplished by deflating the cuff; this can be complicated if the plastic sheath covering the foam is perforated. If perforation occurs, the foam may not be deflatable because the air cannot be totally aspirated.[21]

Subglottic Secretion Removal. The cuff has also been implicated in the development of ventilator-associated pneumonia. Fluids can leak around the cuff into the airway, resulting in microaspiration. Bacteria-laden oral secretions trickle down the larynx and pool above the cuff of the artificial airway. These secretions are referred to as *subglottic secretions*. Subglottic secretions can then leak into the lower airways around the cuff via the longitudinal folds in that form in the cuff as it accommodates for the shape of the airway, an underinflated cuff that fails to form a proper seal in the airway, or inadvertent movement of the endotracheal tube within airway. Thus, the use of established cuff inflation techniques, monitoring of cuff pressures, using an appropriate method of tube stabilization, and oral hygiene are important interventions for preventing this problem.[29] Deep oropharyngeal suctioning to remove subglottic secretions should be performed at least every 12 hours and prior to deflating the cuff or moving the tube.[30]

Specialized tubes are available to allow for the continuous removal of subglottic secretions. These tubes have an additional lumen, with an opening above the cuff, which is connected to continuous (−20 to −30 cm H_2O) suction (Fig. 21-9).[11] These tubes are recommended for patients who are expected to be intubated for longer than 72 hours.[31] One issue with these tubes is that the aspiration lumen can become clogged and, thus, requires a small amount of air to be injected into the aspiration port every 4 hours.

Suctioning

Suctioning is often required to maintain a patent airway in the patient with an ETT or tracheostomy tube. Suctioning is a sterile procedure that is performed only when the patient needs it and not on a routine schedule.[10,32,33] Indications for suctioning include coughing, secretions in the airway, respiratory distress, presence of rhonchi on auscultation, increased peak airway pressures on the ventilator, and decreasing oxygenation saturation.[11] Complications associated with suctioning include hypoxemia, atelectasis, bronchospasms, dysrhythmias, increased intracranial pressure, and airway trauma.[11,32]

Complications. Hypoxemia can result because the oxygen source is disconnected from the patient or the oxygen is removed

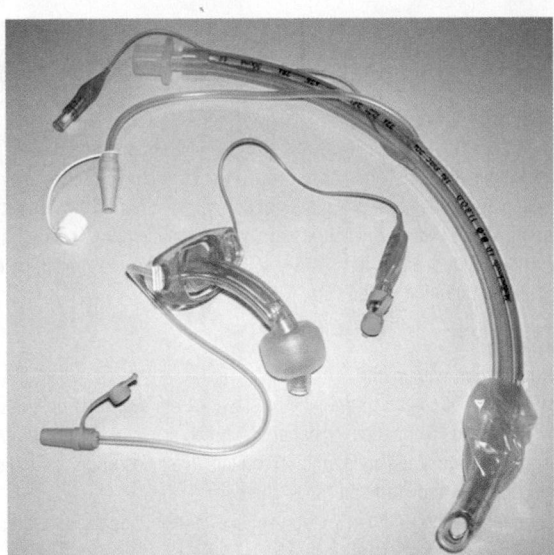

FIGURE 21-9 Endotracheal and tracheostomy tubes with sub-glottic suction ports. (From Altobelli N. Airway management. In: Kacmarek RM, et al, eds. *Egan's Fundamentals of Respiratory Care.* 10th ed. St. Louis: Mosby; 2013.)

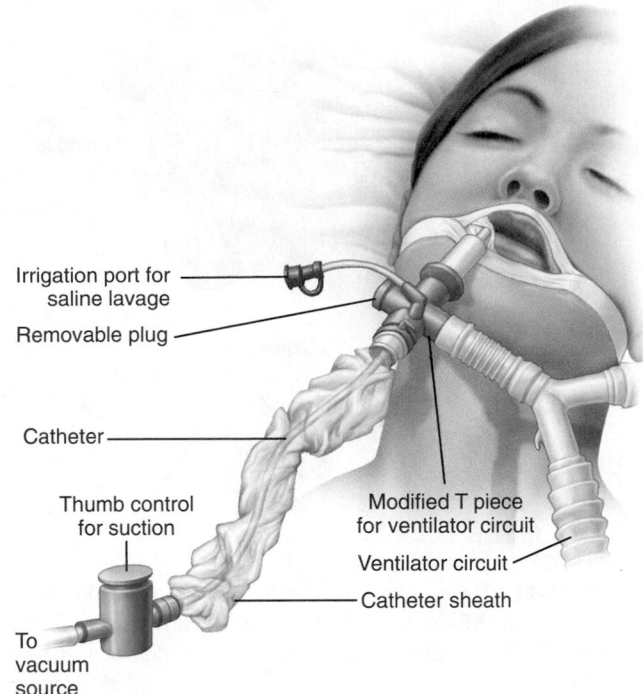

FIGURE 21-10 Closed tracheal suction system. (Modified from Sills JR. *Entry-Level Respiratory Therapist Exam Guide.* St. Louis: Mosby; 2000.)

from the patient's airways when the suction is applied. Atelectasis is thought to occur when the suction catheter is larger than one half of the diameter of the ETT. Excessive negative pressure occurs when suction is applied, promoting collapse of the distal airways. Bronchospasms are the result of stimulation of the airways with the suction catheter. Cardiac dysrhythmias, particularly bradycardias, are attributed to vagal stimulation. Airway trauma occurs with impaction of the catheter in the airways and excessive negative pressure applied to the catheter.[10,11,32]

Suctioning Protocol. A number of protocols regarding suctioning have been developed. Several practices have been found helpful in limiting the complications of suctioning. Hypoxemia can be minimized by giving the patient three hyperoxygenation breaths (breaths at 100% Fio_2) with the ventilator before the procedure begins and again after each pass of the suction catheter.[10,33,34] If the patient exhibits signs of desaturation, hyperinflation (breaths at 150% tidal volume) should be added to the procedure.[10] Atelectasis can be avoided by using a suction catheter with an external diameter of less than one half of the internal diameter of the ETT.[32,33] Using no greater than 120 mm Hg of suction decreases the chances of hypoxemia, atelectasis, and airway trauma.[10,33] Limiting the duration of each suction pass to 10 to 15 seconds;[10,32,33] and the number of passes to a maximum of three also helps minimize hypoxemia, airway trauma, and cardiac dysrhythmias.[35] The process of applying intermittent (instead of continuous) suction has been shown to be of no benefit.[33,36] The instillation of normal saline to help remove secretions has not proved to be of any benefit;[32,33,37] and it may actually contribute to the development of hypoxemia, as well as lower airway colonization, resulting in ventilator-associated pneumonia (VAP).[10,38,39]

Closed Tracheal Suction System. One device to facilitate the suctioning of a patient on a ventilator is the closed tracheal suction system (CTSS) (Fig. 21-10). This device consists of a suction catheter in a plastic sleeve that attaches directly to the ventilator tubing. It allows the patient to be suctioned while remaining on the ventilator. Advantages of the CTSS include maintenance of oxygenation and PEEP during suctioning, reduction of hypoxemia-related complications, and protection of staff members from the patient's secretions. The CTSS is convenient to use, requiring only one person to perform the procedure.[11]

Concerns related to the CTSS include autocontamination, inadequate removal of secretions, and increased risk of unintentional extubation resulting from the extra weight of the system on the ventilator tubing. Autocontamination has been shown not to be an issue if the catheter is cleaned properly after every use. Inadequate removal of secretions may or may not be a problem, and further investigation is required to settle this issue.[11] Although recommendations for changing the catheter vary, one study indicated that the catheter could be changed on an as-needed basis without increasing the incidence of VAP.[40] Once recent study found that suctioning with the CTSS caused massive aspiration of fluid around the tracheal tube cuff as a result of a significant drop in airway pressure.[41]

Communication

One of the major stressors for the patient with an artificial airway is impaired communication. This is related to the inability to speak, insufficient explanations from staff members, inadequate understanding, fear of being unable to communicate, and difficulty with communication methods.[42] A number of interventions can facilitate communication in the patient with an ETT or tracheostomy tube. These include establishing an environment that fosters communication, performing a complete assessment of the patient's ability to communicate,

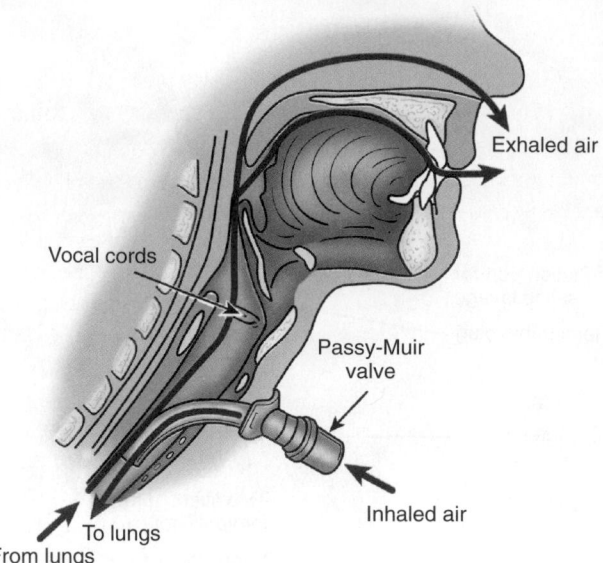

FIGURE 21-11 Passy-Muir valve mechanism of action. (From Hodder RV. A 55-year-old patient with advanced COPD, tracheostomy tube, and sudden respiratory distress. *Chest.* 2002;121[1]:279.)

BOX 21-3 SAMPLE ORAL CARE PROTOCOL

Standard of Care
1. The oral cavity is assessed initially and daily by a registered nurse.
2. Unconscious patients and those with artificial airways (endotracheal or tracheostomy tubes) are provided oral care every 4 hours and as needed.
3. Patients with cuffed artificial airways have oropharyngeal and subglottic secretions suctioned at least every 12 hours and before repositioning of the tube or deflation of the cuff.

Procedure
1. Set up suction equipment.
2. Position patient's head to the side or place in semi-Fowler's position.
3. Provide suction, as needed, to patients with an artificial airway to remove any oropharyngeal and subglottic secretions (those secretions that migrate down the tube and settle on top of the cuff).
4. Brush teeth using suction toothbrush and small amounts of water and alcohol-free antiseptic oral rinse.
   - Brush for approximately 1 to 2 minutes.
   - Exert gentle pressure while moving in short horizontal or circular strokes.
5. Gently brush surface of tongue.
6. Use suction swab to clean the teeth and tongue if brushing causes discomfort or bleeding.
   - Place swab perpendicular to gum line, applying gentle mechanical action for 1 to 2 minutes.
   - Turn swab in clockwise rotation to remove mucus and debris.
7. Swab mouth with 15 mL of 0.12% chlorhexidine every 12 hours.
8. Apply mouth moisturizer inside mouth.
9. Apply lip balm, if needed.

---

anticipating the patient's needs, teaching the patient and family how to communicate, using a variety of methods to communicate, and facilitating the patient's ability to communicate by providing the patient with his or her eyeglasses or hearing aid.[43]

Methods to facilitate communication in this patient population include the use of verbal and nonverbal language and a variety of devices to assist the patient on short-term and long-term ventilator assistance. Nonverbal communication may include the use of sign language, gestures, lip reading, pointing, facial expressions, or eye blinking. Simple devices available include pencil and paper; Magic Slates; magnetic boards with plastic letters; picture, alphabet, or symbol boards; and flash cards. More sophisticated devices include typewriters, computers, talking ETT and tracheostomy tubes, and external handheld vibrators. Regardless of the method selected, the patient must be taught how to use the device.[10,43]

Passy-Muir Valve. One device used to assist the mechanically ventilated patient with a tracheostomy to speak is the Passy-Muir valve. This one-way valve opens on inhalation, allowing air to enter the lungs through the tracheostomy tube, and closes on exhalation, forcing air over the vocal cords and out the mouth, permitting the patient to speak (Fig. 21-11). Before the valve can be placed on a tracheostomy tube, the cuff must be deflated to allow air to pass around the tube, and the tidal volume of the ventilator must be increased to compensate for the air leak. In addition to aiding communication, the Passy-Muir valve can assist the ventilator-dependent patient with relearning normal breathing patterns. The valve is contraindicated in patients with laryngeal or pharyngeal dysfunction, excessive secretions, or poor lung compliance.[43]

Oral Hygiene

Patients with artificial airways are extremely susceptible to developing VAP because of microaspiration of subglottic secretions. These secretions are full of microorganisms from the patient's mouth. Because the cuff of the artificial airway does not form a tight seal in the patient's airway, these secretions seep around the cuff into the patient's lungs, promoting the development of VAP.[44] Although bacteria are normally present in a patient's mouth, in the critically ill patient, increased amounts of bacteria and more resistant bacteria are present. Decreased salivary flow, poor mucosal status, and dental plaque all contribute to this problem.[45]

Proper oral hygiene has the potential to decrease the incidence of VAP.[30,45] However, recent studies have shown that routine oral care is not a priority intervention for many nurses.[46] Currently, no evidence-based protocol exists for oral care. Research studies are lacking, particularly with regard to frequency and effectiveness of different procedures.[47] Most experts agree, however, that oral care should consist of brushing the patient's teeth with a soft toothbrush to reduce plaque, brushing the patient's tongue and gums with a foam swab to stimulate the tissue, and performing deep oropharyngeal suctioning to remove any secretions that have pooled above the patient's cuff.[30,48] A sample oral care protocol is outlined in Box 21-3. One intervention that has evidence supporting its use is rinsing or swabbing the patient's mouth with 15 mL of 0.12% chlorhexidine every 12 hours.[49] This procedure has been shown to reduce oral colonization of bacteria and to decrease the incidence of ventilator-associated pneumonia, particularly in patients who have undergone cardiac surgery or trauma.[39,50]

Endotracheal Extubation

Definition
Purposeful removal of the endotracheal tube from the nasopharyngeal or oropharyngeal airway

Activities
- Position patient for best use of ventilatory muscles, usually with head of bed elevated 75 degrees.
- Instruct patient about procedure.
- Hyperoxygenate patient and suction endotracheal airway.
- Suction oral airway.
- Deflate endotracheal cuff and remove endotracheal tube.
- Encourage patient to cough and expectorate sputum.
- Administer oxygen, as ordered.
- Encourage coughing and deep breathing.
- Suction airway, as needed.
- Monitor for respiratory distress.
- Observe for signs of airway occlusion.
- Monitor vital signs.
- Encourage voice rest for 4 to 8 hours, as appropriate.
- Monitor ability to swallow and talk.

From Bulechek GM, et al. *Nursing Interventions Classification (NIC)*, 6th ed. St. Louis: Mosby; 2013.

Extubation and Decannulation

After the airway is no longer needed, it is removed. Extubation is the process of removing an ETT. It is a simple procedure that can be accomplished at the bedside (Box 21-4).[10,11] Before the cuff of an ETT or tracheostomy tube is deflated in preparation for removal, it is very important to ensure that secretions are cleared from above the tube cuff. Complications of extubation include sore throat, stridor, hoarseness, odynophagia, vocal cord immobility, pulmonary aspiration, and cough.[17] Decannulation is the process of removing a tracheostomy tube. It is also a simple process that can be performed at the bedside. After removal of the tracheostomy tube, the stoma is usually covered with a dry dressing, with the expectation that it will close within several days.[10,11] Difficulty removing the tracheostomy tube because of a tight stoma is usually the only complication associated with decannulation.[17]

INVASIVE MECHANICAL VENTILATION

Indications

Mechanical ventilation is the process of using an apparatus to facilitate the transport of oxygen and CO_2 between the atmosphere and the alveoli for the purpose of enhancing pulmonary gas exchange. It is indicated for physiologic and clinical reasons. Physiologic objectives include supporting cardiopulmonary gas exchange (alveolar ventilation and arterial oxygenation), increasing lung volume (end-expiratory lung inflation and functional residual capacity), and reducing the work of breathing. Clinical objectives include reversing hypoxemia and acute respiratory acidosis, relieving respiratory distress, preventing or reversing atelectasis and respiratory muscle fatigue, permitting sedation and neuromuscular blockade, decreasing oxygen consumption, reducing intracranial pressure, and stabilizing the chest wall.[51,52]

Use of Mechanical Ventilators
Types of Ventilators

The two main types of ventilators currently available are: 1) positive-pressure ventilators and 2) negative-pressure ventilators. Negative-pressure ventilators are applied externally to the patient and decrease the atmospheric pressure surrounding the thorax to initiate inspiration. They generally are not used in the critical care environment. Positive-pressure ventilators use a mechanical drive mechanism to force air into the patient's lungs through an ETT or tracheostomy tube.[53]

Ventilator Mechanics

The ventilator must complete four phases of ventilation to properly ventilate the patient: 1) change from exhalation to inspiration; 2) inspiration; 3) change from inspiration to exhalation; and 4) exhalation. The ventilator uses four different variables to begin, sustain, and terminate each of these phases. These variables are described in terms of *volume, pressure, flow,* and *time.*[7,51,54,55]

Trigger. The phase variable that initiates the change from exhalation to inspiration is called the *trigger.* Breaths may be pressure triggered or flow triggered, depending on the sensitivity setting of the ventilator and the patient's inspiratory effort; or they may be time triggered, depending on the rate setting of the ventilator. A breath that is initiated by the patient is known as a *patient-triggered* or *patient-assisted* breath, whereas a breath that is initiated by the ventilator is known as a *machine-triggered* or *machine-controlled* breath.[54]

A *time-triggered breath* is a machine-controlled breath that is initiated by the ventilator after a preset length of time has elapsed. It is controlled by the rate setting on the ventilator (e.g., a rate of 10 breaths per minute yields 1 breath every 6 seconds). *Flow-triggered* and *pressure-triggered* breaths are patient-assisted breaths that are initiated by decreased flow or pressure, respectively, within the breathing circuit. Flow triggering (also known as *flow-by*) is controlled by adjusting the flow-sensitivity setting of the ventilator, whereas pressure triggering is controlled by adjusting the pressure-sensitivity setting. Many ventilators offer the various types of triggers in combination. For example, a breath may be time triggered and flow triggered, depending on the patient's ability to interact with the ventilator and initiate a breath.[7,53,54]

Limit. The variable that maintains inspiration is called the *limit* or *target.* Inspiration can be pressure limited, flow limited, or volume limited. A *pressure-limited breath* is one in which a preset pressure is attained and maintained during inspiration. A *flow-limited breath* is one in which a preset flow is reached before the end of inspiration. A *volume-limited breath* is one in which a preset volume is delivered during the inspiration. However, the limit variable does not end inspiration; it only sustains it.[7,53,54]

Cycle. The variable that ends inspiration is called the *cycle.* The classification of positive-pressure ventilators is based on this variable: volume-cycled, pressure-cycled, flow-cycled, and time-cycled ventilators. *Volume-cycled ventilators* are designed to deliver a breath until a preset volume is delivered. *Pressure-cycled ventilators* deliver a breath until a preset pressure is reached within the patient's airways. *Flow-cycled ventilators* deliver a breath until a preset inspiratory flow rate is achieved. *Time-cycled ventilators* deliver a breath over a preset time interval.[7,53,54]

Baseline. The variable that is controlled during exhalation is called the *baseline*. Pressure is almost always used to adjust this variable. The patient exhales to a certain baseline pressure that is set on the ventilator. It may be set at zero (i.e., atmospheric pressure) or above atmospheric pressure (i.e., PEEP).[7,53,54]

Modes of Ventilation

The term *ventilator mode* refers to how the machine ventilates the patient. Selection of a particular mode of ventilation determines how much the patient will participate in his or her own ventilatory pattern. The choice depends on the patient's situation and the goals of treatment. The mode is determined by the combination of phase variables selected. Many modes are available (Table 21-5), and some may be used in conjunction with others.[7,51-55] Because brands of ventilators vary in their ability to perform certain functions, not all modes are available on all ventilators.[54]

Ventilator Settings

Settings on the ventilator allow the ventilator parameters to be individualized to the patient and also allow selection of the desired ventilation mode (Table 21-6). Each ventilator has a patient-monitoring system that allows all aspects of the

TABLE 21-5 MODES OF MECHANICAL VENTILATION

MODE OF VENTILATION	CLINICAL APPLICATION	NURSING IMPLICATIONS
Continuous mandatory (volume or pressure) ventilation (CMV), also known as assist-control (AC) ventilation: delivers gas at preset tidal volume or pressure (depending on selected cycling variable) in response to patient's inspirator or efforts and initiates breath if patient fails to do so within preset time.	Volume-controlled (VC) CMV is used as the primary mode of ventilation in spontaneously breathing patients with weak respiratory muscles. Pressure-controlled (PC) CMV is used in patients with decreased lung compliance or increased airway resistance, particularly when the patient is at risk for volutrauma.	Hyperventilation can occur in patients with increased respiratory rates. Sedation may be necessary to limit the number of spontaneous breaths. Patient on VC-CMV should be monitored for volutrauma. Patient on PC-CMV should be monitored for hypercapnia.
Pressure-regulated volume control ventilation (PRVCV): a variation of CMV that combines volume and pressure features; delivers a preset tidal volume using the lowest possible airway pressure; airway pressure will not exceed preset maximum pressure limit.	PRVCV is used in patients with rapidly changing pulmonary mechanics (airway resistance and lung compliance), limiting potential complications.	
Pressure-controlled inverse ratio ventilation (PC-IRV): PC-CMV mode in which the inspiratory-to-expiratory (I : E) time ratio is greater than 1 : 1.	PC-IRV is used in patients with hypoxemia refractory to positive end-expiratory pressure (PEEP); the longer inspiratory time increases functional residual capacity and improves oxygenation by opening collapsed alveoli, and the shorter expiratory time induces auto-PEEP that prevents alveoli from recollapsing.	Requires sedation or pharmacologic paralysis, or both because of discomfort. Increased intrathoracic pressure can result in excessive air trapping and decreased cardiac output.
Intermittent mandatory (volume or pressure) ventilation (IMV), also known as synchronous intermittent mandatory ventilation (SIMV): delivers gas at preset tidal volume or pressure (depending on selected cycling variable) and rate while allowing patient to breathe spontaneously; ventilator breaths are synchronized to patient's respiratory effort.	VC-IMV is used as a primary mode of ventilation in many clinical situations and as a weaning mode. PC-IMV is used in patients with decreased lung compliance or increased airway resistance when the need to preserve the patient's spontaneous effects is important.	May increase the work of breathing and promote respiratory muscle fatigue. Patient should be monitored for hypercapnia, particularly with PC-IMV.
Adaptive support ventilation (ASV): ventilator automatically adjusts settings to maintain 100 mL/min/kg of minute ventilation; pressure support.	ASV is a computerized mode of ventilation that increases or decreases ventilatory support based on patient needs; can be used with any patient requiring volume-controlled ventilation.	Not intended as a weaning mode. Adapts to changes in patient position.
Constant positive airway pressure (CPAP): positive pressure applied during spontaneous breaths; patient controls rate, inspiratory flow, and tidal volume.	CPAP is a spontaneous breathing mode used in patients to increase functional residual capacity and improve oxygenation by opening collapsed alveoli at end expiration; it is also used for weaning.	Side effects include decreased cardiac output, volutrauma, and increased intracranial pressure. No ventilator breaths are delivered in PEEP or CPAP mode unless used with CMV or IMV.
Airway pressure release ventilation (APRV): two different levels of CPAP (inspiratory puland expiratory) are applied for set periods of time, allowing spontaneous breathing to occur at both levels.	APRV is a spontaneous breathing mode used to maintain alveolar recruitment without imposing additional peak inspiratory pressures that could lead to barotrauma.	Patient needs to be monitored for hypercapnia.

TABLE 21-5 MODES OF MECHANICAL VENTILATION—cont'd

MODE OF VENTILATION	CLINICAL APPLICATION	NURSING IMPLICATIONS
Pressure support ventilation (PSV): preset positive pressure used to augment patient's inspiratory efforts; patient controls rate, inspiratory flow, and tidal volume.	PSV is a spontaneous breathing mode used as the primary mode of ventilation in patients with stable respiratory drive to overcome any imposed mechanical resistance (e.g., artificial airway). PSV can also be used with IMV to support spontaneous breaths.	Patient should be monitored for hypercapnia. Advantages include reduced patient work of breathing and improved patient-ventilator synchrony.
Volume-assured pressure support ventilation (VAPSV), also known as pressure augmentation (PA): a variation of PSV with a set tidal volume to ensure that patient receives minimum tidal volume with each pressure support breath.	VAPSV is a spontaneous breathing mode used to treat acute respiratory illness and to facilitate weaning.	Advantages include increased patient comfort, decreased work of breathing, decreased respiratory muscle fatigue, and promotion of respiratory muscle conditioning.
Neurally adjusted ventilatory assist (NAVA): a partial ventilatory support mode that uses the electrical activity of the diaphragm (Edi) to control patient ventilator interaction.	NAVA delivers an assisted breath in proportion to and in synchrony with the patient's respiratory effort.	Requires an esophageal catheter (similar to an nasogastric tube) that measures the electrical signal to the diaphragm (Edi).
Independent lung ventilation (ILV): each lung is ventilated separately.	ILV is used in patients with unilateral lung disease, bronchopleural fistulas, or bilateral asymmetric lung disease.	Requires a double-lumen endotracheal tube, two ventilators, sedation, pharmacologic paralysis, or all.
High-frequency ventilation (HFV): delivers a small volume of gas at a rapid rate. *High-frequency positive-pressure ventilation (HFPPV):* delivers 60-100 breaths/mm. *High-frequency jet ventilation (HFJV):* delivers 100-600 cycles/min. *High-frequency oscillation (HFO):* delivers 900-3000 cycles/min.	HFV is used in situations in which conventional mechanical ventilation compromises hemodynamic stability, in patients with bronchopleural fistulas, during short-term procedures, and with diseases that create a risk of volutrauma.	Patients require sedation, pharmacologic paralysis, or both. Inadequate humidification can compromise airway patency. Assessment of breath sounds is difficult.

TABLE 21-6 VENTILATOR SETTINGS

PARAMETER	DESCRIPTION	TYPICAL SETTINGS
Respiratory rate or Frequency (f)	Number of breaths the ventilator delivers per minute	6-20 breaths/min
Tidal volume (Vt)	Volume of gas delivered to patient during each ventilator breath	6-10 mL/kg 4-8 mL/kg in acute respiratory distress syndrome (ARDS)
Oxygen concentration (FiO_2)	Fraction of inspired oxygen delivered to patient	May be set between 21% and 100%; adjusted to maintain PaO_2 (arterial partial pressure of oxygen) level greater than 60 mm Hg or SpO_2 (oxygen saturation based on pulse oximeter) level greater than 92%
Positive end-expiratory pressure (PEEP)	Positive pressure applied at the end of expiration of ventilator breaths	3-5 cm H_2O
Pressure support (PS)	Positive pressure used to augment patient's inspiratory efforts	5-10 cm H_2O
Inspiratory flow rate and time	Speed with which the tidal volume is delivered	40-80 L/min Time: 0.8-1.2 sec
I : E ratio	Ratio of duration of inspiration to duration of expiration	1 : 2 to 1 : 1.5 unless inverse ratio ventilation is desired
Sensitivity	Determines the amount of effort the patient must generate to initiate a ventilator breath; it may be set for pressure-triggering or flow-triggering	Pressure trigger: 0.5-1.5 cm H_2O below baseline pressure Flow trigger: 1-3 L/min below baseline flow
High pressure limit	Regulates the maximal pressure the ventilator can generate to deliver the tidal volume; when the pressure limit is reached, the ventilator terminates the breath and spills the undelivered volume into the atmosphere	10-20 cm H_2O above peak inspiratory pressure

patient's ventilatory pattern to be assessed, monitored, and displayed.[51,53,56]

Complications

Mechanical ventilation is often life saving, but, like other interventions, it is not without complications. Some complications are preventable, whereas others can be minimized but not eradicated. Physiologic complications associated with mechanical ventilation include ventilator-induced lung injury, cardiovascular compromise, gastrointestinal disturbances, patient-ventilator dyssynchrony, and HAP.

Ventilator-Induced Lung Injury

Mechanical ventilation can cause two different types of injury to the lungs: 1) air leaks and 2) biotrauma.[55,57] Air leaks related to mechanical ventilation are the result of excessive pressure in the alveoli (barotrauma), excessive volume in the alveoli (volutrauma), or shearing due to repeated opening and closing of the alveoli (atelectrauma).[55,58] Barotrauma, volutrauma, and atelectrauma can lead to excessive alveolar wall stress and damage to the alveolar–capillary membrane, resulting in air leakage into the surrounding spaces. The air then travels out through the hilum and into the mediastinum (pneumomediastinum), pleural space (pneumothorax), subcutaneous tissues (subcutaneous emphysema), pericardium (pneumopericardium), peritoneum (pneumoperitoneum), and retroperitoneum (pneumoretroperitoneum). The resultant disorders vary from the fairly benign to the potentially lethal—the most lethal of which is a pneumothorax or pneumopericardium resulting in cardiac tamponade.[55,59]

Barotrauma, volutrauma, and atelectrauma can also cause the release of cellular mediators and initiation of the inflammatory-immune response. This type of ventilator-induced injury is known as *biotrauma*.[55,60] Biotrauma can result in the development of ARDS.[61] To limit ventilator-induced lung injury, the plateau pressure (pressure needed to inflate the alveoli) should be kept at less than 32 cm H_2O, PEEP should be used to avoid end-expiratory collapse and reopening, and the tidal volume should be set at 6 to 10 mL/kg.[57,60]

Cardiovascular Compromise

Positive-pressure ventilation increases intrathoracic pressure, which decreases venous return to the right side of the heart. Impaired venous return decreases preload, which results in a decrease in cardiac output. As a secondary consequence, hepatic and renal dysfunction may occur. Positive-pressure ventilation impairs cerebral venous return. In patients with impaired autoregulation, positive-pressure ventilation can result in increased intracranial pressure.[55,62]

Gastrointestinal Disturbances

Gastrointestinal disturbances can occur as a result of positive-pressure ventilation. Gastric distention occurs when air leaks around the ETT or tracheostomy tube cuff and overcomes the resistance of the lower esophageal sphincter.[7] Vomiting can occur as a result of pharyngeal stimulation from the artificial airway.[17] These problems can be prevented by inserting a nasogastric tube and ensuring appropriate cuff inflation.

Hypomotility and constipation may occur as a result of immobility and the administration of paralytic agents, analgesics, and sedatives.[7]

Patient-Ventilator Dyssynchrony

Because the ventilatory pattern is normally initiated by the establishment of negative pressure within the chest, the application of positive pressure can lead to patient difficulties in breathing while on the ventilator. To achieve optimal ventilatory assistance, the patient should breathe in synchrony with the machine. The selected mode of ventilation, the settings, and the type of ventilatory circuitry used can increase the work of breathing and lead to breathing out of synchrony with the ventilator. Patient–ventilator dyssynchrony can result in decreased effectiveness of mechanical ventilation, the development of auto-PEEP, and psychologic distress. Patients who are not breathing in synchrony with the ventilator appear to be fighting or "bucking" the ventilator. To minimize this problem, the ventilator is adjusted to accommodate the patient's spontaneous breathing pattern and to work with the patient. If this is not possible, the patient may need to be sedated or pharmacologically paralyzed.[63-65]

Ventilator-Associated Pneumonia

Ventilator-associated pneumonia (VAP) is a subgroup of hospital-acquired pneumonia that refers to the development of pneumonia 48 to 72 hours after endotracheal intubation.[66] A great potential for the development of pneumonia exists after placement of an artificial airway because the tube bypasses or impairs many of the lung's normal defense mechanisms. After an artificial airway has been placed, contamination of the lower airways follows within 24 hours. This results from a number of factors that directly and indirectly promote airway colonization. The use of respiratory therapy devices (e.g., ventilators, nebulizers, intermittent positive-pressure breathing machines) also can increase the risk of pneumonia. The severity of the patient's illness and the presence of ARDS or malnutrition significantly increase the likelihood that an infection will ensue. Therapeutic measures such as nasogastric intubation and gastric alkalization with enteral feedings or medications facilitate the development of pneumonia. Nasogastric tubes promote aspiration by acting as a wick for stomach contents, whereas enteral feedings, antacids, histamine inhibitors, and proton-pump inhibitors increase the pH level of the stomach, promoting the growth of bacteria that can then be aspirated (Fig. 21-12).[66,67] Additional information on managing the patient with pneumonia is provided in Chapter 20.

Prevention of VAP is critical. The Institute for Healthcare Improvement (IHI) identified five interventions that when consistently implemented together have shown to improve patient outcomes. Known as the "IHI Ventilator Bundle" these interventions are: 1) elevation of the head of the bed; 2) daily "sedation vacations" and assessment of readiness to extubate; 3) peptic ulcer disease prophylaxis; 4) deep venous thrombosis prophylaxis; and 5) daily oral care with chlorhexidine.[68]

Semirecumbency. Positioning of the patient who requires mechanical ventilation is very important. Semirecumbent positioning (elevation of the head of the bed 30 to 45 degrees)

Pathogenesis of VAP

Common Sources of VAP Pathogens:

- ☐ Aspiration
- ☐ Intubation Procedure
- ☐ Biofilm Formation
- ☐ Contaminated Secretions
- ☐ Contaminated Respiratory Equipment

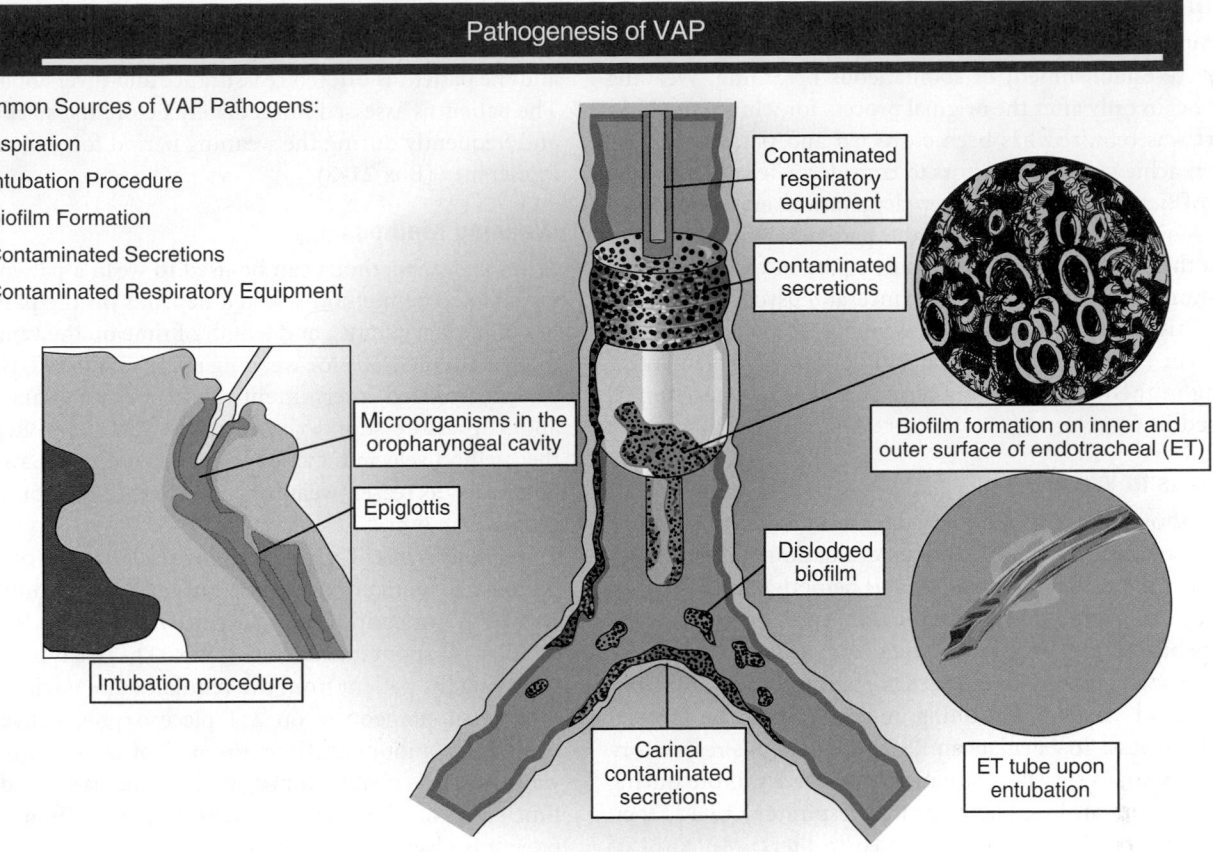

Contaminated respiratory equipment

Contaminated secretions

Biofilm formation on inner and outer surface of endotracheal (ET)

Microorganisms in the oropharyngeal cavity

Epiglottis

Dislodged biofilm

Intubation procedure

Carinal contaminated secretions

ET tube upon entubation

FIGURE 21-12 Pathogenesis of ventilator-associated pneumonia. (Redrawn from Sachdev G, Napolitano LM. Postoperative pulmonary complications: pneumonia and acute respiratory failure. *Surg Clin N Am.* 2012;92:321.)

reduces the incidence of gastroesophageal reflux and subsequent aspiration and decreases the incidence of VAP. The head of the patient's bed should be elevated to 30 to 45 degrees at all times unless contraindicated (e.g., hemodynamic instability, presence of intra-aortic balloon pump, physician's order to the contrary). However, this intervention does increase the risk of skin shear on the coccyx, and extra surveillance is mandatory for prevention of pressure ulcers.[69,70]

Sedation Vacation. Many patients receiving mechanical ventilation require sedation to ameliorate symptoms of anxiety and stress associated with critical illness. However, the prolonged use of sedation has been shown to contribute to the development of complications, including oversedation, prolonged mechanical ventilation, and delirium. To decrease the incidence of these complications the concept of a "sedation vacation" has been developed. A "sedation vacation" is simply the daily interruption of sedation to evaluate the patient and their need for continued sedation and mechanical ventilation. Not every patient is a candidate for this procedure. Contraindications include hemodynamic instability, increased intracranial pressure, ongoing agitation, seizures, or alcohol withdrawal, and patient's receiving neuromuscular blocking agents. If the patient is able to tolerate being off the sedation for more than 4 hours (this number varies depending on the protocol being used), then the sedation is discontinued. Signs of intolerance include

ongoing agitation, increased respiratory rate, decreasing oxygen saturation, cardiac dysrhythmias, and signs of respiratory distress.[71]

Other Measures to Reduce the Incidence of Ventilator-Associated Pneumonia. Recent studies have shown that use of an ETT with a polyurethane cuff may decrease the incidence of VAP. A traditional ETT has a polyvinyl low-pressure high-volume cuff. When the cuff is inflated, folds form in the cuff, allowing fluids and air to leak around the cuff and into the lungs. This is why subglottic secretion removal is so important. Polyurethane cuffs are much thinner than the traditional polyvinyl cuffs and do not form folds when they are inflated. No leakage of fluids into the lungs occurs.[72,73] In addition, some evidence suggests that the shape of the cuff may also impact this issue. A taper-shaped cuff appears to better prevent fluid leakage when compared with a cylindrical cuff commonly found on most tubes.[74]

Another recent study found that the use of silver-coated ETTs significantly reduced the incidence and delayed the onset of VAP, compared with a regular ETT. The tube decreased the incidence of VAP by preventing bacterial colonization and biofilm formation.[75] Biofilm is formed when bacteria cling to the inner lumen of the ETT and then secrete an exopolysaccharide substance. This substance forms a gelatinous matrix that allows bacteria to thrive on a nonbiologic surface.[72]

Weaning

Weaning is the gradual withdrawal of the mechanical ventilator and the re-establishment of spontaneous breathing. Weaning should begin only after the original process for which ventilator support was required has been corrected and patient stability has been achieved. Other factors to consider when weaning are length of time on ventilator, sleep deprivation, and nutritional status. Major factors that affect the patient's ability to wean include the ability of the lungs to participate in ventilation and respiration, cardiovascular performance, and psychologic readiness.[76] This discussion focuses on weaning of the patient from short-term (≤3 days) mechanical ventilation. Management of weaning in the patient on long-term mechanical ventilation is discussed in Chapter 20.

Readiness to Wean

Patients should be screened every day for their readiness to be weaned. The screen should include an evaluation of the patient's level of consciousness, physiologic and hemodynamic stability, adequacy of oxygenation and ventilation, spontaneous breathing capability, and respiratory rate and pattern.[76] Routine parameters that are usually assessed are presented in Table 21-7.

The rapid, shallow breathing index (RSBI) can predict weaning success. To calculate an RSBI, the patient's respiratory rate and minute ventilation are measured for 1 minute during spontaneous breathing. The measured respiratory rate is then divided by the tidal volume (expressed in liters). An RSBI of less than 105 is considered predictive of weaning success. If the patient is receiving sedation, the medication should be discontinued at least 1 hour before the RSBI is measured. If the patient meets criteria for weaning readiness and has an RSBI of less than 105, a spontaneous breathing trial can be performed.[77] One study showed that implementation of a weaning program that incorporated daily spontaneous breathing trials (SBT) had a positive impact on extubation rates and no effect on reintubation rates.[78] Figure 21-13 outlines one approach for an SBT.

After the patient's readiness to be weaned has been established, the patient is prepared for the weaning trial. The patient

is positioned upright to facilitate breathing and suctioned to ensure airway patency. The process is explained to the patient, and the patient is offered reassurance and diversional activities. The patient is assessed immediately before the start of the trial and frequently during the weaning period for signs of weaning intolerance (Box 21-5).[76,77,79,80]

Weaning Methods

A number of methods can be used to wean a patient from the ventilator. The method selected depends on the patient, his or her pulmonary status, and length of time on the ventilator. The three main methods for weaning are: 1) T-tube (T-piece) trials, 2) synchronized intermittent mandatory ventilation (SIMV), and 3) pressure support ventilation (PSV).[76,79,81] Regardless of the method selected, evidence shows that using a standardize approach decreases weaning time and length of stay in the critical care unit.[82]

T-Piece Trials. T-piece weaning trials consist of alternating periods of ventilatory support (usually assist-control ventilation [ACV] or continuous mandatory ventilation [CMV]) with periods of spontaneous breathing. The trial is initiated by removing the patient from the ventilator and having the patient breathe spontaneously on a T-piece oxygen delivery system. After a set amount of time, the patient is placed back on the ventilator. The goal is to progressively increase the duration of time spent off the ventilator. During the weaning process, the patient is observed closely for respiratory muscle fatigue.[76-79,81] Constant positive airway pressure (CPAP) may be added to prevent atelectasis and improve oxygenation.[79,81]

Synchronized Intermittent Mandatory Ventilation Trials. The goal of SIMV weaning is the gradual transition from ventilatory support to spontaneous breathing. It is initiated by placing the ventilator in the SIMV mode and slowly decreasing the rate, usually one to three breaths at a time, until a rate of zero or near-zero is reached. An arterial blood gas (ABG) sample is usually obtained 30 minutes after the trial. This method of weaning can increase the work of breathing, and the patient must be closely monitored for signs of respiratory muscle fatigue.[76,79,81]

Pressure Support Ventilation Trials. PSV weaning consists of placing the patient on the pressure support mode and setting the pressure support at a level that facilitates the patient's achieving a spontaneous tidal volume of 10 to 12 mL/kg. PSV augments the patient's spontaneous breaths with a positive-pressure boost during inspiration. During the weaning process, the level of pressure support is gradually decreased in increments of 3 to 6 cm H_2O, while the tidal volume is maintained at 10 to 15 mL/kg, until a level of 5 cm H_2O is achieved. If the patient is able to maintain adequate spontaneous respirations at this level, extubation is considered. PSV also can be used with SIMV weaning to help overcome the resistance in the ventilator system.[76,79,81]

Nursing Management

Nursing management of the patient receiving mechanical ventilation is outlined in Box 21-6. Routine assessment of these patients includes monitoring for patient-related and ventilator-related complications.

TABLE 21-7	CONVENTIONAL WEANING PARAMETERS	
PARAMETERS	**WEANABLE VALUES**	**NORMAL RANGES**
NIF (cm of water)	<−20	<−50
VC (mL/kg)	>10	>65-75
V_T (mL/kg)	<5	>5-7
RR (breaths/min)	<32	12-20
V_E (L/min)	>10	>10
Rapid shallow breathing index (RSBI) (RR/V_T)	<105	<40

From Casserly B, Rounds S. Essentials in critical care medicine. In: Andreoli TE, ed. *Andreoli and Carpenter's Cecil Essentials of Medicine.* 8th ed. Philadelphia: Saunders; 2010.

NIF, Negative inspiratory force; *RR,* respiratory rate; *VC,* vital capacity; *V_E,* minute ventilation; *V_T,* tidal volume.

Approach to Discontinuing Ventilation/Extubation

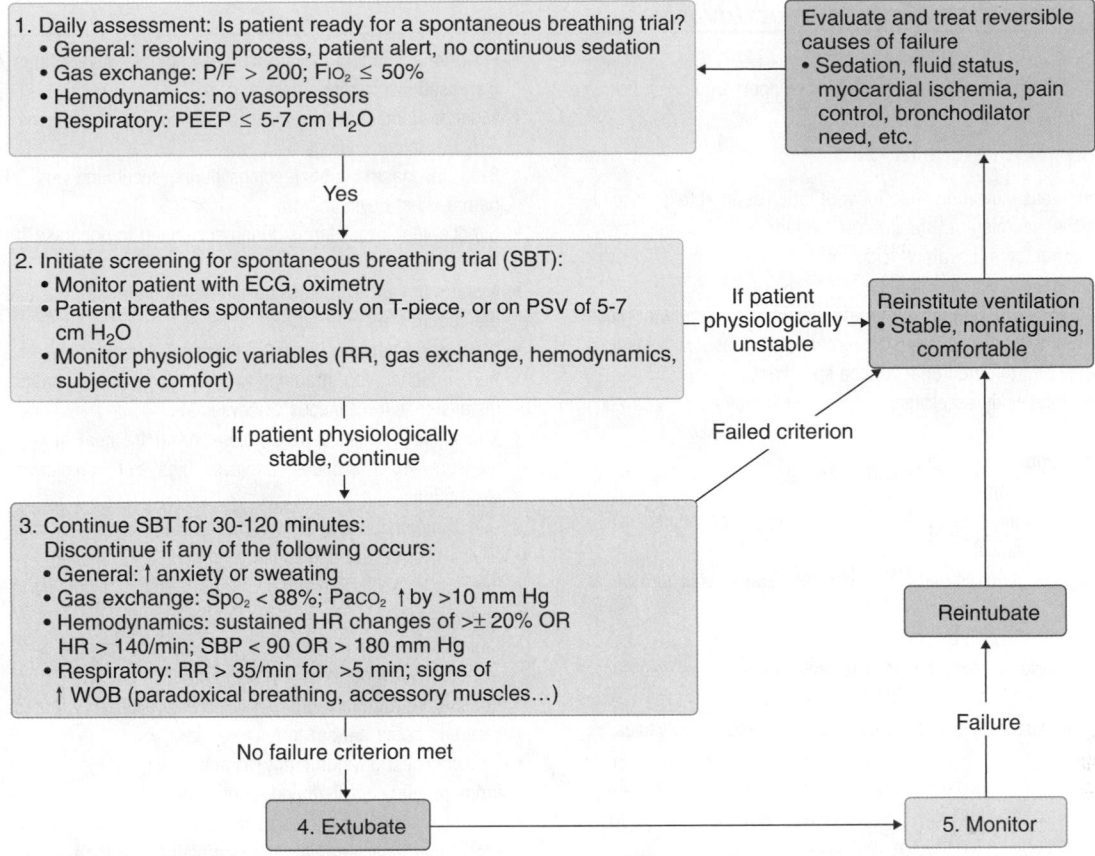

FIGURE 21-13 Algorithm for assessing whether a patient is ready to be liberated from mechanical ventilation and extubated. *ECG*, Electrocardiogram; *HR*, heart rate; *P/F*, PaO$_2$/FIO$_2$ ratio; *PSV*, pressure support ventilation; *RR*, respiratory rate; *SBP*, systolic blood pressure; *Spo$_2$*, oxygen saturation based on pulse oximeter; *WOB*, work of breathing. (From Slutsky AS, Hudson LD. Mechanical ventilation. In: Goldman L, Scharfer AI, eds. *Goldman's Cecil Medicine*. 24th ed. Philadelphia: Elsevier; 2012.)

BOX 21-5 WEANING INTOLERANCE INDICATORS

- Decrease in level of consciousness
- Systolic blood pressure increased or decreased by 20 mm Hg
- Diastolic blood pressure greater than 100 mm Hg
- Heart rate increased by 20 beats per minute
- Premature ventricular contractions greater than 6 per minute, couplets, or runs of ventricular tachycardia
- Changes in ST segment (usually elevation)
- Respiratory rate greater than 30 breaths per minute or less than 10 breaths per minute
- Respiratory rate increased by 10 breaths per minute
- Spontaneous tidal volume less than 250 mL
- Arterial partial pressure of carbon dioxide (PaCO$_2$) increased by 5 to 8 mm Hg, pH less than 7.30, or both
- Oxygen saturation based on pulse oximeter (SpO$_2$) less than 90%
- Use of accessory muscles of ventilation
- Complaints of dyspnea, fatigue, or pain
- Paradoxical chest wall motion or chest abdominal asynchrony
- Diaphoresis
- Severe agitation or anxiety unrelieved by reassurance

Patient Assessment

It includes a total patient assessment, with particular emphasis on the pulmonary system, placement of the ETT or tracheostomy tube, and observation for subcutaneous emphysema and dyssynchrony with the ventilator. Bedside evaluation of vital capacity, minute ventilation, ABG values, and other pulmonary function tests may be warranted, according to the patient's condition. The use of pulse oximetry can facilitate continuous, noninvasive assessment of oxygenation. The use of capnography may facilitate continuous noninvasive assessment of ventilation. Static and dynamic compliance should also be monitored to assess for changes in lung compliance (see Appendix B).[83]

Symptom Management

Patients requiring mechanical ventilation may present with a variety of disturbing symptoms, including anxiety, pain, shortness of breath, confusion and agitation, and sleep disturbances. These symptoms are often managed with sedation and analgesic medications. As discussed earlier, these medications could contribute to prolonged mechanical ventilation and delirium.

BOX 21-6 NIC

Mechanical Ventilation Management: Invasive

Definition

Assisting the patient receiving artificial breathing support through a device inserted into the trachea

Activities

- Monitor for conditions indicating need for ventilation support (e.g., respiratory muscle fatigue, neurologic dysfunction secondary to trauma, anesthesia, drug overdose, refractory respiratory acidosis).
- Monitor for impending respiratory failure.
- Consult with other health care personnel in selection of a ventilator mode (initial mode usually volume control with breath rate, fraction of inspired oxygen (FiO_2) level and targeted tidal volume specified).
- Obtain baseline total body assessment of patient initially and with each change of caregiver.
- Initiate setup and application of the ventilator.
- Ensure that ventilator alarms are on.
- Instruct patient and family about rationale and expected sensations associated with use of mechanical ventilators.
- Routinely monitor ventilator settings, including temperature and humidification of inspired air.
- Check all ventilator connections regularly.
- Monitor for decrease in exhaled volume and increase in inspiratory pressure.
- Administer muscle paralyzing agents, sedatives, and narcotic analgesics, as appropriate.
- Monitor for activities that increase oxygen consumption (e.g., fever, shivering, seizures, pain, or basic nursing activities), which may supersede ventilator support settings and cause oxygen desaturation.
- Monitor for factors that increase patient or ventilator work of breathing (e.g., morbid obesity, pregnancy, massive ascites, lowered head of bed, biting of ET, condensation in ventilator tubes, clogged filters).
- Monitor for symptoms that indicate increased work of breathing (e.g., increased heart or respiratory rate, increased blood pressure, diaphoresis, changes in mental status).
- Monitor effectiveness of mechanical ventilation on patient's physiologic and psychologic status.
- Initiate relaxation techniques, as appropriate.
- Provide care to alleviate patient distress (e.g., positioning, tracheobronchial toileting, bronchodilator therapy, sedation and/or analgesia, frequent equipment checks).
- Provide patient with a means for communication (e.g., paper and pencil, alphabet board).
- Empty condensed water from water traps.
- Ensure change of ventilator circuits every 24 hours.
- Use aseptic technique in all suctioning procedures and as appropriate.
- Monitor ventilator pressure readings, patient–ventilator synchronicity and patient breath sounds.
- Perform suctioning based on presence of adventitious breath sounds, increased inspiratory pressure, or both.
- Monitor pulmonary secretions for amount, color, and consistency and regularly document findings.
- Stop nasogastric tube feedings during suctioning and 30 to 60 minutes before chest physiotherapy.
- Silence ventilator alarms during suctioning to decrease frequency of false alarms.
- Monitor patient's progress on current ventilator settings and make appropriate changes, as ordered.
- Monitor for adverse effects of mechanical ventilation (e.g., tracheal deviation, infection, barotrauma, volutrauma, reduced cardiac output, gastric distension, subcutaneous emphysema).
- Monitor for mucosal damage to oral, nasal, tracheal, or laryngeal tissue from pressure from artificial airways, high cuff pressures, or unplanned extubations.
- Use commercial tube holders, rather than tape or strings, to fix artificial airways to prevent unplanned extubations.
- Position to facilitate ventilation–perfusion matching ("good lung down"), as appropriate.
- Collaborate with physician to use pressure support or PEEP to minimize alveolar hypoventilation, as appropriate.
- Collaborate routinely with physician and respiratory therapist to coordinate care and assist patient to tolerate therapy.
- Perform chest physiotherapy, as appropriate.
- Promote adequate fluid and nutritional intake.
- Promote routine assessments for weaning criteria (e.g., hemodynamic, cerebral, metabolic stability, resolution of condition prompting intubation, ability to maintain patent airway, ability to initiate respiratory effort).
- Provide routine oral care with soft moist swabs, antiseptic agent, and gentle suctioning.
- Monitor effects of ventilator changes on oxygenation: ABG, SaO_2, SvO_2, end-tidal CO_2, Qsp/Qt, $A\text{-}aDO_2$, patient's subjective response.
- Monitor degree of shunt, vital capacity, V_d/V_t, MVV, inspiratory force, and FEV_1 for readiness to wean from mechanical ventilation based on agency protocol.
- Document all changes to ventilator settings with rationale for changes.
- Document all patient responses to ventilator and ventilator changes (e.g., chest movement observation or auscultation, changes in x-ray, changes in ABGs).
- Monitor for postextubation complications (e.g., stridor, glottic swelling, laryngospasm, tracheal stenosis).
- Ensure emergency equipment at bedside at all times (e.g., manual resuscitation bag connected to oxygen, masks, suction equipment or supplies) including preparations for power failures.

From Bulechek GM, et al. *Nursing Interventions Classification (NIC)*, 6th ed. St. Louis: Mosby; 2013.
A-aDO₂, Alveolar-arterial difference in partial pressure of oxygen; *ABG*, arterial blood gases; *CO₂*, carbon dioxide; *CPAP*, continuous positive airway pressure; *ET*, endotracheal tube; *FEV₁*, forced expiratory volume in 1 second; *MMV*, mandatory minute ventilation; *PEEP*, positive end-expiratory pressure; *Qs/Qt*, measurement of pulmonary shunt that describes the percentage of blood reaching the left side of the heart without picking up oxygen; *SaO₂*, arterial oxygen saturation, *SVO₂*, venous oxygen saturation; *Vₒ/Vₜ*, dead space volume-tidal volume ratio.

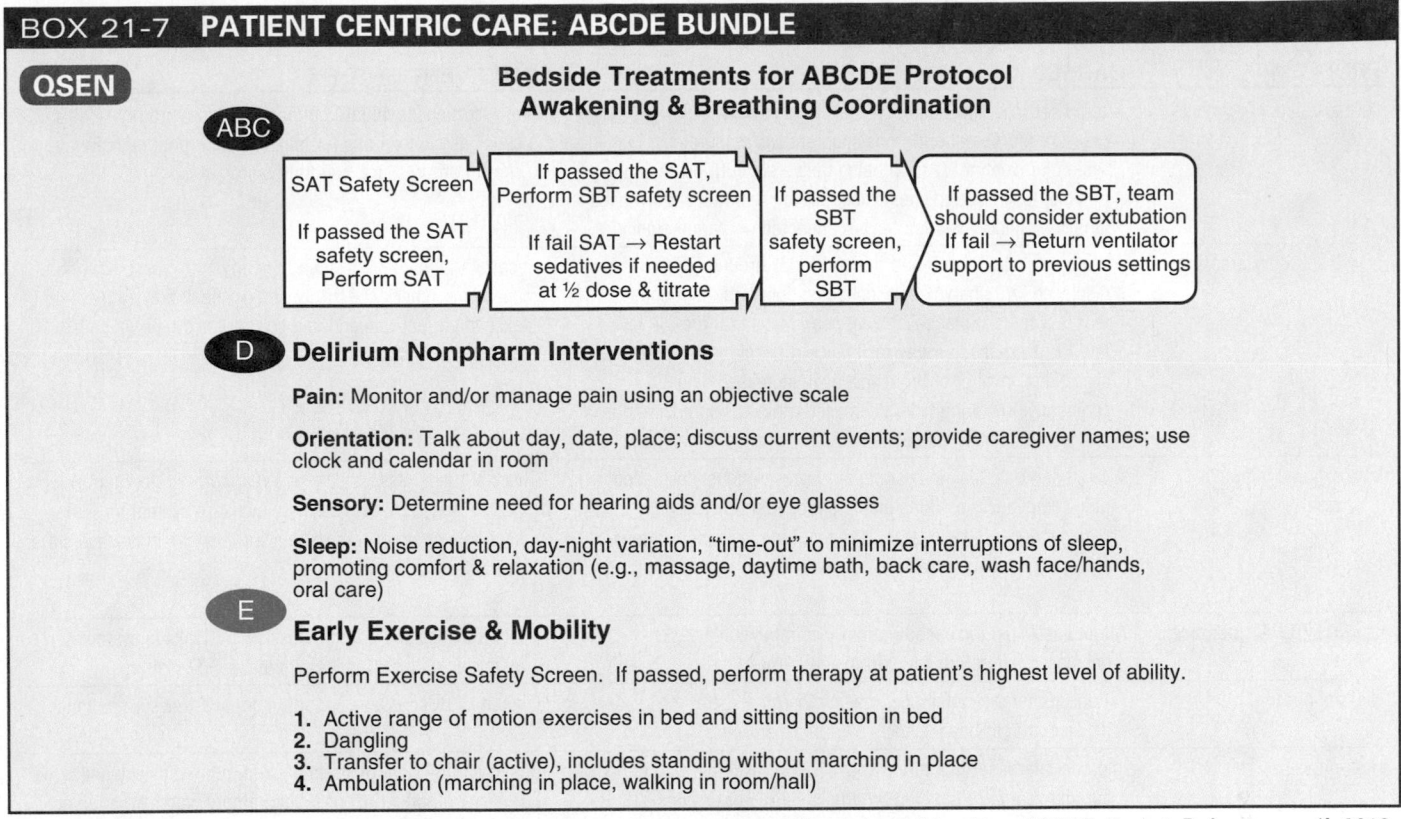

BOX 21-7 PATIENT CENTRIC CARE: ABCDE BUNDLE

QSEN

Bedside Treatments for ABCDE Protocol
Awakening & Breathing Coordination

ABC

SAT Safety Screen

If passed the SAT safety screen, Perform SAT

If passed the SAT, Perform SBT safety screen

If fail SAT → Restart sedatives if needed at ½ dose & titrate

If passed the SBT safety screen, perform SBT

If passed the SBT, team should consider extubation
If fail → Return ventilator support to previous settings

D Delirium Nonpharm Interventions

Pain: Monitor and/or manage pain using an objective scale

Orientation: Talk about day, date, place; discuss current events; provide caregiver names; use clock and calendar in room

Sensory: Determine need for hearing aids and/or eye glasses

Sleep: Noise reduction, day-night variation, "time-out" to minimize interruptions of sleep, promoting comfort & relaxation (e.g., massage, daytime bath, back care, wash face/hands, oral care)

E Early Exercise & Mobility

Perform Exercise Safety Screen. If passed, perform therapy at patient's highest level of ability.

1. Active range of motion exercises in bed and sitting position in bed
2. Dangling
3. Transfer to chair (active), includes standing without marching in place
4. Ambulation (marching in place, walking in room/hall)

From *ICU Delirium and Cognitive Impairment Study Group.* http://www.mcvanderbilt.edu/icudelirium/docs/ABCDE_Pocket_References.pdf. 2012. Accessed July 2012.
SAT, Spontaneous awakening trial; *SBT,* spontaneous breathing trial.

Nonpharmacologic interventions have been shown to be of benefit to these patients. These interventions include promoting a healing environment, promoting sleep (see Chapter 7), and interventions to lessen anxiety (e.g., music therapy, guided imagery, nursing presence, and animal-assisted therapy). Nursing activities to promote a healing environment include minimizing noise levels, ensuring the patient has access to natural light, establishing a method of communication with the patient, and providing the patient with explanations of what is occurring around them.[84] Referral to a complementary and alternative therapy specialist (if one available) is also appropriate.

ABCDE Bundle

Another bundle that has recently been proposed is the Awakening and Breathing Coordination, Delirium Monitoring, and Early Mobility (ABCDE) bundle. This bundle focuses on enhancing communication between team members in the critical care unit, standardizing patient care processes, and decreasing the incidence of delirium and prolonged weakness associated with critical illness.[85] The ABCDE bundle activities are presented in Box 21-7.

Ventilator Assessment

Assessment of the ventilator includes a review of all the ventilator settings and alarms. A clear understanding of the alarms and their related problems is important (Table 21-8). The peak inspiratory pressure, exhaled tidal volume, and ABGs are also monitored.

Patient Safety

Several measures are required to maintain a trouble-free ventilator system. These include maintaining a functional manual resuscitation bag connected to oxygen at the bedside, ensuring that the ventilator tubing is free of water, positioning the ventilator tubing to avoid kinking, maintaining the patency of ventilator tubing and connections, changing ventilator tubing per hospital policy, and monitoring the temperature of the inspired air. If the ventilator malfunctions, the patient is removed from the ventilator and ventilated manually with a manual resuscitation bag. Alarms should be sufficiently audible with respect to distance and competing noise within the unit. Issues regarding patient transport are addressed Box 21-8.

NONINVASIVE VENTILATION

Noninvasive ventilation (NIV) is an alternative method of ventilation that uses a mask instead of an ETT to deliver the therapy. Advantages of this type of ventilation include decreased frequency of hospital-acquired pneumonia, increased comfort, and the noninvasive nature of the procedure, which allows easy application and removal. It is indicated in type I and type II acute respiratory failure, cardiogenic pulmonary edema, and other situations in which intubation is not an option.

TABLE 21-8 TROUBLESHOOTING VENTILATOR ALARMS

PROBLEM	CAUSES	INTERVENTIONS
Low exhaled V_T	Altered settings; any condition that triggers high- or low-pressure alarm; patient stops spontaneous respirations; leak in system preventing V_T from being delivered; cuff insufficiently inflated; leak through chest tube; airway secretions; decreased lung compliance; spirometer disconnected or malfunctioning	Check settings; evaluate patient, check respiratory rate; check all connections for leaks; suction patient's airway; check cuff pressure; calibrate spirometer.
Low inspiratory pressure	Altered settings; unattached tubing or leak around ETT; ETT displaced into pharynx or esophagus; poor cuff inflation or leak; tracheoesophageal fistula; peak flows that are too low; low V_T; decreased airway resistance resulting from decreased secretions or relief of bronchospasm; increased lung compliance resulting from decreased atelectasis; reduction in pulmonary edema; resolution of ARDS; change in position	Reset alarm; reconnect tubing; modify cuff pressures; tighten humidifier; check chest tube; adjust peak flow to meet or exceed patient demand and correct for the patient's V_T; reposition or change ETT.
Low exhaled minute volume	Altered settings; leak in system; airway secretions; decreased lung compliance; malfunctioning spirometer; decreased patient-triggered respiratory rate resulting from medications, sleep, hypocapnia, alkalosis, fatigue, change in neurologic status	Check settings; assess patient's respiratory rate, mental status, and work of breathing; evaluate system for leaks; suction airway; assess patient for changes in disease state; calibrate spirometer.
Low PEEP/CPAP pressure	Altered settings; increased patient inspirator/flows; leak; decreased expiratory flows from ventilator	Check settings and correct; observe for leaks in system; if unable to correct problem, increase PEEP settings.
High respiratory rate	Increased metabolic demand; medication administration; hypoxia; hypercapnia; acidosis; shock; pain; fear; anxiety	Evaluate ABGs; assess patient; calm and reassure patient.
High-pressure limit	Improper alarm setting; airway obstruction resulting from patient fighting ventilator (holding breath as ventilator delivers V_T); patient circuit collapse; tubing kinked; ETT in right main stem bronchus or against carina; cuff herniation; increased airway resistance resulting from bronchospasm, airway secretions, plugs, and coughing; water from humidifier in ventilator tubing; decreased lung compliance resulting from tension pneumothorax, change in patient position, ARDS, pulmonary edema, atelectasis, pneumonia, or abdominal distention	Reset alarms; clear obstruction from tubing; unkink and reposition patient off of tubing; empty water from tubing; check breath sounds; reassure patient and sedate if necessary; check ABGs for hypoxemia; observe for abdominal distention that would put pressure on the diaphragm; check cuff pressures; obtain chest radiograph and evaluate for ETT position, pneumothorax, and pneumonia; reposition ETT; give bronchodilator therapy.
Low-pressure oxygen inlet	Improper oxygen alarm setting; oxygen not connected to ventilator; dirty oxygen intake filter	Correct alarm setting; reconnect or connect oxygen line to a 50-psi source; clean or replace oxygen filter.
I:E ratio	Inspiratory time longer than expiratory time; use of an inspiratory phase that is too long with a fast rate; peak flow setting too low while rate too high; machine too sensitive	Change inspiratory time or adjust peak flow; check inspiratory phase, or hold; check machine sensitivity.
Temperature	Sensor malfunction; overheating resulting from too low or no gas flow; sensor picking up outside airflow (from heater, open door or window, air conditioner); improper water levels	Test or replace sensor; check gas flow; protect sensor from outside source that would interfere with readings; check water levels.

Modified from Flynn JBM, Bruce NP. *Introduction to Critical Care Nursing Skills.* St. Louis: Mosby; 1993.
ABGs, Arterial blood gases; *ARDS,* acute respiratory distress syndrome; *CPAP,* constant positive airway pressure; *ETT,* endotracheal tube; *PEEP,* positive end-expiratory pressure; *Vt,* tidal volume.

Contraindications to NIV include hemodynamic instability, dysrhythmias, apnea, uncooperativeness, intolerance of the mask, recent upper airway or esophageal surgery, and inability to maintain a patent airway, clear secretions, or properly fit the mask.[86]

NIV can be applied with a total face, nasal or facial mask and ventilator or with a BiPAP machine (Respironics Inc., Murrysville, PA) (Fig. 21-14). One study found that a full-face mask is better tolerated than a nasal mask.[87] This type of ventilation uses a combination of PSV and PEEP supplied by a ventilator, or inspiratory and expiratory positive airway pressure (IPAP and EPAP, respectively) supplied by a BiPAP machine, to assist the spontaneously breathing patient with ventilation. On inspiration, the patient receives PSV or IPAP to increase tidal volume and minute ventilation, resulting in increased alveolar ventilation, a decreased $Paco_2$ level, relief of dyspnea, and reduced accessory muscle use. On expiration, the patient receives PEEP or EPAP to increase functional residual capacity, resulting in an increased PaO_2 level. Humidified supplemental oxygen is administered to maintain a clinically acceptable Pao_2 level, and timed breaths may be added, if necessary.[52]

Nursing Management

Nursing management of the patient receiving noninvasive ventilation is outlined in Box 21-9. Routine assessment of these patients includes monitoring for patient-related and

⚡ BOX 21-8 PATIENT SAFETY ALERT

Intrahospital Transport of Critically Ill Patients

QSEN The following is an excerpt from the *Guidelines for The Inter- and Intrahospital Transport of Critically Ill Patients*:

1. Pretransport Coordination and Communication
   - Confirm receiving unit readiness to receive patient
   - Nurse to nurse handoff (if patient care responsibility is being transferred to a nurse in the receiving area)
   - Notify respiratory therapist and/or other members of the health care team of timing of transport and request equipment support, as needed
   - Mechanical ventilator in receiving unit (for mechanically ventilated patients)
2. Accompanying Personnel
   - A minimum of two people should accompany a critically ill patient (one of which should be a critical care nurse)
   - Unstable patients should be accompanied by a physician
3. Accompanying Equipment
   - Blood pressure monitor or cuff
   - Pulse oximeter
   - Cardiac monitor with defibrillator
   - Basic resuscitation medications (emergency cart should be readily available in receiving unit)
   - Additional sedatives and narcotic analgesics
   - Additional intravenous fluids and medications
   - Oxygen delivery device attached to oxygen source with at least a 30-minute reserve or manual resuscitation bag and/or transport ventilator (for mechanically ventilated patients)
   - Transport ventilator must have alarms and back up battery
4. Monitoring During Transport
   - Continuous electrocardiographic monitoring
   - Continuous pulse oximetry
   - Periodic measurement of blood pressure, pulse rate, and respiratory rate

From Warren J, et al. Guidelines for the inter- and intrahospital transport of critically ill patients. *Crit Care Med.* 2004;32:256.

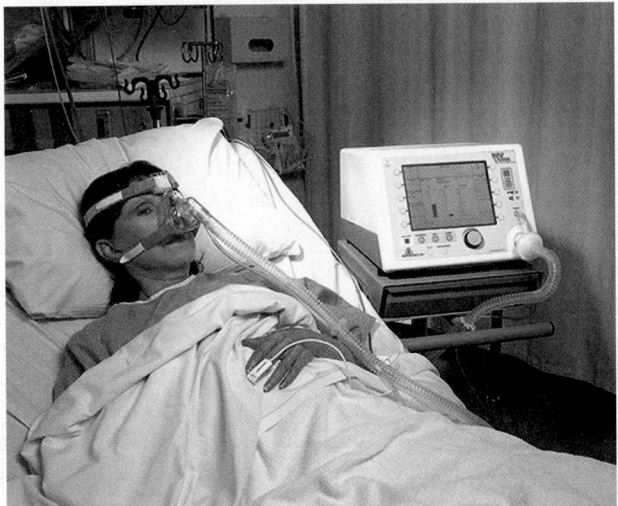

FIGURE 21-14 BiPAP via face mask. (Courtesy Respironics Inc., Murrysville, PA.)

ventilator-related complications. As with invasive mechanical ventilation, the patient must be closely monitored. Respiratory rate, accessory muscle use, and oxygenation status are continually assessed to ensure that the patient is tolerating this method of ventilation. Continuous pulse oximetry is also used.[88,89]

The key to ensuring adequate ventilatory support is a properly fitted mask. A nasal mask, face mask, or a full-face mask may be used, depending on the patient. A properly fitted mask minimizes air leakage and discomfort for the patient. Transparent dressings placed over the pressure points of the face help minimize air leakage and prevent facial skin necrosis caused by the mask. The BiPAP machine is able to compensate for air leaks.[89]

The patient is positioned with the head of the bed elevated at 45 degrees to minimize the risk of aspiration and to facilitate breathing. Insufflation of the stomach is a complication of this mode of therapy and places the patient at risk for aspiration. The patient is closely monitored for gastric distention, and a nasogastric tube is placed for decompression, as necessary. Often, patients are very anxious and have high levels of dyspnea before the initiation of noninvasive mechanical ventilation. After adequate ventilation has been established, anxiety and dyspnea are usually sufficiently relieved. Heavy sedation should be avoided, but if it is needed, it would constitute the need for intubation and invasive mechanical ventilation. It is important to spend 30 minutes with the patient after initiation of noninvasive ventilation because the patient needs reassurance and must learn how to breathe on the machine.[87,89] The patient who requires noninvasive ventilation with a face mask should never be restrained. The patient must be able to remove the mask if it becomes displaced or the patient vomits. A displaced mask can force the patient's bottom jaw inward and occlude the patient's airway.

POSITIONING THERAPY

Positioning therapy can help match ventilation and perfusion through the redistribution of oxygen and blood flow in the lungs, which improves gas exchange. On the basis of the concept that preferential blood flow occurs to the gravity-dependent areas of the lungs, positioning therapy is used to place the least damaged portion of the lungs into a dependent position. The least damaged portions of the lungs receive preferential blood flow, resulting in less ventilation–perfusion mismatch.[69] The current two approaches to position therapy are: 1) prone positioning and 2) rotation therapy.

Prone Positioning

Prone positioning is a therapeutic modality that is used to improve oxygenation in patients with ARDS.[90-92] It involves turning the patient completely over onto his or her stomach in the face-down position. Although a number of theories have been proposed to explain how prone positioning improves oxygenation, the discovery that ARDS causes greater damage to the dependent areas of the lungs probably provides the best explanation. It was originally thought that ARDS was a diffuse, homogeneous disease that affected all areas of the lungs equally. It is now known that the dependent lung areas are more heavily damaged than the nondependent lung areas. Turning the patient to the prone position improves perfusion to the less damaged areas of the lungs, improves ventilation–perfusion match, and decreases intrapulmonary shunting. Prone positioning can be used to facilitate the mobilization of secretions and provide

BOX 21-9 NIC

Mechanical Ventilation Management: Noninvasive

Definition

Assisting the patient receiving artificial breathing support that does not necessitate a device inserted into the trachea

Activities

- Monitor for conditions indicating appropriateness of noninvasive ventilation support (e.g., acute exacerbations of chronic obstructive pulmonary disease, asthma, noncardiogenic and cardiogenic pulmonary edema, acute respiratory failure due to community acquired pneumonia, obesity hypoventilation syndrome, obstructive sleep apnea).
- Monitor for contraindications to noninvasive ventilation support (e.g., hemodynamic instability, cardiovascular or respiratory arrest, unstable angina, acute myocardial infarction, refractory hypoxemia, severe respiratory acidosis, decreased level of consciousness, problems with securing or placing noninvasive equipment, facial trauma, inability to cooperate, morbidly obese, thick secretions, or bleeding).
- Consult with other health care personnel in selection of a noninvasive ventilator type (e.g., pressure limited [bilevel positive airway pressure], volume-cycled flow-limited, or constant positive airway pressure [CPAP]).
- Consult with other health care personnel and patient in selection of noninvasive device (e.g., nasal or face mask, nasal plugs, nasal pillow, helmet, oral mouthpiece).
- Obtain baseline total body assessment of patient initially and with each change of caregiver.
- Instruct patient and family about rationale and expected sensations associated with use of noninvasive mechanical ventilators and devices.
- Place patient in semi-Fowler position.
- Apply noninvasive device assuring adequate fit and avoidance of large air leaks (take particular care with edentulous or bearded patients).
- Apply facial protection, as needed, to avoid pressure damage to skin.
- Initiate setup and application of the ventilator.
- Observe patient continuously in first hour after application to assess tolerance.
- Ensure that ventilator alarms are on.
- Routinely monitor ventilator settings, including temperature and humidification of inspired air.
- Check all ventilator connections regularly.
- Monitor for decrease in exhaled volume and increase in inspiratory pressure.
- Monitor for activities that increase oxygen consumption (e.g., fever, shivering, seizures, pain, or basic nursing activities), which may supersede ventilator support settings and cause oxygen desaturation.

- Monitor for symptoms that indicate increased work of breathing (e.g., increased heart or respiratory rate, increased blood pressure, diaphoresis, changes in mental status).
- Monitor the effectiveness of mechanical ventilation on patient's physiologic and psychologic status.
- Initiate relaxation techniques, as appropriate.
- Ensure periods of rest daily (e.g., 15 to 30 minutes every 4 to 6 hours).
- Provide care to alleviate patient distress (e.g., positioning; treat side effects such as rhinitis, dry throat, or epistaxis; give sedation and/or analgesia; frequent equipment checks; cleansing or change of noninvasive device).
- Provide patient with a means for communication (e.g., paper and pencil, alphabet board).
- Empty condensed water from water traps.
- Ensure change of ventilator circuits every 24 hours.
- Use aseptic technique, as appropriate.
- Monitor patient–ventilator synchronicity and patient breath sounds.
- Monitor patient's progress on current ventilator settings and make appropriate changes, as ordered.
- Monitor for adverse effects (e.g., eye irritation, skin breakdown, occluded airway from jaw displacement with mask, dyspnea, anxiety, claustrophobia, gastric distension).
- Monitor for mucosal damage to oral, nasal, tracheal, or laryngeal tissue.
- Monitor pulmonary secretions for amount, color, and consistency, and regularly document findings.
- Collaborate routinely with physician and respiratory therapist to coordinate care and assist patient to tolerate therapy.
- Perform chest physiotherapy, as appropriate.
- Promote adequate fluid and nutritional intake.
- Promote routine assessments for weaning criteria (e.g., resolution of condition prompting ventilation, ability to maintain adequate respiratory effort).
- Provide routine oral care with soft moist swabs, antiseptic agent, and gentle suctioning.
- Document all changes to ventilator settings with rationale for changes.
- Document all patient responses to ventilator and ventilator changes (e.g., chest movement observation or auscultation, changes in radiograph, changes in arterial blood gases).
- Ensure emergency equipment at bedside at all times (e.g., manual resuscitation bag connected to oxygen, masks, suction equipment or supplies), including preparations for power failures.

From Bulechek GM, et al. *Nursing Interventions Classification (NIC)*. 6th ed. St. Louis: Mosby; 2013.

---

pressure relief. Prone positioning is contraindicated in patients with increased intracranial pressure, hemodynamic instability, spinal cord injuries, or abdominal surgery. Patients who are unable to tolerate the face-down position are also not appropriate candidates for this type of therapy.[90-92]

No standard has been established for the length of time a patient should remain in the prone position. A review of the research on this subject revealed a wide variation, anywhere from 30 minutes to 40 hours.[92] The therapy is considered successful if the patient has an improvement in Pao_2 of greater than 10 mm Hg within 30 minutes of being placed in the prone position.[93] The positioning schedule (length of time in the prone position and frequency of turning) is usually based on

the patient's tolerance of the procedure, the success of the procedure in improving the patient's Pao_2, and whether the patient is able to sustain improvements in Pao_2 when turned back to the supine position. Prone positioning is discontinued when the patient no longer demonstrates a response to the position change.[93]

The biggest limitation to prone positioning is the actual mechanics of turning the patient. A number of methods have been discussed in the literature, including manually turning the patient and positioning with pillows to support the patient and use of the RotoProne™ Therapy System (Fig. 21-15).[90,92] Regardless of the method used, the abdomen must be allowed to hang free to facilitate diaphragmatic descent.

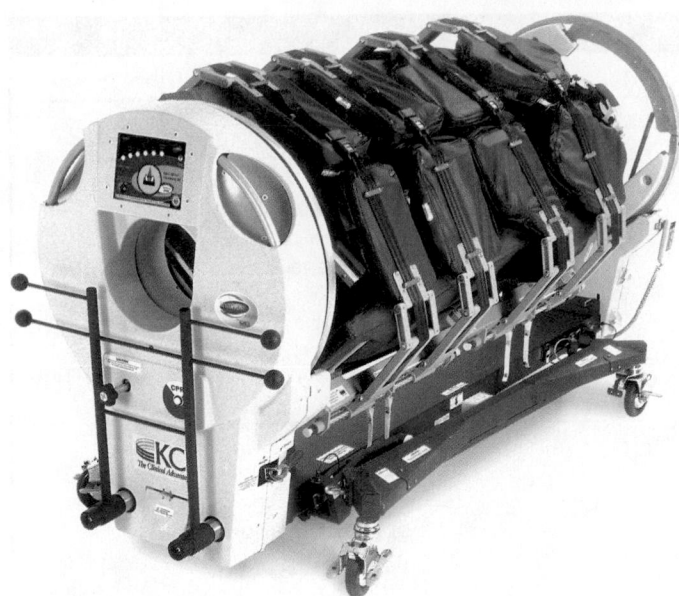

FIGURE 21-15 RotoProne™ therapy system. (Courtesy KCI USA, Inc., San Antonio, TX. RotoProne is a trademark of the ArjoHuntleigh group of companies.)

Before the patient is turned to the prone position, his or her eyes are lubricated and taped closed, tubes and drains are secured, and the procedure is explained to the patient and family. A team is organized to implement the turning procedure, and one member is positioned at the head of the bed to maintain the patient's airway. Complications of the procedure include dislodgment or obstruction of tubes and drains, hemodynamic instability, massive facial edema, pressure ulcers, aspiration, and corneal ulcerations.[90,92]

Rotation Therapy

Automated turning beds to provide rotation therapy are often used in the critical care setting. *Kinetic therapy* and *continuous lateral rotation therapy* (CLRT) are two forms of rotation therapy. The patient is continuously turned from side to side with a rotation of 40 degrees or greater (kinetic therapy) or with a rotation of less than 40 degrees (CLRT).[94] Two types of beds can perform this type of therapy: 1) an oscillation bed, in which the mattress inflates and deflates to provide rotation; and 2) a kinetic bed, in which the entire platform of the bed rotates.[95]

Rotation therapy is thought to improve oxygenation through better matching of ventilation to perfusion and to prevent pulmonary complications associated with bed rest and mechanical ventilation.[96,97] However, to achieve such benefits, rotation must be aggressive, and the patient must be turned at least 40 degrees per side, with a total arc of at least 80 degrees, for at least 18 hours a day.[97,98] CLRT has been shown to be of minimal pulmonary benefit to the critically ill patient.[94] Kinetic therapy decreases the incidence of VAP, particularly in patients with neurologic problems and in those who have undergone surgery.[98] In one study, kinetic therapy decreased the incidence of VAP and lobar atelectasis in medical, surgical, and trauma patients.[97]

Complications of the procedure include dislodgment or obstruction of tubes, drains, and lines; hemodynamic instability; and pressure ulcers. Lateral rotation does not replace manual repositioning to prevent pressure ulcers.[99] Repositioning changes the relationship of the patient's posterior surface to the mattress. This gives the skin a chance to reperfuse and to ventilate. Repositioning shifts weight-bearing points. To prevent pressure ulcers, the patient should be positioned 30 degrees from the surface of the mattress regardless of the degree of rotational turn. One study found that patients receiving rotational therapy still developed pressure ulcers of the sacrum, occiput, and heels.[100]

THORACIC SURGERY

The term *thoracic surgery* refers to a number of surgical procedures that involve opening the thoracic cavity (thoracotomy), the organs of respiration, or both. Indications for thoracic surgery range from tumors and abscesses to repair of the esophagus and thoracic vessels.[101] Table 21-9 describes a variety of thoracic surgical procedures and their indications. This discussion focuses only on the surgical procedures that involve the removal of lung tissue.

Preoperative Care

Before surgery, a complete evaluation of the patient is needed to determine the appropriateness of surgery as a treatment and to determine whether lung tissue can be removed without jeopardizing respiratory function. This is especially important when a lobectomy or pneumonectomy is being considered. When resection is being undertaken for tumor treatment, preoperative care includes evaluation of the type and extent of the tumor and the physical condition of the patient.[102]

The evaluation of the patient's physical status should focus on the adequacy of cardiopulmonary function. The preoperative evaluation should include pulmonary function tests to determine the patient's ability to manage with less lung tissue. Cardiac function also should be evaluated. Uncontrolled dysrhythmias, acute myocardial infarction, severe chronic heart failure, and unstable angina are all contraindications to surgery.[103,104]

Surgical Considerations

The type and location of surgery will dictate the type of surgical approach that is used. The most common approach is the posterolateral thoracotomy, which allows for exposure of both the lung and mediastinum. Other approaches that are used include anterolateral thoracotomy and median sternotomy.[101]

Special care is taken to avoid drainage of blood or secretions into the unaffected lung during surgery (Fig. 21-16) because such an occurrence could cause hypoxemia and cardiac dysfunction. A double-lumen endotracheal tube is used during the surgery to protect the unaffected lung from secretions and necrotic tumor fragments. To decrease the incidence of hypoxemia during the procedure, 5 to 10 cm H_2O of PEEP is maintained to the deflated lung. In addition, the deflated lung is intermittently ventilated during the procedure.[105]

TABLE 21-9 THORACIC SURGERIES

PROCEDURE	DEFINITION	INDICATIONS
Pneumonectomy	Removal of entire lung with or without resection of the mediastinal lymph nodes	Malignant lesions Unilateral tuberculosis Extensive unilateral bronchiectasis Multiple lung abscesses Massive hemoptysis Bronchopleural fistula
Lobectomy	Resection of one or more lobes of lung	Lesions confined to a single lobe Pulmonary tuberculosis Bronchiectasis Lung abscesses or cysts Trauma
Segmental resection	Resection of bronchovascular section of lung lobe	Small peripheral lesions Bronchiectasis Congenital cysts or blebs
Wedge resection	Removal of small wedge-shaped section of lung tissue	Small, peripheral lesions (without lymph node involvement) Peripheral granulomas Pulmonary blebs
Bronchoplastic reconstruction (also called *sleeve resection*)	Resection of lung tissue and bronchus with end-to-end reanastomosis of bronchus	Small lesions involving the carina or major bronchus without evidence of metastasis May be combined with lobectomy

TABLE 21-9 **THORACIC SURGERIES—cont'd**

PROCEDURE	DEFINITION	INDICATIONS
Lung volume reduction surgery	Resection of the most damaged portions of lung tissue, allowing more normal chest wall configuration	Severe emphysema
Bullectomy	Resection of a large bulla (an airspace that is greater than 1 cm in diameter that formed as a result of pulmonary tissue destruction)	Severe emphysema with large bullae compressing surrounding tissue
Open lung biopsy	Resection of a small portion of the lung for biopsy	Failure of closed lung biopsy Removal of small lesions
Decortication	Removal of fibrous membrane from pleural surface of lung	Fibrothorax resulting from hemothorax or empyema
Drainage of empyema	Drainage of pus in the pleural space	Acute and chronic infections
Partial rib resection	Removal of one or more ribs to allow healing of underlying lung tissue	Chronic empyemic infections
Video-assisted thoracoscopy (VATS)	Endoscopie procedure performed through small incisions in the chest	Evaluation of pulmonary, pleural, mediastinal, or pericardial conditions Biopsy of lung, pleural, or mediastinal lesions Recurrent spontaneous pneumothorax Evacuation of emphysema, hemothorax, pleural effusion, or pericardial effusion Blebectomy or bullectomy Pleurodesis Sympathectomy Closure of bronchopleural fistula Lysis of adhesions

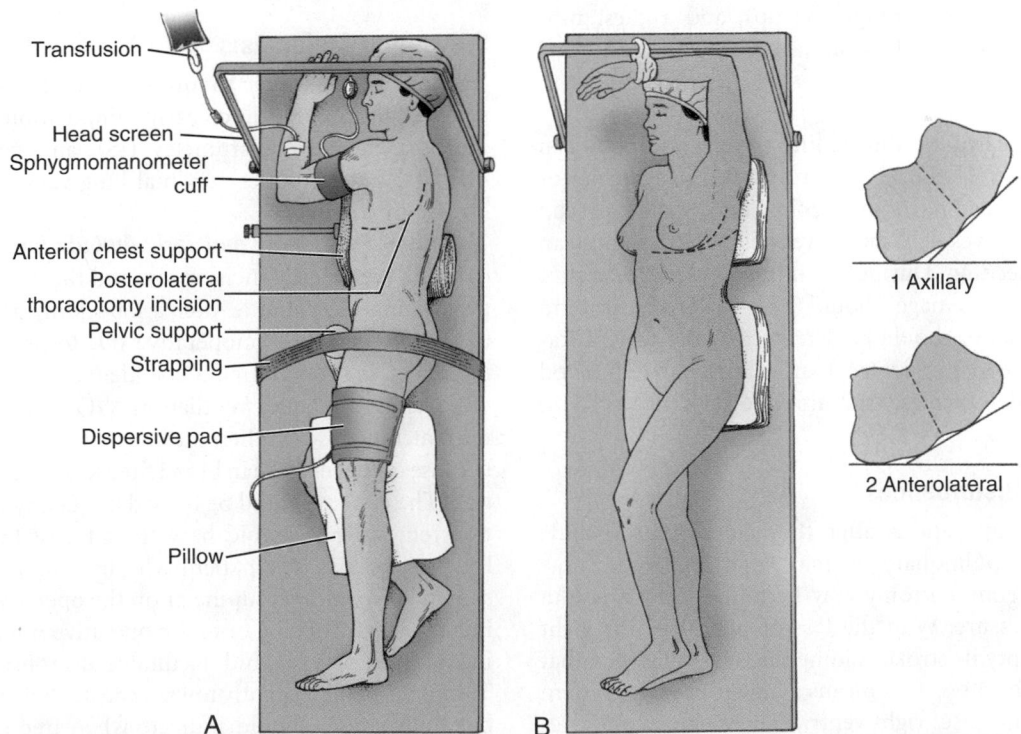

FIGURE 21-16 **Positions for thoracotomy incisions.** *A,* Lateral position for posterolateral incision. *B,* Semilateral position for axillary or anterolateral position. (From Blanchard B. Thoracic surgery. In: Rothrock JC, McEwen DR, eds. *Alexander's Care of the Patient in Surgery.* 14th ed. St. Louis: Elsevier; 2011.)

Complications and Medical Management

A number of complications are associated with a lung resection. These include acute respiratory failure, bronchopleural fistula, hemorrhage, cardiovascular disturbances, and mediastinal shift.

Acute Lung Failure

In the postoperative period, acute respiratory failure may result from atelectasis or pneumonia. Atelectasis can occur as a result of anesthesia, the surgical procedure, immobilization, and pain. Treatment should be aimed at correcting the underlying problems and supporting gas exchange. Supplemental oxygen and mechanical ventilation with PEEP may be necessary.[106]

Bronchopleural Fistula

Development of a postoperative bronchopleural fistula is a major cause of mortality after a lung resection. A bronchopleural fistula develops when the suture line fails to secure occlusion of the bronchial stump, and an opening develops into the pleural space.[107] This can result from an imperfect stump closure, perforation of the stump (e.g., with a suction catheter), high pressure within the airways (e.g., caused by mechanical ventilation), or infection.[108,109] During surgery, careful attention is given to isolating and closing the bronchus in an attempt to secure a lasting seal with subsequent stump healing.[101] In addition, early extubation is encouraged to eliminate the possibility of perforation of the stump and high airway pressures.[108] Clinical manifestations of a bronchopleural fistula include shortness of breath and coughing up serosanguineous sputum. Immediate surgery is usually necessary to close the stump and prevent flooding of the remaining lung with fluid from the residual space.[109] If this occurs, the patient should be placed with the operative side down (remaining lung up), and a chest tube should be inserted to drain the residual space.[101]

Hemorrhage

Hemorrhage is an early, life-threatening complication that can occur after a lung resection. It can result from bronchial or intercostal artery bleeding or disruption of a suture or clip around a pulmonary vessel.[108] Excessive chest tube drainage can signal excessive bleeding. During the immediate postoperative period, chest tube drainage should be measured every 15 minutes; this frequency should be decreased as the patient stabilizes. If chest tube loss is greater than 100 mL/hr, fresh blood is noted, or a sudden increase in drainage occurs, hemorrhage should be suspected.

Cardiovascular Disturbances

Cardiovascular complications after thoracic surgery include dysrhythmias and pulmonary edema. Resections of a large lung area or a pneumonectomy may be followed by a rise in central venous pressure. With the loss of one lung, the right ventricle must empty its stroke volume into a vascular bed that has been reduced by 50%. This means a higher pressure system is created, which increases right ventricular workload and precipitates right ventricular failure. Depending on previous heart function, acute decompensation of both ventricles can result. Measures are aimed at supporting cardiac function and avoiding intravascular volume excess. These measures include

---

optimizing preload, afterload, and contractility with vasoactive agents.[108]

Postoperative Nursing Management

Nursing care of the patient who has had thoracic surgery incorporates a number of nursing diagnoses (Box 21-10). Nursing interventions include optimizing oxygenation and ventilation, preventing atelectasis, monitoring chest tubes, assisting the patient to return to an adequate activity level, providing comfort and emotional support, and maintaining surveillance for complications.

Optimizing Oxygenation and Ventilation

Nursing interventions to optimize oxygenation and ventilation include positioning, preventing desaturation during procedures, and promoting secretion clearance.

Preventing Atelectasis

Nursing interventions to prevent atelectasis include proper patient positioning and early ambulation, deep-breathing exercises, incentive spirometry (IS), and pain management. The goal is to promote maximal lung ventilation and prevent hypoventilation.

Patient Positioning and Early Ambulation. The nurse should consider the surgical incision site and the type of surgery when positioning the patient. After a lobectomy, the patient should be turned onto the nonoperative side to promote V/Q matching. When the good lung is dependent and blood flow is greater to the area with better ventilation, V/Q matching is better. V/Q mismatching results when the affected lung is positioned down because of the increase in blood flow to an area with less ventilation. The patient should be turned frequently to promote secretion removal but should have the affected lung dependent as little as possible. The patient who has had a pneumonectomy should be positioned supine or on the operative side during the initial period. Turning onto the operative side promotes splinting of the incision and facilitates deep-breathing exercises. Tilting the patient slightly toward the unaffected side is possible, but the surgeon should indicate when free side-to-side positioning is safe.[109]

When sitting at the bedside or ambulating, patients must be encouraged to keep the thorax in straight alignment while they breathe deeply. This position best accommodates diaphragmatic descent and intercostal muscle action. The sitting or standing position provides enhanced ventilation to areas of the lung that are dependent in the supine position, thus accommodating maximal inflation and promoting gas exchange. Ambulation is essential in restoring lung function and should be initiated as soon as possible.

Deep Breathing and Incentive Spirometry. Deep breathing and incentive spirometry should be performed regularly by patients who have undergone a thoracotomy. Deep breathing involves having the patient take a deep breath and holding it for approximately 3 seconds or longer. Incentive spirometry involves having the patient take at least 10 deep, effective breaths per hour using an incentive spirometer. These activities help re-expand collapsed lung tissue, thus promoting early resolution of the pneumothorax in patients with partial lung resections. The chest should be auscultated during inflation to ensure that all dependent parts of the lung are well ventilated and to help the patient understand the depth of breath necessary for optimal effect. Coughing, which should be encouraged only when secretions are present, assists in mobilizing secretions for removal.[110]

Pain Management. Pain can be a major problem after thoracic surgery. Pain can increase the workload of the heart, precipitate hypoventilation, and inhibit mobilization of secretions. Clinical manifestations of pain include tachypnea, tachycardia, elevated blood pressure, facial grimacing, splinting of the incision, hypoventilation, moaning, and restlessness. Several alternatives for pain management after thoracic surgery can be used. The two most common methods are systemic narcotic administration and epidural narcotic administration. Opioids can be administered intravenously or via the patient-controlled analgesia (PCA) method. In addition, the patient should be assisted with splinting the incision with a pillow or blanket when deep breathing and coughing. Splinting stabilizes the area and reduces pain when moving, deep breathing, or coughing.[106]

Maintaining the Chest Tube System

Chest tubes are placed after most thoracic surgery procedures to remove air and fluid. The drainage will initially appear bloody, becoming serosanguineous and then serous over the first 2 to 3 days postoperatively. Approximately 100 to 300 mL of drainage will occur during the first 2 hours postoperatively, which will decrease to less than 50 mL/hr over the next several hours. Routine stripping of chest tubes is not recommended because excessive negative pressure can be generated in the chest. If blood clots are present in the drainage tubing or an obstruction is present, the chest tubes may be carefully milked. The chest tube may be placed to suction or water seal.[111]

During auscultation of the lungs, air leaks should be evaluated. In the early phase, an air leak is commonly heard over the affected area because the pleura have not yet tightly sealed. As healing occurs, this leak should disappear. An increase in an air leak or the appearance of a new air leak should prompt investigation of the chest drainage system to discover whether air is leaking into the system from outside or whether the leak is originating from the incision. Increased air leaks not related to the thoracic drainage system may indicate disruption of sutures.[108]

Assisting Patient to Return to Adequate Activity Level

Within a few days after surgery, range-of-motion exercises for the shoulder on the operative side should be performed. The patient frequently splints the operative side and avoids shoulder movement because of pain. If immobility is allowed, stiffening of the shoulder joint can result. This is referred to as *frozen shoulder* and may require physical therapy and rehabilitation to regain satisfactory range of motion of the shoulder joint.[109]

Usually on the day after surgery, the patient is able to sit in a chair. Activity should be systematically increased, with attention to the patient's activity tolerance. With adequate pulmonary function before surgery and a surgical approach designed to preserve respiratory function, full return to previous activity levels is possible. This may take as long as 6 months to 1 year, depending on the tissue resected and the patient's general condition.[101]

PHARMACOLOGY

A number of pharmacologic agents are used in the care of the patient with pulmonary dysfunction who is critically ill. Table 21-10 reviews these agents and the special considerations necessary for administering them.

Bronchodilators and Adjuncts

Medications to facilitate removal of secretions and dilate airways are of major benefit in the treatment of pulmonary disorders. Mucolytics are administered to help liquefy secretions, which facilitates their removal. Bronchodilators such as beta$_2$-agonists and anticholinergic agents aid in smooth muscle relaxation and are of particular benefit to patients with airflow limitations. Steroids are often used in conjunction with beta$_2$-agonists to enhance their effects and to decrease airway inflammation.[112-114]

Neuromuscular Blocking Agents

Sedation is necessary in many patients to assist with maintaining adequate ventilation. It can be used to comfort the patient and to decrease the work of breathing, particularly if the patient is fighting the ventilator. More information about sedation is provided in Chapter 10. In some patients, sedation does not decrease spontaneous respiratory efforts enough to allow adequate ventilation, and patient–ventilator dyssynchrony may develop. Neuromuscular paralysis may be necessary to facilitate optimal ventilation. Paralysis also may be necessary to decrease oxygen consumption in the patient who is severely compromised.[115-117]

Nursing management of the patient receiving a neuromuscular blocking agent should incorporate a number of additional interventions. Because paralytic agents only halt skeletal muscle movement and do not inhibit pain or awareness, they must be administered together with a sedative or anxiolytic agent. Pain medication is administered if the patient has a pain-producing illness or surgery. Providing reorientation and explanations for all procedures is critical because the patient can still hear but cannot move or see. The patient is also at high risk for developing the complications of immobility, so

TABLE 21-10 PHARMACOLOGIC MANAGEMENT

Pulmonary Disorders

MEDICATION	DOSAGE	ACTIONS	SPECIAL CONSIDERATIONS
Neuromuscular Blocking Agents (NMBAs)			
Vecuronium (Norcuron)	Loading dose: 0.08-0.1 mg/kg IV IV infusion: 0.8-1.2 mcg/kg/min	Used to paralyze patient to decrease oxygen demand and avoid ventilator dyssynchrony	Boxed Warning from FDA: Risk of anaphylactic and anaphylactoid type adverse reactions, including fatalities reported in association with use of neuromuscular blockers.
Pancuronium (Pavulon)	Loading dose: 0.06-0.1 mg/kg IV infusion: 0.02-0.04 mg/kg/hr		Administer sedative and analgesic agents concurrently, because NMBAs have no sedative or analgesic properties.
Rocuronium (Zemuron)	Loading dose: 0.6 mg/kg IV IV infusion: 10-12 mcg/kg/min		Evaluate level of paralysis q4h using a peripheral nerve stimulator.
Atracurium (Tracrium)	Loading dose: 0.30-0.50 mg/kg IV IV infusion: 4-12 mcg/kg/min		Protect patients from the environment because they are unable to respond.
Cisatracurium (Nimbex)	Loading dose: 0.15-0.2 mg/kg IV IV Infusion: 0.5-10.2 mcg/kg/min)		Prolonged muscle paralysis may occur after discontinuation of the paralytic agent.
Mucolytics			
Acetylcysteine (Mucomyst)	Nebulizer, 20% solution: 3-5 mL tid–qid Nebulizer, 10% solution: 6-10 mL tid–qid	Used to decrease viscosity and elasticity of mucus by breaking down disulfide bonds within mucus	May be administered with a bronchodilator because medication can cause bronchospasms and inhibit ciliary function. Treatment is considered effective when bronchorrhea develops and coughing occurs. Antidote for acetaminophen overdose.
B₂-Agonists			
Epinephrine (Adrenalin) Racemic epinephrine	Nebulizer, 1% solution: 2.5-5 mg (0.25-0.5 mL) qid Nebulizer, 2.25% solution: 5.625-11.25 mg (0.25-0.5 mL) qid	Used to relax bronchial smooth muscle and dilate airways to prevent bronchospasms	May cause skeletal muscle tremors. Higher doses may cause tachycardia, palpitations, increased blood pressure, dysrhythmias, and angina.
Isoetharine 1% (Bronkosol)	Nebulizer, 1% solution: 2.5-5 mg (0.25-0.5 mL) qid		May increase serum glucose and decrease serum potassium levels.
Terbutaline	MDI, 340 mcg/puff: 1-2 puffs qid MDI, 200 mcg/puff: 2 puffs q4-6h		Treatment is considered effective when breath sounds improve and dyspnea is lessened.
Metaproterenol (Alupent, Metaprel)	Nebulizer, 5% solution: 15 mg (0.3 mL) tid–qid MDI, 650 mcg/puff: 2-3 puffs tid–qid		Only approximately 10% of the administered dose reaches the site of action within the lungs.
Albuterol (Proventil, Ventolin)	Nebulizer, 5% solution: 2.5 mg (0.5 mL) tid–qid MDI, 90 mcg/puff: 2 puffs tid–qid		
Levalbuterol (Xopenex)	Nebulizer: 0.63 mg q6-8h		
Anticholinergic Agents			
Ipratropium (Atrovent)	Nebulizer, 0.02% solution: 0.5 mg (2.5 mL) q6-8h	Used to block the constriction of bronchial smooth muscle and reduce mucus production	There are relatively few adverse effects because systemic absorption is poor.
Xanthines			
Theophylline	Loading dose: 4.6 mg/kg IV IV infusion: 0.4-0.8 mg/kg/hr	Used to dilate bronchial smooth muscle and reverse diaphragmatic muscle fatigue	Administer loading dose over 30 minutes. Monitor serum blood levels; therapeutic level is 10-20 mg/dL.

TABLE 21-10 PHARMACOLOGIC MANAGEMENT
Pulmonary Disorders—cont'd

MEDICATION	DOSAGE	ACTIONS	SPECIAL CONSIDERATIONS
Aminophylline	Loading dose: 5.7 mg/kg IV IV infusion: 0.5-1 mg/kg/hr		Administer with caution to patients with cardiac, renal, or hepatic disease. Signs of toxicity include central nervous system excitation, seizures, confusion, irritability, hyperglycemia, headache, nausea, hypotension, and dysrhythmias.
Inhaled Corticosteroids			
Beclomethasone (Vanceril, Beclovent)	MDI, 42 meg/puff: 2 puffs tid-qid	Used to decrease airway inflammation and enhance effectiveness of beta-agonists	Suppresses inflammatory response and interferes with ability to fight infection.
Flunisolide (AeroBid)	MDI, 250 meg/puff: 2 puffs bid		Oral candidiasis is a side effect that can be minimized by having patients rinse their mouths after treatment.
Triamcinolone (Azmacort)	MDI, 100 meg/puff: 2 puffs tid-qid		

Data from *Elsevier/Gold Standard.* http://www.mdconsult.com/das/pharm/lookup/340530070-12?type=alldrugs. Accessed July 9, 2012.
FDA, U.S. Food and Drug Agency; *MDI,* metered-dose inhaler, *NMBAs,* neuromuscular blocking agents.

interventions related to the prevention of skin breakdown, atelectasis, and deep vein thrombosis are also implemented. Patient safety is another concern because the patient cannot react to the environment. Special precautions are taken to protect the patient at all times.[118]

Peripheral Nerve Stimulator

Long-term use of neuromuscular blocking agents can result in prolonged neuromuscular blockade and skeletal muscle weakness. To avoid this complication, the patient's level of paralysis is carefully monitored with the use of a peripheral nerve stimulator (PNS). The PNS delivers an electrical stimulus (single twitch, post-tetanic count, double-burst stimulation, or train-of-four [TOF]) to a preselected nerve (ulnar, facial, posterior tibial, or peroneal) by electrodes (needle, ball, or pregelled), and the response is monitored to gauge the level of paralysis.[118]

In most cases, the ulnar nerve is used, with pregelled electrodes being placed 2 to 3 inches proximal to the crease of the wrist (Fig. 21-17). The TOF stimulation test, which delivers four electrical stimuli in a row, is the most common test used. When the ulnar nerve is stimulated with TOF, the expected response is four twitches (adduction) of the thumb medially across the palm of the hand. The number of twitches correlates with the level of paralysis: 4 twitches indicates less than 75% blockade; 3 twitches is approximately 75% blockade; 2 twitches is approximately 80% blockade; 1 twitch is approximately 90% blockade; and 0 twitch indicates 100% blockade. Usually, the neuromuscular blocking agent is titrated to maintain an 80% blockade (two twitches). The goal is to administer the smallest dose possible of the paralytic agent, to avoid prolonged weakness after the therapy is discontinued.[118]

Use of the PNS for estimating the degree of paralysis is not without its problems. Poor skin contact, improper electrode

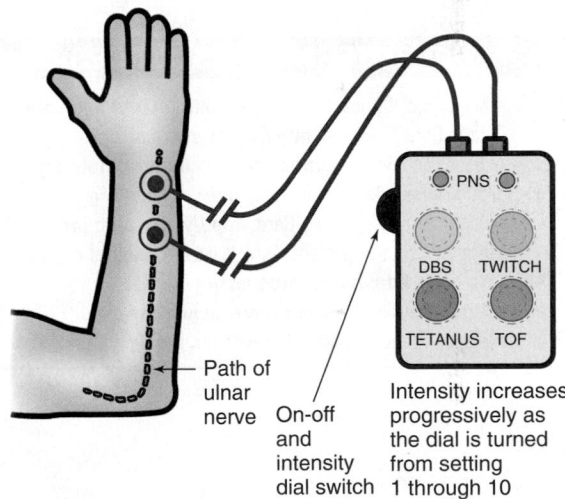

FIGURE 21-17 Peripheral nerve stimulator (PNS). Note the placement of electrodes along the ulnar nerve. *DBS,* Double-burst stimulation; *TOF,* train-of-four.

placement, edema in the extremity being monitored, and malfunction of the device can lead to overestimation of the degree of blockade. The patient appears to have a zero-twitch TOF response, but evidence of muscle movement is present. More problematic is underestimation of the degree of blockade. Direct stimulation of the muscle or mistaking finger responses for those of the thumb can result in a false-positive twitch response. This can result in unnecessary administration of additional doses of the paralytic agent. It is imperative that the patient's twitch response be correlated with clinical observations of patient movement.[118]

BOX 21-11   CASE STUDY

Patient with Acute Respiratory Failure

Brief Patient History

Mr. B is a 63-year-old man who is clinically obese. He has a long history of chronic obstructive pulmonary disease (COPD) associated with smoking two packs of cigarettes a day for 40 years. During the past week, Mr. B has experienced a flulike illness with fever, chills, malaise, anorexia, diarrhea, nausea, vomiting, and a productive cough with thick, brownish, purulent sputum.

Clinical Assessment

Mr. B is admitted to the intermediate care unit from the emergency department with acute respiratory insufficiency. He is sitting up in bed, leaning forward, with his elbows resting on the over-the-bed table. Mr. B is breathing through his mouth, taking rapid shallow breaths, using his accessory muscles to ventilate. On inhalation, his nostrils flare and his accessory muscles retract. During exhalation, Mr. B uses pursed-lip breathing, and his intercostal muscles bulge. He appears anxious and irritable and is able to speak only one or two barely audible words between each breath. Auscultation reveals crackles posteriorly over the right and left lower lung fields.

Diagnostic Procedures

His admission chest radiograph reveals infiltrates in the right lower lobe and left lower lobe. Gram stain of Mr. B's sputum shows numerous gram-positive diplococci. His baseline vital signs are as follows: blood pressure of 110/60 mm Hg, heart rate of 108 beats/min (sinus tachycardia), respiratory rate of 30 breaths/min, and temperature of 101.3°F. His baseline arterial blood gas (ABG) values on a 28% Venturi face mask are as follows: PaO_2 of 58 mm Hg, $PaCO_2$ of 33 mm Hg, pH of 7.52, HCO_3^- level of 28, and O_2 saturation of 88%.

Medical Diagnosis

Mr. B is diagnosed with community-associated pneumococcal pneumonia.

Questions

1. What major outcomes do you expect to achieve for this patient?
2. What problems or risks must be managed to achieve these outcomes?
3. What interventions must be initiated to monitor, prevent, manage, or eliminate the problems and risks identified?
4. What interventions should be initiated to promote optimal functioning, safety, and well-being of the patient?
5. What possible learning needs do you anticipate for this patient?
6. What cultural and age-related factors may have a bearing on the patient's plan of care?

BOX 21-12   INTERNET RESOURCES

American Association of Critical-Care Nurses: **http://www.aacn.org**
Society for Critical Care Medicine: **http://www.sccm.org**
Respiratory Nursing Society: **http://respiratorynursingsociety.org**
American Holistic Nurses Association: **http://www.ahna.org**
American Association of Respiratory Care: **http://www.aarc.org**
American College of Chest Physicians: **http://www.chestnet.org/accp**
NHLBI ARDS Network: **http://www.ardsnet.org**
American College of Physicians: **http://www.acponline.org**
American College of Surgeons: **http://www.facs.org**

American Lung Association: **http://www.lung.org**
American Medical Association: **http://www.ama-assn.org**
American Thoracic Society: **http://www.thoracic.org**
American Holistic Medical Association: **http://www.holisticmedicine.org**
ICU Delirium and Cognitive Impairment Study Group:
  http://www.mc.vanderbilt.edu/icudelirium
Centers for Disease Control and Prevention: **http://www.cdc.gov**
National Institutes for Health: **http://www.nih.gov**
PubMed Health: **http://www.ncbi.nlm.nih.gov/pubmedhealth**

SUMMARY

Oxygen Therapy

- Oxygen is a medication, and the primary indication for its use is hypoxemia.
- Oxygen can be delivered by various methods, including low-flow systems, reservoir systems, and high-flow systems.
- Complications of oxygen therapy include oxygen toxicity, CO_2 retention, and absorption atelectasis.

Artificial Airways

- Artificial airways (oropharyngeal and nasopharyngeal) are used to maintain airway patency by keeping the tongue from obstructing the upper airway.
- ETTs (oral and nasal) are used to maintain airway patency, to protect the airway from aspiration, to facilitate access to invasive positive-pressure ventilation, and to aid in secretion removal.

- Complications of ETTs include tube obstruction, tube displacement, sinusitis and nasal injury, tracheoesophageal fistula, mucosal lesions, laryngeal or tracheal stenosis, and cricoid abscess.
- Tracheostomy tubes provide the best method of long-term airway maintenance.
- Complications of tracheostomy tubes include hemorrhage, wound infection, subcutaneous emphysema, tube obstruction, tube displacement, tracheal stenosis, tracheoesophageal fistula, tracheoinnominate artery fistula, and tracheocutaneous fistula.
- Cuff pressure should be monitored every shift and should be maintained at 20 to 25 mm Hg (24 to 30 cm H_2O).
- Humidification is required for all ETTs and tracheostomy tubes.

- Complications associated with suctioning can be minimized if hyperoxygenation is initiated before the start of the procedure, each suction pass is limited to 10 to 15 seconds, and normal saline is not instilled.
- Oral care should consist of brushing the patient's teeth with a soft toothbrush to reduce plaque, brushing the patient's tongue and gums with a foam swab to stimulate the tissue, and performing deep oropharyngeal suction to remove any secretions that have pooled above the cuff.
- After an artificial airway is no longer needed, it should be removed.

Invasive Mechanical Ventilation
- Indications for mechanical ventilation include supporting cardiopulmonary gas exchange (alveolar ventilation and arterial oxygenation), increasing lung volume (end-expiratory lung inflation and functional residual capacity), and reducing the work of breathing.
- Complications associated with mechanical ventilation include ventilator-induced lung injury, cardiovascular compromise, gastrointestinal disturbances, patient–ventilator dyssynchrony, and VAP.
- Strategies to prevent VAP ("VAP Bundle") include elevation of the head of the bed, daily "sedation vacations" and assessment of readiness to extubate, peptic ulcer disease prophylaxis, deep venous thrombosis prophylaxis, and daily oral care with chlorhexidine.
- Weaning is the gradual withdrawal of the mechanical ventilator and the re-establishment of spontaneous breathing; it should begin only after the original process for which ventilator support was required has been corrected and patient stability has been achieved.

Noninvasive Mechanical Ventilation
- Noninvasive mechanical ventilation uses a mask instead of an ETT to administer positive-pressure ventilation and is indicated in type I and type II acute respiratory failure, cardiogenic pulmonary edema, and other situations in which intubation is not an option.
- Respiratory rate, accessory muscle use, and oxygenation status are continually assessed to ensure that the patient is tolerating this method of ventilation.

Positioning Therapy
- On the basis of the concept that preferential blood flow occurs to the gravity-dependent areas of the lungs, positioning therapy is used to place the least damaged portion of the lungs into a dependent position.
- Prone positioning involves turning the patient completely over onto his or her stomach in the face-down position; it is used to improve oxygenation in ARDS.

- Kinetic therapy (continuous turning of a patient from side to side with a 40-degree or greater rotation) and CLRT (continuous turning with a less than 40-degree rotation) are two forms of rotation therapy.
- Rotation therapy is thought to improve oxygenation through better matching of ventilation to perfusion and to prevent pulmonary complications associated with bed rest and mechanical ventilation.

Thoracic Surgery
- The term *thoracic surgery* refers to a number of surgical procedures that involve opening the thoracic cavity (thoracotomy) or the organs of respiration, or both; indications for thoracic surgery range from tumors and abscesses to repair of the esophagus and of thoracic vessels.
- Before surgery, a complete evaluation of the patient is needed to determine the appropriateness of surgery as a treatment and whether lung tissue can be removed without jeopardizing respiratory function.
- The most common approach is the posterolateral thoracotomy, which allows for exposure of the lung and the mediastinum.
- Complications of a lung resection include acute respiratory failure, bronchopleural fistula, hemorrhage, cardiovascular disturbances, and mediastinal shift.
- Nursing actions include optimizing oxygenation and ventilation, preventing atelectasis, monitoring chest tubes, assisting the patient to return to an adequate activity level, providing comfort and emotional support, and maintaining surveillance for complications.

Pharmacology
- Mucolytics are administered to help liquefy secretions, which facilitates their removal.
- Bronchodilators, such as beta$_2$-agonists and anticholinergic agents, aid in smooth muscle relaxation and are of particular benefit to patients with airflow limitations.
- Steroids are often used in conjunction with beta$_2$-agonists to enhance their effects and to decrease airway inflammation.
- Sedation is necessary in many patients to assist with maintaining adequate ventilation; it can be used to comfort the patient and to decrease the work of breathing, particularly if the patient is fighting the ventilator.
- Neuromuscular paralysis may be necessary to facilitate optimal ventilation and to decrease oxygen consumption in the severely compromised patient.
- To avoid prolonged neuromuscular blockade, the patient's level of paralysis is carefully monitored by means of a PNS.

REFERENCES

1. Henderson Y. Delivering oxygen therapy to acutely breathless adults. *Nurs Stand*. 2008;22(35):46.
2. O'Driscoll BR, et al. BTS guideline for emergency oxygen use in adult patients. *Thorax*. 2008;63(suppl 6):vi1.
3. Heuer AJ. Medical gas therapy. In: Kacmarek RM, et al, eds. *Egan's Fundamentals of Respiratory Care*. 10th ed. St. Louis: Mosby; 2013.
4. Kernick J, Magarey J. What is the evidence for the use of high flow nasal cannula oxygen in adult patients admitted to critical care units? A systematic review. *Aust Crit Care*. 2010;23:53.
5. White AC. The evaluation and management of hypoxemia in the chronic critically ill patient. *Clin Chest Med*. 2001;22:123.
6. Barnes TA. Emergency cardiovascular life support. In: Kacmarek RM, et al, eds. *Egan's Fundamentals of Respiratory Care*. 10th ed. St. Louis: Mosby; 2013.
7. Pierce LNB. *Management of the Mechanically Ventilated Patient*. 2nd ed. St. Louis: Saunders; 2007.
8. McCorstin P, et al. Management of the mechanically ventilated patient in the emergency department. *J Emerg Nurs*. 2008;34:121.
9. Walz JM, Zayaruzny M, Heard SO. Airway management in critical illness. *Chest*. 2007;131:608.
10. St John RE, Seckel MA. Airway management. In: Burns SM, ed. *AACN Protocols for Practice: Care of the Mechanically Ventilated Patient*. 2nd ed. Sudbury, MA: Jones and Bartlett; 2007.
11. Altobelli N. Airway management. In: Kacmarek RM, et al, eds. *Egan's Fundamentals of Respiratory Care*. 10th ed. St. Louis: Mosby; 2013.
12. Chethan DB, Hughes RC. Tracheal intubation, tracheal tubes and laryngeal mask airways. *J Perioper Pract*. 2008;18:88.
13. Colice GL. Technical standards for tracheal tubes. *Clin Chest Med*. 1991;12:433.
14. Mace SE. Challenges and advances in intubation: rapid sequence intubation. *Emerg Med Clin N Am*. 2008;26:1043.
15. Kabrhel C, et al. Orotracheal intubation. *N Eng J Med*. 2007;356:e15.
16. Miñambres E, et al. Tracheal rupture after endotracheal intubation: a literature systematic review. *Eur J Cardiothorac Surg*. 2009;35:1056.
17. Feller-Kopman D. Acute complications of artificial airways. *Clin Chest Med*. 2003;24:445.
18. Gaissert HA, Burns J. The compromised airway: tumors, strictures, and tracheomalacia. *Surg Clin N Am*. 2010;90:1065.
19. Durbin CG. Tracheostomy: why, when, and how? *Respir Care*. 2010;55:1056.
20. St John RE, Malen JF. Contemporary issues in adult tracheostomy management. *Crit Care Nurs Clin North Am*. 2004;16:413.
21. Morris LL, Afifi MS. *Tracheostomies: The Complete Guide*. New York: Springer; 2010.
22. Vallamkondu V, Visvanathan V. Clinical review of adult tracheostomy. *J Perioper Pract*. 2011;21:172.
23. Cabrini L, et al. Percutaneous tracheostomy, a systematic review. *Acta Anaesthesiol Scand*. 2012;56:270.
24. Samuelson KAM. Adult intensive care patients' perception of endotracheal tube-related discomforts: a prospective evaluation. *Heart Lung*. 2011;40:49.
25. Züchner K. Humidification: measurement and requirements. *Respir Care Clin N Am*. 2006;12:149.
26. Fink J, Ari A. Humidity and bland aerosol therapy. In: Kacmarek RM, et al, eds. *Egan's Fundamentals of Respiratory Care*. 10th ed. St. Louis: Mosby; 2013.
27. Schulze A. Respiratory gas conditioning and humidification. *Clin Perinatol*. 2007;34(1):19.
28. Wright SE, VanDahm K. Long-term care of the tracheostomy patient. *Clin Chest Med*. 2003;24:473.
29. Hamilton VA, Grap MJ. The role of the endotracheal tube cuff in microaspiration. *Heart Lung*. 2012;41:167.
30. Browne JA, et al. Pursuing excellence: development of an oral hygiene protocol for mechanically ventilated patients. *Crit Care Nurs Q*. 2011;34:25.
31. Muscedere J, et al. Comprehensive evidence-based clinical practice guidelines for ventilatory-associated pneumonia: prevention. *J Crit Care*. 2008;23:126.
32. American Association for Respiratory Care. AARC Clinical Practice Guidelines. Endotracheal suctioning of mechanically ventilated patients with artificial airways 2010. *Respir Care*. 2010;55:758.
33. Pedersen CM, et al. Endotracheal suctioning of the adult intubated patient–what is the evidence. *Intensive Crit Care Nurs*. 2009;25:21.
34. Grap MJ, et al. Endotracheal suctioning: ventilator vs. manual delivery of hyperoxygenation breaths. *Am J Crit Care*. 1996;5:192.
35. Stone KS. Ventilator versus manual resuscitation bag as the method of delivering hyperoxygenation before endotracheal suctioning. *AACN Clin Issues Crit Care Nurs*. 1990;1:289.
36. Czarnik RE, et al. Differential effects of continuous versus intermittent suction on tracheal tissue. *Heart Lung*. 1991;20:144.
37. Raymond SJ. Normal saline instillation before suctioning: helpful or harmful? A review of the literature. *Am J Crit Care*. 1995;4:267.
38. Kinloch D. Instillation of normal saline during endotracheal suctioning: effects on mixed venous oxygen saturation. *Am J Crit Care*. 1999;8:231.
39. Hagler DA, Traver GA. Endotracheal saline and suction catheters: sources of lower airway contamination. *Am J Crit Care*. 1994;3:444.
40. Jelic S, Cunningham JA, Factor P. Clinical review: airway hygiene in the intensive care unit. *Crit Care*. 2008;12:209.
41. Dave MH, et al. Massive aspiration past the tracheal tube cuff caused by closed trachael suction system. *J Intensive Care Med*. 2011;26:326.
42. Jenabzadeh NE, Chlan L. A nurse's experience being intubated and receiving mechanical ventilation. *Crit Care Nurse*. 2011;31(6):51.
43. Grossbach I, et al. Promoting effective communication for patients receiving mechanical ventilation. *Crit Care Nurse*. 2011;31:46.
44. Scherzer R. Subglottic secretion aspiration in the prevention of ventilator-associated pneumonia. *Dimens Crit Care Nurs*. 2010;29:276.
45. Stonecypher K. Ventilator-associated pneumonia: the importance of oral care in intubated adults. *Crit Care Nurs Q*. 2010;33:339.
46. Binkley C, et al. Survey of oral care practices in U.S. intensive care units. *Am J Infect Control*. 2004;32:161.
47. Garcia R. A review of the possible role of oral and dental colonization on the occurrence of health-care associated pneumonia: underappreciated risk and a call for interventions. *Am J Infect Control*. 2005;33:527.
48. Roberts N, Moule P. Chlorhexidine and tooth-brushing as prevention strategies in reducing ventilator-associated pneumonia. *Nurs Crit Care*. 2011;16:295.

49. Chlebicki MP, Safdar N. Topical chlorhexidine for prevention of ventilator-associated pneumonia: a meta-analysis. *Crit Care Med.* 2007;35(2):595.

50. Grap JM, et al. Early, single chlorhexidine application reduces ventilator-associated pneumonia in trauma patients. *Heart Lung.* 2011;40:e115.

51. Kracz M, et al. State-of-the-art mechanical ventilation. *J Cardiothorac Vasc Anesth.* 2012;26:486.

52. Archambault PM, St-Onge M. Invasive and noninvasive ventilation in the emergency department. *Emeg Med Clin N Am.* 2012;30:421.

53. Chatburn RL, Volsko TA. Mechanical ventilators. In: Kacmarek RM, et al, eds. *Egan's Fundamentals of Respiratory Care.* 10th ed. St. Louis: Mosby; 2013.

54. Cairo JM. *Pilbeam's Mechanical Ventilation: Physiological and Clinical Applications.* 5th ed. St. Louis: Elsevier; 2012.

55. MacIntyre NR, Branson RD. *Mechanical Ventilation.* 2nd ed. St. Louis: Saunders; 2009.

56. Kacmarek RM. Initiating and adjusting invasive ventilatory support. In: Kacmarek RM, et al, eds. *Egan's Fundamentals of Respiratory Care.* 10th ed. St. Louis: Mosby; 2013.

57. Gattinoni L, et al. Ventilator-induced lung injury: the anatomical and physiological framework. *Crit Care Med.* 2010;38:S539.

58. Sarge T, Talmor D. Targeting transpulmonary pressure to prevent ventilator induced lung injury. *Minerva Anestesiol.* 2009;75:293.

59. Wahla AS, Khan FZ. Development of massive pneumopericardium after intubation and positive pressure ventilation. *J Coll Physicians Surg Pak.* 2012;22:401.

60. Sarge T, Talmor D. Transpulmonary pressure: its role in preventing ventilator-induced lung injury. *Minerva Anestesiol.* 2008;74:335.

61. Oeckler RA, Hubmayr RD. Cell wounding and repair in ventilator injured lungs. *Respir Physiol Neurobiol.* 2008;163:44.

62. Frazier SK. Cardiovascular effects of mechanical ventilation and weaning. *Nurs Clin North Am.* 2008;43:1.

63. Unroe M, MacIntyre N. Evolving approaches to assessing and monitoring patient-ventilator interactions. *Curr Opin Crit Care.* 2010;16:261.

64. Haas CF, Bauser KA. Advanced ventilator modes and techniques. *Crit Care Nurs Q.* 2012;35:27.

65. Grossbach I, et al. Overview of mechanical ventilator support and management of patient- and ventilator-related responses. *Crit Care Nurse.* 2011;31(3):30.

66. Rebmann T, Green LR. Preventing ventilator-associated pneumonia: An executive summary of the Association for Professionals in Infection Control and Epidemiology, Inc, Elimination Guide. *Am J Infect Control.* 2010;38:647.

67. Kieninger AN, Lipsett PA. Hospital-acquired pneumonia: pathophysiology, diagnosis, and treatment. *Surg Clin N Am.* 2009;89:439.

68. *Institute for Healthcare Improvement.* Implement the IHI ventilator bundle. http://www.ihi.org/knowledge/pages/changes/implementtheventilatorbundle.aspx. 2012. Accessed July 29, 2012.

69. Johnson KL, Meyenburg T. Physiological rationale and current evidence for therapeutic positioning of critically ill patients. *AACN Adv Crit Care.* 2009;20:228.

70. Niël-Weise B, et al. An evidenc-based recommendation on bed head elevation for mechanically ventilated patients. *Crit Care.* 2011;15:R111.

71. Berry E, Zecca H. Daily interruptions of sedation: a clinical approach to improve outcomes in critically ill patients. *Crit Care Nurse.* 2012;32(1):43.

72. Ramirez P, et al. Measures to prevent nosocomial infections during mechanical ventilation. *Curr Opin Crit Care.* 2012;18:86.

73. Lorente L, et al. Influence of an endotracheal tube with polyurethane cuff and subglottic secretion drainage on pneumonia. *Am J Respir Crit Care Med.* 2007;176:1079.

74. Blot S, et al. What is new in the prevention of ventilator-associated pneumonia? *Curr Opin Pulm Med.* 2011;17:155.

75. Kollef MH, et al. Silver-coated endotracheal tubes and incidence of ventilator-associated pneumonia: the NASCENT randomized trial. *JAMA.* 2008;300:805.

76. Kacmarek RM. Discontinuing ventilatory support. In: Kacmarek RM, et al, eds. *Egan's Fundamentals of Respiratory Care.* 10th ed. St. Louis: Mosby; 2013.

77. MacIntyre N. Discontinuing mechanical ventilatory support. *Chest.* 2007;132:1049.

78. Robertson TE, et al. Improved extubation rates and earlier liberation from mechanical ventilation with implementation of a daily spontaneous-breathing trial protocol. *J Am Coll Surg.* 2008;206:489.

79. Burns SM. Weaning from mechanical ventilation. In: Burns SM, ed. *AACN Protocols for Practice: Care of the Mechanically Ventilated Patient.* 2nd ed. Sudbury, MA: Jones and Bartlett; 2007.

80. Siner JM, Manthous CA. Liberation from mechanical ventilation: what monitoring matters? *Crit Care Clin.* 2007;23:613.

81. Caroleo S, et al. Weaning from mechanical ventilation: an open issue. *Minerva Anestesiol.* 2007;73:417.

82. Blackwood B, et al. Use of weaning protocols for reducing duration of mechanical ventilation in critically ill adult patients: Cochrane systematic review and meta-analysis. *BMJ.* 2011;342:c7237.

83. Bekos V, Marini JJ. Monitoring the mechanically ventilated patient. *Crit Care Clin.* 2007;23:575.

84. Tracy MF, Chlan L. Nonpharmacological interventions to management common symptoms in patient receiving mechanical ventilation. *Crit Care Nurse.* 2011;31(3):19.

85. Balas MC, et al. Critical care nurse's role in implementing the "ABCDE Bundle" into practice. *Crit Care Nurse.* 2012;32(2):35.

86. McNeill GBS, Glossop AJ. Clinical applications of non-invasive ventilation in critical care. *Cont Edu Anaesth Crit Care & Pain.* 2012;12:33.

87. Holanda MA, et al. Influence of total face, facial and nasal masks on short-term adverse effects during noninvasive ventilation. *J Bras Pneumol.* 2009;35:164.

88. Williams PF. Noninvasive ventilation. In: Kacmarek RM, et al, eds. *Egan's Fundamentals of Respiratory Care.* 10th ed. St. Louis: Mosby; 2013.

89. Pierce LNB. Invasive and noninvasive modes and methods of mechanical ventilation. In: Burns SM, ed. *AACN Protocols for Practice: Care of the Mechanically Ventilated Patient.* 2nd ed. Sudbury, MA: Jones and Bartlett; 2007.

90. Dirkes S, et al. Prone positioning: is it safe and effective? *Crit Care Nurs Q.* 2012;35:64.

91. Alsaghir AH, Martin CM. Effect of prone positioning in patients with acute respiratory distress syndrome: a meta-analysis. *Crit Care Med.* 2008;36:603.

92. Dickinson S, et al. Prone positioning therapy in ARDS. *Crit Care Clin.* 2011;27:511.

93. Wright AD, Flynn M. Using the prone position for ventilated patients with respiratory failure: a review. *Nurs Crit Care.* 2011;16:19.

94. Goldhill DR, et al. Rotational bed therapy to prevent and treat respiratory complications: a review and meta-analysis. *Am J Crit Care.* 2007;16:50.

95. Stiller K. Physiotherapy in intensive care: towards an evidence-based practice. *Chest.* 2000;118:1801.

96. Ranee M. Kinetic therapy positively influences oxygenation in patients with ALI/ARDS. *Nurs Crit Care.* 2005;10:35.

97. Ahrens T, et al. Effect of kinetic therapy on pulmonary complications. *Am J Crit Care.* 2004;13:376.

98. Collard HR. Prevention of ventilator-associated pneumonia: an evidence-based systematic review. *Ann Intern Med.* 2003;138:494.

99. Powers J, Daniels D. Turning points: implementing kinetic therapy in the ICU. *Nurs Manage.* 2004;35:1.

100. Russell T, Logsdon A. Pressure ulcers and lateral rotation beds: a case study. *J Wound Ostomy Continence Nurs.* 2003;30:143.

101. Blanchard B. Thoracic surgery. In: Rothrock JC, McEwen DR, eds. *Alexander's Care of the Patient in Surgery.* 14th ed. St. Louis: Elsevier; 2011.

102. Banki F. Pulmonary assessment for general thoracic surgery. *Surg Clin N Am.* 2010;90:969.

103. Sweitzer BJ, Smetana GW. Identification and evaluation of the patient with lung disease. *Med Clin N Am.* 2009;93:1017.

104. von Groote-Bidlingmaier F, et al. Functional evaluation before lung resection. *Clin Chest Med.* 2011;32:773.

105. Della Rocca G, Coccia C. Ventilatory management of one-lung ventilation. *Minerva Anestesiol.* 2011;77:534.

106. Sachdev G, Napolitano LM. Postoperative pulmonary complications: pneumonia and acute respiratory failure. *Surg Clin N Am.* 2012;92:321.

107. Shekar K, et al. Bronchopleural fistula: an update for intensivists. *J Crit Care.* 2010;25:47.

108. Kopec SE, et al. The postpneumonectomy state. *Chest.* 1998;114:1158.

109. Brenner Z, Addona C. Caring for the pneumonectomy patient: challenges and changes. *Crit Care Nurse.* 1995;15(5):65.

110. Hirsch CA. Airway clearance therapy. In: Kacmarek RM, et al, eds. *Egan's Fundamentals of Respiratory Care.* 10th ed. St. Louis: Mosby; 2013.

111. Cerfolio RJ. Advances in thoracostomy tube management. *Surg Clin North Am.* 2002;82:833.

112. Grimes GC, et al. Medications for COPD: a review of effectiveness. *Am Fam Physician.* 2007;76:1141.

113. Gardenhire DS. Airway pharmacology. In: Kacmarek RM, et al, eds. *Egan's Fundamentals of Respiratory Care.* 10th ed. St. Louis: Mosby; 2013.

114. Hanania NA, Sharafkhaneh A. Update on the pharmacologic therapy for chronic obstructive pulmonary disease. *Clin Chest Med.* 2007;28:589.

115. Bennett S, Hurford WE. When should sedation or neuromuscular blockade be used during mechanical ventilation? *Respir Care.* 2011;56:168.

116. Honiden S, Siegel MD. Analytic reviews: managing the agitated patient in the ICU: sedation, analgesia, and neuromuscular blockade. *J Intensive Care Med.* 2010;25:187.

117. Luer J. Sedation and neuromuscular blockade in mechanically ventilated patients. In: Burns SM, ed. *AACN Protocols for Practice: Care of the Mechanically Ventilated Patient.* 2nd ed. Sudbury, MA: Jones & Bartlett; 2007.

118. Loyola R, Dreher HM. Management of pharmacologically induced neuromuscular blockade using peripheral nerve stimulation. *Dimens Crit Care Nurs.* 2003;22:157.

Neurologic Anatomy and Physiology

Kathleen M. Stacy

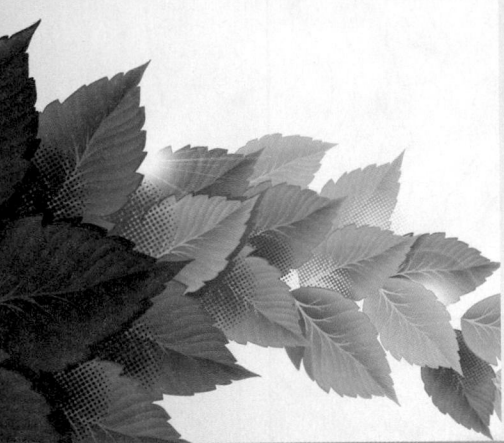

The nervous system is the "executive suite" of the human body. It directs all other systems and provides the unique ability for thought, emotion, understanding of complex information, and integration of numerous stimuli. As the recipient of all sensory information for analysis, the nervous system generates intellectual and motor responses aimed at maintaining the integrity of life structures. Critical care nurses must attain a basic understanding of the anatomy and physiology of this complex system because it serves as the basis for innervation and proper functioning of all other systems. This chapter reviews the anatomic divisions and functions of the central nervous system (CNS), including the cellular microstructure, protective encasement, networked functions, and mechanisms aimed at maintenance of structural and physiologic integrity. The cranial nerves, a component of the peripheral nervous system (PNS), are presented in tabular form.

DIVISIONS OF THE NERVOUS SYSTEM

The nervous system is the most highly organized system of the body, with all of its parts functioning as an inseparable unit. This system is usually classified by anatomic function.

Anatomic Divisions

The CNS is made up of the brain and the spinal cord. The PNS comprises 12 pairs of cranial nerves, 31 pairs of spinal nerves, and all other nerves serving a variety of functions throughout the body.[1,2]

Physiologic Divisions

The somatic, or voluntary, nervous system is composed of fibers that connect the CNS with structures of the skeletal muscles and the skin. The autonomic, or involuntary, nervous system is composed of fibers that connect the CNS with smooth muscle, cardiac muscle, internal organs, and glands. It includes sympathetic and parasympathetic branches.[1,2]

Most activities of the nervous system originate from sensory receptors such as visual, auditory, or tactile receptors. This sensory information is transmitted to the CNS by afferent fibers (sensory fibers). Efferent fibers (motor fibers) transmit the CNS response to the periphery to produce a motor response such as contraction of skeletal muscles, contraction of the smooth muscles of organs, or secretion by endocrine glands. To better understand the macrostructure and functions of the nervous system, it helps to study the microstructure, or the cellular level.[1-4]

MICROSTRUCTURE OF THE NERVOUS SYSTEM

Two types of cells make up the nervous system: 1) neurons and 2) neuroglia. Neurons are the cells primarily charged with the functional work of the nervous system, including receipt of information, integration, and transmission or conduction of nerve impulses to recipient cells. Neuroglial cells serve as the support infrastructure of the nervous system, providing protection and a structural foundation for neurons and participating in neuronal repair.[1-4]

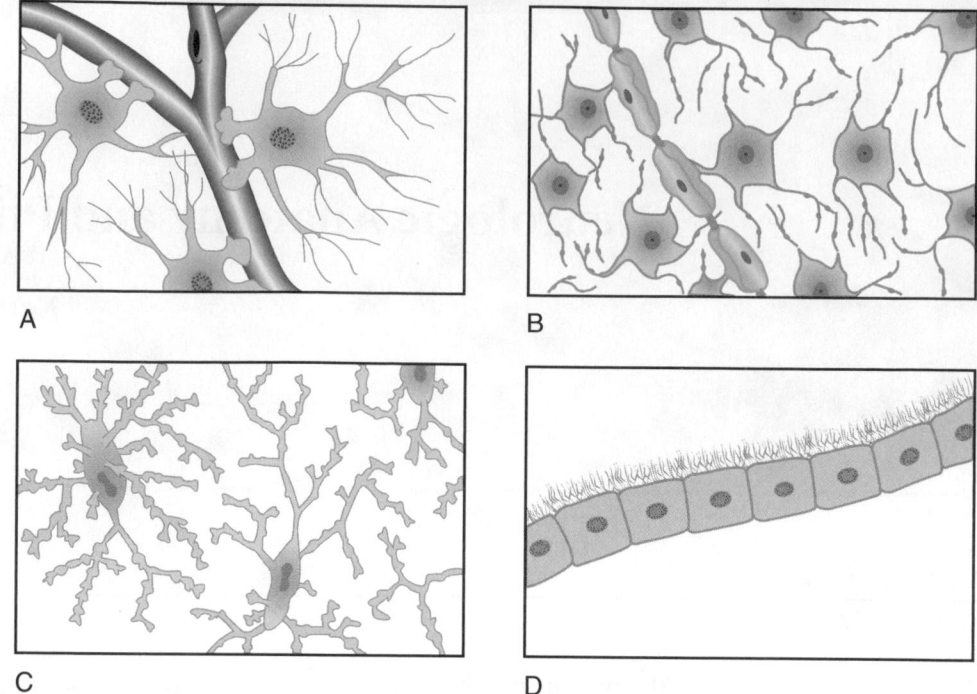

FIGURE 22-1 Neuroglial Cells. *A,* Astrocytes along the capillary. *B,* Oligodendrocytes along the nerves. *C,* Microglia (phagocytes). *D,* Ependymal cells form a sheet that lines fluid cavities in the brain. (From Black JM, Hawks JH. *Medical-Surgical Nursing: Clinical Management for Positive Outcomes.* 8th ed. Philadelphia: Saunders; 2009.)

TABLE 22-1	TYPES OF NEUROGLIAL CELLS
CELL TYPE	**FUNCTION**
Astroglia (astrocyte)	Supplies nutrients to neuron structure and to support framework for neurons and capillaries; forms part of the blood–brain barrier
Oligodendroglia	Forms the myelin sheath in the central nervous system
Ependyma	Lines the ventricular system; forms the choroid plexus, which produces cerebrospinal fluid
Microglia	Occurs mainly in the white matter; phagocytizes waste products from injured neurons

Neuroglia

In the nervous system, 6 to 10 times more neuroglial cells exist than do neurons. Neuroglial cells consist of four types: 1) *astroglia (astrocytes),* 2) *oligodendroglia,* 3) *ependyma,* and 4) *microglia* (Fig. 22-1). These cells provide the neuron with structural support, nourishment, and protection (Table 22-1).[1-4] They retain the ability to replicate, but they can replicate abnormally and therefore are the primary source of CNS neoplasms.[3,4]

Neurons

Neurons are the basic functional unit within the CNS, and they are charged with the highly specialized task of data integration and signal transmission. The CNS is made up of more than 10 billion neurons.[1,2] The cellular appearance of neurons varies, but each cell contains three basic components: 1) the cell body, 2) dendrites, and 3) an axon (Fig. 22-2). Neurons are structurally classified as *unipolar,* a cell body with one process that divides into a central branch (one axon) and a peripheral branch (one dendrite); as *bipolar,* a cell body with two processes (one axon and one dendrite); or *multipolar,* a cell body with one axon and several dendrites. The cell body (soma) controls the metabolic activity of the neuron and contains the organelles such as the nucleus, mitochondria, endoplasmic reticulum, Golgi apparatus, and liposomes, which are necessary for cellular metabolism and maintenance.[1-3] Compared with other body cells, the neuron's protein-embedded membrane with its phospholipid bilayer is unique, consisting of specialized pores that work as ion-specific channels or pumps to promote passage of ions through an otherwise impermeable plasma membrane.[4]

The neuronal cell body is the life support unit of the neuron. The metabolic demands of these specialized units necessitate uninterrupted perfusion with glucose and oxygen to maintain neuronal life and optimal functioning. Until recently, it was believed that CNS neuronal repair was impossible, but research has validated that neurons are more *plastic* than was previously thought, although rates of repair (plasticity) or restoration of neuronal function are driven by factors that remain largely unknown.[5-7] Within the brain and the spinal cord, neuronal cell bodies make up regions of gray matter. Outside the CNS, *ganglia* are cell bodies within the PNS that reside near and work closely with CNS neurons.[1-4]

Dendrites form the receptive component of the neuron; they are branched fibers extending only a short distance from the cell body. Each neuron may have several dendrites, which function as impulse receivers for the cell body.[1,2,7] The axon is the part of the neuron concerned with transmission of impulses away from the cell body to other neurons, muscle cells, endocrine glands, or some other effector organ.[8] Neurons contain only one axon, whose length may be microscopic or, in some cases, may extend up to 4 feet. Some axons are protected by a

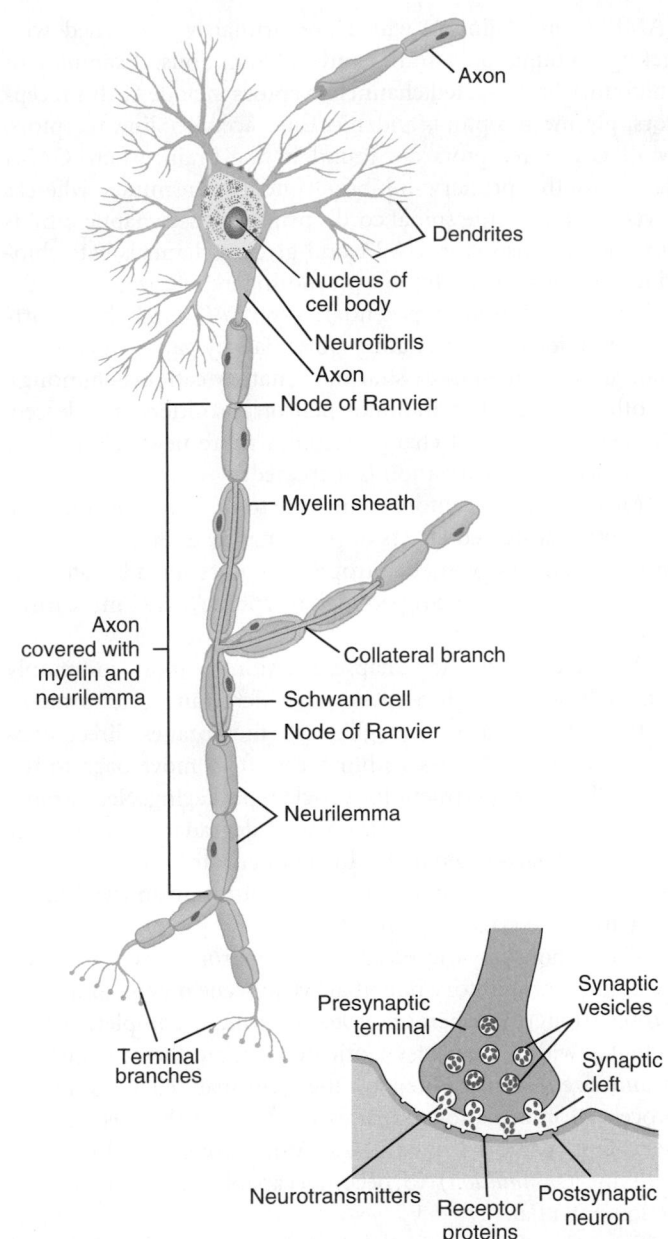

FIGURE 22-2 A neuron (the basic element of the nervous system) and a chemical synapse. (From Black JM, Hawks JH. *Medical-Surgical Nursing: Clinical Management for Positive Outcomes.* 8th ed. Philadelphia: Saunders; 2009.)

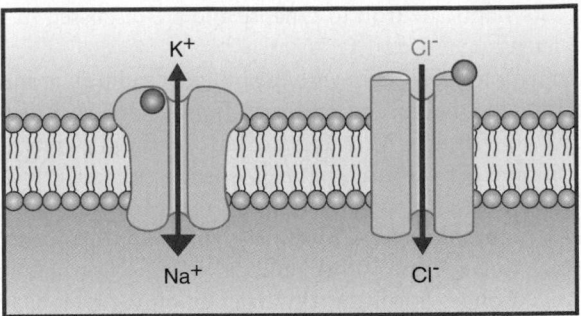

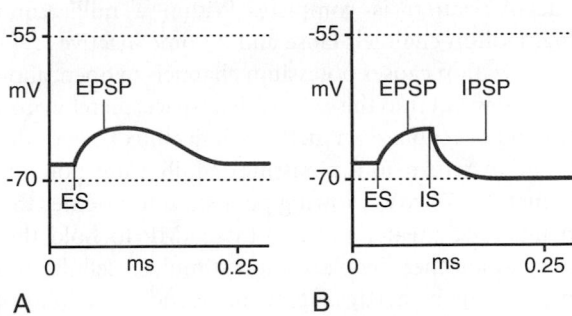

FIGURE 22-3 *A,* A transmitter-gated excitatory ionotropic receptor. Binding of the transmitter (red, in this example representing glutamate) has opened the pore of a "mixed" Na+–K+ cation channel. A large influx of sodium ions has depolarized the membrane, as shown by the excitatory postsynaptic potential (EPSP). *B,* A transmitter-gated inhibitory ionotropic receptor. Binding of the transmitter (*blue,* representing GABAA) has opened the pore of a chloride channel. Inward chloride conductance has been increased, and the inhibitory postsynaptic potential (IPSP) restores the membrane potential to its resting state. Neuronal voltage-gated channel selectivity. K^+, Potassium ion; Na^+, sodium ion. (From Fitzgerald MJT, et al. *Clinical Neuroanatomy and Neuroscience.* 5th ed. Philadelphia: Saunders; 2007.)

myelin sheath, a white phospholipid complex laid down by Schwann cells in the PNS and by oligodendroglia in the CNS. Myelin sheathes protect neuronal axons and provide insulation for the conduction of nerve impulses.[1,2,9] Fibers enclosed in the sheath are called *myelinated fibers;* those not enclosed are called *unmyelinated fibers.* The white matter of the CNS is composed of myelinated fiber tracts.[1,2]

Myelinated fibers use a process called *saltatory conduction* to support rapid axonal transmission of nerve impulses.[3,4,9] Structurally, axons participating in this form of impulse transmission are laid out with a noncontinuous myelin cover, interrupted with 2 micrometer bare segments called the *nodes of Ranvier.* These nodes are packed with sodium channels, making them extremely sensitive to membrane depolarization. Because segments of the axon covered by myelin are impervious to sodium influx, impulse transmission is pulled down the length of the

axon to the next node of Ranvier. Saltatory conduction increases transmission velocity up to 100-fold, allowing transmission at rates as high as 120 meters per second (m/s).[1,4]

Neuronal function is driven by depolarization–repolarization cycles, similar to that described for cardiac physiology (see Chapter 12), but what makes the nervous system so exceptional is its ability to undergo the depolarization–repolarization cycle up to 1000 times per second to ensure optimal receipt, integration, and transmission of information throughout the body.[3] The movement of ions across the neuronal membrane generates electrical action potentials (Fig. 22-3). Neuronal resting membrane potential (RMP) is –65 millivolts (mV), approximating the equilibrium potential for potassium; on depolarization, sodium channels open, shifting the equilibrium potential in the positive direction.[1,3,4]

Mechanisms for ionic movement involve two types of neuronal channels: 1) *voltage-gated* and 2) *ligand-gated.* Many pharmaceutical and therapeutic agents currently in use or undergoing testing manipulate these ionic transport mechanisms. Voltage-gated channels become activated with changes in transmembrane electrical potential, promoting sodium and calcium influx and potassium efflux. These channels are the primary drivers of cellular action potentials.[1,2] Ligand-gated channels are primarily concerned with mitigating the response of a postsynaptic neuron to synapse and are discussed in more detail later.[1,2]

Action potentials begin with the influx of sodium, producing a focal zone of membrane depolarization at some level between −55 mV to −35 mV. After this critical threshold is reached, a large number of sodium channels open, resulting in fast and massive localized depolarization of the plasma membrane. Rapid sodium influx (upstroke phase) increases the membrane potential to between 70 mV and 90 mV. As the membrane potential changes locally, it stimulates adjoining regions in the neuron to begin depolarization in a self-propagating fashion until depolarization is complete. Within a millisecond of opening, sodium channels close and become inactive.[1-4]

Depolarization causes potassium channels to open, allowing this ion to flow out into the extracellular space, thereby promoting the onset of repolarization. Potassium efflux triggers the cell membrane to return to a potassium equilibrium potential of approximately −75 mV, allowing potassium to re-enter the cell but maintaining greater polarity than RMP to hold the cell refractory to another depolarization stimulus. Cellular pumps that depend on a steady supply of adenosine triphosphate (ATP) are also activated to remove sodium and restore the −65 mV RMP, allowing the cycle to begin anew.[1-4]

After an action potential reaches the axon terminal, it initiates a cascade of events that promote interneuronal communication, or *synapse*. Two types of synapse exist: 1) electrical and 2) chemical. In an electrical synapse, gap junctions made up of narrow (3.5-nm) bridges allow cytoplasm and intracellular metabolites to pass in an essentially continuous fashion between neurons, facilitating impulse conduction from one neuron to the next.[1,2,4] In a chemical synapse, which is involved in most synaptic events, no physical bridge exists between neurons. Instead, a large synaptic cleft of 20 to 40 nanometers (nm) prevents direct action potential transmission from one neuron to another. When the wave of depolarization reaches the presynaptic terminal, it signals the release of neurotransmitters into the synaptic cleft.[1,2]

The two classifications of neurotransmitters are: 1) small-molecule transmitters and 2) neuroactive peptides. Examples of small-molecule transmitters include acetylcholine, dopamine, norepinephrine, epinephrine, serotonin, histamine, gamma-aminobutyric acid (GABA), glycine, and glutamate. Neuroactive peptides include such substances as pituitary peptides, hypothalamic-releasing hormones, and neurohypophyseal hormones. This chapter is primarily concerned with the small-molecule transmitters, which are stored in vesicles within the axon terminal and released into the synapse through a process called *exocytosis*. Exocytosis is stimulated by arrival of the action potential in the axon terminal and results in release of neurotransmitters into the synaptic cleft, where these molecules rapidly diffuse to interact with postsynaptic receptors.[1,2,4]

Ligand-gated channels are activated by binding of ligand agonists to receptors on the postsynaptic neuron. Ions passing through ligand-gated channels promote an excitatory or inhibitory response within postsynaptic neurons. Examples of excitatory ligand-gated channel receptors include the inotropic glutamate receptors (N-methyl-D-aspartate [NMDA], alpha-amino-3-hydroxyl-5-methyl-4-isoxazolepropionic acid [AMPA], and kainite), which are primarily concerned with gating sodium, potassium, and calcium ions. Examples of inhibitory ligand-gated channel receptors include GABA receptors, glycine receptors, and nicotinic acetylcholine receptors. Most GABA receptors are found in the brain, where GABA serves as the primary inhibitory neurotransmitter, whereas glycine serves as the spinal cord's primary postsynaptic inhibitory neurotransmitter. GABA and glycine channels gate chloride ions, which inhibit by promoting repolarization to the chloride equilibrium potential (−60 mV) and by short-circuiting incoming excitatory potentials by gating anions and clamping the membrane shut to excitatory cations (shunting). In other words, when inhibitor neurotransmitters are released, the neuron's internal charge becomes more negative, and the resistance to depolarization is increased.[1]

Metabotropic receptors contribute to impulse transmission, promoting sustained effects of postsynaptic excitation or inhibition. Examples of metabotropic receptors include catecholamine receptors, neuropeptide receptors, and muscarinic receptors.[1,4]

Termination of the synapse reaction is most commonly accomplished through reuptake, in which transporter proteins embedded in neuron and glial cell membranes direct neurotransmitter molecules within the cleft to move back to the intracellular compartment for vesicle repackaging. Neurotransmitters may also go through enzyme degradation, with their component parts taken up for further neurotransmitter synthesis and storage. Ultimately, remaining neurotransmitter diffuses away from the synaptic cleft.[1,2,4]

The response in the postsynaptic neuron to synapse is an excitatory or inhibitory potential. Membrane potentials are not strong enough by themselves to generate a complete action potential within the postsynaptic neuron, but they are, instead, summarized or integrated by the neuronal cell body in the process of information transmission.[9] When the postsynaptic neuron is bombarded with excitatory potentials, they may combine (*summation*) to become capable of stimulating an action potential.[1-4]

Examples of disease-induced or chemically-induced mechanisms that alter neuronal transmission are provided in Figure 22-4.

CENTRAL NERVOUS SYSTEM

The CNS consists of the brain and the spinal cord. Serving as the control unit for all body systems, the remarkably delicate CNS requires significant protection to preserve normal function. This section addresses the anatomy and physiology of the brain and the spinal cord, supporting the critical care nurse's understanding of pathophysiologic changes that contribute to clinical examination findings.

Cranial Protective Mechanisms
Bony Structures
The outermost protective measures underneath the integument are the bony structures that encase the CNS. The skull, or cranium, surrounds the brain and is composed of eight flat, irregular bones fused at sutures during early childhood

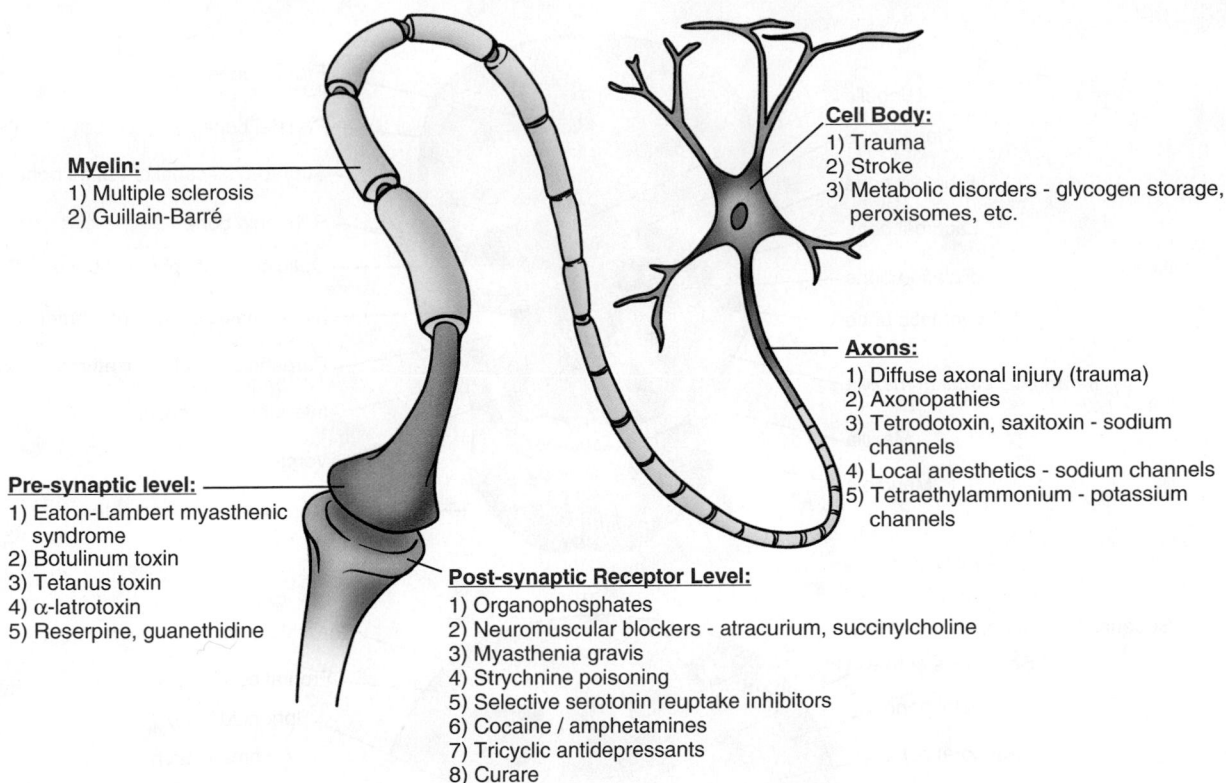

Myelin:
1) Multiple sclerosis
2) Guillain-Barré

Cell Body:
1) Trauma
2) Stroke
3) Metabolic disorders - glycogen storage, peroxisomes, etc.

Axons:
1) Diffuse axonal injury (trauma)
2) Axonopathies
3) Tetrodotoxin, saxitoxin - sodium channels
4) Local anesthetics - sodium channels
5) Tetraethylammonium - potassium channels

Pre-synaptic level:
1) Eaton-Lambert myasthenic syndrome
2) Botulinum toxin
3) Tetanus toxin
4) α-latrotoxin
5) Reserpine, guanethidine

Post-synaptic Receptor Level:
1) Organophosphates
2) Neuromuscular blockers - atracurium, succinylcholine
3) Myasthenia gravis
4) Strychnine poisoning
5) Selective serotonin reuptake inhibitors
6) Cocaine / amphetamines
7) Tricyclic antidepressants
8) Curare

FIGURE 22-4 Neuronal Pathophysiology. (Modified from Layon AJ, et al. *Textbook of Neurointensive Care.* Philadelphia: Sanders; 2004.)

(Fig. 22-5).[1,2] The skull protects the brain from direct force and superficial trauma, although excessive force may fracture the skull, destroying this protective mechanism and driving bony fragments into fragile brain tissue.[10]

If the skull is seen from the inside, the superior surfaces form a smooth inner wall, whereas the basilar skull contains ridges and folds with sharp edges.[1,2] Traumatic impact to the head often results in fracture of the basilar skull as a result of gravitational forces that displace energy in a downward fashion toward the skull base.

The cranium is a solid, nonexpanding bony vault with only one large opening at the base called the *foramen magnum*, through which the brainstem projects and connects to the spinal cord. Several other very small openings in the base of the skull allow entrance and exit of blood vessels and nerve fibers.[1,2]

Meninges

Directly beneath the skull lie the meninges, which form another source of protection for the CNS. The meninges consist of three layers: 1) the *dura mater*, 2) the *arachnoid mater*, and 3) the *pia mater* (Fig. 22-6).[1,2,11]

Dura Mater. The outermost layer of meninges directly beneath the skull is the dura mater. *Dura* is the Latin term for "tough," and true to its name, this layer is made up of fibrous tissue that is double-folded to support the CNS, nerves, and vascular structures.[1,3] Within the dura mater's double layers lie venous sinuses that collect blood from intracranial and meningeal veins for drainage into the internal jugular veins.[11]

Four extensions of the dura mater directly support and separate specific areas of the brain: 1) the falx cerebri, 2) the tentorium cerebelli, 3) the falx cerebelli, and 4) the diaphragma sellae. The falx cerebri divides the right and left hemispheres of the brain vertically through the longitudinal fissures extending from the frontal lobe to the occipital lobe. The tentorium cerebelli forms a tent between the occipital lobes and the cerebellum and separates the cerebral hemispheres from the brainstem and the cerebellum. Structures within the brain that are located above the tentorium are often referred to as *supratentorial*, whereas those located below the tentorium are referred to as *infratentorial* and make up the region of the brain called the *posterior fossa*. The falx cerebelli forms the division between the two lateral lobes of the cerebellum, and the diaphragma sellae forms a roof over the sella turcica, which houses the pituitary gland.[1,2]

The main blood supply for the dura mater is the middle meningeal artery. This artery lies on the surface of the dura in the epidural space and within grooves formed on the inside of the parietal bone. Traumatic disruption of the parietal bone may result in tearing of the middle meningeal artery and development of an epidural hematoma.[12] A potential space exists between the dura mater and the arachnoid mater. This area contains a large number of unsupported small veins that may become disrupted and torn when traumatic head injury occurs, leading to development of a subdural hematoma.[12]

Arachnoid Mater. The arachnoid membrane is a delicate, fragile membrane that loosely surrounds the brain. Fine threads of elastic tissue called *trabeculae* connect the arachnoid to the pia mater, creating a spongy, weblike structure called the *subarachnoid space*.[11] Cerebrospinal fluid (CSF) circulates freely in the subarachnoid space, which also contains the origins of the

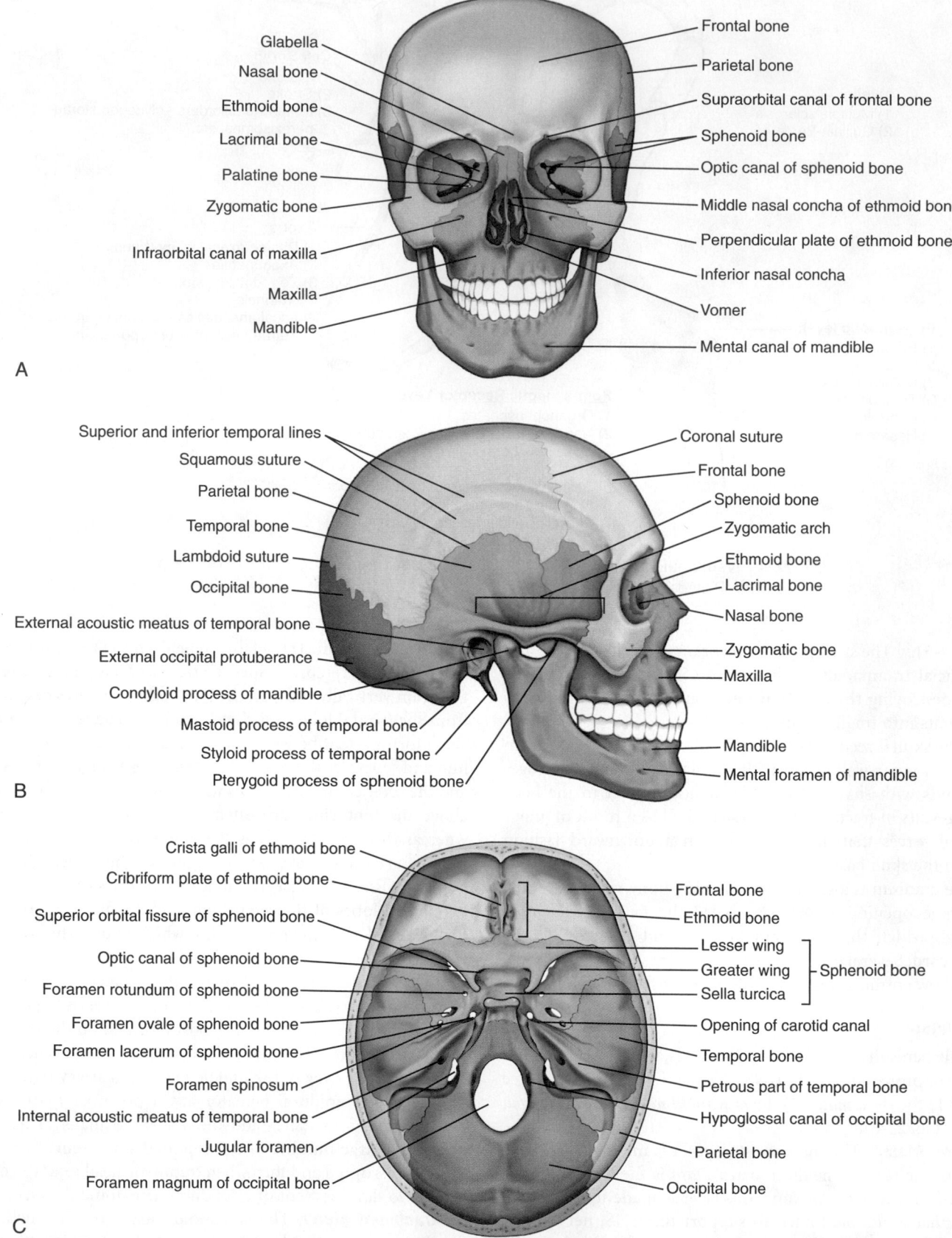

FIGURE 22-5 Skull. *A,* Anterior view. *B,* Skull viewed from the right side. *C,* Floor of the cranial cavity viewed from above. (From Patton KT, Thibodeau GF. *Anatomy and Physiology.* 8th ed. St. Louis: Mosby; 2013.)

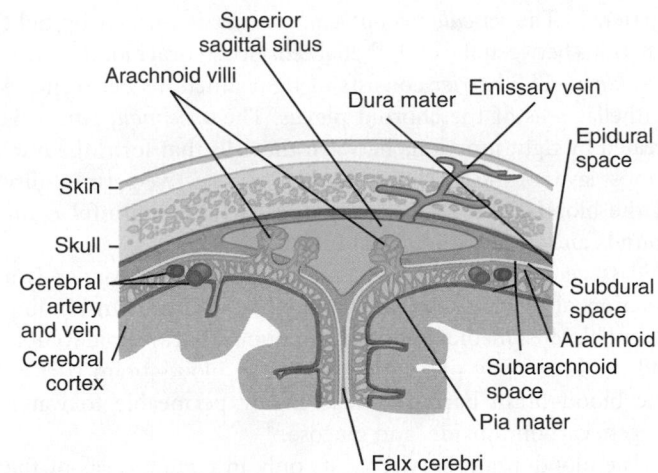

FIGURE 22-6 The meninges (coronal section through the superior sagittal sinus). (From Black JM, Hawks JH. *Medical-Surgical Nursing: Clinical Management for Positive Outcomes.* 8th ed. Philadelphia: Saunders; 2009.)

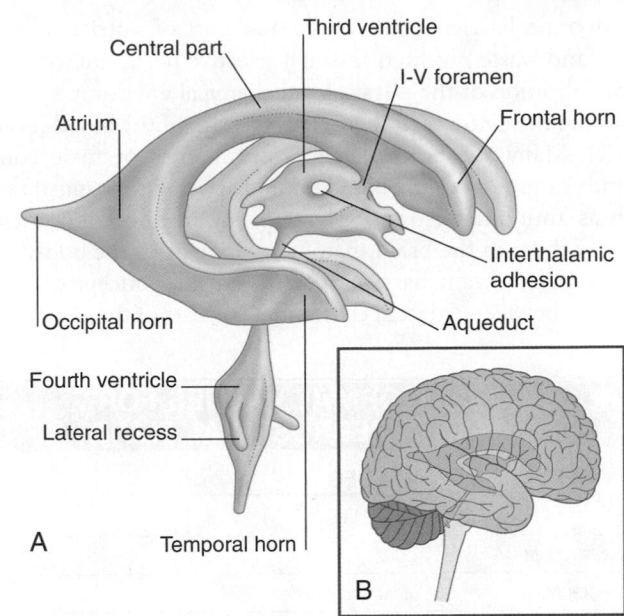

FIGURE 22-7 Ventricular System. *A,* Isolated cast. *B,* Ventricular system in situ. (From Fitzgerald MJT, et al. *Clinical Neuroanatomy and Neuroscience.* 5th ed. Philadelphia: Saunders; 2007.)

brain's large arteries where they enter the skull and differentiate into anterior and posterior circulatory branches.[1,2,13] Rupture of an artery within the subarachnoid space allows for blood to mix with CSF, producing a *subarachnoid hemorrhage.*[12]

At the base of the brain, widened areas of subarachnoid space form cisterns, or spaces, that are filled with CSF. The largest of these cisterns, the cisterna magna, lies between the medulla and the cerebellum, and it communicates with the fourth ventricle.[1,2]

Tufts of arachnoid membrane, called *arachnoid villi,* or granulations, project into the superior sagittal and transverse venous sinuses. Absorption of CSF by arachnoid villi allows its removal by the venous drainage system.[1,2,4] The delicate structure of the arachnoid villi places them at risk for obstruction by blood in subarachnoid hemorrhage, resulting in *obstructive hydrocephalus.*[14]

Pia Mater. The pia mater adheres directly to brain tissue. Rich in small blood vessels that supply a large volume of arterial blood to the CNS, this membrane closely follows all folds and convolutions of the brain's surface. Tufts or folds of the pia mater in the lateral, third, and fourth ventricles form a portion of the choroid plexus that is responsible for the production of CSF.[1,3]

Ventricular System

The *ventricular system* consists of four CSF-filled canals lined with ependymal cells, a type of neuroglial cell (Fig. 22-7). This system is made up of two large *lateral ventricles* that each lie within a hemisphere of the cerebral cortex. Extending from the frontal lobes to the occipital lobe, the lateral ventricles consist of a body, an atrium, and frontal, temporal, and occipital horns.[1-3,13] When cannulation of the ventricular system is required for intracranial pressure monitoring, CSF drainage, or placement of a CSF shunt, the frontal horn of the lateral ventricle on the nondominant side of the brain is most often selected.[15,16]

The foramen of Monro connects the two lateral ventricles with a central cavity, the *third ventricle.* Located directly above the midbrain, the walls of the third ventricle are formed by the

thalami. The *cerebral aqueduct* (aqueduct of Sylvius) is the canal between the third and *fourth ventricle,* which lies between the brainstem and the cerebellum. At the base of the fourth ventricle, two openings—the *foramen of Luschka* and the *foramen of Magendie*—open into the subarachnoid space.[1,2] Blockage of CSF flow occurring within the ventricular system obstructs the normal circulation of CSF, causing dilation of the ventricles, a condition called *obstructive hydrocephalus.*[14]

Cerebrospinal Fluid

CSF fills the ventricular system and surrounds the brain and spinal cord in the subarachnoid space. Protection of the CNS is further provided by CSF, which acts as a shock absorber when energy is displaced in traumatic injury. CSF is normally clear, colorless, and odorless. It is secreted by the choroid plexuses of the ventricular system, although small amounts are also synthesized by capillaries of the pia mater. Believed to be a filtrate of blood, CSF contains some unique properties that make its synthesis a mystery (Table 22-2).[1,2,13]

The production of CSF occurs at a rate of approximately 20 milliliters per hour (mL/hr), or 500 mL/day. With a circulating volume of 135 to 150 mL, CSF must be regularly resorbed to prevent development of hydrocephalus. Resorption through intact arachnoid villi is favored by increased hydrostatic pressure mechanics that maintain CSF volume within normal limits. The flow of CSF begins in the lateral ventricles, moves through the foramina of Monro into the third ventricle, moves through the cerebral aqueduct into the fourth ventricle, and moves out the foramen of Magendie and the foramina of Luschka into the subarachnoid space of the brain and spinal cord (Fig. 22-8).[1,2,3,13]

Blood–Brain Barrier

The blood–brain barrier is a physiologic mechanism that helps maintain the delicate metabolic balance in the CNS. The blood–brain barrier regulates the transport of nutrients, ions, water, and waste products through selective permeability.[1,2,17]

Stabilization of the physical and chemical environment surrounding the neurons of the CNS is the task of the blood–brain barrier. Many substances such as metabolites or toxic compounds cannot cross the blood–brain barrier. Other substances such as antibiotics cross slowly, resulting in lower concentrations of them in the brain than in other areas of the body.[17]

The blood–brain barrier operates on the concept of *tight junctions* between adjacent cells, and it consists of three separate

barriers.[1,3] The *vascular endothelial barrier* is formed by tight junctions between the endothelial cells of cerebral blood vessels. The *blood–CSF barrier* consists of tight junctions between the epithelial cells of the choroid plexus. The *arachnoid barrier* is created by tight junctions between the cells that form the outermost layer of the arachnoid mater. The selective permeability of the blood–brain barrier keeps out toxic or harmful compounds and protects neuronal function.[18]

Passage of substances across the blood–brain barrier is a function of particle size, lipid solubility, and protein-binding potential. Most medications or compounds that are lipid soluble and stable at body pH rapidly cross the blood–brain barrier. The blood–brain barrier is also highly permeable to water, oxygen, carbon dioxide, and glucose.[18]

The blood–brain barrier exists only in certain areas of the CNS. The areas in which it does not exist—the pineal region, the basal hypothalamus, and the floor of the fourth ventricle—require contact with plasma to sense changes in concentration of glucose and carbon dioxide and the changes in serum osmolality.[1] Initiation of feedback mechanisms by the hypothalamus in response to these changes regulates the internal environment of the remainder of the body.[4]

Of clinical significance, disruption or alteration of blood–brain barrier permeability occurs with injury to brain tissue from trauma, toxic insults, and ischemic injury. Brain irradiation also may alter the permeability of the blood–brain barrier, although intravenously administered chemotherapeutic agents

TABLE 22-2	NORMAL VALUES FOR CEREBROSPINAL FLUID
PROPERTY	**VALUES**
pH	7.35-7.45
Specific gravity	1.007
Appearance	Clear and colorless
Cells	0 white blood cells (WBCs)/mm³; 0 red blood cells (RBCs)/mm³; 0-10 lymphocytes/mm³
Glucose	50-75 mg/dL (two thirds of blood sugar value)
Protein	5-25 mg/dL
Volume	135-150 mL
Pressure	70-200 mm H₂O (lumbar puncture); 3-15 mm Hg (ventricular)

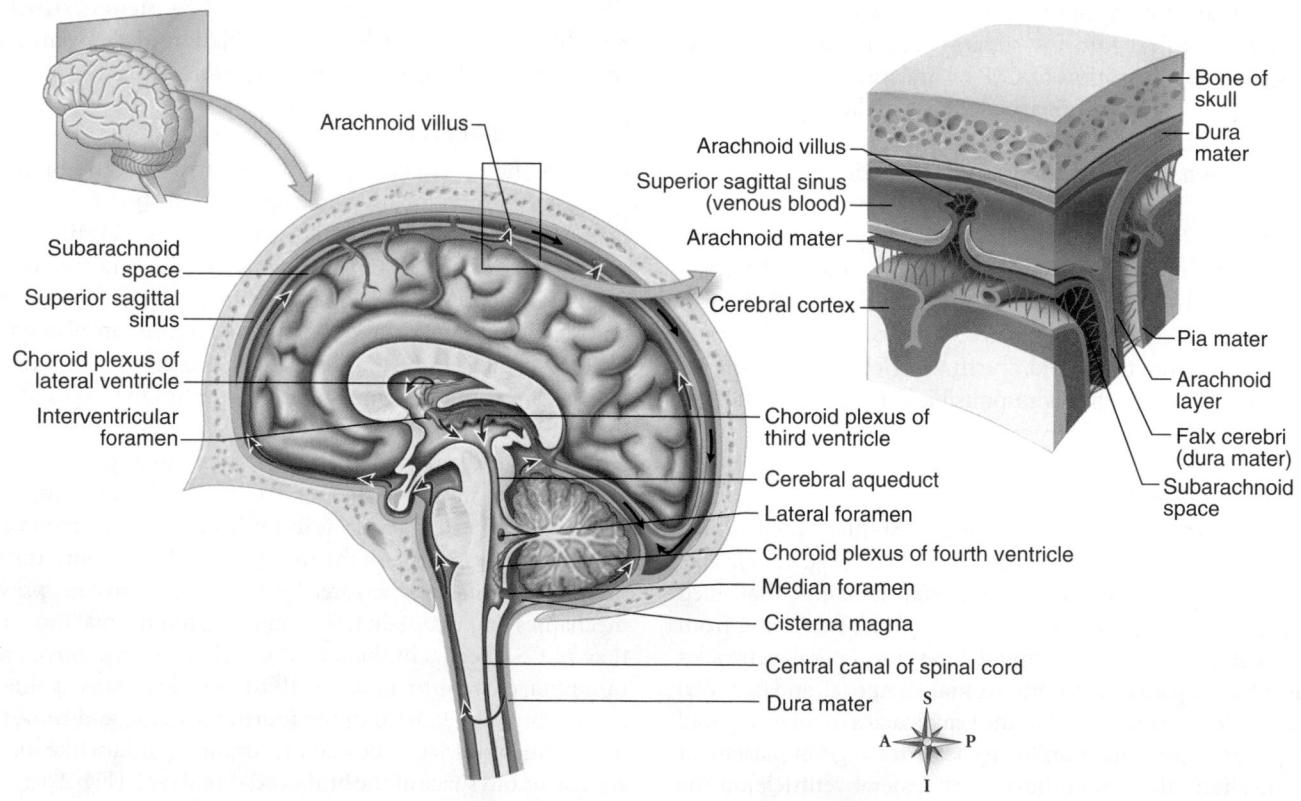

FIGURE 22-8 **Flow of Cerebrospinal Fluid.** The fluid produced by filtration of blood by the choroid plexus of each ventricle flows inferiorly through the lateral ventricles, interventricular foramen, third ventricle, cerebral aqueduct, fourth ventricle, and subarachnoid space and to blood. (From Patton KT, Thibodeau GF. *Anatomy and Physiology.* 8th ed. St. Louis: Mosby; 2013.)

have been shown to have little effect on blood–brain barrier permeability.[19]

Cerebrum

The cerebrum is the largest portion of the brain, comprising 80% of its weight. It is composed of two cerebral hemispheres (right and left), separated by the longitudinal fissure and connected at the base by the *corpus callosum* (Fig. 22-9B).[1,2,20]

The outermost aspect of the cerebrum is called the *cerebral cortex* and is made up of *gray matter*, consisting of neuronal cell bodies. Directly below the cerebral cortex lies *white matter*, consisting of myelinated axons, which communicate impulses from the cerebral cortex to other areas of the brain. White matter tracts consist of three types of fibers: 1) *commissural* (transverse), 2) *projection*, and 3) *association*.[1,2,20] Commissural fibers are tracts that communicate between the two cerebral hemispheres, and the corpus callosum is the largest commissural tract. Projection fibers communicate between the cerebral cortex and the lower regions of the brain and the spinal cord. Association fibers communicate between various regions of the same hemisphere.[1,2,20]

The cerebral hemispheres are divided into the *frontal, parietal, temporal,* and *occipital* lobes (see Fig. 22-9A). The *rhinencephalon* is often labeled the fifth lobe of the cerebral cortex. Lying deep inside the cerebrum and anatomically associated with the temporal lobe, the rhinencephalon is sometimes referred to as the *limbic lobe*.[1,2,20]

The primary functions of the cerebral cortex include sensory, motor, and intellectual (cognitive) functions, making this area of the brain vital to normal human functioning and providing capabilities that make humans unique as a species.[3,4,20] Brodmann's classification of cerebral cortical cytoarchitecture identifies more than 100 unique areas and provides a useful way to localize specific cortical functions within the brain (see Fig. 22-9C).[3] This section covers the areas within Brodmann's classification that are commonly assessed in relation to the development of specific neurologic pathology.

Frontal Lobe

The frontal lobe lies underneath the frontal bone of the skull and is separated posteriorly from the parietal lobe by the central sulcus (fissure of Rolando) and inferiorly from the temporal lobe by the lateral fissure (Sylvian fissure) (see Fig. 22-9A). The major functions of the frontal lobe are voluntary motor function, cognitive function (orientation, memory, insight, judgment, arithmetic, and abstraction), and expressive language (verbal and written).[1,2,20]

The prefrontal areas (see Fig. 22-9C), located just behind the frontal bone's distribution over the forehead, are concerned with cognition.[3,4] These areas work in concert with other areas of the brain to intellectually appraise and respond to environmental information or stimuli. They augment the intellect with socially trained emotional responses learned over the course of childhood and young adulthood, and they participate in triggering autonomic nervous system responses such as tachycardia in relation to situational needs.[3,4] The location of the prefrontal cortex makes it vulnerable to traumatic injury, often resulting in profound changes in cognitive capacity and social responses to environmental stimuli after brain injury.[21]

The motor strip of the frontal cortex is represented by Brodmann area 4 (see Fig. 22-9C) and consists of cell bodies for neurons associated with *voluntary (pyramidal) motor* functions. Because most voluntary motor tracts cross over to the opposite side as they descend through the brainstem, the right motor strip represents voluntary motor function for the left side of the body, and vice versa.[3,4] The motor *homunculus* (Fig. 22-10B) is a graphic representation of the distribution of voluntary motor function throughout area 4. Appearing as an upside-down man, the foot of the homunculus is illustrated on the superior medial aspects of the frontal lobes, with the knees, hips, trunk, and shoulders extending along the lateral surfaces and with the hands, thumb, head, face, and tongue represented in a lateral inferior distribution extending to the Sylvian fissure. The homunculus demonstrates larger body part size to denote areas with greater representation because of the amount of dexterity associated with the part's function. The large surface area of the trunk occupies a relatively small part of the motor strip, whereas smaller body areas such as the thumb or tongue, which involve a great deal of dexterity and fine motor movement, occupy a larger area of the motor strip.[3] Damage to the motor strip results in compromise of motor function on the opposite side of the body.[22]

Broca area (Brodmann areas 44 and 45) is located at the inferior frontal gyrus close to the motor strip's facial distribution (see Fig. 22-9C). Most commonly, Broca area is located on the left side of the frontal lobe, although it occasionally is located in the right frontal hemisphere. Broca area is responsible for expressive language, and it is used in the formation of verbal and written communication.[3,4,23] Damage occurring to this area results in disability ranging from difficulties with word finding to an expressive or nonfluent aphasia, in which verbal and written communication are significantly compromised, although verbal language reception and comprehension may remain intact.[22,23]

Parietal Lobe

The parietal lobe lies directly behind the frontal lobe on the opposite side of the central sulcus. The posterior border of the parietal lobe is the parieto-occipital fissure, which separates it from the occipital lobe (see Fig. 22-9A). The parietal lobes are primarily concerned with sensory functions, including integration of sensory information; awareness of body parts; interpretation of touch, pressure, and pain; and recognition of object size, shape, and texture.[1]

The parietal lobe contains a sensory strip (Brodmann areas 1, 2, and 3) that lies opposite the motor strip of the frontal lobe (see Fig. 22-9C). Similar to the homunculus of the motor strip, a sensory homunculus recreates a caricature of an upside-down man (see Fig. 22-10A) representing areas that account for receipt and initial analyses of sensory information from different areas of the body. Areas of the body with greater sensory needs occupy larger areas on the sensory strip, which is concerned with deep or internal sensations and with cutaneous sensations such as touch, pressure, position, and vibration. Injury to these areas may result in tactile sensory loss on the opposite side of the body.

The somatic sensory associative area of the parietal lobe (see Fig. 22-9C) facilitates further assessment of sensory stimuli,

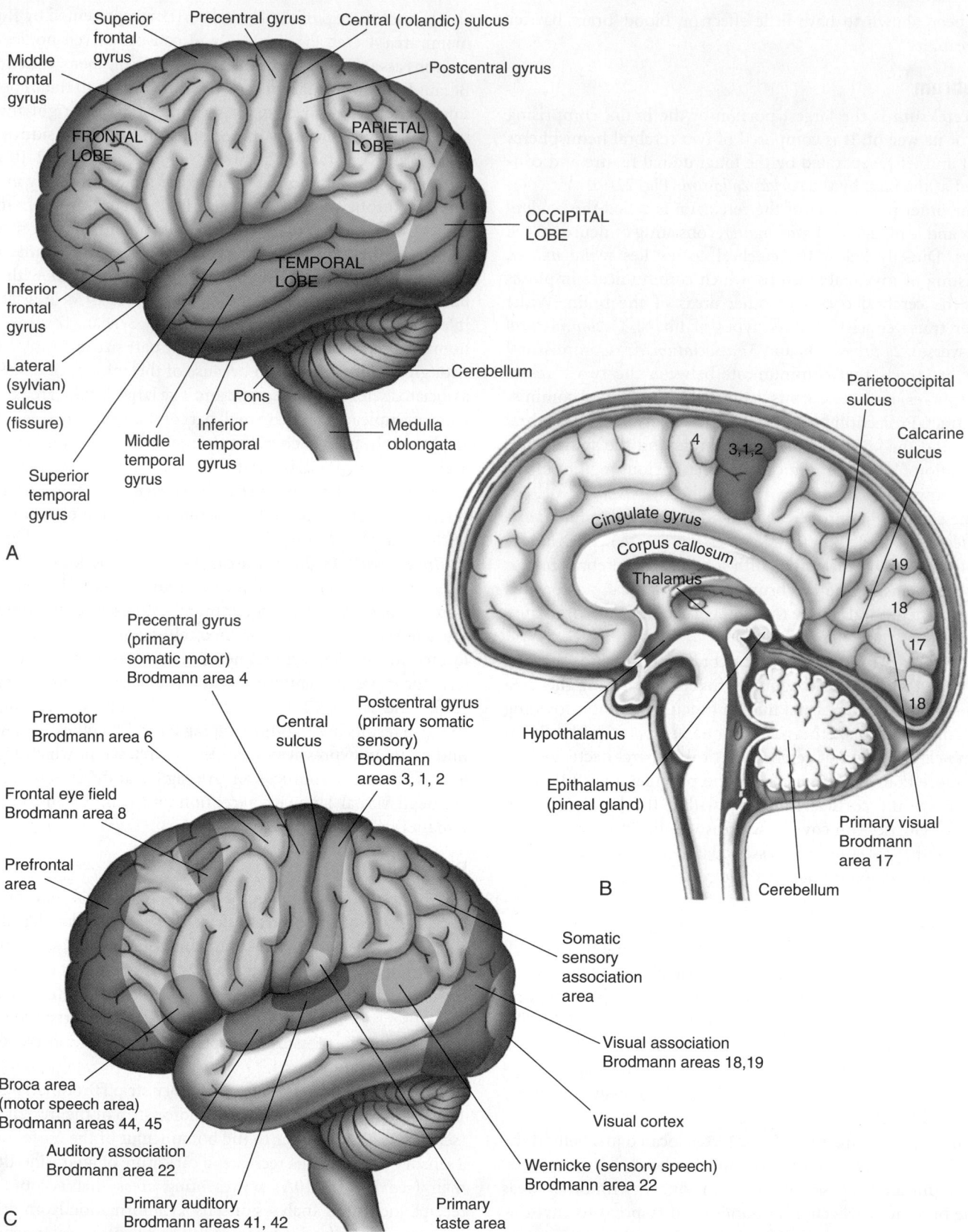

FIGURE 22-9   **The Cerebral Hemispheres.** *A,* Left hemisphere of cerebrum, lateral view. *B,* Functional areas of the cerebral cortex, midsagittal view. *C,* Functional areas of the cerebral cortex, lateral view. (From Huether SE, et al. *Understanding Pathophysiology.* 4th ed. St. Louis: Mosby; 2008.)

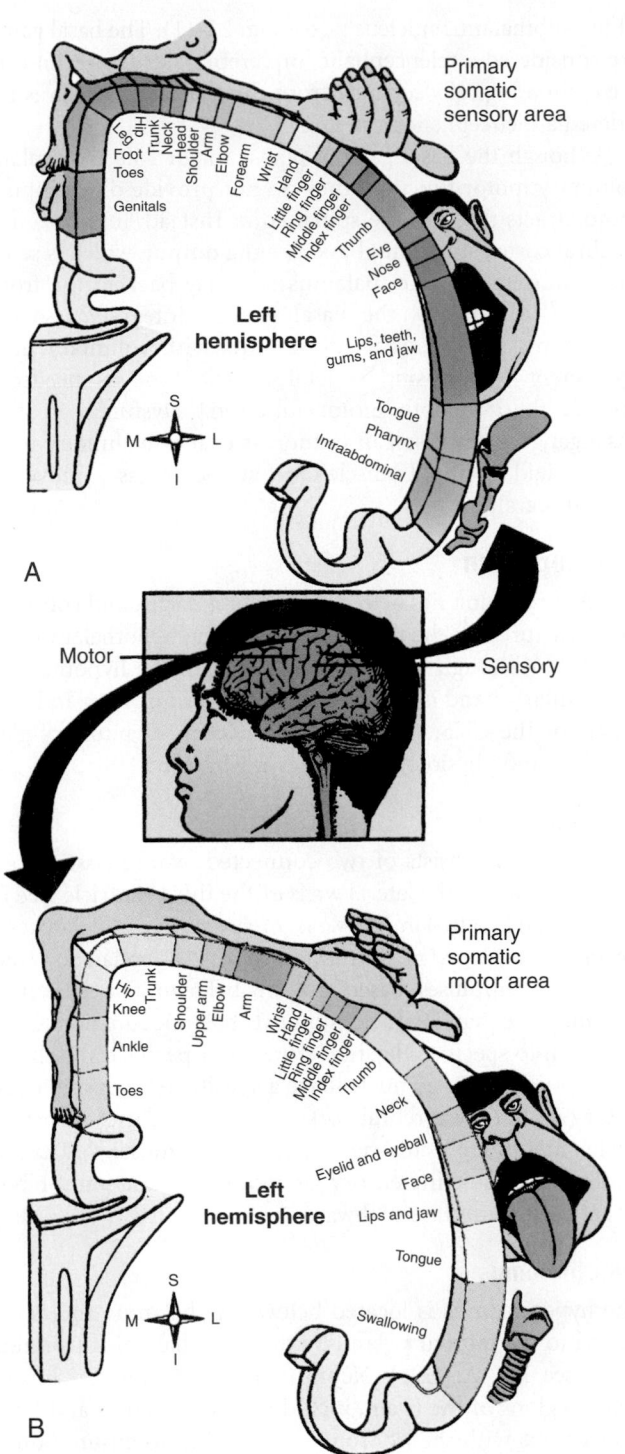

FIGURE 22-10 Primary somatic sensory *(A)* and motor *(B)* areas of the cortex. (From Patton KT, Thibodeau GF. *Anatomy and Physiology.* 8th ed. St. Louis: Mosby; 2013.)

Wernicke area (Brodmann area 22) is partially located within the parietal lobe and partially in the temporal lobe, most commonly on the left side of the cerebral cortex (see Fig. 22-9C). This area is concerned with reception of written and verbal language and includes many intricate connections to other parts of the brain associated with auditory and visual functions, cognitive appraisal, and expressive language.[1] Injury to this area of the brain may result in disability ranging from minor receptive language dysfunction to *receptive* or *fluent aphasia*, in which expressive language function remains but is illogical in content or a "word salad." When brain injury includes the areas important to language reception and expression, *global aphasia* may result, significantly limiting receipt and expression of language.[11,15]

Temporal Lobe

The temporal lobe lies beneath the temporal bone in the lateral portion of the cranium (see Fig. 22-9A). The anterior, lower border of the temporal lobe is encased in the sphenoid wing. With a strong blow to the head, the temporal lobe is easily contused and lacerated as it moves against this hard, irregular surface. Separated from the frontal and parietal lobes by the lateral fissure, this lobe has the primary functions of hearing, speech, behavior, and memory.[1,2,20]

The primary auditory areas (Brodmann areas 41 and 42) receive sound impulses and assist in determining the source of sound and the meaning of sound (see Fig. 22-9C).[3,4] Injury to these areas may result in auditory perceptual loss.[24] Auditory centers in the temporal lobe are closely linked with Wernicke area.[4]

In the superior portion of the temporal lobe, where the frontal, parietal, and temporal lobes meet, is an essential interpretive area in which auditory, visual, and somatic association areas are integrated into complex thought and memory.[3,4] Seizures in this region of the temporal lobe cause auditory, visual, and sensory hallucinations.[25]

Occipital Lobe

The occipital lobe forms the most posterior aspects of the cerebral cortex (see Fig. 22-9A) and is concerned with interpretation of visual stimuli.[1,2,20] The primary visual cortex (see Fig. 22-9C) receives impulses from projections of the optic nerve (cranial nerve II). These impulses are then referred to the visual associative areas (Brodmann areas 18 and 19) for interpretation and integration (see Fig. 22-9C).[3,4] Injury to the occipital lobes may result in cortical blindness, in which the eye structures remain intact but the ability to receive and interpret visual stimuli is lost.[26]

Limbic Lobe

The rhinencephalon, or limbic lobe, lies medially along the inner aspects of the temporal lobe. The core of the limbic system consists of the hippocampus and the amygdaloid nucleus.[1,2,20] Compared with animals living in the wild, the limbic lobe is poorly developed in humans as a result of the sophisticated cognitive capabilities of the frontal lobe, which mediate many of the protective strategies used by humans in everyday life. The limbic lobe's primary functions are related to

promoting an ability to determine size, shape, texture, locality of stimuli, temperature, vibration, and precise purpose of familiar objects based solely on tactile discrimination. Interpretive aspects of the parietal lobe's response to stimuli include awareness of body parts, perceptual orientation in space, and recognition of environmental spatial relationships.[1] Injury to these areas may result in perceptual neglect or inattention.[11,15]

self-preservation and include functions such as recall of pleasurable as well as unpleasant or potentially dangerous events, modification of mood and emotional responses in relation to perceived events, interpretation of smell, and augmentation of visceral processes (e.g., heart rate, respiration) associated with emotion. When the injured prefrontal cortex results in cognitive disability, this controversial area of the brain may take on increased control to support self-preservation needs. Unfortunately, this may result in significantly aberrant behavior that is frequently judged as socially unacceptable.[27]

Internal Capsule

Fiber tracts from many portions of each half of the cerebrum converge in the area of the brain known as the *internal capsule* as they progress toward the brainstem and the spinal cord. The internal capsule contains afferent and efferent fibers (Fig. 22-11). Afferent (sensory) impulses destined for the cortex travel through the internal capsule in the following succession: brainstem to thalamus to internal capsule to cerebral cortex. Efferent (motor) fibers leaving the cortex also pass through the internal capsule.[1,2] Injury to a portion of the internal capsule may result in pure sensory loss, motor loss, or both on the opposite side of the body with preservation of cortical function.[28]

Basal Ganglia

The basal ganglia participate in regulating extrapyramidal (involuntary) motor function.[1-4] Located deep within the white matter of the cerebral hemispheres, the basal ganglia consist of four nuclei: 1) the corpus striatum (caudate nucleus and putamen); 2) the globus pallidus; 3) the substantia nigra; and

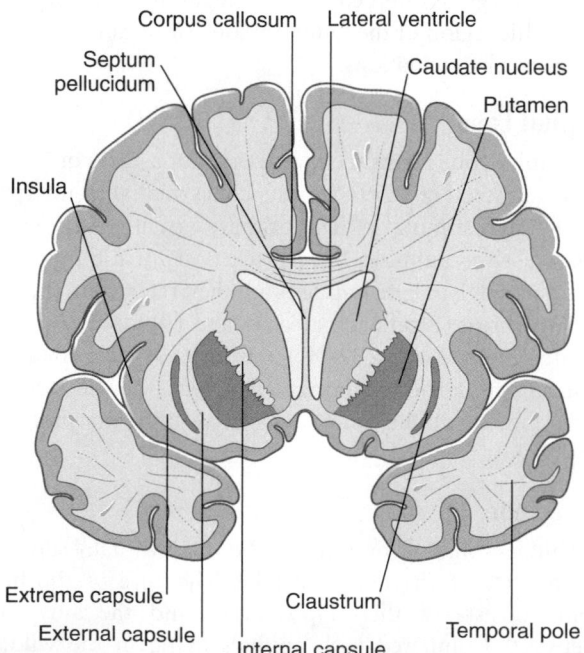

Corpus callosum   Lateral ventricle
Septum pellucidum
Caudate nucleus
Putamen
Insula
Extreme capsule
External capsule
Claustrum
Internal capsule
Temporal pole

FIGURE 22-11 A coronal section through the anterior limb of the internal capsule. (From Fitzgerald MJT, et al. *Clinical Neuroanatomy and Neuroscience.* 5th ed. Philadelphia: Saunders; 2007.)

4) the subthalamic nucleus[1,2] (see Fig. 22-11). The basal ganglia are considered a telencephalic, or cerebral, structure, and they are embryologically separate from the thalamus, which is considered a diencephalic structure.[1,2]

Although the basal ganglia play a major role in regulating voluntary motor function, they do not provide direct input to motor tracts through the spinal cord. Instead, input from the cerebral cortex stimulates basal ganglia output, which is sent to the brainstem and the thalamus for relay back to the frontal cortex.[4,29] Ultimately, the basal ganglia integrate associated movements and postural adjustments with voluntary motor movement, suppressing skeletal muscle tone as needed to provide fluid, smooth motor function.[4] Dysfunction of the basal ganglia may result in tremor or other involuntary movements; rigid, nonfluid muscle tone; and slowness of movement without paralysis.[29]

Diencephalon

The diencephalon lies below the cerebral cortex and consists of two structures: 1) the thalamus and 2) the hypothalamus (Fig. 22-12).[1,2] Although structurally wedded to the hypothalamus, the pituitary gland is considered an endocrine organ and is not a part of the CNS. A complete discussion of pituitary gland anatomy and physiology is found in Chapter 31.

Thalamus

The thalamus consists of two connected ovoid masses of gray matter and forms the lateral walls of the third ventricle (see Fig. 22-12). The two thalami serve as a relay station and gatekeeper for motor and sensory stimuli, preventing or enhancing transmission of impulses based on the behavioral needs of the person. More than 50 nuclei support thalamic function and are divided into specific relay nuclei and nonspecific diffusely projecting nuclei.[1,2] Relay nuclei have a specific relationship or trajectory within the cerebral cortex, whereas diffusely projecting nuclei are thought to mediate cortical arousal.[3,4] Thalamic injury may result in sensory or motor dysfunction, or both, when normal impulse pathways are interrupted.[30]

Hypothalamus

The hypothalamus is located below the thalamus and is connected to the pituitary gland by the hypothalamic or pituitary stalk (see Fig. 22-12).[1,2] Neural control of emotion involves many regions of the brain, including the amygdala and limbic associations with the prefrontal cortex, but to ensure homeostasis, these systems all work through the hypothalamus to coordinate the body's behavioral responses to emotion. The hypothalamus maintains internal homeostasis through its ability to stimulate autonomic nervous system response and endocrine system function in relation to body needs, giving the hypothalamus a role in temperature regulation, regulation of food and water intake, control of pituitary hormone release, and augmentation of overall autonomic nervous system output to a sympathetic or parasympathetic state.[3,4]

Cerebellum

The cerebellum (Fig. 22-13), or hindbrain, is separated from the cerebrum by the dural fold called the *tentorium cerebelli.*

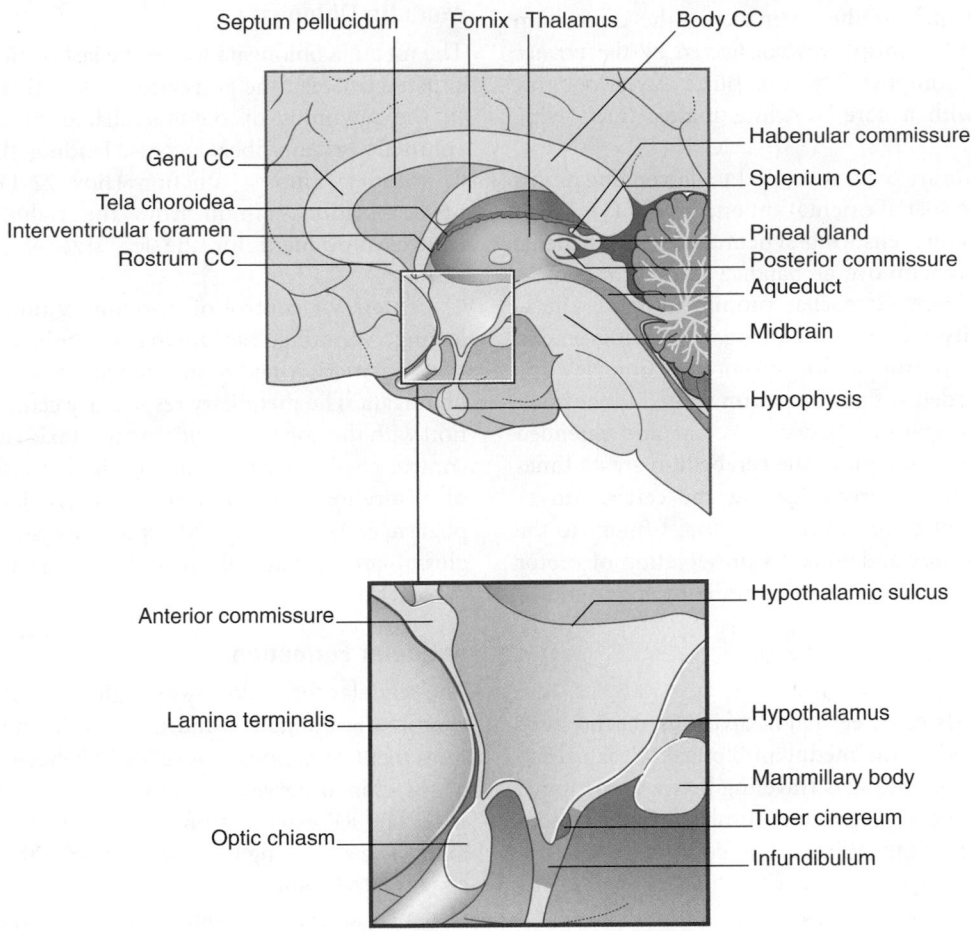

FIGURE 22-12 The diencephalon and its boundaries. *CC*, Corpus callosum. (From Fitzgerald MJT, et al. *Clinical Neuroanatomy and Neuroscience*. 5th ed. Philadelphia: Saunders; 2007.)

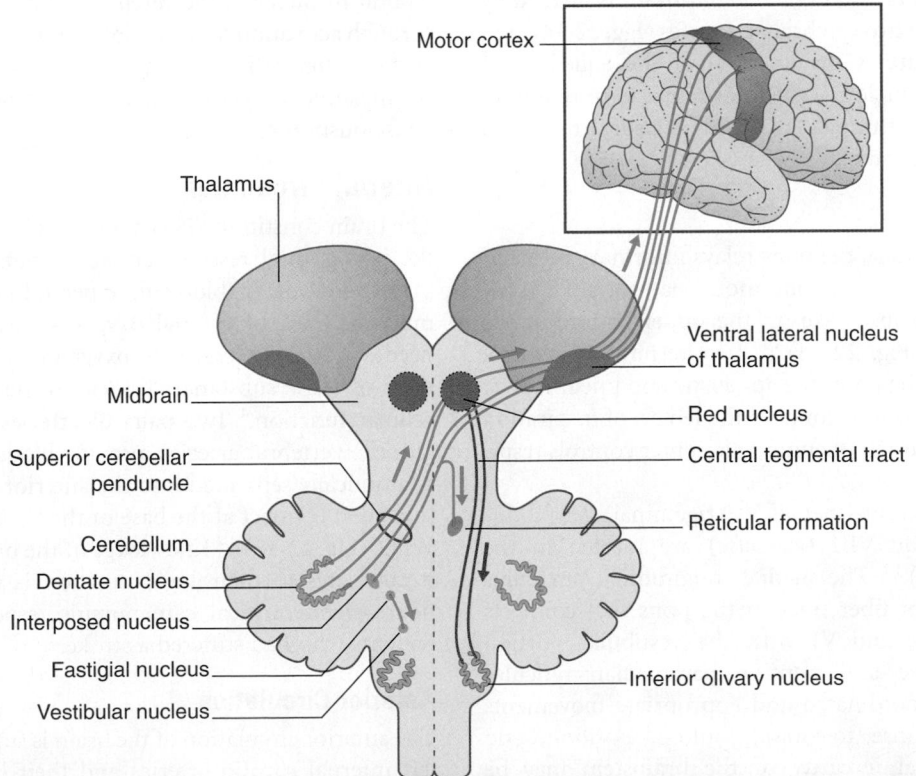

FIGURE 22-13 Principal cerebellar efferents. Arrows indicate directions of impulse conduction. (From Fitzgerald MJT, et al. *Clinical Neuroanatomy and Neuroscience*. 5th ed. Philadelphia: Saunders; 2007.)

Accounting for one fifth of the brain's size, the cerebellum consists of two lateral hemispheres connected by the *vermis*. The cerebellum is composed of an outer layer of gray matter, or cortex, with a core of white matter tracts lying beneath.[1,2]

Cerebellar impulses are communicated to descending motor pathways to integrate spatial orientation and equilibrium with posture and muscle tone, ensuring synchronized adjustments in movement that maintain overall balance and motor coordination (see Fig. 22-13).[3,4] Cerebellar monitoring and adjustment of motor activity occurs simultaneously with movement, enabling significant control of fine motor function.[3,4,31] The cerebellum is bombarded with information related to the goals of movement and disparities between actual and intended movements. Axons projecting into the cerebellum are 40 times more numerous than the axons leaving the cerebellum to ensure adequate receipt of motor information.[31] Injury to the cerebellum produces *ataxia*, defined as preservation of motor strength with lack of control (coordination) over fine motor function.[32]

Brainstem

The brainstem consists of three major divisions: 1) the midbrain, 2) the pons, and 3) the medulla oblongata. It is packed with sensory and motor pathways traveling between the spinal cord and the brain, and it contains a number of centers that regulate vital mechanisms throughout the body.[1,2]

Midbrain

The midbrain forms the junction between the pons and the diencephalon. The cell bodies of cranial nerves III and IV originate in the midbrain (Table 22-3). The midbrain is divided by a sagittal plane into the two cerebral peduncles (Fig. 22-14), and anatomically, it constitutes the location of the aqueduct of Sylvius.[1,2] The major function of the midbrain is to relay stimuli to and from the brain through ascending sensory tracts and descending motor pathways.[3,4]

Pons

Located above the medulla, the pons relays information to and from the brain through sensory and motor pathways. The posterior aspects of the pons make up the upper surface of the fourth ventricle (see Fig. 22-14).[1,2] Two respiratory control centers are located in the pons: the apneustic and pneumotaxic centers. The apneustic center controls the length of inspiration and expiration, whereas the pneumotaxic center controls respiratory rate.[3,4]

The cell bodies of cranial nerves V (trigeminal), VI (abducens), VII (facial), and VIII (acoustic) are located in the pons (see Table 22-3).[1,2] The medial longitudinal fasciculus (MLF) is an important fiber tract in the pons that connects cranial nerves III, IV, and VI with the vestibular portion of the acoustic nerve and pontine paramedian reticular formation, allowing coordinated and appropriate movements of the eyes in response to noise, motion, position, and arousal. The structural integrity of the brainstem may be assessed through clinical stimulation of the MLF in caloric testing.[3,4]

Medulla Oblongata

The medulla oblongata forms the last section of the brainstem, situated between the pons and the spinal cord (see Fig. 22-14). In the pyramids of the medulla, decussation (crossing) of voluntary motor fibers occurs, lending the name *pyramidal* to voluntary motor function (Box 22-1). Below the point of decussation, stimuli from the right side of the brain control movement for the left side of the body, and vice versa.[1,2]

Centers for control of involuntary functions such as swallowing, vomiting, hiccupping, coughing, heart rate, arterial vasoconstriction, and respiration are located within the medulla oblongata. The medullary respiratory center works in conjunction with the apneustic and pneumotaxic centers in the pons to control respiratory function and is responsible for the rhythm of respiration.[3,4] The cell bodies of cranial nerves IX (glossopharyngeal), X (vagus), XI (spinal accessory), and XII (hypoglossal) are located in the medulla oblongata (see Fig. 22-14 and Table 22-3).[1,2]

Reticular Formation

The reticular formation (RF) of the brainstem is located at the core of the brainstem and is active in modulating sensation, movement, consciousness, reflexive behaviors, and the activities of the cranial nerves arising from the brainstem (III through XII). The RF extends from the upper pons to the diencephalon.[1,2] The ascending RF is referred to as the reticular activating system (RAS), and it is responsible for increasing wakefulness, vigilance, and responsiveness of cortical and thalamic neurons to sensory stimuli.[30] In the thalamus, the RAS activates relay and diffuse projection nuclei to increase distribution of sensory stimuli throughout the cerebral cortex.[3,4] The RAS also works through activation of the hypothalamus, which results in diffuse cortical stimulation and autonomic stimulation.[1] Damage to the thalamic or hypothalamic RAS pathways results in impaired consciousness.[33]

Arterial Circulation

The brain constitutes 2% of the body's weight but uses 20% of the body's total resting cardiac output.[4] It requires approximately 750 mL of blood flow per minute and can extract as much as 45% of arterial oxygen to meet normal metabolic needs.[4] It has no reserve of oxygen or glucose, making reductions of these substances critical to the disruption of normal cellular function.[4] Two pairs of arteries, the internal carotids and the vertebral arteries, provide blood to the brain and are anatomically separated into the anterior and posterior circulations that connect at the base of the brain to form the circle of Willis (Fig. 22-15).[1,2] Knowledge of the brain's arterial supply as it correlates to neurologic function is an essential aspect of neuroscience critical care nursing, especially in the care of patients who had suffered a stroke.

Anterior Circulation

The anterior circulation of the brain is supplied by the right and left internal carotid arteries and their branches (Fig. 22-16). Originating as the common carotids, the left common carotid

Text continued on page 609.

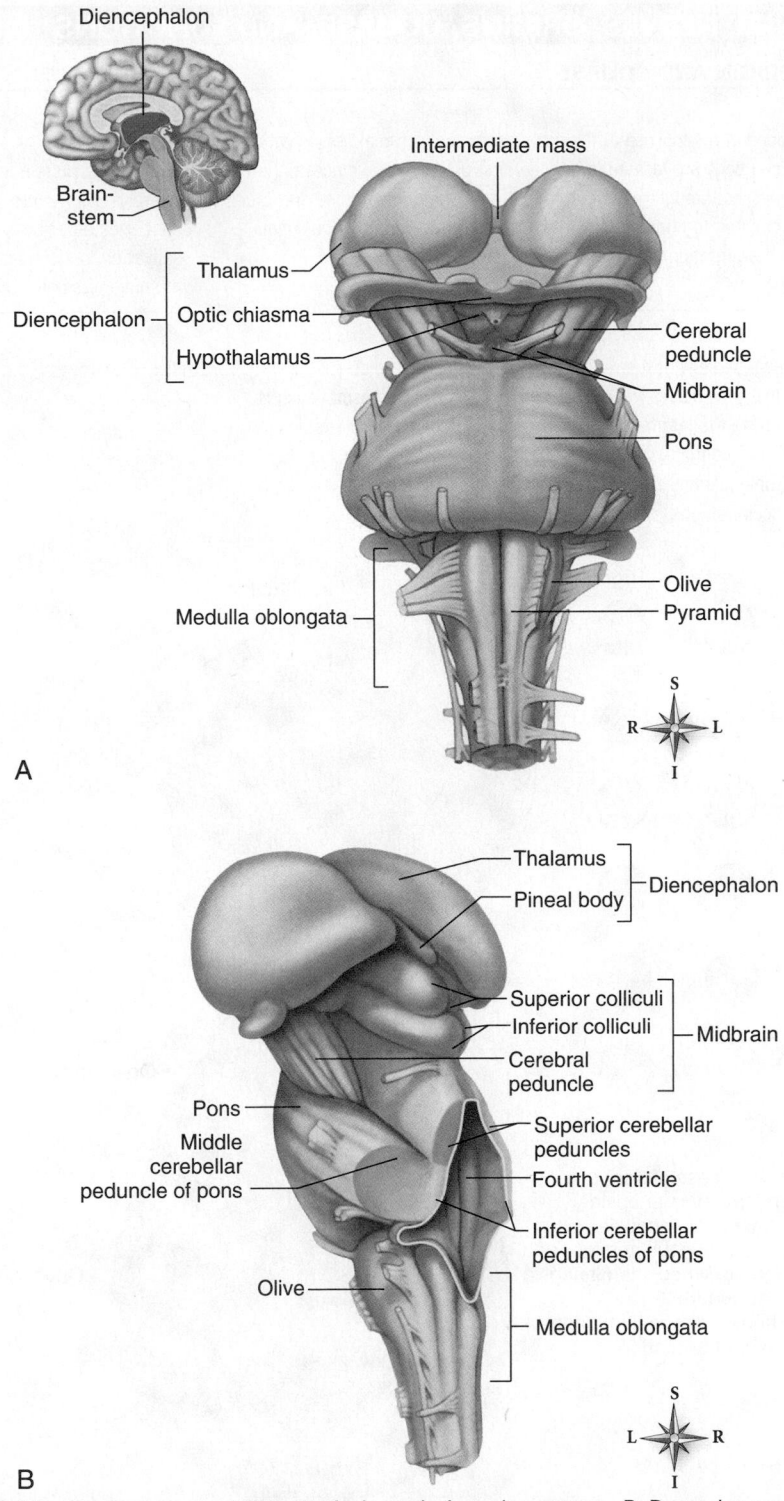

Diencephalon

Brain-
stem

Diencephalon
— Thalamus
— Optic chiasma
— Hypothalamus

Intermediate mass

Cerebral
peduncle
— Midbrain
— Pons

Olive
Pyramid

Medulla oblongata

S
R — L
I

A

Thalamus
Pineal body
Diencephalon

Superior colliculi
Inferior colliculi
Midbrain
Cerebral
peduncle

Pons
Superior cerebellar
peduncles
Middle
cerebellar
peduncle of pons
Fourth ventricle

Inferior cerebellar
peduncles of pons

Olive

Medulla oblongata

S
L — R
I

B

FIGURE 22-14 **Brainstem and Diencephalon.** *A,* Anterior aspect. *B,* Posterior aspect (shifted slightly to lateral). (From Patton KT, Thibodeau GF. *Anatomy and Physiology.* 8th ed. St. Louis: Mosby; 2013.)

TABLE 22-3 CRANIAL NERVES, ORIGINS, COURSE, AND FUNCTIONS

CRANIAL NERVE	ORIGIN AND COURSE	FUNCTION
I Olfactory Sensory	Found in the mucosa of the nasal cavity; only cranial nerves with cell body are located in peripheral structure (nasal mucosa). It passes through the cribriform plate of the ethmoid bone and goes on to olfactory bulbs at the floor of the frontal lobe. Final interpretation is in the temporal lobe.	Smell However, the system is more than receptor and interpreter for odors; perception of smell also sensitizes other body systems and responses, such as salivation, peristalsis, and even sexual stimulus. Loss of sense of smell is called *anosmia*.
II Optic Sensory	Ganglion cells of the retina converge to the optic disc and form the optic nerve. Nerve fibers pass to the optic chiasm, which is above the pituitary gland. Some fibers decussate; others do not. The two tracts go to the lateral geniculate body near the thalamus and then on to the end station for interpretation in the occipital lobe.	Vision

Left   Right

Visual Fields

A
B
C
D
E
F

Left   Right

A-Total blindness of right eye
B-Bitemporal hemianopsia
C-Left nasal hemianopsia
D-Left homonymous hemianopsia
E-Left homonymous hemianopsia
  inferior quadrant
F-Left homonymous hemianopsia
  superior quadrant

Optic nerve
Optic tract
Optic radiation
Visual cortex

G.J.Wassilchenko

TABLE 22-3	CRANIAL NERVES, ORIGINS, COURSE, AND FUNCTIONS—cont'd	
CRANIAL NERVE	**ORIGIN AND COURSE**	**FUNCTION**
III Oculomotor		
Motor	Originates in the midbrain and emerges from the brainstem at the upper pons.	Extraocular movement of eyes
Motor	Motor fibers go to superior, medial, and inferior recti and to the inferior oblique for eye movement and levator muscle of the eyelid.	Raising of eyelid
Parasympathetic	Parasympathetic fibers go to ciliary muscles and iris of eye.	Constriction of pupil; changing shape of lens

Superior rectus tested
by gaze up and out

Inferior oblique tested
by gaze up and in

Medial rectus tested
by gaze directed in
toward nose (medial)

Inferior rectus tested
by gaze down and out

G.J.Wassilchenko

A   B   C

Continued

TABLE 22-3 **CRANIAL NERVES, ORIGINS, COURSE, AND FUNCTIONS—cont'd**

CRANIAL NERVE	ORIGIN AND COURSE	FUNCTION
IV Trochlear Motor	Midbrain origin near oculomotor nerve, emerges at upper pons near cerebral peduncle; motor fibers go to superior oblique muscle of the eyeball.	Extraocular movement of eyes

Superior oblique tested
by gaze down and in

A   B   C

G.J. Wassilchenko

CRANIAL NERVE	ORIGIN AND COURSE	FUNCTION
V Trigeminal Sensory	Originates in the fourth ventricle and emerges at lateral parts of the pons; has three branches to face: ophthalmic, maxillary, and mandibular.	*Ophthalmic branch:* sensation to cornea, ciliary body, iris, lacrimal gland, conjunctiva, nasal mucosal membranes, eyelids, eyebrows, forehead, and nose *Maxillary branch:* sensation to skin of cheek, lower lid, side of nose and upper jaw, teeth, mucosa of mouth, sphenopalatine-pterygoid region, and maxillary sinus *Mandibular branch:* sensation to skin of lower lip, chin, ear, mucous membrane, teeth of lower jaw, and tongue
Motor	Goes to temporalis, masseter, pterygoid gland, anterior part of digastric muscles (all for mastication), and the tensor tympani and tensor veli palatine muscles (clench jaw).	Supplies muscles for chewing (mastication) and opening jaw

Ophthalmic branch

Trigeminal nerve

Maxillary branch

Mandibular branches

G.J. Wassilchenko

TABLE 22-3 **CRANIAL NERVES, ORIGINS, COURSE, AND FUNCTIONS—cont'd**

CRANIAL NERVE	ORIGIN AND COURSE	FUNCTION
VI Abducens Motor	Posterior part of pons goes to lateral rectus muscle for eye movement. Lateral rectus tested by gaze directed outward away from nose (lateral).	Extraocular eye movement; rotates eyeball outward

Lateral rectus tested by gaze directed outward away from nose (lateral)

G.J.Wassilchenko

A   B   C

VII Facial Sensory	Lower portion of pons goes to anterior two thirds of tongue and soft palate.	Taste in anterior two thirds of tongue; sensation to soft palate
Motor	Pons to muscles of forehead, eyelids, checks, lips, ears, nose, and neck.	Movement of facial muscles to produce facial expressions, close eyes
Parasympathetic	Pons to salivary gland and lacrimal glands.	Secretory for salivation and tears
VIII Acoustic Sensory	Nerve has two divisions. *Cochlear division* originates in spinal ganglia of the cochlea, with peripheral fibers to the organ of Corti in the internal ear. It goes to the pons, and impulses are transmitted to the temporal lobe. *Vestibular division* originates in the otolith organs of the semicircular canals in the inner ear and in the vestibular ganglion. It terminates in the pons, with some fibers continuing to cerebellum. It is the only cranial nerve that originates wholly within a bone, the petrous portion of the temporal bone.	Hearing Equilibrium
IX Glossopharyngeal Sensory	Posterior one third of tongue for taste sensation and sensations from soft palate, tonsils, and opening to mouth in back of oral pharynx (fauces). Fibers go to the medulla and then to the temporal lobe for taste and sensory cortex for other sensations.	Taste in posterior one third of tongue; sensation in back of throat; stimulation elicits gag reflex
Motor	Medulla to constrictor muscles of pharynx and stylopharyngeal muscles.	Voluntary muscles for swallowing and phonation
Parasympathetic	Medulla to parotid salivary gland through the otic ganglia.	Secretory, salivary glands; carotid reflex

Continued

TABLE 22-3 CRANIAL NERVES, ORIGINS, COURSE, AND FUNCTIONS—cont'd

CRANIAL NERVE	ORIGIN AND COURSE	FUNCTION
X Vagus		
Sensory	Sensory fibers in back of the ear and posterior wall of the external ear go to the medulla oblongata and on to the sensory cortex.	Sensation behind ear and part of external ear meatus
Motor	Fibers go from the medulla oblongata through the jugular foramen with glossopharyngeal nerve and on to the pharynx, larynx, esophagus, bronchi, lungs, heart, stomach, small intestine, liver, pancreas, and kidneys.	Voluntary muscles for phonation and swallowing; involuntary activity of visceral muscles of heart, lungs, and digestive tract
Parasympathetic	Medulla oblongata to the larynx, trachea, lungs, aorta, esophagus, stomach, small intestines, and gallbladder.	Carotid reflex; autonomic activity of respiratory tract and digestive tract, including peristalsis and secretion from organs
XI Spinal Accessory		
Motor	The nerve has two roots: cranial and spinal. Cranial portion arises at several rootlets at the side of medulla, runs below the vagus, and is joined by the spinal portion from motor cells in cervical cord. Some fibers go along with vagus nerve to supply motor impulse to the pharynx, larynx, uvula, and palate. Major portion goes to the sternomastoid and trapezius muscles, branches to cervical spinal nerves C2-C4.	Some fibers for swallowing and phonation; turning head and shrugging shoulders
XII Hypoglossal		
Motor	Arises in the medulla oblongata and goes to the muscles of the tongue.	Movement of tongue necessary for swallowing and phonation

BOX 22-1 DECUSSATION OF VOLUNTARY MOTOR FIBERS

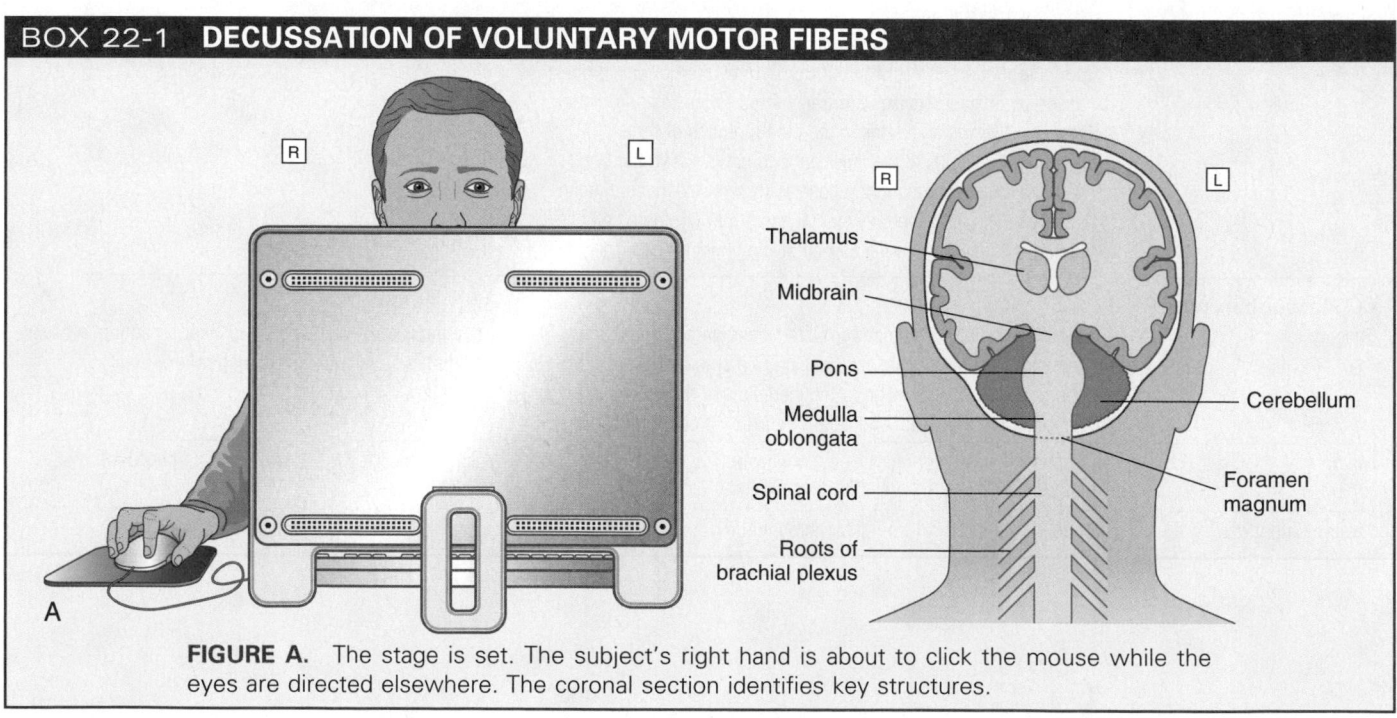

FIGURE A. The stage is set. The subject's right hand is about to click the mouse while the eyes are directed elsewhere. The coronal section identifies key structures.

BOX 22-1   **DECUSSATION OF VOLUNTARY MOTOR FIBERS—cont'd**

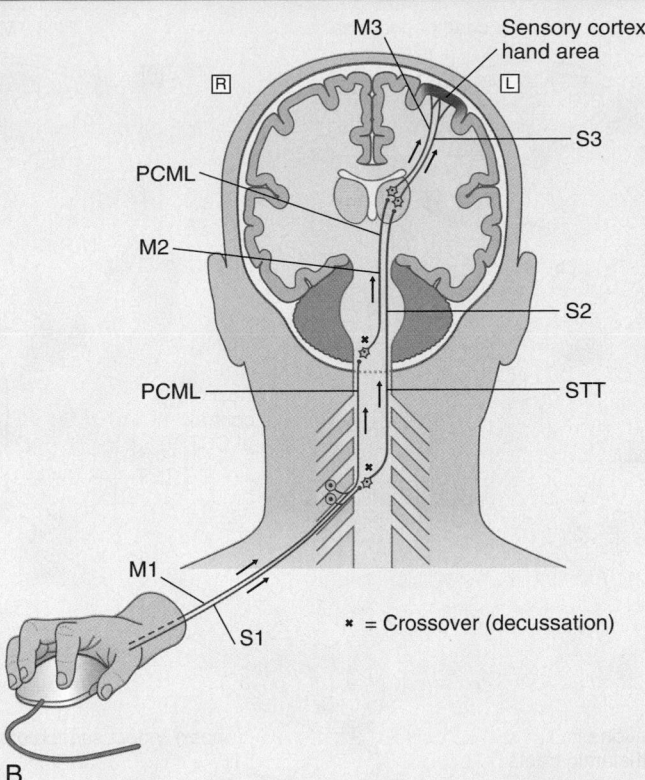

FIGURE B. **Afferents.** The left parietal lobe constructs a map of the right hand in relation to the mouse, based on information sent to the left somatic sensory cortex (postcentral gyrus) from the skin and deep tissues. The information is relayed by three successive sets of neurons from the skin and by another set of three from the deep tissues. The first set in each case is composed of first-order or primary afferent neurons. These neurons are called unipolar, because each axon emerges from a single point (or pole) of the cell body and divides in a T-shaped manner to provide continuity of impulse conduction from tissue to central nervous system. The primary afferent neurons terminate by forming contacts known as synapses on the multipolar (more or less star-shaped) cells of the second-order (secondary) set. The axons of the second-order neurons project across the midline before turning up to terminate on third-order (tertiary) multipolar neurons projecting to the postcentral gyrus.

Primary afferents activated by contacts with the skin of the hand (S1) terminate in the posterior horn of the gray matter of the spinal cord. Second-order cutaneous afferents (S2) cross the midline in the anterior white commissure and ascend to the thalamus within the spinothalamic tract (STT), to be relayed by third-order neurons to the hand area of the sensory cortex.

The most significant deep tissue sensory organs are neuromuscular spindles (muscle spindles) contained within skeletal muscles. The primary afferents supplying the muscle spindles of the intrinsic muscles of the hand belong to large unipolar neurons whose axons (labeled M1) ascend ipsilaterally (on the same side of the spinal cord) within the posterior funiculus. They synapse in the nucleus cuneatus in the medulla oblongata. The multipolar second-order neurons send their axons across the midline in the sensory decussation. The axons ascend (M2) through pons and midbrain before synapsing on third-order neurons (M3) projecting from thalamus to sensory cortex. *PCML,* Posterior column–medial lemniscal pathway; *STT,* spinothalamic tract.

Continued

BOX 22-1   DECUSSATION OF VOLUNTARY MOTOR FIBERS—cont'd

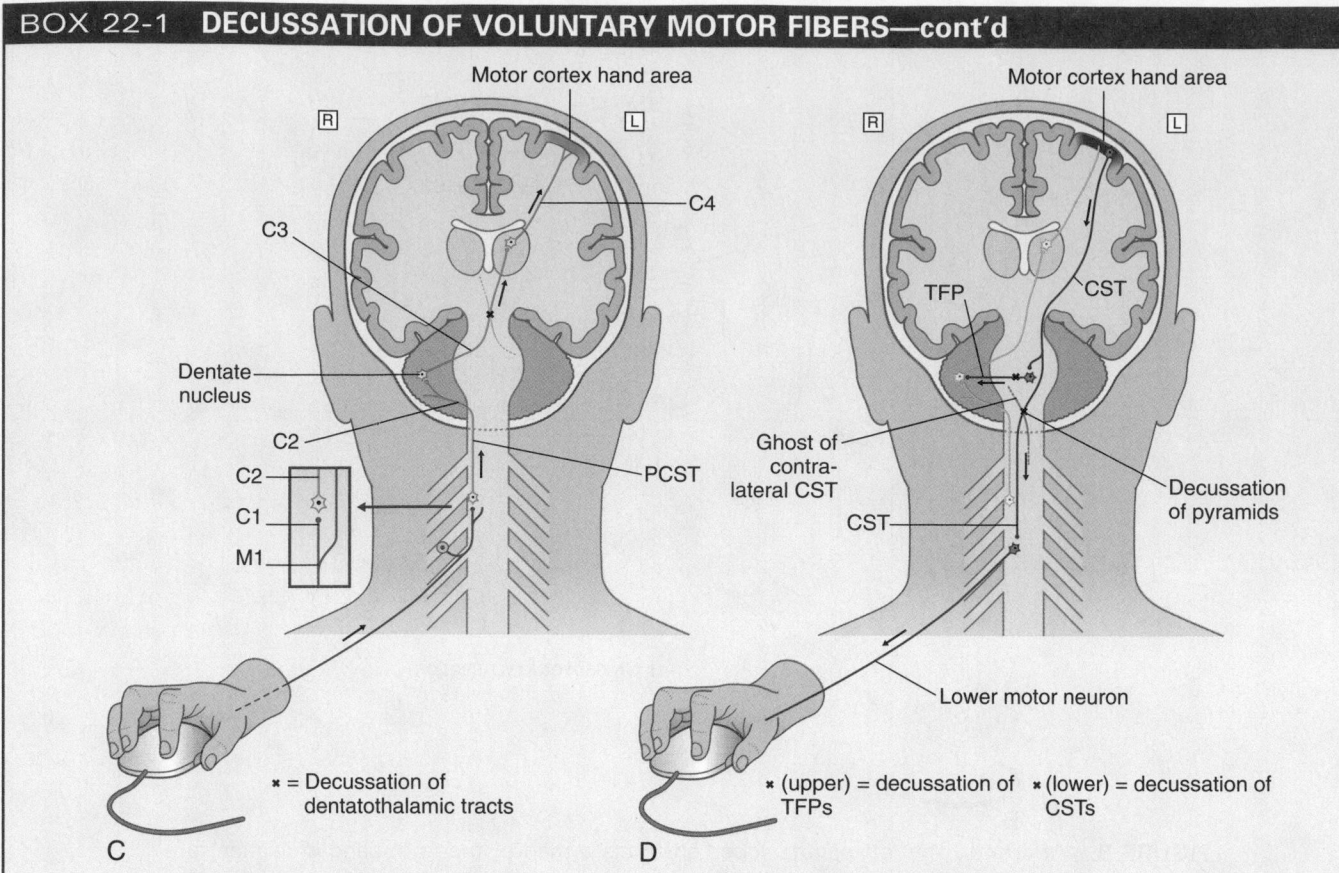

Motor cortex hand area

R   L   C4

C3

Dentate nucleus

C2

C2
C1
M1

PCST

Motor cortex hand area

R   L

TFP   CST

Ghost of contra-lateral CST

CST

Decussation of pyramids

Lower motor neuron

✗ = Decussation of dentatothalamic tracts

✗ (upper) = decussation of TFPs   ✗ (lower) = decussation of CSTs

C

D

FIGURE C.   Cerebellar Control. Before the brain sends an instruction to click the mouse, it requires information on the current state of contraction of the muscles. This information is constantly being sent from the muscles to the cerebellar hemisphere on the same side. As indicated in the diagram, M1 neurons are dual-purpose sensory neurons. At their point of entry to the posterior funiculus, they give off a branch, here labeled C1, to a spinocerebellar neuron that projects (C2) to the ipsilateral cerebellum. From here, a cerebellothalamic neuron (C3) is shown projecting across the midbrain to the contralateral thalamus, where a further neuron (C4) relays information to the hand area of the motor cortex in the precentral gyrus.

FIGURE D.   Motor Output. Multipolar neurons in the left motor cortex now fire impulses along the upper motor neurons that constitute the corticospinal tract (CST), which crosses to the opposite side in the motor decussation. The CST synapses on lower motor neurons projecting from the anterior horn of the spinal gray matter to activate flexor muscles of the index finger and local stabilizing muscles.

Note that a copy of the outgoing message is sent to the right cerebellar hemisphere by way of transverse fibers of the pons (TFP) originating in multipolar neurons located on the left side of the pons.

Modified from Fitzgerald MJT, et al. *Clinical Neuroanatomy and Neuroscience.* 5th ed. Philadelphia: Saunders; 2007.

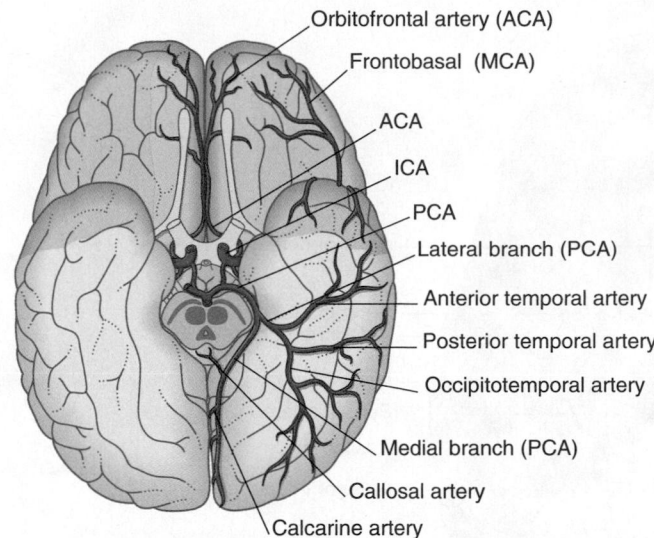

FIGURE 22-15 View from below the cerebral hemispheres, showing the cortical branches and territories of the three cerebral arteries. *ACA*, Anterior cerebral artery; *ICA*, internal carotid artery; *MCA*, middle cerebral artery; *PCA*, posterior cerebral artery. (From Fitzgerald MJT, et al. *Clinical Neuroanatomy and Neuroscience*. 5th ed. Philadelphia: Saunders; 2007.)

Labels in figure:
Orbitofrontal artery (ACA)
Frontobasal (MCA)
ACA
ICA
PCA
Lateral branch (PCA)
Anterior temporal artery
Posterior temporal artery
Occipitotemporal artery
Medial branch (PCA)
Callosal artery
Calcarine artery

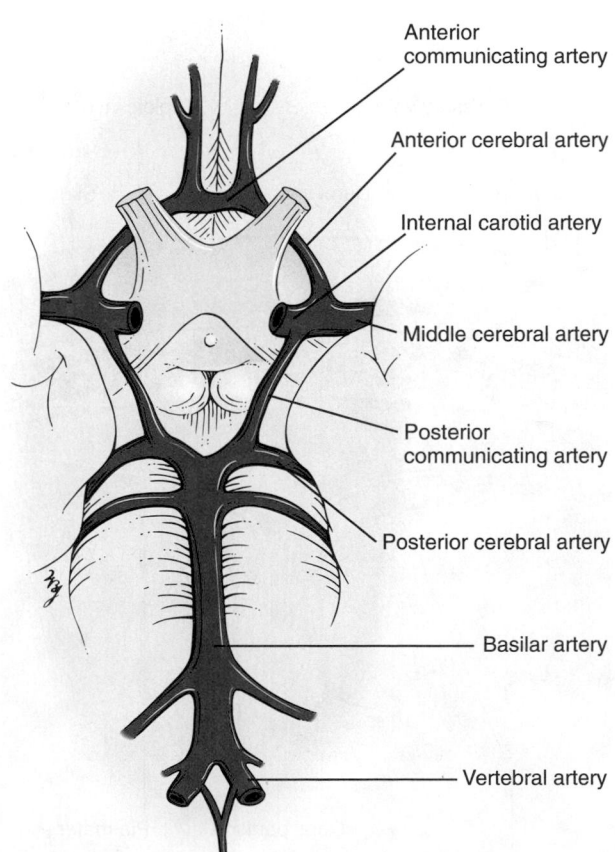

FIGURE 22-16 Circle of Willis. (From Swartz MH. *Textbook of Physical Diagnosis: History and Examination*. 6th ed. Philadelphia: Saunders; 2009.)

Labels in figure:
Anterior communicating artery
Anterior cerebral artery
Internal carotid artery
Middle cerebral artery
Posterior communicating artery
Posterior cerebral artery
Basilar artery
Vertebral artery

takes off from the arch of the aorta, whereas the right common carotid originates from the innominate artery. At the level of the cricothyroid junction, the common carotid splits to form the external and internal carotid arteries. The external carotid feeds the face, the scalp, and the skull and includes the branch called the *middle meningeal artery*, which lies between the skull and the dura.[1,2]

The internal carotid artery continues upward through the carotid siphon and enters the base of the skull through an opening in the petrous bone. At the base of the brain, the internal carotid gives off the right and left middle cerebral arteries (MCAs); the right and left anterior cerebral arteries (ACAs), which are connected by the anterior communicating artery (ACoA); and the two posterior communicating arteries (PCoAs). The anterior circulation provides 80% of the blood flow to the cerebral hemispheres, covering the needs of the frontal lobes and most of the parietal and temporal lobes and supplying the subcortical structures residing above the brainstem. The internal carotid artery gives rise to the ophthalmic artery at the siphon before bifurcating into the anterior cerebral and middle cerebral arteries. The ophthalmic artery supplies blood to the optic nerve and eye and may reverse its course to supplement the anterior circulation's arterial blood volume in the case of internal carotid artery occlusion.[1,2]

Posterior Circulation

The posterior circulation begins with the two vertebral arteries (Fig. 22-17), which originate from the subclavian arteries and travel posteriorly through small openings in the lateral spinous processes of the cervical spine. They enter the skull through the foramen magnum, and at the level of the pons, the two vertebral arteries fuse to form the basilar artery. The terminal portion of the vertebral arteries gives rise to two important arterial branches before basilar artery fusion: the posterior inferior cerebellar arteries (PICAs). Two major infratentorial branches of the basilar artery include the anterior inferior cerebellar arteries (AICAs) and the superior cerebellar arteries (SCAs), which together with the PICAs supply the cerebellum. The distal basilar artery gives rise to the two posterior cerebral arteries (PCAs), which emerge in the supratentorial region to supply the posterior aspects of the cerebral cortex.[1,2]

Circle of Willis

The circle of Willis is a vascular supply system unique to the brain's circulation (see Fig. 22-14). Located above the optic chiasm in the subarachnoid space, the circle is fed by branches of the internal carotid and basilar arteries. The anterior circulation is connected between the two ACAs by the ACoA and to the posterior circulation by the two PCoAs.[1,2] Approximately 50% of the population has a complete or "ideal" circle of Willis. In others, atretic (small and nonfunctional or hypoplastic) segments often are found in the first branch of the ACAs, called A1; in the first branch of the PCAs, called P1; and in the PCoAs. When complete, the circle of Willis is capable of supporting some degree of collateral blood flow in the case of arterial occlusion, although a sufficient arterial supply in the face of arterial obstruction is not guaranteed.[34]

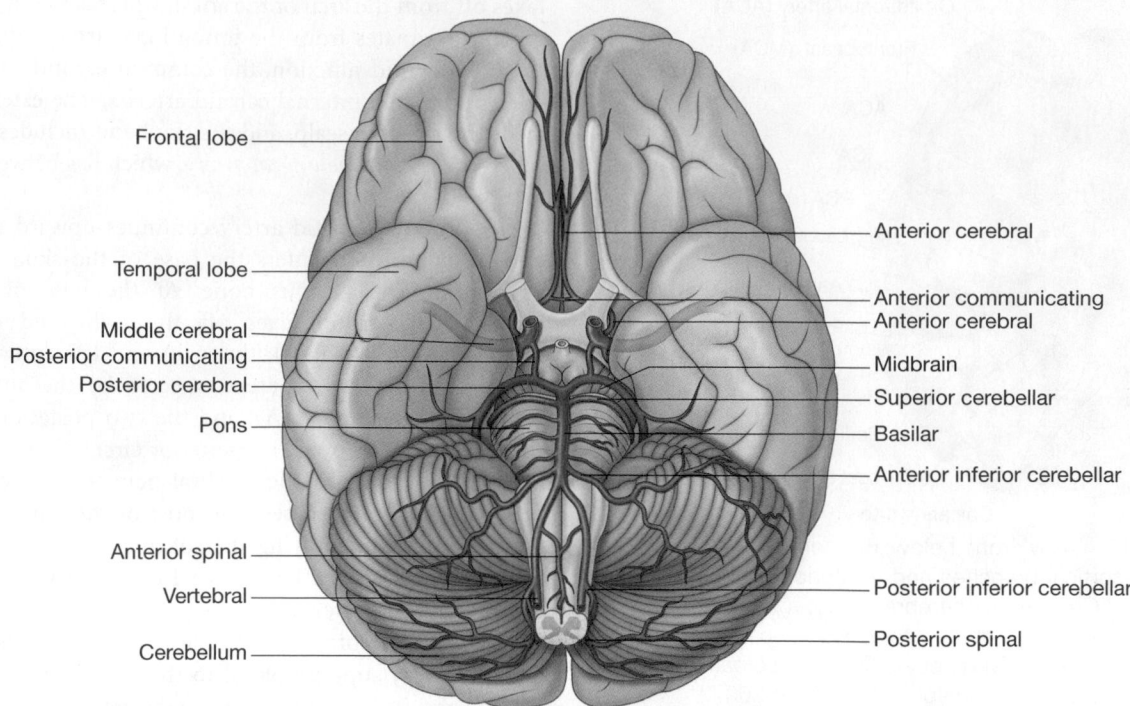

FIGURE 22-17 Posterior arterial distribution. (From Drake RL, et al. *Gray's Anatomy for Students*. 2nd ed. London: Churchill Livingstone; 2009.)

Venous Circulation

Venous drainage occurs through venous sinuses, many of which are housed in the double-folded membrane of the dura mater (Fig. 22-18). Capillaries drain into venules, which then flow into cerebral veins, ultimately emptying into sinuses located throughout the cranium. Blood from these sinuses empties into the internal jugular vein, which empties into the superior vena cava (Fig. 22-19). Cerebral veins have thinner walls relative to veins in the general circulation and lack a muscular layer or valves.[1,2]

Spinal Cord

The spinal cord, one division of the CNS, extends from the medulla below the foramen magnum. Similar to the brain, the spinal cord is composed of gray and white matter, although the cord's gray matter is located internally and the white matter on its surface. The distal end of the spinal cord tapers to the *conus medullaris*, which is situated at the level of the first or second lumbar vertebra. Exiting from the spinal cord are 31 pairs of spinal nerves, which exit through intervertebral foramina. Because the spinal cord ends at vertebrae L1 and the final nerve roots do not exit until the coccyx, long lengths of nerves, called the *cauda equina*, extend below the conus medullaris toward their associated intervertebral foramina to exit the spinal canal (Fig. 22-20).[1,2]

Spinal Protective Mechanisms

Protective mechanisms similar to those listed for the brain provide protection to the spinal cord.[1,2]

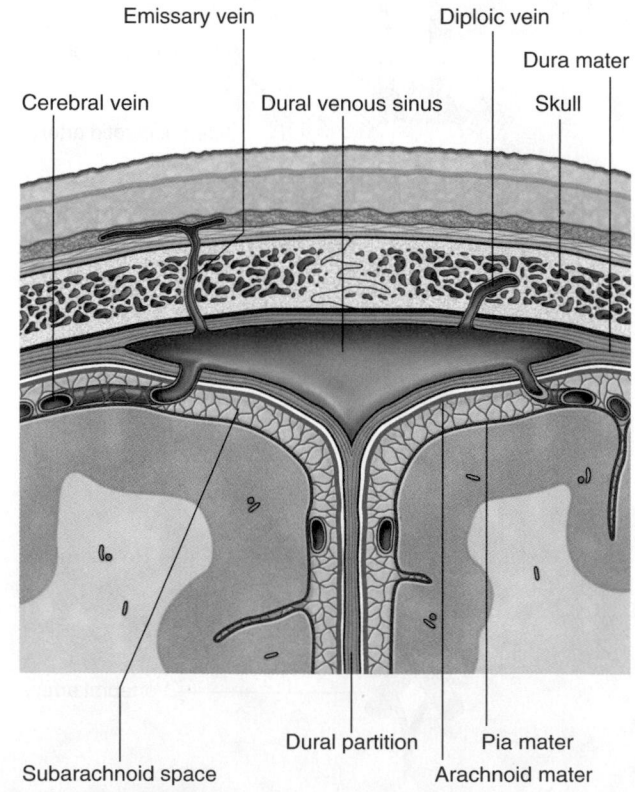

FIGURE 22-18 Dural venous sinuses. (From Drake RL, et al. *Gray's Anatomy for Students*. 2nd ed. London: Churchill Livingstone; 2009.)

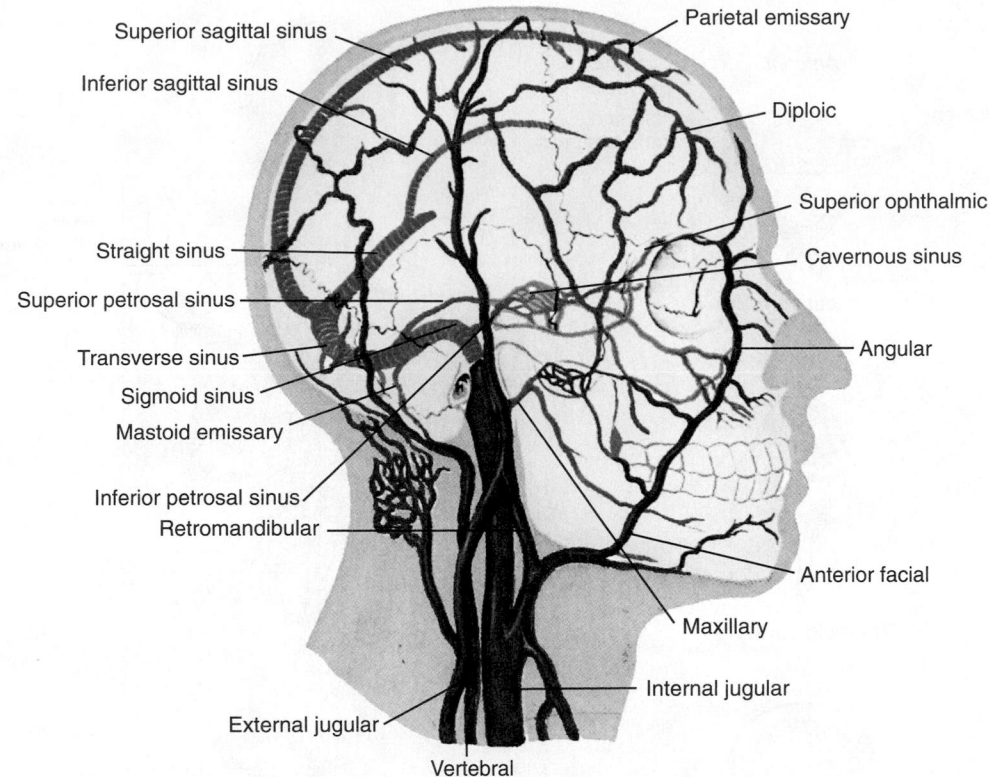

FIGURE 22-19 Venous Circulation.

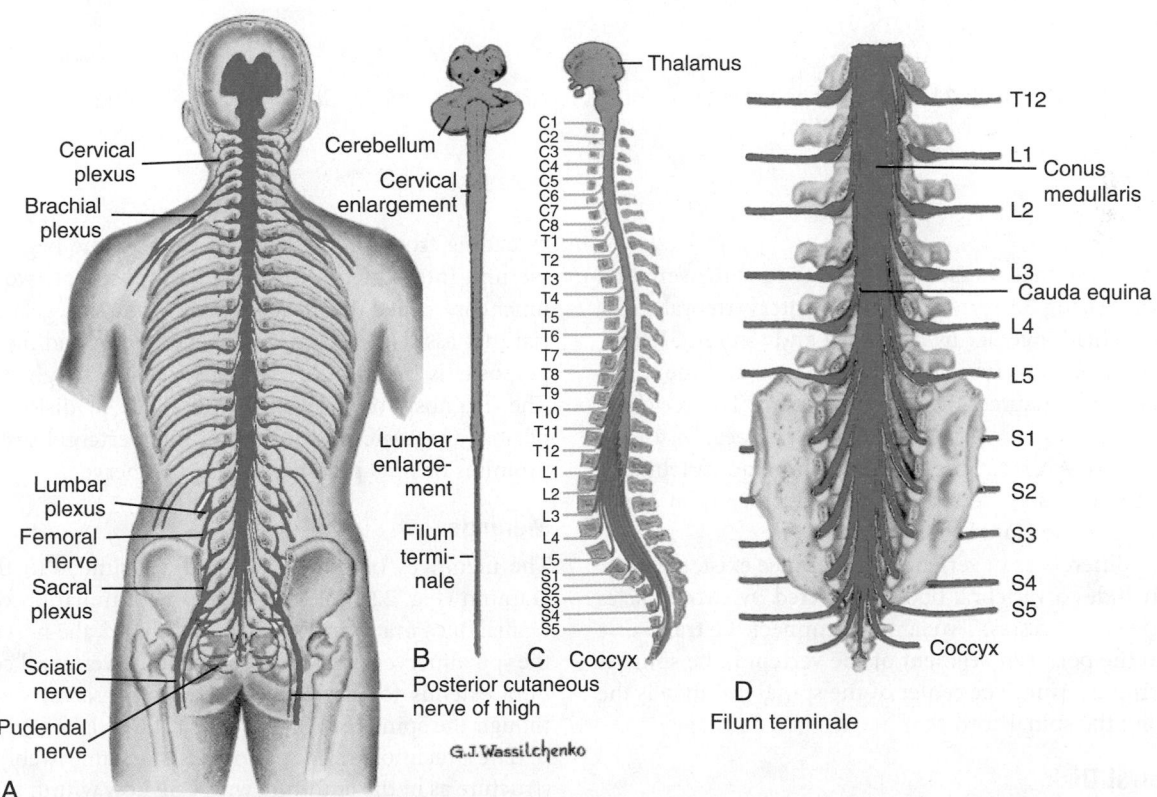

FIGURE 22-20 Spinal Cord within the Vertebral Canal and Exiting Spinal Nerves. *A,* Posterior view in situ. *B,* Anterior view. *C,* Lateral view. *D,* Cauda equina.

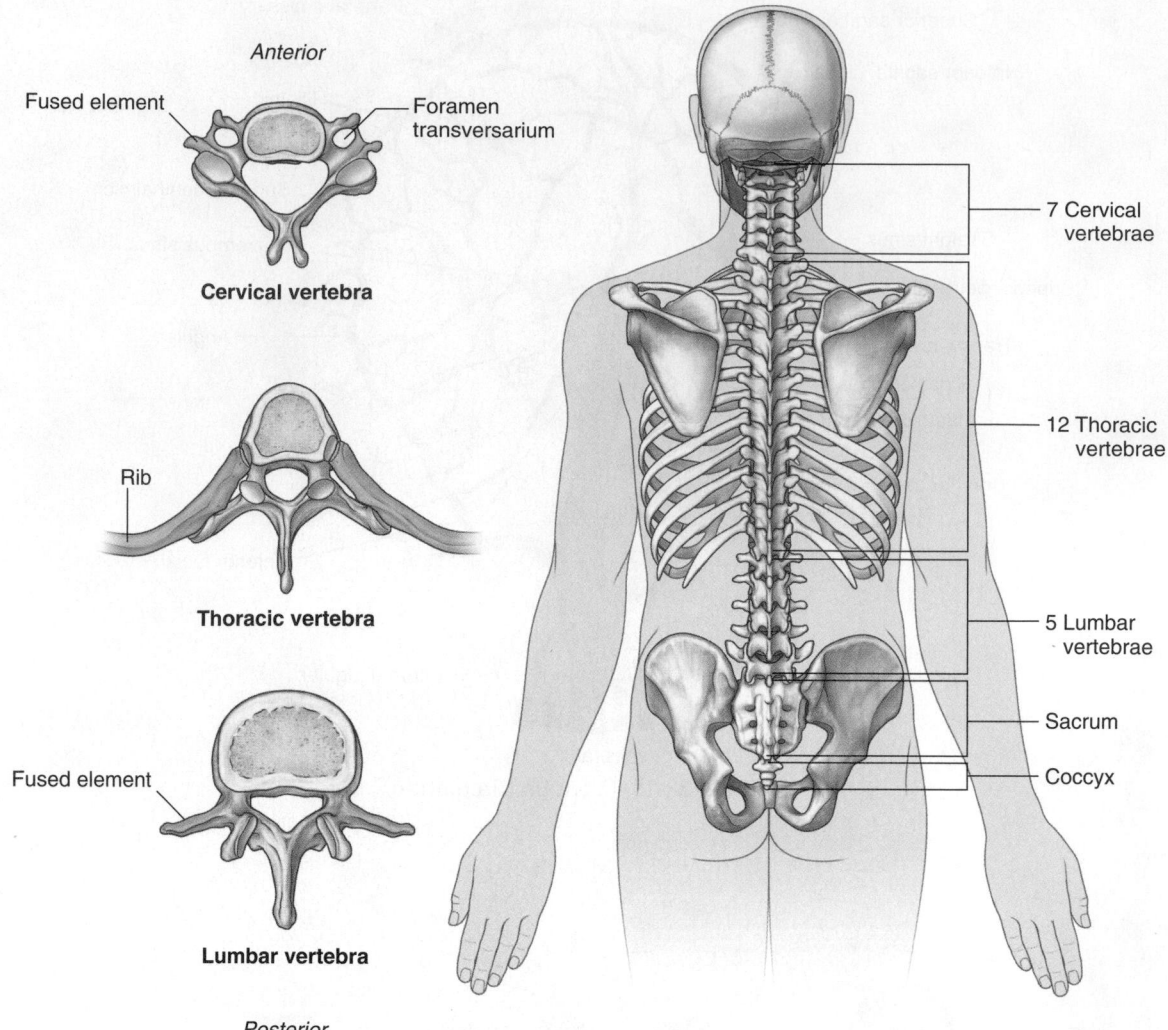

Anterior

Fused element — — Foramen transversarium

Cervical vertebra

Rib —

Thoracic vertebra

Fused element —

Lumbar vertebra

Posterior

7 Cervical vertebrae

12 Thoracic vertebrae

5 Lumbar vertebrae

Sacrum

Coccyx

FIGURE 22-21 **Vertebrae.** (From Drake RL, et al. *Gray's Anatomy for Students.* 2nd ed. London: Churchill Livingstone; 2009.)

Bony Structures

The bony structure that encases the spinal cord is the vertebral column. Comprising 33 vertebrae and 24 intervertebral disks, this column is held together by ligaments and tendons. It provides support and protection for the spinal cord and the structure and flexibility required for body movement. The vertebrae are divided into sections in relation to their appearance (Fig. 22-21). There are 7 cervical vertebrae, 12 thoracic vertebrae, 5 lumbar vertebrae, 5 sacral vertebrae (fused together as one), and 4 coccygeal vertebrae (fused together as one).[1,2]

Although differences in vertebral appearance exist, the basic structure includes a vertebral body connected by two pedicles to the transverse processes. Two laminae connect the transverse processes to the posterior segment of the vertebra, the spinous process, forming a ring. The center of the spinal foramen is the canal housing the spinal cord.[1,2]

Intervertebral Disk

Vertebral bodies are separated by an intervertebral disk. These fibrocartilaginous structures lie between each vertebral body,

extending from the cervical vertebra to the beginning of the sacrum. Intervertebral disks are composed of two layers. The inner core, called the *nucleus pulposus*, is a soft, gelatinous material that assists in shock absorbency. Surrounding the nucleus pulposus is the annulus fibrosus, a thick, tough outer layer.[1,2] The diagnosis of herniated disk refers to dislocation of the normal anatomic position of an intervertebral disk that compromises or puts pressure on a spinal nerve.[35]

Meninges

The meninges of the spinal cord are similar to those in the cranium (Fig. 22-22). The dura is a continuation of the intracranial dura mater, and it encases the cord, the nerve roots, and the spinal nerves until they exit from the vertebral column. The dura extends to the level of the second sacral vertebra, even though the spinal cord itself ends at the L1 or L2 level.[1,2]

The arachnoid mater provides the same weblike, delicate structure as in the cranium, with CSF flow within the subarachnoid space. Because the spinal cord terminates at L2 and the meninges continue to S2, a volume of CSF is contained in the

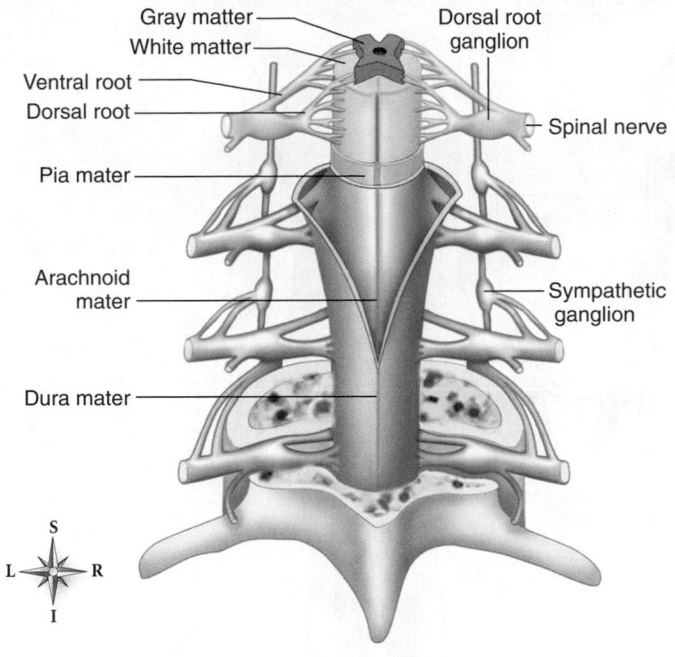

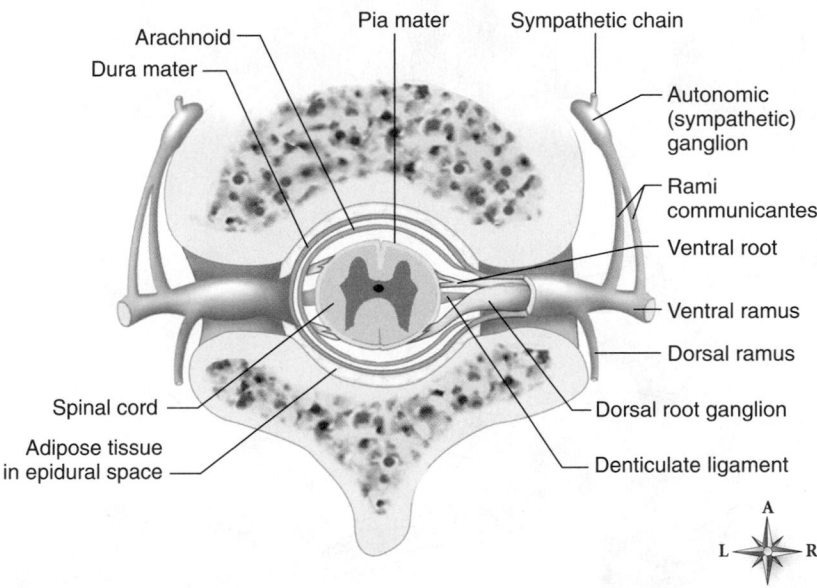

FIGURE 22-22 **Coverings of the Spinal Cord.** The dura mater is shown in purple. Note how it extends to cover the spinal nerve roots and nerves. The arachnoid is highlighted in pink and the pia mater in orange. (From Patton KT, Thibodeau GF. *Anatomy and Physiology*. 8th ed. Philadelphia: Mosby; 2013.)

lumbar cistern, and it constitutes the site targeted for a lumbar puncture. The pia mater of the spinal cord is a thicker, firmer, less vascular membrane than that in the cranium.[1,2]

Spinal Nerves

The 31 pairs of spinal nerves comprise: 8 cervical, 12 thoracic, 5 lumbar, 5 sacral, and 1 coccygeal (see Fig. 22-20). In the cervical region, the first seven pairs of nerves exit the cord above the corresponding vertebrae. The C8 nerve pair exits the spinal cord below the C7 vertebra. From this point on, all thoracic, lumbar, and sacral nerves exit below the corresponding vertebrae.[1,2] In

other words, spinal cord segments associated with each spinal nerve and the corresponding vertebra do not directly line up.

The spinal nerve has two roots: 1) the dorsal root and 2) the ventral root. The dorsal root is an afferent pathway that carries sensory impulses from the body into the spinal cord. The ventral root is an efferent pathway that carries motor information from the spinal cord to the body. The dorsal and ventral roots join together as they exit the spinal foramen and become a spinal nerve (see Fig. 22-22).[1,2] Distribution of the sensory components of each spinal nerve are illustrated as dermatomes. Dermatome diagrams facilitate identification of sensory innervation throughout the body (Fig. 22-23).[1]

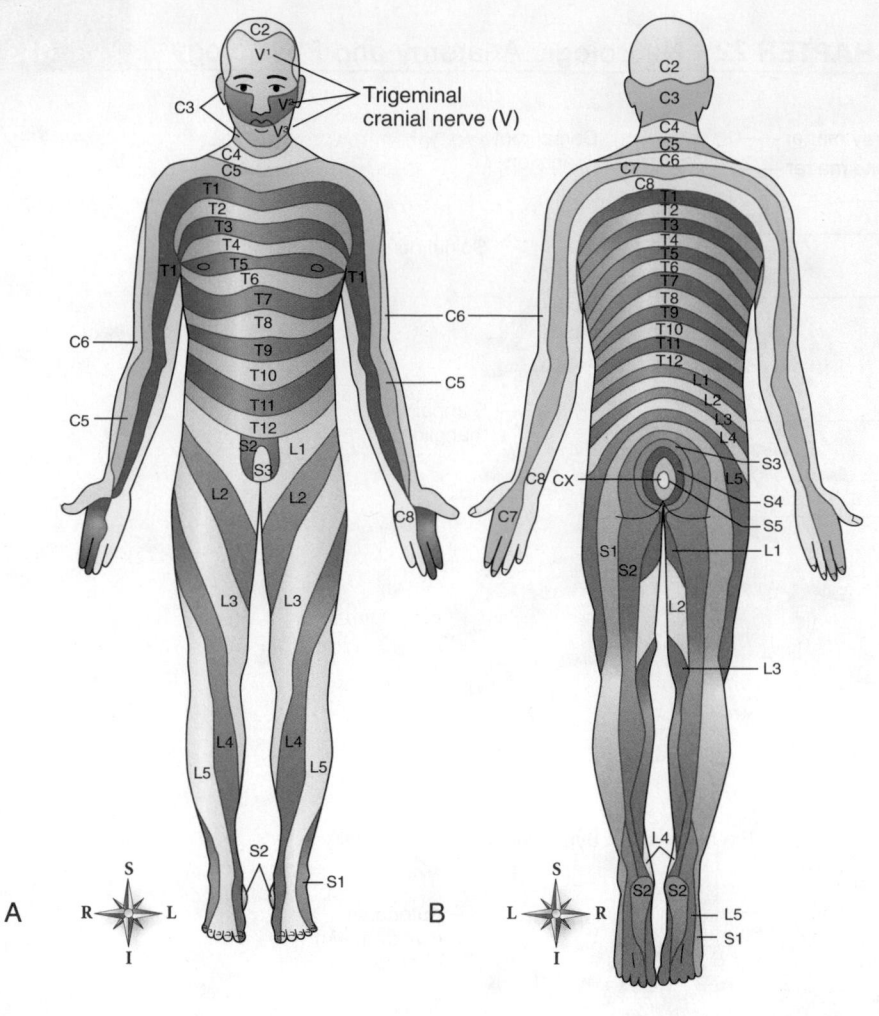

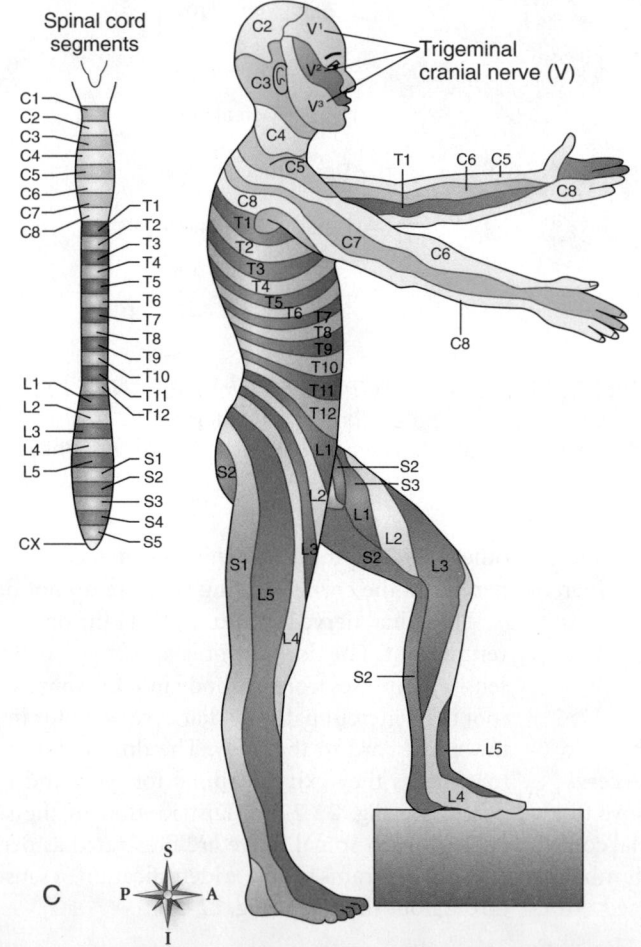

FIGURE 22-23 Dermatome Distribution of Spinal Nerves. *A,* The front of the body's surface. *B,* The back of the body's surface. *C,* The side of the body's surface. The inset shows the segments of the spinal cord connected with each of the spinal nerves associated with the sensory dermatomes shown. *C,* Cervical segments and spinal nerves; *L,* lumbar segments and spinal nerves; *S,* sacral segments and spinal nerves; *T,* thoracic segments and spinal nerves. (From Patton KT, Thibodeau GA. *Anatomy and Physiology.* 8th ed. St. Louis: Mosby; 2013.)

Cross-Section of the Spinal Cord

The spinal cord is composed of gray matter and white matter. The central gray matter, which appears in the shape of an H, consists of cell bodies, small projection fibers, and glial support cells. The gray matter of the spinal cord has been divided into areas based on cell body type and location. The three main divisions are: 1) the anterior horn, 2) the lateral horn, and 3) the posterior horn. The anterior horn contains motor neurons and is the final junction for motor information before it exits the CNS. The lateral horn contains preganglionic fibers of the autonomic nervous system: sympathetic fibers T1 to L2 and parasympathetic fibers S2 to S4. The posterior horn contains sensory neurons and becomes the entry point for afferent impulses to the CNS.[1,2]

The white matter, which surrounds the gray matter, contains the myelinated ascending and descending tracts, which carry information to and from the brain (Fig. 22-24). Spinal tracts are named in such a way that the prefix denotes the origin of the tract and the suffix is the destination, promoting easy identification of sensory or motor tracts.[1,2] Sensory tracts begin with the prefix *spino-* and motor tracts end with the suffix *-spinal* (Tables 22-4 and 22-5). The complexity of spinal cord tracts is beyond the scope of this chapter, which is limited to the tracts that are most clinically significant and easily tested.

Vascular Supply

Arterial blood supply to the spinal cord is provided by branches of the vertebral arteries and small radicular arteries that enter through intervertebral foramina. They combine to form the anterior spinal and two posterior spinal arteries. These three arteries, along with some additional radicular arterial flow from cervical, intercostal, lumbar, and sacral arteries, feed the entire length of the spinal cord (Fig. 22-25).[1,2]

Arterial supply to the spinal cord is segmented at best, making portions of the spinal cord that receive blood supply from two separate sources vulnerable to low-flow states. The most vulnerable of these areas are C2 to C3, T1 to T4, and L1 to L2. Evidence of this tenuous blood supply is occasionally evident after surgical procedures that involve cross-clamping of the aorta, resulting in spinal cord infarction.[36]

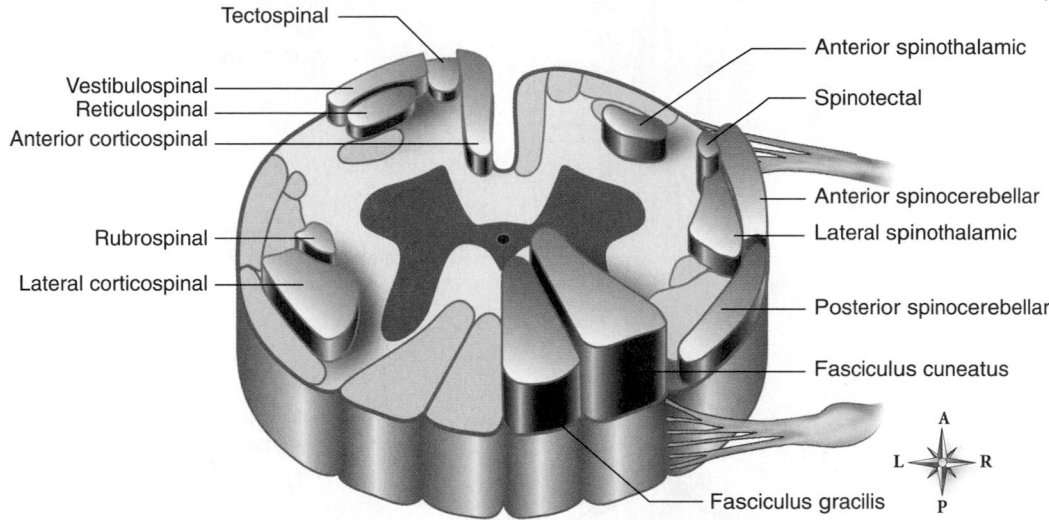

FIGURE 22-24 Spinal cord tracts of the white matter. (From Patton KT, Thibodeau GF. *Anatomy and Physiology.* 8th ed. St. Louis: Mosby; 2013.)

TABLE 22-4 MAJOR ASCENDING TRACTS OF SPINAL CORD

NAME	FUNCTION	LOCATION	ORIGIN*	TERMINATION†
Lateral spinothalamic	Pain, temperature, and crude touch on opposite side	Lateral white columns	Posterior gray column on opposite side	Thalamus
Anterior spinothalamic	Crude touch and pressure	Anterior white columns	Posterior gray column on opposite side	Thalamus
Fasciculi gracilis and cuneatus	Discriminating touch and pressure sensations, including vibration, stereognosis, and two-point discrimination; also conscious kinesthesia	Posterior white columns	Spinal ganglia on same side	Medulla
Anterior and posterior spinocerebellar	Unconscious kinesthesia	Lateral white columns	Anterior or posterior gray column	Cerebellum
Spinotectal	Touch related to visual reflexes	Lateral white columns	Posterior gray columns	Superior colliculus (midbrain)

From Patton KT, Thibodeau GA. *Anatomy and Physiology.* 8th ed. St. Louis: Mosby; 2013.
*Location of cell bodies of neurons from which axons of tract arise.
†Structure in which axons of tract terminate.

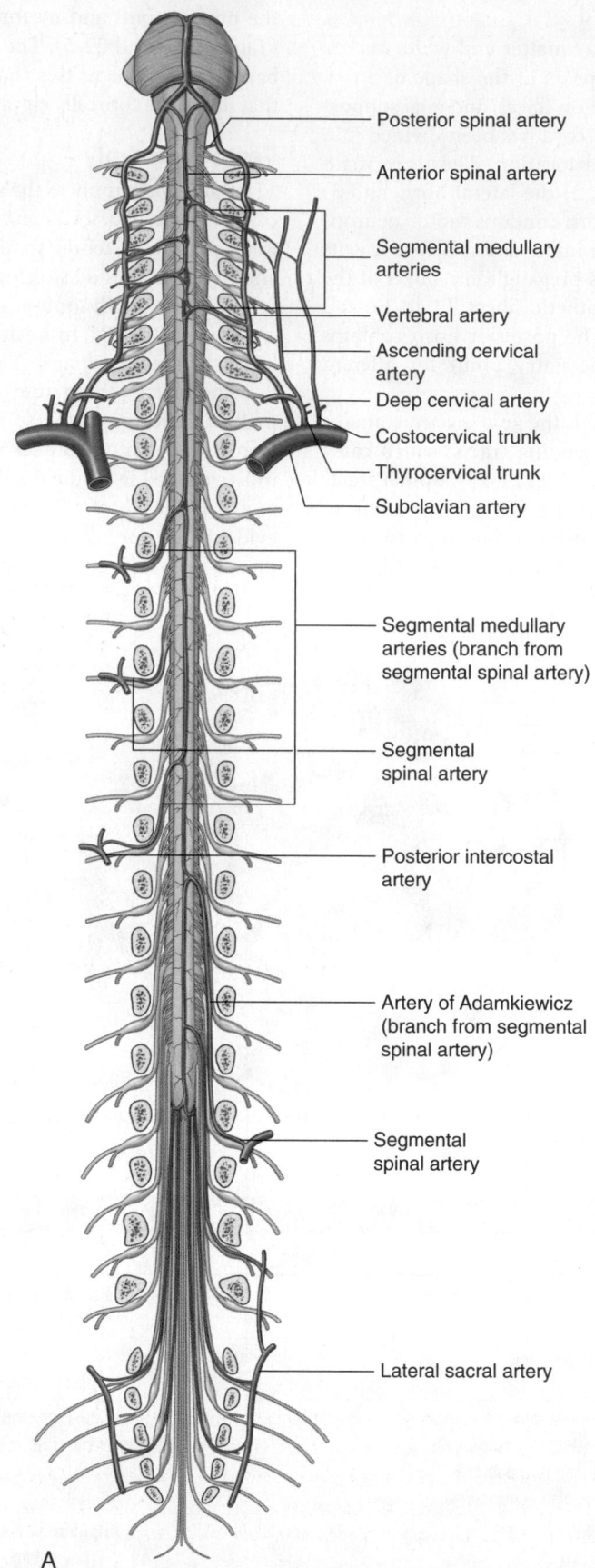

Posterior spinal artery

Anterior spinal artery

Segmental medullary arteries

Vertebral artery

Ascending cervical artery

Deep cervical artery

Costocervical trunk

Thyrocervical trunk

Subclavian artery

Segmental medullary arteries (branch from segmental spinal artery)

Segmental spinal artery

Posterior intercostal artery

Artery of Adamkiewicz (branch from segmental spinal artery)

Segmental spinal artery

Lateral sacral artery

A

FIGURE 22-25   **Arteries That Supply the Spinal Cord.** *A,* Anterior view of spinal cord (not all segmental spinal arteries are shown).

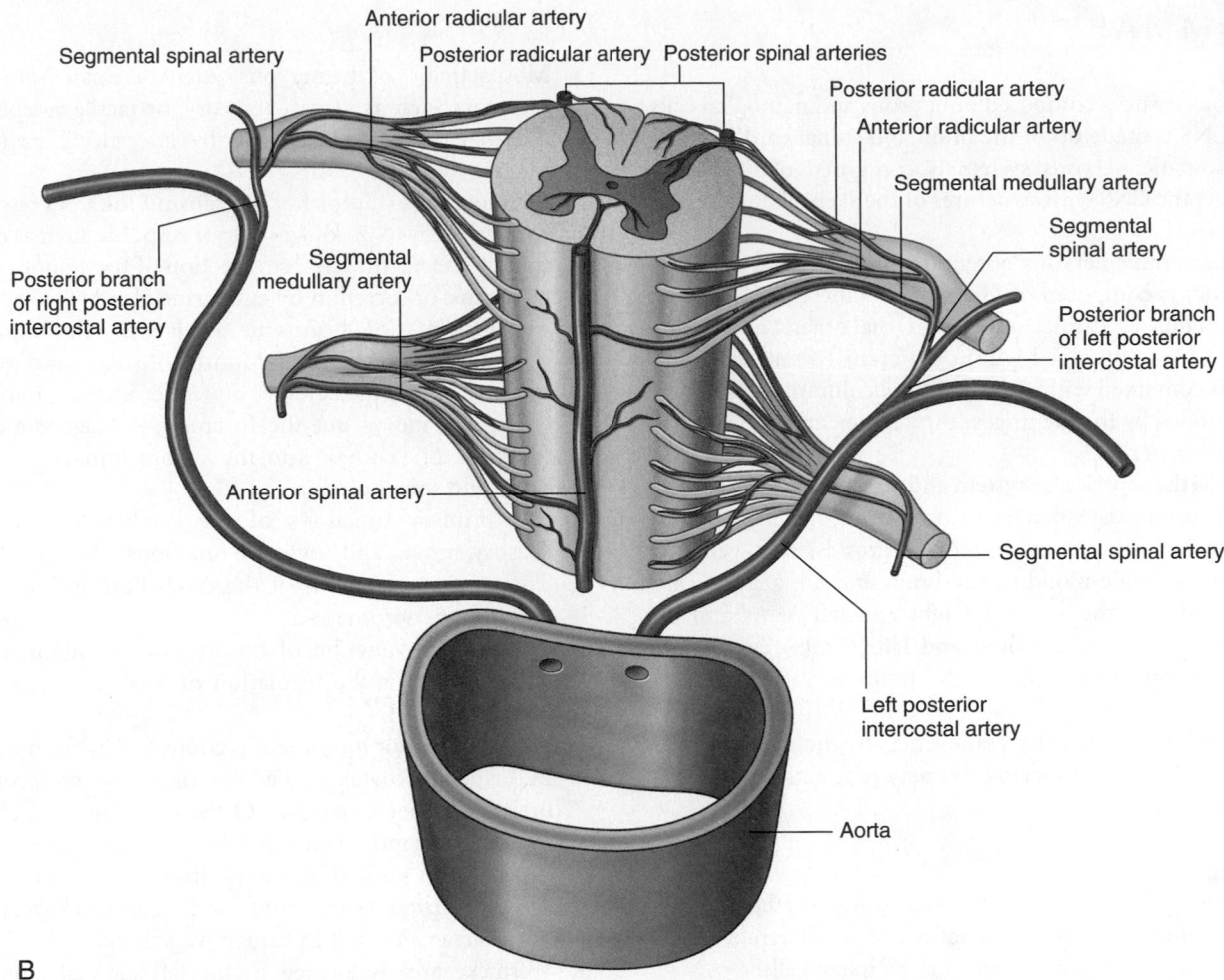

Anterior radicular artery
Segmental spinal artery
Posterior radicular artery Posterior spinal arteries
Posterior radicular artery
Anterior radicular artery
Segmental medullary artery
Segmental spinal artery
Posterior branch of right posterior intercostal artery
Segmental medullary artery
Posterior branch of left posterior intercostal artery
Anterior spinal artery
Segmental spinal artery
Left posterior intercostal artery
Aorta

B

FIGURE 22-25, cont'd. *B,* Segmental supply of spinal cord. (From Drake RL, et al. *Gray's Anatomy for Students.* 2nd ed. London: Churchill Livingstone; 2009.)

TABLE 22-5 MAJOR DESCENDING TRACTS OF SPINAL CORD

NAME	FUNCTION	LOCATION	ORIGIN*	TERMINATION†
Lateral corticospinal (or crossed pyramidal)	Voluntary movement, contraction of individual or small groups of muscles, particularly those moving hands, fingers, feet, and toes of opposite side	Lateral white columns	Motor areas or cerebral cortex of opposite side from tract location in cord	Lateral or anterior gray columns
Anterior corticospinal (direct pyramidal)	Same as lateral corticospinal except mainly muscles of same side	Anterior white columns	Motor cortex but on same side as location in cord	Lateral or anterior gray columns
Reticulospinal	Maintain posture during movement	Anterior white columns	Reticular formation (midbrain, pons, medulla)	Anterior gray columns
Rubrospinal	Coordination of body movement and posture	Lateral white columns	Red nucleus (of midbrain)	Anterior gray columns
Tectospinal	Head and neck movement during visual reflexes	Anterior white columns	Superior colliculus (midbrain)	Medulla and anterior gray columns
Vestibulospinal	Coordination of posture or balance	Anterior white columns	Vestibular nucleus (pons, medulla)	Anterior gray columns

*Location of cell bodies of neurons from which axons of tract arise.
†Structure in which axons of tract terminate.

SUMMARY

Anatomy

- Nervous tissue is composed of neurons and neuroglial cells.
- The CNS is made up of the brain and spinal cord.
- The somatic nervous system is composed of fibers that connect the CNS with structures of the skeletal muscles and the skin.
- The autonomic nervous system (sympathetic and parasympathetic) is composed of fibers that connect the CNS with smooth muscle, cardiac muscle, internal organs, and glands.
- The brain is contained within the cranial vault, the spinal cord is contained within the vertebral column, and both are surrounded by the meninges (dura mater, arachnoid mater, and pia mater).
- CSF fills the ventricular system and surrounds the brain and spinal cord in the subarachnoid space.
- Two pairs of arteries (internal carotids and vertebral arteries) provide blood to the brain and are anatomically separated into the anterior (right and left ACAs and the ACoA) and posterior (right and left PCoAs) circulations that connect at the base of the brain to form the circle of Willis.
- The PNS comprises the cranial nerves, the spinal nerves, and all other nerves serving a variety of functions throughout the body.

Physiology

- Neurons perform the functional work of the nervous system, including receipt of information, integration, and transmission of nerve impulses to recipient cells.
- Neuroglial cells (astrocytes, oligodendroglia, ependyma, and microglia) serve as the support infrastructure of the nervous system, providing protection, structural support, and neuronal repair.

- Most activities of the nervous system originate from sensory receptors such as visual, auditory, or tactile receptors and are transmitted to the CNS by afferent fibers (sensory fibers).
- Efferent fibers (motor fibers) transmit the CNS response to the periphery to produce a motor response such as contraction of skeletal muscles, contraction of the smooth muscles of organs, or secretion by endocrine glands.
- The flow of CSF begins in the lateral ventricles, moves through the foramina of Monro into the third ventricle, moves through the cerebral aqueduct into the fourth ventricle, and moves out the foramen of Magendie and the foramina of Luschka into the subarachnoid space of the brain and spinal cord.
- The primary functions of the cerebral cortex include sensory, motor, and cognitive functions.
- The primary functions of the cerebellum include balance and motor coordination.
- The primary function of the brainstem (midbrain, pons, and medulla) is the regulation of vital functions such as breathing.
- Voluntary motor movement is controlled by the motor strip in the frontal cortex, and as the tracts descend through the brainstem, they cross over to the opposite side. The right motor strip controls the left side of the body, and vice versa.
- Broca area is located in the left frontal lobe and is responsible for expression of written and verbal language. Damage to the area can result in expressive aphasia.
- Wernicke area is located in the left parietal lobe and is responsible for reception of written and verbal language. Damage to the area can result in receptive aphasia.
- The circle of Willis provides collateral blood flow to the brain.

REFERENCES

1. Patton KT, Thibodeau GA. *Anatomy and Physiology*. ed. 8. St. Louis: Mosby; 2013.
2. FitzGerald MJT, et al. *Clinical Neuroanatomy and Neuroscience*. 5th ed. Philadephia: Elsevier; 2007.
3. Koeppen BM, Stanton BA. *Berne and Levy: Physiology*. 6th ed. Philadelphia: Mosby; 2010.
4. Hall JE. *Guyton and Hall Textbook of Medical Physiology*. 12th ed. Philadelphia: Saunders; 2011.
5. Fouad K, Tse A. Adaptive changes in the injured spinal cord and their role in promoting functional recovery. *Neurol Res*. 2008;30:17.
6. Chopp M, et al. Plasticity and remodeling of the brain. *J Neurol Sci*. 2008;265(1-2):97.
7. Nudo RJ. Neural bases of recovery after brain injury. *J Commun Disord*. 2011;44:515.
8. Stuart G, et al. *Dendrites*. 2nd ed. New York: Oxford University Press; 2008.
9. Aggarwal S, et al. Central nervous system myelin: structure, synthesis and assembly. *Trends Cell Biol*. 2011;21:585.
10. Mohindra S, et al. Importance of an intact dura in management of compound elevated fractures; a short series and literature review. *Brain Inj*. 2012;26:194.
11. Patel N, Kirmi O. Anatomy and imaging of the normal meninges. *Semin Ultrasound CT MR*. 2009;30:559.
12. Dainer HM, Smirniotopoulos JG. Neuroimaging of hemorrhage and vascular malformations. *Semin Neurol*. 2008;28:533.
13. Sakka L, et al. Anatomy and physiology of cerebrospinal fluid. *Eur Ann Otorhinolaryngol Head Neck Dis*. 2011;128:309.
14. Rekate HL. A consensus on the classification of hydrocephalus: its utility in the assessment of abnormalities of cerebrospinal fluid dynamics. *Childs Nerv Syst*. 2011;27:1535.
15. Bergsneider M, et al. Surgical management of adult hydrocephalus. *Neurosurgery*. 2008;62(Suppl 2):643.
16. American Association of Neuroscience Nurses. *Guide to the care of the patient undergoing intracranial pressure monitoring/external ventricular drainage or lumbardrainage: AANN clinical practice guideline series*. Glenview: The Association; 2011.
17. Mahringer A, et al. The ABC of the blood-brain barrier-regulation of drug efflux pumps. *Curr Pharm Des*. 2011;17:2762.

18. Bednarczyk J, Lukasiuk K. Tight junctions in neurological diseases. *Acta Neurobiol Exp (Wars).* 2011;71:393.

19. Palmer AM. The role of the blood-CNS barrier in CNS disorders and their treatment. *Neurobiol Dis.* 2010;37:3.

20. Rhoton AL Jr. The cerebrum. Anatomy. *Neurosurgery.* 2007;61(1 Suppl):37.

21. Stuss DT. Traumatic brain injury: relation to executive dysfunction and the frontal lobes. *Curr Opin Neurol.* 2011;24:584.

22. Samara A, Tsangaris GT. Brain asymmetry: both sides of the story. *Expert Rev Proteomics.* 2011;8:693.

23. Fadiga L, et al. Broca's area in language, action, and music. *Ann N Y Acad Sci.* 2009;1169:448.

24. Gainotti G. What the study of voice recognition in normal subjects and brain-damaged patients tells us about models of familiar people recognition. *Neuropsychologia.* 2011;49:2273.

25. Ono T, Galanopoulou AS. Epilepsy and epileptic syndrome. *Adv Exp Med Biol.* 2012;724:99.

26. Flanagan C. Cerebral blindness. *Int Ophthalmol Clin.* 2009;49:15.

27. Roxo MR. The limbic system conception and its historical evolution. *Scientific World J.* 2011;11:2428.

28. Hiraga A. Pure motor monoparesis due to ischemic stroke. *Neurologist.* 2011;17:301.

29. Rothwell JC. The motor functions of the basal ganglia. *J Integr Neurosci.* 2011;10:303.

30. Amici S. Thalamic infarcts and hemorrhages. *Front Neurol Neurosci.* 2012;30:132.

31. Timmann D, et al. The human cerebellum contributes to motor, emotional and cognitive associative learning. A review. *Cortex.* 2010;46:845.

32. Bastian AJ. Moving, sensing and learning with cerebellar damage. *Curr Opin Neurobiol.* 2011;21:596.

33. Young GB. Coma. *Ann N Y Acad Sci.* 2009;1157:32.

34. Zivin JA. Approach to cerebrovascular disease. In: Goldman L, Schafer AI, eds. *Goldman's Cecil Medicine.* 2nd ed. Philadelphia: Elsevier; 2012.

35. Rhee JM, et al. Radiculopathy and the herniated lumbar disk: controversies regarding pathophysiology and management. *Instr Course Lect.* 2007;56:287.

36. Setacci F. Endovascular thoracic aortic repair and risk of spinal cord ischemia: the role of previous or concomitant treatment for aortic aneurysm. *J Cardiovasc Surg (Torino).* 2010;51:169.

CHAPTER

23

Neurologic Clinical Assessment and Diagnostic Procedures

Darlene M. Burke

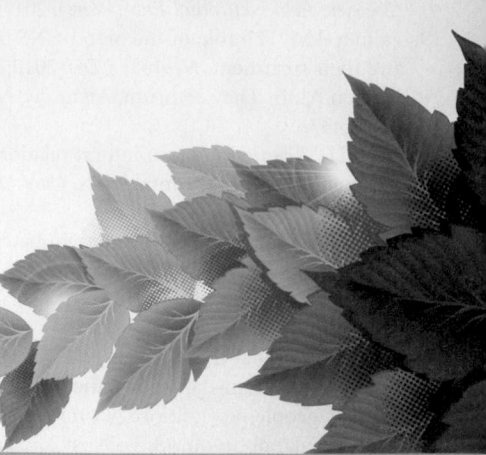

evolve WEBSITE

http://evolve.elsevier.com/Urden/criticalcare/

Evolve features:
- NCLEX Review Questions
- CCRN Review Questions
- PCCN Review Questions
- Mosby's Nursing Skills Procedures
- Animations
- Video Clips
- Glossary

Assessment of the critically ill patient with neurologic dysfunction includes a review of the patient's health history, a thorough physical examination, and an analysis of the patient's laboratory data. Numerous invasive and noninvasive diagnostic procedures may also be performed to assist in the identification of the patient's disorder. This chapter focuses on clinical assessments, laboratory studies, and diagnostic procedures for the critically ill patient with a neurologic dysfunction.

CLINICAL ASSESSMENT

A thorough clinical assessment of the critically ill patient with neurologic dysfunction is imperative for the early identification and treatment of a neurologic disorder and serves as source of comparison for ongoing assessments of the patient. The most important finding in any neurologic assessment is change, which should be reported promptly. Early identification of neurologic deterioration is vital to preventing secondary brain injury.[1] Other medical conditions, as well as the administration of medications, can affect the clinical assessment and should be taken into consideration when the results of the neurologic examination are abnormal.

HISTORY

Common to all neurologic assessments is the need to obtain a comprehensive history of events preceding hospitalization. An adequate neurologic history includes information about clinical manifestations, associated complaints, precipitating factors, progression, and familial occurrences (Box 23-1).[2] The ideal historian for recounting this information is someone who is able to provide a detailed description and chronology of events. If the patient is incapable of serving as the historian, family members or significant others who have contact with the patient on a daily basis should be contacted as soon as possible. Through history taking, the caregiver gains valuable information that directs him or her to focus on certain aspects of the patient's clinical assessment.[3]

PHYSICAL EXAMINATION

Five major components make up the neurologic evaluation of the critically ill patient: 1) level of consciousness, 2) motor function, 3) pupillary function, 4) respiratory function, and 5) vital signs. A complete neurologic examination requires assessment of all five components.[3,4]

Level of Consciousness

Assessment of the level of consciousness is the most important aspect of the neurologic examination. In most situations, a patient's level of consciousness deteriorates before any other neurologic changes are noticed. These deteriorations often are subtle and must be monitored carefully. Assessment of level of consciousness focuses on two areas: 1) evaluation of arousal or alertness and 2) appraisal of content of consciousness or awareness.[3,5] Although universally accepted definitions for various levels of consciousness do not exist, the categories outlined in Box 23-2 are often used to describe the patient's level of consciousness.[3,4,6]

BOX 23-1 DATA COLLECTION

Neurologic History

Common Neurologic Symptoms
- Fainting
- Dizziness
- Blackouts
- Seizures
- Headache
- Memory loss
- Weakness
- Paralysis
- Tremors or other involuntary movements
- Pain
- Numbness
- Tingling
- Speech disturbances
- Vision disturbances

Events Preceding Onset of Symptoms
- Travel
- Animal contact
- Falls
- Infection
- Dental problems or procedures
- Sinus or middle ear infections
- Prodromal symptoms
- Food or drugs ingested

Progression of Symptoms
- Initial onset
- Evolution
- Frequency
- Severity
- Duration
- Associated activities or aggravating factors

Family History
- Stroke (arteriovenous malformation, aneurysm)
- Diabetes mellitus
- Hypertension
- Seizures
- Tumors
- Headaches
- Emotional problems or depression

Medical History
Child
- Birth injuries, congenital defects, encephalitis, meningitis, bedwetting, fainting, seizures, trauma

Adult
- Diabetes; hypertension; cardiovascular, pulmonary, kidney, liver, or endocrine disease; tuberculosis; tropical infection; sinusitis; visual problems; tumors; psychiatric disorders

Surgical History
- Neurologic, ear-nose-throat, dental, eye surgery

Traumatic History
- Motor vehicle accidents, falls, blows to the head, neck or back, being knocked out

Allergies
- Drug, food, environment

Patient Profile
- Personal habits
  - Use of alcohol, recreational drugs, over-the-counter medications, smoking, dietary habits, sleeping patterns, elimination patterns, exercise habits
- Recent life changes
- Living conditions
- Working conditions
- Exposure to toxins, chemicals, fumes; occupational duties
- General temperament

Current Medication Use
- Sedatives, tranquilizers
- Anticonvulsants
- Psychotropics
- Anticoagulants
- Antibiotics
- Calcium channel blockers
- Beta-blockers
- Nitrates
- Oral contraceptives

Evaluation of Arousal

Assessment of the arousal component of consciousness is an evaluation of the reticular activating system and its connection to the thalamus and the cerebral cortex. Arousal is the lowest level of consciousness, and observation centers on the patient's ability to respond to verbal or noxious stimuli in an appropriate manner.[5] To stimulate the patient, the nurse should begin with verbal stimuli in a normal tone. If the patient does not respond, the nurse should increase the stimuli by talking very loudly to the patient. If the patient still does not respond, the nurse should further increase the stimuli by shaking the patient. Noxious stimuli should follow if previous attempts to arouse the patient are unsuccessful. To assess arousal, central stimulation techniques should be used (Box 23-3).[3]

Appraisal of Awareness

Content of consciousness is a higher-level function, and appraisal of awareness is concerned with assessment of the patient's orientation to person, place, time, and situation.[5] Assessment of content of consciousness requires the patient to give appropriate answers to a variety of questions. Changes in the patient's answers that indicate increasing degrees of confusion and disorientation may be the first sign of neurologic deterioration.[2,3]

Glasgow Coma Scale

The most widely recognized tool for assessing level of consciousness tool is the Glasgow Coma Scale (GCS).[7] This scored scale is based on evaluation of three categories: 1) eye opening,

BOX 23-2	**CATEGORIES OF CONSCIOUSNESS**
Alert	Patient responds immediately to minimal external stimuli.
Confused	Patient is disoriented to time or place but usually oriented to person, with impaired judgment and decision making and decreased attention span.
Delirious	Patient is disoriented to time, place, and person, with loss of contact with reality, and often has auditory or visual hallucinations.
Lethargic	Patient displays a state of drowsiness or inaction, in which the patient needs an increased stimulus to be awakened.
Obtunded	Patient displays dull indifference to external stimuli, and response is minimally maintained. Questions are answered with a minimal response.
Stuporous	Patient can be aroused only by vigorous and continuous external stimuli. Motor response is often withdrawal or localizing to stimulus.
Comatose	Vigorous stimulation fails to produce any voluntary neural response.

From Barker E. *Neuroscience Nursing: A Spectrum of Care.* 3rd ed. St. Louis: Mosby; 2008.

BOX 23-3 STIMULATION TECHNIQUES IN PATIENT AROUSAL

Central Stimulation
- *Trapezius pinch:* Squeeze trapezius muscle between thumb and first two fingers.
- *Sternal rub:* Apply firm pressure to sternum with knuckles, using a rubbing motion.

Peripheral Stimulation
- *Nail bed pressure:* Apply firm pressure, using object such as a pen, to nail bed.
- *Pinching of inner aspect of arm or leg:* Firmly pinch small portion of patient's tissue on sensitive inner aspect of arm or leg.

2) verbal response, and 3) best motor response (Table 23-1). The highest possible score on the GCS is 15, and the lowest score is 3. A score of 7 or less on the GCS usually indicates coma. Originally, the scoring system was developed to assist in general communication concerning the severity of neurologic injury. Recently, however, the usefulness of the GCS has been called into question, particularly because of poor inter-rater reliability.[8] Several points should be kept in mind when the GCS is used for serial assessment. It provides data about level of consciousness only, and it never should be considered a complete neurologic examination. Additionally, it is not a sensitive tool for evaluation of an altered sensorium, and it does not account for possible aphasia or mechanical intubation. It is also a poor indicator of lateralization of neurologic deterioration.[9] *Lateralization* involves decreasing motor response on one side or unilateral changes in pupillary reaction.

Motor Function

Assessment of motor function focuses on muscle size and tone and on an estimation of muscle strength. Each side should be assessed individually and then compared with the other.[3,10]

Evaluation of Muscle Size and Tone

Initially, muscles should be inspected for size and shape. The presence of atrophy is noted. Muscle tone is assessed by evaluating opposition to passive movement. The patient is instructed to relax the extremity while the nurse performs passive range-of-motion movements and evaluates the degree of resistance. Muscle tone is appraised for signs of flaccidity (no resistance), hypotonia (little resistance), hypertonia (increased resistance), spasticity, or rigidity.[6]

Estimation of Muscle Strength

Having the patient perform a number of movements against resistance assesses muscle strength. The strength of the movement is then graded on a six-point scale (Box 23-4). The patient is asked to extend both arms with the palms turned upward and to hold that position with the eyes closed. If the patient has a

TABLE 23-1 GLASGOW COMA SCALE

CATEGORY	SCORE	RESPONSE
Eye Opening	4	Spontaneous: Eyes open spontaneously without stimulation
	3	To speech: Eyes open with verbal stimulation but not necessarily to command
	2	To pain: Eyes open with noxious stimuli
	1	None: No eye opening regardless of stimulation
Verbal Response	5	Oriented: Accurate information about person, place, time, reason for hospitalization, and personal data
	4	Confused: Answers not appropriate to question, but use of language is correct
	3	Inappropriate words: Disorganized, random speech, no sustained conversation
	2	Incomprehensible sounds: Moans, groans, and incomprehensible mumbles
	1	None: No verbalization despite stimulation
Best Motor Response	6	Obeys commands: Performs simple tasks on command; able to repeat performance
	5	Localizes to pain: Organized attempt to localize and remove painful stimuli
	4	Withdraws from pain: Withdraws extremity from source of painful stimuli
	3	Abnormal flexion: Decorticate posturing spontaneously or in response to noxious stimuli
	2	Extension: Decerebrate posturing spontaneously or in response to noxious stimuli
	1	None: No response to noxious stimuli; flaccid

BOX 23-4 MUSCLE STRENGTH GRADING SCALE

- 0/5 –No movement or muscle contraction
- 1/5 –Trace contraction
- 2/5 –Active movement with gravity eliminated
- 3/5 –Active movement against gravity
- 4/5 –Active movement with some resistance
- 5/5 –Active movement with full resistance

BOX 23-5 CLASSIFICATION OF ABNORMAL MOTOR FUNCTION

Spontaneous	Occurs without regard to external stimuli and may not occur by request
Localization	Occurs when the extremity opposite the extremity receiving pain crosses midline of the body in an attempt to remove the noxious stimulus from the affected limb
Withdrawal	Occurs when the extremity receiving the painful stimulus flexes normally in an attempt to avoid the noxious stimulus
Decortication	Abnormal flexion response that may occur spontaneously or in response to noxious stimuli (see Fig. 23-1A and C)
Decerebration	Abnormal extension response that may occur spontaneously or in response to noxious stimuli (see Fig. 23-1B and C)
Flaccid	No response to painful stimuli

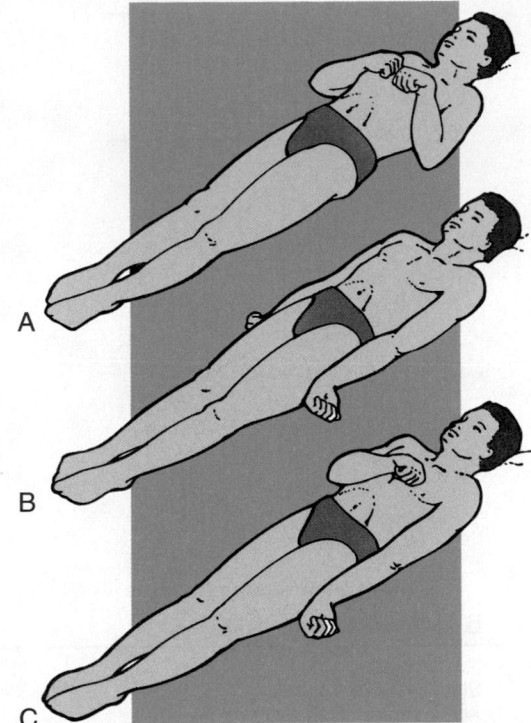

FIGURE 23-1 Abnormal Motor Responses. *A*, Decorticate posturing. *B*, Decerebrate posturing. *C*, Decorticate posturing on right side and decerebrate posturing on left side of body.

weaker side, that arm will drift downward and pronate. The lower extremities are tested by asking the patient to push and pull the feet against resistance or to elevate the legs.[6]

Abnormal Motor Responses

If the patient is incapable of comprehending and following a simple command, noxious stimuli are necessary to determine motor responses. The stimulus is applied to each extremity separately to allow evaluation of individual extremity function. Peripheral stimulation is used to assess motor function (see Box 23-2).[3,4] Motor responses elicited by noxious stimuli are interpreted differently from those elicited by voluntary demonstration.[3] These responses may be classified as shown in Box 23-5.

Abnormal flexion also is known as *decorticate posturing* (Fig. 23-1A). In response to painful stimuli, the upper extremities exhibit flexion of the arm, wrist, and fingers, with adduction of the limb. The lower extremity exhibits extension, internal rotation, and plantar flexion. Abnormal flexion occurs with lesions above the midbrain, located in the region of the thalamus or cerebral hemispheres. Abnormal extension also is known as *decerebrate rigidity* or *posturing* (see Fig. 23-1B); when the patient is stimulated, teeth clench, and the arms are stiffly extended, adducted, and hyperpronated. The legs are stiffly extended, with plantar flexion of the feet. Abnormal extension occurs with lesions in the area of the brainstem.[10] Because abnormal flexion and extension appear similar in the lower extremities, the upper extremities are noted to determine the presence of these abnormal movements. It is possible for the patient to exhibit abnormal flexion on one side of the body and

extension on the other (see Fig. 23-1C).[3,4] Outcome studies indicate abnormal flexion, which has a less serious prognosis than does extension, or decerebrate posturing.[10] Onset of posturing or a change from abnormal flexion to abnormal extension requires immediate physician notification.

Evaluation of Reflexes

Deep tendon reflexes (DTRs) are usually evaluated by a physician when a complete neurologic evaluation is performed. DTRs are tested by tapping the appropriate tendon using a reflex or percussion hammer. The muscle needs to be relaxed and the joint at midposition for reflex testing to be accurate.[5] The four reflexes tested are: 1) the Achilles (ankle jerk), 2) the quadriceps (knee jerk), 3) the biceps, and 4) the triceps. DTRs are graded on a scale from 0 (absent) to 4 (hyperactive). A DTR grade of 2 is normal (Fig. 23-2). Hyper-reflexia is associated with upper motor neuron interruption, and areflexia is associated with lesions of the lower motor neurons.[6]

Superficial reflexes are normal if present and abnormal if absent. Superficial reflexes are tested by stimulating cutaneous receptors of the skin, cornea, or mucous membrane. Stroking, scratching, or touching can be used as the stimulus (Table 23-2). The corneal reflex is present if the eyelids quickly close when the cornea is lightly stroked with a wisp of cotton. An alternative approach is to drop a small amount of water or saline onto the cornea.[4,6] The pathway for the corneal reflex is formed by the trigeminal cranial nerve V (CN V), the facial nerve (CN VII), and the pons. The pharyngeal reflex is present if retching or gagging occurs with stimulation of the back of the pharynx.[3,4,6]

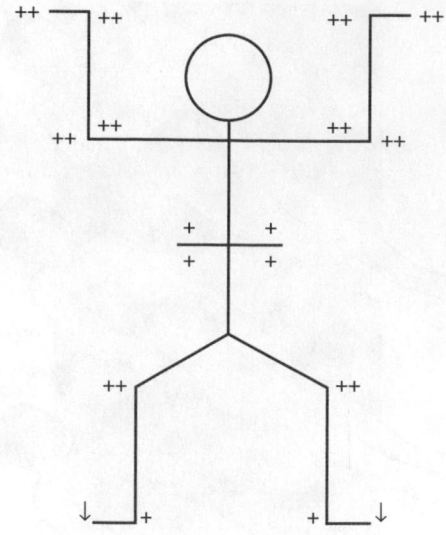

Scoring Deep Tendon Reflexes

Grade	Deep Tendon Reflex Response
0	No response
1+	Sluggish or diminished
2+	Active or expected response
3+	More brisk than expected, slightly hyperactive
4+	Brisk, hyperactive, with intermittent or transient clonus

FIGURE 23-2 The patient's reflex scores are recorded by entering the correct scores at the correct location on the stick figure. (From Barker E. *Neuroscience Nursing: A Spectrum of Care.* 3rd ed. St. Louis: Mosby; 2008.)

TABLE 23-2   SUPERFICIAL REFLEXES

REFLEX	NERVES INVOLVED	NORMAL REACTION
Corneal	CN V and VII	Prompt closure of both eyelids when cornea touched with wisp of cotton
Pharyngeal	CN IX and X	Gagging response to pharyngeal stimulation
Abdominal	Epigastric (T6-T9); midabdominal (T9-T11); hypogastric (T11-L1)	Contraction of abdominal muscle when stroked, so that a brief, brisk movement of umbilicus toward stimulus occurs
Cremasteric	L1, L2	Elevation of testicle when inner aspect of thigh stroked
Anal		Contraction of anal ring as perineum is stroked or scratched
Bulbocutaneous	S4, S5	
Anocutaneous	S5	
Plantar	L5, S1	Flexion of toes from stimulation of sole of foot

From Barker E. *Neuroscience Nursing: A Spectrum of Care.* ed 3. St. Louis: Mosby; 2008.
CN, Cranial nerve.

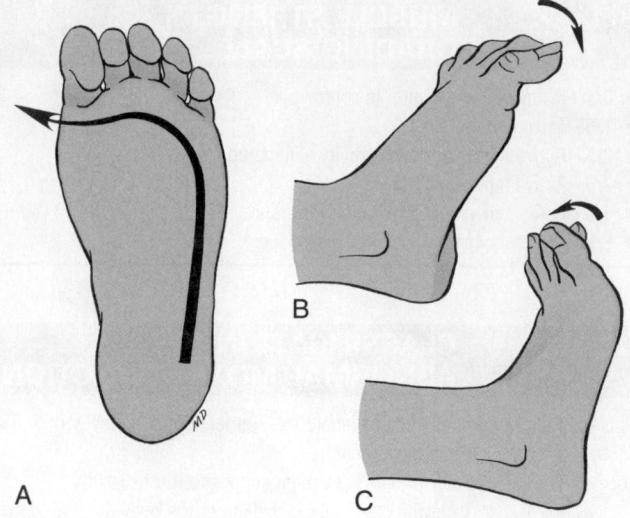

FIGURE 23-3 Babinski Reflex. *A,* Test maneuver: using a blunt point, scratch the sole of the foot as shown. *B,* Normal response (absence of Babinski response) is plantiflexion of the toes. *C,* Abnormal response (presence of Babinski's response) is dorsiflexion of the big toe and often a fanning of the other toes. (From Black JM, Hawks JH. *Medical-Surgical Nursing: Clinical Management for Positive Outcomes.* 8th ed. Philadelphia: Saunders; 2009.)

The presence of pathologic reflexes is an abnormal neurologic finding.[11] The grasp reflex is present when tactile stimulation of the palm of the hand produces a grasp response that is not a conscious voluntary act. The grasp reflex is a primitive reflex that normally disappears with maturational development. Presence of the grasp reflex in the adult indicates cortical damage. Babinski reflex is a pathologic sign in any individual older than 2 years. The presence of this reflex is tested by slow, deliberate stroking of the lateral half of the sole of the foot. Sustained extensor response of the big toe is indicative of a positive Babinski's reflex. This response is sometimes accompanied by the fanning out of the other four toes. Flexor response of all the toes in response to the same stimuli is a normal finding and indicates absence of Babinski reflex (Fig. 23-3). Babinski reflex is a significant neurologic finding because it indicates an upper motor neuron lesion in the brain, brainstem, or spinal cord.[11] The disease may be degenerative, neoplastic, inflammatory, vascular, or posttraumatic. Babinski reflex may also become positive during transtentorial herniation.[3]

Pupillary Function

Assessment of pupillary function focuses on three areas: 1) estimation of pupil size and shape, 2) evaluation of pupillary reaction to light, and 3) assessment of eye movements.

Pupillary function is an extension of the autonomic nervous system. Parasympathetic control of the pupil occurs through innervation of the oculomotor nerve (CN III), which exits from the brainstem in the midbrain area. When the parasympathetic fibers are stimulated, the pupil constricts. Sympathetic control originates in the hypothalamus and travels down the entire length of the brainstem. When the sympathetic fibers are stimulated, the pupil dilates. Pupillary changes provide a valuable assessment tool because of pathway locations. The oculomotor nerve lies at the junction of the midbrain and the tentorial notch. Any increase of pressure that exerts force down through the tentorial notch compresses the oculomotor nerve. Oculomotor nerve compression results in a dilated, nonreactive pupil. Sympathetic pathway disruption occurs with involvement in the brainstem. Loss of sympathetic control leads to pinpoint, nonreactive pupils. Control of eye movements occurs with interaction of three cranial nerves: 1) oculomotor (CN III), 2) trochlear (CN IV), and 3) abducens (CN VI). The pathways for these cranial nerves provide integrated function through the internuclear pathway of the medial longitudinal fasciculus (MLF) located in the brainstem. The MLF provides coordination of eye movements with the vestibular nerve (CN VIII) and the reticular formation.[12]

Estimation of Pupil Size and Shape

Pupil diameter should be documented in millimeters (mm) with the use of a pupil gauge to reduce the subjectivity of description. Most people have pupils of equal size, between 2 and 5 mm. A discrepancy up to 1 mm between the two pupils is normal; it is called *anisocoria* and occurs in 16% to 17% of the human population.[13] Change or inequality in pupil size, especially in patients who previously have not shown this discrepancy, is a significant neurologic sign. It may indicate impending danger of herniation and should be reported immediately. With the location of CN III at the notch of the tentorium, pupil size and reactivity play a key role in the physical assessment of intracranial pressure (ICP) changes and herniation syndromes. In addition to CN III compression, changes in pupil size occur for other reasons. Large pupils can result from the instillation of cycloplegic agents such as atropine or scopolamine or can indicate extreme stress. Extremely small pupils can indicate opioid overdose, lower brainstem compression, or bilateral damage to the pons.[13,14]

Pupil shape is included in the assessment of pupils. Although the pupil is normally round, an irregularly shaped or oval pupil may be observed in patients who have undergone eye surgery. Initial stages of CN III compression from elevated ICP can cause the pupil to have an oval shape.[3,13]

Evaluation of Pupillary Reaction to Light

The pupillary light reflex depends on optic nerve (CN II) and oculomotor nerve (CN III) function (Fig. 23-4).[6,13] The technique for evaluation of the pupillary light response involves use of a narrow-beamed bright light shined into the pupil from the outer canthus of the eye. If the light is shined directly onto the pupil, glare or reflection of the light may prevent the assessor's proper visualization. Pupillary reaction to light is identified as brisk, sluggish, or nonreactive or fixed.[3] Each pupil should be evaluated for direct light response and for consensual response. The consensual pupillary response is constriction in response to a light shined into the opposite eye. This reflex occurs as a result of the crossing of nerve fibers at the optic chiasm.[3] Evaluation of consensual response is necessary to rule out optic nerve dysfunction as a cause for lack of a direct light reflex. Because

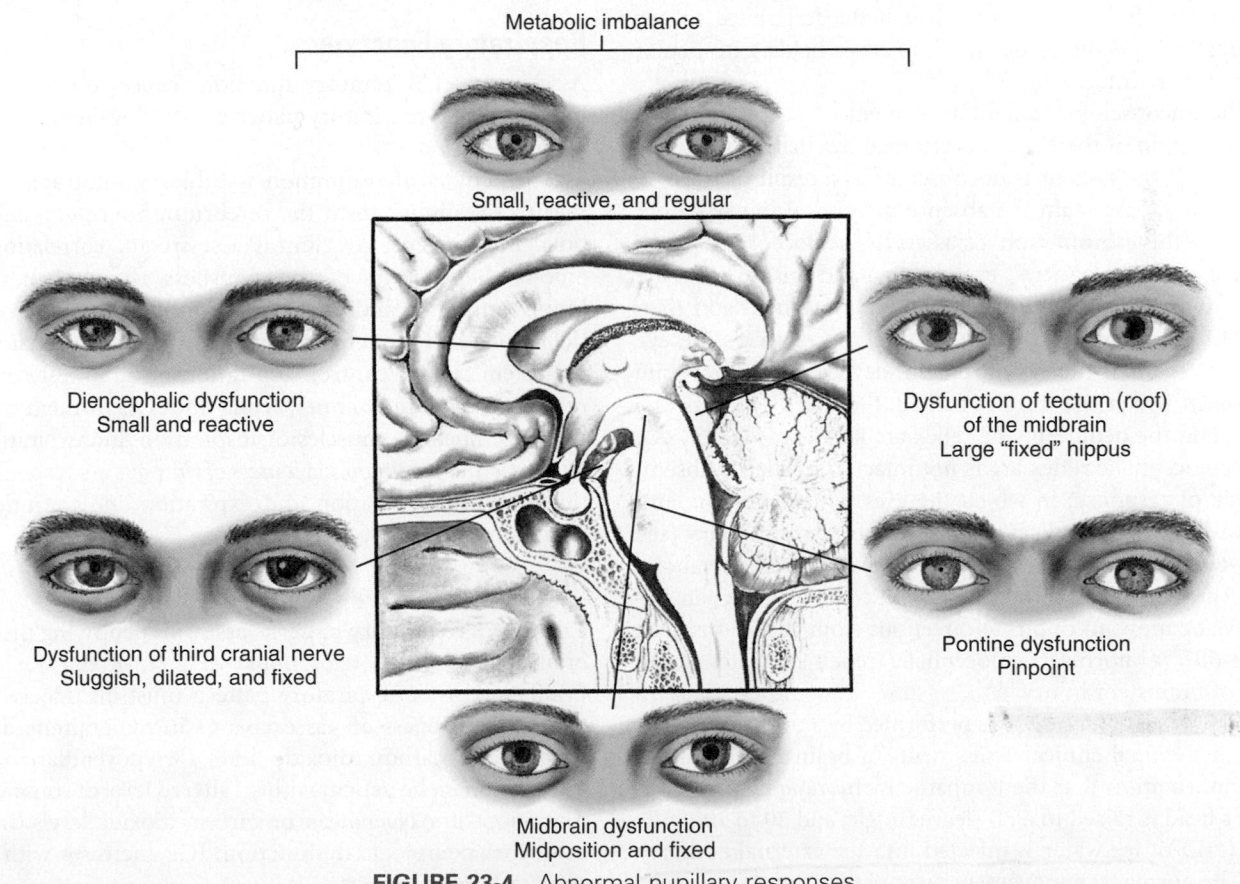

Metabolic imbalance

Small, reactive, and regular

Diencephalic dysfunction
Small and reactive

Dysfunction of tectum (roof)
of the midbrain
Large "fixed" hippus

Dysfunction of third cranial nerve
Sluggish, dilated, and fixed

Pontine dysfunction
Pinpoint

Midbrain dysfunction
Midposition and fixed

FIGURE 23-4 Abnormal pupillary responses.

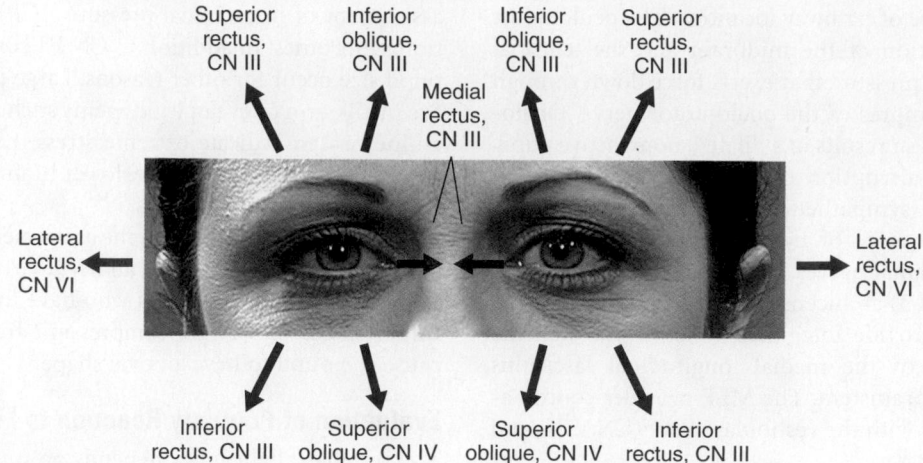

FIGURE 23-5   Extraocular Eye Movements. (From Seidel HM, et al. *Mosby's Guide to Physical Examination.* 7th ed. St. Louis: Mosby; 2011.)

the optic nerve is the afferent pathway for the light reflex, shining a light into a blind eye produces neither a direct light response in that eye nor a consensual response in the opposite eye. A consensual response in the blind eye produced by shining a light into the opposite eye demonstrates an intact oculomotor nerve. Oculomotor compression associated with transtentorial herniation affects the direct light response and the consensual response in the affected pupil.[3,4,12,13]

Assessment of Eye Movement

In the conscious patient, the function of the three cranial nerves of the eye and their MLF innervation can be assessed by asking the patient to follow a finger through the full range of eye motion. If the eyes move together into all six fields, extraocular movements are intact (Fig. 23-5).[3,12]

In the unconscious patient, assessment of ocular function and innervation of the MLF is performed by eliciting the doll's eyes reflex. If the patient is unconscious as a result of trauma, the nurse must ascertain the absence of cervical injury before performing this examination. To assess the oculocephalic reflex, the nurse holds the patient's eyelids open and briskly turns the head to one side while observing the eye movement and then briskly turns the head to the other side and observes the eye movement again. If the eye movement deviates to the opposite direction in which the head is turned, the doll's eyes reflex is present, and the oculocephalic reflex arc is intact (Fig. 23-6A). If the oculocephalic reflex arc is not intact, the reflex is absent. This lack of response, in which the eyes remain midline and move with the head, indicates significant brainstem injury (see Fig. 23-6C). The reflex may also be absent in severe metabolic coma. An abnormal oculocephalic reflex is present when the eyes rove or move in opposite directions from each other (see Fig. 23-6B). Abnormal oculocephalic reflex indicates some degree of brainstem injury.[3,4,12]

The oculovestibular reflex is performed by a physician, often as one of the final clinical assessments of brainstem function. After confirmation that the tympanic membrane is intact, the patient's head is raised to a 30-degree angle, and 20 to 100 milliliters (mL) of ice water is injected into the external auditory canal. The normal eye movement response is a conjugate, slow,

tonic nystagmus, deviating toward the irrigated ear and lasting 30 to 120 seconds. This response indicates brainstem integrity. Rapid nystagmus returns the eye position back to the midline only in a conscious patient with cortical functioning (Fig. 23-7).[3,10] An abnormal response is disconjugate eye movement, which indicates a brainstem lesion, or no response, which indicates little or no brainstem function. The oculovestibular reflex may be temporarily absent in reversible metabolic encephalopathy.[8] This test is an extremely noxious stimulation and may produce a decorticate or decerebrate posturing response in a comatose patient. In the conscious patient, this procedure may produce nausea, vomiting, or dizziness.[3,12,14]

Respiratory Function

Assessment of respiratory function focuses on two areas: 1) observation of respiratory pattern and 2) evaluation of airway status.

The activity of respiration is a highly integrated function that receives input from the cerebrum, brainstem, and metabolic mechanisms. In clinical assessment, correlations exist among altered levels of consciousness, the level of brain or brainstem injury, and the patient's respiratory pattern. Under the influence of the cerebral cortex and the diencephalon, three brainstem centers control respirations. The lowest center, the *medullary respiratory center*, sends impulses through the vagus nerve to innervate muscles of inspiration and expiration. The *apneustic* and *pneumotaxic centers of the pons* are responsible for the length of inspiration and expiration and the underlying respiratory rate.[3,4,10]

Observation of Respiratory Pattern

Changes in respiratory patterns assist in identifying the level of brainstem dysfunction or injury (Fig. 23-8 and Table 23-3). Evaluation of the respiratory pattern must include assessment of the effectiveness of gas exchange in maintaining adequate oxygen and carbon dioxide levels. Hypoventilation is not uncommon in the patient with an altered level of consciousness. Alterations in oxygenation or carbon dioxide levels can result in further neurologic dysfunction. ICP increases with hypoxemia or hypercapnia.[3,4,10]

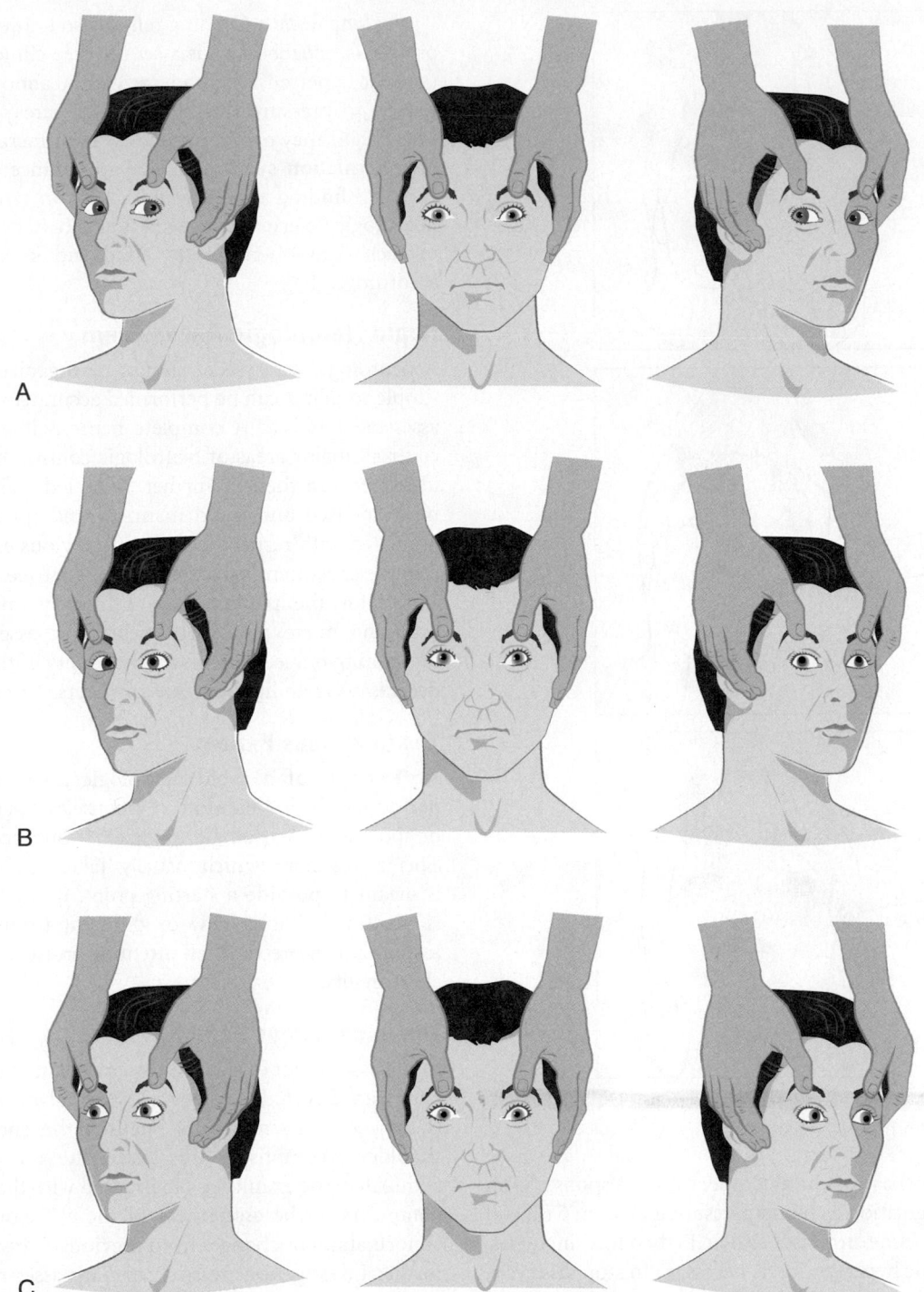

FIGURE 23-6 Oculocephalic Reflex (Doll's Eyes). *A*, Normal. *B*, Abnormal. *C*, Absent.

Evaluation of Airway Status

Evaluation of the respiratory function in a patient with a neurologic deficit must include assessment of airway maintenance and secretion control. Cough, gag, and swallow reflexes responsible for protection of the airway may be absent or diminished.[15]

Vital Signs

Assessment of vital signs focuses on two areas: 1) evaluation of blood pressure and 2) observation of heart rate and rhythm. As a result of the brain and brainstem influences on cardiac, respiratory, and body temperature functions, changes in vital signs could be signs of deterioration in neurologic status.[3,4]

Evaluation of Blood Pressure

A common manifestation of intracranial injury is systemic hypertension. Cerebral autoregulation, responsible for the control of cerebral blood flow (CBF), frequently is lost with any type of intracranial injury. After cerebral injury, the body often is in a hyperdynamic state (increased heart rate, blood pressure,

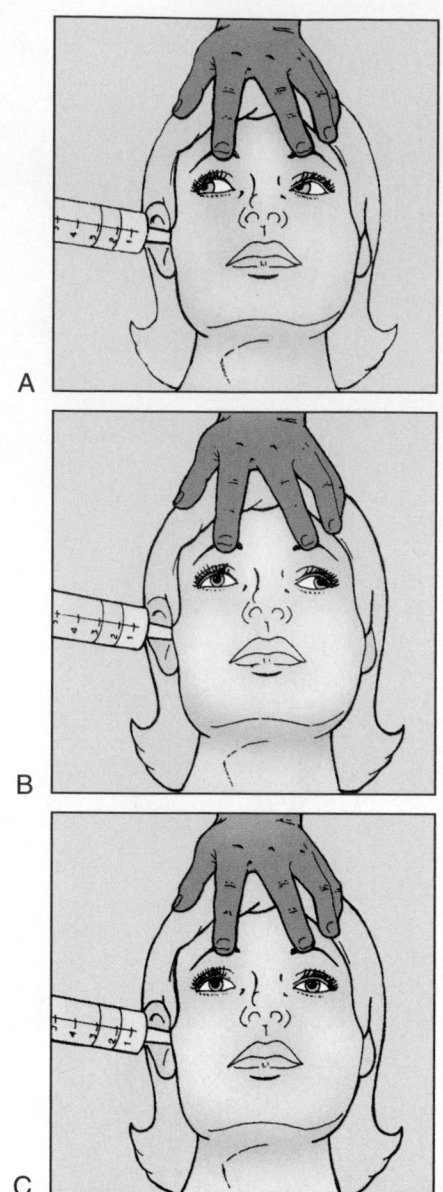

FIGURE 23-7 Oculovestibular Reflex (Cold Caloric Test). *A*, Normal. *B*, Abnormal. *C*, Absent.

and cardiac output) as part of a compensatory response. With the loss of autoregulation as blood pressure increases, CBF and cerebral blood volume increase, and ICP therefore increases. Control of systemic hypertension is necessary to stop this cycle, but caution must be exercised. The mean arterial pressure must be maintained at a level sufficient to produce adequate CBF in the presence of elevated ICP. Attention must also be paid to the pulse pressure because widening of this value may occur in the late stages of intracranial hypertension.[15,16]

Observation of Heart Rate and Rhythm

The medulla and the vagus nerve provide parasympathetic control to the heart. When stimulated, this lower brainstem system produces bradycardia. Sympathetic stimulation increases the rate and contractility. Various intracranial pathologies and abrupt ICP changes can produce bradycardia, premature ventricular contractions (PVCs), QT changes, and myocardial damage.[17]

Cushing Reflex. Cushing reflex, also known as *Cushing triad* or *Cushing phenomena*, is a set of three clinical manifestations (systolic hypertension, bradycardia, and abnormal respirations) related to pressure on the medullary area of the brainstem. These signs may occur in response to intracranial hypertension or a herniation syndrome. The appearance of Cushing reflex is a late finding that may be absent in patients with severe neurologic deterioration. Attention should be paid to alteration in each component of the triad and intervention initiated accordingly.[18]

Rapid Neurologic Assessment

A neurologic assessment should be organized, thorough, and simple so that it can be performed accurately and easily at each assessment point.[3] A complete neurologic assessment should cover all major areas of neurologic control. Any abnormalities identified can then be further evaluated and investigated in a more focused and rapid manner. Findings should always be evaluated with respect to those of previous examinations. One critical assessment point is handoff between nurses who are caring for the patient. It is extremely important that the off-going nurse perform a neurologic assessment with the on-coming nurse. This ensures reliability of the assessment and decreases variability between caregivers.

The Conscious Patient

An example of a rapid neurologic assessment that can be performed during handoff of a conscious patient with known or potential neurologic deficit is outlined in Box 23-6. This assessment, which usually takes less than 4 minutes, is meant to provide a starting point. If any neurologic deficit is identified that is new or different from that of the last assessment, more detailed attention must be focused on that abnormality.

The Unconscious Patient

In the assessment of the unconscious patient (Box 23-7), initial efforts are directed at achieving maximal arousal of the patient. Calling the patient's name, patting the chest, or shaking a shoulder accomplishes this task. After the patient has been stimulated, the examiner can proceed with the neurologic evaluation. As in the assessment of the conscious patient, if any abnormalities or changes from previous assessment are noticed, further investigation must occur. This assessment takes 3 to 4 minutes.

Neurologic Changes Associated with Intracranial Hypertension

Assessment of the patient for signs of increasing ICP is an important responsibility of the critical care nurse. Increasing ICP can be identified by changes in level of consciousness, pupillary reaction, motor response, vital signs, and respiratory patterns (Fig. 23-9).[10,19]

DIAGNOSTIC PROCEDURES

The nursing management of a patient undergoing a neurodiagnostic procedure involves a variety of interventions. Nursing

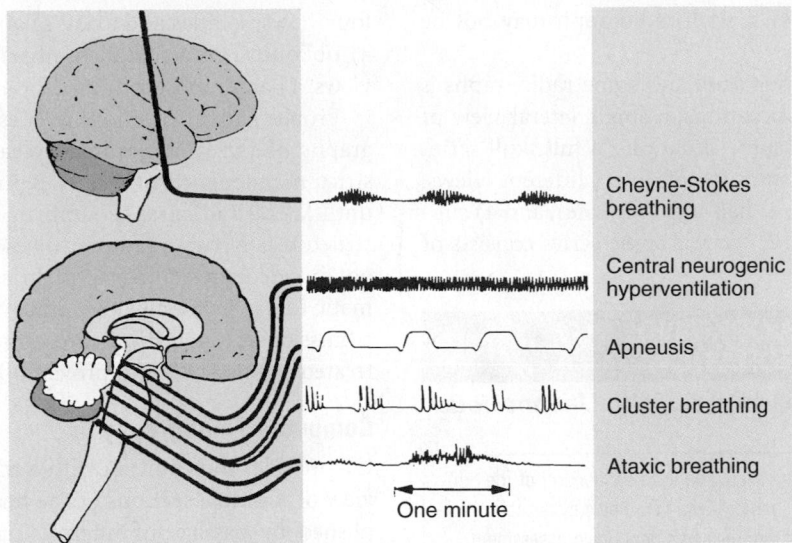

FIGURE 23-8 Abnormal respiratory patterns with corresponding levels of central nervous system activity.

TABLE 23-3 RESPIRATORY PATTERNS

PATTERN OF RESPIRATION	DESCRIPTION OF PATTERN	SIGNIFICANCE
Cheyne-Stokes breathing	Rhythmic crescendo and decrescendo of rate and depth of respiration; includes brief periods of apnea	Usually seen with bilateral deep cerebral lesions or some cerebellar lesions
Central neurogenic hyperventilation	Very deep, very rapid respirations with no apneic periods	Usually seen with lesions of the midbrain and upper pons
Apneustic breathing	Prolonged inspiratory and/or expiratory pause of 2-3 seconds	Usually seen in lesions of the middle to lower pons
Cluster breathing	Clusters of irregular, gasping respirations separated by long periods of apnea	Usually seen in lesions of the lower pons or upper medulla
Ataxic respirations	Irregular, random pattern of deep and shallow respirations with irregular apneic periods	Usually seen in lesions of the medulla

BOX 23-6 TEAM WORK AND COLLABORATION

Rapid Neurologic Assessment of the Conscious Patient

QSEN The following outline should be used for handoff of the critically ill conscious patient with neurologic dysfunction:

1. *Level of consciousness:* Address the patient and ask a variety of orientation questions; avoid the obvious, overused questions about name, date, and place, and focus on questions about recent and past events from the patient's experiences such as spouse's name, home address, what was eaten at the previous meal. As examiner, you should be aware of the correct answers to all questions asked.
2. *Facial movements:* During assessment of level of consciousness, observe the patient's facial movements for symmetry and listen to speech patterns for evidence of slurred speech.
3. *Pupillary function and eye movements:* Perform pupil check and assess extraocular eye movements.
4. *Motor assessment:* Assess movement and strength in upper and lower extremities.
5. *Sensory:* With a finger, stroke the patient bilaterally on the face, upper aspect of the arm, hand, leg, and foot; ask the patient to identify what is touched and any difference in sensation between the two sides.
6. *Vital signs:* Observe alterations in blood pressure, heart rate or rhythm, respiratory pattern, or temperature.
7. *Change in status:* Ask the patient if he or she feels any differences between this and the previous examination.

activities are directed toward preparing the patient psychologically and physically for the procedure, monitoring the patient's responses to the procedure, and assessing the patient after the procedure. Preparation includes teaching the patient about the procedure, answering questions, and transporting and positioning the patient for the procedure. During the procedure, the nurse observes the patient for signs of pain, anxiety, or hemorrhage and monitors vital signs. After the procedure, the nurse observes for complications of the procedure and medicates the patient for any postprocedure discomfort. Any evidence of increasing ICP should be immediately reported to the physician, and emergency measures to maintain circulation must be initiated.

Radiologic Procedures

The following discussion focuses on the more commonly performed radiologic procedures that are used for the diagnosis of the critically ill patient with a neurologic dysfunction.

Skull and Spine Films

The purpose of radiographs of the skull or spine is to identify fractures, anomalies, or possible tumors. The role of skull radiographs in trauma has diminished with the advent of computed tomography (CT). If the patient is to undergo a CT scan during the initial assessment process, a skull radiograph may not be necessary.[20]

The procedure for obtaining skull and spine radiographs is relatively painless. In many situations, a single lateral view of the skull is adequate, but in some situations, a full skull series is required. A skull series consists of four different views: 1) lateral, 2) posteroanterior, 2) half-axial (Towne), and 4) submentovertical (base) views.[20] A cervical spine series consists of four views: 1) atlas and axial, 2) anteroposterior, 3) lateral, and 4) oblique. Thoracic and lumbar spine series consists of two views: 1) anteroposterior and 2) lateral.[20]

Proper patient positioning is essential, especially for radiographs of the spine. Spinal precautions (e.g., cervical collar, strict maintenance of head alignment) must be maintained until lateral radiographs confirm the integrity of the cervical structures. Nursing care involves positioning the patient to obtain adequate radiographs. In any situation in which traumatic injury, especially head injury, is the cause of the patient's admission to the critical care unit, the cervical spine must be treated as unstable until proven otherwise.[21]

Computed Tomography

CT provides the clinician with a mathematically reconstructed view of multiple sections of the head and body. This is accomplished by passage of intersecting x-ray beams through the examined area and measurement of the density of substances through which the x-ray beams pass. The denser the substance through which an x-ray beam passes, the whiter it appears on the finished film. The less dense a substance is, the blacker it appears. With normal findings for a CT scan of the head, bone appears white, blood appears off-white, brain tissue appears shaded gray, cerebrospinal fluid (CSF) appears off-black, and air appears black (Fig. 23-10).[22]

CT offers rapid, convenient, noninvasive visualization of structures and is the diagnostic study of choice for an acute

---

BOX 23-7   TEAM WORK AND COLLABORATION

Rapid Neurologic Assessment of the Unconscious Patient

QSEN   The following outline should be used for handoff of the critically ill unconscious patient with neurologic dysfunction:

1. *Level of consciousness:* Perform the Glasgow Coma Scale assessment.
2. *Pupillary assessment:* Perform pupillary assessment with special attention to size, reactivity, and shape of pupil compared with the opposite eye.
3. *Motor examination:* Assess each extremity individually by means of a predetermined coding score of motor movement.
4. *Respiratory pattern:* If the patient is not receiving mechanical ventilation, observe respiratory patterns for evidence of deteriorating level of function.
5. *Vital signs:* Include a comparison of preassessment vital signs with postassessment vital signs, paying special attention to arterial blood pressure and intracranial pressure, if these parameters are being monitored.

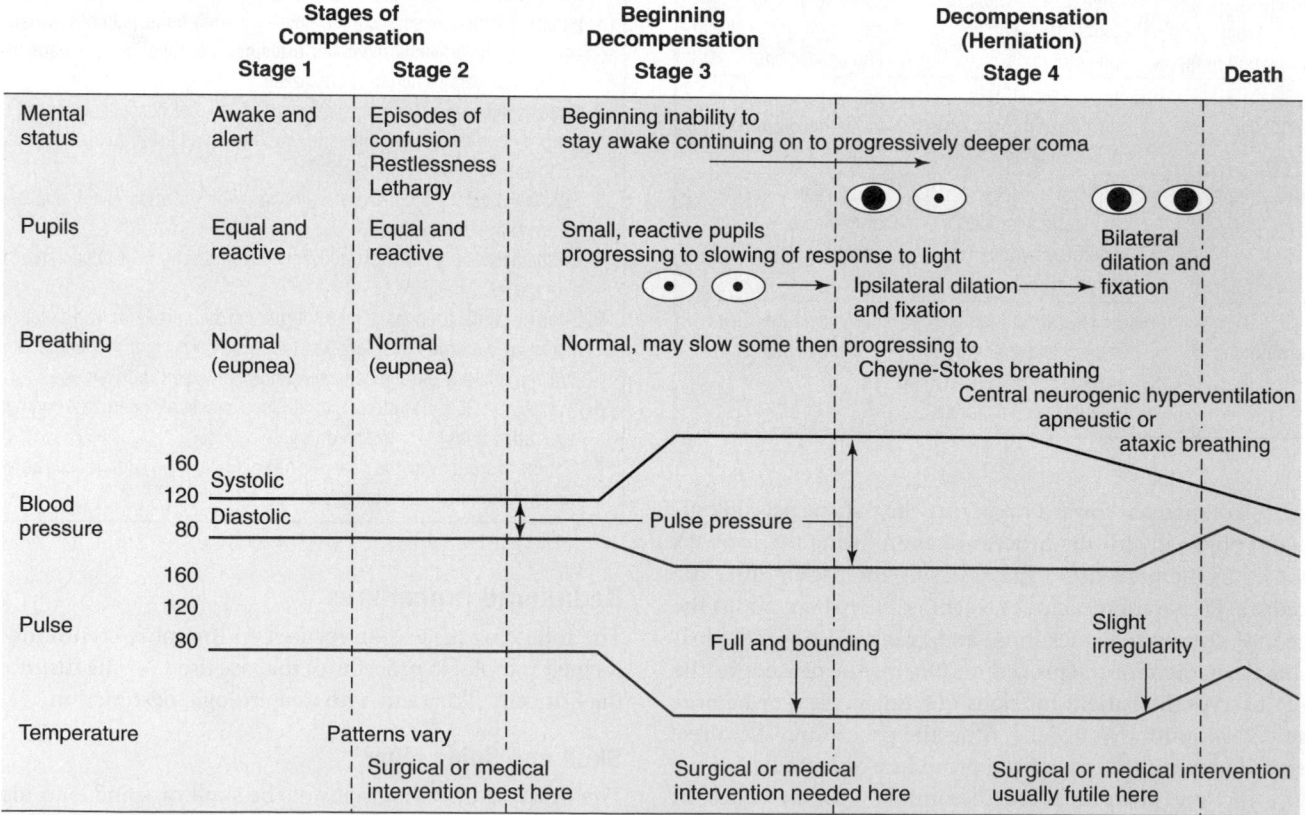

FIGURE 23-9 Clinical correlates of compensated and decompensated phases of intracranial hypertension. (From Beare PG, Myers JL. *Principles and Practice of Adult Health Nursing.* 3rd ed. St. Louis: Mosby; 1998.)

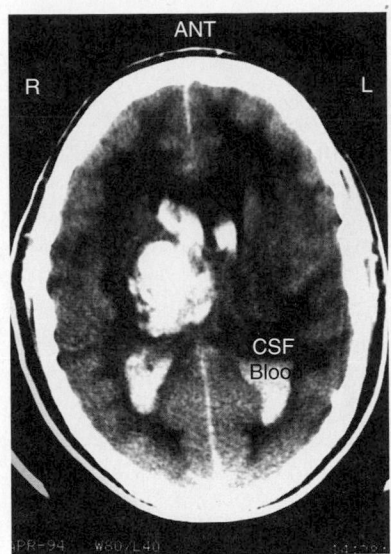

FIGURE 23-10 Computed Tomography Scan of the Brain Demonstrating an Intracerebral Hemorrhage. In this patient with hypertension and an acute severe headache, the noncontrast computed tomography scan shows a large area of fresh blood in the region of the right thalamus. Blood also is seen in the anterior and posterior horns of the lateral ventricles. Because blood is denser than cerebrospinal fluid, it is layered dependently. (From Mettler FA. *Essentials of Radiology*. 2nd ed. Philadelphia: Elsevier; 2005.)

head injury. Serial evaluations may be obtained to verify midline shift and increasing ICP.[23] CT also is used in the diagnostic work-up of space-occupying lesions, hemorrhage, and vascular abnormalities; cerebral edema; hydrocephalus; and severe headache. CT is the preferred method for diagnosing subarachnoid hemorrhage and for differentiating intracranial hemorrhage and infarction.[22,23]

CT can be performed with and without the use of a contrast medium. Without contrast, the scan is noninvasive, requires no premedication of the patient, and is effective for analysis and location of normal brain structures. A non–contrast-enhanced CT scan of the head is appropriate for trauma patients when the goal is to view the intracranial area for evidence of intracranial hemorrhage, cerebral edema, or shift of structures. Non–contrast-enhanced CT also is appropriate in the diagnosis of hydrocephalus.[23] The use of an intravenously injected contrast medium enhances the vascular areas and enables detection of vascular lesions or further definition of lesions identified on a non–contrast-enhanced scan. The letter *C* is evident on the radiograph when contrast has been used.[22]

Nursing management of the patient undergoing CT can be divided into two areas of focus: 1) observation of the patient's tolerance of the procedure and 2) observation of the patient's reaction to the dye used in contrast-enhanced scanning. Because of the associated activity and positioning, transporting and scanning of a critically ill patient with known or suspected intracranial hypertension can cause deterioration in the patient's condition. The nurse must always remain with the patient during CT scanning and closely observe the neurologic status, vital signs, and, if monitored, ICP.[21]

If the patient is scheduled to receive contrast for CT scanning, questions about possible sensitivity to iodine-based dye must be asked beforehand, if possible. During infusion of the dye and for 10 to 30 minutes afterward, the patient is observed closely for an anaphylactic reaction. Less than 1% of all patients undergoing contrast-enhanced CT have severe anaphylactic reactions, shock, or cardiac arrest. Another potential complication of the dye is acute kidney failure. Two measures reported to reduce the incidence and severity of renal dysfunction after contrast-enhanced CT are: 1) antihistamine administration and 2) adequate hydration before and after the study.[20]

Magnetic Resonance Imaging

Magnetic resonance imaging (MRI) has replaced CT as the diagnostic study of choice for many conditions. MRI produces images with greater detail than CT and provides views of several planes (sagittal, coronal, axial, and oblique) not possible with CT. No ionizing radiation is used. For MRI, the patient is placed in a large magnetic field that stimulates the nuclei of the atoms of the body. Introduction of radiofrequency waves causes resonance of the nuclei, which is emitted as the nuclei relax. A computer then constructs an image of the tissue (Fig. 23-11). Intravenous administration of a non–iodine-based contrast medium enhances the images by influencing the magnetic environment and signal intensity.[20,22]

With MRI, small tumors, whose tissue densities are different from those of the surrounding cells, can be identified before they could be visualized through any other radiographic test. MRI also can identify small hemorrhages deep in the brain that are invisible on CT. MRI can detect areas of cerebral infarct within a few hours of the incident and can identify small areas of plaque in patients with multiple sclerosis. MRI with contrast is the preferred study for detection of infectious and inflammatory processes of the central nervous system, malignancy, and metastatic lesions; cervical spine imaging; and postoperative evaluation of tumor recurrence. MRI also is the diagnostic study of choice in the evaluation of spinal cord injury.[23]

Nursing management for the patient undergoing MRI is focused on the patient's tolerance of the procedure. Concerns related to transport of the patient with neurologic problems for MRI are identical to those discussed for CT. Teaching and preparation of the patient are essential for successful performance of MRI. The procedure is lengthy and requires the patient to lie motionless in a tight, enclosed space. Many patients experience anxiety, panic, and an acute sense of claustrophobia. Mild sedation, a blindfold, or both may be necessary. The patient with neurologic impairment may not be able to comprehend the instructions, and sedation, possibly combined with neuromuscular blockade, is required. Removal of all metal from the patient's body and clothing is essential because the basis of MRI is a strong magnetic field. In the past, it was thought that any metallic material such as dental filling, prostheses, or internal clips or staples would prevent scanning. Further study and changes in the type of metals used for many procedures have made the test safer. Any questions about specific devices or metals must be directed to the neuroradiologist before the test. The test is considered relatively safe and noninvasive, but all risks of this procedure have not been identified.[21]

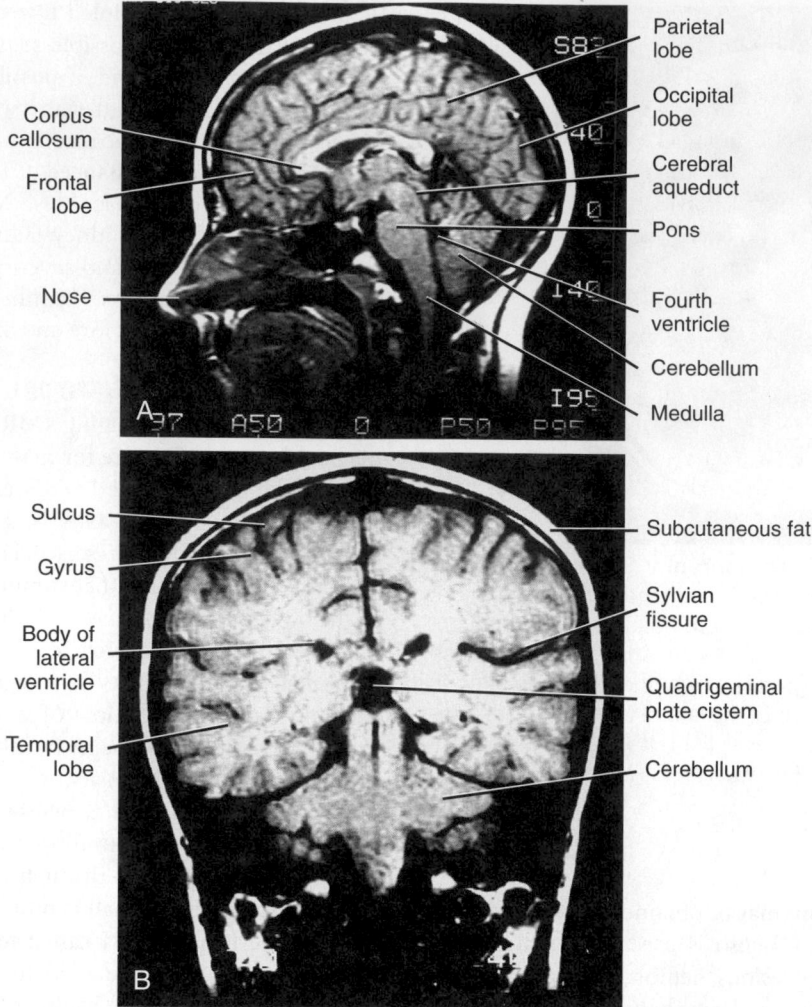

FIGURE 23-11 Normal Magnetic Resonance Imaging Anatomy of the Brain. *A,* Coronal projection. *B,* Sagittal projection. (From Mettler FA. *Essentials of Radiology.* 2nd ed. Philadelphia: Elsevier; 2005.)

Cerebral Angiography

The following discussion focuses on the more commonly performed angiography procedures that are used for the diagnosis of the critically ill patient with a neurologic dysfunction.

Conventional Angiography. Conventional angiography involves the injection of radiopaque contrast medium into the intracranial or extracranial vasculature (Fig. 23-12). With the use of serial radiologic filming, an angiogram traces the flow of blood from the arterial circulation through the capillary bed to the venous circulation. Cerebral angiography allows visualization of the lumen of vessels to provide information about patency, size (narrowing or dilation), irregularities, or occlusion. Angiography is used in the diagnosis of cerebral aneurysm, vasospasm, arteriovenous malformation (AVM), carotid artery disease, and some vascular tumors. Angiography also is used to evaluate cerebral vasculature in the patient who had suffered a stroke. Information obtained from the angiogram guides the surgeon in choosing the operative approach or provides information on which to make medical management decisions other than surgery.[24]

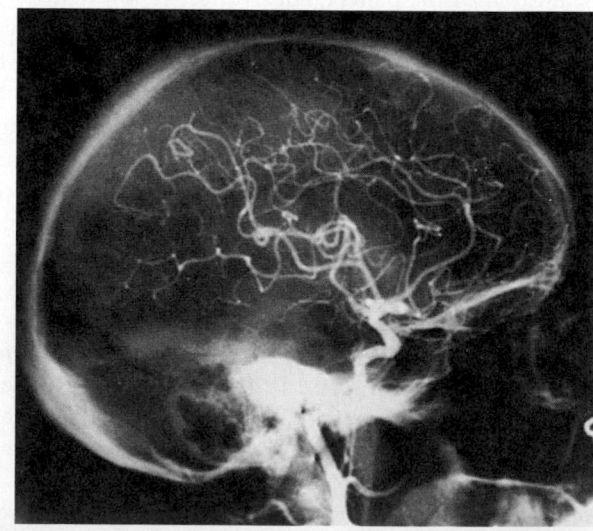

FIGURE 23-12 Cerebral angiography. (From Ehrlich RA, Daly JA. *Patient Care in Radiography.* 8th ed. St. Louis: Mosby; 2013.)

The procedure involves placement of a catheter in the femoral artery and threading it up the aorta and into the origin of the cerebral circulation. Other injection sites include direct carotid or vertebral artery puncture or placement of a catheter in the brachial, the axillary, or the subclavian artery. Several views of vessels can be studied by means of angiography. A four-vessel angiogram involves injections into the right and left internal carotid arteries and the right and left vertebral arteries. If the area of suspected disease already has been identified, a single-vessel study may be all that is required. This is particularly true when angiography is used as a follow-up in the evaluation of intracranial vascular surgery. If carotid artery disease is a working diagnosis, the angiographic study may include views of the arch of the aorta and of the external and internal carotid arteries.[20]

After the catheter is appropriately placed, the contrast medium is injected. A rapid succession of radiographs is taken as the contrast medium progresses through the cerebral circulation. Separate injections of the contrast medium are administered for each vessel being studied.[24]

Nursing management associated with this invasive procedure is comprehensive. Renal insufficiency, bleeding, and cardiac instability are contraindications to cerebral angiography and must be assessed before the procedure. As with contrast-enhanced CT, the nurse must assess the patient for possible sensitivity to iodine-based contrast before angiography. Instruction and education of the patient are essential to patient preparation. The patient's complete understanding of the role this procedure plays in diagnosis, as well as the process itself, relieves anxiety about the unknown and ensures cooperation in what is commonly an uncomfortable procedure.[21]

Before the procedure, the patient has no oral intake (NPO status) for at least 4 hours. Sedation is administered immediately before the procedure. Discomforts during the procedure include the need to lie still on a cold, hard table and the possibility of pain during preparation and insertion of the groin catheter. The patient often experiences a hot, burning sensation when the contrast medium is injected, especially if it is injected into the external carotid system. Preparation of patients for this burning sensation assures them that it is not an abnormal occurrence.[21]

The patient must be made aware of the postprocedure assessment. After the procedure, adequate hydration is necessary to assist the kidneys in clearing the heavy dye load. Inadequate hydration may lead to renal dysfunction and possibly shutdown. If the patient cannot tolerate oral fluids, an intravenous line is placed before the procedure is begun. Postprocedure assessment involves measurement of vital signs, neurologic evaluation, observation of the puncture site, and assessment of neurovascular integrity distal to the puncture site every 15 minutes for the first hour. Any abnormalities must be reported immediately. The patient should be kept on bed rest for 8 to 12 hours.[21]

Complications associated with cerebral angiography include: 1) cerebral embolus caused by the catheter dislodging a segment of atherosclerotic plaque in the vessel, 2) hemorrhage or hematoma formation at the insertion site, 3) vasospasm of a vessel caused by the irritation of catheter placement, 4) thrombosis of the extremity distal to the injection site, and 5) allergic or adverse reaction to the contrast medium, including renal impairment.[20]

Digital Subtraction Angiography. Digital subtraction angiography (DSA) eliminates the shadows and distortions of bone or other material that sometimes block the viewing of the cerebral vessels.[20] Radiographs taken before and after intravenous or intra-arterial dye injection are superimposed on each other, and all matching digital images are subtracted by the computer. Only the dye-enhanced cerebral vessels are left for study and evaluation.[24] Intra-arterial two dimensional DSA is particularly useful in detecting ruptured intracranial aneurysms and three-dimensional DSA technique offers an even more precise demonstration of the aneurysm anatomy.[25] In addition, an advantage of DSA over conventional arteriography is that significantly less dye is utilized. The major disadvantage of DSA is that the patient must remain motionless during the entire procedure. Even swallowing interferes significantly with the imaging process. Complications and nursing management for DSA are similar to those described for cerebral angiography.[21]

Magnetic Resonance Angiography. Magnetic resonance angiography (MRA) is a technique that offers noninvasive visualization of the cerebrovascular system.[23] It uses MRI technology to evaluate CBF and provide details about cerebral vessels. MRA of the carotid arteries has become an established complement to preoperative ultrasound evaluation. It helps determine the area of salvageable tissue (or penumbra) after acute stroke and head injury.[23] MRA is also being used to identify intracranial aneurysms, AVMs, and vasospasm.[23] Contrast-enhanced MRA (CEMRA) may be performed to improve image resolution and reduce artifact. The most commonly used agent is gadolinium, a non-nephrotoxic contrast medium that is injected intravenously.[22]

Computed Tomography Angiography. Computed tomography angiography (CTA) is a technique that uses high-speed helical CT technology with the administration of contrast to visualize the cerebrovascular system. It is used to assess the carotid arteries for stenosis and to evaluate cerebral aneurysms. CTA is becoming a well-accepted substitute for conventional cerebral angiography. The downside to this procedure is that it requires large doses of contrast and radiation.[26]

Myelography

Myelography is radiographic examination of the spinal cord and vertebral column after injection of a contrast material into the subarachnoid space through the lumbar region of the spine between L2 and L3 or L3 and L4 or by cisternal puncture. Myelography allows visualization of the spinal canal, the subarachnoid space around the spinal cord, and the spinal nerve roots (Fig. 23-13). MRI has replaced myelography in most cases, but myelography may be necessary in postoperative patients with multiple clips or metallic hardware. Possible risks involved in the use of myelography include injection of the dye outside the subarachnoid space, arachnoiditis as a result of irritation of the arachnoid membranes from a foreign material, and allergic reaction. Other adverse reactions include confusion, hallucinations, headache, grand mal seizure, chest pain, and dysrhythmias.[27] Postprocedure care includes keeping the patient's head

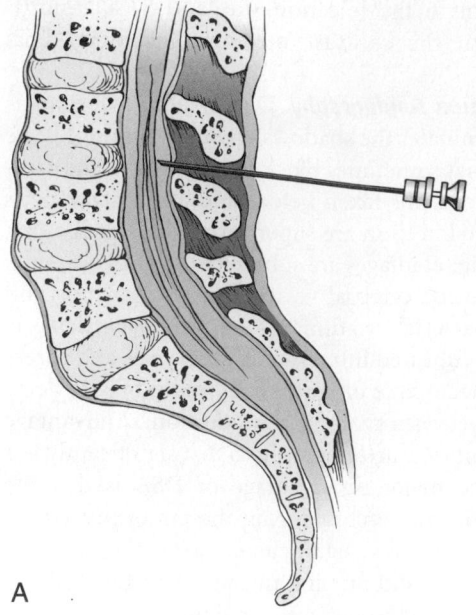

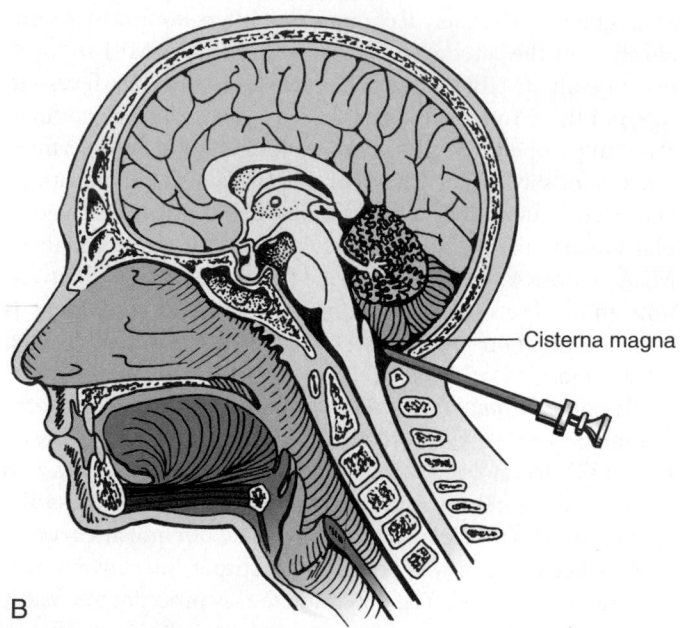

Cisterna magna

FIGURE 23-13   *A,* Lumbar puncture. *B,* Cisternal puncture. (Modified from Phipps WJ, et al. *Medical-Surgical Nursing: Health and Illness Perspectives.* 7th ed. St. Louis: Mosby; 2003.)

elevated 45 degrees for 8 hours, monitoring neurologic status, and encouraging intake of oral fluids.[21]

Cerebral Blood Flow and Metabolism Imaging

Measurement of cerebral blood flow (CBF) provides valuable information for clinical management of critical care patients with neurologic problems.[28] The average CBF in a human is 55 mL/100 g of brain per minute, but actual values may vary widely across gray and white matter. The ischemic threshold for CBF is approximately 18 mL/100 g/min, with 10 mL/100 g/min often considered the threshold for irreversible injury.[29] CBF is influenced by mean arterial pressure, ICP, and the partial

pressure of carbon dioxide and oxygen.[30] The measurements of CBF and CPP do not, however, address the brain's metabolic need for oxygen. Neuronal demand for oxygen is governed by the metabolic rate. The rate at which the brain consumes oxygen is known as the cerebral metabolic rate of oxygen ($CMRO_2$), the normal value of which is 3.4 mL/100 g/min. Measurement of $CMRO_2$ is a valuable tool for assessing brain vitality and function and has been shown to be a better marker of injury severity in hypoxia-ischemia than CBF alone.[31]

The following discussion focuses on the more commonly performed imaging studies that assess cerebral blood flow and cerebral metabolism in the critically ill patient with a neurologic dysfunction.

Perfusion Computed Tomography

Perfusion CT allows rapid evaluation of cerebral perfusion. A perfusion CT scan is made by passing x-rays through the brain, as in a regular CT scan; however, in addition to revealing the structure of brain tissue, perfusion CT measures CBF, cerebral blood volume, and mean transit time. This is done by scanning the patient several times every few seconds before, during, and after the intravenous delivery of an iodine-containing contrast agent that absorbs the x-rays. Perfusion CT has been found to be useful for diagnosis of cerebral ischemia and infarction associated with stroke and for evaluation of cerebral ischemia associated with vasospasm after subarachnoid hemorrhage.[32]

Xenon Computed Tomography

Xenon CT is used to study regional CBF. The scan is a computerized radiographic study of the brain that is performed while the patient breathes a carefully regulated flow of xenon, which is a colorless, odorless gas. It has higher resolution in blood flow measurements than other techniques such as positron emission tomography (PET). Xenon CT has been used in the evaluation of a wide variety of disorders and has been most useful in the evaluation of cerebrovascular disease and brain metabolism. Xenon CT studies are occasionally used to determine brain death.[33]

Perfusion Magnetic Resonance Imaging

Perfusion MRI provides a relative measurement of the parameters of cerebral microvascularization, an absolute measurement of the parameters of cerebral microvascularization, or both: regional blood volume, mean transit time, and regional blood flow. The two most common methods for imaging perfusion are: 1) the dynamic susceptibility contrast approach, which detects the first passage of an intravascular contrast agent such as gadolinium, and 2) arterial spin labeling (ASL), which utilizes magnetically labeled arterial blood water as a diffusible flow tracer.[34] The main applications of first-pass perfusion MRI are identification of vascular pathologies (ischemic strokes, vasospasm) and tumoral pathologies. Progress in sequences and the very high fields are expected to lead to improvements in the spin labeling technique.[35]

Carotid Ultrasonography

Ultrasound technology, although not an absolute measure of CBF, uses a noninvasive technique to provide information about the flow velocity of blood through the carotid vessels. Carotid duplex studies are used as a routine screening procedure for intraluminal narrowing of the common and internal carotid arteries as a result of atherosclerotic plaques. A Doppler probe is placed externally over the vessel, where high-frequency sound waves (ultrasound) are generated and blood flow velocities calculated. As the diameter of the vessel changes, the velocity of the flow of blood through the vessel changes; the higher the flow velocity, the narrower is the vessel. Carotid duplex studies are noninvasive, relatively inexpensive, and painless.[21] When changes in flow velocities that may indicate significant occlusion of the vessel are identified, CTA or MRA may be used to verify the degree of severity of the narrowed vessel. If necessary, cerebral angiography is performed to confirm ambiguous or equivocal findings.[36]

Emission Tomography Studies

The following discussion focuses on two different nuclear medicine studies that may be used to evaluate the critically ill patient with a neurologic dysfunction.

Positive Emission Tomography. A positive emission tomography (PET) scan is a nuclear medicine study that uses CT technology to produce a three-dimensional image of detailed biochemical changes in brain tissue, as it traces the brain's metabolic activity.[37] Oxygen-15 (^{15}O)-labeled water is injected into the patient, and the PET camera measures the amount of the radiotracer as it flows through the brain, which allows for the measurement of CBF, the fraction of oxygen extracted from the arterial blood by the cerebral tissue (OEF), and $CMRO_2$.[38] During the procedure, the patient will need to lie still and may be asked to think, reason, and remember.[21] The amount of radiation the patient will be exposed to is very small, about one to three times the normal human annual exposure to background radiation. One consideration with regard to cerebral PET is the long scan time during which a patient's physiologic condition must remain stable.[36]

Single-Photon Emission Computed Tomography. Another nuclear medicine scanning procedure that integrates CT and a radioactive tracer to produce a three-dimensional measurement of regional CBF is single-photon emission computed tomography (SPECT). The test differs from PET in that tracer stays in the bloodstream rather than being absorbed by surrounding tissue, thereby limiting the images to areas where blood flows. SPECT is cheaper and more readily available than higher-resolution PET. The major clinical uses of SPECT are to detect cerebrovascular disease, seizures, and tumors.[39]

Electrophysiology Studies

The following discussion focuses on the two of the frequently performed electrophysiology studies that are used in the diagnosis and management of the critically ill patient with a neurologic dysfunction.

Electroencephalography

Electroencephalography (EEG) records electrical impulses, commonly called *brain waves*, generated by the brain. The nurse caring for a patient with a neurologic dysfunction must be aware of the appropriate indications for use and the limitations

TABLE 23-4	TYPES OF ELECTRICAL BRAIN WAVES	
WAVE	**DURATION**	**DESCRIPTION**
Delta	1-4 cycles/second	Normal; seen in stages 3 and 4 of sleep
Alpha	8-13 cycles/second	Normal; relaxed state with eyes closed; often seen in occipital leads
Theta	4-7 cycles/second	Less common in adults than in children; characteristic of coma in brain injury
Beta	12-40 cycles/second	Fast waves indicating mental or physical activity
Sleep spindles	12-14 cycles/second	Seen in stage 2 sleep, not rapid eye movement
Spike and slow waves	Variable	Seen in irritable brain tissue (e.g., seizure)

of this diagnostic procedure. The purpose of EEG is to detect and localize abnormal electrical activity. This abnormal activity can be defined as *slowing*, which occurs in areas of injury or infarct, or as the *spikes* and *waves* seen in irritated tissue. Indications for the use of EEG include suspected seizure activity, cerebral infarct, metabolic encephalopathies, altered consciousness, infectious disease, some head injuries, and confirmation of brain death.[21,40]

Noninvasive electrodes are placed on the head, and the electrical impulses detected are transferred to a central recording device that records the information in wave form. Six types of waves or rhythms may be present (Table 23-4). Intermittent slowing with triphasic wave morphology is associated with metabolic encephalopathy. Continuous, generalized slowing in the delta or theta range is associated with anoxic damage. The combination of alpha-waves that do not change with stimulation and a coma state is called *alpha-coma*, and it is associated with a poor prognosis.[41]

Other EEG abnormalities associated with poor prognosis are *burst suppression* (occasional generalized bursts of activity with intervening inactivity or severe voltage depression) and *periodic patterns* (generalized spikes at fixed intervals of one to two per second). Absence of electrical activity on EEG, *electrocerebral silence*, can occur transiently in the period immediately after cardiopulmonary resuscitation, severe hypothermia, and central nervous system depressant overdose. Enduring electrocerebral silence provides evidence for the clinical determination of brain death.[41]

The limitations of EEG are significant. Only electrical activity involving large areas of cortex is recorded on EEG. Accuracy of EEG depends on the location of electrophysiologic activity. Abnormal EEG findings are not cause specific. Similar EEG changes occur with a variety of conditions. The EEG result can be normal even when significant pathology is present.[40]

In preparing the patient for an EEG, the nurse must stress the noninvasive aspects of this procedure. During the procedure, the awake patient may be asked to perform certain simple tasks such as blinking, closing the eye, or swallowing. Occasionally, testing must be performed during sleep or after a period of sleep deprivation.[21]

Evoked Potentials

Evoked potentials are cerebral electrical impulses generated in response to a sensory stimulus. Impulses are recorded as they travel through the brainstem and into the cerebral cortex. Measuring evoked potentials is a sophisticated way of observing the status of sensory pathways as they enter the central nervous system, travel through the brainstem, and reach the cerebral cortex. Evoked potential studies are used in the determination of prognosis in coma and the existence and extent of brainstem or spinal cord injury in the traumatically injured patient. Evaluation of evoked potentials is valuable during therapeutically induced comas such as barbiturate coma inasmuch as these sensory pathways are unaffected by the depressive activity of such medications. Evoked potentials are monitored intraoperatively during spinal surgery and cerebral tumor dissection.[40]

The four types of evoked potential tests are: 1) visual evoked responses (VERs), 2) brainstem auditory evoked responses (BAERs), 3) somatosensory evoked responses (SSERs), and 4) motor evoked potentials (MEPs). VERs involve monitoring the visual pathways through the brainstem and cortex in response to the patient's viewing a shifting geometric pattern on a screen or a flashing light stimulus emitted from a mask placed over the eye.[40] BAERs involve monitoring the auditory pathway through the brainstem and cortex in response to a rhythmic clicking sound sent through earphones placed over the patient's ears. BAERs are useful in assessing brainstem integrity in the critical care unit when cranial nerve testing cannot be performed or is inconclusive.[40] SSERs involve monitoring of sensory pathways from the extremities ascending the spinal cord through the brainstem and into the cortex. This is performed by administering a small electrical shock to a nerve root in the periphery such as the ulnar or radial nerve. SSERs can be used to evaluate cortical functioning after cardiac arrest or head trauma. SSERs also are used routinely during spinal surgery.[40] MEPs assess the functional integrity of descending motor pathways. The motor cortex is stimulated by direct high-voltage electrical stimulation through the scalp or use of a magnetic field to induce an electrical current within the brain. Electrical stimulation is a painful procedure and must be reserved for anesthetized patients. Magnetic stimulation is painless.[40]

LABORATORY STUDIES

The major laboratory study performed in the patient with neurologic dysfunction is analysis of CSF obtained by a lumbar puncture or a ventriculostomy.[3,4]

Cerebrospinal Fluid Analysis

The main purpose of a lumbar puncture is to obtain CSF for analysis. CSF opening pressure may also be obtained. CSF samples are evaluated for the presence of subarachnoid blood or infection, or they are sent for laboratory analysis (Table 23-5).[42]

A lumbar puncture involves the introduction of a 20- to 22-gauge hollow needle into the subarachnoid space at L3 to L4 or L4 to L5, below the end of the spinal cord, which usually is at L1 or L2 (see Fig. 23-13A). The patient can be placed in the lateral decubitus position, with the knees and head tightly tucked, or in the sitting position, leaning over a bedside table or some other support. Before initiating the procedure, the patient's coagulation profile should be checked for abnormalities.[43]

Two life-threatening risks associated with lumbar puncture include: 1) possible brainstem herniation, if the ICP is elevated and 2) respiratory arrest associated with neurologic deterioration. During the procedure, the nurse must monitor the patient's neurologic and respiratory status. If the patient is not fully alert and cooperative, the nurse may need to assist the patient in maintaining the position necessary for the lumbar puncture. The longstanding routine of keeping the patient flat in bed for several hours after a lumbar puncture to prevent a headache has been refuted by scientific study.[43]

Cisternal puncture, which is the introduction of a needle into the cisterna magna between C1 and C2 (see Fig. 23-13B), is another method for obtaining access to the subarachnoid space. Risks of cisternal puncture are slightly higher than those associated with a lumbar puncture, but cisternal puncture is necessary if the lumbar space cannot be entered because of scar tissue or some other physical barrier or if the CSF pathway is totally blocked somewhere along the spinal column.[44]

MULTIMODAL BEDSIDE MONITORING

Monitoring for secondary injury is a fundamental aspect of caring for the critically ill patient with a neurologic dysfunction. By utilizing more than one monitoring technique, the observer is more likely to determine whether a genuine change in cerebral physiology has occurred and what the most appropriate intervention should be.[15,45] The following discussion focuses on both commonly used and emerging multimodal techniques to monitor intracranial pressure, cerebral perfusion pressure, brain oxygenation, cerebral blood flow, cerebral metabolism, and brain function.

Intracranial Pressure Monitoring

In the patient with suspected intracranial hypertension, a device may be placed within the cranium to quantify and monitor ICP, and possibly drain excess CSF. Under normal physiologic conditions, mean ICP is maintained below 15 mm Hg.[46] An increase in ICP can decrease blood flow to the brain, causing brain damage. Persistent ICP elevation above 20 mm Hg remains the most significant factor associated with a fatal outcome.[46,47]

Types of Catheters

A variety of catheters are available to monitor ICP. They can be separated into two categories: 1) those that facilitated drainage and 2) those that do not allow for drainage. Catheters that allow for drainage are attached to a fluid-filled pressure monitoring system and an external transducer. Catheters that do not allow for drainage are of two types: 1) fiberoptic (using a light sensor to facilitate measurement of ICP), and 2)

TABLE 23-5 ANALYSIS OF CEREBROSPINAL FLUID

CHARACTERISTIC	NORMAL FINDINGS	ABNORMAL FINDINGS	POSSIBLE CAUSES AND COMMENTS
Pressure	<200 mm H$_2$O	<60 mm H$_2$O	Faulty needle placement
			Dehydration
			Spinal block along subarachnoid space
			Block of foramen magnum
			Hydrocephalus
		>200 mm H$_2$O	Muscle tension
			Abdominal compression
			Brain tumor
			Subdural hematoma
			Brain abscess
			Brain cyst
			Cerebral edema (any cause)
Color	Clear, colorless	Cloudy or turbid	Cloudy as a result of microorganisms (e.g., WBCs)
			Turbid as a result of increased cell count
		Yellow (xanthochromic)	Breakdown of RBCs with RBC pigments, high protein count
		Smoky	RBCs
Blood	None	Red blood cells: blood tinged	Traumatic tap: Bloody in first sample
		Grossly bloody	Traumatic tap: Bloody in all samples
Volume	150 mL	Increase	Hydrocephalus
Specific gravity	1.007	Increase	Infection, presence of cells or protein
WBCs	0-5 cells/mm^3	<500 cells/mm^3	Bacterial or viral infections of meninges, neurosyphilis, subarachnoid hemorrhage, infarction, abscess, tuberculous meningitis, metastatic lesions
		>500 cells/mm^3	Purulent infection
Glucose	50-75 mg/dL or 60%–70% of blood glucose	<40 mg/dL	Bacterial meningitis, tuberculosis, parasitic, fungal carcinomatous, subarachnoid hemorrhage
		>80 mg/Dl	May not be of neurologic significance
Chloride	700-750 mg/dL	Decreased (<625 mg/dL)	Meningeal infection, tuberculosis meningitis, hypochloremia
		Increased (>800 mg/dL)	May not be of neurologic significance; correlated with blood levels of chloride and not routine; done only on request
Culture and sensitivity	No organisms present	*Neisseria* or *Streptococcus*	Identify organisms to begin therapy; Gram stain for some cultures may take several weeks.
Serology for syphilis	Negative	Positive	Syphilis
Protein*	15-50 mg/dL	Increased (>60 mg/dL)	Bacterial meningitis, brain tumors (benign and malignant), complete spinal block, ALS, Guillain-Barré syndrome, subarachnoid hemorrhage, infarction, CNS trauma, CNS degenerative diseases, herniated disk, DM with polyneuropathy
		Decreased (<10 mg/dL)	May not be of neurologic significance
Osmolality	295 Osm/L	Increased	Protein, WBCs, microorganisms, RBCs
Lactate	10-20 mg/dL	Increased	Bacterial, seizure activity, fungal meningitis, CNS trauma, coma related to toxic or metabolic causes

From Barker E. *Neuroscience Nursing: A Spectrum of Care.* 3rd ed. St. Louis: Mosby; 2008.
*Blood in the CSF will raise the protein level.
ALS, Amyotrophic lateral sclerosis; *CNS*, central nervous system; *CSF*, cerebrospinal fluid; *DM*, diabetes mellitus; *RBC*, red blood cell; *WBC*, white blood cell.

microsensor (using a microchip on the end of the catheter to facilitate measurement of ICP).[48] A combination device that includes both intraventricular drainage and fiberoptic catheterization is also available for ICP monitoring. A new hybrid device that combines external ventricular drainage of cerebrospinal fluid and monitoring of intracranial pressure can be used to monitor ICP and drain cerebrospinal fluid both intermittently or continuously.[49]

Monitoring Sites

The five sites for monitoring ICP are: 1) the intraventricular space, 2) the subarachnoid space, 3) the epidural space, 4) the subdural space, and 5) the parenchyma (Fig. 23-14). Each site has advantages and disadvantages for monitoring ICP (Table 23-6). The type of monitor and site chosen depends on the suspected pathologic condition and the physician's preference.[15,50,51]

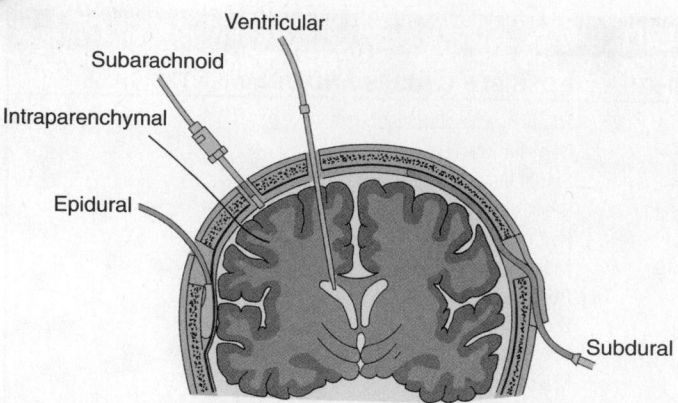

FIGURE 23-14 Intracranial pressure monitoring sites. (From Lewis SL, et al. *Medical-Surgical Nursing: Assessment and Management of Clinical Problems.* 8th ed. St. Louis: Elsevier; 2011.)

Intraventricular Space. ICP monitoring is accomplished by placing a small catheter into the ventricular system; this procedure is known as a *ventriculostomy*. With the patient under local anesthesia, the catheter is inserted through a burr hole and usually placed in the anterior horn of the lateral ventricle. If possible, the side chosen for placement of the ventriculostomy is the nondominant hemisphere.[50] Any of the catheters mentioned above can be used in the intraventricular space.[52]

Subarachnoid Space. ICP monitoring is accomplished by placing a small hollow bolt or screw with a sensor at the tip into the subarachnoid space. With the patient under local anesthesia, it is inserted through a burr hole and usually placed in the front of the skull behind the hairline. Inserting this device is easier than inserting the ventriculostomy catheter.[51,52]

Epidural Space. ICP monitoring is accomplished by placing a small fiberoptic sensor into the epidural space. It is inserted

TABLE 23-6	ADVANTAGES, DISADVANTAGES, AND NURSING CONSIDERATIONS OF ICP MONITORING TECHNIQUES		
MONITORING DEVICE	**ADVANTAGES**	**DISADVANTAGES**	**NURSING CONSIDERATIONS**
Intraventricular catheter (ventriculostomy)	Allows accurate ICP measurement	Provides an additional site for infection	Provide appropriate sedatives or analgesics during catheter insertion.
	Provides access to CSF for drainage or sampling	Is most invasive ICP monitoring technique	Do baseline and serial neurologic assessments.
	Provides access for instillation of contrast media	Requires frequent transducer balancing or recalibration	Measure patient's temperature at least every 4 hours. Note character, amount, and turbidity of CSF drainage.
	Allows reliable evaluation of intracranial compliances (volume–pressure relationships)	Catheter may be occluded by blood clot or tissue debris	Document ICP and CPP measurements, response to stimulation, and nursing care activities per hospital or unit protocol.
		Insertion difficult if ventricles are small, compressed, or displaced	Monitor quality of ICP waveform. Monitor system and tubing for air bubbles, and flush or purge system, as appropriate.
		Is associated with risk for CSF leakage around insertion site	Drain CSF, as indicated for treatment of ICP elevation. Notify physician if CSF drainage is not within prescribed parameters.
		Is associated with increased risk for infection	Monitor insertion site for bleeding, drainage, swelling, and CSF leakage.
			Set to zero, or calibrate device per hospital or unit protocol.
			Level transducer at the foramen of Monro.
			External landmarks include the tragus of the patient's ear and the external auditory canal, among others.
			All ICP measurements should be made with the transducer at a consistent level relative to external landmarks.
			Administer sedatives or analgesics as appropriate to decrease risk of catheter being dislodged by patient's movements.
			Educate patient's family, as indicated.
			Notify physician if ICP or CPP is not within specified parameters.
Subarachnoid bolt or screw	Is associated with lower infection rates than is ventriculostomy	Has potential for dampened waveform (cerebral edema, blood or tissue debris)	Administer appropriate sedatives or analgesics during insertion.
		Is quickly and easily placed	Do baseline and serial neurologic assessments. Measure patient's temperature at least every 4 hours.
	Can be used with small or collapsed ventricles	Is less accurate at high ICP elevations	Monitor insertion site for bleeding, drainage, swelling, and CSF leakage.

TABLE 23-6 ADVANTAGES, DISADVANTAGES, AND NURSING CONSIDERATIONS OF ICP MONITORING TECHNIQUES—cont'd

MONITORING DEVICE	ADVANTAGES	DISADVANTAGES	NURSING CONSIDERATIONS
	Requires no penetration of brain tissue	Requires frequent balancing or recalibration (e.g., with position changes) Provides no access for CSF sampling	Monitor quality of ICP waveform. Document ICP and CPP measurements and response to stimulation per hospital or unit protocol. Administer sedatives or analgesics as appropriate to decrease risk of catheter being dislodged by patient's movements. Set to zero, or calibrate device per hospital or unit protocol. Level transducer at the foramen of Monro. External landmarks include the tragus of the patient's ear and the external auditory canal, among others. All ICP measurements should be made with the transducer at a consistent level relative to external landmarks. Educate patient's family as indicated. Notify physician if ICP or CPP is not within specified parameters.
Subdural or epidural catheter or sensor	Is least invasive Is associated with decreased risk of infection Is easily and quickly placed	Increase in baseline drift over time means possible loss of reliability or accuracy Provides no access for CSF drainage or sampling	Administer appropriate sedatives or analgesics during insertion. Do baseline and serial neurologic assessments. Measure patient's temperature at least every 4 hours. Monitor insertion site for bleeding, drainage, and swelling. Monitor quality of ICP waveform and drift over time. Document ICP and CPP measurements and response to stimulation per hospital or unit protocol. Administer sedatives or analgesics, as appropriate to decrease risk of catheter being dislodged or damaged by patient's movements. Educate patient's family as indicated. Notify physician if ICP or CPP is not within specified parameters.
Fiberoptic transducer–tipped catheter	Can be placed in subdural or subarachnoid space, in a ventricle, or directly within brain tissue Is easily transported	Provides no access for CSF sampling or drainage	Administer appropriate sedatives or analgesics during insertion. Do baseline and serial neurologic assessments.
		Cannot be recalibrated after placement	Measure patient's temperature at least every 4 hours.
	Requires setting to zero only once (during insertion) Has baseline drift of up to 1 mm Hg per day Is associated with decreased risk for infection when brain tissue is not penetrated	Requires periodic replacement of probe Is easily damaged	Monitor insertion site for bleeding, drainage, swelling, and CSF leakage. Monitor quality of ICP waveform and drift over time.
			Document ICP and CPP measurements and response to stimulation per hospital or unit protocol.
	Provides good-quality ICP waveforms (less artifact than with other devices) Requires no adjustment in level of transducer with patient's change of position		Administer sedatives or analgesics as appropriate to decrease risk of catheter being dislodged or damaged by patient's movements. Educate patient's family, as indicated. Notify physician if ICP or CPP is not within specified parameters.

From Arbour R. Intracranial hypertension: monitoring and nursing assessment. *Crit Care Nurse.* 2004;24(5):19.
CPP, Cerebral perfusion pressure; *CSF,* cerebrospinal fluid; *ICP,* intracranial pressure.

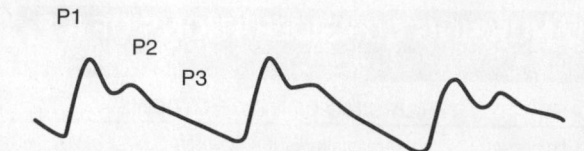

FIGURE 23-15 Normal Intracranial Pressure Waveform. (From Bader MK, Littlejohns LR. *AANN Core Curriculum for Neuroscience Nursing.* 4th ed. St. Louis: Elsevier; 2004.)

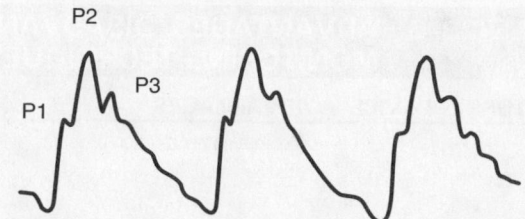

FIGURE 23-16 Abnormal Intracranial Pressure Waveform. (From Bader MK, Littlejohns LR. *AANN Core Curriculum for Neuroscience Nursing.* 4th ed. St. Louis: Elsevier; 2004.)

through a burr hole while the patient is under local anesthesia. The physician strips the dura away from the inner table of the skull before inserting the epidural monitor.[51,52]

Subdural Space. ICP monitoring is accomplished by placing a fiberoptic or microsensor catheter into the subdural space. It is inserted through a burr hole while the patient is under local anesthesia.[51,52]

Intraparenchymal Site. ICP monitoring is accomplished by placing a fiberoptic catheter or microsensor catheter into the parenchymal tissue. After placing a subarachnoid bolt (as previously described), a hole is punched in the dura, and the catheter is inserted approximately 1 cm into the brain's white matter.[51,52]

The intraventricular space is considered the gold standard for monitoring of ICP, since it is the most accurate of all methods.[50] However, a recent study found that an intraparenchymal catheter was better than an intraventricular catheter unless CSF drainage was required. The intraparenchymal catheter was associated with decreased monitoring time, decreased length of stay, and decreased device-related complications.[53]

Nursing considerations for each type of device are discussed in Table 23-6.

Intracranial Pressure Waves

The ICP pulse waveform is observed on a continuous, real-time pressure display, and it corresponds to each heartbeat. The waveform arises primarily from pulsations of the major intracranial arteries but also receives retrograde venous pulsations.[50]

Normal Intracranial Pressure Waveform. The normal ICP wave has three or more defined peaks (Fig. 23-15). The first peak (P1) is called the *percussion wave.* Originating from the pulsations of the choroid plexus, it has a sharp peak and is fairly consistent in its amplitude. The second peak (P2) is called the *tidal wave.* The tidal wave varies more in shape and amplitude, ending on the dicrotic notch. The P2 portion of the pulse waveform has been most directly linked to the state of decreased compliance. When the P2 component is equal to or higher than P1, decreased compliance occurs (Fig. 23-16). Immediately after the dicrotic notch is the third wave (P3), which is called the *dicrotic wave.* After the dicrotic wave, the pressure usually tapers down to the diastolic position unless retrograde venous pulsations add a few more peaks.[50,54,55]

A, B, and C pressure waves are not true waveforms (Fig. 23-17). Rather, they are the graphically displayed trend data of ICP over time. These waves reflect spontaneous alterations in

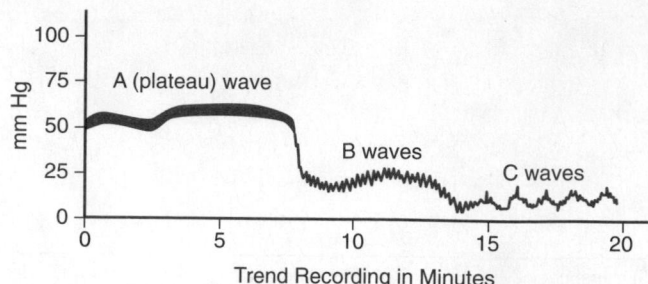

FIGURE 23-17 Intracranial Pressure Waves. Composite diagram of A-waves (plateau waves), B-waves (sawtooth waves), and C-waves (small rhythmic waves). (From Barker E. *Neuroscience Nursing: A Spectrum of Care.* 3rd ed. St. Louis: Mosby; 2008.)

ICP associated with respiration, systemic blood pressure, and deteriorating neurologic status.

A-Waves. Also called *plateau waves* because of their distinctive shape, A-waves are the most clinically significant of the three types. They usually occur in an already elevated baseline ICP (>20 mm Hg) and are characterized by sharp increases in ICP of 30 to 69 mm Hg, which plateau for 2 to 20 minutes and then return to baseline. The cause of A-waves is unknown, but they may result from vasodilation and increased CBF, decreased venous outflow (and, therefore, increased cerebral blood volume), fluctuations in $Paco_2$ (and, therefore, changes in cerebral blood volume), or decreased CSF absorption. B-waves often precede A-waves. Plateau waves are considered significant because of the reduced cerebral perfusion pressure associated with ICP, in the range of 50 to 100 mm Hg. Transient signs of intracranial hypertension such as a decreased level of consciousness, bradycardia, pupillary changes, or respiratory changes may accompany these waves. Some research suggests that prolonged increases in ICP associated with plateau waves may result in transient and permanent cell damage from ischemia.[4,50]

B-Waves. B-waves are sharp, rhythmic oscillations with a sawtooth appearance that occur every 30 seconds to 2 minutes and that can raise the ICP from 5 to 70 mm Hg. They are a normal physiologic phenomenon that can occur in any patient, but they are amplified in states of low intracranial compliance. B-waves appear to reflect fluctuations in cerebral blood volume.[4,50]

C-Waves. C-waves are small, rhythmic waves that occur every 4 to 8 minutes at normal levels of ICP. They are related to normal fluctuations in respiration and systemic arterial pressure.[4,50]

Pupillometry

Quantitative measurement and classification of pupillary reactivity using a handheld pupillometer, and the Neurological Pupil index (NPi) is an emerging technique to trend increased ICP in patients with severe traumatic brain injury (TBI), aneurysmal subarachnoid hemorrhage, or intracerebral hemorrhage (ICH). The pupillometer is a handheld infrared system, which automatically tracks and analyzes pupil dynamics over a 3-second period.[56] A detachable headrest facilitates the correct and consistent placement of the pupillometer in front of the eye. The device has been specifically designed to minimize possible interobserver variability in the pupillary evaluation.[57] NPi classifies pupil reactivity through the use of an algorithm. An inverse relationship between decreasing pupil reactivity and increasing ICP has been identified with the use of pupillometry and NPi.[57]

Cerebral Perfusion Pressure Monitoring

Measurement of ICP allows for an estimation of cerebral perfusion pressure (CPP). CPP is the blood pressure gradient across the brain, and it is calculated as the difference between the incoming mean arterial pressure (MAP) and the opposing ICP on the arteries: (CPP = MAP − ICP). Over the last two decades, treatment approaches have emphasized maintaining the CPP near 80 mm Hg, to provide an adequate of supply to the brain and, thus, avoid secondary cerebral ischemia.[58] However, recent studies have emphasized that individual patients may have different CPP thresholds, depending on the degree of autoregulation and intracranial compliance.[59] The 2007 Brain Trauma Foundation guidelines now recommend a CPP in the range of 50 to 70 mm Hg and consideration of cerebral autoregulation status when selecting a CPP target in a specific patient.[60]

Cerebral Blood Flow Monitoring
Transcranial Doppler Studies

Transcranial Doppler (TCD) studies monitor CBF velocity through cranial windows (thinned areas) of the skull. Three areas commonly used are: 1) the temporal bone (transtemporal), 2) the eye (transorbital), and 3) the foramen magnum (transoccipital). Depending on the angle of the Doppler probe, flow velocities can be measured in the anterior, middle, or posterior cerebral arteries and the vertebral and basilar arteries. Numerous clinical applications for TCD have been identified.[61]

TCD studies often are used in critical care for patients after an intracranial aneurysm rupture when vasospasm development is a concern. The noninvasive technique and portability of the equipment allow frequent bedside monitoring of flow velocity and, therefore, of vascular diameter. Use of serial TCD studies for the detection of cerebral vasospasm greatly reduces the need for cerebral angiograms to verify and follow postsubarachnoid hemorrhage vasospasm.[61]

Additional uses of TCD include identification of intracranial lesions in the patient with stroke, evaluation of flow-velocity changes during carotid endarterectomy, and detection of CBF changes associated with increased ICP. TCD has been used to detect cerebral circulatory arrest in brain death determination, but it must be accompanied by clinical evaluation and additional diagnostic tests because intracranial circulation may be preserved in patients who are brain dead.[61]

The limitations of the TCD study must be understood. Its accuracy is operator dependent. Correct location and angle of the probe are essential. A few patients have temporal bones too thick for ultrasound penetration. A normal TCD study does not completely rule out the presence of vasospasm because vasospasm may not be evident in the particular vessel examined. TCD results are always evaluated in conjunction with clinical assessment findings.[61]

During the TCD study, the patient experiences only mild pressure at the transducer site. No pain is involved. The patient must remain still during the study, which lasts 15 to 90 minutes.[61]

Transcranial Color-Coded Duplex Sonography. Transcranial color-coded duplex sonography (TCCS) is a noninvasive ultrasound study that enables the visualization of the intracranial structures and basal cerebral arteries and the measurement of blood flow velocities through the arteries. The color component of the study provides more reliable data compared with the traditional TCD. TCCS is becoming a reliable tool for detecting narrowing or occlusion of cerebral arteries, screening for vasospasm, and monitoring changes in intracranial dynamics. AVMs can also be detected with TCCS.[62]

Thermal Diffusion Flowmetry

A relatively new method for continuous, real-time CBF monitoring is thermal diffusion flowmetry (TDF). Thermal diffusion therapy allows the quantitative measurement of regional cerebral blood flow (rCBF), which is considered an important upstream monitoring parameter indicative of tissue viability.[56] With this method, a TD-rCBF microprobe is placed 20 to 25 mm below the cortical surface via a small burr hole and is secured by tightening a metal bolt. Once the microprobe is in place, the nurse attaches it to an umbilical cord and monitor to begin calibration.[56] The microprobe includes a heated distal thermistor and a proximal thermistor. The distal thermistor measures blood flow via heat transfer to the capillaries. A microprocessor then converts this information in to a measure of CBF in mL/100 g/min, which is represented as the K-value on the monitor. As a general rule, mean TD-rCBF values range between 18 and 25 mL/100 g/min.[63]

It is important to consider, however, that CBF values measured by TD-rCBF vary, depending on the placement of the probe.[63] Another important consideration with the use of TDF is that the monitor only provides CBF parameters within a temperature range of 25° C to 39.5° C.[56] Patient cooling should, therefore, be considered if the temperature of the brain is greater than 38.5° C.[56] Other considerations with the use of TDF are that the probe can be viewed on CT or with radiography and is not compatible with MRI. Also, as the TDF monitor does not run on battery power, the probe must be disconnected from the umbilical cord and secured to the patient's head dressing prior to patient transport. Additionally, if the probe is used in conjunction with a microdialysis catheter, the two catheters must be separated by 2 mm for accurate results.[56]

Laser Doppler Flowmetry

Another new method being used for CBF monitoring is laser Doppler flowmetry (LDF). With LDF, a probe directly inserted into the brain parenchyma detects density measurements of moving blood, thereby providing momentary percentage changes in local CBF. LDF does not provide absolute quantitative values of CBF, but rather relative change—which currently limits its utility in the context of neuromonitoring.[30]

Cerebral Oxygenation and Metabolic Monitoring

The following methods may be used in the critical care unit to monitor the patient cerebral oxygenation status and cerebral metabolic state.

Jugular Venous Oxygen Saturation

Jugular venous oxygen saturation ($SjvO_2$) is an indicator of global oxygen extraction of the brain. Jugular venous desaturation suggests an increase in cerebral oxygen extraction, which indirectly implies that a decrease has occurred in cerebral oxygen delivery, and hence perfusion.[45] Any disorder that increases $CMRO_2$ or decreases oxygen delivery may decrease $SjvO_2$, and conversely, any disorder that decreases $CMRO_2$ or increases oxygen delivery may increase $SjvO_2$.[64,65]

To measure $SjvO_2$, a fiberoptic catheter is placed retrograde through the internal jugular vein into the jugular bulb and attached to a bedside monitor. The normal value is 55% to 75%. Patients with values less than 54% are hypoxemic or oligemic (low CBF compared with metabolic rate). Oligemia occurs as a result of decreased blood flow due to hypotension, vasospasm, or intracranial hypertension or as a result of increased brain metabolic requirements due to fever or seizures. $SjvO_2$ values below 45% are indicative of severe cerebral hypoxia. Patients with values above 75% are considered hyperemic (high CBF compared with metabolic need).[45] $SjvO_2$ also increases if the brain is so severely injured the neurons are unable to extract oxygen. As a global measure, $SjvO_2$ monitoring is complementary to focal monitoring of brain tissue oxygen pressure ($PbtO_2$).[58]

$SjvO_2$ monitoring has several limitations. The most significant limitation is that $SjvO_2$ does not reflect metabolic inadequacies in the focal areas of brain injury and, therefore, may miss regional areas of ischemia.[45] Another limitation is that $SjvO_2$ readings are affected by the position and movement of the patient's head.[65] Inaccuracies with $SjvO_2$ monitoring can occur with catheter misplacement, contamination with extra cerebral blood, when the catheter abuts the blood vessel wall, or if thrombosis occurs around the catheter tip.[45]

Near Infrared Spectroscopy

$SjvO_2$ is representative of global cerebral oxygenation, whereas infrared spectroscopy (NIRS) is an emerging bedside diagnostic technique, similar to pulse oximetry, that measures regional cerebral oxygenation. The major advantage of NIRS is that it is a noninvasive method for measuring $CMRO_2$. The major

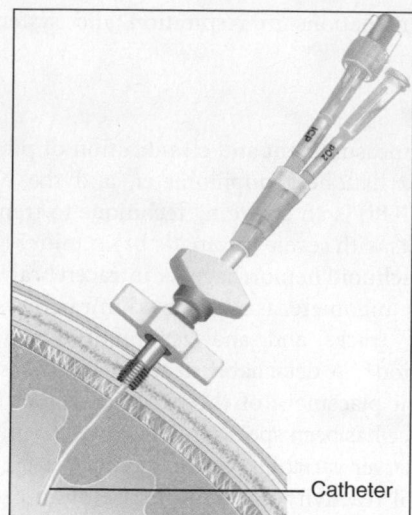

FIGURE 23-18 The LICOX brain tissue oxygen system involves a catheter inserted through an intracranial bolt. The system measures oxygen in the brain, brain tissue temperature, and intracranial pressure. (From Lewis SL, et al. *Medical-Surgical Nursing: Assessment and Management of Clinical Problems.* 8th ed. St. Louis: Elsevier; 2011.)

limitations of NIRS include its inability to distinguish between intracranial and extracranial changes in blood flow, and the difficulty associated with NIRS data interpretation.[45,66]

Brain Tissue Oxygen Pressure

Monitoring $PbtO_2$ has been shown to be a reliable and sensitive diagnostic method to monitor cerebral oxygenation. $PbtO_2$ uses a device similar to pulse oximetry that allows continuous monitoring of regional tissue oxygenation and, in particular, areas of high ischemic risk.[45,67] The device consists of a monitoring probe on the end of a catheter, which is inserted into the brain parenchyma and attached to a bedside monitor (Fig. 23-18). The probe may be inserted into the damaged portion of the brain to measure regional oxygenation or inserted into the undamaged portion of the brain to measure global oxygenation. One risk associated with insertion of the catheter is bleeding and hematoma formation.[68] Although no consensus on normal values exists because values vary from device to device, it has been concluded that the probability of death increases with prolonged periods of $PbtO_2$ less than 15 mm Hg and any episode of $PbtO_2$ less than 6 mm Hg.[67]

In the patient with head injury, the goal of treatment is to maintain the $PbtO_2$ greater than 20 mm Hg. Factors that decrease $PbtO_2$ include tissue hypoxia, hypocapnia, hypovolemia, decreased blood pressure, low hemoglobin levels, intracranial hypertension, and hyperthermia.[68] Treatment is directed at the underlying cause.

Cerebral Microdialysis

Cerebral microdialysis is a neuromonitoring method that measures the concentration of chemicals found in the brain parenchyma, with the goal of detecting neurochemical changes indicative of primary and secondary brain injury.[30] Cerebral microdialysis involves placement of a small catheter into the brain parenchyma, either during surgery or through a burr hole, which is secured by a cranial bolt. This microdialysis catheter has a 10-mm semipermeable distal membrane.[56] When fluid isotonic to the tissue interstitium is pumped into the catheter, the catheter acts likes an artificial blood capillary. It is, therefore, through diffusion that the metabolic markers glucose, pyruvate, lactate, glutamate, and glycerol are collected from the interstitial fluid and analyzed hourly.[30] Lactate and pyruvate are ischemic metabolites and the ratio of lactate to pyruvate is currently the best early biomarker of secondary ischemic injury.[56] A lactate-to-pyruvate ratio greater than 40 is indicative of cerebral metabolic crisis.[58] Glycerol, a marker of cell membrane damage, and glutamate, an excitatory amino acid, provide additional evidence of developing brain injury.[58] Despite its increasing use in the clinical management of patients with TBI, cerebral microdialysis is still generally considered a research tool.[29]

Continuous Electroencephalography Monitoring

Continuous electroencephalography (cEEG) in the critical care unit is increasingly recognized as an important diagnostic and prognostic tool.[69] Continuous EEG monitoring provides dynamic information about brain function, permitting early detection of changes in neurologic status. This is especially useful when the clinical examination is limited. The principal applications for cEEG are monitoring for seizures and ischemia, guiding therapy for seizures and ischemia (especially vasospasm), adjusting levels of sedation for paralyzed or delirious patients, and charting trends in brain function and prognosis.[70] The drawbacks to the use of cEEG are that it is an expensive, labor-intensive program that requires expertise for interpretation, and is subject to artifact from the ICU environment.[70,71] More research on cEEG is needed to determine its cost-saving potential and impact on outcome.

SUMMARY

Clinical Assessment

- A neurologic history includes information about clinical manifestations, associated complaints, precipitating factors, progression of symptoms, familial occurrences, and events preceding the onset of symptoms.
- The five major components of a neurologic examination are evaluation of: 1) level of consciousness, 2) motor function, 3) pupillary function, 4) respiratory function, and 5) vital signs.
- Assessment of the level of consciousness focuses on evaluation of arousal and appraisal of awareness.
- Assessment of motor function focuses on the evaluation of muscle size and tone and estimation of muscle strength.
- Assessment of papillary function focuses on estimation of pupil size and shape, evaluation of papillary reaction to light, and appraisal of eye movements.
- Assessment of respiratory functions focuses on observation of respiratory pattern and evaluation of airway status.
- Assessment of vital signs focuses on evaluation of blood pressure and observation of heart rate.
- Increasing ICP can be identified by changes in the level of consciousness, pupillary reaction, motor response, vital signs, and respiratory patterns.

Diagnostic Procedures

- Radiologic procedures are often performed to identify abnormalities of the brain, spinal cord, and the surrounding bone and tissue. These tests include skull and spine radiography, CT, MRI, cerebral angiography, and myelography.
- Imaging of cerebral blood flow and metabolism can help to define the cause and extent of brain injury, identify appropriate treatments, and predict the outcome. These tests include perfusion CT, xenon CT, perfusion MRI, carotid duplex sonography, PET, and SPECT.
- Electrophysiology studies are often performed to evaluate the electrical impulses of the brain. These tests include EEG, VERs, BAERs, SSERs, and MEPs.

Laboratory Studies

- CSF analysis is performed (by lumbar puncture or ventriculostomy) to look for the presence of blood or infection in the subarachnoid space.

Multimodal Monitoring

- ICP monitoring is used in the patient with suspected intracranial hypertension. The use of pupillometry and NPi is a new technique for trending increased ICP. Measurement of ICP allows for an estimation of CPP, which is the blood pressure gradient across the brain.
- CBF monitoring plays an important role in neurologic care because the brain depends on continuous blood flow to supply glucose and oxygen. TCD, TCCS, TDF, and LDF are techniques to monitor CBF.
- Measurements of brain oxygenation and metabolism provide insight into understanding acute brain injury and ways to manage secondary brain injury. Techniques to monitor brain oxygenation, metabolism, or both include $SjvO_2$, NIRS, $PbtO_2$, and cerebral microdialysis.
- cEEG is used to detect epileptic seizures and cerebral ischemia.

REFERENCES

1. McGlinsey A, Kirk A. Neurological assessment: early identification of neurological deterioration is vital to preventing secondary brain injury. Available at: http://nursing.advanceweb.com/Continuing-Education/CE-Articles/Neurological-Assessment.aspx. Accessed July 6, 2012.
2. Daroff RB, et al. Diagnosis of neurological disease. In: Daroff RB, et al, eds. *Bradley's Neurology in Clinical Practice.* 6th ed. Philadelphia: Elsevier; 2012.

3. Barker E. *Neuroscience Nursing: A Spectrum of Care*. 3rd ed. St. Louis: Mosby; 2008.

4. Bader MK, Littlejohns LR, eds. *AANN Core Curriculum for Neuroscience Nursing*. 5th ed. Glenview: American Association of Neuroscience Nurses; 2010.

5. Koita J, et al. The mental status examination in emergency practice. *Emerg Med Clin North Am*. 2010;28:439.

6. Seidel HM, et al. *Mosby's Guide to Physical Examination*. 7th ed. St. Louis: Mosby; 2011.

7. Teasdale G, Jennett W. Assessment of coma and impaired consciousness—a practical scale. *Lancet*. 1974;2:81.

8. Green SM. Cheerio, laddie! Bidding farewell to the Glasgow Coma Scale. *Ann Emer Med*. 2011;58:427.

9. Kornbluth J, Bhardwaj A. Evaluation of coma: a critical appraisal of popular scoring systems. *Neurocrit Care*. 2011;14:134.

10. Berger JR. Stupor and coma. In: Daroff RB, et al, eds. *Bradley's Neurology in Clinical Practice*. 6th ed. Philadelphia: Elsevier; 2012.

11. McGee S. *Evidence-Based Physical Diagnosis*. 3rd ed. Philadelphia: Elsevier; 2012.

12. Rucker JC. Pupillary and eyelid abnormalities. In: Daroff RB, et al, eds. *Bradley's Neurology in Clinical Practice*. 6th ed. Philadelphia: Elsevier; 2012.

13. Adoni A, McNett M. The pupillary response in traumatic brain injury: a guide for trauma nurses. *Trauma Nurs*. 2007;14:191.

14. Bishop BS. Pathologic papillary signs: self-learning module. Part II. *Crit Care Nurs*. 1991;11(7):58.

15. Haddad SH, Arabi YM. Critical care management of severe traumatic brain injury in adults. *Scand J Trauma Resusc Emerg Med*. 2012;20:12.

16. Saiki RL. Current and evolving management of traumatic brain injury. *Crit Care Nurs Clin North Am*. 2009;21:549.

17. Samuels MA. The brain-heart connection. *Circulation*. 2007;116:77.

18. Fodstad H. History of the Cushing reflex. *Neurosurgery*. 2006;59:1132.

19. Yuh EL, Dillon WP. Intracranial hypotension and intracranial hypertension. *Neuroimaging Clin N Am*. 2010;20:597.

20. Saunders D. Skull and brain: methods of examination and anatomy. In: Adam A, Dixon AK, eds. *Grainger & Allison's Diagnostic Radiology: A Textbook of Medical Imaging*. 5th ed. London: Elsevier Churchill Livingstone; 2008.

21. Chernecky CC, Berger BJ. *Laboratory Tests and Diagnostic Procedures*. 5th ed. St. Louis: Saunders; 2008.

22. Cogbill TH, Ziegelbein KJ. Computed tomography, magnetic resonance, and ultrasound imaging: basic principles, glossary of terms, and patient safety. *Surg Clin N Am*. 2011;91:1.

23. Ajtai B, et al. Neuroimaging: structural imaging: magnetic resonance imaging, computed tomography. In: Daroff RB, et al, eds. *Bradley's Neurology in Clinical Practice*. 6th ed. Philadelphia: Elsevier; 2012.

24. McInnis LA, et al. Angiography: from a patient's perspective. *Crit Care Nurs Clin N Am*. 2010;22:51.

25. Ahn SS, Kim YD. Three-dimensional digital subtraction angiographic evaluation of aneurysm remnants after clip placement. *J Korean Neurosurg Soc*. 2010;47:185.

26. Ledezma CJ, Wintermark M. Multimodal CT in stroke imaging: new concepts. *Radiol Clin North Am*. 2009;47:109.

27. Stevens JM, et al. The spine. In: Adam A, Dixon AK, eds. *Grainger & Allison's Diagnostic Radiology: A Textbook of Medical Imaging*. 5th ed. London: Churchill Livingstone; 2008.

28. Kim N, et al. Noninvasive measurement of cerebral blood flow and blood oxygenation using near-infrared and diffuse correlation spectroscopies in critically brain-injured adults. *Neurocrit Care*. 2010;12:173.

29. Noble K. Traumatic brain injury and increased intracranial pressure. *J Perianesth Nurs*. 2010;25:242.

30. Barazangi N, Hemphill JC. Advanced cerebral monitoring in neurocritical care. *Neurol India*. 2008;56:405.

31. Jain V, et al. MRI estimation of global brain oxygen consumption rate. *J Cereb Blood Flow Metab*. 2010;30:1598.

32. Hoeffner EG, et al. Cerebral perfusion CT: technique and clinical applications. *J Neuroradiol*. 2008;35:252.

33. Carlson AP, et al. Xenon-enhanced cerebral blood flow at 28% xenon provides uniquely safe access to quantitative, clinically useful cerebral blood flow information: a multicenter study. *AJNR Am J Neuroradiol*. 2011;32:1315.

34. Van Boven RW, et al. Advances in neuroimaging of traumatic brain injury and posttraumatic stress disorder. *J Rehabil Res Develop*. 2009;46:717.

35. Hoa D. Brain perfusion imaging. Available at: http://www.imaios.com/en/e-Courses/e-MRI/Cerebral-perfusion-imaging/introduction. Accessed July 8, 2012.

36. Adamczyk P, Liebeskind DS. Neuroimaging: vascular imaging: computed tomographic angiography, magnetic resonance angiography, and ultrasound. In: Daroff RB, et al, eds. *Bradley's Neurology in Clinical Practice*. 6th ed. Philadelphia: Elsevier; 2012.

37. Miletich RS. Positron emission tomography for neurologists. *Neurol Clin*. 2009;27:61.

38. Derdeyn CP. Positron emission tomography imaging of cerebral ischemia. *PET Clinics*. 2007;2:35.

39. Zukotynski K, et al. In: Christain PE, Waterstram-Rich KM, eds. *Nuclear Medicine and PET/CT: Technology and Techniques*. 7th ed. St. Louis: Elsevier; 2012.

40. Emercon RG, Pedley TA. Clinical neurophysiology: electroencephalography and evoked potentials. In: Daroff RB, et al, eds. *Bradley's Neurology in Clinical Practice*. 6th ed. Philadelphia: Elsevier; 2012.

41. Andraus ME, Alves-Leon SV. Non-epileptiform EEG abnormalities: an overview. *Arq Neuropsiquiatr*. 2011;69:829.

42. Welch H, Hasbun R. Lumbar puncture and cerebrospinal fluid analysis. *Handb Clin Neurol*. 2010;96:31.

43. Shlamovitz GZ. Lumbar puncture. Available at http://emedicine.medscape.com/article/80773-overview. Accessed July 6, 2012.

44. Euerle BD. Spinal puncture and cerebrospinal fluid examination. In: Roberts JR, Hedges JR, eds. *Clinical Procedures in Emergency Medicine*. Philadelphia: Saunders; 2010.

45. Kitchener N, et al. The flying publisher guide to critical care in neurology. Available at: http://www.operationflyingpublisher.com/pdf/FPG_007_CriticalCareinNeurology_2012.pdf. Accessed July 8, 2012.

46. Balasteri M, et al. Impact of intracranial pressure and cerebral perfusion pressure on severe disability and mortality after head injury. *Neurocritical Care*. 2006;4:8.

47. Narotam PK, et al. Brain tissue monitoring in traumatic brain injury and major trauma: Outcome analysis of a brain tissue oxygen-directed therapy. *J Neurosurg*. 2009;111:672.

48. Chin LS. ICP monitors. Available at: http://emedicine.medscape.com/article/1983045-overview#a3. Accessed July 8, 2012.

49. Slazinski T. Combination intraventricular/fiberoptic catheter insertion (assist), monitoring, nursing care, troubleshooting, and removal. In: Lynn-McHale Wiegand DJ, ed. *AACN Procedure Manual for Critical Care*. 6th ed. St. Louis: Saunders; 2011.

50. American Association of Neuroscience Nurses. *Guide to the Care of the Patient Undergoing Intracranial Pressure Monitoring/External Ventricular Drainage or Lumbar Drainage: AANN Clinical Practice Guideline Series.* Glenview: The Association; 2011.

51. Arbour R. Intracranial hypertension: monitoring and nursing assessment. *Crit Care Nurse.* 2004;24(5):19.

52. Brain Trauma Foundation, et al. Guidelines for the management of severe traumatic brain injury. VII. Intracranial pressure monitoring. *J Neurotrauma.* 2007;24(Suppl 1):S45.

53. Kasotakis G, et al. Intraperechymal vs extracranial ventricular drain intracranial pressure monitors in traumatic brain injury: less is more? *J Am Coll Surg.* 2012;214:950.

54. Rangel-Castillo L, Robertson CS. Management of intracranial hypertension. *Crit Care Clin.* 2006;22:713.

55. Bhatia A, Gupta AK. Neuromonitoring in the intensive care unit. I. Intracranial pressure and cerebral blood flow monitoring. *Intensive Care Med.* 2007;33:1263.

56. Cecil S, et al. Traumatic brain injury: advanced multimodal neuromonitoring from theory to practice. *Crit Care Nurse.* 2011;31(2)25.

57. Chen JW, et al. Pupillary reactivity as an early indicator of increased intracranial pressure: The introduction of the Neurological Pupil Index. *Surg Neurol Int.* 2011;2:82.

58. Hemphill JC, et al. Mulitmodal monitoring and neurocritical care bioinformatics. *Nat Rev Neurol.* 2011;7:451.

59. Naval NS, et al. Controversies in the management of aneurysmal subarachnoid hemorrhage. *Crit Care Med.* 2006;34:511.

60. Brain Trauma Foundation, et al. Guidelines for the management of severe traumatic brain injury. IX. Cerebral perfusion thresholds. *J Neurotrauma.* 2007;24(Suppl. 1):S59.

61. Kassab MY, et al. Transcranial Doppler: an introduction for primary care physicians. *J Am Board Fam Med.* 2007;20:65.

62. Krejza J. Clinical applications of transcranial color-coded duplex sonography. *J Neuroimaging.* 2004;14:215.

63. Vajkoczy P, et al. Monitoring cerebral blood flow in neurosurgical intensive care, Available at: http://www.touchneurology.com/articles/monitoring-cerebral-blood-flow-neurosurgical-intensive-care-0?page=0,4. Accessed July 8, 2012.

64. Smith M. Perioperative uses of transcranial perfusion monitoring. *Anesthesiol Clin.* 2007;25:557.

65. Slazinski T. Jugular venous oxygen saturation monitoring: insertion (assist), patient care, troubleshooting, and removal. In: Lynn-McHale Wiegand DJ, ed. *AACN Procedure Manual for Critical Care.* 6th ed. St. Louis: Saunders; 2011.

66. Murkin JM, Arango M. Near-infrared spectroscopy as an index of brain and tissue oxygenation. *Br J Anaesth.* 2009;103(suppl 1):i3.

67. Bader MK. Recognizing and treating ischemic insults to the brain: the role of brain tissue oxygen monitoring. *Crit Care Nurs Clin North Am.* 2006;18:243.

68. Wartenberg KE, et al. Multimodality monitoring in neurocritical care. *Crit Care Clin.* 2007;23:507.

69. Vulliemoz S, et al. Imaging compatible electrodes for continuous electroencephalogram monitoring in the intensive care unit. *J Clin Neurophysiol.* 2009;26:236.

70. Young GB. Continuous EEG monitoring in the ICU: challenges and opportunities. *Can J Neurol Sci.* 2009;2:89.

71. Wijdicks E, Rabinstein AA. Critical care neurology: five new things. *Neurol Clin Pract.* 2011;1:34.

Neurologic Disorders and Therapeutic Management

Lourdes Januszewicz, Barbara Buesch

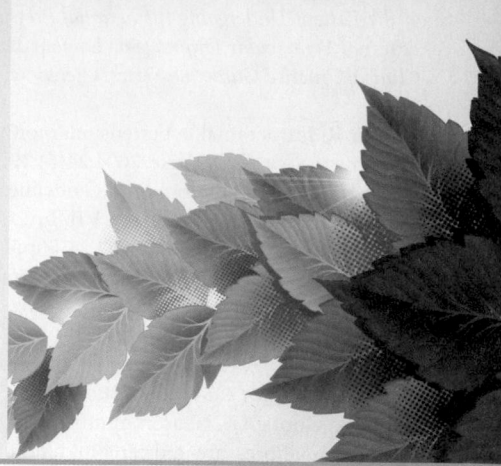

evolve WEBSITE

http://evolve.elsevier.com/Urden/criticalcare/

Evolve features:

- NCLEX Review Questions
- CCRN Review Questions
- PCCN Review Questions
- Mosby's Nursing Skills Procedures
- Animations
- Video Clips
- Glossary

To accurately anticipate and plan nursing interventions, the critical care nurse must have an understanding of the disease pathology, determine the areas of focused assessment, and be well acquainted with the medical management of the patient with neurologic disorders. Fortunately, despite a wide array of neurologic disorders, only a few routinely require the critical care environment.

COMA

Description

Normal consciousness requires awareness and arousal. Awareness is the combination of cognition (mental and intellectual) and affect (mood) that can be construed based on the patient's interaction with the environment.[1] Alterations of consciousness may be the result of deficits in awareness, arousal, or both.[2] The four discrete disorders of consciousness are: 1) coma, 2) vegetative state, 3) minimally conscious state, and 4) locked-in syndrome. *Coma* is characterized by the absence of both wakefulness and awareness, whereas a *vegetative state* is characterized by the presence of wakefulness with the absence of awareness. In the *minimally conscious state*, wakefulness is present, and awareness is severely diminished but not absent. *Locked-in syndrome* is characterized by the presence of wakefulness and awareness, but with quadriplegia and the inability to communicate verbally; thus, the patient appears to be unconscious.[3] Box 24-1 lists the disorders of consciousness in descending order of wakefulness.

Coma is the deepest state of unconsciousness; arousal and awareness are lacking.[1-3] The patient cannot be aroused and does not demonstrate any purposeful response to the surrounding environment.[4] Coma is a symptom rather than a disease, and it occurs as a result of some underlying process.[1,2] The incidence of coma is difficult to ascertain because a wide variety of conditions can induce coma.[1,2] This state of unconsciousness is, unfortunately, very commonly encountered in the critical care unit, and it is the focus of the following discussion.

Etiology

The causes of coma can be divided into two general categories: 1) structural or surgical and 2) metabolic or medical. Structural causes of coma include ischemic stroke, intracerebral hemorrhage (ICH), trauma, and brain tumors.[5] Metabolic causes of coma include drug overdose, infectious diseases, endocrine disorders, and poisonings.[5] Coma demands immediate attention, resulting in a high percentage of admissions to all hospital services.[6] Box 24-2 provides a list of the possible causes of coma.

Pathophysiology

Consciousness involves arousal, or wakefulness, and awareness. Neither of these functions is present in the patient in coma. Ascending fibers of the reticular activating system (ARAS) in the pons, hypothalamus, and thalamus maintain arousal as an autonomic function. Neurons in the cerebral cortex are responsible for awareness. Diffuse dysfunction of both cerebral hemispheres and diffuse or focal dysfunction of the reticular activating system can produce coma.[1,6,7] Structural causes usually produce compression or dysfunction in the area of the ARAS, whereas most medical causes lead to general dysfunction of both cerebral hemispheres.[8] Trauma, hemorrhage, and tumor

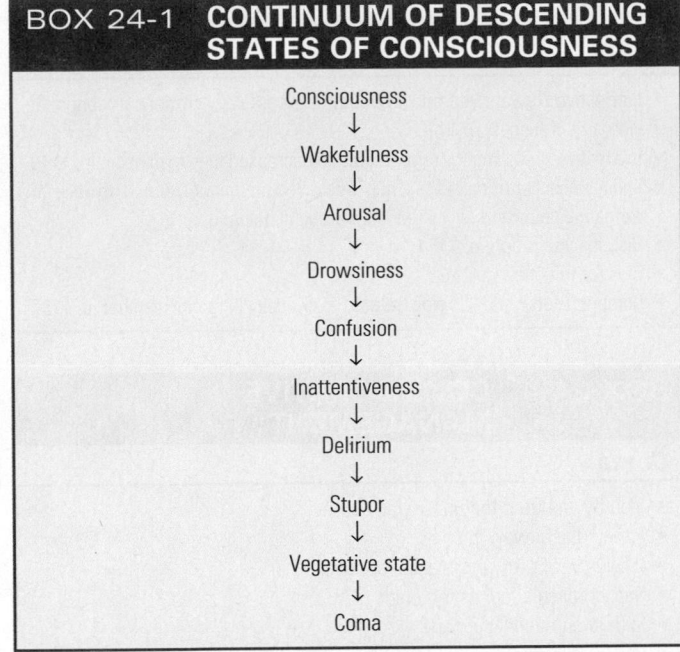

BOX 24-1   CONTINUUM OF DESCENDING STATES OF CONSCIOUSNESS

Consciousness
↓
Wakefulness
↓
Arousal
↓
Drowsiness
↓
Confusion
↓
Inattentiveness
↓
Delirium
↓
Stupor
↓
Vegetative state
↓
Coma

BOX 24-2   CAUSES OF COMA

Structural or Surgical Coma	Metabolic or Medical Coma
Trauma	Infection
Epidural hematoma	Meningitis
Subdural hematoma	Encephalitis
Diffuse axonal injury	Metabolic encephalopathy
Brain contusion	Metabolic conditions
Intracerebral hemorrhage	Hypoglycemia
Subarachnoid hemorrhage	Hyperglycemia
Posterior fossa hemorrhage	Hyperosmolar states
Supratentorial hemorrhage	Uremia
Hydrocephalus	Hepatic encephalopathy
Ischemic stroke	Hypertensive encephalopathy
Tumor	Hypoxic encephalopathy
Other causes	Hyponatremia
	Hypercalcemia
	Myxedema
	Intoxication
	Opioid overdose
	Alcohol
	Poisonings
	Psychogenic causes

and the coma is profound, the response of the patient to emergent treatment may provide clues to the underlying diagnosis; for example, the patient who becomes responsive with the administration of naloxone can be presumed to have ingested some type of opiate.[6]

Detailed serial neurologic examinations are essential for all patients in coma. Assessment of pupillary size and reaction to light (normal, sluggish, or fixed), extraocular eye movements (normal, asymmetric, or absent), motor response to pain (normal, decorticate, decerebrate, or flaccid), and breathing pattern yields important clues for determining whether the cause of coma is structural or metabolic.[1,6]

The areas of the brainstem that control consciousness and pupillary responses are anatomically adjacent. The sympathetic and parasympathetic nervous systems control pupillary dilation and constriction, respectively. The anatomic directions of these pathways are known, and changes in pupillary responses can help identify where a lesion may be located (see Fig. 23-4 in Chapter 23). For example, if damage occurs in the midbrain region, pupils will be slightly enlarged and unresponsive to light. Lesions that compress the third nerve result in a fixed and dilated pupil on the same side as the neurologic insult. Pupillary responses are usually preserved when the cause of coma is metabolic in origin. Pupillary light responses are often the key to differentiating between structural and metabolic causes of coma.[1,6,7,9]

Areas of the brainstem adjacent to those responsible for consciousness also control the oculomotor eye movement. The ability to maintain conjugate gaze requires preservation of the internuclear connections of cranial nerves III, VI, and VIII by means of the medial longitudinal fasciculus (MLF).[8] As with pupillary responses, structural lesions that impinge on these pathways cause oculomotor dysfunction such as a disconjugate gaze. Deficits in extraocular eye movements usually accompany a structural cause.[1,5,9]

Focal or asymmetric motor deficits usually indicate structural lesions.[1,5] Abnormal motor movements may also help pinpoint the location of a lesion. Decorticate posturing (abnormal flexion) can be seen with damage to the diencephalon. Decerebrate posturing (abnormal extension) can be seen with damage to the midbrain and pons. Flaccid posturing is an ominous sign and can be seen with damage to the medulla.[9]

Abnormal breathing patterns may also assist in differentiating structural from metabolic causes of coma. Cheyne-Stokes respirations are seen in patients with cerebral hemispheric dysfunction or metabolic suppression. Central neurogenic hyperventilation, or Kussmaul breathing, occurs with metabolic acidosis or damage to the midbrain and upper pons. Apneustic breathing may occur with damage to the pons, hypoglycemia, and anoxia. Ataxic breathing occurs with damage to the medulla. Agonal breathing occurs with failure of the respiratory centers in the medulla.[6,9]

In addition to physical assessment, laboratory studies and diagnostic procedures are done. Structural causes of coma are usually readily apparent with computed tomography (CT) or magnetic resonance imaging (MRI).[4,8] Laboratory studies are also used to identify metabolic or endocrine abnormalities.[7] Evoked potentials are also useful in facilitating a differential

can damage the ARAS, leading to coma. Destruction of large regions of bilateral cerebral hemispheres can be the result of seizures or viral agents. Toxic drugs, toxins, or metabolic abnormalities can suppress cerebral function.[5-7]

Assessment and Diagnosis

The clinical diagnosis of the comatose state is readily established by assessment of the level of consciousness. However, determining the full nature and cause of coma requires a thorough history and physical examination. A medical history is essential because events immediately preceding the change in the level of consciousness can often provide valuable clues to the origin of the coma. When limited information is available diagnosis between the disorders of consciousness and in evaluating a patient's prognosis. Generally, a patient in coma, with absence of brainstem auditory evoked responses (BAERs), is considered to have a poor prognosis of recovery.[3] Occasionally, the cause of coma is never clearly determined.

Medical Management

The goal of medical management of the patient in coma is identification and treatment of the underlying cause of the condition. Initial medical management includes emergency measures to support vital functions and prevent further neurologic deterioration. Protection of the airway and ventilatory assistance are often needed. Administration of thiamine (at least 100 milligrams [mg]), glucose, and a opioid antagonist is suggested when the cause of coma is not immediately known.[1,6] Thiamine is administered before glucose because the coma produced by thiamine deficiency, Wernicke encephalopathy, can be precipitated by a glucose load.[1]

The patient who remains in coma after emergent treatment requires supportive measures to maintain physiologic body functions and prevent complications. Intubation for continued airway protection and nutritional support are essential. Fluid and electrolyte management is often complex because of alterations in the neurohormonal system. Anticonvulsant therapy may be necessary to prevent further ischemic damage to the brain.[1,5,6]

The health care team and the patient's family make decisions jointly regarding the level of medical management to be provided. Family members require informational support in terms of the probable cause of coma and the prognosis for recovery of consciousness and function. Prognosis depends on the cause of coma and the length of time unconsciousness persists. Only 15% of patients in nontraumatic coma make a satisfactory recovery.[7] Metabolic coma usually has a better prognosis compared with coma caused by a structural lesion, and traumatic coma usually has a better outcome compared with nontraumatic coma.[5,7]

Much research has been directed toward identifying the prognostic indicators for the patient in coma after a cardiopulmonary arrest. In a meta-analysis, the best predictors of poor outcome after cardiac arrest were lack of corneal or papillary response at 24 hours and lack of motor movement at 72 hours. However, regardless of the cause or duration of coma, outcome for an individual cannot be predicted with 100% accuracy.[10] Research has focused on induced hypothermia in patients after cardiac arrest. The use of hypothermia has demonstrated improved neurologic outcomes and survival rates. When a patient remains comatose after return of spontaneous circulation, the body is cooled to 32° C to 34° C for up to 24 hours.[11,12]

Nursing Management

Nursing management of the patient in coma incorporates a variety of nursing diagnoses (Box 24-3) and is directed by the specific cause of the coma, although some common interventions are used. The patient in coma totally depends on the health care team. Nursing interventions focus on monitoring for changes in neurologic status and clues to the origin of the coma, supporting all body functions, maintaining surveillance

---

BOX 24-3   NURSING DIAGNOSES

Coma

- Ineffective Airway Clearance, related to excessive secretions or abnormal viscosity of mucus, p. 1148
- Ineffective Breathing Pattern, related to decreased lung expansion, p. 1149
- Imbalanced Nutrition: Less Than Body Requirements, related to lack of exogenous nutrients or increased metabolic demand, p. 1143
- Risk for Aspiration, p. 1154
- Risk for Infection, p. 1160
- Compromised Family Coping, related to critically ill family member, p. 1127

BOX 24-4   COLLABORATIVE MANAGEMENT

Coma

- Identify and treat the underlying cause.
- Protect the airway.
- Provide ventilatory assistance, as required.
- Support circulation, as required.
- Initiate nutritional support.
- Provide eye care.
- Protect skin integrity.
- Initiate range-of-motion exercises.
- Maintain surveillance for complications:
  - Infections
  - Metabolic alterations
  - Cardiac dysrhythmias
  - Temperature alterations
- Provide comfort and emotional support.
- Plan for the rehabilitation program.

---

for complications, providing comfort and emotional support, and initiating rehabilitation measures.[1] Measures to support body functions include promoting pulmonary hygiene, maintaining skin integrity, initiating range-of-motion exercises, managing bowel and bladder functions, and ensuring adequate nutritional support.[1]

Eye Care

The blink reflex is often diminished or absent in the patient in coma. The eyelids may be flaccid and may depend on body positioning to remain in a closed position, and edema may prevent complete closure. Loss of these protective mechanisms results in drying and ulceration of the cornea, which can lead to permanent scarring and blindness.[1]

Two interventions that are commonly used to protect the eyes are instilling saline or methylcellulose lubricating drops and taping the eyelids in the shut position. Evidence suggests that an alternative technique may be more effective in preventing corneal epithelial breakdown. In addition to instilling saline drops every 2 hours, a polyethylene film is taped over the eyes, extending beyond the orbits and eyebrows. The film creates a moisture chamber around the cornea and assists in keeping the eyes moist and in the closed position. This technique also prevents damage to the eyes that results from tape or gauze being placed directly on the delicate skin of the eyelids.[13]

Collaborative management of the patient in coma is outlined in Box 24-4.

STROKE

Stroke is a descriptive term for the sudden onset of acute neurologic deficit persisting for more than 24 hours and caused by the interruption of blood flow to the brain. Stroke is the fourth leading cause of death in the United States, preceded by heart disease, cancer, and chronic respiratory disease. Each year, approximately 795,000 people have a stroke; 610,000 of these are first attacks, and 185,000 are recurrent attacks.[14]

Strokes are classified as ischemic and hemorrhagic (Fig. 24-1). Hemorrhagic strokes can be further categorized as subarachnoid hemorrhages (SAHs) and intracerebral hemorrhages (ICHs). Approximately 87% of all strokes are ischemic, 10% are ICHs, and 3% are SAHs. Although less common, hemorrhagic strokes (ICHs and SAHs) have a higher mortality rate compared with ischemic strokes. Approximately 8% to 12% of ischemic strokes and 37% to 38% of hemorrhagic strokes result in death within 30 days.[14] The annual cost for care and loss of productivity was estimated to be $76.6 billion in 2012.[14]

The national concern for the incidence and effects of stroke is illustrated by the inclusion of emergent stroke care in the American Heart Association (AHA) guidelines for basic and advanced life support. Major public education programs, stroke appraisal screening programs, development of stroke centers, and algorithms for stroke management are based on the success that these same approaches have had with coronary artery disease.

Ischemic Stroke

Description

Ischemic stroke results from interruption of blood flow to the brain and accounts for 80% to 85% of all strokes. The interruption can be the result of a thrombotic or embolic event. Thrombosis can form in large vessels (large-vessel thrombotic strokes) or small vessels (small-vessel thrombotic strokes). Embolic sources include the heart (cardioembolic strokes) and atherosclerotic plaques in larger vessels (atheroembolic strokes). In 30% of the cases, the underlying cause of the stroke is unknown (cryptogenic strokes).[15]

Strokes are preventable. Most thrombotic strokes are the result of the accumulation of atherosclerotic plaque in the vessel lumen, especially at the bifurcations or curves of the vessel. The pathogenesis of cerebrovascular disease is identical to that of coronary vasculature. The greatest risk factor for ischemic stroke is hypertension.[15,16] Other risk factors are dyslipidemia, diabetes, smoking, and carotid atherosclerotic disease.[14,17] Common sites of atherosclerotic plaque are the bifurcation of the common carotid artery, the origins of the middle and anterior cerebral arteries, and the origins of the vertebral arteries.[16] Ischemic strokes resulting from vertebral artery dissection have been reported after chiropractic manipulation of the cervical spine.[18]

Etiology

An embolic stroke occurs when an embolus from the heart or lower circulation travels distally and lodges in a small vessel, obstructing the blood supply. At least 20% of ischemic strokes are attributed to a cardioembolic phenomenon.[15] The most common cause of cardiac emboli is atrial fibrillation. It is responsible for about 50% of all cardiac emboli.[19] Other sources of cardiac emboli are from mitral stenosis, mechanical valves, atrial myxoma, endocarditis, and recent myocardial infarction.[16] Researchers hypothesize that a patent foramen ovale or atrial septal aneurysms may be the cause of cryptogenic stroke.[20]

Pathophysiology

Ischemic stroke is a cerebral hemodynamic insult. When cerebral blood flow is reduced to a level insufficient to maintain neuronal viability, ischemic injury occurs. In focal stroke, an area of hypoperfused tissue, the ischemic penumbra, surrounds a core of ischemic cells. The ischemic penumbra can be salvaged with return of blood flow. However, sustained anoxic insult initiates a chain of biochemical events leading to apoptosis, or cellular death.[21]

The phenomenon of a focal ischemic stroke is identical to that associated with myocardial infarction, which is why the term *brain attack* is used in public education strategies. Often, a history of transient ischemic attacks (TIAs), brief episodes of neurologic symptoms that last less than 24 hours, offers a warning that stroke is likely to occur. Sudden onset indicates embolism as the final insult to flow.[15,16] The size of the stroke depends on the size and location of the occluded vessel and the availability of collateral blood flow. Global ischemia results when severe hypotension or cardiopulmonary arrest provokes a transient drop in blood flow to all areas of the brain.[21]

Cerebral edema sufficient to produce clinical deterioration develops in 10% to 20% of patients with ischemic stroke and can result in intracranial hypertension. The edema results from a loss of normal metabolic function of the cells and peaks at 4 days.[15] This process is commonly the cause of death during the first week after a stroke.[22] Secondary hemorrhage at the site of the stroke lesion, known as *hemorrhagic conversion*, and seizures are the two other major acute neurologic complications of ischemic stroke.[22,23]

Assessment and Diagnosis

The characteristic sign of an ischemic stroke is the sudden onset of focal neurologic signs persisting for more than 24 hours.[15] These signs usually occur in combination. Box 24-5 lists common patterns of neurologic symptoms associated with an ischemic stroke. Hemiparesis, aphasia, and hemianopia are common. Changes in the level of consciousness usually occur only with brainstem or cerebellar involvement, seizure, hypoxia, hemorrhage, or elevated intracranial pressure (ICP). These changes may be exhibited as stupor, coma, confusion, and agitation.[1] The reported frequency of seizures in patients with ischemic stroke ranges from 3% to 8%. If seizures occur, they are usually seen within 24 hours of an insult.[23]

The National Institutes of Health Stroke Scale (NIHSS) is often used as the basis of the focused neurologic examination. The score ranges from 0 to 42 points; the higher the score, the more neurologically impaired the patient is. A change of 4 points on the scale indicates significant neurologic change. The components of the NIHSS include level of consciousness (LOC); LOC questions; LOC commands; gaze; visual fields; face, arm, and leg strength; sensation; limb ataxia; and language

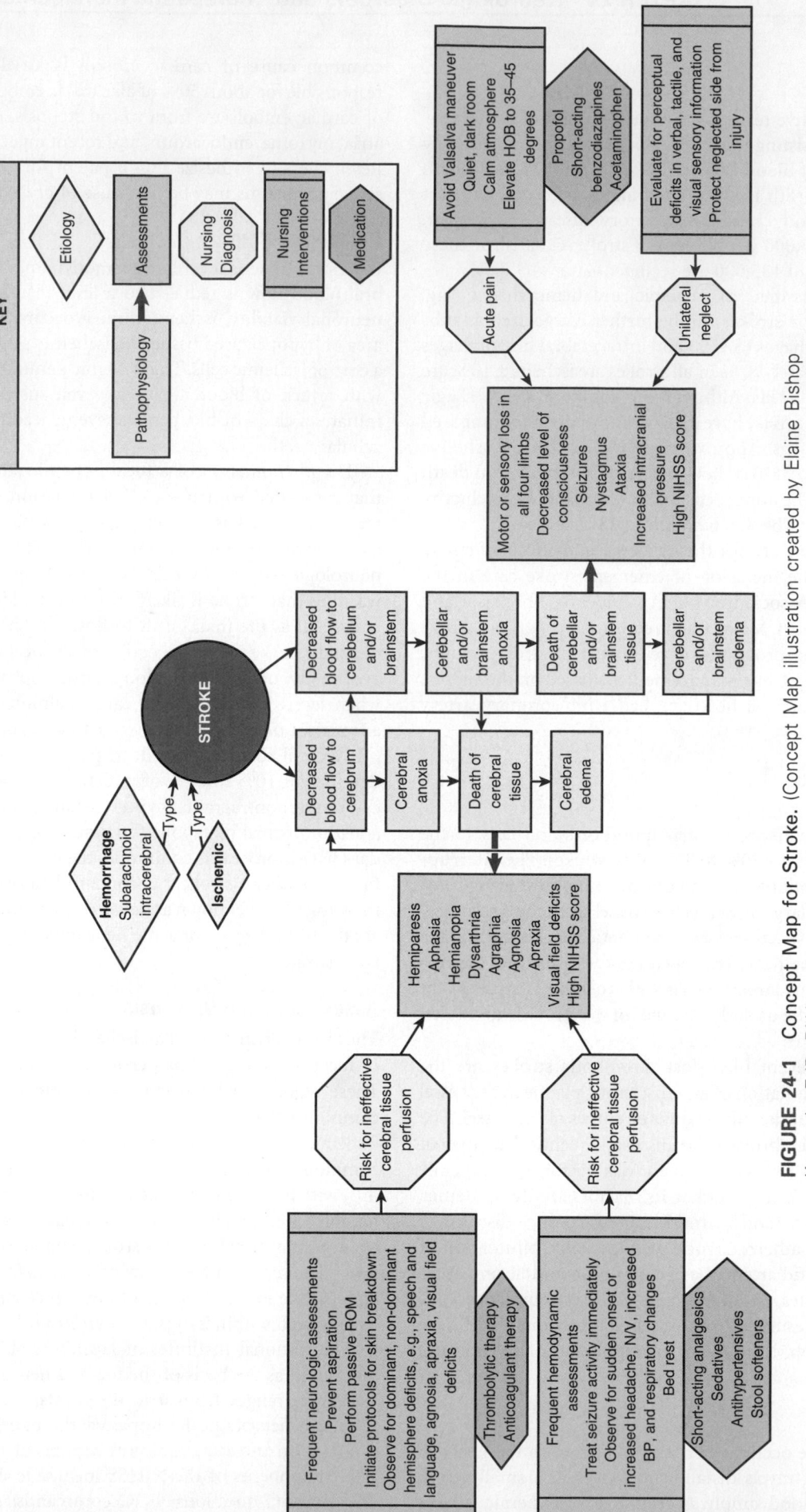

FIGURE 24-1 Concept Map for Stroke. (Concept Map illustration created by Elaine Bishop Kennedy, EdD, RN.)

BOX 24-5 NEUROLOGIC ABNORMALITIES IN ACUTE ISCHEMIC STROKES

Left (Dominant) Hemisphere

Aphasia, right hemiparesis, right-sided sensory loss, right visual field defect, poor right conjugate gaze, dysarthria, difficulty in reading, writing, or calculating

Right (Nondominant) Hemisphere

Neglect of the left visual space, left visual field defect, left hemiparesis, left-sided sensory loss, poor left conjugate gaze, extinction of left-sided stimuli, dysarthria, spatial disorientation

Brainstem, Cerebellum, and Posterior Hemisphere

Motor or sensory loss in all four limbs, crossed signs, limb or gait ataxia, dysarthria, disconjugate gaze, nystagmus, amnesia, bilateral visual field defects

Small Subcortical Hemisphere or Brainstem (Pure Motor Stroke)

Weakness of face and limbs on one side of the body without abnormalities of higher brain function, sensation, or vision

Small Subcortical Hemisphere or Brainstem (Pure Sensory Stroke)

Decreased sensation of face and limbs on one side of the body without abnormalities of higher brain function, motor function, or vision

From Adams HP, et al. Guidelines for the management of patients with acute ischemic stroke: a statement for healthcare professionals from a special writing group of the Stroke Council, American Heart Association. *Circulation.* 1994;90(3):1588.

BOX 24-6 CHARACTERISTICS OF PATIENTS WITH ISCHEMIC STROKE WHO COULD BE TREATED WITH RTPA

Diagnosis of Ischemic Stroke Causing Measurable Neurologic Deficit

- The neurologic signs should not be clearing spontaneously.
- The neurologic signs should not be minor and isolated.
- Caution should be exercised in treating a patient with major deficits.
- The symptoms of stroke should not be suggestive of subarachnoid hemorrhage.
- Onset of symptoms less than 3 hours before beginning treatment.
- No head trauma or prior stroke in previous 3 months.
- No myocardial infarction in the previous 3 months.
- No gastrointestinal or urinary tract hemorrhage in previous 21 days.
- No major surgery in the previous 14 days.
- No arterial puncture at a noncompressible site in the previous 7 days.
- No history of previous intracranial hemorrhage.
- Blood pressure not elevated (systolic <185 mm Hg and diastolic <110 mm Hg).
- No evidence of active bleeding or acute trauma (fracture) on examination.
- Not taking an oral anticoagulant or, if anticoagulant being taken, international normalized ratio (INR) 1.7 or less.
- If receiving heparin in previous 48 hours, aPTT must be in normal range.
- Platelet count 100 000 mm^3 or greater.
- Blood glucose concentration 50 mg/dL (2.7 mmol/L) or greater.
- No seizure with postictal residual neurologic impairments.
- Computed tomography does not show a multilobar infarction (hypodensity >1/3 cerebral hemisphere).
- The patient or family members understand the potential risks and benefits from treatment.

aPTT, Activated partial thromboplastin time; *INR,* international normalized ratio.
From Adams HP, Jr. et al. Guidelines for the early management of adults with ischemic stroke: a guideline from the American Heart Association/American Stroke Association Stroke Council, Clinical Cardiology Council, Cardiovascular Radiology and Intervention Council, and the Atherosclerotic Peripheral Vascular Disease and Quality of Care Outcomes in Research Interdisciplinary Working Groups: the American Academy of Neurology affirms the value of this guideline as an educational tool for neurologists. *Stroke.* 2007;38:1655.

function.[15] A copy of the NIHSS with complete instructions is available at http://www.ninds.nih.gov/disorders/stroke/strokescales.htm.

Confirmation of the diagnosis of ischemic stroke is the first step in the emergent evaluation of these patients. Differentiation from intracranial hemorrhage is vital. Noncontrast computed tomography (CT) scanning is the method of choice for this purpose, and it is considered the most important initial diagnostic study. In addition to excluding intracranial hemorrhage, CT can assist in identifying early neurologic complications and the cause of the insult.[15] Magnetic resonance imaging (MRI) can demonstrate infarction of cerebral tissue earlier than can CT but is less useful in the emergent differential diagnosis.[24] Because of the strong correlation between acute ischemic stroke and heart disease, 12-lead electrocardiography (ECG), chest radiography, and continuous cardiac monitoring are suggested to detect a cardiac cause or coexisting condition. Echocardiography is valuable in identifying a cardioembolic phenomenon when a sufficient index of suspicion warrants its use.[1] Laboratory evaluation of hematologic function, electrolyte and glucose levels, and renal and hepatic function is also recommended. Arterial blood gas analysis is performed if hypoxia is suspected, and electroencephalography (EEG) is performed if seizures are suspected. Lumbar puncture is performed only if SAH is suspected and the CT scan is normal.[1]

Medical Management

Major changes have taken place in the medical management of ischemic stroke since 1996. Based on results of the National

Institute of Neurologic Disorders and Stroke (NINDS) recombinant tissue plasminogen activator (rtPA) Stroke Study, fibrinolytic therapy with intravenous rtPA is recommended within 3 hours of onset of ischemic stroke.[20] This time frame has now been expanded from 3 hours to 4.5 hours.[25] Patients who should be considered for fibrinolysis are listed in Box 24-6. Confirmation of diagnosis with CT must be accomplished before rtPA administration. The recommended dose of rtPA is 0.9 milligram per kilogram (mg/kg) up to a maximum dose of 90 mg. Ten percent of the total dose is administered as an initial intravenous bolus, and the remaining 90% is administered by intravenous infusion over 60 minutes.[20,24]

The desired result of fibrinolytic therapy is to dissolve the clot and reperfuse the ischemic brain. The goal is to reverse or minimize the effects of stroke. The major risk and complication of rtPA therapy is bleeding, especially intracranial hemorrhage. Unlike fibrinolytic protocols for acute myocardial infarction, subsequent therapy with anticoagulant or antiplatelet agents is not recommended after rtPA administration in ischemic stroke. Patients receiving fibrinolytic therapy for stroke should not receive aspirin, heparin, warfarin, ticlopidine, or any other anti-thrombotic or antiplatelet medications for at least 24 hours after treatment.[15,20]

The major barriers to effective application of fibrinolytic therapy for ischemic stroke are prehospital and in-hospital delays.[26] To help decrease delays, the public needs to be educated about stroke symptoms and activation of emergency medical system (EMS). EMS responders need adequate education and training on managing a patient with an acute ischemic stroke, focusing on stabilization and transport of the patient quickly to the emergency department. The receiving hospital should ideally have certification for primary stroke treatment and have expert staff and the infrastructure to care for the patient with complex stroke.[20,24]

Other emergent care of the patient with ischemic stroke must include airway protection and ventilatory assistance to maintain adequate tissue oxygenation.[22] Hypertension is often present in the early period as a compensatory response, and in most cases, blood pressure (BP) must not be lowered (Table 24-1). For the patient who has not received fibrinolytic therapy, antihypertensive therapy is considered only if the diastolic blood pressure is greater than 120 mm Hg or the systolic blood pressure is greater than 220 mm Hg.[15,20] Criteria are different for patients who have received rtPA. Their blood pressure is kept below 180/105 mm Hg to prevent intracranial hemorrhage. Intravenous labetalol or nicardipine is used to achieve blood pressure control. If these agents are not effective, nitroprusside, hydralazine, or enalaprilat should be considered.[15] Body temperature and glucose levels also must be normalized.[15,22]

Medical management also includes the identification and treatment of acute complications such as cerebral edema or seizure activity. Prophylaxis for these complications is not recommended. Deep vein thrombosis (DVT) prophylaxis, however, should be initiated to decrease the risk of pulmonary embolism.[15] One study demonstrated that improved outcomes for patients with ischemic stroke can be achieved by managing swallowing issues, initiating DVT prophylaxis, and treating hypoxemia.[27] Surgical decompression is recommended if a large cerebellar infarction compresses the brainstem.[22]

Subarachnoid Hemorrhage
Description
Subarachnoid hemorrhage (SAH) is bleeding into the subarachnoid space, which usually is caused by rupture of a cerebral

TABLE 24-1	BLOOD PRESSURE MANAGEMENT FOR STROKE ACCORDING TO THE AMERICAN STROKE ASSOCIATION GUIDELINES
BLOOD PRESSURE*	**TREATMENT**
Nonthrombolytic Candidates	
DBP >140 mm Hg	Sodium nitroprusside (0.5 mcg/kg/min); aim for 10%-20% reduction in DBP
SBP >220 mm Hg, DBP 121-140 mm Hg, or MAP[†] >130 mm Hg	10-20 mg of labetalol[‡] given by IVP over 1-2 min; may repeat or double labetalol every 20 min to a maximum dose of 300 mg
SBP <220 mm Hg, DBP = 120 mm Hg, or MAP[†] <130 mm Hg	Emergency antihypertensive therapy is deferred in the absence of aortic dissection, acute myocardial infarction, severe congestive heart failure, or hypertensive encephalopathy
Thrombolytic Candidates *Pretreatment*	
SBP >185 mm Hg or DBP >110 mm Hg	1-2 inches of nitroglycerine paste (Nitropaste) or 1-2 doses of 10-20 mg of labetalol[‡] given by IVP; if BP is not reduced and maintained to <185/110 mm Hg, the patient should not be treated with tPA
During and After Treatment Monitor BP	BP is monitored every 15 min for 2 hr, then every 30 min for 6 hr, and then hourly for 16 hr
DBP >140 mm Hg	Sodium nitroprusside (0.5 mcg/kg/min)
SBP >230 mm Hg or DBP 121-140 mm Hg	10 mg of labetalol[‡] given by IVP over 1-2 min; may repeat or double labetalol every 10 min to a maximum dose of 300 mg or give initial labetalol bolus and then start a labetalol drip at 2-8 mg/min. If BP not controlled by labetalol, consider sodium nitroprusside
SBP 180-230 mm Hg or DBP 105-120 mm Hg	10 mg of labetalol[‡] given by IVP; may repeat or double labetalol every 10-20 min to a maximum dose of 300 mg or give initial labetalol bolus and then start a labetalol drip at 2-8 mg/min

*All initial blood pressures should be verified before treatment by repeating reading in 5 minutes.
[†]As estimated by one third of the sum of systolic and double diastolic pressure.
[‡]Labetalol should be avoided in patients with asthma, cardiac failure, or severe abnormalities in cardiac conduction. For refractory hypertension, alternative therapy may be considered with sodium nitroprusside or enalapril.
BP, Blood pressure; *DBP*, diastolic blood pressure; *IVP*, intravenous push; *MAP*, mean arterial pressure; *SBP*, systolic blood pressure; *tPA*, tissue-type plasminogen activator.
From Bader MK, Littlejohns LR. *AANN Core Curriculum for Neuroscience Nursing.* 4th ed. St. Louis: Elsevier; 2004.

aneurysm or arteriovenous malformation (AVM).[22] At the time of autopsy, approximately 4% of the population has been found to have one or more aneurysms.[28] With improvements in imaging techniques, an increased number of incidental intracranial aneurysms has been found. Computed tomographic angiography (CTA) and magnetic resonance angiography (MRA) can detect up to 95% of all aneurysms. Among people younger than 40 years, more men than women are likely to have SAHs, whereas among those older than 40 years, more women have SAHs. Aneurysmal SAH is associated with a mortality rate of 25% to 50%, with most patients dying on the first day after the insult.[28] Hemorrhage from AVM rupture has a better chance of survival and is associated with an overall mortality rate of 10% to 15%.[29] Known risk factors for SAH include hypertension, smoking, and alcohol or stimulant use.[30]

Etiology

Cerebral aneurysm rupture accounts for approximately 85% of all cases of spontaneous SAH.[28] An aneurysm is an outpouching of the wall of a blood vessel that results from weakening of the wall of the vessel (Table 24-2).[28] Ninety percent of aneurysms are congenital—the cause of which is unknown. The other 10% can be the result of traumatic injury (that stretches and tears the muscular middle layer of the arterial vessel) or infectious material (most often from infectious vegetation on valves of the left side of the heart after bacterial endocarditis) that lodges against a vessel wall and erodes the muscular layer, or they are of undetermined cause.[30] Multiple aneurysms occur in approximately 30% of the cases and often are bilateral, occurring in the same location on both sides of the cerebral vascular system.[31]

AVM rupture is responsible for roughly 6% of all SAHs.[31] An AVM is a tangled mass of arterial and venous blood vessels that shunt blood directly from the arterial side into the venous side, bypassing the capillary system. AVMs may be small, focal lesions or large, diffuse lesions that occupy almost an entire hemisphere.[30] They are always congenital, although the exact embryonic cause for these malformations is unknown. They also

TABLE 24-2	ANEURYSM CLASSIFICATION ACCORDING TO TYPE, SHAPE, LOCATION, AND COMMON CHARACTERISTICS

TYPES OF ANEURYSMS	CHARACTERISTICS	TYPES OF ANEURYSMS	CHARACTERISTICS
Berry or saccular	Most common type, usually congenital; appears at a bifurcation in the anterior circulation, primarily at the base of the brain or the circle of Willis and its branches; grows from the base of the arterial wall with a neck or stem; contains blood; thinned dome is usually the site of rupture	Dissecting	May occur during angiography; caused by trauma, syphilis, arteriosclerosis, or when blood is forced between layers of the arterial wall; intima is pulled away from the medial layer, allowing blood to enter
Giant or fusiform	Can have an irregular shape and be larger than 2.5 cm and atherosclerotic; involves mainly the internal carotid or vertebrobasilar artery; rarely ruptures; has no stem; may act like a space-occupying lesion in the brain; difficult to manage	Traumatic	Sometimes called a *pseudoaneurysm*, which may resolve after trauma
		Charcot-Bouchard	Small aneurysm that can be seen in the area of the basal ganglia or the brainstem in individuals with a history of hypertension; chronic hypertension causes fibrinoid necrosis in the penetrating and subcortical arteries, weakening the arterial walls and causing formation of small aneurysmal outpouching
Mycotic	Rare form; usually occurs from septic emboli, usually results from bacterial infection, which weaken the vessel wall, causing dilation involving the distal branches of the middle cerebral arteries		

occur in the spinal cord and the renal, gastrointestinal, and integumentary systems.[31] Small, superficial AVMs are seen as port-wine stains of the skin. In contrast to the SAH from an aneurysm in the middle-aged population, SAH from an AVM usually occurs in the second to fourth decades of life.[30,31]

Pathophysiology

The pathophysiologies of the two most common causes of SAH, cerebral aneurysm and AVM, are distinctly different.

Cerebral Aneurysm. As the individual with a congenital cerebral aneurysm gets older, blood pressure rises, and more stress is placed on the poorly developed and thin vessel wall. Ballooning of the vessel occurs, giving the aneurysm a berrylike appearance. Most cerebral aneurysms are saccular or berrylike, with a stem or neck. Aneurysms are usually small, are 2 to 7 millimeters (mm) in diameter, and often occur at the base of the brain on the circle of Willis.[29] Figure 24-2 illustrates the usual distribution between the vessels. Most cerebral aneurysms occur at the bifurcation of blood vessels.[28,29,32]

The aneurysm becomes clinically significant when the vessel wall becomes so thin that it ruptures, sending arterial blood at a high pressure into the subarachnoid space. For a brief moment after the aneurysm ruptures, ICP is thought to approach mean arterial pressure, and cerebral perfusion decreases.[32] In other situations, the unruptured aneurysm expands and places pressure on surrounding structures. This is particularly true with posterior communicating artery aneurysms because they put pressure on the oculomotor nerve (cranial nerve III), causing ipsilateral pupil dilation and ptosis.[31]

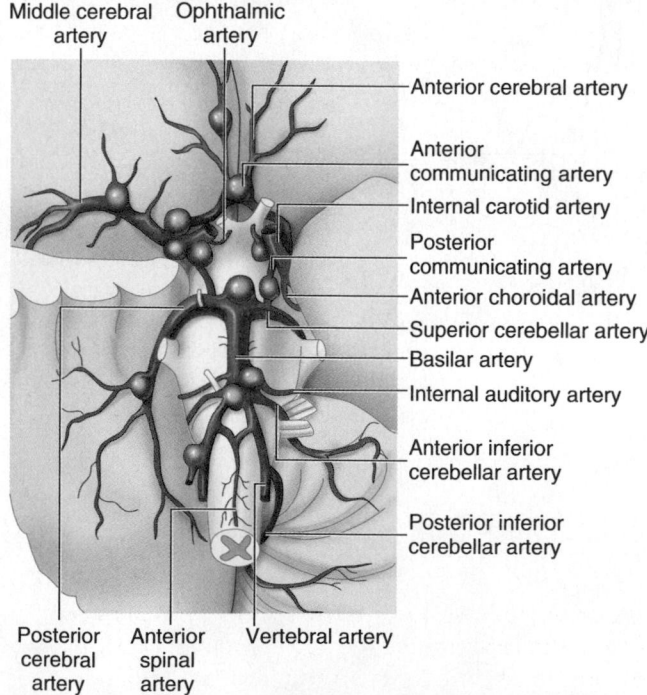

Middle cerebral artery
Ophthalmic artery
Anterior cerebral artery
Anterior communicating artery
Internal carotid artery
Posterior communicating artery
Anterior choroidal artery
Superior cerebellar artery
Basilar artery
Internal auditory artery
Anterior inferior cerebellar artery
Posterior inferior cerebellar artery
Posterior cerebral artery
Anterior spinal artery
Vertebral artery

FIGURE 24-2 **Common Sites of Berry Aneurysms.** The size of the aneurysm in the drawing is proportional to the frequency of occurrence at the various sites. (From Zivin JA. Hemorrhagic cerebrovascular disease. In: Goldman L, Schafer AI, eds. *Goldman's Cecil Medicine.* 24th ed. St. Louis: Elsevier; 2012.)

Arteriovenous Malformation. The pathophysiologic features of an AVM are related to the size and location of the malformation. One or more cerebral arteries, also known as *feeders,* supply an AVM. These feeder arteries tend to enlarge over time and increase the volume of blood shunted through the malformation and increase the overall mass effect. Large, dilated, tortuous draining veins develop as a result of increasing arterial blood flow being delivered at a higher-than-normal pressure. Normal vascular flow has a mean arterial pressure of 70 to 80 mm Hg, a mean arteriole pressure of 35 to 45 mm Hg, and a mean capillary pressure that drops from 35 to 10 mm Hg as it connects with the venous side. Lack of this capillary bridge allows blood with a mean pressure of 35 to 45 mm Hg to flow into the venous system. Unlike arteries, veins have no muscular layer and become extremely engorged and rupture easily. Some patients with AVMs also have cerebral atrophy. It is the result of chronic ischemia because of the shunting of blood through the AVM and away from normal cerebral circulation.[33]

Assessment and Diagnosis

The patient with an SAH characteristically has an abrupt onset of pain, described as the "worst headache of my life." A brief loss of consciousness, nausea, vomiting, focal neurologic deficits, and a stiff neck may accompany the headache.[28-32] The SAH may result in coma or death.

The patient's history may reveal one or more incidences of sudden onset of headache with vomiting in the weeks preceding a major SAH. These are small "warning leaks" of an aneurysm in which small amounts of blood ooze from the aneurysm into the subarachnoid space. The presence of blood is an irritant to the meninges, particularly the arachnoid membrane, and the irritation causes headache, stiff neck, and photophobia. These warning leaks seldom are detected because the condition is not severe enough for the patient to seek medical attention.[32] If a neurologic deficit such as third cranial nerve palsy develops before aneurysm rupture, medical intervention is sought, and the aneurysm may be surgically secured before the devastation of a rupture can occur. Symptoms of unruptured AVM—headaches with dizziness or syncope or fleeting neurologic deficits—also may be found in the history.[31]

Diagnosis of SAH is based on clinical presentation, CT findings, and lumbar puncture results. Noncontrast CT is the cornerstone of definitive SAH diagnosis.[30-34] In 95% of the cases, CT demonstrates blood in the subarachnoid space if performed within 48 hours the hemorrhage.[28,32] On the basis of the appearance and the location of the SAH, diagnosis of the cause—aneurysm or AVM—may be made from the CT scan. MRI is not routinely used, but it may provide greater sensitivity for detecting the areas of SAH clot and the potential location of the bleed.[32]

If the initial CT finding is negative, a lumbar puncture is performed to obtain cerebrospinal fluid (CSF) for analysis. CSF after SAH appears bloody and has a red blood cell count greater than 1000 cells/mm³. If the lumbar puncture is performed more than 5 days after the SAH, the CSF fluid is xanthochromic (dark amber) because the blood products have broken down.[33] Cloudy CSF usually indicates some type of infectious process such as bacterial meningitis, not SAH.[31]

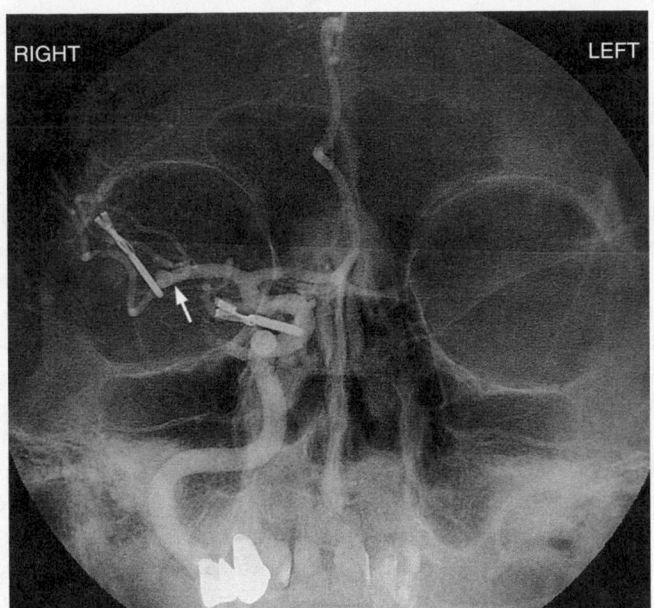

FIGURE 24-3 Cerebral angiography shows the location of aneurysm *(arrow)* at the posterior communicating artery. (From Tortorici M. *Fundamentals of Angiography.* St. Louis: Mosby; 1982.)

BOX 24-7   HUNT AND HESS CLASSIFICATION OF SUBARACHNOID HEMORRHAGE

- *Grade I:* Asymptomatic or minimal headache and slight nuchal rigidity
- *Grade II:* Moderate to severe headache, nuchal rigidity, but no neurologic deficit other than cranial nerve palsy
- *Grade III:* Drowsiness, confusion, or mild focal deficit
- *Grade IV:* Stupor, moderate to severe hemiparesis, possible early decerebrate rigidity, and vegetative disturbances
- *Grade V:* Deep coma, decerebrate rigidity, moribund appearance

From Hunt WE, Hess RM. Surgical risks as related to time of intervention in the repair of intracranial aneurysms. *J Neurosurg.* 1968;28:14.

After the SAH has been documented, cerebral angiography is necessary to identify the exact cause of the hemorrhage (Fig. 24-3). If a cerebral aneurysm rupture is the cause, angiography is essential for identifying the exact location of the aneurysm in preparation for surgery.[31,33,34] After the aneurysm has been located, it is graded using the Hunt and Hess classification scale. This scale categorizes the patient on the basis of the severity of the neurologic deficits associated with the hemorrhage (Box 24-7).[35] If AVM rupture is the cause, angiography is necessary to identify the feeding arteries and draining veins of the malformation.[30]

Medical Management

SAH is a medical emergency, and time is of the essence. Preservation of neurologic function is the goal, and early diagnosis is crucial. Initial treatment must always support vital functions. Airway management and ventilatory assistance may be necessary.[22] A ventriculostomy is performed to control ICP if the patient's level of consciousness is depressed.[32,34]

Evidence suggests that only 19% of the deaths attributable to aneurysmal SAH are related to the direct effects of the initial hemorrhage.[36] Rebleeding accounts for 22% of deaths from aneurysmal SAH, cerebral vasospasm for 23%, and non-neurologic medical complications for 23%.[36] Principal non-neurologic causes of death are systemic inflammatory response syndrome (SIRS) and secondary organ dysfunction.[37] After initial intervention has provided the necessary support for vital physiologic functions, medical management of acute SAH is aimed primarily toward the prevention and treatment of the complications of SAH, which may produce further neurologic damage and death.[32]

Rebleeding. Rebleeding is the occurrence of a second SAH in an unsecured aneurysm or, less commonly, an AVM.[28] The incidence of rebleeding during the first 24 hours after the first bleed is 4%, with a 1% to 2% chance per day in the following month. The mortality rate associated with aneurysmal rebleeding is approximately 70%.[30,31]

Historically, conservative measures to prevent rebleeding have included blood pressure control and SAH precautions (see "Nursing Management"). An elevation in blood pressure is a normal compensatory response to maintain adequate cerebral perfusion after a neurologic insult. In the belief that hypertension contributes to rebleeding, nitroprusside, metoprolol, or hydralazine has been commonly used to maintain a systolic blood pressure no greater than 140 mm Hg.[32] Individualized guidelines must be determined on the basis of the clinical condition and pre-existing values of the patient. Evidence suggests that rebleeding has more to do with variations in blood pressure than it does with absolute values and that blood pressure control does not lower the incidence of rebleeding.[34]

Surgical Clipping of Aneurysms. Definitive treatment for the prevention of rebleeding is surgical clipping or endovascular coiling with complete obliteration of the aneurysm.[31,32] Timing of the operation is a key medical management issue. Since the introduction of microsurgery and improved surgical techniques, patients commonly are taken to the operating room within the first 48 hours after rupture.[32] This early surgical intervention to secure the aneurysm eliminates the risk of rebleeding and allows more aggressive therapy to be used in the postoperative period for the treatment of vasospasm.[31,32] Early surgery also allows the neurosurgeon to flush out the excess blood and clots from the basal cisterns (reservoir of CSF around the base of the brain and circle of Willis) to reduce the risk of vasospasm.[37] Careful consideration of the patient's clinical situation is necessary in determining the optimal time for surgery.

The surgical procedure involves a craniotomy to expose and isolate the area of aneurysm. A clip is placed over the neck of the aneurysm to eliminate the area of weakness (Fig. 24-4). This is a technically difficult procedure that requires the skill of an experienced neurosurgeon. It is not uncommon, particularly in early surgery, for the clot to break away from the aneurysm as it is surgically exposed. Extensive hemorrhage into the craniotomy site results, and cessation of the hemorrhage often causes increased neurologic deficits. Deficits also may occur as a result of surgical manipulation to gain access to the site of the aneurysm.[32]

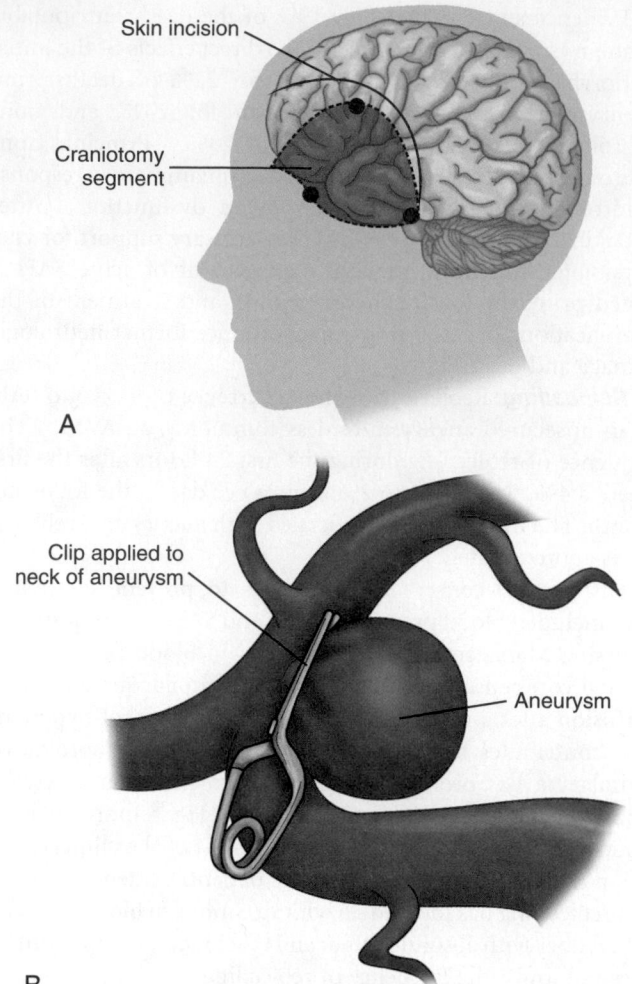

Skin incision

Craniotomy
segment

A

Clip applied to
neck of aneurysm

Aneurysm

B

FIGURE 24-4 Clipping of a Posterior Communicating Artery Aneurysm. *A,* The *solid curved line* shows the typical skin incision, and the *dashed lines* show the craniotomy location. *B,* Application of the clip to the aneurysm.

Surgical Excision of Arteriovenous Malformations. Management of AVM has traditionally involved surgical excision or conservative management of such symptoms as seizures and headache. The decision for surgical excision depends on the location and size of the AVM. Some malformations are located so deep in the cerebral structures (thalamus or midbrain) that attempts to remove the AVM would cause severe neurologic deficits. History of a previous hemorrhage and the patient's age and overall condition are also taken into account when making the decision regarding surgical intervention.[32]

Surgical excision of large AVMs includes the risk of reperfusion bleeding. As feeding arteries of the AVM are clamped off, the arterial blood that usually flowed into the AVM is diverted into the surrounding circulation. In many cases, the surrounding tissue has been in a state of chronic ischemia, and the arterial vessels feeding these areas are maximally dilated. As arterial blood begins to flow at a higher volume and pressure into these dilated arteries, blood may seep from the vessels. Evidence of reperfusion bleeding in the operating room is an indication that no more arterial blood can be diverted from the AVM without risk of serious ICH. In the postoperative phase, a low blood pressure is maintained to prevent further reperfusion bleeding.

For large AVMs, two to four stages of surgery may be required over 6 to 12 months.[32]

Embolization. Embolization is used to secure a cerebral aneurysm or AVM that is surgically inaccessible because of size, location, or medical instability of the patient. Embolization involves several new interventional neuroradiology techniques. All of the techniques use a percutaneous transfemoral approach in a manner similar to an angiography. Under fluoroscopy, the catheter is threaded up to the internal carotid artery. Specially developed microcatheters are then manipulated into the area of the vascular anomaly, and embolic materials are placed endovascularly. Three embolization techniques are used, depending on the underlying pathologic derangement.[30]

The first type of embolization is used to embolize an AVM. Small polymeric silicone (Silastic) beads or glue is slowly introduced into the vessels feeding the AVM. Blood flow carries the material to the site, and embolization is achieved. This procedure may be used in combination with surgery. One to three sessions of embolization of the feeding vessels are performed to reduce the size of the lesion before a craniotomy is performed for total excision. The primary risk of this procedure is lodging of the embolic substance in a vessel that feeds normal tissue, which creates an embolic stroke with the immediate onset of neurologic symptoms.[30]

The second type of embolization involves placement of one or more detachable coils into an aneurysm to produce an endovascular thrombus (Fig. 24-5). The advantage of this technique is that an electrical current creates a positive charge on the coil, which induces electrothrombosis. Complications include embolic stroke, coil migration, overproduction of the clot, subtotal occlusion and intraprocedural rupture of the vasculature, and death.[30]

Cerebral Vasospasm. The presence or absence of cerebral vasospasm significantly affects the outcome of aneurysmal SAH. This complication does not occur with SAH resulting from AVM rupture. Cerebral vasospasm is a narrowing of the lumen of the cerebral arteries, possibly in response to subarachnoid blood clots coating the outer surface of the blood vessels. Because aneurysms usually occur at the circle of Willis, the major vessels responsible for feeding the cerebral circulation are affected by vasospasm. Depending on the arterial vessels involved in the vasospasm reaction, decreased arterial flow occurs in large areas of the cerebral hemispheres.[30]

It is estimated that 70% of all SAH patients develop vasospasm, which is demonstrable by angiography.[38] Thirty-two percent of these patients develop symptomatic vasospasm, resulting in ischemic stroke or death for up to 23% of them despite the use of maximal therapy.[38] The onset of vasospasm is usually 3 to 12 days after the initial hemorrhage.[22] Three treatments are commonly used: 1) induced hypertensive, hypervolemic, hemodilution (HHH) therapy; 2) oral nimodipine; and 3) transluminal cerebral angioplasty.[34,38]

Hypertensive, Hypervolemic, Hemodilution Therapy. HHH therapy involves increasing the patient's blood pressure and cardiac output with vasoactive medications and diluting the patient's blood with fluid and volume expanders. Systolic blood pressure is maintained between 150 and 160 mm Hg. The increase in volume and pressure forces blood through

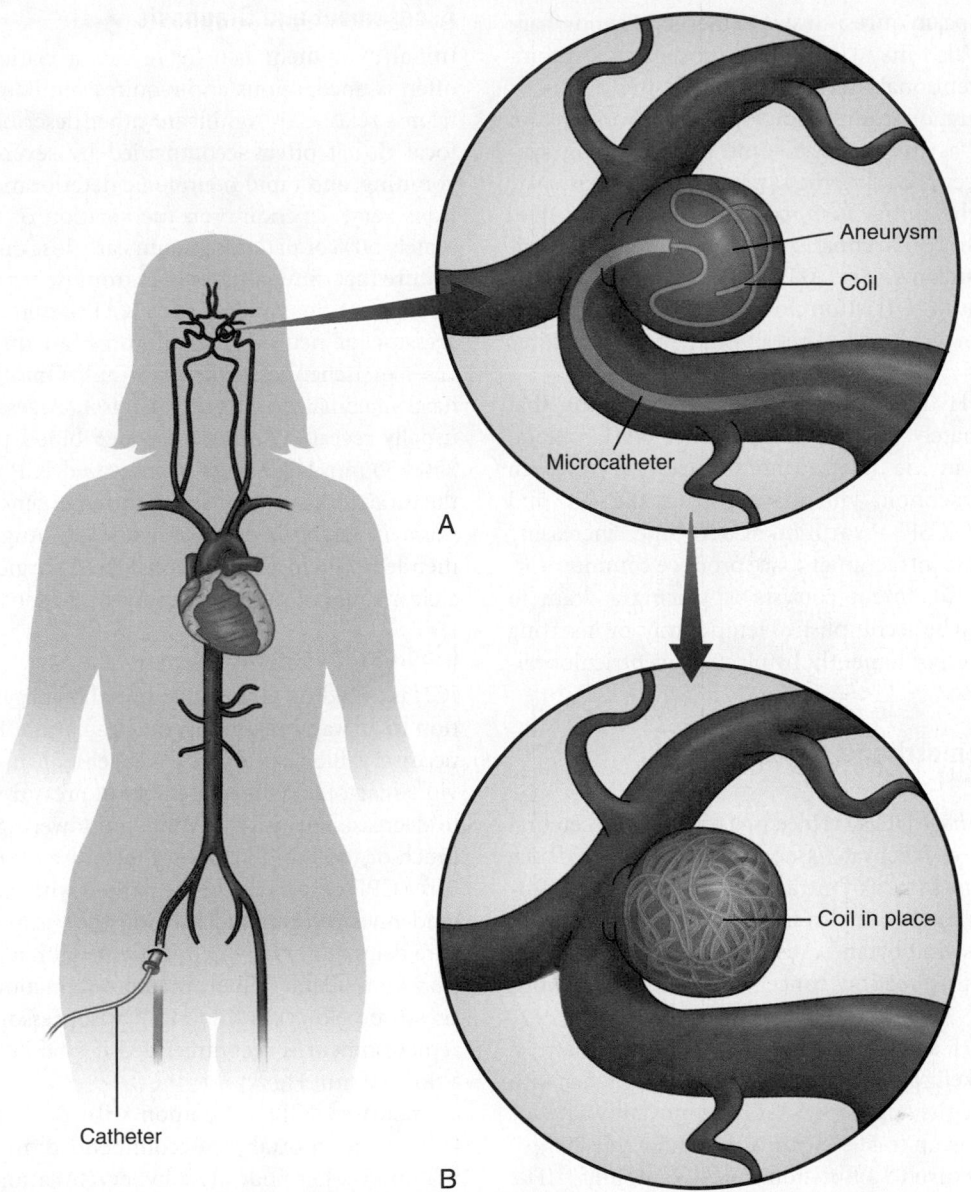

FIGURE 24-5 Endovascular Occlusion of a Posterior Communicating Artery Aneurysm. *A,* Insertion of the microcatheter into the aneurysm through the right femoral artery, aorta, and left carotid artery. *B,* Occlusion of the aneurysm with coils.

the vasospastic area at higher pressures. Hemodilution facilitates flow through the area by reducing blood viscosity. Many anecdotal reports exist of patients' neurologic deficits improving as systolic pressure increases from 130 mm Hg to between 150 and 160 mm Hg.[39] The Stroke Council of the AHA has recommended this therapy for prevention and treatment of vasospasm.[34]

The obvious deterrent to the use of induced hypertension is the risk of rebleeding in an unsecured aneurysm. Surgical clipping of the aneurysm before HHH therapy is preferred. Cerebral edema, elevated ICP, heart failure, and electrolyte imbalance are also risks of HHH therapy. Careful monitoring of the patient's neurologic status, hemodynamic parameters, ICP, and serum electrolytes is necessary.[32]

Nimodipine. Nimodipine is strongly recommended to reduce the poor outcomes associated with vasospasm. The exact

nature of the effect of nimodipine is not clear, but the use of the medication has demonstrated consistently positive effects on outcome without any demonstrable effect on the incidence or severity of vasospasm.[34,38] A dose of 60 mg of nimodipine is given orally every 4 hours for 21 days. Nimodipine may produce hypotension, especially when administered concurrently with other antihypertensive agents.[38]

Cerebral Angioplasty. Cerebral angioplasty is used when pharmacologic management of cerebral vasospasm has failed. It is performed only when CT or MRI provides evidence that infarction has not occurred. An interventional neuroradiologist performs the procedure, and the patient is placed under local, general, or neuroleptic analgesia. The technique of cerebral angioplasty is very similar to that used in the coronary vasculature. Risks include intimal perforation or rupture, cerebral artery thrombosis or embolism, recurrence of stenosis, and severe, diffuse vasospasm unresponsive to therapy. Hemorrhage at the femoral site also may occur. This procedure is recommended when conventional therapy is unsuccessful.[34,38]

Hyponatremia. Hyponatremia develops in 10% to 43% of patients with SAH as the result of central salt-wasting syndrome. It usually occurs during the same period as vasospasm, several days after the initial hemorrhage.[29] The use of fluid restriction to treat hyponatremia in the SAH patient is associated with a poor outcome. The AHA Stroke Council strongly recommends that fluid restriction not be used in this instance and instead recommends sodium replenishment with isotonic fluids.[34]

Hydrocephalus. Hydrocephalus is a late complication that occurs in approximately 25% of patients after SAH.[30] Blood that has circulated in the subarachnoid space and has been absorbed by the arachnoid villi may obstruct the villi and reduce the rate of CSF absorption. Over time, increasing volumes of CSF in the intracranial space produce communicating hydrocephalus. Treatment consists of placing a drain to remove CSF. This can be accomplished temporarily, by inserting a ventriculostomy, or permanently, by placing a ventriculoperitoneal shunt.[26,31,34]

Intracerebral Hemorrhage
Description

Intracerebral hemorrhage (ICH) is bleeding directly into cerebral tissue.[40] ICH destroys cerebral tissue, causes cerebral edema, and increases ICP. The source of intracerebral bleeding is usually a small artery, but it can result also from rupture of an AVM or aneurysm. The most important cause of spontaneous ICH is hypertension, and this section concentrates on spontaneous hypertensive ICH.[41]

Spontaneous ICH accounts for at least 10% of all stroke admissions.[40] The likelihood of death or disability is higher with ICH than with ischemic stroke or SAH. The mortality rate for hemorrhagic stroke is up to 50% within 1 month. Only 20% of patients with ICH return to a functional life at 6 months.[42] The key risk factors for ICH are age-associated cerebral amyloid angiopathy and hypertension.[40]

Etiology

ICH is most often caused by hypertensive rupture of a cerebral vessel, resulting from a longstanding history of hypertension.[40] Other possible causes of spontaneous ICH are anticoagulation or fibrinolytic therapy, coagulation disorders, drug abuse, and hemorrhage into a cerebral infarct or brain tumors.[31,43] Often, on questioning, the patient with a hypertensive hemorrhage admits to having discontinued antihypertensive medication 2 to 3 weeks before the hemorrhage.

Pathophysiology

The pathophysiology of ICH is caused by continued elevated blood pressure exerting force against smaller arterial vessels that have become damaged from arteriosclerotic changes. Eventually, these arteries break, and blood bursts from the vessels into the surrounding cerebral tissue, creating a hematoma. ICP rises precipitously in response to the increase in overall intracranial volume.[43]

Assessment and Diagnosis

Initial assessment usually reveals a critically ill patient who often is unconscious and requires ventilatory support. History from a relative or significant other describes a sudden onset of focal deficit often accompanied by severe headache, nausea, vomiting, and rapid neurologic deterioration. Signs and symptoms vary, depending on the location of the ICH.[43] Approximately 50% of patients sustain early loss of consciousness, a key feature that differentiates ICH from ischemic stroke. More than one half of the patients with ICH present with a smooth progression of neurologic symptoms, an uncommon finding in cases of ischemic stroke or SAH.[44] One third of the patients have maximal symptoms at onset. Assessment of vital signs usually reveals a severely elevated blood pressure (200/100 to 250/150 mm Hg). Signs of increased ICP are often present by the time the patient arrives in the emergency department. Diagnosis is established easily with CT. Angiography is recommended only in patients considered surgical candidates and if a clear cause of hemorrhage is not evident.[40-44]

Medical Management

ICH is a medical emergency. Initial management requires attention to airway, breathing, and circulation. Intubation is usually necessary. Blood pressure management must be based on individual factors. Reduction in blood pressure is usually necessary to decrease ongoing bleeding, but lowering blood pressure too much or too rapidly may compromise cerebral perfusion pressure (CPP), especially in the patient with elevated ICP. National guidelines recommend keeping the *mean* arterial blood pressure below 130 mm Hg in patients with a history of hypertension by moderate blood pressure reduction to a mean arterial pressure below 110 mm Hg.[44] Vasopressor therapy after fluid replenishment is recommended if systolic blood pressure falls below 90 mm Hg.[41]

Increased ICP is common with ICH and is a major contributor to mortality. Recommended management includes mannitol, when indicated; hyperventilation; and neuromuscular blockade with sedation. Steroids are avoided. CPP must be kept higher than 70 mm Hg.[41,42]

The goal for fluid management is euvolemia, with a recommended pulmonary artery occlusion pressure (PAOP) of 10 to 14 mm Hg. Body temperature is maintained at less than 38.5° C by using acetaminophen or cooling blankets. Euglycemia, a blood glucose level less than 140 milligram per deciliter (mg/dL), is maintained by using insulin therapy, but hypoglycemia should be avoided. Use of short-acting benzodiazepines or propofol is recommended to treat agitation or hyperactivity. Pneumatic compression devices are used to decrease risk of pulmonary embolism. Prophylactic anticonvulsant therapy is sometimes used.[41,44]

The benefit of surgical treatment for spontaneous ICH is unclear. Recommendations for surgical removal of the clot depend on the size and location of the hematoma, the patient's ICP, and other neurologic symptoms.[44] Medical treatment is recommended if the hemorrhage is small (<10 cm) or neurologic deficit is minimal.[41,44] Likewise, surgery offers no improvement in outcome for patients with a Glasgow Coma Scale (GCS) score of 4 or less. Surgical evacuation of the

BOX 24-8   EVIDENCE-BASED PRACTICE

Spontaneous Intracerebral Hemorrhage Management Guidelines

QSEN   The following are class 1 recommendations from the American Heart Association and American Stroke Association. Class 1 recommendations are conditions for which evidence and general agreement exist that the procedure or treatment is useful and effective.

- Rapid neuroimaging with CT or MRI is recommended to distinguish ischemic stroke from ICH.
- Patients with a severe coagulation factor deficiency or severe thrombocytopenia should receive appropriate factor replacement therapy or platelets, respectively.
- In patients with ICH whose INR is elevated owing to OAC-therapy, warfarin should be withheld, and they should be given therapy to replace vitamin K–dependent factors and correct the INR and should receive intravenous vitamin K.
- Patients with ICH should receive intermittent pneumatic compression for prevention of venous thromboembolism in addition to elastic stockings.
- Initial monitoring and management of patients with ICH should take place in an intensive care unit, preferably one with physician and nursing neuroscience intensive care expertise.
- Blood glucose levels should be monitored, and normoglycemia is recommended.
- Patients with clinical seizures should be treated with antiepileptic medications. Patients with a change in mental status who are found on EEG to have electrographic seizures should be treated with antiepileptic medications.
- Patients with cerebellar hemorrhage who are deteriorating neurologically or who have brainstem compression, hydrocephalus, or both from ventricular obstruction should undergo surgical removal of the hemorrhage as soon as possible.
- After the acute ICH, absent medical contraindications, blood pressure should be well controlled, particularly for patients with ICH location typical of hypertensive vasculopathy.

CT, Computed tomography; *EEG,* electroencephalography; *ICH,* intracerebral hemorrhage; *INR,* international normalized ratio; *MRI,* magnetic resonance imaging; *OAC,* oral anticoagulant. Modified from Morgenstern LB, et al. American Heart Association and American Stroke Council on cardiovascular nursing: guidelines for the management of spontaneous intracerebral hemorrhage: a guideline for healthcare professionals from the American Heart Association/American Stroke Association. *Stroke.* 2010;41:2108.

⊚ BOX 24-9   NURSING DIAGNOSES

Stroke

- Risk for Ineffective Cerebral Tissue Perfusion, p. 1156
- Acute Pain, related to transmission and perception of cutaneous, visceral, muscular, or ischemic impulses, p. 1123
- Unilateral Neglect, related to perceptual disruption, p. 1162
- Impaired Verbal Communication, related to cerebral speech center injury, p. 1147
- Impaired Swallowing, related to neuromuscular impairment, fatigue, and limited awareness, p. 1146
- Risk for Aspiration, p. 1154
- Risk for Infection, p. 1160
- Anxiety, related to threat of biologic, psychologic, or social integrity, p. 1125
- Disturbed Body Image, related to actual change in body structure, function, or appearance, p. 1136
- Compromised Family Coping, related to critically ill family member, p. 1127
- Deficient Knowledge: Discharge Regimen, related to lack of previous exposure to information, p. 1134 (see Box 24-10, Patient Education for Stroke)

Monitoring for Changes in Neurologic and Hemodynamic Status

The goal of frequent assessments is early recognition of neurologic or hemodynamic deterioration. Close monitoring of the patient's neurologic signs and vital signs is essential and requires almost continuous observation. Automatic noninvasive devices such as a blood pressure cuff and a pulse oximeter are helpful. Seizure activity must be identified and treated immediately. It is essential that all personnel working with the patient be aware of the desired hemodynamic and neurologic parameters set by the physician and that the physician be notified at the first sign of any changes.

Maintaining Surveillance for Complications

The patient with stroke should be monitored closely for signs of bleeding, vasospasm, and increased ICP. Other complications of stroke include aspiration, malnutrition, pneumonia, DVT, pulmonary embolism, pressure ulcers, contractures, and joint abnormalities.[29] Nursing measures to prevent these complications are well known.

Additional complications that may be seen in the patient with stroke are related to the area of the brain that has been damaged. Damage to the temporoparietal area can create a variety of disturbances that affect the patient's ability to interpret sensory information. Damage to the dominant hemisphere (usually left) produces problems with speech and language and abstract and analytic skills. Damage to the nondominant hemisphere (usually right) produces problems with spatial relationships. The resulting deficits include agnosia, apraxia, and visual field defects. Perceptual deficits are not as readily noticeable as are motor deficits, but they may be more debilitating and may lead to inability to perform skilled or purposeful tasks. The patient also may experience impaired swallowing.[30,33]

Bleeding and Vasospasm. In the patient with a cerebral aneurysm, sudden onset of, or an increase in, headache and nausea and vomiting, increased blood pressure, and changes in respiration herald the onset of rebleeding. The first indication

clot is recommended for patients with cerebellar hemorrhage greater than 3 cm with neurologic deterioration or hydrocephalus with brainstem compression, as well as for young patients with moderate or large lobar hemorrhage with clinical deterioration.[41,44] Numerous techniques are being investigated to lessen the risk of brain damage associated with craniotomy for ICH.

Evidence-based guidelines for the management of the patient with ICH are listed in Box 24-8.

Nursing Management

Nursing management of the patient with stroke incorporates a variety of nursing diagnoses (Box 24-9). Nursing interventions focus on monitoring for changes in neurologic and hemodynamic status, maintaining surveillance for complications, providing comfort and emotional support, and educating the patient and family.

of vasospasm is usually the appearance of new focal or global neurologic deficits.

SAH precautions must be implemented to prevent any stress or straining that could potentially precipitate rebleeding. Precautions include blood pressure control; bed rest; a dark, quiet environment; and stool softeners. Short-acting analgesics and sedatives are used to relieve pain and anxiety. The patient must be kept calm. Limb restraints cause straining and must therefore be avoided. The head of the bed should be elevated to 35 to 45 degrees at all times. The patient is taught to avoid any activities that correspond to performance of the Valsalva maneuver, such as pushing with the legs to move up in bed, straining for a bowel movement, or holding his or her breath during procedures or discomfort. DVT precautions are routinely implemented. Collaboration with the patient and family is used to establish a visitation plan to meet patient and family needs. Often, family members at the bedside can assist the patient to remain calm.[30,32,33]

Increased Intracranial Pressure. Numerous signs and symptoms of increased ICP can be observed. A change in the level of consciousness is the most sensitive indicator. Others include unequal pupil size, decreased pupillary response to light, headache, projectile vomiting, altered breathing patterns, Cushing triad (bradycardia, systolic hypertension, and bradypnea), diminished brainstem reflexes, papilledema, and abnormal extension (decerebrate posturing) or flexion (decorticate posturing).[30,32,33]

Damage to the Nondominant Hemisphere. Patients with nondominant hemispheric pathologic conditions may exhibit emotional lability, with periods of euphoria, impulsiveness, and inattention. A short attention span, lack of insight, and poor judgment may lead to injuries as the patient attempts to perform activities beyond his or her capabilities. These patients also may suffer from agnosia, visual field defects, and apraxia.[30,32,33]

Agnosia. *Agnosia* is a disturbance in the perception of familiar sensory (e.g., verbal, tactile, visual) information. Unilateral neglect is a form of agnosia characterized by an unawareness or denial of the affected half of the body. This denial may range from inattention to refusing to acknowledge a paralysis by neglecting the involved side of the body or by denying ownership of the side, attributing the paralyzed arm or leg to someone else. The neglect also may extend to extrapersonal space. This defect most often results from right hemispheric brain damage that causes left hemiplegia.

Other types of agnosia exist in addition to unilateral neglect. Some patients are unable to recognize objects visually (visual object agnosia), whereas others cannot recognize faces (prosopagnosia) and may have to rely on the voice or characteristic mannerisms of a familiar person to identify that person. Tactile agnosia is a perceptual disorder in which a patient is unable to recognize an object that has been placed in his or her hand by touch alone. This may occur even in the presence of an intact sense of touch. If allowed to see or hear the object, the patient usually recognizes it.

Spatial orientation is affected, resulting in interference with the patient's ability to judge position, distance, movement, form, and the relationship of his or her body parts to surrounding objects. Patients may confuse concepts such as "up and down" or "forward and backward." They may have difficulty following a route from one place to another and may even get lost in areas that were once familiar. Stroke patients may also experience reading and writing problems related to visual perception and visuospatial deficits. One type of spatial dyslexia is related to unilateral spatial neglect. The patient may not look at the beginning of a line of written material that appears on the left. Instead, the patient fixes attention on a point to the right of the beginning of the line and reads to the end of the line. If asked to draw a design, the person completes only half of a design or drawing.

Visual Field Defects. *Visual field defects* may accompany agnosia, although they do not cause it. A hemispheric lesion can interrupt the visual pathways, with the resulting visual defect dependent on the location and extent of the lesion. At the optic chiasm, nerve fibers coming from the nasal half of each retina cross to the opposite side, whereas fibers coming from the temporal half of each retina do not cross. This partial crossing allows binocular vision. In the optic chiasm, fibers from the nasal half of each retina join the uncrossed fibers from the temporal half of the retina to form the optic tract. Impulses conducted to the right hemisphere by the right optic tract represent the left field of vision, and those conducted to the left hemisphere by the left optic tract represent the right field of vision. Optic radiations extend back to the occipital lobes. Visual defects restricted to a single field, right or left, are called *homonymous hemianopsia*.

The nurse may be the first person to notice that the patient has this defect. The patient with hemianopsia may neglect all sensory input from the affected side and initially may appear unresponsive if approached from the affected side. If the nurse approaches the patient from the healthy side, the patient actually may be quite alert. Another clue to hemianopsia is the patient eating food only from one half of the tray. Hemianopsia may recede gradually with time. Many patients can learn to scan their environment visually to compensate for the defect, although in the acute stage of stroke, the patient may be too lethargic to follow instructions in methods of visual scanning. This visual defect can lead to fear and confusion and can present a risk to the patient's safety.

Apraxia. Lesions in the parietal lobe and in other cortical structures can result in *apraxia*, an inability to perform a learned movement voluntarily. Even though the patient may understand the task to be performed and may have intact motor ability, he or she cannot perform the task and often fumbles and makes mistakes. The patient suffering from dressing apraxia, for example, may not be able to orient clothing in space, becoming tangled in his or her clothes when attempting to dress.

Damage to the Dominant Hemisphere. Damage to the dominant hemisphere produces problems with speech and language. Impaired communication is a condition that results from a patient's difficulty in expressing and exchanging thoughts, ideas, or desires.[30,32,33] The posterior temporoparietal area contains the receptive speech center known as *Wernicke area*. The center for the perception of written language lies anterior to the visuoreceptive areas. Located at the base of the frontal lobe's motor strip and slightly anterior to it is *Broca area*, also known as the *motor speech center*. These sensory and motor areas are connected by a large bundle of nerve fibers. Rather than receptive and motor language functions being entirely within discrete areas, it is thought that language is an integrated sensorimotor process, control of which is roughly located in these areas in the dominant cerebral hemisphere. It also is recognized that the elaborately complex functions of speech and language depend on other associative areas of the cerebrum and their thalamic connections. Consequently, much inconsistency exists in the degree of communication impairment among patients with lesions located in the same area of the brain.

Aphasia is a loss of language abilities caused by brain injury, usually to the dominant hemisphere. It involves more than just understanding speech or expressing oneself through verbal means. *Language* is a much broader term, referring to what the individual is attempting to interpret or convey through listening, speaking, reading, writing, and gesturing. Most cases of aphasia are partial rather than complete. The severity of the disorder depends on the area and the extent of the cerebral damage.

Receptive Aphasia. *Receptive aphasia*, also referred to as *sensory*, *Wernicke*, or *fluent aphasia*, occurs when the connection between the primary auditory cortex in the temporal lobe and the angular gyrus in the parietal lobe is destroyed. The patient's comprehension of speech is impaired, but he or she can still talk if the motor area for speech (Broca area) is intact. The patient may talk excessively, with many errors in the use of words. The patient can hear the examiner but cannot comprehend what is being said and cannot repeat the examiner's words. These patients may talk nonsense, with rambling speech that gives little information. Patients with receptive aphasia also cannot read words, although they can see them.

Expressive Aphasia. *Expressive aphasia*, also known as *motor*, *Broca*, or *nonfluent aphasia*, is primarily a deficit in language output or speech production. Depending on the lesion's size and exact location, wide variation in the motor deficit can result. Expressive aphasia can range from a mild dysarthria (imperfect articulation as a result of weakness or lack of coordination of speech musculature) to incorrect intonation and phrasing and, in its most severe form, to complete loss of ability to communicate through verbal and written means. In this severe form of aphasia, the patient also experiences a loss of ability to communicate through conventional gestures such as nodding or shaking the head for *yes* or *no*. In most cases of expressive aphasia, the muscles of articulation are intact. If speech is possible at all, the words *yes* and *no* are occasionally uttered, sometimes appropriately. Some patients may sing the words of well-known songs. Other patients, when excited or angered, may utter expletives. Some patients with expressive aphasia struggle or hesitate in trying to express words. They struggle to form words while using motor musculature (*verbal apraxia*), an articulatory disorder that is a feature of some expressive types of aphasia. All these difficulties lead to exasperation and despair in the patient. Most patients with expressive aphasia also have severely impaired writing ability. Even though penmanship may be intact, they are unable to express themselves through writing—a deficit called *agraphia*. If the right hand is paralyzed, as is often the case, the patient still cannot write or print with the left hand. In the recovery phase of severe expressive aphasia, patients become able to speak aloud to some degree, although words are uttered slowly and laboriously. Many patients, however, are able to learn to communicate ideas to some extent.

Global Aphasia. *Global aphasia* results when a massive lesion affects the motor and sensory speech areas. The patient cannot transform sounds into words and cannot comprehend spoken words. All language modalities are affected, and impairment may be so severe that the patient may be unable to communicate on any level. These patients usually have severe hemiplegia and homonymous hemianopsia. Their language function rarely recovers to a significant degree unless the lesion is caused by some transient disorder such as cerebral edema or a metabolic derangement.

Impaired Swallowing. Normal swallowing occurs in four phases that are controlled by the cranial nerves. Damage to the brain, brainstem, or cranial nerves may result in a variety of swallowing deficits that could place the patient at risk for aspiration. The stroke patient is observed for signs of dysphagia, including drooling; difficulty handling oral secretions; absence of gag, cough, or swallowing reflexes; moist, gurgling voice quality; decreased mouth and tongue movements; and the presence of dysarthria. A speech therapy consult is initiated if any of these signs are present, and the patient must not be orally fed. In the absence of these warning signs, the patient may be fed, as ordered by the physician, although he or she must be continually monitored for signs of aspiration.[30,32,33]

Educating the Patient and Family

Rehabilitation starts in the critical care area, with a multidisciplinary team designing and implementing an individualized plan for maximizing the patient's potential for neurologic rehabilitation. Early in the patient's hospital stay, the patient and family must be taught about stroke, its causes, and its treatment (Box 24-10). As the patient moves toward discharge, teaching focuses on the interventions necessary for preventing the recurrence of the event and on maximizing the patient's rehabilitation potential. The patient's family must be encouraged to participate in the patient's care; learn how to feed, dress, and bathe the patient; and learn some basic rehabilitation

---

BOX 24-10 PATIENT EDUCATION

Stroke

- Pathophysiology of disease
- Specific cause
- Risk factor modification
- Importance of taking medications
- Activities of daily living
- Measures to prevent injuries of impaired limbs
- Measures to compensate for residual deficits
- Basic rehabilitation techniques
- Importance of participating in neurologic rehabilitation program or support group

Additional information for the patient and family can be found at the National Stroke Association website (http://www.stroke.org) and the American Stroke Association website (http://www.strokeassociation.org/STROKEORG).

techniques. The importance of participating in a neurologic rehabilitation program or a support group, or both, must be stressed.

Collaborative management of the patient with a stroke is outlined in Box 24-11.

GUILLAIN-BARRÉ SYNDROME

Description

Guillain-Barré syndrome (GBS), once thought to be a single entity characterized by inflammatory peripheral neuropathy, is a combination of clinical features with various forms of presentation and multiple pathologic processes. A full discussion of this complex condition is beyond the scope of this chapter. Most cases of GBS do not require admission to the critical care unit. However, the prototype of GBS, known as *acute inflammatory demyelinating polyradiculoneuropathy* (AIDP), involves a rapidly progressive, ascending peripheral nerve dysfunction, which leads to paralysis that may produce respiratory failure. Because of the need for ventilatory support, AIDP is one of the few peripheral neurologic diseases that necessitates care in a critical care environment.[45] In this discussion, all references to GBS pertain to the AIDP prototype.

The annual incidence of GBS is 1.8 cases per 100,000 persons.[45] It occurs more often in males and is the most commonly acquired demyelinating neuropathy. Occasionally, clusters of cases are reported, as occurred following the 1977 swine flu vaccinations.[45]

Etiology

The precise cause of GBS remains unknown, but the syndrome involves an immune-mediated response involving cell-mediated immunity and development of immunoglobulin G (IgG) antibodies. Most patients report a viral infection 1 to 3 weeks before the onset of clinical manifestations, usually involving the upper respiratory tract.[45,46]

Numerous antecedent causes, or triggering events, have been associated with GBS. They include viral infections (e.g., influenza virus; cytomegalovirus; hepatitis A, B, or C virus; Epstein-Barr virus; human immunodeficiency virus), bacterial infections (e.g., gastrointestinal *Campylobacter jejuni, Mycoplasma pneumoniae*), vaccines (e.g., rabies, tetanus, influenza), lymphoma, surgery, and trauma.[45,46]

Pathophysiology

GBS affects the motor and sensory pathways of the peripheral nervous system as well as the autonomic nervous system functions of the cranial nerves. The major finding in AIDP-type GBS is a segmental demyelination process of the peripheral nerves. GBS is thought to be an autoimmune response to antibodies formed in response to a recent physiologic event. T cells migrate to the peripheral nerves, resulting in edema and inflammation. Macrophages then invade the area and break down the myelin. Inflammation around this demyelinated area causes further dysfunction. Some axonal damage also occurs.[45,46]

The myelin sheath of the peripheral nerves is generated by Schwann cells and acts as an insulator for the peripheral nerve. Myelin promotes rapid conduction of nerve impulses by allowing the impulses to jump along the nerve by means of the nodes of Ranvier. Disruption of the myelin fiber slows and may eventually stop the conduction of impulses along the peripheral nerves. In GBS, the more thickly myelinated fibers of motor pathways and the cranial nerves are more severely affected than are the thinly myelinated sensory fibers of cutaneous pain, touch, and temperature.[45,46]

After the temporary inflammatory reaction stops, myelin-producing cells begin the process of reinsulating the demyelinated portions of the peripheral nervous system. When remyelination occurs, normal neurologic function should return. In some instances, the axon may be damaged during the inflammatory process. The degree of axonal damage is responsible for the degree of neurologic dysfunction that persists after recovery.[45,46]

Assessment and Diagnosis

Symptoms of GBS include motor weakness, paresthesias and other sensory changes, cranial nerve dysfunction (especially oculomotor, facial, glossopharyngeal, vagal, spinal accessory, and hypoglossal), and some autonomic dysfunction. The usual course of GBS begins with an abrupt onset of lower extremity weakness that progresses to flaccidity and ascends over a period of hours to days. Motor loss usually is symmetric, bilateral, and ascending. In the most severe cases, complete flaccidity of all peripheral nerves, including spinal and cranial nerves, occurs.[46-48]

The patient is admitted to the hospital when lower extremity weakness prevents mobility. Admission to the critical care unit is necessary when progression of the weakness threatens respiratory muscles. As the patient's weakness progresses, close observation is essential. Frequent assessment of the respiratory system, including ventilatory parameters such as inspiratory force and tidal volume, is necessary. The most common cause of death of patients with GBS is respiratory arrest. As the disease progresses and respiratory effort weakens, intubation and mechanical ventilation are necessary. Frequent assessment of neurologic deterioration is continued until the patient reaches the peak of the disease, and a plateau occurs.[46,47]

The diagnosis of GBS is based on clinical findings plus CSF analysis and nerve conduction studies. The diagnostic finding is elevated CSF protein with normal cell count.[46] The increased protein count usually occurs after the first week but does not occur in approximately 10% of all cases. Nerve conduction studies that test the velocity at which nerve impulses are conducted show significant reduction, as the demyelinating process of the disease suggests.[47]

Medical Management

With no curative treatment available, the medical management of GBS is limited. The disease must run its course, which is characterized by ascending paralysis that advances over 1 to 3 weeks and then remains at a plateau for 2 to 4 weeks.[46] The plateau stage is followed by descending paralysis and return to normal or near-normal function. The main focus of medical management is the support of bodily functions and the prevention of complications.[47]

Plasmapheresis and intravenous immune globulin (IVIG) are used to treat GBS.[45,46,49,50] They have been shown to be equally effective.[45] Plasmapheresis involves the removal of venous blood through a catheter, separation of plasma from blood cells, and reinfusion of the cells plus autologous plasma or another replacement solution. Although the number of exchanges may vary, four to six exchanges usually are performed over a 5- to 8-day period.[45] IVIG has emerged as the preferred therapy because of convenience and availability. The usual dose is 0.4 mg/kg for 5 days.[47]

Nursing Management

The nursing management of the patient with GBS incorporates a variety of nursing diagnoses and interventions (Box 24-12). The goal of nursing management is to support all normal body functions until the patient can do so on his or her own. Although the condition is reversible, the patient with GBS requires extensive long-term care because recovery can be a long process. Nursing interventions focus on maintaining surveillance for complications, initiating rehabilitation, facilitating nutritional support, providing comfort and emotional support, and educating the patient and family.

Maintaining Surveillance for Complications

Continuous assessment of the progressive paralysis associated with GBS is essential to timely intervention and the prevention of respiratory arrest and further neurologic insult. After the patient is intubated and placed on mechanical ventilation, close observation for pulmonary complications such as atelectasis, pneumonia, and pneumothorax is necessary. Autonomic

---

BOX 24-12 NURSING DIAGNOSES
Guillain-Barré Syndrome

- Ineffective Breathing Pattern, related to musculoskeletal fatigue or neuromuscular impairment, p. 1149
- Acute Pain, related to transmission and perception of cutaneous, visceral, muscular, or ischemic impulses, p. 1123
- Activity Intolerance, related to prolonged immobility or deconditioning, p. 1119
- Risk for Aspiration, p. 1154
- Imbalanced Nutrition: Less Than Body Requirements, related to lack of exogenous nutrients or increased metabolic demand, p. 1143
- Risk for Infection, p. 1160
- Anxiety, related to threat of biologic, psychologic, or social integrity, p. 1125
- Powerlessness related to lack of control over current situation or disease progression, p. 1152
- Ineffective Coping, related to situational crisis and personal vulnerability, p. 1150
- Compromised Family Coping, related to critically ill family member, p. 1127
- Deficient Knowledge: Discharge Regimen, related to lack of previous exposure to information, p. 1134 (see Box 24-13, Patient Education for Guillain-Barré Syndrome)

---

dysfunction (dysautonomia) in the GBS patient can produce variations in heart rate and blood pressure that can reach extreme values.[46,51] Hypertension and tachycardia may require beta-blocker therapy. All patients with GBS must be observed for this phenomenon.[48]

Initiating Rehabilitation

In patients with GBS, immobility may last for months. The usual course of GBS involves an average of 10 days of symptom progression and 10 days of maximal level of dysfunction, followed by 2 to 48 weeks of recovery. Although GBS usually is completely reversible, the patient will require physical and occupational rehabilitation because of the problems of long-term immobility. Rehabilitation starts in the critical care area, with a multidisciplinary team designing and implementing an individualized plan for maximizing the patient's potential for rehabilitation.[51]

Facilitating Nutritional Support

Nutritional support is implemented early in the course of the disease. Because recovery from GBS is a long process, adequate nutritional support will remain a problem for an extended period. Nutritional support usually is accomplished through the use of enteral feeding.

Providing Comfort and Emotional Support

Pain control is another important component in the care of the patient with GBS. Although patients may have minimal to no motor function, most sensory functions remain, causing patients considerable muscle ache and pain. Because of the length of this illness, a safe, effective, long-term solution to pain management must be identified.[51] These patients also require extensive psychologic support. Although the illness is almost 100% reversible, lack of control over the situation, constant pain or discomfort, and the long-term nature of the disorder

Guillain-Barré Syndrome

- Pathophysiology of disease
- Importance of taking medications
- Measures to compensate for residual deficits
- Basic rehabilitation techniques
- Importance of participating in neurologic rehabilitation program, if necessary

Additional information for the patient and family can be found at the GBS/CIDP Foundation International website (http://www.gbs-cidp.org).

BOX 24-14 **COLLABORATIVE MANAGEMENT**

Guillain-Barré Syndrome

- Support bodily functions.
  - Protect airway.
  - Provide ventilatory assistance, as required.
- Initiate treatments to limit duration of the syndrome.
  - Plasmapheresis
  - Intravenous immunoglobulin
- Initiate nutritional support.
- Maintain surveillance for complications.
  - Infections
  - Cardiac dysrhythmias
  - Blood pressure alterations
  - Temperature alterations
- Provide comfort and emotional support.
- Design and implement appropriate rehabilitation program.
- Educate patient and family.

TABLE 24-3 **TYPES OF BRAIN TUMORS OCCURRING IN ADULTS**

TYPE	PATHOLOGY
Gliomas	
Astrocytomas (grades I to III) Glioblastoma multiforme (also called astrocytoma grade IV) Oligodendroglioma (grades I to III) Ependymoma (grades I to IV) Medulloblastoma	Nonencapsulated, tend to infiltrate brain tissue; arise in any part of brain connective tissue; infiltrate primarily cerebral hemisphere tissue; not well outlined so difficult to excise completely; grow rapidly—most persons live months to years after diagnosis; tumors assigned grade from I to IV, with IV being most malignant
Tumors from Support Structures	
Meningiomas	Arise from meningeal coverings of brain; usually benign but may undergo malignant changes; usually encapsulated, and surgical cure possible; recurrence possible
Neuromas (acoustic neuroma, schwannoma)	Arise from Schwann cells inside auditory meatus on vestibular portion of eighth cranial nerve; usually benign but may undergo cellular change and become malignant; will regrow if not completely excised; surgical resection often difficult because of location
Pituitary adenoma	Arise from various tissues; surgical approach usually successful; recurrence possible
Developmental (Congenital) Tumors	
Dermoid, epidermoid, craniopharyngioma	Arise from embryonic tissue in various sites in brain; success of surgical resection dependent on location and invasiveness
Angiomas	Arise from vascular structures; usually difficult to resect
Metastatic Tumors	
	Cancer cells spreading to brain via circulatory system; surgical resection difficult; even with treatment, prognosis poor; survival beyond 1-2 yr uncommon

From Forsyth LW, Garnett JC. Traumatic and neoplastic problems. In: Monahan FD, et al, eds. *Phipps' Medical-Surgical Nursing: Health and Illness Perspective*. 8th ed. St. Louis: Mosby; 2007.

create coping difficulties for the patient. GBS does not affect the level of consciousness or cerebral function. Patient interaction and communication are essential elements of the nursing management plan.

Educating the Patient and Family

Early in the patient's hospital stay, the patient and family must be taught about GBS and its different treatments (Box 24-13). As the patient moves toward discharge, teaching focuses on the interventions to maximize the patient's rehabilitation potential. The patient's family must be encouraged to participate in the patient's care and to learn some basic rehabilitation techniques. The importance of participating in a neurologic rehabilitation program (if necessary) must be stressed.

Collaborative management of the patient with GBS is outlined in Box 24-14.

CRANIOTOMY

Types of Surgery

A craniotomy is performed to gain access to portions of the central nervous system (CNS) inside the cranium, usually to allow removal of a space-occupying lesion such as a brain tumor (Table 24-3). Common procedures include tumor resection or removal, cerebral decompression, evacuation of hematoma or abscess, and clipping or removal of an aneurysm or AVM. Most patients who undergo craniotomy for tumor

resection or removal do not require care in a critical care unit. Patients who do usually need intensive monitoring or are at greater risk for complications because of underlying cardiopulmonary dysfunction or the surgical approach used.[52] Box 24-15 provides definitions of common neurosurgical terms.

Preoperative Care

Protection of the integrity of the CNS is a major priority of care for the patient awaiting a craniotomy. Optimal arterial oxygenation, hemodynamic stability, and cerebral perfusion are essential for maintaining adequate cerebral oxygenation. Management of seizure activity is essential for controlling metabolic needs.

BOX 24-15	**OPERATIVE TERMS**

- *Burr hole:* Hole made into the cranium using a special drill
- *Craniotomy:* Surgical opening of the skull
- *Craniectomy:* Removal of a portion of the skull without replacing it
- *Cranioplasty:* Plastic repair of the skull
- *Supratentorial:* Above the tentorium, separating the cerebrum from the cerebellum
- *Infratentorial:* Below the tentorium; includes the brainstem and the cerebellum; an infratentorial surgical approach may be used for temporal or occipital lesions
- *Stereotactic:* Minimally invasive surgical intervention that uses a three-dimensional coordinate system to localize a specific area of the brain for ablation, biopsy, dissection, or radiosurgery

Detailed assessment and documentation of the patient's preoperative neurologic status are imperative for accurate postoperative evaluation. Attention is focused on identifying and describing the nature and extent of any preoperative neurologic deficits. When pituitary surgery is planned, a thorough evaluation of endocrine function is necessary to prevent major intraoperative and postoperative complications.[53]

Trends in health care demand judicious use of routine preoperative studies. Depending on the type of surgery to be performed and the general health of the patient, preoperative screening may include a complete blood cell count (CBC); tests for blood urea nitrogen (BUN), creatinine, and fasting blood sugar (FBS); chest radiography; and ECG. A blood type and cross-match may also be ordered.[54]

Preoperative teaching is necessary to prepare the patient and family for what to expect in the postoperative period. A description of the intravascular lines and intracranial catheters used during the postoperative period allows the family to focus on the patient and not be overwhelmed by masses of tubing. Some or all of the patient's hair is shaved off in the operating room, and a large, bulky, turban-like craniotomy dressing is applied. Most patients experience some degree of postoperative eye or facial swelling and periorbital ecchymosis. An explanation of these temporary changes in appearance helps alleviate the shock and fear many patients and families experience in the immediate postoperative period.[54]

All craniotomy patients require instruction to avoid activities known to provoke sudden changes in ICP. These activities include bending, lifting, straining, and the Valsalva maneuver. Patients commonly elicit the Valsalva maneuver during repositioning in bed by holding their breath and straining with a closed epiglottis. This is prevented effectively by teaching the patient to continue to breathe deeply through the mouth during all position changes.[54]

The patient undergoing trans-sphenoidal surgery requires preparation for the sensations associated with nasal packing. The patient often awakens with alarm because of the inability to breathe through the nose. Preoperative instruction in mouth breathing and avoidance of coughing, sneezing, or blowing of the nose facilitates postoperative cooperation.[53]

The psychosocial issues associated with the prospect of neurosurgery cannot be overemphasized. Few procedures are as threatening as those involving the brain or spinal cord. For some patients, the fear of permanent neurologic impairment may be as ominous as or more ominous than the fear of death. Steps to meet the needs of the patient and the family include collaboration with religious and social services personnel, patient-controlled visitation, and provision of as much privacy as the patient's condition permits. The patient and family must be provided with the opportunity to express their fears and concerns jointly and apart from each other.[52]

Surgical Considerations

Whereas the emphasis in the surgical approach for most other types of surgery is to gain adequate exposure of the surgical site, the neurosurgeon must select a route that also produces the least amount of disruption to the intracranial contents. Neural tissue is unforgiving. A significant portion of neurologic trauma and postoperative deficits is related to the surgical pathway through the brain tissue, rather than to the procedure performed at the site of pathology. Depending on the location of the lesion and the surgical route chosen, a transcranial or a trans-sphenoidal approach is used to open the skull.

Transcranial Approach

In the transcranial approach, a scalp incision is made, and a series of burr holes is drilled into the skull to form an outline of the area to be opened (Fig. 24-6). A special saw is then used to cut between the holes. In most cases, the bone flap is left attached to the muscle to create a hinge effect. In some cases, the bone flap is removed completely and placed in the abdomen for later retrieval and implantation or discarded and replaced with synthetic material. Next, the dura is opened and retracted. After the intracranial procedure, the dura and the bone flap are closed, the muscles and scalp are sutured, and a turbanlike dressing is applied.[52]

Trans-sphenoidal Approach

The trans-sphenoidal approach is the technique of choice for removal of a pituitary tumor without extension into the intracranial vault (Fig. 24-7).[53,54] This approach involves making a microsurgical entrance into the cranial vault through the nasal cavity. The sphenoid sinus is entered to reach the anterior wall of the sella turcica. The sphenoid bone and the dura are then opened to gain intracranial access. After removal of the tumor, the surgical bed is packed with a small section of adipose tissue grafted from the patient's abdomen or thigh. After closure of the intranasal structures, nasal splints and soft packing or nasal tampons impregnated with antibiotic ointment are placed in the nasal cavities. Occasionally, epistaxis balloons are used instead. A nasal drip pad or mustache-type dressing is placed at the base of the nose to catch surgical drainage.[52]

The patient may be placed in the supine, prone, or sitting position for a craniotomy procedure. A skull clamp connected to skull pins is used to position and secure the patient's head throughout the operation. During a trans-sphenoidal approach or a transcranial approach into the infratentorial area, the patient's head is elevated during surgery. This position places the patient at risk for an air embolism. Air can enter the vascular system through the edges of the dura or a venous opening. Continuous monitoring of the patient's heart sounds

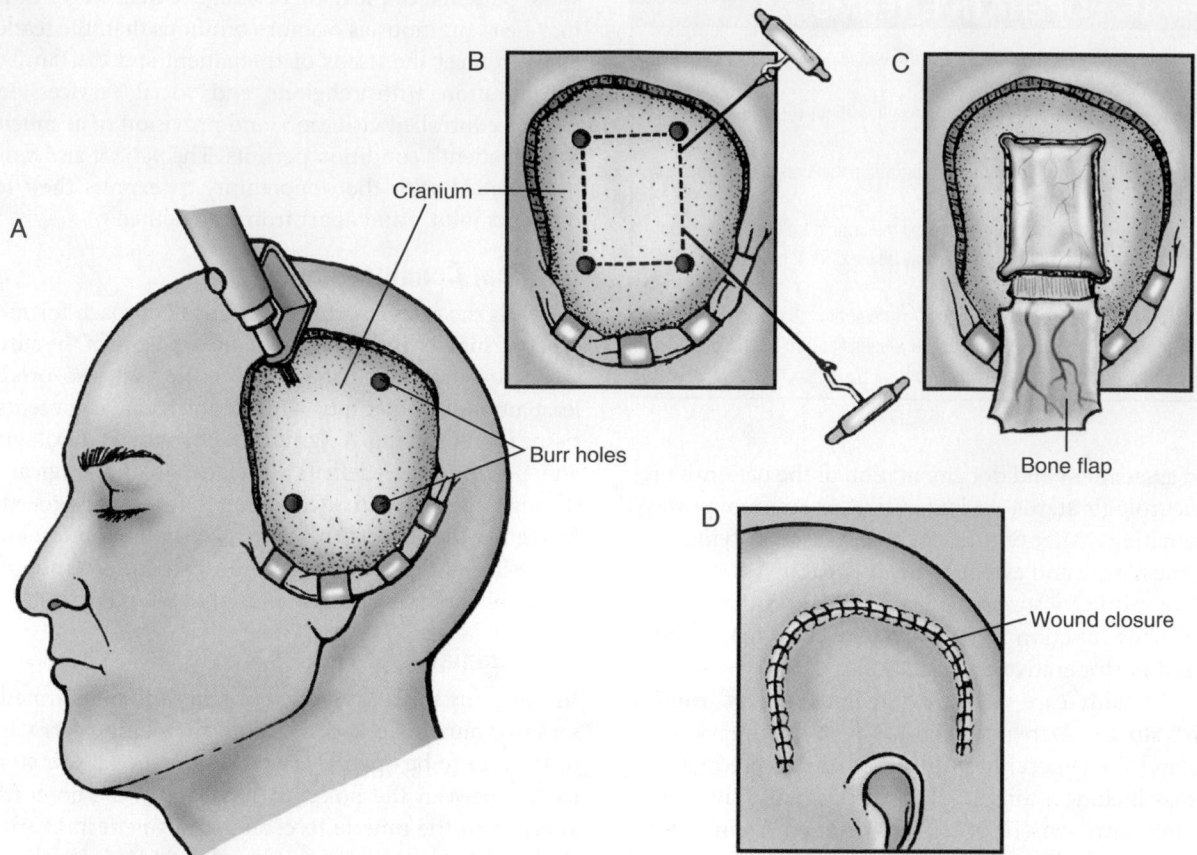

FIGURE 24-6 Craniotomy Procedure. *A,* Burr holes are drilled into skull. *B,* Skull is cut between burr holes with a surgical saw. *C,* Bone flap is turned back to expose cranial contents. *D,* After surgery, bone flap is replaced and wound is closed. (From Forsyth LW, Garnett JC. Traumatic and neoplastic problems of the brain. In: Monahan FD, et al, eds. *Phipps' Medical-Surgical Nursing: Health and Illness Perspectives.* 8th ed. St. Louis: Mosby; 2007.)

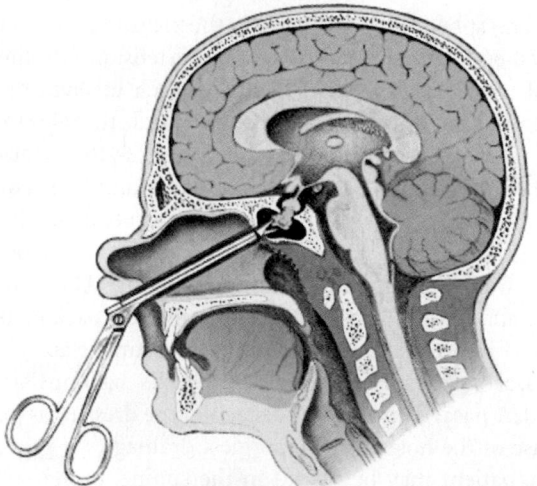

FIGURE 24-7 Trans-sphenoidal hypophysectomy.

by Doppler signal allows immediate recognition of this complication. If it occurs, an attempt may be made to withdraw the embolus from the right atrium through a central line. Flooding the surgical field with irrigation fluid and placing a moistened sterile surgical sponge over the surgical site creates an immediate barrier to any further air entrance.[52]

Postoperative Medical Management

Definitive management of the postoperative neurosurgical patient varies, depending on the underlying reason for the craniotomy. During the initial postoperative period, management is usually directed toward the prevention of complications. Complications associated with a craniotomy include intracranial hypertension, surgical hemorrhage, fluid imbalance, cerebrospinal fluid leak, and DVT.

Intracranial Hypertension

Postoperative cerebral edema is expected to peak 48 to 72 hours after surgery. If the bone flap is not replaced at the time of surgery, intracranial hypertension will produce bulging at the surgical site. Close monitoring of the surgical site is important so that integrity of the incision can be maintained. Postcraniotomy management of intracranial hypertension is usually accomplished through CSF drainage, patient positioning, and steroid administration.[54]

Surgical Hemorrhage

Surgical hemorrhage after a transcranial procedure can occur in the intracranial vault and manifests as signs and symptoms of increasing ICP. Hemorrhage after a trans-sphenoidal craniotomy may be evident from external drainage, the patient's complaint of persistent postnasal drip, or excessive swallowing. Loss of vision after pituitary surgery indicates an evolving hemorrhage. Postoperative hemorrhage requires surgical reexploration.[55]

Fluid Imbalance

Fluid imbalance in the postcraniotomy patient usually results from a disturbance in production or secretion of antidiuretic hormone (ADH). ADH is secreted by the posterior pituitary (neurohypophysis) gland. It stimulates the renal tubules and collecting ducts to retain water in response to low circulating blood volume or increased serum osmolality. Inoperative trauma or postoperative edema of the pituitary gland or hypothalamus can result in insufficient ADH secretion. The outcome is unabated renal water loss even when blood volume is low and serum osmolality is high. This condition is known as *diabetes insipidus* (DI). The polyuria associated with DI is often more than 200 milliliters per hour (mL/hr). Urine specific gravity of 1.005 or less and elevated serum osmolality provide evidence of insufficient ADH. The loss of volume may provoke hypotension and inadequate cerebral perfusion. DI is usually self-limiting, and fluid replacement is the only required therapy. In some cases, however, it may be necessary to administer vasopressin intravenously to control the loss of fluid.[56]

The syndrome of inappropriate antidiuretic hormone (SIADH) commonly occurs with neurologic insult and results from excessive ADH secretion. SIADH manifests as inappropriate water retention with hyponatremia in the presence of normal renal function. Urine specific gravity is elevated, and urine osmolality is greater than serum osmolality. The dangers associated with SIADH include circulating volume overload and electrolyte imbalance, both of which may impair neurologic functioning. SIADH is usually self-limiting, with the mainstay of treatment being fluid restriction.[56]

Cerebrospinal Fluid Leak

Leakage of CSF results from an opening in the subarachnoid space, as evidenced by clear fluid draining from the surgical site. When this complication occurs after trans-sphenoidal surgery, it is evidenced by excessive, clear drainage from the nose or persistent postnasal drip.[57] To differentiate CSF drainage from postoperative serous drainage, a specimen is tested for glucose content. A CSF leak is confirmed by glucose values of 30 mg/dL or greater. Management of the patient with a CSF leak includes bed rest and head elevation. Lumbar puncture or placement of a lumbar subarachnoid catheter may be used to reduce CSF pressure until the dura heals. The risk of meningitis associated with CSF leak often necessitates surgical repair to reseal the opening.[58]

Deep Vein Thrombosis

Patients who have undergone neurosurgery are at particularly high risk for the development of DVT. Research has demonstrated that these patients have a variety of additional risk factors including preoperative leg weakness, longer preoperative and postoperative stay in the critical care unit, longer operative procedure time, prone positioning on frames with flexion of the hips or knees, longer time in the postanesthesia care unit, more days on bed rest, lengthy operative procedures, and delay of postoperative mobility and activity.[59,60] Clinical manifestations of DVT include leg or calf pain and erythema, warmth, and swelling of the affected limb. Unfortunately, the patient with a DVT is often asymptomatic, and the diagnosis is not made until the patient experiences a pulmonary embolus.[61] The primary treatment for DVT is prophylaxis. Following neurosurgery, sequential (intermittent) pneumatic compression boots or stockings are effective in reducing the incidence of DVT. Effectiveness is enhanced when these devices are initiated in the preoperative period. Low-dose unfractionated heparin or low-molecular-weight heparin may also be used prophylactically in high-risk patients once the risk of bleeding has decreased.[62]

Postoperative Nursing Management

The nursing management of the patient following neurosurgery incorporates a variety of nursing diagnoses (Box 24-16). As in preoperative care, the primary goal of postcraniotomy nursing management is protection of the integrity of the CNS. Nursing interventions focus on preserving adequate CPP, promoting arterial oxygenation, providing comfort and emotional support, maintaining surveillance for complications, initiating early rehabilitation, and educating the patient and family. Frequent neurologic assessment is necessary to evaluate accomplishment of these objectives and to identify problems and quickly intervene if complications do arise. Often, a ventriculostomy is placed to facilitate ICP monitoring and CSF drainage.

Preserving Adequate Cerebral Perfusion

Nursing interventions to preserve cerebral perfusion include patient positioning, fluid management, and avoidance of postoperative vomiting and fever.

Positioning. Patient positioning is an important component of care for the craniotomy patient. The head of the bed should be elevated 30 to 45 degrees at all times to reduce the incidence of hemorrhage, facilitate venous drainage, and control ICP. Other positioning measures to control ICP include maintaining the patient's head in a neutral position at all times and avoiding neck or hip flexion. These rules of positioning must be followed throughout all nursing activities, including linen changes and transporting the patient for diagnostic evaluation.

◎ BOX 24-16 NURSING DIAGNOSES
Craniotomy

- Decreased Intracranial Adaptive Capacity, related to failure of normal intracranial compensatory mechanisms, p. 1131
- Ineffective Cerebral Tissue Perfusion, related to decreased blood flow, p. 1156
- Ineffective Cerebral Tissue Perfusion, related to hemorrhage, p. 1156
- Acute Pain, related to transmission and perception of cutaneous, visceral, muscular, or ischemic impulses, p. 1123
- Disturbed Body Image, related to actual change in body structure, function, or appearance, p. 1136
- Deficient Knowledge: Discharge Regimen, related to lack of previous exposure to information, p. 1134 (see Box 21-17, Patient Education for Craniotomy)

Most craniotomy patients can be turned from side to side within these restrictions, using pillows for support, except in some cases of extensive tumor removal, cranioplasty, and when the bone flap is not replaced. Specific orders from the surgeon must be obtained in these instances. The patient with an infratentorial incision may be restricted to only a very small pillow under the head to prevent strain on the incision. Avoidance of anterior or lateral neck flexion also protects the integrity of this type of incision.

Fluid Management. Fluid management is another important component of postcraniotomy care. Hourly monitoring of fluid intake and output facilitates early identification of fluid imbalance. Urine specific gravity must be measured if DI is suspected. Fluid restriction may be ordered as a routine measure to lessen the severity of cerebral edema or as treatment for the fluid and electrolyte imbalances associated with SIADH.[56]

Avoidance of Vomiting and Fever. Postoperative vomiting must be avoided to prevent sharp spikes in ICP and possibly surgical hemorrhage. Antiemetics are administered as soon as nausea is apparent. Early nutrition in the patient is beneficial. If the patient is unable to eat, enteral hyperalimentation delivered through a feeding tube is the preferred method of nutritional support and can be initiated as early as 24 hours after surgery. Postoperative fever may also adversely affect ICP and increase the metabolic needs of the brain. Acetaminophen is administered orally, rectally, or through a feeding tube. External cooling measures such as a hypothermia blanket may be necessary.

Promoting Arterial Oxygenation

Routine pulmonary care is used to maintain airway clearance and prevent pulmonary complications. To prevent dangerous elevations in ICP, this care measure must be performed using proper technique and at time intervals that are adequately spaced from other patient care activities. If pulmonary complications do arise, consideration must be given to maintaining adequate oxygenation during repositioning. It may be necessary to restrict turning to only the side that places the good lung down.

Providing Comfort and Emotional Support

Pain management in the patient after craniotomy primarily involves control of headache. Small doses of intravenous morphine are used in the critical care setting. Oral analgesics should be started as soon as can be tolerated. Nonopioid medications such as tramadol may be used as an adjunct medication.[63] As opioid analgesics cause constipation, administration of stool softeners and initiation of a bowel program are important components of postcraniotomy care. Constipation is hazardous because straining to have a bowel movement can create significant elevations in blood pressure and ICP.

Maintaining Surveillance for Complications

Following neurosurgery, the patient is at risk for infection, corneal abrasions, and injury from falls or seizures.

Infection. After neurosurgery, patients are at risk for a variety of infections, including meningitis, cerebral abscesses, bone flap infections, and subdural empyema.[64] Care of the incision and surgical dressings is specific to the institution and the physician. The rule of thumb for a craniotomy dressing is to reinforce it, as needed, and change it only on a physician's order. Often, a drain is left in place to facilitate decompression of the surgical site. If a ventriculostomy is present, it is treated as a component of the surgical site. All drainage devices must be secured to the dressing to prevent unintentional displacement with patient movement. Sterile technique is required to prevent infection. Postoperatively, infection should be suspected if the patient exhibits signs of mental status changes, headache, fever, and purulent drainage and swelling around the incision site.[64]

Corneal Abrasions. Routine eye care may be necessary to prevent corneal drying and ulceration. Periorbital edema interferes with normal blinking and eyelid closure, which are essential to adequate corneal lubrication. Saline drops are instilled every 2 hours. If the patient remains in a comatose state, covering the eyes with a polyethylene film extending over the orbits and eyebrows may be beneficial.[13,65]

Injury. After craniotomy, the patient may experience periods of altered mentation. Protection from injury may require the use of restraint devices. The side rails of the bed must be padded to protect the patient from injury. Having a family member stay at the bedside or the use of music therapy is often helpful to keep the patient calm during periods of restlessness. In rare circumstances, continuous sedation with or without neuromuscular blockade may be necessary to control patient activity and metabolic needs on a short-term basis.

Initiating Early Rehabilitation

Increased activity, including ambulation, is begun as soon as tolerated by the patient in the postoperative period. Rehabilitation measures and discharge planning may begin in the critical care unit but are beyond the scope of this chapter. Transfer to a general care or rehabilitation unit is usually accomplished as soon as the patient is deemed stable and free of complications.

Educating the Patient and Family

Preoperatively, the patient and family should be taught about the precipitating event necessitating the need for the craniotomy and its expected outcome (Box 24-17). The severity of the disease and the need for critical care management postoperatively must be stressed. As the patient moves toward discharge, teaching focuses on medication instructions; incisional care, including the signs of infection; and the signs and symptoms of increased ICP. If the patient has neurologic deficits, teaching focuses on the interventions to maximize the patient's rehabilitation potential, and the patient's family members must be encouraged to participate in the patient's care and to learn some basic rehabilitation techniques. The importance of participating in a neurologic rehabilitation program must be stressed.

INTRACRANIAL HYPERTENSION

Pathophysiology

The intracranial space comprises three components: 1) brain substance (80%), 2) CSF (10%), and 3) blood (10%). Under normal physiologic conditions, the mean ICP is maintained below 15 mm Hg.[33,66] Essential to understanding the pathophysiology of ICP, the Monro-Kellie hypothesis proposes that an increase in volume of one intracranial component must be compensated by a decrease in one or more of the other components so that total volume remains fixed. This compensation, although limited, includes displacing CSF from the intracranial vault to the lumbar cistern, increasing CSF absorption, and compressing the low-pressure venous system.[67,68] Pathophysiologic alterations that can elevate ICP are outlined in Table 24-4.

BOX 24-17 PATIENT EDUCATION

Craniotomy

Before Surgery

- Pathophysiology and expected outcome of underlying disease
- Need for intensive care management after surgery
- Routine preoperative surgical care

After Surgery

- Routine postoperative surgical care
- Discharge medications—purpose, dose, and side effects
- Incisional care
- Signs and symptoms of infection
- Signs and symptoms of increased intracranial pressure
- Measures to compensate for residual deficits
- Basic rehabilitation techniques
- Importance of participating in neurologic rehabilitation program

---

Additional information for the patient and family can be found at the National Brain Tumor Society website (www.braintumor.org).

Volume-Pressure Curve

When capable of compliance, the brain can tolerate significant increases in intracranial volume without much increase in ICP. The amount of intracranial compliance, however, does have a limit. After this limit has been reached, a state of decompensation with increased ICP results. As the ICP rises, the relationship between volume and pressure changes, and small increases in volume may cause major elevations in ICP (Fig. 24-8).[33,67] The exact configuration of the volume–pressure curve and the point at which the steep rise in pressure occurs vary among patients. The configuration of this curve is also influenced by the cause and the rate of volume increases within the intracranial vault; for example, neurologic deterioration occurs more rapidly in a patient with an acute epidural hematoma than in a patient with a meningioma of the same size.[66] Regardless of how fast the pressure increases, intracranial hypertension occurs when ICP is greater than 20 mm Hg.[67]

Cerebral Blood Flow and Autoregulation

Cerebral blood flow (CBF) corresponds to the metabolic demands of the brain and is normally 50 mL/100 g of brain tissue/min. Although the brain makes up only 2% of body weight, it requires 15% to 20% of the resting cardiac output and 15% of the body's oxygen demands. The normal brain has a complex capacity to maintain constant CBF, despite wide ranges in systemic arterial pressure—an effect known as *autoregulation*. A mean arterial pressure of 50 to 150 mm Hg does not alter CBF when autoregulation is functioning. Outside the limits of this autoregulation, CBF becomes passively dependent on the perfusion pressure.[67]

TABLE 24-4 MECHANISMS OF INTRACRANIAL PRESSURE ELEVATION

PATHOPHYSIOLOGY	EXAMPLE	TREATMENT
Disorders of CSF Space		
Overproduction of CSF	Choroid plexus papilloma	Diuretics, surgical removal
Communicating hydrocephalus from obstructed arachnoid	Old subarachnoid hemorrhage	Surgical drainage from lumbar drain
Noncommunicative hydrocephalus	Posterior fossa tumor obstructing aqueduct	Surgical drainage by ventricular drain
Interstitial edema	Any of above	Surgical drainage of CSF
Disorders of Intracranial Blood		
Intracranial hemorrhage causing increased ICP	Epidural hematoma	Surgical drainage
Vasospasm	Subarachnoid hemorrhage	Hypervolemia and hypertensive therapy
Vasodilation	Elevated $Paco_2$	Hyperventilation
Increasing cerebral blood volume and ICP	Hypoxia	Adequate oxygenation
Disorders of Brain Substance		
Expanding mass lesion with local vasogenic edema causing increased ICP	Brain tumor	Steroids Surgical removal
Ischemic brain injury with cytotoxic edema increasing ICP	Anoxic brain injury from cardiac or respiratory arrest	Resistant to therapy
Increased cerebral metabolic rate increasing cerebral blood flow and ICP	Seizures, hyperthermia	Anticonvulsant medications to control fever

Modified from Helfaer MA, Kirsch JR. Intracranial vault pathophysiology. *Crit Care Rep.* 1989;1:12.
CSF, Cerebrospinal fluid; *ICP,* intracranial pressure.

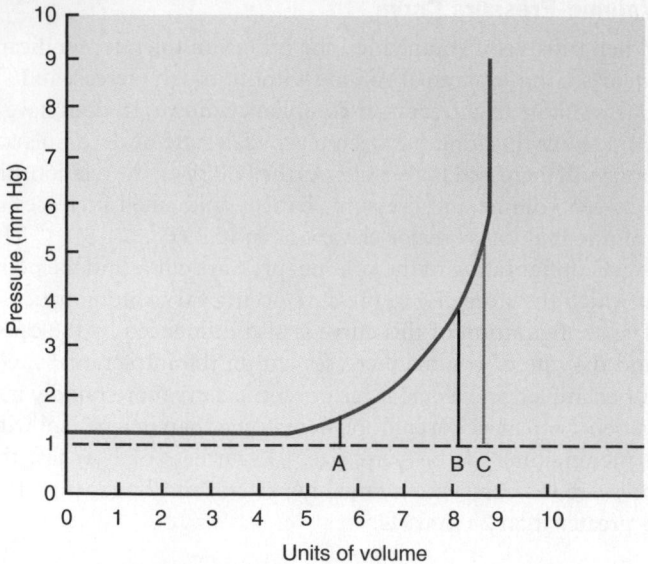

FIGURE 24-8 Intracranial Volume–Pressure Curve. Pressure is normal *(A)* and increases in intracranial volume are tolerated without increases in intracranial pressure. Increases in volume *(B)* may cause increases in pressure. Small increases in volume *(C)* may cause larger increases in pressure.

Factors other than arterial blood pressure that affect CBF are conditions that result in acidosis, alkalosis, and changes in metabolic rate. Conditions that cause acidosis (e.g., hypoxia, hypercapnia, ischemia) result in cerebrovascular dilation. Conditions causing alkalosis (e.g., hypocapnia) result in cerebrovascular constriction. Normally, a reduction in metabolic rate (e.g., from hypothermia or barbiturates) decreases CBF, and increases in metabolic rate (e.g., from hyperthermia) increase CBF.[66,69]

Arterial blood gases exert a profound effect on CBF. Carbon dioxide, which affects the pH of the blood, is a potent vasoactive substance. Carbon dioxide retention (hypercapnia) leads to cerebral vasodilation, with increased cerebral blood volume, whereas hypocapnia leads to cerebral vasoconstriction and a reduction in cerebral blood volume. Prolonged hypocapnia, however, especially at an arterial partial pressure of carbon dioxide ($Paco_2$) level lower than 20 mm Hg, can lead to cerebral ischemia. Low arterial partial pressure of oxygen (Pao_2) levels, especially below 40 mm Hg, lead to cerebral vasodilation, which increases the intracranial blood volume and can contribute to increased ICP. High Pao_2 levels have not been shown to affect CBF in either direction.[66,69]

Assessment and Diagnosis

The numerous signs and symptoms of increased ICP include decreased level of consciousness, Cushing triad (bradycardia, systolic hypertension, and widening pulse pressure), diminished brainstem reflexes, papilledema, decerebrate posturing (abnormal extension), decorticate posturing (abnormal flexion), unequal pupil size, projectile vomiting, decreased pupillary reaction to light, altered breathing patterns, and headache.[33,70] Patients may exhibit one or all of these symptoms, depending on the underlying cause of the elevation in ICP. One of the earliest and most important signs of increased ICP is a decrease in the level of consciousness. This change must be reported immediately to the physician.[69,70]

In the patient with suspected intracranial hypertension, a monitoring device may be placed within the cranium to quantify ICP. Under normal physiologic conditions, the mean ICP is maintained below 15 mm Hg. The device is used to monitor serial ICPs and assist with the management of intracranial hypertension. An increase in ICP can decrease blood flow to the brain, causing brain damage. The monitoring device can also provide a sterile access for draining excess CSF. The four sites for monitoring ICP are the intraventricular space, the subarachnoid space, the epidural space, and the parenchyma. Each site has advantages and disadvantages for monitoring ICP. The type of monitor chosen depends on the suspected pathologic condition and the physician's preferences.[69-72] Chapter 23 provides a more detailed discussion of ICP monitoring.

Medical and Nursing Management

After intracranial hypertension is documented, therapy must be prompt to prevent secondary insults (Fig. 24-9). Although the exact pressure level denoting intracranial hypertension remains uncertain, most current evidence suggests that ICP generally must be treated when it exceeds 20 mm Hg.[33,66,69] All therapies are directed toward reducing the volume of one or more of the components (e.g., blood, brain, CSF) that lie within the intracranial vault. A major goal of therapy is to determine the cause of the elevated pressure and, if possible, to remove the cause.[33,66,69] In the absence of a surgically treatable mass lesion, intracranial hypertension is treated medically. Nurses play an important role in rapid assessment and implementation of appropriate therapies for reducing ICP. Nursing interventions for the promotion of cerebral perfusion and management of cerebral edema are outlined in Boxes 24-18 and 24-19.

Positioning and Other Nursing Activities

Positioning of the patient is a significant factor in the prevention and treatment of intracranial hypertension. Head elevation has long been advocated as a conventional nursing intervention to control ICP, presumably by increasing venous return. However, this may decrease CPP. Close monitoring of ICP and CPP should be done with positioning, customizing positioning to maximize CPP, and minimize ICP.[68]

Positions that impede venous return from the brain cause elevations in ICP. Obstruction of jugular veins or an increase in intrathoracic or intra-abdominal pressure is communicated as increased pressure throughout the open venous system, thereby impeding drainage from the brain and increasing ICP. Positions that decrease venous return from the head (e.g., Trendelenburg, prone, extreme flexion of the hips, angulation of the neck) must be avoided if possible. If changes to positions such as Trendelenburg are necessary to provide adequate pulmonary care, critical care nurses must closely monitor ICP and vital signs.[66]

Some routine nursing activities do affect ICP and may be harmful. Use of positive end-expiratory pressures (PEEP) greater than 20 cm H_2O, coughing, suctioning, tight tracheostomy tube ties, and the Valsalva maneuver have been associated with increases in ICP. Cumulative increases in ICP have been

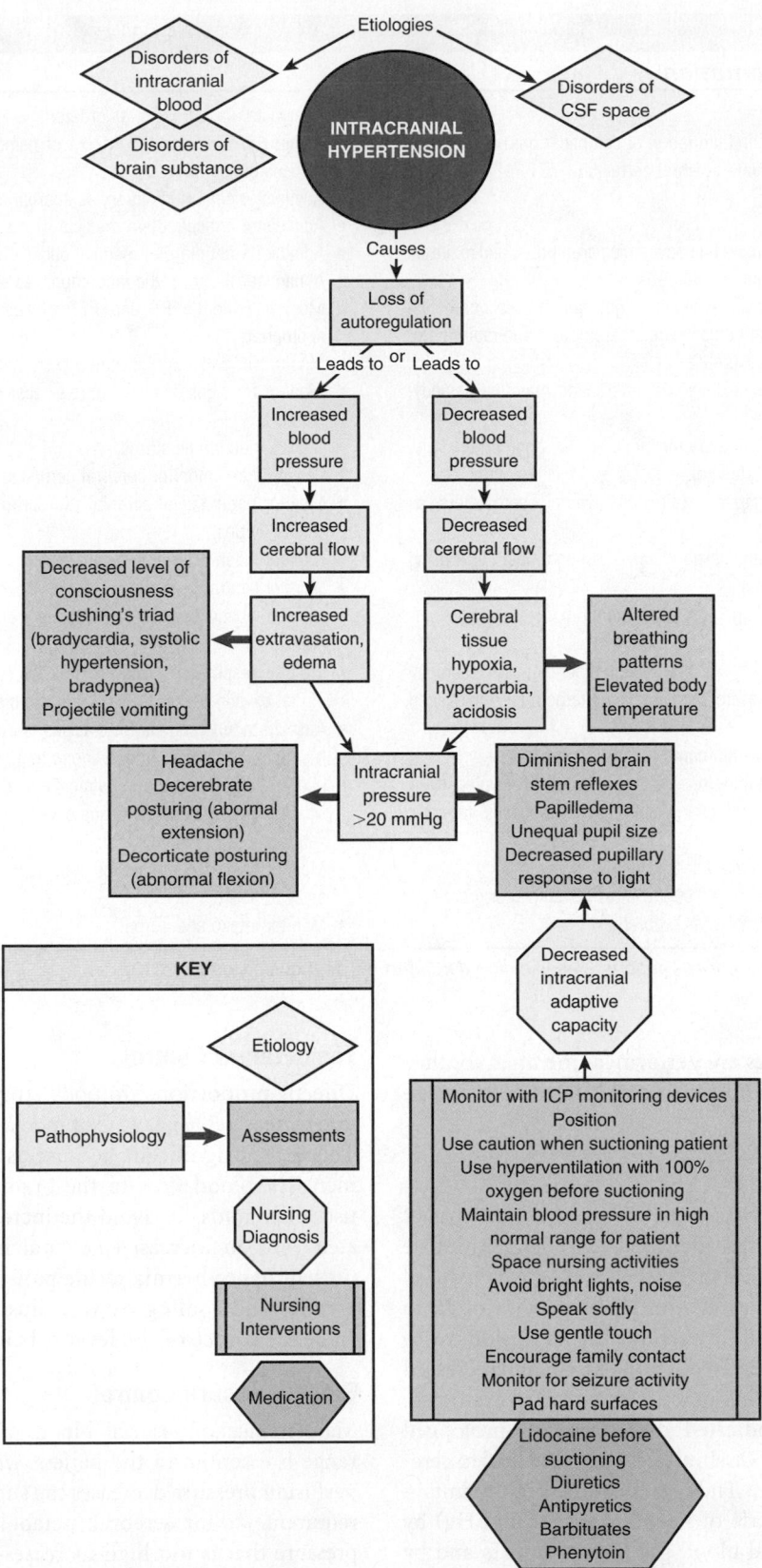

FIGURE 24-9 Concept Map for Intracranial Hypertension. (Concept map illustration created by Elaine Bishop Kennedy, EdD, RN.)

BOX 24-18 NIC

Cerebral Perfusion Promotion

Definition

Promotion of adequate perfusion and limitation of complications for a patient experiencing or at risk for inadequate cerebral perfusion

Activities

- Consult with physician to determine hemodynamic parameters, and maintain hemodynamic parameters within this range.
- Induce hypertension with volume expansion or inotropic or vasoconstrictive agents, as ordered, to maintain hemodynamic parameters and maintain or optimize cerebral perfusion pressure (CPP).
- Administer and titrate vasoactive drugs, as ordered, to maintain hemodynamic parameters.
- Administer agents to expand intravascular volume, as appropriate (e.g., colloid, blood products, and crystalloid).
- Administer volume expanders to maintain hemodynamic parameters, as ordered.
- Monitor prothrombin time (PT) and partial thromboplastin time (PTT), if using hetastarch as a volume expander.
- Administer rheologic agents (e.g., low-dose mannitol or low-molecular-weight dextrans), as ordered.
- Keep hematocrit level around 33% for hypervolemic hemodilution therapy.
- Phlebotomize patient, as appropriate, to maintain hematocrit level in desired range.
- Maintain serum glucose level within normal range.
- Consult with physician to determine optimal head of bed (HOB) placement (e.g., 0, 15, or 30 degrees) and monitor patient's responses to head positioning.
- Avoid neck flexion or extreme hip or knee flexion.
- Keep partial carbon dioxide pressure (PCO_2) level at 25 mm Hg or greater.
- Administer calcium channel blockers, as ordered.

- Administer vasopressin, as ordered.
- Administer and monitor effects of osmotic and loop-active diuretics and corticosteroids.
- Administer pain medication, as appropriate.
- Administer anticoagulant medication, as ordered.
- Administer antiplatelet medications, as ordered.
- Administer thrombolytic mediations, as ordered.
- Monitor patient's PT and PTT to keep one to two times normal, as appropriate.
- Monitor for anticoagulant therapy side effects.
- Monitor for signs of bleeding (e.g., test stool and nasogastric drainage for blood).
- Monitor neurologic status.
- Calculate and monitor cerebral perfusion pressure (CPP).
- Monitor patient's intracranial pressure (ICP) and neurologic responses to care activities.
- Monitor mean arterial pressure (MAP).
- Monitor central venous pressure (CVP).
- Monitor pulmonary artery wedge pressure (PAWP) and pulmonary artery pressure (PAP).
- Monitor respiratory status (e.g., rate, rhythm, and depth of respirations; partial oxygen pressure, PCO_2, pH, and bicarbonate levels).
- Auscultate lung sounds for crackles or other adventitious sounds.
- Monitor for signs of fluid overload (e.g., rhonchi, jugular venous distention [JVD], edema, increase in pulmonary secretions).
- Monitor determinants of tissue oxygen delivery (e.g., $PaCO_2$, arterial oxygen saturation [SaO_2], hemoglobin levels, cardiac output), if available.
- Monitor laboratory values for changes in oxygenation or acid–base balance, as appropriate.
- Monitor intake and output.

From Bulechek GM, et al. *Nursing Interventions Classification (NIC)*. 6th ed. St. Louis: Mosby; 2013.

---

reported when care activities are performed one after another. Conversely, family contact and gentle touch have been associated with decreases in ICP.[66,72]

Hyperventilation

Controlled hyperventilation has been an important adjunct of therapy for the patient with increased ICP. The rationale employed in hyperventilation is that if the $PaCO_2$ can be reduced from its normal level of 35 to 40 mm Hg to a range of 25 to 30 mm Hg in the patient with intracranial hypertension, vasoconstriction of cerebral arteries, reduction of CBF, and increased venous return will result. This practice is being re-examined. Additional research has indicated that severe or prolonged hyperventilation can reduce cerebral perfusion and lead to cerebral ischemia and infarction. The current trend is to maintain $PaCO_2$ levels on the lower side of normal (35 ± 2 mm Hg) by carefully monitoring arterial blood gas measurements and by adjusting ventilator settings.[67,71,72]

Although hypoxemia must be avoided, excessively high levels of oxygen offer no benefits, and increasing inspired oxygen concentrations above 60% may lead to toxic changes in lung tissue. The use of pulse oximetry has led to greater awareness of the circumstances, such as pain and anxiety, that can cause oxygen desaturation and thus elevate ICP.[33,66]

Temperature Control

Directly proportional to body temperature, cerebral metabolic rate increases 7% per 1° C of increase in body temperature.[68,69,72] This fact is significant because as the cerebral metabolic rate increases, blood flow to the brain must increase to meet the tissue demands. To avoid the increase in blood volume associated with an increased cerebral metabolic rate, nurses must prevent hyperthermia in the patient with a brain injury. Antipyretics and cooling devices must be used when appropriate while the source of the fever is being determined.[68,69]

Blood Pressure Control

Maintenance of arterial blood pressure in the high-normal range is essential in the patient with brain injury. Inadequate perfusion pressure decreases the supply of nutrients and oxygen requirements for cerebral metabolic needs. However, a blood pressure that is too high increases cerebral blood volume and may increase ICP.[69] Figure 24-10 shows the relationship between blood pressure and ICP.

Control of systemic hypertension may require nothing more than the administration of a sedative agent. Small, frequent doses may be sufficient to blunt noxious stimuli and prevent them from triggering increases in blood pressure. When sedation proves inadequate in controlling systemic arterial

BOX 24-19 NIC

Cerebral Edema Management

Definition

Limitation of secondary cerebral injury resulting from swelling of brain tissue

Activities

- Monitor for confusion, changes in mentation, complaints of dizziness, syncope.
- Monitor neurologic status closely, and compare to baseline.
- Monitor vital signs.
- Monitor CSF drainage characteristics: color, clarity, consistency.
- Record CSF drainage.
- Monitor CVP, PAWP, and PAP, as appropriate.
- Monitor ICP and CPP.
- Analyze ICP waveform.
- Monitor respiratory status: rate, rhythm, and depth of respirations; Pao_2, Pco_2, pH, bicarbonate levels.
- Allow ICP to return to baseline between nursing activities.
- Monitor patient's ICP and neurologic responses to care activities.
- Decrease stimuli in patient's environment.
- Plan nursing care to provide rest periods.
- Give sedation, as needed.
- Note patient's change in response to stimuli.
- Screen conversation within patient's hearing.
- Administer anticonvulsants, as appropriate.
- Avoid neck flexion or extreme hip or knee flexion.
- Avoid Valsalva maneuvers.
- Administer stool softeners.
- Position with head of bed up 30 degrees or greater.
- Avoid use of PEEP.
- Administer paralyzing agent, as appropriate.
- Encourage family or significant other to talk to patient.
- Restrict fluids.
- Avoid use of hypotonic IV fluids.
- Adjust ventilator settings to keep $Paco_2$ at prescribed level.
- Limit suction passes to less than 15 seconds.
- Monitor laboratory values: serum and urine osmolality, sodium, and potassium.
- Monitor volume pressure indices.
- Perform passive range-of-motion exercises.
- Monitor intake and output.
- Maintain normothermia.
- Administer loop-active or osmotic diuretics.
- Implement seizure precautions.
- Titrate barbiturate to achieve suppression or burst-suppression of EEG, as ordered.
- Establish means of communication: ask yes-or-no questions, and provide magic slate, paper and pencil, picture board, flashcards, VOCAID device.

From Bulechek GM, et al. *Nursing Interventions Classification (NIC)*. 6th ed. St. Louis: Mosby; 2013.
CPP, Cerebral perfusion pressure; *CSF*, cerebrospinal fluid; *CVP*, central venous pressure; *EEG*, electroencephalogram; *ICP*, intracranial pressure; *IV*, intravenous; *PAP*, pulmonary artery pressure; *PAWP*, pulmonary artery wedge pressure; *PEEP*, positive end-expiratory pressure.

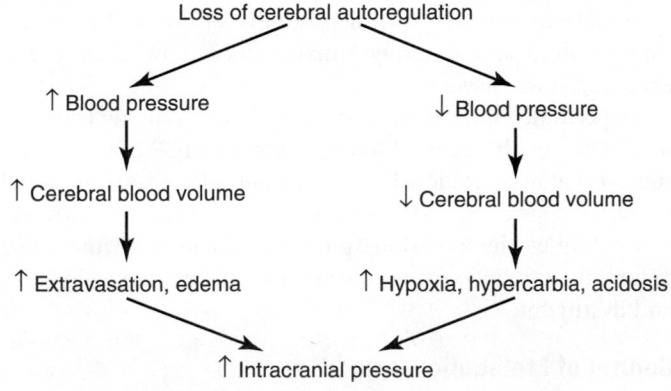

FIGURE 24-10 Loss of pressure autoregulation.

hypertension, antihypertensive agents are used. Care must be taken in choosing these agents because many of the peripheral vasodilators (e.g., nitroprusside, nitroglycerin) also are cerebral vasodilators. All antihypertensives are believed to cause some degree of cerebral vasodilation. To reduce this vasodilating effect, concurrent treatment with beta-blockers (e.g., metoprolol, labetalol) may be beneficial.[66,69]

Systemic hypotension should be treated aggressively with fluids to maintain a systolic blood pressure greater than 90 mm Hg. Crystalloids, colloids, and blood products can be used, depending on the patient's condition. Studies have demonstrated a positive effect on ICP and CPP with hypertonic saline.[73] If fluids fail to adequately elevate the patient's blood pressure, the use of inotropic agents may be necessary.[66]

Seizure Control

The incidence of post-traumatic seizures in the patient population with head injury has been estimated at 15% to 20%. Because of the risk of a secondary ischemic insult associated with seizures, many physicians prescribe anticonvulsant medications prophylactically. Seizures cause metabolic requirements to increase, which results in elevation of CBF, cerebral blood volume, and ICP, even in paralyzed patients. If blood flow cannot match demand, ischemia develops, cerebral energy stores are depleted, and irreversible neuronal destruction occurs.[69,74] Phenytoin is the recommended mediation for seizure prophylaxis. A loading dose of 15 to 20 mg/kg is administered intravenously (IV) over 30 minutes followed by 100 mg IV every 8 hours, titrated to therapeutic level, for 7 days.[75] Fast-acting, short-duration agents such as lorazepam may be indicated for breakthrough seizures until therapeutic medication levels can be achieved.

Cerebrospinal Fluid Drainage

CSF drainage for intracranial hypertension may be used with other treatment modalities (Figs. 24-11 and 24-12). CSF drainage is accomplished by the insertion of a pliable catheter into the anterior horn of the lateral ventricle (ventriculostomy), preferably on the nondominant side. This drainage can help support the patient through periods of cerebral edema by controlling spikes in ICP. One of the major advantages of the ventriculostomy is its dual role as a monitoring device and a treatment modality. Care should be taken to avoid infection. However, cleansing ointment such as bacitracin or

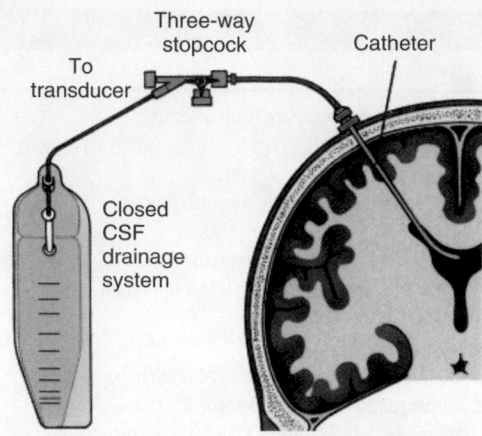

INTRAVENTRICULAR CATHETER

FIGURE 24-11 Intermittent Drainage System. Intermittent drainage involves draining cerebrospinal fluid (CSF) through a ventriculostomy when intracranial pressure exceeds the upper pressure parameter set by the physician. Intermittent drainage is achieved by opening the three-way stopcock to allow CSF to flow into the drainage bag for brief periods (30 to 120 seconds) until the pressure is below the upper pressure parameter. (From Barker E. *Neuroscience Nursing*. 3rd ed. St. Louis: Mosby; 2008.)

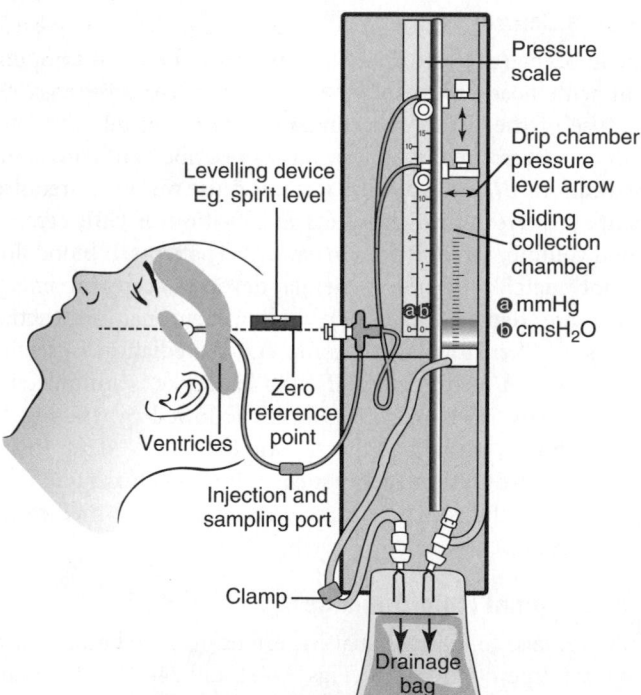

FIGURE 24-12 Continuous Drainage System. Continuous drainage involves placing the drip chamber of the drainage system at a specified level above the foramen of Monro (usually 15 cm). The system is left open to allow continuous drainage of cerebrospinal fluid into the chamber (which drains into a collection bag) against a pressure gradient that prevents excessive drainage and ventricular collapse.

povidone is not recommended. Ventriculitis occurs in 10% to 17%.[71,76]

Hyperosmolar Therapy

Osmotic diuretics and hypertonic saline have also been used to reduce increased ICP. In the presence of an intact blood–brain barrier, hyperosmolar therapy is used to draw water from brain tissue into the intravascular compartment. The direction of flow is from the hypoconcentrated tissue to the hyperconcentrated cerebral vasculature. If the situation becomes reversed and the tissue becomes hyperconcentrated in relation to the cerebral vasculature, a rebound phenomenon may occur. These agents have little direct effect on edematous cerebral tissue situated in an area of a defective blood–brain barrier; instead, they require an intact blood–brain barrier for osmosis to occur.[69,75]

The most widely used osmotic diuretic is mannitol, a large-molecule agent that is retained almost entirely in the extracellular compartment and has little of the rebound effect observed with other osmotic diuretics. Administration of mannitol increases cerebral blood flow and thus induces cerebral vasoconstriction as part of the brain's autoregulatory response to keep blood flow constant.[69,74]

Perhaps the most common difficulty associated with the use of osmotic agents is the provocation of electrolyte disturbances. Careful attention must be paid to body weight and fluid and electrolyte stability. Serum osmolality must be kept between 300 and 320 milliosmoles per liter (mOsm/L). Hypernatremia and hypokalemia often are associated with repeated administration of osmotic agents. Central venous pressure readings must be monitored to prevent hypovolemia. Smaller doses of mannitol simplify fluid and electrolyte management, and their use is encouraged whenever possible.[74,75]

Hypertonic saline, given in concentrations ranging from 3% to 23.4%, can also be used to treat increased ICP. Some studies suggest that hypertonic saline is as equally effective as mannitol for reducing increased ICP.[77] Adverse effects include electrolyte abnormalities, hypotension, pulmonary edema, acute renal failure, hemolysis, central pontine myelinolysis, coagulopathy, and dysrhythmias.[75]

Control of Metabolic Demand

Any treatment modality that increases the incidence of noxious stimulation to the patient carries with it the potential for increasing ICP. Noxious stimuli include pain, the presence of an endotracheal tube, coughing, suctioning, repositioning, bathing, and many other routine nursing interventions. Agents used to reduce metabolic demands include the use of benzodiazepines such as midazolam and lorazepam, intravenous sedative–hypnotics such as propofol, opioid narcotics such as fentanyl and morphine, and neuromuscular blocking agents such as vecuronium and atracurium. These agents may be administered separately or in combination via continuous drip or as an intravenous bolus on an as-needed basis.[66]

The preferred treatment regimen begins with the administration of benzodiazepines for sedation and narcotics for analgesia. If these agents fail to blunt the patient's response to noxious stimuli, propofol or a neuromuscular blocking agent is added. The use of these medications is recommended only in patients who have an ICP monitor in place because sedatives, opioids, and neuromuscular blocking agents affect the reliability of neurologic assessment. The use of neuromuscular blocking agents without sedation is not recommended because these agents can cause skeletal muscle paralysis and because they have no analgesic effect and do not adequately protect the patient from pain and the physiologic responses that can occur from pain-producing procedures.[69,78] If these agents fail to control the patient's ICP, barbiturate therapy is considered.

Barbiturate Therapy. Barbiturate therapy is a treatment protocol developed for the management of uncontrolled intracranial hypertension that has not responded to the conventional treatments previously described.[69] The two most commonly used medications in high-dose barbiturate therapy are: 1) pentobarbital and 2) thiopental. The goal with either medication is a reduction of ICP to 15 to 20 mm Hg while a mean arterial pressure of 70 to 80 mm Hg is maintained. Patients are maintained on high-dose barbiturate therapy until ICP has been controlled within the normal range for 24 hours. Barbiturates must never be stopped abruptly; they are tapered slowly over approximately 4 days. Despite the theoretical reasons for barbiturate use, clinical trials of its use have not shown improved outcome.[66,74]

Complications of high-dose barbiturate therapy can be disastrous unless a specific and organized approach is used. The most common complications are hypotension, hypothermia, and myocardial depression. If any complications occur and are allowed to persist unchecked, they may cause secondary insults to an already damaged brain. Hypotension, the most common complication, results from peripheral vasodilation and can be compounded in an already dehydrated patient who has received large doses of an osmotic diuretic in an attempt to control ICP. Careful monitoring of fluid status by central venous pressure or a pulmonary artery catheter can help prevent this complication. Myocardial depression results from cardiac muscle suppression and can be avoided by frequent monitoring of fluid status, cardiac output, and serum drug levels. If an adequate cardiac output cannot be maintained in the presence of normothermia, barbiturates must be reduced, regardless of serum levels.[66,69]

Collaborative management of the patient's intracranial hypertension is outlined in Box 24-20.

BOX 24-20 COLLABORATIVE MANAGEMENT

Intracranial Hypertension

- Position patient to achieve maximal intracranial pressure (ICP) reduction.
- Reduce environmental stimulation.
- Maintain normothermia.
- Control ventilation to ensure a normal $PaCO_2$ level (35 ± 2 mm Hg).
- Administer diuretic agents, anticonvulsants, sedation, analgesia, paralytic agents, and vasoactive medications to ensure cerebral perfusion pressure (CPP) greater than 70 mm Hg.
- Drain cerebrospinal fluid for ICP greater than 20 mm Hg.

Herniation Syndromes

The goal of neurologic evaluation, ICP monitoring, and treatment of increased ICP is to prevent herniation. Herniation of intracerebral contents results in the shifting of tissue from one compartment of the brain to another and places pressure on cerebral vessels and vital function centers of the brain. If unchecked, herniation rapidly causes death as a result of the cessation of CBF and respirations.[66]

Supratentorial Herniation

The four types of supratentorial herniation syndrome are: 1) uncal; 2) central, or transtentorial; 3) cingulate; and 4) transcalvarial (Fig. 24-13).

Uncal Herniation. Uncal herniation is the most common herniation syndrome. In uncal herniation, a unilateral, expanding mass lesion, usually of the temporal lobe, increases ICP, causing lateral displacement of the tip of the temporal lobe (uncus). Lateral displacement pushes the uncus over the edge of the tentorium, puts pressure on the oculomotor nerve (cranial nerve III) and the posterior cerebral artery ipsilateral to the lesion, and flattens the midbrain against the opposite side. Clinical manifestations of uncal herniation include ipsilateral pupil dilation, decreased level of consciousness, respiratory pattern changes leading to respiratory arrest, and contralateral hemiplegia leading to abnormal flexion (decorticate) or abnormal extension (decerebrate) posturing. If no intervention occurs, uncal herniation results in fixed and dilated pupils, flaccidity, and respiratory arrest.[66,79]

Central Herniation. In *central, or transtentorial, herniation,* an expanding mass lesion of the midline, frontal, parietal, or occipital lobe results in downward displacement of the hemispheres, basal ganglia, and diencephalon through the tentorial notch. Central herniation often is preceded by uncal and cingulate herniation. Clinical manifestations of central herniation include loss of consciousness; small, reactive pupils progressing to fixed, dilated pupils; respiratory changes leading to

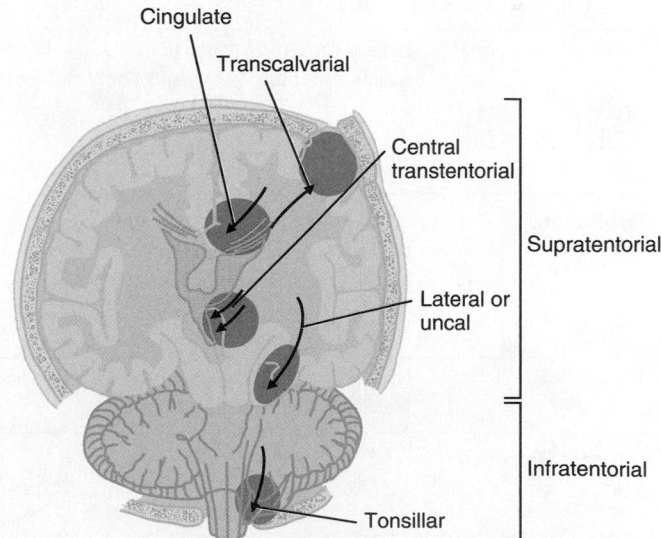

FIGURE 24-13 Types of intracranial herniation. (From Goddard L. Neurological disorders. In: Linton AD. *Introduction to Medical-Surgical Nursing.* St. Louis: Elsevier; 2012.)

respiratory arrest; and abnormal flexion (decorticate) posturing progressing to flaccidity. In the late stages, uncal and central herniation syndromes affect the brainstem similarly.[66,79]

Cingulate Herniation. *Cingulate herniation* occurs when an expanding lesion of one hemisphere shifts laterally and forces the cingulate gyrus under the falx cerebri. Cingulate herniation occurs often. When a lateral shift is observed on the CT scan, cingulate herniation has occurred. Little is known about the effects of cingulate herniation, and no accompanying clinical manifestations exist to assist in its diagnosis. Cingulate herniation is not in itself a life-threatening condition, but if the expanding mass lesion that caused cingulate herniation is not controlled, uncal or central herniation will follow.[66,79]

Transcalvarial Herniation. *Transcalvarial herniation* is the extrusion of cerebral tissue through the cranium. In the presence of severe cerebral edema, transcalvarial herniation occurs through an opening from a skull fracture or craniotomy site.[66]

Infratentorial Herniation

The two infratentorial herniation syndromes are: 1) upward transtentorial herniation and 2) downward cerebellar herniation.

Upward Transtentorial Herniation. *Upward transtentorial herniation* occurs when an expanding mass lesion of the cerebellum causes protrusion of the vermis (central area) of the cerebellum and the midbrain upward through the tentorial notch. Compression of the third cranial nerve and diencephalon occurs. Blockage of the central aqueduct and distortion of the third ventricle obstruct CSF flow. Deterioration progresses rapidly.[66,79]

Downward Cerebellar Herniation. *Downward cerebellar herniation* occurs when an expanding lesion of the cerebellum exerts pressure downward, sending the cerebellar tonsils through the foramen magnum. Compression and displacement of the medulla oblongata occur, rapidly resulting in respiratory and cardiac arrest.[66,79]

PHARMACOLOGIC AGENTS

Many pharmacologic agents are used in the care of patients with neurologic disorders. Table 24-5 reviews the various agents used and any special considerations necessary for administering them.

TABLE 24-5 PHARMACOLOGIC MANAGEMENT
Neurologic Disorders

MEDICATION	DOSAGE	ACTION	SPECIAL CONSIDERATIONS
Anticonvulsants			
Phenytoin (Dilantin)	Loading dose: 10-20 mg/kg IV Maintenance dose: 100 mg q6-8h IV	Prevents the influx of sodium at the cell membrane	Monitor serum levels closely; therapeutic level is 10-20 mg/L (if hypoalbuminuria, monitor free phenytoin serum levels: therapeutic level of 0.1-0.2 mg/L) Infuse phenytoin no faster than 50 mg/min; administer with normal saline only because it precipitates with other solutions
Fosphenytoin (Cerebyx)	Loading dose: 15-20 mg/kg IV Maintenance dose: 4-6 mg/kg/24 hr IV	Prevents the influx of sodium at the cell membrane	Monitor serum levels closely; therapeutic level is 10-20 mg/L Dosage, concentration, and infusion rate of fosphenytoin is expressed as phenytoin sodium equivalents (FE)
Barbiturates			
Phenobarbital	Loading dose: 6-8 mg/kg IV Maintenance dose: 1-3 mg/kg/24 hr IV	Produces central nervous system depression and reduces the spread of an epileptic focus	May depress cardiac and respiratory function Administer phenobarbital at a rate of 60 mg/min; monitor serum level closely; therapeutic level is 15-40 mcg/mL
Pentobarbital	Loading dose: 3-10 mg/kg over 30 min Maintenance dose: 0.5-3 mg/kg/hr IV	Induces barbiturate coma	Monitor serum level of pentobarbital closely; therapeutic level for coma is 15-40 mg/L
Osmotic Diuretics			
Mannitol	1-2 g/kg IV	Treats cerebral edema by pulling fluid from the extravascular space into the intravascular space; requires intact blood–brain barrier	Side effects include hypovolemia and increased serum osmolality Monitor serum osmolality and notify the physician if >310 mOsm/L Warm and shake before administering to ensure crystals are dissolved

TABLE 24-5 PHARMACOLOGIC MANAGEMENT: NEUROLOGIC DISORDERS

Neurologic Disorders—cont'd

MEDICATION	DOSAGE	ACTION	SPECIAL CONSIDERATIONS
Calcium Channel Blockers			
Nimodipine (Nimotop)	60 mg q4h NG or PO for 21 days	Decreases cerebral vasospasm	Side effects include hypotension, palpitations, headache, and dizziness Monitor blood pressure frequently when implementing therapy
Local Anesthetics			
Lidocaine	50-100 mg IV or 2 mL of 4% solution	Blunts the effects of tracheal stimulation on intracranial pressure	Must be administered not longer than 5 minutes before suctioning
Thrombolytics			
Tissue-type plasminogen activator (tPA)	0.9 mg/kg total, with 10% of the dose administered as IV bolus over 1 min and 90% of the dose administered as continuous IV infusion over 1 hr	Converts plasminogen to plasmin to dissolve clot	Treatment must start within 4.5 hr of the onset of the symptoms Do not exceed 90 mg Do not use anticoagulants during the first 24 hr Monitor patient for bleeding

Data from *Elsevier/Gold Standard.* http://www.mdconsult.com/das/pharm/lookup/340530070-12?type=alldrugs. Accessed August 12, 2012.
IV, Intravenous; *NG*, nasogastric; *PO*, by mouth.

BOX 24-21 INTERNET RESOURCES

American Association of Critical-Care Nurses: **http://www.aacn.org**
American Association of Neuroscience Nurses: **http://www.aann.org**
Society for Critical Care Medicine: **http://www.sccm.org**
American Academy of Neurology: **http://www.aan.com**
American College of Physicians: **http://www.acponline.org**
American Association of Neurological Surgeons: **http://www.aans.org**
American College of Surgeons: **http://www.facs.org**

American Stroke Association: **http://www.strokeassociation.org**
National Stroke Association: **http://www.stroke.org**
The Internet Stroke Center: **http://www.strokecenter.org**
Society for Neuroscience: **http://www.sfn.org**
American Medical Association: **http://www.ama-assn.org**
National Institutes for Health: **http://www.nih.gov**
PubMed Health: **http://www.ncbi.nlm.nih.gov/pubmedhealth**

BOX 24-22 CASE STUDY

Patient with a Neurologic Problem

Brief Patient History

Mr. P is a 24-year-old man. While he was water skiing, he was hit by a boat. He was rescued from the water by friends. He was immobilized and transported to the hospital by paramedics called to the scene.

Clinical Assessment

Mr. P is admitted to the emergency department with abrasions and bruising to his head and shoulders. He is having difficulty breathing and is unable to move his extremities. He complains of neck pain, and he has a cervical collar in place. He has urinary and fecal incontinence. He does not have motor, sensory, or deep tendon reflexes from the neck to the feet. He is awake and able to talk.

Diagnostic Procedures

The admission magnetic resonance imaging (MRI) showed an incomplete spinal cord transection. Baseline vital signs include the following: blood pressure of 85/60 mm Hg, heart rate of 48 beats/min (sinus bradycardia), respiratory rate

of 8 breaths/min, temperature of 99.3° F, and O_2 saturation of 88%. The Glasgow Coma Scale score was 10.

Medical Diagnosis

Mr. P is diagnosed with an incomplete spinal cord transection and neurogenic shock.

Questions

1. What major outcomes do you expect to achieve for this patient?
2. What problems or risks must be managed to achieve these outcomes?
3. What interventions must be initiated to monitor, prevent, manage, or eliminate the problems and risks identified?
4. What interventions should be initiated to promote optimal functioning, safety, and well-being of the patient?
5. What possible learning needs do you anticipate for this patient?
6. What cultural and age-related factors may have a bearing on the patient's plan of care?

SUMMARY

Coma

- The two main causes of coma are structural (e.g., ischemic stroke, ICH, trauma, brain tumors) and metabolic (e.g., drug overdose, infectious diseases, endocrine disorders, poisonings).
- Coma is the deepest state of unconsciousness; arousal and awareness are lacking as a result of diffuse dysfunction of both cerebral hemispheres or diffuse or focal dysfunction of the reticular activating system.
- Medical management focuses on identification and treatment of the underlying cause of the condition and support of vital functions.
- Nursing interventions focus on supporting all body functions, maintaining surveillance for complications, providing comfort and emotional support, initiating rehabilitation measures and educating the patient and family.

Stroke

- The sudden onset of an acute neurologic deficit persisting for more than 24 hours is known as a *stroke*, and it is caused by the interruption of blood flow to the brain.
- Strokes are classified as ischemic or hemorrhagic. Hemorrhagic strokes can be further categorized as SAHs (cerebral aneurysms and AVMs) and ICHs.
- Nursing interventions focus on monitoring for changes in neurologic status, maintaining surveillance for complications, providing comfort and emotional support, initiating rehabilitation measures, and educating the patient and family.

Ischemic Stroke

- The two main causes of ischemic stroke are thrombosis and embolism, and it results in a neuronal tissue injury from decreased or absent blood flow.
- The characteristic sign of an ischemic stroke is the sudden onset of focal neurologic signs persisting for more than 24 hours. The signs depend on the affected portion of the brain.
- Medical management focuses on preservation of brain tissue through fibrinolytic therapy, management of blood pressure, and treatment of complications.

Subarachnoid Hemorrhage

- SAH is bleeding into the subarachnoid space, and it is usually caused by rupture of a cerebral aneurysm or AVM.
- Medical management focuses on preservation of neurologic function, support of vital functions, and treatment of complications (rebleeding, vasospasm, hyponatremia, and hydrocephalus).

Intracerebral Hemorrhage

- ICH is bleeding directly into cerebral tissue, and it is usually caused by rupture of a small artery in the brain resulting from hypertension.
- Medical management focuses on preservation of neurologic function, control of blood pressure, support of vital functions, and management of intracranial hypertension.

Guillain-Barré Syndrome

- Guillain-Barré syndrome involves a rapidly progressive, ascending peripheral nerve dysfunction leading to paralysis that may produce respiratory failure.
- Medical management focuses on support of vital functions and the administration of treatments to limit the duration of the syndrome.
- Nursing interventions focus on maintaining surveillance for complications, initiating rehabilitative measures, providing comfort and emotional support, and educating the patient and family about the disorder.

Craniotomy

- A craniotomy is performed to gain access to portions of the CNS inside the cranium for the purposes of tumor resection or removal, cerebral decompression, evacuation of hematoma or abscess, or repair of an aneurysm or AVM.
- Postoperative medical management focuses on preventing complications, including intracranial hypertension, hemorrhage, fluid imbalances, CSF leaks, and DVT.
- Nursing interventions focus on positioning the patient's head in accordance with the physician's orders, monitoring the patient's intake and output, administering medications to control vomiting and fever, promoting postoperative pulmonary care, providing comfort and emotional support, maintaining surveillance for complications, initiating rehabilitative measures, and education of the patient and family.

Intracranial Hypertension

- One of the earliest signs of increased ICP is a decrease in level of consciousness.
- ICP can be measured using an ICP monitor, and it should be treated when it exceeds 20 mm Hg.
- Medical and nursing management is directed toward reducing the volume of one or more of the components (e.g., blood, brain, CSF) that lie within the intracranial vault.
- Herniation of intracerebral contents results in the shifting of tissue from one compartment of the brain to another and places pressure on cerebral vessels and vital function centers of the brain. If unchecked, it rapidly causes death.

REFERENCES

1. Barker E. Altered states of consciousness and sleep. In: Barker E, ed. *Neuroscience Nursing: A Spectrum of Care*. 3rd ed. St. Louis: Mosby; 2008.

2. Hoesch RE, et al. Coma after global ischemic brain injury: pathophysiology and emerging therapies. *Crit Care Clin.* 2008;24:25.

3. Gawryluk JR, et al. Improving the clinical assessment of consciousness with advances in electrophysiological

and neuroimaging techniques. *BMC Neurol*. 2010; 10:11.

4. Rosenberg RN. Consciousness, coma, and brain death 2009. *JAMA*. 2009;301:1172.

5. Hocker S, Rabinstein AA. Management of the patient with diminished responsiveness. *Neurol Clin*. 2012;30:1.

6. Ropper AH. Coma. In: Longo DL, et al, eds. *Harrison's Principles of Internal Medicine*. 18th ed. Philadelphia: McGraw-Hill; 2012.

7. Bleck TP. Levels of consciousness and attention. In: Goetz CG, ed. *Textbook of Clinical Neurology*. 3rd ed. St. Louis: Saunders; 2007.

8. Berger JR. Stupor and coma. In: Daroff RB, et al, eds. *Bradley's Neurology in Clinical Practice*. 6th ed. Philadelphia: Elsevier; 2012.

9. Boss BJ. Alteration in cognitive systems, cerebral hemodynamics, and motor function. In: McCance KL, et al, eds. *Pathophysiology: The Biologic Basis for Disease in Adults and Children*. 6th ed. St. Louis: Mosby; 2010.

10. Bruno MA, et al. From unresponsive wakefulness to minimally conscious PLUS and functional locked-in syndromes: recent advances in our understanding of disorders of consciousness. *J Neurol*. 2011;258:1373.

11. Weng Y, Sun S. Therapeutic hypothermia after cardiac arrest in adults: mechanism of neuroprotection, phases of hypothermia, and methods of cooling. *Crit Care Clin*. 2012;28:231.

12. Delhaye C, et al. Hypothermia therapy: neurological and cardiac benefits. *J Am Coll Cardiol*. 2012;59:197.

13. Cortese D, et al. Moisture chamber versus lubrication for the prevention of corneal epithelial breakdown. *Am J Crit Care*. 1995;4:425.

14. Roger VL, et al. Heart disease and stroke statistics-2012 update: a report from the American Heart Association. *Circulation*. 2012;125:E2.

15. American Association of Neuroscience Nurses. *Guide to the Care of the Hospitalized Patient with Ischemic Stroke: AANN Clinical Practice Guideline Series*. 2nd ed. Chicago: The Association; 2009.

16. Biller J, et al. Vascular diseases of the nervous system. In: Daroff RB, et al, eds. *Bradley's Neurology in Clinical Practice*. 6th ed. Philadelphia: Elsevier; 2012.

17. Romano JG, Sacco RL. Progress in secondary stroke prevention. *Ann Neurol*. 2008;63:418.

18. Murphy DR. Current understanding of the relationship between cervical manipulation and stroke: what does it mean for the chiropractic profession? *Chiropr Osteopat*. 2010;18:22.

19. Babarro EG, et al. Cardioembolic stroke: Call for a multidisciplinary approach. *Cerebrovasc Dis*. 2009;27:(suppl 1)82.

20. Albers GW, et al. Antithrombotic and thrombolytic therapy for ischemic stroke: American College of Chest Physicians Evidence-Based Clinical Practice Guidelines (8th Edition). *Chest*. 2008;133(suppl 6):630S.

21. Boss BJ. Disorders of central and peripheral nervous system and the neuromuscular junction. In: McCance KL, Huether SE, eds. *Pathophysiology: The Biologic Basis for Disease in Adults and Children*. 6th ed. St. Louis: Mosby; 2010.

22. Seder DB, Mayer SA. Critical care management of subarachnoid hemorrhage and ischemic stroke. *Clin Chest Med*. 2009;30:103.

23. Szaflarski JP, et al. Incidence of seizures in the acute phase of stroke: a population-based study. *Epilepsia*. 2008;49:974.

24. Alexandrov AW. Hyperacute ischemic stroke management: reperfusion and evolving therapies. *Crit Care Nurs Clin N Am*. 2009;21:451.

25. Del Zoppo GJ, et al. Expansion of the time window for treatment of acute ischemic stroke with intravenous tissue plasminogen activator: a science advisory from the American Heart Association/American Stroke Association. *Stroke*. 2009;40:2945.

26. Advisory Working Group on Stroke Center Identification Options of the American Stroke Association. Recommendations for improving the quality of care through stroke centers and systems: an examination of stroke center identification options: multidisciplinary consensus recommendations from the Advisory Working Group on Stroke Center Identification Options of the American Stroke Association. *Stroke*. 2002;33:e1.

27. Bravata DM, et al. Processes of care associated with acute stroke outcomes. *Arch Intern Med*. 2010;170:804.

28. Anderson T. Current and evolving management of subarachnoid hemorrhage. *Crit Care Nurs Clin N Am*. 2009;21:529.

29. Venti M. Subarachnoid and intraventricular hemorrhage. *Front Neurol Neurosci*. 2012;30:149.

30. Pillai P, et al. Management of aneurysms, subarachnoid hemorrhage, and arteriovenous malformations. In: Barker E, ed. *Neuroscience Nursing: A Spectrum of Care*. 3rd ed. St. Louis: Mosby; 2008.

31. Lindsay KW, et al. *Neurology and Neurosurgery Illustrated*. 5th ed. London: Churchill Livingstone; 2010.

32. American Association of Neuroscience Nurses. *Care of the Patient With Aneurysmal Subarachnoid Hemorrhage: AANN Clinical Practice Guideline Series*. Chicago: The Association; 2009.

33. Bader MK, Littlejohns LR, eds. *AANN Core Curriculum for Neuroscience Nursing*. 5th ed. Glenview: American Association of Neuroscience Nurses; 2010.

34. Benderson JB, et al. Guidelines for the management of aneurysmal sub-arachnoid hemorrhage: a statement for healthcare professionals from a special writing group of the Stroke Council, American Heart Association. *Circulation*. 2009;40:994.

35. Hunt WE, Hess RM. Surgical risks as related to time of intervention in the repair of intracranial aneurysms. *J Neurosurg*. 1968;28:14.

36. Solenski NJ, et al. Medical complications of aneurysmal subarachnoid hemorrhage: a report of the multicenter, cooperative aneurysm study. *Crit Care Med*. 1995;23:1007.

37. Classen J, et al. Effect of acute physiologic derangements on outcome after subarachnoid hemorrhage. *Crit Care Med*. 2004;32:832.

38. Keyrouz SG, Diringer MN. Clinical review: prevention and therapy vasospasm in subarachnoid hemorrhage. *Crit Care*. 2007;11:220.

39. Treggiari MM, et al. Hemodynamic management of subarachnoid hemorrhage. *Neurocrit Care*. 2011;15:329.

40. Rincon F, Mayer SA. Clinical review: critical care management of spontaneous intracerebral hemorrhage. *Crit Care*. 2008;12:237.

41. Hsieh PC, et al. Current updates in perioperative management of intracerebral hemorrhage. *Neurol Clin*. 2006;24:745.

42. Naval NS, Nyquist PA, Carhuapoma JR. Management of spontaneous intracerebral hemorrhage. *Neurol Clin*. 2008;26:373.

43. Zivin JA. Hemorrhagic cerebrovascular disease. In: Goldman L, Schafer AI, eds. *Goldman's Cecil Medicine*. 24th ed. St. Louis: Elsevier; 2012.

44. Morgenstern LB, et al. American Heart Association Stroke Council and Council on Cardiovascular Nursing: Guidelines for the management of spontaneous intracerebral hemorrhage: A Guideline for Healthcare Professionals From the American Heart

Association/American Stroke Association. *Stroke.* 2010;41(9): 2108.

45. Yuki N, Hartung HP. Guillain-Barré syndrome. *N Engl J Med.* 2012;366:2294.

46. Van Doorn PA, et al. Clinical features, pathogenesis, and treatment of Guillain-Barré syndrome. *Lancet Neurol.* 2008;7:939.

47. Randall DP. Guillain-Barré syndrome. *Dis Mon.* 2010;56:256.

48. Shah DN. The spectrum of Guillain-Barré syndrome. *Dis Mon* 2010;56:262.

49. Cortese I, et al. Evidence-based guideline update: plasmapheresis in neurologic disorders: report of the Therapeutics and Technology Assessment Subcommittee of the American Academy of Neurology. *Neurology.* 2011;76:294.

50. Patwa HS, et al. Evidence-based guideline: intravenous immunoglobulin in the treatment of neuromuscular disorders: report of the Therapeutics and Technology Assessment Subcommittee of the American Academy of Neurology. *Neurology.* 2012;78:1009.

51. Mullings KR, et al. Rehabilitation of Guillain-Barré syndrome. *Dis Mon.* 2010;56:288.

52. Ferrara-Hoffman DL, Krizman SJ. Neurosurgery. In: Rothrock JC, ed. *Alexander's Care of the Patient in Surgery.* 14th ed. St. Louis: Elsevier; 2011.

53. Swearingen B. Update on pituitary surgery. *J Clin Endocrinol Metab.* 2012;97:1073.

54. Delaune A, et al. Cranial surgery. In: Barker E, ed. *Neuroscience Nursing: A Spectrum of Care.* 3rd ed. St. Louis: Mosby; 2008.

55. Seifman MA, et al. Postoperative intracranial haemorrhage: a review. *Neurosurg Rev.* 2011;34:393.

56. Hannon MJ, et al. Clinical review: disorders of water homeostasis in neurosurgical patients. *J Clin Endocrinol Metab.* 2012;97:1423.

57. Ausiello JC, et al. Postoperative assessment of the patient after transsphenoidal pituitary surgery. *Pituitary.* 2008;11:391.

58. Daele JJ, et al. Traumatic, iatrogenic, and spontaneous cerebrospinal fluid (CSF) leak: endoscopic repair. *B-ENT.* 2011;7(Suppl 17):47.

59. Collen JF, et al. Prevention of venous thromboembolism in neurosurgery: a metaanalysis. *Chest.* 2008;134:237.

60. Chibbaro S, Tacconi L. Safety of deep venous thrombosis prophylaxis with low-molecular-weight heparin in brain surgery. Prospective study on 746 patients. *Surg Neurol.* 2008;70:117.

61. Osinbowale O, et al. Venous thromboembolism: a clinical review. *Postgrad Med.* 2010;122:54.

62. Gould MK, et al. Prevention of VTE in nonorthopedic surgical patients: Antithrombotic Therapy and Prevention of Thrombosis, 9th ed: American College of Chest Physicians Evidence-Based Clinical Practice Guidelines. *Chest.* 2012; 141(Suppl 2):e227S.

63. Nemergut EC, et al. Pain management after craniotomy. *Best Pract Res Clin Anaesthesiol.* 2007;21:557.

64. Dashti SR, et al. Operative intracranial infection following craniotomy. *Neurosurg Focus.* 2008;24(6):E10.

65. Hang Mui So, et al. Comparing the effectiveness of polyethylene covers (Gladwrap™) with lanolin (Duratears®) eye ointment to prevent corneal abrasions in critically ill patients: a randomized controlled study. *Internat J Nurs Studies.* 2008;45:1565.

66. Barker E. Intracranial pressure and monitoring. In: Barker E, ed. *Neuroscience Nursing: A Spectrum of Care.* 3rd ed. St. Louis: Mosby; 2008.

67. Eigsti J, Henke K. Anatomy and physiology of neurological compensatory mechanisms. *Dimens Crit Care Nurs.* 2006;25:197.

68. March K, Madden L. Intracranial pressure management. In: Littlejohns LR, Bader MK, eds. *AACN-ANNA Protocols for Practice: Monitoring Technologies in Critically Ill Neuroscience Patients.* Sudbury, MA: Jones & Bartlett; 2009.

69. Rangel-Castillo L, Gopinath S, Robertson CS. Management of intracranial hypertension. *Neurol Clin.* 2008;26:521.

70. Latorre JG, Greer DM. Management of acute intracranial hypertension: a review. *Neurologist.* 2009;15:193.

71. Bhatia A, Gupta AK. Neuromonitoring in the intensive care unit. I. Intracranial pressure and cerebral blood flow monitoring. *Intens Care Med.* 2007;33:1263.

72. American Association of Neuroscience Nurses. *Guide to the Care of the Patient with Intracranial Pressure Monitoring: AANN Reference Series for Clinical Practice.* Chicago: The Association; 2005.

73. Rauen CA, et al. Seven evidence-based practice habits: putting some sacred cows out to pasture. *Crit Care Nurse.* 2008;28(2):98.

74. Curley G, Kavanagh BP, Laffey JG. Hypocapnia and the injured brain: more harm than benefit. *Crit Care Med.* 2010;38:1348.

75. Strandvik GF. Hypertonic saline in critical care: a review of the literature and guidelines for use in hypotensive states and raised intracranial pressure. *Anaesthesia.* 2009;64:990.

76. Saiki RL. Current and evolving management of traumatic brain injury. *Crit Care Nurs Clin N Am.* 2009;21:549.

77. Haddad SH, Arabi YM. Critical care management of severe traumatic brain injury in adults. *Scand J Trauma Resusc Emerg Med.* 2012;20:12, 75.

78. Leeper B, Lovasik D. Cerebrospinal drainage systems: external ventricular and lumbar drains. In: Littlejohns LR, Bader MK, eds. *AACN-ANNA Protocols for Practice: Monitoring Technologies in Critically Ill Neuroscience Patients.* Sudbury, MA: Jones & Bartlett; 2009.

79. Mortazavi MM, et al. Hypertonic saline for treating raised intracranial pressure: literature review with meta-analysis. *Neurosurg.* 2012;116:210.

80. Cook AM, Weant KA. Pharmacologie strategies for the treatment of elevated intracranial pressure: focus on metabolic suppression. *Adv Emerg Nurs J.* 2007;29:309.

81. Morrison CAM. Brain herniation syndromes. *Crit Care Nurs.* 1987;7(5):34.

Kidney Anatomy and Physiology

Mary E. Lough

The kidneys are complex organs responsible for numerous functions and substances necessary to maintain homeostasis. The primary roles of the kidneys are to remove metabolic wastes, maintain fluid and electrolyte balance, and help achieve acid–base balance. Hormones produced by the kidneys have an important role in blood pressure control, red blood cell production, and bone metabolism. The kidneys are important in maintaining the intracellular and extracellular environment required by all cells to function effectively. When a patient experiences kidney dysfunction, some or all of the functions of the kidneys may be decreased or absent, leading to altered homeostasis.

This chapter provides an overview of the anatomy and physiologic processes of the kidneys. An understanding of normal kidney function is essential to understanding the pathophysiology, symptoms, and therapeutic management of kidney disease and failure.

MACROSCOPIC ANATOMY

The kidneys are paired organs located retroperitoneally, one on each side of the vertebral column between T12 and L3.[1] The right kidney is slightly lower than the left because of the position of the liver. Each kidney is approximately 12 centimeters (cm) long, 6 cm wide, and 2.5 cm thick in the adult. Kidney size and weight varies between men and women; 125 to 170 grams in men, and 115 to 155 grams in women.[1] The kidneys are protected anteriorly and posteriorly by the rib cage and by a tough fibrous capsule that encloses each kidney. Additional protection is provided by a cushion of perirenal fat and the support of the kidney fascia.

Internally, the kidneys are made up of two distinct areas: the cortex and the medulla. The kidney *cortex* is the outer layer and contains the glomeruli, proximal tubules, cortical portions of the loops of Henle, distal tubules, and cortical collecting ducts. The kidney cortex is about 1 cm in thickness. The kidney *medulla* is the inner kidney layer, made up of the pyramids, which contain the medullary portions of the loops of Henle, the vasa recta, and the medullary portions of the collecting ducts. Numerous pyramids taper and join to form a minor calyx; several minor calyces join to form a major calyx. The major calyces then join and enter the funnel-shaped *kidney pelvis*, a 5- to 10-mL conduit that directs urine into the ureter (Fig. 25-1).

The kidney system also includes the urinary drainage system—the ureters, bladder, and urethra (Fig. 25-2). The ureters are fibromuscular tubes that exit the central part of the kidney pelvis. The ureters are 28 to 34 cm in length and enter the urinary bladder at an oblique angle. As urine is formed by the kidneys, the urine flows through the ureters by peristalsis. The peristaltic action of the ureters and the angle at which the ureters enter the bladder help prevent reflux of urine from the bladder back up into the kidneys. The bladder is a muscular sac within the pelvis and has a capacity of 280 to 500 mL. Urine leaves the bladder through the urethral orifice and is excreted from the body through the urethra. The male urethra is about 20 cm long; the female urethra is 3 to 5 cm long.

VASCULAR ANATOMY

The kidneys are highly vascular and receive up to 20% of the cardiac output—about 1 liter to 1.2 L/min of blood flow.[2]

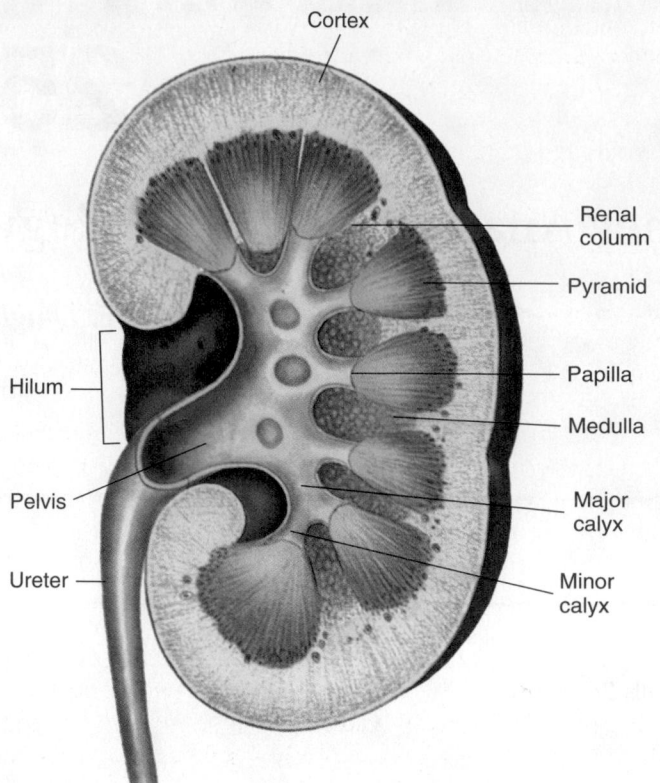

Blood enters the kidneys through the renal arteries, which branch bilaterally from the abdominal aorta. The renal artery divides into arterial branches that become progressively smaller vessels, eventually ending with the afferent arterioles. A single *afferent arteriole* supplies blood to each glomerulus, a tuft of capillaries that is the first structure of the nephron. The nephron is often described as the *functional unit* of the kidneys.[1]

Blood exits the glomerulus by the *efferent arteriole*, which connects with the peritubular capillary network, also known as the *vasa recta* (straight vessels), that parallel the long loops of Henle. The intricate capillary network maintains the intracapillary pressure that allows water and solutes to move between the tubules and the capillaries for urine formation and the concentration and dilution of urine. The capillaries then rejoin and form gradually enlarging venous vessels, until the blood leaves each kidney through the renal vein and returns to the general circulation by the inferior vena cava.[2]

MICROSCOPIC STRUCTURE AND FUNCTION

Each kidney is made up of about one million nephrons, the functional units of the kidneys. Because of the vast number of nephrons, the kidneys can continue to function even when several thousand nephrons are damaged or destroyed by disease or injury. Each nephron has the ability to perform all of the individual functions of the kidneys. The nephron is made up of several distinct structures: the glomerulus, the Bowman capsule, the proximal tubule, the loop of Henle, the distal tubule, and the collecting duct (Fig. 25-3).

FIGURE 25-1 **Cross Section of the Kidney.** (From Thompson JM, et al. *Mosby's Clinical Nursing.* 5th ed. St. Louis: Mosby; 2002.)

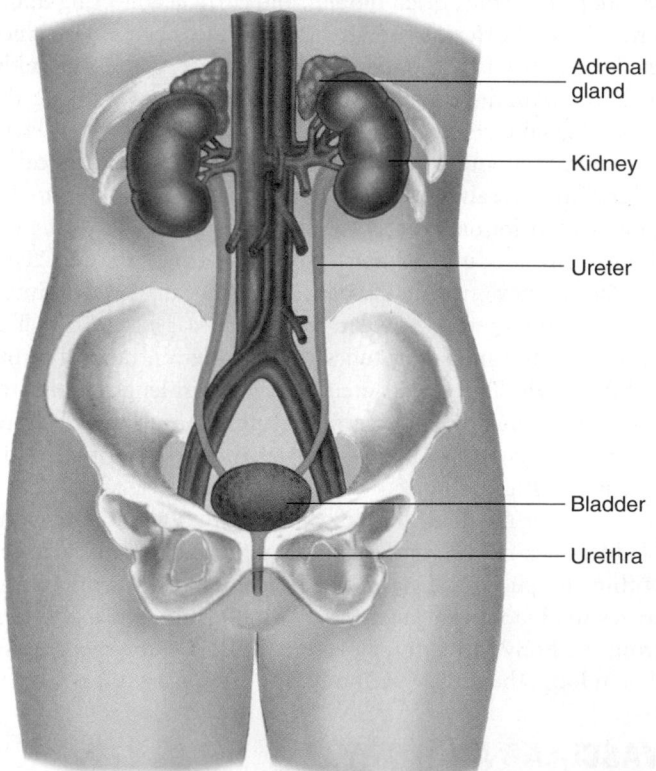

FIGURE 25-2 **Structures of the Urinary System.** (From Thompson JM, et al. *Mosby's Clinical Nursing.* 5th ed. St. Louis: Mosby; 2002.)

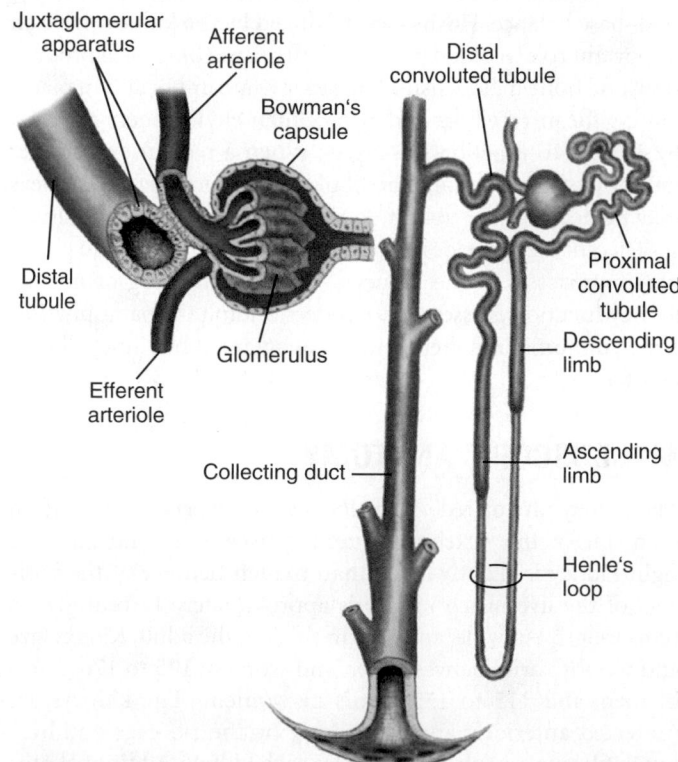

FIGURE 25-3 **Components of the Nephron.** (From Thompson JM, et al. *Mosby's Clinical Nursing.* 5th ed. St. Louis: Mosby; 2002.)

Two types of nephrons make up each kidney: the cortical nephrons and the juxtamedullary nephrons. Most are cortical nephrons. These superficial cortical nephrons have glomeruli located in the outer cortex and have short loops of Henle. The midcortical nephrons are located lower in the cortex and have loops of Henle that may be short or long. Both types of cortical nephrons perform excretory and regulatory functions. The remaining nephrons are juxtamedullary nephrons with glomeruli located deep in the cortex and extending into the medullary layer of the kidney. The juxtamedullary nephrons have long loops of Henle that have an important role in the concentration and dilution of urine. The peritubular capillaries, known as the vasa recta, surround the juxtamedullary nephrons maintaining a concentration gradient to concentrate the urine.

Glomerulus

The first structure of each nephron is the glomerulus, a high-pressure capillary bed that serves as the filtering point for the blood. Positive filtration pressure in the glomerulus is achieved as a result of the high arterial pressure as the blood enters the *afferent arteriole* and the resistance created by the smaller *efferent arteriole* as the blood exits the glomerulus. As a result of the positive-pressure gradient, fluid and solutes are filtered through the glomerular capillary walls. The glomerulus has three layers: the endothelium, the basement membrane, and the epithelium. The inner endothelial layer lines the glomerulus and contains numerous pores that allow filtration of fluid and small solutes from the blood. The middle basement membrane layer also controls filtration according to the size, electrical charge, protein-binding capability, and shape of the molecules. This complex is also described as the *glomerular filtration barrier* (GFB). It is freely permeable to water and small or midsized molecules but large molecules such as albumin and red blood cells are prevented from entering the filtrate.[3] The presence of large molecules in the urine is a signal that the glomerular membrane is damaged. The outer epithelium layer contains pores that allow the filtered blood, or filtrate, into the Bowman space.

The Bowman Capsule

A filtrate of plasma, usually called the *ultrafiltrate*, enters the Bowman space, which is surrounded by the Bowman capsule, a tough, membranous layer of epithelial cells that completely surrounds the glomerular capillary bed. The Bowman space is located between the capillary walls of the glomerulus and the inner layer of the Bowman capsule and contains the initial filtrate from the blood. Fluid, solutes, and other substances filtered by the glomerulus collect in the space. The Bowman space is a continuous structure that joins the first portion of the nephron's tubular system—the proximal tubule.[1]

Proximal Tubule

The *proximal tubule* is located in the cortex of the kidney and has a large surface area available for solute and fluid transportation. The proximal tubule resorbs (takes back) most of the filtered water and sodium and many of the solutes the body does not routinely excrete in the urine. Solutes that are usually resorbed include all of the glucose, some of the water-soluble vitamins, most phosphate and bicarbonate, and much of the potassium, chloride, and calcium that is filtered by the glomerulus. Proteins are resorbed in the proximal tubule by two specialized receptors known as megalin and cubilin that bind albumin and vitamin-binding proteins.[1] Creatinine is minimally resorbed and is excreted in the urine.

In addition to its major role in resorbing water and solutes from the filtrate, the proximal tubule secretes organic anions and cations into the tubular lumen. Ammonia is produced from the metabolism of glutamine in the mitochondria of the proximal tubule cells, where ammonia (NH_3) combines with hydrogen (H^+) to form ammonium (NH_4^+), which is secreted into the proximal tubule lumen.[1]

Because of the large amount of solutes in the glomerular filtrate, the fluid that enters the proximal tubule is hyperosmotic. When the filtrate leaves the proximal tubule and enters the loop of Henle, it is isosmotic (equivalent to plasma) as a result of the resorption of solutes and water.

Loop of Henle

After selective resorption in the proximal tubule, the isosmotic filtrate enters the loop of Henle. The *loop of Henle* consists of a thin descending limb, a thin ascending limb, and a thick ascending limb. There are two types of nephrons: the cortical nephrons with short loops of Henle and the juxtamedullary nephrons with long loops of Henle. The nephrons with short loops of Henle do not have a thin ascending limb. As a result, the cortical nephrons perform excretory and regulatory functions but play only a minor role in the concentration or dilution of urine. The juxtamedullary nephrons have glomeruli that are next to (juxtaposed to) the medulla near where the cortex and medulla sections of the kidney join and contain a thin ascending limb. These nephrons with the thin ascending limbs are critical for concentrating and diluting the urine by means of the countercurrent mechanism. The thin descending limb is very permeable to water but fairly impermeable to urea, sodium, and other solutes. As a result, water (but not solute) is resorbed into the general circulation, and a more concentrated filtrate is produced. The filtrate then moves up the thin ascending limb, which is impermeable to water but allows movement of sodium, chloride, and urea back into the filtrate. The thick ascending limb is also impermeable to water but allows resorption of sodium, chloride, potassium, calcium, and bicarbonate. Because of the low water and high solute resorption in the loop of Henle, the filtrate leaves the ascending limb hypo-osmotic (more dilute than plasma).

Distal Tubule

The hypo-osmotic filtrate enters the distal tubule located in the cortex of the kidney. The first portion of the distal tubule contains the cells of the *macula densa*, which are specialized cells that are a component of the juxtaglomerular apparatus important in blood pressure control. The first section of the distal tubule is impermeable to water and transports solutes such as sodium, bicarbonate, calcium, and potassium. The later section of the distal tubule further regulates sodium, bicarbonate, potassium, and calcium according to hormonal influences and the acid–base and electrolyte balance needs of the body. The

---

BOX 25-1   TUBULAR RESORPTION AND SECRETION

Glomerulus
- Filters fluid and solutes from blood

Proximal Tubule
- Resorbs Na^+, K^+, Cl^-, HCO_3^-, urea, glucose, and amino acids
- Filtrate leaves isosmotic

Loop of Henle
- Resorbs Na^+, K^+, Cl^-
- Blocks resorption of H_2O from ascending limb
- Countercurrent mechanism dilutes or concentrates urine
- Filtrate leaves hypo-osmotic

Distal Tubule
- Na^+, K^+, Ca^{2+}, PO_4^{3-} selectively resorbed
- H_2O resorbed in the presence of antidiuretic hormone (ADH)
- Na^+ resorbed in the presence of aldosterone
- Filtrate leaves hypo-osmotic

Collecting Duct
- Resorption similar to that in distal tubule
- H_2O resorbed in the presence of ADH
- HCO_3^- and H^+ resorbed or secreted to acidify urine
- Filtrate leaves hyperosmotic or hypo-osmotic, depending on body needs

---

permeability of the late distal tubule is influenced by antidiuretic hormone (ADH). In the presence of ADH, the late distal tubule is impermeable to water but resorbs some solutes, and the filtrate remains hypo-osmotic. In the absence of ADH, the late distal tubule is more permeable to water, and the filtrate may become isosmotic.

Collecting Duct

Several distal tubules join to form a collecting duct that begins in the cortex and extends through the medulla to empty into the papilla. The final composition of the urine occurs in the collecting duct, primarily because of the transport of potassium, sodium, and water. Water permeability is determined by the absence or presence of ADH. In the absence of, or with small amounts of ADH, the urine becomes dilute, whereas larger amounts of ADH result in concentrated urine. The filtrate usually is more concentrated when it leaves the collecting duct than it was when it entered. Acidification of the urine is accomplished by the transport of bicarbonate and hydrogen in the collecting duct. Several collecting ducts then combine to form the pyramids. After the urine leaves the collecting ducts, no change in the composition of the filtrate occurs. Box 25-1 summarizes tubular resorption and secretion in the various structures of the nephron.

NERVOUS SYSTEM INNERVATION

The autonomic nervous system provides the primary innervation to the kidneys and the urinary drainage system. Kidney neural innervation is derived from the celiac plexus and the sympathetic plexuses of the abdominal viscera to form the renal plexus. The renal plexus enters the kidneys along the path of the renal arteries. The inferior mesenteric plexus, the hypogastric plexus, and the pudic nerve from the sacral region serve the urinary bladder, the ureters, and the urethra.

Nervous system control in the urinary tract is reflected in the process of micturition, or the release of urine. Bladder fullness stimulates stretch receptors in the bladder wall and a portion of the urethra. Signals are carried through nerves in the sacral area and return as parasympathetic messages to contract the detrusor muscle of the bladder. With a full bladder, contractions usually are powerful enough to relax the external sphincter. Sympathetic stimulation returns the external sphincter to contraction after the urine is released. The cerebral cortex and brainstem portions of the central nervous system also exert control over the urinary bladder. The central nervous system regulates the micturition reflex, frequency, and external sphincter tone and allows conscious control over release of urine from the bladder.

URINE FORMATION

The nephrons are responsible for removing metabolic substances and waste products from the blood and retaining essential electrolytes and water as needed by the body. The entire blood volume of an individual is filtered by the kidneys 60 to 70 times each day, resulting in about 180 L of filtrate. The glomerular filtration rate (GFR), or the amount of filtrate formed in the nephrons, is therefore about 125 mL/min. The kidneys must reduce the 180 L of filtrate to an average of 1 to 2 L of urine per day. Although 180 L of filtrate is formed, 99% of it is resorbed, and only 1% is excreted as urine. The three processes necessary for changing the 180 L of filtrate into 1 to 2 L of urine are glomerular filtration, tubular resorption, and tubular secretion.

Glomerular Filtration

The first process in urine formation is glomerular filtration, which depends on glomerular blood flow, pressure in the Bowman space, and plasma oncotic pressure.[2] Glomerular blood flow is the most important of these three factors and is maintained through an autoregulatory mechanism within the kidneys.[2] The autoregulatory mechanism maintains consistent kidney blood flow and perfusion at a constant level as long as the mean arterial pressure (MAP) remains between 80 and 180 mm Hg. The afferent and efferent arterioles of the glomeruli have the ability to increase or decrease the glomerular blood flow rate through selective dilation and constriction. When the mean arterial blood pressure is decreased, the afferent arteriole dilates, and the efferent arteriole constricts to maintain a higher pressure in the glomerular capillary bed and maintain the GFR at 125 mL/min. The ability of the kidneys to autoregulate blood flow begins to fail when the mean arterial blood pressure is less than 80 mm Hg or greater than 180 mm Hg.

The second factor that influences the GFR is the pressure in the Bowman space. An increase in pressure in this space decreases filtration because the increased pressure resists the movement of solutes and water from the capillaries into the space. For example, if the tubules of the nephrons are blocked by cellular debris, backward pressure is exerted on the Bowman space, the GFR drops below 125 mL/min, and urine output decreases.

The third factor that influences GFR is plasma oncotic pressure. When the oncotic pressure in the blood is decreased (as in disease states that result in low plasma protein levels), pressure in the glomerular capillary bed is decreased. Although the mean arterial pressure in the glomerulus favors filtration, decreased amounts of fluid and solutes leave the capillaries and enter the Bowman space because the oncotic pressure gradient in the plasma that encourages movement of fluid and solutes out of the plasma is less favorable. Filtration still occurs, but it is decreased from the normal 125 mL/min, resulting in a decrease in the amount of filtrate and therefore urine.

The status of the glomerular filtration system is assessed by measuring the GFR. Creatinine is used as a measure of the GFR because it is a waste product produced at a fairly constant rate by the muscles, is freely filtered by the glomerulus, and is minimally resorbed or secreted by the tubules. Most of the creatinine produced by the body is excreted by the kidneys, making the creatinine clearance a good screening and follow-up test for estimating the GFR. Creatinine clearance usually mirrors the GFR, so that a normal creatinine clearance rate is approximately 125 mL/min. A creatinine clearance rate less than 100 mL/min reflects a GFR of less than 100 mL/min and is a signal of decreased kidney function. A creatinine clearance rate (and GFR) less than 20 mL/min results in symptoms of kidney failure.

Tubular Resorption

The second process in the formation of urine is tubular resorption—the movement of a substance from the tubular lumen (filtrate) into the peritubular capillaries (blood). Tubular resorption allows the 180 L of solutes and water filtered by the glomerulus to be taken back into the circulation, decreasing the 180 L of filtrate to 1 to 2 L of urine per day. Most tubular resorption takes place in the proximal tubule and occurs by passive and active transport processes.

Passive Transport

Passive transport of substances in the tubule depends on changes in concentration gradients and does not require energy. Diffusion and osmosis are the primary passive transport processes in the nephrons. Diffusion is the spontaneous movement of molecules or solutes from an area of higher concentration to an area of lower concentration across a semipermeable membrane (not all substances cross, particularly large molecules). For example, when water is resorbed by the tubules, the concentration of urea in the tubules is increased. Urea then diffuses across the semipermeable membrane of the tubule and re-enters the plasma to achieve balance in the concentration gradient.

Osmosis is the movement of water from an area of lower solute concentration to an area of higher solute concentration. Osmosis occurs any time the concentration of solutes on one side of a semipermeable membrane is greater than the concentration of solutes on the other side of the membrane. For example, when the concentration of sodium is greater in the peritubular capillaries than in the tubules, water passively

moves from the tubules into the capillaries to balance the concentration gradient.

Active Transport

Active transport of substances into or out of the tubules requires substances to move against an electrochemical gradient, and it takes energy in the form of adenosine triphosphate (ATP). In active transport, the substance combines with a carrier and then diffuses across the semipermeable tubular membrane. Substances that are actively resorbed include glucose, amino acids, calcium, potassium, and sodium. The rate at which substances can be actively resorbed depends on the availability of the carriers, saturation of the carriers, and availability of energy. The transport maximum refers to the maximum rate at which substances can be resorbed and varies according to each substance.

The threshold concentration of a substance is important in active transport. The threshold of a substance is the plasma level of a substance at which none of the substance appears in the urine.[2] When the threshold of a substance in the plasma is exceeded, progressively larger amounts of the substance appear in the urine because the large amounts cannot be resorbed. For example, the serum threshold concentration for glucose is about 180 mg/dL. At or below a plasma glucose concentration of 180 mg/dL, all glucose is actively resorbed from the kidney tubules back into the circulation, and none is excreted in the urine. When the plasma glucose concentration is above 180 mg/dL, the threshold concentration is exceeded, and some of the glucose cannot be resorbed from the tubules and is excreted in the urine.

Tubular Secretion

The third process in urine formation is tubular secretion, the transport of substances from the peritubular capillaries into the lumen of the tubules. Tubular secretion allows the body to remove excess substances; it occurs by diffusion and by active transport, and it depends on the needs of the body. For example, potassium, hydrogen, medications, or medication metabolites are secreted into the tubules to decrease their concentration in the body. Tubular secretion plays a lesser role than tubular resorption in changing the filtrate into urine.

FUNCTIONS OF THE KIDNEYS

The formation of urine through the processes previously described is a major function of the kidneys. The kidneys are also responsible for other functions essential to maintaining homeostasis, including the elimination of metabolic wastes, blood pressure regulation, the regulation of erythrocyte production, the activation of vitamin D, prostaglandin synthesis, acid–base balance, and fluid–electrolyte balance.

Elimination of Metabolic Wastes

Metabolic processes in the body produce waste products that are selectively filtered out of the circulation by the kidneys. Urea, uric acid, and creatinine are byproducts of protein metabolism that the kidneys filter out of the circulation and excrete in the urine. Metabolic acids, bilirubin, and medication metabolites are also eliminated as waste products.

Urea

Urea and creatinine are the primary waste products that are measured in determining kidney function. Urea is measured as blood urea nitrogen (BUN) and is the end product of protein metabolism and results from the breakdown of ammonia in the liver. The level of urea in the blood is influenced by protein breakdown, the amount of protein in the diet, fluid volume, and excretion from the kidneys. The body forms approximately 25 to 28 g of urea per day. More urea is formed if protein intake is high or if the individual is in a catabolic state and is breaking down body protein stores. Urea is primarily excreted in the urine and therefore accumulates if the glomerulus is unable to filter it from the blood.

Creatinine

Creatinine is an end product of protein metabolism produced by the muscles. Creatinine is normally completely filtered and minimally resorbed by the kidneys. As a result, creatinine is excreted in the urine. Like urea, creatinine accumulates when the glomerulus is unable to filter it from the blood. The level of creatinine in the blood provides an indicator of kidney function.

Blood Pressure Regulation

The kidneys regulate arterial blood pressure by maintaining the circulating blood volume by means of fluid balance and by altering peripheral vascular resistance through the renin-angiotensin-aldosterone system (RAAS). Regulation by the RAAS occurs in the *juxtaglomerular apparatus* (JGA), a group of specialized cells located around the afferent arteriole where the distal tubule and afferent arteriole make contact[4,5] (see Fig. 25-3). Another group of specialized cells is located near the distal tubule; known as the *macula densa*, these cells control a feedback mechanism from the distal tubule to the afferent arteriole to control blood flow through the afferent arteriole.[4]

An increase in tubular filtrate in the macula densa causes the afferent arteriole to constrict and therefore decrease the GFR and the amount of filtrate produced. Conversely, a decrease in the amount of tubular filtrate results in afferent arteriole dilation, an increased GFR, and an increased amount of filtrate.

The JGA synthesizes, stores, and releases renin.[5] *Renin* is released in response to reduced pressure in the glomerulus, sympathetic stimulation of the kidneys, and a decrease in the amount of sodium in the distal tubule.[5] Renin enters the lumen of the afferent arteriole and is released into the general circulation. Renin is then converted to angiotensin I, which is further converted to angiotensin II as the blood circulates through the lungs. *Angiotensin II* is an active compound that causes afferent and efferent arteriole vasoconstriction, resulting in an increased vascular resistance, and it therefore maintains hydrostatic pressure within the kidneys. A powerful vasoconstrictor, angiotensin II also causes increased systemic vascular resistance and therefore increased arterial blood pressure. Intracellular actions of angiotensin II constitute an emerging area of research.[6,7] Angiotensin II also stimulates the release of aldosterone by the adrenal cortex.

Aldosterone acts on the distal tubule to facilitate sodium and water resorption, resulting in an expanded circulating blood

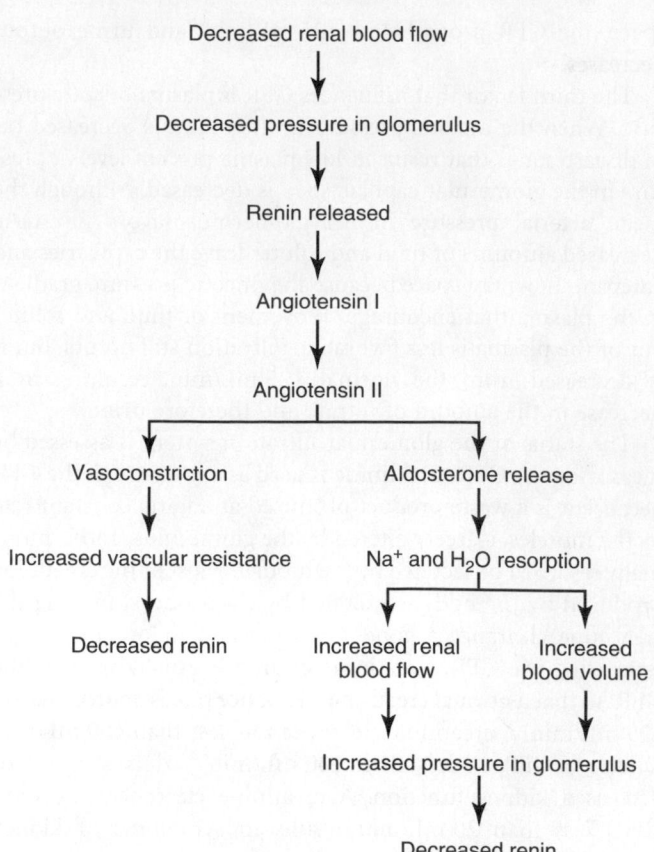

FIGURE 25-4 Renin-angiotensin-aldosterone system.

volume and increased blood pressure. When the arterial blood pressure increases, the JGA reduces the release of renin, and the RAAS is less active. Figure 25-4 summarizes the major aspects of the renin-angiotensin-aldosterone mechanism.

Erythrocyte Production

The kidneys secrete erythropoietin, the hormone that controls erythrocyte (red blood cell) production in the bone marrow. Erythropoietin is released in response to a decrease in the amount of oxygen delivered to the kidneys, such as in anemia or prolonged hypoxia.[8] The hormone remains active for about 24 hours after release and stimulates the bone marrow to increase the production of erythrocytes. The absence of erythropoietin, which occurs in individuals with kidney failure, results in a profound anemia that is treated by administering synthetic erythropoietin or by blood transfusion therapy.[8,9]

Vitamin D Activation

The kidneys convert vitamin D from food sources into an active form for use by the body. Active vitamin D stimulates the absorption of calcium by the intestine and resorption of calcium by the tubules so that calcium is available for bone and tooth metabolism and blood clotting functions. When the kidneys fail, the body is unable to convert dietary vitamin D to its active form, calcium is poorly absorbed, and bone disease and other immunologic deficiencies result.[10] Lack of vitamin D may also be responsible for changes in the immune system that increase the risk of infection in patients with chronic kidney disease (CKD).[11]

Prostaglandin Synthesis

Prostaglandins are vasoactive substances that dilate or constrict the arteries. The kidney produces two vasodilatory prostaglandins (PGs): E and I; they are typically abbreviated *PGE$_1$* and *PGI$_2$*.[12] The prostaglandins produced by the kidneys have only local blood flow effects with minimal or no systemic effects. The primary prostaglandins produced by the kidneys are the vasodilators PGE$_1$ and PGI$_2$, which act on the afferent arteriole to maintain blood flow and glomerular perfusion and filtration. The vasodilating effects of the prostaglandins also counteract the effects of angiotensin II and the sympathetic nervous system on the kidneys and maintain blood flow to the kidney despite systemic vasoconstriction. Another prostaglandin that may affect kidney function is PGF$_2$, which contributes to vasoconstriction in times of volume depletion. Box 25-2 lists the effects of prostaglandins.

Acid–Base Balance

The kidneys are actively involved in acid–base regulation by resorbing or excreting acids and bases in the kidney tubules. For example, bicarbonate, the principal blood buffer, is resorbed from the tubules, and hydrogen, a potent organic acid, is secreted into the tubules. However, the tubules do not function as rapidly in altering acid–base concentrations as do the lungs; the kidneys therefore regulate the day-to-day balance rather than coping with emergencies requiring an immediate physiologic response.

FLUID BALANCE

Regulation of the total amount of water in the body is vital for homeostasis, and it is one of the most important functions of the kidneys. In the absence of effective kidney function, fluid volume overload occurs and threatens homeostasis. Similarly, if the kidneys are unable to preserve adequate amounts of fluid, a severe volume deficit occurs that also disrupts homeostasis.

Fluid Compartments

The fluid of the body is present in distinct internal spaces or compartments. The compartments are separated from each other by semipermeable membranes with openings (pores) that allow molecules of specific size and molecular weight to pass through while preventing larger, heavier molecules from doing so. As a result of the semipermeable membrane, fluid movement between the compartments is dynamic and constant.

Between 45% and 60% of body weight is made up of water.[13] The body has two main fluid compartments: intracellular and

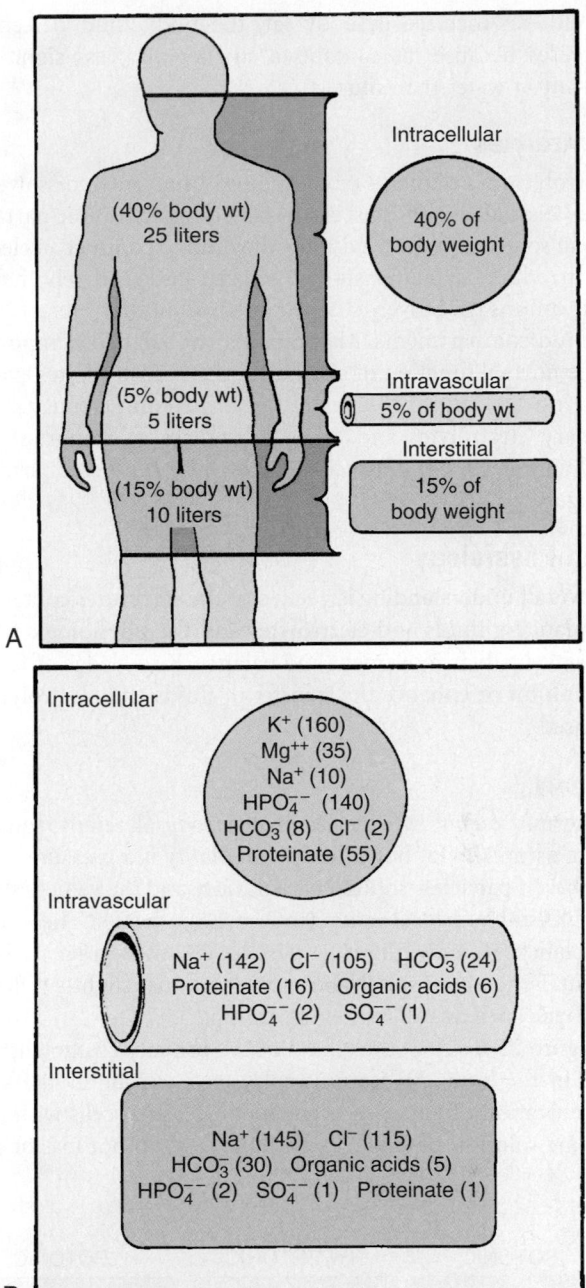

FIGURE 25-5 *A,* Fluid compartments. *B,* Electrolytes by fluid compartment.

extracellular. The *intracellular compartment* is the fluid inside each of the body's cells, and it accounts for 40% of the total body water content.[13] The remaining fluid is outside the body's cells and makes up the *extracellular compartment.* The extracellular compartment is composed of two distinct subcompartments: *intravascular* and *interstitial.* The *intravascular compartment,* meaning the fluid within the blood vessels, accounts for 5% of the body water. The interstitial compartment corresponds to the fluid in the tissue spaces outside of the body cells and the blood vessels and accounts for 15% of body water. Approximate amounts of fluid contained in each compartment are shown in Figure 25-5A.

With an increase in body fat, the body fluid percentage decreases because fat contains a smaller and less significant amount of water than muscle.

Electrolytes

Electrolytes are elements or compounds that, when dissolved in water, dissociate into ions, electrically charged atomic particles. Ions in solution in the fluid allow the fluid to conduct an electrical current. A balance exists between cations (positively charged ions), anions (negatively charged ions), and other substances in the fluid compartments. Maintaining this balance is important to the normal function of all body systems. Electrolytes exist in differing amounts in each of the fluid compartments. The primary electrolytes and other substances of importance in fluid and electrolyte balance are shown by fluid compartment in Figure 25-5B.

Fluid Physiology

An overall understanding is needed of the structures containing or balancing fluids and electrolytes and the physiologic forces that govern their movement and balance. Knowledge of factors that inhibit or enhance the transfer of fluids and electrolytes is required.

Tonicity

The terms *isotonic, hypotonic,* and *hypertonic* all refer to tonicity, or the osmolality of body fluids. *Osmolality* is a measure of the number of particles (solute) in a solution, and the value is stated in milliosmoles per kilogram (mOsm/kg) of water. The normal osmolality of body fluids is 275 to 295 mOsm/kg of body weight. Different hospital laboratories may use slightly different numbers, such as 280 to 300 mOsm/kg.[13]

Figure 25-6 shows the effects of the tonicity (osmolality) of fluid in the body. An isotonic solution has roughly the same concentration of particles as the blood plasma; cells within an isotonic solution maintain consistency and do not lose or gain

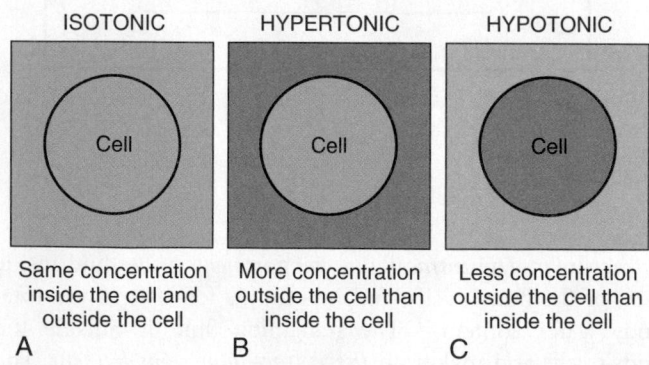

ISOTONIC	HYPERTONIC	HYPOTONIC
Cell	Cell	Cell
Same concentration inside the cell and outside the cell	More concentration outside the cell than inside the cell	Less concentration outside the cell than inside the cell
A	B	C

FIGURE 25-6 *A,* Isotonic solution. The extracellular solute concentration is the same as the intracellular concentration, with no movement of water into or out of the cell. *B,* Hypertonic solution. The extracellular solute concentration is greater than the intracellular concentration. Water moves from the cell into the extracellular compartment. *C,* Hypotonic solution. The extracellular solute concentration is less than the intracellular concentration. Water moves from the extracellular compartment into the cell.

fluid to their surroundings. A *hypertonic solution* contains a greater concentration of particles than that inside the cell and causes fluid to be drawn out of the cells. Used inappropriately, too much fluid may be withdrawn, causing a withering of the cell (crenation). A *hypotonic solution* contains a lesser concentration of particles than that inside the cell and causes fluid to be drawn into the cells. If used incorrectly, a hypotonic solution can cause too much fluid to enter the cell, causing the cells to swell and burst (hemolysis).

Hydrostatic Pressure

The force of left ventricular contraction of the heart propels the blood through the circulatory system, causing the blood to exert pressure against the vessel walls. This hydrostatic pressure creates the tendency for fluids and dissolved substances to move into the interstitial spaces by filtration (movement of fluid and substances from an area of high pressure to one of low pressure). Without opposing forces counteracting the hydrostatic pressure, fluid would leave the intravascular space until the space was depleted. Whereas hydrostatic pressure favors fluid and electrolyte movement out of the intravascular compartment, the colloid osmotic pressure of the plasma holds the fluid and substances in the intravascular space.

Osmotic Pressure

Osmotic pressure is created by solutes and other substances (e.g., albumin, globulin, fibrinogen) suspended in fluid. Colloid osmotic pressure is created primarily by the presence of plasma proteins in the intravascular space. Plasma proteins exert a pull on water molecules and therefore produce osmotic pressure, which retains fluid within the intravascular compartment. This force is maintained because proteins are large and cannot move or be transported across the semipermeable membrane unless the permeability of the membrane is changed by disease or other assaults on the body (e.g., burns, infections). Similarly, the solute and protein content of the interstitium results in interstitial colloid osmotic pressure. A decrease in serum protein lessens the osmotic pressure in the intravascular space so that the interstitial oncotic pressure is greater than the intravascular pressure and pulls fluid from the vascular space into the interstitial space, causing edema.

Diffusion, Osmosis, and Active Transport

Fluid balance within the compartments is achieved through the processes of diffusion, osmosis, and active transport. Just as in the kidney tubule cells, these three processes are constantly at work in other parts of the body to facilitate the movement of water and solutes to maintain homeostasis between the intracellular and extracellular compartments.

Movement of Water

The combined effects generated by ventricular contraction, colloid osmotic pressure in the intravascular space, solute content of the extracellular fluid (ECF), and solutes in the intracellular fluid (ICF), cause constant movement between the ICF and ECF compartments.[13] Ultimately, a state of equilibrium is established, with a balance of fluid throughout the fluid compartments. An increase in plasma volume results in increased capillary hydrostatic pressure, forcing fluid into the interstitial space and creating edema. A decrease in plasma volume causes the movement of fluid from the interstitium into the vascular space because the interstitial hydrostatic pressure is greater than the capillary hydrostatic pressure.

Factors Controlling Fluid Balance
Antidiuretic Hormone and Aquaporins
ADH, also known as *vasopressin*, is secreted by the posterior pituitary gland and functions as the primary controller of ECF volume. Feedback messages for release of ADH are sent by osmoreceptors (water receptors) located in the hypothalamus. As serum osmolality rises above 285 mOsm/kg (normal range, 275 to 295 mOsm/kg), ADH is released and carried through the circulation to the nephrons. The kidney distal tubules, connecting tubules, and the collecting ducts alter their permeability to water by the action of three *aquaporins*. These are aquaporin-2 (AQP2), aquaporin-3 (AQP3), and aquaporin-4 (AQP4).[14] ADH acts via the aquaporin-2 receptor (AQP2) on the distal tubule and collecting ducts to resorb water.[14] ADH action in the kidney is predominantly mediated through the aquaporins.

The normal range of urinary osmolality is from 500 to 800 mOsm/kg. Box 25-3 identifies several additional mechanisms that stimulate the release of ADH. In addition to the usual stimuli, the presence of severe emotional or physical stress can initiate ADH release through the limbic system that surrounds the hypothalamus.

Aldosterone
Box 25-4 shows several factors that stimulate the release of aldosterone. The relationship between sodium and water plays an important role in the influence of the RAAS on body water regulation (see Fig. 25-4). A reduction in vascular volume stimulates the release of renin. Renin is converted to angiotensin I, which is converted to the powerful vasoconstrictor angiotensin

II. Angiotensin II stimulates the adrenal glands to secrete aldosterone, which acts on the distal tubules to resorb sodium from the tubular lumen into the circulation. When sodium is retained, so is water. Angiotensin II also constricts the renal vasculature, reducing kidney blood flow and available glomerular filtrate, sending a signal to the posterior pituitary to release ADH. The two systems intertwine to maintain fluid and electrolyte balance.

Atrial Natriuretic Peptide
An additional influence on fluid and electrolyte regulation comes from the synthesis of atrial natriuretic peptide (ANP). This hormone is secreted from cells in the atria of the heart in response to hypernatremia, stimulation of stretch receptors as a result of increased volume, and increased pressure in the heart (Box 25-5). ANP affects sodium and water balance by blocking aldosterone and ADH production, initiating vasodilation, and stimulating increased sodium and water excretion by the collecting ducts of the kidneys. The physiologic effects of ANP include a reduction in fluid overload through diuresis, decreased cardiac workload, and reduction in cardiac preload and afterload.

ELECTROLYTE BALANCE

Potassium
Potassium is the primary intracellular electrolyte and is responsible for numerous physiologic functions (Box 25-6). As with many solutes, diffusion and active transport across the cell membrane maintain potassium balance. Potassium leaves the cell by diffusion, moving toward the area of lesser concentration outside the cell, but it must be actively transported back into the cell to maintain cellular stability.[13] One of the most important potassium functions in the body—that of aiding nervous impulse conduction and muscle contraction—is accomplished with the movement of potassium across the cell membrane. The

---

BOX 25-3 FACTORS STIMULATING RELEASE OF ANTIDIURETIC HORMONE

- Hyperosmolality of extracellular fluid (ECF)
- Hypovolemia
- Increased body temperature
- Medications
  - Opioids
  - Antineoplastics
  - Oral hypoglycemics
  - Beta-adrenergics
- Severe emotional or physical stress

BOX 25-4 FACTORS STIMULATING RELEASE OF ALDOSTERONE

- Hypovolemia
- Hyponatremia
- Hyperkalemia
- Stress—emotional, physical

BOX 25-5 FACTORS STIMULATING RELEASE OF ATRIAL NATRIURETIC PEPTIDE

- Hypernatremia
- Hypervolemia
- Vasoconstriction
- Decreased cardiac output
- Increased cardiac preload and afterload
- Increased systemic vascular resistance

BOX 25-6 FUNCTIONS OF POTASSIUM

Normal Serum Value
- 3.5-4.5 mEq/L

Functions
- Transmission of nerve impulses
- Intracellular osmolality
- Enzymatic reactions
- Acid–base balance
- Myocardial, skeletal, and smooth muscle contractility

gastrointestinal tract and skin excrete small amounts of potassium, but the major controllers of potassium stores are the kidneys.[13] Potassium is resorbed by the proximal tubules and secreted into the distal tubules as needed to maintain balance. Resorption and secretion of potassium are influenced by many factors (Box 25-7). Of the estimated 60 to 100 mEq/day ingested by an individual, 90% of the potassium is resorbed before arriving at the distal tubule, where the remainder is usually excreted.

Potassium and sodium are in a constant state of competition within the body despite the need for electrolytes and their different functions. Because both electrolytes are cations, one intracellular and one extracellular, potassium and sodium must remain in balance to preserve electrical neutrality at the cell membrane. In the presence of aldosterone, potassium is excreted by the tubules, and sodium is retained. Potassium wasting therefore may occur despite the body's need for potassium. If potassium stores are low within the cell, the other intracellular electrolytes (magnesium and phosphorus) are often similarly depleted.

Sodium

Sodium is the most abundant extracellular electrolyte in the body and is associated with fluid balance and the amount of water retained or excreted by the kidneys.[13] Along the length of the nephron sodium is resorbed from the filtrate. This is an active metabolic process that is regulated by site-specific sodium transporters.[15] When diuretics are administered, sodium absorption is inhibited and consequently sodium is eliminated in the urine.[15] Sodium plays an essential role in the transmission of nerve impulses through the sodium pump, or active transport mechanism, at the cellular level. Sodium is key to a number of physiologic functions (Box 25-8).

The body contains a complex system of safeguards and feedback mechanisms to protect the level of sodium in the ECF. Sodium balance is regulated by the kidneys, the adrenal glands (aldosterone secretion), and the posterior pituitary gland (ADH secretion). Most sodium resorption occurs in the proximal tubule under the influence of aldosterone. Because of the extremely sensitive mechanism for retaining sodium, ingestion of large amounts of sodium is unnecessary.

Calcium

Calcium is the electrolyte of greatest quantity in the body, with stores estimated at 1200 g. Of the total body calcium, 99% is contained in the bones.[16] The remaining 1% is contained primarily in the ECF in the vascular space. The calcium contained within bone is in an inactive form that maintains bone strength and is a ready storehouse for mobilization of calcium to the serum in cases of depletion.[16] In addition to bone metabolism, calcium is responsible for numerous other important functions, including myocardial contractility, coagulation, and neuromuscular activity (Box 25-9).

The mobilization of calcium from bone stores is accomplished through the influence of *parathyroid hormone* (PTH). The calcium in the intravascular space (plasma calcium) exists in three forms: ionized, protein bound, or complexed. *Ionized calcium* is the active form and functions in cell membrane stability and blood clotting. Protein-bound calcium, which ionizes more quickly than the calcium in the bone, is readily put to use during an immediate crisis. Complexed calcium is combined with other anions such as chloride, citrate, or phosphate and is available for filtration by the glomerulus for potential removal in the urine. Ionized calcium not needed for physiologic functions is returned to the bone under the influence of the hormone *calcitonin*.

In the ionized (active) form, calcium plays an important role in maintaining the internal integrity of the cell. The amount of ionized calcium in the serum depends on changes in serum pH and on the availability of plasma protein, primarily albumin. Because changes in pH and albumin levels occur with relative frequency, the measurement of total serum calcium alone can be deceptive. To accurately determine the ionized calcium, it is necessary to measure it with a laboratory test because the results of calculated values are unreliable. Estimation of ionized calcium levels—calculated from the serum albumin and total serum calcium—have been found to be inaccurate in critically ill patients. Often, the total serum calcium and the

---

BOX 25-7 FACTORS AFFECTING RESORPTION AND SECRETION OF POTASSIUM

- Sodium balance: sodium deficit results in potassium loss
- Acid–base balance: acidosis moves hydrogen into the cell and potassium out, with potassium being excreted in the urine
- Diuretics: increased loss of potassium in distal tubule
- Gastrointestinal losses: vomiting, gastric suction may remove potassium
- Insulin: promotes movement of potassium into the cell
- Epinephrine: enhances potassium resorption from distal tubule

---

BOX 25-8 FUNCTIONS OF SODIUM

Normal Serum Value
- 135-145 mEq/L

Functions
- Body fluid movement and retention
- Extracellular osmolality
- Active transport mechanism (with potassium)
- Neuromuscular activity
- Enzyme activities
- Acid–base balance

BOX 25-9 FUNCTIONS OF CALCIUM

Normal Serum Value
- 8.5-10.5 mg/dL

Functions
- Hardness of bone and teeth
- Skeletal muscle contraction
- Blood coagulation
- Cellular permeability
- Heart muscle contraction

BOX 25-10 FUNCTIONS OF PHOSPHORUS

Normal Serum Value
- 2.5-4.5 mg/dL

Functions
- Intracellular energy production (ATP)
- Bone hardness
- Structure of cellular membrane
- Oxygen delivery to tissues
- Enzyme regulation (ATPase)

BOX 25-11 FUNCTIONS OF MAGNESIUM

Normal Serum Value
- 1.3-2.1 mEq/L

Functions
- Neuromuscular transmission
- Contraction of heart muscle
- Activation of enzymes for cellular metabolism
- Active transport at cellular level
- Transmission of hereditary information

BOX 25-12 FUNCTIONS OF CHLORIDE

Normal Serum Value
- 97-110 mEq/L

Functions
- Body fluid osmolality (with sodium)
- Body water balance (with sodium)
- Acid–base balance
- Acidity of body fluids, especially gastric secretions
- Red blood cell oxygenation and carbon dioxide transport

ionized calcium values are measured. Increasingly, the ionized calcium value is the one used to accurately guide calcium management in critically ill patients.

Calcium levels depend on individual dietary intake and on a variety of physiologic mechanisms related to absorption. The uptake of calcium is influenced by the levels of phosphorus, magnesium, vitamin D, and its breakdown products, PTH, and calcitonin.

Phosphorus

As with calcium and magnesium, the serum values of phosphorus represent a minute portion of the actual body stores.[16] Approximately 80% of the phosphorus is found in the bones.[16] Most of the remaining phosphorus is intracellular, with only a small amount in the ECF. The primary function of phosphorus is the formation of ATP, which provides intracellular energy for active transport mechanisms across the cell membrane. Additional functions of phosphorus include cell membrane structure, acid–base balance, oxygen delivery to the tissues, cellular immunity, and bone strength (Box 25-10).

Absorption of phosphorus takes place in the gastrointestinal tract, and serum phosphorus levels change frequently and dramatically, particularly in response to the ingestion of phosphate-rich foods such as milk, red meats, poultry, and fish. Most excretion occurs in the kidneys. More than 90% of the phosphorus in the plasma is filtered by the glomerulus, and about 80% is resorbed by the proximal tubules. Resorption by the kidneys is increased when body stores are low, and it is combined with sodium and excess hydrogen ions to maintain acid–base balance.

Phosphorus abnormalities are evident early in the course of kidney failure.[17] The Third National Health and Nutrition Examination Survey (NHANES III, 1988-1994, which included 14,722 adults) revealed that people with mild or moderate kidney dysfunction—defined as a urinary creatinine clearance rate (CrCl) between 50 and 60 mL/min—already have elevations of serum phosphorus and potassium levels.[17,18] In contrast, serum ionized calcium remains relatively unchanged until the creatinine clearance rate is extremely low (CrCl less than 20 mL/min) and kidney failure is advanced.

Magnesium

Magnesium is the second most important and abundant intracellular electrolyte; about 60% of it is located in the bone.[13] The ECF contains only about 1% of the body's magnesium, and the remaining amount resides in the ICF. The levels of other intracellular electrolytes, such as calcium and potassium, are affected by the level of magnesium. For example, calcium and magnesium compete for absorption in the gastrointestinal tract. If the dietary intake of calcium is higher than that of magnesium, calcium is preferentially resorbed and vice versa. The most important functions of magnesium are ensuring the transport of sodium and potassium across the cell membrane and as a cofactor in many intracellular enzyme reactions. Depletion of magnesium liberates potassium to the ECF, which causes an increase in the excretion of potassium by the kidney and hypokalemia. Magnesium also plays a role in maintaining neuromuscular activity, protein synthesis, and intracellular energy production (Box 25-11).

Chloride

Chloride is predominantly found in the ECF. Changes in serum chloride levels usually indicate changes in the other electrolytes or in acid–base balance. Chloride plays a major role in maintaining serum osmolality, water balance, and acid–base balance. Additional functions of chloride are listed in Box 25-12.

Chloride is usually ingested with sodium in the form of salt and is resorbed or excreted in the proximal tubules of the kidney. Chloride is actively transported out of the tubules into the interstitium with sodium to help maintain the high tubular interstitial osmolality and the mechanism for concentrating the urine.

Bicarbonate

Bicarbonate (HCO_3^-) is an anion in the ECF, and it performs the essential function of maintaining the acid–base balance.[13] Although bicarbonate is not solely responsible for the acid–base balance, it is the major ECF buffer. Bicarbonate levels in the body are in balance with carbonic acid (H_2CO_3) levels. The ratio between the two must remain proportional at 1 mEq of carbonic acid to 20 mEq of bicarbonate; otherwise, acid–base disturbances will result. When the carbonic acid level is elevated, acidosis results. When the bicarbonate level is high, alkalosis results.

The kidneys regulate the amount of bicarbonate available in the ECF. Resorption of bicarbonate occurs primarily from the proximal tubule into the peritubular capillaries. Bicarbonate is also produced in the distal tubule and resorbed into the blood in response to acid–base balance and body requirements. The kidneys resorb or excrete bicarbonate in response to the number of hydrogen ions present as part of the body's buffer system. More bicarbonate is resorbed when a large number of hydrogen ions are present, and more is excreted when few hydrogen ions are present.

Effects of Aging

Kidney function declines gradually with age, but this usually does not affect homeostasis in the healthy older adult unless proteinuria is present.[19,20] Proteinuria is associated with complication in both the kidney and cardiovascular systems.[19] With aging, the GFR declines by about 0.75 mL/min/year.[19] However, despite the gradual decrease in the GFR and the associated reduction in clearance of creatinine, serum creatinine levels may not rise. This occurs because the reduced muscle mass associated with aging produces less creatinine to be excreted by the kidneys, essentially masking the overall effects of aging on the kidneys. As a result, relatively low levels of serum creatinine in older adults may be associated with reductions in the GFR and creatinine clearance. The gradual decline in kidney function that occurs with aging usually is not a threat to homeostasis because the remaining GFR is adequate. The Cockcroft-Gault formula is used to estimate GFR and includes age in the formula[19] (see Chapter 26). However, when older adults become ill, the decline in kidney function can be accelerated, making older adults especially susceptible to acute and chronic kidney dysfunction.

The kidneys carry out many functions. Although fluid balance is perhaps the most obvious function, an understanding of the numerous other roles of the kidneys provides crucial information for the care of any critically ill patient.

■ SUMMARY

Anatomy

- The kidneys are paired organs located retroperitoneally, one on each side of the vertebral column between T12 and L3.
- The nephron is the functional unit of the kidney; comprised of the glomerulus, proximal tubule, loop of Henle, distal tubule, and the collecting ducts.

Physiology

- The kidneys play a major role in maintaining homeostasis.
- Important functions of the kidneys include waste product removal, fluid electrolyte balance, and acid–base balance.

- Hormone functions of the kidneys support red blood cell production, blood pressure regulation, and bone metabolism.
- Kidney function declines gradually with age, making older adults more susceptible to kidney dysfunction during illness.

REFERENCES

1. Nielsen S, et al. Anatomy of the kidney. In: Taal MW, et al., eds. *Brenner & Rector's The Kidney*. Vol 1. 9th ed. Philadelphia: Saunders; 2011.
2. Munger KA, et al. The renal circulations and glomerular ultrafiltration. In: Taal MW, et al., eds. *Brenner & Rector's The Kidney*. vol 2. 9th ed. Philadelphia: Saunders; 2011.
3. Menon MC, Chuang PY, He CJ. The glomerular filtration barrier: components and crosstalk. *Internat J Nephrol*. Epub August 14, 2012.
4. Kurtz A. Renin release: sites, mechanisms, and control. *Annu Rev Physiol*. 2011;73:377.
5. Perlewitz A, Persson AE, Patzak A. The juxtaglomerular apparatus. *Acta Physiologica*. 2012;205(1):6.
6. Velez JC. The importance of the intrarenal renin-angiotensin system. *Nat Clin Pract Nephrol*. 2009;5(2):89.
7. Kumar R, et al. The intracrine renin-angiotensin system. *Clin Sci*. 2012;123(5):273.
8. Moore E, Bellomo R. Erythropoietin (EPO) in acute kidney injury. *Ann Intens Care*. 2011;1(1):3.
9. Ramanath V, et al. Anemia and chronic kidney disease: making sense of the recent trials. *Rev Recent Clin Trials*. 2012;7(3):187.
10. Kandula P, et al. Vitamin D supplementation in chronic kidney disease: a systematic review and meta-analysis of observational studies and randomized controlled trials. *Clin J Am Soc Nephrol: CJASN*. 2011;6(1):50.
11. Sterling KA, et al. The immunoregulatory function of vitamin D: implications in chronic kidney disease. *Nat Rev Nephrol*. 2012;8(7):403.
12. Wang H, et al. Prostaglandin E1 for preventing the progression of diabetic kidney disease. *Cochrane Database System Rev*. 2010;(5):CD006872.
13. Rhoda KM, Porter MJ, Quintini C. Fluid and electrolyte management: putting a plan in motion. *JPEN J Parent Enteral Nutr*. 2011;35(6):675.
14. Knepper MA. Systems biology in physiology: the vasopressin signaling network in kidney. *Amer J Physiol Cell Physiol*. 2012;303(11):C1115.
15. Bernstein PL, Ellison DH. Diuretics and salt transport along the nephron. *Semin Nephrol*. 2011;31(6):475.

16. Bonjour JP. Calcium and phosphate: a duet of ions playing for bone health. *J Amer Coll Nutr.* 2011;30(5 Suppl 1):438S.

17. O'Seaghdha CM, et al. Serum phosphorus predicts incident chronic kidney disease and end-stage renal disease. *Nephrol Dial Transplant.* 2011;26(9):2885.

18. Hsu CY, Chertow GM. Elevations of serum phosphorus and potassium in mild to moderate chronic renal insufficiency. *Nephrol Dial Transplant.* 2002;17(8):1419.

19. Verma V, Kant R, Sunnoqrot N, Gambert SR. Proteinuria in the elderly: evaluation and management. *Internat Urol Nephrol.* 2012;44(6):1745.

20. Peters R, et al. Kidney function in the very elderly with hypertension: data from the hypertension in the very elderly (HYVET) trial. *Age Ageing.* 2013;42(2):253.

Kidney Clinical Assessment and Diagnostic Procedures

Mary E. Lough

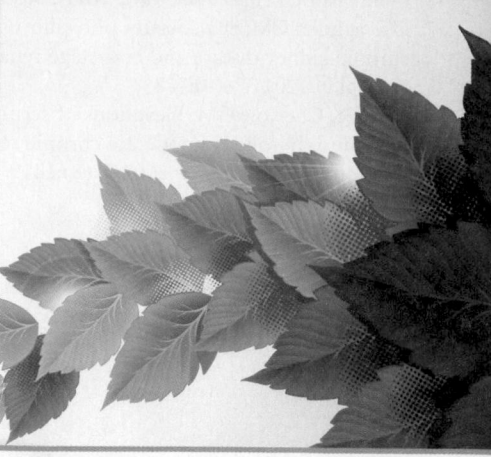

Understanding the anatomic structures and physiologic workings of the kidneys provides the basis for understanding the clinical manifestations that signal kidney or renal vascular dysfunction. The body produces many clinical signs and symptoms that indicate kidney disorders. However, these signs and symptoms are often subtle, and although some symptoms point directly to the kidneys, many are exhibited by other body systems. A detailed history and careful physical examination help focus on the kidneys as the source of symptoms and often uncover the cause of the problem.

HISTORY

The history begins with a description of the chief complaint, stated in the patient's own words. A description of the chief complaint includes the onset, location, duration, and factors or strategies that lessen or aggravate the problem.[1] The individual should be encouraged to describe the effects of any treatment for the problem, prescription and nonprescription medications taken to alleviate symptoms, efforts taken to determine the cause of the problem, and procedures performed to improve the problem. A careful history that explores symptoms fully is an essential component of the clinical assessment.

Predisposing factors for acute kidney dysfunction are obtained during the history, including the use of over-the-counter medicines, recent infections requiring antibiotic therapy, antihypertensive medicines, and any diagnostic procedures performed using radiopaque contrast.[2] Nonsteroidal anti-inflammatory medications (e.g., ibuprofen), antibiotics (especially aminoglycosides), antihypertensives (especially medicines that block angiotensin),[3] and iodine-based dyes may cause an acute or chronic decline in kidney function. A history of recent onset of nausea and vomiting or appetite loss caused by taste changes (uremia often causes a metallic taste) may provide clues to the rapid onset of kidney problems.[2] Symptoms that indicate rapid fluid volume gains are explored. For example, weight gains of more than 2 pounds per day, sleeping on additional pillows, and sitting in a chair to sleep are signals of volume overload and potential cardiac stress related to kidney dysfunction.

In addition to determining the immediate reason for admission to the critical care unit, compiling a complete medical and social history is important. Similar symptoms, problems, or treatment for similar complaints in the past may help establish the cause of the current problem or provide clues for treatment. For example, a history of obstructive urologic problems, frequent kidney infections, or previous acute kidney injury or failure may signal risk factors for current kidney problems. The patient, family member, or significant other should be encouraged to provide as much detail as possible during the history.

The family history may provide important information that points to the kidneys as the source of the patient's symptoms. For example, the patient may reveal that one or two close family members have always had swelling of the extremities or high blood pressure. These symptoms should lead to questions about a history of kidney problems in the family. Box 26-1 summarizes the information gained from a kidney history.

PHYSICAL EXAMINATION

In the critical care area, nursing assessment does not routinely include a full physical examination of the kidneys and urologic

BOX 26-1 DATA COLLECTION

Kidney History

Common Kidney-Related Symptoms
- Dyspnea
- Peripheral dependent edema
- Nocturia
- Nausea
- Metallic taste in mouth
- Loss of appetite
- Headache
- Rapid weight gain
- Itching
- Dry, scaly skin
- Weakness, fatigue
- Cognitive function changes
- Mental status changes

Patient Profile
- Personal habits
- Use of over-the-counter medications, herbs, vitamins, and dietary supplements
- Illicit drug use
- Change in employment caused by illness
- Financial problems resulting from illness (e.g., cost, time off work)
- Sexual function (e.g., decreased libido, amenorrhea)

Risk Factors
- Family history
- Hypertension
- Diabetes mellitus
- Prior acute kidney failure

Medical History
Child
- Nephrotic syndrome, streptococcal infection, hypoplastic kidneys, obstructive uropathy

Adult
- Frequent urinary tract infections
- Calculi
- Vasculitis
- Use of iodine-based radiographic contrast media
- Use of nonsteroidal anti-inflammatory medications

Family History
- Hypertension
- Diabetes mellitus
- Polycystic kidney disease
- Kidney disease
- Chronically swollen extremities

Current Medication Use
- Nonsteroidal anti-inflammatory medications
- Antibiotics
- Antihypertensives
- Diuretics

Past Kidney Studies
- Urinalysis with proteinuria
- Creatinine clearance
- Kidney-ureter-bladder (KUB) radiograph
- Intravenous pyelogram
- Kidney ultrasound
- Renal arteriography
- Kidney biopsy

system. However, many of the assessment parameters for the kidneys provide information related to the volume status of the individual and are helpful in a large number of patients regardless of kidney function or status. Although not often performed in the depth described in the following sections, the critical care nurse must be aware of how to perform a thorough kidney assessment in stable patients and as needed in patients with kidney dysfunction.

Inspection

Bleeding

Visual inspection related to the kidneys focuses on the patient's flank and abdomen. Kidney trauma is suspected if a purplish discoloration is present on the flank (Grey-Turner sign) or near the posterior 11th or 12th ribs.[1] Bruising, abdominal distention, and abdominal guarding may also signal kidney trauma or a hematoma around a kidney. Individuals who have experienced a traumatic injury should be carefully assessed for signs of kidney trauma.

Volume

Inspection is especially helpful in looking for signs of volume depletion or overload that may signal or lead to kidney problems. Fluid volume assessment begins with an inspection of the patient's jugular neck veins. The supine position facilitates normal jugular venous distention. An absence of distention (flat neck veins) indicates hypovolemia. Assessment continues with the head of the bed elevated 45 to 90 degrees.[1] Fluid overload exists when the neck veins remain distended more than 2 cm above the sternal notch when the bed is at 45 degrees.[4]

Hand vein inspection may be helpful in assessing volume status, and is performed by observing for venous distention when the hand is held in the dependent position. Venous filling that takes longer than 5 seconds suggests hypovolemia. When the hand is elevated, the distention should disappear within 5 seconds. If distention does not disappear within 5 seconds after the hand is elevated, fluid overload is suspected.

Assessment of skin turgor provides additional data for identifying fluid-related problems. To assess turgor, the skin over the forearm is picked up and released.[5] Normal elasticity and fluid status allow an almost immediate return to shape after the skin is released. In fluid volume deficit, however, the skin remains raised and does not return to its normal position for several seconds.[5] Because of the loss of skin elasticity in older persons, skin turgor assessment may not be as accurate a fluid assessment measure for this age group.

Inspection of the oral cavity provides clues to fluid volume status. When a fluid volume deficit exists, the mucous membranes of the mouth become dry. However, mouth breathing and some medicines (e.g., antihistamines) can also dry the mucous membranes temporarily. The most accurate way to assess the oral cavity is to inspect the mouth using a tongue blade and light. Dryness of the oral cavity is more indicative of fluid volume deficit than are complaints of a dry mouth.[4]

Edema

Edema is the presence of excess fluid in the interstitial space, and it can be a sign of volume overload. In the presence of volume excess, edema may develop in dependent areas of the body, such as the feet and legs of an ambulatory person or the sacrum of an individual confined to bed. However, edema does not always indicate fluid volume overload. A loss of albumin from the vascular space can cause peripheral edema despite hypovolemia or normal fluid states. A critically ill patient may have a low serum albumin level (hypoalbuminemia) because of inadequate nutrition after surgery, a burn, or a head injury and may exhibit edema as a result of the loss of plasma oncotic pressure and not as a result of volume overload. Edema also may signal circulatory difficulties. An individual who is fluid balanced but who has poor venous return may experience pedal edema after prolonged sitting in a chair with the feet dependent. Similarly, an individual with heart failure may experience edema because the left ventricle is unable to pump blood effectively through the vessels. A key feature that distinguishes edema due to excess volume or hypoalbuminemia from circulatory compromise is that the edema does not reverse with elevation of the extremity.

Edema can be assessed by applying fingertip pressure on the swollen area over a bony prominence, such as the ankles, pretibial areas (shins), and sacrum. If the indentation made by the fingertip does not disappear within 15 seconds, pitting edema exists. Pitting edema indicates increased interstitial volume, and it usually is not evident until significant weight gain has occurred. Edema also may appear in the hands and feet, around the eyes, and in the cheeks. Dependent areas, such as the feet and sacrum, are the areas most likely to demonstrate edema in patients confined to a wheelchair or bed. One way of measuring the extent of edema is by using a subjective scale of 1 to 4, with 1 indicating only minimal pitting and 4 indicating severe pitting (Table 26-1).[1] Other scales for assessing and measuring edema can be used (see Table 13-3).

Auscultation

Auscultation of the kidneys yields virtually no useful information. However, the renal arteries are auscultated for a bruit, a blowing or swishing sound that resembles a cardiac murmur (Fig. 26-1). The examiner listens for bruits above and to the left and right of the umbilicus.[1] A renal artery bruit usually indicates stenosis, which may lead to acute or chronic kidney dysfunction due to compromised blood flow to one or both kidneys. A bruit over the upper portion of the abdominal aorta may indicate an aneurysm or a stenotic area that can decrease blood flow to the kidneys.

Auscultation is especially helpful in providing information about extracellular fluid (ECF) volume status. Listening for specific sounds in the heart and lungs provides information about the presence or absence of increased fluid in the interstitium or vascular space.

Heart

Auscultation of the heart requires assessing the rate and rhythm and listening for extra sounds. Fluid overload is often accompanied by a third or fourth heart sound, which is best heard with the bell of the stethoscope.[1] Increased heart rate alone provides little information about fluid volume, but combined with a low blood pressure, it may indicate hypovolemia.

The heart is auscultated for the presence of a pericardial friction rub. A rub can best be heard at the third intercostal space to the left of the sternal border while the individual leans slightly forward.[1] A pericardial friction rub indicates pericarditis, and it may result from uremia in a patient with kidney failure.

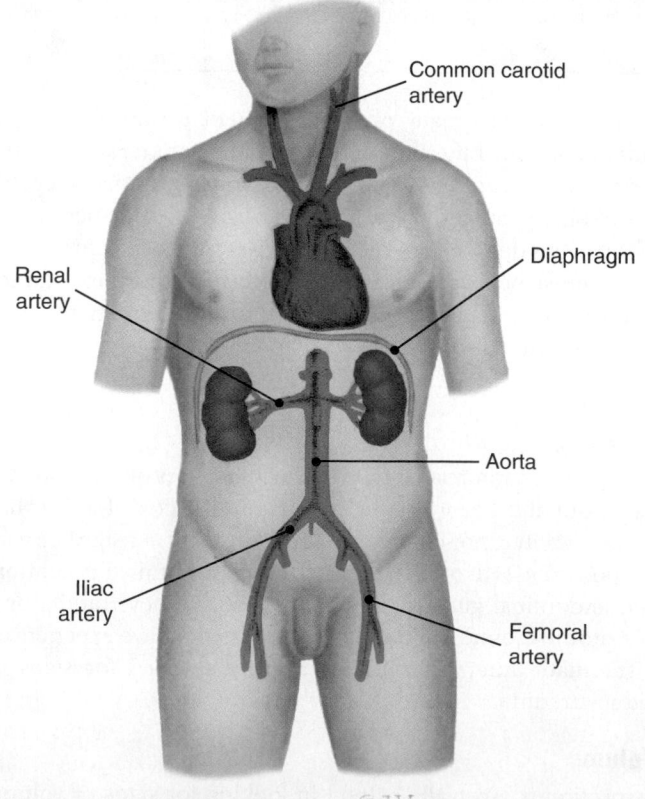

FIGURE 26-1   Sites for auscultation of bruits.

TABLE 26-1	**PITTING EDEMA SCALE**
RATING	**APPROXIMATE EQUIVALENT**
+1	2-mm depth
+2	4-mm depth (lasting up to 15 sec)
+3	6-mm depth (lasting up to 60 sec)
+4	8-mm depth (lasting longer than 60 sec)

Blood Pressure

Blood pressure and heart rate changes are very useful in assessing fluid volume deficit.[3] In stable critically ill patients or in patients on a telemetry unit, orthostatic vital sign measurements provide clues to blood loss, dehydration, unexplained syncope, and the effects of some antihypertensive medications. A drop in systolic blood pressure of 20 mm Hg or more, a drop in diastolic blood pressure of 10 mm Hg or more, or a rise in pulse rate of more than 15 beats/min from lying to sitting or from sitting to standing indicates orthostatic hypotension. Box 26-2 describes how to assess for orthostatic hypotension. The drop in blood pressure occurs because a sufficient preload is not immediately available when the patient changes position. The heart rate increases in an attempt to maintain cardiac output and circulation. Orthostatic hypotension produces subjective feelings of weakness, dizziness, or faintness. Orthostatic hypotension occurs with hypovolemia, prolonged bed rest, or as a side effect of medications that affect blood volume or blood pressure.

Lungs

Lung assessment is essential in gauging fluid status. Crackles indicate fluid overload. Dyspnea with mild exertion, dyspnea at night that prevents sleeping in a supine position (orthopnea), or dyspnea that awakens the individual from sleep (paroxysmal nocturnal dyspnea) may indicate pooling of fluid in the lungs. Shallow, gasping breaths with periods of apnea reflect severe acid–base imbalances.

Palpation

Although rarely performed in critically ill patients, palpation of the kidneys in stable patients provides information about the kidneys' size and shape. Palpation of the kidneys is achieved through the bimanual capturing approach. Capturing is accomplished by placing one hand posteriorly under the flank of the supine patient with the examiner's fingers pointing to the midline and placing the opposite hand just below the rib cage anteriorly.[1,2] The patient is asked to inhale deeply while pressure is exerted to bring the hands together (Fig. 26-2). As the patient exhales, the examiner may feel the kidney between the hands. After each kidney is palpated in this manner, the two should be compared for size and shape. Each kidney should be firm and smooth, and the two organs should be of equal size. The examiner is usually unable to palpate a normal left kidney. The right kidney is more easily palpated because of its lower position,

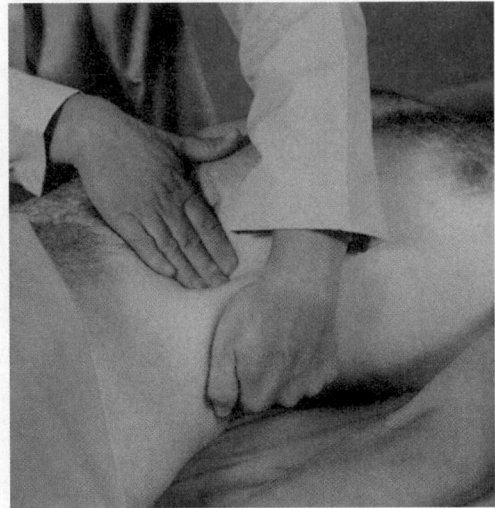

FIGURE 26-2 Palpation of the kidney. (From Barkauskas V, et al. *Health and Physical Assessment.* 3rd ed. St. Louis: Mosby; 2002.)

caused by downward displacement by the liver. Problems should be suspected if a mass (cancer) or an irregular surface (polycystic kidneys) is palpated, a size difference is detected, the kidney extends significantly lower than the rib cage on either side, or there is evidence of recent blunt trauma.[1]

Percussion

Percussion is performed to detect pain in the area of a kidney or to determine excess accumulation of air, fluid, or solids around the kidneys. Percussion of the kidneys also provides information about kidney location, size, and possible problems. Like palpation, percussion of the kidneys is not a routine part of a nursing assessment in critical care. However, the information gained through percussion can provide important patient-care data.

Kidneys

Percussion of a kidney is performed with the patient in a side-lying or sitting position, with the examiner's hand placed over the costovertebral angle (lower border of the rib cage on the flank).[1] Striking the back of the hand with the opposite fist produces a dull thud, which is normal. Pain may indicate infection (e.g., urinary tract infection that has extended into the kidneys) or injury resulting from trauma. Traumatic injury to the kidneys should be assessed in the presence of a penetrating abdominal wound, with blunt abdominal trauma, or with a fractured pelvis or ribs.

Abdomen

Observation and percussion of the abdomen may help in assessing fluid status. Percussing the abdomen with the patient in the supine position generally yields a dull sound (solid bowel contents or fluid) or a hollow sound (gaseous bowel).[1]

Ascites, or excess fluid accumulation and distention of the abdominal cavity, is an important observation in determining fluid overload. Differentiating ascites from distortion caused by solid bowel contents is accomplished by producing a fluid wave.

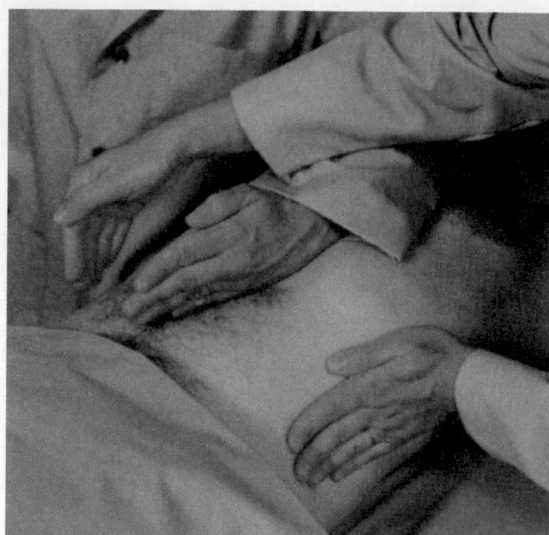

FIGURE 26-3   Test for the presence of a fluid wave. (From Barkauskas V, et al. *Health and Physical Assessment.* 3rd ed. St. Louis: Mosby; 2002.)

A fluid wave is elicited by exerting pressure to the abdominal midline while one hand is placed on the right or left flank.[1] Tapping the opposite flank produces a wave in the accumulated fluid that can be felt under the hands (Fig. 26-3). Other signs of ascites include a protuberant, rounded abdomen and abdominal striae.[1]

Individuals with kidney failure may have ascites caused by volume overload, which forces fluid into the abdomen due to increased capillary hydrostatic pressures. However, ascites may or may not represent fluid volume excess. Severe ascites in persons with compromised liver function may result from decreased plasma proteins. The ascites occurs because the increased vascular pressure associated with liver dysfunction forces fluid and plasma proteins from the vascular space into the interstitial space and abdominal cavity. Although the individual may exhibit marked edema, the intravascular space is volume depleted, and the patient is hypovolemic.

ADDITIONAL ASSESSMENTS

Weight Monitoring

One of the most important assessments of kidney and fluid status is the patient's weight. In the critical care unit, weight is monitored for each patient every day and is an important vital signs measurement. Significant fluctuations in body weight over a 1- to 2-day period indicate fluid gains and losses. Rapid weight gains or losses of more than 2 pounds per day usually indicate fluid rather than nutritional factors. One liter of fluid equals 1 kg, or approximately 2.2 pounds.

Whenever possible, the patient is weighed during admission to the critical care unit. It is important to document whether the current weight differs significantly from the weight 1 to 2 weeks before admission to the hospital. The patient is weighed daily for comparison with the previous day's weight. The weight is obtained at the same time each day, with the patient wearing the same amount of clothing and using the same scales. The individual's weight is of critical importance to the dialysis nurse

caring for a patient with acute or chronic kidney failure. The differences in weight from day to day are used to calculate the amount of fluid to remove during a dialysis treatment.[6]

Intake and Output Monitoring

Like patient weight, intake and output are monitored for all patients in the critical care unit. Intake and output can be compared with the patient's weight to more accurately evaluate fluid gains or losses. Urinary output plus insensible fluid losses (perspiration, stool, and water vapor from the lungs) can vary by 750 to 2400 mL/day. When intake exceeds output (e.g., excessive intravenous fluid, decreased urine output), a positive fluid balance exists. In impaired kidney function, the positive fluid balance results in fluid volume overload. Conversely, if output exceeds intake (e.g., fever, increased respiration, profuse sweating, vomiting, diarrhea, gastric suction, diuretic therapy), a negative fluid balance exists, and volume deficit results. During a 24-hour period, fever can increase skin and respiratory losses by as much as 75 mL per 1° F increase in temperature.

Individuals with *acute kidney injury* (AKI) often exhibit a decrease in urine output, or oliguria (less than 0.5 mL/kg/hr in adults; less than 1 mL/kg/hr in infants and young children). However, there may be a fairly normal or only slightly decreased urine output that reflects water removal without solute removal in the early phases of AKI. Although urine output is a sensitive indicator, kidney function cannot be accurately determined by urine output alone. For additional information on AKI see Chapter 27.

Abnormal output of body fluids creates fluid imbalances and causes electrolyte and acid–base disturbances. For example, gastrointestinal suction or loss by diarrhea can result in fluid deficit, sodium and potassium deficits, and metabolic acidosis from excessive loss of bicarbonate.

In maintaining daily records of intake and output, all gains or losses must be recorded. A standard list of the fluid volume held in various containers (e.g., milk cartons, juice containers) expedites this process. Discussions about the importance of accurate intake and output with the patient and family or friends are necessary and can improve the accuracy of intake and output volumes assessment.

Hemodynamic Monitoring

Body fluid status is accurately reflected in measurements of cardiovascular hemodynamics. Measurements such as central venous pressure (CVP), pulmonary artery occlusion pressure (PAOP), cardiac index (CI), and mean arterial pressure (MAP) provide a clear picture of the increases or decreases in vascular volume returning to and being ejected from the heart.[7] Volume depletion and volume overload are easily detected by use of central venous or arterial catheters, from which pressure measurements can be obtained (Table 26-2).

A central venous catheter often is inserted to evaluate fluid volume status and to measure the CVP. The CVP represents the filling pressure of the right atrium and is a measurement of right ventricular preload. The CVP changes with fluctuations in volume status. A normal CVP is 2 to 5 mm Hg. In volume depletion, the CVP is less than 2 mm Hg, whereas volume overload is reflected by readings of more than 5 mm Hg (see

TABLE 26-2 HEMODYNAMIC ASSESSMENT OF FLUID STATUS

MEASUREMENT	VOLUME DEPLETION	VOLUME OVERLOAD
Central venous pressure (CVP)	<2 mm Hg	>5 mm Hg
Pulmonary artery occlusion pressure (PAOP)	<5 mm Hg	>12 mm Hg
Cardiac index (CI)	<2.2 L/min/m^2	>4 L/min/m^2
Mean arterial pressure (MAP)	Decreased	Increased

BOX 26-3 FLUID AND ELECTROLYTE ASSESSMENT

Fluid Status
- Skin turgor
- Mucous membranes
- Intake and output
- Presence of edema or ascites
- Neck and hand vein engorgement
- Lung sounds (crackles)
- Dyspnea
- Central venous pressure (CVP) <2 mm Hg or >5 mm Hg
- Pulmonary artery occlusive pressure (PAOP) <5 mm Hg or >12 mm Hg
- Tachycardia
- Hypertension, hypotension
- Cardiac index (CI) <2.2 L/min/m^2
- S_3, S_4 heart sounds
- Headache
- Blurred vision
- Vertigo on rising
- Papilledema
- Mental changes
- Serum osmolality

Electrolyte and Waste Product Status
- Complete blood cell count (CBC)
- Serum electrolyte levels
- Nitrogen waste products (BUN)
- Electrocardiogram tracings (potassium, calcium, magnesium levels)
- Behavioral and mental changes (sodium, BUN levels)
- Chvostek and Trousseau signs (calcium levels)
- Changes in peripheral sensation (numbness, tremor—sodium, potassium, calcium levels)
- Muscle strength (potassium, BUN)
- Gastrointestinal changes (nausea and vomiting—BUN)
- Itching (calcium, phosphorus, BUN)
- Therapies that can alter electrolyte status (gastrointestinal suction, diuretics, antihypertensives, calcium channel blockers)

"Bedside Hemodynamic Monitoring" in Chapter 14 for more information on CVP interpretation).

If the patient has coexisting cardiopulmonary disease or if more information about hemodynamic function is required, a pulmonary artery catheter may be inserted. This catheter provides information about left ventricular filling pressures and cardiac output. The PAOP represents the left atrial pressure required to fill the left ventricle. When the left ventricle is full at the end of diastole, it represents the volume of blood available for ejection. It is also known as left ventricular preload and is measured by the PAOP. The normal PAOP is 5 to 12 mm Hg. In fluid volume excess, the PAOP increases. In fluid volume deficit, the PAOP is low.[7]

The CI demonstrates the cardiac output, or amount of blood ejected by the left ventricle over 1 minute, standardized for body size. The normal CI is 2.2 to 4 L/min/m^2. Compensatory mechanisms in early hypovolemic shock maintain the CI at or near normal. With prolonged fluid loss, the CI decreases. Fluid volume overload increases heart rate, which increases cardiac output, but only to a point. Left ventricular failure may result from massive volume overload, such as with acute heart failure resulting from kidney failure, in which case the CI decreases. The most common cause of AKI in which hemodynamic monitoring is indicated is severe sepsis.[7]

MAP is regulated by cardiac output and systemic vascular resistance (SVR), and it represents an averaged blood pressure within the arterial system. Changes in cardiac output or SVR inevitably result in corresponding MAP changes. For example, an increase in SVR during the early stages of hypovolemic shock leads to elevation of the MAP. Ongoing fluid losses eventually lead to a decreased cardiac output, which leads to a reduction in MAP. The net effect of a decreased MAP to the kidneys is a reduction in effective blood flow, which may lead to AKI.

Other Observations

Kidney system dysfunction often leads to fluid and electrolyte imbalances and the retention of metabolic waste products. Some of the disturbances in fluid, electrolyte, and waste product levels are accompanied by clinical manifestations less observable or measurable than those previously mentioned but that indicate a change from normal function. Box 26-3 summarizes important aspects to consider during kidney and fluid and electrolyte assessment.

Sudden or slowly developing changes in cognitive function and mental status must be investigated. For example, acidosis often results in disorientation. Lethargy, decreased attention or memory, coma, and confusion may result from sodium, calcium, or magnesium excess or deficit or retained waste products. Apprehension or anxiety may result from sodium deficit, a shift of fluid from the plasma to the interstitium, or respiratory changes caused by fluid volume overload. In older adults, new-onset confusion or a fall incurred by a previously mobile, alert individual may signal volume deficit in the absence of apparent acute illness.[8]

Apathy and withdrawal may accompany hypovolemic states. Patients with kidney failure and the accompanying systemic increases in electrolytes, fluids, and nitrogenous waste products may exhibit apathy, restlessness, confusion, and withdrawal.[2] The speed of onset depends on how rapidly or slowly the kidney failure progresses and alters homeostasis.

LABORATORY ASSESSMENT

There is no single or ideal laboratory test or marker that detects a decrease in kidney function.[11] Laboratory tests (serum and urine) used to detect and diagnose kidney dysfunction have limitations, but when reviewed daily for changes or trends, they provide valuable information concerning the status of the kidneys. Small changes in kidney function are associated with short- and long-term outcomes for hospitalized patients.[9] In addition to the history and physical examination, laboratory data are extremely helpful in the diagnosis, management, and ongoing evaluation of kidney system dysfunction.

Serum Components
Blood Urea Nitrogen

Blood urea nitrogen (BUN) is a byproduct of protein and amino acid metabolism. The normal value for BUN is 5 to 20 mg/dL, which is increased when kidney function deteriorates. With kidney dysfunction, the BUN is elevated because of a decrease in the glomerular filtration rate (GFR) and resulting decrease in urea excretion. Elevations in the BUN can be correlated with the clinical manifestations of uremia; as the BUN rises, symptoms of uremia become more pronounced.[2] However, a drop in the GFR with an increase in the BUN also may be caused by hypovolemia and dehydration, nephrotoxic medications, or a sudden hypotensive episode. In these cases, the rise in BUN is caused by a decreased GFR in the presence of normal kidney function. BUN is also increased by changes in protein metabolism that occur with excessive protein intake and catabolism. A catabolic state may occur with starvation (or chronic poor nutrition in a critically ill patient), severe infection, surgery, or trauma. The BUN level also may be elevated as the result of hematoma resorption, gastrointestinal bleeding, excessive licorice ingestion, or steroid or tetracycline therapy. A decrease in the BUN level may indicate volume overload, liver damage, severe malnutrition (as a result of depleted protein stores), use of phenothiazines, or pregnancy.

Creatinine

Creatinine is a byproduct of muscle and normal cell metabolism, and it appears in serum in amounts generally proportional to the body muscle mass. Although slightly higher in males than females, the normal serum creatinine level is about 0.5 to 1.2 mg/dL. Creatinine is freely filtered by the glomerulus, easily excreted by the kidney tubules, and minimally resorbed or secreted in the tubules.[2] Creatinine levels are fairly constant and are affected by fewer factors than BUN. As a result, the serum creatinine level is a more sensitive and specific indicator of kidney function than BUN. Creatinine excess occurs most often in persons with kidney failure resulting from impaired excretion. However, the body's production and release of creatinine may vary during muscle wasting in acute illness, leading to a falsely low serum level of creatinine. Elevated levels of creatinine are seen in muscle growth disorders such as acromegaly, with traumatic skeletal muscle injury, and with some medications that decrease creatinine removal (e.g., trimethoprim, cimetidine) in the absence of kidney dysfunction. Malnutrition can result in transient increases in creatinine levels as the rapid muscle catabolism associated with malnutrition releases increased amounts of creatinine into the circulation.

BUN to Creatinine Ratio. Another useful diagnostic parameter in kidney disease is the ratio of blood urea nitrogen (BUN) to creatinine. The usual ratio of BUN to creatinine is 10 to 1,

and a change in the ratio may indicate kidney dysfunction. For example, if BUN and creatinine levels are elevated and maintained at an approximate ratio of 10 to 1, the disorder is intrarenal, or affecting the tubules of the kidneys. If the ratio of BUN to creatinine levels is greater than 10 to 1, the cause is most likely prerenal (e.g., hypovolemia). In prerenal kidney failure, the creatinine is excreted by functioning tubules, but the urea nitrogen is retained because of the poor GFR and hemoconcentration, leading to the increased ratio. In the diagnosis of prerenal kidney failure, the ratio is a more useful indicator of kidney function than the separate tests of BUN and creatinine.

Creatinine Clearance

The urine creatinine clearance is a measure of how well the kidneys remove creatinine. Because of the relatively constant rate at which creatinine is produced and the nearly complete removal of creatinine by normal kidneys, the ability of the kidneys to remove (clear) creatinine from the blood is an indication of how well the glomeruli and tubules are working. Measuring the creatinine clearance—the amount of creatinine in the excreted urine and the amount of creatinine in the blood over 24 hours—provides a reliable and accurate estimate of glomerular filtration and therefore of kidney function.[2] The normal value for creatinine clearance is 110 to 120 mL/min; values less than 50 mL/min indicate significant kidney dysfunction. The creatinine clearance is traditionally measured using a 12- or 24-hour urine collection and blood sample. Newer methods use a random, smaller-volume urine specimen and blood sample. Creatinine clearance can also be estimated from the serum creatinine level (Box 26-4), a method commonly

---

BOX 26-4 CREATININE CLEARANCE CALCULATIONS*

Measured: 24-Hour Urine
(Urine creatinine × Volume of urine)/Serum creatinine

Estimated: Adults—Cockcroft-Gault Formula
[[(140 − Age) × Body weight (kg)]/[72 × Plasma creatinine (mg/dL)]]

For women, multiply the result by 0.85.

Estimated: Adults—Modification of Diet in Renal Disease (MDRD) Formula
186 × (Plasma creatinine) − 1.154 × (Age in years) − 0.203

For women, multiply the result by 0.742.
For African Americans, multiply the result by 1.210.†

Estimated: Children
≤10 kg: 0.45 × Height (cm)/Serum creatinine (mg/dL)
>10, <70 kg: 0.55 × Height (cm)/Serum creatinine (mg/dL)
≥70 kg: [1.55 × Age (yr) + 0.5 × Height (cm)/Serum creatinine (mg/dL)]

*Online calculators available from the *National Kidney Foundation* at http://www.kidney.org/professionals.
†Both risk factor assessments apply for African American women. The number would be multiplied by both 0.742 (woman) and 1.210 (African American).

used in the critical care unit. The estimated or calculated creatinine clearance is widely used to determine changes in medication dosing with kidney dysfunction because of the many medications excreted by the kidneys.

Cystatin C

Although not widely used in practice, cystatin C is another serum marker for kidney function. Cystatin C is a substance synthesized and released by most cells in the body at a constant rate.[10] Like creatinine, cystatin C is filtered easily by the glomerulus and not secreted or resorbed by the tubules. The advantage of cystatin C is that it is metabolized by the tubules. In normal kidney function, cystatin C levels are very low because the glomerulus filters it and the tubules metabolize it. In kidney dysfunction, the glomerular filtration of cystatin C is reduced and therefore not provided to the tubules for metabolism. Cystatin C is affected by fewer factors (e.g., age, gender, muscle mass) than creatinine, and a change in its level can be detected earlier during AKI than creatinine.[10] Cystatin C and other kidney-related biomarkers may become more widely used as a kidney function marker as additional clinical validation studies are completed.[10]

Osmolality

The serum osmolality reflects the concentration or dilution of vascular fluid and measures the dissolved particles in the serum. The normal serum osmolality is 275 to 295 mOsm/L.[3] An elevated osmolality level indicates hemoconcentration or dehydration, and a decreased osmolality level indicates hemodilution or volume overload. When the serum osmolality level increases, antidiuretic hormone (ADH) is released from the posterior pituitary gland and stimulates increased water resorption in the kidney tubules. This expands the vascular space, returns the serum osmolality level back to normal, and results in more concentrated urine and an elevated urine osmolality level. The opposite occurs with a decreased serum osmolality level, which inhibits the production of ADH. The decreased ADH results in increased excretion of water in the tubules, producing dilute urine with a low osmolality, and returns the serum osmolality level back to normal. Sodium accounts for 85% to 95% of the serum osmolality value; doubling the serum sodium level gives an estimate of the serum osmolality level in healthy individuals. Other particles in the serum can increase the osmolality and need to be considered in individuals with common comorbid conditions. A more precise estimation of serum osmolality can be calculated from the following formula:

$$2 \times Na \, (mEq/L) + BUN/3 \, (mg/dL) + Glucose/18 \, (mg/dL)$$

The calculated serum osmolality level is a useful tool while awaiting full laboratory results. Measured serum osmolality is a useful parameter in determining fluid balance and fluid replacement therapy for critically ill patients. Serum osmolality is also a useful parameter in determining disorders of ADH secretion that may occur in critically ill patients. A decreased serum osmolality level may indicate syndrome of inappropriate ADH secretion (SIADH), or too much ADH, whereas an elevation of the serum osmolality level may indicate diabetes insipidus (DI), or too little ADH.

Anion Gap

The *anion gap* is a calculation of the difference between the measurable extracellular plasma cations (sodium and potassium) and the measurable anions (chloride and bicarbonate).[3] In plasma, sodium is the predominant cation and chloride is the predominant anion. Extracellular potassium concentration in plasma is so small that it is generally ignored, leaving the following equation for calculation of the anion gap:

$$[Na^+] - ([Cl^-] + [HCO_3^-])$$

The normal anion gap is 8 to 16 mEq/L, a range that has been verified in a healthy population of adults.[11] The "gap" represents the unmeasurable ions present in the ECF (phosphates, sulfates, ketones, lactate). An increased anion gap level usually reflects overproduction or decreased excretion of acid products and indicates metabolic acidosis; a decreased anion gap indicates metabolic alkalosis.

Acute and chronic kidney failure can increase the anion gap because of retention of acids and altered bicarbonate resorption.[12] The anion gap is also increased in diabetic ketoacidosis caused by ketone production. The measurement of the anion gap is a rapid method for identifying acid–base imbalance but cannot be used to pinpoint the source of the acid–base disturbance specifically.

Hemoglobin and Hematocrit

The hemoglobin and hematocrit levels can indicate increases or decreases in intravascular fluid volume. Hemoglobin and hematocrit values vary between genders; the hemoglobin level in males is normally 13.5 to 17.5 g/dL, and in females, it is 12 to 16 g/dL. The hematocrit level is 40% to 54% in males and 37% to 47% in females. Hematocrit levels are higher in newborns (up to 65%) and decrease to adult ranges between the ages of 4 and 10 years. Hemoglobin transports oxygen and carbon dioxide and is important in maintaining cellular metabolism and acid–base balance.[3]

The hematocrit value is the proportion or concentration of red blood cells (RBCs) in a volume of whole blood and is expressed as a percentage. The hematocrit level is approximately three times the hemoglobin level if the individual is in a normal fluid balance. An increase in the hematocrit value often indicates a fluid volume deficit, which results in hemoconcentration. Although rare, true disorders of RBC production, such as polycythemia, can result in an increased hematocrit level.

Conversely, a decreased hematocrit value can indicate fluid volume excess because of the dilutional effect of the extra fluid load. Decreases also can result from anemias, blood loss, liver damage, or hemolytic reactions. In individuals with acute kidney failure, anemia may occur early in the disease.[13] A decreased hematocrit level may indicate the anemia of kidney failure or may reflect fluid volume overload. If the hematocrit value is decreasing but the hemoglobin concentration remains constant, the cause is fluid volume overload. Decreased hematocrit values and hemoglobin concentrations indicate a true loss of RBCs. The history and bedside assessment, including hemodynamic monitoring data, aid in determining whether fluid imbalances or disease states, or both, are responsible for changes in hematocrit levels in the critically ill patient.

Albumin

Slightly more than 50% of the total plasma protein is serum albumin. It is manufactured in the liver, and a normal blood level is 3.5 to 5 g/dL. Albumin is primarily responsible for the maintenance of colloid osmotic pressure, which functions to hold fluid in the vascular space. The blood vessel walls, because of their impermeability to plasma proteins, prevent albumin from leaving the vascular space. However, in some disease states such as severe burns (cell membrane destruction) or nephrotic syndrome (increased glomerular capillary permeability to protein and protein loss in the urine), albumin is lost from the vascular space.

Decreased albumin levels in the vascular space result in a fluid shift from the plasma to the interstitium, creating peripheral edema. A decreased albumin level can result from protein-calorie malnutrition, which occurs in many critically ill patients in whom available stores of albumin are depleted. A decrease in the plasma oncotic pressure results, and fluid shifts from the vascular space to the interstitial space. Liver disease or severe injury to the liver also causes a decrease in albumin levels as the diseased liver fails to synthesize sufficient albumin. Severe portal hypertension can force albumin and other plasma proteins into the abdominal cavity, resulting in ascites.

Increased albumin levels are rare. The body uses a fixed amount of protein for energy and body cell replacement and converts excess protein into stored fat. If all plasma protein levels are elevated, fluid volume deficit (hemoconcentration) is suspected.

Urinalysis

Analysis of the urine provides excellent information about the patient's kidney function and condition relative to fluids and electrolytes. Specific tests and abnormal indications are presented in Table 26-3. In the critically ill patient a routine urinalysis specimen may be obtained to rule out the presence of urinary protein or glucose. A sterile urine culture may be obtained if a urinary tract infection (UTI) is suspected.

Urine Appearance

Physical examination of the urine focuses on a general inspection of the urine's color, clarity, and odor. Normal urine is pale yellow, but it may vary due to food intake (carrots, beets, rhubarb), medications (phenytoin, nitrofurantoin, phenazopyridine), or metabolic byproducts (bilirubin, methemoglobin). Clarity of the urine may be affected by bacteria, white blood cells (WBCs), or urates. Normal urine has minimal odor; a strong odor may be caused by concentrated urine (as in dehydrated states), infection, medicines (especially vitamins), or foods (broccoli, asparagus).[14]

Urine pH

Urine pH indicates the acidity or alkalinity of the urine. The normal urinary pH is acidic but has a range from 4.5 to 8.[14] The kidneys regulate acid–base balance; more hydrogen ions are excreted than bicarbonate ions, causing the acidity of the urine. Changes in metabolic function and kidney function produce changes in urinary pH.

An increase in urinary acidity (decreased pH) indicates retention of sodium and acids by the body, which occurs in intrarenal AKI. A decrease in urinary acidity (increased pH or more alkaline) means the body is retaining bicarbonate. In the presence of normal kidney function, urinary pH levels are greatly affected by diet and medications. Certain food groups, such as citrus fruits and vegetables, lead to alkaline urine, whereas a diet high in protein can produce acidic urine. In the critical care unit, patients receiving total parenteral nutrition or a high-protein tube-feeding formula may have acidic urine because of high protein intake.

Urine Specific Gravity

Specific gravity measures the density or weight of urine compared with that of distilled water. The normal urinary specific gravity is 1.005 to 1.025.[14] For comparison, the specific gravity of distilled water is 1.000. Because urine is composed of many solutes and substances suspended in water, the specific gravity should always be higher than that of water.

The specific gravity reflects hydration status and indicates the ability of the kidneys to dilute or concentrate the urine. Decreases in specific gravity reflect the inability of the kidneys to excrete the usual solute load into the urine (less dense with fewer solutes). Increases in specific gravity are caused by dehydration (more concentrated urine), or with additional glucose (diabetes) or protein (glomerular dysfunction) that increase urine density.[14] A fixed specific gravity (does not vary with fluid intake) suggests early kidney dysfunction because the kidneys are unable to excrete or resorb water and solutes.

Urine Osmolality

The urine osmolality may be measured in tandem with the serum osmolality value. The simultaneous measurement of the serum and urine osmolality levels provides an accurate assessment of fluid status. The normal urine osmolality level is 500 to 1200 mOsm/kg and depends on resorption or excretion of water in the kidney tubules. The urine osmolality level increases (and urine output decreases) during fluid volume deficit because of the retention of fluid by the body. The urine osmolality level decreases (and urine output increases) during volume excess because fluid is excreted by the kidneys.

Urine Protein

Protein normally is absent from urine because protein molecules are too large to be filtered across the intact glomerular capillary membrane. Protein amounts greater than 150 mg/day signal compromise of the glomerular membrane and intrinsic kidney damage.[14]

Traditionally, quantitative measurement of the amount of protein in the urine required a 24-hour urine collection.[14] A "spot" or random urine sample can also be used as the correlation between the two tests is very strong.[14] Both the amount of

TABLE 26-3 URINALYSIS RESULTS

TEST	NORMAL	POSSIBLE CAUSES FOR INCREASED VALUES	POSSIBLE CAUSES FOR DECREASED VALUES
pH	4.5-8.0	Alkalosis	Acidosis Intrarenal AKI
Specific gravity	1.003-1.030*	Volume deficit Glycosuria Proteinuria Prerenal AKI (>1.020)	Volume overload Intrarenal AKI
Osmolality	300-1200 mOsm/kg	Volume deficit Prerenal AKI (urine > serum osmolality)	Volume excess Intrarenal AKI (urine < serum osmolality)
Protein	30-150 mg/24 hr†	Trauma Infection Intrarenal AKI Transient with exercise Glomerulonephritis	
Sodium	40-220 mEq/24 hr	High-sodium diet Intrarenal AKI	Prerenal AKI
Creatinine	1-2 g/24 hr		Intrarenal AKI Chronic kidney failure
Urea	6-17 g/24 hr		Intrarenal AKI Chronic kidney failure
Myoglobin	Absent	Crush injury Rhabdomyolysis	
RBCs	0-5‡	Trauma Intrarenal AKI Infection Strenuous exercise Renal artery thrombus	
WBCs	0-5‡	Infection	
Bacteria	None to few	Infection	
Casts	None to few	RBC: glomerular disease WBC: pyelonephritis Glomerular disease Nephrotic syndrome Epithelial: glomerular disease	

*Adult value; newborn value is slightly lower at 1.001-1.020.
†Higher values usually apply for persons after exercise; lower values apply for persons at rest.
‡Cells per low-power field.
AKI, Acute kidney injury; *RBCs,* red blood cells; *WBCs,* white blood cells.

protein and the amount of creatinine in the urine specimen are measured. A normal *urine protein to urine creatinine ratio* is less than 0.2; a protein-to-creatinine ratio of 3.5 indicates approximately 3.5 grams of protein are being excreted per day, indicating severe protein loss by the kidneys.

Urine Glucose

Glycosuria is defined as glucose in the urine. Glucose normally is completely resorbed by the kidney tubules, and the urine should be free of glucose. Urinary glucose should not exceed 130 mg per day.[14] In the presence of acute or chronic kidney failure, glycosuria may not be a reliable indicator of the level of hyperglycemia because of the damaged nephrons. In the critical care unit, the serum glucose is measured, not urine values.

Urine Ketones

Ketones in the urine are abnormal and signal hyperglycemia caused by type 1 diabetes or starvation ketosis.[14]

Urine Electrolytes

Levels of electrolytes in the urine are not measured as often as levels in serum, but they can yield information about kidney function. To measure urinary electrolyte levels, a 24-hour urine sample may be needed, although potassium and sodium can be measured in a randomly collected specimen.

Urine Sodium. The most commonly measured electrolyte in the urine is sodium. Urinary sodium is a reflection of the action of aldosterone and subsequent retention or excretion of sodium by the kidney tubules to maintain fluid balance. In the presence of hypovolemia, the kidney tubules retain sodium (and therefore water), and the amount of sodium in the urine and the fractional excretion of sodium are very low. The opposite is true with volume overload and with kidney diseases that cause sodium wasting. The amount of sodium in the urine can help in determining the pathology of AKI as long as diuretics have not been administered. In prerenal AKI due to ineffective circulation reaching the kidneys, the urine sodium level is low. If the AKI results from damage to the kidney tubules, the urine sodium level is normal or elevated.

Urine Sediment

The presence of sediment such as epithelial cells and casts in urine aids in identifying problems related to the kidneys.[14] A fresh urine specimen, tested 30 to 60 minutes following collection, is important.[14] Urine becomes more alkaline after it has been collected, resulting in a change in the urine sediment (e.g., casts dissolve, cells lyse). The presence or absence of urine sediment can be helpful in identifying the cause of AKI. In prerenal AKI, the kidneys are not injured, and urinary sediment is absent. However, in intrarenal AKI, the kidney glomeruli or tubules are damaged, allowing urinary sediment containing casts and epithelial cells in the urine.[14]

Casts are cylindrical structures composed mainly of mucoprotein (Tamm-Horsfall protein), which is secreted by epithelial cells lining the loops of Henle, the distal tubules, and the collecting ducts. Casts may form in the presence of epithelial cells, RBCs, or WBCs in the tubular lumen. These cells or clumps of cellular breakdown products can adhere to and be surrounded by the fibrillar mucoprotein matrix, and the resulting casts are washed out of the kidney tubular system in the urinary flow. Casts differ in composition and size and correlate with the severity and type of kidney damage. For example, WBC casts indicate pyelonephritis, or they may occur during acute glomerulonephritis. RBC casts indicate glomerulonephritis. Hyaline casts, which consist of Tamm-Horsfall protein, are associated with kidney parenchymal disease and glomerular capillary membrane inflammation. Consistent appearance of epithelial cells shed by the lining of the nephron may indicate nephritis. Although small numbers of epithelial cells normally appear in the urine and an occasional cast may be found, their consistent appearance is abnormal.[14]

Hematuria

Obvious and microscopic hematuria may signal kidney damage. Although a few RBCs in the urine are normal, discernibly bloody urine usually indicates bleeding within the urinary tract or kidney trauma. Microscopic hematuria may occur normally after strenuous exercise or the insertion of a retention catheter but should disappear within 48 hours.

The presence of myoglobin can make the urine appear red. Microscopic examination of the urine fails to reveal RBCs, with myoglobin being present instead. Myoglobin in the urine may result from skeletal muscle damage (e.g., traumatic crush injury) or rhabdomyolysis. Rhabdomyolysis may develop in patients admitted to a critical care unit for many reasons, including traumatic injury, cocaine abuse, status epilepticus, heat prostration, or collapse during intense physical exercise (e.g., running a marathon race on a hot day). Myoglobin is released by the muscle cells and blocks the tubules that can result in intrarenal AKI.

URINE TOXICOLOGY SCREEN

Urine can be screened to detect the presence of alcohol, illegal drugs, prescription and nonprescription medications, and other substances that are excreted via the kidneys.[15] The is often referred to as a Urine Drug Screen (UDS).[15] Urine toxicology tests conducted in the emergency department or the critical care unit are considered screening tests and are not diagnostic of a disease state.[15] These analyses are typically undertaken to provide information about causes of an altered level of consciousness rather than to identify kidney-related problems.

IMAGING STUDIES

Although laboratory assessment is used most often in diagnosing kidney problems in the critically ill patient, imaging studies can confirm or clarify causes of particular disorders. Imaging assessment includes the use of ultrasound and radiologic techniques. Ultrasound is a noninvasive imaging technique that is available in most hospitals. Kidney ultrasound is especially useful in determining the size, shape, and contour of the kidneys, the presence of masses or cysts, and the presence of renal artery stenosis.[16] Radiologic assessment ranges from basic to more complex (Table 26-4) and provides information about abnormal masses, abnormal fluid collections, obstructions, vascular supply alterations, and other disorders of the kidneys and urinary tract.[16]

Some radiologic studies require the use of contrast or injection of a radiopaque dye. Because many of the dyes used in radiology are potentially nephrotoxic, they must be used carefully in patients with AKI or chronic kidney disease.[17,18] To prevent contrast induced nephrotoxicity (CIN), adequate hydration before and after the test and careful monitoring of kidney function are always indicated.[17,18]

KIDNEY BIOPSY

Kidney biopsy is the definitive tool for diagnosing disease processes involving the parenchyma of the kidney. Percutaneous needle biopsy involves inserting a needle through the flank to obtain a specimen of cortical and medullary kidney tissue.[19,20] An open biopsy is a surgical procedure and is rarely done in critically ill patients. In either case, biopsy is the last choice for diagnostic assessment in the critically ill patient because of the periprocedural risks of bleeding, hematoma, and infection.[19,20]

TABLE 26-4	KIDNEY IMAGING TESTS
TEST	**COMMENTS**
Kidney-ureter-bladder (KUB) radiograph	Flat-plate radiograph of the abdomen; determines position, size, and structure of the kidneys, urinary tract, and pelvis; useful for evaluating the presence of calculi and masses; usually followed by additional tests
Intravenous pyelogram (IVP)	Intravenous injection of contrast with radiography; allows visualization of internal kidney tissues
Angiography	Injection of contrast into arterial blood perfusing the kidneys; allows visualization of renal blood flow; may also visualize stenosis, cysts, clots, trauma, and infarctions
Computed tomography (CT)	Radioisotope is administered by intravenous route and absorbed by the kidneys; scintillation photography is then performed in several planes; spiral or helical CT allows rapid imaging; density of the image helps evaluate kidney vessels, perfusion, tumors, cysts, stones/calculi, hemorrhage, necrosis, and trauma
Ultrasound	High-frequency sound waves are transmitted to the kidneys and urinary tract, and the image is viewed on an oscilloscope; noninvasive; identifies fluid accumulation or obstruction, cysts, stones/calculi, and masses; useful for evaluating kidney before biopsy
Magnetic resonance imaging (MRI)	A scanner produces three-dimensional images in response to the application of high-energy radiofrequency waves to the tissues; produces clear images; density of the image may indicate trauma, cysts, masses, malformation of the vessels or tubules stones/calculi, and necrosis

SUMMARY

Clinical Assessment

- Predisposing factors for acute kidney dysfunction are obtained during the history, including the use of over-the-counter medicines, recent infections requiring antibiotic therapy, antihypertensive medicines, and any diagnostic procedures performed using radiopaque contrast.
- Urine output may be decreased or normal, depending on the cause of the kidney dysfunction but low urine output is insufficient to identify acute kidney injury (AKI).

Laboratory Studies

- Blood urea nitrogen (BUN) is a byproduct of protein and amino acid metabolism. BUN is increased when kidney function deteriorates.
- Serum creatinine is used to trend kidney function in critical illness as creatine is not resorbed by the kidney tubules and rises when kidney function deteriorates.

- Cystatin C is a newer serum biomarker for early identification of acute kidney injury.
- Electrolyte derangements are frequent in kidney failure including: sodium, potassium, phosphate, calcium, chloride, and bicarbonate.
- Anion gap is increased in kidney failure in association with electrolyte and acid–base changes.
- Urinalysis can provide valuable information about kidney function, but results are not reliable if the patient has recently been administered diuretics.

Diagnostic Procedures

- Ultrasound, computed tomography (CT), and magnetic resonance imaging (MRI) are noninvasive tests used to obtain images of the kidney.
- Kidney biopsy is rarely performed in the critically ill patient.

REFERENCES

1. Seidel HM, et al. *Mosby's Guide to Physical Examination.* 7th ed. St. Louis: Mosby; 2010.
2. Schira M. Assessment of kidney structure and function. In: Counts C, ed. *Core Curriculum for Nephrology Nursing.* 5th ed. Pitman, NJ: American Nephrology Nurses Association; 2008.
3. Wadel HM, Textor SC. The role of the kidney in regulating arterial blood pressure. *Nat Rev Nephrol.* 2012;8(10):602.
4. Parker K. Alterations in fluid, electrolyte, and acid–base balance. In: Molzahn A, Butera E, eds. *Contemporary Nephrology Nursing: Principles and Practice.* 2nd ed. Pitman, NJ: American Nephrology Nurses Association; 2006.
5. de Vries Feyens C, de Jager CP. Images in clinical medicine: decreased skin turgor. *New Engl J Med.* 2011;364:e6.

6. Purcell W, et al. Accurate dry weight assessment: reducing the incidence of hypertension and cardiac disease in patients on hemodialysis. *Nephrol Nurs J.* 2004;31(6):631.
7. Davison DL, Patel K, Chawla LS. Hemodynamic monitoring in the critically ill: spanning the range of kidney function. *Amer J Kidney Dis.* 2012;59:715.
8. Faes M, et al. Dehydration in geriatrics. *Geriatr Aging.* 2007;10(9):590.
9. Bellomo R. Acute renal failure. *Semin Respir Crit Care Med.* 2011;32:639
10. Weekley CC, Peralta CA. Advances in the use of multimarker panels for renal risk stratification. *Curr Opin Nephrol Hypertens.* 2012;21:301.
11. Farwell WR, Taylor EN. Serum anion gap, bicarbonate and biomarkers of inflammation in healthy individuals in a national survey. *CMAJ.* 2010;182:137.

12. Abramowitz MK, Hostetter TH, Melamed ML. The serum anion gap is altered in early kidney disease and associates with mortality. *Kidney Internat.* 2012;82:701.

13. Ramanath V, et al. Anemia and chronic kidney disease: making sense of the recent trials. *Recent Clin Trials.* 2012;7:187.

14. Lerma EV, Rosner MH. Urinalysis. In: Lerna EV, Nisenson AR. eds. *Nephrology Secrets.* 3rd ed. Philadelphia: Elsevier; 2012.

15. Markway EC, Baker SN. A review of the methods, interpretation, and limitations of the urine drug screen. *Orthopedics.* 2011;34:877.

16. Rosen A, Simpson WL. Renal imaging techniques. In: Lerna EV, Nisenson AR, eds. *Nephrology Secrets.* 3rd ed. Philadelphia: Elsevier; 2012.

17. Isaac S. Contrast-induced nephropathy: nursing implications. *Crit Care Nurs.* 2012;32:41.

18. Stacul F, et al. Contrast induced nephropathy: updated ESUR Contrast Media Safety Committee guidelines. *Eur Radiol.* 2011;21:2527.

19. Whittier WL. Complications of the percutaneous kidney biopsy. *Adv Chronic Kidney Dis.* 2012;19(3):179.

20. Corapi KM, et al. Bleeding complications of native kidney biopsy: a systematic review and meta-analysis. *Amer J Kidney Dis.* 2012;60(1):62.

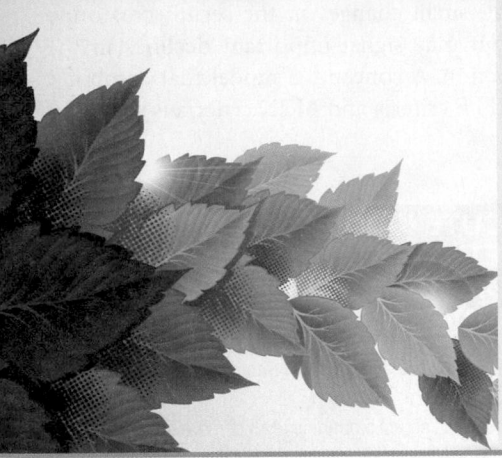

Kidney Disorders and Therapeutic Management

Mary E. Lough

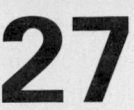 **WEBSITE**

http://evolve.elsevier.com/Urden/criticalcare/

Evolve Features:
- NCLEX Review Questions
- CCRN Review Questions
- PCCN Review Questions
- Mosby's Nursing Skills Procedures
- Animations
- Video Clips
- Glossary

ACUTE KIDNEY INJURY

Acute kidney injury (AKI) is a relatively new term used to describe the spectrum of acute-onset kidney disorders that can range from mild impairment of kidney function through acute kidney failure that requires renal replacement therapy (dialysis).[1,2] Severe AKI is characterized by a sudden decline in glomerular filtration rate (GFR), with subsequent retention of products in the blood that are normally excreted by the kidneys; this disrupts electrolyte balance, acid–base homeostasis, and fluid volume equilibrium. A transition to greater use of the word *kidney* rather than *renal* reflects a trend in the nephrology literature that emphasizes the vulnerability of the kidney during critical illness.[1,2]

Critical Illness and Acute Kidney Injury

Critical care patients with AKI have a longer length of hospital stay, more complications and higher mortality.[1,2] AKI-associated mortality ranges from 15% to 60%.[2] One of the reasons for poor survival is that critical care patients often have coexisting non-kidney conditions that increase their susceptibility to the development of AKI. High-risk diagnoses include heart failure, shock, respiratory failure, and sepsis. An observational study that examined the incidence and course of severe AKI in 618 patients in six academic medical centers in the United States found that AKI was accompanied by multiorgan failure in most patients, even those who did not require dialysis.[3] In this observational study 64% of patients required dialysis, the in-hospital mortality rate was 37%, and the rate of nonrecovery of kidney function (permanent dialysis) or death was 50%.[3] The mortality

rate exceeded 50% when four or more body systems had failed.[3] Other clinical studies report similar findings with equally high mortality.[2] Today the most frequent causes of AKI in the critically ill are associated with sepsis and cardiac surgery.[1]

Typically, a patient is not admitted to the critical care unit with a diagnosis of AKI alone; there is always coexisting hemodynamic, cardiac, pulmonary, or neurologic compromise. Many patients come into the hospital with underlying changes in kidney function, such as an elevated serum creatinine level, although they have no symptoms and are often unaware of their compromised kidney function. The lack of kidney reserve places these patients at increased risk for AKI if complications occur in any other organ systems. As a result, the picture of AKI in the modern critical care unit has changed to encompass patients with kidney injury who also have multisystem dysfunction that complicates their clinical course.

Definitions of Acute Kidney Injury

One of the challenges of estimating the incidence of AKI in the critical care unit has been the wide variation in definitions that have been used. Measurement of kidney function is indirect, and the diagnosis of AKI is predominantly derived from changes in urine output and elevation of serum creatinine level, with the understanding that changes in these values reflect a decline in the GFR.[1,2] Urine output is sometimes a problematic measure to use because diuretics artificially increase the urine output but may not alter the course of kidney failure. The clinical insult may have direct effects on the kidney, such as the inflammation associated with sepsis, which accounts for almost 50% of the AKI seen in critical care units.[1]

RIFLE Criteria

The risk of critically ill patients developing AKI has been classified by a multinational group of nephrologists.[1,2] The classification uses the acronym RIFLE—*risk, injury, failure, loss,* and *end*-stage kidney disease (ESKD).[2] The *RIFLE* system classifies AKI in three categories of increasing severity (R, I, F) and two outcome criteria (L, E) based on GFR status reflected by the change in urine output or loss of kidney function[2] (Table 27-1). If AKI is superimposed on a kidney that is already compromised, the term *chronic* is added to the RIFLE criteria to denote the cause as acute-on-chronic kidney failure.[2]

Acute Kidney Injury Network Criteria

The *Acute Kidney Injury Network* (AKIN) criteria are listed in Box 27-1. These criteria are similar to those proposed by the RIFLE group, and both groups intend to make the point that in the acutely ill patient, small changes in the serum creatinine level and urine output may signal important declines in the GFR and kidney function. A conceptual model that combines the features of the RIFLE criteria and AKIN criteria is shown in Figure 27-1.[2]

TABLE 27-1	**RIFLE CRITERIA FOR ACUTE KIDNEY DYSFUNCTION**	
RIFLE	**SERUM CREATININE CRITERIA***	**URINE OUTPUT CRITERIA**
*R*isk	Serum Cr increased 1.5 times above normal *or* Serum Cr increase ≥0.3 mg/dL	UO <0.5 mL/kg/hr for 6 hr
*I*njury	Serum Cr increased 2 times above normal	UO <0.5 mL/kg/hr for 12 hr
*F*ailure	Serum Cr increased 3 times above normal *or* Serum Cr ≥4 mg/dL *or* Serum Cr acute rise ≥0.5 mg/dL	UO <0.3 mL/kg/hr for 24 hr *or* anuria for 12 hr (oliguria)
*L*oss	Persistent AKI = complete loss of kidney function for more than 4 wk	
*E*SKD	End-stage kidney disease	

Data from Kellum JA, et al. Definition and classification of acute kidney injury. *Nephron Clin Pract.* 2008;109(4):c182.
*All serum creatinine references are based on changes from baseline.
AKI, Acute kidney injury; *Cr,* creatinine; *UO,* urine output.

BOX 27-1	**ACUTE KIDNEY INJURY NETWORK (AKIN) CRITERIA FOR THE DIAGNOSIS OF ACUTE KIDNEY INJURY**

- *Definition:* Acute kidney injury (AKI) is an abrupt (within 48 hours) reduction in kidney function defined as:
  - An absolute increase in the serum creatinine level of more than or equal to 0.3 mg/dL (≥26.4 µmol/L)
  - A percentage increase in serum creatinine of more than or equal to 50% (1.5-fold from baseline)
  - A reduction in urine output (documented oliguria of less than 0.5 mL/kg/hr for more than 6 hours)

Explanatory Notes

- *Serum creatinine:* These criteria include an absolute and a percentage change in creatinine to accommodate variations related to age, gender, and body mass index and to reduce the need for a baseline creatinine level, but they do require at least two serum creatinine values within 48 hours.
- *Urine output:* The urine output criterion was included based on the predictive importance of this measure but with the awareness that urine outputs may not be measured routinely in non-critical care unit settings. It is assumed that the diagnosis based on the urine output criterion alone will require exclusion of urinary tract obstructions that reduce urine output or of other easily reversible causes of reduced urine output.
- *Clinical context:* These criteria should be used in the context of the clinical presentation and after adequate fluid resuscitation when applicable. Many acute kidney diseases exist, and some may result in AKI. Because diagnostic criteria are not documented, some cases of AKI may not be diagnosed.
- *Physiologic state:* AKI may be superimposed on or lead to chronic kidney disease.

Data from Mehta RL, et al. for the Acute Kidney Injury Network. Report of an initiative to improve outcomes in acute kidney injury. *Crit Care.* 2007;11(2):R31.

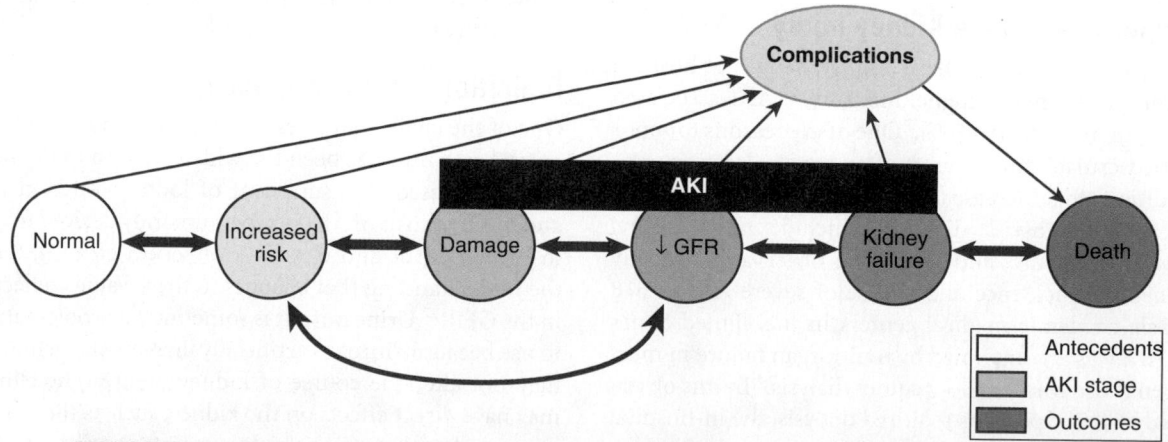

FIGURE 27-1   Model of the components of acute kidney injury. (Modified from Acute Kidney Injury Network. AKI Conceptual Model, developed at the Vancouver Summit 2006. http://www.akinet.org.)

BOX 27-2 ACUTE KIDNEY INJURY

Prerenal Acute Kidney Injury
- Prolonged hypotension (sepsis, vasodilation)
- Prolonged low cardiac output (heart failure, cardiogenic shock)
- Prolonged volume depletion (dehydration, hemorrhage)
- Renovascular thrombosis (thromboemboli)

Intrarenal Acute Kidney Injury
- Kidney ischemia (advanced stage of prerenal acute kidney injury)
- Endogenous toxins (rhabdomyolysis, tumor lysis syndrome)
- Exogenous toxins (radiocontrast dye, nephrotoxic medications)
- Infection (acute glomerulonephritis, interstitial nephritis)

Postrenal Acute Kidney Injury
- Obstruction (urethra, prostate, or bladder)
- Rare as a cause of acute kidney injury in critical care

TABLE 27-2 NORMAL SERUM ELECTROLYTE VALUES

ELECTROLYTE	NORMAL VALUE
Sodium	135-145 mEq/L
Potassium	3.5-4.5 mEq/L
Chloride	98-108 mEq/L
Calcium	8.5-10.5 mg/dL or 4.5-5.8 mEq/L
Phosphorus	2.7-4.5 mg/dL
Magnesium	1.5-2.5 mEq/L
Bicarbonate	24-28 mEq/L

Types of Acute Kidney Injury

Previously, ARF was predominantly classified by the location of the insult relative to the kidney: *prerenal* (before), *intrarenal* (within), and *postrenal* (after) (Box 27-2). This remains a useful way to imagine the relationship between anatomy and functional insults to the kidney, although it is not evident that insults classified in this manner have any impact on outcomes of patients with AKI.

Prerenal Acute Kidney Injury

Any condition that decreases blood flow, blood pressure, or kidney perfusion before arterial blood reaches the renal artery that supplies the kidney may be anatomically described as *prerenal* AKI.[1] When arterial hypoperfusion due to low cardiac output, hemorrhage, vasodilation, thrombosis, or other cause reduces the blood flow to the kidney, glomerular filtration decreases, and consequently, urine output decreases (see Box 27-2). This is a major reason the critical care nurse monitors the urine output on an hourly basis.[4,5] Initially, in prerenal states, the integrity of the kidney's nephron structure and function may be preserved. If normal perfusion and cardiac output are restored quickly, the kidney will recover and not suffer permanent injury. However, if the prerenal insult is not corrected, the GFR will decline, the blood urea nitrogen (BUN) concentration will rise (prerenal azotemia),[1] and the patient will develop oliguria and be at risk for significant kidney damage. *Oliguria*, defined as urine output less than 400 mL/day, or urine output less than 0.5 mL/kg/hr,[4] with an elevated serum creatinine, is a classic finding in AKI. Prerenal azotemia is associated with a lower mortality than other forms of AKI.[6]

Intrarenal Acute Kidney Injury

Any condition that produces an ischemic or toxic insult directly at parenchymal nephron tissue places the patient at risk for development of *intrarenal* AKI[1] (see Box 27-2). Ischemic damage may be caused by prolonged hypotension or low cardiac output. Toxic injury reaction may occur in response to substances that damage the kidney tubular endothelium, such as some antimicrobial medications and the contrast dye used in radiologic diagnostic studies. The insult may involve the glomeruli and the tubular epithelium. When the internal filtering structures are pathologically affected, the condition was previously known as *acute tubular necrosis* (ATN), although the newer term of AKI is now more often used.[1]

Postrenal Acute Kidney Injury

Any obstruction that hinders the flow of urine from beyond the kidney through the remainder of the urinary tract may lead to *postrenal* AKI. This is not a common cause of kidney failure in the critically ill.[1] When monitoring of the urine output reveals a sudden decrease in the patient's urine output from the urinary catheter, a blockage may be responsible. Sudden development of *anuria* (urine output less than 100 mL/24 hr) should prompt verification that the urinary catheter is not occluded.

Azotemia

The term *azotemia* is used to describe an acute rise in the BUN level often associated with prerenal AKI.[1,6] *Uremia* is another term used to describe an elevated BUN value.

ASSESSMENT AND DIAGNOSIS

Laboratory Assessment

After AKI is suspected, the degree of injury is assessed using blood analysis. Most serum levels of electrolytes become increasingly elevated as AKI develops (Table 27-2). Urinalysis values are also altered by AKI although these values are not predictive of outcome in critical illness. Consequently urinary electrolytes are rarely measured[1] (Table 27-3). Clinical findings associated with AKI are listed in Table 27-4. Normal and abnormal urinalysis findings and reasons for their significance are summarized in Chapter 26.

Acidosis

Acidosis (pH less than 7.35) is one of the trademarks of severe acute kidney insult. Metabolic acidosis occurs as a result of the accumulation of unexcreted waste products. The acid waste products consist of strong negative ions (anions), elevated serum phosphorus levels (hyperphosphatemia), and other normally unmeasured ions (e.g., sulfate, urate, lactate) that decrease the serum pH. A low serum albumin concentration, which often occurs in AKI, has a slight alkalinizing effect, but it is not enough to offset the metabolic acidosis. Even respiratory compensation and mechanical ventilatory support are rarely

TABLE 27-3 INITIAL URINE LABORATORY ANALYSIS FINDINGS IN ACUTE KIDNEY INJURY*

ASSESSMENT	PRERENAL[†]	INTRARENAL[‡]	POSTRENAL[§]
Urine volume	Normal	Oliguria or nonoliguria	Oliguria to anuria
Urine specific gravity	>1.020	1.010	1.000-1.010
Urine osmolality (mOsm/kg)	>350	<300	300-400
Urine sodium (mEq/L)	<20	>30	20-40
FENa (%)	<1%	>2%-3%	1%-3%
BUN/Cr ratio	20:1	Ischemic: 20:1 Toxic: 10:1	10:1
Urine microscopy (sediment)	Normal	Dark granular casts, hyaline casts, kidney epithelial cells	Normal

*Results of urine laboratory tests are valid only in the absence of diuretics.
[†]Urine in prerenal failure is concentrated, with low sodium.
[‡]Urine in intrarenal failure shows kidney damage because the nephron cannot concentrate urine or conserve sodium, and evidence of kidney damage (casts) is seen.
[§]Urine test results in postrenal failure vary because the findings initially depend on the hydration status of the patient rather than the status of the kidney.
Anuria, Urine volume less than 100 mL/24 hr; *BUN*, blood urea nitrogen; *Cr*, creatinine; *FENa*, fractional excretion of sodium; *oliguria*, urine volume of 100-400 mL/24 hr; *polyuria*, urine volume excessive over 24 hours.

sufficient to reverse the metabolic acidosis. Acidosis in AKI is complex, as evidenced by the fact that many AKI patients maintain a normal anion gap. The reasons for this remain unknown. Information on acidosis and arterial blood gas interpretation is presented in Chapter 19. Anion gap measurement is discussed in Chapter 26.

Blood Urea Nitrogen

The BUN level is not a reliable indicator of kidney injury as an individual test.[1] The BUN concentration is changed by protein intake, blood in the gastrointestinal tract, and cell catabolism, and it is diluted by fluid administration. A BUN-to-creatinine ratio may be calculated to determine the cause of the AKI (see Table 27-3). The BUN-to-creatinine ratio is most useful in diagnosing prerenal AKI (often described as prerenal azotemia), in which the BUN level is greatly elevated relative to the serum creatinine value.[6]

Serum Creatinine

Creatinine is a byproduct of muscle metabolism that is formed nonenzymatically from creatine in muscles.[7] Creatinine is completely excreted when kidney function is normal.[7] Consequently, when the kidneys are not working, the serum creatinine level rises. Even small increases in serum creatinine represent a significant decrease in GFR.[7] Serum creatinine level is assessed daily to follow the trend of kidney function and to determine whether it is stable, getting better, or getting worse.

Creatinine Clearance

If the patient is making sufficient urine, the urinary creatinine clearance can be measured. A normal urinary creatinine clearance rate is 120 mL/min, but this value decreases with kidney failure. Critical care patients with severe AKI will manifest elevated serum creatinine and may be oliguric. Consequently, the urinary creatinine clearance rate is rarely measured during critical illness.[7]

Fractional Excretion of Sodium

The fractional excretion of sodium (FENa) in the urine can be measured early in the AKI course to differentiate between prerenal AKI and inter-renal AKI (parenchymal). A FENa value below 1% (in the absence of diuretics) suggests prerenal compromise, because *resorption* of almost all the filtered sodium is an appropriate response to decreased perfusion to the kidneys. If diuretics are administered, the test is meaningless. A FENa value above 2% implies the kidney cannot concentrate the sodium and that the damage is intrarenal (ATN). FENa values do not have any predictive benefit in critical illness and are rarely measured.[1]

Urinary sodium is measured in milliequivalents per liter (mEq/L). The interpretation of results is similar to the FENa. A urinary sodium concentration less than 10 mEq/L (low) suggests a prerenal condition. A urinary sodium level greater than 40 mEq/L (in the presence of an elevated serum creatinine and the absence of a high sodium load) suggests intrarenal damage has occurred (see Table 27-2). As with other urinalysis tests, the use of diuretics invalidates any results. Because the diuretics alter resorption of water and produce dilute urine, the test result will not reflect actual kidney function.

AT-RISK DISEASE STATES AND ACUTE KIDNEY INJURY

Many patients come into the critical care unit with disease states that predispose them to the development of AKI. Many others already have kidney damage but are unaware of this condition (Fig. 27-2).

Underlying Chronic Kidney Disease

The incidence of chronic kidney disease (CKD) in United States is about 10%, or 1 in 10 people.[8] Clinical practice guidelines for the management of ESKD categorize kidney dysfunction into five stages. Because of the large numbers of adults with kidney

TABLE 27-4 SERUM ELECTROLYTES IN ACUTE KIDNEY FAILURE

ELECTROLYTE DISTURBANCE	SERUM VALUE	CLINICAL FINDINGS	ELECTROLYTE DISTURBANCE	SERUM VALUE	CLINICAL FINDINGS
Potassium			Hypercalcemia	>10.5 mg/dL or >5.8 mEq/L	Deep bone pain Excessive thirst Anorexia Lethargy, weakened muscles
Hypokalemia	<3.5 mEq/L	Muscular weakness Cardiac irregularities on ECG Abdominal distention and flatulence Paresthesia Decreased reflexes Anorexia Dizziness, confusion Increased sensitivity to digitalis	**Magnesium**		
			Hypomagnesemia	<1.4 mEq/L	Choroid or athetoid muscle activity Facial tics, spasticity Cardiac dysrhythmias
Hyperkalemia	>4.5 mEq/L	Irritability and restlessness Anxiety Nausea and vomiting Abdominal cramps Weakness Numbness and tingling (fingertips and circumoral) Cardiac irregularities on ECG	Hypermagnesemia	>2.5 mEq/L	CNS depression Respiratory depression Lethargy Coma Bradycardia Changes on ECG
Sodium			**Phosphorus**		
Hyponatremia	<135 mEq/L	Disorientation Muscle twitching Nausea, vomiting, abdominal cramps Headaches, dizziness Seizures, postural hypotension Cold, clammy skin Decreased skin turgor Tachycardia Oliguria	Hypophosphatemia	<3.0 mg/dL	Hemolytic anemias Depressed white blood cell function Bleeding (decreased platelet aggregation) Nausea, vomiting Anorexia
			Hyperphosphatemia	>4.5 mg/dL	Tachycardia Nausea, diarrhea, abdominal cramps Muscle weakness, flaccid paralysis Increased reflexes
Hypernatremia	>145 mEq/L	Extreme thirst Dry, sticky mucous membranes Altered mentation Seizures (later stages)	**Chloride**		
			Hypochloremia	<98 mEq/L	Hyperirritability Tetany or muscular excitability Slow respirations
Calcium			Hyperchloremia	>108 mEq/L	Weakness, lethargy Deep, rapid breathing Possible unconsciousness (later stages)
Hypocalcemia	<8.5 mg/dL or <4.5 mEq/L	Irritability Muscular tetany, muscle cramps Decreased cardiac output (decreased contractions) Bleeding (decreased ability to coagulate) Changes on ECG Positive Chvostek or Trousseau signs	**Albumin**		
			Hypoalbuminemia	<3.8 g/dL	Muscle wasting Peripheral edema (fluid shift) Decreased resistance to infection Poorly healing wounds

CNS, Central nervous system; *ECG,* electrocardiogram.

dysfunction (diagnosed or not), kidney function must be assessed on all critically ill patients at risk for fluid and electrolyte imbalance. The GFR associated with each stage and the numeric population estimates for each stage of kidney dysfunction are shown in Table 27-5.

Most people in the early stages of kidney disease are unaware of their condition.[9] A national health survey queried individuals about whether they had ever been told by their physician that they had "weak or failing kidneys." The answer to this question was correlated with the individual's GFR and the presence of albuminuria by urine test to stratify them according to the five stages of CKD (see Table 27-5). The results showed that more

than one half of the respondents were unaware that they had kidney dysfunction until they reached stage 5 or ESKD, when they would become dialysis dependent.[9] In contrast, the prevalence of CKD in individuals between 18 and 39 years of age is only 0.5%.[8] CKD results, categorized by stage of CKD, are listed in Table 27-5.

Older Age and Acute Kidney Injury

Among adults older than 60 years, the prevalence of CKD in the United States is close to 25%.[8] The numbers of older adults with CKD is increasing in tandem with the increase in diabetes and hypertension in the U.S. population.[10]

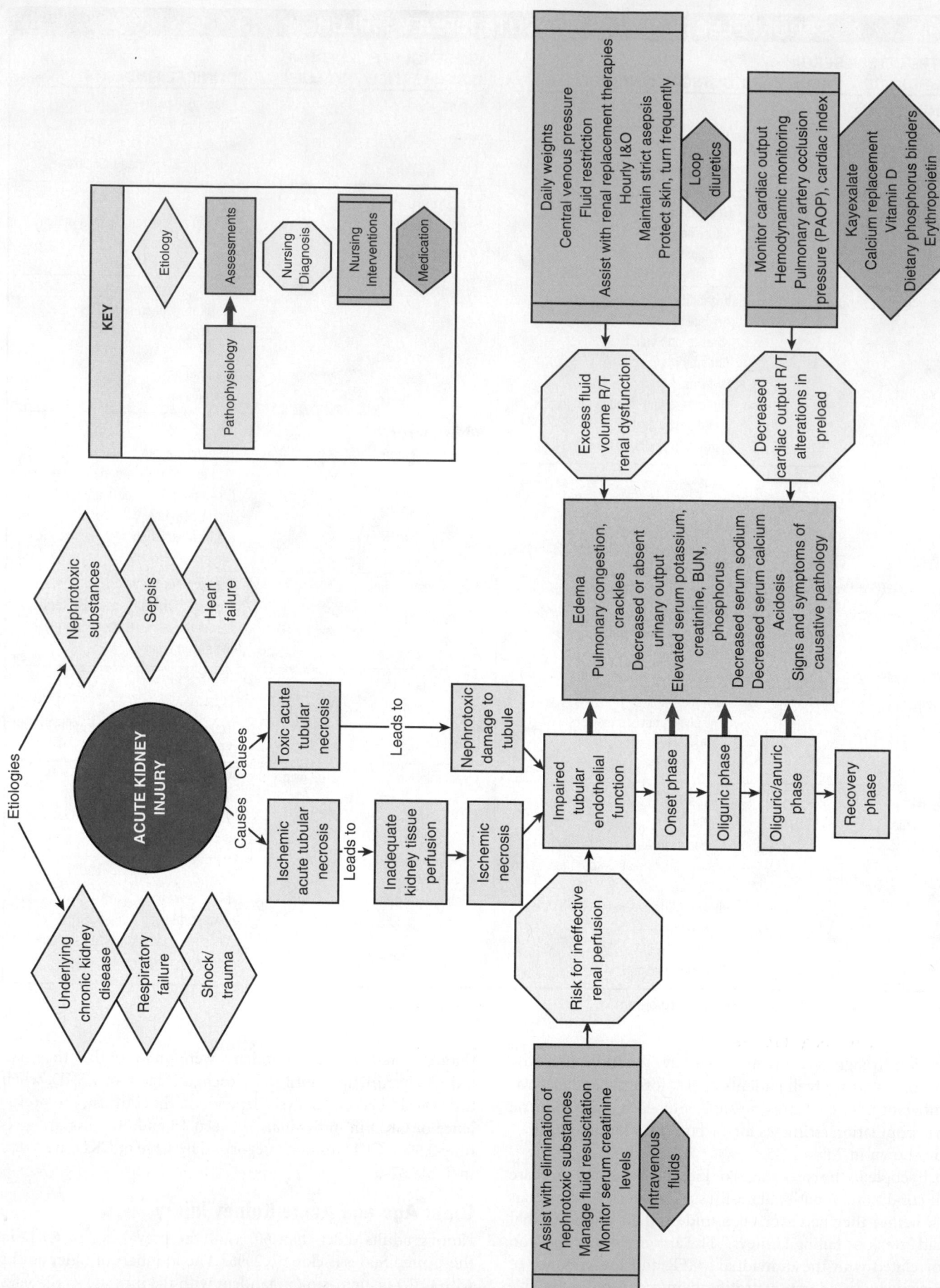

FIGURE 27-2   Concept Map for Acute Kidney Injury. (Concept map illustration created by Elaine Bishop Kennedy, EdD, RN.)

TABLE 27-5	DECREASED KIDNEY FUNCTION BY STAGE IN ADULT U.S. POPULATION		
STAGE*	POPULATION AFFECTED*	GFR AND DIAGNOSIS*	PERCENTAGE WHO KNOW THEY HAVE KIDNEY DYSFUNCTION (%)[†]
1	9 million (3.3%)	Normal; persistent albuminuria	40.5
2	5.3 million (3.0%)	60 to 89; persistent albuminuria	29.3
3	7.6 million (4.3%)	30 to 59	22.0
4	400,000 (0.2%)	15 to 29	44.5
5	300,000 (0.2%)	Below 15: ESKD	100

*Data from Coresh J, et al. Prevalence of chronic kidney disease and decreased kidney function in the adult US population: Third National Health and Nutrition Examination Survey. *Am J Kidney Dis.* 2003;41(1):1.
[†]Data from Nickolas TL, et al. Awareness of kidney disease in the US population: findings from the National Health and Nutrition Examination Survey (NHANES) 1999 to 2000. *Am J Kidney Dis.* 2004;44(2):185.
ESKD, End-stage kidney disease; *GFR,* glomerular filtration rate (mL/min/1.73 m² of body surface area).

Heart Failure and Acute Kidney Injury

There is a strong association between kidney failure and heart failure.[11] In studies of critically ill patients with AKI, 54%[3] have acute kidney failure and heart failure. Not all patients with kidney failure and heart failure have the same pathology, and this variation has been recognized. Heart-kidney interactions have been categorized into five subtypes under the term *cardiorenal syndromes.*[12] The purpose of the new classification system is to identify relevant biomarkers, treatments, and future avenues for research.[12]

Several of the risk factors for atherosclerotic cardiovascular disease are also detrimental to the kidney over the long term, notably hypertension and diabetes. Maintenance of a BP below 130/80 mm Hg and a blood glucose within the normal range decrease the risk of both developing CKD and the atherosclerotic cardiac diseases such as coronary artery disease or peripheral arterial disease.

Respiratory Failure and Acute Kidney Injury

There is a significant association between respiratory failure and kidney failure. In studies of critically ill patients with kidney failure, over 50% have respiratory failure.[3] Mechanical ventilation can alter kidney function. Positive-pressure ventilation reduces blood flow to the kidney, lowers the GFR, and decreases urine output.[13] These effects are intensified with the addition of positive end-expiratory pressure (PEEP).[13] AKI increases inflammation, causes the lung vasculature to become more permeable, and contributes to the development of acute respiratory distress syndrome (ARDS). Patients with AKI are more likely to require prolonged mechanical ventilatory support.[14,15]

Sepsis and Acute Kidney Injury

Sepsis causes almost half of the cases of AKI in the critically ill.[1] Sepsis and septic shock create hemodynamic instability and reduce perfusion to the kidney. Immunologic, toxic, and inflammatory factors may alter the function of the kidney microvasculature and tubular cells. Clinical guidelines for hemodynamic support in sepsis emphasize the need for adequate fluid resuscitation, because reversal of hypotension and restoration of hemodynamic stability can often be achieved with fluids alone.[16] Unfortunately, in severely septic patients, inflammation increases vascular permeability, and much of this fluid may move into the third space (interstitial space). If the blood pressure remains low, the use of vasopressors is recommended to raise refractory low blood pressure after volume resuscitation.[16] Vasopressors raise blood pressure and increase systemic vascular resistance (SVR), but they also may raise the vascular resistance within the kidney microvasculature. Other practices aimed at reversing the deleterious effects of sepsis include maintaining the patient's hemoglobin level at 7 to 9 g/dL and blood glucose level below 150 mg/dL and ensuring optimal hydration as evidenced by a central venous pressure above 8 mm Hg.[16]

Trauma and Acute Kidney Injury
Trauma Admissions

Trauma patients have different demographics from those of other critical care populations. They are always emergency admissions, are younger, are more often male, and have fewer coexisting illnesses.[17] A 5-year retrospective study of 9449 trauma admissions to critical care units in Australia and New Zealand used the RIFLE criteria to determine incidence of AKI in the first 24 hours after admission; 18% of trauma patients developed AKI.[17] However, if patients were older or had preexisting comorbid illnesses, their risk of AKI rose to 35%.[17] Although these AKI numbers are high, they likely underestimate the true incidence because the study did not include patients who developed AKI later than 24 hours after admission to the critical care unit.[17]

Rhabdomyolysis

Trauma patients with major crush injuries have an elevated risk of kidney failure because of the release of creatine and myoglobin from damaged muscle cells, a condition called *rhabdomyolysis.*[18] Myoglobin in large quantities is toxic to the kidney. A major goal of treatment is to prevent rhabdomyolysis-induced AKI. Mortality rate is low, provided adequate crystalloid volume is administered early in the course of treatment.[19] It is important to trend the serum potassium levels. Life-threatening hyperkalemia can occur as cell lysis permits intracellular potassium to be released into the bloodstream.[20]

The level of creatine kinase (CK), a marker of systemic muscle damage, increases in patients with rhabdomyolysis. One trauma service reported that of 2083 critical care trauma admissions, 85% had elevated CK levels, and 10% developed AKI resulting from rhabdomyolysis.[21] A CK level of 5000 units/L was the lowest abnormal value in patients who developed AKI associated with rhabdomyolysis.[21]

Crystalloid volume resuscitation is the primary treatment for preservation of adequate kidney function and prevention of AKI. In many hospitals, the intravenous (IV) fluids are alkalinized by the addition of sodium bicarbonate, and the urine output is increased by IV administration of the diuretic mannitol. A bicarbonate and mannitol regimen is instituted to prevent acidosis and hyperkalemia, because both are frequent complications of rhabdomyolysis. Close attention is paid to hourly urine output that can be dark brown or tea-colored,[19] CK levels, serum creatinine levels, serum potassium levels, and any signs of compartment syndrome in all patients admitted with this diagnosis.

Contrast-Induced Nephrotoxic Injury and Acute Kidney Injury

More than 1 million radiologic studies or procedures that involve use of IV radiopaque contrast are performed every year. Approximately 1% of those patients will require dialysis as a result of contrast-induced nephrotoxicity (CIN).[22] Patients at highest risk are those with pre-existing CKD, baseline serum creatinine levels more than 1.5 mg/dL, dehydration, diabetes, heart failure, or advanced age (older than 75 years).[23,24] The clinical definition of CIN is an increase in serum creatinine concentration of 0.5 mg/dL or more, or a 25% increase from the patient's baseline within 3 days of contrast medium exposure, without an alternative clinical explanation for development of AKI.[23] The effects of reversible, contrast-induced AKI may not be limited to the immediate hospitalization; it has been linked to increased mortality in the 5-year period after the reversible AKI, compared with similar patients who did not have kidney injury.[25]

Radiopaque Contrast

High–molecular-weight contrast medium is a potential cause of nephrotoxicity. A recommended strategy to prevent CIN involves use of a lower quantity of contrast per study and use of nonionic, low-osmolar or iso-osmolar (iohexol) contrast media that are less nephrotoxic.[23]

Promote Hydration and Avoid Dehydration

The best method of prevention is aggressive hydration with IV normal saline during and after the procedure.[23] After some diagnostic intravascular catheterization procedures, the alert patient is asked to drink several liters of water over a 12-hour period to protect the kidney. Avoiding dehydration is vital.

Medications

The addition of sodium bicarbonate, because of its alkalinizing effect, may confer protection to the vulnerable kidney beyond hydration with normal saline only.[23] Other strategies such as adjunctive use of N-acetylcysteine or hemofiltration have shown conflicting results in research studies and are not recommended.[23]

Potentially nephrotoxic medications are also stopped before the procedure. Metformin, a medication that decreases insulin resistance in type 2 diabetes, has been associated with lactic acidosis in rare instances.[23] For patients with elevated serum creatinine, Metformin is stopped the day before any procedure involving contrast and not started again for 48 hours when serum creatinine has returned to baseline.[24]

In summary, the mainstay measures to protect the kidney from contrast-induced AKI are to use the smallest dose of low- or iso-osmolar contrast media possible, provide vigorous fluid volume expansion, stop all nephrotoxic medications, and avoid repeat contrast media injections within 48 hours.

Catheter-Associated Urinary Tract Infection

The majority of critically ill patients have a urinary drainage catheter inserted to accurately record urine output.[26] This is an appropriate use of a urinary catheter. However, because of the risk of catheter-associated urinary tract infection (CAUTI), the catheter should be removed as soon as clinically feasible.[27] Critically ill patients who have a protracted illness have a significant risk of contracting a CAUTI, especially if the catheter is required for several days.[28] Additionally, critically ill patients who have developed a CAUTI have a higher mortality and longer lengths of stay.[29]

The focus on prevention of CAUTI has gained considerable momentum. The Centers for Medicare and Medicaid Services (CMS) will no longer provide reimbursement for hospital-acquired CAUTI because it is considered a preventable infection. The Joint Commission has added prevention of CAUTI as a 2012 patient safety goal.[30] Currently only 40% of hospitals routinely collect data on the rates of CAUTI in critical care units as part of a prevention and monitoring program.[31,32] Prevention is the best cure, and many critical care units have adopted a "bundle" approach to eliminate CAUTI.[33,34] The key components of CAUTI prevention are listed below[26]:

1. Avoid unnecessary use of urinary catheters
2. Insert urinary catheters using aseptic technique
3. Adopt evidence-based standards for maintenance of urinary catheters
4. Review the need for the urinary catheter daily and remove promptly

Interventions to prevent CAUTI are listed in the Box 27-3.

Hemodynamic Monitoring and Fluid Balance

Hemodynamic monitoring is important for the analysis of fluid volume status in the critically ill patient with AKI.

Hemodynamic Monitoring

Hemodynamic monitoring includes surveillance of the central venous pressure, pulmonary artery occlusion pressure, cardiac output, and cardiac index.[35]

Daily Weight

A less high-tech method but also important is a daily weight and focused physical assessment. The daily weight, combined with accurate intake and output monitoring, is a powerful indicator of fluid gains or losses over 24 hours. A 1-kg weight gain over 24 hours represents 1000 mL (1 liter) of additional fluid retention.

⚡ BOX 27-3 PATIENT SAFETY ALERT

Prevention of Catheter-Associated Urinary Tract infections (CAUTI)

QSEN **1. Avoid Unnecessary Use of Indwelling Urinary Catheters**

Critical Care Indications

Accurate measurements of urinary output

Prolonged immobilization (e.g., potentially unstable thoracic or lumbar spine, multiple traumatic injuries such as pelvic fractures)

Perioperative Indications

Urologic or genitourinary tract surgery

Prolonged duration of surgery (catheters inserted for this reason should be removed in the post-anesthesia care unit [PACU])

Large-volume infusions or diuretics administered during surgery

Intraoperative monitoring of urinary output

Other Indications

Acute urinary retention or bladder outlet obstruction

Assist in healing of open sacral or perineal wounds in incontinent patients

Improve comfort for end-of-life care if needed

2. Inset Urinary Catheters Using Aseptic Technique

Hand Hygiene

Wash hands thoroughly before or after any patient-care activity

Use gloves when touching the catheter site or meatus

Sterile Technique and Sterile Equipment

Use standard supply kits that contain all necessary items:

- Sterile gloves, drape, sponges, antiseptic solution for cleaning the meatus, single-use packet of lubricant jelly for insertion
- Use as small a catheter as possible to minimize urethral trauma
- Single attempt to insert urinary catheter
- Use new catheter if second attempt at catheterization is required

3. Adopt Evidence-Based Standards for Maintenance of Urinary Catheters

Maintenance of a Closed Drainage System

Maintain a sterile closed drainage system

Maintain unobstructed urine flow (avoid dependent loops)

Keep drainage bag below the level of the bladder at all times

Do not allow drainage bag to touch the floor

Empty the collection bag regularly, using a separate container for each patient

Do not allow the drainage spigot to touch the collection container

Do not break the system to collect a urine sample. Collect from sampling port in the tubing drainage system, disinfecting the port and aspirating using aseptic technique

Avoid catheter irrigation except in the case of an obstructed catheter; use a bladder ultrasound scan to determine if there is urine in the bladder

Routine scheduled replacement of catheters is not recommended

Catheter Securement and Hygiene

Keep urinary catheter secured to prevent catheter movement and urethral friction

Do not clean periurethral area with antiseptics. Urethral cleaning during a bath is appropriate

4. Review the Need for the Urinary Catheter Daily and Remove Promptly

Documentation and Monitoring

Document when the catheter was inserted

Nurses and physicians should review the need for the urinary catheter for every patient every day

Hospital Strategies to Ensure Early Removal of Urinary Catheters

Ensure clinicians are aware that longer duration of catheter use increases CAUTI risk. This awareness can be reinforced by:

- Alerts in computerized ordering systems
- Automatic stops on catheter orders at 24, 48, 72 hours, depending on the clinical situation
- Development of standardized nursing protocols that allow nurses to remove urinary catheters if predetermined criteria are met

Know Your Own CAUTI Data

Each critical care unit should make sure that all nurses and physicians are aware of their unit/patient statistics on CAUTI per 1000 catheter days

Publicize the strategies used to prevent CAUTI

Based on data from Gould CV, et al. *Guideline for prevention of catheter associated urinary tract infections 2009*. Centers for Disease Control and Prevention. http://www.cdc.gov/hicpac/pdf/cauti/cautiguideline2009final.pdf. 2009. Accessed September 15, 2012.

Physical Assessment

Physical signs and symptoms are used to assess fluid balance. Signs that suggest extracellular fluid (ECF) depletion include thirst, decreased skin turgor, and lethargy. Signs that imply intravascular fluid volume overload include pulmonary congestion, increasing heart failure, and rising blood pressure. The patient with untreated AKI is edematous. Several factors contribute to this state:

1. Fluid retention caused by inadequate urine output.
2. Low serum albumin levels create a lower oncotic pressure in the vasculature, and more fluid seeps out into the interstitial spaces to cause peripheral edema.
3. Inflammation associated with AKI or a coexisting nonrenal disease increases vascular permeability, facilitating fluid movement from the vessels into interstitial spaces.

In critical illness, even though there is peripheral edema, and the patient may have gained 8 L of fluid over his or her "dry-weight" baseline, the patient may remain "intravascularly dry"

and hemodynamically unstable, because the retained fluid is not inside a vascular compartment and cannot contribute to maintenance of hemodynamic stability. The patient with AKI is assessed frequently for pitting edema over bony prominences and in dependent body areas.

Electrolyte Balance

Potassium

Electrolyte levels require frequent observation, especially in the critical phases of AKI when potassium can quickly reach levels of 6.0 mEq/L or higher (see Table 27-4). Specific electrocardiographic changes are associated with hyperkalemia: peaked T waves, a widening of the QRS interval, and ultimately, ventricular tachycardia or fibrillation.[36] If hyperkalemia is identified, all potassium supplements are stopped. If the patient is producing urine, IV diuretics can be administered. Acute hyperkalemia can be treated temporarily by IV administration of insulin and glucose. An infusion of 50 mL of 50% dextrose accompanied by 10 units of regular insulin forces potassium out of the serum and into the cells.

To treat smaller increases in serum potassium, nonabsorbable potassium-binding resins may be used.[37] The binding resins can be administered orally, through a nasogastric tube, or rectally, to treat hyperkalemia. Cation exchange resins employ either sodium (Kayexalate) or calcium (Sorbisterit, Ca-Resonium, Argamate) and exchange the cation for potassium across the gastrointestinal wall.[38] The potassium is contained in the lower gastrointestinal tract and is eliminated with the stool. Potassium-binding resins and dialysis are the only permanent methods of potassium removal to treat hyperkalemia.

Sodium

Alterations in sodium level are an expected finding in kidney failure (see Table 27-4). Both hypernatremia (elevated serum sodium) and hyponatremia (low serum sodium) are associated with increased mortality with kidney failure[39]; this is unrelated to whether the patient has a diagnosis of heart failure or not.[39]

Calcium and Phosphorus

Serum calcium levels are reduced (hypocalcemia) in kidney failure (see Table 27-4). This reduction results from multiple factors, including hyperphosphatemia. Chronically elevated serum phosphorus levels, above 5.5 mg/dL, are associated with higher mortality rates for patients with kidney failure.[40,41] Calcium and phosphorus levels are regulated by a complex physiologic feedback mechanism involving parathyroid hormone (PTH) and fibroblast growth factor (FGF-23).[42] Normally, PTH helps calcium be resorbed back into the bloodstream at the proximal tubule and distal nephron, and it promotes excretion of phosphorus by the kidney to maintain homeostasis. In kidney failure, this mechanism is nonfunctional; the serum phosphorus level rises, and the serum calcium level falls.[40,41]

Calcium Replacement

Most calcium in the bloodstream is bound to protein. Calcium levels can be measured in two ways: total calcium (tCa) or ionized calcium (iCa). Unfortunately, protein–calcium binding confounds the measurement of accurate calcium levels. In the past, calculations were used to estimate the amounts of protein-bound versus unbound calcium, but these calculations have been shown to produce inaccurate results. The metabolically active, non–protein-bound portion is known as the *ionized calcium* and is the preferred method of measurement.[43] Without adequate levels of serum calcium, a compensatory mechanism "steals" calcium from the bones, making the patient with kidney failure more vulnerable to fractures. Maintaining adequate calcium stores in the body is important and is achieved by administration of calcium supplements and vitamin D.[41]

Dietary–Phosphorus-Binding Medications

A second method used in tandem with calcium supplements to achieve normal calcium levels is to lower the level of phosphorus in the bloodstream.[40] Phosphorus occurs in many foods, especially those with a high protein content or food additives such as dairy products, processed meats, some carbonated drinks, and nuts.[44] After eating these foods, free phosphorus passes from the gastrointestinal tract into the bloodstream and raises the serum level. Medications that bind dietary phosphorus in the gastrointestinal tract are administered orally or by nasogastric tube. The binding agent must be taken at the same time as a meal. After the dietary phosphorus is bound to the binding substance in the bowel, it is eliminated from the intestine with stool.[40] This lowers the serum phosphorus level.

The types of dietary-phosphorus binders used have changed over the years. The original binders were aluminum salts (aluminum hydroxide) that bound dietary phosphorus effectively in the gastrointestinal tract but conferred aluminum toxicity because some of the aluminum metal was also absorbed. For this reason, aluminum binders have largely been abandoned.[40]

The second generation of dietary–phosphorus-binding agents that are widely prescribed use calcium salts: calcium carbonate, or calcium acetate (PhosLo), to bind dietary phosphorus in the gastrointestinal tract. Calcium-based medications are safer, but elevated serum calcium levels and calcium deposits in other areas of the body (extraosseous calcification) are a problem.

A third generation of nonabsorbable dietary–phosphorus-binding medications is available. These are non-aluminum-, non–calcium-based medications. They include sevelamer hydrochloride (RenaGel) and lanthanum carbonate (Fosrenol). These medications have a good safety profile and are frequently prescribed to lower serum phosphorus levels in CKD.[40]

Medical Management
Treatment Goals

Treatment goals for patients with AKI focus on prevention, compensation for the deterioration of kidney function, and regeneration of kidney functional capacity. Key treatment areas include prevention strategies, fluid balance, anemia, medications, and electrolyte imbalance.

Prevention

The only truly effective remedy for AKI is prevention. Effective prevention requires assessment of the patient's risk for AKI. Knowledge of the most frequent causes of AKI in the critically ill is essential if prevention strategies are to be enacted. The critical care team collaborates closely with the clinical pharmacist to avoid medications with nephrotoxic side effects in patients with AKI or CKD.[23] Nonsteroidal anti-inflammatory medications (NSAIDs) for pain relief are avoided in patients with elevated creatinine levels. The use of intravascular contrast dye is preferably delayed until the patient is fully rehydrated.

Fluid Resuscitation

Prerenal failure is caused by decreased perfusion and flow to the kidney. It is often associated with trauma, hemorrhage, hypotension, and major fluid losses. If contrast dye is used, aggressive fluid resuscitation with normal saline (NaCl) is recommended. The objectives of volume replacement are to replace fluid and electrolyte losses and to prevent ongoing loss. Maintenance IV fluid therapy is initiated when oral fluid intake is inadvisable. Maintenance fluids are calculated with consideration for individual body surface area. Adults require approximately 1500 mL/ m^2/24 hr; fever, burns, and trauma significantly increase fluid requirements. Other important criteria when calculating fluid volume replacement include baseline metabolism, environmental temperature, and humidity. The rate of replacement depends on cardiopulmonary reserve, adequacy of kidney function, urine output, fluid balance, ongoing loss, and type of fluid replaced.

Crystalloids and Colloids. Crystalloids and colloids refer to two different types of IV fluids used for volume management in critically ill patients. These IV solutions are used on all types of patients, not just those with acute kidney failure. Adequacy of IV fluid replacement depends on strict, ongoing evaluation and frequent adjustment. Frequent monitoring of serum electrolyte levels is required, and strictly regulated intake and output are correlated with daily weight records. In septic shock, hemodynamic readings are frequently undertaken. After a fluid challenge, a merely minimal increase in central venous pressure implies that additional fluid replacement is required. Continued decreases in central venous pressure, pulmonary artery occlusion pressure, and the cardiac index indicate ongoing volume losses.

Which IV fluid to select to successfully resuscitate hemodynamically unstable patients has been a controversial topic in critical care. The debate centers on the differences between crystalloid and colloid solutions.

Crystalloids. Crystalloid solutions, which are balanced salt solutions, are in widespread use for maintenance infusion and replacement therapy. Crystalloid fluids include normal saline solution (0.9 NaCl), half-strength saline solution (0.45 NaCl), and lactated Ringer (LR) solution (Table 27-6). LR solution usually is avoided in patients with kidney failure because it contains potassium. A noncrystalloid solution that may be infused is dextrose (5% or 10%) in water (D_5W, $D_{10}W$).

Colloids. Colloids are solutions containing oncotically active particles that are used to expand intravascular volume to achieve and maintain hemodynamic stability. Albumin (5% and 25%)

TABLE 27-6   FREQUENTLY USED INTRAVENOUS SOLUTIONS

SOLUTION	ELECTROLYTES	INDICATIONS
Crystalloids*		
Dextrose in water (D_5W), isotonic	None	Maintain volume Replace mild loss Provide minimal calories
Normal saline solution (0.9% NaCl)	Sodium: 154 mEq/L Chloride: 154 mEq/L Osmolality: 308 mEq/L	Maintain volume Replace mild loss Correct mild hyponatremia
Half-strength saline solution (0.45% NaCl)	Sodium: 77 mEq/L Chloride: 77 mEq/L	Free water replacement Correct mild hyponatremia Free water and electrolyte replacement (fluid- and electrolyte-restricted conditions)
Lactated Ringer solution	Sodium: 130 mEq/L Potassium: 4 mEq/L Calcium: 2.7 mEq/L Chloride: 107 mEq/L Lactate: 27 mEq/L pH: 6.5	Fluid and electrolyte replacement (contraindicated for patients with kidney or liver disease or in lactic acidosis)
Colloids		
5% Albumin (Albumisol)	Albumin: 50 g/L Sodium: 130-160 mEq/L Potassium: 1 mEq/L Osmolality: 300 mOsm/L Osmotic pressure: 20 mm Hg pH: 6.4 to 7.4	Volume expansion Moderate protein replacement Achievement of hemodynamic stability in shock states
25% Albumin (salt-poor)	Albumin: 240 g/L Globulins: 10 g/L Sodium: 130-160 mEq/L Osmolality: 1500 mOsm/L pH: 6.4 to 7.4	Concentrated form of albumin sometimes used with diuretics to move fluid from tissues into the vascular space for diuresis
Hetastarch	Sodium: 154 mEq/L Chloride: 154 mEq/L Osmolality: 310 mOsm/L Colloid osmotic pressure: 30-35 mm Hg	Synthetic polymer (6% solution) used for volume expansion Hemodynamic volume replacement after cardiac surgery, burns, sepsis
Low–molecular-weight dextran (LMWD)	Glucose polysaccharide molecules with average molecular weight of 40,000; no electrolytes	Volume expansion and support (contraindicated for patients with bleeding disorders)
High–molecular-weight dextran (HMWD)	Glucose polysaccharide molecules with average molecular weight of 70,000; no electrolytes	Used prophylactically in some cases to prevent platelet aggregation; available in saline and glucose solutions

*For crystalloid solutions that contain electrolytes, specific concentrations of electrolytes and pH vary according to the manufacturer.

and hetastarch are colloid solutions (see Table 27-6). Colloids expand intravascular volume, and the effect can last as long as 24 hours, although the use of colloids in critical care volume resuscitation is discouraged because of increased cost without evidence of increased benefit.[45]

The controversy over whether colloids or crystalloid IV fluids are most effective for volume resuscitation appears to have been put to rest by a series of randomized clinical trials and meta-analytic reviews. The SAFE study (*saline versus albumin fluid evaluation*) was a randomized, prospective, double-blind trial that examined whether the selection of resuscitation fluid in the critical care unit affected survival at 28 days.[45] This was a huge study, with almost 7000 critical care patients randomized to two similar groups. One group received 4% albumin, and the other group received 0.9 normal saline (NaCl) for fluid resuscitation.[45] The patients in both groups were similar in terms of organ dysfunction, mechanical ventilator support (64% of patients), and renal replacement therapy (1% of patients). The SAFE results showed that there was no difference in the mortality rate, time in the critical care unit, ventilator days, or renal replacement therapy days.[45] The researchers concluded that albumin and saline should be considered clinically equivalent treatments for intravascular volume expansion in critically ill patients.[45] The exception was for patients with traumatic brain injury (TBI), in which case albumin was associated with a higher mortality rate.[46]

The findings of the SAFE study investigators have been validated by a systematic review of randomized trials of crystalloids versus colloids that reported no difference in mortality rates for the critically ill and injured based on resuscitation fluid.[47] Consequently, colloids are not favored because of their higher cost, and crystalloids are the recommended fluid to use for resuscitation in critical care.

Fluid Restriction. Fluid restriction constitutes a large part of the medical treatment for acute kidney failure. Fluid restriction is used to prevent circulatory overload and the development of interstitial edema when the kidneys cannot remove excess volume. The fluid requirements are calculated on the basis of daily urine volumes and insensible losses. Obtaining daily weight measurements and keeping accurate intake and output records is essential. Patients with kidney failure are usually restricted to 1 L of fluid per 24 hours if the urine output is 500 mL or less. Insensible losses range from 500 to 750 mL/day.

Fluid Removal. Acute kidney failure results in retention of water, solutes, and potential toxins in the circulation, and prompt measures are needed to decrease their levels. Diuretics are used to stimulate the urine output in the early stages of AKI. Renal replacement therapy (hemodialysis or hemofiltration) is another choice, particularly if volume overload exacerbates pulmonary edema or heart failure.

Pharmacologic Management

The first step is to stop all nephrotoxic medications. Second, if medications are eliminated through the kidneys, it is important to decrease the frequency of administration (e.g., from every 6 hours to every 12 or 24 hours) or to decrease the dose and to monitor the concentration by measuring serum medication levels.

Diuretics

Diuretics are used to stimulate urinary output in the fluid overloaded patient with functioning kidneys. Care must be taken in their use to avoid the creation of secondary electrolyte abnormalities (Table 27-7). Diuretics reduce volume overload and are helpful for symptoms such as pulmonary edema, but they have not been shown to prevent AKI.[48] Diuretics are used in many patient populations other than those with incipient kidney failure.

Loop Diuretics. Loop diuretics include furosemide (Lasix), bumetanide (Bumex), and torsemide (Torsemide).[49] Furosemide is the most frequently used diuretic in critical care patients. It may be administered orally, as an IV bolus, or as a continuous IV infusion. Electrolytic abnormalities are frequently encountered, and close monitoring of serum potassium, magnesium, and sodium is essential. Loop diuretics block the Na-K-2Cl transporter in the nephron on ascending limb of the loop of Henle, where most sodium is reabsorbed (Fig. 27-3). This diuresis is also a *natriuresis* as sodium is excreted in the urine. Diuretic resistance can develop over time in patients with chronic heart failure or kidney failure who were taking loop diuretics at home before they were admitted to the hospital.[50] Their higher diuretic medication dosages are a reflection of diuretic resistance.[50]

Thiazide Diuretics. Diuretics from different classes may be prescribed in combination. A thiazide diuretic such as chlorothiazide (Diuril) or metolazone (Zaroxolyn) may be administered and followed by a loop diuretic to take advantage of the fact that these medications work on different parts of the nephron[51] (see Fig. 27-3). Creatinine clearance impacts the efficacy of thiazide diuretics. Metolazone is a more effective diuretic in kidney failure when the creatinine clearance is below 30 mL/min. A normal creatinine clearance is 120 mL/min (see Table 27-7). Sometimes a thiazide diuretic is added to a loop diuretic to compensate for the development of loop diuretic resistance.[50]

Osmotic Diuretics. Osmotic diuretics, such as mannitol, are prescribed to increase urine output and decrease fluid overload. It is important to use an in-line 5-micron filter when administering this IV medication. Mannitol is frequently administered for patients with brain injury and increased intracranial pressure (ICP). More information on the use of mannitol in the neuroscience population can be found in Chapter 24. Mannitol is filtered by the glomerulus, not absorbed by the nephron, and works in the proximal tubule and the descending section of the loop of Henle via aquaporin water channels[49] (see Fig. 27-3).

Carbonic Anhydrase Inhibitor Diuretics. Only one carbonic anhydrase inhibitor acts as a diuretic and it is used in very specific clinical circumstances. Acetazolamide (Diamox) acts on the proximal tubule where it inhibits the carbonic anhydrase enzyme allowing more bicarbonate (HCO_3^-) to be released into the filtrate resulting in an alkaline diuresis (see Fig. 27-3). Acetazolamide is administered to treat the metabolic alkalosis that sometimes occurs following aggressive diuresis with loop diuretics.[52] Acid–base balance and serum bicarbonate levels are frequently monitored when acetazolamide is used to treat metabolic alkalosis (see Table 27-7).

TABLE 27-7 PHARMACOLOGIC MANAGEMENT

Kidney-Related Medications

MEDICATION	DOSAGE	ACTION	SPECIAL CONSIDERATIONS
Diuretics			
Loop Diuretics			
Furosemide	20-80 mg/day (Lasix)	Acts on loop of Henle to inhibit sodium and chloride resorption (natriuresis)	Ototoxicity if administered too rapidly or with other ototoxic medications
Bumetanide	0.5-2 mg/day (Bumex)		Monitor intake and output, hydration; monitor for hypotension
Thiazide Diuretics			
Chlorothiazide (Diuril)	500 mg-1 g/day PO/IV	Inhibits sodium, chloride resorption in distal tubule	Enhanced with low-sodium diet
			Synergistic effect with loop diuretics
Metolazone (Zaroxolyn)	2.5-10 mg/day PO initial dose May increase to 20 mg/day with edema	Inhibits sodium, chloride resorption in distal tubule	Effective to a creatinine clearance of 10 mL/min
Osmotic Diuretics			
Mannitol	0.25-1.0 g/kg IV infusion as a 15%-20% solution over 30-90 min	Increases urine output because higher plasma osmolality	Often used in head injury to decrease cerebral edema
		Increases flow of water from tissues, causing increased GFR	Can be used to promote urinary secretion of toxic substances
		Increases serum sodium, potassium levels	At low temperatures mannitol may crystallize, use in-line 5-micron IV filter with >15% (>15 g/100 mL) solutions
Potassium-Sparing Diuretics			
Spironolactone (Aldactone)	100 mg/day for 5 days PO	Exert effects on collecting duct; retains potassium, increases sodium diuresis	Weak diuretic effect
			Potassium supplements not required; monitor for hyperkalemia
			Used as an aldosterone blocker to treat heart failure
Vaptans			
Conivaptan (Vaprisol)	Loading dose: 20 mg IV as 30 min infusion Continuous IV infusion: 20 mg over 24 hours After first day, can be increased to 40 mg/24 hours Maximum infusion is 4 days	Blocks V2 aquaporin channels in collecting tubules	Used only in hyponatremia with hypervolemia
			Monitor volume status and serum sodium frequently

BP, Blood pressure; *ECG*, electrocardiogram; *GFR*, glomerular filtration rate; *GI*, gastrointestinal; *IV*, intravenous; *PO*, by mouth.

Potassium Sparing Diuretics. Spironolactone (Aldactone) is a "potassium sparing" diuretic. Spironolactone inhibits the aldosterone mineralocorticoid receptor in the late distal tubule and collecting duct of the kidneys causing potassium to be retained and sodium to be excreted (see Fig. 27-3). At high dosages it has a diuretic action, although that is rarely the rationale behind its use today. Spironolactone is most often administered as an *aldosterone antagonist* in the management of heart failure.

Vaptans. A new class of medications collectively described as *vaptans* inhibit the effect of antidiuretic hormone (vasopressin) on the V2 aquaporin channels in the collecting ducts of the kidney (see Fig. 27-3). Blockage of the aquaporin channels renders the collecting ducts impermeable, resulting in solute-free water excretion or *aquadiuresis.*[53] Vaptans are used to correct symptomatic hypervolemic hyponatremic (dilutional) states. The clinical intent is to eliminate water and retain sodium. These medications must not be administered for hypovolemic hyponatremia or anuria. Conditions that can cause dilutional hyponatremia include *Syndrome of Inappropriate Antidiuretic Hormone Secretion* (SIADH) described in Chapter 33, liver cirrhosis with ascites, and heart failure. Only two vaptans are FDA approved in the United States. Conivaptan (Vaprisol), which is administered IV, is approved for short-term use in the hospital only (see Table 27-7). Tolvaptan (Samsca) is only available as an oral medication.[53]

Dopamine

Low-dose dopamine (2 to 3 mcg/kg/min), previously known as renal-dose dopamine, is frequently infused to stimulate blood flow to the kidney. Dopamine is effective in increasing urine output in the short term, but tolerance of the dopamine renal receptor to the medication is theorized to develop in the critically ill patients who are most at risk for AKI. Renal-dose dopamine does not prevent onset of AKI, decrease the need for dialysis or reduce mortality.[1] At this point, the support for routine use of low-dose dopamine for the prevention of AKI remains anecdotal only. Although low-dose dopamine

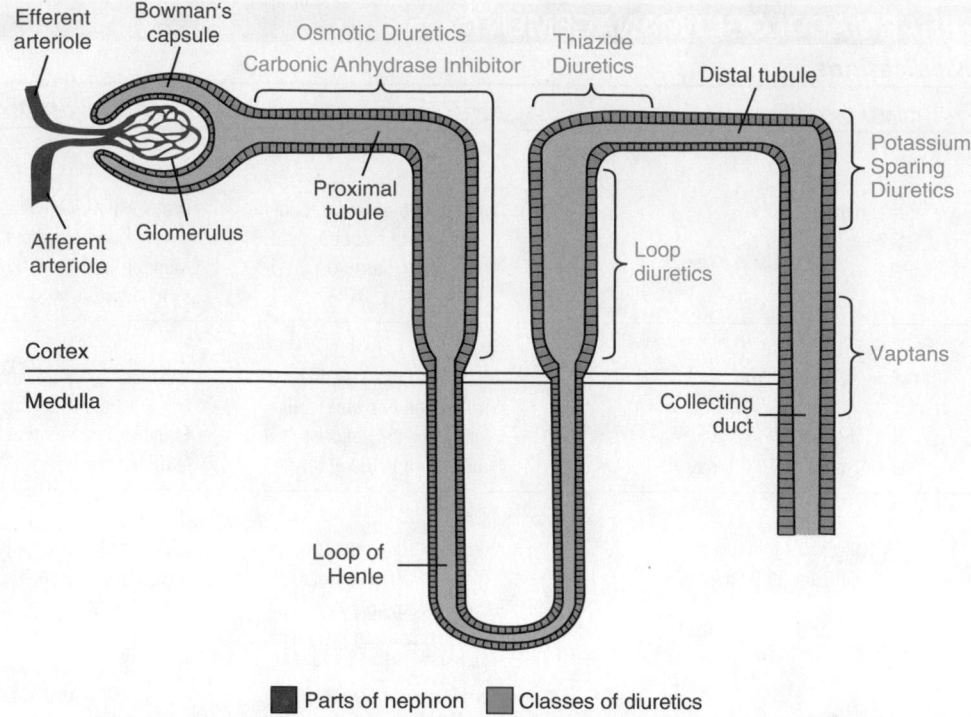

■ Parts of nephron   ■ Classes of diuretics

FIGURE 27-3   Pharmacologic site of action of diuretics in the nephron.

infusions may have other therapeutic uses, such as increasing urine output, in combination with furosemide, in heart failure patients.[54]

Acetylcysteine

N-Acetylcysteine (Mucomyst, Mucosil) is an *N*-acetyl derivative of the amino acid l-cysteine. It has been used for many years as a mucolytic agent to assist with expectoration of thick pulmonary secretions. It is also frequently prescribed for patients with mildly elevated serum creatinine levels before a radiologic study using contrast dye.[24] In research trials, the addition of *N*-acetylcysteine to normal saline hydration did not reduce the incidence of contrast-induced AKI.[23]

Dietary-Phosphorus Binders

Many patients with kidney failure are prescribed a dietary–phosphorus-binding medication (see earlier section on Dietary–Phosphorus-Binding Medications).[40,41] Many dietary-phosphorus binders are available, and some important issues concern all of them. The dietary-phosphorus binder must be taken at the time of the meal. If it is taken 2 hours later, it will increase only the level of the binding substance (e.g., calcium) in the bloodstream and will not lower the serum phosphorus level. Related issues such as the quantity of phosphorus in the diet should be discussed with a clinical nutritionist (dietitian).

Nutrition

Diet or nutritional supplementation for the patient with AKI in the critical care unit is designed to account for the diminished excretory capacity of the kidney. The recommended energy intake is between 20 and 30 kilocalories/kg per day, with 1.2 to 1.5 grams/kg of protein per day to control azotemia (increased BUN level).[55] Oral nutrition is preferred, and if the patient

cannot eat, enteral nutrition is recommended over parenteral (intravenous) nutrition.[56] Fluids are limited, and monitoring of blood glucose levels is recommended. The electrolytes potassium, sodium, and phosphorus are strictly limited.

Nursing Management

Nursing management of the patient with AKI patients involves a variety of nursing diagnoses (Box 27-4). "Prevention is the best cure" is an old saying that captures the role of the critical care nurse, who evaluates all patients for level of kidney function, risk of infection, fluid imbalance, electrolyte disturbances, anemia, readiness to learn, and need for education.

Risk Factors for Acute Kidney Injury

Some individuals are at increased risk for AKI as a complication during hospitalization, and the alert critical care nurse

◎ **BOX 27-4   NURSING DIAGNOSES**

Acute Kidney Injury

- Excess Fluid Volume related to kidney dysfunction, p. 1139
- Risk for Ineffective Renal Perfusion, p. 1159
- Anxiety related to threat to biologic, psychological, or social integrity, p. 1125
- Decreased Cardiac Output related to alterations in preload, p. 1128
- Risk for Infection, p. 1160
- Disturbed Body Image related to functional dependence on life-sustaining technology, p. 1136
- Ineffective Coping related to situational crisis and personal vulnerability, p. 1150
- Disturbed Sleep Pattern related to fragmented sleep, p. 1137
- Deficient Knowledge related to lack of previous exposure to information, p. 1134 (see Box 27-5, Patient Education for Acute Kidney Injury)

recognizes potential risk factors and acts as a patient advocate. Patients at risk include older persons because their GFR may be decreased, dehydrated patients with kidney hypoperfusion, patients with increased creatinine levels before their hospitalization, and patients undergoing a radiologic procedure involving contrast dye.

Infectious Complications

The critical care patient with infectious complications is at risk for AKI. Signs of infection such as an increased white blood cell (WBC) count, redness at a wound or IV line site, or increased temperature are always a cause for concern. A urinary catheter is inserted to facilitate accurate urine measurement and patient comfort. However, any indwelling catheter is a potential source for infection. When the patient no longer makes large quantities of urine and is hemodynamically stable, the catheter must be removed promptly. If the patient cannot void urine spontaneously, a scheduled intermittent urinary catheterization is performed to minimize the risk of infection from an indwelling catheter and drainage system. This method allows the patient's bladder to be emptied, but the catheter does not remain in place.

Fluid Balance

Intravascular fluid balance is often assessed on an hourly basis for the critically ill patient who has hemodynamic lines inserted. Hemodynamic values (heart rate, blood pressure, central venous pressure, pulmonary artery occlusion pressure, cardiac output, and cardiac index) and daily weight measurements are correlated with the intake and output. Urine output is measured hourly by means of a urinary catheter and drainage bag throughout all phases of AKI, particularly in response to diuretics. Any fluid removed with dialysis is included the daily fluid balance. Recognition of the clinical signs and symptoms of fluid overload is important. Excess fluid moves from the vascular system into the peripheral tissues (dependent edema), abdomen (ascites), and lungs (crackles, pulmonary edema, and pulmonary effusions); around the heart (pericardial effusions); and into the brain (increased intracranial swelling).

Electrolyte Imbalance

Hyperkalemia, hypocalcemia, hyponatremia, hyperphosphatemia, and acid–base imbalances occur during AKI (see Table 27-4). Clinical manifestations of these electrolyte imbalances must be prevented and their associated side effects controlled. The more likely imbalances are hyperkalemia and hypocalcemia, which can result in life-threatening cardiac dysrhythmias.[36] Dilutional hyponatremia may develop as fluid overload worsens in the patient with oliguria. Monitoring the serum sodium level is important to prevent this complication. Hyperphosphatemia results in severe pruritus. Nursing care is directed at soothing the itching by performing frequent skin care with emollients, discouraging scratching, and administering phosphate-binding medications. The acid–base imbalances that occur with AKI are monitored by arterial blood gas (ABG) analyses. The goal of treatment is to maintain the pH within the normal range.

Preventing Anemia

Anemia is an expected side effect of kidney failure that occurs because the kidney no longer produces the hormone *erythropoietin*.[57] As a result, the bone marrow is not stimulated to produce erythrocytes, also known as red blood cells (RBCs). Additionally, the normal erythrocyte survival of 80 to 120 days is decreased, in CKD patients on dialysis, to 70 to 80 days increasing their risk for anemia.[57] Care is taken to prevent blood loss in patients with AKI, and blood withdrawal is minimized as much as possible. Irritation of the gastrointestinal tract from metabolic waste accumulation is expected, and stress ulcer prophylaxis must be prescribed. Gastrointestinal bleeding remains a possibility. Stool, nasogastric tube drainage, and emesis are routinely tested for occult blood.

Erythropoiesis-Stimulating Medications. Anemia associated with CKD may be treated pharmacologically by the administration of recombinant human erythropoietin. Three medications are FDA approved for treatment of CKD-associated anemia in the United States: epoetin alfa (Procrit, Epogen), darbepoetin alfa (Aranesp), and methoxy polyethylene glycol-epoetin beta (Mircera).[57] These agents stimulate erythrocyte production by the bone marrow.[57] Adjunctive treatments include administration of iron supplements, vitamin B_{12}, vitamin B_6, and folate. With symptomatic anemia, RBC transfusion may be required.[57,58]

Patient Education

Accurate and uncomplicated information must be provided to the patient and family about AKI, including its prognosis, treatment, and possible complications.[9] Education of the patient can be challenging because elevations of BUN and creatinine levels can negatively affect the level of consciousness. Sleep-rest disorders and emotional upset often occur as complications of AKI and can disrupt short-term memory. Encouraging the patient and family to voice concerns, frustrations, or fears and allowing the patient to control some aspects of the acute care environment and treatment also are essential (Box 27-5).

BOX 27-5   PATIENT EDUCATION

Acute Kidney Injury

- Explain the pathophysiology.
  - Severe acute kidney injury (AKI) is a sudden decline in kidney function that causes an acute buildup of toxins in the blood.
- Explain the cause.
  - Prerenal (before the kidney)
  - Intrarenal (within the kidney)
  - Postrenal (after the kidney)
- Identify predisposing factors; explain the level of kidney function after the acute phase is over.
- Explain diet and fluid restrictions.
- Demonstrate how to check blood pressure, pulse, respirations, and weight.
- Discuss personal hygiene and how to avoid infections.
- Emphasize need for exercise and rest.
- Describe medications and adverse effects.
- Explain need for ongoing follow-up with health care professional.
- Explain purpose of dialysis and importance of regular treatments.

RENAL REPLACEMENT THERAPY: DIALYSIS

Two types of renal replacement therapy are available for the treatment of AKI. They are intermittent hemodialysis (IHD) therapy and continuous renal replacement therapy (CRRT).

Hemodialysis

Hemodialysis roughly translates as "separating from the blood." Indications and contraindications for hemodialysis are listed in Box 27-6. As a treatment, hemodialysis separates and removes

---

BOX 27-6   INDICATIONS AND CONTRAINDICATIONS FOR HEMODIALYSIS

Indications
- Blood urea nitrogen (BUN) level exceeds 90 mg/dL
- Serum creatinine level of 9 mg/dL
- Hyperkalemia
- Medication toxicity
- Intravascular and extravascular fluid overload
- Metabolic acidosis
- Symptoms of uremia
  - Pericarditis
  - Gastrointestinal bleeding
- Changes in mentation
- Contraindications to other forms of dialysis

Contraindications
- Hemodynamic instability
- Inability to anticoagulate
- Lack of access to circulation

---

from the blood the excess electrolytes, fluids, and toxins by means of a hemodialyzer (Fig. 27-4). Hemodialysis is efficient in removing solutes. Because levels of electrolytes, toxins, and fluids increase between treatments, hemodialysis occurs on a regular basis. Traditional hemodialysis treatments last for 3 to 4 hours. A newer option is the use of *Sustained Low-Efficiency Dialysis* (SLED) that is run daily for 8 hours or 12 hours. Sometimes in critical illness this mode is run continuously (C-SLED). In the acute phase of kidney failure, hemodialysis is performed daily. The dialysis frequency gradually decreases to three times per week should the patient's condition progress to chronic kidney failure.

Hemodialyzer

Hemodialysis works by circulating blood outside the body through synthetic tubing to a dialyzer, which consists of hollow-fiber tubes. The dialyzer is sometimes described as an artificial kidney (Fig. 27-5). While the blood flows through the membranes, which are semipermeable, a fluid (dialysate bath) bathes the membranes and, through osmosis and diffusion, performs exchanges of fluid, electrolytes, and toxins from the blood to the bath, where toxins and dialysate then pass out of the artificial kidney. The blood and the dialysate bath are shunted in opposite directions (countercurrent flow) through the dialyzer to match the osmotic and chemical gradients at the most efficient level for effective dialysis.

Ultrafiltration

To remove fluid, a positive hydrostatic pressure is applied to the blood, and a negative hydrostatic pressure is applied to the dialysate bath. The two forces together, called *transmembrane*

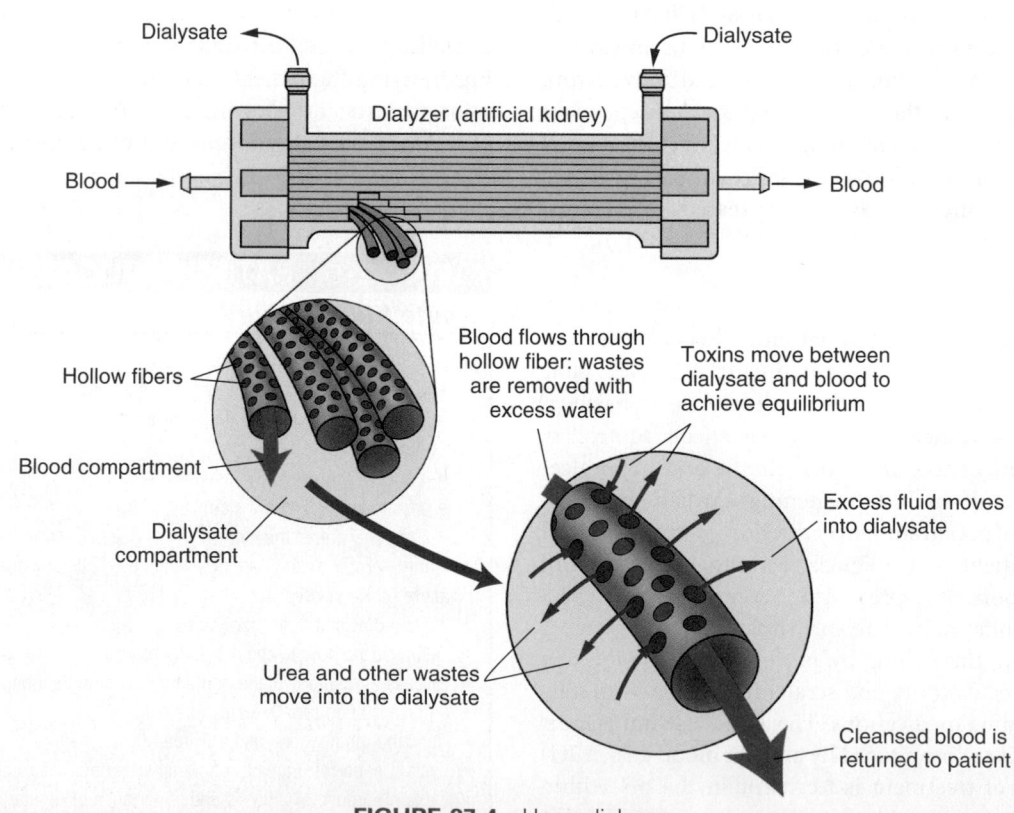

FIGURE 27-4   Hemodialyzer.

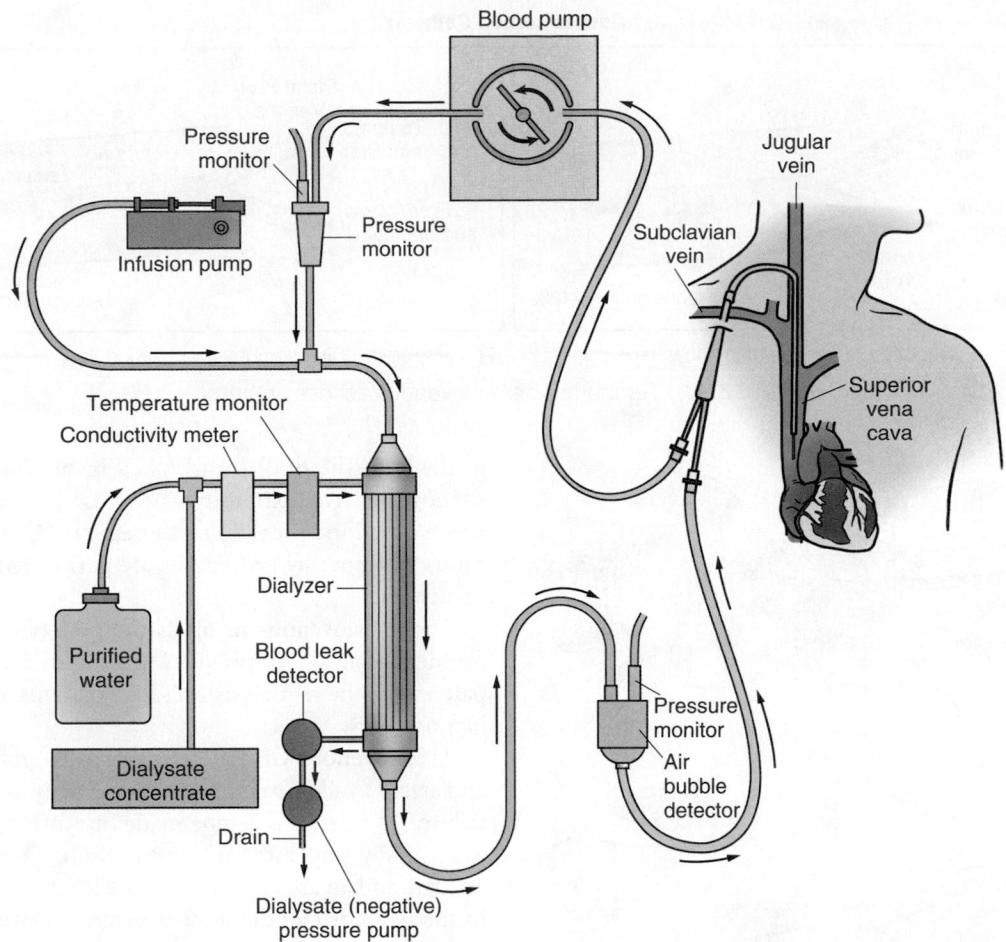

FIGURE 27-5 Components of a hemodialysis system.

pressure, pull and squeeze the excess fluid from the blood. The difference between the two values, expressed in millimeters of mercury (mm Hg) represents the transmembrane pressure and results in fluid extraction, known as *ultrafiltration*, from the vascular space.

Anticoagulation

Heparin or sodium citrate is added to the system just before the blood enters the dialyzer to anticoagulate the blood within the dialysis tubing.[59] Without an anticoagulant, the blood clots because its passage through the foreign tubular substances of the dialysis machine activates the clotting mechanism. Heparin can be administered by bolus injection or intermittent infusion. It has a short half-life, and its effects subside within 2 to 4 hours. If necessary, the effects of heparin are easily reversed with the antidote protamine sulfate. When there is concern about the development of heparin-induced thrombocytopenia (HIT), alternative anticoagulants can be used. Citrate can be infused as an anticoagulant by intermittent bolus or continuous infusion.

Vascular Access

Hemodialysis requires access to the bloodstream. Various types of temporary and permanent devices are in clinical use. It is important for patient safety to be able to recognize these different vascular access devices and to properly care for them. The

following section discusses temporary vascular access catheters used in the acute care hospital environment and permanent methods used for long-term hemodialysis.

Temporary Vascular Access. *Subclavian* and *femoral* veins are catheterized when short-term access is required or when a graft or fistula vascular access is nonfunctional in a patient requiring immediate hemodialysis. Subclavian and femoral catheters are routinely inserted at the bedside. Most temporary catheters are venous lines only. Blood flows out toward the dialyzer and flows back to the patient through the same catheterized vein. A dual-lumen venous catheter is most commonly used. It has a central partition running the length of the catheter. The outflow catheter section pulls the blood flow through openings that are proximal to the inflow openings on the opposite side (Fig. 27-6). This design helps prevent dialyzing the same blood just returned to the area (recirculation), which would severely reduce the procedure's efficiency. A silicone rubber, dual-lumen catheter with a polyester cuff designed to decrease catheter-related infections is also available.

Permanent Vascular Access. The common denominator in permanent vascular access devices is a conduit connection between the arterial circulation and the venous circulation.

Arteriovenous Fistula. The arteriovenous fistula is created by surgically exposing a peripheral artery and vein, creating a side-by-side opening in the artery and the vein to join the two vessels together. The high arterial flow creates a swelling of the

Double Lumen Catheter

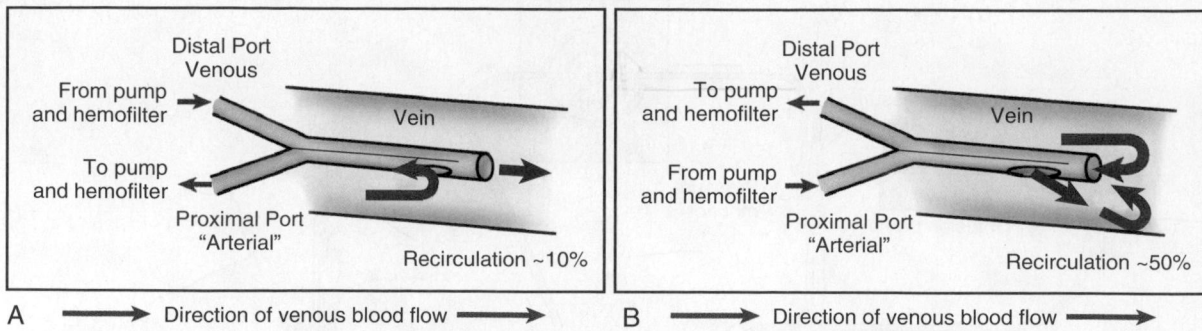

FIGURE 27-6 Temporary dialysis venous access catheter.

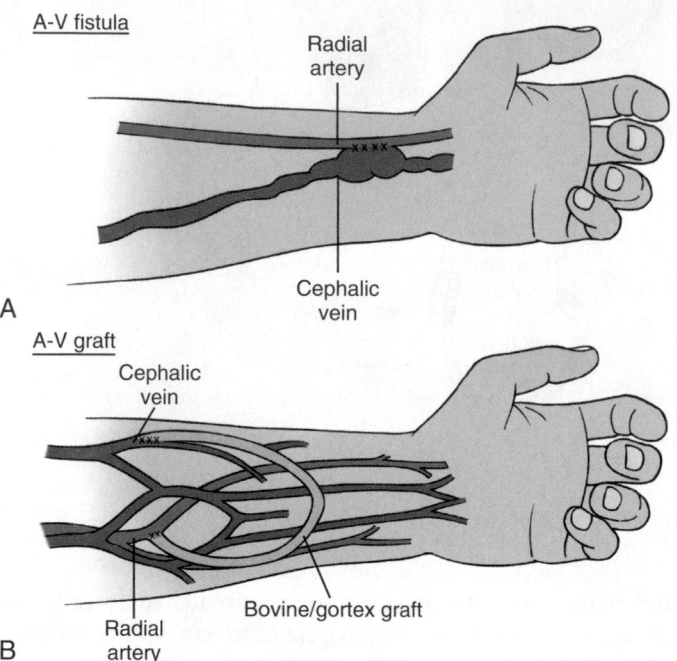

FIGURE 27-7 Vascular access for hemodialysis. *A,* Arteriovenous fistula between the vein and artery. *B,* Internal synthetic graft corrects the artery and vein.

vein, or a pseudoaneurysm, at which point (when healed) a large-bore needle can be inserted to obtain arterial outflow to the dialyzer. Inflow is accomplished through a second large-bore needle inserted into a peripheral vein distal to the fistula (Fig. 27-7A). Fistulas are the preferred mode of access because of the durability of blood vessels, relatively few complications, and less need for revision compared with other access methods. An initial disadvantage of a fistula concerns the time required for development of sufficient arterial flow to enlarge the new access. The minimum reported length of time before a fistula can be cannulated for dialysis is 14 days, but the time lag for many patients can be longer. Ideally the fistula should be established 6 months before the requirement for hemodialysis to ensure it is usable for dialysis when required.[60]

In caring for a patient with a fistula, there are some important nursing priorities to ensure the ongoing viability of the vascular access and safety of the limb (Table 27-8). The critical care nurse frequently assesses the quality of blood flow through the fistula. A patent fistula has a thrill when palpated gently with the fingers and has a bruit if auscultated with a stethoscope. The extremity should be pink and warm to the touch. No blood pressure measurements, IV infusions, or laboratory phlebotomy procedures are performed on the arm with the fistula.

The arteriovenous fistula is the preferred long-term access for hemodialysis. It provides the most favorable long-term patency for hemodialysis access if patients require long-term hemodialysis.

Arteriovenous Grafts. Arteriovenous grafts connect a vein and artery to allow vascular access for dialysis in chronic kidney failure.[61] The graft is a tube made of synthetic material, which is surgically implanted inside the limb. The area is surgically opened, and an artery and a vein are located. A tunnel is created in the tissue where the graft is placed. Anastomoses are made with the graft ends connected to the artery and vein. The blood is allowed to flow through the graft, and the surgical area is closed. The graft creates a raised area that looks like a large peripheral vein just under the skin (see Fig. 27-7B). Two large-bore needles are used for outflow from and inflow to the graft during dialysis. For grafts and fistulas, after needle removal at the end of the hemodialysis treatment, firm pressure must be applied to stop any bleeding (see Table 27-8).

Tunneled Catheters. While waiting for the fistula or graft to mature to be ready for access, some patients with CKD may have a tunneled, cuffed catheter placed in either the internal or external jugular vein.[62,63] The cuff and tunneling are physical barriers to reduce central venous line infections. Modern catheters are made of silicone or silastic elastomers making them more pliable than temporary catheters.[64]

Medical Management

Medical management involves the decision to place a vascular access device and then to choose the most appropriate type and location for each patient. Patients in the critical care setting who require vascular access for hemodialysis typically use a temporary hemodialysis catheter. The exact quantity of fluid and solute removal to be achieved by hemodialysis is determined individually for each patient by clinical examination and review of all relevant laboratory results.

Nursing Management

A non-critical care nurse who is specially trained in dialysis manages the IHD. The dialysis nurse typically comes to the

TABLE 27-8 COMPLICATIONS AND NURSING MANAGEMENT OF ARTERIOVENOUS FISTULA/GRAFT

TYPE	COMPLICATIONS	NURSING MANAGEMENT
Fistula	Thrombosis Infection Pseudoaneurysm Vascular steal syndrome Venous hypertension Carpal tunnel syndrome Inadequate blood flow	Teach patients to avoid wearing constrictive clothing on limbs containing access. Teach patients to avoid sleeping on or bending accessed limb for prolonged periods. Use aseptic technique when cannulating access. Avoid repetitious cannulation of one segment of access. Offer comfort measures, such as warm compresses and ordered analgesics, to lessen pain of vascular steal. Teach patients to develop blood flow in the fistulas through exercises (squeezing a rubber ball) while applying mild impedance to flow just distal to the access (at least once per day for 10-15 min). Avoid too-early cannulation of new access.
Graft	Bleeding Thrombosis False aneurysm formation Infection Arterial or venous stenosis Vascular steal syndrome	Teach patients to avoid wearing constrictive clothing on accessed limbs. Avoid repeated cannulation of one segment of access. Use aseptic technique when cannulating access. Monitor for changes in arterial or venous pressure while patients are on dialysis. Provide comfort measures to reduce pain of vascular steal (e.g., warm compresses, analgesics as ordered).

◎ BOX 27-7   NIC

Hemodialysis Therapy

Definition

Management of extracorporeal passage of the patient's blood through a dializer

Activities

Draw blood sample and review blood chemistries (e.g., blood urea nitrogen, serum creatinine, serum Na, K, and PO$_4$ levels) before treatment

Record baseline vital signs: weight, temperature, pulse, respirations, and blood pressure

Explain hemodialysis procedure and its purpose

Check equipment and solutions, according to protocol

Use sterile technique to initiate hemodialysis and for needle insertions and catheter connections

Use gloves, eye shield, and clothing to prevent direct contact with blood

Initiate hemodialysis, according to protocol

Anchor connections and tubing securely

Check system monitors (e.g., flow rate, pressure, temperature, pH level, conductivity, clots, air detector, negative pressure for ultrafiltration, and blood sensor) to ensure patient safety

Monitor blood pressure, pulse, respirations, temperature, and patient response during dialysis

Administer heparin, according to protocol

Monitor clotting times and adjust heparin administration appropriately

Adjust filtration pressures to remove an appropriate amount of fluid

Institute appropriate protocol, if patient becomes hypotensive

Discontinue hemodialysis according to protocol

Compare postdialysis vital signs and blood chemistries with predialysis values

Avoid taking blood pressure or doing intravenous punctures in arm with fistula

Provide catheter or fistula care according to protocol

Work collaboratively with patient to adjust diet regulations, fluid limitations, and medications to regulate fluid and electrolyte shifts between treatments

Teach patient to self-monitor signs and symptoms that indicate need for medical treatment (e.g., fever, bleeding, clotted fistula, thrombophlebitis, irregular pulse)

Work collaboratively with patient to relieve discomfort from side effects of the disease and treatment (e.g., cramping, fatigue, headaches, itching, anemia, bone demineralization, body image changes, and role disruption)

Work collaboratively with patient to adjust length of dialysis, diet regulations, and pain and diversion needs to achieve optimal benefit of the treatment

From Bulechek GM, et al. *Nursing Interventions Classification (NIC)*. 6th ed. St. Louis: Mosby; 2013.

patient's bedside with the hemodialysis machine. During the acute phase of treatment, hemodialysis occurs daily. The frequency is reduced to 3 days per week as the patient becomes hemodynamically stable. The essential nursing elements to manage a patient on hemodialysis are listed in Box 27-7. The essential role of the critical care nurse during dialysis is to monitor the patient's hemodynamic status and ensure the patient remains hemodynamically stable. The AKI patient on hemodialysis depends on a viable venous access catheter. When not in use, the catheter is "heparin-locked" to preserve patency.

The critical care nurse provides education about the disease process and treatment plan to patient and family.

Continuous Renal Replacement Therapy

CRRT is a newer mode of dialysis that has many similarities to traditional hemodialysis. CRRT is a continuous therapy that is monitored by the critical care nurse, and it may continue over many days. The venous blood is circulated through a highly porous hemofilter. As with traditional hemodialysis, access and return of blood are achieved through a large venous catheter

TABLE 27-9 COMPARISON OF CONTINUOUS RENAL REPLACEMENT THERAPY MODES

TYPE	ULTRAFILTRATION RATE	FLUID REPLACEMENT	MODE OF SOLUTE REMOVAL	INDICATION
SCUF	100-300 mL/hr	None	None	Fluid removal
CVVH	500-800 mL/hr	Predilution or postdilution, calculating hourly net loss	Convection	Fluid removal, moderate solute removal
CVVHD	500-800 mL/hr	Predilution or postdilution, subtracting dialysate, then calculating hourly net loss	Diffusion	Fluid removal, maximum solute removal
CVVHDF		Predilution or postdilution, subtracting dialysate, then calculating hourly net loss	Convection and diffusion	Maximal fluid removal, maximal solute removal

CVVH, Continuous venovenous hemofiltration; *CVVHD,* continuous venovenous hemodialysis; *CVVHDF,* continuous venovenous hemodiafiltration; *SCUF,* slow continuous ultrafiltration.

BOX 27-8 INDICATIONS AND CONTRAINDICATIONS FOR CONTINUOUS RENAL REPLACEMENT THERAPY

Indications
- Need for large fluid volume removal in hemodynamically unstable patient
- Hypervolemic or edematous patients unresponsive to diuretic therapy
- Patients with multiple organ dysfunction syndrome
- Ease of fluid management in patients requiring large daily fluid volume
  - Replacement for oliguria
  - Administration of total parenteral nutrition
- Contraindication to hemodialysis and peritoneal dialysis
- Inability to be anticoagulated

Contraindications
- Hematocrit >45%
- Terminal illness

(venovenous). The CRRT system allows the continuous removal of fluid from the plasma. The patient's blood flow is 100 to 200 mL/min, and the dialysate flow ranges from 20 to 40 mL/min. The fluid removal rate varies depending on the particular CRRT method used and removal of solutes (urea, creatinine, and electrolytes), as listed in Table 27-9. The removed fluid is described as *ultrafiltrate*. In an ideal situation, the hydrostatic pressure exerted by a mean arterial pressure (MAP) greater than 70 mm Hg would propel a continuous flow of blood through the hemofilter to remove fluid and solute. However, because many critically ill patients are hypotensive and cannot provide adequate flow through the hemofilter, an electric roller pump "milks" the tubing to augment flow. If large amounts of fluid are to be removed, IV replacement solutions are infused. Indications and contraindications for CRRT are described in Box 27-8.

Controversy exists about when CRRT should be started, the optimal dialysis dose, which patients can derive the greatest benefit, and when CRRT should be discontinued. The debate over the optimal "dose" of dialysis is likely to continue because although two recent clinical trials showed no difference in mortality between critically ill patients receiving intensive or nonintensive dialysis regimens,[65,66] the amount of dialysis in the research studies was greater than that normally achieved in clinical practice.[67] Therefore, the debate continues.

Because controlled removal and replacement of fluid is possible over many hours or days with CRRT, hemodynamic stability is maintained. This makes CRRT highly advantageous for use in the hemodynamically unstable patient with multisystem problems. Several modes of CRRT are used in critical care units, a partial list is provided below[68]:
1. Slow continuous ultrafiltration (SCUF)
2. Continuous venovenous hemofiltration (CVVH)
3. Continuous venovenous hemodialysis (CVVHD)
4. Continuous venovenous hemodiafiltration (CVVHDF)

The decision about which type of therapy to initiate is based on clinical assessment, metabolic status, severity of uremia, whether a particular treatment modality is available at that institution, and other factors.

Continuous Renal Replacement Therapy Terminology

In CRRT, solutes are removed from the blood by *diffusion* or *convection*. Both processes remove fluid, and the two methods remove molecules of different sizes.

Diffusion. Diffusion describes the movement of solutes along a *concentration gradient* from a high concentration to a low concentration across a semipermeable membrane. This is the main mechanism used in hemodialysis. Solutes such as creatinine and urea cross the dialysis membrane from the blood to the dialysis fluid compartment.

Convection. Convection occurs when a pressure gradient is set up so that the water is pushed or pumped across the dialysis filter and carries the solutes from the bloodstream with it. This method of solute removal is known as *solvent drag*, and it is commonly employed in CRRT.

Absorption. The filter attracts solute, and molecules attach (adsorb) to the dialysis filter. The size of solute molecules is measured in *daltons*. The different sizes of molecules that can be removed by convection or diffusion methods are shown in Table 27-9. Tiny molecules such as urea and creatinine are removed by diffusion and convection (all methods). As the molecular size increases above 500 daltons, convection is the more efficient method (Table 27-10).

Ultrafiltrate Volume. The fluid that is removed each hour is not called *urine*; it is known as *ultrafiltrate*.

Replacement Fluid. Typically, some of the ultrafiltrate is replaced through the CRRT circuit by a sterile replacement fluid. The replacement fluid can be added before the filter

TABLE 27-10	SIZE OF MOLECULES CLEARED BY CONTINUOUS RENAL REPLACEMENT THERAPY		
TYPE OF MOLECULE	SIZE OF MOLECULE	SOLUTES	SOLUTE REMOVAL METHOD
Small	<500 daltons	Urea, creatinine	Convection, diffusion
Middle	500-5000 daltons	Vancomycin	Convection better than diffusion
Low–molecular-weight (small) proteins	5000-50,000 daltons	Cytokines, complement	Convection or absorption onto hemofilter
Large proteins	>50,000 daltons	Albumin	Minimal removal

(prefilter dilution) or after the filter (postfilter dilution). The purpose is to increase the volume of fluid passing through the hemofilter and improve convection of solute.

Anticoagulation. Because the blood outside the body is in contact with artificial tubing and filters, the coagulation cascade and complement cascades are activated. To prevent the hemofilter from becoming obstructed by clotting, or clotting off, low-dose anticoagulation must be used. The dose should be low enough to have no effect on patient anticoagulation parameters. Systemic anticoagulation is not the goal. Typical anticoagulant choices include unfractionated heparin (UFH) and sodium citrate. Citrate is an effective prefilter anticoagulant, which has the side effect that it *chelates* (binds to and removes) calcium from the blood. Consequently, iCa levels are verified, and calcium is replaced per protocol when sodium citrate is the anticoagulant.

Modes of Continuous Renal Replacement

Because of the design of the CRRT machine, it is not possible to look at the outside and follow the flow of blood and, if used, dialysate. Each of the CRRT modes is described, and diagrams are employed to clarify the mode of CRRT that is used.

Slow Continuous Ultrafiltration. SCUF slowly removes fluid (100 to 300 mL/hr) through a process of ultrafiltration (Fig. 27-8A). This consists of a movement of fluid across a semipermeable membrane. SCUF has minimal impact on solute removal. However, SCUF is an infrequent clinical choice because it requires both arterial and venous access for effective functioning and the circuit is more likely to thrombose (clot off) than other CRRT methods that use higher flows. Because small amounts of fluid are gently removed, initially it was hoped that SCUF would be a suitable choice for edematous patients with acute heart failure and diminished perfusion to the kidneys that were unresponsive to diuretics. Currently, intermittent *ultrafiltration* using a peripheral venous catheter is more likely to be used to remove excess volume from patients with acute decompensated heart failure when the kidneys are unresponsive to diuretics.[69,70]

Continuous Venovenous Hemofiltration. CVVH is indicated when the patient's clinical condition warrants removal of significant volumes of fluid and solutes. Fluid is removed by ultrafiltration in volumes of 5 to 20 mL/min or up to 7 to 30 L/24 hr. Removal of solutes such as urea, creatinine, and other small non–protein-bound toxins is accomplished by convection. The replacement fluid rate of flow through the CRRT circuit can be altered to achieve desired fluid and solute removal without causing hemodynamic instability. Replacement fluid can be added by the addition of a prehemofilter replacement fluid (see Fig. 27-8B) or posthemofilter replacement fluid.

As with other CRRT systems, the blood outside the body is anticoagulated, and the ultrafiltrate is drained off by gravity or by the addition of negative-pressure suction into a large drainage bag. Because large volumes of fluid may be removed in CVVH, some of the removed ultrafiltrate volume must be replaced hourly with a continuous infusion (replacement fluid) to avoid intravascular dehydration. Replacement fluids may consist of standard solutions of bicarbonate, potassium-free LR solution, acetate, or dextrose. Electrolytes such as potassium, sodium, calcium chloride, magnesium sulfate, and sodium bicarbonate may be added. The formula used to calculate the volume removed from the patient follows with an example:

Ultrafiltrate in bag + Other output
  − (CVVH replacement fluid + IV/oral/NG intake) = Output

$$1000\,mL - 800\,mL = 200\,mL/hr\ output$$

Continuous Venovenous Hemodialysis

CVVHD is technically like traditional hemodialysis, and it removes solute by diffusion because of a slow (15 to 30 mL/min) countercurrent drainage flow on the membrane side of the hemofilter (see Fig. 27-8C). Blood and fluid move by countercurrent flow through the hemofilter. *Countercurrent* means the blood flows in one direction and the dialysate flows in the opposite direction. As with other types of CRRT and hemodialysis, although arterial access is always possible, venovenous vascular access is the most common choice.

CVVHD is indicated for patients who require large-volume removal for severe uremia or critical acid–base imbalances or for those who are resistant to diuretics. A MAP of at least 70 mm Hg is desirable for effective volume removal and dialysis, and it is most effective when used over days, not hours. The use of replacement fluid is optional and depends on the patient's clinical condition and plan of care. The critical care nurse is responsible for calculating the hourly intake and output, identifying fluid trends, and replacing excessive losses. This therapy is ideal for hemodynamically unstable patients in the critical care setting because they do not experience the abrupt fluid and solute changes that can accompany standard hemodialysis treatments.

Continuous Venovenous Hemodiafiltration. Another CRRT option is CVVHDF, which combines two of the previously described methods (CVVH and CVVHD) to achieve maximal fluid and solute removal. A strong transmembrane pressure is applied to the hemofilter to push water across the filter, and a negative pressure is applied at the other side to pull fluid across the membrane and produce large volumes of ultrafiltrate and to create a "solvent drag" (CVVH method). The blood and the dialysate are circulated in a countercurrent flow pattern to remove fluid and solutes by diffusion (hemodialysis method). CVVHDF can remove large volumes of fluid and solute because it employs diffusion gradients and convection.

Complications

Potential problems associated with CRRT and appropriate nursing interventions are listed in Table 27-11. Complications are often related to the rate of flow through the system. If the patient becomes hypotensive or the access lines remain kinked, the ultrafiltration rate will decrease. This can lead to increased clot formation within the hemofilter. As the surface of the hemofilter becomes more clotted, it will not provide effective fluid or solute clearance, and CRRT will be stopped; a new CRRT circuit must then be set up. The most common reasons for interruption in CRRT are clotting and patient clinical issues.[71]

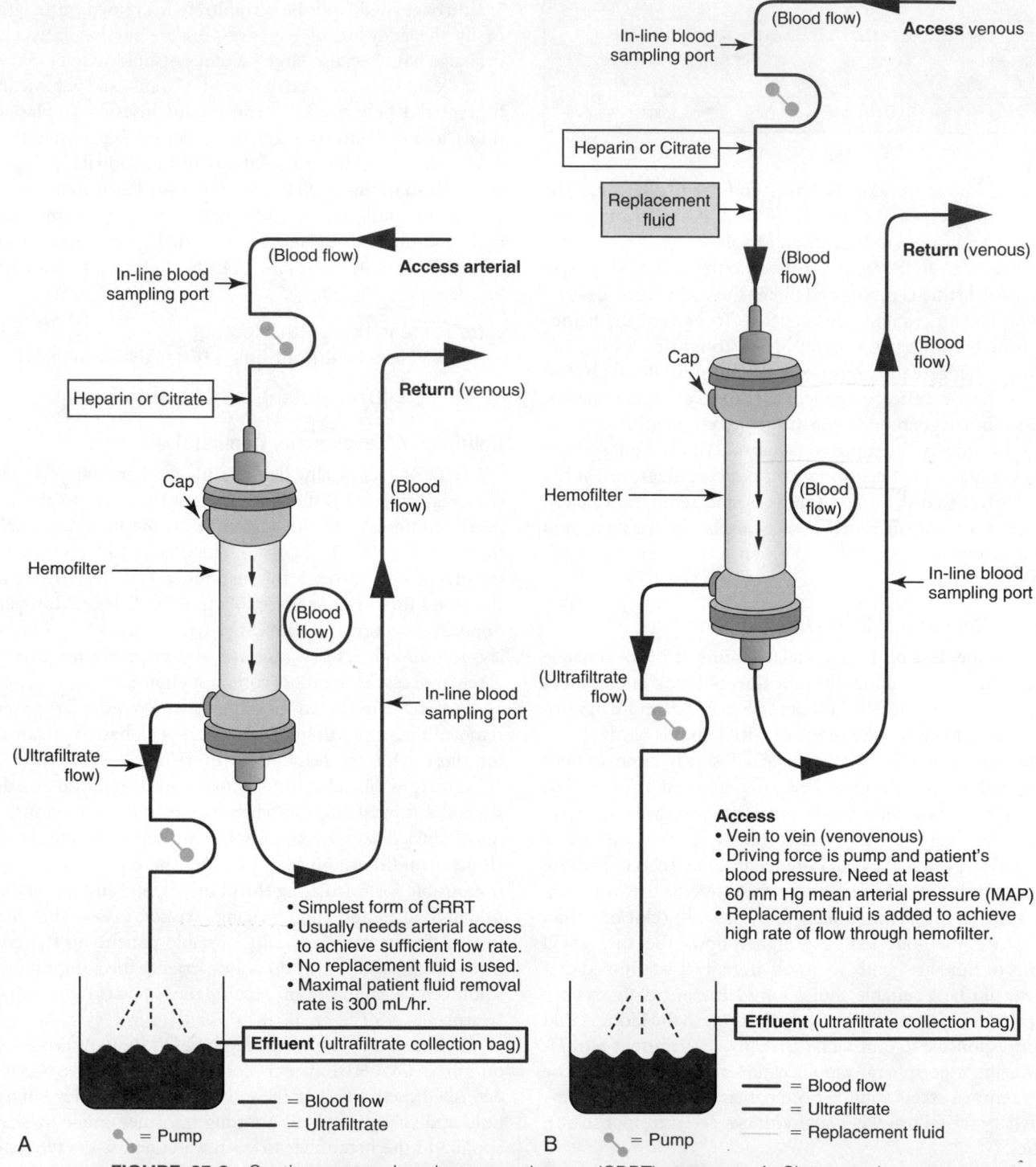

FIGURE 27-8 Continuous renal replacement therapy (CRRT) systems. *A,* Slow, continuous ultrafiltration (SCUF). *B,* Continuous venovenous hemofiltration (CVVH).

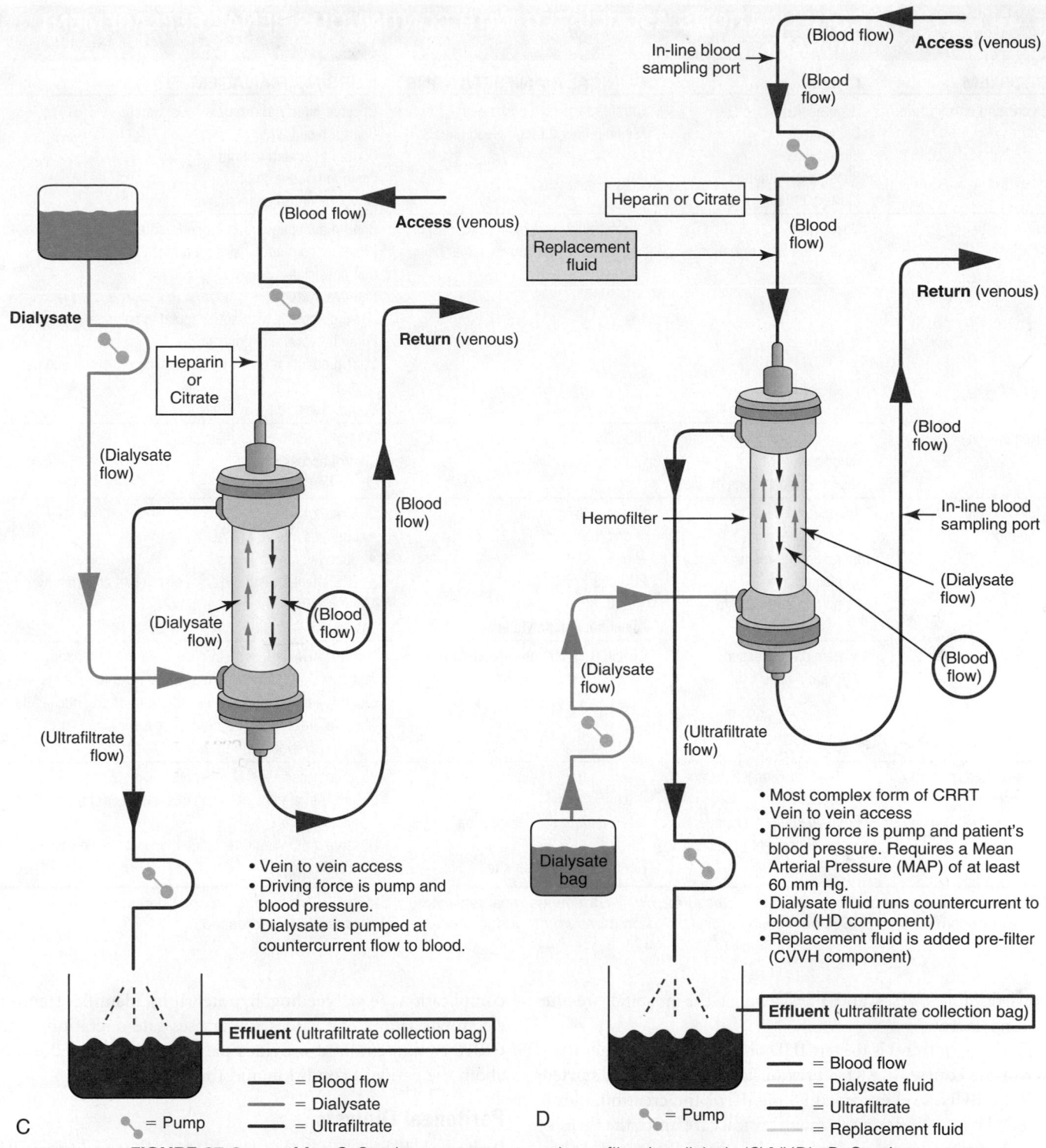

FIGURE 27-8, cont'd. *C,* Continuous venovenous hemofiltration dialysis (CVVHD). *D,* Continuous venovenous hemodiafiltration (CVVHDF).

The critical care nurse monitors the pressures displayed on the CRRT machine screen to monitor the positive pressure of fluid going into the hemofilter (inflow) and the pressures coming out of the hemofilter to ensure that resistance to the negative-pressure pull of the fluid across the hemofilter membrane has not developed. Other patient-related complications include fluid and electrolyte alterations, bleeding because of anticoagulation, or problems with the access site, such as dislodgement or infection.[72]

Medical Management

The choice of the method of blood purification to use to treat AKI is a medical decision. There is no clinical or research consensus about whether IHD or CRRT is the most beneficial, and no difference in outcomes has been shown in clinical research trials.[73,74] Age, gender, and pre-existing chronic conditions are of little help in determining whether to select IHD or CRRT. Often, the acute clinical diagnosis, physician's preference, availability of the CRRT machine, and

TABLE 27-11 **COMPLICATIONS ASSOCIATED WITH CONTINUOUS RENAL REPLACEMENT THERAPY**

PROBLEM	CAUSE	CLINICAL MANIFESTATIONS	NURSING MANAGEMENT
Decreased ultrafiltration rate	Hypotension Dehydration Kinked lines Bending of catheters Clotting of filter	Ultrafiltration rate decreased Minimal flow through blood lines	Observe filter and arteriovenous system Control blood flow Control coagulation time Position patient on back Lower height of collection container
Filter clotting	Obstruction Insufficient heparinization	Ultrafiltration rate decreased, despite height of collection container being lower	Control anticoagulation (heparin/citrate) Maintain continuous system anticoagulation Call physician Remove system Prime catheters with anticoagulated solution Prime new system; connect it Start predilution with 1000 mL saline 0.9% solution per hour Do not use three-way stopcocks
Hypotension	Increased ultrafiltration rate Blood leak Disconnection of one of lines	Bleeding Call physician	Control amount of ultrafiltration Control access sites Clamp lines
Fluid and electrolyte changes	Too much or too little removal of fluid Inappropriate replacement of electrolytes Inappropriate dialysate	Changes in mentation ↑ or ↓ CVP ↑ or ↓ PAOP ECG changes ↑ or ↓ BP and heart rate Abnormal electrolyte levels	Observe for • Changes in CVP or PAOP • Changes in vital signs • ECG change resulting from electrolyte abnormalities Monitor output values every hour Control ultrafiltration
Bleeding	System disconnection ↑ Heparin dose	Oozing from catheter insertion site or connection	Monitor ACT no less than once every hour (heparin) Adjust heparin dose within specifications to maintain ACT Monitor serum calcium if using citrate as an anticoagulant Observe dressing on vascular access for blood loss Observe for blood in filtrate (filter leak)
Access dislodgement or infection	Catheter or connections not secured Break in sterile technique Excessive patient movement	Bleeding from catheter site or connections Inappropriate flow or infusion Fever Drainage at catheter site	Observe access site at least once every 2 hours Ensure that clamps are available within easy reach at all times Observe strict sterile technique when dressing vascular access

ACT, Activated coagulation time; *BP*, blood pressure; *CRRT*, continuous renal replacement therapy; *CVP*, central venous pressure; *ECG*, electrocardiogram; *PAOP*, pulmonary artery occlusion pressure or wedge pressure; ↑, increased; ↓, decreased.

knowledgeable nurses and physicians at the hospital are the deciding factors.

The current trend is to start IHD or CRRT earlier rather than later in the course of AKI.[75] Previously dialysis was not started until the BUN level exceeded 90 mg/dL or the creatinine level exceeded 9 mg/dL. Today, in many critical care units, the threshold to begin treatment is considerably lower.[75] If the patient has severe electrolyte imbalance or fluid overload, even earlier intervention may be required.

Nursing Management

Critical care nurses play a vital role in monitoring the patient receiving CRRT. In many critical care units, the CRRT system is set up by the dialysis staff but is run on a 24-hour basis by critical care nurses with additional training. Complications may be related to the CRRT circuit, the CRRT pump, or to the patient, as shown in Box 27-9. The critical care nurse monitors fluid intake and output, prevents and detects potential complications (e.g., bleeding, hypotension), identifies trends in electrolyte laboratory values, supervises safe operation of the CRRT equipment, and provides patient and family education about the patient's condition and the use of CRRT.

Peritoneal Dialysis

Peritoneal dialysis (PD) is a less high-tech modality used in patients with CKD.[76] When a PD-dependent patient is admitted to the critical care unit with a nonrenal acute illness, PD may be continued, but the patient is more often converted to hemodialysis or CRRT because of the critical illness. PD involves the introduction of sterile dialyzing fluid through an implanted catheter into the abdominal cavity. The dialysate bathes the peritoneal membrane, which covers the abdominal organs and overlies the capillary beds that support the organs. By the processes of osmosis, diffusion, and active transport, excess fluid and solutes travel from the peritoneal capillary fluid through the capillary walls, through the peritoneal membrane, and into the dialyzing fluid. After a selected period, the fluid is drained out of the abdomen by gravity (Fig. 27-9). The process is then repeated at regular, prescribed intervals.

The peritoneal membrane's structure and capillary blood flow to the peritoneum account for the relatively slow nature of PD. The small capillary pores, the capillary membrane, the interstitium, the mesothelium of the peritoneum, and the fluid film layers in the capillary and the peritoneal cavity provide formidable barriers to fluid and solute passage.[77] If needed, a *peritoneal equilibration test* (PET) can be performed to determine the level of solute clearance for a specific patient.

The volume of dialysate instilled into the abdomen affects the clearance. Normally the PD-dependent patients are well versed in the amount, type, and frequency of dialysate to be

infused into the abdomen, with subsequent drainage by gravity into a waste bag. The primary nursing consideration is to avoid contamination of the access point and monitor the patient's vital signs during this process. The dialysate should be instilled at body temperature to be comfortable, provide some vasodilation, and provide increased solute transport in the peritoneum. The length of time the solution remains in the peritoneal cavity, called the *dwell time*, and the solution composition affect the outcome. The dwell time affects the amount of fluid removed from the peritoneal capillaries, although a longer dwell time does not remove proportionately more fluid because of osmotic equilibration across the membranes. The various glucose concentrations of the dialysate provide different rates of fluid removal.

Catheter Placement

Most catheters have four segments: an external segment outside the abdomen, a tunnel segment that passes through subcutaneous tissue and muscle, a cuff for stabilization at the peritoneal membrane, and an internal segment with numerous holes for fast delivery and drainage of dialysate (Fig. 27-10). The infusion and removal of the dialysate fluid are sterile procedures.

Infection

The most significant risk to the patient with the use of PD is development of peritonitis from catheter contamination and infection. Serious infection is also a reason for admitting a patient who uses PD to the hospital.[78] The critical care nurse must be acutely aware of the signs and symptoms of systemic infection, such as a sudden rise in the WBC count, increased temperature, and malaise. Clinicians must remain vigilant for signs of localized catheter or abdominal infection manifested by catheter-site redness, site swelling, cloudy dialysis effluent after the dwell time, and abdominal tenderness or pain.

BOX 27-9 COMPLICATIONS OF CONTINUOUS RENAL REPLACEMENT THERAPY

The Circuit
- Air embolism
- Clotted hemofilter
- Poor ultrafiltration
- Blood leaks
- Broken filter
- Recirculation or disconnection
- Access failure
- Catheter dislodgment

The Pump
- Circuit pressure alarm
  - Decreased inflow pressure
  - Decreased outflow pressure
  - Increased outflow resistance
- Air bubble detector alarm
- Power failure
- Mechanical dysfunction

The Patient
- Code or emergency situation
- Dehydration
- Hypotension
- Electrolyte imbalances
- Acid–base imbalances
- Blood loss or hemorrhage
- Hypothermia
- Infection

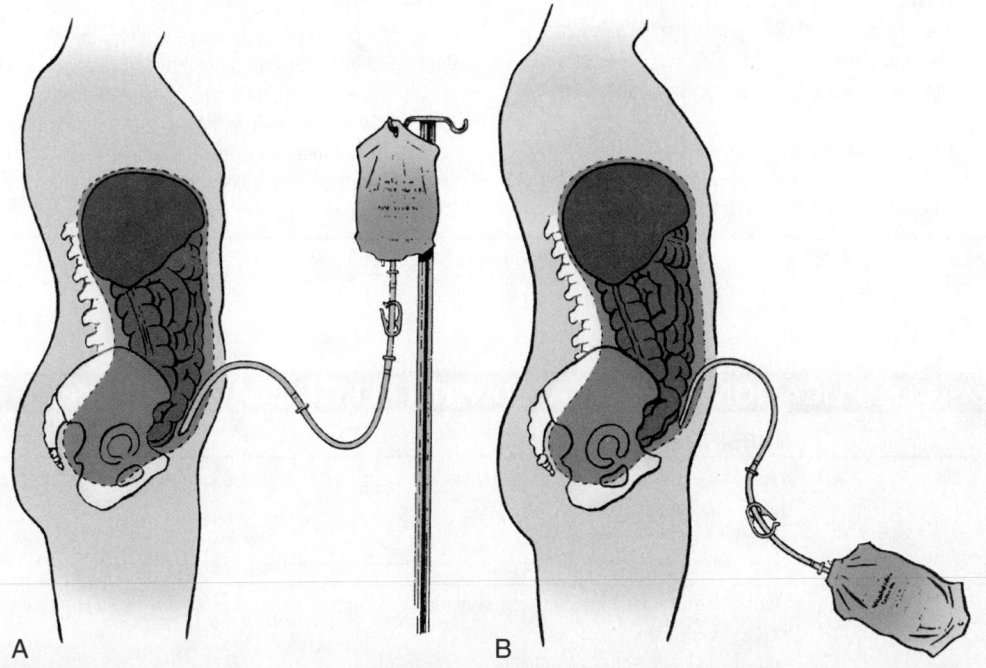

FIGURE 27-9 Peritoneal dialysis. *A*, Inflow. *B*, Outflow (drains by gravity). (From Thompson JM, et al. *Mosby's Clinical Nursing.* 5th ed. St. Louis: Mosby; 2002.)

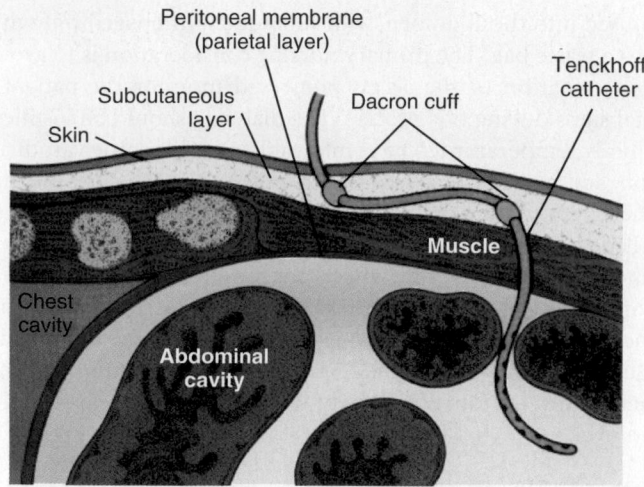

FIGURE 27-10 Tenckhoff catheter used in peritoneal dialysis. (From Lewis SL, et al. *Medical-Surgical Nursing Assessment and Management of Clinical Problems.* 7th ed. St. Louis: Mosby; 2007.)

Medical Management

PD is used for long-term end-stage kidney failure. It is never used as a first-line acute care intervention. If a patient uses PD at home, the dialysis method will continue to be used during the acute care hospitalization, provided the condition precipitating the admission is unrelated to the kidneys or abdomen.

Nursing Management

Nursing management of the patient receiving PD is complex. A comprehensive list of nursing interventions while caring for the patients with PD is provided in Box 27-10. Nurses are vigilant about prevention and detection of complications related to PD (Table 27-12). The critical care nurse observes for signs and symptoms of infection, monitors fluid volume status, infuses the dialysate fluid, observes drainage of the ultrafiltrate fluid, prevents complications associated with the PD catheter, and provides patient and family education. Patients who use PD are knowledgeable partners in the maintenance of their health because of the huge commitment they make in daily management of their PD care.[76]

BOX 27-10 NIC

Peritoneal Dialysis Therapy

Definition

Administration and monitoring of dialysis solution into and out of the peritoneal cavity

Activities

Explain the selected peritoneal dialysis procedure and purpose

Warm the dialysis fluid before instillation

Assess patency of catheter, noting difficulty in inflow/outflow

Maintain record of inflow/outflow volumes and individual/cumulative fluid balance

Have patient empty bladder before peritoneal catheter insertion

Avoid excess mechanical stress on peritoneal dialysis catheters (e.g., coughing, dressing change, infusing large volumes)

Monitor blood pressure, pulse, respirations, temperature, and patient response during dialysis

Ensure aseptic handling of peritoneal catheter and connections

Draw laboratory samples and review blood chemistries (e.g., blood urea nitrogen; serum creatinine; serum Na, K, and PO_4 levels)

Obtain cell count cultures of peritoneal effluent, if indicated

Record baseline vital signs: weight, temperature, pulse, respirations, and blood pressure

Measure and record abdominal girth

Measure and record daily weight

Anchor connections and tubing securely

Check equipment and solutions according to protocol

Administer dialysis exchanges (inflow, dwell, and outflow) according to protocol

Monitor for signs of infection (e.g., peritonitis, exit-site inflammation/drainage)

Monitor for signs of respiratory distress

Monitor for bowel perforation or fluid leaks

Work collaboratively with patient to adjust length of dialysis, diet regulations, and pain and diversion needs to achieve optimal benefit of the treatment

Teach patient to monitor self for signs and symptoms that indicate need for medical treatment (e.g., fever, bleeding, respiratory distress, irregular pulse, cloudy outflow, and abdominal pain)

Teach procedure to patient requiring home dialysis

From Bulechek GM, et al. *Nursing Interventions Classification (NIC).* 6th ed. St. Louis: Mosby; 2013.

TABLE 27-12 COMPLICATIONS ASSOCIATED WITH PERITONEAL DIALYSIS

COMPLICATION	NURSING MANAGEMENT
Peritonitis	Assess for signs and symptoms: cloudy effluent, abdominal pain, rebound tenderness, nausea and vomiting, fever. Obtain effluent sample for culture. Administer antibiotics as ordered. Teach the patient and family about signs and symptoms and prevention.
Exit site infection	Monitor the site daily for signs and symptoms of infection: induration, erythema, purulence, hyperthermia. Increase daily cleaning of site. Apply topical antibiotics as ordered (controversial). Teach the patient and family to avoid creams and lotions around exit site.

TABLE 27-12 COMPLICATIONS ASSOCIATED WITH PERITONEAL DIALYSIS—cont'd

COMPLICATION	NURSING MANAGEMENT
Catheter-tunnel infection	Assess for signs and symptoms of infection: pain along tunnel, induration for several centimeters away from catheter, erythema leading away from exit site, drainage at exit site or as tunnel is "milked" toward exit site. Teach the patient and family about the signs and symptoms of infection. Teach the patient and family to avoid pulling on the PF catheter or trauma to exit site. Emphasize the need to maintain the cleansing regimen at exit site.
Fluid obstruction	Change the position of the patient (standing, lying, side-lying, knee-chest). Relieve the patient's constipation. Irrigate the catheter. Ensure that sufficient fluid is in the abdomen (sometimes requires a residual reservoir of approximately 50 mL).
Rectal pain	Ensure a sufficient reservoir of fluid. Use a slow infusion rate.
Shoulder pain	Ensure that all air is primed from infusion tubing. Attempt draining the effluent with the patient in a knee-chest position. Administer mild analgesics as ordered.
Hernia	Monitor for an increase in size of or pain in the area of the hernia. Dialyze with patient in the supine position. Use an abdominal binder or support for the hernia (as long as not binding on catheter exit site).
Fluid overload	Increase the use of hypertonic solutions. Decrease oral (PO) fluid intake. Shorten dwell times. Weigh patients daily and before and after PD. Monitor lung sounds and peripheral edema.
Dehydration	Assess patients for decreased skin turgor, muscle cramps, hypotension, tachycardia, and dizziness. Discontinue hypertonic solutions. Increase oral fluid intake. Lengthen dwell times.
Blood-tinged effluent	Monitor for a change in effluent color (clear yellow to pink or rust). Administer heparin, as ordered, to prevent fibrin formation. Obtain a patient history about catheter trauma and patient activity before appearance of complication.

BOX 27-11 CASE STUDY

Patient with a Kidney Problem

Brief Patient History

Ms. L is a 32-year-old woman found down in the street near the hospital. She is awake but confused. She is unable to give any medical history and has no idea how long she has been in the street.

Clinical Assessment

Ms. L is admitted to the critical care unit with muscle pain and minimal dark urine output. She continues to be confused, but her neurologic examination results are otherwise normal. She repeatedly tells the nurses that she is tired, has pain everywhere, and just wants to sleep. She is able to move all her extremities and has no signs of injury on skin examination.

Diagnostic Procedures

Laboratory tests show the following results: creatinine phosphokinase (CPK) level of 40,400 U/L, serum myoglobin level of 2.5 mg/L, urinary myoglobin level of 300 mg/L, and serum potassium level of 4.8 mEq/dL. Baseline vital signs were as follows: blood pressure of 85/60 mm Hg, heart rate of 128 beats/min (sinus tachycardia), respiratory rate of 18 breaths/min, temperature of 101.3° F, and O_2 saturation of 98%.

The toxicology screen showed that the patient tested positive for cocaine. The Glasgow Coma Scale score was 14.

Medical Diagnosis

Ms. L is diagnosed with rhabdomyolysis.

Questions

1. What major outcomes do you expect to achieve for this patient?
2. What problems or risks must be managed to achieve these outcomes?
3. What interventions must be initiated to monitor, prevent, manage, or eliminate the problems and risks identified?
4. What interventions should be initiated to promote optimal functioning, safety, and well-being of the patient?
5. What possible learning needs do you anticipate for this patient?
6. What cultural and age-related factors may have a bearing on the patient's plan of care?

SUMMARY

Acute Kidney Injury

- Risk factors for development of AKI include sepsis, cardiac surgery, and diabetes.
- Many critically ill patients have AKI as a complication of their illness. The initial reason for admission to the critical care unit might have been sepsis, hypovolemic shock, trauma, or major surgery. If AKI develops, mortality and morbidity rates increase.
- Vigorous hydration with normal saline remains the most effective intervention to prevent contrast-induced nephrotoxicity (CIN) and AKI.

Catheter-Associated Urinary Tract Infection

- Catheter-associated urinary tract infection (CAUTI) remains a significant risk in critical illness. Prevention strategies include: avoiding unnecessary use of urinary catheters; insertion of urinary catheters using aseptic technique; adoption of evidence-based standards for maintenance of urinary catheters; daily clinical review of the need for the urinary catheter and, if not needed, prompt removal.

Diuretics and Renal Replacement Therapies

- Diuretics increase urine output but do not protect against the development of kidney failure. Diuretics are categorized into different groups based on their pharmacology and site of action in the nephron. The most frequently used diuretics are: loop diuretics, thiazide diuretics, and osmotic diuretics. Two diuretics from different classes can act synergistically to increase urine output when the pharmacologic action of each diuretic is on a different part of the nephron.
- Acute care renal replacement therapies include IHD and CRRT. Both are valuable in acute kidney failure, and one method is not superior to the other in terms of mortality outcomes or recovery of kidney function.

REFERENCES

1. Bellomo R. Acute renal failure. *Semin Respir Crit Care Med*. 2011;32(5):639.
2. Singbartl K, Kellum JA. AKI in the ICU: definition, epidemiology, risk stratification, and outcomes. *Kidney Internat*. 2012;81(9):819.
3. Mehta RL, et al. Spectrum of acute renal failure in the intensive care unit: the PICARD experience. *Kidney Internat*. 2004;66(4):1613.
4. Prowle JR, et al. Oliguria as predictive biomarker of acute kidney injury in critically ill patients. *Crit Care*. 2011;15(4):R172.
5. Macedo E, et al. Defining urine output criterion for acute kidney injury in critically ill patients. *Nephrol Dial Transplant*. 2011;26(2):509.
6. Rachoin JS, et al. The fallacy of the BUN:creatinine ratio in critically ill patients. *Nephrol Dial Transplantat*. 2012;27(6):2248.
7. Endre ZH, Pickering JW, Walker RJ. Clearance and beyond: the complementary roles of GFR measurement and injury biomarkers in acute kidney injury (AKI). *Am J Physiol Renal Physiol*. 2011;301(4):F697.
8. National Kidney and Urologic Diseases Information Clearinghouse (NKUDIC). http://kidney.niddk.nih.gov/kudiseases/pubs/kustats/ Accessed September 15, 2012.
9. Nickolas TL, et al. Awareness of kidney disease in the US population: findings from the National Health and Nutrition Examination Survey (NHANES) 1999 to 2000. *Am J Kidney Dis*. 2004;44(2):185.
10. Coresh J, et al. Prevalence of chronic kidney disease in the United States. *JAMA*. 2007;298(17):2038.
11. Carubelli V, et al. Renal dysfunction in acute heart failure: epidemiology, mechanisms and assessment. *Heart Failure Rev*. 2012;17(2):271.
12. Ronco C, et al. Cardio-renal syndromes: report from the consensus conference of the acute dialysis quality initiative. *Eur Heart J*. 2010;31(6):703.
13. Koyner JL, Murray PT. Mechanical ventilation and the kidney. *Blood Purif*. 2010;29(1):52.
14. Vieira Jr, JM, et al. Effect of acute kidney injury on weaning from mechanical ventilation in critically ill patients. *Crit Care Med*. 2007;35(1):184.
15. Pan SW, et al. Acute kidney injury on ventilator initiation day independently predicts prolonged mechanical ventilation in intensive care unit patients. *J Crit Care*. 2011;26(6):586.
16. Dellinger RP, et al. Surviving Sepsis Campaign: international guidelines for management of severe sepsis and septic shock: 2012. *Crit Care Med*. 2013;41(2):580.
17. Bagshaw SM, George C, Gibney RT, Bellomo R. A multi-center evaluation of early acute kidney injury in critically ill trauma patients. *Ren Fail*. 2008;30(6):581.
18. Delaney KA, Givens ML, Vohra RB. Use of RIFLE criteria to predict the severity and prognosis of acute kidney injury in emergency department patients with rhabdomyolysis. *J Emerg Med*. 2012;42(5):521.
19. Shapiro ML, Baldea A, Luchette FA. Rhabdomyolysis in the intensive care unit. *J Intens Care Med*. 2011.
20. Parekh R, Care DA, Tainter CR. Rhabdomyolysis: advances in diagnosis and treatment. *Emerg Med Pract*. 2012;14(3):1.
21. Brown CV, et al. Preventing renal failure in patients with rhabdomyolysis: do bicarbonate and mannitol make a difference? *J Trauma*. 2004;56(6):1191.
22. Weisbord SD, et al. The incidence of clinically significant contrast-induced nephropathy following non-emergent coronary angiography. *Catheter Cardiovasc Interv*. 2008;71(7):879.
23. Stacul F, et al. Contrast induced nephropathy: updated ESUR Contrast Media Safety Committee guidelines. *Eur Radiol*. 2011;21(12):2527.
24. Isaac S. Contrast-induced nephropathy: nursing implications. *Crit Care Nurse*. 2012;32(3):41.
25. Goldenberg I, Chonchol M, Guetta V. Reversible acute kidney injury following contrast exposure and the risk of long-term mortality. *Am J Nephrol*. 2008;29(2):136.
26. Institute for Healthcare Improvement. Getting started kit: prevent catheter-associated urinary tract infections how-to guide. http://www.bestcare.org.za/file/view/CAUTI-IHI-howtoguide.pdf. Accessed September 15, 2012.

27. Centers for Disease Control and Prevention. Guideline for prevention of catheter associated urinary tract infections 2009. http://www.cdc.gov/hicpac/pdf/cauti/cautiguideline2009final.pdf. Accessed September 15, 2012.

28. Burton DC, et al. Trends in catheter-associated urinary tract infections in adult intensive care units-United States, 1990-2007. *Infect Control Hosp Epidemiol.* 2011;32(8):748.

29. Chant C, Smith OM, Marshall JC, Friedrich JO. Relationship of catheter-associated urinary tract infection to mortality and length of stay in critically ill patients: a systematic review and meta-analysis of observational studies. *Crit Care Med.* 2011;39(5):1167.

30. The Joint Commission. National Patient Safety Goals 2012. http://www.jointcommission.org/standards_information/npsgs.aspx Accessed September 15, 2012.

31. Rosenthal VD, et al. International Nosocomial Infection Control Consortium (INICC) report, data summary of 36 countries, for 2004-2009. *Am J Infect Control.* 2012;40(5):396.

32. Conway LJ, Pogorzelska M, Larson E, Stone PW. Adoption of policies to prevent catheter-associated urinary tract infections in United States intensive care units. *Am J Infect Control.* 2012;40(8):705.

33. Titsworth WL, et al. Reduction of catheter-associated urinary tract infections among patients in a neurological intensive care unit: a single institution's success. *J Neurosurg.* 2012;116(4):911.

34. Marra AR, et al. Preventing catheter-associated urinary tract infection in the zero-tolerance era. *Am J Infect Control.* 2011;39(10):817.

35. Davison DL, Patel K, Chawla LS. Hemodynamic monitoring in the critically ill: spanning the range of kidney function. *Am J Kidney Dis.* 2012;59(5):715.

36. El-Sherif N, Turitto G. Electrolyte disorders and arrhythmogenesis. *Cardiol J.* 2011;18(3):233.

37. Kessler C, Ng J, Valdez K, Geiger B. The use of sodium polystyrene sulfonate in the inpatient management of hyperkalemia. *J Hosp Med.* 2011;6(3):136.

38. Charmot D. Non-systemic drugs: a critical review. *Curr Pharm Des.* 2012;18(10):1434.

39. Kovesdy CP, et al. Hyponatremia, hypernatremia, and mortality in patients with chronic kidney disease with and without congestive heart failure. *Circulation.* 2012;125(5):677.

40. Hutchison AJ, Smith CP, Brenchley PE. Pharmacology, efficacy and safety of oral phosphate binders. *Nature Rev Nephrol.* 2011;7(10):578.

41. Molony DA, Stephens BW. Derangements in phosphate metabolism in chronic kidney diseases/endstage renal disease: therapeutic considerations. *Adv Chronic Kidney Dis.* 2011;18(2):120.

42. Jüppner H. Phosphate and FGF-23. *Kidney Internat* (suppl). 2011;(121):S24.

43. Gauci C, et al. Pitfalls of measuring total blood calcium in patients with CKD. *J Am Soc Nephrol.* 2008;19(8):1592.

44. Kalantar-Zadeh K, et al. Understanding sources of dietary phosphorus in the treatment of patients with chronic kidney disease. *Clin J Am Soc Nephrol.* 2010;5(3):519.

45. The SAFE Study Investigators. A comparison of albumin and saline for fluid resuscitation in the intensive care unit. *N Engl J Med.* 2004;350(22):2247.

46. Investigaors TSS. Saline or albumin for fluid resuscitation in patients with traumatic brain injury. *N Engl J Med.* 2007;357(9):874.

47. Perel P, Roberrts I. Colloids versus crystalloids for fluid resuscitation in critically ill patients. *Cochrane Database Syst Rev.* 2007;Issue 4. Art. No.: CD000567.

48. Nigwekar SU, Waikar SS. Diuretics in acute kidney injury. *Semin Nephrol.* 2011;31(6):523.

49. Wile D. Diuretics: a review. *Ann Clin Biochem.* 2012;49(5):419.

50. Felker GM. Loop diuretics in heart failure. *Heart Fail Rev.* 2012;17(2):305.

51. Asare K. Management of loop diuretic resistance in the intensive care unit. *Am J Health Syst Pharm.* 2009;66(18):1635.

52. Kassamali R, Sica DA. Acetazolamide: a forgotten diuretic agent. *Cardiol Rev.* 2011;19(6):276.

53. Lehrich RW, Greenberg A. Hyponatremia and the use of vasopressin receptor antagonists in critically ill patients. *J Intens Care Med.* 2012;27(4):207.

54. Giamouzis G, et al. Impact of dopamine infusion on renal function in hospitalized heart failure patients: results of the Dopamine in Acute Decompensated Heart Failure (DAD-HF) Trial. *J Cardiac Failure.* 2010;16(12):922.

55. Casaer MP, Mesotten D, Schetz MR. Bench-to-bedside review: metabolism and nutrition. *Crit Care.* 2008;12(4):222.

56. Gervasio JM, Garmon WP, Holowatyj M. Nutrition support in acute kidney injury. *Nutr Clin Pract.* 2011;26(4):374.

57. Ramanath V, et al. Anemia and chronic kidney disease: making sense of the recent trials. *Rev Recent Clin Trials.* 2012;7(3):187.

58. Besarab A. Anemia and iron management. *Semin Dial.* 2011;24(5):498.

59. Oudemans-van Straaten HM, Kellum JA, Bellomo R. Clinical review: anticoagulation for continuous renal replacement therapy–heparin or citrate? *Crit Care.* 2011;15(1):202.

60. Kimball TA, et al. Efficiency of the kidney disease outcomes quality initiative guidelines for preemptive vascular access in an academic setting. *J Vasc Surg.* 2011;54(3):760.

61. Schild AF, et al. Arteriovenous fistulae vs. arteriovenous grafts: a retrospective review of 1,700 consecutive vascular access cases. *J Vasc Access.* 2008;9(4):231.

62. Coryell L, et al. The case for primary placement of tunneled hemodialysis catheters in acute kidney injury. *J Vasc Interv Radiol.* 2009;20(12):1578.

63. Vats HS, et al. A comparison between blood flow outcomes of tunneled external jugular and internal jugular hemodialysis catheters. *J Vasc Access.* 2012;13(1):51.

64. Vats HS. Complications of catheters: tunneled and nontunneled. *Adv Chronic Kidney Dis.* 2012;19(3):188.

65. Palevsky PM, et al. Intensity of renal support in critically ill patients with acute kidney injury. *N Engl J Med.* 2008;359(1):7.

66. Bellomo R, et al. Intensity of continuous renal-replacement therapy in critically ill patients. *N Engl J Med.* 2009;361(17):1627.

67. Kellum JA, Ronco C. Dialysis: results of RENAL–what is the optimal CRRT target dose? *Nat Rev Nephrol.* 2010;6(4):191.

68. Cerdá J, Ronco C. Modalities of continuous renal replacement therapy: technical and clinical considerations. *Semin Dial.* 2009;22(2):114.

69. Felker GM, Mentz RJ. Diuretics and ultrafiltration in acute decompensated heart failure. *JACC.* 2012;59(24):2145.

70. Freda BJ, Slawsky M, Mallidi J, Braden GL. Decongestive treatment of acute decompensated heart failure: cardiorenal implications of ultrafiltration and diuretics. *Am J Kidney Dis.* 2011;58(6):1005.

71. Vesconi S, et al. Delivered dose of renal replacement therapy and mortality in critically ill patients with acute kidney injury. *Crit Care.* 2009;13(2):R57.

72. Finkel KW, Podoll AS. Complications of continuous renal replacement therapy. *Semin Dial.* 2009;22(2):155.

73. Lins RL, et al. Intermittent versus continuous renal replacement therapy for acute kidney injury patients admitted to the intensive care unit: results of a randomized clinical trial. *Nephrol Dial Transplant.* 2009;24(2):512.

74. Karvellas CJ, et al. A comparison of early versus late initiation of renal replacement therapy in critically ill patients with acute kidney injury: a systematic review and meta-analysis. *Crit Care.* 2011;15(1):R72.

75. Macedo E, Mehta RL. When should renal replacement therapy be initiated for acute kidney injury? *Semin Dial.* 2011;24(2):132.

76. Sinnakirouchenan R, Holley JL. Peritoneal dialysis versus hemodialysis: risks, benefits, and access issues. *Adv Chron Kidney Dis.* 2011;18(6):428.

77. Bargman JM. Advances in peritoneal dialysis: a review. *Semin Dial.* 2012;25(5):545.

78. Lafrance JP, et al. Association of dialysis modality with risk for infection-related hospitalization: a propensity score-matched cohort analysis. *Clin J Amer Soc Nephrol.* 2012;7(10):1598.

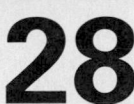

Gastrointestinal Anatomy and Physiology

Kathleen M. Stacy

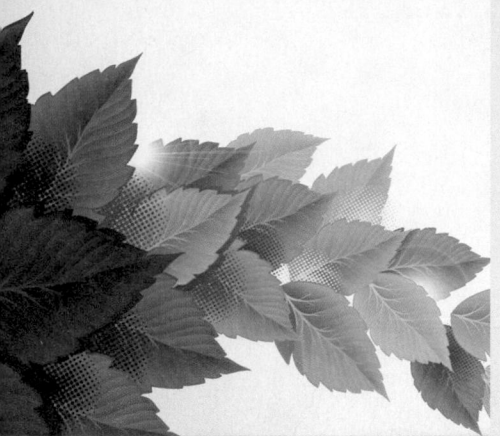

evolve WEBSITE

http://evolve.elsevier.com/Urden/criticalcare/

Evolve features:
- NCLEX Review Questions
- CCRN Review Questions
- PCCN Review Questions
- Mosby's Nursing Skills Procedures
- Animations
- Video Clips
- Glossary

The major function of the gastrointestinal (GI) tract is digestion. It converts ingested nutrients into simpler forms that can be transported from the tract's lumen to the portal circulation and then used in metabolic processes. The GI system also plays a vital role in the detoxification and elimination of bacteria, viruses, chemical toxins, and drugs. Disturbances of the GI system itself or of the complex hormonal and neural controls that regulate it can severely upset homeostasis and compromise the overall nutritional status of the patient. Any circumvention of the normal feeding mechanism can alter digestive processes or contribute to malabsorption.

The critical care nurse must have a comprehensive knowledge of the anatomy and normal function of the GI tract to facilitate assessment, diagnosis, and intervention in patients with GI dysfunction. The GI tract consists of the mouth, the esophagus, the stomach, the small intestine, and the large intestine (Fig. 28-1).

MOUTH

The mouth and accessory organs, which include the lips, cheeks, gums, tongue, palate, and salivary glands, perform the initial phases of digestion, which are ingestion, mastication, and salivation.[1]

Ingestion and Mastication

The mouth is the beginning of the alimentary canal (see Fig. 28-1) and is the means for ingestion and entry of nutrients. The teeth cut, grind, and mix food, transforming it into a form suitable for swallowing and increasing the surface area of food available to mix with salivary secretions. Healthy dentition is vital for this process. Mucous glands located behind the tip of the tongue and serous glands located at the back of the tongue aid in the lubrication of food and in its distribution over the taste buds.[2]

Salivation

Salivation has an important role in the first stage of digestion because saliva lubricates the mouth, facilitates the movement of the lips and the tongue during swallowing, and washes away bacteria. Saliva consists of approximately 99.5% water,[3] which contains a large amount of ions such as potassium, chloride, bicarbonate,[1] thiocyanate, and hydrogen;[3] immunoglobulin A, which is vital for destroying oral bacteria;[1] and mucus. Approximately 1000 to 1500 milliliters (mL) of saliva is produced each day by three pairs of major salivary glands: (1) the submandibular glands, (2) the sublingual glands, and (3) the parotid glands. Parotid gland secretions are enzymatic, containing amylase (ptyalin), which begins the chemical breakdown of large polysaccharides into dextrins and sugars. The mouth and pharynx also are lined with minor salivary glands that provide additional lubrication.[3]

The salivary glands are regulated by the autonomic nervous system, with parasympathetic effects being predominant. Increased parasympathetic stimulation results in profuse secretions of watery saliva, whereas decreased parasympathetic stimulation results in inhibition of salivation.[1,3]

ESOPHAGUS

The esophagus is a hollow muscular tube that lacks cartilage. In adults, it is 23 to 25 cm (9 to 10 inches) long and 2 to 3 cm

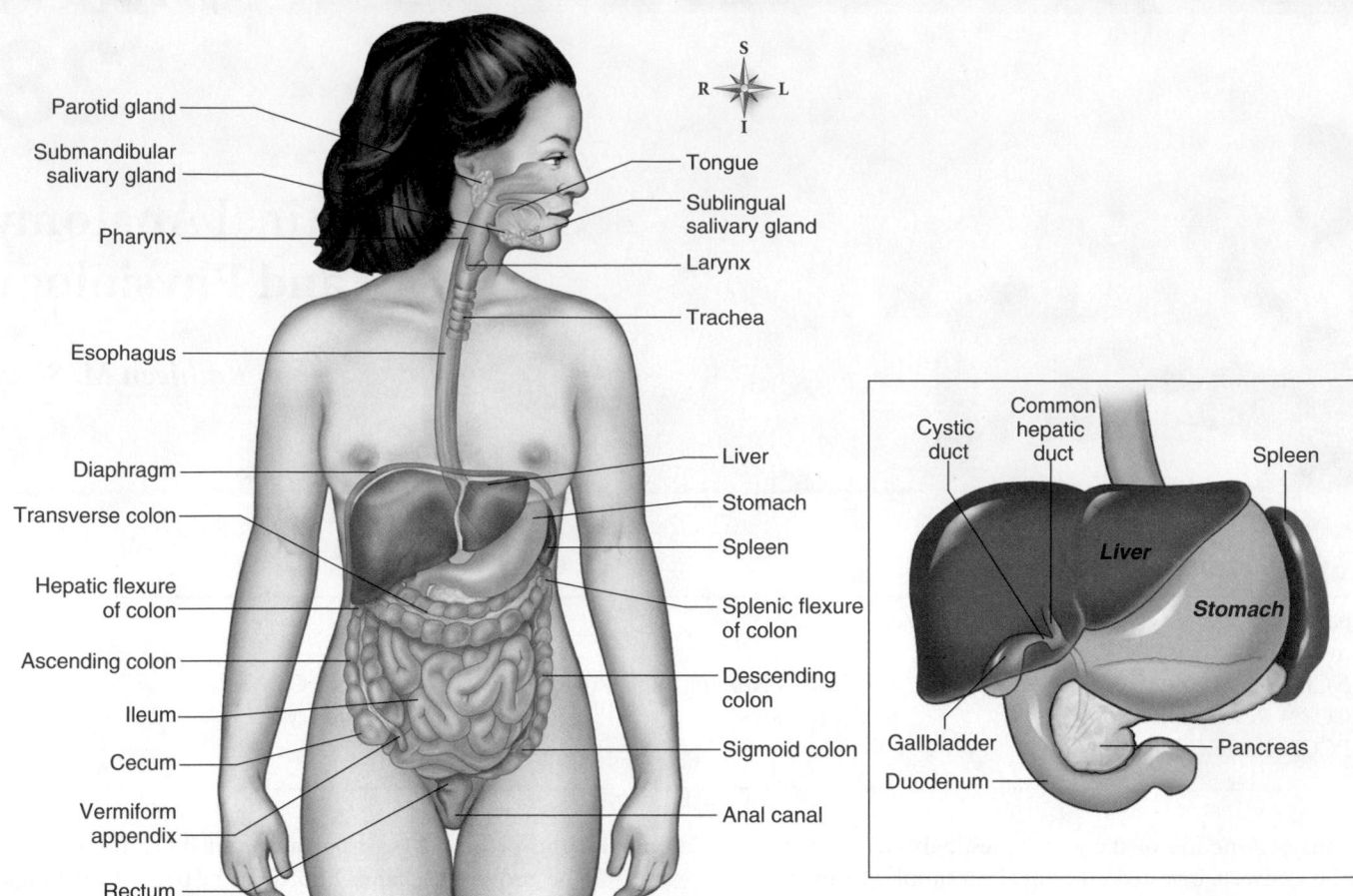

FIGURE 28-1 Anatomy of the gastrointestinal system. (From Patton KT, Thibodeau GA. *Anatomy & Physiology.* 8th ed. St. Louis: Mosby; 2013.)

(1 inch) wide. It is the narrowest part of the digestive tube and lies posterior to the trachea and the heart, with attachments at the hypopharynx and at the cardiac portion of the stomach below the diaphragm. It begins at the level of the C6 to T1 vertebrae and extends vertically through the mediastinum and diaphragm to the level of T11.[4]

The esophagus has two sphincters: (1) the upper esophageal sphincter (also known as *hypopharyngeal sphincter*) and (2) the lower esophageal sphincter (also known as *cardioesophageal* or *gastroesophageal sphincter*).[4] The upper esophageal sphincter inhibits air from entering the esophagus during respiration. The lower esophageal sphincter controls the passage of food into the stomach and prevents reflux of gastric contents.[1]

Swallowing

The functions of the esophagus are to accept a bolus of food from the oropharynx, to transport the bolus through the esophageal body by gravity and peristalsis, and to release the bolus into the stomach through the lower esophageal sphincter. This process is known as *swallowing.*[5] Peristalsis consists of waves of circular muscle contractions and relaxations. Peristalsis that is initiated by swallowing is known as *primary peristalsis,* whereas peristalsis that is initiated by esophageal distention is known as *secondary peristalsis.* Peristaltic waves begin in the pharynx and move distally at a rate of 2 to 6 cm per second.[1]

STOMACH

The stomach is an elongated pouch that is approximately 25 to 30 cm (10 to 12 inches) long and 10 to 15 cm (4 to 6 inches) wide at the maximal transverse diameter (Fig. 28-2). It lies obliquely beneath the cardiac sphincter at the esophagogastric junction and above the pyloric sphincter, next to the small intestine. The anatomic divisions of the stomach are the cardia (proximal end), the fundus (portion above and to the left of the cardiac sphincter), the body (middle portion), the antrum (elongated, constricted portion), and the pylorus (distal end connecting the antrum to the duodenum) (Fig. 28-3). The greater curvature, which begins at the cardiac orifice and arches backward and upward around the fundus, is in contact with the transverse colon and the pancreas at the posterior edge. The lesser curvature extends from the cardia to the pylorus. Two sphincters control the rate of food passage: (1) the lower esophageal sphincter at the esophagogastric junction and (2) the pyloric sphincter at the gastroduodenal junction.[6]

The stomach wall has four layers (Fig. 28-4). The outermost layer, the *serous layer (serosa),* consists of squamous epithelial tissue and continues as a double fold from the lower edge of the stomach to cover the intestine. The second layer, the *muscular layer (muscularis),* extends from the fundus to the antrum and consists of three smooth muscle layers, which are the

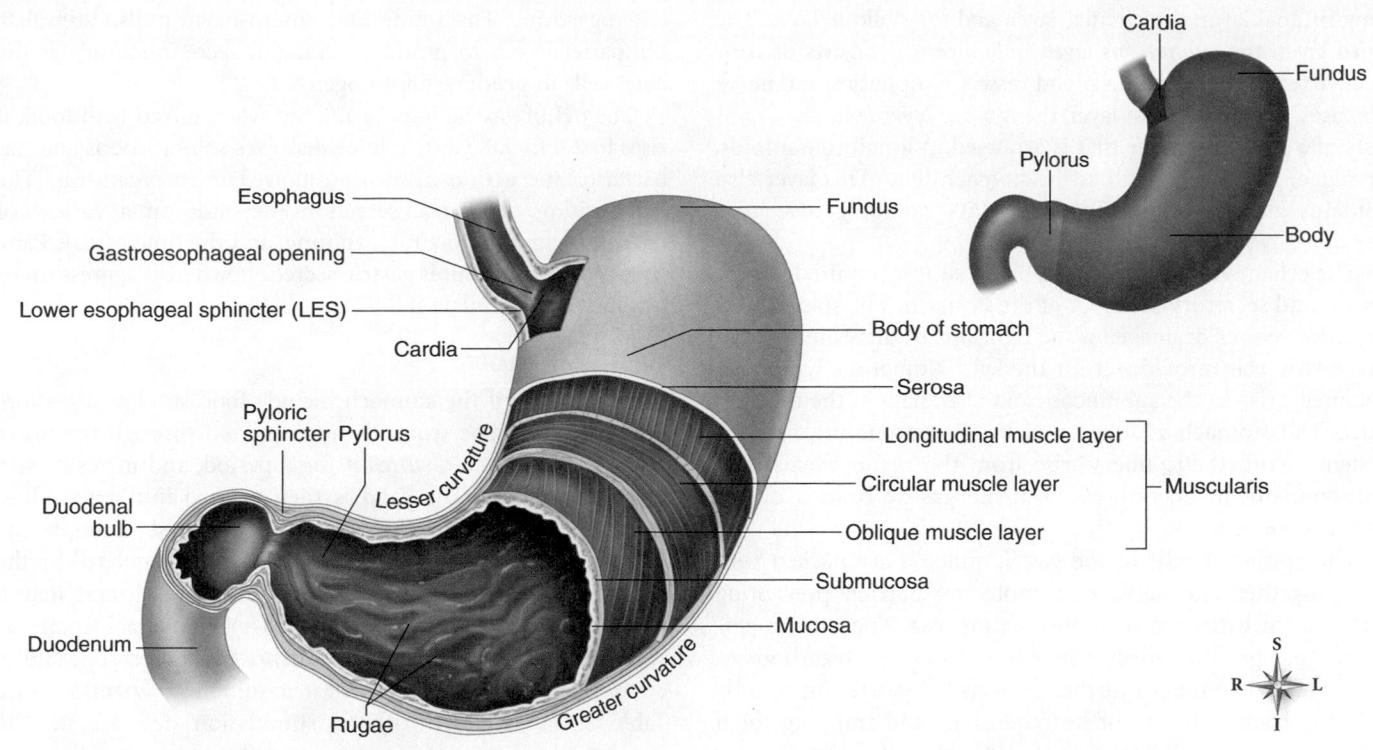

FIGURE 28-2 Gross anatomy of the stomach. (From Patton KT, Thibodeau GA. *Anatomy & Physiology.* 8th ed. St. Louis: Mosby; 2013.)

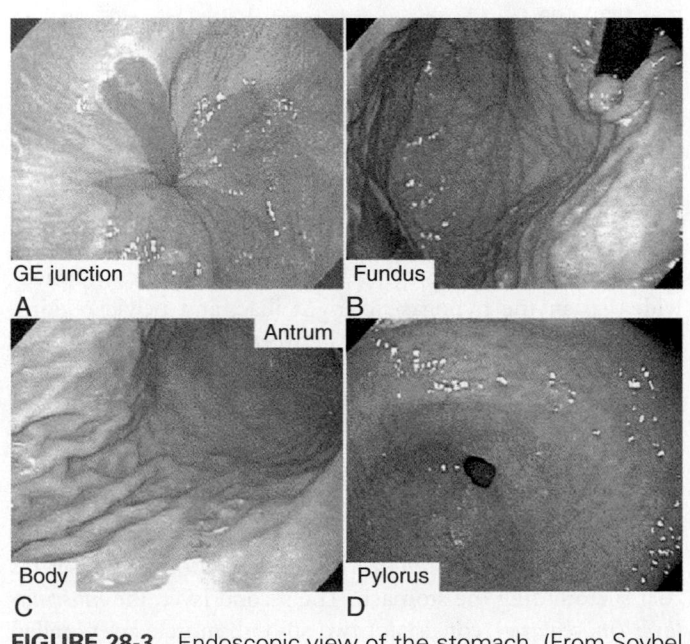

FIGURE 28-3 Endoscopic view of the stomach. (From Soybel DI. Anatomy and physiology of the stomach. *Surg Clin North Am.* 2005;85:875.)

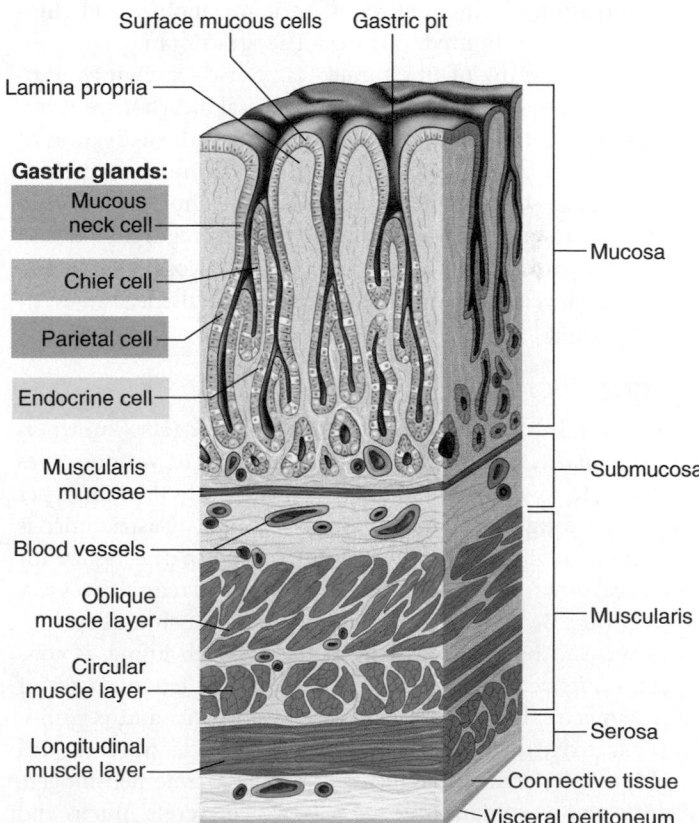

FIGURE 28-4 Structure of the gastric mucosa. (From Patton KT, Thibodeau GA. *Anatomy & Physiology.* 8th ed. St. Louis: Mosby; 2013.)

longitudinal layer, the circular layer, and the oblique layer. The third layer, the *submucous layer (submucosa)*, consists of connective tissue that contains blood vessels, lymphatics, and nerve plexuses. The innermost layer, the *mucous layer (mucosa)*, consists of a muscular layer that is arranged in longitudinal folds, or rugae, that can expand as the stomach fills.[6] This layer also contains glands that secrete about 1500 mL of gastric juice per day.[7]

The celiac artery provides the blood supply required for the motor and secretory activities of the stomach. The splenic vein provides venous drainage for the right side of the stomach, and the gastric vein provides it for the left.[1] Numerous lymphatic channels arise in the submucosa and terminate in the thoracic duct. The stomach is innervated by the autonomic nervous system. Sympathetic fibers arise from the celiac plexus, and parasympathetic fibers arise from the gastric branch of the vagus nerve.[6]

The epithelial cells of the gastric mucosa are packed very close together and serve as a protective barrier, preventing diffusion of hydrogen ions into the mucosa. The surface epithelial cells produce alkaline mucus and secrete a bicarbonate-laden fluid. The mucus further protects the gastric mucosa by delaying back-diffusion of hydrogen ions and trapping them for neutralization by the secreted bicarbonate.[7] The gastric mucosal cells can compensate for cell destruction. Epithelial cells are in a constant state of growth, migration, and desquamation, and they are shed at a rate of one half million cells per minute. The gastric mucosa also has the ability to increase blood flow, providing an additional buffer for acid neutralization and aiding in the removal of toxic metabolites and chloride ions from injured mucosa. The gastric mucosal cells synthesize a family of unsaturated fatty acids known as *prostaglandins*. Prostaglandins facilitate mucosal bicarbonate secretion and inhibit acid secretion by preventing the activation of parietal cells by histamine (a local biochemical mediator). Certain lipid-soluble substances such as alcohol, aspirin, and other nonsteroidal anti-inflammatory drugs, regurgitated bile, and uremic toxins, can break through the mucosal barrier and penetrate the cells, causing their destruction, edema, and eventual bleeding.[7]

Gastric Secretion

The stomach has two types of glands—*oxyntic* (also known as *gastric glands*), and *pyloric*—that contain cells of various types that secrete 1500 to 2400 mL of gastric juice into the lumen per day, depending on the diet and other stimuli.[7] Gastric juice is composed of hydrochloric acid (HCl), pepsin (necessary for the breakdown of protein), mucus, intrinsic factor (necessary for vitamin B_{12} absorption), sodium, and potassium. Pepsinogen, secreted by the chief cells of the stomach lining, is converted to its active form, pepsin, in the acidic environment of the stomach.[1] The cardiac glands secrete mucus and pepsinogen. The oxyntic glands contain parietal cells, which secrete HCl and intrinsic factor, and chief cells, which secrete pepsinogen. Pyloric glands contain mucous cells, which secrete mucus and pepsinogen, and G-cells, which secrete gastrin (Table 28-1).[6] Gastric glands are stimulated by the parasympathetic stimulation and gastrin and inhibited by gastric-inhibitory peptide and

enterogastrone. Histamine and entero-oxyntin also stimulate the parietal cells to produce acid, and secretin stimulates the chief cells to produce pepsinogen.[1]

The pH of gastric juice is 1.0, but when mixed with food, it rises to 2.0 to 3.0. Gastric juice dissolves soluble foods and has bacteriostatic action against swallowed microorganisms. The composition of gastric secretions depends on a variety of factors, including flow rate, volume, and the time of day. Pain, fear, or rage can inhibit gastric secretion, whereas aggression or hostility can stimulate it.[1]

Gastric Motility

The functions of the stomach include food storage, digestion, and emptying. The stomach receives food through the lower esophageal sphincter, stores it for a period, and mixes it with gastric secretions. The food is then ground into a semifluid consistency called *chyme*, which is delivered through the pylorus to the duodenum. Gastric motility is regulated by the autonomic nervous system, digestive hormones, and neural reflexes. Gastrin, motilin (see Table 28-1), and parasympathetic stimulation increase gastric motility, whereas secretin, cholecystokinin, enterogastrone, gastric-inhibitory peptide (see Table 28-1), and sympathetic stimulation decrease it. The ileogastric reflex inhibits gastric motility when the ileum is distended.[8]

SMALL INTESTINE

The small intestine, a coiled, folded tube that is approximately 7 m (22 to 23 feet) long, extends from the pyloric sphincter to the cecum and fills most of the abdominal cavity. It has three anatomic divisions: (1) the duodenum, (2) the jejunum, and (3) the ileum. The duodenum, shaped like the letter C, begins at the pyloric sphincter of the stomach and ends at the ligament of Treitz. It is 30 cm (12 inches) long and 4 cm (1 to 1.5 inches) wide.[9] The jejunum, which is 250 cm (8 to 9 feet) long and 4 cm (1 to 1.5 inches) wide, lies in the left iliac and umbilical regions. The ileum, which is 375 cm (12 feet) long and 2.5 cm (1 inch) wide, lies in the hypogastric, right iliac, and pelvic regions. Although the demarcating line between the jejunum and the ileum is somewhat arbitrary, the ileum is narrower than the jejunum. The ileocecal valve, located at the terminal end of the ileum at the junction of the cecum and colon, controls the flow of small bowel contents into the large intestine and prevents reflux (Fig. 28-5).[1]

The small intestine has four layers (Fig. 28-6). The outermost layer, the *serous layer (serosa)*, is a continuation of the serous coat surrounding the stomach. The second layer, the *muscular layer (muscularis)*, consists of two smooth muscle layers called the *longitudinal* and *circular layers*. The third layer, the *submucous layer (submucosa)*, consists of connective tissue that contains blood vessels, lymphatics, glands, and nerve plexuses. The innermost layer, the *mucous layer (mucosa)*, consists of simple columnar epithlelium.[5] The mucosa and submucosa are arranged in circular folds (plicae circulares),[5] which are largest and most numerous in the jejunum and upper ileum.[1] These folds are covered by a second series of projectile-like folds called *villi*, which are in constant motion—constricting, lengthening,

TABLE 28-1	DIGESTIVE HORMONES		
SOURCE	**HORMONE**	**STIMULUS FOR SECRETION**	**ACTION**
Mucosa of the stomach	Gastrin	Presence of partially digested proteins in the stomach	Stimulates gastric glands to secrete hydrochloric acid and pepsinogen; growth of gastric mucosa; promotes gastric motility
	Histamine	Acid in the stomach	Stimulates acid secretion
	Somatostatin	Acid in the stomach	Inhibits acid and pepsinogen secretion and release of gastrin
	Acetylcholine	Vagus and local nerves in stomach	Stimulates release of pepsinogen and acid secretion
	Gastrin-releasing peptide (bombesin)	Vagus and local nerves in stomach	Stimulates gastrin and release of pepsinogen and acid secretion
Mucosa of the small intestines	Motilin	Presence of acid and fat in the duodenum	Increases gastrointestinal (GI) motility
	Secretion	Presence of chyme (acid, partially digested proteins, and fats) in the duodenum	Stimulates pancreas to secrete alkaline pancreatic juice and liver to secrete bile; decreases GI motility; inhibits gastrin and gastric acid secretion
	Cholecystokinin	Presence of chyme (acid, partially digested proteins, and fats) in the duodenum	Stimulates gallbladder to eject bile and pancreas to secrete alkaline fluid; decreases gastric motility; constricts pyloric sphincter; inhibits gastrin; delays gastric emptying
	Enteroglucogon	Intraluminal fats and carbohydrates	Weakly inhibits gastric and pancreatic secretion and enhances insulin release, lipolysis, ketogenesis, and glycogenolysis; delays gastric emptying
	Gastric-inhibitory peptide (GIP)	Fat and glucose in small intestine	Inhibits gastric secretion and gastric emptying, stimulates insulin release
	Peptide YY	Intraluminal fat and bile acids	Inhibits postprandial gastric acid and pancreatic secretion and delays gastric and small bowel emptying
	Pancreatic polypeptide	Protein, fat, and glucose in small intestine	Decreases pancreatic bicarbonate
	Vasoactive intestinal peptide	Intestinal mucosa and muscle	Relaxes intestinal smooth muscle, increases blood flow

NOTE: The digestive hormones are not secreted into the gastrointestinal lumen but rather into the bloodstream, in which they travel to target tissues. There are more than 30 peptide hormone genes expressed in the gastrointestinal tract and more than 100 hormonally active peptides.
Modified from Johnson LR. *Gastrointestinal Physiology*. 7th ed. St. Louis: Mosby; 2007.
Data from Schubert ML, Peura DA. Control of gastric acid secretion in health and disease. *Gastroenterology*. 2008;134(7):1842-1860; Wren AM, Bloom SR. Gut hormones and appetite control. *Gastroenterology*. 2007;132(6):2116-2130.

and shortening (villous movement). The four to five million villi (see Fig. 28-5) give the intestine a velvety appearance; they are more numerous and larger in the jejunum than in the ileum. Villi contain a network of capillaries and blind lymphatic vessels called *lacteals*. The outer layer of the villus is composed of microvilli. The circular folds of the small intestine, along with the villi and microvilli, increase the digestive-absorptive surface of the small intestine 600 times.[9,10]

The gastroduodenal artery provides the blood supply for the duodenum, and branches of the superior mesenteric artery provide for the jejunum and the ileum. The superior mesenteric vein provides for venous drainage of the small intestine.[11] Numerous lymphatic channels arise in the submucosa and terminate in the thoracic duct. The small intestine is extrinsically innervated by the autonomic nervous system. Sympathetic fibers arise from the celiac plexus, whereas parasympathetic fibers arise from the gastric branch of the vagus nerve. Intrinsic innervation, which initiates motor functions, is provided by Auerbach's plexus and Meissner's plexus, which are located in the intestinal wall.[1]

Intestinal Secretion

The small intestine has two major types of glands: (1) Brunner's glands and (2) intestinal glands. Brunner's glands lie in the mucosa of the duodenum and secrete mucus, an alkaline fluid (pH of 9) that neutralizes chyme and protects the mucosa.[10] Intestinal glands are found in pits of the submucosa and are called the *crypts of Lieberkühn*. These crypts secrete 2 to 3 liters (L) per day of yellow fluid containing enzymes that assist in nutrient digestion.[7]

Intestinal Motility

Intestinal motility consists of two separate motions: (1) peristalsis and (2) haustral segmentation. Peristalsis is sequential contraction and relaxation of short segments of the small intestine that facilitate digestion and absorption. Haustral segmentation is rhythmic contractions that facilitate the mixing and forward movement of chyme. It is controlled by Auerbach's plexus. Intestinal motility is also affected by neural reflexes located along the length of the small intestine. Motility is inhibited by the intestino-intestinal reflex, which is activated

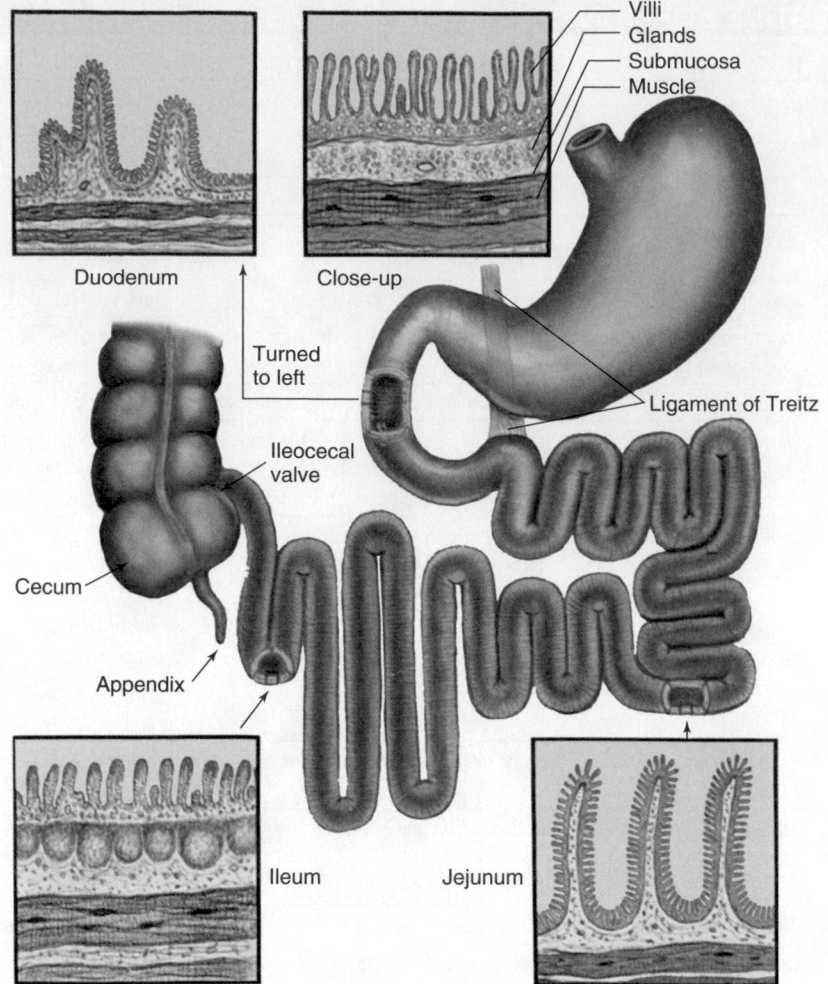

FIGURE 28-5   Clinical anatomy of the small intestine. (From Thompson JM, et al. *Mosby's Clinical Nursing.* 5th ed. St. Louis: Mosby; 2002.)

by distention of the small intestine, and is stimulated by the gastroileal reflux, which is initiated by an increase in gastric motility.[12]

Digestion and Absorption

The functions of the small intestine include digestion and absorption. Digestion, which involves breaking down large molecules into small ones, is essential for nutrient absorption from the small intestine (Fig. 28-7). Maintenance of pH and osmolality is crucial for digestion in the small intestine. The entry of chyme into the duodenum stimulates the production of secretin, which stimulates the pancreas to secrete a highly alkaline fluid into the duodenum. In the small intestine, chyme mixes with pancreatic enzymes, intestinal enzymes, and bile from the liver and gallbladder, and it is then reduced to absorbable elements of proteins, fats, and carbohydrates. The nutrients are absorbed through the villi and transported to the liver by the portal system for further processing. The small intestine absorbs up to 8 L of fluid per day, passing only a small part of this fluid into the large intestine. In addition to the nutrients, electrolytes, water, components of saliva, gastric juice, and bile, intestinal and pancreatic secretions are also absorbed.[1]

LARGE INTESTINE

The large intestine, which extends from the ileocecal valve to the anus, is approximately 90 to 150 cm (4 to 5 feet) long and 4 to 6 cm (2 inches) in diameter. It is divided into the ascending colon, the hepatic flexure, the transverse colon, the splenic flexure, the descending colon, the sigmoid colon, the rectum, and the anal canal (Fig. 28-8).[10]

The colon has four layers. The outermost layer, the *serous layer (serosa)*, is formed from the visceral peritoneum and covers most of the large intestine, with the exclusion of the sigmoid colon. The second layer, the *muscular layer (muscularis)*, consists of two smooth muscle layers: the *longitudinal* and the *circular* muscles. These muscles work together to propel fecal matter through the colon and to "knead" the stool into a compact bolus. The longitudinal muscle consists of three muscular bands that stretch from the cecum to the distal sigmoid colon. These muscular bands create sacculations of haustra, important clinical features that normally are apparent on a barium enema radiograph. Haustra aid segmentation so that absorption of fluid from the fecal bolus is achieved. The third layer, the *submucous layer (submucosa)*, consists of connective

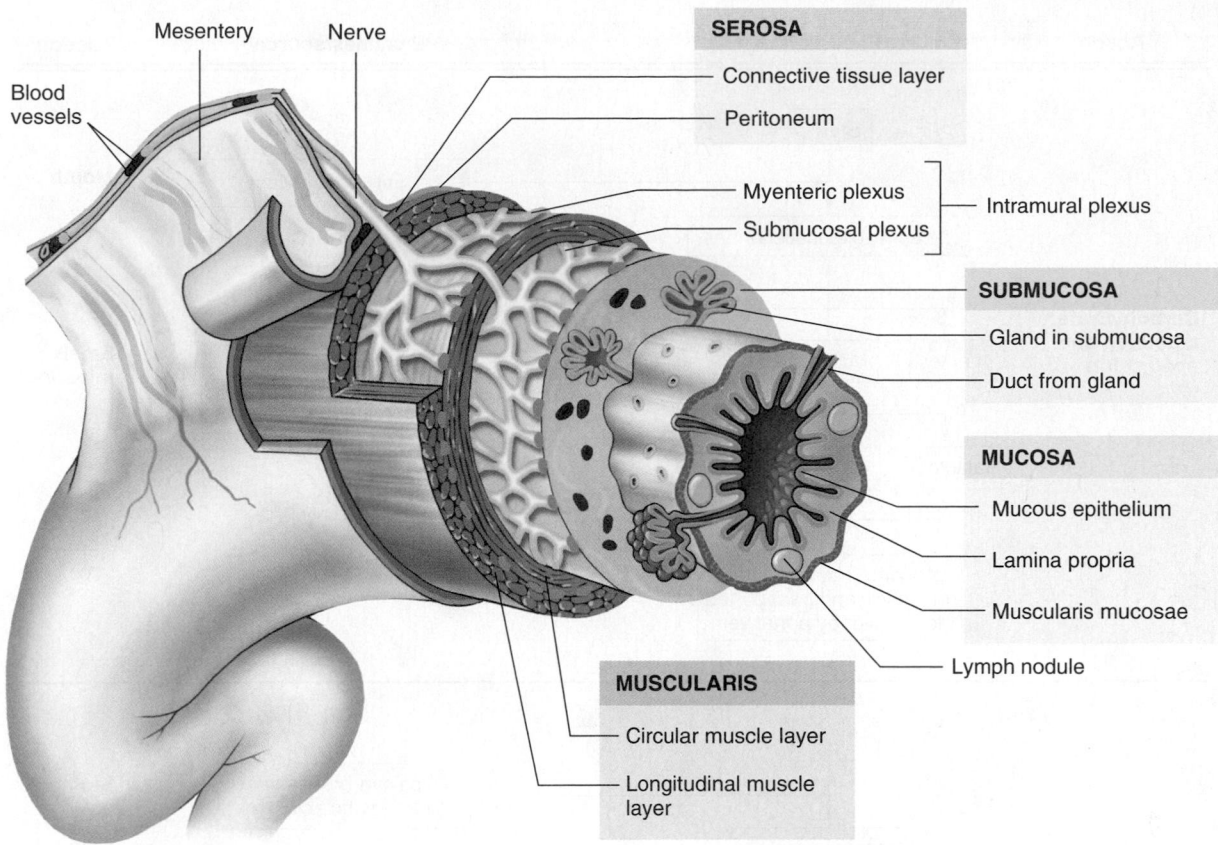

FIGURE 28-6 Cross-section of the gastrointestinal wall. (From Patton KT, Thibodeau GA. *Anatomy & Physiology*. 8th ed. St. Louis: Mosby; 2013.)

tissue that contains blood vessels, lymphatics, glands, and nerve plexuses. The innermost layer, the *mucous layer (mucosa)*, is lined with simple columnar epithelial cells and contains deep crypts of Lieberkühn that are lined with mucus-producing goblet cells. The mucus eases the passage of the fecal material and protects the mucosal surface from trauma.[10]

The rectum begins at the midsacrum, is 12 to 15 cm (5 inches) long, and is quite angulated. These angles, also known as *Houston's valves*, are important in the defecation process because they tend to slow the passage of fecal material in the rectal vault, assisting the continence mechanism.

Arterial blood is supplied to the colon from branches of the superior and inferior mesenteric arteries. Venous drainage occurs through the branches of the superior and inferior mesenteric veins into the portal system. The colon is intrinsically innervated by Auerbach's plexus, which controls secretion and motility and is extrinsically innervated by the autonomic nervous system. The sympathetic and parasympathetic branches of the autonomic system innervate the colon, regulating motility. Sympathetic stimulation inhibits colonic activity and constricts the anal sphincters, whereas parasympathetic stimulation increases colonic activity and secretion and relaxes the anal sphincters.[9]

Colonic Motility

Colonic motility consists of haustral shuttling and peristalsis. Haustral shuttling, a variation of haustral segmentation,

consists of the contraction and relaxation of the circular muscle. It moves the contents of the colon back and forth to facilitate the grinding of food masses and fluid absorption. Peristalsis is produced primarily by the longitudinal muscles and propels the fecal bolus forward. Mass peristalsis is a strong, slow contraction in which the distal left colon contracts en masse to move the fecal bolus into the rectum.[13]

Resorption

The major functions of the colon are resorption of water, sodium, chloride, glucose, and urea; dehydration of undigested residue; putrefaction of contents by bacteria; movement of the fecal bolus through the colon; and elimination of the fecal mass. The colon receives approximately 1000 to 2000 mL of chyme per day, and all but 50 to 250 mL of it is absorbed in the ascending and transverse colon.[5]

The colon contains billions of anaerobic bacteria that putrefy remaining proteins and indigestible residue; synthesize folic acid, vitamin K, nicotinic acid, riboflavin, and some B vitamins; and convert urea salts to ammonium salts and ammonia for absorption into the portal circulation.[1] Common colonic bacteria include *Bacteroides, Lactobacillus*, and *Clostridium*.[14]

ACCESSORY ORGANS

The accessory organs of digestion are the liver, the biliary system, and the pancreas (Fig. 28-9).

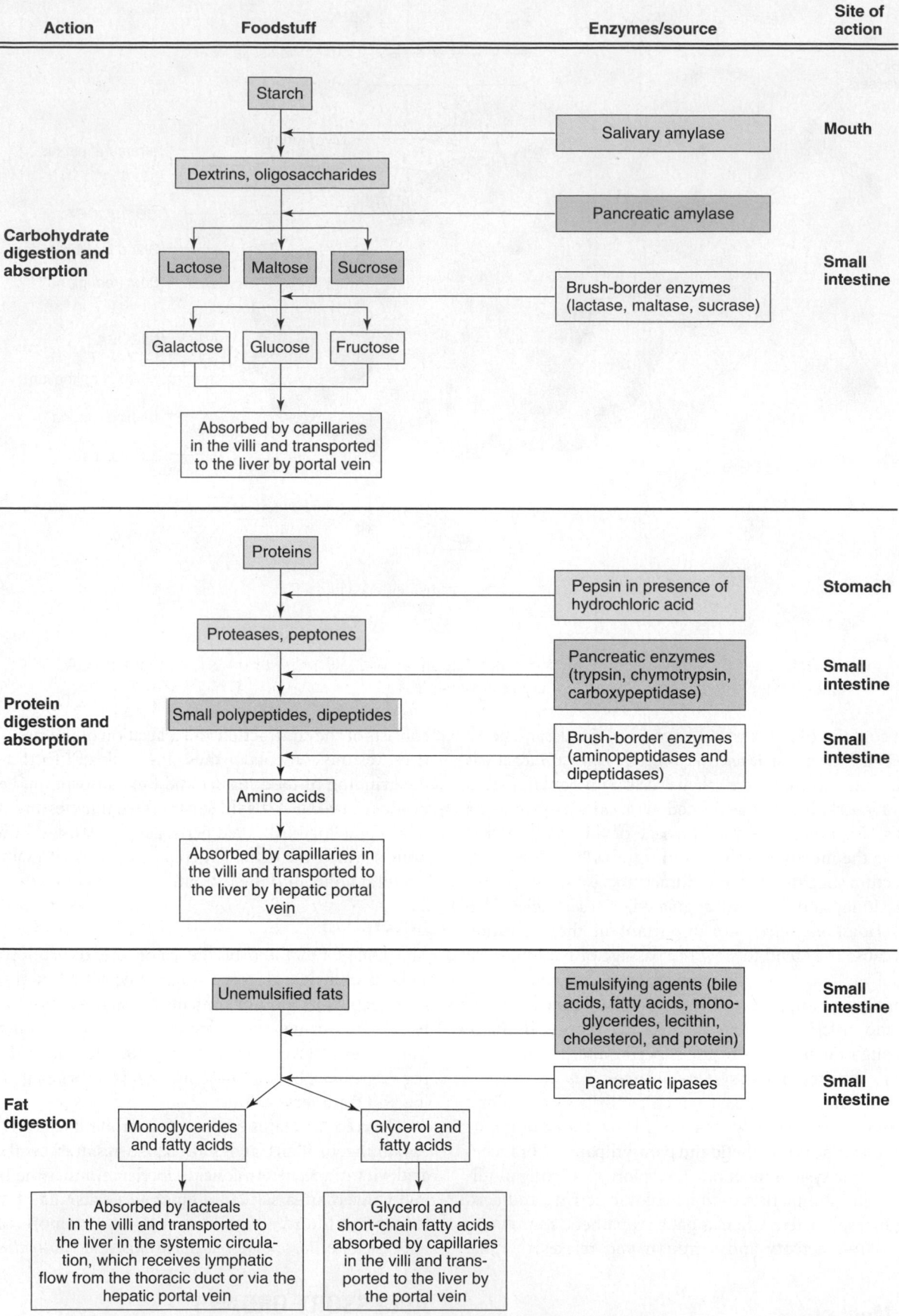

FIGURE 28-7 Digestion and absorption of foodstuffs. (From McCance KL, et al., eds. Pathophysiology. *The Biologic Basis for Disease in Adults and Children.* 6th ed. St. Louis: Mosby; 2010.)

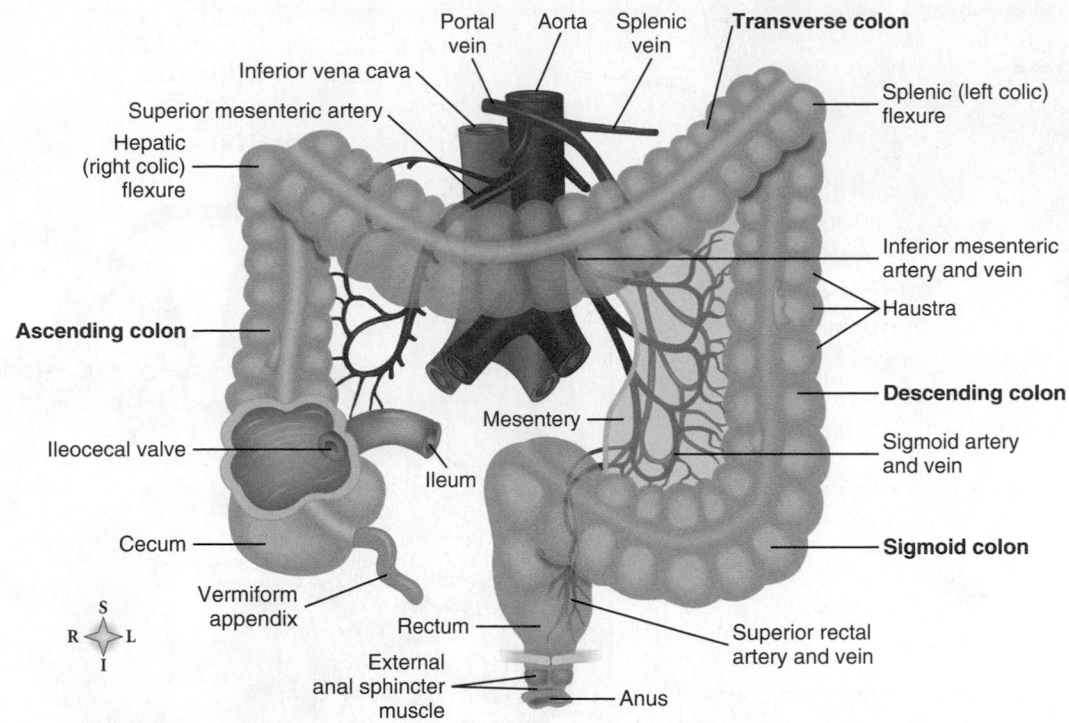

FIGURE 28-8 Large intestine. (Modified from Patton KT, Thibodeau GA. *Anatomy & Physiology.* 8th ed. St. Louis: Mosby; 2013.)

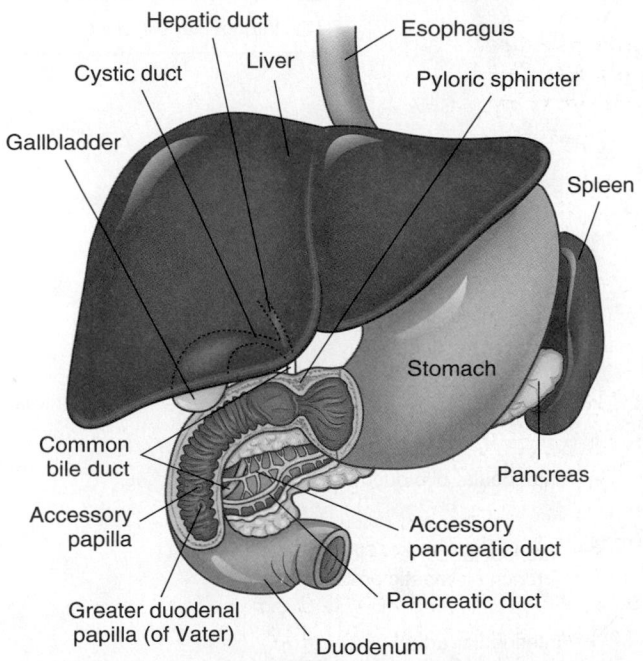

FIGURE 28-9 Liver, gallbladder, and pancreas. (From McCance KL, et al., eds. Pathophysiology: *The Biologic Basis for Disease in Adults and Children*, 6th ed. St. Louis: Mosby; 2010.)

Liver

The liver is the largest internal organ in the body. Weighing 1200 to 1600 g (3 to 4 pounds), it is friable and dark red in color and has a soft-solid consistency. Located in the right upper abdominal quadrant, it fits snugly against the right interior diaphragm. The liver is surrounded by connective tissue known as *Glisson's capsule*, which is covered by serosa and contains blood vessels and lymphatics. The peritoneum covering the liver forms the falciform ligament, which attaches the liver to the anterior portion of the abdomen between the diaphragm and umbilicus and divides the liver into two main lobes, right and left (see Fig. 28-8). The right lobe, which is six times larger than the left, has three sections: the right lobe proper, the caudate lobe, and the quadrate lobe. The left lobe is divided into two sections. Each lobe is divided into numerous lobules.[10,15]

The liver receives one third of the total cardiac output from two major sources: (1) the hepatic artery, which provides oxygenated blood; and (2) the portal vein, which is supplied with nutrient-rich blood from the gut, pancreas, spleen, and stomach (Fig. 28-10). The portal vein, which accounts for 75% of the total liver blood flow, branches into sinusoids to transport blood to each lobule. Unlike capillaries, sinusoids lack a definite cell wall but contain a lining of phagocytic (Kupffer) cells and some nonphagocytic cells of modified epithelium. Sinusoids empty blood into an intralobular vein in the center of the lobule. Intralobular veins empty into larger veins and then into the hepatic vein, which empties on the posterior surface of the liver and eventually into the vena cava. The hepatic artery also divides and subdivides between the lobules, supplying sinusoids with oxygenated blood before emptying into the hepatic vein. Lymphatic spaces are located between liver cells. Lymph drains into lymphatic vessels that surround the hepatic vein and bile ducts.[15]

Nutrient Metabolism

The liver plays a key role in metabolizing and storing carbohydrates, fats, proteins, and vitamins. Glycogen, the stored form of glucose, can be synthesized from glucose or from protein, fat, or lactic acid. Glycogen is broken down to glucose by the liver

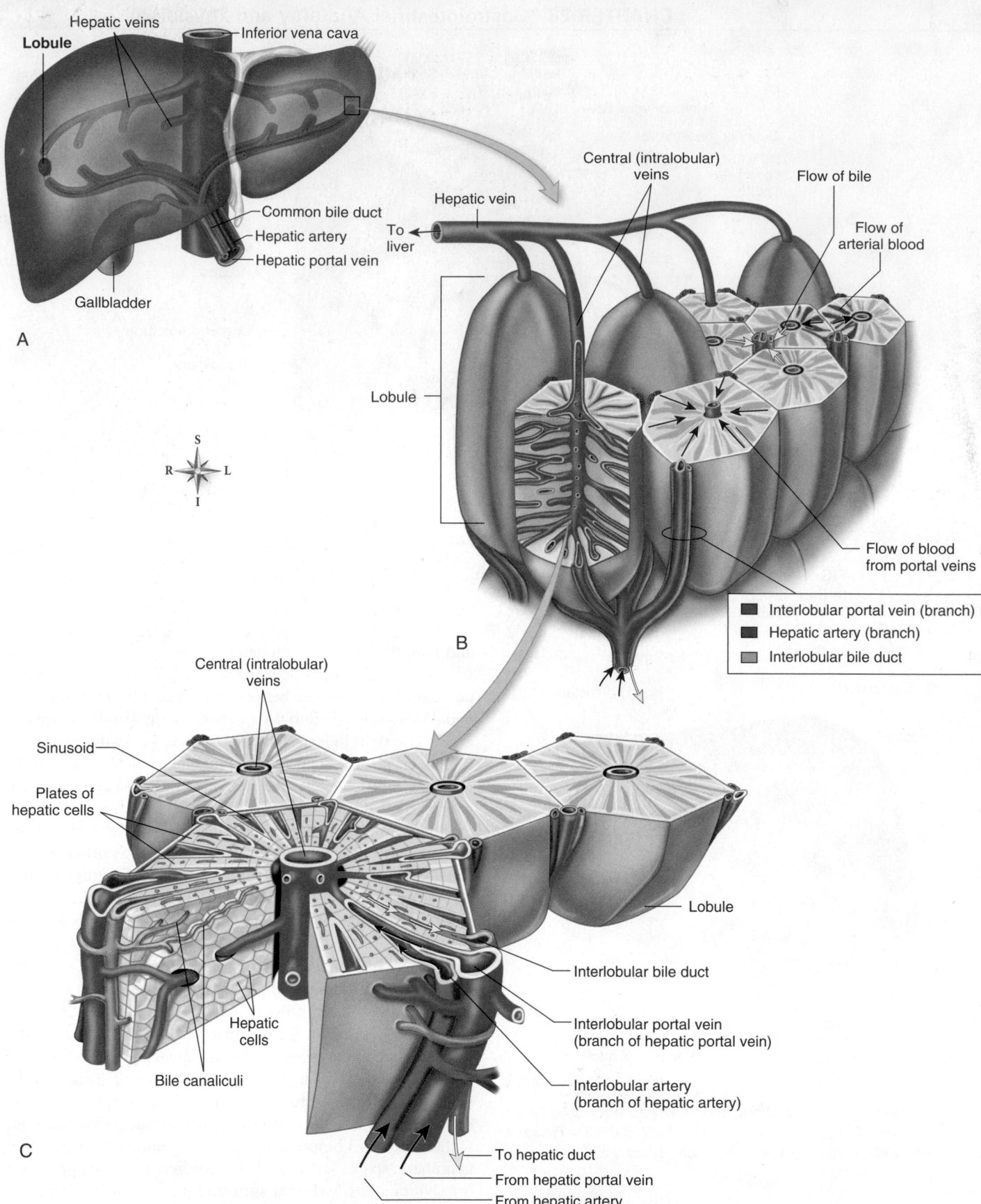

FIGURE 28-10 **Microscopic Structure of the Liver.** *A,* This diagram shows the location of liver lobules relative to the overall circulatory scheme of the liver. *B* and *C,* Enlarged views of several lobules show how blood from the hepatic portal veins and hepatic arteries flows through sinusoids and, thus, past plates of hepatic cells toward a central vein in each lobule *(black arrows).* Hepatic cells form bile, which flows through bile canaliculi toward hepatic ducts that eventually drain the bile from the liver *(yellow arrows).* (From Patton KT, Thibodeau GA. *Anatomy & Physiology.* 8th ed. St. Louis: Mosby; 2013.)

to maintain normal blood glucose levels. The liver also has a vital role in amino acid metabolism and can synthesize amino acids from metabolites of carbohydrates and fats or can deaminate amino acids to produce ketoacids and ammonia, from which urea is formed. In fat metabolism, the liver hydrolyzes triglycerides to glycerol and fatty acids in the process of ketogenesis and synthesizes phospholipids, cholesterol, and lipoproteins.[10,15]

Hematologic Function

The liver synthesizes plasma proteins such as globulins and albumin, which are important in maintaining the normal osmotic balance of blood. It also synthesizes a number of clotting factors, including fibrinogen and prothrombin. Kupffer cells destroy worn red blood cells, and hepatocytes conjugate bilirubin (byproduct of red cell destruction) for excretion.[10,15]

Detoxification and Storage

Steroid hormones are conjugated and polypeptide hormones are inactivated by the liver. The liver stores fat-soluble vitamins, vitamin B_{12}, and the minerals iron and copper. Detoxification of drugs and toxins occurs in Kupffer cells.[10,15]

Bile

The production of bile makes the liver a vital organ in digestion and absorption. The major components of bile are bile pigments, bile salts, cholesterol, neutral fats, phospholipids, inorganic salts, fatty acids, mucin, conjugated bilirubin, lecithin, and water. Traces of albumin, gammaglobulin, urea, nitrogen, and glucose are also present in bile. The principal electrolytes of bile are sodium, chloride, and bicarbonate.[15]

Bile emulsifies fat globules and absorbs fat-soluble vitamins. Bile salts also serve as an excretion route for bilirubin, cholesterol, and various hormones. Approximately 80% of bile salts are actively resorbed in the distal ileum and are recycled to the liver through the enterohepatic circulation; only 20% are lost in feces.[1]

Bilirubin

The primary bile pigment, bilirubin, is formed from the heme portion of hemoglobin during the degradation of red blood cells by Kupffer cells. When released into the bloodstream, bilirubin binds to albumin as fat-soluble, unconjugated bilirubin. Taken up by liver hepatocytes, unconjugated bilirubin is conjugated with glucuronic acid to form water-soluble, conjugated bilirubin, which is then excreted through hepatic ducts into the large intestine. If the amount of bilirubin sent to the liver is in excess, the ability of the liver to conjugate the bilirubin may be taxed; free, unconjugated or indirect bilirubin appears in the blood. High levels of unconjugated bilirubin in the blood suggest hepatocellular dysfunction, whereas high levels of conjugated bilirubin suggest biliary tract obstruction.[1]

Biliary System

The biliary system (Fig. 28-11) consists of the gallbladder and its related ductal system, including the hepatic, cystic, and common bile ducts. The hepatic duct, from the liver, joins the cystic duct, from the gallbladder, to form the common bile duct, which empties into the duodenum. The common bile duct is surrounded by Oddi's sphincter, which pierces the wall of the duodenum and controls the flow of bile into the duodenum. The gallbladder is a pear-shaped organ that is 7 to 10 cm (3 to 4 inches) long and 2.5 to 3.5 cm (approximately 1 inch) wide, lying on the underside of the liver (see Fig. 28-9). It is attached to the liver by connective tissue, peritoneum, and blood vessels.[10,16]

Bile

The main functions of the gallbladder are to collect, concentrate, acidify, and store bile. Bile is continuously formed in the liver and excreted into the hepatic duct for transport to the gallbladder through the cystic duct. The gallbladder can store up to 90 mL of bile and concentrate it approximately 15 to 29 times by removing approximately 90% of the water. Cholesterol and pigment are likewise concentrated. Bile, which is golden or orange-yellow in the liver, becomes dark brown when concentrated in the gallbladder. By altering its shape and volume, the gallbladder regulates pressure within the biliary system. Relaxation of the sphincter of Oddi is coordinated with gallbladder contraction through the regulatory action of cholecystokinin. Such factors as sight, smell, and taste can stimulate gallbladder contraction, whereas fear or excitement can decrease contraction. After a meal, the amount of bile entering the duodenum increases as a result of enhanced liver secretion and gallbladder contraction. Intestinal secretion of cholecystokinin and secretin, high levels of bile salts in the blood, and vagal stimulation increase biliary secretion.[15]

Pancreas

The pancreas is a soft, lobulated, fish-shaped gland (see Fig. 28-11) lying beneath the duodenum and the spleen (see Fig. 28-9). The pinkish-yellow organ is 15 to 20 cm (6 to 8 inches) long and 5 cm (1 to 1.5 inches) wide. Its anatomic divisions include the *head*, which lies in the C-shaped curve of the duodenum to which it is attached; the *body*, the main part of the gland, which extends horizontally across the abdomen and is largely hidden behind the stomach; and the *tail*, a thin, narrow portion in contact with the spleen. The main pancreatic duct, called the *duct of Wirsung*, traverses the entire length of the organ. The duct of Wirsung empties exocrine secretions into the ampulla of Vater, which is the same lumen draining the common bile duct, at the entrance to the duodenum.[10]

The internal structural unit of the pancreas is the lobule, consisting of numerous small ducts with secretory cells called *tubuloacinar* cells. Each acinus has a small duct that empties into lobular ducts. Lobules are joined by connective tissue into lobes, which unite to form the gland. The ducts from each lobule empty into the duct of Wirsung.[10]

Arterial blood supply to the pancreas is provided by branches of the superior mesenteric artery and celiac arteries. Venous drainage of the head of the pancreas occurs through the portal vein, and drainage of the body and tail occurs through the splenic vein. The pancreas is innervated by the autonomic nervous system. Sympathetic stimulation decreases pancreatic secretion, and parasympathetic stimulation increases it.[10]

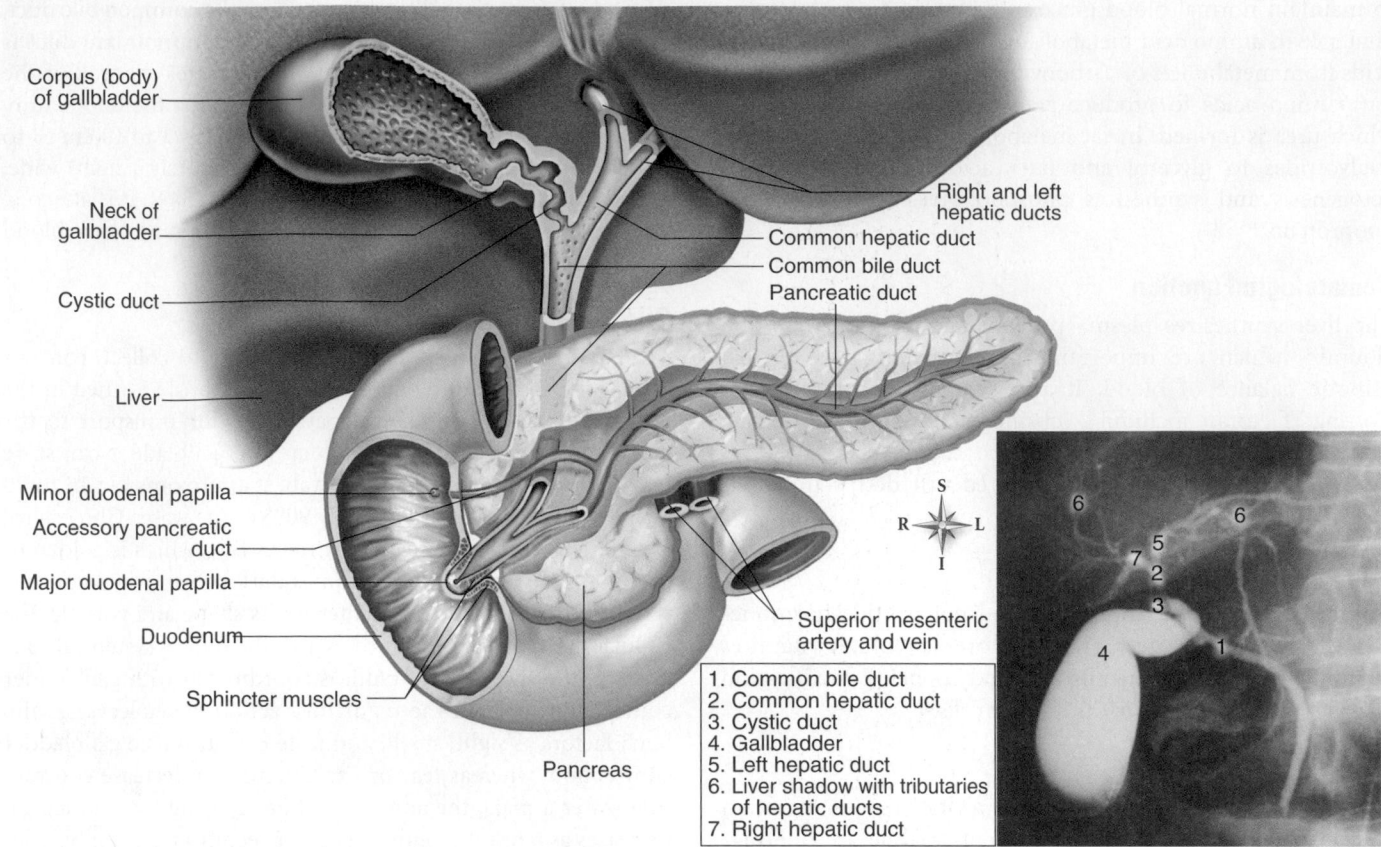

Corpus (body) of gallbladder

Neck of gallbladder

Cystic duct

Liver

Minor duodenal papilla

Accessory pancreatic duct

Major duodenal papilla

Duodenum

Sphincter muscles

Pancreas

Right and left hepatic ducts

Common hepatic duct

Common bile duct

Pancreatic duct

Superior mesenteric artery and vein

1. Common bile duct
2. Common hepatic duct
3. Cystic duct
4. Gallbladder
5. Left hepatic duct
6. Liver shadow with tributaries of hepatic ducts
7. Right hepatic duct

FIGURE 28-11 Gallbladder and pancreas. (From Patton KT, Thibodeau GA. Anatomy & *Physiology.* 8th ed. St. Louis: Mosby; 2013.)

Exocrine Functions

Exocrine functions of the pancreas are limited to digestion. Acinar cells secrete pancreatic juice, which consists of water, sodium bicarbonate, and electrolytes at a highly alkaline pH. Enzymes produced in the pancreas include trypsin, chymotrypsin, carboxypeptidase, amylase, and lipase. The pancreas also produces a trypsin inhibitor that prevents activation of trypsinogen (inactive form of trypsin), which inhibits autodigestion. Autodigestion is the underlying cause of acute pancreatitis. Pancreatic exocrine function is regulated by digestive hormones. Signals provided primarily by the intestinal hormones *secretin* and *cholecystokinin* stimulate the pancreas to secrete pancreatic juice. The two hormones potentiate each other's effects on the pancreas.[17]

Endocrine Functions

Endocrine tissue in the pancreas consists of spherical islets called *islets of Langerhans*, which are embedded within the lobules of acinar tissue throughout the pancreas, especially in the distal body and tail. Endocrine products include *insulin*, which is produced in beta cells; *glucagon*, which is produced in alpha cells; and *gastrin*. All of these hormones are secreted directly into the bloodstream.[17]

▌ S U M M A R Y

Anatomy

- The gastrointestinal (GI) tract consists of the mouth (lips, cheeks, gums, tongue, palate, and salivary glands), the esophagus, the stomach, the small intestine, and the large intestine.
- The accessory organs of digestion are the liver, the biliary system, and the pancreas.

Physiology

- The major function of the GI tract is digestion.
- Digestion is the conversion of ingested nutrients into simpler forms that can be transported from the tract's

lumen to the portal circulation and then used in metabolic processes.

- The mouth and accessory organs perform the initial phases of digestion, which are ingestion, mastication, and salivation.
- The functions of the stomach include food storage, digestion, and emptying.
- Gastric motility is regulated by the autonomic nervous system, digestive hormones, and neural reflexes.
- The functions of the small intestine include digestion and absorption.

- Intestinal motility consists of peristalsis and haustral segmentation.
- The major functions of the colon include resorption of water, sodium, chloride, glucose, and urea; dehydration of undigested residue; putrefaction of contents by bacteria; movement of the fecal bolus through the colon; and elimination of the fecal mass.
- Colonic motility consists of haustral shuttling and peristalsis.

- The functions of the liver include metabolism and storage of carbohydrates, fats, proteins, and vitamins; synthesis of plasma proteins; detoxification of drugs and toxins; and the production of bile.
- The main functions of the gallbladder are to collect, concentrate, acidify, and store bile.
- The main functions of the pancreas are digestion and glucose regulation.

REFERENCES

1. Huether SE. Structure and function of the digestive system. In: McCance KL, et al., eds. *Pathophysiology: The Biologic Basis for Disease in Adults and Children.* 6th ed. St. Louis: Mosby; 2010.
2. Canaan TJ. Variations of structure and appearance of the oral mucosa. *Dent Clin North Am.* 2005;49:1.
3. Mandel L. Salivary gland disorders. *Dent Clin North Am.* 2011;55:121.
4. Oezcelik A, DeMeester SR. General anatomy of the esophagus. *Thorac Surg Clin.* 2011;21:289.
5. Matsuo K, Palmer JB. Anatomy and physiology of feeding and swallowing: normal and abnormal. *Phys Med Rehabil Clin North Am.* 2008;19:691.
6. Soybel DI. Anatomy and physiology of the stomach. *Surg Clin North Am.* 2005;85:875.
7. Hall JE. *Guyton and Hall Textbook of Medical Physiology.* 12th ed. Philadelphia: Saunders; 2011.
8. Rostas JL, et al. Gastric motility physiology and surgical intervention. *Surg Clin North Am.* 2011;91:983.
9. Androulakis J, et al. Embryologic and anatomic basis of duodenal surgery. *Surg Clin North Am.* 2000;80:171.
10. SGNA. *Gastroenterology Nursing: A Core Curriculum.* 4th ed. St. Louis: Society of Gastroenterology Nurses and Associates; 2008.
11. Lin PH, Chaikof EL. Embryology, anatomy, and surgical exposure of the great abdominal vessels. *Surg Clin North Am.* 2000;80:417.
12. Smout A, Fox M. Weak and absent peristalsis. *Neurogastroenterol Motil.* 2012;24(suppl 1):40.
13. Wald A. Motility disorders of the colon and rectum. *Curr Opin Gastroenterol.* 2012;28:52.
14. Macfarlane GT, Macfarlane S. Bacteria, colonic fermentation, and gastrointestinal health. *J AOAC Int.* 2012;95:50.
15. Misdraji J. Anatomy, histology, embryology, and developmental anomalies of the liver. In: Feldman M, et al., eds. *Sleisenger & Fordtran's Gastrointestinal and Liver Disease: Pathophysiology, Diagnosis, and Management.* 9th ed. Philadelphia: Saunders; 2010.
16. Adkins RB, et al. Embryology, anatomy, and surgical applications of the extrahepatic biliary system. *Surg Clin North Am.* 2000;80:363.
17. Chen N, et al. The complex exocrine-endocrine relationship and secondary diabetes in exocrine pancreatic disorders. *J Clin Gastroenterol.* 2011;45:850.

Gastrointestinal Clinical Assessment and Diagnostic Procedures

Kathleen M. Stacy

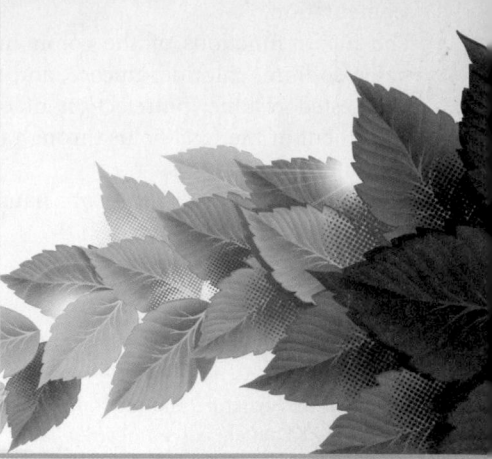

evolve WEBSITE

http://evolve.elsevier.com/Urden/criticalcare/

Evolve features:

- NCLEX Review Questions
- CCRN Review Questions
- PCCN Review Questions
- Mosby's Nursing Skills Procedures
- Animations
- Video Clips
- Glossary

Assessment of the critically ill patient with gastrointestinal (GI) dysfunction includes a review of the patient's history, a thorough physical examination, and analysis of the patient's laboratory data. Numerous invasive and noninvasive diagnostic procedures may also be performed to identify the disorder.

CLINICAL ASSESSMENT

A thorough clinical assessment of the patient with GI dysfunction is imperative for the early identification and treatment of GI disorders. The completed assessment serves as the foundation for developing the management plan for the patient. The assessment process can be brief or can involve a detailed history and examination, depending on the nature and immediacy of the patient's situation.[1,2]

HISTORY

Taking a thorough and accurate history is extremely important to the assessment process. The patient's history provides the foundation and direction for the rest of the assessment. The overall goal of the patient interview is to expose key clinical manifestations that will facilitate the identification of the underlying cause of the illness. This information can then assist in the development of an appropriate management plan.

The initial presentation of the patient determines the rapidity and direction of the interview. For a patient in acute distress, the history should be curtailed to a few questions about the patient's chief complaint and the precipitating events. For a patient in no obvious distress, the history should focus on

current symptoms, the patient's medical history, and the family's history. Specific items regarding each of these areas are outlined in Box 29-1, Data Collection.[3,4]

PHYSICAL EXAMINATION

The physical examination helps establish baseline data about the physical dimensions of the patient's situation.[3] The abdomen is divided into four quadrants (left upper, right upper, left lower, and right lower), with the umbilicus as the middle point, to specify the location of examination findings (Fig. 29-1 and Box 29-2). The assessment should proceed when the patient is as comfortable as possible and in the supine position; however, the position may need readjustment if it elicits pain. To prevent stimulation of GI activity, the order for the assessment should be changed to inspection, auscultation, percussion, and palpation.[4]

Inspection

Inspection should be performed in a warm, well-lit environment, and the patient should be in a comfortable position, with the abdomen exposed. Although assessment of the GI system classically begins with inspection of the abdomen, the patient's oral cavity also must be inspected to determine any unusual findings. Abnormal findings of the mouth include temporomandibular joint tenderness, inflammation of gums, missing teeth, dental caries, ill-fitting dentures, and mouth odor.

Observe the skin for pigmentation, lesions, striae, scars, petechiae, signs of dehydration, and venous pattern. Pigmentation may vary considerably and still be within normal limits because

BOX 29-1   DATA COLLECTION

Gastrointestinal History

Common Gastrointestinal Symptoms
- Oral lesions
- Digestion or indigestion (heartburn)
- Dysphagia
- Nausea
- Vomiting
- Hematemesis
- Change in stool color or contents (e.g., clay-colored, tarry, fresh blood, mucus, undigested food)
- Constipation
- Diarrhea
- Abdominal pain
- Jaundice
- Anal discomfort
- Fecal incontinence

Patient Lifestyle
- Usual height and weight
- Dietary habits
  - Usual number of meals or snacks per day
  - Usual fluid intake per day
- Nutrient intake
  - Types of food usually eaten at each meal or snack
  - Food likes and dislikes
  - Religious or medical food restrictions
  - Food intolerances
  - Patient's perceptions and concerns about adequacy of diet and appropriateness of weight
  - Effects of lifestyle on food intake, weight gain or loss
  - Vitamins or nutritional supplements (e.g., type, amount, frequency)
- Bowel elimination
  - Usual frequency of bowel movements
  - Usual consistency and color of stool
  - Ability to control elimination of gas and stool
  - Any changes in bowel elimination patterns
  - Use of enemas or laxatives (e.g., reason for use, frequency, type, response)
- Alcohol intake (e.g., frequency, usual amounts)
- Exercise patterns

Medical History
- Chronic illnesses
- Previous weight gain or loss
- Tooth extractions or orthodontic work
- Gastrointestinal (GI) disorders (e.g., peptic ulcer, inflammatory bowel disease, polyps, cholelithiasis, diverticular disease, pancreatitis, intestinal obstruction)
- Hepatitis or cirrhosis
- Abdominal surgery
- Abdominal trauma
- Cancer affecting GI system
- Spinal cord injury
- Women: episiotomy or fourth-degree laceration during delivery
- Exposure to infectious agents (e.g., foreign travel, water source)

Family History
- Investigate for history of following disorders, and document (+ or −) responses
- Hirschsprung disease
- Obesity
- Metabolic disorders
- Inflammatory disorders
- Malabsorption syndromes
- Familial Mediterranean fever
- Rectal polyps
- Polyposis syndromes
- Cancer of the GI tract

Current Medication Use
- Laxatives
- Stool softeners
- Antiemetics
- Antidiarrheals
- Antacids
- Aspirin
- Acetaminophen
- Nonsteroidal anti-inflammatory drugs
- Corticosteroids

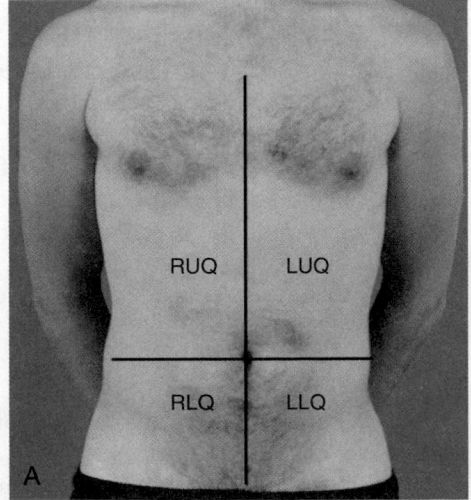
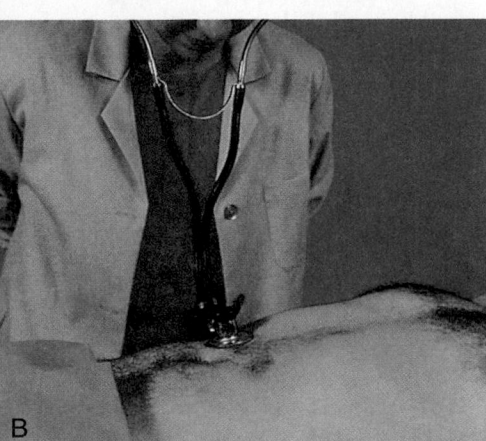

FIGURE 29-1   *A,* Anatomic mapping of the four quadrants of the abdomen. *B,* Auscultation for bowel sounds. (From Barkauskas V, et al. *Health & Physical Assessment.* 3rd ed. St. Louis: Mosby; 2002.)

BOX 29-2 ANATOMIC CORRELATES OF THE FOUR QUADRANTS OF THE ABDOMEN

Right Upper Quadrant
- Liver and gallbladder
- Pylorus
- Duodenum
- Head of pancreas
- Right adrenal gland
- Portion of right kidney
- Hepatic flexure of colon
- Portion of ascending and transverse colon

Left Upper Quadrant
- Left lobe of liver
- Spleen
- Stomach
- Body of pancreas
- Left adrenal gland
- Portion of left kidney
- Splenic flexure of colon
- Portions of transverse and descending colon

Right Lower Quadrant
- Lower pole of right kidney
- Cecum and appendix
- Portion of ascending colon
- Bladder (if distended)
- Ovary and salpinx
- Uterus (if enlarged)
- Right spermatic cord
- Right ureter

Left Lower Quadrant
- Lower pole of left kidney
- Sigmoid colon
- Portion of descending colon
- Bladder (if distended)
- Ovary and salpinx
- Uterus (if distended)
- Left spermatic cord
- Left ureter

From Barkauskas V, et al. *Health & Physical Assessment*. 3rd ed. St. Louis: Mosby; 2002.

TABLE 29-1 ABNORMAL ABDOMINAL SOUNDS

SOUND	CAUSE
Hyperactive bowel sounds (borborygmi), loud and prolonged	Hunger, gastroenteritis, or early intestinal obstruction
High-pitched, tinkling sounds	Intestinal air and fluid under pressure; characteristic of early intestinal obstruction
Decreased (hypoactive) bowel sounds Infrequent and abnormally faint sounds	Possible peritonitis or ileus
Absence of bowel sounds (confirmed only after auscultation of all four quadrants and continuous auscultation for 5 minutes)	Temporary loss of intestinal motility, as occurs with complete ileus
Friction rubs	Pathologic conditions such as tumors or infection that cause inflammation of organ's peritoneal covering
High-pitched sounds heard over liver and spleen (RUQ and LUQ), synchronous with respiration	
Bruits	Abnormality of blood flow (requires additional evaluation to determine specific disorder)
Audible swishing sounds that may be heard over aortic, iliac, renal, and femoral arteries	
Venous hum	Increased collateral circulation between portal and systemic venous systems
Low-pitched, continuous sound	

LUQ, Left upper quadrant; *RUQ,* right upper quadrant.
From Doughty DB, Jackson DB. *Gastrointestinal Disorders*. St. Louis: Mosby; 1993.

of race and ethnic background, although the abdomen usually is of a lighter color than other exposed areas of the skin. Abnormal findings include jaundice, skin lesions, and a tense and glistening appearance of the skin. Old striae (stretch marks) usually are silver, whereas pinkish purple striae may indicate Cushing syndrome.[4] A bluish discoloration of the umbilicus (Cullen sign) and of the flank (Grey-Turner sign) indicates retroperitoneal bleeding.[1]

Observe the abdomen for contour, noting whether it is flat, slightly concave, or slightly round; observe for symmetry and for movement. Marked distention is an abnormal finding. In particular, ascites may cause generalized distention and bulging flanks. Asymmetric distention may indicate organ enlargement or a mass. Peristaltic waves should not be visible except in very thin patients. In the case of intestinal obstruction, hyperactive peristaltic waves may be observed. Pulsation in the epigastric area is often a normal finding, but increased pulsation may indicate an aortic aneurysm. Symmetric movement of the abdomen with respirations is usually seen in men.[4,5]

Auscultation

Auscultation of the abdomen provides clinical data regarding the status of the bowel's motility. Initially, listen with the diaphragm of the stethoscope below and to the right of the umbilicus. The examination proceeds methodically through all four quadrants, lifting and then replacing the diaphragm of the stethoscope lightly against the abdomen (see Fig. 29-1). Normal bowel sounds include high-pitched, gurgling sounds that occur approximately every 5 to 15 seconds or at a rate of 5 to 34 times per minute. Colonic sounds are low pitched and have a rumbling quality. A venous hum may be audible sometimes.[6] Table 29-1 provides a list of abnormal abdominal sounds.

Abnormal findings include the absence of bowel sounds throughout a 5-minute period, extremely soft and widely separated sounds, and increased sounds with a high-pitched, loud rushing sound (peristaltic rush). Absent bowel sounds may result from inflammation, ileus, electrolyte disturbances, and ischemia. Bowels sounds may be increased with diarrhea and early intestinal obstruction.[6]

The abdomen should be auscultated for the presence of bruits, using the bell of the stethoscope (Fig. 29-2). Bruits are created by turbulent flow over a partially obstructed artery and are always considered an abnormal finding. The aorta, the right and left renal arteries, and the iliac arteries should be auscultated.[5,6]

Percussion

Percussion is used to elicit information about deep organs such as the liver, spleen, and pancreas (Fig. 29-3). Because the abdomen is a sensitive area, muscle tension may interfere with this part of the assessment. Percussion often helps relax tense muscles, and it is performed before palpation. Percussion in the absence of disease helps delineate the position and size of the

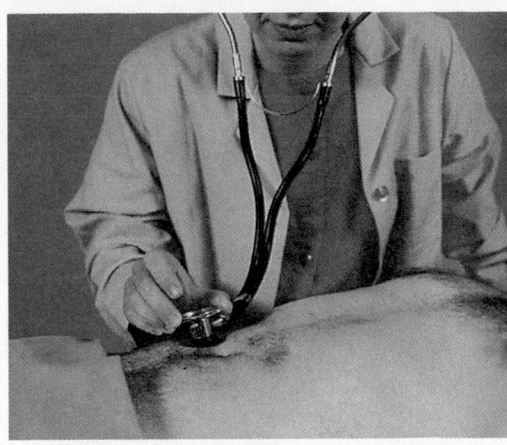
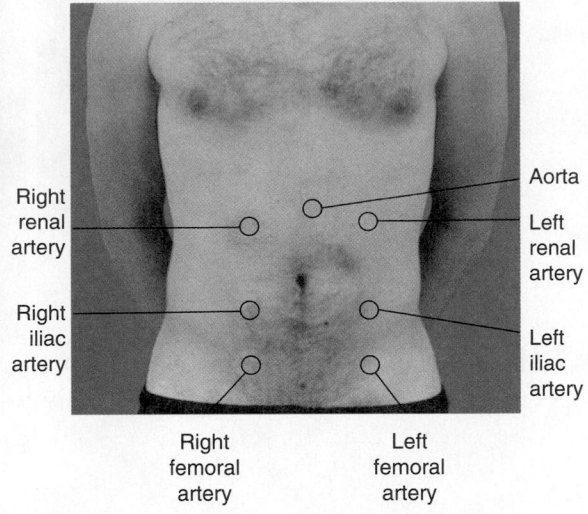

Right renal artery

Right iliac artery

Right femoral artery

Aorta

Left renal artery

Left iliac artery

Left femoral artery

FIGURE 29-2   Auscultation for bruits. The left illustration shows the correct placement of the stethoscope. (From Barkauskas V, et al. *Health & Physical Assessment*. 3rd ed. St. Louis: Mosby; 2002.)

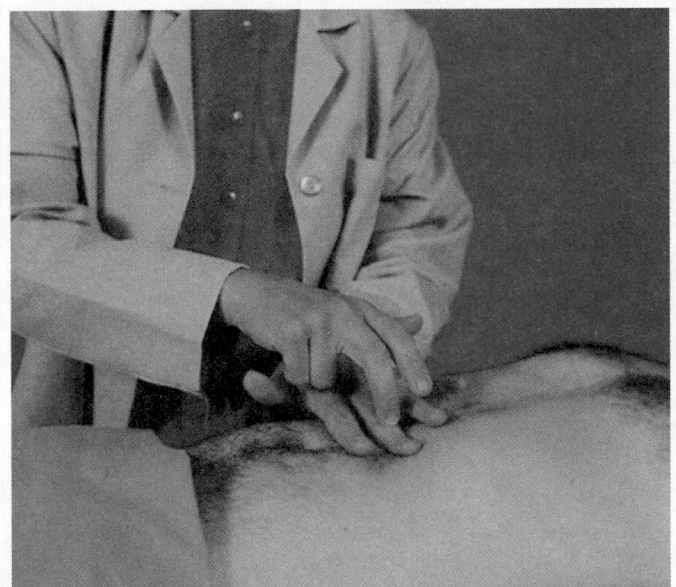

FIGURE 29-3   Percussion of the abdomen. (From Barkauskas V, et al. *Health & Physical Assessment*. 3rd ed. St. Louis: Mosby; 2002.)

liver and spleen, and it assists in the detection of fluid, gaseous distention, and masses in the abdomen.[5]

Percussion should proceed systematically and lightly in all four quadrants. Normal findings include tympany over the empty stomach, tympany or hyper-resonance over the intestine, and dullness over the liver and spleen. Abnormal areas of dullness may indicate an underlying mass. Solid masses, enlarged organs, and a distended bladder also produce areas of dullness. Dullness over both flanks may indicate ascites and necessitates further assessment.[6]

Palpation

Palpation is the assessment technique most useful in detecting abdominal pathologic conditions. Light and deep palpation

of each organ and quadrant should be completed. Light palpation, which has a palpation depth of approximately 1 cm, assesses to the depth of the skin and fascia (Fig. 29-4A). Deep palpation assesses the rectus abdominis muscle and is performed bimanually to a depth of 4 to 5 cm (see Fig. 29-4B). Deep palpation is most helpful in detecting abdominal masses. Areas in which the patient complains of tenderness should be palpated last.[6]

Normal findings include no areas of tenderness or pain, no masses, and no hardened areas. Persistent involuntary guarding may indicate peritoneal inflammation, particularly if it continues even after relaxation techniques are used. Rebound tenderness, in which pain increases with quick release of a palpated area, indicates an inflamed peritoneum.[4]

Assessment Findings for Common Disorders

Table 29-2 presents a variety of common GI disorders and their associated assessment findings.

LABORATORY STUDIES

The value of various laboratory studies used to diagnose and treat diseases of the GI system has been emphasized often. However, no single study provides an overall picture of the various organs' functional state, and no single value is predictive by itself. Laboratory studies used in the assessment of GI function, liver function, and pancreatic function are found in Tables 29-3, 29-4, and 29-5, respectively.

DIAGNOSTIC PROCEDURES

To complete the assessment of the critically ill patient with GI dysfunction, the patient's diagnostic tests are reviewed. Although many procedures exist for diagnosing GI disease, their application in the critically ill patient is limited. Only procedures that are currently used in the critical care setting are presented here.

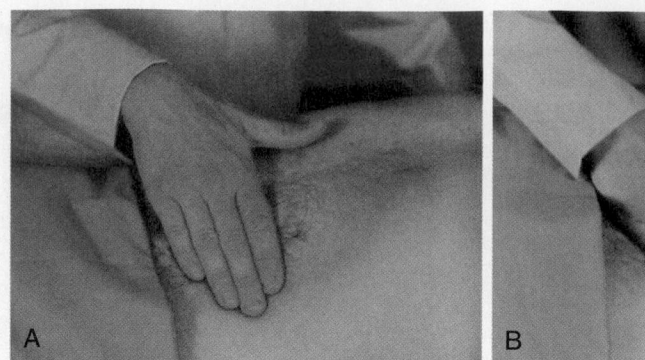
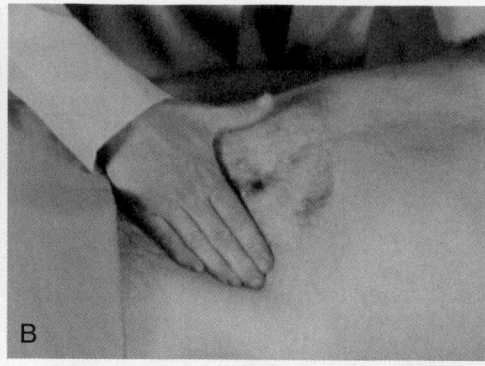

FIGURE 29-4 Palpation of the abdomen. *A,* Light. *B,* Deep. (From Barkauskas V, et al. *Health & Physical Assessment.* 3rd ed. St. Louis: Mosby; 2002.)

TABLE 29-2 ASSESSMENT FINDINGS OF COMMON GASTROINTESTINAL DISORDERS

CONDITION	HISTORY	SYMPTOMS	SIGNS
Right Lower Quadrant (RLQ) of the Abdomen			
Appendicitis	Children (except infants) and young adults	Anorexia	Signs may be absent early
		Nausea	Vomiting
		Early vague epigastric, periumbilical, or generalized pain after 12-24 hours; RLQ at McBurney point	Localized RLQ guarding and tenderness after 12-24 hours
			Rovsing sign: pain in RLQ with application of pressure, iliopsoas sign
			Obturator sign
			White blood cell count of 10,000/mm^3 or shift to left
			Low-grade fever
			Cutaneous hyperesthesia in RLQ
			Signs highly variable
Perforated duodenal ulcer	Prior history	Abrupt onset pain in epigastric area or RLQ	Tenderness in epigastric area or RLQ
			Signs of peritoneal irritation
			Heme-positive stool
			Increased white blood cell count
Cecal volvulus	Seen most often in older adults	Abrupt severe abdominal pain	Distention
			Localized tenderness
			Tympany
Strangulated hernia	Any age Women: femoral Men: inguinal	Severe localized pain If bowel obstructed, generalized pain	If bowel obstructed, distention
Right Upper Quadrant (RUQ) of the Abdomen			
Liver hepatitis	Any age, often young blood product user Drug addict	Fatigue Malaise Anorexia Pain in RUQ Low-grade fever May have severe fulminating disease with liver failure	Hepatic tenderness Hepatomegaly Bilirubin elevated Jaundice Lymphocytosis in one third of cases Liver enzymes elevated Hepatitis A or B or antibodies to the viruses may be found
Acute hepatic congestion	Usually older adults with acute heart failure Pericardial disease Pulmonary embolism	Symptoms of acute heart failure	Hepatomegaly Acute heart failure

TABLE 29-2 ASSESSMENT FINDINGS OF COMMON GASTROINTESTINAL DISORDERS—cont'd

CONDITION	HISTORY	SYMPTOMS	SIGNS
Biliary stones, colic	"Fair, fat, forty" (90%) but can be 30 to 80 years old	Anorexia Nausea Pain severe in RUQ or epigastric area Episodes lasting 15 minutes to hours	Tenderness in RUQ Jaundice
Acute cholecystitis	"Fair, fat, forty" (90%) but may be 30 to 80 years old	Severe RUQ or epigastric pain Episodes prolonged up to 6 hours	Vomiting Tenderness in RUQ Peritoneal irritation signs Increased white blood cell count
Perforated peptic ulcer	Any age	Abrupt RUQ pain	Tenderness in epigastrium, right quadrant, or both Peritoneal irritation signs Free air in abdomen
Left Upper Quadrant (LUQ) of the Abdomen			
Splenic trauma	Blunt trauma to LUQ of abdomen	Pain: LUQ pain of the abdomen often referred to the left shoulder (Kehr sign)	Hypotension Syncope Increased dyspnea Radiographic studies show enlarged spleen
Pancreatitis	Alcohol abuse Pancreatic duct obstruction Infection Cholecystitis	Pain in LUQ or epigastric region radiating to the back or chest	Fever Rigidity Rebound tenderness Nausea Vomiting Jaundice Cullen sign Turner sign Abdominal distention Diminished bowel sounds
Pyloric obstruction	Duodenal ulcer	Weight loss Gastric upset Vomiting	Increasing dullness in LUQ Visible peristaltic waves in epigastric region
Left Lower Quadrant (LLQ) of the Abdomen			
Ulcerative colitis	Family history Jewish ancestry Cachexia	Chronic, watery diarrhea with bloody mucus Anorexia Weight loss Fatigue	Fever Anemia Leukocytosis
Colonic diverticulitis	Older than 39 years Low-residue diet	Pain that recurs in LUQ	Fever Vomiting Chills Diarrhea Tenderness over descending colon

Modified from Barkauskas V, et al. *Health & Physical Assessment*. 3rd ed. St. Louis: Mosby; 2002.

The nursing management of a patient undergoing a diagnostic procedure involves a variety of interventions. Nursing actions include preparing the patient psychologically and physically for the procedure, monitoring the patient's responses to the procedure, and assessing the patient after the procedure. Preparing the patient includes teaching the patient about the procedure, answering any questions, and transporting and positioning the patient for the procedure. Monitoring the patient's responses to the procedure includes observing the patient for signs of pain, anxiety, or hemorrhage and monitoring vital signs. Assessing

TABLE 29-3 SELECTED LABORATORY STUDIES OF GASTROINTESTINAL FUNCTION

TEST	NORMAL FINDINGS	CLINICAL SIGNIFICANCE OF ABNORMAL FINDINGS
Stool studies	Resident microorganisms: clostridia, enterococci, *Pseudomonas*, a few yeasts	Detection of *Salmonella typhi* (typhoid fever), *Shigella* (dysentery), *Vibrio cholerae* (cholera), *Yersinia* (enterocolitis), *Escherichia coli* (gastroenteritis), *Staphylococcus aureus* (food poisoning), *Clostridium botulinum* (food poisoning), *Clostridium perfringens* (food poisoning), *Aeromonas* (gastroenteritis)
	Fat: 2-6 g/24 hr	Steatorrhea (increased values) resulting from intestinal malabsorption or pancreatic insufficiency
	Pus: none	Large amounts of pus associated with chronic ulcerative colitis, abscesses, and anorectal fistula
	Occult blood: none (ortho-toluidine or guaiac test)	Positive test results associated with bleeding
	Ova and parasites: none	Detection of *Entamoeba histolytica* (amebiasis), *Giardia lamblia* (giardiasis), and worms
D-Xylose absorption	5-hr urinary excretion: 4.5 g/L Peak blood level: >30 mg/dL	Differentiation of pancreatic steatorrhea (normal D-xylose absorption) from intestinal steatorrhea (impaired D-xylose absorption)
Gastric acid stimulation	11-20 mEq/hr after stimulation	Detection of duodenal ulcers, Zollinger-Ellison syndrome (increased values), gastric atrophy, gastric carcinoma (decreased values)
Manometry*	Values vary at different levels of the intestine	Inadequate swallowing, motility, sphincter function
Culture and sensitivity of duodenal contents	No pathogens	Detection of *Salmonella typhi* (typhoid fever)
Breath tests		
Glucose or D-xylose breath test	Negative for hydrogen or carbon dioxide	May indicate intestinal bacterial overgrowth
Urea breath test	Negative for isotopically labeled carbon dioxide	Presence of *Helicobacter pylori* infection
Lactose breath test	Negative for exhaled hydrogen	Lactose intolerance

*Use of water-filled catheters connected to pressure transducers passed into the esophagus, stomach, colon, or rectum to evaluate contractility.
From McCance KL, Huether SE, eds. *Pathophysiology: The Biologic Basis for Disease in Adults and Children.* 6th ed. St. Louis: Mosby; 2010.

the patient after the procedure includes observing for complications of the procedure and medicating the patient for any post-procedural discomfort. Any evidence of GI bleeding should be immediately reported to the physician, and emergency measures to maintain circulation must be initiated.

Endoscopy

Available in several forms, fiberoptic endoscopy is a diagnostic procedure for the direct visualization and evaluation of the GI tract. Endoscopy can provide information about lesions, mucosal changes, obstructions, and motility dysfunction, and a biopsy specimen can be obtained during the procedure. The main difference between the various diagnostic forms is the length of the anatomic area that can be examined. Esophagogastroduodenoscopy (EGD) permits viewing of the upper GI tract from the esophagus to the upper duodenum, and it is used to evaluate sources of upper GI bleeding (Fig. 29-5). Colonoscopy permits viewing of the lower GI tract from the rectum to the distal ileum, and it is used to evaluate sources of lower GI bleeding. Enteroscopy permits viewing of the small bowel beyond the ligament of Treitz, and it is used to evaluate sources of GI bleeding that have not been identified previously with EGD or colonoscopy. Endoscopic retrograde cholangiopancreatography (ERCP) enables viewing of the biliary and pancreatic ducts, and it is used in the evaluation of

pancreatitis. During this procedure, contrast is injected into the ducts through the endoscope, and radiographs are obtained.[7] Endoscopy also provides therapeutic benefits for a variety of conditions, including GI bleeding.[8]

Nursing Management

The patient should take nothing by mouth (NPO) for 6 to 12 hours before endoscopy of the upper GI tract. The patient should receive a bowel preparation before endoscopy of the lower GI tract.[7] In some cases, the procedure is performed at the patient's bedside, particularly if the patient is actively bleeding and too unstable to be moved to the GI suite. Fiberoptic endoscopy may present risks for the patient. Although rare, potential complications include perforation of the GI tract, hemorrhage, aspiration, vasovagal stimulation, and oversedation.[7] Signs of perforation include abdominal pain and distention, GI bleeding, and fever.[9]

Angiography

Angiography is used as a diagnostic and a therapeutic procedure. Diagnostically, it is used to evaluate the status of the GI circulation (Fig. 29-6).[7] Therapeutically, it is used to achieve transcatheter control of GI bleeding.[10] Angiography is used in the diagnosis of upper gastrointestinal (UGI) bleeding only when endoscopy fails, and it is used to treat patients

TABLE 29-4 COMMON LABORATORY STUDIES OF LIVER FUNCTION

TEST	NORMAL VALUE	INTERPRETATION
Serum Enzymes		
Alkaline phosphatase	13-39 units/L Male 12-39 units/L Female 9-31 units/L	Increases with biliary obstruction and cholestatic hepatitis
Aspartate aminotransferase (AST; previously serum glutamate oxaloacetate transaminase [SGOT])	5-40 units/L	Increases with hepatocellular injury (and injury in other tissues, i.e., skeletal and cardiac muscle)
Alanine aminotransferase (ALT; previously serum glutamate pyruvate transaminase [SGPT])	5-35 units/L	Increases with hepatocellular injury and necrosis
Lactate dehydrogenase (LDH)	0-250 units/L	Isoenzyme lactate dehydrogenase (LD_5) is elevated with hypoxic and primary liver injury
5'-Nucleotidase	2-11 units/L	Increases with increase in alkaline phosphatase and cholestatic disorders
Bilirubin Metabolism Serum bilirubin		
Indirect (unconjugated)	0-1.0 mg/dL	Increases with hemolysis (lysis of red blood cells)
Direct (conjugated)	0-0.3 mg/dL	Increases with hepatocellular injury or obstruction
Total	0-1.0 mg/dL	Increases with biliary obstruction
Urine bilirubin	0.2-1.3 mg/dL	Increases with biliary obstruction
Urine urobilinogen	0.3-2.1 mg/2 hr (male) 0.1-1.1 mg/2 hr (female)	Increases with hemolysis or shunting or portal blood flow
Serum Proteins Albumin	4.0-6.0 g/dL	Decreases with hepatocellular injury
Globulin	2.0-4.0 g/dL	Increases with hepatitis
Total	6-8 g/dL	
Albumin-to-globulin (A/G) ratio	1.5-2.5:1	Ratio reverses with chronic hepatitis or other chronic liver disease
Transferrin	250-300 mcg/dL	Liver damage with decreased values, iron deficiency with increased values
Alpha-fetoprotein	<10 ng/dL	Elevated values in primary hepatocellular carcinoma
Blood Clotting Functions Prothrombin time	10-14 sec or 90% of control	Increases with chronic liver disease (cirrhosis) or vitamin K deficiency
International normalized ratio (INR)	0.9-1.3	Increased values indicate high chance of bleeding; useful for monitoring effects of drugs such as warfarin
Partial thromboplastin time (PTT)	25-40 sec	Increases with severe liver disease or heparin therapy
Bromsulphalein (BSP) excretion	<6% retention in 45 min	Increased retention with hepatocellular injury

From McCance KL, Huether SE, eds. *Pathophysiology: The Biologic Basis for Disease in Adults and Children.* 6th ed. St. Louis: Mosby; 2010.

TABLE 29-5 COMMON LABORATORY STUDIES OF PANCREATIC FUNCTION

TEST	NORMAL VALUE	CLINICAL SIGNIFICANCE
Serum amylase	60-180 Somogyi units/mL	Elevated levels with pancreatic inflammation
Serum lipase	1.5 Somogyi units/mL	Elevated levels with pancreatic inflammation (may be elevated with other conditions; differentiates with amylase, isoenzyme study)
Urine amylase	35-260 Somogyi units/hr	Elevated levels with pancreatic inflammation
Secretin test	Volume 1.8 mL/kg/hr Bicarbonate concentration: >80 mEq/L Bicarbonate output: >10 mEq/L/30 sec	Decreased volume with pancreatic disease because secretin stimulates pancreatic secretion
Stool fat	2-5 g/25 hr	Measures fatty acids: decreased pancreatic lipase increases stool fat

From McCance KL, Huether SE, eds. *Pathophysiology: The Biologic Basis for Disease in Adults and Children.* 6th ed. St. Louis: Mosby; 2010.

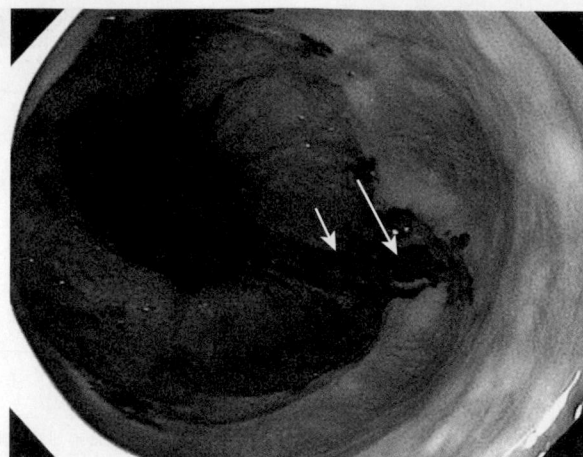

FIGURE 29-5 Endoscopic appearance of a Mallory-Weiss tear with mild oozing. Note that the tear starts at the gastroesophageal junction *(large arrow)* and extends distally into the hiatal hernia *(small arrow)*. (From Feldman M, et al. *Sleisenger and Fordtran's Gastrointestinal and Liver Disease.* 9th ed. Philadelphia: Saunders; 2010.)

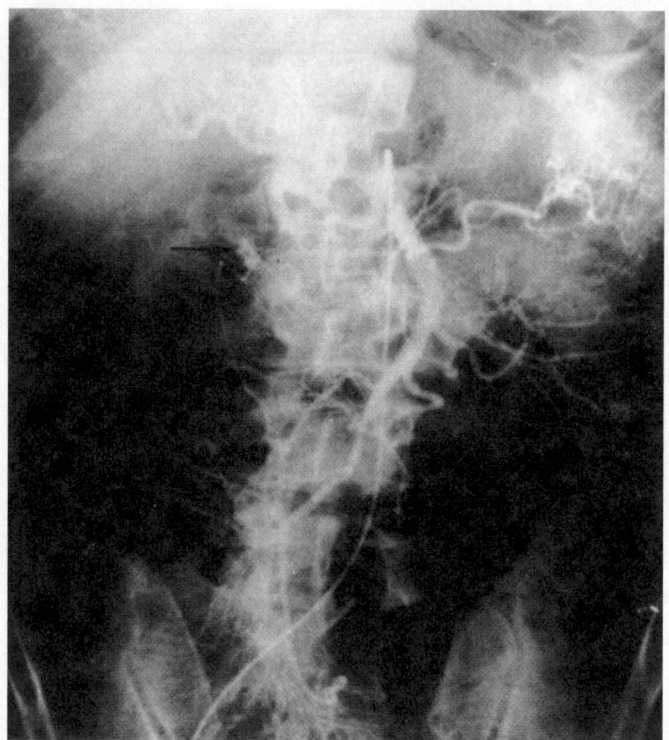

FIGURE 29-6 Arteriogram of superior mesenteric artery shows diverticular bleeding. Note the area of contrast extravasation. (From Doughty DB, Jackson DB. *Gastrointestinal Disorders.* St. Louis: Mosby; 1993.)

(approximately 15%) whose GI bleeding is not stopped with medical measures or endoscopic treatment.[10] Angiography also is used to evaluate cirrhosis, portal hypertension, intestinal ischemia, and other vascular abnormalities.[7]

The radiologist cannulates the femoral artery with a needle and passes a guidewire through it into the aorta. The needle is removed, and an angiographic catheter is inserted over the guidewire. The catheter is advanced into the vessel supplying the portion of the GI tract that is being studied. After the

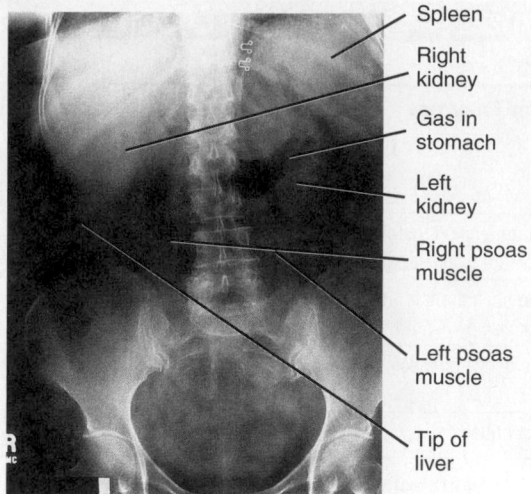

Spleen
Right kidney
Gas in stomach
Left kidney
Right psoas muscle
Left psoas muscle
Tip of liver

FIGURE 29-7 Abdominal flat plate radiograph. Note the air in the patient's stomach. (From Mettler F. *Essentials of Radiology.* 2nd ed. Philadelphia: Saunders; 2005.)

catheter is in place, contrast medium is injected, and serial radiographs are obtained. If the procedure is undertaken to control bleeding, vasopressin (Pitressin Synthetic) or embolic material (Gelfoam) is injected after the site of the bleeding is located.[10]

Nursing Management

Complications include overt and covert bleeding at the femoral puncture site, neurovascular compromise of the affected leg, and sensitivity to the contrast medium. Before the procedure, the patient should be asked about any sensitivity to contrast. Postprocedural assessment involves monitoring vital signs, observing the injection site for bleeding, and assessing neurovascular integrity distal to the injection site every 15 minutes for the first 1 to 2 hours. Depending on how the puncture site is stabilized after the procedure, the patient may have to remain flat in bed for a specified length of time. Any evidence of bleeding or neurovascular impairment must be immediately reported to the physician.[11]

Plain Abdominal Series

Although numerous radiologic studies are available to investigate GI dysfunction further, many of these studies are not performed on the critically ill patient. The radiologic study that is performed most often is the plain abdominal series (Fig. 29-7). An abdominal radiograph is useful in the diagnosis of a bowel obstruction and perforation.[12]

Air in the bowel serves as a contrast medium to aid in the visualization of the bowel. Gas patterns (the presence of gas inside or outside the bowel lumen and the distribution of gas in dilated and nondilated bowel) are best revealed by plain radiographs. Common radiologic signs of free air in the abdomen include the presence of air on both sides of the bowel wall and the presence of air in the right upper quadrant anterior to the liver.[12] Table 29-6 lists common radiologic findings. Abdominal radiographs are used to verify nasogastric or feeding tube placement.

TABLE 29-6 PLAIN FILM FINDINGS

FINDING	APPEARANCE	ASSOCIATIONS
Pneumoperitoneum	Air seen under diaphragm on upright chest or overlying right lobe of liver on left lateral decubitus films	Most commonly associated with bowel perforation, although other causes exist
Peritoneal fluid	Medial displacement of colon separated from flank stripes by fluid density on flat plate	Ascites or hemorrhage
Adynamic ileus	Dilatation of entire intestinal tract, including stomach	Many causes, including trauma, infection (intra-abdominal and extra-abdominal), metabolic disease, and medications (e.g., narcotics)
Sentinel loop	Single distended loop of small bowel containing an air-fluid level	Represents localized ileus associated with localized inflammatory process such as cholecystitis, appendicitis, or pancreatitis
Small bowel obstruction	Dilated loops of small bowel (distinguished by valvulae conniventes, thin, transverse linear densities that extend completely across diameter of bowel) with air-fluid levels	Can be associated with other serious pathology such as incarcerated hernia, appendicitis, or mesenteric ischemia
Large bowel obstruction	Dilated loops, usually more peripheral in the abdomen (distinguished by haustra—short, thick indentations that do not completely cross-bowel and are less frequently spaced than valvulae conniventes)	Can be associated with diverticulitis and malignancy
Cecal volvulus	Usually found in middle or upper abdomen to the left; often kidney shaped	
Sigmoid volvulus	Dilated loop of colon arising from left side of pelvis and projecting obliquely upward toward right side of abdomen	
Early ischemic bowel findings	May resemble mechanical obstruction with dilated loops and air-fluid levels	
Later ischemic bowel findings	May resemble a dynamic ileus; thumbprinting (edema of bowel wall with convex indentations of lumen) and pneumatosis intestinalis (linear or mottled gas pattern in bowel wall)	
Gallbladder emergency findings	Ring of air outlining the gallbladder Air in biliary tree combined with signs of small bowel obstruction, possibly with visible calculus in pelvis	Emphysematous cholecystitis Gallstone ileus
Abdominal aortic aneurysm (AAA)	Usually appears left of midline on supine film and anterior to spine in lateral projection; calcification in wall of aneurysm is variable	Ruptured or leaking AAA may reveal loss of psoas shadows or large soft tissue mass

From Hendrickson M, Naparst TR. Abdominal surgical emergencies in the elderly. *Emerg Med Clin North Am.* 2003;21:937.

Nursing Management

An abdominal radiographic series can be obtained at the patient's bedside using a portable x-ray machine. The series includes two views of the abdomen: one in the supine position and one in the upright position. For patients unable to sit upright, a lateral decubitus radiograph may be obtained with the patient's left side down. No special interventions are required before or after the procedure.[11]

Abdominal Ultrasound

Abdominal ultrasound is useful in evaluating the status of the gallbladder and biliary system, the liver, the spleen, and the pancreas. It plays a key role in the diagnosis of many acute abdominal conditions such as acute cholecystitis and biliary obstructions because it is sensitive in detecting obstructive lesions and ascites. Ultrasound is used to identify gallstones and hepatic abscesses, candidiasis, and hematomas. Intestinal gas, ascites, and extreme obesity can interfere with transmission of the sound waves and limit the usefulness of the procedure.[13]

The procedure uses sound waves to produce echoes that are converted into electrical energy and transferred to a screen for viewing. A transducer, which emits and receives sound waves, is moved slowly over the area of the abdomen being studied. Tissues with various densities produce different echoes, which translate into the different structures on the viewing screen.[14]

Nursing Management

An ultrasound scan can be obtained at the patient's bedside using a portable scanning unit. Ultrasound is easily performed, noninvasive, and well tolerated even by critically ill patients. The procedure requires only that the patient lie still for 20 to 30 minutes. No special interventions are required before or after the procedure.[11]

Computed Tomography of the Abdomen

Computed tomography (CT) is a radiographic examination that provides cross-sectional images of internal anatomy (Fig. 29-8). It may be used to evaluate abdominal vasculature and identify focal points found on nuclear scans as solid, cystic, inflammatory, or vascular.[14] CT detects mass lesions more than 2 cm in diameter and allows visualization and evaluation of many different aspects of GI disease. It is particularly useful in identifying pancreatic pseudocysts, abdominal abscesses, biliary obstructions, and a variety of GI neoplastic lesions.[15]

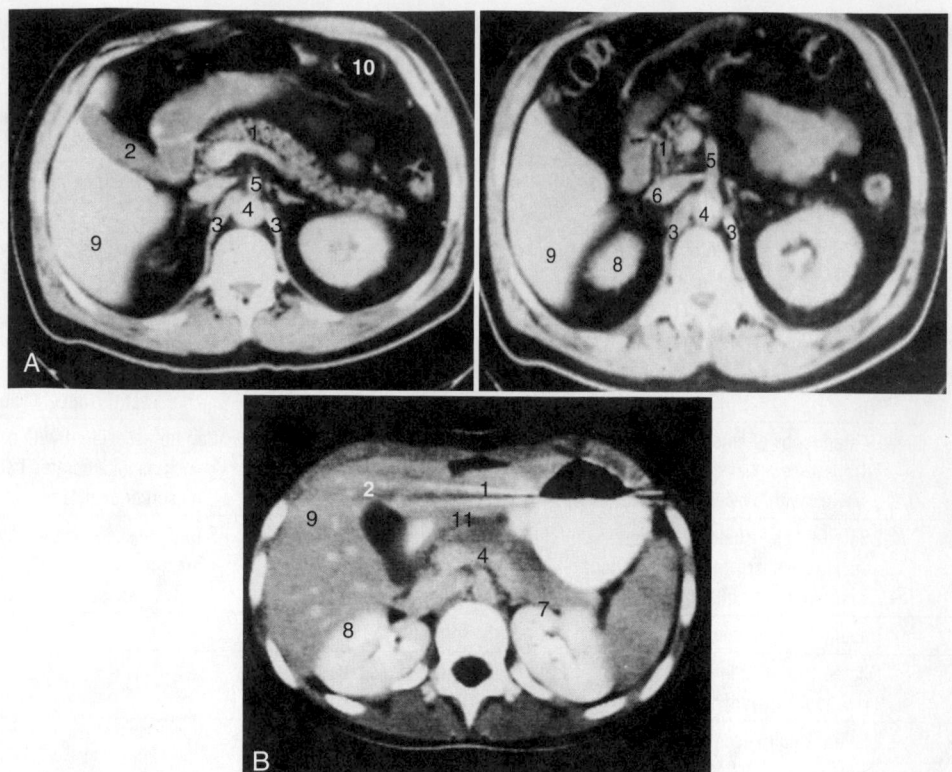

FIGURE 29-8 Abdominal computed tomography (CT) in patient with abundant *(A)* and little *(B)* intra-abdominal fat. *1,* Pancreas; *2,* gallbladder; *3,* crus of the diaphragm; *4,* aorta; *5,* superior mesenteric artery; *6,* inferior vena cava with left renal vein; *7,* left kidney; *8,* right kidney; *9,* liver; *10,* bowel; *11,* splenoportal confluence. (From Seeram E. *Computed Tomography: Physical Principles, Clinical Applications, and Quality Control.* 3rd ed. St. Louis: Saunders; 2009.)

The procedure involves taking the patient to the CT scanner, placing the patient on the table, and inserting the area to be studied into the opening of the scanner. Multiple scans are obtained at various angles, and a computer synthesizes images of the structures being studied. Intravenous or GI contrast may be used to facilitate the imaging of the blood vessels or the GI tract, respectively.[14]

Nursing Management

Before the procedure, the patient should be asked about any sensitivity to contrast. The procedure usually takes 30 minutes without contrast and 60 minutes with contrast, during which time the patient must lie very still. No special interventions are required before or after the procedure.[11]

Hepatobiliary Scintigraphy

A hepatobiliary scan is a nuclear scan that is used to assess the status of the liver and the biliary system. It is valuable in detecting GI abnormalities such as acute and chronic cholecystitis, biliary obstruction, and bile leaks, and it yields additional information about organ size.[16]

The scan involves injecting an intravenous technetium 99m (^{99m}Tc)–labeled iminodiacetic agent (radiotracer), such as disofenin (DISIDA) or mebrofenin (TMBIDA). Serial images are then obtained using a gamma (scintillation) camera. The liver cells take up 80% to 90% of the radiotracer, which is then secreted into the bile and transported throughout the biliary system, allowing visualization of the biliary tract, the gallbladder, and the duodenum.[7] Pooling of the iminodiacetic agent around the liver indicates poor uptake and hepatocellular dysfunction.[16]

Nursing Management

The hepatobiliary scan is relatively noninvasive and safe, although the patient must be transported to the nuclear medicine department. The patient may need to maintain NPO status for 2 to 4 hours before the procedure. Sedation is usually not required, but the patient must be able to lie flat and remain still for 60 minutes during the scanning procedure. No special interventions are required after the procedure.[11]

Gastrointestinal Bleeding Scan

A GI bleeding scan is used to evaluate the presence of an active bleed, to identify the site of the bleed, and to assess the need for an arteriogram.[17] The GI bleeding scan is sensitive to low rates of bleeding (0.1 milliliters per minute [mL/min]), but it is reliable only when the patient is actively bleeding.[7,17]

The scan is usually performed with intravenous ^{99m}Tc-labeled sulfur colloid or ^{99m}Tc-labeled red blood cells (radiotracers). To tag the red blood cells, a blood sample is taken from the patient. The red blood cells are separated, tagged with ^{99m}Tc, and then returned to the patient. Serial images are obtained using a gamma (scintillation) camera. Extravasation and accumulation or pooling of radiotracers in the bowel lumen indicates active bleeding is occurring and facilitates identification of the site.[7,17]

Nursing Management

The GI bleeding scan is relatively noninvasive and safe, although the patient must be transported to the nuclear medicine department. Sedation usually is not required, but the patient must be able to lie flat and remain still for 60 minutes or longer during the scanning procedure. No special interventions are required after the procedure.[11]

Magnetic Resonance Imaging

Magnetic resonance imaging (MRI) is used to identify tumors, abscesses, hemorrhages, and vascular abnormalities. Small tumors, whose tissue densities are different from those of the surrounding cells, can be identified before they would be visible on any other radiographic test.[7] Magnetic resonance angiography (MRA) is a form of MRI that is used to assess blood vessels and blood flow.[14] Magnetic resonance cholangiopancreatography (MRCP) is a form of MRI used to evaluate the biliary and pancreatic ducts.[18]

During MRI, the patient is placed in a large magnetic field that stimulates the protons of the body. Introduction of radiofrequency waves causes resonance of these protons, which then emit an image that a computer is able to reconstruct for viewing. Intravenous administration of a non–iodine-based contrast medium enhances the image by influencing the magnetic environment and signal intensity.[14]

Nursing Management

The MRI procedure is lengthy and requires that the patient be transported to the scanner. The patient must lie motionless in a tight, enclosed space (if a closed MRI scanner is used), and sedation may be necessary. Removal of all metal from the patient's body is essential because the basis of MRI is a magnetic field. Patients with implanted metal objects are not candidates for the procedure. No special interventions are required after the procedure.[11]

Percutaneous Liver Biopsy

Liver biopsy is a diagnostic procedure that is used to evaluate liver disease. Morphologic, biochemical, bacteriologic, and immunologic studies are performed on the tissue sample to diagnose liver disorders such as cirrhosis, hepatitis, infections, or cancer. A biopsy can also yield information about the progression of the patient's disease and response to therapy.[7,19]

Percutaneous liver biopsy can be performed at the bedside or in the imaging department and involves the use of an imaging-guided needle.[20] Before the test, the patient should maintain NPO status for 6 hours and have blood drawn for coagulation studies. The procedure is performed by anesthetizing the pericapsular tissue, inserting a coring or suction needle between the eighth and ninth intercostal space into the liver while the patient holds his or her breath on exhalation, withdrawing the needle with the sample, and applying pressure to stop the bleeding.[7]

Nursing Management

During liver biopsy, the patient may experience a deep pressure sensation or dull pain that radiates to the right shoulder. After the procedure, the patient is positioned on the right side for 2 hours and kept on complete bed rest for the next 6 to 8 hours.[7,19] Hemorrhage is the major complication associated with liver biopsy, although it occurs in less than 1% of patients. Other complications include damage to neighboring organs (e.g., kidney, lung, colon, gallbladder), bile peritonitis, hemothorax, and infection at the needle site. Puncturing of the gallbladder can cause leakage of bile into the abdominal cavity, resulting in peritonitis.[19]

▌ S U M M A R Y

History

- A review of the patient's current illness and symptoms, including the presence or absence of bleeding, abdominal pain, and dysphagia, is an important part of obtaining the patient's history.
- If the patient's condition permits, additional information regarding the patient's personal and social status, general health status, and family history, including nutritional intake, oral hygiene, and bowel elimination, should be obtained.

Clinical Assessment

- To prevent stimulation of GI activity, the order for the assessment should be changed to inspection, auscultation, percussion, and palpation.
- Inspection should focus on the oral cavity, skin, and abdomen.
- Auscultation provides clinical data on the status of the bowel's motility.
- Normal bowel sounds are high-pitched, gurgling sounds that occur approximately every 5 to 15 seconds, and colonic sounds are low pitched and have a rumbling quality.

- Percussion is used to elicit information about deep organs such as the liver, spleen, and pancreas.
- Light and deep palpation methods are used to detect pathologic conditions of the abdomen.

Laboratory Studies

- No single laboratory study provides an overall picture of the various organs' functional state.

Diagnostic Procedures

- Fiberoptic endoscopy is a diagnostic procedure for the direct visualization and evaluation of the GI tract.
- Angiography is used diagnostically to evaluate the status of GI circulation and therapeutically to achieve control of GI bleeding.
- An abdominal radiograph is useful in the diagnosis of a bowel obstruction and perforation.
- Abdominal ultrasound is used to evaluate the status of the gallbladder and biliary system, the liver, the spleen, and the pancreas.
- CT provides cross-sectional images of the internal anatomy of the abdomen and is used to evaluate abdominal

vasculature and identify focal points found on nuclear scans as solid, cystic, inflammatory, or vascular.

- A hepatobiliary scan is a nuclear scan that is used to assess the status of the liver and the biliary system.
- A gastrointestinal bleeding scan is used to evaluate the presence of an active GI bleed, to identify the site of the bleed, and to assess the need for an arteriogram.

- MRI is used to identify tumors, abscesses, hemorrhages, and vascular abnormalities.
- Liver biopsy is a diagnostic procedure that is used to evaluate liver disease.

REFERENCES

1. O'Toole MT. Advanced assessment of the abdomen and gastrointestinal problems. *Nurs Clin North Am*. 1990;24:771.
2. Baid H. The process of conducting a physical assessment: a nursing perspective. *Br J Nurs*. 2006;15:710.
3. Seidel HM, et al. *Mosby's Guide to Physical Examination*. 7th ed. St. Louis: Mosby; 2010.
4. Barkauskas V, et al. *Health and Physical Assessment*. 3rd ed. St. Louis: Mosby; 2002.
5. Thompson JM, et al. *Mosby's Clinical Nursing*. 5th ed. St. Louis: Mosby; 2002.
6. O'Hanlon-Nicholas T. Basic assessment series: gastrointestinal system. *Am J Nurs*. 1998;98(4):48.
7. SGNA. *Gastroenterology Nursing: A Core Curriculum*. 4th ed. St. Louis: Society of Gastroenterology Nurses and Associates; 2008.
8. Hwang JH, et al. Guideline: the role of endoscopy in the management of acute non-variceal upper GI bleeding. *Gastrointest Endosc*. 2012;75:1135.
9. Ginzburg L. Complications of endoscopy. *Gastrointest Endosc Clin North Am*. 2007;17:405.
10. Walker TG, et al. Angiographic evaluation and management of acute gastrointestinal hemorrhage. *World J Gastroenterol*. 2012;18:1191.
11. Pangana KD, Pangana TJ. *Mosby's Diagnostic and Laboratory Test Reference*. 10th ed. St. Louis: Mosby; 2011.
12. Yeh EL, McNamara RM. Abdominal pain. *Clin Geriatr Med*. 2007;23:255.
13. Godfrey EM, et al. Endoscopic ultrasound: a review of current diagnostic and therapeutic applications. *Postgrad Med J*. 2010;86:346.
14. Cogbill TH, Ziegelbein KJ. Computed tomography, magnetic resonance and untrasound imaging: basic principles, glossary of terms and patient safety. *Surg Clin North Am*. 2011;91:1.
15. McSweeney SE, et al. Current and emerging techniques in gastrointestinal imaging. *J Postgrad Med*. 2010;56:109.
16. Lambie H, et al. Tc99m-hepatobiliary iminodiacetic acid (HIDA) scintigraphy in clinical practice. *Clin Radiol*. 2011;66:1094.
17. Mellinger JD, et al. Imaging of gastrointestinal bleeding. *Surg Clin North Am*. 2011;91:92.
18. Maccioni F, et al. Magnetic resonance cholangiography: past, present and future: a review. *Eur Rev Med Pharmacol Sci*. 2010;14:721.
19. Rustagi T, et al. Percutaneous liver biopsy. *Trop Gastroenterol*. 2010;31:199.
20. Karamshi M. Performing a percutaneous liver biopsy in parenchymal liver diseases. *Br J Nurs*. 2008;17:746.

Gastrointestinal Disorders and Therapeutic Management

Sheryl Leary

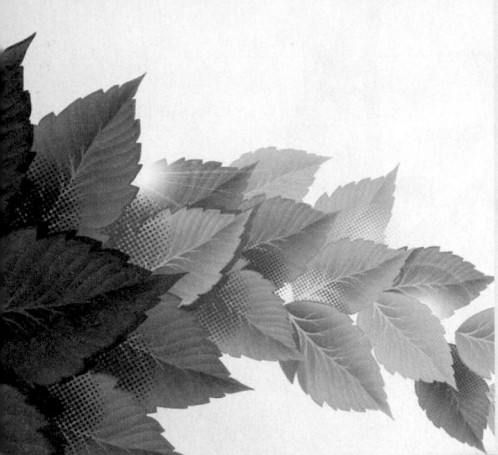

evolve WEBSITE

http://evolve.elsevier.com/Urden/criticalcare/

Evolve features:

- NCLEX Review Questions
- CCRN Review Questions
- PCCN Review Questions
- Mosby's Nursing Skills Procedures
- Animations
- Video Clips
- Glossary

Understanding the pathology of a disease, the areas of assessment on which to focus, and the usual medical management allows the critical care nurse to accurately anticipate and plan nursing interventions. This chapter focuses on gastrointestinal (GI) disorders commonly seen in the critical care environment.

ACUTE GASTROINTESTINAL HEMORRHAGE

Description

GI hemorrhage is a potentially life-threatening emergency that remains a common complication of critical illness and results in over 300,000 hospital admissions yearly.[1] Despite advances in medical knowledge and nursing care, the mortality rate for patients with acute GI bleeding remains at 10% per annum in the United States.[1]

Etiology

GI hemorrhage occurs from bleeding in the upper or lower GI tract. The ligament of Treitz is the anatomic division used to differentiate between the two areas. Bleeding proximal to the ligament is considered to be from the upper GI tract, and bleeding distal to the ligament is considered to be from the lower GI tract.[1-3] The various causes of acute GI hemorrhage are listed in Box 30-1.[4] Only the three main causes of GI hemorrhage commonly seen in the critical care unit are discussed further.

Peptic Ulcer Disease

Peptic ulcer disease (i.e., gastric and duodenal ulcers), which results from the breakdown of the gastromucosal lining, is the leading cause of upper GI hemorrhage, accounting for approximately 40% of cases.[5,6] Normally, protection of the gastric mucosa from the digestive effects of gastric secretions is accomplished in several ways. First, the gastroduodenal mucosa is coated by a glycoprotein mucous barrier that protects the surface of the epithelium from hydrogen ions and other noxious substances present in the gut lumen.[6-8] Adequate gastric mucosal blood flow is necessary to maintain this mucosal barrier function. Second, gastroduodenal epithelial cells are protected structurally against damage from acid and pepsin because they are connected by tight junctions that help prevent acid penetration. Third, prostaglandins and nitric oxide protect the mucosal barrier by stimulating the secretion of mucus and bicarbonate and inhibiting the secretion of acid.[6-8]

Peptic ulceration occurs when these protective mechanisms cease to function, allowing gastroduodenal mucosal breakdown. After the mucosal lining is penetrated, gastric secretions autodigest the layers of the stomach or duodenum, leading to injury of the mucosal and submucosal layers. This results in damaged blood vessels and subsequent hemorrhage. The two main causes of disruption of gastroduodenal mucosal resistance are the bacterial action of *Helicobacter pylori* and nonsteroidal anti-inflammatory drugs (NSAIDs).[9]

Stress-Related Mucosal Disease

Stress-related mucosal disease (SRMD) is an acute erosive gastritis that covers both types of mucosal lesions that are often found in the critically ill patient: stress-related injury and discrete stress ulcers.[10-12] Additional terms used to describe this condition include *stress ulcers, stress erosions, stress gastritis,*

Upper Gastrointestinal Tract	Lower Gastrointestinal Tract
• Peptic ulcer disease	• Diverticulosis
• Stress-related erosive syndrome	• Angiodysplasia
• Esophagogastric varices	• Neoplasm
• Mallory-Weiss tear	• Inflammatory bowel disease
• Esophagitis	• Trauma
• Neoplasm	• Infectious colitis
• Aortoenteric fistula	• Radiation colitis
• Angiodysplasia	• Ischemia
	• Aortoenteric fistula
	• Hemorrhoids

hemorrhagic gastritis, and *erosive gastritis.* These abnormalities develop within hours of admission.[11] They range from superficial mucosal erosions to deep focal lesions and usually affect the upper GI tract.[11] SRMD occurs by means of the same pathophysiologic mechanisms as peptic ulcer disease, but the main cause of disruption of gastric mucosal resistance is increased acid production and decreased mucosal blood flow, resulting in ischemia and degeneration of the mucosal lining.[11] Patients at risk include those in situations of high physiologic stress, as occurs with mechanical ventilation, extensive burns, severe trauma, major surgery, shock, sepsis, coagulopathy, or acute neurologic disease.[13] SRMD is decreasing in incidence because of advances in therapeutic techniques and prevention of hypoperfusion of the mucosa.[14]

Esophagogastric Varices

Esophagogastric varices are engorged and distended blood vessels of the esophagus and proximal stomach that develop as a result of portal hypertension caused by hepatic cirrhosis, a chronic disease of the liver, which results in damage to the liver sinusoids (Fig. 30-1). Without adequate sinusoid function, resistance to portal blood flow is increased, and pressures within the liver are elevated. This leads to increased portal venous pressure (portal hypertension), causing collateral circulation to divert portal blood from areas of high pressure within the liver to adjacent areas of low pressure outside the liver, such as into the veins of the esophagus, the spleen, the intestines, and the stomach. The tiny, thin-walled vessels of the esophagus and proximal stomach that receive this diverted blood lack sturdy mucosal protection. The vessels become engorged and dilated, forming esophagogastric varices that are vulnerable to damage from gastric secretions and that may result in subsequent rupture and massive hemorrhage.[15] The risk of variceal bleeding increases with disease severity and variceal size, but overall, bleeding occurs in 25% to 30% of patients within 2 years of diagnosis, and 20% to 30% mortality from each bleeding episode.[16,17]

Pathophysiology

GI hemorrhage is a life-threatening disorder that is characterized by acute, massive bleeding. Regardless of the cause, acute

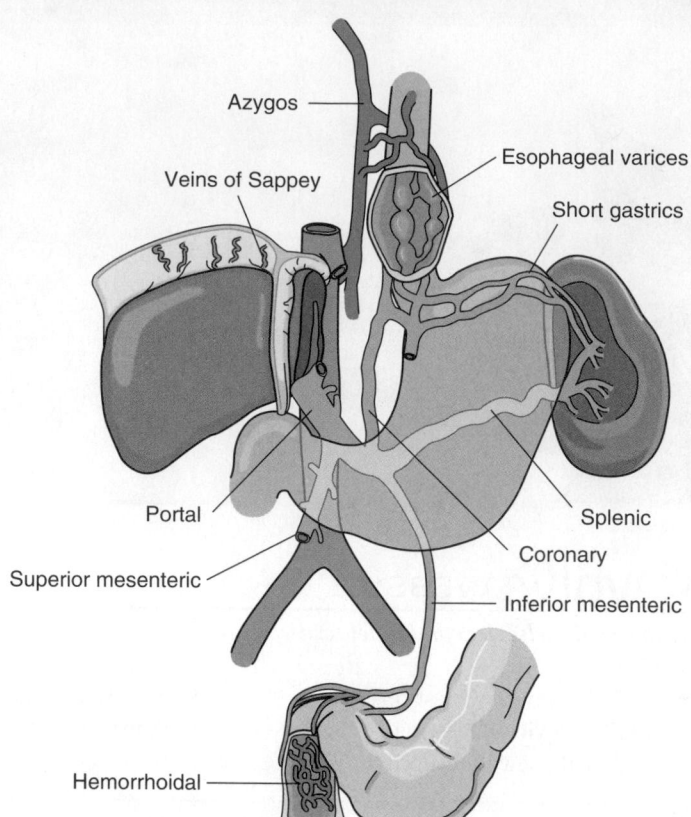

FIGURE 30-1 Varices related to portal hypertension. Portal vein, its major tributaries, and the most important shunts (collateral veins) between the portal and caval systems. (From Monahan FD, et al. *Phipps' Medical-Surgical Nursing: Concepts and Clinical Practice.* 8th ed. St. Louis: Mosby; 2007.)

GI hemorrhage results in hypovolemic shock, initiation of the shock response, and development of multiple organ dysfunction syndrome if left untreated (see Concept Map, Fig. 30-2).[7] However, the most common cause of death in cases of GI hemorrhage is exacerbation of the underlying disease, not intractable hypovolemic shock.

Assessment and Diagnosis

The initial clinical presentation of the patient with acute GI hemorrhage is that of a patient in hypovolemic shock, and the clinical presentation depends on the amount of blood lost (Table 30-1).[7] Hematemesis (bright red or brown, "coffee grounds" emesis), hematochezia (bright red stools), and melena (black, tarry, or dark red stools) are the hallmarks of GI hemorrhage.[5,18]

Hematemesis

The patient who is vomiting blood is usually bleeding from a source above the duodenojejunal junction; reverse peristalsis is seldom sufficient to cause hematemesis if the bleeding point is below this area. The hematemesis may be bright red or look like coffee grounds, depending on the amount of gastric contents at the time of bleeding and the length of time the blood has been in contact with gastric secretions. Gastric acid converts bright red hemoglobin to brown hematin, accounting for the coffee grounds appearance of the emesis. Bright red emesis results

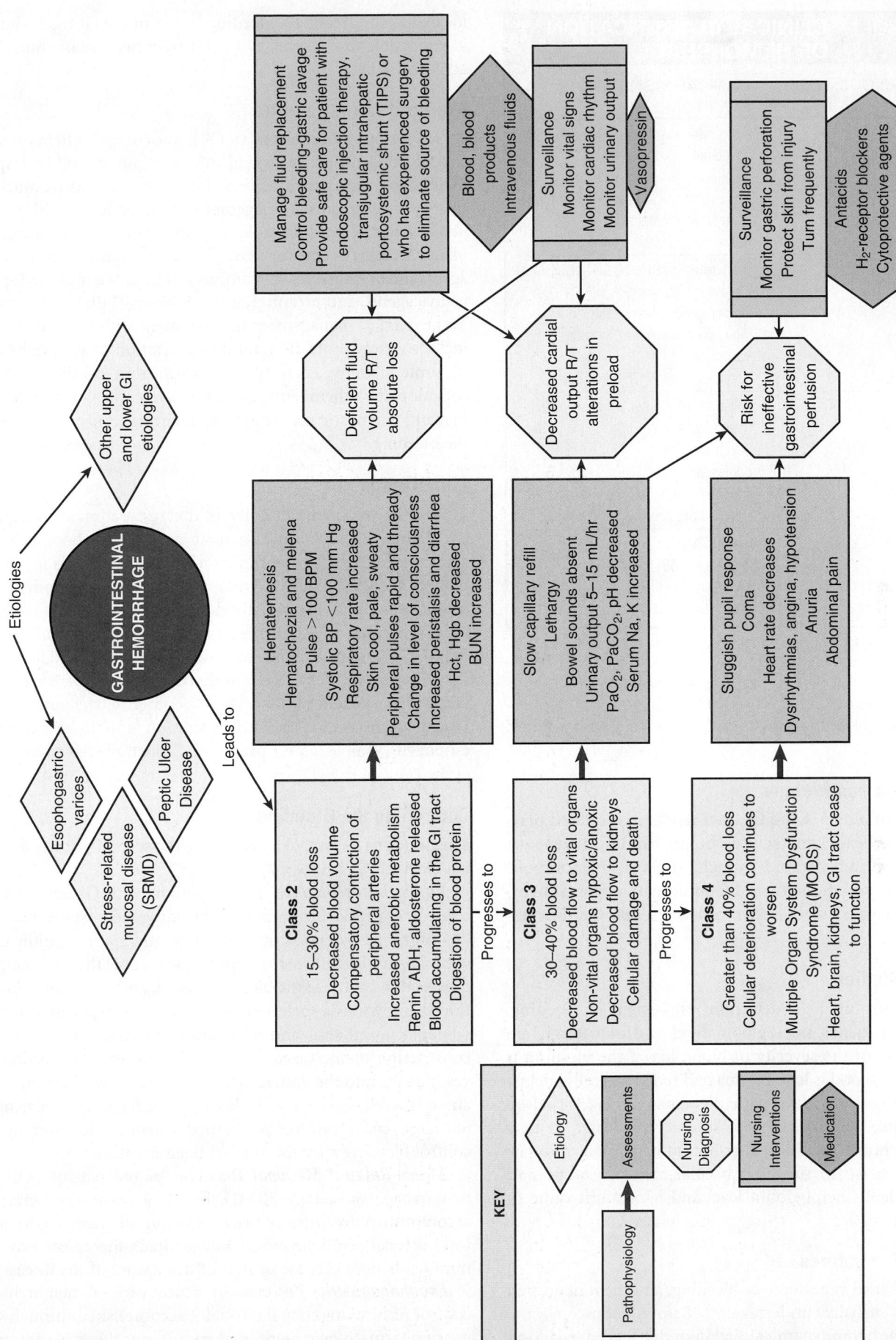

FIGURE 30-2   Concept Map for Gastrointestinal Hemorrhage. (Illustrated by Elaine B. Kennedy, EdD, RN.)

TABLE 30-1 CLINICAL CLASSIFICATION OF HEMORRHAGE

CLASS	BLOOD LOSS (%)	CLINICAL SIGNS AND SYMPTOMS
1	≤15	Pulse rate: normal or <100 beats/min (supine) Capillary refill <3 seconds Urine output: adequate (30-35 mL/hr) Orthostatic hypotension Apprehensive
2	15-30	Pulse rate: increased (>100 beats/min) Capillary refill: sluggish Pulse pressure: decreased Blood pressure: normal (supine) Tachypnea Urine output: low (25-30 mL/hr)
3	30-40	Pulse rate: 120+ beats/min (supine) Hypotension Skin: cool, pale Confused Hyperventilating Urine output: low (5-15 mL/hr)
4	≥40	Profoundly hypotensive Pulse rate: 140+ beats/min Confused, lethargic Urine output minimal

From Klein DG. Physiologic response to traumatic shock. *AACN Clin Issues Crit Care Nurs.* 1990;1:505.

from profuse bleeding with little contact with gastric secretions.[19]

Hematochezia and Melena

The presence of blood in the GI tract results in increased peristalsis and diarrhea. Hematochezia occurs from massive lower GI hemorrhage and, if rapid enough, upper GI hemorrhage. Melena occurs from digestion of blood from an upper GI hemorrhage and may take several days to clear after the bleeding has stopped.

Laboratory Studies

Laboratory tests can help determine the extent of bleeding, although the patient's hemoglobin level and hematocrit are poor indicators of the severity of blood loss if the bleeding is acute. As whole blood is lost, plasma and red blood cells are lost in the same proportion; if the patient's hematocrit is 45% before a bleeding episode, it will be 45% several hours later.[7] It may take 24 to 72 hours for the redistribution of plasma from the extravascular space to the intravascular space to occur and cause the patient's hemoglobin level and hematocrit value to decrease.[19]

Diagnostic Procedures

To isolate and treat the source of bleeding, an urgent fiberoptic endoscopy is usually undertaken.[20] Before endoscopy, the patient must be hemodynamically stabilized.[21] Tagged red blood cell scanning, angiography, or both, may be done to assist with localizing and treating a bleeding lesion in the GI tract when it is impossible to clearly view the GI tract because of continued active bleeding.[19]

Medical Management

To reduce mortality related to GI hemorrhage, patients at risk should be identified early, and interventions should be implemented to reduce gastric acidity and support the gastric mucosal defense mechanisms. Management of the patient at risk for GI hemorrhage should include prophylactic administration of pharmacologic agents for neutralization of gastric acids. These agents include antacids, histamine-2 (H_2) antagonists, cytoprotective agents, and proton pump inhibitors (PPIs).[5,22] Priorities in the medical management of the patient with GI hemorrhage include airway protection, fluid resuscitation to achieve hemodynamic stability, correction of co-morbid conditions (e.g., coagulopathy), therapeutic procedures to control or stop bleeding, and diagnostic procedures to determine the exact cause of the bleeding.[5,21]

Stabilization

The initial treatment priority is the restoration of adequate circulating blood volume to treat or prevent shock. This is accomplished with the administration of intravenous infusions of crystalloids, blood, and blood products.[22] Hemodynamic monitoring can help guide fluid replacement therapy, particularly in patients at risk for heart failure.[7] Supplemental oxygen therapy is initiated to increase oxygen delivery and improve tissue perfusion.[7,22] A large nasogastric tube may be inserted to confirm the diagnosis of active bleeding, to facilitate gastric lavage, decrease the risk for aspiration and to prepare the esophagus, stomach, and proximal duodenum for endoscopic evaluation.[5]

Controlling the Bleeding

Interventions to control bleeding are the second priority for the patient with GI hemorrhage.

Peptic Ulcer Disease. In the patient with GI hemorrhage related to peptic ulcer disease, bleeding hemostasis may be accomplished by endoscopic injection therapy in conjunction with thermal or hemostatic clips.[20] Endoscopic thermal therapy uses heat to cauterize the bleeding vessel, and endoscopic injection therapy uses a variety of agents such as hypertonic saline, epinephrine, ethanol, and sclerosants to induce localized vasoconstriction of the bleeding vessel.[6] Intra-arterial infusion of vasopressin into the gastric artery or intra-arterial injection of an embolizing agent (e.g., Gelfoam pledgets, polyvinyl alcohol particles, coils) can be performed during arteriography to control bleeding after the site has been identified.[19]

Stress-Related Mucosal Disease. In the patient with GI hemorrhage caused by SRMD, bleeding hemostasis may be accomplished by intra-arterial infusion of vasopressin and intra-arterial embolization. Endoscopic therapies provide minimal benefit because of the diffuse nature of the disease.[19]

Esophagogastric Varices. In acute variceal hemorrhage, control of bleeding may be initially accomplished through the use of pharmacologic agents and endoscopic therapies. Intravenous vasopressin, somatostatin, and octreotide can reduce

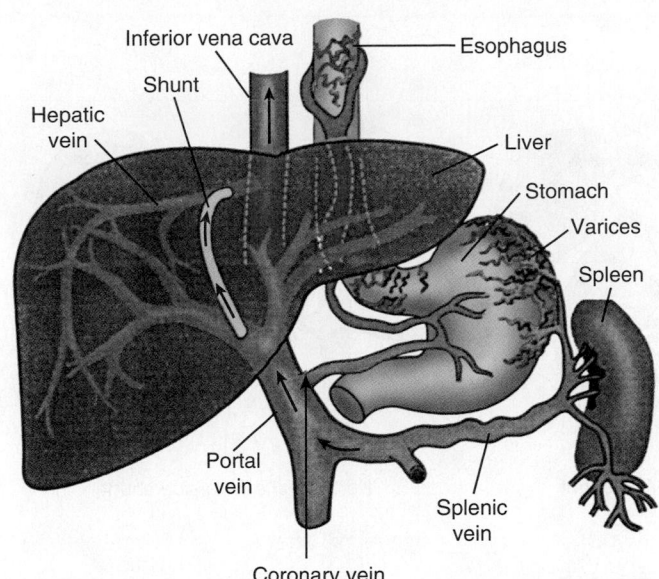

FIGURE 30-3 Anatomic location of the transjugular intrahepatic portosystemic shunt (TIPS). (From Vargas HE, et al. Management of portal hypertension-related bleeding. *Surg Clin North Am.* 1999;79:1.)

portal venous pressure and slow variceal hemorrhaging by constricting the splanchnic arteriolar bed.[16] Two commonly used endoscopic therapies are endoscopic injection sclerotherapy (EIS) and endoscopic variceal ligation (EVL).[23] EIS controls bleeding by the injection of a sclerosing agent in or around the varices. This creates an inflammatory reaction that induces vasoconstriction and results in the formation of a venous thrombosis. During EVL, bands are placed around the varices to create an obstruction to stop the bleeding.[24]

If these initial therapies fail, transjugular intrahepatic portosystemic shunting (TIPS) may be necessary. In a TIPS procedure, a channel between the systemic and portal venous systems is created to redirect portal blood, thereby reducing portal hypertension and decompressing the varices to control bleeding (Fig. 30-3).[23,24]

Surgical Intervention

The patient who remains hemodynamically unstable despite volume replacement may need urgent surgery.

Peptic Ulcer Disease. Surgical intervention is required to control bleeding in a minority of patients.[25] The operative procedure of choice to control bleeding from peptic ulcer disease is a vagotomy and pyloroplasty. During this procedure, the vagus nerve to the stomach is severed, eliminating the autonomic stimulus to the gastric cells and reducing hydrochloric acid production. Because the vagus nerve also stimulates motility, a pyloroplasty is performed to provide for gastric emptying.[26]

Stress-Related Mucosal Disease. In the past, several operative procedures were used to control bleeding from SRMD. Because of the advent of stress ulcer prophylaxis, a marked decrease occurs in the incidence of hemorrhage from SRMD.[22]

Esophagogastric Varices. If medical treatment is unsuccessful and angiographic interventional TIPS procedure is not available, operative procedures to control bleeding gastroesophageal

varices may be undertaken. Though rarely performed, operative interventions focus on some form of shunting (Fig 30-4).[25] These shunt procedures are also referred to as *decompression procedures* because they result in the diversion of portal blood flow away from the liver and decompression of the portal system. The portacaval shunt procedure has two variations: (1) an *end-to-side portacaval shunt procedure*, which involves the ligation of the hepatic end of the portal vein with subsequent anastomosis to the vena cava; and (2) a *side-to-side portacaval shunt procedure*, during which the side of the portal vein is anastomosed to the side of the vena cava. A *mesocaval shunt procedure* involves the insertion of a graft between the superior mesenteric artery and the vena cava. During a *distal splenorenal shunt procedure*, the splenic vein is detached from the portal vein and anastomosed to the left renal vein.[27]

Nursing Management

All critically ill patients should be considered at risk for stress ulcers and, therefore, GI hemorrhage. Routine assessment of gastric fluid pH monitoring is controversial.[12,28] Maintaining the pH between 3.5 and 4.5 is a goal of prophylactic therapy. Gastric pH measurements made with litmus paper or direct nasogastric tube probes may be used to assess gastric fluid pH and the effectiveness or need for prophylactic agents.[28] Patients at risk also should be assessed for the presence of bright red or coffee grounds emesis, bloody nasogastric aspirate, and bright red, black, or dark red stools.[4] Any signs of bleeding should be promptly reported to the physician.

Nursing management of a patient experiencing acute GI hemorrhage incorporates a variety of nursing diagnoses (Box 30-2). Nursing interventions include administering volume replacement, controlling the bleeding, providing comfort and emotional support, maintaining surveillance for complications, and educating the patient and family.

Administering Volume Replacement. Measures to facilitate volume replacement include obtaining intravenous access and administering prescribed fluids and blood products. Two large-diameter peripheral intravenous catheters should be inserted to facilitate the rapid administration of prescribed fluids.[1]

Controlling the Bleeding. One measure to control active bleeding is gastric lavage. It is used to decrease gastric mucosal blood flow and evacuate blood from the stomach. Gastric lavage is performed by inserting a large-bore nasogastric tube into the stomach and irrigating it with normal saline or water until the returned solution is clear. It is important to keep accurate records of the amount of fluid instilled and aspirated to ascertain the true amount of bleeding.[1] Historically, iced saline was favored as a lavage irrigant. Research has shown, however, that low-temperature fluids shift the oxyhemoglobin dissociation curve to the left, decrease oxygen delivery to vital organs, and prolong bleeding time and prothrombin time. Iced saline also may further aggravate bleeding; therefore, room-temperature water or saline is the preferred irrigant for use in gastric lavage.[29]

Maintaining Surveillance for Complications. The patient should be continuously observed for signs of gastric perforation. Although a rare complication, gastric perforation

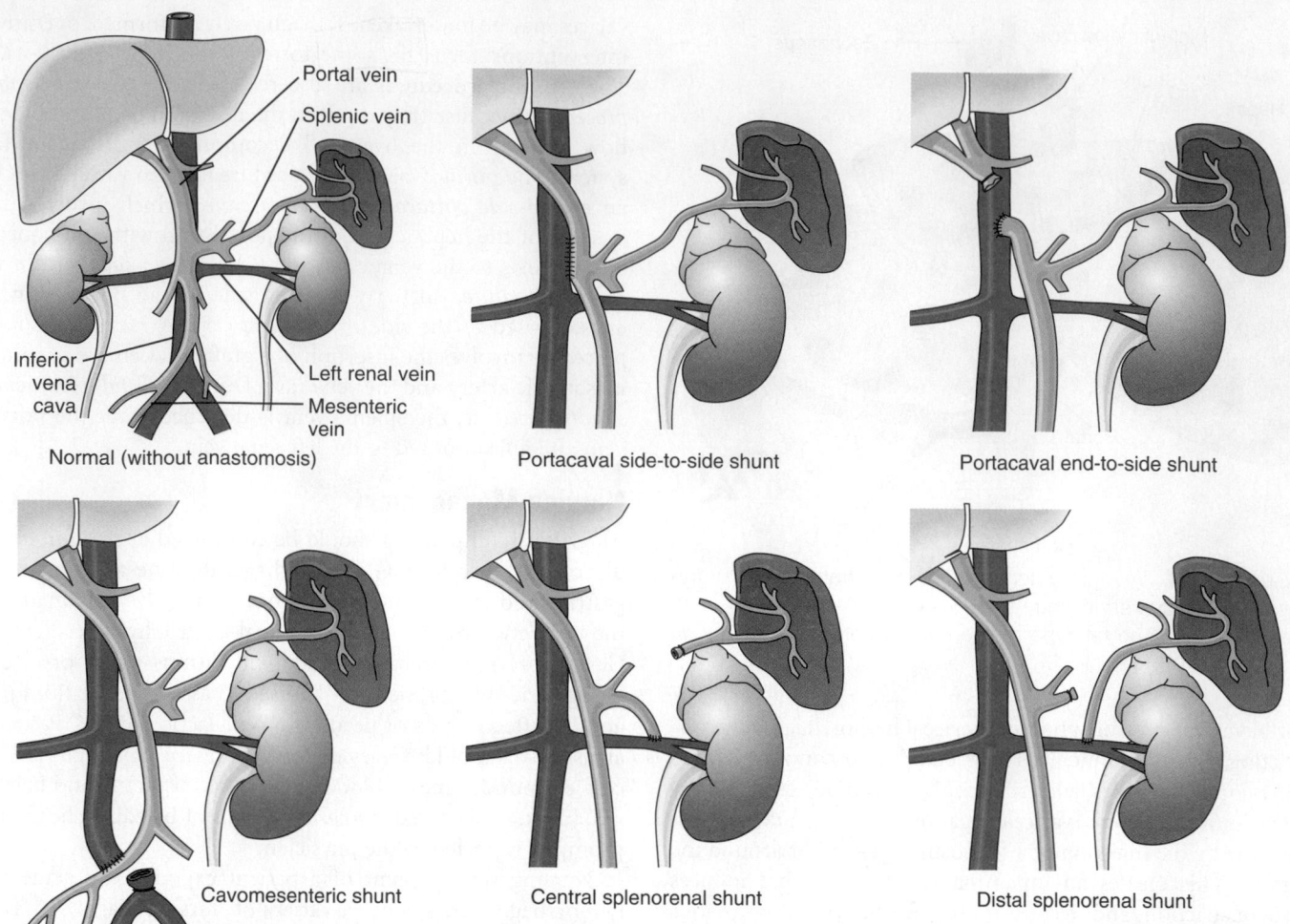

FIGURE 30-4 Portosystemic shunt operative procedures. (From Copstead LC, Banasik JL. *Pathophysiology*. 4th ed. St. Louis: Saunders; 2010.)

Labels in figure:
Normal (without anastomosis) — Portal vein, Splenic vein, Inferior vena cava, Left renal vein, Mesenteric vein
Portacaval side-to-side shunt
Portacaval end-to-side shunt
Cavomesenteric shunt
Central splenorenal shunt
Distal splenorenal shunt

BOX 30-2 NURSING DIAGNOSES

Acute Gastrointestinal Hemorrhage

- Deficient Fluid Volume, related to absolute loss, p. 1132
- Decreased Cardiac Output, related to alterations in preload, p. 1128
- Risk for Aspiration, p. 1154
- Imbalanced Nutrition: Less Than Body Requirements, related to lack of exogenous nutrients and increased metabolic demand, p. 1143
- Risk for Infection, p. 1160
- Powerlessness, related to health care environment or illness-related regimen, p. 1152
- Compromised Family Coping, related to critically ill family member, p. 1127
- Deficient Knowledge, related to lack of previous exposure to information, p. 1134 (see Patient Education, Box 30-3)

---

constitutes a surgical emergency. Signs and symptoms include sudden, severe, generalized abdominal pain with significant rebound tenderness and rigidity. Perforation should be suspected when fever, leukocytosis, and tachycardia persist despite adequate volume replacement.[30]

Educating the Patient and Family. Early in the hospital stay, the patient and family should be taught about acute GI hemorrhage and its causes and treatments. As the patient moves toward discharge, teaching should focus on the interventions

necessary for preventing the recurrence of the precipitating disorder. If an alcohol abuser, the patient should be encouraged to stop drinking and be referred to an alcohol cessation program (Box 30-3).

Collaborative management of the patient with acute GI hemorrhage is outlined in Box 30-4.

ACUTE PANCREATITIS

Description

Acute pancreatitis is an inflammation of the pancreas that produces exocrine and endocrine dysfunction that may also involve surrounding tissues, remote organ systems, or both. The clinical course can range from a mild, self-limiting disease to a systemic process characterized by organ failure, sepsis, and death. In approximately 80% of patients, it takes the milder form of *edematous interstitial pancreatitis*, whereas the other 20% develop severe *acute necrotizing pancreatitis*.[31] Reported mortality rates for acute pancreatitis range from 2% to 15% overall, with a steadily increasing rate of about 20,000 deaths per year in the United States.[32,33] Several prognostic scoring systems have been developed to predict the severity of acute pancreatitis. One of the most commonly used is Ranson criteria[34] (Box 30-5). If the patient has 0 to 2 factors present, the predicted mortality

BOX 30-3 PATIENT EDUCATION

Acute Gastrointestinal Hemorrhage

- Gastrointestinal hemorrhage
- Specific cause
- Precipitating factor modification
- Interventions to reduce further bleeding episodes
- Importance of taking medications
- Lifestyle changes
- Stress management
- Diet modifications
- Alcohol cessation
- Smoking cessation
  Additional information for the patient can be found at the following websites:
- Alcoholics Anonymous: http://www.aa.org
- International Foundation for Functional Gastrointestinal Disorders: http://www.iffgd.org
- Healthfinder – U.S. Department of Health and Human Services: http://healthfinder.gov
- Web MD: http://www.webmd.com

BOX 30-4 COLLABORATIVE MANAGEMENT

Acute Gastrointestinal Hemorrhage

- Initiate fluid resuscitation to achieve hemodynamic stability.
  - Crystalloids
  - Colloids
  - Blood and blood products
- Determine the cause of the bleeding.
  - Gastric lavage
- Control bleeding.
  - Endoscopic interventions
  - Vasopressin, somatostatin, octreotide
  - Transjugular intrahepatic portosystemic shunting
  - Surgery (last resort)
- Provide comfort and emotional support.
- Maintain surveillance for complications.
  - Hypovolemic shock
  - Gastric perforation

BOX 30-5 RANSON'S CRITERIA FOR ESTIMATING THE SEVERITY OF ACUTE PANCREATITIS

At Admission

- Age >55 years
- Hypotension
- Abnormal pulmonary findings
- Abdominal mass
- Hemorrhagic or discolored peritoneal fluid
- Increased serum LDH levels (>350 units/L)
- AST >250 units/L
- Leukocytosis (>16,000/mm^3)
- Hyperglycemia (>200 mg/dL; no diabetes history)
- Neurologic deficit (confusion, localizing signs)

During Initial 48 Hours of Hospitalization

- Fall in hematocrit >10% with hydration or hematocrit <30%
- Necessity for massive fluid and colloid replacement
- Hypocalcemia (<8 mg/dL)
- Arterial PO$_2$ <60 mm Hg with or without acute respiratory distress syndrome
- Hypoalbuminemia (<3.2 mg/dL)
- Base deficit >4 mEq/L
- Azotemia

From Latifi R, et al. Nutritional management of acute and chronic pancreatitis. *Surg Clin North Am.* 1991;71:583.
AST, Aspartate aminotransferase; *LDH,* lactate dehydrogenase; *PO$_2$,* partial pressure of oxygen.

BOX 30-6 CAUSES OF ACUTE PANCREATITIS

- Biliary disease (stones, sludge, common bile duct obstruction)
- Toxins (ethyl alcohol, methyl alcohol, scorpion, venom, parathion)
- Smoking
- Medications
- Hypercalcemia (hyperparathyroidism)
- Hyperlipidemia
- Tumors
- Infections (bacterial, viral, parasitic)
- Trauma (abdominal, surgical, endoscopic)
- Hypoperfusion
- Vasculitis
- Pregnancy
- Hypothermia
- Sphincter of Oddi dysfunction
- Autoimmune diseases
- Ampullary stenosis
- Idiopathic cause

rate is 2%; with 3 to 4 factors, the rate is 15%; with 5 to 6 factors, the rate is 40%; and with 7 to 8 factors, predicted mortality rate is 100%.[34-36]

Etiology

The two most common causes of acute pancreatitis are gallstone migration and alcoholism.[36] Together, they account for approximately 80% of cases.[19] Less common causes are quite diverse and include surgical trauma, hypercalcemia, various toxins, ischemia, infections, and the use of certain medications (Box 30-6). In up to 20% of patients with acute pancreatitis, no etiologic factor can be determined.[19,31]

Pathophysiology

In acute pancreatitis, the normally inactive digestive enzymes become prematurely activated within the pancreas itself, leading to autodigestion of pancreatic tissue. The enzymes become activated through various mechanisms, including obstruction of or damage to the pancreatic duct system, alterations in the secretory processes of the acinar cells, infection, ischemia, and other unknown factors.[7,36]

Trypsin is the enzyme that becomes activated first. It initiates the autodigestion process by triggering the secretion of proteolytic enzymes such as kallikrein, chymotrypsin, elastase, phospholipase A, and lipase. Release of kallikrein and chymotrypsin results in increased capillary membrane permeability, leading to leakage of fluid into the interstitium and the development of edema and relative hypovolemia. Elastase is the most harmful enzyme in terms of direct cell damage. It dissolves the elastic fibers of blood vessels and ducts, leading to hemorrhage. Phospholipase A, in the presence of bile, destroys the phospholipids of cell membranes, causing severe pancreatic and adipose tissue necrosis. Lipase flows into the damaged tissue and is absorbed into the systemic circulation, resulting in fat necrosis of the pancreas and surrounding tissues.[7,37]

The extent of injury to the pancreatic cells determines the type of acute pancreatitis that develops. If injury to the pancreatic cells is mild and without necrosis, edematous pancreatitis develops. The acinar cells appear structurally intact, and blood flow is maintained through small capillaries and venules. This form of acute pancreatitis is self-limiting. If injury to the pancreatic cells is severe, acute necrotizing pancreatitis develops.[32,37] Cellular destruction in pancreatic injury results in the release of toxic enzymes and inflammatory mediators into the systemic circulation and causes injury to vessels and other organs distant from the pancreas; this may result in systemic inflammatory response syndrome (SIRS), multiorgan failure, and death.[19,36] Local tissue injury results in infection, abscess and pseudocyst formation, disruption of the pancreatic duct, and severe hemorrhage and shock.[19]

Assessment and Diagnosis

The clinical manifestations of acute pancreatitis range from mild to severe and often mimic those of other disorders (Box 30-7). Acute onset of abdominal pain, nausea, and vomiting are hallmark symptoms.[19,32,37] Epigastric to periumbilical pain may vary from mild and tolerable to severe and incapacitating. Many patients report a twisting or knifelike sensation that radiates to the low dorsal region of the back. The patient may obtain some comfort by leaning forward or assuming a semifetal position.

BOX 30-7 **PRESENTING CLINICAL MANIFESTATIONS OF ACUTE PANCREATITIS**

- Pain
- Vomiting
- Nausea
- Fever
- Abdominal distention
- Abdominal guarding
- Abdominal tympany
- Hypoactive or absent bowel sounds
- Severe disease
- Peritoneal signs
- Ascites
- Jaundice
- Palpable abdominal mass
- Grey-Turner sign
- Cullen sign
- Signs of hypovolemic shock

From Krumberger JM. Acute pancreatitis. *Crit Care Nurs Clin North Am.* 1993;5:185.

Other clinical findings include fever, diaphoresis, weakness, tachypnea, hypotension, and tachycardia. Depending on the extent of fluid loss and hemorrhage, the patient may exhibit signs of hypovolemic shock.[19,37]

Physical Examination

The results of physical assessment usually reveal hypoactive bowel sounds and abdominal tenderness, guarding, distention, and tympany. Findings that may indicate pancreatic hemorrhage include Grey Turner sign (gray-blue discoloration of the flanks) and Cullen sign (discoloration of the umbilical region); however, they are rare and usually seen several days into the illness.[19] A palpable abdominal mass indicates the presence of a pseudocyst or abscess.[19]

Laboratory Studies

Assessment of laboratory data usually demonstrates elevated levels of serum amylase and lipase. Serum lipase is more pancreas specific than amylase and a more accurate marker for acute pancreatitis. Amylase is present in other body tissues, and other disorders (e.g., intra-abdominal emergencies, renal insufficiency, salivary gland trauma, liver disease) may contribute to an elevated level. Unlike other serum enzymes, however, amylase is excreted in urine, and this clearance increases with acute pancreatitis. Measurement of urinary versus serum amylase should be considered in light of the patient's creatinine clearance. The serum amylase level may be elevated for only 3 to 5 days; if the patient delays seeking treatment, a normal level (false-negative result) may be detected. A marker of severity may be determined with a serum cross-reactive (C-reactive) protein level.[19,38] Leukocytosis, hypocalcemia, hyperglycemia, hyperbilirubinemia, and hypoalbuminemia may also be present (Table 30-2).[19,36,38]

Diagnostic Procedures

An abdominal ultrasound scan is obtained as part of the diagnostic evaluation to determine the presence of biliary stones. Contrast-enhanced computed tomography (CT) is considered the gold standard for diagnosing pancreatitis and for ascertaining the overall degree of pancreatic inflammation and necrosis.[19,32]

Medical Management

Initial management of the patient with severe acute pancreatitis includes ensuring adequate fluid and electrolyte replacement, providing nutritional support, and correcting metabolic alterations.[35] Careful monitoring for systemic and local complications is critical.

Fluid Management

Because pancreatitis if often associated with massive fluid shifts, intravenous crystalloids and colloids are administered immediately to prevent hypovolemic shock and maintain hemodynamic stability. Electrolytes are monitored closely, and abnormalities such as hypocalcemia, hypokalemia, and hypomagnesemia are corrected.[37] If hyperglycemia develops, exogenous insulin may be required.

TABLE 30-2 LABORATORY TESTS AND DIAGNOSTIC PROCEDURES FOR ACUTE PANCREATITIS

STUDY	FINDING IN PANCREATITIS
Laboratory Studies	
Serum amylase	Elevated
Serum isoamylase	Elevated
Urine amylase	Elevated
Serum lipase (if available)	Elevated
Serum triglycerides	Elevated
Cross-reactive protein	Elevated
Glucose	Elevated
Calcium	Decreased
Magnesium	Decreased
Potassium	Decreased
Albumin	Decreased or increased
White blood cell count	Elevated
Bilirubin	May be elevated
Liver enzymes	May be elevated
Prothrombin time	Prolonged
Arterial blood gases	Hypoxemia, metabolic acidosis
Diagnostic Procedures	

- Abdominal ultrasonography
- Computed tomography scan
- Magnetic resonance imaging
- Endoscopic retrograde cholangiopancreatography
- Abdominal radiographs (flat plate and upright or decubitus)
- Chest radiographs (posteroanterior and lateral)

Modified from Krumberger JM. Acute pancreatitis. *Crit Care Nurs Clin North Am.* 1993;5:185.

Nutritional Support

Over the past three decades, nutritional support has shifted. Previously, conventional nutritional management was to place the patient on a nothing-by-mouth (NPO) regimen and institute intravenous hydration. The rationale was to rest the inflamed pancreas and prevent enzyme release. Enteral or parental support should be initiated if oral intake is withheld more than 5 to 7 days.[39] Randomized clinical trials have demonstrated that enteral feeding (gastric or jejunal) is safe and cost effective and that it is associated with fewer septic and metabolic complications than other methods.[40-42] Enteral feeding enhances immune modulation and maintenance of the intestinal barrier, and it avoids complications associated with parental nutrition. Early initiation of enteral feeding is preferred over TPN.[39] However, TPN still has a role for the critically ill patient with acute pancreatitis who does not tolerate enteral feeding or when nutritional goals are not reached within 2 days.[37,41,42] In the past, nasogastric suction was also recommended, but this intervention has not been shown to be beneficial and should be instituted only if the patient has persistent vomiting, obstruction, or gastric distention.[37]

Systemic Complications

Acute pancreatitis can affect every organ system, and recognition and treatment of systemic complications are crucial to management of the patient (Box 30-11). The most serious complications are hypovolemic shock, acute respiratory distress syndrome (ARDS), acute kidney injury (AKI), and GI hemorrhage. Hypovolemic shock is the result of relative hypovolemia resulting from third spacing of intravascular volume and vasodilation caused by the release of inflammatory immune mediators. These mediators also contribute to the development of ARDS and AKI. Other possible pulmonary complications include pleural effusions, atelectasis, and pneumonia.[37]

Local Complications

Local complications include the development of infected pancreatic necrosis and pancreatic pseudocyst.[19,32,38] The necrotic areas of the pancreas can lead to development of a widespread pancreatic infection (infected pancreatic necrosis), which significantly increases the risk of death.

Prophylactic antibiotics may not reduce mortality in patients suspected of having necrotizing pancreatitis.[43] The use of IV antibiotics should not be used prophylactically but if sepsis, abscess, or biliary calculi is evident.[37] After the patient develops infected necrosis, however, surgical débridement is necessary.[36] The procedure of choice is a minimal invasive necrosectomy, which entails careful débridement of the necrotic tissue in and around the pancreas. A pancreatic pseudocyst is a collection of pancreatic fluid enclosed by a nonepithelialized wall. Cyst formation may result from liquefaction of a pancreatic fluid collection or from direct obstruction in the main pancreatic duct.[37] A pancreatic pseudocyst may (1) resolve spontaneously; (2) rupture, resulting in peritonitis; (3) erode a major blood vessel, resulting in hemorrhage; (4) become infected, resulting in abscess; or (5) invade surrounding structures, resulting in obstruction. Treatment involves drainage of the pseudocyst surgically, endoscopically, or percutaneously.[36,37,44]

Nursing Management

Nursing management of the patient with pancreatitis incorporates a variety of nursing diagnoses (Box 30-8). Nursing interventions include providing pain relief and emotional support, maintaining surveillance for complications, and educating the patient and family.

Providing Comfort and Emotional Support

Pain management is a major priority in acute pancreatitis. Administration of around-the-clock analgesics to achieve pain relief is essential. Morphine, fentanyl, or hydromorphine are the commonly used narcotics for pain control.[37] Relaxation techniques and the knee-chest position can also assist in pain control.

BOX 30-8 NURSING DIAGNOSES

Acute Pancreatitis

- Acute Pain, related to transmission and perception of cutaneous, visceral, muscular, ischemia impulses, p. 1123
- Deficient Fluid Volume, related to relative fluid loss, p. 1132
- Decreased Cardiac Output, related to alterations in preload, p. 1128
- Ineffective Breathing Pattern, related to decreased lung expansion, p. 1149
- Imbalanced Nutrition: Less Than Body Requirements, related to lack of exogenous nutrients or increased metabolic demand, p. 1143
- Anxiety, related to threat to biologic, psychologic, and/or social integrity, p. 1125
- Compromised Family Coping, related to critically ill family member, p. 1127
- Deficient Knowledge, related to lack of previous exposure to information, p. 1134 (see Patient Education, Box 30-9)

Maintaining Surveillance for Complications

The patient must be routinely monitored for signs of local or systemic complications (Box 30-10). Intensive monitoring of each of the organ systems is imperative because organ failure is a major indicator of the severity of the disease.[19] The patient must be closely monitored for signs and symptoms of pancreatic infection, which include increased abdominal pain and tenderness, fever, and increased white blood cell count (see Box 30-10).[19]

Educating the Patient and Family

Early in the patient's hospital stay, the patient and family should be taught about acute pancreatitis and its causes and treatment. As the patient moves toward discharge, teaching should focus on the interventions necessary for preventing the recurrence of the precipitating disorder. If sustained, permanent damage to the pancreas has occurred, the patient will require teaching specific to diet modification and supplemental pancreatic enzymes. Diabetes education may also be necessary. If an alcohol abuser, the patient should be encouraged to stop drinking and be referred to an alcohol cessation program (Box 30-9). Collaborative management of the patient with pancreatitis is outlined in Box 30-12.

ACUTE LIVER FAILURE

Description

Acute liver failure (ALF), is a life-threatening condition characterized by severe and sudden liver cell dysfunction, coagulopathy, and hepatic encephalopathy.[45] Although uncommon, ALF is associated with a mortality rate as high as 40%, and it usually occurs in patients without pre-existing liver disease.[45] Because liver transplantation is one of the few definitive treatments, the patient with ALF should be transferred to a critical care unit and strongly considered for referral to a major medical center where transplantation services are available.[45]

Etiology

The causes of ALF include infections, medications, toxins, hypoperfusion, metabolic disorders, and surgery (Box 30-13); however, viral hepatitis and medication-induced liver damage are the predominant causes in North America. Patients are

BOX 30-9 PATIENT EDUCATION

Acute Pancreatitis

- Pancreatitis
- Specific cause
- Precipitating factor modification
- Interventions to reduce further episodes
- Importance of taking medications
- Lifestyle changes
- Diet modification
- Stress management
- Alcohol cessation
- Diabetes management, if needed

   Additional information for the patient can be found at the following websites:
- The Pancreatitis Association, Inc.: http://pancassociation.org
- Alcoholics Anonymous: http://www.aa.org
- International Foundation for Functional Gastrointestinal Disorders: http://www.iffgd.org
- Healthfinder—U.S. Department of Health and Human Services: http://healthfinder.gov
- Web MD: http://www.webmd.com

BOX 30-10 COMPLICATIONS OF ACUTE PANCREATITIS

Respiratory
- Early hypoxemia
- Pleural effusion
- Atelectasis
- Pulmonary infiltration
- Acute respiratory distress syndrome
- Mediastinal abscess

Cardiovascular
- Hypotension and shock
- Pericardial effusion
- ST-T changes

Renal
- Acute tubular necrosis
- Oliguria
- Renal artery or vein thrombosis

Hematologic
- Disseminated intravascular coagulation
- Thrombocytosis
- Hyperfibrinogenemia

Endocrine
- Hypocalcemia
- Hypertriglyceridemia
- Hyperglycemia

Neurologic
- Fat emboli
- Psychosis
- Encephalopathy and coma

Ophthalmic
- Purtscher's retinopathy (sudden blindness)

Dermatologic
- Subcutaneous fat necrosis

Gastrointestinal or Hepatic
- Hepatic dysfunction
- Obstructive jaundice
- Stress ulceration
- Erosive gastritis
- Paralytic ileus
- Duodenal obstruction
- Pancreatic
  - Pseudocyst
  - Phlegmon
  - Abscess
  - Ascites
- Bowel infarction
- Massive intraperitoneal bleed
- Perforation
  - Stomach
  - Duodenum
  - Small bowel
  - Colon

BOX 30-11 SIGNS AND SYMPTOMS OF PANCREATIC INFECTION

Symptoms
- Persistent abdominal pain
- Abdominal tenderness

Signs
- Prolonged fever
- Abdominal distention
- Palpable abdominal mass
- Vomiting

Diagnostics
- Laboratory findings
  - Increased white blood cell count
  - Persistent elevation of serum amylase
  - Hyperbilirubinemia
  - Elevated alkaline phosphatase level
  - Positive culture and Gram stain
- Radiography or computed tomography findings
  - Pancreatic inflammation or enlargement
  - Necrosis
  - Cystic or mass lesions
  - Fluid accumulations
  - Pseudocyst abscess

Modified from Krumberger JM. Acute pancreatitis. *Crit Care Nurs Clin North Am.* 1993;5:185.

BOX 30-12 COLLABORATIVE MANAGEMENT

Acute Pancreatitis

- Ensure adequate circulating volume.
- Provide nutritional support.
- Correct metabolic alterations.
- Minimize pancreatic stimulation.
- Provide comfort and emotional support.
- Maintain surveillance for complications.
- Multiple organ dysfunction syndrome.

BOX 30-13 CAUSES OF ACUTE LIVER FAILURE

Infections
- Hepatitis A, B, C, D, E, non-A, non-B, non-C
- Herpes simplex virus (types 1 and 2)
- Epstein-Barr virus
- Varicella zoster
- Dengue fever virus
- Rift Valley fever virus

Medications or Toxins
- Industrial substances (chlorinated hydrocarbons, phosphorus)
- *Amanita phalloides* (mushrooms)
- Aflatoxin (a toxic metabolite of fungus)
- Medications (isoniazid, rifampin, halothane, methyldopa, tetracycline, valproic acid, monoamine oxidase inhibitors, phenytoin, nicotinic acid, tricyclic antidepressants, isoflurane, ketoconazole, trimethoprim-sulfamethoxazole, sulfasalazine, pyrimethamine, octreotide)
- Acetaminophen toxicity
- Cocaine

Hypoperfusion
- Venous obstructions
- Budd-Chiari syndrome
- Veno-occlusive disease
- Ischemia

Metabolic Disorders
- Wilson disease
- Tyrosinemia
- Heat stroke
- Galactosemia

Surgery
- Jejunoileal bypass
- Partial hepatectomy
- Liver transplantation failure

Other Causes
- Reye syndrome
- Acute fatty liver of pregnancy
- Massive malignant infiltration
- Autoimmune hepatitis

---

usually healthy before the onset of symptoms because ALF tends to occur in patients with no known liver history. A thorough medication and health history is imperative to determine a possible cause. The patient should be questioned about exposure to environmental toxins, hepatitis, intravenous drug use, sexual history, viral hepatitis, medication toxicity, and poisoning. Additional vascular causes such as thrombosis, ischemia, and Budd-Chiari syndrome and metabolic disorders such as Reye syndrome, Wilson disease, galactosemia, and fructose intolerance should be considered.[45]

Pathophysiology

ALF is a syndrome characterized by the development of acute liver failure over 1 to 3 weeks, followed by the development of hepatic encephalopathy within 8 weeks, in a patient with a previously healthy liver. The interval between the failure of the liver and the onset of hepatic encephalopathy usually is less than 2 weeks. The underlying cause is massive necrosis of the hepatocytes.[46]

Acute liver failure results in a number of derangements, including impaired bilirubin conjugation, decreased production of clotting factors, depressed glucose synthesis, and decreased lactate clearance. This results in jaundice, coagulopathies, hypoglycemia, and metabolic acidosis. Other effects of acute liver failure include increased risk of infection and altered carbohydrate, protein, and glucose metabolism. Hypoalbuminemia, fluid and electrolyte imbalances, and acute portal hypertension contribute to the development of ascites.[45] Hepatic encephalopathy is thought to result from failure of the liver to detoxify various substances in the bloodstream, and it may be worsened by metabolic and electrolyte imbalances.[46]

The patient may experience a variety of other complications, including cerebral edema, cardiac dysrhythmias, acute respiratory failure, sepsis, and AKI. Cerebral edema and increased intracranial pressure (ICP) develop as a result of breakdown of the blood–brain barrier and astrocyte swelling. Circulatory failure that mimics sepsis is common in ALF and may exacerbate low cerebral perfusion pressure (CPP).[47] Hypoxemia, acidosis, electrolyte imbalances, and cerebral edema can precipitate the development of cardiac dysrhythmias. Acute respiratory failure, progressing to ARDS, intrapulmonary shunting, ventilation–perfusion mismatch, sepsis, and aspiration may attribute to the universal arterial hypoxemia.[47]

Assessment and Diagnosis

Early recognition of ALF is essential. The diagnosis should include potentially reversible conditions (e.g., autoimmune hepatitis) and should differentiate ALF from decompensating chronic liver disease. Prognostic indicators such as coma grade, serum bilirubin, prothrombin time, coagulation factors, and pH should be assessed and potential causes investigated.[45]

Signs and symptoms of ALF include headache, hyperventilation, jaundice, mental status changes, palmar erythema, spider nevi, bruises, and edema. The patient should be evaluated for the presence of asterixis, or "liver flap," best described as the inability to voluntarily sustain a fixed position of the extremities. Asterixis is best recognized by downward flapping of the hands when the patient extends the arms and dorsiflexes the wrists. Hepatic encephalopathy is assessed by using a grading system that stages the encephalopathy according to the patient's clinical manifestations (Box 30-14). Diagnostic findings include prolonged prothrombin times, elevated levels of serum bilirubin, aspartate aminotransferase (AST), alkaline phosphatase, and serum ammonia and decreased levels of serum albumin.[46] Arterial blood gases (ABGs) reveal respiratory alkalosis, metabolic acidosis, or both. Hypoglycemia, hypokalemia, and hyponatremia also may be present.[46,47]

Factors I (fibrinogen), II (prothrombin), V, VII, IX, and X are produced exclusively by the liver. Prothrombin time may be the most useful of tests of these in the evaluation of acute ALF because levels may be 40 to 80 seconds above control values. Test results show decreased levels of plasmin and plasminogen and increased levels of fibrin and fibrin-split products. Platelet counts may be less than 100,000/mm^3.[46]

Medical Management

Medical interventions are directed toward management of the multiple system impact of ALF.

Ammonia Levels

Antibiotics such as neomycin, metronidazole, rifaximin, or lactulose, which is the gold standard, are administered to remove or decrease production of nitrogenous wastes in the large intestine. Antibiotics reduces bacterial flora of the colon. This aids in decreasing ammonia formation by decreasing bacterial action on the protein in feces. Side effects include renal toxicity and hearing impairment. Lactulose, a synthetic ketoanalogue of lactose split into lactic acid and acetic acid in the intestine, is given orally through a nasogastric tube or as a retention enema. The result is the creation of an acidic environment that results in ammonia being drawn out of the portal circulation. Lactulose has a laxative effect that promotes expulsion.[46,47]

Complications

Bleeding is best controlled through prevention. If an invasive procedure (e.g., central line placement, ICP monitor) will be performed or the patient develops active bleeding, vitamin K, fresh-frozen plasma (to maintain a reasonable prothrombin time), and platelet transfusions are necessary.[25] Metabolic disturbances such as hypoglycemia, metabolic acidosis, hypokalemia, and hyponatremia should be monitored and treated appropriately. Prophylactic antibiotic administration may be initiated because the patient is at high risk for an infection.[25] The development of cerebral edema necessitates ICP monitoring. Treatment with mannitol has been shown to be of benefit in managing ICP in the patient with ALF, but it must be used with caution in patients with renal failure to avoid hyperosmolarity.[47] Other interventions to control ICP include elevating the head of the bed (HOB) to 30 degrees, treating fever and hypertension, minimizing noxious stimulation, and correcting hypercapnia and hypoxemia.[25] Renal failure develops in 70% of patients with ALF and continuous renal replacement therapy (CRRT) provides renal support.[25] Hemodynamic instability is a common complication necessitating fluid administration and vasoactive medications to prevent prolonged episodes of hypotension. A pulmonary artery catheter may be used to guide clinical management.[46]

If ALF continues and the patient shows no immediate signs of improvement or reversal, the patient should be considered for a liver transplantation. Prompt referral to a transplantation center should be a high priority for patients experiencing ALF.[25,45]

Nursing Management

Nursing management of the patient with ALF incorporates a variety of nursing diagnoses (Box 30-15). Nursing interventions include protecting the patient from injury, providing comfort and emotional support, maintaining surveillance for complications, and educating the patient and family.

Protecting the Patient from Injury

Use of benzodiazepines and other sedatives is discouraged in the patient with ALF because pertinent neurologic changes may be masked and hepatic encephalopathy may be exacerbated.[47] These patients are often very difficult to manage because they may be extremely agitated and combative. Physical restraint may be necessary to prevent injury to the patient.

Maintaining Surveillance for Complications

As the neurologic condition worsens, respiratory depression and arrest can occur quickly. Continuous pulse oximetry

---

BOX 30-14 STAGING OF HEPATIC ENCEPHALOPATHY

I. Euphoria or depression, mild confusion, slurred speech, disordered sleep rhythm; slight asterixis and normal electroencephalogram (EEG)

II. Lethargy, moderate confusion; marked asterixis and abnormal EEG

III. Marked confusion, incoherent speech, sleeping but arousable; asterixis present and abnormal EEG

IV. Coma; initially responsive to noxious stimuli, later unresponsive; asterixis absent and abnormal EEG

BOX 30-15 NURSING DIAGNOSES

Acute Liver Failure

- Ineffective Breathing Pattern, related to decreased lung expansion, p. 1149
- Impaired Gas Exchange, related to ventilation/perfusion mismatching or intrapulmonary shunting, p. 1144
- Decreased Cardiac Output, related to alterations in preload, p. 1128
- Decreased Cardiac Output, related to alterations in heart rate, p. 1128
- Decreased Intracranial Adaptive Capacity, related to failure of normal compensatory mechanisms, p. 1131
- Risk for Infection, p. 1160
- Imbalanced Nutrition: Less Than Body Requirements, related to lack of exogenous nutrients or increased metabolic demand, p. 1143
- Disturbed Body Image, related to actual change in body structure, function, or appearance, p. 1136
- Compromised Family Coping, related to critically ill family member, p. 1127
- Deficient Knowledge, related to lack of previous exposure to information, p. 1134 (see Patient Education, Box 30-16)

BOX 30-16 PATIENT EDUCATION

Acute Liver Failure

- Specific cause
- Precipitating factor modification
- Interventions to reduce further episodes
- Importance of taking medications
- Lifestyle changes
- Diet modification
- Alcohol cessation
  Additional information for the patient can be found at the following websites:
- American Liver Foundation: http://www.liverfoundation.org
- National Liver Foundation: http://www.nlfindia.com
- Alcoholics Anonymous: http://www.aa.org
- International Foundation for Functional Gastrointestinal Disorders: http://www.iffgd.org
- Healthfinder – U.S. Department of Health and Human Services: http://healthfinder.gov
- Web MD: http://www.webmd.com

BOX 30-17 COLLABORATIVE MANAGEMENT

Acute Liver Failure

- Decrease ammonia levels.
- Control bleeding.
- Correct metabolic alterations.
- Prevent infection.
- Prepare patient for liver transplantation, if necessary.
- Protect patient from injury.
- Provide comfort and emotional support.
- Maintain surveillance for complications:
  - Cerebral edema
  - Renal failure

Collaborative management of the patient with ALF is outlined in Box 30-17.

GASTROINTESTINAL SURGERY

Types of Surgery

GI surgery refers to a wide variety of surgical procedures that involve the esophagus, the stomach, the intestine, the liver, the pancreas, or the biliary tract. Indications for GI surgery are numerous and include bleeding or perforation from peptic ulcer disease, obstruction, trauma, inflammatory bowel disease, and malignancy. Patients may be admitted to the critical care unit for monitoring after GI surgery as a result of their underlying medical condition; however, this portion of the chapter focuses only on several surgical procedures that commonly require postoperative critical care.

Esophagectomy

Esophagectomy is usually performed for cancer of the distal esophagus and gastroesophageal junction. The technically difficult procedure involves the removal of part or all of the esophagus, part of the stomach, and lymph nodes in the surrounding area. The stomach is then pulled up into the chest and connected to the remaining part of the esophagus. If the entire esophagus and stomach must be removed, part of the bowel may be used to form the esophageal replacement (Figs. 30-5 and 30-6).[48]

Pancreaticoduodenectomy

The standard operation for pancreatic cancer is a pancreaticoduodenectomy, also called the *Whipple procedure*. In the Whipple procedure, the pancreatic head, the duodenum, part of the jejunum, the common bile duct, the gallbladder, and part of the stomach are removed. The continuity of the GI tract is restored by anastomosing the remaining portion of the pancreas, the bile duct, and the stomach to the jejunum (Fig. 30-7).[48]

Bariatric Surgery

Bariatric surgery refers to surgical procedures of the GI tract that are performed to induce weight loss. Bariatric procedures are divided into three broad types: (1) restrictive, (2) malabsorptive, and (3) combined restrictive and malabsorptive.[49]

monitoring and ABG analysis are helpful in assessing adequacy of respiratory efforts. A thorough neurologic assessment should be performed at least every hour.

Educating the Patient and Family

Early in the patient's hospital stay, the patient and family should be taught about ALF and its causes and treatment. As patient discharge is imminent, teaching should focus on the interventions necessary for preventing the recurrence of the precipitating cause. If the patient is considered a candidate for liver transplantation, the patient and family will need specific information regarding the procedure and care. Evaluation for liver transplantation may include screening for medical contraindications, human immunodeficiency virus (HIV) serology, anticipated compliance, and assessment of the social support system. Psychiatric and other specialty team consultations are necessary for a thorough evaluation of the patient's suitability for a liver transplantation (Box 30-16).

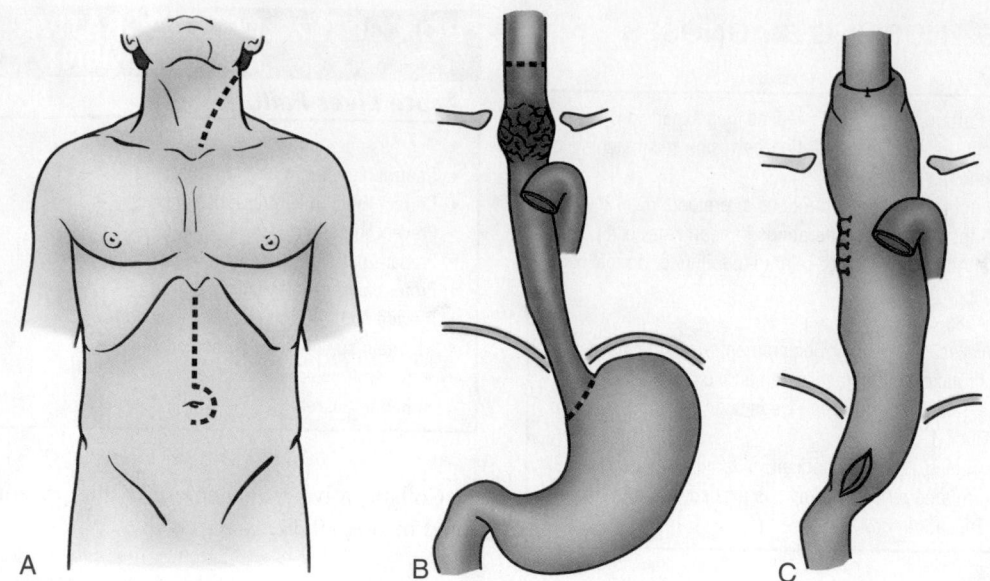

FIGURE 30-5 Overview of transhiatal esophagectomy: *(A)* with gastric mobilization *(B)* and gastric pull-up *(C)* for cervical esophagogastric anastomosis. (Modified from Ellis F. Esophagogastrectomy for carcinoma: technical considerations based on anatomic location of lesion. *Surg Clin North Am.* 1980;60:265.)

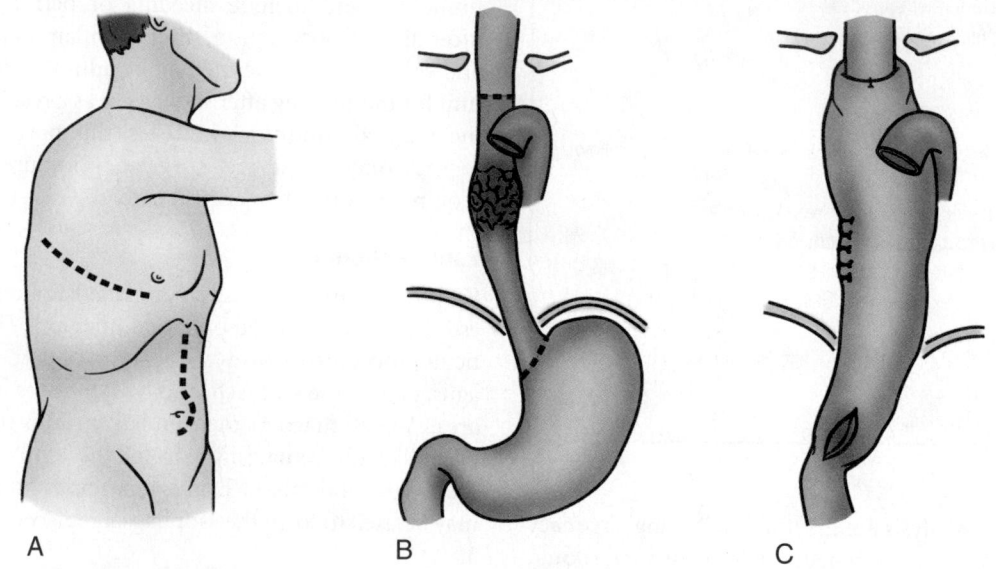

FIGURE 30-6 Overview of transthoracic esophagectomy: *(A)* with esophageal resection, gastric mobilization *(B)*, and intrathoracic anastomosis *(C)* for a midesophageal tumor. (Modified from Ellis FH. Esophagogastrectomy for carcinoma: technical considerations based on anatomic location of lesion. *Surg Clin North Am.* 1980;60:265.)

Restrictive procedures such as vertical banded gastroplasty (VBG) (Fig. 30-8A) and gastric banding (see Fig. 30-8B) reduce the capacity of the stomach and limit the amount of food that can be consumed. Malabsorptive procedures such as the biliopancreatic diversion (BPD) (see Fig. 30-8C) alter the GI tract to limit the digestion and absorption of food. The Roux-en-Y gastric bypass (RYGBP) (see Fig. 30-8D) combines both strategies by creating a small gastric pouch and anastomosing the jejunum to the pouch. Food then bypasses the lower stomach

and duodenum, resulting in decreased absorption of digestive materials.[49]

Preoperative Care

A thorough preoperative evaluation should be conducted to evaluate the patient's physical status and identify risk factors that may affect the postoperative course. Because obesity is associated with a higher incidence of co-morbidities such as cardiovascular disease, hypertension, diabetes, gastroesophageal

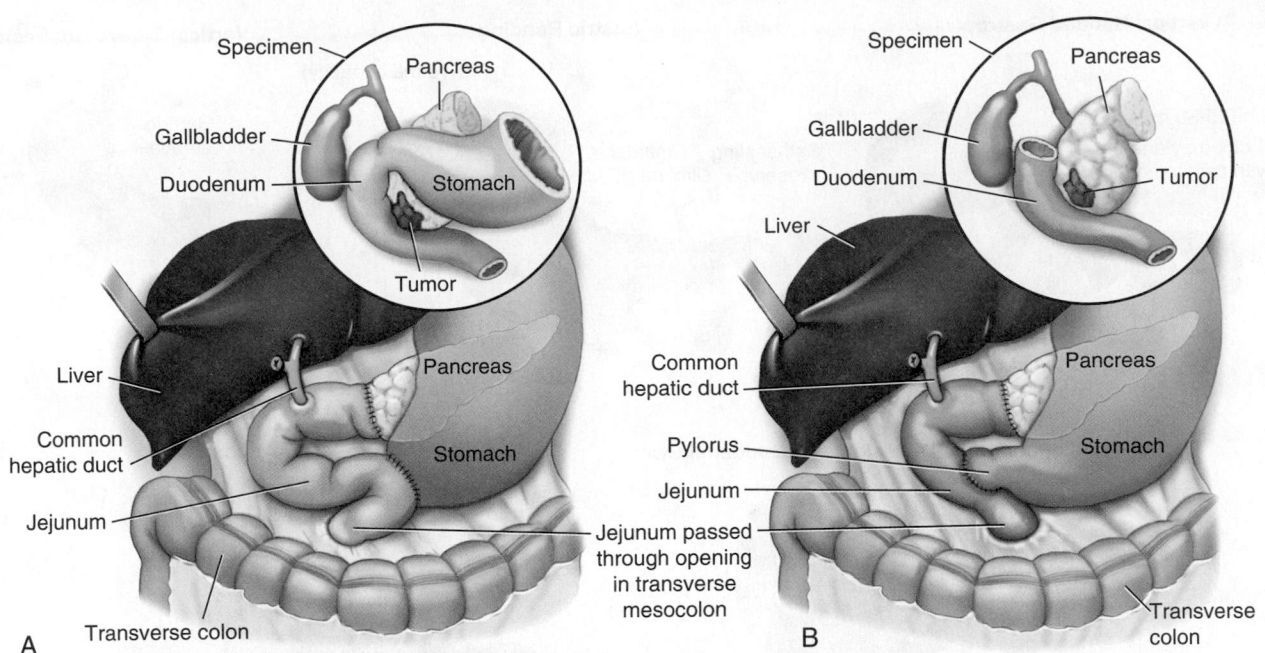

FIGURE 30-7 Standard and Pylorus-Preserving Whipple Procedures. *A,* The standard Whipple procedure involves resection of the gastric antrum, head of pancreas, distal bile duct, and entire duodenum with reconstruction as shown. *B,* The pylorus-preserving Whipple procedure does not include resection of the distal stomach, pylorus, or proximal duodenum.

reflux, obstructive sleep apnea, and heart failure, an extensive workup may be required for the patient who underwent bariatric surgery.[48,50]

Surgical Considerations

Two approaches may be used for esophageal resection: *transhiatal* or *transthoracic* (see Figs. 30-5 and 30-6). In both approaches, the stomach is mobilized through an abdominal incision and then transposed into the chest. The anastomosis of the stomach to the esophagus is performed in the chest (transthoracic) or in the neck (transhiatal). The approach selected depends on the location of the tumor, the patient's overall health and pulmonary function, and the experience of the surgeon. After surgery, the patient has a nasogastric tube in place, and it should not be manipulated because of the potential to damage the anastomosis. Those who undergo transthoracic esophagectomy have chest tubes.[48]

Most bariatric procedures can be performed using an open or laparoscopic surgical technique. Although laparoscopic approaches are more technically difficult to perform, they have largely replaced open procedures because they are associated with decreased pulmonary complications, less postoperative pain, reduced length of hospital stay, fewer wound complications (e.g., infections, incisional hernia), and an earlier return to full activity.[48,49] Open procedures are performed on patients who have had prior upper abdominal surgery, are morbidly obese, or who may not be able to tolerate the increased abdominal pressure associated with laparoscopic procedures.[48]

Complications and Medical Management

Several complications are associated with GI surgery, including respiratory failure, atelectasis, pneumonia, anastomotic leak, deep vein thrombosis, pulmonary embolus, and bleeding. The morbidly obese patient is at even greater risk for many postoperative complications.[49]

Pulmonary Complications

The risk for pulmonary complications is substantial after GI surgery, and adverse respiratory events such as atelectasis and pneumonia are twice as likely to occur in the patient who is obese.[50] Aggressive pulmonary exercise should be initiated in the immediate postoperative period. Early ambulation and adequate pain control assist in reducing the risk of atelectasis development. Suctioning, chest physiotherapy, or bronchodilators may be needed to optimize pulmonary function. Patients should be closely monitored for the development of oxygenation problems. Treatment should be aimed at supporting adequate ventilation and gas exchange. Mechanical ventilation may be required in the event of respiratory failure.

Anastomotic Leak

An anastomotic leak is a severe complication of GI surgery. It occurs when there is a breakdown of the suture line in a surgical anastomosis and results in leakage of gastric or intestinal contents into the abdomen or mediastinum (transthoracic esophagectomy).[48] The clinical signs and symptoms of a leak can be subtle and often go unrecognized. They include tachycardia,

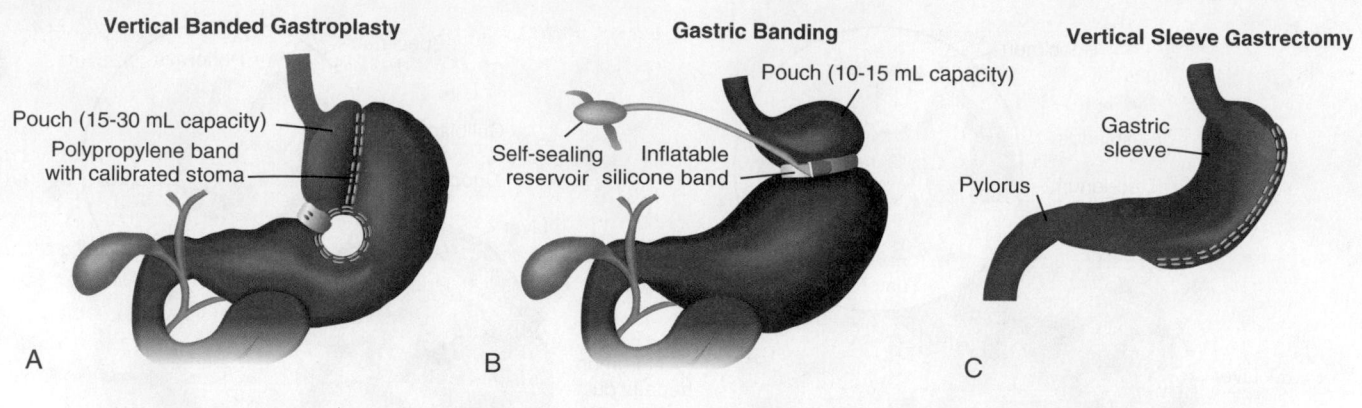

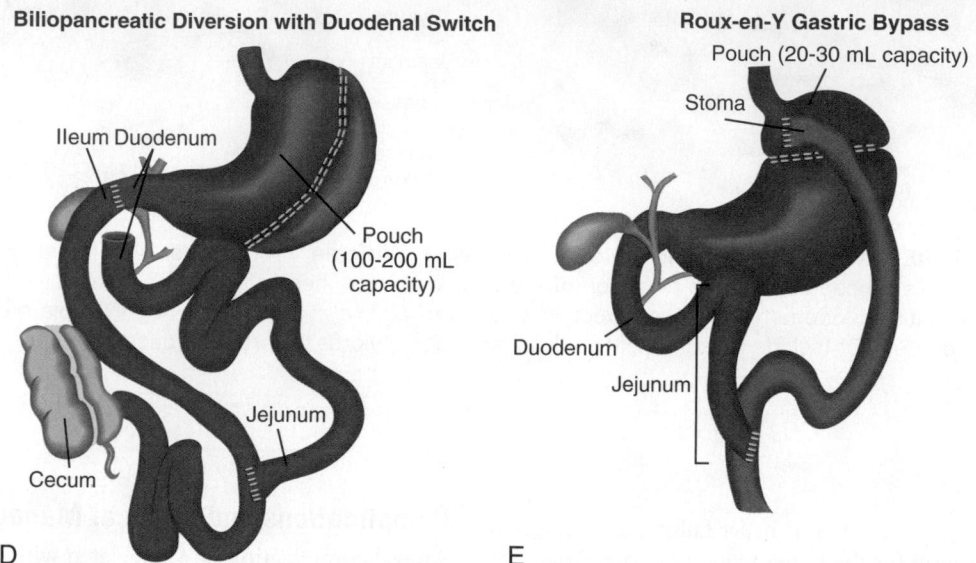

FIGURE 30-8 **Bariatric Surgical Procedures.** *A,* Vertical banded gastroplasty involves creating a small gastric pouch. *B,* Adjustable gastric banding uses a band to create a gastric pouch. *C,* Vertical sleeve gastrectomy involves creating a sleeve-shaped stomach by removing about 80% of the stomach. *D,* Biliopancreatic diversion with duodenal switch procedure creates an anastomosis between the stomach and intestine. *E,* Roux-en-Y gastric bypass procedure involves constructing a gastric pouch whose outlet is a Y-shaped limb of small intestine. (From Lewis SL, et al. *Medical-Surgical Nursing: Assessment and Management of Clinical Problems.* 8th ed. St. Louis: Mosby; 2011.)

tachypnea, fever, abdominal pain, anxiety, and restlessness.[48] In the patient who had an esophagectomy, a leak of the esophageal anastomosis may manifest as subcutaneous emphysema in the chest and neck.[48] If undetected, a leak can result in sepsis, multiorgan failure, and death. Patients with progressive tachycardia and tachypnea should have a radiologic study (upper GI study with Gastrografin or CT scan with contrast) to rule out an anastomotic leak.[50] The type of treatment depends on the severity of the leak. If the leak is small and well contained, it may be managed conservatively by maintaining the NPO status, administering antibiotics, and draining the fluid percutaneously. If the patient is deteriorating rapidly, an urgent laparotomy is indicated to repair the defect.[48,50]

Deep Vein Thrombosis and Pulmonary Embolism

Pulmonary embolism (PE) is a very serious complication of any surgical procedure. Deep vein thrombosis (DVT) prophylaxis

should be initiated before surgery and continued until the patient is fully ambulatory to reduce the risk of clot development. Typically, a combination of sequential compression devices and subcutaneous unfractionated heparin or low–molecular-weight heparin is used. Patients determined to be at high risk for PE may benefit from prophylactic inferior vena cava filter placement.[48]

Bleeding

Upper GI bleeding is an uncommon but life-threatening complication of GI surgery. Early bleeding usually occurs at the site of the anastomosis and can usually be treated through endoscopic intervention. Surgical revision may be needed for persistent, uncontrolled bleeding. Late bleeding is usually a result of ulcer development. Medical therapy is aimed at the prevention of this complication through administration of histamine 2 (H_2)–antagonists or PPIs.[5]

Postoperative Nursing Management

Nursing care of the patient who has had GI surgery incorporates a number of nursing diagnoses (Box 30-18). Nursing management involves interventions aimed at optimizing oxygenation and ventilation, preventing atelectasis, providing comfort and emotional support, and maintaining surveillance for complications.

Pulmonary Management

Nursing interventions in the postoperative period are focused on promoting ventilation and adequate oxygenation and preventing complications such as atelectasis and pneumonia. After the patient is extubated, deep-breathing exercises and incentive spirometry should be initiated, and the patient should perform them regularly. Early ambulation is encouraged to promote

maximal lung inflation, thereby reducing the risk of pulmonary complications and the potential for pulmonary embolus.

Pain Management

It is imperative to appropriately manage the patient's pain after GI surgery. Adequate analgesia is necessary to promote the mobility of the patient and decrease pulmonary complications. Initial pain management may be accomplished by intravenous opioid (morphine, hydromorphone) administration by means of a patient-controlled analgesia (PCA) pump, or through continuous epidural infusion of an opioid and local anesthetic (bupivacaine).[48] Oral pain medications can be started after an anastomosis leak is ruled out. Nonpharmacologic interventions such as positioning, application of heat or cold, and distraction may also be used. If the patient's pain is not being sufficiently relieved, the pain management service should be consulted.[48,50]

THERAPEUTIC MANAGEMENT

Gastrointestinal Intubation

Because GI intubation is used so often in critical care units, it is important for nurses to know the clinical indications and responsibilities inherent in tube use. The three categories of GI tubes are based on function: (1) nasogastric suction tubes, (2) long intestinal tubes, and (3) feeding tubes (Box 30-19).

Nasogastric Suction Tubes

Nasogastric tubes remove fluid regurgitated into the stomach, prevent accumulation of swallowed air, may partially

---

◎ BOX 30-18 NURSING DIAGNOSES

Gastrointestinal Surgery

- Ineffective Breathing Pattern, related to decreased lung expansion, p. 1149
- Impaired Gas Exchange, related to alveolar hypoventilation, p. 1144
- Decreased Cardiac Output, related to alterations in preload, p. 1128
- Acute Pain, related to transmission and perception of cutaneous, visceral, muscular, or ischemic impulses, p. 1123
- Anxiety, related to threat to biologic, psychologic, or social integrity, p. 1125
- Disturbed Body Image, related to actual change in body structure, function, or appearance, p. 1136
- Deficient Knowledge, related to lack of previous exposure to information, p. 1134

⚡ BOX 30-19 PATIENT SAFETY ALERT

Tubing Misconnections—A Persistent and Potentially Deadly Occurrence

QSEN Tubing and catheter misconnection errors are an important and under-reported problem in health care organizations. These errors often are caught and corrected before any injury to the patient occurs. Given the reality of and potential for life-threatening consequences, increased awareness and analysis of these errors—including averted errors—can lead to dramatic improvement in patient safety.

Nine cases involving tubing misconnections have been reported to The Joint Commission's Sentinel Event Database. These errors resulted in 8 deaths and 1 instance of permanent loss of function, and they affected 7 adults and 2 infants. Reports in the media and to such organizations as the ECRI Institute, the U.S. Food and Drug Administration (FDA), the Institute for Safe Medication Practices (ISMP), and the United States Pharmacopeia (USP) indicate that misconnection errors occur with significant frequency and, in a number of instances, lead to deadly consequences.

Types of Misconnections

The types of tubes and catheters involved in the cases reported to The Joint Commission included central intravenous (IV) catheters, peripheral IV catheters, nasogastric feeding tubes, percutaneous enteric feeding tubes, peritoneal dialysis catheters, tracheostomy cuff inflation tubes, and automatic blood pressure cuff insufflation tubes. The specific misconnections involved an enteric tube feeding into an IV catheter; injection of barium sulfate (gastrointestinal contrast medium) into a central venous catheter; an enteric tube feeding into

a peritoneal dialysis catheter; a blood pressure insufflator tube connected to an IV catheter; and injection of IV fluid into a tracheostomy cuff inflation tube.

A review by the USP of more than 300 cases reported to its databases found misconnection errors involving the following:

- IV infusions connected to epidural lines and epidural solutions (intended for epidural administration) connected to peripheral or central IV catheters
- Bladder irrigation solutions using primary IV tubing connected as secondary infusions to peripheral or central IV catheters
- Infusions intended for IV administration connected to an indwelling bladder (Foley) catheter
- Infusions intended for IV administration connected to nasogastric tubes
- IV solutions administered with blood administration sets and blood products transfused with primary IV tubing
- Primary IV solutions administered through various other functionally dissimilar catheters such as external dialysis catheters, a ventriculostomy drain, an amnioinfusion catheter, and the distal port of a pulmonary artery catheter

Many of the misconnection cases involved Luer connectors, which are small devices used in the connection of many medical components and accessories. There are two types of Luer connectors: slips and locks. A Luer slip connector consists of a tapered "male" fitting that slips into a wider "female" fitting to create a secure connection. The Luer lock connector has a threaded collar on

Continued

⚡ BOX 30-19   PATIENT SAFETY ALERT—cont'd

the male fitting and a flange on the female fitting that screw together to create a more secure connection.

Examples of misconnections involving Luer connectors include the following:

- Capnography sampling tube to an IV cannula
- Enteral feeding set to a central venous catheter
- Enteral feeding set to a hemodialysis line
- Noninvasive blood pressure (NIBP) insufflation tube to a needleless IV port
- Oxygen tubing to a needleless IV port
- Sequential compression device (SCD) hose to a needleless "piggyback" port of an IV administration set

Root Causes Identified

The basic lesson from these cases is that if it *can* happen, it *will* happen. Luer connectors are implicated in or contribute to many of these errors because they enable functionally dissimilar tubes or catheters to be connected. Other causes include the routine use of tubes or catheters for unintended purposes such as using IV extension tubing for epidurals, irrigation, drains, and central lines; using them to extend enteric feeding tubes; and positioning functionally dissimilar tubes used in patient care close to one another. In the cases reported to the Sentinel Event Database, contributing factors included movement of the patient from one setting or service to another and staff fatigue associated with working consecutive shifts.

Risk Reduction Strategies

No standards that specifically restrict the use of Luer connectors to certain medical devices have been published. Consequently, a broad range of medical devices, which have different functions and access the body through different routes, are often outfitted with Luer fittings that can be easily misconnected. Organizations in Europe and the United States are developing standards to restrict the types of devices that use Luer fittings in an attempt to mitigate misconnection hazards. According to Jim Keller, vice-president of the Health Technology Evaluation and Safety for the ECRI Institute, and Stephanie Joseph, project engineer for the ECRI Institute, the solution for reducing or eliminating misconnection errors lies in engineering controls respecting how products and devices are designed ("incompatibility by design") and in re-engineering work practices.

"A well-designed device should prevent misconnections and should prompt the user to take the correct action," explained Joseph, author of a guidance article published in the March 2006 issue of the ECRI Institute's *Health Devices* journal. As a first step in prevention, Joseph urges hospitals to avoid buying non-IV equipment (e.g., nebulizers, NIBP devices, enteral feeding sets) that can mate with the Luer connectors on patient IV lines. Joseph also emphasizes that the single most important work practice solution for clinicians is to trace all lines back to their origin before connecting or disconnecting any devices or infusions.

Other solutions include specific education and training regarding this problem for all clinicians and having practitioners take simple precautions such as turning on the light in a darkened room before connecting or reconnecting tubes or devices. The risk of waking a sleeping patient is minimal by comparison. Errors have occurred when patients or family members attempted to disconnect and reconnect equipment themselves. Staff should emphasize to all patients the importance of contacting a clinical staff member for assistance when an need to disconnect or reconnect devices is identified.

Some approaches to reducing the risk of misconnections have significant potential for unintended consequences:

- Labeling all tubes and catheters may not always be practical and may therefore lead to inconsistent implementation. However, labeling certain high-risk catheters (e.g., epidural, intrathecal, arterial) should always be done.
- Color-coding tubes and catheters can lead users to rely on the color coding rather than having a clear understanding of which tubes and catheters are connected correctly to which body inlets. Training or educating all staff (including temporary agency and travel staff) about the institution's color-coding system requires ongoing attention. Color-coding schemes often vary across institutions in the same community, creating increased risk when agency and travel staff are used.

Joint Commission Recommendations

The Joint Commission offers the following recommendations and strategies to health care organizations to reduce tubing misconnection errors:

1. Do not purchase non-IV equipment that is equipped with connectors that can physically mate with a female Luer IV line connector.
2. Conduct acceptance testing (for performance, safety, and usability) and, as appropriate, risk assessment (e.g., failure mode and effect analysis) on new tubing and catheter purchases to identify the potential for misconnections, and take appropriate preventive measures.
3. Always trace a tube or catheter from the patient to the point of origin before connecting any new device or infusion.
4. Recheck connections, and trace all patient tubes and catheters to their sources on the patient's arrival to a new setting or service as part of the handing-off process. Standardize this "line reconciliation" process.
5. Route tubes and catheters having different purposes in different, standardized directions (e.g., IV lines routed toward the head; enteric lines toward the feet). This is especially important in the care of neonates.
6. Inform nonclinical staff, patients, and their families that they must get help from clinical staff in case of a real or perceived need to connect or disconnect devices or infusions.
7. For certain high-risk catheters (e.g., epidural, intrathecal, arterial), label the catheter, and do not use catheters that have injection ports.
8. Never use a standard Luer syringe for oral medications or enteric feedings.
9. Emphasize the risk of tubing misconnections in orientation and training curricula.
10. Identify and manage conditions and practices that may contribute to health care worker fatigue, and take appropriate action.

The Joint Commission also urges product manufacturers to implement "designed incompatibility," as appropriate, to prevent dangerous misconnections of tubes and catheters.

Resources

- The ECRI Institute. Fatal air embolism caused by the misconnection of a medical device hoses to needleless Luer ports on IV administration sets [hazard report]. *Health Devices*. 2004;33(6):223.
- The ECRI Institute. Misconnected flowmeter leads to two deaths [special report]. *Health Devices Alerts*. January 25, 2003.
- The ECRI Institute. Preventing misconnections of lines and cables. *Health Devices*. 2006;35(3):81.
- Safe systems, safe patients: common connectors pose a threat to safe practice. *Texas Board Nurs Bull*. 2006;37(2):6.
- U.S. Food and Drug Administration. FDA patient safety news, Show #31, September 2004; Show #20, October 2003; Show #46, December 2005. Available at www.accessdata.fda.gov/psn/index.cfm. Accessed May 2009.

Modified from The Joint Commission: Sentinel Event Alert, no. 36, April 3, 2006. Available at http://www.jointcommission.org/sentinel_event_alert_issue_36_tubing_misconnections—a_persistent_and_potentially_deadly_occurrence. Accessed June 2012.

decompress the bowel, and reduce the patient's risk for aspiration. Nasogastric tubes also can be used for collecting specimens, assessing the presence of blood, and administering tube feedings. The most common nasogastric tubes are the single-lumen Levin tube and the double-lumen Salem sump. The Salem sump has one lumen that is used for suction and drainage and another that allows air to enter the patient's stomach and prevents the tube from adhering to the gastric wall and damaging the mucosa. The tube is passed through the nose into the nasopharynx and then down through the pharynx into the esophagus and stomach. The length of time the nasogastric tube remains in place depends on its use. The tube is then placed to gravity, low intermittent suction, or low continuous suction, and in rare instances, it is clamped.[51]

Nursing management focuses on preventing complications common to this therapy, for example, ulceration and necrosis of the nares, esophageal reflux, esophagitis, esophageal erosion and stricture, gastric erosion, and dry mouth and parotitis from mouth breathing. Interference with ventilation and coughing, aspiration, and loss of fluid and electrolytes can be critical problems. Interventions include irrigating the tube every 4 hours with normal saline, ensuring the blue air vent of the Salem sump is patent and maintained above the level of the patient's stomach, and providing frequent mouth and nares care (Box 30-20).[51]

Long Intestinal Tubes

Miller-Abbott, Cantor, and Andersen tubes are examples of long, weighted-tip intestinal tubes that are placed preoperatively or intraoperatively. Their considerable length allows

removal of the contents of the intestine to treat an obstruction that cannot be managed by a nasogastric tube. These tubes can decompress the small bowel and can splint the small bowel intraoperatively or postoperatively. Because progression of the tubes depends on bowel peristalsis, their use is contraindicated in patients with paralytic ileus and severe mechanical bowel obstructions.

Interventions used in the care of the patient with a long intestinal tube are similar to those with a nasogastric tube. The patient should be observed for (1) gaseous distention of the balloon section, which makes removal difficult; (2) rupture of the balloon; (3) overinflation of the balloon, which can lead to intestinal rupture; and (4) reverse intussusception if the tube is removed rapidly. Intestinal tubes should be removed slowly; usually 6 inches of the tube is withdrawn every hour.[51]

Feeding Tubes

Small-diameter (8- to 12-Fr [French]) flexible feeding tubes, such as Dobhoff tubes, are commonly placed at the bedside for patients who cannot take nourishment orally. The feeding tube may be inserted orally or nasally so that the tip ends up in the stomach or duodenum. To facilitate passage into the GI tract, these tubes have a weighted tungsten tip, and a guidewire is needed to prevent them from curling up in the back of the patient's throat. A radiograph must be obtained to verify correct placement of the tube before initiating feeding.[52] The tube should also be marked with indelible ink where it exits the mouth or nares so that tube location can be checked at 4-hour intervals.[52]

Nursing management of the patient with a feeding tube includes prevention of complications and monitoring the tolerance of feeding. Tracheobronchial aspiration of gastric contents is a serious potential complication.[52-54] Before administering medications or feedings, it is important to ensure that the tube is in the patient's stomach or duodenum. Assessing the exit point marked on the tube helps determine whether the tube has maintained the same position. Looking for coiling in the mouth or throat can help detect upward displacement that may have occurred as a result of vomiting. The traditional practice of confirming placement by auscultating air inserted through the tube over the epigastrium is not reliable and is not recommended.[52-55] If any doubt exists about the tube's position, a repeat radiograph should be obtained. During feedings, the head of bed should be elevated at least 30 degrees to minimize the risk of aspiration, and gastric residuals should be checked at least every 4 to 6 hours.[53,54] Large gastric residuals, cramping, and abdominal distention may indicate intolerance of feeding, and the physician should be notified.[54] Other interventions include nares and oral care and flushing the tube with water before and after medication administration to maintain patency.[54]

Endoscopic Injection Therapy

Endoscopic injection therapy is used to control bleeding of ulcers. It may be performed emergently, electively, or prophylactically. An endoscope is introduced through the patient's mouth, and endoscopy of the esophagus and stomach is performed to identify the bleeding varices or ulcers. An injector

---

◎ BOX 30-20 NIC

Tube Care: Gastrointestinal

Definition
Management of a patient with a gastrointestinal tube

Activities
Monitor for correct placement of the tube per agency protocol.
Verify placement with radiograph per agency protocol.
Connect tube to suction, if indicated.
Secure tube to appropriate body part with consideration for patient comfort and skin integrity.
Irrigate tube per agency protocol.
Monitor for sensations of fullness, nausea, and vomiting.
Monitor bowel sounds.
Monitor for diarrhea.
Monitor fluid and electrolyte status.
Monitor amount, color, and consistency of nasogastric output.
Replace the amount of gastrointestinal output with the appropriate intravenous solution, as ordered.
Provide nose and mouth care three to four times daily or as needed.
Provide hard candy or chewing gum to moisten the mouth, as appropriate.
Initiate and monitor delivery of enteral tube feedings per agency protocol.
Teach patient and family how to care for tube, when indicated.
Provide skin care around tube insertion site.
Remove tube, when indicated.

From Bulechek GM, et al. *Nursing Interventions Classification (NIC)*. 6th ed. St. Louis: Mosby; 2013.

with a retractable 23- to 25-gauge needle is introduced through the biopsy channel of the endoscope. The needle then is inserted in or around the varices or into the area around the ulcer, and a liquid agent is injected (Fig. 30-9). The most commonly used agent is epinephrine, which results in localized vasoconstriction and enhanced platelet aggregation. Sclerosing agents such as ethanolamine, alcohol, and polidocanol also may be used. These agents cause an inflammatory reaction in the vessel that results in thrombosis and eventually produces a fibrous band. Repeated sclerotherapy results in the development of supportive scar

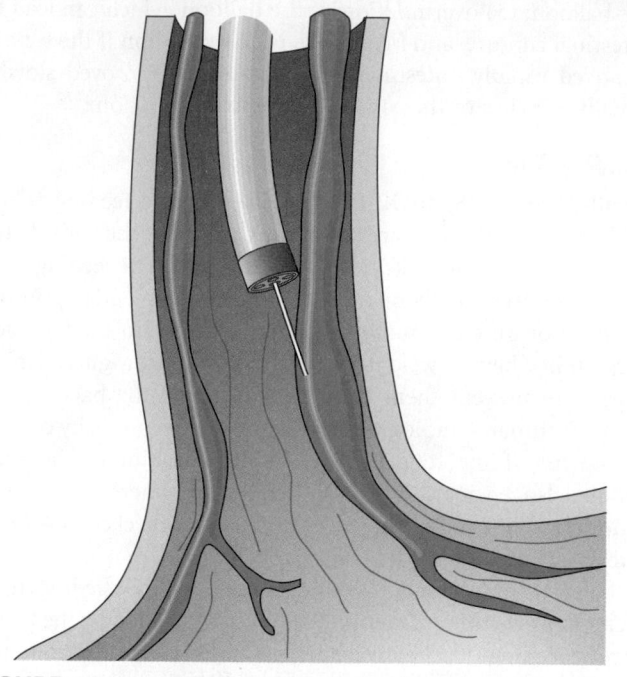

FIGURE 30-9 Endoscopic sclerosis of varices. (From Copstead LC, Banasik JL. *Pathophysiology.* 4th ed. St. Louis: Saunders; 2010.)

tissue around the varices. Other embolic agents are used, including fibrinogen and thrombin, which when injected together react to form an active fibrin clot, and "glues" (n-butyl cyanoacrylate), which are used as a sealant to stop the bleeding.[20,24,56]

Endoscopic Variceal Ligation

Endoscopic variceal ligation (EVL) involves applying bands or metal clips around the circumference of the bleeding varices to induce venous obstruction and control bleeding. EVL has replaced endoscopic sclerotherapy of variceal hemorrhage (Fig. 30-10). Between 1 and 2 days after the procedure, necrosis and scar formation promote band and tissue sloughing. Fibrinous deposits within the healing ulcer potentiate vessel obliteration. Band ligation is accomplished through endoscopy, with multiple bands placed per session.[16] The procedure may be repeated on an inpatient or outpatient basis every 1 to 2 weeks until all the varices are obliterated.[56] Endoscopic variceal ligation controls bleeding in approximately 80% to 90% of the time.[56] The most common complication of endoscopic variceal ligation is the development of superficial mucosal ulcers. Varices may reoccur as local banding does not affect portal pressure.[16,57]

Transjugular Intrahepatic Portosystemic Shunt

TIPS is an angiographic interventional procedure for decreasing portal hypertension. TIPS is advocated for (1) patients with portal hypertension who are also experiencing active bleeding or have poor liver reserve, (2) transplant recipients, and (3) patients with other operative risks.[25,57] The TIPS procedure is usually performed by a gastroenterologist, vascular surgeon, or interventional radiologist.

Portal hypertension is confirmed by direct measurement of the pressure in the portal vein (gradient greater than 10 mm Hg). Cannulation is achieved through the internal jugular vein, and an angiographic catheter is advanced into the middle or right

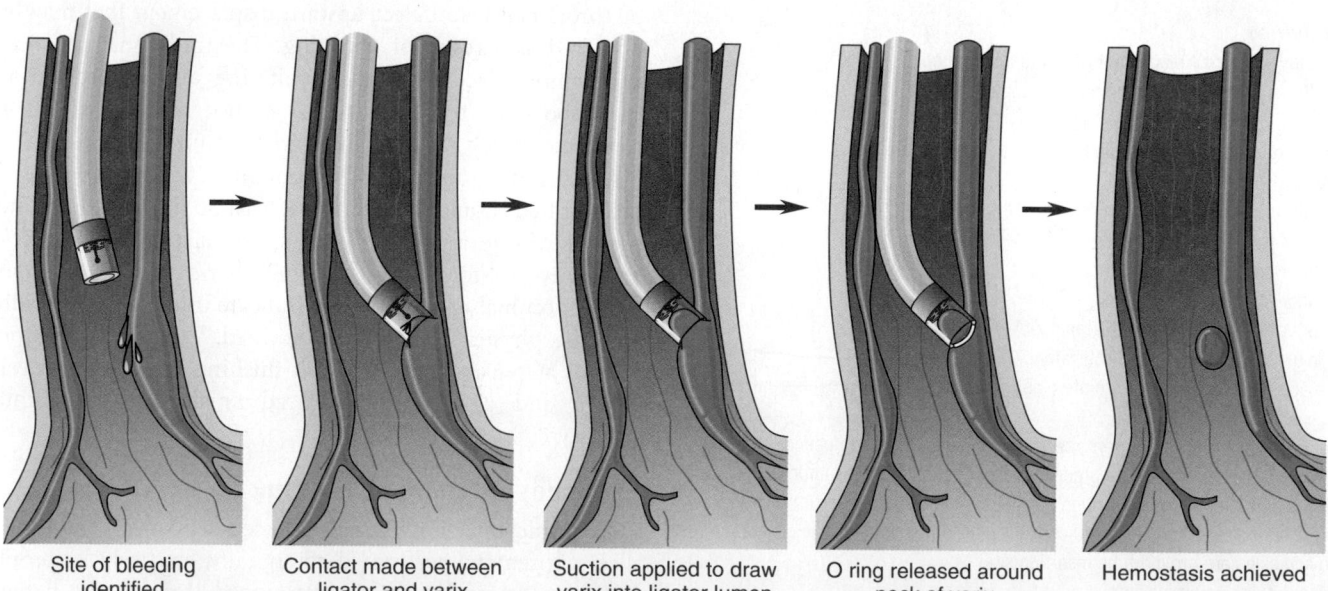

| Site of bleeding identified | Contact made between ligator and varix | Suction applied to draw varix into ligator lumen | O ring released around neck of varix | Hemostasis achieved |

FIGURE 30-10 Endoscopic band ligation. (From Copstead LC, Banasik JL. *Pathophysiology.* 4th ed. St. Louis: Saunders; 2010.)

hepatic vein. The midhepatic vein is then catheterized, and a new route is created connecting the portal and hepatic veins using a needle and guidewire with a dilating balloon. A polytetrafluoroethylene (PTFE)–coated stent is then placed in the liver parenchyma to maintain that connection (Fig. 30-11). The increased resistance in the liver is bypassed.[25,58] TIPS may be performed on patients with bleeding varices, with refractory bleeding varices, or as a bridge to liver transplantation if the candidate becomes hemodynamically unstable. Postprocedural care should include observation for overt (cannulation site) or covert (intrahepatic site) bleeding, hepatic or portal vein laceration (resulting in rapid loss of blood volume), and inadvertent puncture of surrounding organs. Other complications include hepatic encephalopathy, liver failure, bacteremia, and stent stenosis.[25,58]

Pharmacologic Agents

Many pharmacologic agents are used in the care of patients with GI disorders. Table 30-3 reviews the various agents and any special considerations necessary for administering them.

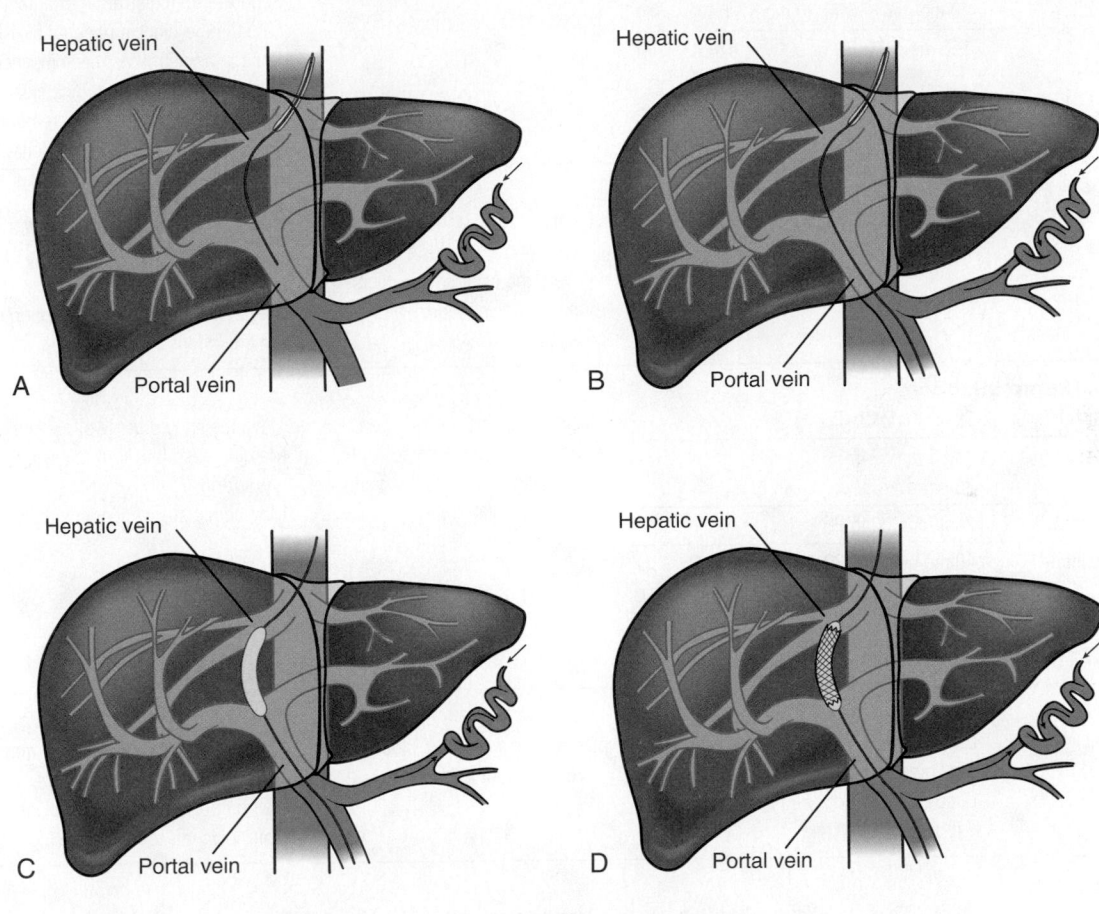

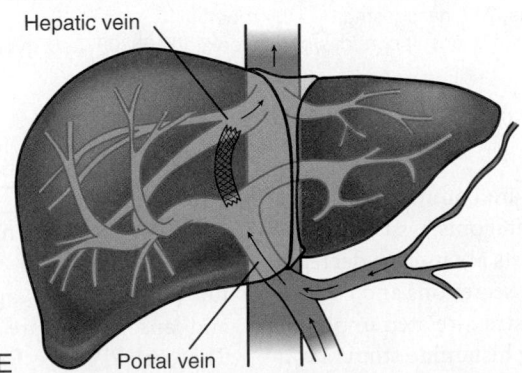

FIGURE 30-11 Transjugular Intrahepatic Portosystemic Shunt (TIPS). *A,* Needle directed though liver parenchyma to portal vein. *B,* Needle and guidewire passed down to midportal vein. *C,* Balloon dilation. *D,* Deployment of stent. *E,* Intrahepatic shunt from portal to hepatic vein. (From Urder LU, et al. *Priorities in Critical Care Nursing.* 6th ed. St. Louis: Mosby; 2012.)

TABLE 30-3   PHARMACOLOGIC MANAGEMENT

Gastrointestinal Disorders

MEDICATION	DOSAGE	ACTIONS	SPECIAL CONSIDERATIONS
Antacids	30-90 mL q1-2h PO or NG; possibly titrated to NG pH	Used to buffer stomach acid and raise gastric pH	Can cause diarrhea or constipation and electrolyte disturbances Irrigate NG tube with water after administration because antacids can clog tube
Histamine₂ (H₂) Antagonists			
Cimetidine (Tagamet)	300 mg q6h IV or PO	Used to reduce volume and concentration of gastric secretions	Side effects include CNS toxicity (confusion or delirium) and thrombocytopenia
Ranitidine (Zantac)	150 mg q12h PO or 50 mg q8h IV		Separate administration of antacids and PO histamine blocking agents by 1 hour
Famotidine (Pepcid)	40 mg daily PO or 20 mg q12h IV		Dosage adjustments recommended for patients with moderate (creatinine clearance <50 mL/min) or severe (creatinine clearance <10 mL/min) renal insufficiency
Nizatidine (Axid)	150 mg q12h PO or 300 mg q24h		
Gastric Mucosal Agents			
Sucralfate (Carafate)	1 g q6h NG or PO, given 1 hour before meals and at bedtime	Forms an ulcer-adherent complex with proteinaceous exudates Covers the ulcer and protects against acid, pepsin, and bile salts	Requires an acid medium for activation; do not administer within 30 minutes of an antacid May cause severe constipation May cause decreased absorption of certain medications
Gastric Proton-Pump Inhibitors			
Omeprazole (Prilosec)	20-40 mg q12h PO	Inactivates acid, or hydrogen, acid pump, blocking secretion of hydrochloric acid by gastric parietal cells	Capsules should be swallowed intact
Lansoprazole (Prevacid)	15-30 mg q24h PO 30 mg over 30 min q24h IV		May increase levels of phenytoin, diazepam, warfarin
Rabeprazole (Aciphex)	20-40 mg q24h PO		May administer concomitantly with antacids
Esomeprazole (Nexium)	40 mg q12-24h PO 20-40 mg q24h IV		
Pantoprazole (Protonix)	20-40 mg q24h PO 80 mg q8-12h IV		
Vasopressin (Pitressin Synthetic)	Loading dose of 20 units over 20 min IV, followed by 0.2-0.4 unit/min IV infusion Doses can be increased to 0.9 unit/min, if necessary	Decreases splanchnic blood flow, reducing portal pressure	Side effects include coronary, mesenteric, and peripheral vasoconstriction May be administered concurrently with nitroglycerin to minimize side effects
Somatostatin Octreotide (Sandostatin)	Bolus dose of 25-50 mcg followed by IV infusion of 25-50 mcg/hr for 48 hours	Decreases splanchnic blood flow, reducing portal pressure	May cause hyperglycemia or hypoglycemia when initiating the drip and changing dosages

CNS, Central nervous system; *IV*, intravenous; *NG*, nasogastric; *PO*, by mouth.
From Gold Standard. Available at: http://www.mdconsult.com/das/pharm/lookup/340530070-12?type=alldrugs. Accessed June 14, 2012.

Antiulcer Agents

A number of different antiulcer agents are commonly used in the critical care setting, including H₂-antagonists, gastric PPIs, and gastric mucosal agents. H₂-antagonists are used to decrease the volume and concentration of gastric secretions and control gastric pH, decreasing the incidence of stress-related upper GI bleeding. These agents work by blocking histamine stimulation of the H₂-receptors on the gastric parietal cells, reducing acid production.[59] Although these medications may be administered orally, intramuscularly, or intravenously, they usually are given intravenously in the critical care setting.

PPIs decrease gastric acid secretion by binding to the proton pump, blocking the release of acid from the gastric parietal cells. PPIs are potent acid inhibitors and have greater suppressive ability and efficacy to consistency reduce rebleeding rates than the H₂-agonists.[59-61] Esomeprazole, pantoprazole, and lansoprazole are available for intravenous administration. The oral PPIs are formulated as enteric-coated tablets or as delayed-release capsules containing enteric-coated granules. Absorption occurs in an alkaline environment and begins only after the granules leave the stomach and enter the duodenum.

Unlike H$_2$-antagonists or PPIs, sucralfate does not affect gastric acid concentration but rather exerts its action locally. Sucralfate reacts with hydrochloric acid to form a sticky, paste-like substance that adheres to the surface of the ulcer and shields it from pepsin, acid, and bile. Sucralfate predominantly binds to damaged GI mucosa, with minimal adherence to normal tissue.[59] It is administered orally or through a gastric tube. Sucralfate should not be crushed but may be dissolved in 10 mL of water to form a slurry. It is also available as a suspension.

Vasopressin

Vasopressin is used to control gastric ulcer and variceal bleeding. It is administered intra-arterially, through a catheter inserted into the right or left gastric artery (through the femoral artery, aorta, and celiac trunk) or intravenously. It causes splanchnic and systemic vasoconstriction, subsequently reducing portal blood flow and pressure.[24,62-64]

A major side effect of the medication is systemic vasoconstriction, which can result in cardiac ischemia, chest pain, hypertension, acute heart failure, dysrhythmias, phlebitis, bowel ischemia, and cerebrovascular accident. These side effects can be offset with concurrent administration of nitroglycerin.[24,62,63] Other complications include bradycardia and fluid retention. Nursing responsibilities associated with the use of this therapy include maintenance of a patent infusion line and continuous monitoring for vasoconstrictive complications of therapy. Because of the known adverse effects, vasopressin is not the first choice of treatment.[62,63]

Octreotide

Octreotide, a long-acting synthetic analog of somatostatin, is a peptide that is administered parenterally in the patient with acute bleeding and cirrhosis. It reduces splanchnic vasodilation and portal pressure through the inhibition of secretion of various vasodilator hormones, and it is as effective as vasopressin in treating variceal bleeding with minimal side effects. Combined with endoscopic therapy, octreotide is the preferred treatment for achieving hemostasis.[16]

BOX 30-21 INTERNET RESOURCES

American Association of Critical-Care Nurses: **http://www.aacn.org**
Society for Critical Care Medicine: **http://www.sccm.org**
SGNA – Society of Gastroenterology Nurses and Associates, Inc.: **http://www.sgna.org**
American Gastroenterological Association: **http://www.gastro.org**
American College of Gastroenterology: **http://gi.org**
American Society for Gastrointestinal Endoscopy: **http://www.asge.org**
American Liver Foundation: **http://www.liverfoundation.org**
American Association for the Study of Liver Diseases: **http://www.aasld.org**

American College of Physicians: **http://www.acponline.org**
American College of Surgeons: **http://www.facs.org**
American Medical Association: **http://www.ama-assn.org**
National Digestive Diseases Information Clearinghouse (NDDIC): **http://digestive.niddk.nih.gov**
National Institutes for Health: **http://www.nih.gov**
PubMed Health: **http://www.ncbi.nlm.nih.gov/pubmedhealth**
American Society for Parenteral and Enteral Nutrition: **http://www.nutritioncare.org**

BOX 30-22 CASE STUDY

Patient with Gastrointestinal Issues

Brief Patient History
Mrs. S is a 70-year-old woman with a long history of chronic back pain. She has been taking nonsteroidal anti-inflammatory drugs (NSAIDs) for several years. She was recently started on warfarin for atrial fibrillation.

Clinical Assessment
Mrs. S is admitted to the critical care unit because she is vomiting bright red blood. She is pale and diaphoretic and complains of epigastric pain.

Diagnostic Procedures
Mrs. S's vital signs include the following: blood pressure of 70/40 mm Hg, heart rate of 130 beats/min (sinus tachycardia), respiratory rate of 30 breaths/min, and temperature of 101.3°F. Her urine output is 15 mL/hr, hemoglobin level is 9 g/dL, and international normalized ratio (INR) is 5.3.

Medical Diagnosis
Mrs. S is diagnosed with upper gastrointestinal bleeding.

Questions
1. What major outcomes do you expect to achieve for this patient?
2. What problems or risks must be managed to achieve these outcomes?
3. What interventions must be initiated to monitor, prevent, manage, or eliminate the problems and risks identified?
4. What interventions should be initiated to promote optimal functioning, safety, and well-being of the patient?
5. What possible learning needs do you anticipate for this patient?
6. What cultural and age-related factors may have a bearing on the patient's plan of care?

SUMMARY

Acute Gastrointestinal Hemorrhage

- Acute GI hemorrhage can be caused by peptic ulcer disease or stress-related erosive syndrome, and it can result in hypovolemic shock.
- Medical management focuses on restoration of hemodynamic stability and control of bleeding. Nursing actions include administering volume replacement, controlling the bleeding, and maintaining surveillance for complications.

Acute Pancreatitis

- Acute pancreatitis can be caused by gallstones and alcoholism, and it can result in autodigestion of the pancreas.
- Medical management focuses on fluid management, nutritional support, and control of systemic and local complications.
- Nursing actions include providing comfort and emotional support and maintaining surveillance for complications.

Acute Liver Failure

- ALF is a life-threatening condition characterized by severe and sudden liver cell dysfunction, coagulopathy, and hepatic encephalopathy.
- Medical management focuses on treatment of elevated ammonia levels and control of complications such as bleeding, metabolic disturbances, and cerebral edema.
- Nursing actions include protecting the patient from injury and maintaining surveillance for complications.

Gastrointestinal Surgery

- Complications of GI surgery include atelectasis, pneumonia, anastomosis leak, deep vein thrombosis, and bleeding.
- Postoperative nursing actions include managing pain and preventing complications.

Therapeutic Management

- Nasogastric suction tubes and long intestinal tubes are often used in the management of GI disorders.
- Endoscopic procedures to control bleeding include endoscopic injection therapy and endoscopic variceal ligation.
- TIPS is an angiographic interventional procedure for decreasing portal hypertension.
- Common pharmacologic agents used in the management of GI disorders include antacids, H_2-antagonists, gastric mucosal agents, PPIs, vasopressin, and octreotide.

REFERENCES

1. Cappell MS, Friedel D. Initial management of acute upper gastrointestinal bleeding: from initial evaluation up to gastrointestinal endoscopy. *Med Clin North Am.* 2008;92:491.
2. Tariq SH, Mekjian G. Gastrointestinal bleeding in older adults. *Clin Geriatr Med.* 2007;23:769.
3. Acosta R, Wong R. Differential diagnosis of upper gastrointestinal bleeding proximal to the ligament of Trietz. *Gastrointest Endosc Clin North Am.* 2011;21:555.
4. Manning-Dimmitt LL, et al. Diagnosis of gastrointestinal bleeding in adults. *Am Fam Physician.* 2005;71:1339.
5. Ghassemi KA, et al. Gastric acid inhibition in the treatment of peptic ulcer hemorrhage. *Curr Gastroenterol Rep.* 2009;11:462.
6. Schubert ML. Gastric secretion. *Curr Opin Gastroenterol.* 2010;26:598.
7. Huether SE. Alterations of digestive function. In: McCance KL, et al, eds. *Pathophysiology: The Biologic Basis for Disease in Adults and Children.* 6th ed. St. Louis: Mosby; 2010.
8. Schubert ML, Peura DA. Control of gastric acid secretion in health and disease. *Gastroenterology.* 2008;134:1842.
9. Ferri FF. *Ferri's Clinical Advisor 2013.* Philadelphia: Mosby; 2013.
10. Marik P, et al. Stress ulcer prophylaxis in the new millennium: a systematic review and meta-analysis. *Crit Care Med.* 2010;38:2222.
11. Porath A. Does stress ulcer prophylaxis explain the association between *Clostridium difficile*-associated disease and mechanical ventilation? *Chest.* 2010;137:1001.
12. Ali T. Stress-induced ulcer bleeding in critically ill patients. *Gastroenterol Clin North Am.* 2009;38:245.
13. Pilkington KB, et al. Prevention of gastrointestinal bleeding due to stress ulceration: a review of current literature. *Anaesth Intensive Care.* 2012;40:253.
14. Laine L, et al. Gastric mucosal defense and cytoprotection: bench to bedside. *Gastroenterology.* 2008;135:60.
15. Stevens A, et al. *Core Pathology.* 3rd ed. St. Louis: Mosby; 2009.
16. Cat TB, Liu-DeRyke X. Medical management of variceal hemorrhage. *Crit Care Nurs Clin North Am.* 2010;22:381.
17. Bambha K, et al. Predictors of early re-bleeding and mortality after acute variceal haemorrhage in patients with cirrhosis. *Gut.* 2008;57:814.
18. Jessee MA. Stool studies: tried, true, and new. *Crit Care Nurs Clin Am.* 2010;22:129.
19. Goldman L, Schafer A. *Goldman's Cecil Medicine.* 24th ed. Philadelphia: Saunders; 2012.
20. Huang JH, et al. Guideline: the role of endoscopy in acute non-variceal upper GI bleeding. *Gastrointest Endosc.* 2012;75:1132.
21. Sudheendra D. Radiologic techniques and effectiveness of angiography to diagnose and treat acute upper gastrointestinal bleeding. *Gastrointest Endosc Clin North Am.* 2011;21:697.
22. Jairath V, Barkun AN. The overall approach to the management of upper gastrointestinal bleeding. *Gastrointest Endosc Clin N Am.* 2011;21:657.
23. Yoshida H, et al. Treatment modalities for bleeding esophagogastric varices. *J Nihon Med Sch.* 2012;79:19.
24. Opio CK, Garcia-Tsao G. Managing varices: drugs, bands, and shunts. *Gastroenterol Clin North Am.* 2011;40:561.
25. Garcia-Tsao G, Bosch J. Management of varices and variceal hemorrhage in cirrhosis. *N Engl J Med.* 2010;362:823.
26. Lundell L. Acid secretion and gastric surgery. *Dig Dis.* 2011;29:487.
27. Costa G, et al. Surgical shunt versus TIPS for treatment of variceal hemorrhage in the current era of liver and multivisceral transplantation. *Surg Clin North Am.* 2010;90:891.
28. Ghosh T. Review article: methods of measuring gastric acid secretion. *Aliment Pharmacol Ther.* 2011;33:768.
29. Gilbert DA, Saunders DR. Iced saline lavage does not slow bleeding from experimental canine gastric ulcers. *Dig Dis Sci.* 1981;26:1065.
30. Milosavljevic T, et al. Complications of peptic ulcer disease. *Dig Dis.* 2011;29:491.
31. Khan AS, et al. Controversies in the etiologies of acute pancreatitis. *JOP.* 2010;11:545.
32. Tonsi AF, et al. Acute pancreatitis at the beginning of the 21st century: the state of the art. *World J Gastroenterol.* 2009;15:2945.
33. Singla A, et al. National hospital volume in acute pancreatitis: analysis of the Nationwide Inpatient Sample 1998-2006. *HPB (Oxford).* 2009;11:391.
34. Ranson JH, et al. Prognostic signs and the role of operative management in acute pancreatitis. *Surg Gynecol Obstet.* 1974;139:69.

35. Munsell MA, Buscaglia JM. Acute pancreatitis. *J Hosp Med.* 2010;5:241.

36. Wang G, et al. Acute pancreatitis: etiology and common pathogenesis. *World J Gastroenterol.* 2009;15:1427.

37. Muniraj T, et al. Acute pancreatitis. *Dis Mon.* 2012;58:98.

38. Chernecky CC, Berger BJ, eds. *Laboratory Tests and Diagnostic Procedures.* 5th ed. St. Louis: Saunders; 2008.

39. ASPEN Board of Directors and the Clinical Guidelines Taskforce. Guidelines for the use of parenteral and enteral nutrition in adult and pediatric patients. *JPEN J Parenter Enteral Nutr.* 2009;33:259.

40. Siow E. Enteral versus parental nutrition for acute pancreatitis. *Crit Care Nurse.* 2008;28(4):19.

41. Al-Omran M, et al. Enteral versus parenteral nutrition for nutrition for acute pancreatitis. *Cochrane Database Syst Rev.* 2010;20(1):CD002837.

42. Moraes JM, et al. A full solid diet as the initial meal in mild acute pancreatitis is safe and results in a shorter length of hospitalization: results from a prospective, randomized, controlled, double-blind clinical trial. *J Clin Gastroenterol.* 2010;44:517.

43. Dellinger EP, et al. Early antibiotic treatment for severe acute necrotizing pancreatitis. A randomized, double-blind, placebo-controlled study. *Ann Surg.* 2007;245:674.

44. Stevens T, et al. Acute pancreatitis: problems in adherence to guidelines. *Cleve Clin J Med.* 2009;76:697.

45. Foston TP, Carpentar D. Acute liver failure. *Crit Care Nurs Clin North Am.* 2010;22:395.

46. Mahajan A, Lat I. Correction of coagulopathy in the setting of acute liver failure. *Crit Care Nurs Clin North Am.* 2010;22:315.

47. Ginès P, et al. Management of critically-ill cirrhotic patients. *J Hepatol.* 2012;56(Suppl 1):S13.

48. Smith CE. Gastrointestinal surgery. In: Rothrock JC, ed. *Alexander's Care of the Patient in Surgery.* 14th ed. St. Louis: Mosby; 2011.

49. Apau D, Whiteing N. Pre- and post-operative nursing considerations of bariatric surgery. *Gastrointest Nurs.* 2011;9(3):44.

50. Cannon-Diehl R. Emerging issues for the postbariatric surgical patient. *Crit Care Nurs Q.* 2010;33:361.

51. Noble KA. Name that tube. *Nursing.* 2003;33:56.

52. Bourgault AM, Halm MA. Feeding tube placement in adults: safe verification method for blindly inserted tubes. *Am J Crit Care.* 2009;18:73.

53. McClave SA, et al. Guidelines for the provision and assessment of nutrition support therapy in the adult critically ill patient: Society of Critical Care Medicine and American Society for Parenteral and Enteral Nutrition: executive summary. *Crit Care Med.* 2009;37:1757.

54. Guenter P. Safe practices for enteral nutrition in critically ill patients. *Crit Care Nurs Clin North Am.* 2010;22:197.

55. Bankhead R, et al. Enteral nutrition practice recommendations. *JPEN J Parenter Enteral Nutr.* 2009;33:122.

56. Holster IL, Kuipers EJ. Update on the endoscopic management of peptic ulcer bleeding. *Curr Gastroenterol Rep.* 2011;13:525.

57. Cárdenas A. Management of acute variceal bleeding: emphasis on endoscopic therapy. *Clin Liver Dis.* 2010;14:251.

58. Riggio O, et al. Hepatic encephalopathy after transjugular intrahepatic portosystemic shunt. *Clin Liver Dis.* 2012;16:133.

59. Quenot JP, et al. When should stress ulcer prophylaxis be used in the ICU? *Curr Opin Crit Care.* 2009;15:139.

60. Leontiadis GI, Howden CW. The role of proton pump inhibitors in the management of upper gastrointestinal bleeding. *Gastroenterol Clin North Am.* 2009;38:199.

61. Bardou M, et al. Intravenous proton pump inhibitors: an evidence-based review of their use in gastrointestinal disorders. *Drugs.* 2009;69:435.

62. Foster KJ, et al. Current and emerging strategies for treating hepatic encephalopathy. *Crit Care Nurs Clin North Am.* 2010;22:341.

63. Walker TG, et al. Angiographic evaluation and management of acute gastrointestinal hemorrhage. *World J Gastroenterol.* 2012;18:1191.

64. Miñano C, Garcia-Tsao G. Clinical pharmacology of portal hypertension. *Gastroenterol Clin North Am.* 2010;39:681.

Endocrine Anatomy and Physiology

Mary E. Lough

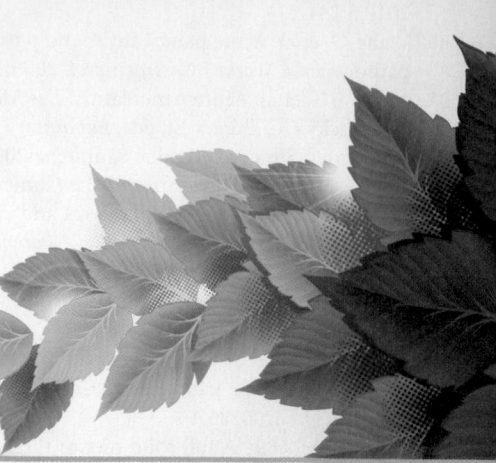

Maintaining dynamic equilibrium among the various cells, tissues, organs, and systems of the human body is a highly complex and specialized process. Two systems regulate these critical relationships: the nervous system and the endocrine system. The nervous system communicates by nerve impulses that control skeletal muscle, smooth muscle tissue, and cardiac muscle tissue. The endocrine system controls and communicates by distributing potent hormones throughout the body. Figure 31-1 lists the endocrine glands and their hormones, target tissues, and actions. When stimulated, the endocrine glands secrete hormones into surrounding body fluids. In the circulation, these hormones travel to specific target tissues, where they exert a pronounced effect. Receptors found on or within these specialized target tissue cells are equipped with molecules that recognize the hormone and bind it to the cell, producing a specific response.

PANCREAS

Anatomy

The pancreas is a long, triangular organ. It is clinically described as consisting of a *head, neck, body,* and *tail.* The head of the organ lies in the C-shaped curvature of the duodenum, and the tail extends behind and below the stomach toward the spleen. The pancreas is approximately 15 cm (6 inches) long and 4 cm (1.5 inches) wide.

Pancreas Blood Supply

The pancreas receives arterial blood supply from many sources. The head of the pancreas receives its blood supply from both

pancreaticoduodenal arteries: the superior pancreaticoduodenal artery, which is a branch of the common hepatic (which comes from the celiac trunk), and the inferior pancreaticoduodenal artery, which branches from the superior mesenteric artery. These two blood supplies anastomose. The neck, body, and tail of the pancreas receive their blood supply from multiple branches of the splenic artery (another branch of the celiac trunk). Venous drainage occurs through the veins that correspond to the arteries and that ultimately empty into the portal vein. The pancreas has two major functions: *digestive* and *hormonal.*

Exocrine Cells

Specialized exocrine cells within the pancreas secrete digestive enzymes into a duct that is 3 mm wide and transverses the length of the pancreas. The pancreatic duct joins with the cystic duct, carrying bile from the liver and gallbladder, before it empties into the duodenum at the major duodenal papilla. This common ductal exit for the two organs raises the danger of a gallstone lodging at the duodenal papilla and blocking the outflow of pancreatic enzymes. Pancreas exocrine anatomy is illustrated in Figure 28-9 in Chapter 28, and pancreatic digestive juices are discussed as part of the physiology of the gastrointestinal (GI) system. Most pancreatic tissue is devoted to production of exocrine digestive juices.

Endocrine Cells

The pancreas contains specialized endocrine cells that secrete hormones directly into the bloodstream. The endocrine tissue is less than 5% of the total volume of the pancreas. The function

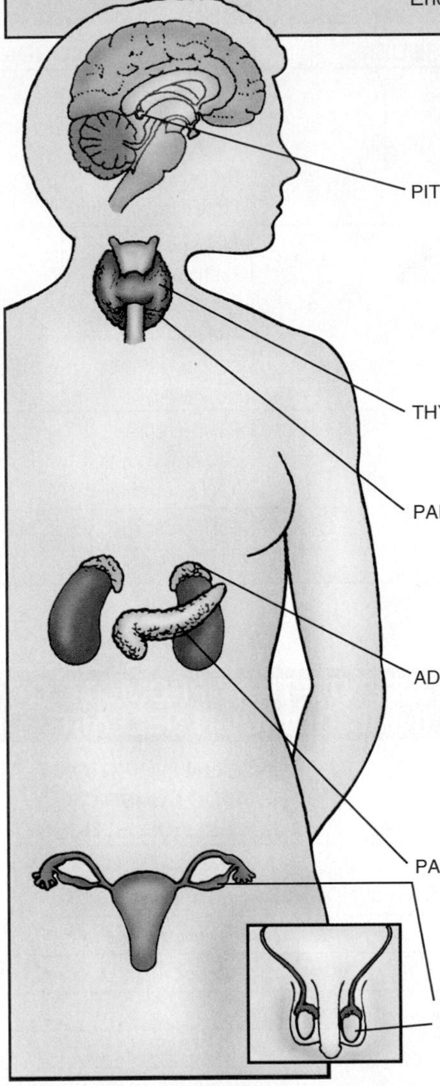

Endocrine gland		Hormone	Target cell/organ	Action
PITUITARY	ANTERIOR PITUITARY	Corticotropin hormone	Adrenal cortex	Stimulates adrenal cortex functioning
		Somatotropin hormone	All body cells	Promotes general body growth
		Thyrotropic hormone	Thyroid	Controls thyroid gland hormones
		Gonadotropic hormones	Gonads	Stimulate primary and secondary sex characteristics
		Prolactin	Mammary glands	Breast development and lactation
	POSTERIOR PITUITARY	Oxytocin	Breast and uterus	Stimulates milk ejection and uterine contraction
		Antidiuretic hormone (arginine vasopressin)	Kidney tubules, collecting ducts	Controls permeability to water
			Arterial wall smooth muscle	Vasoconstriction
THYROID		Thyroxine	All body cells	Stimulates metabolism and increased oxygen use
		Triiodothyronine	All body cells	
		Thyrocalcitonin	Bone cells	
PARATHYROID		Parathormone	Bones, kidneys, gastrointestinal tract	Stimulates use of calcium and phosphorus
		Calcitonin	Bone cells	Stimulates use of calcium and phosphorus
ADRENAL	CORTEX	Glucocorticoids	All body cells	Increase gluconeogenesis
		Mineralcorticoids	Renal tubules	Retain sodium, excrete potassium
		Androgens	Facial, pectoral hair, vocal cords	Stimulate secondary sex traits
	MEDULLA	Epinephrine	Heart muscle, smooth muscle, arterioles	Increases heart rate, muscle contraction, vasoconstriction, glycogenolysis
		Norepinephrine	Blood vessels	Vasoconstriction
PANCREAS		Glucagon	Hepatic muscle tissue	Gluconeogenesis, glycogenolysis
		Insulin	Skeletal, muscle, cardiac cell	Promotes utilization of glucose, fat and protein anabolism
		Somatostatin	Pancreatic A and B cells	Inhibits secretion of both insulin and glucagon
		Pancreatic polypeptide	Gallbladder smooth muscle	Contraction
OVARY TESTIS		Estrogen	Accessory sex organs, breasts	Stimulates secondary sex characteristics
		Progesterone	Uterus	Prepares uterus for fertilized ovum
		Testosterone	Male organs, accessory sex organs	Primary and secondary sex characteristics

FIGURE 31-1 Location of endocrine glands with the hormones they produce, target cells or organs, and hormonal actions.

of the endocrine hormones is the focus of the following discussion.

Physiology

The physiology of glucose metabolism has traditionally focused exclusively on the pancreas. With increases in knowledge, glucose metabolism physiology has expanded to include cellular glucose transport (GLUT) proteins and also incretin proteins from the GI system.

In the pancreas, clusters of cells that appear to form tiny islands among the exocrine cells accomplish the pancreatic endocrine functions. These clusters are known as the *islets of Langerhans* and are composed of four distinct cell types: *alpha, beta, delta,* and *PP*. The locations of the cells that produce these hormones are shown in Figure 31-2. Alpha cells secrete *glucagon*, beta cells secrete *insulin*, delta cells secrete *somatostatin*, and PP cells secrete *pancreatic polypeptide hormone*. Glucagon, insulin, somatostatin, and polypeptide hormones are released into the surrounding capillaries to empty into the portal vein, where they are distributed to target cells in the liver. The

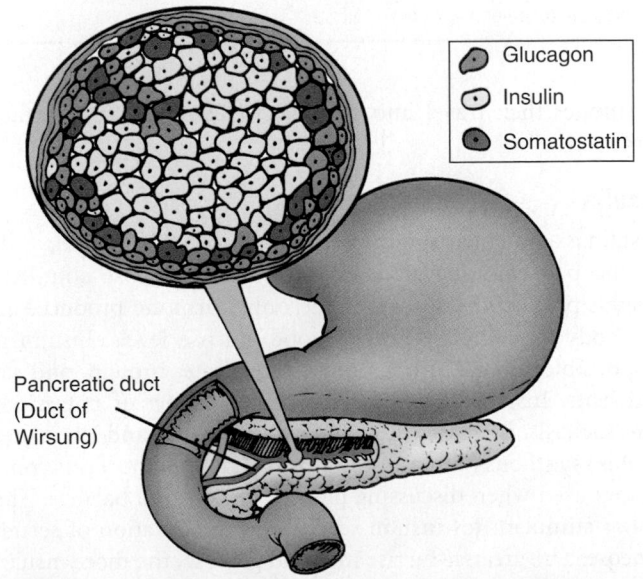

Glucagon
Insulin
Somatostatin

Pancreatic duct (Duct of Wirsung)

FIGURE 31-2 Macroscopic and microscopic structures of the pancreas and the islets of Langerhans.

TABLE 31-1　PANCREATIC ENDOCRINE CELLS, HORMONES, STIMULANT RELEASE FACTOR, TARGET TISSUE, AND RESPONSE OR ACTION

CELL	HORMONE	STIMULANT RELEASE FACTOR	TARGET TISSUE	RESPONSE OR ACTION
Alpha	Glucagon	↓ Glucose Exercise ↑ Amino acids SNS stimulation	Hepatocyte Myocyte	↑ Glucose in bloodstream ↑ Gluconeogenesis ↑ Glycogenolysis ↑ Fat mobilization ↑ Protein mobilization
Beta	Insulin	Glucose	Skeletal cells Muscle cells Cardiac cells	↓ Blood glucose ↓ Fat mobilization ↑ Fat storage ↓ Protein mobilization ↑ Protein synthesis ↑ Glucogenesis
Delta	Somatostatin	Hyperglycemia	Alpha cells Beta cells	↓ Blood glucose ↓ Glycogen secretion ↓ Insulin secretion
PP	Pancreatic polypeptide	Acute hypoglycemia	Gallbladder Smooth muscle	↑ Gallbladder contraction ↓ Pancreatic enzyme

SNS, Sympathetic nervous system; ↑, increases; ↓, decreases.

BOX 31-1　TERMS USED FOR INSULIN AND GLUCOSE IMBALANCE

- **Anabolism**—constructive phase of metabolism in which the body converts simple substances into more complex compounds in the presence of energy
- **Catabolism**—destructive phase of metabolism in which the body breaks down complex substances to form simpler substances in the presence of energy
- **Gluconeogenesis**—formation of glucose from noncarbohydrate nutrients (e.g., fats, protein), which occurs in the liver
- **Glycogen**—storage form of glucose in liver and muscles
- **Glycogenesis**—formation of glycogen from glucose and adenosine triphosphate after a meal when both are plentiful
- **Glycogenolysis**—conversion of glycogen stored in the liver and muscles into usable glucose
- **Osmolality**—measurement of the number of particles in a solution or the concentration of a solution

TABLE 31-2　AGENTS THAT PROMOTE OR INHIBIT INSULIN RELEASE

INSULIN RELEASE (MAJOR STIMULANT: HIGH BLOOD GLUCOSE)	INSULIN INHIBITION (MAJOR INHIBITOR: LOW BLOOD GLUCOSE)
Hormones	
Glucagon	Somatostatin
Corticotropic hormone	Norepinephrine
Thyrotropin	Epinephrine
Somatotropin	
Glucocorticoids	
Incretins	
Medications	
Beta-adrenergic stimulators	Beta-adrenergic blocking agents
Sulfonylurea	Diazoxide
Theophylline	Phenytoin
Acetylcholine	Thiazide or sulfonamide diuretics

hormones then travel into general circulation to reach other target cells.

Insulin

Insulin is a potent anabolic hormone produced by the beta cells of the pancreas. Elevated levels of blood glucose stimulate insulin production. Insulin is the only hormone produced in the body that directly lowers blood glucose levels. Insulin is responsible for the storage of carbohydrate, protein, and fat nutrients. Insulin also augments the transport of potassium into the cells, decreases the mobilization of fats, and stimulates protein synthesis (Table 31-1). Box 31-1 defines the terms commonly used when discussing glucose and insulin balance. The major stimulant for insulin secretion is an elevation of serum glucose. The greater the rise in blood glucose, the more insulin the normal pancreas produces. Other hormones inhibit the release of insulin (Table 31-2).

Blood Glucose

Blood glucose is reported in millimoles per liter (mmol/L), which is the System International (SI) unit of measure used throughout the world. In the United States, blood glucose is measured in milligrams per deciliter (mg/dL). The normal blood glucose range is 70 to 100 mg/dL (3.9 to 5.6 mmol/L). To convert mmol/L of glucose to mg/dL, multiply the mmol/L value by 18. To convert mg/dL of glucose to mmol/L, divide the mg/dL value by 18.

In patients who have symptoms of diabetes, pancreatic beta cell destruction has already occurred. In type 1 diabetes, all of the beta cells are nonfunctional. In type 2 diabetes, about 50% of the beta cells are destroyed by the time the patient exhibits signs and symptoms of diabetes. The destruction of the beta cells disrupts homeostatic ability to regulate blood glucose.

Carbohydrate Anabolism. Glucose is admitted to the skeletal, cardiac, and adipose cells for use as energy in the presence of effective insulin facilitated by the glucose transporter 4 (GLUT4), as described below. The movement of glucose from the circulation into the intracellular compartment reduces the concentration of glucose in the bloodstream and helps preserve the blood's osmolality. Simultaneously, glucose is available to the cell as its main energy source. Excess glucose in the form of *glycogen* is stored in the hepatic and muscle cells for use as fuel at a later time. In skeletal muscle, 90% of the glucose in the cell is converted to *glycogen* for longer-term storage.[1] Liver glycogen contributes up to 10% of total liver weight when fully replete.[1]

Fat Anabolism. Adequate, effective insulin levels affect fat metabolism. Dyslipidemias are strongly associated with type 2 diabetes. Type 2 diabetes is characterized by overproduction of large, triglyceride-rich, *very-low-density lipoproteins* (VLDLs).[2] Disorders of carbohydrate and fat metabolism are also associated with metabolic syndrome, a precursor to diabetes and cardiovascular disease.[3]

Protein Conservation. Insulin and the GLUTs (see below) together facilitate the transfer of glucose across the cell wall. By having glucose (carbohydrate) available as the body's fuel source, protein is spared from use as energy. Protein is then available for critical protein synthesis and for amino acid transport into the cells. Protein metabolism also benefits from an adequate insulin supply. Only in acute hyperglycemia of diabetic ketoacidosis (DKA) or in starvation states does the body use protein for energy sources.

Glucagon

Glucagon, synthesized by alpha cells in the pancreas, has the opposite effect of insulin. Glucagon is released during hypoglycemia to induce hepatic glucose output. Because glucagon counter-regulates insulin levels and raises blood glucose levels, it is a potent *gluconeogenic hormone.* By means of *gluconeogenesis*, glucagon can form glucose from noncarbohydrate sources such as fat and protein when required. Glucagon release from the pancreas is stimulated by low blood glucose levels, starvation, exercise, or stimulation of the sympathetic nervous system (SNS), as listed in Box 31-2.[4,5] Glucagon release protects the brain from the consequences of hypoglycemia.[5]

To meet short-term energy requirements, glucagon stimulates the release of *glycogen* stores from liver and muscle cells. Through a process called *glycogenolysis*, the glycogen stored in the liver is converted into a glucose form that can be used by the cells.[5]

For long-term energy needs, glucagon stimulates glucose release through the more complex process of *gluconeogenesis*. In gluconeogenesis, fat and protein nutrients are rapidly broken down into end products that are then changed into glucose.[5]

A normal blood glucose level is maintained in the healthy body by the insulin-to-glucagon ratio. When the blood glucose level is high, insulin is released, and glucagon is inhibited. When blood glucose levels are low, glucagon rather than insulin is

---

BOX 31-2   EFFECTS OF THE INSULIN-TO-GLUCAGON RATIO ON CARBOHYDRATE, FAT, AND PROTEIN METABOLISM

BALANCED INSULIN AND GLUCAGON	DECREASED INSULIN AND INCREASED GLUCAGON
↑ Use of glucose by cells	↓ Use of glucose by cells
↑ Movement of potassium intracellularly	↓ Movement of potassium intracellularly
↑ Carbohydrate metabolism	↑ Blood glucose
↓ Gluconeogenesis	↑ Gluconeogenesis
↑ Glycogen storage	↓ Glycogen storage
↓ Glycogenolysis	↑ Glycogenolysis
↓ Lipolysis	↑ Lipolysis
↓ Fat mobilization	↑ Fat mobilization
↑ Fat storage	↓ Fat stores
↓ Protein mobilization	↑ Hepatic metabolism fats
↑ Protein synthesis	↑ Ketogenesis
	↑ Mobilization of protein
	↑ Proteolysis
	↑ Lipoprotein

---

released to raise the blood glucose level. The brain has a very limited supply of glucose, and glucagon release is essential to protect the brain from the effects of hypoglycemia.[6]

Somatostatin

Somatostatin is a hormone that is produced in the pancreatic delta cells. Somatostatin decreases glucagon secretion, and in high quantities, it decreases insulin release (see Table 31-1). Hyperglycemia stimulates the activity of the delta cells. It is theorized that the release of insulin enables somatostatin to control beta cell activity. Somatostatin may be involved in the regulation of the postprandial influx of glucose into cells.

Pancreatic Polypeptide

The role of pancreatic polypeptide, synthesized by the PP cells within the islets of Langerhans, is not completely understood. Pancreatic polypeptide release can be stimulated by acute hypoglycemia or by an intake that is high in protein and low in carbohydrate. The effect of hypersecretion or hyposecretion of this hormone has not been identified. The hormone represses pancreatic enzyme secretion and relaxes the smooth muscle tissue of the gallbladder.

Glucose Transporters

Human cells take up glucose by means of facultative glucose-transport proteins known by the term *glucose transporter (GLUT)*. These proteins are specialized by tissue distribution and function as described in Table 31-3.[7] At the cellular level, glucose crosses the cell plasma membrane through *aqueous pores* formed by GLUT transporters. At this time, 14 GLUTs have been identified.[8] The GLUT number indicates the order in which the molecular sequence and GLUT tissue locations were identified.[8] The functions of a few key GLUTs are described in more detail below.

TABLE 31-3 GLUCOSE TRANSPORTERS

GLUCOSE TRANSPORTER (GLUT)	ANATOMIC LOCATIONS	FUNCTION
GLUT1	Erythrocytes, endothelial cells of brain Transport across blood–brain barrier	Basal glucose uptake
GLUT2	Pancreatic beta bells, liver, kidney, small intestine	High-capacity, low-affinity GLUT Can transport fructose
GLUT3	Brain cells, nerve cells	Transports glucose into neural tissue
GLUT4	Striated muscle and adipose tissue	Insulin-regulated transport in muscle and fat
GLUT5	Intestine, kidney, testis	Transports fructose
GLUT6	Spleen, leukocytes, brain	
GLUT7	Small intestine, colon, testis	Transports fructose
GLUT8	Testis, brain, muscle, adipocytes	Fuel supply of mature spermatozoa
GLUT9	Liver, kidney	
GLUT10	Liver, pancreas	Muscle-specific fructose transporter
GLUT11	Heart, muscle	
GLUT12	Heart, prostate, mammary gland	

GLUT1 and GLUT3. The central nervous system (CNS) is freely permeable to glucose transported by GLUT1 and GLUT3.[6,9] The CNS does not rely on insulin for transport of glucose across the neural cell membrane. The brain and other CNS cells require a constant source of glucose because they retain minimal glucose and glycogen stores.

GLUT2. The GLUT2 proteins are associated with glucose sensing and facilitate rapid entry of glucose into specialized cells such as the pancreatic beta cells and into the glucose-sensing cells in the hepatoportal vein area.[8] In the intestine, in the presence of a high-glucose meal, GLUT2 proteins may translocate to the apical cell surface to increase glucose absorption from the gut to the bloodstream.[8]

GLUT4. The GLUT4 protein plays a pivotal role in the way glucose moves from the bloodstream into the cell.[10] After a meal, the levels of sugars and amino acids in the bloodstream rise. This increase signals pancreatic beta cells to release insulin into the bloodstream. As the insulin circulates in the vascular system, it activates an insulin receptor on the plasma membrane of cells, primarily peripheral muscle and adipose cells. This receptor initiates signaling cascades inside the cell to activate GLUT4, which resides within the cells in clathrin-coated pits until needed. GLUT4 translocates (travels) from intracellular storage sites to the plasma membrane in response to the signal from the insulin receptor.[10,11] At the cell surface, GLUT4 facilitates the passive transport of glucose along a concentration gradient into striated muscle and fat cells.

In the baseline state (between meals with normal blood glucose) only 4% to 10% GLUT4 are on the cell surface, whereas 90% are within the cell.[12] Within 10 to 15 minutes of insulin stimulation of muscle cells, GLUT4 levels at the cell surface double as rapid translocation from the interior to the cell surface occurs.[12] Between meals, the liver normally provides sufficient glucose output to maintain constant circulating blood glucose levels within the normal range.

GLUT5. Fructose absorption is the target for GLUT5 proteins, which are found on the apical membrane of intestinal cells.[8] GLUT5 is of interest because of the high levels of fructose in many modern processed foods and the link between high-fructose foods and obesity.

Incretins

The *incretins*, which are hormones that are released from the GI tract after a meal, increase the production of insulin from the pancreatic beta cells. Two incretins are of particular clinical importance: 1) *glucagon-like-peptide 1* (GLP-1) and 2) *glucose-dependent insulinotropic polypeptide* (GIP). The physiology of the incretins has been used to develop new medicines that reduce postprandial blood glucose levels in type 2 diabetes as listed in Table 33-3 in Chapter 33. More insulin is released following oral glucose ingestion than in response to the same amount of intravenous glucose because of release of the gut incretins.[13,14] The increase in insulin section caused by stimulation from the incretins may make up to 70% of the insulin response, depending on the size of the meal.[13,14] This incretin-effect is impaired in patients with type 2 diabetes.[13,14] The physiologic effects of GIP and GLP-1 are listed in Table 31-4.

The incretins have other beneficial physiologic effects, including proliferation of pancreatic beta cells, decrease in beta cell death (apoptosis), and increase in GLUT2 proteins in the islets of Langerhans. Incretins augment the effects of insulin to increase glucose and fatty-acid uptake and storage in triglycerides.[15]

Glucose-Dependent Insulinotropic Polypeptide. GIP is synthesized and predominantly released from the K-cells of the duodenum. GIP acts directly on pancreatic beta cells to increase insulin secretion.

Glucagon-Like-Peptide 1. GLP-1 is synthesized and released from the L-cells of the ileum and colon.[13] When blood glucose levels are high, GLP-1 stimulates insulin release from the pancreas and inhibits glucagon release from the liver. GLP-1 has a short half-life of less than 2 minutes because it is rapidly broken down by the enzyme *dipeptidyl peptidase-4* (DPP-4).[16] *Gliptins* are medicines that have been developed to inhibit the DPP-4 enzyme and slow the inactivation of endogenous GLP-1 to reduce postprandial glucose elevation after a meal.

GLP-I exerts other beneficial effects, including decreased gastric emptying and the feeling of satiety (feeling of being full) after a meal. When blood glucose levels are within normal range, GLP-1 inhibits the release of somatostatin from the pancreatic delta cells and glucagon from the liver.[14]

TABLE 31-4 INCRETINS IMPACT ON METABOLISM

ACTIONS	GIP	GLP-1
Pancreas	Stimulates insulin synthesis and release from pancreatic beta cells after a meal when BG is elevated	Stimulates insulin synthesis and release from pancreatic beta cells after a meal when BG is elevated
	Maintains beta cell mass and function Decreases beta cell death (apoptosis)	Maintains beta cell mass and function Decreases beta cell death (apoptosis)
	Increases GLUT2 expression in pancreas	Increases GLUT2 expression in pancreas
		Increases somatostatin release from the pancreatic delta cells
		Decreases glucagon release from the pancreas
Liver		Decreases release of glucose from the liver
Gastrointestinal system		Delays gastric emptying
Central nervous system		Decreases appetite, sense of satiety after a meal
Muscle		Increases glucose uptake in muscle
Adipose tissue		Increases glucose uptake and free fatty acid synthesis to triglycerides
Bone	Increases bone formation Decreases bone resorption	Increases bone formation Decreases bone resorption

BG, Blood glucose; *GIP*, glucose-dependent insulinotropic polypeptide; *GLP-1*, glucagon-like-peptide 1; *GLUT2*, glucose transporter 2.

PITUITARY GLAND AND HYPOTHALAMUS

Anatomy

The hypothalamus is linked to the pituitary gland in two distinct ways: 1) a vascular network connects the anterior portion of the pituitary with the hypothalamus and 2) a separate pathway of nerve fibers connects the posterior pituitary with the hypothalamus. Understanding the proximity of the hypothalamus and the pituitary gland to each other is necessary to appreciate the correlation that exists between these organs.

The hypothalamus lies in the base of the brain, superior to the pituitary gland. It is composed of specialized nervous tissue responsible for the integrated functioning of the nervous system and endocrine system, which is called *neuroendocrine control*. The hypothalamus weighs approximately 4 grams (g) and forms the walls and lower portion of the third ventricle of the brain. The area composing the floor of the ventricle thickens in the center and elongates. It is from this funnel-shaped portion, called the *infundibular stalk* or *stem*, that the pituitary gland is suspended, as illustrated in Figure 31-3. The infundibular stalk contains a rich vascular supply and a network of communicating neurons that travel from the hypothalamus to the pituitary. The vascular network and neural pathways transport chemical and neural signals and maintain constant communication between the nervous system and the endocrine system.

The pituitary gland is also called the *hypophysis*. It is attached below the hypothalamus and is found recessed in the base of the cranial cavity in a hollow depression of the sphenoid bone known as the *sella turcica*. Secured in such a protected environment, the pituitary is one of the most inaccessible endocrine glands in humans. However, because of this location, the pituitary gland is susceptible to injury from surgical and accidental trauma to the face and head. The pituitary is composed of the anterior lobe and the posterior lobe (see Fig. 31-3). Each component within the pituitary has its own origin, morphology, and function.

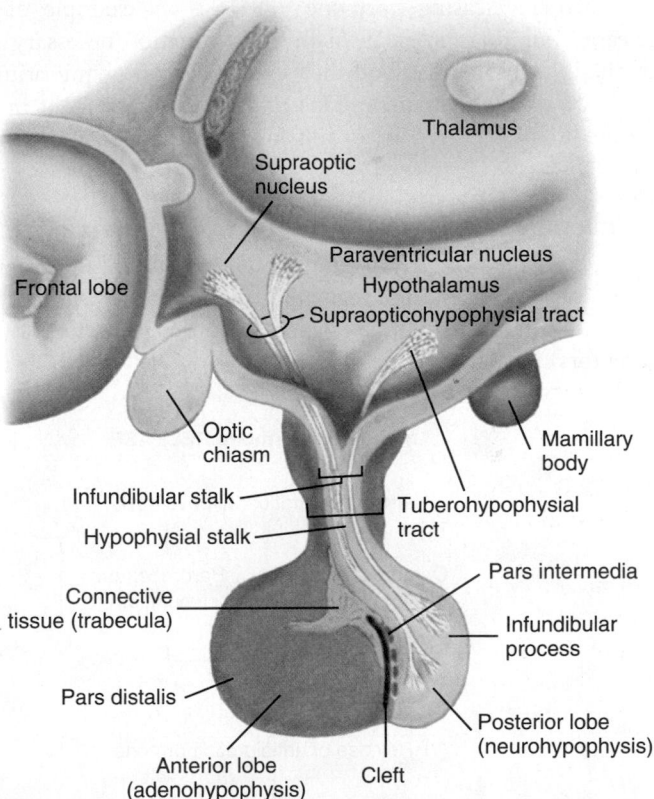

FIGURE 31-3 Anatomy of the hypothalamus and the pituitary gland and their locations in the skull. (From Thompson JM, et al. *Mosby's Clinical Nursing*. 5th ed. St. Louis: Mosby; 2002.)

Anterior Pituitary

The anterior lobe of the pituitary, also called the *adenohypophysis*, is the largest portion of the gland. It communicates with the hypothalamus by means of a vascular network. The glandular tissue of the anterior pituitary produces several hormones, including adrenocorticotropic hormone (ACTH), thyroid-stimulating hormone (TSH), follicle-stimulating hormone (FSH), luteinizing hormone (LH), growth hormone (GH), and prolactin. Information about all the hormones, their target tissues, and their actions is found in Figure 31-1.

Posterior Pituitary

The posterior lobe of the pituitary gland is also known as the *neurohypophysis*. It retains its continuity with the hypothalamus by means of neural fibers running through the infundibular stalk. The neurohypophysis has no glandular properties but functions as an extension of the hypothalamus. It collects, stores, and later releases hormones that are produced in the hypothalamus. Oxytocin and antidiuretic hormone (ADH) are manufactured in the hypothalamus and stored in the posterior pituitary.

Physiology

The hypothalamus gland is known as the "master gland" because of the influence it has over all areas of body functioning. The hypothalamus controls pituitary gland action and response by secreting substances called *release-inhibiting factors.* These factors control the release or inhibition of hormones. Thyrotropin-releasing hormone (TRH) is an example of a release-inhibiting factor. Virtually every function necessary to maintaining the human body in a state of dynamic equilibrium is regulated in this manner. One of the most important hormones to understand in caring for the critically ill patient is ADH.

Antidiuretic Hormone

ADH, known also as *arginine vasopressin*, is an important hormone responsible for regulating fluid balance within the body. ADH acts through specialized vasopressin receptors (V receptors) in specific target tissue:

V_1 receptors in arterial walls
V_2 receptors in kidney collecting ducts
V_3 receptors in pituitary tissue

ADH has two functions: 1) by means of the V_1 receptors, it constricts smooth muscles within the arterial wall and 2) through V_2 receptors, it regulates fluid balance by altering the permeability of the kidney tubule to water. ADH also contributes to control of the sodium level in the extracellular fluid by control of plasma osmolality. The sodium ion concentration in the plasma largely determines plasma osmolality. Osmoreceptors, located in the hypothalamus are sensitive to changes in the circulating plasma osmolality.[17]

Disorders of water metabolism are divided into *hyperosmolar* and *hypo-osmolar* states. Hyperosmolar disorders have a deficit of body water relative to body solute. Hypo-osmolar disorders have an excess of body water relative to total body solute.[18]

Sodium and water metabolism are regulated by different but complementary systems within the body. Sodium metabolism is predominately regulated by the renin–angiotensin–aldosterone system (RAAS), and water metabolism is primarily controlled by arginine vasopressin.

A low sodium level is associated with a low serum osmolality (hypo-osmolar state). When sodium levels rise, plasma osmolality increases (hyperosmolar state). ADH is then released to stimulate water resorption at the nephron to maintain sodium balance. This process decreases water loss from the body and subsequently concentrates and reduces urine volume. Fluid conserved in this manner is returned to the circulating plasma, where it dilutes the concentration (osmolality) of plasma, as shown in Figure 31-4.

The release of ADH increases with hypovolemia. Primarily, the plasma osmotic pressure and the volume of circulating blood regulate the release of ADH. Stretch receptors located in the left atrium are sensitive to volume changes in the plasma

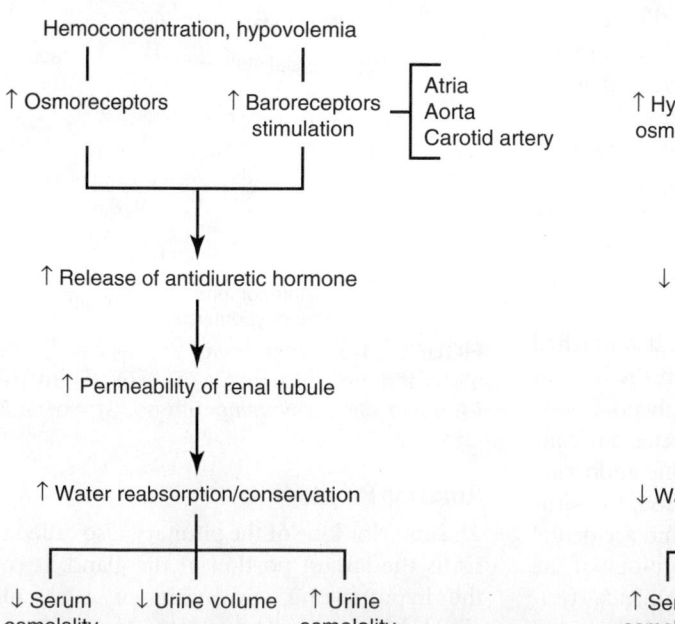
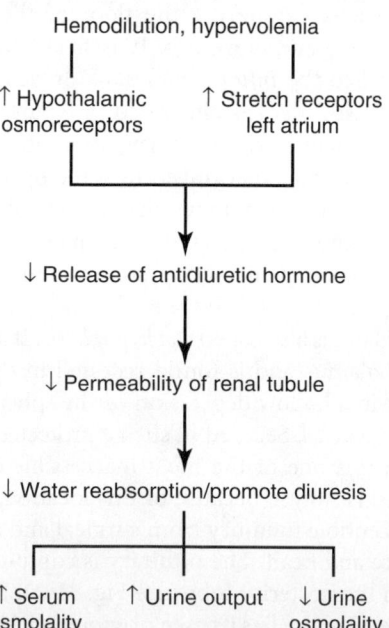

FIGURE 31-4 Physiology of the release and restriction of antidiuretic hormone.

TABLE 31-5 FACTORS AFFECTING ANTIDIURETIC HORMONE

ANTIDIURETIC HORMONE STIMULATION	ANTIDIURETIC HORMONE RESTRICTION
Increased serum osmolality	Decreased serum osmolality
Emesis	Hypervolemia
Hypovolemia	Water intoxication
Hemorrhage	Cold
Pain	Congenital defect
	Carbon dioxide inhalation
Hypothalamic-Pituitary System Damage	
Accidental trauma	Accidental trauma
Surgical trauma	Surgical trauma
Pathologic trauma	Pathologic trauma
Stress: physical and emotional	
Acute infections	
Malignancies	
Nonmalignant pulmonary disorders	
Stimulated pulmonary baroreceptors	
Nocturnal sleep	
Medications	
Nicotine	Phenytoin
Barbiturates	Chlorpromazine
Oxytocin	Reserpine
Glucocorticoids	Norepinephrine
Anesthetics	Ethanol
Acetaminophen	Opioids
Amitriptyline	Lithium
Carbamazepine	Demeclocycline
Cyclophosphamide	Tolazamide
Chlorpropamide	
Potassium-depleting diuretics	
Vincristine	
Isoproterenol	

that may be caused by vomiting, diarrhea, or blood loss. Hemorrhage that is sufficient to lower the blood pressure or emesis that is sufficient to reduce fluid volume stimulates the release of ADH. Other factors capable of influencing ADH secretion are pain, stress, malignant disease, surgical intervention, alcohol, and some medications. Table 31-5 lists additional factors that affect ADH levels.

THYROID GLAND

Anatomy

The thyroid gland weighs 15 to 25 g in the adult human.[19] The size of the adult gland varies according to the availability of dietary iodine in different geographic regions. The gland partially encases the trachea, is wrapped around the second to fourth tracheal rings anteriorly and laterally, and is located at the level of the sixth and seventh cervical vertebrae posteriorly. The thyroid gland lies inferior the thyroid cartilage and the articulating surface of the *cricoid cartilage*. This bow tie–shaped gland has two lateral lobes that are partially covered by the sternohyoid and sternothyroid muscles. The thyroid isthmus, the band of narrow thyroid tissue that connects the lateral lobes, lies directly inferior to the cricoid cartilage, as shown in Figure 31-5.

Two important nerves associated with speech and swallowing pass close to the thyroid gland. The *recurrent laryngeal nerve* and *superior laryngeal nerve* are branches of the *vagus nerve*. The considerable anatomic variety in the location of these nerves increases the risk of injury during surgical procedures such as thyroidectomy.[19]

The thyroid gland has a rich blood supply from the superior and inferior thyroid arteries. The superior thyroid artery is the first branch of the external carotid artery.[19] Venous drainage is from the superior, middle, and inferior thyroid veins. Lymphatic drainage follows the route of the thyroid veins.[19] The functional units of the thyroid gland are spherical cells called *follicles*. Follicles are filled with the protein *thyroglobulin*.[20]

The parathyroid glands (usually four) are intimately associated with the posterior surface of the thyroid gland. The parathyroid glands derive their name from their anatomic proximity to the thyroid, although they have a completely different function. The parathyroid glands maintain calcium homeostasis.

Physiology

Functioning of the thyroid gland depends on many factors that respond to a delicate hormonal interplay; the hypothalamus, anterior pituitary, dietary intake of iodine, and circulating protein bodies in the blood all affect thyroid gland function.

Pituitary Gland and Thyroid-Stimulating Hormone

The anterior lobe of the pituitary gland secretes TSH, also known as *thyrotropin*. TSH then stimulates the thyroid gland to produce thyroid hormones.

Iodine and Iodide

Through a complex process, dietary iodine is absorbed and concentrated in the thyroid follicles. About 100 microgram (mcg) of iodide is needed on a daily basis to generate sufficient quantities of thyroid hormone. In the United States, dietary ingestion of iodide ranges from 200 to 500 mcg per day. The iodine is oxidized to iodide by the enzyme *thyroid peroxidase*. Through active transport, the amino acid tyrosine binds the iodide to thyroglobulin, eventually yielding triiodothyronine (T_3) and thyroxine (T_4). More than 99% of T_3 and T_4 circulates in the bloodstream bound to transport proteins: thyroxin-binding globulin, prealbumin, and albumin. The minute amount of free thyroid hormone that is not protein bound is responsible for activating thyroid responses throughout the body.

Thyroglobulin

Thyroglobulin (Tg) is a key precursor in the biosynthesis of thyroid hormone. Thyroglobulin is stored in the thyroid

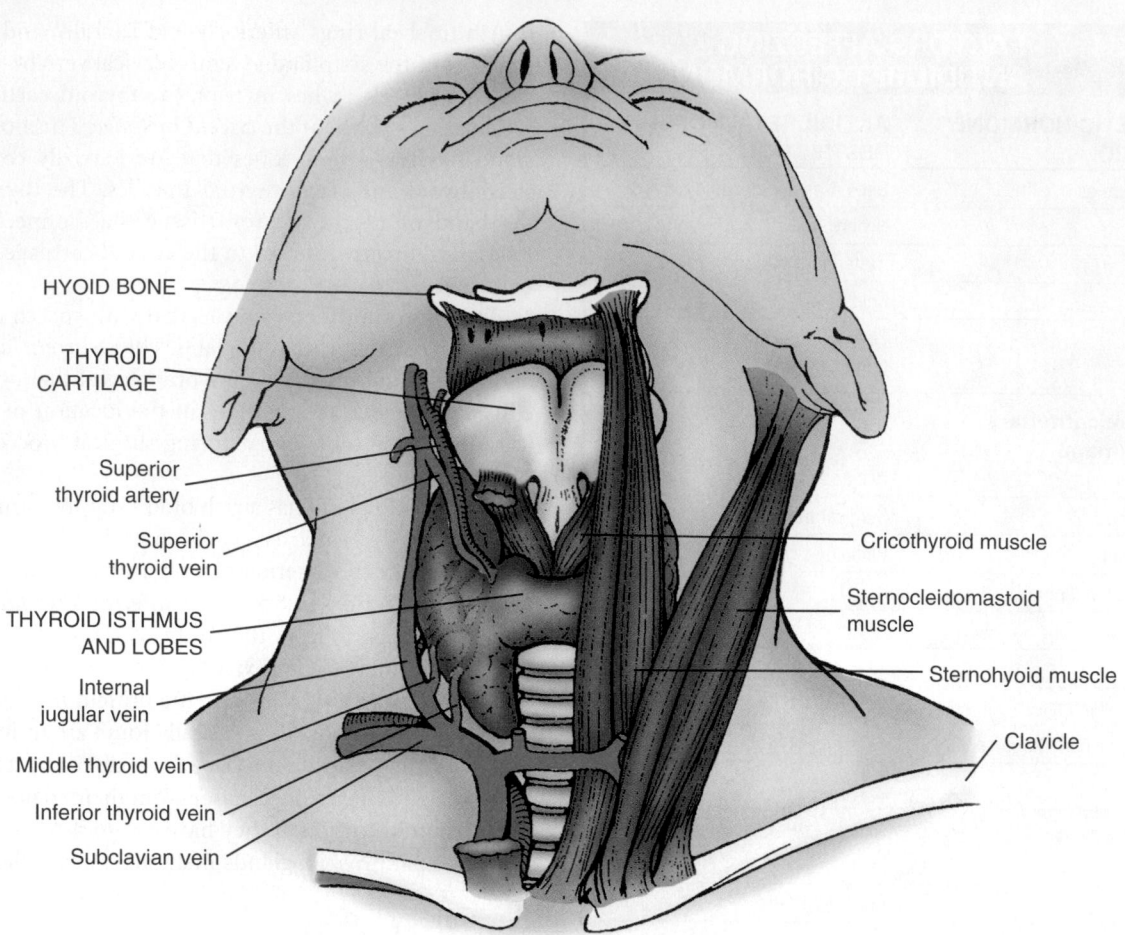

HYOID BONE

THYROID
CARTILAGE

Superior
thyroid artery

Superior
thyroid vein

THYROID ISTHMUS
AND LOBES

Internal
jugular vein

Middle thyroid vein

Inferior thyroid vein

Subclavian vein

Cricothyroid muscle

Sternocleidomastoid
muscle

Sternohyoid muscle

Clavicle

FIGURE 31-5   Gross anatomy of the human thyroid.

follicles until needed. TSH release stimulates thyroglobulin secretion into the bloodstream.[20]

Triiodothyronine and Thyroxine

TSH prompts the thyroid cells to produce thyroid hormones (T_3 and T_4) in the presence of iodine in the thyroid follicles. In the normal thyroid gland, 90% of the thyroid hormone that is produced is in the form of *thyroxine* (T_4) and 10% as *triiodothyronine* (T_3). These hormones are named according to the number of iodine atoms in their structure; T_3 has three iodine atoms and T_4 has four iodine atoms.[20]

Most T_4 is subsequently converted into the more biologically active T_3. Most T_3 in the bloodstream is the result of the conversion of T_4 to T_3 in the peripheral tissues, liver, and kidneys. T_3 acts more rapidly on target tissues compared with T_4, and it is more actively potent. Both thyroid hormones impact the rate at which oxygen is used in the body and, thus, affect all metabolic processes in the body.

Calcitonin

The thyroid gland produces a third hormone, *thyrocalcitonin*, also called *calcitonin*. This hormone is produced by the parafollicular cells, or C-cells, found scattered among the thyroid follicular cells. Calcitonin acts in concert with parathyroid hormone to maintain normal calcium blood levels. Calcitonin lowers calcium levels in the blood through urinary excretion

and by promoting calcium absorption in the bone. In contrast, parathyroid hormone limits urinary loss and stimulates bones to release calcium. Throughout the remainder of this discussion, thyroid hormone refers collectively to T_3 and T_4, not calcitonin.

Hypothalamic–Pituitary–Thyroid Axis Feedback Loop

The hypothalamic–pituitary–thyroid axis regulates the mechanism for the synthesis and secretion of thyroid hormone. The production and secretion of thyroid hormone is regulated by a feedback mechanism that limits the amount of hormone circulating to the cellular need at that time, as illustrated in Figure 31-6.

In response to decreased circulating levels of T_3 and T_4, the hypothalamus releases TRH. TRH activates TSH in the anterior pituitary and TSH stimulates the thyroid gland to manufacture and release the thyroid hormones T_3 and T_4 in the presence of iodine.[20] When serum blood levels of T_3 and T_4 become high, the pituitary inhibits the production of additional TSH. When levels of T_3 and T_4 become too low, the pituitary is stimulated to secrete additional TSH.

T_4 prompts the activation of beta-adrenergic receptors in widespread areas of the body. These receptors trigger an SNS response and release norepinephrine at sympathetic nerve endings.[21] The effect is stimulation of the cardiac tissue, nervous tissue, and smooth muscle tissue, as well as an increase in

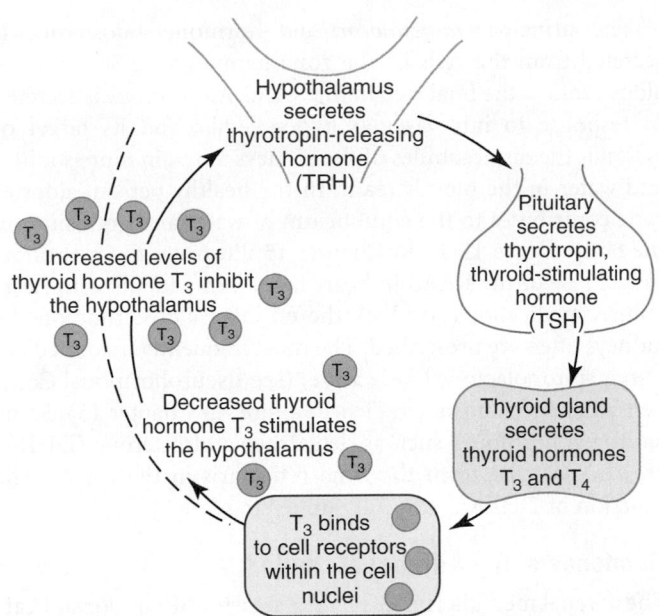

FIGURE 31-6 Hypothalamus-pituitary-thyroid axis feedback loop.

BOX 31-3 MAJOR FUNCTIONS OF THYROID HORMONES

- Interact with growth hormone
  - Maturation of skeletal system
  - Development of central nervous system
- Stimulate carbohydrate metabolism
  - Increase the rate of glucose absorption from the gastrointestinal tract
  - Increase the rate of glucose use by the cells
- Accelerate the rate of fat metabolism
  - Increase cholesterol degradation in the liver
  - Decrease serum cholesterol levels
- Increase protein anabolism and catabolism
  - Mobilize protein and release amino acids into circulation
  - Increase energy from protein nutrients through gluconeogenesis
- Increase the body's demand for vitamins
- Increase oxygen consumption and use
- Increase basal metabolic rate
- Have marked chronotropic and inotropic effects on heart
- Increase cardiac output
- Stimulate contractility and excitability of myocardium
- Increase blood volume
- Expand respiratory rate and depth necessary for normal hypoxic and hypercapnic drive
- Promote sympathetic overactivity
- Boost erythropoiesis
- Increase metabolism and clearance of various hormones and pharmacologic agents
- Stimulate bone resorption

---

metabolism and thermogenesis (increased body heat). Box 31-3 lists the major actins of thyroid hormones in more detail.

ADRENAL GLAND

Anatomy

The adrenal glands, also called *suprarenal glands*, are small, yellowish, bilateral, pyramidal or semilunar-shaped organs located at the superior pole of the kidney. As a neighbor to the kidney, they are retroperitoneal and embedded in the fat pad of the kidney. The normal adrenal gland is 3 to 4 cm in its longest axis and weighs approximately 5 g in the adult (Fig. 31-7). Functionally and histologically, two glands exist within the suprarenal gland: 1) the outer cortex and 2) the inner medulla. Both regions secrete hormones that are integral to the body's response to stress.

Adrenal Cortex

The adrenal cortex is the thicker outer region, and it makes up 85% of the gland. The cortex is composed of three different layers of cells, each with a specific endocrine function: 1) the zona glomerulosa, 2) the zona fasciculata, and 3) the zona reticularis. The cortex secretes cortisol, it regulates fluid homeostasis by means of aldosterone, and it secretes androgens.

Adrenal Medulla

The inner region is called the *adrenal medulla*. The inner medulla is a part of the SNS, and it resembles a cluster of neurons more than an endocrine gland. The adrenal medulla contains clusters of specialized *chromaffin cells*, which are modified preganglionic sympathetic neurons.[22,23] Different sets of chromaffin cells contain chromaffin granules that are specific for each of catecholamines epinephrine or norepinephrine.[22] The granules for each catecholamine appear in different sets of cells within the adrenal medulla. A chromaffin cell usually contains granules only for one catecholamine or the other.[22]

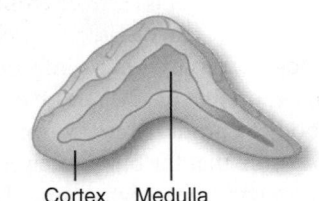

Cortex   Medulla

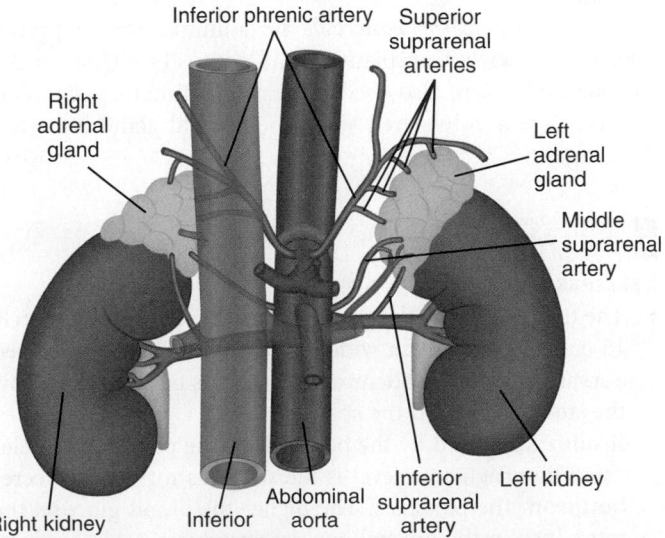

FIGURE 31-7 Adrenal Gland. *A,* Cross section of the adrenal gland showing the outer cortex and inner medulla. *B,* Anatomical relationship of the adrenal glands to the kidneys.

The adrenal medulla is stimulated by the SNS by preganglionic bundles of sympathetic nerve fibers that originate in the spinal cord.[22] The role of the chromaffin cells is to secrete the catecholamines epinephrine and norepinephrine. Under physiologic stress, these hormones produce a widespread excitatory effect described as a "surge of adrenaline" or as the "fight-or-flight response."[23]

Adrenal Blood Supply

The rich arterial blood supply comes to the adrenal gland from three sources (see Fig. 31-7): (1) the superior suprarenal artery is a branch of the inferior phrenic artery; (2) the middle suprarenal artery branches directly off of the aorta; and (3) the inferior suprarenal artery branches off the renal artery.

Venous drainage is usually achieved through a single vein from each adrenal gland. The vein from the right adrenal gland drains into the inferior vena cava, and the vein from the left adrenal gland empties into the left renal vein.

Physiology

The adrenal cortex and the adrenal medulla secrete important and very different hormones. Each part of the gland is functionally independent.

Hormones of the Adrenal Cortex

The adrenal cortex (outer layer) secretes three different classes of hormone, all of which are lipid-based steroid hormones: 1) glucocorticoid, 2) corticosteroid, and 3) mineralocorticoid. The *glucocorticoid* hormone cortisol is secreted from the cells of the zona fasciculata and zona reticularis. Cortisol is released in response to physiologic stress caused by infection, trauma, and the fasting state. In hypoglycemia, the release of cortisol triggers other cells in the body to produce energy from fats and amino acids (proteins) to ensure that the brain receives a steady supply of glucose. Pharmacologic doses (high doses) of glucocorticoids are used to depress the inflammatory response and inhibit the immune system.

Pharmacologic *corticosteroids* are administered to prevent rejection of newly transplanted solid organs (see Chapter 37). Corticosteroids are also used to treat inflammatory disorders, and they are administered when the adrenal gland is cortisol deficient.

The principal *mineralocorticoid* hormone aldosterone is secreted from the cells of the zona glomerulosa. Secretion of aldosterone is the final step in the RAAS. Aldosterone is secreted in response to intravascular hypovolemia, and its target of action is the distal tubules of the kidneys to retain more sodium and water in the bloodstream. In the healthy person, aldosterone contributes to the equilibrium of water and potassium in the body. Figure 15-18 in Chapter 15 illustrates the neurohormonal role of the RAAS in heart failure. In patients with heart failure, medications to block the effect of aldosterone on the kidneys often are prescribed. The most frequently used medication is spironolactone (Aldactone) (see "Neurohormonal Compensatory Mechanisms in Heart Failure" in Chapter 15). Some androgen hormones such as dehydroepiandrosterone (DHEA) are also secreted from the zona reticularis in the cortex. The function of DHEA is not fully understood.

Hormones of the Adrenal Medulla

The adrenal medulla (inner region) secretes two important catecholamines: *epinephrine*, also known as *adrenaline*, and *norepinephrine*, also known as *noradrenaline*. The adrenal medulla acts as a functional extension of the SNS. Stimulation of the SNS stimulates the chromaffin cells in the adrenal medulla to secrete predominantly epinephrine and some norepinephrine into the bloodstream. This results in an epinephrine surge described as the fight-or-flight response. In the critical care unit, intravenous infusions of epinephrine and norepinephrine are used in shock states to raise the blood pressure. The pharmacologic effects of these catecholamines are described in Chapter 16, Table 16-18.

Hypothalamic–Pituitary–Adrenal Axis

The adrenal glands are physiologically linked to the hypothalamus and the pituitary gland. When the brain perceives a stressful or threatening situation, the hypothalamus releases *corticotropin-releasing hormone* (CRH), which acts on the anterior pituitary to release *adrenocorticotrophic hormone* (ACTH), which circulates in the bloodstream to reach the adrenal cortex and stimulate glucocorticoid hormone release. Under stress-free conditions, cortisol is secreted in a diurnal pattern, and levels are highest in the early morning and lowest in the late evening.[24] Illness or trauma disrupts this normal physiology with resultant loss of the diurnal pattern.[24]

■ SUMMARY

Pancreas

- The pancreas is a long, triangular organ approximately 15 cm long and 4 cm wide. It is situated in the C-shaped curvature of the duodenum and extends behind and below the stomach toward the spleen.
- Insulin is released by the beta cells of the pancreas. An elevated blood glucose level is the stimulus for insulin secretion from the pancreas. The higher the blood glucose, the more insulin the normal pancreas produces.
- Glucagon is synthesized from the alpha cells in the pancreas. Its effect is the opposite of the effect of insulin. Glucagon release is stimulated by hypoglycemia, and it stimulates glucose output from the liver.

- In addition to insulin, human cells take up glucose by means of facultative glucose-transport proteins known as GLUTs.
- Incretins are hormones released from the GI tract after a meal that increase the production of insulin from the pancreatic beta cells.

Pituitary

- The pituitary gland is attached below the hypothalamus and recessed in the base of the skull in a hollow depression known as the *sella turcica*.
- The anterior pituitary gland secretes ACTH, TSH, and other hormones.

- The posterior pituitary gland secretes ADH, also known also as *arginine vasopressin.*
- Sodium and water metabolism are regulated by two complementary systems within the body; sodium metabolism by the RAAS and water metabolism by arginine vasopressin (ADH).

Thyroid

- The thyroid gland has a "bow-tie" shape. It is wrapped around the trachea anteriorly and laterally at the level of the sixth and seventh cervical vertebrae. The thyroid isthmus, the band of narrow thyroid tissue that connects the lateral lobes, lies directly below to the cricoid cartilage.

- The thyroid hormones are T_4 and T_3. Most T_4 is converted to the more potent and biologically active T_3 in the peripheral tissues, liver, and kidneys.
- The thyroid gland produces a third hormone, *thyrocalcitonin* (calcitonin), which acts in concert with parathyroid hormone to maintain normal calcium blood levels.

Adrenal

- The adrenal glands are small, pyramid-shaped organs located at the superior pole of the kidneys.
- The adrenal gland contains a cortex and medulla that represent two functionally different endocrine zones. The adrenal cortex secretes cortisol and aldosterone. The adrenal medulla secretes epinephrine and norepinephrine.

REFERENCES

1. Greenberg CC, Jurczak MJ, Danos AM, Brady MJ. Glycogen branches out: new perspectives on the role of glycogen metabolism in the integration of metabolic pathways. *Am J Physiol Endocrinol Metab.* 2006;291(1):E1.
2. Adiels M, Olofsson SO, Taskinen MR, Boren J. Overproduction of very low-density lipoproteins is the hallmark of the dyslipidemia in the metabolic syndrome. *Arterioscler Thromb Vasc Biol.* 2008;28(7):1225.
3. Brunzell JD, et al. Lipoprotein management in patients with cardiometabolic risk: consensus statement from the American Diabetes Association and the American College of Cardiology Foundation. *Diabetes Care.* 2008;31(4):811.
4. Taborsky Jr GJ. The physiology of glucagon. *J Diabetes Sci Technol.* 2010;4(6):1338.
5. Cryer PE. Minireview: glucagon in the pathogenesis of hypoglycemia and hyperglycemia in diabetes. *Endocrinology.* 2012;153(3):1039.
6. Thorens B. Brain glucose sensing and neural regulation of insulin and glucagon secretion. *Diabetes Obes Metab.* 2011;13(suppl 1):82.
7. Thorens B. Sensing of glucose in the brain. *Handb Exp Pharmacol.* 2012;(209):277.
8. Thorens B, Mueckler M. Glucose transporters in the 21st Century. *Am J Physiol Endocrinol Metabol.* 2010;298(2):E141.
9. Simpson IA, Carruthers A, Vannucci SJ. Supply and demand in cerebral energy metabolism: the role of nutrient transporters. *J Cereb Blood Flow Metab.* 2007;27(11):1766.
10. Rowland AF, Fazakerley DJ, James DE. Mapping insulin/GLUT4 circuitry. *Traffic.* 2011;12(6):672.
11. Leto D, Saltiel AR. Regulation of glucose transport by insulin: traffic control of GLUT4. *Nat Rev Mol Cell Biol.* 2012;13(6):383.
12. Zaid H, Antonescu CN, Randhawa VK, Klip A. Insulin action on glucose transporters through molecular switches, tracks and tethers. *Biochem J.* 2008;413(2):201.
13. Ahrén B, Carr RD, Deacon CF. Incretin hormone secretion over the day. *Vitam Horm.* 2010;84:203.
14. Phillips LK, Prins JB. Update on incretin hormones. *Ann New York Academy of Sciences.* 2011;1243:E55.
15. Kim W, Egan JM. The role of incretins in glucose homeostasis and diabetes treatment. *Pharmacol Rev.* 2008;60(4):470.
16. Campbell RK. Clarifying the role of incretin-based therapies in the treatment of type 2 diabetes mellitus. *Clin Ther.* 2011;33(5):511.
17. Sinke AP, Deen PM. The physiological implication of novel proteins in systemic osmoregulation. *FASEB J.* 2011;25(10):3279.
18. Adler SM, Verbalis JG. Disorders of body water homeostasis in critical illness. *Endocrinol Metab Clin North Am.* 2006;35(4):873.
19. Mohebati A, Shaha AR. Anatomy of thyroid and parathyroid glands and neurovascular relations. *Clin Anat.* 2012;25(1):19.
20. Stathatos N. Thyroid physiology. *Med Clin North Am.* 2012;96(2):165.
21. Silva JE, Bianco SD. Thyroid-adrenergic interactions: physiological and clinical implications. *Thyroid.* 2008;18(2):157.
22. Díaz-Flores L, et al. Histogenesis and morphofunctional characteristics of chromaffin cells. *Acta Physiol (Oxf).* 2008;192(2):145.
23. Pérez-Alvarez A, Hernández-Vivanco A, Albillos A. Past, present and future of human chromaffin cells: role in physiology and therapeutics. *Cell Mol Neurobiol.* 2010;30(8):1407.
24. Mesotten D, Vanhorebeek I, Van den Berghe G. The altered adrenal axis and treatment with glucocorticoids during critical illness. *Nat Clin Pract Endocrinol Metab.* 2008;4(9):496.

Endocrine Clinical Assessment and Diagnostic Procedures

Mary E. Lough

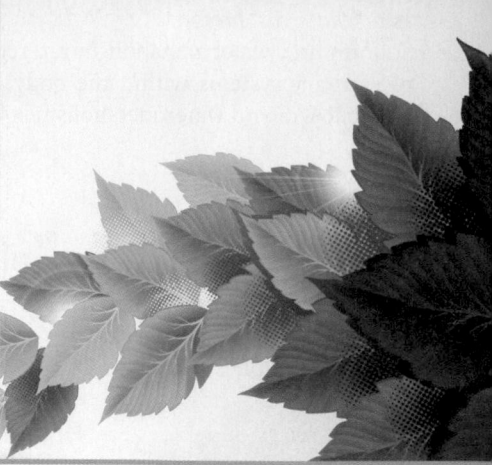

evolve WEBSITE

http://evolve.elsevier.com/Urden/criticalcare/

Evolve Features:
- NCLEX Review Questions
- CCRN Review Questions
- PCCN Review Questions
- Mosby's Nursing Skills Procedures
- Animations
- Video Clips
- Glossary

Assessment of the patient with endocrine dysfunction is a systematic process that incorporates history taking and physical examination. Most of the endocrine glands are deeply encased in the human body. Although the placement of the glands provides security for the glandular functions, their resulting inaccessibility limits clinical examination. Nevertheless, the endocrine glands may be assessed indirectly. The critical care nurse who understands the metabolic actions of the hormones produced by endocrine glands assesses the physiology of the gland by monitoring that gland's target tissue as listed in Figure 31-1 in Chapter 31. This chapter describes clinical and diagnostic evaluation of the pancreas, the posterior pituitary, and the thyroid gland.

HISTORY

The initial presentation of the patient determines the rapidity and direction of the interview. For a patient in acute distress, the history is curtailed to only a few questions about the patient's chief complaint and precipitating events. For the patient without obvious distress, the endocrine history focuses on four areas: 1) current health status, 2) description of the current illness, 3) medical history and general endocrine status, and 4) family history. Data collection in the endocrine history for diabetes complications is outlined in Box 32-1.

PANCREAS

Physical Assessment

Insulin, which is produced by the pancreas, is responsible for glucose metabolism. The clinical assessment provides information about pancreatic functioning. Clinical manifestations of abnormal glucose metabolism often include hyperglycemia, which is the initial assessment priority for the patient with pancreatic dysfunction.[1,2] Patients with hyperglycemia may ultimately be diagnosed with type 1 or type 2 diabetes or be hyperglycemic in association with a severe critical illness.[1,2] All of these conditions have specific identifying features.[1,2] More information on the specific pathophysiology and management of each condition is available in Chapter 33.

Hyperglycemia

Because severe hyperglycemia affects a variety of body systems, all systems are assessed. The patient may complain of blurred vision, headache, weakness, fatigue, drowsiness, anorexia, nausea, and abdominal pain. On *inspection*, the patient has flushed skin, polyuria, polydipsia, vomiting, and evidence of dehydration. Progressive deterioration in the level of consciousness, from alert to lethargic or comatose, is observed as the hyperglycemia exacerbates. If ketoacidosis occurs, the patient's breathing becomes deep and rapid (Kussmaul respirations), and the breath may have a fruity odor. *Auscultation* of the abdomen may reveal hypoactive bowel sounds. *Palpation* elicits abdominal tenderness. *Percussion* may reveal diminished deep tendon reflexes. Because hyperglycemia results in osmotic diuresis, the patient's fluid volume status is assessed. Signs of dehydration include tachycardia, orthostatic hypotension, and poor skin turgor. The key laboratory tests that assist in assessment are discussed in the following section.

Laboratory Studies

Pertinent laboratory tests for pancreatic function measure short-term and long-term blood glucose levels, which can identify and diagnose diabetes.

BOX 32-1 DATA COLLECTION

Complications of Diabetes

Current Health Status

- The body may not be able to adjust to increased insulin needs resulting from sudden physiologic changes such as infection, injury, or surgery. The nurse assesses whether the patient has a severe infection, surgical wound, or traumatic injury.
- Recent or current signs and symptoms:
  - Unexplained changes in weight, thirst, hunger
  - Headache, blurred vision
  - Longstanding, unhealed infection
  - Vaginitis, pruritus
  - Leg pain, numbness
- Unexplained change in urinary patterns (e.g., daytime and nighttime, frequency, volume)
- Energy or stamina changes
- Endurance level
- Weakness
- Unexplained, excessive fatigue
- Behavior or mental changes (also ask family member or significant other for input):
  - Memory loss
  - Orientation

Assessment of Current Illness: Onset, Characteristics, and Course

- Chronic illness: Physiologic or psychologic stress may increase endogenous glucose.

- Recent treatments that could be a source of exogenous glucose:
  - Hyperalimentation
  - Peritoneal dialysis
  - Hemodialysis
- Medications, including prescription and over-the-counter preparations: Pharmacologic agents may alter pancreatic function by increasing or decreasing the release of endocrine hormones. Medications also may interfere with hormonal action at the receptor site on the target cell.

Medical History: Questions

- Have you had prior pancreatic surgery?
- Have you ever been told that any of the following applied to you:
  - Too much sugar in the urine?
  - Too much sugar in the blood?
  - Will probably develop too much sugar later in life?
- If you answered yes to any of these questions, what treatment, if any, was prescribed?
- Are you currently following such a treatment?

Family History: Questions

- Has a family member ever been diagnosed with diabetes or "sugar in the blood"?
- If so, how did he or she treat the condition?

TABLE 32-1 BLOOD GLUCOSE LEVELS

PATIENT STATUS	FASTING BG (mg/dL)	FASTING BG (mmol/L)
Hypoglycemia	<70	< 3.9
Normal	70-100	>3.9-5.6
Prediabetes	100-125	5.6-6.9
Diabetes	≥126	≥7.0

Data from American Diabetes Association. Standards of medical care in diabetes—2012, *Diabetes Care.* 2012;35(suppl 1):S11.

BG, Blood glucose; *mg/dL,* milligram per deciliter; *mmol/L,* millimole per liter.

Blood Glucose

The fasting plasma glucose (FPG) level is assessed by a simple blood test after the person has not eaten for 8 hours. A normal FPG level is between 70 and 100 milligrams per deciliter (mg/dL).[1] A fasting glucose level between 100 and 125 mg/dL identifies a person who is *prediabetic.*[1] Even these individuals are at increased risk for complications of diabetes, such as coronary heart disease and stroke. A FPG level of 126 mg/dL (7 millimoles per liter [mmol/L]) or higher is diagnostic of diabetes (Table 32-1). In nonurgent settings, the test is repeated on another day to ensure that the result is accurate. After a meal, the concentration of glucose increases in the bloodstream. Recommended postprandial blood glucose levels should not exceed 180 mg/dL (10 mmol/L).[1]

All critically ill patients must have their blood glucose levels monitored frequently while in the hospital. Clinical practice guidelines from the American Association of Clinical Endocrinologists (AACE) and the American Diabetes Association (ADA) recommend instituting insulin therapy when the blood glucose is greater than 180 mg/dL in critical illness.[3] A target blood glucose range of 140 to 180 mg/dL is recommended.[3]

When a continuous insulin infusion is administered, point-of-care blood glucose testing is performed hourly or according to hospital protocol by the critical care nurse to achieve and maintain the blood glucose within the target range.[3]

Hypoglycemia is defined as a blood glucose level below 70 mg/dL (3.9 mmol/L).[1,3] A complication of intensive glucose control is that hypoglycemic episodes may occur more frequently both in the hospital and with self-management of glucose levels in diabetes.[3]

Before discharge to home, patients with diabetes should be taught to monitor their blood glucose levels.[4] Maintaining blood glucose within the normal range is associated with fewer long-term diabetes related complications.[4] Laboratory blood tests and point-of-care or self-monitoring of blood glucose represent the standard of care for management of diabetes. Unfortunately, home monitoring of blood glucose is not the norm despite research evidence that maintaining blood glucose levels as close to normal as possible prolongs life and reduces complications.

Urine Glucose

Testing the urine for glucose is not recommended for patients with diabetes because too much variation exists in the threshold for glucose when diabetes-related kidney damage has occurred. Urine glucose measurements are affected by variation in fluid intake, reflect an average glucose level, not a specific point in time, and are altered by some medications. Urine glucose testing does not offer any help in the identification of hypoglycemia. For all of these reasons, urine glucose testing is never to be used.

Glycated Hemoglobin

Blood testing of glucose is useful for daily management of diabetes. However, a different blood test is used to achieve an objective measure of blood glucose over an extended period. The *glycated hemoglobin test*, also known as *glycosylated hemoglobin (HbA$_{1C}$ or A$_{1C}$)* provides information about the average amount of glucose that has been present in the patient's bloodstream over the previous 3 to 4 months. During the 120-day life span of red blood cells (RBCs; erythrocytes), the hemoglobin within each cell binds to the available blood glucose through a process known as *glycosylation*. Typically, 4% to 6% of hemoglobin contains the glucose group A$_{1C}$. A normal A$_{1C}$ value is less than 5.4%, with an acceptable target level for diabetic patients below 6.5%.[1,2,5] The A$_{1C}$ value correlates with specific blood glucose levels as shown in Table 32-2.[1,2] The American Diabetes Association recommends use of the A$_{1C}$ value both during initial assessment of diabetes mellitus, and for follow-up to monitor treatment effectiveness.[1]

Blood Ketones

Ketone bodies are a byproduct of rapid fat breakdown. Ketone blood levels rise in acute illness, fasting, and with sustained elevation of blood glucose in type 1 diabetes in the absence of insulin. In diabetic ketoacidosis (DKA), fat breakdown (*lipolysis*) occurs so rapidly that fat metabolism is incomplete, and the ketone bodies (acetone, beta-hydroxybutyric acid, and acetoacetic acid) accumulate in the blood (*ketonemia*) and are excreted in the urine (*ketonuria*). It is recommended that all patients with diabetes perform self-test, or have their blood or urine tested, for the presence of ketones during any alteration

TABLE 32-2	CORRELATION BETWEEN HEMOGLOBIN A$_{1c}$ CONCENTRATION AND PLASMA GLUCOSE LEVEL	
HbA$_{1c}$ (%)	MEAN PLASMA GLUCOSE LEVEL (mg/dL)	MEAN PLASMA GLUCOSE LEVEL (mmol/L)
6	126	7.0
7	154	8.6
8	183	10.2
9	212	11.8
10	240	13.4
11	269	14.9
12	298	16.5

Data from American Diabetes Association. Standards of medical care in diabetes—2012. *Diabetes Care*. 2012;35(suppl 1):S11.
HbA$_{1c}$, Glycosylated hemoglobin; *mg/dL*, milligram per deciliter; *mmol/L*, millimole per liter.

in level of consciousness or acute illness with an elevated blood glucose.[6] A blood test that measures *beta-hydroxybutyrate*, the primary metabolite of ketoacidosis, provides the most accurate measurement.[6,7] Self-test meters to measure blood ketones from a fingerstick are now available.[6]

Elevated levels of ketones (ketonemia) may be detected by a fruity, sweet-smelling odor on the exhaled breath. This distinctive breath odor derives from the elimination of acetone as part of the compensatory response to maintain a normal pH.

Urine Ketones

Ketones are eliminated in the urine, and urine may be tested for ketones. Ketonuria is retrospective and indicates that blood ketones were or are elevated.[6,7] Ketonuria may also occur in fasting and starvation states.

PITUITARY GLAND

The pituitary gland, recessed in the base of the cranium, is not accessible to physical assessment. The critical care nurse must, therefore, be aware of the systemic effects of a normally functioning pituitary to be able to identify dysfunction. One essential hormone formed in the hypothalamus but secreted through the posterior pituitary gland is *antidiuretic hormone* (ADH), also known as *vasopressin*.

Physical Assessment

ADH controls the amount of fluid lost and retained within the body. Acute dysfunction of the posterior pituitary or the hypothalamus may result in insufficient or excessive ADH production. The clinical signs of posterior pituitary dysfunction often manifest as fluid volume deficit (insufficient ADH production) or fluid volume excess (excessive ADH production).

Hydration Status

The nurse determines the effectiveness of ADH production by conducting a hydration assessment. A hydration assessment includes observations of skin integrity, skin turgor, and buccal membrane moisture. Moist, shiny buccal membranes indicate satisfactory fluid balance. Skin turgor that is resilient and returns to its original position in less than 3 seconds after being pinched or lifted indicates adequate skin elasticity. The skin over the forehead, clavicle, and sternum is the most reliable for testing tissue turgor because it is less affected by aging and more easily assessed for changes related to fluid balance. The skin in the groin and axilla is slightly moist to touch in a well-hydrated patient. In older patients, these typical assessment findings may be absent.

Other indicators that the patient's hydration status is adequate for metabolic demands include a balanced intake and output and absence of thirst. Absence of thirst, however, is not a reliable indicator of dehydration in those with decreased thirst mechanisms such as the older or critically ill patients. Absence of abrupt changes in mental status may also indicate normal hydration. Other indicators of normal hydration include absence of edema, stable weight, and urine specific gravity that falls within the normal range (1.005 to 1.030).

Vital Signs

Changes in heart rate, blood pressure, and central venous pressure (when available) are useful to determine fluid volume status. Blood pressure and pulse are monitored frequently. Decreased blood pressure with increased pulse is characteristic of hypovolemia, whereas elevated blood pressure and a rapid, bounding pulse may indicate hypervolemia. Orthostatic hypotension, which occurs when intravascular fluid volume decreases, is identified by a drop in systolic blood pressure of 20 mm Hg or a drop in diastolic blood pressure of 10 mm Hg when the patient changes position from lying to standing.

Weight Changes and Intake and Output

Daily weight changes coincide with fluid retention and fluid loss. Sudden changes in weight can result from a change in fluid balance; 1 L of fluid lost or retained is equal to approximately 2.2 pounds (lb), or 1 kilogram (kg), of weight gained or lost. To use weight as a true determinant of the fluid balance, all extraneous variables are eliminated, and the same scale is used at the same time each day. Precise measurement and notation of intake and output are used as criteria for fluid replacement therapy.

Laboratory Assessment

No single diagnostic test identifies dysfunction of the posterior pituitary gland. Diagnosis usually is made through the patient's clinical presentation and history. Although serum measurement of ADH is available, it is rarely obtained in critical illness.

Serum Antidiuretic Hormone

The normal serum ADH range is 1 to 5 picogram per milliliter (pg/mL). Prior to ADH measurement, all medications that may alter the release of ADH are withheld for a minimum of 8 hours. Common medications that affect ADH levels include morphine sulfate, lithium carbonate, chlorothiazide, carbamazepine, oxytocin, and selective serotonin reuptake inhibitors (SSRIs). Nicotine, alcohol, positive-pressure and negative-pressure ventilation, and emotional stress also influence ADH.

Serum ADH levels are then compared with the blood and urine osmolality to differentiate *syndrome of inappropriate antidiuretic hormone* (SIADH) from central *diabetes insipidus* (DI). Increased ADH levels in the bloodstream compared with a low serum osmolality and elevated urine osmolality confirms the diagnosis of SIADH. Reduced levels of serum ADH in a patient with high serum osmolality, hypernatremia, and reduced urine concentration signal central DI. Chapter 33 provides more information about SIADH and DI.

Serum and Urine Osmolality

Values for serum osmolality in the bloodstream range from 275 to 295 milliosmole per kilogram of water (mOsm/kg H_2O). *Osmolality* measurements determine the concentration of dissolved particles in a solution. In a healthy person, a change in the concentration of solutes triggers a chain of events to maintain adequate serum dilution. The most accurate measures of the body's fluid balance are obtained when urine and blood samples are collected simultaneously.

Increased serum osmolality stimulates the release of ADH, which reduces the amount of water lost through the kidney. Body fluid is thus retained at the kidney tubules and collecting ducts to dilute the particle concentration in the bloodstream.

Decreased serum osmolality inhibits the release of ADH. The kidney tubules increase their permeability, and fluid is eliminated from the body in an attempt to regain normal concentration of particles in the bloodstream. Urine osmolality in the person with normal kidneys depends on fluid intake. With high fluid intake, particle dilution is low but will increase if fluids are restricted. The expected range for urine osmolality is, therefore, wide, ranging from 50 to 1400 mOsm/kg.

Antidiuretic Hormone Test

The ADH test is used to differentiate *neurogenic* DI (central) from *nephrogenic* (kidney) DI. The patient is challenged with 0.05 to 1.0 mL of intranasally administered ADH in the form of desmopressin (1-deamino-8-D-arginine vasopressin, commonly abbreviated as DDAVP). An intravenous line is inserted before ADH administration, and urine volume and osmolality are measured every 30 minutes for 2 hours before and after the ADH challenge. The patient with normal posterior pituitary function responds to the exogenous ADH by resorbing water at the kidney tubule and raising the urine osmolality slightly. In cases of severe central DI, in which the pituitary is affected, the urine osmolality shows a significant increase (becomes more concentrated), which indicates that the cell receptor sites on the kidney tubules are responsive to vasopressin. Test results in which urine osmolality remains unchanged indicate nephrogenic DI, suggesting kidney dysfunction because the kidneys are no longer responsive to ADH. This test is rarely performed in the critical care unit because of the unstable hemodynamic and volume status of most patients.

Diagnostic Procedures

In addition to laboratory tests, radiographic examination, computed tomography (CT), and magnetic resonance imaging (MRI) are used to diagnose structural lesions such as cranial bone fractures, tumors, or blood clots in the region of the pituitary. Although these procedures do not diagnose DI or SIADH, they are useful in uncovering the likely underlying cause.

Radiographic Examination

A basic radiographic examination of the inferior skull views the sella turcica and surrounding bone formation. Bone fractures or tissue swelling at the base of the brain, which are apparent on a radiograph, suggest interference with the vascular supply and nerve impulses to the hypothalamic–pituitary system. Dysfunction may occur if the hypothalamus, infundibular stalk, or pituitary gland is impaired.

Computed Tomography

CT of the base of the skull identifies pituitary tumors, blood clots, cysts, nodules, or other soft tissue masses. This rapid procedure causes no discomfort except that it requires the patient to lie perfectly still. CT studies can be performed with radiopaque contrast or without contrast. The contrast dye is given intravenously to highlight the hypothalamus, infundibular stalk, and pituitary gland. This dye may cause allergic reactions in iodine-sensitive persons, and the patient must be carefully questioned about iodine allergy before the test. The size and shape of the sella turcica and the position of the hypothalamus, infundibular stalk, and pituitary are identified.[8]

Magnetic Resonance Imaging

MRI enables the radiologist to visualize internal organs and cellular characteristics of specific tissues. MRI uses a magnetic field rather than radiation to produce high-resolution, cross-sectional images. The soft brain tissue and surrounding cerebrospinal fluid (CSF) make the brain especially suited to MRI especially in cases of DI or SIADH.[8]

THYROID GLAND

Clinical Assessment

History

The history of a patient in the critical care unit should be as detailed as possible. Information regarding the clinical manifestations of hypothyroidism or hyperthyroidism must be obtained from the patient, family, or others with knowledge about the patient. Sample questions considered pertinent to detection of thyroid disease are provided in Box 32-2.

Physical Examination

The thyroid is palpated for tenderness, nodules, and enlargement and is auscultated for bruits. The normal-size thyroid gland usually is neither visible nor palpable in the anterior neck.[9] Palpation may be done from an anterior or posterior approach. Auscultation of the thyroid is accomplished by use of the bell portion of the stethoscope to identify a bruit or blowing noise from the circulation through the thyroid gland. The presence of a bruit indicates enlargement of the thyroid, as evidenced by increased blood flow through the glandular tissue.

Laboratory Studies

Controversy exists about routine measurement of thyroid function in adults without clinical symptoms. The American Thyroid Association recommends thyroid function measurement in all adults beginning at age 35 years and every 5 years thereafter; more frequent screening is recommended for high-risk or symptomatic individuals. The U.S. Preventive Services Task Force (USPSTF) found the research evidence insufficient to either recommend or recommend against routine screening for thyroid disease in asymptomatic adults.[10] No specific recommendations have been made with regard to thyroid function screening for critically ill patients.

Thyroid hormone blood tests measure the levels of circulating thyroid hormone and assess the integrity of the hormonal negative feedback response within the hypothalamic–pituitary axis. An inverse, linear relationship exists between TSH and T_4.[11] When the hypothalamic–pituitary axis is normal, TSH production is inhibited by the presence of normal thyroid hormone and the TSH value will be normal.[11] Laboratory diagnosis of hyperthyroidism and hypothyroidism usually is based on the simultaneous measurement of thyroid-stimulating hormone (TSH) and free thyroxine (T_4).[12]

- Hypothyroidism: high TSH and low serum T_4
- Hyperthyroidism (thyrotoxicosis): very low TSH, high serum T_4, and an increased T_3:T_4 ratio[13]

BOX 32-2 DATA COLLECTION

Thyrotoxicosis (Hyperthyroidism) and Myxedema (Hypothyroidism)

The patient is the best source for the following information. If the patient is unable to respond, the following questions can be directed to family, friends, a significant other, or those involved in admission of the patient to the critical care unit.

- Have you ever been diagnosed with overactive thyroid, increased metabolism, or hyperthyroidism? What about underactive thyroid, slowed metabolism, or hypothyroidism?
- Have you ever been treated for hyperthyroidism or hypothyroidism?
- Have you ever had an operation for thyroid disease?
- Have you ever received radioactive iodine for thyroid disease?
- Were you taking any medicine for thyroid disease? If so, what is the name of the medicine, and what is the prescribed dose and frequency?
- When did you first notice the constant restlessness or extreme fatigue?
- Has your weight been the same or changed over the past year?
- Has your appetite changed over the past 6 months?
- Have you lost weight even though your appetite has increased (may indicate hyperthyroidism)?
- Have you gained weight or stayed at the same weight even though you have not felt like eating over the past 6 months (may indicate hypothyroidism)?
- Do you always feel warm (may indicate hyperthyroidism)?
- Do you open windows in house, even in winter months?
- Do you wear lightweight clothing, even when others are wearing layers of heavier clothing?
- Do you always feel cold (may indicate hypothyroidism)?

- Do you wear multiple layers of clothing despite warm weather or the use of a heater or furnace?
- Do you use several blankets and keep windows closed, even in warm weather?
- Do you complain about never being able to "warm up"?
- Over the past 6 months to 1 year, have you developed any of the following?

INDICATORS FOR HYPOTHYROIDISM	INDICATORS FOR HYPERTHYROIDISM
Loss of coarse, dry scalp hair and outer edge of eyebrow	Hair thinning
Sleepiness, lethargy, depression	Swelling (face, eyes, legs)
Weight gain despite decreased appetite	Insomnia, nervousness, anxiety
Severe constipation	Weight loss despite increased appetite
Muscle and joint pain (hands, wrists, feet)	Diarrhea
Dry, itchy skin	Muscle weakness or wasting; tremors
Increased sensitivity to cold	Warm, moist skin
Bradycardia	Heat intolerance, sweating
Menstruation changes; impaired fertility	Tachycardia, atrial fibrillation
	Menstruation changes; impaired fertility

TABLE 32-3 THYROID TESTS

NAME OF TEST	ABBREVIATION	REFERENCE VALUE*	REFERENCE VALUE*
Total serum thyroxine	TT_4	58-160 nmol/L	4.5-12.6 mcg/dL
Free thyroxine	T_4	9-23 pmol/L	0.7-1.8 ng/dL
Total serum triiodothyronine	TT_3	1.2-2.7 nmol/L	80-180 ng/dL
Free triiodothyronine	T_3	3.5-7.7 pmol/L	0.2-0.5 ng/dL
Thyroid-stimulating hormone (thyrotropin)	TSH	0.4-4.0 mIU/L	
Thyroglobulin†	Tg	3.0-40 mcg/L	

mcg/L, Microgram per liter; *mIU/L*, milli-international unit per liter; *nmol/L*, nanomole per liter; *pmol/L*, picomole per liter.
*Some tests are reported with more than one reference value because different laboratories report results using several reference scales.
†Thyroglobulin (Tg) reference values should be determined locally because serum Tg concentrations are influenced by iodide intake.
Reference values from Demers LM, et al. Laboratory medicine practice guidelines. Laboratory support for the diagnosis and monitoring of thyroid disease. *Thyroid.* 2003;13(1):3.

Thyroid Stimulating Hormone

Over the past decade, laboratory tests developed to analyze TSH have become much more sensitive, allowing more accurate measurement of low levels of thyroid hormone. Thyroid hormone reference ranges in adults are listed in Table 32-3.[14] Because serum values vary slightly among laboratory methods, it is imperative to know the normal reference values used by the hospital laboratory.

The upper limit of normal for some of these values is under scrutiny. A U.S. national survey found the average level of TSH in the population in all ages to be only 1.49 milli-international unit per liter (mIU/L), considerably lower than most cited laboratory norms.[11] The serum level of TSH increases as people grow older, which may signal declining thyroid function as more stimulation of the thyroid gland is required.[11] The average TSH level varies by age:[14]

1.60 mIU/L after age 50 years
1.79 mIU/L after age 60 years
1.98 mIU/L after age 70 years
2.08 mIU/L for those older than 80 years

Because this age-adjusted increase is predictable, it is not recommended that laboratories use age-adjusted reference values when assessing thyroid function.[11] Most asymptomatic people with a normal thyroid gland have a TSH level between 0.4 and 2.5 mIU/L.[15]

Thyroid Tests in the Critically Ill

Thyroid hormone testing in patients with nonthyroidal critical illness may be inconclusive because of the hormonal disruption caused by the illness.[16] In critical illness, measurement of TSH is usually the first thyroid-related laboratory test that is obtained.

Medications and Thyroid Testing

Additional measurement difficulties involve concomitant use of certain medications that interfere with thyroid function and lower serum levels.[17]

TSH secretion is affected by several medications routinely administered in critical care units. Glucocorticoids in large doses may lower the serum level of T_3 and inhibit TSH secretion.[11] Dopamine infusions at greater than 1 mcg/kg/min directly blocks TSH release.[17] Amiodarone, an antidysrhythmic medication is an iodine-rich compound that is structurally similar to T_3 and T_4. At usual doses, amiodarone contains 35 to 140 times the iodine recommended daily allowance (RDA) of 150 mcg per day.[18]

Several medications increase the serum level of T_4 by displacing protein-bound T_4.[17] Medications that displace T_4, including unfractionated and low-molecular-weight heparins, cause an increase in serum T_4 levels.[17] Salicylates (aspirin) and furosemide (Lasix) raise T_4 serum levels by the same mechanism.[17] A more complete list of medications that alter thyroid hormone serum levels is provided in Table 32-4. It is not clear whether it is necessary to adjust management of the critically ill patient in response to these laboratory findings.

Diagnostic Procedures

Diagnostic tests often begin with ultrasonography to visualize a nodule or tumor.[19,20] To diagnose hypothyroidism, a nuclear medicine scan using an oral iodine radioactive isotope may be requested.[21] The thyroid-scanning procedure may also detect the presence of ectopic thyroid tissue, thyroid carcinomas, and the amount of viable thyroid glandular tissue after therapeutic irradiation.

ADRENAL GLAND

Primary Adrenal Disorders

Admission to the critical care unit with a primary adrenal disorder is rare. The term *primary* indicates that the principal problem lies within the adrenal gland. Secondary adrenal dysfunction is caused by dysfunction in another gland or by a clinical condition such as sepsis.

The adrenal gland is actually two glands in one, as described in Chapter 31, and this may make the history and presentation complex. The adrenal cortex (outer layer) secretes two classes of hormones, and if deficient or released in excess, they may cause clinical symptoms. Two hormones relevant to care of the critically ill are: 1) the glucocorticoid hormone cortisol and 2) the mineralocorticoid hormone aldosterone. *Cortisol* is secreted in response to physiologic stress as a result of infection, trauma, and hypoglycemia. *Aldosterone* is secreted in response to intravascular hypovolemia. It is the final step in renin–angiotensin–aldosterone system (RAAS) pathway.

TABLE 32-4 MEDICATIONS THAT INFLUENCE DIAGNOSTIC THYROID LEVELS

Triiodothyronine (T$_3$)

Increase	Decrease
Methadone	Anabolic steroid
Estrogens	Androgens
Progestins	Salicylates
Amiodarone	Phenytoin
	Lithium
	Reserpine
	Propranolol
	Sulfonamides
	Propylthiouracil
	Methylthiouracil

Thyroxine (T$_4$)

Increase	Decrease
Oral contraceptives	Phenytoin
Heparin	Steroids
Aspirin	Diphenylhydantoin
Furosemide	Chlorpromazine
Clofibrate	Lithium
Phenylbutazone	Sulfonylurea
Some nonsteroidal anti-inflammatory drugs (NSAIDs)	Sulfonamides
	Reserpine

Propranolol	Chlordiazepoxide
Corticosteroids	
Amiodarone	

Thyroid-Stimulating Hormone (TSH)

Increase TSH	Decrease TSH and TSH Response to TRH
Metoclopramide	Glucocorticoids
Iodides	Dopamine
Lithium	Heparin
Potassium iodide	Aspirin
Morphine sulfate	Carbamazepine

Thyroxine-Binding Globulin (TBG)

Increase	Decrease
Opiates	Androgen therapy
Oral contraceptives	L-Asparaginase
Estrogens	
Clofibrate	
5-Fluorouracil (5-FU)	
Perphenazine	

TRH, Thyrotropin-releasing hormone.

The adrenal medulla (inner layer) also secretes two hormones that cause clinical symptoms if they are deficient or released in excess. They are *epinephrine* (also known as *adrenalin*), and *norepinephrine* (*noradrenalin*), and both are secreted from the adrenal gland in response to stress.

Clinical Assessment

History

A detailed history may help to identify conditions or medications that may affect adrenal gland function. Primary endocrine disorders are rare, but a history of uncontrolled hypertension despite three or more oral medications may indicate whether endocrine-related hypertension should be investigated. The medication history may help determine whether the patient takes glucocorticoid tablets, and the patient or family should be asked about using steroid creams for dermatologic conditions and about using steroid-based inhalers for chronic obstructive lung disease (COPD).

Physical Examination

The physical examination is related to the effects of adrenal dysfunction, and the signs depend on the hormone involved and whether the problem is related to excess or deficiency. This means that the signs and symptoms are very diverse. A methodic approach to assessing all signs and symptoms is important because adrenal disease is often missed or misdiagnosed.

Adrenal Cortex

Primary Cushing Syndrome. Cushing syndrome is caused by the excess release of the glucocorticoid hormone *cortisol.* Excess cortisol produces the classic signs and symptoms listed

in Box 32-3. Primary Cushing disease is rare, but if a patient is not taking exogenous steroids, it becomes a diagnosis of exclusion when the relevant constellation of signs and symptoms are present.[22]

Secondary Cushing Syndrome. Symptoms identical to those of primary Cushing syndrome (see Box 32-3) occur in patients with the secondary form who chronically take pharmacologic doses of glucocorticoids, for example, transplant recipients who take steroids to prevent solid organ rejection; patients with COPD, or those with chronic inflammatory conditions. When patients are admitted to the critical care unit, it is important to ascertain whether they are steroid dependent to avoid the deleterious effects of abrupt steroid withdrawal.

Primary Aldosteronism

In patients with primary aldosteronism, the adrenal cortex secretes excess mineralocorticoid (aldosterone) unrelated to the renin–angiotensin system.[23] Several subtypes of this rare condition exist, but all may cause the patient to present emergently with severe hypertension and critically low serum level of potassium (hypokalemia), which can be lethal if not identified and effectively treated.

Addison Disease

Addison disease is a rare disorder of the adrenal cortex that involves hyposecretion of glucocorticoids (cortisol), sometimes occurring with hyposecretion of mineralocorticoids (aldosterone). Physiologically, it may be envisioned as the opposite of the disorders described previously, and the signs and symptoms are the inverse of the conditions with excess hormone secretion. An *addisonian crisis* is a life-threatening condition in which the

<table>
<tr><td colspan="2">

BOX 32-3 CAUSES OF CUSHING SYNDROME

Primary Cushing Syndrome
Cushing syndrome is divided into adrenocorticotropin-dependent and adrenocorticotropin-independent types. Adrenocorticotropin is also known as *adrenocorticotropic hormone (ACTH)* or *corticotropin.*

ACTH-Dependent Cushing Syndrome
Most cases (80%) result from a pituitary adenoma that causes the pituitary gland to produce excess ACTH. Excess secretion of ACTH stimulates the adrenal cortex to release supraphysiologic amounts of *cortisol* into the bloodstream, circumventing the normal inhibitory feedback loop.
   The other 20% of cases are caused by ectopic ACTH secretion from small-cell cancers of the lung, metastases, and endocrine tumors.

ACTH-Independent Cushing Syndrome
It is usually caused by a unilateral adrenal tumor: adrenal adenoma (60%) or adrenal carcinoma (40%).

Secondary or Iatrogenic Cushing Syndrome
The patient takes pharmacologic doses of glucocorticoids, which may be prescribed to prevent rejection after solid organ transplantation or for the treatment of chronic inflammatory conditions.

Clinical Signs and Symptoms of Cushing Syndrome
- Emotional lability (can range from depression to psychosis)
- Hyperglycemia and poorly controlled type 2 diabetes
- Obesity or weight gain in abdomen
- Rounded face
- Acne
- Thin skin, bruises easily, poor wound healing
- Hypertension
- Hirsutism (excess hair growth)
- Dorsocervical fat pad ("buffalo hump")
- Decreased libido
- Fatigue, weakness

</td></tr>
</table>

BOX 32-4 PHEOCHROMOCYTOMA: SIGNS AND SYMPTOMS

SIGNS*	SYMPTOMS*
Hypertension	Headaches
Tachycardia	Dizziness or faintness
Tachypnea	Palpitations, chest pain
Pallor or flushing	Anxiety and nervousness
Hyperglycemia or poorly controlled type 2 diabetes	Excessive sweating
Decreased gastrointestinal motility	Weakness, fatigue
	Weight loss
	Constipation

*Not all patients have all signs and symptoms.

adrenal gland is almost nonfunctional, usually because of destruction of adrenal tissue. The patient presents acutely with critical hypotension, an elevated serum potassium level (hyperkalemia), a low serum sodium level (hyponatremia), and hypoglycemia.

Critical Illness-Related Corticosteroid Insufficiency

The adrenal gland is designed to respond to acute physiologic stress. However, evidence suggests that the adrenal gland may become exhausted and no longer secrete adequate amounts of stress hormones in prolonged critical illness and in septic shock. The Society of Critical Care Medicine (SCCM) recommends that this condition be called *critical illness–related corticosteroid insufficiency* (CIRCI).[24] Differentiating the signs and symptoms of adrenal insufficiency caused by shock from other causes by clinical examination alone is almost impossible in the critically ill, and CIRCI was probably an overlooked diagnosis in the past. The routine use of the corticotropin stimulation test in the presence of refractory vasopressor-dependent hypotension helps to make this diagnosis.[24]

Adrenal Medulla

Pheochromocytoma. Pheochromocytomas are rare tumors that arise from the catecholamine-producing *chromaffin cells* of the adrenal medulla.[25,26] Most produce norepinephrine, but some produce both norepinephrine and epinephrine.[26] These tumors produce a far greater quantity of catechols than normal adrenal medullary tissue. The concentrations of catecholamines are so high within the tumor that it has have been likened to a volcano that can erupt at any time.[26] When huge amounts of norepinephrine or epinephrine are released into the bloodstream, it creates a *catecholamine storm* that could be life threatening. The body responds as if to a severe fight-or-flight threat by hypertension, tachycardia, increased respiratory rate, and hyperglycemia. The patient may describe symptoms of headache, dizziness, palpitations, chest pain, anxiety, nervousness, and fatigue (Box 32-4).[25,26] Because the body perceives the catecholamine onslaught to be a signal for the person to be ready to escape a threatening situation, it slows down the GI tract, and constipation is another symptom. Most pheochromocytomas are detected on autopsy rather than during life.[27] The patients at greatest risk are those who are admitted to a critical care unit for another reason or are admitted in shock with an undiagnosed adrenal tumor.

Laboratory Studies
Adrenal Insufficiency and Critical Illness

For critically ill patients with refractory hypotension, especially if septic and hypotensive while on vasopressors after adequate fluid resuscitation, a diagnosis of CIRCI should be considered. To determine whether the adrenal gland can to respond to stress, the diagnosis is facilitated by the *cosyntropin stimulation test* (CST). *Cosyntropin* is the name for synthetic adrenocorticotropic hormone (ACTH). An initial measurement of total serum cortisol is obtained to establish a baseline value. If the baseline value is below 10 mcg/dL (in the presence of the clinical signs described previously), the patient is considered to have adrenal insufficiency. If after intravenous administration of a stimulation dose of 250 mcg of cosyntropin, the rise from baseline is less than 9 mcg/dL, the patient is considered to have adrenal insufficiency related to critical illness.[24] This test is invalid if the patient has recently received steroids.[24]

Diagnostic Procedures

CT is the most widely used test to image the adrenal glands.[28] Percutaneous adrenal biopsy is rare in all cases, and unlikely to be performed in critical illness.[28]

SUMMARY

Assessment of the patient with endocrine dysfunction is a systematic process that incorporates the medical and family history, physical examination, and laboratory test results.

Pancreas

- Normal fasting blood glucose is 70 and 100 mg/dL. A fasting glucose between 110 and 126 mg/dL identifies prediabetes. A blood glucose level greater than 126 mg/dL is diagnostic of diabetes. Hyperglycemia is a frequent finding in the critically ill patient.

Pituitary

- Normal serum ADH range is 1 to 5 pg/mL. Prior to ADH measurement, all medications that may alter ADH release are withheld for a minimum of 8 hours.
- Serum osmolality ranges from 275 to 295 mOsm/kg H_2O. Urine osmolality ranges from 50 to 1400 mOsm/kg.

- Serum ADH levels are compared with blood and urine osmolality to differentiate SIADH from central DI.

Thyroid

- Hypothyroidism is identified by high TSH and low T_4 values.
- Hyperthyroidism is identified by low TSH and high T_4 values.

Adrenal

- The adrenal gland is designed to respond to acute physiologic stress. In prolonged critical illness and in septic shock, the adrenal gland may not secrete adequate amounts of cortisol. The cosyntropin stimulation test is used to evaluate adrenal gland function.

REFERENCES

1. American Diabetes Association. Standards of medical care in diabetes-2012. *Diabetes Care*. 2012;35(suppl 1):S11.
2. American Diabetes Association. Diagnosis and classification of diabetes mellitus. *Diabetes Care*. 2012;35(Suppl 1):S64.
3. Moghissi ES, et al. American Association of Clinical Endocrinologists and American Diabetes Association consensus statement on inpatient glycemic control. *Diabetes Care*. 2009;32(6):1119.
4. Cryer PE, et al. Evaluation and management of adult hypoglycemic disorders: an Endocrine Society Clinical Practice Guideline. *J Clin Endocrinol Metabol*. 2009;94(3):709.
5. Handelsman Y, et al. American Association of Clinical Endocrinologists Medical Guidelines for Clinical Practice for developing a diabetes mellitus comprehensive care plan. *Endocr Pract*. 2011;17(suppl 2):1.
6. Kitabchi AE, Umpierrez GE, Miles JM, Fisher JN. Hyperglycemic crises in adult patients with diabetes. *Diabetes Care*. 2009;32(7):1335.
7. Arora S, Henderson SO, Long T, Menchine M. Diagnostic accuracy of point-of-care testing for diabetic ketoacidosis at emergency-department triage: β-hydroxybutyrate versus the urine dipstick. *Diabetes Care*. 2011;34(4):852.
8. Ouyang T, Rothfus WE, Ng JM, Challinor SM. Imaging of the pituitary. *Radiol Clin North Am*. 2011;49(3):549, vii.
9. Ellis H. The clinical examination of the thyroid gland. *Br J Hosp Med (Lond)*. 2007;68(9):M154.
10. U.S. Preventative Services Task Force. Screening for thyroid disease: recommendation statement. *Ann Intern Med*. 2004;140(2):125.
11. Demers LM. Thyroid disease: pathophysiology and diagnosis. *Clin Lab Med*. 2004;24(1):19.
12. Hepburn S, Farid S, Dawson J, Goodall S. Thyroid function testing. *Br J Hospital Med*. 2012;73(8):C114.
13. Seigel SC, Hodak SP. Thyrotoxicosis. *Med Clin North Am*. 2012;96(2):175.
14. Ross DS. Serum thyroid-stimulating hormone measurement for assessment of thyroid function and disease. *Endocrinol Metab Clin North Am*. 2001;30(2):245.
15. Almandoz JP, Gharib H. Hypothyroidism: etiology, diagnosis, and management. *Med Clin North Am*. 2012;96(2):203.
16. Mebis L, Van den Berghe G. Thyroid axis function and dysfunction in critical illness. *Best Pract Res Clin Endocrinol Metab*. 2011;25(5):745.
17. Kundra P, Burman KD. The effect of medications on thyroid function tests. *Med Clin North Am*. 2012;96(2):283.
18. Cohen-Lehman J, Dahl P, Danzi S, Klein I. Effects of amiodarone therapy on thyroid function. *Nat Rev Endocrinol*. 2010;6(1):34.
19. Sholosh B, Borhani AA. Thyroid ultrasound part 1: technique and diffuse disease. *Radiol Clin North Am*. 2011;49(3):391.
20. Henrichsen TL, Reading CC. Thyroid ultrasonography. Part 2: nodules. *Radiol Clin North Am*. 2011;49(3):417.
21. Intenzo CM, Dam HQ, Manzone TA, Kim SM. Imaging of the thyroid in benign and malignant disease. *Semin Nucl Med*. 2012;42(1):49.
22. Nieman LK, et al. The diagnosis of Cushing's syndrome: an Endocrine Society Clinical Practice Guideline. *J Clin Endocrinol Metab*. 2008;93(5):1526.
23. Funder JW, et al. Case detection, diagnosis, and treatment of patients with primary aldosteronism: an Endocrine Society Clinical Practice Guideline. *J Clin Endocrinol Metabol*. 2008;93(9):3266.
24. Marik PE, et al. Recommendations for the diagnosis and management of corticosteroid insufficiency in critically ill adult patients: consensus statements from an international task force by the American College of Critical Care Medicine. *Crit Care Med*. 2008;36(6):1937.
25. Zuber SM, Kantorovich V, Pacak K. Hypertension in pheochromocytoma: characteristics and treatment. *Endocrinol Metabol Clin North Am*. 2011;40(2):295.
26. Pacak K. Preoperative management of the pheochromocytoma patient. *J Clin Endocrinol Metab*. 2007;92(11):4069.
27. Mannelli M, et al. Subclinical phaeochromocytoma. *Best Pract Res Clin Endocrinol Metab*. 2012;26(4):507.
28. Boland GW. Adrenal imaging: from Addison to algorithms. *Radiol Clin North Am*. 2011;49(3):511.

Endocrine Disorders and Therapeutic Management

Mary E. Lough

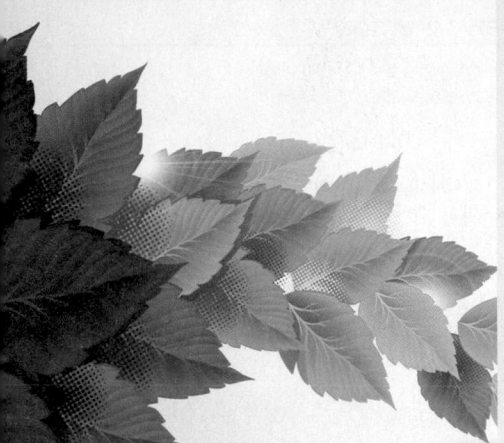

evolve WEBSITE

http://evolve.elsevier.com/Urden/criticalcare/

Evolve features:

- NCLEX Review Questions
- CCRN Review Questions
- PCCN Review Questions
- Mosby's Nursing Skills Procedures
- Animations
- Video Clips
- Glossary

The endocrine system is almost invisible when it functions well, but it causes widespread upset when an organ is suppressed, hyperstimulated, or under physiologic stress. This results in a wide spectrum of possible disorders; some are rare, and others are frequently encountered in the critical care unit. This chapter focuses on the neuroendocrine stress associated with critical illness and on disorders of three major endocrine glands: the pancreas, the posterior pituitary gland, and the thyroid gland.

NEUROENDOCRINOLOGY OF STRESS AND CRITICAL ILLNESS

Major neurologic and endocrine changes occur when an individual is confronted with physiologic stress caused by any critical illness, sepsis,[1] trauma, major surgery, or underlying cardiovascular disease.[2] The normal "fight or flight" response that is initiated in times of physiologic or psychologic stress is exacerbated in critical illness through activation of the neuroendocrine system, specifically the hypothalamic-pituitary-adrenal axis (HPA).[3] All endocrine organs are affected by acute critical illness, as shown in Table 33-1.

Acute Neuroendocrine Response to Critical Illness

The fight or flight acute response to physiologic threat is a rapid discharge of the catecholamines *norepinephrine* and *epinephrine* into the bloodstream.[3] Norepinephrine is released from the nerve endings of the sympathetic nervous system (SNS).

Hypothalamic-Pituitary-Adrenal Axis in Critical Illness

Epinephrine (adrenalin) is released from the medulla of the adrenal glands. Epinephrine increases cerebral blood flow and cerebral oxygen consumption and may be the trigger for recruitment of the hypothalamic-pituitary axis.[3]

The pituitary gland has two parts (anterior and posterior) that function under control of the hypothalamus, as described in Chapter 31.

The *posterior pituitary gland* releases antidiuretic hormone (ADH), also known as *vasopressin* (pitressin), as a component of the physiologic stress response. This hormone is an antidiuretic with a powerful vasoconstrictive effect on blood vessels.[3] The combination of epinephrine and vasopressin quickly raises blood pressure; it also decreases gastric motility.[3] Epinephrine increases heart rate, causes ventricular dysrhythmias in susceptible patients, and provides some analgesia or lack of pain awareness during acute physical stress.[3]

The *anterior pituitary gland* produces several hormones including *corticotropin* (also called ACTH), which stimulates release of *cortisol* from the adrenal cortex.[4] Cortisol release is an important protective response to stress. Increased cortisol levels alter carbohydrate, fat, and protein metabolism so that energy is immediately and selectively available to vital organs such as the brain. However, if critical illness is prolonged, the HPA may not be able to respond adequately to prolonged physiologic stress.

The *adrenal gland* produces cortisol from the cortex and the epinephrine from the medulla. Diminished adrenal gland function may result from a variety of causes during critical illness:

- *Primary hypoadrenalism* describes an intrinsic failure of the adrenal gland to produce normal endogenous glucocorticosteroid hormones (e.g., cortisol) and mineralocorticosteroid hormones (e.g., aldosterone). Primary adrenal failure is rare.

TABLE 33-1   ENDOCRINE RESPONSES TO STRESS

GLAND OR ORGAN	HORMONE	RESPONSE OR PHYSICAL EXAMINATION
Adrenal cortex	Cortisol	↑ Insulin resistance → ↑ glycogenolysis → ↑ glucose circulation
		↑ Hepatic gluconeogenesis → ↑ glucose available
		↑ Lipolysis
		↑ Protein catabolism
		↑ Sodium → ↑ water retention to maintain plasma osmolality by movement of extravascular fluid into the intravascular space
	Glucocorticoid	↓ Connective tissue fibroblasts → poor wound healing
		↓ Histamine release → suppression of immune system
		↓ Lymphocytes, monocytes, eosinophils, basophils
		↑ Polymorphonuclear leukocytes → ↑ infection risk
		↑ Glucose
		↓ Gastric acid secretion
	Mineralocorticoids	↑ Aldosterone → ↓ sodium excretion → ↓ water excretion → ↑ intravascular volume
		↑ Potassium excretion → hypokalemia
		↑ Hydrogen ion excretion → metabolic acidosis
Adrenal medulla	Epinephrine	↑ Endorphins → ↓ pain
	Norepinephrine, epinephrine	↑ Metabolic rate to accommodate stress response
		↑ Live glycogenolysis → ↑ glucose
		↑ Insulin (cells are insulin resistant)
		↑ Cardiac contractility
		↑ Cardiac output
		↑ Dilation of coronary arteries
		↑ Blood pressure
		↑ Heart rate
		↑ Bronchodilation → ↑ respirations
		↑ Perfusion to heart, brain, lungs, liver, and muscle
		↓ Perfusion to periphery of body
		↓ Peristalsis
	Norepinephrine	↑ Peripheral vasoconstriction
		↑ Blood pressure
		↑ Sodium retention
		↑ Potassium excretion
Pituitary	All hormones	↑ Endogenous opioids → ↓ pain
Anterior pituitary	Corticotropin	↑ Aldosterone → ↓ sodium excretion → ↓ water excretion → ↑ intravascular volume
		↑ Cortisol → ↑ blood volume
	Growth hormones	↑ Protein anabolism of amino acids to protein
		↑ Lipolysis → ↑ gluconeogenesis
Posterior pituitary	Antidiuretic hormone	↑ Vasoconstriction
		↑ Water retention → restoration of circulating blood volume
		↓ Urine output
		↑ Hypo-osmolality
Pancreas	Insulin	↑ Insulin resistance → hyperglycemia
	Glucagon	↑ Glycolysis (directly opposes action of insulin)
		↑ Glucose for fuel
		↑ Glycogenolysis
		↑ Gluconeogenesis
		↑ Lipolysis
Thyroid	Thyroxine	↓ Routine metabolic demands during stress
Gonads	Sex hormones	Energy and oxygen supply diverted to brain, heart, muscles, and liver

↑, Increased; →, causes; ↓, decreased.

- *Secondary adrenal dysfunction,* or *Cushing syndrome,* occurs as a result of the administration of therapeutic steroids. In response to exogenous glucocorticosteroids, the adrenal glands stop production of intrinsic hormones. Patients who have taken steroids before their admission to the hospital need their dosage increased during illness.

- *Critical illness—related corticosteroid insufficiency* (CIRCI) describes a situation in which the adrenal gland produces glucocorticosteroids but the quantity is insufficient for the disease process. Peripheral cortisol resistance occurs as inflammatory cytokines induce cellular resistance to cortisol.[5]

Serum Cortisol Level

Clinical assessment of adrenal dysfunction is difficult in the critically ill, and a specialized laboratory assay is necessary for an accurate diagnosis. First, a baseline serum cortisol level is obtained. Adrenal failure is likely if the cortisol level is less than 10 mcg/dL.[5]

Cosyntropin Stimulation Test

Further confirmation of adrenal dysfunction may be obtained by performance of a corticotropin stimulation test *(cosyntropin test)*. Cosyntropin is a medication made from the first 24 amino acids of corticotropin. In the test, 250 mcg cosyntropin is administered by the intravenous (IV) route, and serum blood levels are measured 30 minutes later. A serum cortisol rise from baseline of less than 9 mcg/dL after 30 minutes denotes inability of the adrenal gland to respond to a stress stimulus (nonresponder).[5] If the cortisol rise is greater than 9 mcg/dL in response to corticotropin stimulation, the adrenal glands are functioning normally (responder).[5] Corticosteroids are given only to nonresponders. The combination of a low baseline cortisol value (less than 10 mcg/dL) with minimal or no rise (less than 9 mcg/dL) after cosyntropin stimulation is evidence of adrenal gland dysfunction with corticosteroid deficiency.[5]

Corticosteroid Replacement

Clinical practice guidelines[5] recommend short-term provision of low-dose hydrocortisone for patients who have a diagnosis of septic shock with refractory vasopressor-dependent hypotension. Hydrocortisone is the recommended replacement because it is the pharmacologic steroid that most resembles endogenous cortisol.

The guidelines recommend use of the cosyntropin stimulation test as described previously. However, the test is not recommended as a stand-alone method to identify patients who might receive low-dose steroids. This apparent contradiction is explained by the fact that several clinical trials of low-dose steroid replacement in sepsis have demonstrated a faster resolution of the shock symptoms but no difference in overall mortality compared with placebo.[5] High-dose steroid replacement is never recommended in the management of sepsis. Corticosteroids are never discontinued abruptly and must be tapered gradually over several days.[5]

Liver and Pancreas in Critical Illness

The liver releases the hormone *glucagon* to stimulate the liver to pour additional glucose into the bloodstream in response to physiologic stress. Glucagon rapidly raises blood glucose levels. Peripheral tissues may become *insulin resistant*, meaning the tissues are unable to use the available insulin to transport glucose inside the cells. This further raises blood glucose levels, causing persistent stress-induced hyperglycemia.[6] There is a second metabolic system that enables insulin to enter the cell (see Chapter 31). The insulin-independent *glucose transporters* (GLUT 1, GLUT 2, and GLUT 3) are active during physiologic stress, but may be unable to keep up with the massive increase in glucose production by the liver. Continuous infusion of insulin to return and maintain blood glucose levels within a safe, near-normal range reduces morbidity and mortality.[2]

Hyperglycemia in Critical Illness

Normal fasting blood glucose levels range between 70 and 100 mg/dL in a healthy person. Critically ill patients frequently have much higher blood glucose levels, and several retrospective analyses have reported that hyperglycemic patients have a higher mortality rate than patients with normal blood glucose values. In 2001, a landmark prospective, randomized study showed a significant reduction in morbidity and mortality among critically ill surgical patients whose blood glucose concentration was maintained between 80 and 110 mg/dL with a continuous insulin infusion, compared with those whose blood glucose was only treated if it was greater than 180 mg/dL.[7] A study of medical critical care patients by the same group with the same protocol demonstrated a survival benefit after 3 days of tight glucose control with a continuous insulin infusion.[8] These initial studies were greeted with tremendous enthusiasm and many critical care units adopted stringent glucose control standards to reduce hyperglycemia-associated morbidity and mortality. However, achievement of such tight glucose control outside of a research trial can be challenging as shown by the results of more recent clinical trials.

The NICE-SUGAR trial was a prospective randomized trial of 6014 critically ill patients. It compared continuous insulin infusion to achieve tight glucose control (target 81 to 108 mg/dL) with a conventional glucose control range (target below 180 mg/dL).[9] In the tight glucose control group 6.8% had episodes of severe hypoglycemia (below 40 mg/dL); in the conventional control group only 0.5% experienced severe hypoglycemia.[9] There was a 2.6% higher risk of death in the intensive glucose control group (27.5% died) compared with the conventional control group (24.9% died).[9]

Clinical Practice Guidelines Related to Blood Glucose Management in Critically Ill Patients

As a result of the studies just described, clinical practice guidelines were developed by the American Association of Clinical Endocrinologists (AACE) and the American Diabetes Association (ADA) that recommend the use of continuous insulin infusions to maintain blood glucose in critical care patients between 140 and 180 mg/dL, with frequent monitoring of blood glucose.[2] The 140 to 180 mg/dL level was selected to minimize the risk of hypoglycemia.

Other glucose-control guidelines relevant to critical illness have also been published. The Society of Critical Care Medicine (SCCM) recommends initiating glycemic control when the blood glucose rises above 150 mg/dL.[1,10] Insulin management must be initiated if the blood glucose level is above 180 mg/dL.[2,10] More liberal glucose control represents the current trend of targeted values.

Insulin Management in the Critically Ill

As a result of the research that has highlighted the deleterious effects of hyperglycemia in critical illness, most hospitals have developed an institution-specific glucose–insulin algorithm to lower blood glucose into the targeted range.[11] The vigilance of the critical care nurse is pivotal to the success of any intervention to lower blood glucose using a continuous insulin infusion. As discussed earlier, many glucose control protocols are using less restrictive ranges due to concerns about iatrogenic hypoglycemia.

Frequent Blood Glucose Monitoring

Monitoring the blood glucose with a point-of-care glucometer is the basis of targeted glucose control. As part of the comprehensive initial assessment, the blood sugar is measured by a standard laboratory sample or by a finger-stick capillary blood sample. In many institutions, if the blood sugar is greater than 180 mg/dL, the patient is started on a continuous IV insulin infusion. While the glucose is elevated, blood sample measurements are usually obtained hourly, to allow titration of the insulin drip to lower blood glucose.[11] After the patient is stable, blood glucose measurements can be spaced approximately every 2 hours, based on individual hospital protocols.

Several different blood-sampling methods are available. A capillary finger-stick is perhaps the easiest initial option, although the fingers can become noticeably marked if there are numerous sticks over several days. Trauma to the fingers is also exacerbated if peripheral perfusion is diminished. If a central venous catheter (CVC) or an arterial line with a blood conservation system attached is in place, this can be a highly efficient system for sampling, because there is no blood wastage. If a blood conservation setup is not attached, use of the venous or arterial catheter for access is unacceptable because of the quantity of "waste" blood that would be discarded.

Continuous Insulin Infusion

Many hospitals use insulin infusion protocols for management of stress-induced hyperglycemia that are implemented by the critical care nurse.[2,11] Effective glucose protocols gauge the insulin infusion rate based on two parameters: 1) the immediate blood glucose result and 2) the rate of change in the blood glucose level since the last hourly measurement. The following three examples illustrate this concept:

- Patient A receives 3 units of continuous IV regular insulin per hour and has a blood glucose measurement of 110 mg/dL, but 1 hour ago it was 190 mg/dL; the insulin rate must be decreased to avoid sudden hypoglycemia.
- Patient B receives 3 units of continuous IV regular insulin per hour and has a blood glucose measurement of 110 mg/dL, but 1 hour ago it was 112 mg/dL; in this situation, no change is made in the insulin infusion rate.
- Patient C receives 3 units of continuous IV regular insulin per hour and has a blood glucose measurement of 190 mg/dL, and 1 hour ago it was 197 mg/dL; the insulin rate must be increased to more rapidly move the patient's blood sugar toward the targeted glucose range (i.e., 140 to 180 mg/dL, although this range will vary by individual hospital protocol).

The important point to emphasize is that the *rate of change* of the blood glucose is as important as the *most recent* blood glucose measurement.[11] Each of the patients described in the examples may have the same insulin infusion rate, depending on their catabolic state, but individualization among patients with different diagnoses can be safely achieved as long as the rate of change is also considered.

A person's insulin requirement often fluctuates over the course of an illness. This occurs in response to changes in the clinical condition, such as development of an infection, caloric alterations caused by stopping or starting enteral or parenteral nutrition, administration of therapeutic steroids, or because the person is less catabolic. A method to allow for corrective incremental changes (up or down) to adapt to the reality of clinical developments and maintain the glucose within the target range is essential. Some protocols alter only the infusion rate, whereas others incorporate bolus insulin doses if the glucose concentration is greater than a pre-established threshold (e.g., 180 mg/dL). Typically, after the blood glucose has remained within the target range for a number of hours (varies according to the hospital protocol), the time interval between measurements for blood glucose monitoring may be extended to every 2 hours.

Transition from Continuous to Intermittent Insulin Coverage

The transition from a continuous insulin infusion to intermittent insulin coverage must be handled with care to avoid large fluctuations in blood glucose levels. Before the conversion, the regular insulin infusion should be at a stable and preferably low rate, and the patient's blood glucose level should be maintained consistently within the target range. The transition from IV to subcutaneous administration depends on numerous factors, including whether the patient is able to eat a consistent amount of dietary carbohydrate.[12]

Clinicians use various methods to calculate the quantity of insulin to prescribe during the transition from IV to subcutaneous insulin to maintain stable blood glucose levels. Figure 33-1 depicts hypothetical examples of how a combination of basal and bolus insulin regimens (prandial insulin) can work in clinical practice. The following paragraphs describe the application of one calculation method for a 67-year-old patient, Alice Smith, who is recovering from critical illness and has recently been weaned from the ventilator and extubated.

1. Ms. Smith is in stable condition on a regular insulin drip at 1 unit per hour. She is ready to be transitioned to subcutaneous insulin and will be taking food and liquids by mouth. Her total insulin requirement over the previous 24 hours was 32 units. Ms. Smith will now require basal coverage (provided by subcutaneous intermediate or long-acting insulin) and *prandial* coverage for mealtimes (provided by short-acting subcutaneous insulin).

2. The 30 units of insulin infused during the previous 24 hours is Ms. Smith's required daily insulin dose. To transition to subcutaneous insulin, a proportion of this amount (i.e., 75% to 80%) will be divided between basal and prandial components.[2] In this situation, 75% of the 32 units = 24 units. Half of this amount (12 units) will be administered subcutaneously as intermediate or long-acting insulin; the other half will be administered as short-acting insulin to coincide with meals (i.e., 4 units with each of three meals).

3. The options for insulin administration for Ms. Smith are as follows:

Basal insulin: 12 units of glargine once daily, *or* 6 units twice daily of Neutral Protamine Hagedorn (NPH) administered subcutaneously

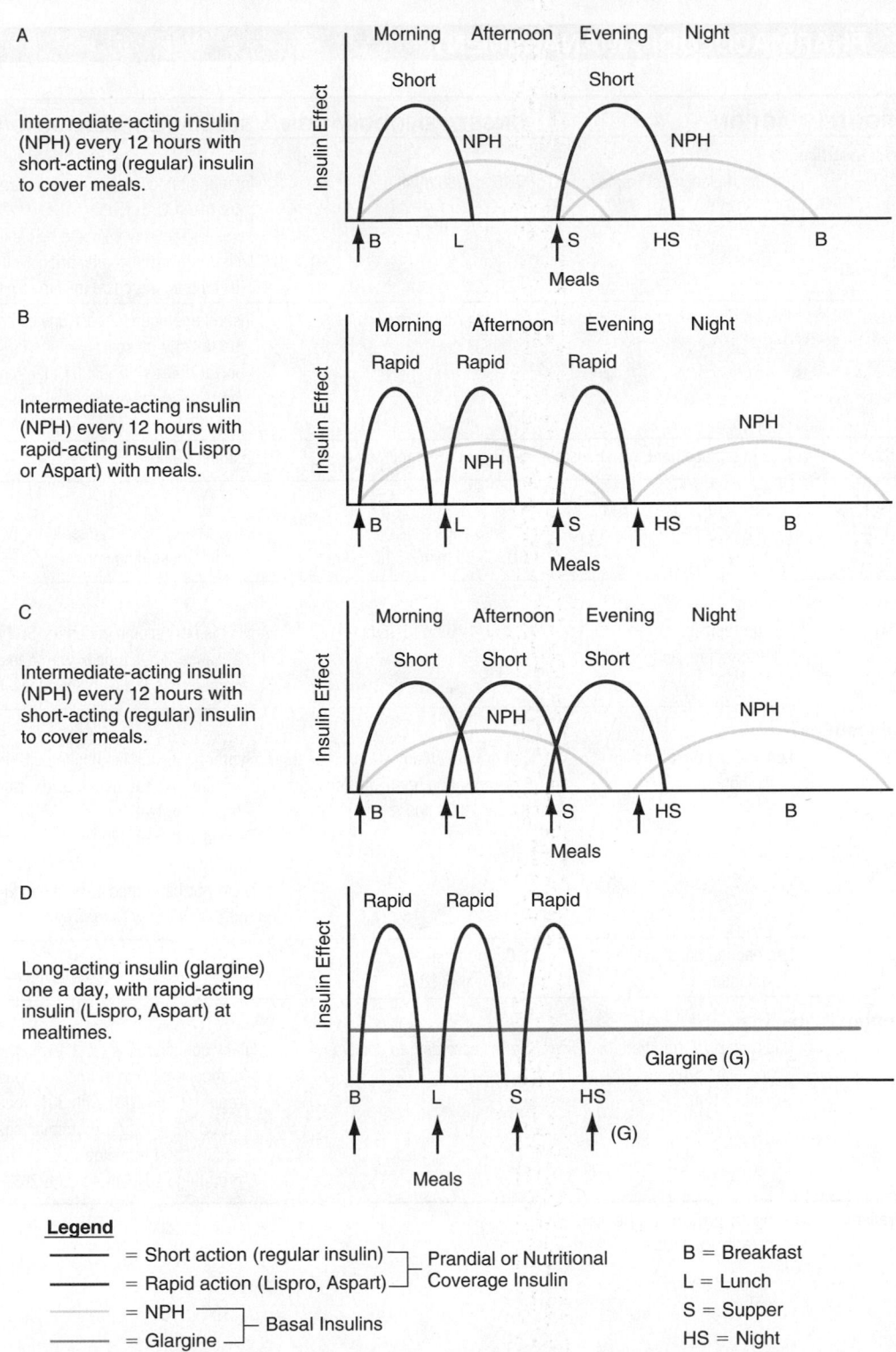

FIGURE 33-1 Basal and nutritional bolus insulin combinations.

Prandial insulin: 4 units regular insulin given subcutaneously before each meal (short-acting), *or* 4 units Lispro or Aspart given subcutaneously with each meal (ultra–short-acting insulin); verify current blood glucose level.

Supplemental corrective insulin: A supplemental correction scale can be used to cover any hyperglycemia above the target range, and administration can be combined with scheduled blood glucose measurements; verify current blood glucose level.

After the transition to subcutaneous insulin, the dosage is adjusted based upon the patient's *insulin sensitivity*, or stated another way, according to how much insulin is needed for each 15 grams of carbohydrate intake. Patients who are *insulin resistant* require more insulin than those who are *insulin sensitive*.

Table 33-2 describes the various types of insulin available for use. These include ultra–short-acting, short-acting, intermediate-acting, long-acting, and combination insulin replacement options.[13] Even after the transition to subcutaneous insulin is

TABLE 33-2 PHARMACOLOGIC MANAGEMENT

Insulin*

INSULIN	ROUTE†	ACTION	ONSET/PEAK/DURATION	SPECIAL CONSIDERATIONS
Ultra–Short-Acting Insulins				
Aspart (NovoLog)	SQ	Insulin replacement, rapid onset	5-15 min/30-90 min/<5 hr	Insulin analogue almost *immediately* absorbed; must be taken with food. Insulin appearance should be clear. Must be used in combination with intermediate-acting or long-acting basal insulin regimen. See Fig. 33-1.
Lispro (Humalog)	SQ	Insulin replacement, rapid onset	5-15 min/30-90 min/<5 hr	Insulin analogue; almost *immediately* absorbed; must be taken with food. Shorter duration of action than regular insulin; should be used with basal longer-acting insulin. See Fig. 33-1.
Glulisine (Apidra)	SQ	Insulin replacement, rapid onset	5-15 min/30-90 min/<5 hr	Insulin analog
Short-Acting Insulin				
Regular	IV or SQ	Insulin replacement therapy	IV: <15 min SQ: 30-60 min/2-3 hr/5-8 hr	Only type of insulin suitable for IV continuous infusion or IV bolus administration
Intermediate-Acting Basal Insulin				
Neutral Protamine Hagedorn (NPH)	SQ	Insulin replacement, intermediate action	2-4 hr/4-10 hr/10-16 hr	NPH is not recommended for SQ basal insulin because it has a peak with a less predictable time course than the long-acting insulin analogs.
Long-Acting Basal Insulins				
Glargine (Lantus)	SQ	Long-acting basal insulin analogue;	2-4 hr until steady state/no peak Concentration relatively constant over 20-24 hours	Synthetic insulin (analogue); differs from human insulin by three amino acids, slow release over 24 hours; no peak. Decrease dose by 20% if switching from NPH to glargine. Must not be diluted or mixed with other insulins. See Fig. 33-1.
Detemir (Levemir)	SQ	Long-acting basal insulin analogue	3-8 hr until steady state/ no peak/5-23 hr	
Combination (Premixed) Insulins				
Various	SQ	Rapid plus intermediate or long-acting insulin combination	Varies according to combination used	Many combinations exist; examples (long-acting component/short-acting component) include 70/30 regular (70% NPH with 30% regular), NovoLog mix 70/30 (70% aspart-protamine suspension with 30% aspart), and Humalog mix 75/25 (75% lispro-protamine suspension with 25% lispro).

*Dosages are individualized according to patient's age and size.
†Only regular insulin is suitable for intravenous use.
IV, Intravenous; *SQ*, subcutaneous.

completed, blood glucose is monitored frequently to maintain blood glucose within the target range and detect hyperglycemia or hypoglycemia.[14]

Corrective Insulin Coverage

A patient may be prescribed supplemental or corrective doses of insulin in addition to the basal/prandial insulin combination. The use of the trio of basal, prandial, and corrective insulin is designed to eliminate the use of the traditional sliding scale. Criticisms of the sliding scale method are that the dosages are rarely re-evaluated or adjusted once established and that the scales treat hyperglycemia only after it has occurred; they are not proactive in the manner of the basal/bolus/corrective insulin method.[11]

Hypoglycemia Management

It is important to have a protocol for the management of hypoglycemia. The major drawback to use of intensive insulin protocols, as described earlier, is the potential for hypoglycemia.[14] Whenever hypoglycemia is detected, it is important to *stop* any continuous infusion of insulin. An example of one protocol to reverse hypoglycemia follows:

Stress of Critical Illness

- Deficient Fluid Volume related to absolute loss, p. 1132
- Imbalanced Nutrition: Less Than Body Requirements related to exogenous nutrients and increased metabolic demand, p. 1143
- Risk For Infection, p. 1160
- Risk for Ineffective Peripheral Tissue Perfusion, p. 1158
- Compromised Family Coping related to critically ill family member, p. 1127

BOX 33-2 **PATIENT EDUCATION**

Stress of Critical Illness

- Even if the patient is unresponsive because of the underlying critical illness or because of sedation and analgesic medications, brief explanations of procedures are quietly and simply given before interventions.
- During the period of acute illness, questions are answered and information is provided to the family and significant others.
- After recovery additional information is provided to the patient concerning their illness.

- Blood glucose level lower than 40 mg/dL (severe hypoglycemia): administer 50 mL dextrose (50%) in water ($D_{50}W$) as an IV bolus.
- Blood glucose level between 40 and 70 mg/dL (hypoglycemia): administer 25 mL of $D_{50}W$ as an IV bolus.

In all cases of hypoglycemia, the blood glucose concentration is monitored every 15 minutes until the blood glucose has risen above 70 mg/dL.

Nursing Management

Nursing management of the patient with neuroendocrine stress resulting from critical illness incorporates a variety of nursing diagnoses (Box 33-1). The goals of nursing management are to monitor the hyperglycemic side effects of vasopressor therapy; administer prescribed corticosteroids; monitor blood glucose and insulin effectiveness; avoid hypoglycemia; provide nutrition; and provide education to the patient's family and supportive others (Box 33-2).

Monitor Hyperglycemic Side Effects of Vasopressor Therapy

Two vasopressors frequently used as continuous infusions to counteract hypotension also raise blood glucose. Epinephrine and norepinephrine stimulate gluconeogenesis (creation of new glucose), increase liver glycogenolysis (glucose production), increase lipolysis (fat breakdown), suppress insulin secretion, and increase peripheral insulin resistance. All of these actions increase blood glucose.

Administer Prescribed Corticosteroids

Critically ill patients with below-normal cortisol levels may be prescribed IV hydrocortisone.[1] Therapeutic steroids raise blood glucose levels and can make glycemic control more difficult. Frequent monitoring of the blood glucose concentration is necessary to guide treatment of hyperglycemia in the patient receiving IV corticosteroids. Ongoing monitoring for the presence of new infection is mandatory.

Monitor Blood Glucose, Insulin Effectiveness, Avoid Hypoglycemia

The critical care nurse is responsible for the hourly monitoring of blood glucose and titration of the insulin infusion according to the hospital's protocol while the patient is hyperglycemic. The use of standardized protocols makes possible a systematic approach to the control of blood glucose. It is essential and recommended that nurses receive effective and ongoing education about the anabolic impact of insulin therapy in critical illness.[2] Hospital protocols to minimize development of hypoglycemia, such as using the 140-180 mg/dL target range,[2] and rapid reversal of any occurrence of severe hypoglycemia (below 40 mg/dL) by provision of IV dextrose ($D_{50}W$) are essential.[10]

Provide Nutrition

Whenever an insulin infusion is started to lower blood glucose, enteral nutritional support should be considered. In the absence of nutrition, a 10% dextrose solution may temporarily be infused. The 10% dextrose offers the advantage of carbohydrate calories for metabolism, limits fluctuations in the blood sugar, and reduces the risk of hypoglycemia. After the patient's metabolic condition is stable, introduction of non-glucose nutrition (protein and fat) is recommended.[15]

Patient Education

While the patient is acutely ill, most of the educational interventions are directed to the family at the bedside. Numerous explications are required to describe the IV medications, the nutritional needs, the purpose of insulin, the role of steroids (if applicable), the ongoing nursing care, prevention of complications, and management of the underlying disease process. Educational issues that may be discussed are listed in the Box 33-2.

Collaborative Management

It is well established that standardized protocols designed to manage the complications of critical illness result in lower morbidity and mortality for patients. Optimally, all disciplines concerned with the endocrine status of the patient will have participated in the hospital's guidelines related to targeted glucose control. Guidelines for blood glucose monitoring in critical illness are described in Box 33-3.[2,16]

DIABETES MELLITUS

Diabetes mellitus is a progressive endocrinopathy associated with carbohydrate intolerance and insulin dysregulation.

Diagnosis of Diabetes

Diabetes mellitus is diagnosed by measurement of the fasting plasma glucose (FPG) or by a glycated hemoglobin above 6.5%.[16] The blood glucose may also be called a fasting blood glucose (FBG). The benchmarks for a normal blood glucose value have been progressively lowered as more knowledge has been gained about the benefits of maintaining the plasma glucose level as close to normal as possible.

Blood glucose values endorsed by the ADA are as follows[16]:
- An FPG level 70 to 100 mg/dL (5.6 mmol/L) signifies normal fasting glucose.

- An FPG level between 100 and 125 mg/dL (5.6 and 6.9 mmol/L) denotes impaired fasting glucose (IFG).
- An FPG level greater than 126 mg/dL (7 mmol/L) provides a diagnosis of diabetes (result is verified by testing more than once).

The benefit and importance of maintaining blood glucose at levels as close to normal as possible has been conclusively demonstrated in patients with type 1 and type 2 diabetes. The Diabetes Control and Complications Trial (DCCT) of 1995 on type 1 diabetes and the United Kingdom Prospective Diabetes Study (UKPDS), published in 1998, on type 2 diabetes demonstrated that lifestyle changes and use of medications that lead to consistently normal glucose levels reduce microvascular diabetes-related complications and decrease mortality.

Types of Diabetes

Two distinct types of diabetes are discussed in this chapter[17]:
- Type 1 diabetes results from beta-cell destruction, usually leading to absolute insulin deficiency.
- Type 2 diabetes results from a progressive insulin secretory defect in addition to insulin resistance.

The two diseases are different in nature, cause, treatment, and prognosis. A further category of *prediabetes* describes patients with impaired fasting glucose (FPG between 100 and 125 mg/dL) who are likely to develop diabetes in the future and who are at increased risk for coronary artery disease and stroke.[16] Other conditions, such as gestational diabetes, are not discussed in this chapter.

Glycated Hemoglobin

For individuals with diabetes, maintenance of blood glucose within a tight normal range is fundamental to avoid the development of microvascular and neuropathic secondary conditions. Although the plasma glucose produces a snapshot of the blood glucose concentration at a single point in time, the *glycated hemoglobin* (HbA_{1C}), also known as a *glycosylated hemoglobin*, measures the percentage of glucose the red cells have absorbed from the plasma over the previous 3-month period. The optimal target for patients with diabetes is an A_{1C} value below 6.5%.[16]

Type 1 Diabetes

Type 1 diabetes mellitus accounts for only about 5% to 10% of the diabetic population.[17] Older names for this condition included insulin-dependent diabetes (IDDM) and juvenile diabetes. Type 1 diabetes is an autoimmune disease that causes progressive destruction of the beta cells of the islets of Langerhans in the pancreas. Autoantibodies that falsely identify self as a foreign invader to be destroyed can now be identified by laboratory analysis. Autoantibodies that contribute to pancreatic destruction include autoantibodies to the islet cell, to insulin, to glutamic acid decarboxylase (GAD_{65}), and to the tyrosine phosphatases IA-2 and IA-2β (beta).[17] One or more of these autoantibodies are present in 85% to 90% of individuals with type 1 diabetes when fasting hyperglycemia is initially detected.[17] Over time, the autoantibodies render the pancreatic beta cells incapable of secreting insulin and regulating intracellular glucose. In type 1 diabetes, the rate of beta-cell destruction is highly variable. It occurs rapidly in some individuals (mainly children) and slowly in others (mainly adults). Some patients, particularly children and adolescents, may have ketoacidosis as the first manifestation of their disease.

Genetic predisposition and unknown environmental factors are also believed to play an important role.[17] Patients with type 1 diabetes are prone to development of other autoimmune disorders such as Graves disease (hyperthyroidism), Hashimoto thyroiditis, Addison disease, autoimmune hepatitis, myasthenia gravis, and pernicious anemia.[17] Lack of insulin impairs carbohydrate, protein, and fat metabolism.

Management of Type 1 Diabetes

Patients with type 1 diabetes must receive IV or subcutaneous insulin therapy. Treatment with exogenous insulin replacement restores normal entry of glucose into the cells. The range of insulin replacements available is expanding, and it is essential that critical care nurses be knowledgeable about this class of medications (see Table 33-2). Without insulin, the rapid breakdown of noncarbohydrate substrate, particularly fat, leads to ketonemia, ketonuria, and diabetic ketoacidosis (DKA), a life-threatening complication associated with type 1 diabetes (see later discussion).

Type 2 Diabetes

Type 2 diabetes accounts for 90% to 95% of those with diabetes.[17] Previously used names for this condition were non–insulin-dependent diabetes, type II diabetes, or adult-onset diabetes.[17] Type 2 diabetes is identified by *insulin resistance* with a relative, versus absolute, insulin deficiency. Most patients with type 2 diabetes are obese, with excess adipose tissue concentrated in the abdominal area. The onset of hyperglycemia occurs gradually and many people are unaware that they have diabetes. Initially, type 2 diabetes is managed by oral medications (non–insulin therapies) because the pancreatic beta cells remain functional. Although, as progressive beta cell dysfunction occurs, a basal long-acting insulin is added to the oral noninsulin medications.[18,19]

Insulin resistance describes a complex metabolic situation in which organ and tissue cells deny entry to insulin and glucose. This creates the clinical paradox in which elevated serum insulin levels and hyperglycemia are present at the same time. Insulin resistance has a strong association with obesity.

Lifestyle Management for Type 2 Diabetes

For most patients with type 2 diabetes, a program of weight reduction, increased physical exercise, and a change in diet pattern is the first step.[18] The diet should contain less than 30% of calories from fat, with an increased quantity of whole grains, vegetables, and fruits. Crash diets are discouraged, and a gradual program of weight loss, if needed, is recommended. The exercise program is tailored to the individual but might start with 30 minutes of brisk walking each day if the person was previously sedentary.

Patients who have type 2 diabetes are prone to a wide range of other complications that increase morbidity and mortality. In addition to medications to control blood glucose, patients often require medications to lower their blood pressure, lower their cholesterol and triglyceride levels, treat ischemic heart disease, and manage symptoms of heart failure.[16,19]

Pharmacologic Management of Type 2 Diabetes

If lifestyle changes are unsuccessful in reversing the pattern of type 2 diabetes, oral noninsulin antihyperglycemic medications are prescribed (Table 33-3).[16] These medications are not oral forms of insulin, because insulin would be destroyed by gastric juices. There are several types of oral agents: sulfonylureas, glinides, biguanides, thiazolidinediones, alpha-glucosidase inhibitors, incretin mimetics, and incretin enhancers. These oral antidiabetic medications work to lower plasma glucose levels by a variety of mechanisms: increasing insulin secretion, increasing sensitivity to insulin, and delaying carbohydrate absorption (Box 33-4). The pharmacologic management of type 2 diabetes is increasingly complex. Current guidelines recommend a patient-focused, individualized approach that includes pharmacologic management and risk factor modification to reduce early mortality from cardiovascular disease.[19]

Insulin secretagogues stimulate the secretion of insulin from the pancreatic beta cells. Two medication classes have this action: the second generation *sulfonylureas* (glyburide, glipizide, glimepiride, and gliclazide), and the *meglitinides* (repaglinide and nateglinide).[16] The sulfonylureas reduce the A_{1C} by 1 to 2 percentage points and have a long duration of action. Side effects include hypoglycemia and weight gain.[18]

Insulin sensitizers work at two locations in the body. They increase insulin sensitivity in the liver, thereby increasing the ability of insulin to suppress endogenous glucose production, and they increase insulin sensitivity at the peripheral cellular level (fat and muscle), to increase glucose uptake. Two separate classes of medications work in different ways to increase insulin sensitivity.

The *biguanides* (metformin) increase insulin sensitivity in the liver and have only a minor effect on skeletal muscle. Metformin is considered first-line therapy for patients with type 2 diabetes.[18,20] Metformin may be used as monotherapy or be combined with basal insulin or with other oral medications that lower blood glucose.[18] Metformin is associated with a rare risk of metabolic acidosis; gastrointestinal side effects are common.

The *thiazolidinediones* (TZDs), also known as *glitazones* (pioglitazone and rosiglitazone), belong to a class of medications called *peroxisome proliferator–activated receptor gamma modulators*, which increase the sensitivity of muscle, fat, and liver cells to endogenous and exogenous insulin (insulin

TABLE 33-3 PHARMACOLOGIC MANAGEMENT

Medications for Type 2 Diabetes

MEDICATION*	DOSAGE	ACTION	ONSET/PEAK/ DURATION	SPECIAL CONSIDERATIONS
Insulin Secretagogues				
Second-Generation Sulfonylureas				
Glipizide (Glucotrol)	*Initial dosage:* Immediate release tablet 5 mg once/day *Maximum dose:* 40 mg bid	Stimulates insulin release	1 hr/1-3 hr/12-24 hr	Administer with breakfast or after first main meal Also available in an extended release formulation (Glucotrol XL); do not cut, crush, or chew. Extended release: *Initial dosage:* 5 mg, once daily; *maximum dose:* 20 mg/day. Adjust dose if creatinine clearance <50 mL/min.
Glyburide (DiaBeta; Micronase)	*Initial dosage:* 2.5 mg once/day *Maintenance dosage:* 1.5–20 mg/day	Stimulates insulin release	1 hr/4 hr/18-24 hr	Administer with breakfast or first main meal
Glimepiride (Amaryl)	*Initial dosage:* 1-2 mg once/day *Maximum dosage:* 8 mg once/day	Stimulates insulin release	Duration 24 hours	Administer with breakfast or first main meal of day Initial dose is lower in patients with kidney dysfunction (1 mg once/day)

Continued

TABLE 33-3 **PHARMACOLOGIC MANAGEMENT**

Medications for Type 2 Diabetes—cont'd

MEDICATION*	DOSAGE	ACTION	ONSET/PEAK/ DURATION	SPECIAL CONSIDERATIONS
Meglitinides				
Nateglinide (Starlix)	*Initial dosage:* 120 mg tid *Maximum dosage:* 120 mg tid	Stimulates insulin release	Peak <1 hour	Administer 15-30 minutes before meals Cut dose in half (i.e., 60 mg tid) for frail older patients and for those near their HA_{1c} target
Repaglinide (Prandin)	*Initial dosage:* 1-2 mg tid *Maximum dosage:* 16 mg per day	Stimulates insulin release		Administer 15-30 minutes before meals Cut dose in half (i.e., 0.5 mg tid) for frail older patients
Insulin Sensitizers **Biguanides**				
Metformin (Glucophage)	*Initial dosage:* 500 mg bid; or 850 mg in morning *Maximum dosage:* 2550 mg tid	Reduces glucose output from liver Increases insulin action by decreasing peripheral insulin resistance	1-3 hr/24 hr/24-48 hr	Temporarily withhold if patient is having contrast radiography Adverse effects: lactic acidosis (rare) GI upset Use extreme caution in patients with creatinine clearance <50 mL/min
Thiazolidinediones (TZDs)				
Pioglitazone (Actos)	*Initial dosage:* 15-30 mg bid *Maximum dosage:* 45 mg once/daily	Increases peripheral insulin sensitivity	Peak 2-3 hours	Associated with weight gain, edema and heart failure Bone fractures
Rosiglitazone (Avandia)	*Initial dosage:* 4 mg once/day or 2 mg bid *Maximum dosage:* 8 mg once/day or 4 mg bid	Increases peripheral insulin sensitivity		Associated with weight gain, edema and heart failure LDL cholesterol increase FDA warnings on cardiovascular safety Bone fractures
Carbohydrate Inhibitors ***Alpha-Glucosidase Inhibitors***				
Acarbose (Precose)	*Initial dosage:* 25 mg tid *Maximum dosage:* 100 mg tid	Delays carbohydrate digestion by blocking absorption of complete carbohydrates in small intestine	Peak 2-3 hours	Administer with first bite of each meal GI side effects (flatulence, abdominal pain, diarrhea) Not recommended in severe kidney dysfunction
Miglitol (Glyset)	*Initial dosage:* 25 mg tid *Maximum dosage:* 100 mg tid		Peak 2-3 hours	Administer with first bite of each meal
Incretin Mimics and Enhancers ***Incretin Mimetics***				
Exenatide (Byetta) Exenatide extended release (Bydureon)	*Initial dosage (immediate release):* 5 mg bid; after 1 month may increase to 10 mg bid *Extended release:* 2 mg once/ week	Activates GLP-1 receptors in pancreatic beta cells		SQ injection, avoid if creatinine clearance <30 mL/min GI side effects (nausea, vomiting diarrhea) Pancreatitis has occurred.
Liraglutide (Victoza)	*Initial dosage:* 0.6 mg SQ once/day (irrespective of meals) for 7 days, then increase to 1.2 mg once/day	Same as above.		Pancreatitis has occurred
Incretin Enhancers				
Sitagliptin: 100 mg oral once/day Saxagliptin: 2.5 to 5 mg oral once/day		Inhibits DPP-4 hormone activity, prolongs survival of endogenously released incretin hormones		Pancreatitis has occurred Reduce dosage with kidney dysfunction for Sitagliptin and Saxagliptin
Linagliptin: 5 mg oral once/day				No dosage adjustment for kidney dysfunction needed with Linagliptin

bid, Twice daily; *DPP-4*, dipeptidyl peptidase-4; *GI*, gastrointestinal; *GLP-1*, glucagon like peptide-1; *LDL*, low-density lipoprotein; *tid*, three times daily.

*Combination medications are too numerous to include in this table.

BOX 33-4 ORAL ANTIHYPERGLYCEMIC MEDICATION ACTIONS

- Medications that stimulate the pancreas to make more insulin (insulin secretagogues)
  - Sulfonylureas
  - Glinides
- Medications that sensitize the body to insulin (insulin sensitizers)
  - Biguanides
  - Thiazolidinediones
- Medications that delay carbohydrate absorption from small intestine
  - Alpha-glucosidase inhibitors
- Medications that augment gut incretin hormone effects
  - Incretin mimetics
  - Incretin enhancers

sensitizers).[21] Caution is recommended when using these medications with patients who have risk factors for heart failure (pioglitazone and rosiglitazone), or risk factors for myocardial infarction (rosiglitazone).[18]

The *alpha-glucosidase inhibitors* slow digestion of ingested carbohydrates in the proximal small intestine.[18] These medications delay glucose absorption and reduce postprandial hyperglycemia following meals.[22] The medications in this class are acarbose and miglitol.[19] A review of the physiology of carbohydrate digestion is helpful to understand how these agents work. Carbohydrates are broken down to absorbable components in the duodenum and upper jejunum. The carbohydrates are digested to oligosaccharides in the small intestine by pancreatic lipase, after which the oligosaccharides are cleaved to monosaccharides by *alpha-glucosidase enzymes*. The monosaccharides are then available to be absorbed from the intestine into the bloodstream. The alpha-glucosidase inhibitor medications work by decreasing the conversion of carbohydrates from oligosaccharides to monosaccharides, thus limiting the rise in blood glucose that occurs after eating. The most frequently prescribed medication in this class is acarbose, which is nonabsorbable.

A newer class of medications lowers blood glucose by acting on gastric *incretin* hormones. The main therapeutic target is the incretin hormone *glucagon-like peptide-1* (GLP-1), which is secreted from the gastric mucosa in response to food ingestion. GLP-1 stimulates the pancreatic beta cells to produce insulin. See Table 31-3 in Chapter 31 for a description of the incretin hormones' physiologic effects.[23]

Pharmacologic incretin therapies have two different mechanisms of action[16]:

- The *incretin mimetics* augment activity of GLP-1. The medications are *GLP-1 receptor agonists* that increase insulin secretion from the pancreatic beta-receptors. The medications in this class are administered by subcutaneous injection (exenatide and liraglutide).
- The *incretin enhancers* inhibit degradation of GLP-1 by dipeptidyl peptidase-4 (DPP-4). The medications are *DPP-4 inhibitors* and they slow the degradation of native GLP-1 hormone by the enzyme DPP-4; this extends the physiologic glucose-lowering activity of GLP-1. The DPP-4 inhibitor oral medications (sitagliptin, saxagliptin, linagliptin) are recommended in current guidelines for management of hyperglycemia in type 2 diabetes.[19]

A serious complication of type 2 diabetes that, when present, mandates admission to a critical care unit, is hyperglycemic hyperosmolar state (HHS). This severe, sustained elevation of glucose levels leads to a serum hyperosmolality, and if left untreated, it progresses toward cellular dehydration, coma, and death (discussed later).

DIABETIC KETOACIDOSIS

Epidemiology and Etiology

DKA is a life-threatening complication of diabetes mellitus. Type 1 diabetics who are dependent on insulin are typically affected.

The diagnostic criteria for DKA are as follows[24]:

- Blood glucose greater than 250 mg/dL
- pH less than 7.3
- Serum bicarbonate less than 18 mEq/L
- Moderate or severe ketonemia or ketonuria

DKA is categorized as mild, moderate, or severe depending on the severity of the metabolic acidosis (assessed by blood pH, bicarbonate, ketones) and by the presence of altered mental status (Table 33-4).[24] Hospitalizations for DKA are increasing.[24] DKA accounts for more than 500,000 hospital days per year, with hospital costs that exceed $2.4 billion per year.[24] Infection is the most common precipitating cause of DKA.[24] Symptoms of fatigue and polyuria may precede full-blown DKA, which can develop in less than 24 hours in a person with type 1 diabetes. In a patient with undiagnosed diabetes, it is unknown how long it may take for DKA to develop as the pancreatic beta cells gradually fail. Hospital admission is generally required for DKA related to new-onset type 1 diabetes. With management by experienced clinicians, the mortality rate from DKA in type 1 diabetics is less than 1%.[24]

Changes in the type of insulin, change in dosage, or increased metabolic demand can precipitate DKA in individuals with type 1 diabetes.[24] Life cycle changes, such as growth spurts in the adolescent, require an increase in insulin intake, as do surgery, infection, and trauma. In young persons with diabetes, psychologic problems combined with eating disorders are a contributing factor in up to 20% of cases of recurrent ketoacidosis.[24]

Ketoacidosis also occurs with acute pancreatitis. In addition to elevated glucose and acidosis, the serum amylase and lipase are abnormally high, which helps to establish pancreatitis as a separate diagnosis from type 1 diabetes. Other nondiabetic causes of ketoacidosis are starvation ketosis and alcoholic ketoacidosis. These cases are distinguished from classic DKA by clinical history and usually by a plasma glucose below 200 mg/dL.[24]

Pathophysiology
Insulin Deficiency

Insulin is the metabolic key to the transfer of glucose from the bloodstream into the cell, where it can be used immediately for energy or stored for use at a later time. Without insulin, glucose remains in the bloodstream, and cells are deprived of their energy source. A complex pathophysiologic chain of events follows (Fig. 33-2). The release of glucagon from the liver is stimulated when insulin is ineffective in providing the cells with

TABLE 33-4   **DIAGNOSTIC CRITERIA FOR DIABETIC KETOACIDOSIS (DKA) AND HYPERGLYCEMIC HYPEROSMOLAR SYNDROME (HHS)**

	DKA			HHS
	MILD (PLASMA GLUCOSE >250 mg/dL)	**MODERATE (PLASMA GLUCOSE >250 mg/dL)**	**SEVERE (PLASMA GLUCOSE >250 mg/dL)**	**PLASMA GLUCOSE >600 mg/dL**
Arterial pH	7.25-7.30	7.00 to <7.24	<7.00	>7.30
Serum bicarbonate (mEq/L)	15-18	10 to <15	<10	>18
Urine ketone*	Positive	Positive	Positive	Small
Serum ketone*	Positive	Positive	Positive	Small
Effective serum osmolality†	Variable	Variable	Variable	>320 mOsm/kg
Anion gap‡	>10	>12	>12	Variable
Mental status	Alert	Alert/drowsy	Stupor/coma	Stupor/coma

Data from Kitabchi AE, et al. Hyperglycemic crises in adult patients with diabetes: a consensus statement from the American Diabetes Association. *Diabetes Care*. 2009;32(7):1335.
*Nitroprusside reaction method.
†Effective serum osmolality: 2[measured Na⁺ (mEq/L)] + glucose (mg/dL)18.
 Anion gap: (Na⁺) − (Cl + HCO₃⁻)mEq/L.

glucose for energy. Glucagon increases the amount of glucose in the bloodstream by breaking down stored glucose (glycogenolysis). Noncarbohydrates (fat and protein) are converted into glucose (gluconeogenesis). Plasma glucose levels for the patient in DKA typically are above 250 mg/dL. Elevated serum glucose levels alone do not define DKA; the other crucial determining factor is the presence of ketoacidosis as listed in Table 33-4.[24] About 10% of patients in DKA present to the hospital with a plasma glucose below 250 mg/dL and with ketoacidosis.[24]

Hyperglycemia

Hyperglycemia increases the plasma osmolality, and the blood becomes hyperosmolar. Cellular dehydration occurs as the hyperosmolar extracellular fluid draws the more dilute intracellular and interstitial fluid into the vascular space in an attempt to return the plasma osmolality to normal. Dehydration stimulates catecholamine production in an effort to provide emergency support. Catecholamine output stimulates further glycogenolysis, lipolysis, and gluconeogenesis, pouring glucose into the bloodstream.

Fluid Volume Deficit

Polyuria (excessive urination) and *glycosuria* (sugar in the urine) occur as a result of the osmotic particle load that occurs with DKA. The excess glucose, filtered at the glomeruli, cannot be resorbed at the renal tubule and spills into the urine. The unresorbed solute exerts its own osmotic pull in the renal tubules, and less water is returned to circulation through the collecting ducts. As a result, large volumes of water, along with sodium, potassium, and phosphorus, are excreted in the urine, causing a fluid volume deficit. The serum sodium concentration may be decreased because of the movement of water from the intracellular to the extracellular (vascular) space.[24]

Ketoacidosis

In the healthy individual, the presence of insulin in the bloodstream suppresses the manufacture of ketones. In insulin deficiency states, fat is rapidly converted into glucose

(gluconeogenesis). *Ketoacidosis* occurs when free fatty acids are metabolized into ketones: acetoacetate, β-hydroxybutyrate, and acetone are the three ketone bodies that are produced. During normal metabolism, the ratio of β-hydroxybutyrate to acetoacetate is 1:1, with acetone present in only small amounts. In insulin deficiency, the quantities of all three ketone bodies increase substantially, and the ratio of β-hydroxybutyrate to acetoacetate increases to as much as 10:1. β-Hydroxybutyrate and acetoacetate are the ketones responsible for acidosis in DKA. Acetone does not cause acidosis and is safely excreted in the lungs, causing the characteristic fruity odor.

Ketones are measurable in the bloodstream (ketonemia). Blood tests that measure the quantity of β-hydroxybutyric acid, the predominant ketone body in the blood, are the most useful.[24] Because ketones are excreted by the kidney, they are also measurable in the urine (*ketonuria*). Ketone blood tests are preferred over urine tests for diagnosis and monitoring of DKA in critical care. When the blood and urine become clear of ketones, the DKA is resolved.

Acid–Base Balance

The acid–base balance varies depending on the severity of the DKA. The patient with mild DKA typically has a pH between 7.25 and 7.30. In severe DKA, the pH can drop below 7.00 (see Table 33-4).[24] Acid ketones dissociate and yield hydrogen ions (H⁺), which accumulate and precipitate a fall in serum pH. The level of serum bicarbonate also decreases, consistent with a diagnosis of metabolic acidosis. Breathing becomes deep and rapid (Kussmaul respirations) to release carbonic acid in the form of carbon dioxide. Acetone is exhaled, giving the breath its characteristic fruity odor.

Gluconeogenesis

Gluconeogenesis is the process of breaking down fat or protein to make new glucose. Fat is metabolized to ketones, as described earlier. Protein used for gluconeogenesis leaves no reserve protein available for synthesis and repair of vital body tissues. Nitrogen accumulates as protein is metabolized to urea. Urea,

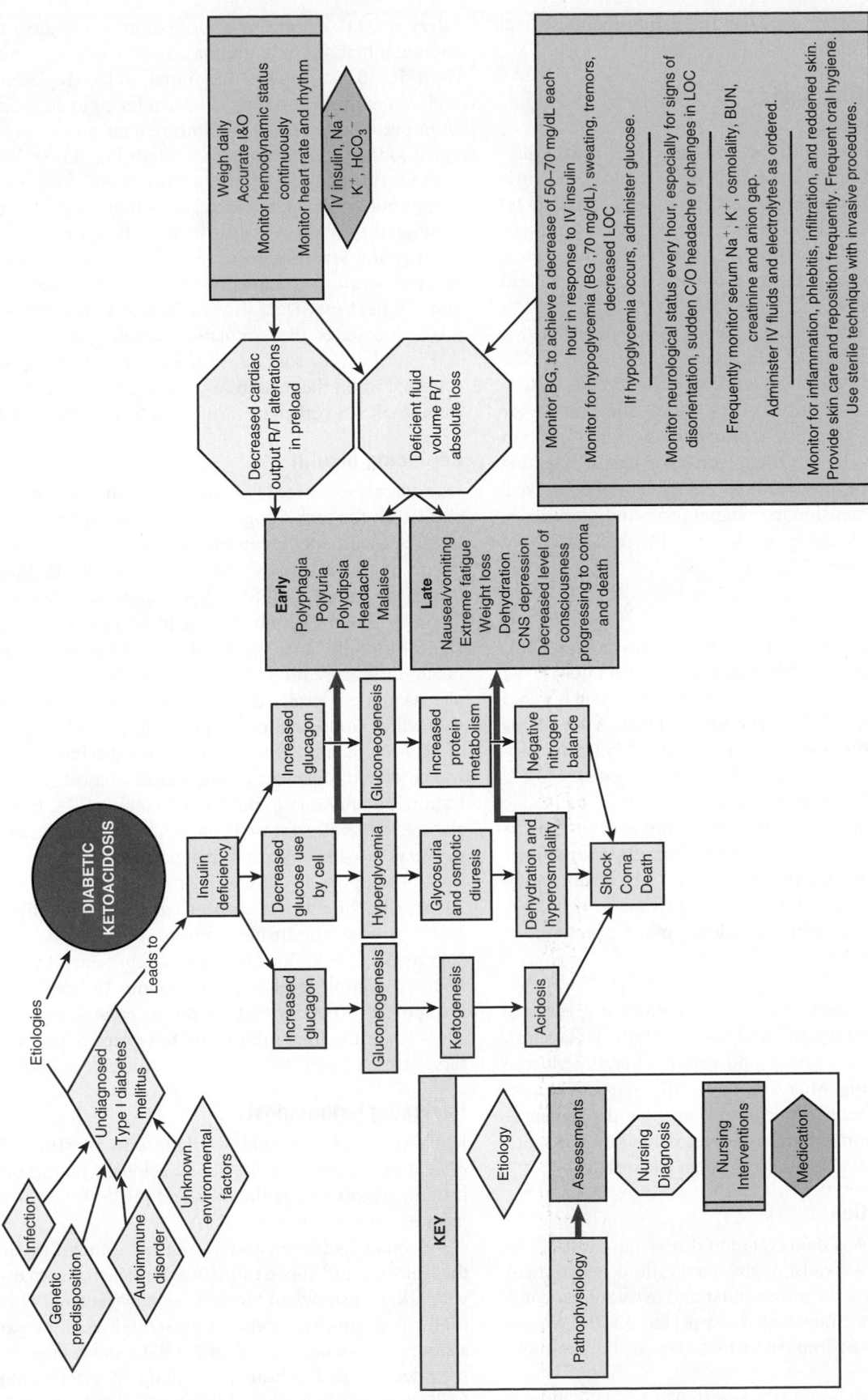

FIGURE 33-2 Concept Map for Diabetic Ketoacidosis. (Concept map illustration created by Elaine Bishop Kennedy, EdD, RN.)

added to the bloodstream, increases the osmotic diuresis and accentuates the dehydration.

Assessment and Diagnosis
Clinical Manifestations

DKA has a predictable clinical presentation. It is usually preceded by patient complaints of malaise, headache, polyuria (excessive urination), polydipsia (excessive thirst), and polyphagia (excessive hunger). Nausea, vomiting, extreme fatigue, dehydration, and weight loss follow. Central nervous system depression, with changes in the level of consciousness, can lead quickly to coma.[16,24]

The patient with DKA may be stuporous or unresponsive, depending on the degree of fluid-balance disturbance. The physical examination reveals evidence of dehydration, including flushed dry skin, dry buccal membranes, and skin turgor that takes longer than 3 seconds to return to its original position after the skin has been lifted. Often, "sunken eyeballs," resulting from lack of fluid in the interstitium of the eyeball, are observed. Tachycardia and hypotension may signal profound fluid losses. Kussmaul respirations are present, and the fruity odor of acetone may be detected.

Laboratory Studies

Considering the complexity and potential seriousness of DKA, the laboratory diagnosis is straightforward. With a known type 1 diabetic patient, the presence of hyperglycemia and ketones provides rapid diagnostic confirmation of DKA. A blood gas sample can confirm the acid–base imbalance. Other clues may be gleaned from the venous blood chemistry panel. CO_2, if measured, is low in the presence of uncompensated metabolic acidosis, and the anion gap is elevated. Serum sodium may be low as a result of the movement of water from the intracellular space into the extracellular (vascular) space.[24] The serum potassium level is often normal; a low serum potassium level in DKA suggests a significant potassium deficiency may be present.[24]

Medical Management

Diagnosis of DKA is based on the combination of presenting symptoms, patient history, medical history (type 1 diabetes), precipitating factors (if known), and results of serum glucose and urine ketone testing. After diagnosis, DKA requires aggressive clinical management to prevent progressive decompensation. The goals of treatment are to reverse dehydration, replace insulin, reverse ketoacidosis, and replenish electrolytes.

Reversing Dehydration

The patient with DKA is dehydrated and may have lost 5% to 10% of body weight in fluids. Aggressive IV fluid replacement is provided to rehydrate the intracellular and extracellular compartments and prevent circulatory collapse (Fig. 33-3).[24] Assessment of hydration is an important first step in the treatment of DKA.

Intravenous isotonic normal saline (0.9% NaCl) is infused to replenish the vascular deficit and to reverse hypotension. For the severely dehydrated patient, 1 L of normal saline is infused immediately. Laboratory assessment of serum osmolality and the serum sodium concentration can help guide the subsequent interventions. If the serum osmolality is elevated and serum sodium is high (hypernatremia), infusions of hypotonic sodium chloride (0.45) follow the initial saline replacement. The replacement infusion typically includes 20 to 30 mEq of potassium per liter to restore the intracellular potassium debt, provided kidney function is normal (see Fig. 33-3).[24] In patients without normally functioning kidneys and in those with cardiopulmonary disease, careful attention must be paid to the volume of fluid replacement to avoid fluid overload.

After the serum glucose level decreases to 200 mg/dL, the infusing solution is changed to a 50/50 mix of hypotonic saline and 5% dextrose. Dextrose is added to replenish depleted cellular glucose as the circulating serum glucose decreases to 200 mg/dL.[24] Dextrose infusion also prevents unexpected hypoglycemia when the insulin infusion is continued but the patient cannot take in sufficient carbohydrate from an oral diet.

Replacing Insulin

In moderate to severe DKA, an initial IV bolus of regular insulin at 0.1 unit for each kilogram of body weight may be administered. Subsequently, a continuous infusion of regular insulin at 0.1 unit/kg/hr is infused simultaneously with IV fluid replacement (see Fig. 33-3).[24] In a 70-kg adult, the infusion would be 7 units of insulin per hour. If the plasma glucose concentration does not fall by 50 to 70 mg/dL during the first hour of treatment, the glucose measurement should be rechecked. When the plasma glucose level is decreasing as expected, the insulin infusion will be increased each hour until a steady glucose decline of between 50 and 70 mg/dL per hour is achieved.[24]

Frequent assessment of the patient's blood glucose concentration is mandatory in moderate to severe DKA. Initially, blood glucose tests are performed hourly. The frequency then decreases to every 2 to 4 hours as the patient's blood glucose level stabilizes and approaches normal. After the level has decreased to 200 mg/dL, the acidosis has been corrected, and rehydration has been achieved, the insulin infusion rate may be decreased to 0.05 to 0.1 unit/kg/hr. This usually represents 3 to 6 units per hour in an adult receiving a continuous IV insulin infusion. It is important to verify that the serum potassium concentration is not lower than 3.3 mEq/L and to replace potassium if necessary, before administering the initial insulin bolus.[24]

Reversing Ketoacidosis

Replacement of fluid volume and insulin interrupts the ketotic cycle and reverses the metabolic acidosis. In the presence of insulin, glucose enters the cells, and the body ceases to convert fats into glucose.

Adequate hydration and insulin replacement usually correct the acidosis, and this treatment is sufficient for many patients with DKA. As shown in Figure 33-3, replacement of bicarbonate is no longer routine except for the severely acidotic patient with a serum pH value lower than 7.0.[24] An indwelling arterial line provides access for hourly sampling of arterial blood gases (ABGs) to evaluate pH, bicarbonate, and other laboratory values in the patient with severe DKA.

Hyperglycemia usually resolves before the ketoacidemia does.[24] Type 1 diabetes patients with DKA can require 6 L of IV fluid replacement even for mild DKA.[25] In one clinical report,

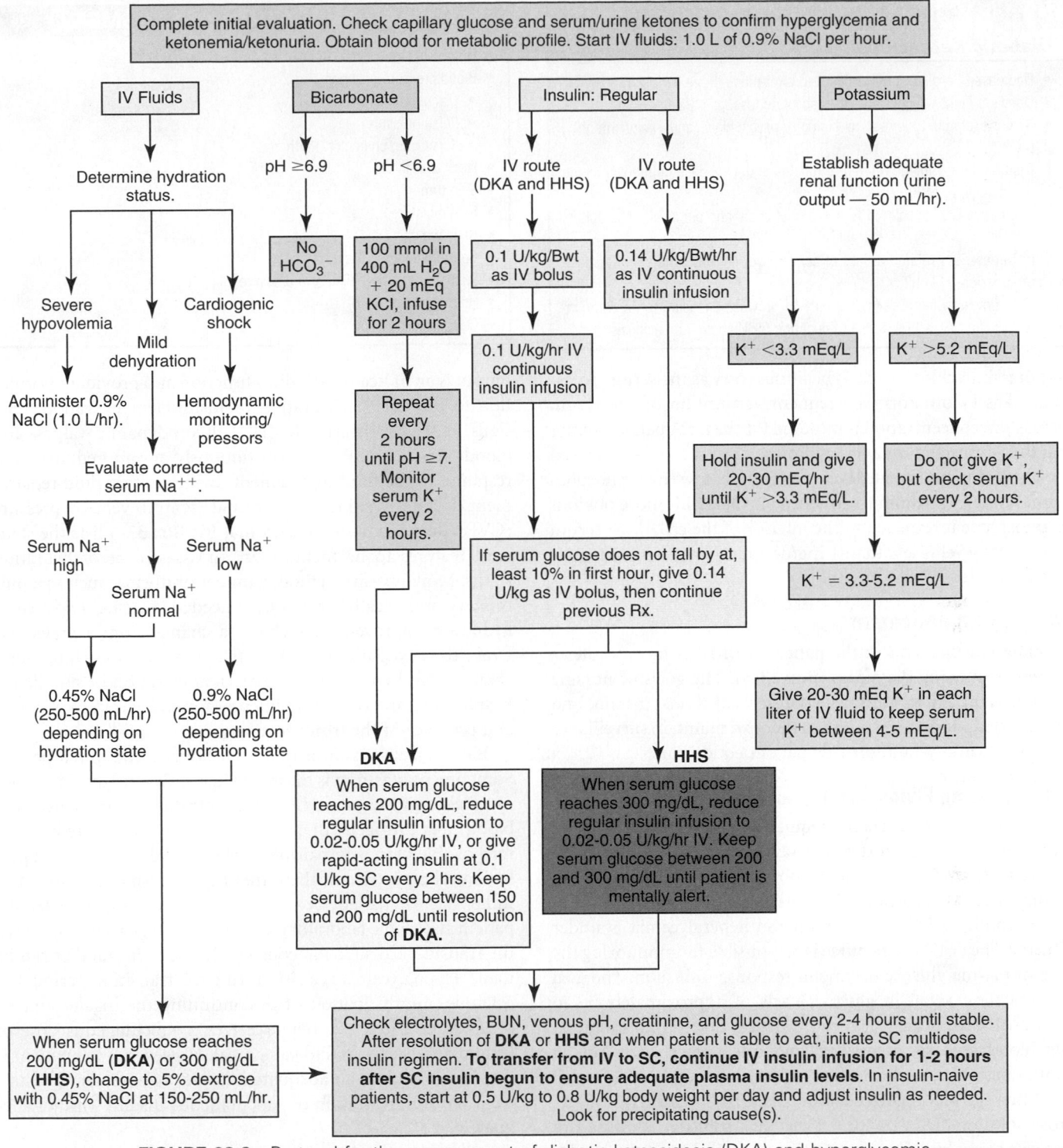

FIGURE 33-3 Protocol for the management of diabetic ketoacidosis (DKA) and hyperglycemic hyperosmolar state (HHS). (From Kitabchi AE, et al. Hyperglycemic crises in adult patients with diabetes: a consensus statement from the American Diabetes Association. *Diabetes Care.* 2009;32[7]:1335.)

patients with previously diagnosed type 1 diabetes in DKA took an average of 21 hours after being started on an IV insulin protocol to clear ketones from the urine. The insulin infusion was continued for 36 hours until the patients could tolerate an oral diet; during this time, the patients received a total of 9.5 L of normal saline for rehydration.[26] Patients who are newly diagnosed with type 1 diabetes take longer to clear urine ketones

and require more insulin to achieve normal glycemic control, compared with long-term diabetics.[26]

Replenishing Electrolytes

Low serum potassium (hypokalemia) occurs as insulin promotes the return of potassium into the cell and metabolic acidosis is reversed. Replacement of potassium by administration

◎ BOX 33-5 NURSING DIAGNOSES
Diabetic Ketoacidosis

- Decreased Cardiac Output related to alterations in preload, p. 1128
- Deficient Fluid Volume related to absolute loss, p. 1132
- Anxiety related to threat to biologic, psychologic, and social integrity, p. 1125
- Disturbed Body Image related to functional dependence on life-sustaining technology, p. 1136
- Ineffective Coping related to situational crisis and personal vulnerability, p. 1150
- Powerlessness related to lack of control over current situation or disease progression, p. 1152
- Deficient Knowledge related to lack of previous exposure to information, p. 1134 (see Box 33-9, Patient Education for Diabetic Ketoacidosis)

BOX 33-6 HYDRATION ASSESSMENT

- Hourly intake
- Blood pressure changes
  - Orthostatic hypotension
  - Pulse pressure
  - Pulse rate, character, rhythm
- Neck vein filling
- Skin turgor
- Skin moisture
- Body weight
- Central venous pressure
- Pulmonary arterial occlusion pressure
- Hourly output
- Complaints of thirst

of potassium chloride (KCl) begins as soon as the serum potassium falls below normal. Frequent verification of the serum potassium concentration is required for the DKA patient receiving fluid resuscitation and insulin therapy.

The serum phosphate level is sometimes low (hypophosphatemia) in DKA. Insulin treatment may make this more obvious as phosphate is returned to the interior of the cell. If the serum phosphate level is less than 1 mg/dL, phosphate replacement is recommended.[24]

Nursing Management

Nursing management of the patient with DKA incorporates a variety of nursing diagnoses (Box 33-5). The goals of nursing management are to administer prescribed fluids, insulin, and electrolytes; monitor response to therapy; maintain surveillance for complications; and provide patient education.

Administering Fluids, Insulin, and Electrolytes

Rapid IV fluid replacement requires the use of a volumetric pump. Insulin is administered intravenously to patients who are severely dehydrated or have poor peripheral perfusion, to ensure effective absorption. Patients with DKA are kept on NPO status (nothing by mouth) until the hyperglycemia is under control. The critical care nurse is responsible for monitoring the rate of plasma glucose decline in response to insulin. The goal is to achieve a fall in glucose levels of approximately 50 to 70 mg/dL each hour.[24] The coordination involved in monitoring blood glucose, potassium, and often blood gases on an hourly basis is considerable.

When the blood glucose level falls to 200 mg/dL, a 5% dextrose solution (D_5W) with 0.45% NaCl solution is infused to prevent hypoglycemia.[24] At this time, it is likely that the insulin dose per hour will also be decreased. The regular insulin drip is not discontinued until the ketoacidosis subsides, as identified by absence of ketones and a normal pH by arterial blood gas analysis.[24]

Insulin is given subcutaneously after glucose levels, dehydration, hypotension, and acid–base balance are normalized; the patient is in stable condition and taking an oral diet.

Monitoring Response to Therapy

Accurate intake and output (I&O) measurements must be maintained to monitor reversal of dehydration. Hourly urine output is an indicator of kidney function and provides information to prevent overhydration or insufficient hydration. Vital signs, especially heart rate (HR), hemodynamic values, and blood pressure (BP), are continuously monitored to assess response to the fluid replacement. Evidence that fluid replacement is effective includes normal central venous pressure (CVP), decreased HR, and normal BP. Box 33-6 lists the standard features to be included in an assessment of hydration status. More invasive hemodynamic monitoring, such as a pulmonary artery catheter, is rarely needed. Further evidence of hydration improvement includes a change from a previously weak, thready pulse to a pulse that is strong and full, and a change from hypotension to a gradual elevation of systolic BP. Respirations are assessed frequently for changes in rate, depth, and presence of the fruity acetone odor.

Blood glucose is measured each hour in the initial period. Sometimes potassium is measured just as frequently. The serum osmolality and serum sodium concentration are evaluated, and blood urea nitrogen (BUN) and creatinine levels are assessed for possible kidney impairment related to decreased renal perfusion. The purpose of these frequent assessments is to determine that the patient's clinical status is improving. After the patient has stable laboratory indicators and is awake and alert, the transition to subcutaneous insulin and an oral diet can be made. Hypoglycemia is a risk during the transition period. For example, in anticipation of discontinuing the insulin and IV dextrose infusion, a patient receives a subcutaneous dose of insulin and is expected to eat a meal. However, if the patient is then unable to eat an adequate amount, hypoglycemia results from the administration of subcutaneous insulin without adequate glucose.

Surveillance for Complications

The patient in DKA can experience a variety of complications, including fluid volume overload, hypoglycemia, hypokalemia or hyperkalemia, hyponatremia, cerebral edema, and infection.

Fluid Volume Overload. Fluid overload from rapid volume infusion is a serious complication that can occur in the patient with a compromised cardiopulmonary system or kidneys. Neck vein engorgement, dyspnea without exertion, and pulmonary crackles on auscultation signal circulatory overload. Reduction in the rate and volume of infusion, elevation of the head of the

◎ **BOX 33-7 NIC**

Hypoglycemia Management

Definition

Preventing and treating low blood glucose levels

Activities

Identify patient at risk for hypoglycemia

Determine recognition of hypoglycemia signs and symptoms

Monitor blood glucose levels, as indicated

Monitor for signs and symptoms of hypoglycemia (e.g., shakiness, tremor, sweating, nervousness, anxiety, irritability, impatience, tachycardia, palpitation, chills, clamminess, lightheadedness, pallor, hunger, nausea, headache, tiredness, drowsiness, weakness, warmth, dizziness, faintness, blurred vision, nightmares, crying out in sleep, paresthesia, difficulty concentrating, difficulty speaking, incoordination, behavior change, confusion, coma, seizure)

Provide simple carbohydrate, as indicated

Provide complex carbohydrate and protein, as indicated

Administer glucagon, as indicated

Contact emergency medical services, as necessary

Administer intravenous glucose, as indicated

Maintain IV access, as appropriate

Maintain patent airway, as necessary

Protect from injury, as necessary

Review events prior to hypoglycemia to determine probable cause

Provide feedback regarding appropriateness of self-management of hypoglycemia

Instruct patient and significant others on signs and symptoms, risk factors, and treatment of hypoglycemia

Instruct patient to have simple carbohydrates available at all times

Instruct patient to obtain and carry/wear appropriate emergency identification

Instruct significant others on the use and administration of glucagon, as appropriate

Instruct on interaction of diet, insulin or oral agents, and exercise

Provide assistance in making self-care decisions to prevent hypoglycemia (e.g., reducing insulin/oral agents and/or increasing food intake for exercise)

Encourage self-monitoring of blood glucose levels

Encourage ongoing telephone contact with diabetes care team for consultation regarding adjustments in treatment regimen

Collaborate with patient and diabetes care team to make changes in insulin regimen (e.g., multiple daily injections), as indicated

Modify blood glucose goals to prevent hypoglycemia in the absence of hypoglycemia symptoms

Inform patient of increased risk of hypoglycemia with intensive therapy and normalization of blood glucose levels

Instruct patient regarding probable changes in hypoglycemia symptoms with intensive therapy and normalization of blood glucose levels

From Bulechek GM, et al. *Nursing Interventions Classification (NIC)*. 6th ed. St. Louis: Mosby; 2013.

bed, and provision of oxygen may be required to manage the increased intravascular volume. Hourly urine measurement is mandatory to assess kidney function and adequacy of fluid replacement.

Hypoglycemia. Hypoglycemia is defined as a serum glucose level lower than 70 mg/dL.[24] Most acute care hospitals have specific procedures for management of the hypoglycemic patient (Box 33-7). For example, if hypoglycemia is detected by finger-stick point-of-care testing at the bedside, a blood sample is sent to the laboratory for verification, the physician is notified immediately, and replacement glucose is given intravenously or orally, depending on the patient's clinical condition, diagnosis, and level of consciousness.

Unexpected behavior change or decreased level of consciousness, diaphoresis, and tremors are physical warning signs that the patient has become hypoglycemic. These symptoms are especially important to recognize if the frequency of glucose testing has lengthened to 2- to 4-hour intervals. A comparison between the physical symptoms expected with hypoglycemia and those of hyperglycemia is provided in Box 33-8.

Hypokalemia and Hyperkalemia. Hypokalemia can occur within the first hours of rehydration and insulin treatment. Continuous cardiac monitoring is required, because low serum potassium (hypokalemia) can cause ventricular dysrhythmias.

Hyperkalemia occurs with acidosis or with overaggressive administration of potassium replacement in patients with renal insufficiency. Severe hyperkalemia is demonstrated on the cardiac monitor by a large, peaked T wave; flattened P wave; and widened QRS complex. See Figure 14-75 in Chapter 14. Ventricular fibrillation can follow.

BOX 33-8 CLINICAL MANIFESTATIONS OF HYPOGLYCEMIA AND HYPERGLYCEMIA

HYPOGLYCEMIA	HYPERGLYCEMIA
• Restlessness	• Excessive thirst
• Apprehension	• Excessive urination
• Irritability	• Hunger
• Trembling	• Weakness
• Weakness	• Listlessness
• Diaphoresis	• Mental fatigue
• Pallor	• Flushed, dry skin
• Paresthesia	• Itching
• Pallor	• Headache
• Headache	• Nausea
• Hunger	• Vomiting
• Difficulty thinking	• Abdominal cramps
• Loss of coordination	• Dehydration
• Difficulty walking	• Weak, rapid pulse
• Difficulty talking	• Postural hypotension
• Visual disturbances	• Hypotension
• Blurred vision	• Acetone breath odor
• Double vision	• Kussmaul respirations
• Tachycardia	• Rapid breathing
• Shallow respirations	• Changes in level of consciousness
• Hypertension	• Stupor
• Changes in level of consciousness	• Coma
• Seizures	
• Coma	

Hyponatremia. Sodium elimination from the body results from the osmotic diuresis and is compounded by the vomiting and diarrhea that can occur during DKA. Clinical manifestations of hyponatremia include abdominal cramping, postural hypotension, and unexpected behavioral changes. Sodium chloride is infused as the initial IV solution. Maintenance of the saline infusion depends on clinical manifestations of sodium imbalance and serum laboratory values.

Risk for Cerebral Edema. Changes in the patient's neurologic status may be insidious. Alterations in level of consciousness, pupil reaction, and motor function may be the result of fluctuating glucose levels and cerebral fluid shifts. Confusion and sudden complaints of headache are ominous signs that may signal cerebral edema. These observations require immediate action to prevent neurologic damage. Neurologic assessments are performed every hour or as needed during the acute phase of hyperglycemia and rehydration. Assessment of level of consciousness serves as the index of the patient's cerebral response to the rehydration therapy.

Risk for Infection. Skin care takes on new dimensions for the patient with DKA. Dehydration, hypovolemia, and hypophosphatemia interfere with oxygen delivery at the cell site and contribute to inadequate perfusion and tissue breakdown. Patients must be repositioned frequently to relieve capillary pressure and promote adequate perfusion to body tissues. The typical patient with type 1 diabetes is of normal weight or underweight. Bony prominences must be assessed for tissue breakdown, and the patient's body weight must be repositioned every 1 to 2 hours. Irritation of skin from adhesive tape, shearing force, and detergents should be avoided. Maintenance of skin integrity prevents unwanted portals of entry for microorganisms.

Oral care, including tooth brushing and use of lip balm, helps keep lips supple and prevents cracking. Prepared sponge sticks or moist gauze pads can be used to moisten oral membranes of the unconscious patient. Swabbing the mouth moistens the tissue and displaces the bacteria that collect when saliva, which has a bacteriostatic action, is curtailed by dehydration. The conscious patient must be provided the means to self-remove oral bacteria by tooth brushing and frequent oral rinsing.

Strict sterile technique is used to maintain all IV systems. All venipuncture sites are checked every 4 hours for signs of inflammation, phlebitis, or infiltration. Strict surgical asepsis is used for all invasive procedures. Sterile technique is used if urinary catheterization is necessary to obtain urine samples for testing. Urinary catheter care is provided every 8 hours.

Patient Education

It is important to be aware of the knowledge level and adherence history of patients with previously diagnosed diabetes to formulate an appropriate teaching plan. Learning objectives include a discussion of target glucose levels, definition of hyperglycemia and its causes, harmful effects, symptoms, and how to manage insulin and diet when one is unwell and unable to eat. Additional objectives include a definition of DKA and its causes, symptoms, and harmful consequences. The patient and family are also expected to learn the principles of diabetes

---

BOX 33-9   PATIENT EDUCATION
Diabetic Ketoacidosis

Acute Phase
- Explain rationale for critical care unit admission
- Reduce anxiety associated with critical care unit

Predischarge
- Assess knowledge level
- Assess compliance history
- Diabetes disease process
- Target glucose levels
- Causes of diabetic ketoacidosis (DKA)
- Pathophysiology of DKA
- Self-care monitoring of blood glucose level
- Insulin regimen
- Sick-day management
- Universal precautions for caregivers
- Signs and symptoms to report to health care practitioner

---

management. Universal precautions must be emphasized for all family caregivers. The patient and family must also learn the warning signs of DKA to report to the attention of a health care practitioner. Education of the patient, family, or other support persons to achieve knowledge-based, independent self-management of blood glucose level and avoidance of diabetes-related complications are the ultimate goals of the teaching process (Box 33-9).

Collaborative Management

In all aspects of patient care management, health care professionals work as a team with the major collaborative goal of providing the best possible outcome for each patient. Current guidelines related to Collaborative Management of patients with hyperglycemia crisis are listed Box 33-10.

HYPERGLYCEMIC HYPEROSMOLAR STATE

Epidemiology and Etiology

HHS is a potentially lethal complication of type 2 diabetes. The hallmarks of HHS are extremely high levels of plasma glucose with resultant elevation in serum hyperosmolality causing osmotic diuresis. Ketosis is absent or mild. Inability to replace fluids lost through diuresis leads to profound dehydration and changes in level of consciousness. The overall mortality rate from HHS ranges from 5% to 20%.[24] Because patients with HHS have type 2 diabetes as an underlying disorder, they are generally older adults with cardiovascular comorbidities.

The diagnostic criteria for HHS are as follows and as shown in Table 33-4[24]:

- Blood glucose greater than 600 mg/dL
- Arterial pH greater than 7.3
- Serum bicarbonate greater than 18 mEq/L
- Serum osmolality greater than 320 mOsm/kg H$_2$O (320 mmol/kg)
- Absent or mild ketonuria

Most patients with this level of metabolic disruption experience visual changes, mental status changes, and potentially hypovolemic shock.

HHS occurs when the pancreas produces a relatively insufficient amount of insulin for the high levels of glucose that flood the bloodstream. HHS primarily affects older, obese persons with underlying cardiovascular conditions. Infection is the primary reason that type 2 diabetics develop HHS; the most common infections are pneumonia and urinary tract infections. The patient may have type 2 diabetes treated with diet and oral hypoglycemic agents that is destabilized by an infection. Other precipitating causes of HHS include stroke, myocardial infarction, trauma, major surgery, and the stress of critical illness.

Differences Between Hyperglycemic Hyperosmolar State and Diabetic Ketoacidosis

Clinically, HHS is distinguished from DKA by the presence of extremely elevated serum glucose, more profound dehydration, and minimal or absent ketosis (Table 33-5). Another major difference is that protein and fats are not used to create new supplies of glucose in HHS as they are in DKA; as a result, the ketotic cycle is never started or does not occur until the glucose level is extremely elevated.

Pathophysiology

HHS represents a deficit of insulin and an excess of glucagon (Fig. 33-4). Reduced insulin levels prevent the movement of glucose into the cells, allowing glucose to accumulate in the plasma. The decreased insulin triggers glucagon release from the liver, and hepatic glucose is poured into the circulation. As the number of glucose particles increases in the blood, serum hyperosmolality increases. In an effort to decrease the serum osmolality, fluid is drawn from the intracellular compartment (inside the cells) into the vascular bed. Profound intracellular volume depletion occurs if the patient's thirst sensation is absent or decreased. HHS may evolve over days or even weeks.[24]

BOX 33-10 EVIDENCE-BASED PRACTICE

Diabetic Ketoacidosis

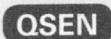 Summary of evidence and evidence-based recommendations for controlling symptoms related to diabetic ketoacidosis (DKA)

Strong Evidence to Support

Regular insulin by continuous infusion is recommended.

Replace serum potassium if level is lower than 3.3 mEq/L.

Replace serum phosphate if level is lower than 1.0 mg/dL.

Very Little Evidence to Support

No support for use of routine bicarbonate to correct low serum pH; use may be considered if pH is below 7.0.

Reference

Kitabchi AE, et al. Hyperglycemic crises in adult patients with diabetes: a consensus statement from the American Diabetes Association. *Diabetes Care.* 2009;32(7):1335.

TABLE 33-5 COMPARISON OF DIABETIC KETOACIDOSIS AND HYPERGLYCEMIC HYPEROSMOLAR STATE

CHARACTERISTICS AND LABORATORY TESTS	DKA	HHS
Cause	Insufficient exogenous glucose for glucose needs	Insufficient exogenous/endogenous insulin for glucose needs
Onset	Sudden (hours)	Slow, insidious (days, weeks)
Precipitating factors	Noncompliance with type 1 diabetes therapy, illness, surgery, decreased activity	Recent acute illness in an older patient; therapeutic procedures
Mortality (%)	9-14	10-50
Population affected	Patients with type 1 diabetes	Patients with type 2 diabetes
Clinical manifestations	Dry mouth, polydipsia, polyuria, polyphagia, dehydration, dry skin, hypotension, weakness	Mental confusion, tachycardia, changes in level of consciousness
	Ketoacidosis; air hunger, acetone breath odor, respirations deep and rapid, nausea, vomiting	No ketosis, no breath odor, respirations rapid and shallow, usually mild nausea/vomiting
Laboratory tests		
Glucose (mg/dL)	300-800	600-2000
Ketones	Strongly positive	Normal or mildly elevated
pH	<7.3	Normal*
Osmolality (mOsm/L)	<350	>350
Sodium	Normal or low	Normal or elevated
Potassium (K+)	Normal, low, or elevated (total body K+ depleted)	Low, normal, or elevated
Bicarbonate	<15 mEq/L	Normal
Phosphorus	Low, normal, or elevated (may decrease after insulin therapy)	Low, normal, or elevated (may decrease after insulin therapy)
Urine acetone	Strong	Absent or mild

*Exception: In severe HHS, lactic acidosis may develop as a result of dehydration and severe tissue hypoperfusion and ischemia.

DKA, Diabetic ketoacidosis; *HHS,* hyperglycemic hyperosmolar state.

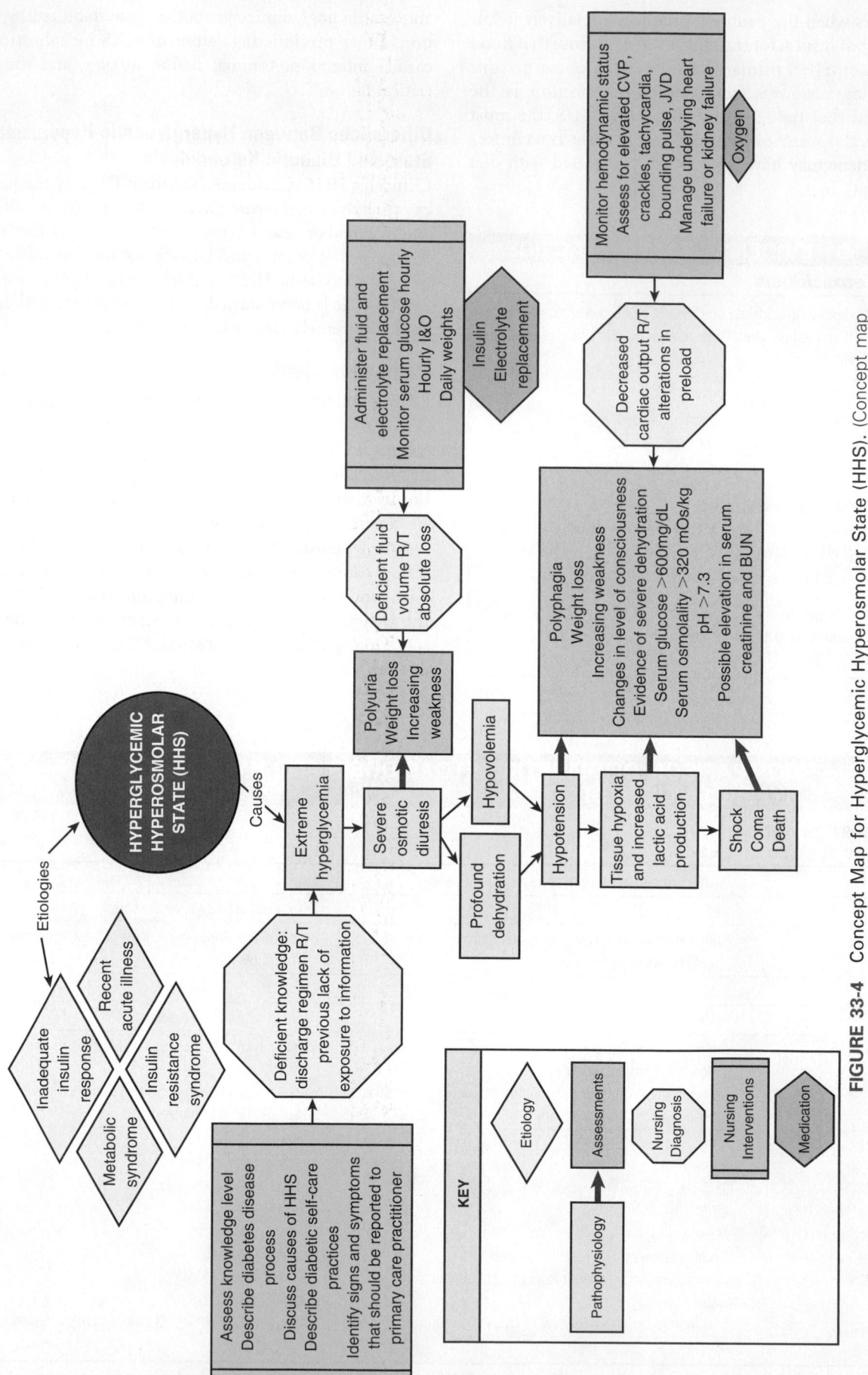

FIGURE 33-4 Concept Map for Hyperglycemic Hyperosmolar State (HHS). (Concept map illustration created by Elaine Bishop Kennedy, EdD, RN.)

Hemoconcentration persists despite removal of large amounts of glucose in the urine (glycosuria). The glomerular filtration and elimination of glucose by the kidney tubules is ineffective in reducing the serum glucose level sufficiently to maintain normal glucose levels. The hyperosmolality and reduced blood volume stimulate release of ADH to increase the tubular resorption of water. ADH, however, is powerless to overcome the osmotic pull exerted by the glucose load. Excessive fluid volume is lost at the kidney tubule, with simultaneous loss of potassium, sodium, and phosphate in the urine. This chain of events results in progressively worsening hypovolemia.

Hypovolemia reduces perfusion to the kidney and oliguria develops. Although this process conserves water and preserves the blood volume, it prevents further glucose loss, and hyperosmolality increases. Ketosis is absent or mild in HHS.

The SNS reacts to the body's stress response to try to restore homeostasis. Epinephrine, a potent stimulus for gluconeogenesis, is released, and additional glucose is added to the bloodstream. Unless the glycemic diuresis cycle is broken by aggressive fluid replacement and insulin administration, intracellular dehydration negatively affects fluid and oxygen transport to the brain cells. Central nervous system dysfunction may result and may lead to coma. Hemoconcentration increases the blood viscosity, which may result in clot formation; thromboemboli; and cerebral, cardiac, and pleural infarcts.

Assessment and Diagnosis
Clinical Manifestations

HHS has a slow, subtle onset and develops over several days. Initially, the symptoms may be nonspecific and may be ignored or attributed to the patient's concurrent disease processes. History reveals malaise, blurred vision, polyuria, polydipsia (depending on the patient's thirst sensation), weight loss, and increasing weakness. Medical attention may not be obtained for these nonspecific, nonacute symptoms until the patient is unable to take sufficient fluids to offset the fluid losses. Progressive dehydration follows and leads to mental confusion, convulsions, and eventually coma, especially in older patients.

The physical examination may reveal a profound fluid deficit. Signs of severe dehydration include longitudinal wrinkles in the tongue, decreased salivation, and decreased CVP, with increases in HR and rapid respirations (Kussmaul air hunger does not occur). In older patients, assessment of clinical signs of dehydration is challenging. Neurologic status is affected as the serum glucose climbs, especially at levels greater than 1500 mg/dL. Without intervention, obtundation and coma occur.

Laboratory Studies

Laboratory findings are used to establish the definitive diagnosis of HHS. Plasma glucose levels are strikingly elevated (greater than 600 mg/dL). Serum osmolality is greater than 320 mOsm/kg. Acidosis is absent (arterial pH greater than 7.3), and the serum bicarbonate concentration is greater than 18 mEq/L. Ketonuria is absent or mild.[24] The patient may have an elevated hematocrit and depleted potassium and phosphorus levels.

Point-of-care finger-stick or arterial-line testing of glucose at the bedside is the usual method for frequent monitoring of the serum blood glucose. Insulin replacement is then prescribed according to the blood glucose result. Some electrolytes also can be tested at the bedside (potassium, sodium, ionized calcium), but usually an arterial line is required for frequent blood access. If point-of-care testing is not available, traditional serial laboratory tests keep the clinician apprised of the fluctuating serum electrolyte levels and provide the basis for electrolyte replacement. Intracellular potassium and phosphate levels usually are depleted as a result of prior osmotic diuresis.[24]

Elevated BUN and creatinine levels suggest kidney impairment as a result of the severe reduction in renal circulation. Metabolic acidosis usually is absent at lower glucose levels. Acidosis may result from starvation ketosis or from an increase in lactic acid production caused by poor tissue perfusion.

Medical Management

The goals of medical management are rapid rehydration, insulin replacement, and correction of electrolyte abnormalities, specifically potassium replacement. The underlying stimulus of HHS must be discovered and treated. The same basic principles used to treat DKA are used for the patient with HHS.

Rapid Rehydration

The primary intervention for HHS is rapid rehydration to restore the intravascular volume. The fluid deficit may be as much as 150 mL/kg of body weight. The average 150-pound adult can lose more than 7 to 10 L of fluid. Physiologic saline solution (0.9%) is infused at 1 L/hr, especially for the patient in hypovolemic shock if there is no cardiovascular contraindication. Several liters of volume replacement may be required to achieve a BP and CVP within normal range. Infusion volumes are adjusted according to the patient's hydration state and sodium level.[24]

The serum sodium concentration is the parameter that is monitored to determine whether to change from isotonic (0.9%) to hypotonic (0.45%) saline. For example, patients with sodium levels equal to or less than 140 mEq/L may be given 0.9% normal saline solution, whereas those with levels greater than 140 mEq/L are given 0.45% saline solution (see Fig. 33-3).[24] It is difficult to assess the serum sodium level in the presence of hemoconcentration. Another recommendation is to calculate a *corrected sodium value*. This involves adding 1.6 mEq to the sodium laboratory value for each 100 mg/dL plasma glucose above normal.[24] Sodium input should not exceed the amount required to replace the losses. Careful monitoring of the serum sodium level is recommended to avoid a sodium-water imbalance and hemolysis as the hemoconcentration is reduced.

To prevent hypoglycemia in HHS, when the serum glucose decreases to 300 mg/dL, the hydrating solution is changed to D_5W with 0.45% NaCl at 150 to 250 mL/hr.[24]

Insulin Administration

Volume resuscitation lowers the serum glucose level and improves symptoms even without insulin administration. However, insulin replacement is recommended in the treatment of HHS because acidosis can develop if insulin is withheld, and insulin will facilitate the cellular use of glucose.

Methods to lower the blood glucose level vary. One method is to administer an IV bolus of regular insulin (0.15 unit/kg of body weight) initially, followed by a continuous insulin drip. Regular insulin, infusing at an initial rate calculated as 0.1 unit/kg hourly (e.g., 7 units/hr for a person weighing 70 kg) should lower the plasma glucose concentration by 50 to 70 mg/dL during the first hour of treatment. If the measured glucose level does not decrease by this amount, the insulin infusion rate may be doubled until the blood glucose is declining at a rate of 50 to 70 mg/dL per hour.[24]

Insulin Resistance. Patients with HHS have underlying type 2 diabetes and may exhibit signs of insulin resistance.[19] In critical illness, the presence of *counter-regulatory hormones*, also known as *stress hormones* (cortisol, glucagon, epinephrine) increases glucose production and induces insulin resistance. Patients with HHS may require supraphysiologic doses of insulin initially to overcome the hyperglycemia and insulin resistance. Hourly serial monitoring of the blood glucose level permits safe glycemic management and avoids the most common complication, which is hypoglycemia caused by overzealous insulin administration.[24] After the patient has recovered from the hyperglycemic crisis and insulin has been discontinued, oral medications designed to decrease insulin resistance in type 2 diabetics will be part of the treatment plan (see Table 33-3).

Electrolyte Replacement

Increasing the circulating levels of insulin with therapeutic doses of IV insulin promotes the rapid return of potassium and phosphorus into the cell. Serial laboratory tests keep the clinician apprised of the serum electrolyte levels and provide the basis for electrolyte replacement. Potassium typically is added to the IV infusion (see Fig. 33-3). If the serum potassium concentration is lower than 3.3 mEq/L, it is essential to replenish the serum potassium before giving insulin.[24] Many hospitals have potassium replacement algorithms that are used to treat hypokalemia. Serum phosphate levels are carefully monitored, and phosphate replaced if the level is lower than 1.0 mg/dL.[24]

Nursing Management

Nursing management of the patient with HHS incorporates a variety of nursing diagnoses (Box 33-11). Nursing management goals are similar to those outlined for DKA. The critical care nurse administers prescribed fluids, insulin, and electrolytes; monitors the response to therapy; maintains surveillance for complications; and provides patient education.

Administering Fluids, Insulin, and Electrolytes

Rigorous fluid replacement and continuous IV insulin replacement must be controlled with an electronic volumetric pump. Accurate I&O measurements are maintained to monitor fluid balance. I&O measurements include the total of all fluids administered minus hourly losses, such as urine output and emesis. Hemodynamic monitoring may include use of an arterial line and measurements of CVP if the patient manifests signs of hypovolemic shock. Arterial line access is very helpful in monitoring serial blood glucose and electrolyte values. The use of a blood conservation system on the arterial line is essential to avoid iatrogenic exsanguination of the patient. Most critical

---

◎ BOX 33-11 NURSING DIAGNOSES
Hyperglycemic Hyperosmolar State

- Decreased Cardiac Output related to alterations in preload, p. 1128
- Deficient Fluid Volume related to absolute loss, p. 1132
- Anxiety related to threat to biologic, psychologic, and social integrity, p. 1125
- Deficient Knowledge related to previous lack of exposure to information, p. 1134 (see Box 33-13, Patient Education for Hyperglycemic Hyperosmolar State)

---

care units have developed protocols or guidelines to ensure that patients in hyperglycemic crisis are managed safely (see Fig. 33-3). The major responsibility for delivery of insulin, hourly monitoring of blood glucose, and infusion of appropriate crystalloid solutions lies with the critical care nurse (Box 33-12). Many hospitals mandate a double-check procedure for medications such as insulin that have the potential to cause harm if wrongly administered.

Monitoring Response to Therapy

The BP, HR, and CVP are monitored to evaluate the degree of dehydration, the effectiveness of hydration therapy, and the patient's fluid tolerance. Because patients with HHS have underlying type 2 diabetes and, if older, are likely have preexisting illnesses such as heart failure and kidney failure, it is important to monitor for symptoms of circulatory overload. Symptoms to anticipate include elevated CVP, tachycardia, bounding pulse, dyspnea, tachypnea, lung crackles, and engorged neck veins. The astute critical care nurse is aware of the clinical manifestations of fluid overload and observes for potential complications when rehydrating the patient with HHS and cardiac, pulmonary, or renal disease.

The serum glucose level should decrease by 50 to 70 mg/dL per hour with insulin administration.[24] This decrease is monitored by hourly blood glucose determinations. Based on the result, the critical care nurse can alter the infusion of insulin according to hospital protocol (see Fig. 33-4).

Surveillance for Complications

The potential complications of HHS are similar to those described for DKA: hypoglycemia, hypokalemia or hyperkalemia, and infection. The patient with HHS is at risk for other complications specific to associated disease entities. A history of cardiovascular, pulmonary, or kidney disease, whether known or latent, places the patient with HHS at high risk for complications.

Patient Education

As the patient's condition improves and the patient demonstrates readiness to learn, education about type 2 diabetes and avoiding a recurrence of HHS becomes a priority (Box 33-13). Most teaching occurs after the patient has left the critical care unit. Teaching topics include a description of type 2 diabetes and how it relates to HHS, dietary restrictions, exercise requirements, medication protocols, home testing of blood glucose, signs and symptoms of hyperglycemia and hypoglycemia, foot care, and lifestyle modifications if cardiovascular disease is present.

BOX 33-12 NIC

Hyperglycemia Management

Definition

Preventing and treating above-normal blood glucose levels

Activities

Monitor blood glucose levels, as indicated

Monitor for signs and symptoms of hyperglycemia: polyuria, polydipsia, polyphagia, weakness, lethargy, malaise, blurring of vision, or headache

Monitor urine ketones, as indicated

Monitor ABG, electrolyte, and beta-hydroxybutyrate levels, as available

Monitor orthostatic blood pressure and pulse, as indicated

Administer insulin, as prescribed

Encourage oral fluid intake

Monitor fluid status (including intake and output)

Maintain IV access, as appropriate

Administer IV fluids, as needed

Administer potassium, as prescribed

Consult physician if signs and symptoms of hyperglycemia persist or worsen

Assist with ambulation if orthostatic hypotension is present

Provide oral hygiene, if necessary

Identify possible causes of hyperglycemia

Anticipate situations in which insulin requirements will increase (e.g., intercurrent illness)

Restrict exercise when blood glucose levels are greater than 250 mg/dL, especially if urine ketones are present

Instruct patient and significant others on prevention, recognition, and management of hyperglycemia

Encourage self-monitoring of blood glucose levels

Instruct on urine ketone testing, as appropriate

Instruct on indications for, and significance of, urine ketone testing, if appropriate

Instruct patient to report moderate or high urine ketone levels to the health professional

Instruct patient and significant others on diabetes management during illness, including use of insulin and/or oral agents, monitoring fluid intake; carbohydrate replacement; and when to seek health professional assistance, as appropriate

Provide assistance in adjusting regimen to prevent and treat hyperglycemia (e.g., increasing insulin or oral agent), as indicated

Facilitate adherence to diet and exercise regimen

Test blood glucose levels of family members

From Bulechek GM, et al. *Nursing Interventions Classification (NIC)*. 6th ed. St. Louis: Mosby; 2013.

ABG, Arterial blood gas; *IV*, intravenous.

BOX 33-13 PATIENT EDUCATION

Hyperglycemic Hyperosmolar State

Acute Phase

- Explain rationale for critical care unit admission

Predischarge

- Assess knowledge level
- Assess compliance history
- Diabetes disease process
- Definition of hyperglycemic hyperosmotic state (HHS)
- Causes of HHS
- Self-care for diabetes
- Signs and symptoms to report to health care practitioner

Collaborative Management

Because HHS is an acute condition superimposed on the chronic health problem of type 2 diabetes, many health professionals provide care and work collaboratively to restore homeostasis for each patient (Box 33-14).

DIABETES INSIPIDUS

Diabetes insipidus (DI) is recognized by the vast quantities of very dilute urine that are produced in susceptible patients. In the critically ill patient, the extreme diuresis is most likely to be caused by a lack of ADH (vasopressin). Any patient who has head trauma,[27] or resection of a pituitary tumor, has an increased risk of developing DI.[28] Normally, ADH is produced in the hypothalamus and stored in the posterior pituitary gland (see Chapter 31). Physiologically, ADH is released primarily in response to even small elevations in serum osmolality and secondarily in reaction to hypovolemia or hypotension. DI can occur if 1) the hypothalamus produces insufficient ADH; 2) the

BOX 33-14 EVIDENCE-BASED PRACTICE

Hyperglycemic Hyperosmolar State

QSEN Summary of evidence and evidence-based recommendations for controlling symptoms related to hyperglycemic hyperosmolar state (HHS)

Strong Evidence to Support

Regular insulin by continuous infusion is recommended to normalize blood glucose

Replace serum potassium if the level is less than 3.3 mEq/L

Replace serum phosphate if the level is less than 1 mg/dL

A multidisciplinary team approach reduces length of stay and improves clinical outcomes

Close follow-up after discharge is recommended to maintain glycosylated hemoglobin (A_{1c}) at less than 6.5% and to prevent diabetes-related complications

Weak Evidence to Support

Use of a sliding insulin scale alone is discouraged, because it is associated with hyperglycemia and hypoglycemia in hospitalized patients.

Reference

Kitabchi AE, et al. Hyperglycemic crises in adult patients with diabetes: a consensus statement from the American Diabetes Association. *Diabetes Care*. 2009;32(7):1335.

posterior pituitary fails to release ADH; or 3) the kidney nephron is resistant (unresponsive) to ADH.

Etiology

DI is divided into three types according to cause: central, nephrogenic, and psychogenic (Box 33-15). Only central DI, also known as neurogenic DI because of its association with the brain, is encountered with any frequency in the critical care unit.

ADH, Antidiuretic hormone.

Central Diabetes Insipidus

In central DI, there is an inability to secrete an adequate amount of ADH (arginine vasopressin) in response to an osmotic or nonosmotic stimuli, resulting in inappropriately dilute urine. The synthesis of ADH is incomplete in the hypothalamus, or the release of ADH from the pituitary is interrupted. Central DI can be congenital or acquired.[29] In critical care, the most likely acute cause of central DI is neurosurgery, traumatic head injury, tumors, increased intracranial pressure, brain death, and infections such as encephalitis or meningitis. Among patients undergoing surgery on the pituitary gland, transient DI occurs in approximately 20% to 30%; permanent DI occurs in 2% to 10% of patients.[29] The degree of hormone replacement required after surgery depends the quantity of pituitary tissue that has been surgically or endoscopically removed.

Nephrogenic Diabetes Insipidus

Nephrogenic DI is a rare congenital or an acquired disorder that occurs when the V_2 receptors on the kidney tubule become nonresponsive to the action of ADH. Some medications cause nephrogenic DI by decreasing the responsiveness of the kidney tubules to ADH. Long-term use of lithium carbonate, prescribed for bipolar disorder, was a frequent culprit in the past.[29]

Primary Polydipsia

Primary polydipsia, previously called psychogenic DI, is a rare form of the disease that occurs with compulsive drinking of more than 5 L of water daily. Long-standing psychogenic DI closely mimics nephrogenic DI because the kidney tubules become less responsive to ADH as a result of prolonged conditioning to hypotonic urine.[29]

Pathophysiology

The purpose of ADH is to maintain normal serum osmolality and circulating blood volume. Normally, ADH binds to the V_2 receptors on the kidney collecting tubules, causing insertion of water channels, known as aquaporins, along the luminal surface. Even small increases in plasma osmolality are sufficient to stimulate ADH release. Although there are several types of DI, this discussion focuses on neurogenic (central) DI, the condition encountered in the critical care unit after neurosurgery or head injury (Fig. 33-5).

In DI, as free water is eliminated, the urine osmolality and specific gravity decrease (dilute urine). At the same time, in the bloodstream, the serum sodium concentration and serum osmolality rise. Normally, a rise in the serum osmolality to greater than 290 mOsm per kilogram of H_2O (290 mmol/L) triggers synthesis and release of ADH. If the thirst mechanism is intact, thirst sensors are activated in the hypothalamus causing a sensation of thirst that leads the person to drink lots of fluids.[30] In central DI, however, no ADH is released, or the ADH released is insufficient. Without ADH, the kidney collecting tubules are incapable of concentrating urine and retaining water.

As extracellular dehydration ensues, hypotension and hypovolemic shock can occur. If the patient is alert, extreme thirst will lead the person to replace lost fluids by drinking lots of water.[30] This excessive intake of water reduces the serum osmolality to a more normal level and prevents dehydration. In the person with decreased level of consciousness, the polyuria leads to severe hypernatremia, dehydration, decreased cerebral perfusion, seizures, loss of consciousness, and death.

Assessment and Diagnosis
Clinical Manifestations

The clinical diagnosis is based on the clinical increase in dilute urine output occurring in the absence of diuretics, a fluid challenge, or hyperglycemia. Central DI is anticipated in conditions in which the underlying disease process is likely to disrupt pituitary function. Central DI that occurs because of increasing intracranial pressure is life threatening. It is imperative that the underlying condition be recognized and treated appropriately. In this situation, medications that treat DI are not sufficient.

Laboratory Studies

The core diagnostic tests used to establish the presence of DI and that evaluate the body's ability to balance fluid and electrolytes are not specific to the endocrine system. The most common tests are serum sodium concentration, serum osmolality, and urine osmolality (Table 33-6). The combination of an obvious clinical picture with high volumes of hypotonic urine, in the presence of the following laboratory criteria, is sufficient to diagnose central DI[29,30]:
- Serum sodium level greater than 145 mEq/L
- Serum osmolality greater than 295 mOsm/kg H_2O (greater than 295 mmol/L)

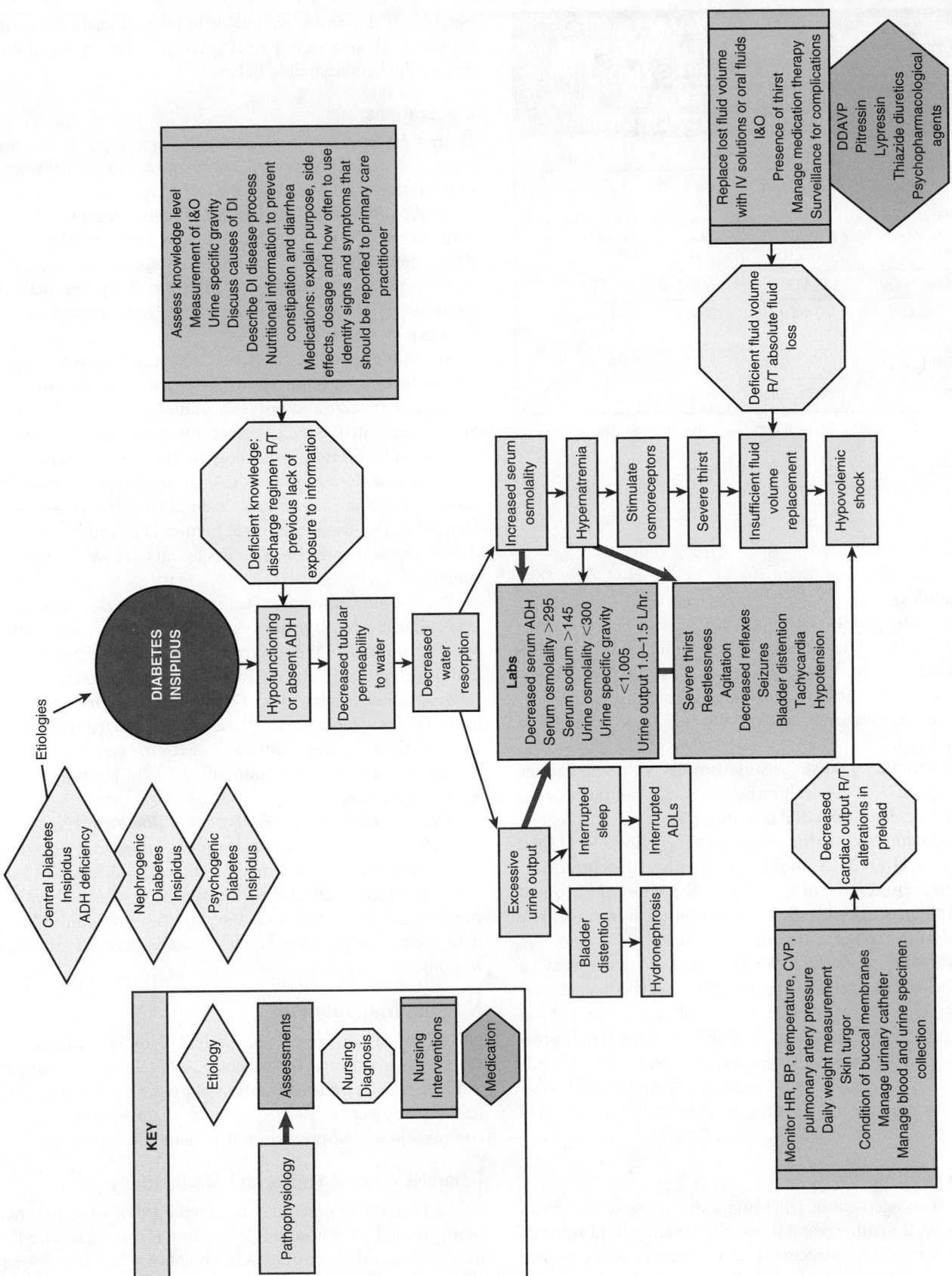

FIGURE 33-5 Concept Map for Diabetes Insipidus (DI). (Concept map illustration created by Elaine Bishop Kennedy, EdD, RN.)

TABLE 33-6   LABORATORY VALUES FOR PATIENTS WITH DIABETES INSIPIDUS AND SYNDROME OF INAPPROPRIATE ANTIDIURETIC HORMONE

VALUE	NORMAL	DI	SIADH
Serum ADH	1-5 pg/mL	Decreased in central DI	Elevated
Serum osmolality (mOsm/L)	275-295*	>295*	<270
Serum sodium (mEq/L)	135-145	>145	<120
Urine osmolality (mOsm/L)	300-1400	<300	Increased
Urine specific gravity	1.005-1.030	<1.005	>1.030
Urine output	1.0-1.5 L/day	1.0-1.5 L/hr	Below normal

*Some hospitals use 280-300 mOsm/L as their normal reference value.
ADH, Antidiuretic hormone; *DI*, diabetes insipidus; *L/day*, liters per day; *pg/mL*, picogram per milliliter; *SIADH*, syndrome of inappropriate antidiuretic hormone.

- Urine osmolality less than 300 mOsm/kg H_2O (less than 200 mmol/L)
- Urine specific gravity less than 1.005

Serum Sodium. The normal serum sodium concentration is 140 mEq/L (range, 135 to 145 mEq/L). In central DI, the serum sodium level can rise precipitously because of the loss of free water. Hypernatremia is usually associated with serum hyperosmolality.

Serum Osmolality Test. Serum osmolality has a narrow normal range, 275 to 295 mOsm/kg. Severe DI can raise serum osmolality to greater than 320 mOsm/kg.

Urine Osmolality. Urine osmolality is low, less than 300 mOsm/kg H_2O (300 mmol/L) in patients with central DI.[29] For greatest accuracy, the urine sample should be collected and tested simultaneously with the blood sample. This test is rarely performed in the critical care unit.

Measurement of Antidiuretic Hormone. Measurement of the baseline serum ADH level is an additional diagnostic step. This is not typically performed in critical care if the clinical circumstances (e.g., head injury with raised intracranial pressure) make further testing unnecessary. Normal ADH levels range from 1 to 5 picogram/mL (pg/mL). With normal hydration the normal morning fasting serum level is lower than 4 pg/mL.

Medical Management

Immediate management of DI requires an aggressive approach. Treatment goals include restoration of circulating fluid volume, pharmacologic ADH replacement, and treatment of the underlying condition.

Volume Restoration

Fluid replacement is provided in the initial phase of the treatment to prevent circulatory collapse. Patients who are able to drink are given voluminous amounts of fluid orally to balance output. For those who are unable to take sufficient fluids orally, hypotonic IV solutions are infused and carefully monitored to restore the hemodynamic balance.

Medications

Central DI requires immediate pharmacologic management. Table 33-7 presents the medications most frequently prescribed to treat central DI and replace ADH.

Medications Used for Central Diabetes Insipidus. Patients with central DI who are unable to synthesize ADH require replacement with ADH (*vasopressin*) or an ADH analogue. The most commonly prescribed medication is the synthetic analogue of ADH, *desmopressin* (DDAVP). It is preferred over vasopressin (Pitressin) because it has a stronger antidiuretic action with little effect on BP. DDAVP can be given IV, subcutaneously, or as a nasal spray. A typical DDAVP dose is 1 to 2 mcg administered IV or subcutaneously every 12 hours.[30] Sometimes only 0.5 mcg is given intravenously. The dosage is subsequently titrated according to the patient's antidiuretic response and close monitoring of urine output is advised.[28] To avoid a medication error, it is important to be aware that DDAVP is also used to control hemorrhage caused by platelet disorders and that the dose ranges for all of these conditions are different.

Vasopressin (Pitressin), 5 units administered subcutaneously every 6 to 8 hours, produces a reduction in urine output.[31] Vasopressin acts on the V_1 receptors in vascular smooth muscle and can elevate systemic BP. Vasopressin can also be prescribed for septic shock states as an IV infusion and for cardiac arrest as an IV push. Dosages for these conditions are very different from that used to treat central DI. Extreme care must be taken to ensure that all medication dosages are accurate for each specific diagnosis.

Medications Used for Nephrogenic Diabetes Insipidus. The mainstay of therapy is to stop any medications that are inducing the ADH resistance. Nephrogenic DI is not a diagnosis encountered in critical care unless the patient is admitted with this condition. It is treated with the diuretic hydrochlorothiazide, with the dosage titration based upon the patient's antidiuretic response.

Nursing Management

Nursing management of the patient with DI incorporates a variety of nursing diagnoses (Box 33-16). Nursing management is directed toward administration of prescribed fluids and medications, evaluation of response to therapy, surveillance for complications, and provision of patient education.

Administration of Fluids and Medications

Rapid IV fluid replacement requires the use of a volumetric pump. Initially, a hypotonic IV solution is used to replace fluids lost and lower the serum hyperosmolality. ADH replacement is accomplished with extreme caution in the patient with a history of heart disease, because ADH may cause hypertension and overhydration. At the first signs of cardiovascular impairment, the medication is discontinued and fluid intake is restricted until urine specific gravity is less than 1.015 and polyuria resumes.

TABLE 33-7 PHARMACOLOGIC MANAGEMENT

Diabetes Insipidus

MEDICATION	DOSAGE*	ACTIONS	SPECIAL CONSIDERATIONS
Central Diabetes Insipidus			
DDAVP (available IV, as nasal spray, Rhinal tube, Rhinyle drops, Stimate)	Nasal: 10-40 mcg before bed or in divided doses Parenteral: 2-4 mcg twice daily	Central DI Antidiuretic Increases water resorption in nephron. Prevents and controls polydipsia, polyuria.	Few side effects Observe for nasal congestion, upper respiratory infection, allergic rhinitis. Monitor intake and output, urine osmolality, serum sodium level.
Vasopressin (Pitressin)	IV, IM, subcutaneous Topical: nasal mucosa	Central DI antidiuretic Promotes resorption of water at kidney tubule. Decreases urine output. Increases urine osmolality. Diagnostic aid Increases gastrointestinal peristalsis.	Monitor fluid volume often, especially in older patients. Assess cardiac status. May precipitate angina, hypertension, or myocardial infarction if increased dose is given to patient with cardiac history. Parenteral extravasation can cause skin necrosis.
Lypressin (Diapid)	Intranasal: 1-2 sprays (7-14 mcg) in each nostril four times daily	Central DI Synthetic ADH Increases resorption of sodium and water in nephron.	Proper instillation is important for absorption and action. Patient sits upright while holding bottle upright for administration. Repeat sprays (>2-3) are ineffective and wasteful; if dose is increased to 2-3 sprays, shorten time between dosing. Cough, chest tightness, shortness of breath
Nephrogenic Diabetes Insipidus			
Thiazide diuretics	Varies according to diuretic chosen, patient's size, and age.	Nephrogenic DI Leads to mild fluid depletion. Increases resorption of water and sodium in proximal nephron; less fluid travels to distal nephron, excreting less water.	Varies according to diuretic chosen.
Psychogenic Diabetes Insipidus			
Anti-compulsive disorder medications, anxiolytics, psychopharmacologic agents	Dosage varies	Psychogenic DI	Varies according to medication chosen.

*Parenteral indicates intravenous or subcutaneous administration.
ADH, Antidiuretic hormone; *DDAVP*, desmopressin acetate; *DI*, diabetes insipidus; *IM*, intramuscular; *IV*, intravenous; *mcg*, microgram.

◎ BOX 33-16   NURSING DIAGNOSES

Diabetes Insipidus

- Decreased Cardiac Output related to alterations in preload, p. 1128
- Deficient Fluid Volume related to absolute fluid loss, p. 1125
- Deficient Knowledge related to lack of previous exposure to information, p. 1134 (see Box 33-17, Patient Education for Diabetes Insipidus)

Evaluation of Response to Therapy

Critical assessment and management of fluid status are the most important initial concerns for the patient with DI. Monitoring of HR, BP, CVP, and pulmonary artery pressures (if a pulmonary artery catheter is in place) provides early indications of response to fluid volume replacement. I&O measurement, condition of buccal membranes, skin turgor, daily weight measurements, presence of thirst, and temperature provide a basic assessment list that is vital for the patient who is unable to regulate fluid needs and losses. Placement of a urinary catheter is essential to accurately monitor the urinary output. Simultaneous urine and blood specimens for determination of osmolality, serum sodium and serum potassium are obtained, and the results are relayed to the physician as necessary. The patient who is unable to satisfy sensations of thirst or to complete any task or self-care activity without the need to urinate may be confused and frightened. For patients who are able to verbalize their fears, having a caring nurse who is interested and nonjudgmental helps to reduce the emotional turmoil associated with their condition.

Surveillance for Complications

The most dangerous potential complication is hypertension and vasospasm of cardiac, cerebral, or mesenteric arterial vessels in response to vasopressin replacement. In most cases, DDAVP is selected for ADH replacement to avoid this complication. A less serious complication of DI is constipation due to fluid loss;

it is treated with dietary fiber, stool softeners, or both. Conversely, diarrhea, abdominal cramping, and intestinal hyperactivity may accompany vasopressin therapy. Untoward effects can be mitigated by modification of the vasopressin dose.

Patient Education

Educating the patient and the family about the disease process and how it affects thirst, urination, and fluid balance encourages patients to participate in their care and reduces the feelings of hopelessness (Box 33-17). For most critical care patients, central DI is a temporary condition that resolves as the underlying medical condition (e.g., brain injury) improves. Patients who are discharged with DI are taught, along with their families, the signs and symptoms of dehydration and overhydration and procedures for accurate daily weight and urine specific gravity measurements. Printed information pertaining to medication actions, side effects, dosages, and timetable is provided, as well as an outline of factors that must be reported to the physician.

Collaborative Management

Central DI is a life-threatening condition. The collaborative assessment and clinical skills of all health care professionals and use of a clear plan of care are essential to achieve optimal outcomes for each patient.

SYNDROME OF INAPPROPRIATE SECRETION OF ANTIDIURETIC HORMONE

The opposing syndrome to DI is the *syndrome of inappropriate secretion of antidiuretic hormone* (SIADH), also known as the *syndrome of inappropriate antidiuresis* (SIAD).[32] The patient with SIADH has an excess of ADH secreted into the bloodstream, more than the amount needed to maintain normal blood volume and serum osmolality. Excessive water is resorbed at the kidney tubule, leading to dilutional hyponatremia.

Etiology

Numerous causes of SIADH are observed in patients who are critically ill (Box 33-18). Central nervous system injury, tumors, and diseases that interfere with the normal functioning of the hypothalamic-pituitary system can cause SIADH.[33] A common cause is malignant bronchogenic small cell carcinoma. This

type of malignant cell is capable of synthesizing and releasing ADH regardless of the body's needs. With much less frequency, other cancers that involve the brain, head and neck, gastroenteral, gynecologic, and hematologic systems are capable of autonomous production of ADH.

Pathophysiology

ADH is a powerful, complex polypeptide compound. When released into the circulation by the posterior pituitary gland, ADH regulates water and electrolyte balance in the body. In SIADH, profound fluid and electrolyte disturbances result from the unsolicited, continuous release of the hormone into the bloodstream (Fig. 33-6). Excessive ADH stimulates the kidney tubules to retain fluid regardless of need. This results in severe overhydration.

Excessive ADH dramatically alters the sodium balance in the extracellular vascular compartment. The overhydration causes a dilutional hyponatremia and reduces the sodium concentration to critically low levels. In the healthy adult, hyponatremia inhibits the release of ADH. In SIADH, however, the increased levels of circulating ADH is unrelated to the serum sodium concentration. Aldosterone production from the adrenal glands is also suppressed. Serum hypo-osmolality leads to a shift of fluid from the extracellular fluid space into the intracellular fluid compartment (inside the cells) in an attempt to equalize osmotic pressure. Because minimal sodium is present in this fluid, edema usually does not result. Without ADH and aldosterone, water is retained, urine output is diminished, and further sodium is excreted in the urine. The urine has an increased osmolality from the decreased water excretion. Urinary concentration is also elevated by excess sodium in the urine. It is believed that, despite the serum hyponatremia, the increased release of ADH promotes sodium loss through the kidneys into the urine.

Assessment and Diagnosis
Clinical Manifestations

The clinical manifestations of SIADH relate to the excess fluids in the extracellular compartment and the proportionate dilution of the circulating sodium. Edema usually is not present, although slight weight gain may occur from the expanded extracellular fluid volume. Early clinical manifestations of dilutional hyponatremia include lethargy, anorexia, nausea, and vomiting. Severe neurologic symptoms usually do not develop until the serum sodium concentration drops to less than 120 mEq/L. Progressively deteriorating neurologic signs of hyponatremia then predominate, and the patient is admitted to the critical care unit. Symptoms of severe hyponatremia include inability to concentrate, mental confusion, apprehension, seizures, decreased level of consciousness, coma, and death.

Laboratory Values

Patients with SIADH present with very dilute serum and very concentrated urine output. Laboratory values confirm this clinical picture. In SIADH, there is decreased plasma osmolality (less than 275 mOsm/kg H_2O), with increased urine osmolality (greater than 100 mOsm/kg).[32] The low serum sodium (less than 125 mEq/L) is associated with increasing severity

BOX 33-18   CAUSES OF SYNDROME OF INAPPROPRIATE SECRETION OF ANTIDIURETIC HORMONE

- *Malignant disease* associated with autonomous production of ADH
  - Bronchogenic small cell carcinoma
  - Pancreatic adenocarcinoma
  - Duodenal, bladder, ureter, and prostatic carcinomas
  - Lymphosarcoma, Ewing sarcoma
  - Acute leukemia, Hodgkin disease
  - Cerebral neoplasm, thymoma
- *Central nervous system diseases* that interfere with the hypothalamic-hypophyseal system and increase the production or release of ADH
  - Head injury
  - Brain abscess
  - Hydrocephalus
  - Pituitary adenoma
  - Subdural hematoma
  - Subarachnoid hemorrhage
  - Cerebral atrophy
  - Guillain-Barré syndrome
- *Neurogenic stimuli* capable of increasing ADH
  - Decreased glomerular filtration rate
  - Physical or emotional stress
  - Pain
  - Fear
  - Trauma
  - Surgery
  - Myocardial infarction
  - Acute infection
  - Hypotension
  - Hemorrhage
  - Hypovolemia
- *Pulmonary diseases* believed to stimulate the baroreceptors and increase ADH
  - Pulmonary tuberculosis
  - Viral and bacterial pneumonia
  - Empyema
  - Lung abscess
- Chronic obstructive lung disease
- Status asthmaticus
- Cystic fibrosis
- *Endocrine disturbances* that hormonally influence ADH
  - Myxedema
  - Hypothyroidism
  - Hypopituitarism
  - Adrenal insufficiency—Addison disease
- *Medications* that mimic, increase the release of, or potentiate ADH
  - Hypoglycemics
    - Insulin
    - Tolbutamide
    - Chlorpropamide
  - Potassium-depleting thiazide diuretics
  - Tricyclic antidepressants
    - Imipramine
    - Amitriptyline
  - Phenothiazine
    - Fluphenazine
    - Thioridazine
  - Thioxanthenes
    - Thiothixene
    - Chlorprothixene
  - Chemotherapeutic agents
    - Vincristine
    - Cyclophosphamide
  - Opiates
  - Carbamazepine
  - Clofibrate
  - Acetaminophen
  - Nicotine
  - Oxytocin
  - Vasopressin
  - Anesthetics

ADH, Antidiuretic hormone.

of neurologic symptoms. The urine sodium concentration is elevated (greater than 40 mEq/L), congruent with the concentrated urine output of SIADH.[32] Use of diuretics negates the reliability of the urine sodium and urine osmolality levels.[32] See Table 33-6 for comparison of the typical laboratory values associated with SIADH with those of DI.

Medical Management

In the critical care unit, SIADH often occurs as a secondary disease. Ideally, recognition and treatment of the primary disease will reduce the production of ADH. If the patient is receiving any of the medications suspected of causing SIADH, discontinuing that medication may return ADH levels to normal.[34] Some of the medications that alter ADH levels are listed in Box 33-18. The goals of medical management are to restore fluid and sodium balance.

Fluid Restriction

Reduction in fluid intake is one component of the treatment plan for SIADH.

Sodium Replacement

Patients with severe hyponatremia (less than 125 mEq/L serum sodium) experience severe neurologic symptoms, even seizures. Too-rapid serum sodium correction must be avoided to reduce the risk of *osmotic demyelination,*[33] which occurs in the white matter of the brain. Severe neurologic damage or death can result.[33] The demyelination complication can be avoided by raising the serum sodium slowly, such as by 8 to 12 mEq/L in 24 hours.[33] Serum sodium levels must be evaluated at least every 4 hours during the acute phase of sodium replacement.

In SIADH an infusion of 3% saline (hypertonic saline) may be used to replenish the serum sodium without adding extra volume. It is imperative to be aware that hypertonic saline solution is dangerous if administered too quickly, as described above. Calculation of the quantity of sodium that will be administered each hour, and over 24 hours, is advised.

Medications

Medications are prescribed when water restriction is ineffective in correcting the SIADH. One pharmacologic action is to

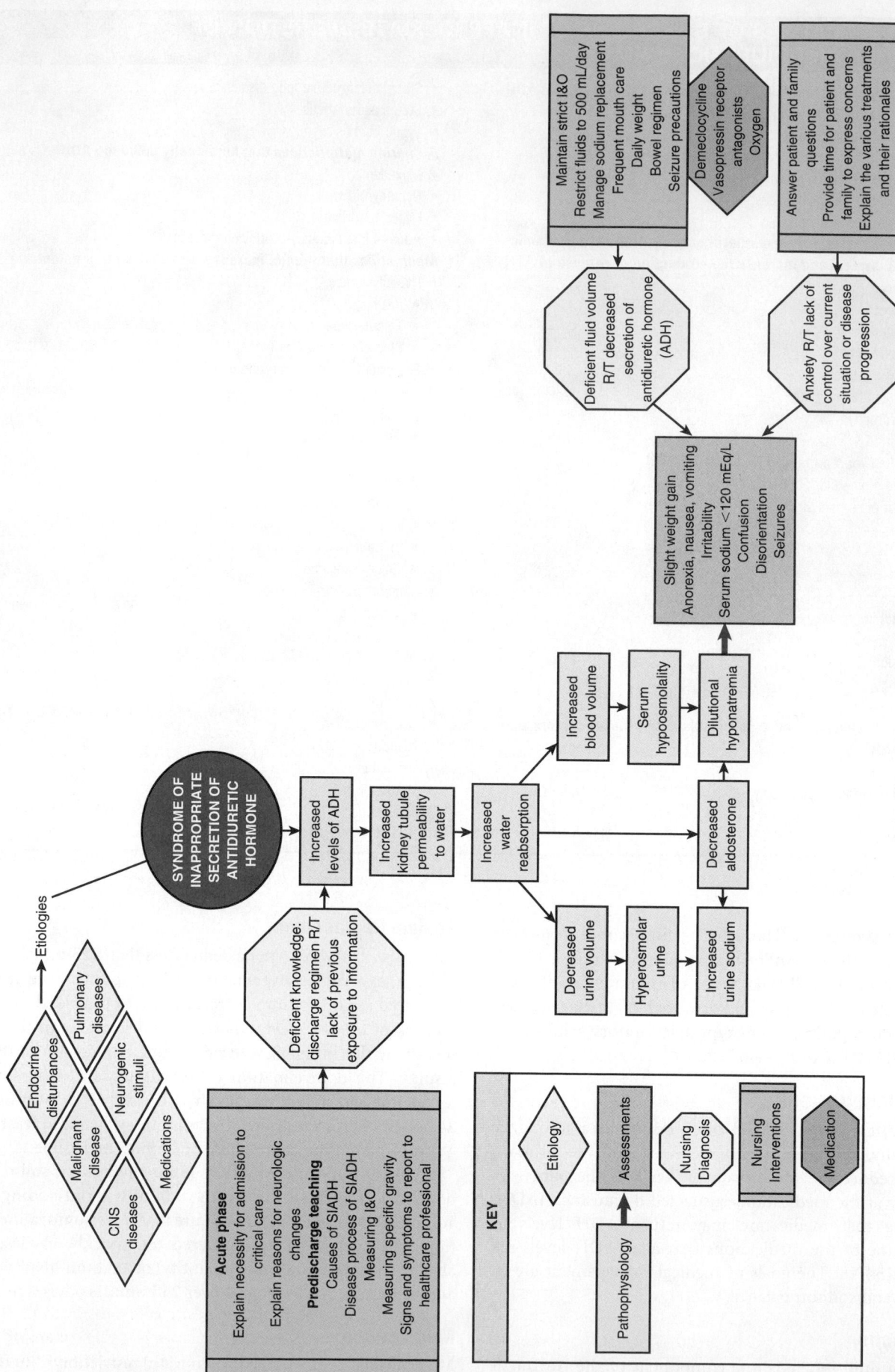

FIGURE 33-6 Concept Map for Syndrome of Inappropriate Secretion of Antidiuretic Hormone (SIADH).

Syndrome of Inappropriate Secretion of Antidiuretic Hormone

- Deficient Fluid Volume related to decreased secretion of antidiuretic hormone (ADH), p. 1139
- Anxiety related to threat to biological, psychologic, or social integrity, p. 1125
- Deficient Knowledge: Discharge Regimen related to lack of previous exposure to information, p. 1134 (see Box 33-20, Patient Education for Syndrome of Inappropriate Secretion of Antidiuretic Hormone)

BOX 33-20 **PATIENT EDUCATION**

Syndrome of Inappropriate Secretion of Antidiuretic Hormone

Acute Phase
- Explain reasons for admission to the critical care unit
- Explain reasons for neurologic changes

Predischarge
- Assess knowledge level
- Causes of inappropriate secretion of antidiuretic hormone (SIADH)
- Disease process of SIADH
- Measuring intake and output
- Measuring urine specific gravity
- Signs and symptoms to report to health care professional

increase the action of ADH on the V_2 kidney tubule receptors so that more water is excreted.

Vasopressin Receptor Antagonists. The *vasopressin receptor antagonists* are used to treat euvolemic hyponatremia such as SIADH. Medications in this class are also described as "vaptans". Conivaptan (Vaprisol) is approved for use only in hospitalized patients. There is an initial 20 mg loading dose IV over 30 minutes, followed by a 20 mg per day continuous infusion for up to 4 days.[33] If the sodium correction is inadequate the infusion dose can be increased to 40 mg per day.[33] Conivaptan is a nonselective vasopressin receptor antagonist, which means that it blocks V_1 receptors in the vasculature and V_2 receptors in the kidney. The patient must be observed carefully to avoid hypotension (caused by V_1 receptor blockade). Hypovolemia is a contraindication. Tolvaptan (Samsca) is an oral medication in the same class. This mediation should be initiated in the hospital, where serum sodium levels can be monitored to avoid a too-rapid rise in serum sodium following aquadiuresis.

Nursing Management

Nursing management of the patient with SIADH incorporates a variety of nursing diagnoses (Box 33-19). Nursing management is directed toward restriction of fluids, surveillance for complications, and provision of patient education.

Restriction of Fluids

Thorough, astute nursing assessments are required for care of the patient with SIADH while an attempt is made to correct the fluid and sodium imbalance; the systemic effects of hyponatremia occur rapidly and can be lethal. Fluids are restricted to between 800 and 1200 mL per day.[35] Accurate measurement of I&O is required. Frequent assessment of the patient's hydration status is accomplished with serial measurements of urine output, serum sodium levels, and serum osmolality. Frequent mouth care (moistening of the buccal membrane) may give comfort during the period of fluid restriction. The patient is weighed daily to gauge fluid retention or loss. Weight gain signifies continual fluid retention, whereas weight loss indicates loss of body fluid.

Patient Education

Rapidly occurring changes in the patient's neurologic status may worry visiting family members. Sensitivity to the family's unspoken fears can be shown by words that express empathy and by providing time for the patient and family to ask questions and express their concerns. The nurse may discuss the

BOX 33-21 **CONDITIONS ASSOCIATED WITH HYPERTHYROIDISM**

- Iodine-induced hyperthyroidism (e.g., related to amiodarone therapy)
- Excessive pituitary production of thyroid-stimulating hormone (TSH) or trophoblastic disease
- Excessive ingestion of thyroid hormone
- Toxic diffuse goiter (Graves disease)
- Toxic adenoma
- Toxic multinodular goiter (Plummer disease)
- Painful subacute thyroiditis
- Silent thyroiditis, including lymphocytic and postpartum variations

course of SIADH, its effect on water balance, and the reasons for fluid restrictions (Box 33-20).

Collaborative Management

At this time, there are no published guidelines that discuss acute collaborative care management of the patient with SIADH. This is a complex condition, and effective clinical management requires the skills of many health care professionals working as a team, with goals that are clearly communicated to all team members.

THYROID STORM

Description

Thyroid storm always occurs as a complication of pre-existing hyperthyroidism. Hyperthyroidism, also called *thyrotoxicosis*, occurs when the thyroid gland produces thyroid hormone in excess of the body's need.[36] Over half the causes of primary hyperthyroidism are due to *Graves disease*, an autoimmune condition that affects 0.5% of the U.S. population, with a 5:1 to 10:1 female to male ratio.[37,38] Graves disease is caused by circulating immunoglobulin-G (IgG) antibodies that attack the thyroid stimulating hormone (TSH) receptor cells on the gland causing release of thyroid hormone unrelated to the normal physiologic feedback mechanisms that are illustrated in Figure 31-6 in Chapter 31.[38] The antidysrhythmic medication amiodarone causes thyroid dysfunction in 10% to 20% of amiodarone-treated patients.[39,40] Conditions associated with hyperthyroidism are presented in Box 33-21.

Thyroid storm, also called *thyroid crisis*, it is a rare and life-threatening exacerbation of hyperthyroidism. The pathophysiology underlying the transition from hyperthyroidism to thyroid storm is not fully understood, as thyroid hormone levels are not necessarily different from patients with hyperthyroidism. Activation of the SNS and enhanced sensitivity to the effects of thyroid hormone are apparent. Stopping antithyroid medications and major stressors, such as infection, surgery, trauma, pregnancy, or critical illness, can precipitate thyroid storm in any patient with pre-existing hyperthyroidism.[36]

Etiology

In thyroid storm, excessive endogenous thyroid hormone increases metabolic activity and stimulates the beta-adrenergic receptors resulting in a heightened SNS response. There is hyperactivity of cardiac tissue, nervous tissue, and smooth muscle tissue and tremendous heat production.[41]

Pathophysiology

Thyroid hormone increases cellular oxygen consumption in almost all metabolically active cells. Excess metabolism generates heat and critically high fever. Cellular oxygen demands are dramatically increased with increased cardiac output to meet tissue demands. The oxygen demands in the hypermetabolic state are so great that the cardiac system cannot compensate adequately. Hypertension and tachycardia follow.

Gastrointestinal peristalsis increases, resulting in diarrhea, nausea, and vomiting. These symptoms all lead to dehydration and compound the problem of malnutrition and weight loss. Muscular weakness occurs and is compounded by the excessive protein breakdown. Metabolic acidosis is a potential problem.

Hypersensitivity to the increased adrenergic-binding sites potentiates the cardiovascular and nervous system responses to the hypermetabolic state. Atrial fibrillation is the most common dysrhythmia in patients with hyperthyroidism, and tachydysrhythmias should be anticipated in thyroid storm, especially in patients with underlying heart disease.[42] Pulmonary edema and acute heart failure also can occur. Increased beta-adrenergic activity manifests in emotional lability, fine muscular tremors, agitation, and even delirium. Clinical manifestations of thyroid storm are listed in Box 33-22.

Assessment and Diagnosis

The clinical presentation of thyroid storm is characterized by a variety of organ systems including:

1. Thermoregulation: fever
2. Heart: atrial fibrillation, supraventricular tachycardia, acute heart failure
3. Central nervous system: agitation, restlessness, delirium
4. Gastrointestinal: nausea, vomiting, diarrhea, unexplained jaundice, stupor, coma

Early manifestations may be insidious or missed, creating a paradoxically abrupt presentation of apparently unrelated signs and symptoms. Using a pre-established thyroid storm scoring system provides one method to systematically diagnose thyroid storm (Table 33-8).[36] A score above 45 is indicative of thyroid storm.

BOX 33-22   CLINICAL MANIFESTATIONS OF THYROID STORM

Cardiovascular System Prompted by Increased Affinity of Beta-Adrenergic Receptors in the Heart
- Tachycardia
- Systolic murmur
- Increased stroke volume
- Increased cardiac output
- Increased systolic blood pressure
- Decreased diastolic blood pressure
- Extra systoles
- Paroxysmal atrial tachycardia
- Premature ventricular contraction
- Palpitations
- Chest pain
- Increased cardiac contractility
- Acute heart failure
- Pulmonary edema
- Cardiogenic shock

Central Nervous System Resulting from an Increased Catecholamine Response
- Hyperkinesis
- Nervousness
- Muscle weakness
- Confusion
- Convulsions
- Heat intolerance
- Fine tremor
- Emotional lability
- Frank psychosis
- Apathy
- Stupor
- Diaphoresis

Gastrointestinal System
- Nausea
- Vomiting
- Diarrhea
- Liver enlargement
- Abdominal pain
- Weight loss
- Increased appetite

Integumentary System
- Pruritus
- Hyperpigmentation of skin
- Fine, straight hair
- Alopecia

Thermoregulatory System
- Hyperthermia
- Heat dissipation
- Diaphoresis

Serum or Urine
- Hypercalcemia
- Hyperglycemia
- Hypoalbuminemia
- Hypoprothrombinemia
- Hypocholesterolemia
- Creatinuria

Laboratory findings are used to confirm the suspicion raised by the clinical signs. The TSH value is extremely low, and thyroid hormones (T_3 and T_4) are high, compared with normal values (see Table 32-3 in Chapter 32 for normal reference values). These results, in combination with the clinical picture, provide the diagnosis.

No laboratory test is available to differentiate thyroid storm from its predecessor, thyrotoxicosis, for which the laboratory values may be similar. Thyroid storm is identified by a combination of the patient's medical history and exacerbation of clinical manifestations.

Medical Management

The goal of acute medical management of thyroid storm is to reduce the clinical effects of thyroid hormone as rapidly as possible. This includes preventing cardiac decompensation, reducing hyperthermia, and reversing dehydration caused by fever or gastrointestinal losses.

Prevent Cardiovascular Collapse

The body's heightened sensitivity to the increased adrenergic and catecholamine receptors must be suppressed. Atrial

TABLE 33-8 THYROID STORM DIAGNOSTIC CRITERIA

CRITERIA	POINTS	CRITERIA	POINTS
Thermoregulatory Dysfunction		**Gastrointestinal-Hepatic Dysfunction**	
Temperature (°F)		Manifestation	
99.0-99.9	5	Absent	0
100.0-100.9	10	Moderate (diarrhea, abdominal pain,	10
101.0-101.9	15	nausea/vomiting)	
102.0-102.9	20	Severe (jaundice)	20
103.0-103.9	25		
≥104.0	30	**Central Nervous System Disturbance**	
		Manifestation	
Cardiovascular		Absent	0
Tachycardia (beats per minute)		Mild (agitation)	10
100-109	5	Moderate (delirium, psychosis, extreme lethargy)	20
110-119	10	Severe (seizure, coma)	30
120-129	15		
130-139	20	**Precipitant History**	
≥140	25	Status	
		Positive	0
Atrial fibrillation		Negative	10
Absent	0		
Present	10	**Scores Totaled:**	
		>45 **Thyroid storm**	
Acute heart failure		25-44 **Impending storm**	
Absent	0	<25 **Storm unlikely**	
Mild	5		
Moderate	10		
Severe	20		

Modified from Burch and Wartofsky. Life-threatening thyrotoxicosis: thyroid storm. *Endocrinol Metal Clin North Am.* 1993;22:263. In Bahn RS, et al. Hyperthyroidism and other causes of thyrotoxicosis: management guidelines of the American Thyroid Association and American Association of Clinical Endocrinologists. *Endocr Pract.* 2011;17(3):456.

dysrhythmias need to be controlled and progression of heart failure halted. Beta-blockers are the mainstay of therapy for cardiac protection.[36]

Reduce Hyperthermia

Reduction in body temperature is achieved by use of a cooling blanket and the antipyretic agent acetaminophen.[36] Salicylates (aspirin) are contraindicated because they inhibit protein binding of T_3 to T_4, increasing the level of free, metabolically active, thyroid hormone.[43]

Reverse Dehydration

Vigorous fluid replacement must be instituted to treat or prevent dehydration. Antibiotic therapy may be warranted in the presence of systemic infection. Dehydration is treated with large volumes of glucose and isotonic sodium solutions to replace circulating fluid and sodium losses from hypermetabolism.

Pharmacologic Management

Pharmacologic treatment is essential in treatment of thyroid storm.[36] A multimodal medication approach is recommended with monitoring in a critical care unit during the acute phase.[36] Beta-blockers are administered to decrease the peripheral cellular sensitivity to catecholamines and antithyroid medications are administered to block the synthesis and release of thyroid hormone into the circulation, and to inhibit peripheral

conversion of T_4 to T_3. Medications used to treat thyroid storm are listed in Table 33-9.

Medications That Block the Catecholamine Effect

To decrease the catecholamine effects of excessive thyroid hormone, beta-adrenergic blocking agents are used. Propranolol is the most frequently used medication (see Table 33-9). Beta-blockers have no effect on thyroid hormone but reduce the exaggerated myocardial stimulation and slow the atrioventricular (AV) conduction rate. Therapeutic doses vary from patient to patient, but higher doses are typically required to effectively control the symptoms. Esmolol, a short-acting IV beta-blocker, may also be used.[36] Non-dihydropyridine calcium channel blockers may be effective in controlling the HR in patients for whom beta-blockers are contraindicated.[36]

Medications That Block Thyroid Synthesis

The synthesis of new thyroid hormone is blocked by the administration of antithyroid medications. Two agents are frequently used: propylthiouracil (PTU) and methimazole (see Table 33-9).[36] These medications are administered by mouth or via a feeding tube. PTU is especially therapeutic because it blocks thyroid synthesis and blocks conversion of T_4 to T_3. Methimazole has a slower rate of action but is more potent than PTU. Both medications act within 1 to 2 hours after absorption from the gastrointestinal tract. These medications have no impact on previously released thyroid hormone.

TABLE 33-9   PHARMACOLOGIC MANAGEMENT
Thyroid Storm

MEDICATION	DOSAGE	ACTIONS	SPECIAL CONSIDERATIONS
Antithyroid Medications			
Propylthiouracil	Loading dose: 500-1000 mg Maintenance dose: 250 mg every 6h	Blocks synthesis of thyroid hormone Blocks conversion of T_3 to T_4	May cause rash, nausea, vomiting, agranulocytosis, skin hyperpigmentation Administer with meals to reduce GI effects
Methimazole	60-80 mg per day	Blocks new hormone synthesis	Monitor signs listed for propylthiouracil May cause rash, agranulocytosis
Iodine (saturated solution of potassium iodide)	5 drops (0.25 mL or 250 mg) orally every 6 hours	Blocks new hormone synthesis	Do not start until 1 hour after antithyroid medications have been administered
Hydrocortisone	Loading: 300 mg IV Maintenance 100 mg every 8 hours	May block conversion of T_4 to T_3	Prophylaxis against adrenal insufficiency Dexamethasone is an alternative medication
Beta-Blockers			
Propranolol	60-80 mg every 4 hours orally	Beta-adrenergic blockade	Monitor HR and BP response to beta blockade
Esmolol	50-100 mcg/kg/min IV pump	Beta-adrenergic blockade	Monitor HR and BP response to beta blockade in the critical care unit

Based on data from Bahn RS, et al. Hyperthyroidism and other causes of thyrotoxicosis: management guidelines of the American Thyroid Association and American Association of Clinical Endocrinologists. *Endocr Pract.* 2011;17(3):456.
BP, Blood pressure; *GI,* gastrointestinal; *HR,* heart rate; *IV,* intravenous; *mcg/kg/min,* micrograms per kilogram per minute; *mg,* milligrams.

BOX 33-23   NURSING DIAGNOSES
Thyroid Storm

- Hyperthermia related to increased metabolic rate, p. 1140
- Imbalanced Nutrition: Less Than Body Requirements related to lack of exogenous nutrients and increased metabolic demand, p. 1143
- Decreased Cardiac Output related to alterations in heart rate or rhythm, p. 1128
- Anxiety related to threat to biologic, psychologic, and social integrity, p. 1125
- Disturbed Sleep Pattern related to fragmented sleep, p. 1137
- Deficient Knowledge related to lack of previous exposure to information, p. 1134 (see Box 33-24, Patient Education for Thyroid Storm)

Medications That Block Release of Thyroid Hormone

Administration of inorganic iodine blocks the release of any preformed thyroxine that is already in the thyroid gland but not yet released.[36] It is essential that iodine therapy not be administered until adequate inhibition of new hormone synthesis has occurred, as described in Table 33-9.[36] The iodide preparations are rapid acting and have a short duration. They are given approximately 1 hour after administration of the antithyroid medications (described in the previous section) to prevent the iodide from being used for thyroid hormone production and possible worsening of the clinical state.

Some patients with thyroid storm have concomitant adrenal insufficiency and may be prescribed hydrocortisone or dexamethasone during the initial stages of thyroid storm management. See Table 33-9 for a list of the most commonly used medications and their nursing implications for the patient in thyroid storm.

Nursing Management

Nursing management of the patient with thyroid storm incorporates a variety of nursing diagnoses (Box 33-23). Nursing interventions are directed toward safe administration and monitoring of the effects of prescribed medications, normalizing body temperature, rehydration with correction of other metabolic derangements, and provision of patient education.

Medication Administration

The timely and ordered sequence of medication administration is essential in the management of thyroid storm (see previous sections on pharmacologic management). The patient in thyroid storm is agitated, anxious, and unable to rest and benefits from an environment that is calm. The effects of the antithyroid medications, iodides, and beta-adrenergic blocking agents gradually decrease the neurologic symptoms related to catecholamine sensitivity. Heart rate should decrease with beta-blockade.

The patient and family need to be reassured that this extreme agitation is the result of the disease process and that the medications will help control the nonstop fidgeting and tremors.

Frequent reassurance and clear, simple explanations of the patient's condition help decrease the fear brought on by the onset of thyroid storm.

Normalize Body Temperature

In thyroid storm, the patient has hyperthermia related to a hypermetabolic state, as evidenced by a critically high body temperature; diaphoresis; hot, flushed skin; intolerance to heat;

tachycardia; and tachypnea. Temperature is assessed frequently until normal body temperature is attained. Nursing measures to provide comfort while the patient is intolerant to heat include a room with a cool environment and a fan to circulate air, and comfortable, nonrestrictive bedclothes. A tepid sponge bath helps to reduce heat by evaporation, and cold-pack applications to the groin and axilla increase heat loss at major blood vessels. If antipyretic medications are required, acetaminophen is the agent of choice, and salicylates are avoided.[43]

Rehydration and Correction of Metabolic Derangements

Hyperthermia, tachypnea, diaphoresis, vomiting, and diarrhea predispose the patient to a fluid volume deficit. Fluids and electrolytes are as vigorously replaced as the decompensated cardiovascular system can tolerate. Glucose solutions are given to replace glycogen stores, which are depleted. Insulin is administered to treat the hyperglycemia that results from mobilization of nutrients and glucocorticoids. Hyponatremia from active loss (e.g., vomiting) is monitored by means of laboratory serum values. Hyponatremia can be prevented or treated with isotonic IV fluid replacement. Additional nursing measures focus on frequent hydration assessments (see Box 33-6).

Patient Education

During the critical events surrounding the thyroid storm, the patient and family are given information according to their emotional state and cognitive level of understanding. The cause of the high fever, anxiety, and cardiac dysrhythmias is explained in understandable terms (Box 33-24). Often, the patient and family are relieved to know that the agitation and nervousness result from circulating hormones that may be decreased by taking daily medications.

Side effects of the specific medication therapy are taught before discharge. Patients treated with beta-blockers are taught to report signs of bradycardia, unexplained fatigue, and orthostatic hypotension, among other untoward effects. Patients discharged with antithyroid medications are alerted to the potential side effect, agranulocytosis (see Table 33-9). Symptoms of *agranulocytosis* include sudden cough, fever, rash, and inflammation. For management or elevated temperature, patients are instructed to use acetaminophen rather than salicylates, because salicylates increase the amount of free thyroid hormone in circulation.

BOX 33-24 PATIENT EDUCATION

Thyroid Storm

Acute Phase
- Explain reasons for critical care unit admission
- Explain reasons for extreme hypermetabolism

Predischarge
- Assess knowledge level
- Disease process of thyrotoxicosis
- Causes of thyrotoxic crisis
- Medications: explain purpose, side effects, dosage, and how often to use
- Signs and symptoms to report to health care professional

Collaborative Management

Management of the patient with thyroid storm is derived from the 2011 guidelines issued by the American Thyroid Association and American Association of Clinical Endocrinologists.[36] The patient with thyroid storm requires interventions by many health care professionals, with clearly communicated goals to facilitate rapid recovery.

MYXEDEMA COMA

Description

A severe deficiency or absence of thyroid hormone produces hypothyroidism. Hypothyroidism, as defined by laboratory tests and clinical symptoms, ranges from mild (subclinical) to severe. Subclinical hypothyroidism has subtle symptoms whereas severe hypothyroidism leads to a comatose state called *myxedema coma*, which can be fatal. Discussion of myxedema coma necessitates frequent reference to its precursor state, hypothyroidism. The term *myxedema* is used only when referring to myxedema coma, as a description of the progressive worsening or terminal stage of hypothyroidism.

Etiology

Hypothyroidism is caused by a deficiency of circulating thyroid hormone. Insufficient thyroid hormone affects all body cells and organs and slows the metabolic rate and response times in every system.

Myxedema coma is rare, more commonly afflicts older patients, and affects many more women than men. Early recognition of symptoms and prompt treatment decrease the mortality rate associated with myxedema, although it remains high compared with many other diseases—35% and 52% in two case series.[44,45] Myxedema coma is rarely seen as a single disease entity in the critical care unit. Its underlying presence often is revealed by an acute primary disease, by surgery, or as a consequence of increased metabolic demands. Cardiopulmonary disease, systemic infection, and exposure to extreme cold are a few of the physiologic stressors that can increase metabolic demand.

Pathophysiology

The effects of hypothyroidism are widespread and varied. When the basal metabolic rate of oxygen consumption is reduced, cells are unable to maintain the processes necessary to sustain life. Without thyroid hormone, protein synthesis is severely curtailed, and amino acid production and repair of tissues are halted. Metabolism of carbohydrate and fat is incomplete, and gluconeogenesis cannot supply additional sources of glucose. Lipolysis is ineffective, and cholesterol collects in the bloodstream. All systems are affected.

Skin

The composition of the skin changes as deposits of *hyaluronic acid* (a gel-like substance capable of holding large amounts of fluid) accumulate in the interstitial spaces, giving rise to a full appearance of face, hands, and feet. The skin is pale, with an overall yellowish appearance resulting from increased carotene deposits. The nails and hair are thin and brittle. Absence of thyroid hormone also leads to decreased or absent sweat production. The hyaluronic acid deposits are evident in heart muscle, skeletal muscles, and muscles of the tongue, pharynx, and proximal esophagus. These striated muscular changes of the tongue, pharynx, and esophagus probably contribute to the hoarse, husky voice and lack of facial expression in patients with hypothyroidism.

Cardiopulmonary System

Interstitial edema impairs cardiac myocytes, resulting in bradycardia and diminished cardiac output. Serous fluid accumulation in the pericardial sac can cause cardiac tamponade.[46] A decreased sensitivity to catecholamines is present even though serum catecholamine levels are elevated. Resting HR and stroke volume are reduced. The force of myocardial contraction is weakened. There is a decrease in the systolic BP and an increase in the diastolic pressure, causing a narrowed pulse pressure. Electrocardiography (ECG) typically reveals low-voltage QRS complexes and low-voltage, flattened, or inverted T waves and prolonged QT interval.[46]

Pulmonary System

Pleural effusions and muscular changes affect gas exchange. The basal rate of oxygen consumption decreases, with a resulting insensitivity to CO_2. Hypoventilation increases the CO_2 serum content, which increases cerebral hypoxia. Hypoxic and hypercapnic ventilatory drives are severely impaired. Respiratory acidosis can occur. Pleural effusion, reduced vital capacity, and shallow respirations occur with any exertion. Respiratory muscle weakness, sleep apnea, and upper airway obstruction may be present.

Patients with myxedema are a high-risk category for any surgical procedure or critical care admission because of their limited ventilatory capacity. Respiratory failure and requirement for mechanical ventilation may be the reason the patient is admitted to the critical care unit.

Kidneys and Fluid and Electrolyte Balance

Renal blood flow is reduced, and the glomerular filtration rate (GFR), urine specific gravity, and urine osmolality are decreased. The ADH level is increased (fluid retention), and sodium is decreased. Urea production is diminished. Elimination of medications by the kidneys is severely slowed in hypothyroidism. Coexisting adrenal insufficiency should also be considered.

Nutrition and Elimination

Decreased gastric motility or even ileus is an expected complication for the patient with severe hypothyroidism. Food utilization and nutrient mobilization decrease with insufficient thyroid hormone. Intestinal hypomotility and abdominal serum cholesterol increases. Abdominal distention, decreased intestinal peristalsis, and eventual paralytic ileus lead to extreme constipation. These findings make the provision of enteral nutrition a challenge. In the more alert patient, a lack of appetite and inability to eat coexist.

Thermoregulation

Heat production decreases as a result of insufficient energy to maintain the base metabolic rate within the cells. The ability to maintain body heat is further restricted by the hypoglycemia.

Anemia

Anemia is present in many patients with hypothyroidism. Symptoms of fatigue and depression are associated. Erythropoiesis (red cell production) is impaired. Coagulation abnormalities may coexist.[46]

Assessment and Diagnosis

The diagnosis of myxedema coma is based on the clinical manifestations of end-stage hypothyroidism. A comparison of severe hyperthyroidism (thyroid storm) and severe hypothyroidism (myxedema) is provided in Box 33-25.

BOX 33-25 CLINICAL MANIFESTATIONS OF HYPERTHYROIDISM COMPARED WITH HYPOTHYROIDISM

HYPERTHYROIDISM (THYROTOXICOSIS, THYROID STORM)	HYPOTHYROIDISM (MYXEDEMA, MYXEDEMA COMA)
• Elevated T_4, T_3	• Decreased T_4, T_3
• Decreased TSH	• Elevated TSH
• Hypercalcemia	• Hyponatremia
• Hyperglycemia	• Hypoglycemia
• Metabolic acidosis	• Respiratory acidosis, metabolic acidosis
• Tachycardia, palpitations, atrial fibrillation	• Hypercholesterolemia
• Angina	• Anemia
• ST wave changes	• Bradycardia
• Shortened QT	• Peripheral vasoconstriction
• Hypertension	• Flattened, inverted T waves
• AV block, acute heart failure	• Prolonged QT and PR intervals
• Hypovolemia	• Decreased stroke volume, decreased cardiac output
• Shortness of breath, tachypnea	• Enlarged heart, pericardial effusion
• Hypermetabolism	• Increased total body fluid with decreased effective arterial blood volume
• Polyphagia	• Hypoventilation, possible CO_2 retention
• Weight loss	• Depressed metabolism
• Nausea, vomiting, increased peristalsis	• Decreased lipolysis, increased cholesterol
• Tremor	• Weight gain
• Extreme restlessness, insomnia, uneasiness, anxiety	• Constipation
• Emotional instability, despondency	• Seizures
• Diaphoresis	• Slowness, depression
• Heat intolerance	• Impaired short-term memory
• Increased DTRs	• Slow, deliberate speech
• Muscle weakness or muscle wasting	• Thickened tongue
• Oligomenorrhea	• Coarse, dry, scaly, edematous skin
	• Hypothermia
	• Delirium (myxedema madness)
	• Lethargy → stupor → coma (myxedema coma)
	• Diminished DTRs
	• Paresthesia of hands
	• Menorrhagia

AV, Atrioventricular; *DTRs,* deep tension reflexes; *TSH,* thyroid-stimulating hormone.

Clinical Presentation

The diagnosis of end-stage hypothyroidism is based on the clinical presentation. Increasing signs of somnolence, depression, and diminished mental acuity signal diminished cellular function. Interstitial edema collects in almost all tissues. Organs become infiltrated with the mucoid-rich mucopolysaccharides, compromising organ function. Patients manifest cardiovascular collapse, hypothermia, decreased kidney function, fluid excess, hypoventilation, and severe metabolic disorders.

Weight gain is attributed to the collection of mucopolysaccharides in the interstitium, the increase in fluid retention, and the decrease in metabolism. Paresthesias of hands and feet are caused by the hyaluronic acid accumulation in the synovial sacs, which leads to compression of nerves and carpal tunnel syndrome. Compression of nerves interferes with the simplest hand grasp and the ability to raise one's hands. Reflexes contract briskly but take extended seconds to relax.

Hypothermia is a very distressing symptom. Most cases of myxedema are diagnosed in the winter months. The myxedematous patient has hypotension, reduced total blood volume, decreased cardiac output, and bradycardia—all related to a decrease in beta-adrenergic stimulation. Neuropsychiatric symptoms of depression, confusion, and decreased mental acuity may degenerate to a psychosis sometimes called *myxedema madness*.[47]

Laboratory Studies

Laboratory test results do not differentiate between hypothyroidism and myxedema coma. The blood test results simply confirm the clinical picture. Typically, patients with myxedema have primary hypothyroidism with a high TSH level and a low T_4 level.[46] If the TSH level is normal or low, other causes of the hypothyroidism must be investigated. TSH is released by the pituitary gland (see Table 32-3 in Chapter 32 for normal reference values); endocrine studies to evaluate the level of pituitary function should be undertaken.

Medical Management

The patient's primary admitting diagnosis may mask an underlying hypothyroidism. However, clinical manifestations can trigger the alert clinician to suspect a hypofunctioning thyroid. The primary disease condition and the myxedema coma must be treated immediately to improve the patient's chances for recovery. Myxedema coma often necessitates ventilator support, correction of fluid and electrolyte imbalance, correction of other multisystem abnormalities, corticosteroid supplementation, and thyroid hormone replacement.[48]

Pharmacologic Management

The type and dose of thyroid hormone replacement to treat end-stage hypothyroidism (myxedema coma) is controversial.[49] One method is to replete T_4 levels with an initial dose of levothyroxine (300 to 400 mcg administered IV) to saturate the previously empty T_4 binding sites, followed by daily administration of 50 to 100 mcg of levothyroxine.[48]

A serum cortisol level is obtained to evaluate adrenal gland function. Glucocorticoids may be necessary to assist the patient

to respond to the stress state of hypothyroidism, until a coexisting adrenal insufficiency is ruled out.[49]

Nursing Management

Nursing care of the patient with myxedema coma focuses on management of the precipitating disease and on the severe impact of hypothyroidism on multiple organ systems. Many nursing diagnoses are associated with management of myxedema coma and are listed in Box 33-26.

Pulmonary Care

The patient with myxedema coma who is admitted to the critical care unit may require intubation and mechanical ventilatory support. Individuals who are not intubated are monitored for development of respiratory failure. Arterial blood gas measurements are evaluated to monitor for CO_2 retention and respiratory acidosis.

Cardiac Concerns

Dysrhythmias are common in the myxedematous patient with impaired myocardial contraction and can quickly be identified by continuous ECG monitoring. Expected signs of myxedema, such as flattened or inverted T waves or prolonged QT and PR intervals, resolve in a positive response to thyroxine replacement therapy.

Thermoregulation

Hypothermia gradually improves as the patient is treated with thyroid hormone. Several warm blankets comfortably wrapped around the patient with mild hypothermia may be sufficient to help raise the body temperature to normal. Active warming devices are also used. Continuous assessments are important to avoid too-rapid heating and vasodilation. Electronic devices that can measure accurately at the extreme lower range of body temperatures are used.

Thyroid Replacement Therapy

Older patients and those with a cardiac history receive IV thyroid hormone replacement with due precautions. Thyroxine can precipitate angina and dysrhythmias. Improvements in the patient's cardiopulmonary and neurologic status, together with changes in T_4 and TSH laboratory values, are used to gauge the success of the thyroid hormone replacement therapy.

Skin Care

Patients with myxedema coma have rough, dry skin. Measures are taken to avoid skin breakdown related to decreased circulation and widespread edema. An emollient for skin hydration follows non-soap baths. Frequent repositioning minimizes pressure against capillary beds over bony prominences.

Elimination

Constipation is managed on a daily basis to avoid impaction. Use of fiber-enriched enteral nutrition may be helpful. Food choices for oral intake include sources of increased fiber, such as fresh fruits and vegetables. Fluids are encouraged as the hypovolemia is corrected and BP stabilizes. Increased fiber is preferable to use of enemas. Enemas are to be avoided, because insertion of the rectal tube may stimulate the vagus nerve.

Patient Education

Patients with myxedema coma have decreased comprehension and mental acuity. All instructions, procedures, and activities are to be explained slowly and provided in written form. The patient and family members may experience myriad emotions with one constant: fear of the unknown. Before any teaching, the nurse evaluates the family's ability to accept the patient's slowed thinking and slowed response time. The family may benefit from a referral to the hospital's social service department for assistance in dealing with the patient's neuropsychiatric symptoms.

All instructions given to the patient or family are given verbally and in writing. A written copy of all schedules is given as a reference for home care before discharge. The nurse discusses the medication schedule and the frequency of the medication doses with the patient and family. Side effects of each medication are described. The patient and family need to know the side effects of medications, including over-the-counter medications, so that they can deal with them at home, and they need to know which signs or symptoms are to be reported to their health care provider (Box 33-27).

Collaborative Management

There are no published guidelines that discuss acute collaborative care management of the patient with myxedema coma. Collaborative management is required to decrease mortality in myxedema coma. Early recognition of symptoms and a willingness to request laboratory tests to confirm the diagnosis allow therapy to be instituted as early as possible.

BOX 33-27 **PATIENT EDUCATION**

Myxedema Coma

Acute Phase
- Explain reasons for critical care unit admission
- Explain reasons for extreme hypermetabolism

Predischarge
- Assess knowledge level
- Disease process of thyrotoxicosis
- Causes of thyrotoxic crisis
- Medications: explain purpose, side effects, dosage, and how often to use
- Signs and symptoms to report to health care professional

BOX 33-28 **CASE STUDY**

Patient with an Endocrine Disorder

Brief Patient History

Ms. S is a 72-year-old woman with a history of hypertension treated with an angiotensin-converting enzyme (ACE) inhibitor and thiazide diuretics. She has a past 100-pack/year history of tobacco abuse, but quit 2 years ago. Ms. S lives independently in a senior apartment. She was brought to the hospital by friends because of a fall. Ms. S states that she has a severe headache but cannot recall whether she hit her head during the fall. She is also having difficulty recalling recent events.

Clinical Assessment

Ms. S is admitted to the critical care unit from the emergency department because of nonspecific ECG changes suggestive of inferior wall ischemia and electrolyte abnormalities. She is awake; alert; oriented to person, time, place; and unable to recall the events leading to her hospitalization. She states that her headache is severe and feels like someone is hitting her head with a hammer. Her skin is warm and dry. Ms. S's gait is visibly unsteady.

Diagnostic Procedures

Ms. S's vital signs include the following: blood pressure of 180/92 mm Hg, heart rate of 100 beats/min (sinus rhythm), respiratory rate of 24 breaths/min, and temperature of 98.8° F.

Ms. S reports that her headache is a 10 on the Baker-Wong faces scale. Laboratory findings include the following: sodium level of 116 mmol/L, potassium level of 3.3 mmol/L, chloride level of 88 mmol/L, carbon dioxide level of 22 mEq/L, magnesium level of 1.8 mg/dL, urinary sodium level of 30 mmol/L, and urine osmolality value of 118 mOsm/L. The test result for troponin I on admission was negative. ECG testing shows a normal sinus rhythm, T-wave inversion in leads II, III, and AVF, and a change from prior ECG findings, suggestive of inferior wall ischemia. Chest radiography identified a mass in the right upper lobe that strongly suggested a neoplasm.

Medical Diagnosis

Ms. S is diagnosed with syndrome of inappropriate diuretic hormone (SIADH).

Questions

1. What major outcomes do you expect to achieve for this patient?
2. What problems or risks must be managed to achieve these outcomes?
3. What interventions must be initiated to monitor, prevent, manage, or eliminate the problems and risks identified?
4. What interventions should be initiated to promote optimal functioning, safety, and well-being of the patient?
5. What possible learning needs do you anticipate for this patient?
6. What cultural and age-related factors may have a bearing on the patient's plan of care?

SUMMARY

Stress of Critical Illness

- The endocrine system is complex, and assessment relies heavily on laboratory tests for confirmation of disease processes. To fully participate in the care of patients with these complex conditions, the critical care nurse must be aware of the intricacies of the endocrine system.
- Physiologic stress associated with critical illness causes increased secretion of stress hormones by the hypothalamic-pituitary-adrenal pathway. This results in secretion of cortisol, stimulation of the SNS, and release of norepinephrine and epinephrine to mobilize glucose. If critical illness is prolonged beyond 7 to 10 days, profound suppression of pituitary, thyroid, and adrenal gland function occurs.

Pancreas: DKA and HHS

- The diagnostic criteria for DKA include a blood glucose concentration greater than 250 mg/dL, an arterial pH value of less than 7.3, a serum bicarbonate level lower than 18 mEq/L, and moderate or severe ketonemia or ketonuria.
- The diagnostic criteria for HHS include a blood glucose concentration greater than 600 mg/dL, an arterial pH value higher than 7.3, a serum bicarbonate level greater than 18 mEq/L, a serum osmolality greater than 320 mOsm/kg H_2O (320 mmol/kg), and absent or mild ketonuria.

Pituitary: DI and SIADH

- Central DI occurs when ADH (vasopressin) is not released from the posterior pituitary gland. The excretion of large quantities of hypotonic urine creates the following alterations in serum and urinary laboratory values: serum sodium greater than 145 mEq/L, serum osmolality greater than 295 mOsm/kg H_2O (295 mmol/L), urine osmolality lower than 200 mOsm/kg H_2O (200 mmol/L), and urine specific gravity lower than 1.005.
- SIADH occurs when excess ADH (vasopressin) is released from the posterior pituitary gland. This stimulates the kidney tubules to retain water, resulting in fluid overload and hyponatremia manifested by alterations in serum and urinary laboratory values: decreased plasma osmolality (less than 275 mOsm/kg H_2O), with increased urine osmolality (greater than 100 mOsm/kg); low serum sodium (less than 125 mEq/L) and elevated urinary sodium (greater than 40 mEq/L).

Thyroid: Thyroid Storm and Myxedema Coma

- Thyroid storm is identified by clinical signs such as high fever, tachycardia, hypertension, and tremor, as evidence of the rapid metabolic rate. The laboratory values are similar to those seen in hyperthyroidism: low TSH and high T_4 levels.
- Myxedema coma is characterized by hypothermia, hypoventilation, bradycardia, depression, and decreased mental acuity, reflecting a slowed metabolic rate. The laboratory values are similar to those seen with hypothyroidism: high TSH and low T_4 levels.

REFERENCES

1. Dellinger RP, et al. Surviving Sepsis Campaign: international guidelines for management of severe sepsis and septic shock: 2012. *Crit Care Med*. 2013;41(2):580.
2. Moghissi ES, et al. American Association of Clinical Endocrinologists and American Diabetes Association consensus statement on inpatient glycemic control. *Diabetes Care*. 2009;32(6):1119.
3. Dünser MW, Hasibeder WR. Sympathetic overstimulation during critical illness: adverse effects of adrenergic stress. *J Intens Care Med*. 2009;24(5):293.
4. Moraes RB, et al. Comparison of low and high dose cosyntropin stimulation tests in the diagnosis of adrenal insufficiency in septic shock patients. *Horm Metab Res*. 2012;44(4):296.
5. Marik PE, et al. Recommendations for the diagnosis and management of corticosteroid insufficiency in critically ill adult patients: consensus statements from an international task force by the American College of Critical Care Medicine. *Crit Care Med*. 2008;36(6):1937.
6. Fahy BG, et al. Glucose control in the intensive care unit. *Crit Care Med*. 2009;37(5):1769.
7. Van den Berghe G, et al. Intensive insulin therapy in critically ill patients. *N Engl J Med*. 2001;345(19):1359.
8. Van den Berghe G, et al. Intensive insulin therapy in the medical ICU. *N Engl J Med*. 2006;354(5):449.
9. Finfer S, et al. Intensive versus conventional glucose control in critically ill patients. *N Engl J Med*. 2009;360(13):1283.
10. Jacobi J, et al. Guidelines for the use of an insulin infusion for the management of hyperglycemia in critically ill patients. *Crit Care Med*. 2012;40(12):3251.
11. McDonnell ME, Umpierrez GE. Insulin therapy for the management of hyperglycemia in hospitalized patients. *Endocrinol Metab Clin North Am*. 2012;41(1):175.
12. Dombrowski NC, Karounos DG. Pathophysiology and management strategies for hyperglycemia for patients with acute illness during and following a hospital stay. *Metabolism*. 2013;62(3):326.
13. Rodbard HW, et al. American Association of Clinical Endocrinologists medical guidelines for clinical practice for the management of diabetes mellitus. *Endocr Pract*. 2007;13(suppl 1):1.
14. McCall AL. Insulin therapy and hypoglycemia. *Endocrinol Metab Clin North Am*. 2012;241(1):57.
15. American Diabetes Association. Nutrition recommendations and interventions for diabetes: a position statement of the American Diabetes Association. *Diabetes Care*. 2008;31(suppl 1):S61.
16. American Diabetes Association. Standards of medical care in diabetes–2012. *Diabetes Care*. 2012;35(suppl 1):S11.

17. American Diabetes Association. Diagnosis and classification of diabetes mellitus. *Diabetes Care*. 2012;35(suppl 1):S64.

18. Nathan DM, et al. Medical management of hyperglycemia in type 2 diabetes: a consensus algorithm for the initiation and adjustment of therapy: a consensus statement of the American Diabetes Association and the European Association for the Study of Diabetes. *Diabetes Care*. 2009;32(1):193.

19. Inzucchi SE, et al. Management of hyperglycemia in type 2 diabetes: a patient-centered approach: position statement of the American Diabetes Association (ADA) and the European Association for the Study of Diabetes (EASD). *Diabetes Care*. 2012;35(6):1364.

20. Qaseem A, et al. Oral pharmacologic treatment of type 2 diabetes mellitus: a clinical practice guideline from the American College of Physicians. *Ann Intern Med*. 2012;156(3):218.

21. Nathan DM, et al. Management of hyperglycemia in type 2 diabetes: a consensus algorithm for the initiation and adjustment of therapy: update regarding thiazolidinediones: a consensus statement from the American Diabetes Association and the European Association for the Study of Diabetes. *Diabetes Care*. 2008;31(1):173.

22. Derosa G, Maffioli P. Efficacy and safety profile evaluation of acarbose alone and in association with other antidiabetic drugs: a systematic review. *Clin Ther*. 2012;34(6):1221.

23. Phillips LK, Prins JB. Update on incretin hormones. *Ann NY Acad Sci*. 2011;1243:E55.

24. Kitabchi AE, et al. Hyperglycemic crises in adult patients with diabetes. *Diabetes Care*. 2009;32(7):1335.

25. Nyenwe EA, Kitabchi AE. Evidence-based management of hyperglycemic emergencies in diabetes mellitus. *Diabetes Res Clin Pract*. 2011;94(3):340.

26. Newton CA, Raskin P. Diabetic ketoacidosis in type 1 and type 2 diabetes mellitus: clinical and biochemical differences. *Arch Intern Med*. 2004;164(17):1925.

27. Hannon MJ, et al. Pituitary dysfunction following traumatic brain injury or subarachnoid haemorrhage. *Best Pract Res Clin Endocrinol Metabol*. 2011;25(5):783.

28. Schreckinger M, et al. Diabetes insipidus following resection of pituitary tumors. *Clin Neurol Neurosurg*. 2013;115(2):121.

29. Fenske W, Allolio B. Current state and future perspectives in the diagnosis of diabetes insipidus: a clinical review. *J Clin Endocrinol Metabol*. 2012;97(10):3426.

30. Loh JA, Verbalis JG. Disorders of water and salt metabolism associated with pituitary disease. *Endocrinol Metab Clin North Am*. 2008;37(1):213.

31. Devin JK. Hypopituitarism and central diabetes insipidus: perioperative diagnosis and management. *Neurosurg Clin North Am*. 2012;23(4):679.

32. Esposito P, et al. The syndrome of inappropriate antidiuresis: pathophysiology, clinical management and new therapeutic options. *Nephron Clin Pract*. 2011;119(1):c62.

33. Verbalis JG, et al. Hyponatremia treatment guidelines 2007: expert panel recommendations. *Am J Med*. 2007; 120(11 suppl 1):S1.

34. Gilbar PJ, et al. Syndrome of inappropriate antidiuretic hormone secretion induced by a single dose of oral cyclophosphamide. *Ann Pharmacother*. 2012;46(9):e23.

35. Crawford A, Harris H. SIADH: fluid out of balance. *Nursing*. 2012;42(9):50.

36. Bahn RS, et al. Hyperthyroidism and other causes of thyrotoxicosis: management guidelines of the American Thyroid Association and American Association of Clinical Endocrinologists. *Endocr Pract*. 2011;17(3):456.

37. Brent GA. Clinical practice. Graves' disease. *N Engl J Med*. 2008;358(24):2594.

38. Seigel SC, Hodak SP. Thyrotoxicosis. *Med Clin North Am*. 2012;96(2):175.

39. Bogazzi F, et al. Amiodarone and the thyroid: a 2012 update. *J Endocrinol Invest*. 2012;35(3):340.

40. Cohen-Lehman J, et al. Effects of amiodarone therapy on thyroid function. *Nat Rev Endocrinol*. 2010;6(1):34.

41. Silva JE, Bianco SD. Thyroid-adrenergic interactions: physiological and clinical implications. *Thyroid*. 2008;18(2):157.

42. Collet TH, et al. Subclinical hyperthyroidism and the risk of coronary heart disease and mortality. *Arch Intern Med*. 2012;172(10):799.

43. Wilkinson JN. Thyroid storm in a polytrauma patient. *Anaesthesia*. 2008;63(9):1001.

44. Dutta P, et al. Predictors of outcome in myxoedema coma: a study from a tertiary care centre. *Crit Care*. 2008;12(1):R1.

45. Rodríguez I, et al. Factors associated with mortality of patients with myxoedema coma: prospective study in 11 cases treated in a single institution. *J Endocrinol*. 2004;180(2):347.

46. Klubo-Gwiezdzinska J, Wartofsky L. Thyroid emergencies. *Med Clin North Am*. 2012;96(2):385.

47. Azzopardi L, et al. Myxoedema madness. *BMJ Case Rep*. 2010;2010.

48. Mathew V, et al. Myxedema coma: a new look into an old crisis. *J Thyroid Res*. 2011;2011:493462.

49. Khandelwal D, Tandon N. Overt and subclinical hypothyroidism: who to treat and how. *Drugs*. 2012;72(1):17.

Trauma

Kara A. Snyder

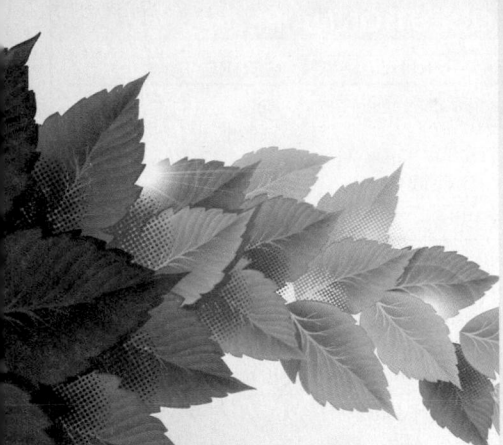

evolve WEBSITE

http://evolve.elsevier.com/Urden/criticalcare/

Evolve features:

- NCLEX Review Questions
- CCRN Review Questions
- PCCN Review Questions

- Mosby's Nursing Skills Procedures
- Animations

- Video Clips
- Glossary

Trauma is the leading cause of death for all age groups younger than 44 years. Injury costs the United States hundreds of billions of dollars annually. It is one of the most pressing health problems in the United States today, but the problem continues to go largely unrecognized.

Injury as a result of trauma is no longer considered to be an accident. The term *motor vehicle accident* (MVA) has been replaced with *motor vehicle crash* (MVC), and the term *accident* has been replaced with *unintentional injury*. Unintentional injury is no accident. Accident traditionally has implied an act of God or an unpredictable event. Domestic violence and alcohol-related issues are priority prevention areas with which health care providers must be actively involved.

Intimate partner violence (IPV) constitutes a major public health issue in the United States. IPV is the leading cause of injury to women, in the United States it is estimated that 4.8 million women and 2.9 million men every year are raped or physically assaulted each year.[1] Up to one third of injuries from IPV result in medical attention being sought and 21% of those who present with acute injuries require emergency surgery.[2]

The Joint Commission has a standard of practice that all patients must be screened for IPV as part of the health history.[3] Studies have shown that screening for IPV in healthcare settings is effective in identifying women who are victims and that patients are not offended when asked about current or past IPV.[4] Key interventions for the victim of IPV are listed in Box 34-1.

In 2010, 10,228 people were killed in alcohol-impaired driving crashes, which account for 31% of the total motor vehicle traffic fatalities in the United States.[5] Each year, alcohol-related crashes in the United States cost about $51 billion.[6]

Alcohol screening and intervention have been recommended as routine components of trauma care.[7] The Alcohol Use Disorders Identification Test (AUDIT) (Table 34-1) is a screening questionnaire that can be used because it can be used to identify frequency of alcoholic drinking and problem drinking.[8]

Over the past few decades, major advances have been made in the management of patients with traumatic injuries in the prehospital, emergency department, and critical care settings. Patients with complex, multisystem trauma are admitted to critical care units, and these patients require complex nursing care. This chapter reviews nursing management of patients with traumatic injuries in the critical care setting.

MECHANISMS OF INJURY

Trauma occurs when an external force of energy impacts the body and causes structural or physiologic alterations, or *injuries*. External forces can be radiation, electrical, thermal, chemical, or mechanical forms of energy. This chapter focuses on trauma from mechanical energy. Mechanical energy can produce blunt or penetrating traumatic injuries. Understanding the mechanism of injury helps health care providers anticipate and predict potential internal injuries.

Blunt Trauma

Blunt trauma is seen most often with MVCs, contact sports, blunt force injuries (e.g., trauma caused by a baseball bat), or falls. Injuries occur because of the forces sustained during a rapid change in velocity (deceleration). To estimate the amount of force sustained in an MVC, multiply the person's weight by the miles per hour (speed) the vehicle was traveling. A 130-pound woman in a vehicle traveling at 60 miles per hour that hits a brick wall, for example, would sustain 7800 pounds of force within milliseconds. As the body stops suddenly, tissues and organs continue to move forward. This sudden change in velocity causes injuries that result in lacerations or crush injuries of internal body structures.

Penetrating Trauma

Penetrating injuries occur with stabbings, firearms, or impalement—injuries that penetrate the skin and result in damage to internal structures. Damage is created along the path of penetration. Penetrating injuries can be misleading inasmuch as the condition of the outside of the wound does not determine the extent of internal injury. Bullets can create internal cavities 5 to 30 times larger than the diameter of the bullet.[9]

Several factors determine the extent of damage sustained as a result of penetrating trauma. Different weapons cause different types of injuries. The severity of a gunshot wound depends on the type of gun, type of ammunition used, and the distance and angle from which the gun was fired. Pellets from a shotgun blast expand on impact and cause multiple injuries to internal structures. Handgun bullets usually damage what is directly in the bullet's path. Inside the body, the bullet can ricochet off bone and create further damage along its pathway. With penetrating stab wounds, factors that determine the extent of injury include the type and length of object used and the angle of insertion.

PHASES OF TRAUMA CARE

Care of trauma victims during wartime enhanced principles of triage and rapid transport of the injured to medical facilities.

TABLE 34-1 AUDIT ALCOHOL SCREENING QUESTIONNAIRE

QUESTION	SCORE*
How often do you have a drink containing alcohol?	Never Monthly or less 2-4 times per month 2-3 times per week 4 or more times per week
How many standard drinks containing alcohol do you have on a typical day when drinking?	1 or 2 3 or 4 5 or 6 7 to 9 10 or more
How often do you have six or more drinks on one occasion?	
During the past year, how often have you found that you were not able to stop drinking once you had started?	Never
During the past year, how often have you failed to do what was normally expected of you because of drinking?	Less than monthly Monthly
During the past year, how often have you needed a drink in the morning to get yourself going after a heavy drinking session?	Weekly Daily or almost daily
During the past year, how often have you had a feeling of guilt or remorse after drinking?	
During the past year, have you been unable to remember what happened the night before because you had been drinking?	
Have you or someone else been injured as a result of your drinking?	No
Has a relative or friend, doctor or other health worker been concerned about your drinking or suggested you cut down?	Yes, but not in the past year Yes, during the past year

*Scores for each question range from 0 to 4, with the first response for each question (never) scoring 0, the second (less than monthly) scoring 1, the third (monthly) scoring 2, the fourth (weekly) scoring 3, and the fifth response (daily or almost daily) scoring 4. For the last two questions, which only have three responses, the scoring is 0, 2, and 4. A score of 8 or more is associated with harmful or hazardous drinking, and a score of 13 or more by women or 15 or more by men is likely to indicate alcohol dependence.
AUDIT, Alcohol Use Disorders Identification Test.

The military experience has demonstrated that more lives can be saved by decreasing the time from injury to definitive care. It also has enhanced incentives and models for improvements in civilian trauma care, such as emergency medical service (EMS) systems and trauma care centers. The goal with critically injured patients is to minimize the time from initial insult to definitive care and to optimize prehospital care so that the patient arrives at the hospital alive.

Statistics demonstrate that deaths as a result of trauma occur in a trimodal distribution (Fig. 34-1).[9] The first peak includes victims who die before medical attention can be provided. The second peak occurs within a few hours after injury. This peak commonly is referred to as the *golden hour* for those

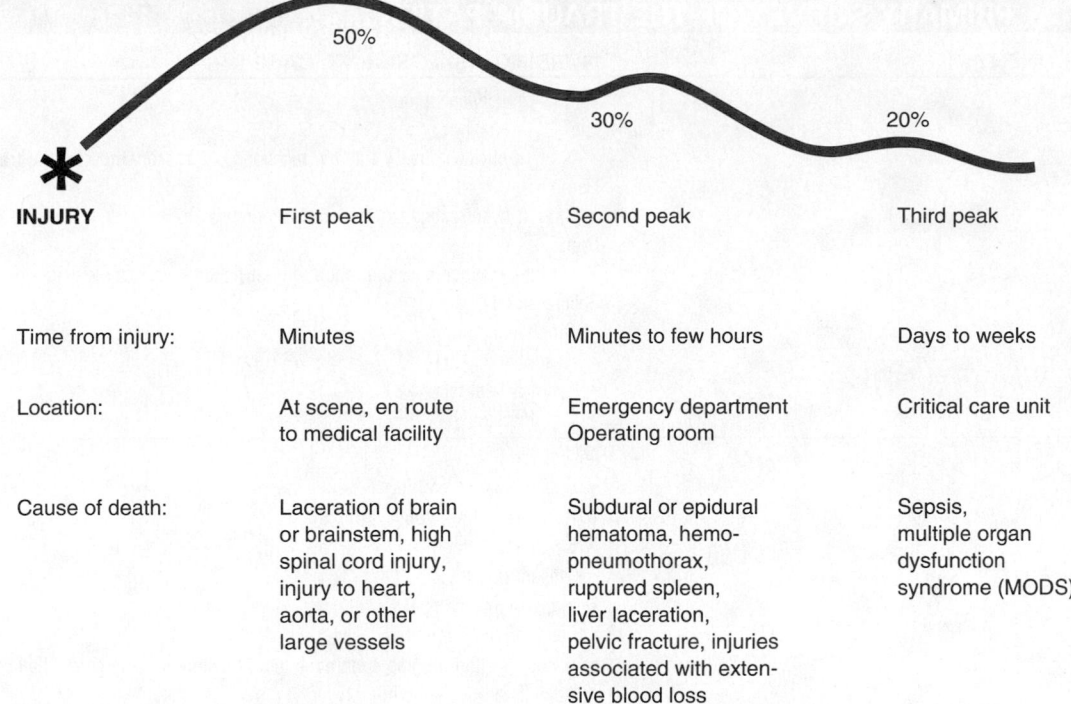

	First peak	Second peak	Third peak
INJURY			
Time from injury:	Minutes	Minutes to few hours	Days to weeks
Location:	At scene, en route to medical facility	Emergency department Operating room	Critical care unit
Cause of death:	Laceration of brain or brainstem, high spinal cord injury, injury to heart, aorta, or other large vessels	Subdural or epidural hematoma, hemo-pneumothorax, ruptured spleen, liver laceration, pelvic fracture, injuries associated with exten-sive blood loss	Sepsis, multiple organ dysfunction syndrome (MODS)

FIGURE 34-1 Trimodal distribution of trauma deaths.

critically injured. The golden hour is a 60-minute time frame that incorporates activation of the EMS system, stabilization in the prehospital setting, transportation to a medical facility, rapid resuscitation on arrival in the emergency department, and provision of definitive care. For the critically injured patient, the primary goal is to minimize the time from injury to definitive care. The third death peak occurs days to weeks after injury as a result of complications, including infection or multiple organ dysfunction syndrome (MODS). It is a nursing challenge to influence the quality of care the trauma patient receives in an attempt to "beat" the trimodal distribution of trauma deaths.

Nursing management of the patient with traumatic injuries begins the moment a call for help is received and continues until the patient's death or return to the community. Care of the trauma patient is seen as a continuum that includes six phases: prehospital resuscitation, hospital resuscitation, definitive care and operative phase, critical care, intermediate care, and rehabilitation.

Prehospital Resuscitation

The goal of prehospital care is immediate stabilization and transportation. This is achieved through airway maintenance, control of external bleeding and shock, immobilization of the patient, and immediate transport (ground or air) to the closest appropriate medical facility.[9] Prehospital personnel should communicate information needed for triage at the hospital. Advanced planning for the injured patient is essential.

Emergency Department Resuscitation

The American College of Surgeons developed guidelines (advanced trauma life support [ATLS]) for rapid assessment, resuscitation, and definitive care for trauma patients in the emergency department.[9] These guidelines delineate a systematic approach to care of the trauma patient: rapid primary survey, resuscitation of vital functions, more detailed secondary survey, and initiation of definitive care. This process constitutes the ABCDEs of trauma care and assists in identifying injuries.

Primary Survey

On arrival of the trauma patient in the emergency department, the primary survey is initiated. During this assessment, life-threatening injuries are discovered and treated. The five steps in the trauma primary survey are performed in ABCDE sequence (Table 34-2):

Airway maintenance with cervical spine protection
Breathing and ventilation
Circulation with hemorrhage control
Disability: neurologic status
Exposure or environmental control

Airway. The patient's airway is assessed for ineffective airway clearance and airway obstruction. The trauma patient is at risk for ineffective airway clearance, especially in the presence of altered consciousness, drugs and alcohol, and maxillofacial or thoracic injuries. Airway obstruction can be caused by foreign bodies, blood clots, or broken teeth. Airway patency should be assessed by inspecting the oropharynx for foreign body obstruc-tion, listening for air movement at the nose and mouth, and auscultation of lung fields. Airway assessment must incorporate cervical spine immobilization. The patient's head should not be rotated, hyperflexed, or hyperextended to establish and main-tain an airway. The cervical spine must be immobilized in all trauma patients until a cervical spinal cord injury has been definitively ruled out. If the patient can verbally communicate, it is likely that the airway is patent. Patients who display non-purposeful motor movements or who have a Glasgow Coma

TABLE 34-2 PRIMARY SURVEY OF THE TRAUMA PATIENT

SURVEY COMPONENT	NURSING ASSESSMENT, CARE
Airway	Immobilize cervical spine Look: • Is there obvious airway trauma, tachypnea, accessory muscle use, tracheal shift? Listen: • Stridor, hyperresonance, dullness to percussion? Feel: • For air exchange over the mouth; insert finger sweep to clear foreign bodies Secure airway: • Oropharyngeal • Nasopharyngeal • Endotracheal tube • Cricothyrotomy
Breathing	Assess for: • Spontaneous breathing • Respiratory rate, depth, symmetry • Chest wall integrity For absent breathing: • Intubate, mechanical ventilation If breathing but ineffective: • Assess life-threatening conditions (e.g., tension pneumothorax, flail chest) • Administer supplemental oxygen • Initiate pulse oximetry
Circulation	Assess pulse quality and rate Use ECG monitoring If no pulse: • Initiate ACLS If pulse but ineffective: • Assess and treat life-threatening conditions (uncontrolled bleeding, shock) Initiate two large-bore IVs or central catheter; obtain serum samples for laboratory tests Provide fluid replacement
Disability	Determine Glasgow Coma Scale score Assess pupil size and reactivity
Exposure or environmental control	Remove all clothing to inspect all body regions Prevent hypothermia

ACLS, Advanced cardiac life support; *ECG*, electrocardiogram; *IV*, intravenous line.

Scale (GCS) score of 8 or less usually require the placement of a definitive airway.[9]

Breathing. The patient is assessed for ineffective breathing patterns and impaired gas exchange; an open, clear airway does not ensure adequate ventilation and gas exchange. Assessment includes chest wall integrity and respiratory rate, depth, and symmetry. Auscultation is performed to assess gas flow in the lungs. Air or blood in the chest may be identified by percussion. Decreased breath sounds or alteration in chest wall integrity necessitate chest tube placement. Endotracheal intubation may be required for patients who have compromised airways caused by mechanical factors, who are unconscious, or who have ventilatory problems.[9] Supplemental oxygen is administered to all injured patients.[9]

Circulation. The next step is to assess for decreased cardiac output, impaired tissue perfusion, and deficient fluid volume. External exsanguination is identified and controlled by direct manual pressure on the wound. Rapid assessment of the circulatory status includes assessment of level of consciousness, skin color, and pulse.[9] Level of consciousness provides data on cerebral perfusion. Ashen, gray facial skin color or white, pale extremities may be ominous signs of hypovolemia.[9] Central pulses (femoral or carotid artery) are assessed bilaterally for rate, regularity, and quality. If a pulse is not present, advanced cardiac life support (ACLS) protocols are instituted. ECG monitoring is initiated to assess for rhythm disturbances. Life-threatening dysrhythmias are treated according to ACLS protocols.

Disability. A rapid neurologic assessment is performed. During this step, the nurse assesses the potential for injury by completing a brief neurologic assessment to establish the patient's level of consciousness and pupil size and reaction. The AVPU method can be used to quickly describe the patient's level of consciousness:

A: **A**lert
V: responds to **V**erbal stimuli
P: responds to **P**ainful stimuli
U: **U**nresponsive

The patient's GCS score can be used (see Table 23-1 in Chapter 23).

Exposure. The final step in the primary survey is exposure and environmental control. All clothing is removed to facilitate a thorough examination of all body surfaces for the presence of injury. After all clothing is removed, the patient must be protected from hypothermia. This can be accomplished through external blankets, warm ambient room temperature, and warmed intravenous fluids.

Resuscitation Phase

After the primary survey the resuscitation phase begins. Hypovolemic shock is the most common type of shock that occurs in trauma patients.[9] Hemorrhage must be identified and treated rapidly. Two large-bore (14- to 16-gauge) peripheral intravenous catheters, intraosseous catheter, or central venous catheter is inserted. During the initiation of intravenous lines, blood samples are drawn (Box 34-2).

Resuscitation is aimed at ensuring adequate perfusion of tissues with oxygen and nutrients to support cellular function. Resuscitation end points (variables or parameters) must be viewed across the continuum of resuscitation from shock. During resuscitation from traumatic hemorrhagic shock, normalization of standard clinical parameters such as blood pressure, heart rate, and urine output are not adequate. The optimal resuscitation end point is a major focus of research in trauma care. During resuscitation, attempts should be made to improve cellular oxygenation. Base deficit and lactate and other assessment parameters have been well-studied to determine adequacy of cellular oxygenation during trauma resuscitation.[10]

Damage Control Resuscitation. Resuscitation practices have been a focus for research in trauma care. *Damage control resuscitation* (DCR) is an emerging concept in trauma care. DCR is a strategy to provide only interventions to control hemorrhage and contamination. The strategy involves permissive hypotension, the use of blood products over isotonic fluid for volume replacement, and the rapid and early correction of coagulopathy with component therapy and begins in the field and continues through the emergency departments, operating rooms, and critical care units.[11]

Massive Transfusion Protocols. Given the emphasis on use of blood products over crystalloids and correction of traumatic coagulopathy, many trauma centers have developed massive transfusion protocols for the 1% to 3% of all trauma patients who require DCR.[12] Having a defined protocol serves as a system-based strategy to facilitate early, timely release of blood products in what can be an often-chaotic situation. The massive transfusion protocol outlines the ratio of packed red blood cells, fresh frozen plasma, platelets, and cryoprecipitate to be administered.[12] The optimal ratio for these blood components has not yet been determined and is a focus for research.

Additional interventions during the resuscitation phase involve placement of urinary and gastric catheters. A gastric tube is inserted to reduce gastric distention and lower the risk of aspiration.[9]

Secondary Survey

The secondary survey begins when the primary survey is completed, resuscitation is well established, and the patient is demonstrating normalization of vital signs. During the secondary survey, a head-to-toe approach is used to thoroughly examine each body region. The history is one of the most important aspects of the secondary survey. Often, head injury, shock, or the use of drugs or alcohol may preclude a good history, so the history must be pieced together from other sources. The prehospital providers (paramedics, emergency medical technicians) usually can provide most of the vital information pertaining to the *unintentional injury.* Specific information that must be elicited pertaining to the mechanism of injury is summarized in Box 34-3. This information can help predict internal injuries and facilitate rapid intervention. The patient's pertinent past history can be assessed by use of the mnemonic AMPLE:
*A*llergies,
*M*edications currently used,
*P*ast medical illnesses/pregnancy,
*L*ast meal, and
*E*vents/environment related to the injury.

BOX 34-2 BLOOD SAMPLES TO OBTAIN WITH INTRAVENOUS PLACEMENT

- Complete blood cell (CBC) count
- Electrolyte profile (Na^+, K^+, Cl^-, CO_2, glucose, blood urea nitrogen [BUN], creatinine [Cr])
- Coagulation parameters: prothrombin time (PT); partial thromboplastin time (PTT)
- Type and screen (ABO compatibility)
- Amylase
- Toxicology screens
- Liver function studies
- Pregnancy test (for females of childbearing age)
- Lactate

BOX 34-3 HISTORY OF MECHANISM OF INJURY

Penetrating Trauma
- Weapon used (handgun, shotgun, rifle, knife)
- Caliber of weapon
- Number of shots fired
- Gender of assailant
- Position of victim and assailant when injury occurred

Blunt Trauma
- Height of fall
- Motor vehicle crash extrication time
- Ejection
- Steering wheel deformation
- Location in automobile (passenger, driver, front seat, back seat)
- Restraint status (lap belt, shoulder harness, or combination; unrestrained)
- Speed of automobiles, direction of impact
- Occupants (number and morbidity status)

BOX 34-4   NURSING REPORT FROM A REFERRING AREA USING THE SBAR METHOD

S: Situation

- Age
- Gender
- Mechanism of injury/injuries sustained
- Admission diagnosis/chief complaint; any loss of consciousness and its duration with current Glasgow Coma Scale score
- Diagnostic tests and procedures completed
- Diagnostic test results and laboratory results
- Medications administered (opiates, sedatives)
- Current issues, including derangements in any physical assessments requiring acute interventions

B: Background

- Significant medical and surgical history
- Home medications

A: Assessments

- Current assessment findings, including vital signs, level of consciousness, established airway, and mechanical ventilation settings
- Family members present and their assessment of coping and current knowledge of nature and extent of injuries and treatment plan

R: Recommendations

- Description of the plan, including fluid volume and blood products

TABLE 34-3   EFFECTS OF TRAUMA RESUSCITATION

ASPECT OF INJURY OR RESUSCITATION	IMPACT ON CRITICAL CARE MANAGEMENT
Prolonged extrication time	Gives an indication of length of time patient may have been hypotensive and/or hypothermic before medical care
Period of respiratory or cardiac arrest	Effects of loss of perfusion to brain (anoxic injury), kidneys, and other vital organs
Time on backboard	Potentiates risk of sacral or occipital breakdown
Number of units of blood; whether any were not fully cross-matched; packed cells versus whole blood used	Potentiates risk of ARDS, MODS

ARDS, Acute respiratory distress syndrome; *MODS*, multiple organ dysfunction syndrome.

TABLE 34-4   FACTORS PREDISPOSING THE TRAUMA PATIENT TO IMPAIRED OXYGENATION

FACTOR	IMPAIRMENT
Impaired ventilation	Injury to airway structures, loss of central nervous system regulation of breathing, impaired level of consciousness
Impaired pulmonary gas diffusion	Pneumothorax, hemothorax, aspiration of gastric contents Shifts to the left of the oxyhemoglobin dissociation curve (can result from infusion of large volumes of banked blood, hypocarbia or alkalosis, or hypothermia)
Decreased oxygen supply	Reduced hemoglobin (from hemorrhage) Reduced cardiac output (cardiovascular injury, decreased preload)
Increased oxygen supply	Increased metabolic demands (associated with the stress response to injury)

During the secondary survey the nurse ensures the completion of special procedures, such as an ECG, radiographic studies (chest, cervical spine, thorax, and pelvis), ultrasonography, and, when required, diagnostic peritoneal lavage. Throughout this survey the nurse continuously monitors the patient's vital signs and response to medical therapies. Emotional support to the patient and family also is imperative.

Definitive Care and Operative Phase

After the secondary survey has been completed, specific injuries usually have been diagnosed. Definitive care related to specific injuries is described throughout this chapter. Trauma is sometimes referred to as a "surgical disease" because the nature and extent of injuries usually requires operative management. After surgery, depending on the patient's status, transfer to the critical care unit may be indicated.

Critical Care Phase

Critically ill trauma patients are admitted into the critical care unit as direct transfers from the emergency department or operating room. Information the nurse must obtain from the emergency department or operating room nurse, or both, is summarized using the **SBAR** method: **S**ituation, **B**ackground, **A**ssessment, and **R**ecommendations (Box 34-4). This information must be obtained before the patient's admission to the critical care unit to ensure availability of needed personnel, equipment, and supplies. This information also helps the nurse to assess the impact of trauma resuscitation on the patient's presentation and course. Table 34-3 summarizes the prehospital, emergency department, and operating room resuscitative measures that can affect the trauma patient's care.

After the patient's arrival in the critical care unit, the nurse uses the primary and secondary surveys and resuscitative measures in accordance with ATLS guidelines to assess the trauma patient's status. Priority nursing care during the critical care phase includes ongoing physical assessments and monitoring the patient's response to medical therapies. The nurse constantly is aware that the third peak of the trimodal distribution of trauma deaths occurs in the critical care setting as a result of complications, including acute respiratory distress syndrome (ARDS), sepsis, prolonged shock states, and MODS. Ongoing nursing assessments are imperative for early detection and treatment of complications.

One of the most important nursing roles is assessment of the balance between oxygen delivery and oxygen demand. Oxygen delivery must be optimized to prevent further system damage. The trauma patient is at high risk for impaired oxygenation as a result of a variety of factors (Table 34-4). Risk factors must be promptly identified and treated to prevent life-threatening sequelae. Prevention and treatment of hypoxemia depend on accurate assessment of the adequacy of pulmonary gas exchange, oxygen delivery, and oxygen consumption.

Frequent and thorough nursing assessments of all body systems are the cornerstone of medical and nursing management of the critically ill trauma patient. The nurse can detect subtle changes and facilitate the implementation of timely therapeutic interventions to prevent complications often associated with trauma. The nurse must be knowledgeable about specific organ injuries and their associated sequelae.

SPECIFIC TRAUMA INJURIES

Traumatic Brain Injuries

More than 1.7 million traumatic brain injuries (TBIs) occur annually; approximately 52,000 Americans die each year of TBI with 275,000 hospitalized as a result of their injury.[13] Children aged 0 to 4 years, older adolescents aged 15 to 19 years, and adults aged 65 years and older are most likely to sustain a TBI.[13]

Mechanism of Injury

TBIs occur when mechanical forces are transmitted to brain tissue. Mechanisms of injury include penetrating or blunt trauma to the head. The leading causes of TBI include falls (35%), MVCs (17%), struck by or against objects (17%), and assaults (10%).[14] Penetrating trauma can result from the penetration of a foreign object such as a bullet, which causes direct damage to cerebral tissue. Blunt trauma can be the result of deceleration, acceleration, or rotational forces. *Deceleration injury* causes the brain to crash against the skull after it has hit a hard surface such as the dashboard of a car. *Acceleration injury* occurs when the brain has been forcefully hit, such as with a baseball bat. In many instances, TBIs can be caused by acceleration and deceleration. Acceleration injuries occur when the skull is hit by a force that causes the brain to move forward to the point of impact, and then as the brain reverses direction and hits the other side of the skull, deceleration injuries occur.

Pathophysiology

Review of the pathophysiology of a TBI can be divided into two categories: primary injury and secondary injury. The critical care nurse must understand this pathophysiology, because goals of care focus on reducing morbidity and mortality from primary and secondary injuries.

Primary Injury. The primary injury occurs at the moment of impact as a result of mechanical forces to the head. The extent of and recovery from injury are related to whether the primary injury was localized to an area or whether it was diffuse (widespread) throughout the brain. Primary injuries may include direct damage to the parenchyma or as injury to the vessels that causes hemorrhage, compressing nearby structures. Examples of primary injuries include contusion, laceration, shearing injuries, and hemorrhage. Primary injury may be mild, with little or no neurologic damage, or severe, with major tissue damage. Immediately after the injury, a cascade of neural and vascular processes is activated.

Secondary Injury. Secondary injury is the biochemical and cellular response to the initial trauma that can exacerbate the primary injury and cause loss of brain tissue not originally damaged. Secondary injury can be caused by ischemia, hypercapnia, hypotension, cerebral edema, sustained hypertension, calcium toxicity, or metabolic derangements. Hypoxia or hypotension, the best known culprits for secondary injury, typically are the result of extracranial trauma.[15] A self-perpetuating cycle develops that may cause the expansion of a relatively focal primary injury as a result of uncontrolled refractory secondary injury.[9,15]

Tissue Ischemia. Tissue ischemia occurs in areas of poor cerebral perfusion as a result of hypotension or hypoxia. The cells in ischemic areas become edematous. Extreme vasodilation of the cerebral vasculature occurs in an attempt to supply oxygen to the cerebral tissue. This increase in blood volume increases intracranial volume and raises intracranial pressure (ICP).

Hypotension. Significant hypotension causes inadequate perfusion to neural tissue. Hypotension rarely is associated with TBI. Hypotension typically is not caused by brain injury unless terminal medullary failure occurs. If a trauma patient is unconscious and hypotensive, a detailed assessment of the chest, abdomen, and pelvis is performed to rule out internal injuries.

Hypercapnia. Hypercapnia is a powerful vasodilator of cerebral vessels. Most often caused by hypoventilation in an unconscious patient, hypercapnia results in cerebral vasodilation, increased cerebral blood volume, and raised ICP.

Brain Edema. Cerebral edema occurs as a result of the changes in the cellular environment caused by contusion, loss of autoregulation, and increased permeability of the blood–brain barrier. Cerebral edema can be focal as it localizes around the area of contusion or diffuse as a result of hypotension or hypoxia. The extent of cerebral edema can be minimized by controlling the other aspects of secondary injury, such as oxygenation, ventilation, and perfusion.

Initial hypertension in the patient with severe TBI is common. As a result of the loss of autoregulation, increased blood pressure results in increased intracranial blood volume and elevates ICP. Every effort must be made to control hypertension to prevent the secondary injury caused by increased ICP (see "Intracranial Pressure Monitoring" in Chapter 24 and "Intracranial Hypertension" in Chapter 25). The effects of increased ICP are varied. As pressure increases inside the closed skull vault, cerebral perfusion decreases, which further compromises the brain. The combined effects of increasing pressure and decreasing perfusion precipitate a downward spiral of events.

Classification of Brain Injuries

Injuries of the brain are described by the functional changes or losses that occur. Some of the major functional abnormalities seen in head injury are described here.

Skull Fracture. Skull fractures are common, but they do not by themselves cause neurologic deficits. Skull fractures can be classified as open (dura is torn) or closed (dura is not torn), or they can be classified as those of the vault or those of the base. Common vault fractures occur in the parietal and temporal regions. Basilar skull fractures usually are not visible on conventional skull films and a computed tomography (CT) is typically required. Assessment findings may include cerebrospinal fluid (CSF) loss—described as rhinorrhea (from nose) or otorrhea (from ear), Battle sign (ecchymosis overlying the mastoid process behind the ear), "raccoon eyes" (subconjunctival and periorbital ecchymosis), or palsy of the seventh cranial nerve.

The significance of a skull fracture is that it identifies the patient with a higher probability of having or developing an intracranial hematoma. Open skull fractures require surgical intervention to remove bony fragments and to close the dura. The major complications of basilar skull fractures are cranial nerve injury and leakage of CSF. CSF leakage may result in a fistula, which increases the possibility of bacterial contamination and resultant meningitis. Because fistula formation may be delayed, patients with a basilar skull fracture are admitted to the hospital for observation and possible surgical intervention.

Concussion. A concussion is a brain injury accompanied by a brief loss of neurologic function, especially loss of consciousness.[14] When loss of consciousness occurs, it may last for seconds to an hour. The neurologic dysfunctions include confusion, disorientation, and sometimes a period of antegrade or retrograde amnesia. Other clinical manifestations that occur after concussion are headache, dizziness, nausea, irritability, inability to concentrate, impaired memory, and fatigue. The diagnosis of concussion is based on the loss of consciousness inasmuch as the brain remains structurally intact despite functional impairment.

Contusion. Contusion, or "bruising" of the brain, usually is related to acceleration–deceleration injuries, which result in hemorrhage into the superficial parenchyma. Frontal or temporal lobe contusions are most common and can be seen in a *coup–contrecoup mechanism of injury* (Fig. 34-2). Coup injury affects the cerebral tissue directly under the point of impact. Contrecoup injury occurs in a line directly opposite the point of impact.

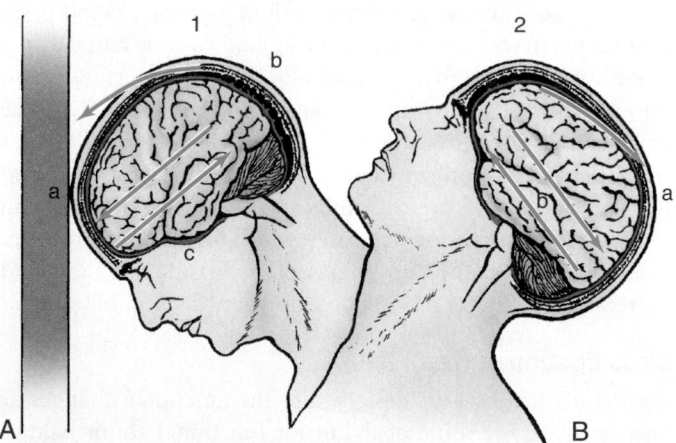

FIGURE 34-2   Coup and contrecoup head injury after blunt trauma. *A*, Coup injury: impact against object, showing the site of impact and direct trauma to brain *(a)*, shearing of subdural veins *(b)*, and trauma to the base of the brain *(c)*. *B*, Contrecoup injury: impact within skull, showing the site of impact from brain hitting opposite side of skull *(a)* and shearing forces throughout brain *(b)*. These injuries occur in one continuous motion; the head strikes the wall (coup) and then rebounds (contrecoup).

The clinical manifestations of contusion are related to the location of the contusion, the degree of contusion, and the presence of associated lesions. Contusions can be small, in which localized areas of dysfunction result in a focal neurologic deficit. Larger contusions can evolve over 2 to 3 days after injury as a result of edema and further hemorrhaging. A large contusion can produce a mass effect that can cause a significant increase in ICP. Contusions are almost always associated with subdural hematoma (SDH).[9]

Contusions of the tips of the temporal lobe are a common occurrence and are of particular concern. Because the inner aspects of the temporal lobe surround the opening in the tentorium where the midbrain enters the cerebrum, edema in this area can cause rapid deterioration in level of consciousness and can lead to herniation. Because of the location, this deterioration can occur with little or no warning at a deceptively low ICP.

Diagnosis of contusion is made by CT. If the CT scan indicates contusion, especially in the temporal area, the nurse must pay specific attention to neurologic assessments and look for subtle changes in pupillary signs or vital signs, irrespective of a stable ICP.

Medical management of cerebral contusions may consist of medical or surgical therapies. Because a contusion can progress over 3 to 5 days after injury, secondary injury may occur. If contusions are small, focal, or multiple, they are treated medically with serial neurologic assessments and possibly with ICP monitoring. Larger contusions that produce considerable mass effect require surgical intervention to prevent the increased edema and elevations in ICP as the contusion matures. Outcome of cerebral contusion varies, depending on the location and the size of the contused area.

Cerebral Hematomas. Extravasation of blood creates a space-occupying lesion within the cranial vault that can lead to increased ICP. Three types of hematomas are discussed here (Fig. 34-3). The first two, epidural and SDH, are extraparenchymal (outside of brain tissue) and produce injury by pressure effect and displacement of intracranial contents. The third type, intracerebral hematoma, directly damages neural tissue and can produce further injury as a result of pressure and displacement of intracranial contents.

Epidural Hematoma. Epidural hematoma (EDH) is a collection of blood between the inner skull and the outermost layer of the dura (Fig. 34-3A). EDHs are most often associated with patients with skull fractures and middle meningeal artery lacerations (two thirds of patients) or skull fractures with venous bleeding.[9] A blow to the head that causes a linear skull fracture on the lateral surface of the head may tear the middle meningeal artery. As the artery bleeds, it pulls the dura away from the skull, creating a pouch that expands into the intracranial space.

The incidence of EDH is relatively low. EDH can occur as a result of low-impact injuries (e.g., falls) or high-impact injuries (e.g., MVCs). EDH occurs from trauma to the skull and meninges rather than from the acceleration–deceleration forces seen in other types of head trauma.

The classic clinical manifestations of EDH include brief loss of consciousness followed by a period of lucidity. Rapid deterioration in the level of consciousness should be anticipated because arterial bleeding into the epidural space can occur

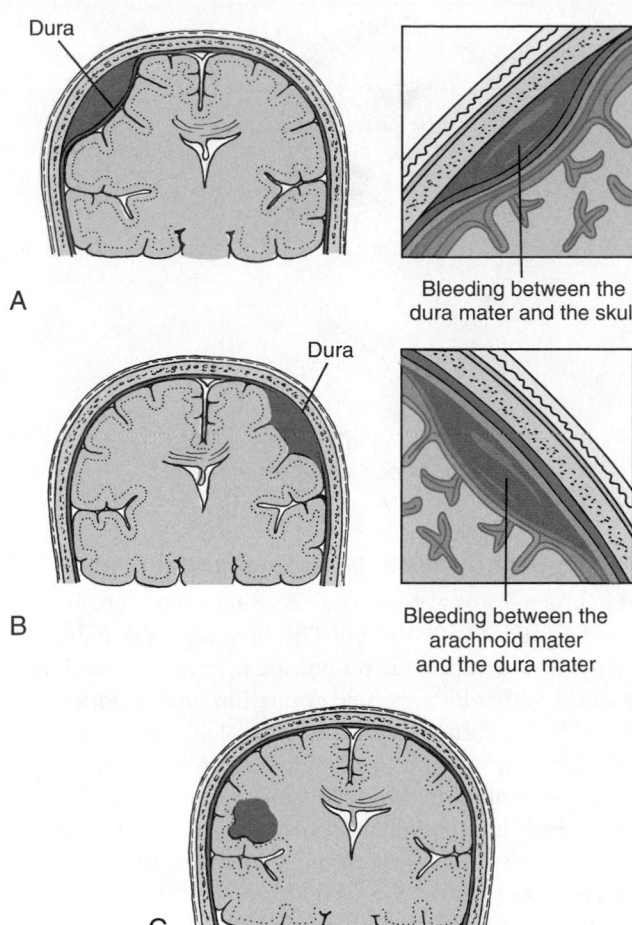

Dura

A

Dura

B

Bleeding between the
dura mater and the skull

Bleeding between the
arachnoid mater
and the dura mater

C

FIGURE 34-3 Types of hematomas. *A,* Epidural hematoma.
B, Subdural hematoma. *C,* Intracerebral hematoma.

quickly. A dilated and fixed pupil on the same side as the impact area is a hallmark of EDH.[9] The patient may complain of a severe, localized headache and may be sleepy. Diagnosis of EDH is based on clinical symptoms and evidence of a collection of epidural blood identified on the CT scan. Treatment of EDH requires surgical intervention to remove the blood and to cauterize the bleeding vessels.

Subdural Hematoma. Subdural hematoma (SDH), which is the accumulation of blood between the dura and underlying arachnoid membrane, most often is related to a rupture in the bridging veins between the cerebral cortex and the dura (Fig. 34-3B). Acceleration–deceleration and rotational forces are the major causes of SDH, which often is associated with cerebral contusions and intracerebral hemorrhage. SDH is common, representing about 30% of severe head injuries. The three types of SDH—acute, subacute, and chronic—are based on the timeframe from injury to clinical symptoms.

Acute Subdural Hematoma. Acute SDHs are hematomas that occur after a severe blow to the head. The clinical presentation of acute SDH is determined by the severity of injury to the underlying brain at the time of impact and the rate of blood accumulation in the subdural space. In other situations, the patient has a lucid period before deterioration. Careful observation for deterioration of the level of consciousness or lateralizing signs, such as inequality of pupils or motor movements, is essential. Rapid surgical intervention, including craniectomy,

craniotomy, or burr hole evacuation, and aggressive medical management can reduce mortality.

Subacute Subdural Hematoma. Subacute SDHs are hematomas that develop symptomatically 2 days to 2 weeks after trauma. In subacute SDHs, the expansion of the hematoma occurs at a rate slower than that in acute SDH, and it takes longer for symptoms to become obvious. Clinical deterioration of the patient with a subacute SDH usually is slower than with an acute SDH, but treatment by surgical intervention, when appropriate, is the same.

Chronic Subdural Hematoma. Chronic SDH is diagnosed when symptoms appear days or months after injury. Most patients with chronic SDH usually are in late middle age or older adults. Individuals at risk for chronic SDH include those with coordination or balance disturbances, and those receiving anticoagulation therapy. Clinical manifestations of chronic SDH are insidious. The patient may report a variety of symptoms such as lethargy, absent-mindedness, headache, vomiting, stiff neck, and photophobia and may show signs of transient ischemic attack, seizures, pupillary changes, or hemiparesis. Because a history of trauma often is not significant enough to be recalled, chronic SDH seldom is seen as an initial diagnosis. CT evaluation can confirm the diagnosis of chronic SDH.

If surgical intervention is required, evacuation of the chronic SDH may occur by craniotomy, burr holes, or catheter drainage. Evacuation by burr hole involves drilling a hole in the skull over the site of the chronic SDH and draining the fluid. Drains or catheters are left in place for at least 24 hours to facilitate total drainage. Outcome after chronic SDH evacuation varies. Return of neurologic status often depends on the degree of neurologic dysfunction before removal. Because this condition is most common in the older or debilitated patient, recovery is a slow process. Recurrence of chronic SDH is not infrequent.

Intracerebral Hematoma. Intracerebral hematoma (ICH) results when bleeding occurs within cerebral tissue. Traumatic causes of ICH include depressed skull fractures, penetrating injuries (bullet, knife), or sudden acceleration–deceleration motion. The ICH can act as a rapidly expanding lesion; however, late ICH into the necrotic center of a contused area also is possible (Fig. 34-3C). Sudden clinical deterioration of a patient 6 to 10 days after trauma may be the result of ICH.

Medical management of ICH may include surgical or nonsurgical management. It is thought that hemorrhages that do not cause significant ICP problems should be treated without surgery. Over time, the hemorrhage may be reabsorbed. If significant problems with ICP occur as a result of the ICH producing a mass effect, surgical removal is necessary. The outcome of a patient with an ICH depends greatly on the location of the hemorrhage. Size, mass effect, and displacement of other intracranial structures also affect the outcome.

Missile Injuries. Missile injuries are caused by objects that penetrate the skull to produce a significant focal damage but little acceleration–deceleration or rotational injury. The injury may be depressed, penetrating, or perforating (Fig. 34-4). Depressed injuries are caused by fractures of the skull, with penetration of bone into cerebral tissue. Penetrating injury is caused by a missile that enters the cranial cavity but does not exit. A low-velocity penetrating injury (knife) may involve only

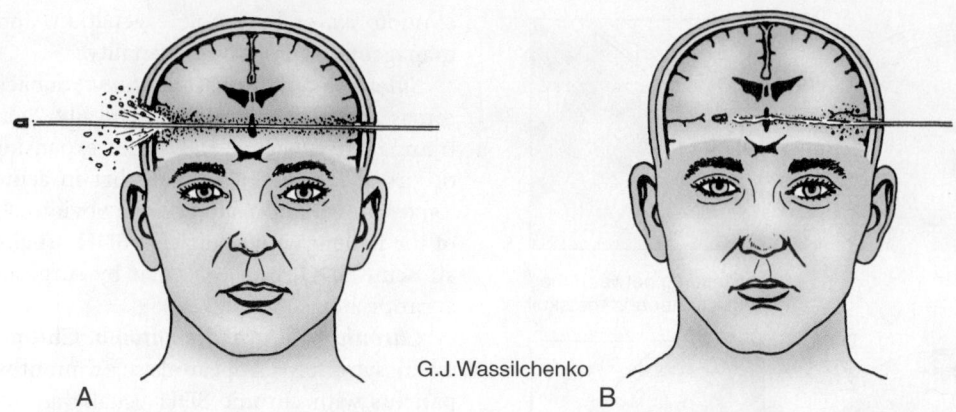

G.J.Wassilchenko

A   B

FIGURE 34-4 Bullet wounds of the head. A bullet wound or other penetrating missile wounds cause an open (compound) skull fracture and damage to brain tissue. Shock wave effects are transmitted throughout the brain. *A,* Perforating injury. *B,* Penetrating injury.

focal damage and no loss of consciousness. A high-velocity missile (bullet) can produce shock waves that are transmitted throughout the brain in addition to the injury caused by the bullet. Perforating injuries are missile injuries that enter and then exit the brain. Perforating injuries have much less ricochet effect but are still responsible for significant injury.

Risk of infection and cerebral abscess is a concern in cases of missile injuries. If fragments of the missile are embedded within the brain, careful consideration of the location and risk of increasing neurologic deficit is weighed against the risk of abscess or infection. The outcome after missile injury is based on the degree of penetration, the location of the injury, and the velocity of the missile.

Diffuse Axonal Injury. Diffuse axonal injury (DAI) is a term used to describe prolonged post-traumatic coma that is not caused by a mass lesion, although DAI with mass lesions has been reported. DAI covers a wide range of brain dysfunction typically caused by acceleration–deceleration and rotational forces. DAI occurs as a result of damage to the axons or disruption of axonal transmission of the neural impulses.

The pathophysiology of DAI is related to the stretching and tearing of axons as a result of movement of the brain inside the cranium at the time of impact. The stretching and tearing of axons result in microscopic lesions throughout the brain, but especially deep within cerebral tissue and the base of the cerebrum. Disruption of axonal transmission of impulses results in loss of consciousness. Unless surrounding tissue areas are significantly injured, causing small hemorrhages, DAI may not be visible on CT or magnetic resonance imaging (MRI). DAI can be classified as one of three grades based on the extent of lesions: mild, moderate, or severe. The patient with mild DAI may be in a coma for 24 hours and may exhibit periods of decorticate and decerebrate posturing. Patients with moderate DAI may be in a coma for longer than 24 hours and exhibit periods of decorticate and decerebrate posturing. Severe DAI usually manifests as a prolonged, deep coma with periods of hypertension, hyperthermia, and excessive sweating. Treatment of DAI includes support of vital functions and maintenance of ICP within normal limits. The outcome after severe DAI is poor because of the extensive dysfunction of cerebral pathways.

Neurologic Assessment of Traumatic Brain Injury

The neurologic assessment is the most important tool for evaluating the patient with a severe TBI, because it can indicate the severity of injury, provide prognostic information, and dictate the speed with which further evaluation and treatment must proceed.[16] The cornerstone of the neurologic assessment is the GCS, although it is not a complete neurologic examination. Pupils and motor strength assessment must be incorporated into the early and ongoing assessments. After injuries are specifically identified, a more thorough, focused neurologic assessment, such as examination of the cranial nerves, is warranted. To assist with the initial assessment, TBIs are divided into three descriptive categories—mild, moderate, or severe—on the basis of the patient's GCS score and duration of the unconscious state.

Degree of Injury

Mild Brain Injury. Mild TBI is described as a GCS score of 13 to 15, with a loss of consciousness that lasts up to 15 minutes. Patients with mild injury often are seen in the emergency department and discharged home with a family member who is instructed to evaluate the patient routinely and to bring the patient back to the hospital if any further neurologic symptoms appear.

Moderate Brain Injury. Moderate TBI is described as a GCS score of 9 to 12, with a loss of consciousness for up to 6 hours. Patients with this type of TBI usually are hospitalized. They are at high risk for deterioration from increasing cerebral edema and ICP, and serial clinical assessments are important. Hemodynamic and ICP monitoring and ventilatory support may not be required for these patients unless other systemic injuries make them necessary. A CT scan usually is obtained on admission. Repeat CT scans are indicated if the patient's neurologic status deteriorates.

Severe Brain Injury. Patients with a GCS score of 8 or less after resuscitation or those who deteriorate to that level within 48 hours of admission have a severe TBI. Patients with severe TBI often receive ventilatory support along with ICP and hemodynamic monitoring. A CT scan is performed to rule out any mass lesions that can be surgically ameliorated. Patients are placed in a critical care setting for continual assessment, monitoring, and management.

Nursing Assessment of the Patient with Traumatic Brain Injury. As in all traumatic injuries, evaluation of the airway, breathing, and circulation (ABCs) is the first step in the assessment of the patient with TBI in the critical care unit. Patients with moderate primary injury may deteriorate as a result of diffuse swelling or bleeding. A patient with severe TBI who is breathing spontaneously may require prophylactic endotracheal or nasotracheal intubation with mechanical ventilatory support to reduce the risk of hypoxia and hypercapnia. After stabilization of the ABCs is assured, a neurologic assessment is performed.

Level of consciousness, motor movements, pupillary response, respiratory function, and vital signs are all part of a complete neurologic assessment of the patient with a TBI. Level of consciousness can be elicited to assess wakefulness. Consciousness is assessed by obtaining the patient's response to verbal and painful stimuli. Determination of orientation to person, place, and time assesses mental alertness. Pupils are assessed for size, shape, equality, and reactivity. Asymmetry must be reported immediately. Pupils are also assessed for constriction to a light source (parasympathetic innervation) or dilation (sympathetic innervation). Because parasympathetic fibers are present in the brainstem, pupils that are slow to react to light may indicate a brainstem injury. A "blown" pupil can be caused by compression of the third cranial nerve or transtentorial herniation. Bilateral fixed pupils can indicate midbrain involvement (see "Pupillary Function" in Chapter 23).

Neurologic assessments are ongoing throughout the patient's critical care stay as part of the initial shift assessment and as part of ongoing assessments to detect subtle deterioration. Serial assessments include monitoring hemodynamic status and ICP. The use of muscle relaxants and sedation for ICP control may mask neurologic signs in the patient with a severe head injury. In these situations, observations for changes in pupils and vital signs become extremely important. Newer shorter-acting sedatives with a very short half-life, such as propofol, can be turned off, and within minutes, a neurologic examination can be performed.

Diagnostic Procedures. The cornerstone of diagnostic procedures for evaluation of TBI is the CT scan. CT is a rapid, noninvasive procedure that can provide invaluable information about the presence of mass lesions and cerebral edema. Serial CT scans may be used over a period of several days to assess areas of contusion and ischemia and to detect delayed hematomas. A nurse must always remain with a TBI patient during a CT scan to provide continued observation and monitoring and during transport to and from the scanner. Transporting the patient, moving the patient from the bed to the CT table, and positioning the head flat during the CT scan are all stressful events and can cause severe increases in ICP. Continuous monitoring of ICP enables rapid intervention during these particularly vulnerable times.

Medical Management

Surgical Management. If a lesion identified on CT is causing a shift of intracranial contents or increasing ICP, surgical intervention is necessary. A craniotomy is performed to remove the EDH, SDH, or large ICH. Patients may also undergo a *decompressive craniectomy* specifically for elevated ICP. This procedure involves removal of the overlying bone flap to allow the underlying brain tissue to expand and swell. This surgical strategy has demonstrated some benefits but remains controversial.[17]

Nonsurgical Management. Most of the management of TBI occurs in the critical care unit. Nonsurgical management includes management of ICP, maintenance of adequate cerebral perfusion pressure (CPP) and oxygenation, and treatment of any complications (e.g., pneumonia, infection). The decision of when to initiate ICP monitoring is critical. ICP monitoring may be required for patients with a GCS score less than 8 and abnormal findings on a head CT scan.[18] Brain tissue oxygen monitoring may also be used.

Nursing Management

Nursing diagnoses for the patient with TBI are listed in Box 34-5. Priority nursing goals include stabilization of vital signs, prevention of further injury, and reduction of increased ICP. Ongoing nursing assessments are the cornerstone to the care of patients with TBI. These assessments are the primary mechanism for determining secondary brain injury from cerebral edema and increased ICP. If secondary injury is to be prevented, the nurse must respond immediately to hypotensive events and, in collaboration with physicians, maximize CPP through reduction of ICP and restoration of mean arterial pressure.[18]

All aspects of care, including hemodynamic management, pulmonary care, maintenance of body temperature, and control of the environment, can impact outcome after TBI.[18] Hemodynamic and fluid management are vital. Arterial blood pressure should be monitored because hypotension in a patient with TBI is rare and may indicate additional injuries. CPP should be maintained at a minimum of 60 mm Hg.[18] In the absence of cerebral ischemia, aggressive attempts to keep CPP above 70 mm Hg with intravenous fluids and vasopressors should be avoided secondary to the risk of ARDS.[18]

Close monitoring of hemodynamic status is of paramount importance in patients with TBI because in addition to fluid management, changes in cardiovascular function and circulating catecholamines contribute to hemodynamic instability.[15]

◎ BOX 34-5   NURSING DIAGNOSES

Traumatic Brain Injury

- Ineffective Breathing Pattern related to neuromuscular impairment, p. 1149
- Risk for Aspiration: impaired laryngeal sensation or reflex; impaired pharyngeal peristalsis or tongue function; impaired laryngeal closure or elevation; increased gastric volume; decreased lower esophageal sphincter pressure, p. 1154
- Impaired Gas Exchange related to ventilation–perfusion mismatching, p. 1144
- Imbalanced Nutrition: Less Than Body Requirements related to lack of exogenous nutrients and increased metabolic demand, p. 1143
- Powerlessness related to lack of control over current situation, p. 1152
- Decreased Intracranial Adaptive Capacity related to failure of normal compensatory mechanisms, p. 1131
- Risk for Ineffective Cerebral Tissue Perfusion, p. 1156

More invasive hemodynamic monitoring may be required to optimize fluid status and cardiac output. *Capnography* (monitoring of exhaled carbon dioxide levels) is suggested to prevent inadvertent hypocapnia or hypercapnia.[18] Aggressive pulmonary care must be instituted. However, endotracheal suctioning can elevate ICP. Techniques to counter elevation in ICP with suctioning are outlined in Box 34-6. Cerebral oxygen consumption is increased during periods of increased body temperature, and therefore euthermia (36° to 37° C) may be achieved with early workup and intervention for infection, use of antipyretics, and cooling measures such as evaporative cooling.

A tremendous catecholamine surge after TBI has been associated with infectious complications and potentially preventable mortality.[19] The use of beta-blockers to suppress this catecholamine surge in patients with TBI has been shown to decrease mortality.[19]

In the early postinjury phase, the patient's environment must be controlled. Stimuli that produce pain, agitation, or discomfort can increase ICP. Analgesics and sedatives should be administered, and patients should be given rest periods. After ICP stabilization, stimulation programs for patients in a coma may be employed. These programs provide stimulation to the tactile, kinesthetic, olfactory, gustatory, auditory, and visual senses. Several methods have been used to stimulate coma patients with various degrees of intensity:

- Intense Multisensory Stimulation Program: stimulatory cycles lasting approximately 15 to 20 minutes, repeated every hour for 12 to 14 hours per day, 6 days per week
- Formalized Not-Intensive Stimulation Program: cycles of stimulation of 10 to 60 minutes twice daily
- Sensory Regulation Program: single brief sessions of stimulation in a quiet environment completely free of noise

Whatever program is used, a stimulation schedule should be established, and accurate documentation of the stimulus and response is essential. Coma stimulation programs should be individualized and family members encouraged to participate.

New pharmacologic agents have started to demonstrate promise in the treatment of patients awakening from head trauma. Amantadine has been prescribed to facilitate awakening. While its full mechanism is only partially understood, it appears to act as an *N*-methyl-D-aspartate antagonist and indirect dopamine agonist.[20] It has been shown to help patients who are undergoing active rehabilitation to awaken faster.[20]

Spinal Cord Injuries

Approximately 12,000 new spinal cord injuries (SCIs) occur annually. As the population has aged since the 1970s, the median age at injury has increased from 28 to the current median age of 41 years.[21] The diagnosis of SCI begins with a detailed history of events surrounding the incident, precise evaluation of sensory and motor function, and radiographic studies of the spine.

Mechanism of Injury

The type of primary injury sustained depends on the mechanism of injury. The greatest cause of SCI is MVCs (39.2%), followed by falls (28.3%), violence (14.6%), other or unknown causes (9.7%), and sports (8.2%).[21]

Hyperflexion. Hyperflexion injury is most often is seen in the cervical area, especially at the level of C5 to C6, because this is the most mobile portion of the cervical spine. This type of injury most often is caused by sudden deceleration motion, as in head-on collisions. Injury occurs from compression of the cord as a result of fracture fragments or dislocation of the vertebral bodies. Instability of the spinal column occurs because of the rupture or tearing of the posterior muscles and ligaments.

Hyperextension. Hyperextension injuries involve backward and downward motion of the head. With this injury, often seen in rear-end collisions or MVCs, the spinal cord is stretched and distorted. Neurologic deficits associated with this injury are often caused by contusion and ischemia of the cord without significant bony involvement. A mild form of hyperextension is the *whiplash* injury.

Rotation. Rotation injuries often occur in conjunction with a flexion or extension injury. Severe rotation of the neck or body results in tearing of the posterior ligaments and displacement (rotation) of the spinal column.

Axial Loading. Axial loading, or vertical compression, injuries occur from vertical force along the spinal cord. This most commonly is seen in a fall from a height in which the person lands on the feet or buttocks. Compression injuries cause *burst fractures* of the vertebral body that often send bony fragments into the spinal canal or directly into the spinal cord (Fig. 34-5).

Penetrating Injuries. Penetrating injury to the spinal cord can be caused by a bullet, knife, or any other object that penetrates the cord. These types of injury cause permanent damage by anatomically transecting the spinal cord.

Pathophysiology

SCIs are the result of a mechanical force that disrupts neurologic tissue or its vascular supply, or both. Much like the pathophysiology of TBI, the injury process includes primary and secondary injury mechanisms. Primary injury is the neurologic damage that occurs at the moment of impact. Secondary injury refers to the complex biochemical processes affecting cellular function. Secondary injury can occur within minutes of injury and can last for days to weeks.

Several events after SCI lead to spinal cord ischemia and loss of neurologic function. A cascade of events is initiated that includes systemic and local vascular changes, electrolyte and biochemical changes, neurotransmitter accumulation, and local edema (Box 34-7). Collectively, these pathophysiologic events result in worsening of the injury, potentially extending the level of functional deficit and worsening long-term outcome. Knowledge of the pathophysiology of secondary processes has led to the development of new medications, which target the cellular changes contributing to injury. Despite ongoing research efforts at repairing the primary injury, minimizing damage by reducing secondary injury has shown the most promise.

Functional Injury of the Spinal Cord

Functional injury of the spinal cord refers to the degree of disruption of normal spinal cord function. This depends on what specific sensory and motor structures within the cord are damaged. SCIs are classified as complete or incomplete. Since 2000, the most frequent category at discharge has been incomplete tetraplegia (34.1%) followed by complete tetraplegia.[21] SCI cannot be classified until spinal shock has resolved.

Complete Injury. Complete SCI results in a total loss of sensory and motor function below the level of injury. Regardless of the mechanism of injury, the result is a complete dissection of the spinal cord and its neurochemical pathways, resulting in one of two conditions: tetraplegia or paraplegia.

Tetraplegia. With tetraplegia, the injury occurs from the C1 to T1 level. Residual muscle function depends on the specific cervical segments involved. The potential functional status resulting from different neurologic levels of injury is described in Table 34-5.

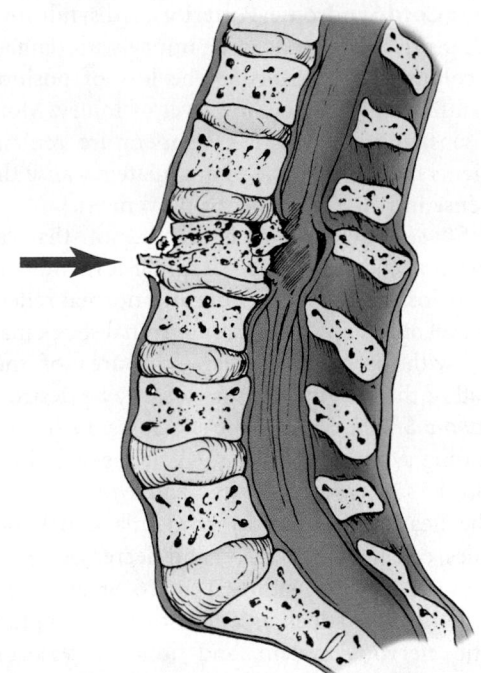

FIGURE 34-5 Spinal cord compression burst fracture. Compression injuries cause burst fractures of the vertebral body that often send bony fragments into the spinal canal or directly into the spinal cord. Include hyperflexion, hyperextension, rotation, axial loading (vertical compression), and missile or penetrating injuries.

BOX 34-7　PRIMARY AND SECONDARY MECHANISMS OF ACUTE SPINAL CORD INJURY

Primary Injury Mechanisms
- Acute compression
- Impact
- Missile
- Distraction
- Laceration
- Shear

Secondary Injury Mechanisms
- Systemic effects
- Heart rate: brief increase, then prolonged bradycardia
- Blood pressure: brief hypertension, then prolonged hypotension
- Decreased
- Peripheral resistance
- Decreased cardiac output
- Increased catecholamines, then decreased
- Hypoxia
- Hyperthermia
- Injudicious movement of the unstable spine leading to worsening compression
- Local vascular changes
- Loss of autoregulation
- Systemic hypotension (neurogenic shock)
- Hemorrhage (especially gray matter)
- Loss of microcirculation

- Reduction in blood flow
- Vasospasm
- Thrombosis
- Electrolyte changes
- Increased intracellular calcium
- Increased intracellular sodium
- Increased sodium permeability
- Increased intracellular potassium

Biochemical Changes
- Neurotransmitter accumulation
- Catecholamines (e.g., norepinephrine, dopamine)
- Excitotoxic amino acids (e.g., glutamate)
- Arachidonic acid release
- Free radical production
- Eicosanoid production
- Prostaglandins
- Lipid peroxidation
- Endogenous opioids
- Cytokines
- Edema
- Loss of energy metabolism
- Decreased adenosine triphosphate production
- Apoptosis

Adapted from Sekhon LHS, Fehlings MG. Epidemiology, demographics, and pathophysiology of acute spinal cord injury. *Spine*. 2001;26(24S):S2.

TABLE 34-5	QUADRIPLEGIA FUNCTIONAL STATUS
NEUROLOGIC LEVEL (VERTEBRAE) OF COMPLETE INJURY	**FUNCTIONAL ABILITY**
C1-C4	Requires electric wheelchair with breath, head, or shoulder controls
C5	Needs electric wheelchair with hand control and/or manual wheelchair with rim projections; may require adaptive devices to assist with ADLs
C6	Independent in manual wheelchair on level surface; may need hand controls; adaptive devices may be needed for ADLs
C7	Requires manual wheelchair on most surfaces
C8-T1	May need adaptive devices

ADLs, Activities of daily living.

Paraplegia. With paraplegia, the injury occurs in the thoracolumbar region (T2 to L1). Patients with injuries in this area may have full use of the arms and may need a wheelchair, although some may have limited ability to ambulate short distances with crutches and orthoses. Thoracic L1 and L2 injuries produce paraplegia with variable innervation to intercostal and abdominal muscles.

Incomplete Injury. Incomplete SCI results in a mixed loss of voluntary motor activity and sensation below the level of the lesion. Incomplete SCI exists if any function remains below the level of injury. Incomplete injuries can result in a variety of syndromes, which are classified according to the degree of motor and sensory loss below the level of injury. Some of the more common syndromes are described here.

Brown-Séquard Syndrome. The Brown-Séquard syndrome is associated with damage to only one side of the cord. This produces loss of voluntary motor movement on the same side as the injury, with loss of pain, temperature, and sensation on the opposite side. Functionally, the side of the body with the best motor control has little or no sensation, whereas the side of the body with sensation has little or no motor control.

Central Cord Syndrome. Central cord syndrome is associated with cervical hyperextension–hyperflexion injury and hematoma formation in the center of the cervical cord. This injury produces a motor and sensory deficit more pronounced in the upper extremities than in the lower extremities. Various degrees of bowel and bladder dysfunction may be present.

Anterior Cord Syndrome. The anterior cord syndrome is associated with injury to the anterior gray horn cells (motor), the spinothalamic tracts (pain), anterior spinothalamic tract (light touch), and the corticospinal tracts (temperature). The result is a loss of motor function and loss of the sensations of pain and temperature below the level of injury. However, below the level of injury, position sense and sensations of pressure and vibrations remain intact. Anterior cord syndrome is commonly caused by flexion injuries or acute herniation of an intervertebral disk.

Posterior Cord Syndrome. Posterior cord syndrome is associated with cervical hyperextension injury with damage to the posterior column. This results in the loss of position sense, pressure, and vibration below the level of injury. Motor function and sensation of pain and temperature remain intact. These patients may not be able to ambulate because the loss of position sense impairs spontaneous movement.

Spinal Shock. Spinal shock is a condition that can occur shortly after traumatic injury to the spinal cord. Spinal shock is the complete loss of all muscle tone and normal reflex activity below the level of injury.[9] Patients with spinal shock may appear completely without function below the area of the injury, although all of the area may not necessarily be destroyed.

Neurogenic Shock. Neurogenic shock results from injury to the descending sympathetic pathways in the spinal cord. This results from loss of vasomotor tone and sympathetic innervation to the heart. A relative hypovolemia and hypovolemic shock ensues, causing hypotension and decreased systemic vascular resistance. Patients with SCI at T6 or above may have profound neurogenic shock as a result of interruption of the sympathetic nervous system and loss of vasoconstrictor response below the level of the injury. Blood vessels cannot constrict, and the heart rate is slow, which results in hypotension, venous pooling, and decreased cardiac output. Cellular oxygenation is threatened as cardiac output declines because of a decrease in stroke volume (hypovolemia) and heart rate (bradycardia). The duration of this shock state can persist for up to 1 month after injury. Blood pressure support may be required with the use of sympathomimetic medications. Because hypotension is a problem, the nurse must be cautious when adjusting backrest position or when repositioning a patient in bed because orthostatic blood pressure changes can occur (see "Neurogenic Shock" in Chapter 35).

Autonomic Dysreflexia. Autonomic dysreflexia is a life-threatening complication that may occur with SCI. This condition is caused by a massive sympathetic response to a noxious stimuli (e.g., full bladder, line insertions, fecal impaction) that results in bradycardia, hypertension, facial flushing, and headache. Immediate intervention is needed to prevent cerebral hemorrhage, seizures, and acute pulmonary edema. Treatment is aimed at alleviating the noxious stimuli. A clinical algorithm for treatment of autonomic dysreflexia is provided in Box 34-8. If symptoms persist, antihypertensive agents can be administered to reduce blood pressure. Prevention of autonomic dysreflexia is imperative and can be accomplished through the use of a good bowel and bladder program.

Assessment

On admission to the critical care unit, attention to the ABCs is imperative in the patient with known or suspected SCI. Stabilization of the spinal cord is mandatory to prevent further injury, and spinal precautions are maintained until the spine is cleared of injury. Stabilization may include the use of bed rest with log-rolling maneuvers and a hard cervical collar until definitive stabilization is achieved. After the ABCs have been evaluated and interventions for life-threatening complications have been initiated, a full physical assessment is made to determine the extent of injury.

BOX 34-8 AUTONOMIC DYSREFLEXIA

- If patient is supine, immediately sit the patient up.
- Begin frequent vital sign monitoring, and perform every 5 minutes.
- Survey for instigating causes; begin with urinary system.
- Loosen clothing, constrictive devices.
- If indwelling catheter is not placed, catheterize the patient.
  - Lidocaine jelly may be instilled 5 minutes before catheter insertion.
- If indwelling catheter is present, do the following:
  - Check system for kinks and obstructions to flow.
  - Irrigate the bladder with small sterile amount of fluid, utilizing strict aseptic technique.
  - If not draining, remove the catheter and replace.
- If systolic blood pressure is greater than 150 mm Hg, consider rapid-onset, short-duration antihypertensive agent.
- If acute symptoms persist, suspect fecal impaction:
  - Instill lidocaine jelly into rectum; wait at least 5 minutes.
  - Perform digital examination to check for presence of stool; if present, gently remove. If signs of autonomic dysreflexia persist, stop examination; instill additional lidocaine jelly, and wait 20 minutes to re-examine.
  - If no stool is found and the abdomen is distended, consider administration of laxative.

TABLE 34-6 EFFECTS OF SPINAL CORD INJURY ON VENTILATORY FUNCTIONS

NEUROLOGIC LEVEL (VERTEBRAE) OF COMPLETE INJURY	RESPIRATORY FUNCTION	COMMENT
C1-C2	Paralysis of diaphragm	Ventilator dependent
C3-C5	Various degrees of diaphragm paralysis	Some diaphragm control; may need ventilatory support; weaning depends on preinjury pulmonary status
C6-T11	Various degrees of impaired intercostal muscles and abdominal muscles	Compromised respiratory function; reduced inspiratory ability; paradoxical breathing patterns; ineffective cough, sneeze

TABLE 34-7 MUSCLE STRENGTH SCALE

Active movement against maximal resistance
Active movement through range of motion against resistance
Active movement through range of motion against gravity
Active movement through range of motion with gravity eliminated
Flicker or trace of contraction
No contraction; total paralysis

Airway. Assessment of ABCs is essential to ensure optimal oxygenation and perfusion to all vital organs, including the spinal cord. Complete cardiovascular and respiratory assessments are essential to the patient's survival and prognosis. The primary assessment begins with an evaluation of airway clearance. In an unresponsive person, an oral airway is inserted while the patient's neck is maintained in a neutral position. The patient must undergo intubation before severe hypoxia can occur, which could further damage the spinal cord.

Breathing. Assessment of breathing patterns and gas exchange is made after an airway has been secured. The level of injury dictates the degree of altered breathing patterns and gas exchange (Table 34-6). Because complete injuries above the C3

level result in paralysis of the diaphragm, patients with these injuries require ventilatory assistance.

Circulation. Assessment of cardiac output and tissue perfusion is imperative to detect life-threatening injuries and promote recovery of injured spinal cord tissue. The patient with SCI is at high risk for developing alterations in cardiac output and tissue perfusion because the cardiovascular system is subjected to a variety of serious and potential physiologic alterations, including dysrhythmias, cardiac arrest, orthostatic hypotension, emboli, and thrombophlebitis.

The patient with SCI is assessed for adequate tissue perfusion by means of invasive and noninvasive hemodynamic monitoring techniques. Cardiac monitoring is required to detect bradycardia and other dysrhythmias that occur in response to reflex vagus activity mediated by the dominant parasympathetic nervous system, as well as changes in ECG rhythm as a result of hypothermia or hypoxia.

Neurologic Assessment for Spinal Cord Injury. The initial neurologic assessment may not be an accurate indication of eventual motor and sensory loss. It focuses on the rapid and accurate identification of present, absent, or impaired functioning of the motor, sensory, and reflex systems that coordinate and regulate vital functions. A detailed motor and sensory examination includes the assessment of all 32 spinal nerves for evidence of dysfunction. Carefully mapped pathways for the sensory portion of the spinal nerves, called *dermatomes*, can assist in localizing the functional sensory level of injury. Motor function may be graded on a 6-point scale (Table 34-7). Initial assessment must be performed correctly and findings thoroughly documented in detail so that subsequent serial assessments can rapidly identify deterioration. The American Spinal Injury Association (ASIA) has developed a form that outlines the required assessments for initial and ongoing classification of SCIs (Fig. 34-6). Ongoing spinal cord assessments must be documented during the critical care phase.

Diagnostic Procedures. Diagnostic radiographic evaluations can identify the severity of damage to the spinal cord. Initial evaluation includes anteroposterior and lateral views for all areas of the spinal cord. CT scan of all seven cervical vertebrae and the top of T1 must be obtained to rule out cervicothoracic junction injury. Flexion and extension views can identify subtle ligament injuries. CT, tomography, myelography, and MRI also may be used.

Screening for Spinal Cord Injury. Screening of the spinal cord for injury becomes an integral part of the assessment for all trauma patients. The degree of trauma, alteration in mentation, intoxication, and distracting injuries dictate the type and extent of examination required to clear the cervical spine. The Eastern Association of Surgeons in Trauma (EAST) developed

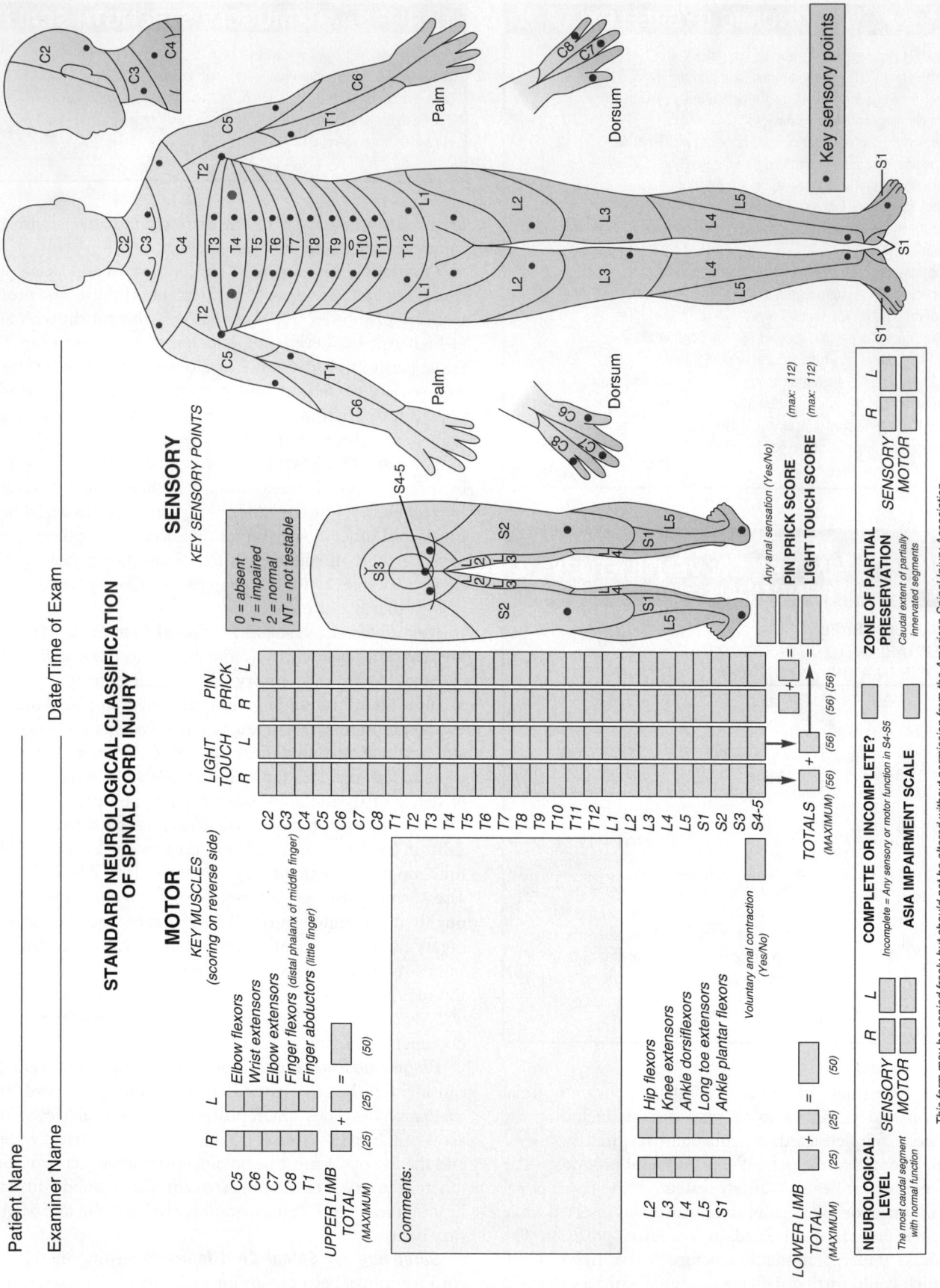

FIGURE 34-6   American Spinal Injury Association classification of spinal cord injuries.

MUSCLE GRADING

0 total paralysis

1 palpable or visible contraction

2 active movement, full range of motion, gravity eliminated

3 active movement, full range of motion, against gravity

4 active movement, full range of motion, against gravity and provides some resistance

5 active movement, full range of motion, against gravity and provides normal resistance

5* muscle able to exert, in examiner's judgement, sufficient resistance to be considered normal if identifiable inhibiting factors were not present

NT not testable. Patient unable to reliably exert effort or muscle unavailable for testing due to factors such as immobilization, pain on effort or contracture.

ASIA IMPAIRMENT SCALE

☐ **A = Complete:** No motor or sensory function is preserved in the sacral segments S4-S5.

☐ **B = Incomplete:** Sensory but not motor function is preserved below the neurological level and includes the sacral segments S4-S5.

☐ **C = Incomplete:** Motor function is preserved below the neurological level, and more than half of key muscles below the neurological level have a muscle grade less than 3.

☐ **D = Incomplete:** Motor function is preserved below the neurological level, and at least half of key muscles below the neurological level have a muscle grade of 3 or more.

☐ **E = Normal:** Motor and sensory function are normal.

CLINICAL SYNDROMES (OPTIONAL)

☐ Central Cord
☐ Brown-Sequard
☐ Anterior Cord
☐ Conus Medullaris
☐ Cauda Equina

STEPS IN CLASSIFICATION

The following order is recommended in determining the classification of individuals with SCI.

1. Determine sensory levels for right and left sides.

2. Determine motor levels for right and left sides.
   Note: in regions where there is no myotome to test, the motor level is presumed to be the same as the sensory level.

3. Determine the single neurological level.
   This is the lowest segment where motor and sensory function is normal on both sides, and is the most cephalad of the sensory and motor levels determined in steps 1 and 2.

4. Determine whether the injury is Complete or Incomplete. (sacral sparing).
   If voluntary anal contraction = **No** *AND all S4-5 sensory scores =* **0** *AND any anal sensation =* **No,** *then injury is COMPLETE. Otherwise injury is incomplete.*

5. Determine ASIA Impairment Scale (AIS) Grade:

   Is injury Complete? If **YES,** AIS=A Record ZPP
          NO ↓   (For ZPP record lowest dermatome or myotome on each side with some (non-zero score) preservation)

   Is injury motor incomplete? If **NO,** AIS=B
          YES ↓   (Yes=voluntary anal contraction OR motor function more than three levels below the motor level on a given side.)

   Are at least half of the key muscles below the (single) neurological level graded 3 or better?
       NO ↓   YES →
     AIS=C   AIS=D

   If sensation and motor function is normal in all segments, AIS=E
   Note: AIS E is used in follow up testing when an individual with a documented SCI has recovered normal function. If at initial testing no deficits are found, the individual is neurologically intact; the ASIA Impairment Scale does not apply.

FIGURE 34-6, cont'd.

TABLE 34-8   EAST GUIDELINES FOR CERVICAL SPINE CLEARANCE

TRAUMA PATIENT POPULATION	RECOMMENDATION
Trauma patients that are awake, alert, not intoxicated, neurologically normal, no complaints of neck pain or tenderness with full range of motion of the cervical spine	Neck is palpated in all directions for tenderness or pain. If physical examination is negative for pain or tenderness, CT imaging of the cervical spine is not required and the cervical collar may be removed.
All other trauma patients with suspected cervical injury must be radiologically evaluated. This includes patients with neck pain or tenderness, whether alert or with altered mental status/ neurological deficit, or distracting injury	Axial CT from occiput to T1 with sagittal and coronal reconstructions. If CT is positive for injury, continue cervical collar, obtain spine consultation, and obtain MRI. In the neurologically intact awake patient with neck pain, if the CT is negative (no injury seen), MRI is negative, and adequate flexion/extension films are negative, discontinue cervical collar.
Trauma patients that are obtunded with gross motor function of extremities	Axial CT from occiput to T1 with sagittal and coronal reconstructions. If the CT is negative (no injury seen), the risk/benefit of an additional MRI must be determined in each hospital. Options are: A. Continue cervical collar until a clinical exam can be performed. B. Remove the cervical collar on the basis of negative CT alone. C. Obtain MRI. If MRI is negative collar can be safely removed. Flexion/extension radiography should not be performed.

From Como, et al. Practice management guidelines for identification of cervical spine injuries following trauma: update from the Eastern Association for the Surgery of Trauma Practice Management Guidelines Committee. *J Trauma.* 2009;67(3):651.
CT, Computed tomography; *EAST,* Eastern Association of Surgeons in Trauma; *MRI,* magnetic resonance imaging.

guidelines for the clearance of the cervical spine (Table 34-8).[22] In these guidelines CT scan has replaced plain radiography as the principal modality for cervical spine assessment following trauma.[22] On admission, the spine is palpated for obvious deformity, and the patient is assessed for the subjective response of pain to palpation.[22] If the patient has distracting injuries, such as rib fractures, is intoxicated, or has received analgesics, examination of the spinal cord may be deferred.[22] MRI may be warranted to definitively diagnose SCI when the patient is stabilized.[22]

Medical Management

After assessment and diagnosis of the SCI, medical management begins. The primary treatment goal is to preserve remaining neurologic function with pharmacologic, surgical, and nonsurgical interventions.

Pharmacologic Management. Methylprednisolone can improve neurologic outcome after SCI, although it has been called into question because of the associated infection risk.[23] Current guidelines cite the use of methylprednisolone as an option for the management of acute cervical spine injury.[24] When it is used, patients receive a methylprednisolone bolus followed by a continuous infusion for at least 24 hours (preferably 48 hours) if their treatment began 3 to 8 hours after their injury.[24] Although the exact mechanism is not completely understood, it is thought that methylprednisolone directly affects the changes that occur within the spinal cord after injury, primarily by preventing post-traumatic spinal cord ischemia, improving energy metabolism, restoring extracellular calcium, and improving nerve impulse conduction.

Surgical Management. Surgical intervention provides spinal column stability in the presence of an unstable injury. Unstable injuries include disrupted ligaments and tendons and a vertebral column that cannot maintain normal alignment. Identification and immobilization of unstable injuries are particularly important for the patient with incomplete neurologic deficit. Without adequate stabilization, movement and dislocation of the vertebral column may cause a complete neurologic deficit. A variety of surgical procedures may be performed to achieve decompression and stabilization. The question of when surgery should be performed remains controversial.

Laminectomy. The laminectomy procedure is the removal of the lamina of the vertebral ring to allow decompression and removal of bony fragments or disk material from the spinal canal.

Spinal Fusion. Spinal fusion entails the surgical fusion of two to six vertebral elements to provide stability and to prevent motion. Fusion is accomplished through the use of bone parts or bone chips taken from the iliac crest or by use of wire or acrylic glue.

Rodding. The rodding procedure stabilizes and realigns larger segments of the spinal column by means of a variety of rodding procedures, such as the use of Harrington rods. The rods are attached by screws and glue to the posterior elements of the spinal column. These types of procedures most often are performed to stabilize the thoracolumbar area.

Nonsurgical Management. If the injury to the spinal cord is stable, nonsurgical management is the treatment of choice. Nonsurgical management for cervical and thoracolumbar injuries is discussed in the following sections.

Cervical Injury. Management of cervical injuries involves the immobilization of the fracture site and realignment of any dislocation. This is accomplished through skeletal traction that involves the use of two-point tongs, which are inserted into the skull through shallow burr holes and are connected to traction weights. Several types of cervical tongs are used. Gardner-Wells and Crutchfield tongs are the most common. These tongs can be applied at the bedside with the use of a local anesthetic.

After the procedure, the patient can be immobilized on a kinetic therapy bed or a regular bed. The kinetic therapy bed is

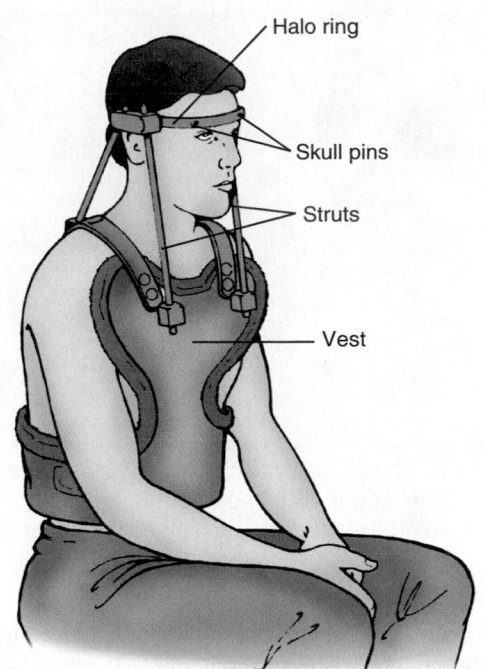

FIGURE 34-7 Halo vest. The halo traction brace immobilizes the cervical spine, which allows the patient to ambulate and participate in self-care.

the most popular method used for cervical immobilization because it maintains spinal column alignment while providing constant turning motion to reduce pulmonary and skin breakdown. Use of cervical skeletal traction on a regular bed makes it difficult to provide adequate care to the pulmonary system and skin because of the extensive degree of immobility.

After the spinal column has been adequately realigned by means of skeletal traction, a halo traction brace often is applied. The halo vest consists of a metal ring secured to the skull with two occipital and two temporal screws. Steel bars anchor the screws to the vest to provide cervical immobilization (Fig. 34-7). The halo traction brace immobilizes the cervical spine, which allows the patient to ambulate and participate in self-care.

Thoracolumbar Injury. Nonsurgical management of the patient with a thoracolumbar injury also involves immobilization. Skeletal traction may be used in high thoracic injury. For the most part, misalignment of the spinal canal does not occur in stable injuries of the thoracolumbar spine. Immobilization to allow fractures to heal is accomplished by bed rest (with the bed flat) and the use of a plastic or fiberglass jacket, a body cast, or a brace.

Nursing Management

Nursing diagnoses and management for the patient with SCI are summarized in Box 34-9. The goal during the critical care phase is to prevent life-threatening complications while maximizing the function of all organ systems. Nursing interventions are aimed at preventing secondary damage to the spinal cord and managing the complications of the neurologic deficit. Because almost all body systems are affected by SCI, nursing management must include interventions that optimize nutrition, elimination, skin integrity, and mobility. Patients with

SCIs have complex psychosocial needs that require a great deal of emotional support from the critical care nurse.

Cardiovascular Complications. The risk for cardiovascular instability is profound in patients with SCI at the C3 to C5 levels, although cardiovascular alterations can occur with most injuries above T6. Alteration in tissue perfusion because of hypotension may require the administration of intravenous fluids. Like management of TBI, the management of acute cervical SCI involves close hemodynamic monitoring. The guidelines for the management of acute cervical SCI cite as an option that hypotension (systolic blood pressure less than 90 mm Hg) should be avoided if possible or corrected as soon as possible after acute SCI.[24] It is also considered an option to maintain the mean arterial blood pressure at 85 to 90 mm Hg for the first 7 days after acute SCI to improve spinal cord perfusion.[24]

Astute assessment of fluid volume is required because pulmonary edema is a threat to SCI patients. Pulmonary artery catheterization may be required to assess for this complication. After the fluid volume status has been optimized, inotropic or vasopressor support, or both, may be implemented.

Another consequence of sympathetic nervous system dysfunction is loss of thermoregulation (*poikilothermy*), in which body temperature is regulated by the external environment. Judicious use of heat or cold for therapeutic or comfort measures is required. Profound changes in body temperature must be avoided. Hypothermia can produce bradydysrhythmias and sinus arrest. This is of concern when the patient has symptoms. Symptomatic bradydysrhythmias may be treated with inotropic medications such as isoproterenol, or the anticholinergic medication atropine. Both medications increase the heart rate but also increase myocardial oxygen consumption. Another option is a temporary transvenous or transcutaneous pacemaker. Before antipyretics are given or a cooling blanket is typically used.

After a prolonged period of bed rest, orthostatic hypotension may become a significant problem. It may be helpful when initially mobilizing the patient with SCI to gradually elevate the head of the bed and dangle the legs over the side of the bed. As with any immobilized patient, the risk for development of deep vein thrombosis (DVT) is high. However, detection of DVT is difficult because pain and tenderness are not applicable to the patient with SCI. Prevention of DVT is imperative and may include a combination of therapies such as low-dose heparin, low–molecular-weight heparin, sequential compression devices, and embolic hose.

Pulmonary Complications. Pulmonary complications are the most common cause of mortality in SCI patients.[24] Initial and ongoing nursing assessments of respiratory status are imperative for identifying actual or potential impairment in ventilation. These evaluations include observation of respiratory rate and rhythm, observation of symmetry of chest expansion and use of accessory muscles, inspection of quantity and character of secretions, and auscultation of breath sounds. Judicious use of serial arterial blood gas (ABG) values provides information on the adequacy of gas exchange.

Depending on the level of SCI, the patient's breathing pattern may be ineffective (see Table 34-6). Intubation and mechanical ventilation may be required. Patients with lesions at C3 to C5 may be able to be weaned from mechanical ventilation. Some patients with C3 injuries may require mechanical ventilation only at night. Weaning can be a complex process because of physical requirements of the diaphragm and the psychologic effects of the fear of the inability to breathe. A variety of weaning methods are available, but a well-coordinated approach by the nurse, physician, respiratory therapist, and patient is essential (see "Invasive Mechanical Ventilation" in Chapter 21). Setbacks are common and reintubation may be required. The critical care nurse must be aware that the neuromuscular blocking agent *succinylcholine* (suxamethonium) must never be administered to an SCI patient any time after 72 hours postinjury. Use of this depolarizing agent can produce hyperkalemic arrest.

Alternative modes of ventilation may include the *pneumobelt,* a corsetlike device that produces ventilation by assisting with expiration. Another assist device is the abdominal binder. It is thought to support the sagging diaphragm in patients with higher-level SCI with loss of abdominal muscle innervation.

Ineffective airway clearance is a particular problem for the SCI patient as a result of hypoventilation (paralysis of respiratory muscles), increased bronchial secretions, and atelectasis secondary to decreased cough. Frequent suctioning for airway clearance is required. Caution must be used with vigorous suctioning because stimulation of the vagus nerve (which runs alongside the trachea) can cause profound bradycardia. Bradycardia exacerbated by hypoxia is likely to develop in patients with cervical SCI. Use of hyperventilation breaths with 100% oxygen before suctioning is recommended. Chest percussion and drainage facilitate removal of secretions. Kinetic therapy beds, which can rotate up to 60 degrees on each side, may provide continual postural drainage and mobilization of secretions. To further aid in mobilizing secretions in the presence of an ineffective cough, a technique of cough assistance can be used (Fig. 34-8). This procedure is similar to abdominal thrusts (formerly known as the Heimlich maneuver). Exact hand placement may vary, and it is important to assess which placement works best for the patient.

Impaired gas exchange can occur in the SCI patient as a result of hypoventilation (paralysis of respiratory muscles), increased bronchial secretions that interfere with adequate gas diffusion, shunting resulting from atelectasis and associated pulmonary injuries, and pulmonary complications (pulmonary

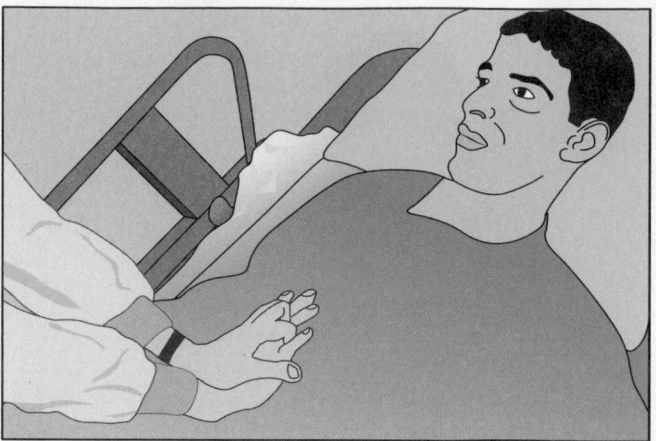

FIGURE 34-8 Cough assistance. A hand or both hands are placed over the upper diaphragm. After the patient inhales, pressure is directed inward and upward as the patient attempts to cough.

embolism). Nursing interventions are directed at improving and maintaining adequate gas exchange.

Musculoskeletal Complications. Immobilized patients are at high risk for contractures. When a muscle is denervated, as in the case of SCI, the muscle fibers shorten and produce a contracture. Irreversible contractures may result in skin breakdown, inability to perform activities of daily living, poor wheelchair posture, and inability to use adaptive devices.[21] Physical therapy and occupational therapy personnel should be consulted early in the patient's course. Range-of-motion exercises are initiated as soon as the spine has been stabilized. Footdrop splints should be applied on admission to prevent contractures and prevent skin breakdown of the heels. Hand splints should be applied for quadriplegics. Hand and foot splints should be removed every 2 hours. Nursing management of the patient in a halo vest includes inspection of pins and traction for security, correct positioning and turning (traction bars or the halo ring must never be used to lift or reposition the patient), placement of wrenches on the front of the vest in case of cardiac arrest, and maintenance of skin integrity inside the halo vest.

Integumentary Complications. Patients with SCI are at high risk for pressure ulcers because of the lack of motor control and sensation. Prevention is the best treatment. Diligent assessments, meticulous skin care, and frequent position changes are required. Specialty surfaces or low-air-loss beds may be necessary for the prevention of pressure ulcers in patients with SCI.[24]

Elimination Complications. Initially after SCI, bowel and bladder tone are flaccid. The degree of bladder and urinary sphincter dysfunction depends on the location and completeness of the injury. A Foley catheter is placed on admission, but it should be removed 3 to 4 days later, at which time the patient is placed on an intermittent catheterization schedule of every 4 to 6 hours. It is not unusual for the male patient with an upper motor neuron injury to experience a reflexogenic erection when being catheterized.[24] An overdistended bladder in the patient with an injury at T6 or above may trigger autonomic dysreflexia. Abdominal distention, constipation, and fecal impaction are major problems encountered in care of the SCI patient. Innervation between the brain and defecation center in the sacral cord has been disrupted. A bowel program to prevent fecal impaction and encourage normal, regular bowel function must be instituted. The patient should not go longer than 3 to 4 days without a bowel movement. Laxatives and stool softeners may be needed, especially if the patient is receiving opiates. Aspects of a successful bowel program include consistent timing of evacuation, proper positioning, physical activity, appropriate fluid intake, a high-fiber diet, and reflex stimulation for those with upper motor neuron injuries.[24]

Maximizing Psychosocial Adaptation. Nursing management of the patient with SCI must include the provision of dedicated emotional support. In the critical care unit, the patient and family experience anxiety, grief, denial, anger, frustration, and hopelessness, because long-term neurologic deficits remain unknown.

Nursing interventions include the promotion of coping mechanisms, support systems, and adaptive skills. Simple, accurate, and consistent information can alleviate fear and anxiety. Feelings of powerlessness may be reduced by including the patient and family in care and decision making. Further psychosocial support can be given by social workers, occupational therapists, psychiatric clinical nurse specialists, and pastors.

Maxillofacial Injuries

Trauma to the face results in complex physiologic and psychologic sequelae. Vital functions that depend on facial integrity include mastication, deglutination, perception of the environment (e.g., vision, hearing, speech, olfaction), and respiration. The face also represents a direct link to self and to expression by playing a major role in personal identity, appearance, and communication. Consequently, maxillofacial trauma has the potential to produce long-term sequelae, with emotional, sensory, and disfigurement implications.

Mechanism of Injury

Maxillofacial injury results from blunt or penetrating trauma. Blunt trauma may occur from motor vehicle, industrial, or athletic injuries; violent blows to the head; or falls. The mechanism for this injury is exemplified by the unbelted driver or passenger who is thrown into the dashboard or windshield. Associated injuries may include concussion, skull fracture, rhinorrhea, SCI, and fractures of other bones. The facial skeleton serves as an energy-absorbing shield to protect the brain, spinal cord, eyes, and pharynx. Nasal bones, the zygoma, and the mandibular condyle are the most susceptible to fracture. Bullet wounds can be life-threatening injuries because of hemorrhage and airway obstruction. Maxillofacial trauma can result in soft tissue injury ranging from abrasions to destruction of most of the face and maxillofacial skeletal fractures. This discussion is limited to maxillofacial skeletal injuries.

Maxillofacial Skeletal Injuries. Fractures of the maxilla are diagnosed according to the *Le Fort classification*. Le Fort fractures are classified in three broad categories, depending on the level of the fracture (Fig. 34-9). The most common, Le Fort I, consists of horizontal fractures in which the entire maxillary arch moves separately from the upper facial skeleton. Le Fort II fractures are an extension of Le Fort I fractures, and they involve the orbit, ethmoid, and nasal bones. Le Fort III

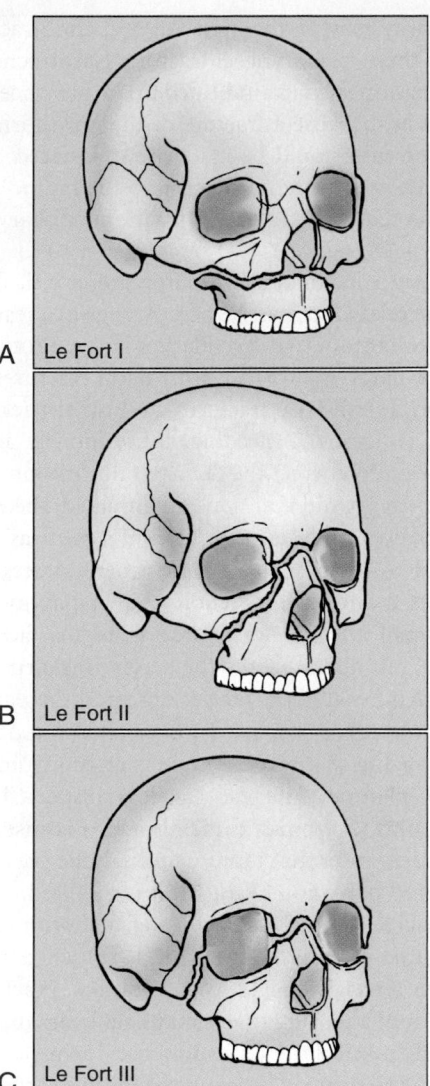

FIGURE 34-9 Fractures of the maxillae are diagnosed according to the Le Fort classification, which consists of three broad categories based on the level of the fracture. *A,* Le Fort I. *B,* Le Fort II. *C,* Le Fort III.

fractures are associated with craniofacial disruption. CSF frequently leaks with Le Fort II and III fractures because there is usually communication between the cranial base and the cribriform plate.

Assessment and Diagnostic Procedures

Patients with maxillofacial trauma are especially prone to ineffective airway clearance, deficient fluid volume related to hemorrhage, and risk for injury. Life-threatening complications associated with maxillofacial trauma include airway obstruction and head and cervical spine injuries. Major or minor facial deformities should not distract the trauma team from the standard assessments and interventions needed to stabilize the ABCs of the patient.

Patients with maxillofacial trauma are at high risk for ineffective airway clearance. The tongue, edema, hemorrhage, foreign objects, vomit, broken teeth, or bone fragments can obstruct the airway. The "look, listen, and feel" methods (see Table 34-2) should be used to assess airway obstruction. An artificial airway may be required. An oral endotracheal tube is used unless there is a laryngeal fracture. Nasotracheal or nasogastric intubation is contraindicated in the presence of unstable facial fractures, because a fracture of the cribriform plate may exist, and the tube could be inadvertently placed through the fractured base of the cranium and into the brain.[9] A tracheostomy may be required for patients with hypopharynx swelling or hemorrhage.

Patients with maxillofacial trauma are at risk for deficient fluid volume related to massive hemorrhage as a result of bleeding from the ethmoid or maxillary sinuses. Profuse bleeding through the nares may occur with nasal fractures, maxillary fractures, or cranial base fractures, and nasal packing may be required to control the bleeding. Intravenously administered fluids are given to correct the deficient fluid volume.

After life-saving interventions are initiated, the comprehensive examination of facial structures is begun as part of the general head-to-toe sequence of assessment. Assessment of the face involves a careful inspection and palpation of the soft tissues. A small abrasion or contusion of the face may seem unobtrusive, but the impact to the underlying structures might have disrupted facial bone integrity, the parotid gland, or facial nerve. The mouth is inspected for traumatic tooth dislodgement, recognizing that some teeth may intrude into the underlying alveolar bone. The ear canal is inspected for occult lacerations of the tympanic membrane. Because specialized facial structures enter the cranium through the eye orbit, careful inspection and palpation of the orbit is required.

Maxillofacial trauma often is associated with cervical SCI. An altered level of consciousness in the presence of maxillofacial fractures strongly suggests neurotrauma. Fractures involving the cranium and dura mater may enable oral bacterial flora to enter CSF, placing the patient at risk for meningitis. Nasal and auditory canals must be inspected for discharge. The drainage also can be tested for glucose inasmuch as CSF has a high glucose content.

The location and displacement of fractures is determined by axonal and coronal CT scans.[9] When true coronal CT is unavailable, CT with facial reconstruction may be substituted.

Medical Management

Treatment of Le Fort fractures includes direct visualization and reduction of the fragments and stabilization with plates and screws.

Nursing Management

Nursing diagnoses for the patient with maxillofacial trauma are listed in Box 34-10. Nursing interventions are aimed at protecting the airway by reducing the risk of emesis and aspiration. Proper orogastric tube functioning must be ensured. Antiemetics may be administered. Unless contraindicated, the head of the bed is elevated 30 degrees. If vomiting occurs, the patient is placed in a side or forward position and oral or nasal suctioning is used. Wire cutters must be available at the bedside in case the vomit cannot clear the wires and occludes the airway. Although this seldom is necessary, the intention in cutting the wires is to cut the vertical attachments, not the horizontal ones.

> **◎ BOX 34-10**   **NURSING DIAGNOSES**
> *Maxillofacial Trauma*
>
> - Risk for Aspiration risk factors: impaired pharyngeal peristalsis or tongue function; impaired laryngeal sensation or reflex; impaired laryngeal closure or elevation, p. 1154
> - Deficient Fluid Volume related to absolute loss, p. 1132
> - Imbalanced Nutrition: Less Than Body Requirements related to lack of exogenous nutrients and increased metabolic demands, p. 1143
> - Acute Pain related to transmission and perception of cutaneous, visceral, muscular, or ischemic impulses, p. 1123

Thoracic Injuries

Thoracic injuries involve trauma to the chest wall, lungs, heart, great vessels, and esophagus. Thoracic trauma most commonly is the result of a violent crime or an MVC. [*motor vehicle collision*]

Mechanism of Injury

Blunt Thoracic Trauma. Blunt trauma to the chest most often is caused by MVCs or falls. Second only to head injury or SCI, thoracic injuries account for 25% of trauma deaths.[25] The underlying mechanism of injury tends to be a combination of acceleration–deceleration injury and direct transfer mechanics, as in a crush injury. Various mechanisms of blunt trauma are associated with specific injury patterns. After head-on collisions, drivers have a higher frequency of injury than do backseat passengers because the driver comes in contact with the steering wheel assembly. Severe thoracic injuries often are seen in patients who are unrestrained. Falls from greater than 20 feet are typically associated with thoracic injury.

Penetrating Thoracic Injuries. The penetrating object involved determines the damage sustained from penetrating thoracic trauma. Low-velocity weapons (e.g., .22-caliber gun, knife) usually damage only what is in the weapon's direct path. Of particular concern, however, are stab wounds that involve the anterior chest wall between the midclavicular lines, the angle of Louis, and the epigastric region because of the proximity of the heart and great vessels.

Specific Thoracic Traumatic Injuries

Chest Wall Injuries

Rib Fractures. Fractures of the ribs can be serious, even life-threatening, particularly when there are three or more rib fractures, there is the presence of pre-existing disease (especially cardiopulmonary disease), or the patient is 65 years old or greater.[26] Fractures of the first and second ribs are associated with intrathoracic vascular injuries (e.g., brachial plexus, great vessels), and because they are protected by the scapula, clavicle, humerus, and muscles, they signify a very high degree of force applied to the thorax. Fractures to the lower ribs (7th to 12th) may be associated with abdominal injuries, such as spleen and liver injuries. Fractures to the middle ribs may be associated with lung injury, including pulmonary contusion and pneumothorax. Lack of bone calcification in pediatric trauma patients means the chest wall is more compliant, and rib fractures need not have occurred for a tremendous amount of force to have been absorbed by the underlying organs.

The pain associated with rib fractures can be aggravated by respiratory excursion. The patient often splints, takes shallow breaths, and refuses to cough, which can result in atelectasis and pneumonia. Localized pain that increases with respiration or that is elicited by rib compression may indicate rib fractures. Definitive diagnosis can be made with a chest radiograph. Interventions include aggressive pulmonary physiotherapy and pain control to improve chest expansion efforts and gas exchange. Pain management interventions must be tailored to the patient's response to therapy. The primary goal of pain management in patients with rib fractures is prevention of pulmonary complications and patient comfort. Nonsteroidal anti-inflammatory drugs (NSAIDs), intercostal nerve blocks, thoracic epidural analgesia, and opiates may be considered to assist with pain control.[25] Epidural analgesia can help increase the functional residual capacity, dynamic lung compliance, and vital capacity; decrease the airway resistance; and increase Pao_2.[25] External splints are not recommended because they further limit chest wall expansion and may add to atelectasis.[25] The patient's pre-existing pulmonary status and age may dictate the course of recovery.[25] Patients should also have incentive spirometry values monitored, as a reduction in volume could indicate increasing pain.[26]

Flail Chest. Flail chest, which is caused by blunt trauma, disrupts the continuity of chest wall structures. Typically, a flail segment occurs when two or more ribs are fractured in two or more places and are no longer attached to the thoracic cage, producing a free-floating segment of the chest wall. A flail chest is a clinical diagnosis wherein the so-called flail segment (or floating segment) moves paradoxically compared to the rest of the chest wall (Fig. 34-10).[25] During inspiration, the intact portion of the chest wall expands while the injured part is sucked in. During expiration, the chest wall moves in, and the flail segment moves out. Although the flail segment increases the work of breathing, the main cause of hypoxemia is the underlying pulmonary contusion.[27] The physiologic effects of the impaired chest wall motion of a flail chest include decreased tidal volume and vital capacity and impaired cough, which lead to hypoventilation and atelectasis.

Inspection of the chest reveals paradoxical movement. Palpation of the chest may indicate crepitus and tenderness near fractured ribs. A chest radiograph that reveals multiple rib fractures and evidence of hypoxia demonstrated by ABG values aids in the diagnosis. Interventions focus on ensuring adequate oxygenation, judicious administration of fluids, and analgesia to improve ventilation.[25] Intubation and mechanical ventilation may be required to prevent further hypoxia.

Ruptured Diaphragm. Diagnosis of a diaphragmatic rupture is often missed in trauma patients because of the subtle and nonspecific symptoms this injury produces. The mechanism of

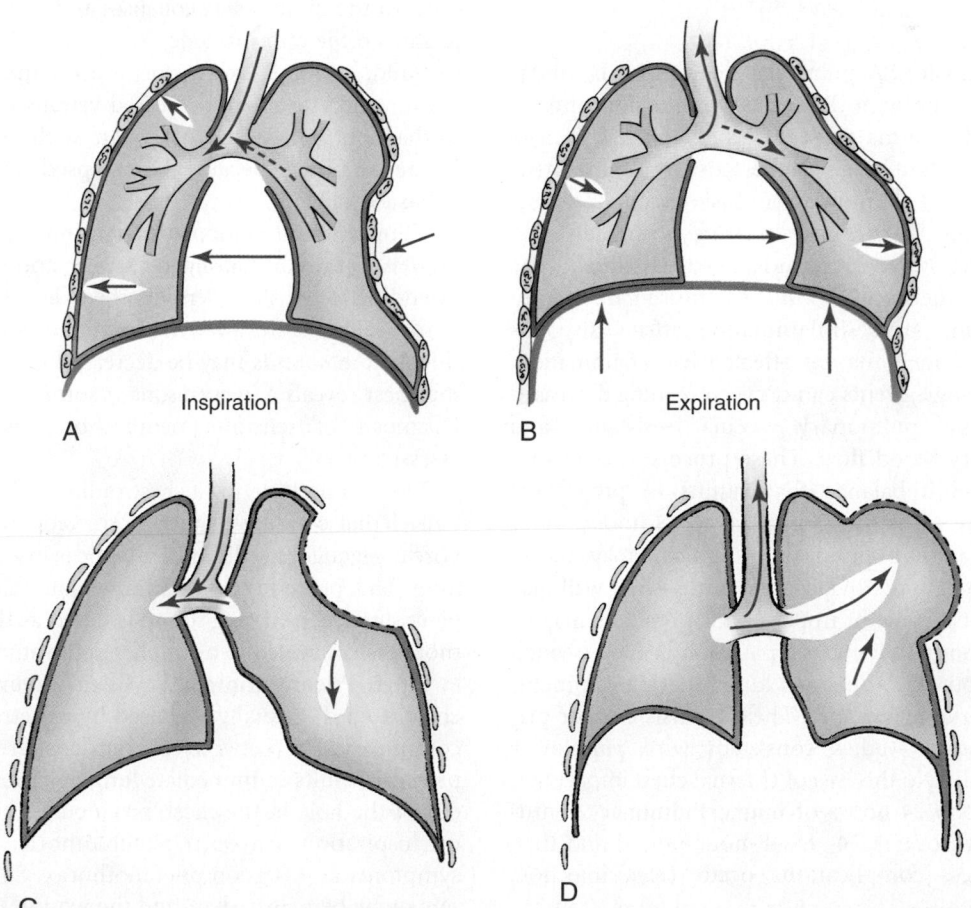

FIGURE 34-10 Flail chest. *A,* Normal inspiration. *B,* Normal expiration. *C,* The area of lung underlying the unstable chest wall sucks in on inspiration. *D,* The same area balloons out on expiration. Notice the movement of mediastinum toward opposite lung on inspiration.

injury appears to be a rapid rise in intra-abdominal pressure as a result of compression force applied to the lower part of the chest or upper region of the abdomen. This injury can occur when a person is thrown forward over the edge of the steering wheel in a high-speed MVC involving deceleration forces. The diaphragm, which offers little resistance to the force, can rupture or tear. Abdominal viscera then can gradually enter the thoracic cavity, moving from the positive pressure of the abdomen to the negative pressure in the thorax. Diaphragmatic rupture can be a life-threatening event. Massive herniation of abdominal contents into the thoracic cavity can compress the lungs and mediastinum, which hampers venous return and leads to decreased cardiac output. Herniated bowel can become strangulated and perforate.

Diaphragmatic herniation may produce significant compromise and changes in respiratory effort. Auscultation of bowel sounds in the chest or unilateral breath sounds may indicate a ruptured diaphragm. The patient may complain of shoulder pain, shortness of breath, or abdominal tenderness. Thoracoscopy may be helpful in evaluating the diaphragm in indeterminate cases, and multidetector CT analysis is a useful diagnostic tool for the evaluation of diaphragmatic injuries.[28] A chest radiograph may reveal the tip of a nasogastric tube above the diaphragm, a unilaterally elevated hemidiaphragm, a hollow or solid mass above the diaphragm, and a shift of the mediastinum away from the affected side. Treatment of a ruptured diaphragm includes its immediate repair.

Pulmonary Injuries

Pulmonary Contusion. A pulmonary contusion is fundamentally a bruise of the lung. Pulmonary contusion often is associated with blunt trauma and other chest injuries, such as rib fractures and flail chest, and it is the most common potentially lethal chest injury.[25] Pulmonary contusions can occur unilaterally or bilaterally. A contusion manifests initially as a hemorrhage, followed by alveolar and interstitial edema. The edema can remain rather localized in the contused area or can spread to other lung areas. Inflammation affects alveolar-capillary units. As more units are affected by inflammation, further pathophysiologic events can occur, including decreased compliance, increased pulmonary vascular resistance, and decreased pulmonary blood flow. These processes result in a ventilation–perfusion imbalance that results in progressive hypoxemia and poor ventilation over a 24- to 48-hour period.

Clinical manifestations of pulmonary contusion may take up to 24 to 48 hours to develop. Inspections of the chest wall may reveal ecchymosis at the site of impact. Moist crackles may be auscultated in the contused lung. The patient may have a cough and blood-tinged sputum. Abnormal lung function can manifest as systemic arterial hypoxemia. The diagnosis is made primarily by radiography studies consistent with pulmonary infiltrate corresponding to the area of external chest impact that manifests within 12 to 24 hours of injury. Pulmonary contusions tend to worsen over a 24- to 48-hour period and then slowly resolve unless complications occur (e.g., infection, ARDS).

Aggressive respiratory care is the cornerstone for care of nonintubated patients with pulmonary contusion. Interventions include ambulation, deep-breathing exercises, turning, and incentive spirometry. Chest physiotherapy is not tolerated if there are coexisting rib fractures. Aggressive removal of airway secretions is important to avoid infection and to improve ventilation. Patients with unilateral contusions are placed with the injured side up and uninjured side down ("down with the good lung"). This positioning maximizes the match between pulmonary ventilation and perfusion. Patients with severe contusions may continue to show decompensation despite aggressive nursing management. Respiratory acidosis, increases in peak airway and plateau pressures, and increased work of breathing may require endotracheal intubation and mechanical ventilation with *positive end-expiratory pressure* (PEEP). Adequate pain control is accomplished with administration of NSAIDs, opiates, intercostal nerve blocks, or thoracic epidural analgesia.[25]

Complications resulting from pulmonary contusions include pneumonia, ARDS, lung abscesses, emphysema, and pulmonary embolism. Factors that contribute to increased mortality rates include shock, coexisting head injury, flail chest, falls from heights greater than 20 feet, advanced age, and pre-existing disease (e.g., coronary artery disease, chronic obstructive pulmonary disease).

Tension Pneumothorax. A tension pneumothorax usually is caused by an injury that perforates the chest wall or pleural space. Air flows into the pleural space with inspiration and becomes trapped. As pressure in the pleural space increases, the lung on the injured side collapses and causes the mediastinum to shift to the opposite side (Fig. 34-11). As pressure continues to build, the shift exerts pressure on the heart and thoracic aorta, which results in decreased venous return and decreased cardiac output. Tissue perfusion with oxygenated blood is further hampered because the collapsed lung cannot participate in gas exchange.

Clinical manifestations of a tension pneumothorax include dyspnea, tachycardia, hypotension, and sudden chest pain extending to the shoulders. Tracheal deviation can be observed as the trachea shifts away from the injured side. On the injured side, breath sounds may be decreased or absent. Percussion of the chest reveals a hyperresonant sound over the affected side. Diagnosis of tension pneumothorax is made by clinical assessment.

There is no time for a chest radiograph because this potentially lethal condition must be treated immediately.[9] A large-bore (14-gauge) needle or chest tube is inserted into the affected lung. This procedure allows immediate release of air from the pleural space. A hissing sound is heard as the tension pneumothorax is converted to a simple pneumothorax.

Open Pneumothorax. An open pneumothorax ("sucking chest wound") usually is caused by penetrating trauma. Open communication between the atmosphere and intrathoracic pressure results in immediate lung deflation. Air moves in and out of the hole in the chest, producing a sucking sound heard on inspiration. An open pneumothorax produces the same symptoms as a tension pneumothorax. Subcutaneous emphysema may be palpated around the wound.

Initial management of an open pneumothorax is accomplished by promptly closing the wound at end expiration with a sterile occlusive dressing (plastic wrap or petroleum gauze)

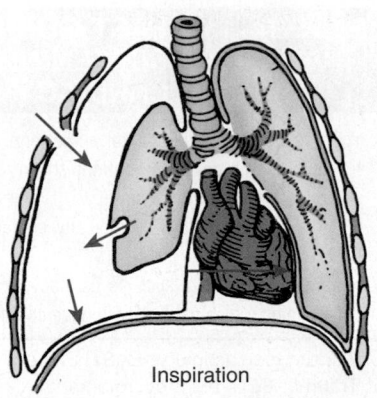 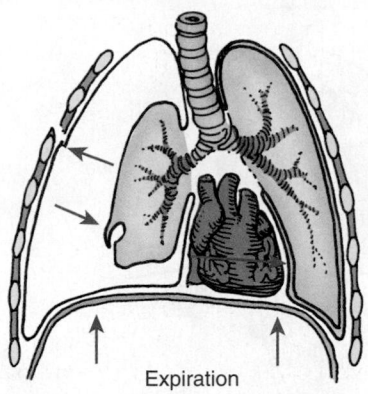

Inspiration   Expiration

FIGURE 34-11   A tension pneumothorax usually is caused by an injury that perforates the chest wall or pleural space. Air flows into the pleural space with inspiration and becomes trapped. As pressure in the pleural space increases, the lung on the injured side collapses and causes the mediastinum to shift to the opposite side. (From Marx J, et al. *Rosen's Emergency Medicine: Concepts and Clinical Practice.* 5th ed. St. Louis: Mosby; 2002.)

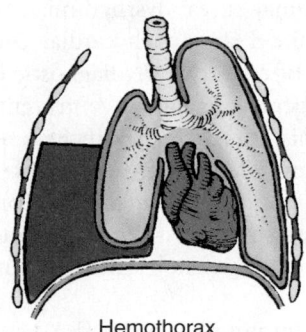

Hemothorax

FIGURE 34-12   Blunt or penetrating thoracic trauma can cause bleeding into the pleural space to form a hemothorax.

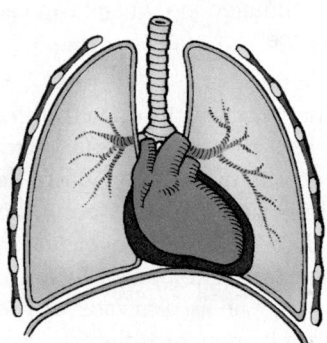

FIGURE 34-13   Cardiac tamponade is the progressive accumulation of blood in the pericardial sac.

large enough to overlap the wound's edges.[9] This dressing should be taped securely on three sides. As the patient breathes in, the dressing gets sucked in to occlude the wound and prevent air from entering. A chest tube is placed as soon as possible. Surgical intervention may be required to close the wound.

Hemothorax. Blunt or penetrating thoracic trauma can cause bleeding into the pleural space, resulting in a hemothorax (Fig. 34-12). A massive hemothorax results from the accumulation of more than 1500 mL of blood in the chest cavity.[29] The source of bleeding may be the intercostal or internal mammary arteries, lungs, heart, or great vessels. Lacerations to the lung parenchyma are low-pressure bleeds and typically stop bleeding spontaneously.[29] Arterial bleeding from hilar vessels usually require immediate surgical intervention.[9] In either case, increasing intrapleural pressure results in a decrease in vital capacity. Increasing vascular blood loss into the pleural space causes decreased venous return and decreased cardiac output.

Assessment findings for patients with a hemothorax include hypovolemic shock. Breath sounds may be diminished or absent over the affected lung. With hemothorax, the neck veins are collapsed, and the trachea is at midline. Massive hemothorax can be diagnosed on the basis of clinical manifestations of hypotension associated with the absence of breath sounds or dullness to percussion on one side of the chest.[9,29]

This life-threatening condition must be treated immediately. Resuscitation with intravenous fluids is initiated to treat the

hypovolemic shock. A chest tube is placed on the affected side to allow drainage of blood. An autotransfusion device can be attached to the chest tube collection chamber. Thoracotomy may be necessary for patients who require persistent blood transfusions or who have significant bleeding (200 mL/hr for 2 to 4 hours or more than 1500 mL on initial tube insertion) or when there are injuries to major cardiovascular structures.[29]

Cardiac and Vascular Injuries

Penetrating Cardiac Injuries. Penetrating cardiac trauma can occur from mechanical injuries as a result of bullets, knives, or impalements. The chest wall offers little protection to the heart from penetrating trauma. The most common site of injury is the right ventricle because of its anterior position. The mortality rate from penetrating trauma to the heart is high. The prehospital mortality rate for penetrating cardiac injuries is very high, and most deaths occur within minutes after injury as a result of exsanguination or tamponade.

Cardiac Tamponade. Cardiac tamponade is the progressive accumulation of blood in the pericardial sac (Fig. 34-13). With cardiac tamponade, progressive accumulation of 120 to 150 mL of blood increases the intracardiac pressure and compresses the atria and ventricles. An increase in intracardiac pressure leads to decreased venous return and decreased filling pressure, which leads to decreased cardiac output, myocardial hypoxia, heart failure, and cardiogenic shock.

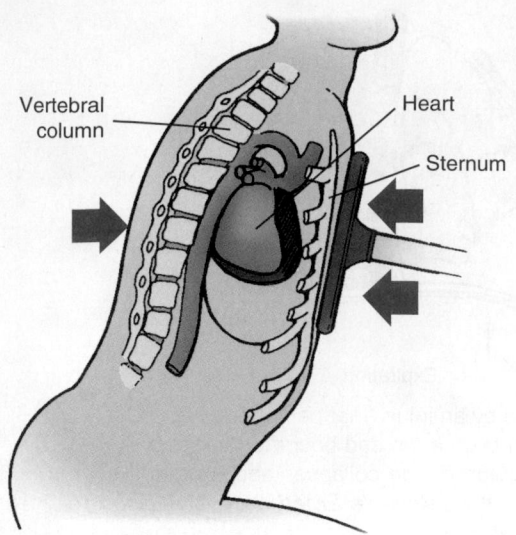

FIGURE 34-14 Blunt cardiac trauma. Sudden acceleration (as from contact with the steering wheel) can cause the heart to be thrown against the sternum.

| BOX 34-11 | EAST GUIDELINES FOR SCREENING OF BLUNT CARDIAC INJURY |

- Obtain an admission ECG for all patients in whom there is suspected BCI.
- If ECG is abnormal, the patient should be admitted for continuous ECG monitoring for 24 to 48 hours.
- If the patient is hemodynamically unstable, an echocardiogram may be performed.
- Cardiac biomarkers such as cardiac troponin T values are not useful in predicting which patients will have complications related to BCI.

BCI, Blunt cardiac injury; *EAST,* Eastern Association for the Surgery of Trauma; *ECG,* electrocardiogram.

Classic assessment findings associated with cardiac tamponade are called *Beck's triad*—presence of elevated central venous pressure with neck vein distention, muffled heart sounds, and hypotension. Pulsus paradoxus may occur. Pulseless electrical activity (PEA) in the absence of hypovolemia and tension pneumothorax suggests cardiac tamponade.[9] Ultrasonography in the emergency setting may be used in cases of penetrating cardiac injuries to identify a hemopericardium.[30]

Immediate treatment is required to remove the accumulation of fluid in the pericardial sac. Pericardiocentesis involves aspiration of fluid from the pericardium by use of a large-bore needle. The inherent risk in this procedure is potential laceration of the coronary artery. Other approaches include surgical procedures such as thoracotomy or median sternotomy. The goal of these procedures is to locate and control the source of bleeding.

Blunt Cardiac Injuries. The most common causes of blunt cardiac trauma include high-speed MVCs, direct blows to the chest, and falls. Because of its mobility and its location between the sternum and thoracic vertebrae, the heart is susceptible to blunt traumatic injury. Sudden acceleration (as from contact with a steering wheel) can cause the heart to be thrown against the sternum (Fig. 34-14). Sudden deceleration can cause the heart to be thrown against the thoracic vertebrae by a direct blow to the chest, such as blows caused by a baseball, animal kick, or fall.

Blunt Cardiac Injury. *Blunt cardiac injury* (BCI), formerly called *myocardial contusion*, covers the spectrum of myocardial contusion, concussion, and rupture. The most often injured chambers include the right atrium and ventricle because of their anterior position in the chest.[31]

Few clinical signs and symptoms are specific for BCI. Evidence of external chest trauma, such as steering wheel imprint or sternal fractures, should raise the suspicion for BCI. However, the presence of a sternal fracture does not predict the incidence of BCI. The patient may complain of chest pain that is similar to anginal pain, but it is not typically relieved with nitroglycerin.[31] The chest pain is usually caused by associated injuries. The EAST guidelines for screening of BCI are listed in Box 34-11. The patient should be monitored for new onset of dysrhythmias and if present, should raise suspicion for BCI.[31] The 12-lead ECG may reveal dysrhythmias, ST changes, heart block, or unexplained sinus tachycardia. Use of biomarkers, such as troponin, offers very little diagnostic help for BCI.[31]

Medical management is aimed at preventing and treating complications. This approach may include administration of antidysrhythmic medications, treatment of heart failure, or insertion of a temporary pacemaker to control conduction abnormalities. Assessment of fluid and electrolyte balance is imperative to ensure adequate cardiac output and myocardial conduction.

Aortic Injury. Blunt aortic injury (BAI) is one of the most lethal blunt thoracic injuries. While BAI occurs in less than 1% of MVCs, it represents 16% of the deaths.[32] Sudden deceleration from speeds of 20 mph are most commonly associated with BAI.[32] Injuries associated with aortic injury include a first or second rib fracture, high sternal fracture, left clavicular fracture at the level of the sternal margin, and massive hemothorax. BAI should be suspected in all victims of trauma with a rapid deceleration or acceleration mechanism of injury.

The thoracic aorta is relatively mobile and tears at fixed anatomic points within the thorax. Sites of aortic disruption (in order of frequency) include the aortic isthmus, just distal to the subclavian artery (where the vessel is fixed to the chest by the ligamentum arteriosum); at the ascending aorta (where the aorta leaves the pericardial sac); at the descending aorta (where the aorta enters the diaphragm); and avulsion of the innominate artery from the aortic arch.[33]

The nurse assesses blood pressure in both arms because a tear in the aortic arch may create a pressure gradient resulting in blood pressure changes between upper extremities. If aortic disruption is suspected, blood pressure is also compared between upper and lower extremities. Baroreceptors are stimulated, resulting in upper extremity hypertension with relative lower extremity hypotension. Additional clinical assessment findings include a pulse deficit at any site, unexplained hypotension, sternal pain, precordial systolic murmur, hoarseness, dyspnea, and lower extremity sensory deficits.

An initial chest radiograph is obtained in the upright position after it is considered safe to do so. Radiograph findings suggesting aortic injury include a widened mediastinum, obscured aortic knob, deviation of the left main stem bronchus or nasogastric tube, and opacification of the aortopulmonary window.[33] Spiral or helical CT is warranted if the initial chest radiograph is inconclusive, but the definitive diagnosis is made by aortography in indeterminate cases.[33]

During the resuscitation phase for a patient with aortic disruption, blood pressure management is the primary goal to minimize injury. Patients with tears at the aortic isthmus are typically hypertensive, and minimizing stress on the vessel is achieved by maintaining the systolic blood pressure less than 90 mm Hg by using antihypertensive agents such as sodium nitroprusside.[32,33] The nurse anticipates definitive surgical intervention early in the resuscitation. Surgical repair may be achieved by a graft, primary anastomosis, and bypass.[32,33]

Postoperative care is directed toward blood pressure stabilization, with the goal of minimizing vessel stress while maintaining tissue perfusion, which typically is accomplished with the use of sodium nitroprusside. Careful assessment of postoperative paraplegia is needed because lack of blood flow to the spinal column might have occurred perioperatively. Paraplegia is closely related to the duration of clamp time intraoperatively. The critical care nurse monitors for signs of bowel ischemia (e.g., tube feeding intolerance, lactic acidosis) and acute kidney injury (e.g., poor urinary output, rising serum creatinine) because blood flow to the mesentery and kidney may have been compromised as a result of the injury or aortic clamp time.

Abdominal Injuries

Abdominal injuries often are associated with multisystem trauma. Abdominal injuries are the third leading cause of traumatic death. Injuries to the abdomen are the result of blunt or penetrating trauma. Two major life-threatening conditions that occur after abdominal trauma are hemorrhage and hollow viscus perforation with associated peritonitis. Death occurring after 48 hours following injury is the result of sepsis and its complications. The critical care nurse must pay particular attention to complication prevention strategies throughout the trauma cycle.

Mechanism of Injury

Blunt Trauma. Blunt abdominal injuries are common. They result most often from MVCs, falls, and assaults. In MVCs, abdominal injury is more likely to occur when a vehicle is struck from the side. In the passenger position of the front seat, liver injury is likely when the point of impact is on the same side as the passenger. A driver is likely to sustain injury to the spleen when the impact is on the driver's side. Pedestrians hit by motor vehicles are at risk for serious abdominal injuries. Blunt trauma to the thorax can produce injuries to the liver, spleen, and diaphragm. Deceleration and direct forces can produce retroperitoneal hematomas. Blunt abdominal injuries often are hidden, requiring careful assessment and reassessment. Unrecognized abdominal trauma is a common cause of preventable death, and blunt abdominal injury deaths are more likely to be fatal than are penetrating abdominal injuries.

Penetrating Trauma. Penetrating abdominal trauma is caused most often by knives or bullets. The danger of penetrating abdominal trauma is that the outside appearance of the wound does not reflect the extent of internal injury. Commonly injured organs from knife wounds are the colon, liver, spleen, and diaphragm. Gunshot wounds to the abdomen usually are more serious than are stab wounds. A bullet destroys tissue along its path. Inside the abdomen, a bullet can travel in erratic paths and ricochet off bone. Death from penetrating injuries depends on the injury to major vascular structures and resultant intra-abdominal hemorrhage. While a majority of patients with gunshot wounds generally receive a laparotomy, selected patients may be managed nonoperatively.[34]

Assessment

The initial assessment of the trauma patient, whether in the emergency department or the critical care unit, follows the primary and secondary survey techniques as outlined by ATLS guidelines.[9] The initial physical assessment may be unreliable given the confounding influences of alcohol, illicit drugs, analgesics, and an altered level of consciousness. Specific assessment findings associated with abdominal trauma are reviewed here.

Physical Assessment. The location of entry and exit sites associated with penetrating trauma are assessed and documented. Inspection of the patient's abdomen may reveal purplish discoloration of the flanks or umbilicus (Cullen sign), which indicates blood in the abdominal wall. Ecchymosis in the flank area (Turner-Grey sign) may indicate retroperitoneal bleeding or a pancreatic injury. A hematoma in the flank area suggests kidney injury. A distended abdomen may indicate the accumulation of blood, fluid, or gas resulting from a perforated organ or ruptured blood vessel. Auscultation of the abdomen may reveal friction rubs over the liver or spleen and may indicate rupture. The abdomen is assessed for rebound tenderness and rigidity. These assessment findings indicate peritoneal inflammation. Referred pain to the left shoulder (Kehr sign) may indicate a ruptured spleen or irritation of the diaphragm from bile or other material in the peritoneum. Subcutaneous emphysema palpated on the abdomen suggests free air as a result of a ruptured bowel.

Diagnostic Procedures. Insertion of a nasogastric tube and urinary catheter serves as a useful diagnostic and therapeutic aid. A nasogastric tube can decompress the stomach, and the contents can be checked for blood. Urine obtained from the urinary catheter can also be tested for the presence of blood.

Serial laboratory test results may be nonspecific for the patient with abdominal trauma. Because of hemoconcentration, hemoglobin and hematocrit results may not reflect actual values. Serial values are more valuable in diagnosing abdominal injuries.

Because of the unreliability of physical examination alone in the patient suspected of having abdominal trauma,[35] diagnostic testing may occur simultaneously during the primary and secondary surveys. Noninvasive tests include bedside ultrasound, CT, and chest and abdominal radiographs.

Diagnostic Peritoneal Lavage. The invasive test *diagnostic peritoneal lavage* (DPL) may also help to exclude or confirm the presence of intra-abdominal injury.[9] After the patient's bladder has been emptied, a small incision is made in the abdomen through the skin and into the peritoneum. A small catheter is inserted. If frank blood is encountered, intra-abdominal injury is evident, and the patient is taken immediately to the operating room. If gross blood is not initially encountered, a liter of fluid (lactated Ringer or 0.9% normal saline) is infused through the catheter into the abdomen. The intravenous bag is then placed in a dependent position, and abdominal fluid is allowed to drain into the intravenous bag. The drainage fluid is sent to the laboratory for analysis. Positive DPL results signal intra-abdominal trauma and usually necessitate surgical intervention (Box 34-12). DPL is invasive, has been associated with complications, and cannot exclude retroperitoneal injuries.

Bedside Ultrasound. The bedside ultrasound, called the *Focused Assessment Sonography for Trauma* (FAST examination) is performed at most trauma centers to evaluate the patient for the presence of intra-abdominal blood.[35] This is a quick and noninvasive means of rapid assessment, but success depends on the skill level of the operator.[36] Bedside ultrasonography is used widely in the United States for the detection of abdominal free fluid and hemoperitoneum. Typically, the right and left upper abdominal quadrant areas are examined: the right upper quadrant (Morrison's pouch); the left upper quadrant splenorenal area; the pericardial sac; and the pelvis (Douglas' pouch)[36] (Fig. 34-15). The primary disadvantage of FAST is the need for free intraperitoneal fluid to produce a positive study result.[36] An initial negative FAST result may be followed by serial ultrasound examinations, abdominal CT, or by DPL.[35] Hemodynamically unstable patients with a positive FAST, specifically free fluid noted in the abdomen, generally undergo emergency surgery to achieve hemostasis.

Although the FAST test has had good sensitivity and specificity, it is not intended to replace DPL or CT. Obese abdomens and patients with ascites may have erroneous results, and further workup for these patients is warranted.[36] Ultrasound is also limited in its ability to diagnose diaphragmatic, intestinal, or pancreas injuries.[36] Abdominal CT scanning is the mainstay of diagnostic evaluation in the hemodynamically stable trauma patient.[35] Abdominal CT provides information about specific organ injury, pelvic injury, and retroperitoneal hemorrhage.

Combined Abdominal Organ Injuries

Patients with multiple visceral injuries may require surgical intervention that uses somewhat nontraditional techniques such as "damage control" surgery. The three phases of this treatment strategy are the *1) initial operation (damage control laparotomy); 2) critical care unit resuscitation;* and *3) definitive reoperation also known as Staged Abdominal Reconstruction or STAR* (Box 34-13).[37] The duration of the initial operation is kept to a minimum. The decision to abbreviate the initial operation is made early during surgery. Damage control laparotomy may be considered if some clinical parameters are met: acidosis (pH less than 7.2), hypothermia (temperature less than 35° C),

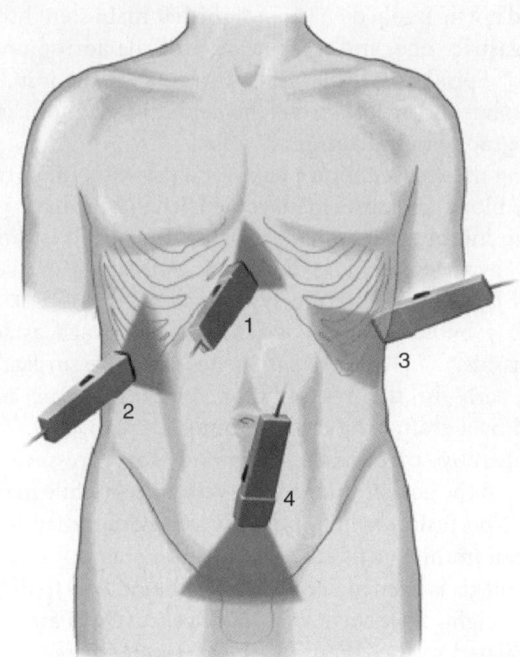

FIGURE 34-15 The Focused Assessment Sonography for Trauma (FAST) quadrants are examined for the presence of free fluid. (From Moore FA, Moore EE. Initial management of life-threatening trauma. In: Ashley SW, editorial chair. *ACS Surgery: Principles and Practice.* Hamilton, Ontario, Canada: Decker Publishing; 2012.)

BOX 34-13   DAMAGE CONTROL SEQUENCE

Initial Operation
- Control contamination
- Control hemorrhage
- Intra-abdominal packing
- Temporary closure

Critical Care Unit Resuscitation
- Correct coagulopathy
- Rewarming
- Maximize hemodynamics
- Ventilatory support
- Injury identification

Planned Reoperation
- Pack removal
- Definitive repair

and clinical coagulopathy and/or if the patient is receiving a massive transfusion.[36] Hypothermia induced by an open visceral cavity in conjunction with massive blood transfusion can lead to coagulopathy and continued bleeding, which results in shock and metabolic acidosis. The triad of hypothermia, coagulopathy, and acidosis creates a self-propagating cycle that can eventually lead to an irreversible physiologic insult. The initial operation must be completed quickly to terminate this self-propagating cycle. Reconstruction and formal closure of the wound may not be completed before the patient is transferred to the critical care unit.

TABLE 34-9 INTERVENTIONS FOR REWARMING THE TRAUMA PATIENT

INTERVENTION	EXTERNAL REWARMING PROCEDURES	INTERNAL REWARMING PROCEDURES
Passive	Maintain a warm room temperature. Remove all wet clothing and linen. Cover the patient with blankets. Avoid bathing patient until normothermia achieved.	Administer warmed, humidified oxygen. Administer warmed intravenous fluids.
Active	Use radiant heat lamps, heating blankets or pads, and hot water bottles.	Perform gastrointestinal irrigation with warmed solutions. Perform extracorporeal rewarming for profound hypothermia. Use esophageal rewarming tubes.

Adapted from Flarity K. Environmental emergencies. In: Kunz Howard P, Steinmann R, eds. *Sheehy's Emergency Nursing: Principles and Practice.* 6th ed. St. Louis: Mosby; 2010.

TABLE 34-10 LIVER INJURY SCALE

GRADE*		INJURY DESCRIPTION
I	Hematoma	Subcapsular, <10% surface area
	Laceration	Capsular tear, <1 cm parenchymal depth
II	Hematoma	Subcapsular, 10%-50% surface area; intraparenchymal <10 cm in diameter
	Laceration	Capsular tear, 1-3 cm parenchymal depth, <10 cm long
III	Hematoma	Subcapsular, >50% surface area or expanding; ruptured subcapsular or parenchymal hematoma; intraparenchymal hematoma >10 cm or expanding
	Laceration	>3 cm parenchymal depth
IV	Laceration	Parenchymal disruption involving 25%-75% of hepatic lobe or 1-3 Couinaud's segments within a single lobe
V	Laceration	Parenchymal disruption involving >75% of hepatic lobe or >3 Couinaud's segments within a single lobe
	Vascular	Juxtahepatic venous injuries (retrohepatic vena cava, central major hepatic veins)
VI	Vascular	Hepatic avulsion

Modified from Trunkey DD. Hepatic trauma: contemporary management. *Surg Clin North Am.* 2004;84:437.
*Advance one grade for multiple injuries up to grade II.

The goal of the critical care phase of this strategy is to continue aggressive resuscitation and correct hypothermia, coagulopathy, and acidosis. Rewarming techniques, described in Table 34-9, are used to correct hypothermia. Coagulation factors and platelets may be administered to correct coagulopathies.

Abdominal Compartment Syndrome. The patient is assessed for additional complications, including ongoing hemorrhage, intra-abdominal hypertension (IAH), and abdominal compartment syndrome. Abdominal compartment syndrome is defined as end-organ dysfunction caused by IAH.[38] Increased pressure can be caused by bleeding, ileus, visceral edema, or a noncompliant abdominal wall. Increased abdominal cavity pressure can impinge on diaphragmatic excursion and can affect ventilation. Clinical manifestations of abdominal compartment syndrome include decreased cardiac output, increased pulmonary vascular resistance, increased peak pulmonary pressures, decreased urine output, and hypoxia.[38] Intra-abdominal pressure can be measured through a urinary catheter after the injection of 25 mL of sterile saline.[38] Intra-abdominal hypertension (IAH) is defined as an intra-abdominal pressure greater than or equal to 12 mm Hg (normal 5 to 7 mm Hg).[37] IAH may be graded: grade I (12 to 15 mm Hg), grade II (16 to 20 mm Hg), grade III (21 to 25 mm Hg), and grade IV (greater than 25 mm Hg).[37] The abdominal perfusion pressure may be calculated (MAP—IAP), with a normal value being greater than 60 mm Hg.

Surgical decompression of the abdomen may be required for abdominal pressures greater than 20 to 25 mm Hg that are associated with signs of organ dysfunction, such as decompensating heart, lung, and kidney status.[37] After surgical decompression is completed and the pressure relieved, the patient may receive a temporary abdominal closure ("open abdomen"), wherein the skin and abdominal fascia are left open. This involves temporarily closing the abdomen with a sterile perforated plastic sheet, clips, vacuum-assisted techniques, and many other options.[37] In some cases closed suction drains are brought out through a sterile plastic drape over the entire wound. The wound is closed permanently in the days, weeks, and months following the surgery or it is allowed to heal by secondary intention and eventual skin grafting.

Specific Organ Injuries

Physical assessment findings, DPL, and CT scanning aid in making a diagnosis of specific abdominal organ injury. The medical and nursing management vary according to specific organ injuries. Liver, spleen, and bowel injuries, which are seen more commonly, are discussed here.

Liver Injuries. The liver is the primary organ injured in penetrating trauma and the second most often injured organ in blunt trauma. Abdominal CT is considered to be the most reliable diagnostic tool to identify and assess the severity of the injury to the liver.[39] The severity of liver injuries is graded to provide a mechanism for determining the amount of trauma sustained by that organ, the care needed, and the possible outcomes (Table 34-10). Nonoperative management is considered the standard of care for hemodynamically stable patients with liver injury.[38] Patients who are admitted to critical care unit are monitored for signs of hemorrhage. Serial serum hematocrit and hemoglobin levels and vital signs are monitored over several days.

Patients with penetrating or blunt liver trauma who are hemodynamically unstable may require surgical intervention to achieve hemostasis. Resection of the devitalized tissue is required for massive injuries. Hemorrhage is common with liver injuries, and ligation of the hepatic arteries or veins may be required to control hemorrhage. Drains may be placed intraoperatively to prevent hematoma development.

Care of the patient with severe liver injuries can be challenging for the critical care nurse. Hemodynamic instability can result from hemorrhage and hypovolemic shock, leading to fluid volume deficit, decreased cardiac output, and decreased tissue perfusion. A massive transfusion protocol may be implemented to restore blood volume and correct coagulopathies. A crucial nursing responsibility is to monitor the patient's response to medical therapies. Continued hemodynamic instability (e.g., hypotension, decreased cardiac output) despite aggressive medical intervention may indicate continued hemorrhage, in which case an exploratory laparotomy may be required to determine and correct the source of bleeding. The patient's postoperative course may be complicated by coagulopathy, acidosis, and hypothermia. Jaundice may occur as a sign of liver dysfunction, but it may also be caused by reabsorption of hematomas or breakdown of transfused red blood cells.

Spleen Injuries. The spleen is the organ most commonly injured by blunt abdominal trauma and is second to the liver as a source of life-threatening hemorrhage. Spleen injuries, like liver injuries, are graded for the purpose of determining the amount of trauma sustained, the care needed, and the possible outcomes (Table 34-11). Hemodynamically stable patients may be monitored in the critical care unit by means of serial hematocrit values and vital signs. Progressive deterioration may indicate the need for operative management.[39]

Patients who exhibit hemodynamic instability require operative intervention with urgent laparotomy.[40] Patients who have had a splenectomy are at risk for the development of overwhelming postsplenectomy sepsis with streptococcal pneumonia. These patients require the polyvalent pneumococcal vaccine (Pneumovax) to help promote immunity against most pneumococcal bacteria. Patients with isolated spleen injuries that require surgical intervention rarely are admitted to the critical care unit. Complications after splenic trauma include wound infection, sepsis, subdiaphragmatic abscess, and fistulas of the colon, pancreas, and stomach.

TABLE 34-11   SPLEEN INJURY SCALE

GRADE*		INJURY DESCRIPTION
I	Hematoma	Subcapsular, <10% surface area
	Laceration	Capsular tear, <1 cm, parenchymal depth
II	Hematoma	Subcapsular, 10%-50% surface area; intraparenchymal <5 cm in diameter
	Laceration	Capsular tear: 1-3 cm parenchymal depth, which does not involve a trabecular vessel
III	Hematoma	Subcapsular, >50% surface area or expanding; ruptured subcapsular or parenchymal hematoma; intraparenchymal hematoma >5 cm or expanding
IV	Laceration	>3 cm parenchymal depth or involving trabecular vessels
	Laceration	Laceration involving segmental or hilar vessels producing major devascularization (>25% of spleen)
V	Laceration	Completely shattered spleen
	Vascular	Hilar vascular injury that devascularizes spleen

*Advance one grade for multiple injuries up to grade II.

Hollow Viscus Injuries. The term *hollow viscus* refers to the hollow organs in the abdomen, such as the stomach, small intestine, and large intestine. Hollow viscus injuries (HVI) can result from blunt or penetrating trauma. The diagnosis of HVI is challenging, as injuries may not show up on CT or ultrasound. A delay in the time to diagnosis contributes to complications.[41] One study demonstrated that serial measurements of the white blood cell (WBC) count can help determine the presence of absence of HVI. Regardless of the mechanism of injury, intestinal contents (e.g., bile, stool, enzymes, bacteria) can leak into the peritoneum and cause peritonitis. Surgical resection and repair is almost always required. The patient's postoperative course is dictated by the amount of spillage of intestinal contents. The patient is observed for signs of sepsis and for abscess or fistula formation.

Genitourinary Injuries

Trauma to the genitourinary tract seldom occurs as an isolated injury. A genitourinary injury must be suspected in any patient with penetrating trauma to the torso; pelvic fracture; blunt trauma to the lower chest or flank; contusions, hematoma, tenderness over the flank, lower abdomen, or perineum; genital swelling or discoloration; blood at the urethral meatus; hematuria after Foley catheter placement; or difficulty with micturition.[9]

Mechanism of Injury

Genitourinary injuries, like all other traumatic injuries, can result from blunt or penetrating trauma. In one study, approximately 5% of patients with pelvic fractures had concomitant genitourinary injury, with men experiencing genitourinary trauma more frequently than women.[42]

Assessment

Evaluation of genitourinary trauma begins after the primary survey has been conducted and immediate life-threatening conditions have been effectively managed. The conscious patient may complain of flank pain or colic pain. Rebound tenderness can be elicited if intraperitoneal extravasation of urine has occurred. Inspection may reveal blood at the urethral meatus. Bluish discoloration of the flanks may indicate retroperitoneal bleeding, whereas perineal discoloration may indicate a pelvic fracture and possible bladder or urethral injury. Hematuria is the most common assessment finding with genitourinary trauma; however, the absence of gross or microscopic hematuria does not exclude a urinary tract injury.[9]

Specific Genitourinary Injuries

Kidney Trauma. The kidney is most often injured by blunt trauma, resulting in contusions or lacerations without urinary extravasation. Injury to the kidneys may be reflected by flank ecchymosis and fracture of inferior ribs or spinous processes. Gross or microscopic hematuria may be present; however, the extent of kidney damage is often incongruous with the degree of hematuria.[43] Gross hematuria can exist with minor injuries and usually clears within a few hours. CT is the most accurate modality available for diagnosing kidney injury because it can assess the extent of parenchymal laceration, urine extravasation, surrounding hemorrhage, and the presence of vascular injury.[43]

Contusions and minor lacerations can usually be treated with observation. The success of nonoperative management may be enhanced by using angiographic embolization. Nonoperative treatment of patients with major lacerations and vascular injuries may be achieved in those who are hemodynamically stable.[44] Operative interventions may be performed in patients with kidney injuries with a devascularized segment of the kidney. Postoperative and postinjury complications can include infection, hemorrhage, infarction, extravasation, calcification, acute kidney injury, and hypertension.

Bladder Trauma. A large percentage of bladder injuries result from pelvic fractures.[42] Physical findings may include lower abdominal bruising, distention, and pain. More definitive findings include difficulty in voiding or incomplete recovery of irrigation fluids from catheterized patients.[43] Bladder injuries are classified as contusions, extraperitoneal ruptures, intraperitoneal ruptures, or combined injuries. The type of injury depends on the location and strength of the blunt force and volume of urine in the bladder at the time of injury. Extraperitoneal rupture of the bladder may be managed conservatively with catheterization and antibiotics for 7 to 10 days.[44] Unresolved extravasation may require surgical intervention.

Nursing Management

Nursing diagnoses that can be applicable in caring for a patient with genitourinary trauma include Risk for Gastrointestinal Perfusion, Risk for Infection, and Deficient Fluid Volume.

After the patient is admitted to the critical care unit, the nurse makes an assessment according to the ATLS guidelines. After the patient's condition has stabilized, nursing management of postoperative kidney trauma is similar to that for genitourinary surgery. The primary nursing interventions include assessment for hemorrhage, maintenance of fluid and electrolyte balance, and maintenance of patency of drains and tubes. Measurement of urinary output includes drainage from the urinary catheter and the nephrostomy or suprapubic tubes. Drainage from these areas is recorded separately. Urine output is measured frequently until bloody drainage and clots have cleared. Gentle irrigation of drainage tubes may be required to clear clots and maintain the patency of the tubes.

Pelvic Fractures

The pelvis is a ring-shaped structure composed of the hip bones, sacrum, and coccyx. Because the pelvis protects the lower urinary tract and major blood vessels and nerves of the lower extremities, pelvic trauma can result in life-threatening hemorrhage and in urologic and neurologic dysfunction. The mortality rate from pelvic trauma ranges from 8% to 40%,[45,46] mostly due to hemorrhagic shock. The volume of blood contained within the pelvis can be compared to volume of a cylinder (similarly shaped to the pelvis) wherein:

$$Volume = \pi \times (radius)^2 \times height$$

Note that the radius plays a large role in determining volume requirements. When the pelvic ring is disrupted, the radius increases, thereby increasing blood volume capacity. There is also loss of the tamponade effect of the retroperitoneal tissues and intrapelvic organs, contributing to further bleeding.[47] Because the pelvic area is a highly vascular compartment already, it can sequester a large volume of blood; death within 24 hours of injury is most often due to hemorrhagic shock.[45]

Mechanism of Injury

Blunt trauma to the pelvis can be caused by MVCs, falls, or a crushing injury. Motorcycle and car crashes have the highest incidence of pelvic fractures. One study found that the biomechanical factors associated with pelvic fractures included no airbag deployment, a smaller vehicle, and lateral deformation location (front vs. rear).[45] Pelvic injuries may be associated with damage to underlying vessels, both arterial and venous.

Assessment

Signs of pelvic fracture include perianal ecchymosis (scrotum or vulva), indicating extravasation of urine or blood, pain on palpation or "rocking" of the iliac crests, lower limb paresis or hypesthesia, hematuria. Lower extremity rotation or leg shortening is also cause for suspicion of a pelvic injury. Patients with a suspected pelvic injury should have a rectal examination to assess for SCI or presence of occult or obvious rectal bleeding.

The diagnosis of pelvic fracture is made by an anteroposterior pelvic radiograph with the patient in the supine position and/or CT scan of the pelvis.[47] Additional radiographs may be required for definitive treatment, but the timing depends on the patient's hemodynamic stability.

Classification of Pelvic Fractures

Pelvic fractures constitute a spectrum of complexity ranging from a single nondisplaced fracture of a pubic ramus to a life-threatening condition in which there are multiple fractures and crush injuries associated with significant hemorrhage and internal injuries.

Lateral Compression Pelvic Injury. Lateral compression (LC) force produces a shortening of the pelvic diameter and typically does not involve ligamentous injury. Although this type of fracture is forgiving to the pelvic ring vessels, localized bleeding may occur, particularly to the posterior pelvis. LC fractures are classified according to severity of injury:

- **Type I LC injury** includes the posterior compression of the sacroiliac joint without ligament disruption or an oblique pubic ramus fracture.
- **Type II LC injury** includes rupture of the posterior sacroiliac ligament or internal rotation of the hemipelvis with a crush injury of the sacrum and an oblique pubic ramus fracture.
- **Type III LC injury** includes the findings of type II LC injury with additional evidence of anteroposterior (AP) compression to the contralateral hemipelvis.

Anteroposterior Compression Pelvic Injury. When force is applied in the AP direction, the pelvic diameter widens. In this case, the injury can be completely ligamentous, which manifests as an open sacroiliac joint or open pubic symphysis. This type of injury is commonly associated with vascular injury. AP compression fractures are classified according to severity of injury:

- **Type I AP injury** includes disruption of the pubic symphysis with less than 2.5 cm of diastasis and with insignificant posterior pelvic involvement.

- **Type II AP injury** includes the disruption of the pubic symphysis of more than 2.5 cm with tearing of associated ligaments.
- **Type III AP injury** is a complete disruption of the pubic symphysis, posterior ligament complexes, and hemipelvic involvement.

Vertical Shear. A vertical shear pelvic injury includes a complete disruption of a hemipelvis associated with a hemipelvic displacement. This type of injury typically occurs in people who fall from a great height and land on one extremity.

Open Fractures. Open pelvic fractures involve an open wound with direct communication between the site of the fracture and a laceration involving the vagina, rectum, or perineum. The mortality rate for these injuries is high, because unlike closed pelvic fractures that bleed into the peritoneum, open pelvic fractures result in external exsanguinations.

Medical Management

The priority of the medical management of pelvic fractures is to prevent or to control life-threatening hemorrhage. Current level 1 guidelines suggest that patients with pelvic fractures and hemodynamic instability or signs of ongoing bleeding after nonpelvic sources of blood loss have been ruled out should be considered for pelvic angiography with contrast, and embolization. Additionally, it is a level 1 guideline that patients who have evidence of arterial extravasation by pelvic CT scan may require angiography and embolization independent of hemodynamic status.[47]

Temporary pelvic binders (TPB) may be applied to help reduce the pelvic ring size and limit the extent of bleeding.[47] These binders may indeed limit hemorrhage, however, improvement in mortality has not been demonstrated.[47] Application of TPBs may be accomplished by wrapping the pelvis with a sheet or commercially available binder between the greater trochanter and the iliac crests. Advantages of this technique are that it is quick, does not involve specialized training, allows continued access to the patient during the resuscitation, and does not require specialized equipment. External pelvic fixation (EPF) with screws and rods placed externally may also be used.[47]

Patients who are hemodynamically stable and have stable closed pelvic fractures may be treated conservatively with ongoing monitoring of vital signs and collaboration with the surgeons for progressive mobility and physical therapy. Definitive management of pelvic fracture may be done with internal screws, nails, and/or plates.

Nursing Management

Initial assessment of the patient with a pelvic fracture in the critical care unit proceeds according to ATLS guidelines.

Massive blood loss contributes to alterations in tissue perfusion. On admission to the critical care unit, the patient may have hemodynamic instability with abnormal coagulation factors. Interventions include intravenously administered blood products and fluids, recognizing that a massive transfusion protocol (MTP) may need to be initiated. The nurse must ensure that an appropriate amount of blood, plasma, and platelets remains cross-matched and available if needed.

The patient is at high risk for injury caused by neurovascular compromise, development of abdominal compartment syndrome, fat embolism syndrome, and wound infection. These syndromes are discussed further later in this chapter. Before the patient is moved, the nurse should know whether the physician has classified the closed pelvic fracture as *stable* or *unstable*. A stable pelvic injury implies that no further pathologic displacement of the pelvis can occur with turning or moving. An unstable pelvic fracture means that further pathologic displacement of the pelvis can occur with turning or moving.

Routine nursing assessments include neurovascular assessments of the lower extremities. Neurologic injury as a result of pelvic fracture may be transient and temporary. Open pelvic fractures may necessitate complex, time-consuming dressing changes. Aggressive pain management strategies should be employed during these dressing changes, because they can be quite painful.

Patients with open pelvic fractures may have a prolonged critical care course with various degrees of complications. The patient with pelvic fractures is at risk for infection because of associated injuries and internal or external fixation devices. Nursing management of external fixation insertion sites is directed at preventing infection. Most institutions have protocols for pin care that require strict compliance.

COMPLICATIONS OF TRAUMA

Deaths from trauma have been historically described as occurring in a trimodal distribution of trauma deaths, meaning that there are three peaks of mortality.[48] The first occurring in the minutes following the event, the second in the subsequent hours and the third peak of death occurring in the critical care unit as a result of complications days to weeks after the initial injury.[49] Due to phenomenal improvements in how complications are prevented in the critical care phase, deaths from trauma are now described in a bimodal distribution, meaning that there are two peaks of mortality occurring in the minutes and hours following trauma.[50] Ongoing nursing assessments are imperative for early detection of complications associated with traumatic injuries. A single complication can increase hospital length of stay and the associated costs of treating the complication.

Hypermetabolism

Nutritional support is an essential component in the care of critically ill trauma patients. Within 24 to 48 hours after traumatic injury, a predictable hypermetabolic response occurs. The metabolic response to injury mobilizes amino acids and accelerates protein synthesis to support wound healing and the immunologic response to invading organisms. Stress hypermetabolism occurs after any major injury and is characterized by increases in metabolic rate and oxygen consumption. Energy requirements accelerate to promote immune function and tissue repair. The goal of early aggressive nutrition is to maintain host defenses by supporting this hypermetabolism and to preserve lean body mass.[51]

Most nutrition experts advocate beginning enteral nutrition as early as possible. Current guidelines recommend enteral feedings be initiated within 72 hours for patients with blunt and penetrating abdominal injuries and those with severe head injuries.[51] Enteral feeding sites can include the gastric route or any site beyond the pylorus of the stomach, including the duodenum and jejunum. Prompt feeding tube placement by the critical care nurse must be a priority, unless contraindicated. Diminished or absent bowel sounds do not mean the small bowel is not working. Small bowel function and the ability to absorb nutrients remain intact, despite the presence of gastroparesis and absent bowel sounds. Because access to the stomach can be obtained more quickly and easily than the duodenum, early gastric feeding is possible.[51] Patients at risk for pulmonary aspiration due to gastric retention or gastroesophageal reflux should receive enteral feedings into the jejunum.[51] If enteral feeding is not successful, parenteral nutrition should be initiated by day 7.[51]

Infection

Infection remains a major source of mortality and morbidity in critical care units. The trauma patient is at risk for infection because of contaminated wounds, invasive therapeutic and diagnostic catheters, intubation and mechanical ventilation, host susceptibility, and the critical care environment. Nursing management must include interventions to decrease and eliminate the trauma patient's risk of infection. The patient with multiple trauma is at risk for infection because of host susceptibility (including pre-existing medical conditions) and the adverse effect of trauma on the immune system.

Wound contamination poses an infection risk for the trauma patient, especially with injuries resulting from deep or penetrating trauma. Exogenous bacteria (from the external environment) can enter through open wounds. Exogenous bacteria can be introduced by dirt, grass, and debris inoculated into the wound at the time of injury, or they can be introduced by personnel during wound care. Endogenous bacteria (from the internal environment) can be released as a result of gastrointestinal or genitourinary perforation, which spills bacteria into the internal environment.

Meticulous wound care is essential. The goals of wound care include minimizing infection risks, removing dead and devitalized tissue, allowing for wound drainage, and promoting wound epithelialization and contraction. Wound healing also is accomplished through interventions that promote tissue perfusion of well-oxygenated blood and that ensure adequate nutritional support for wound healing.

Standard interventions for the prevention of ventilator-associated pneumonia, catheter-associated urinary tract infections, and central–line-associated bloodstream infection apply to the trauma patient. Proper hand hygiene, invasive catheter care, prompt removal of unnecessary tubes and lines, patient positioning, and medical asepsis or sterile technique for all invasive procedures are paramount to optimal to patient outcome.

Sepsis

The patient with multiple injuries is at risk for overwhelming infections and sepsis. The source of sepsis in the trauma patient can be invasive therapeutic and diagnostic catheters or wound contamination with exogenous or endogenous bacteria. The source of the septic nidus must be promptly evaluated. Gram stain and cultures of blood, urine, sputum, invasive catheters, and wounds are obtained (see Chapter 35).

Pulmonary Complications
Respiratory Failure

Post-traumatic respiratory failure is often due to the development of ARDS.[52] ARDS can be caused by direct injury to the lungs or indirect injury (see "Acute Respiratory Distress Syndrome" in Chapter 20).[52] Primary direct injuries in the trauma patient can include aspiration, inhalation, and pulmonary contusion.[50] The indirect injuries include sepsis, massive transfusion, fat emboli, and missed injury. ARDS in the trauma patient can develop 24 to 72 hours after initial injury. The patient receiving multiple blood products, particularly fresh-frozen plasma, must also be monitored for *transfusion-related acute lung injury* (TRALI). Signs of TRALI are similar to those of ARDS, although there is a temporal relationship between the new onset of respiratory distress and the transfusion of blood products.[53]

Fat Embolism Syndrome

Fat embolism syndrome can occur as a complication of orthopedic trauma. The clinical onset of fat embolism syndrome ranges from 12 to 72 hours after injury.[54] Fat embolism syndrome appears to develop as a result of fat droplets that leak from fractured bone and embolize to the lungs. The droplets are broken down into free fatty acids that are toxic to the pulmonary microvascular membranes. Pulmonary fat emboli alter pulmonary hemodynamics and pulmonary vascular permeability. The lung becomes highly edematous and hemorrhagic. The clinical presentation is almost indistinguishable from that of ARDS. Early stabilization of unstable extremity fractures may limit the seeding of fat droplets into the pulmonary system.[54]

Pain

Pain may come from many sources, including surgery, procedures, and trauma. Trauma may contribute to cellular death and inflammation that leads to pain. Relief of pain is a major component in the care of trauma patients.

An issue that often complicates pain management is the high incidence of substance abuse among patients who sustain traumatic injury. Trauma patients, regardless of substance use history require multimodal acute pain management (see Chapters 9 and 10).

Kidney Complications
Acute Kidney Injury

Assessment and ongoing monitoring of kidney function is critical to the survival of the trauma patient. The cause of post-traumatic acute kidney injury is complex and may involve a variety of factors, as listed in Box 34-14.

Prevention of kidney failure is the best treatment, and it begins with ensuring adequate volume to provide adequate renal artery perfusion. Serial assessments of blood urea nitrogen (BUN) and creatinine levels commonly are used to

---

BOX 34-14 ETIOLOGIC FACTORS IN POST-TRAUMATIC ACUTE KIDNEY INJURY

- Pre-existing disease
  - Hypertension
  - Heart failure
  - Diabetes
  - Chronic kidney disease
  - Chronic liver disease
- Prolonged shock states
- Profound acidosis
- SIRS or reperfusion injury
- Abdominal compartment syndrome
- Muscle ischemia; myoglobinuria
- Microemboli
- Nephrotoxic medications
- Radiocontrast dye

SIRS, Systemic inflammatory response syndrome.

---

evaluate kidney function. Progressive kidney failure requires prompt diagnosis and treatment (see "Acute Kidney Injury" in Chapter 27).

Rhabdomyolysis and Myoglobinuria

Patients with a crush injury are susceptible to the development of rhabdomyolysis, with subsequent secondary kidney failure. Crush injuries can compromise blood flow. Loss of arterial blood flow, particularly to the extremities, results in the loss of oxygen transport to distal tissues and ischemia. This initiates a cascade of events that leads to the necrosis of skeletal muscle cells. As cells die, intracellular contents—particularly potassium and myoglobin—are released. Myoglobin, a muscular pigment, is a large molecule that gets lodged in the glomerulus, resulting in presence of myoglobinuria. Circulating myoglobin can lead to the development of kidney failure by three mechanisms: decreased renal perfusion, cast formation with tubular obstruction, and direct toxic effects of myoglobin in the kidney tubules.[55]

Dark tea-colored urine suggests myoglobinuria. Testing for myoglobin in the urine can be done, but may take several days, depending on laboratory resources available for this test. The most rapid screening test is a serum creatine kinase level. Urine output and serial creatine kinase levels should be monitored.

Rhabdomyolysis should be suspected in all patients who experience crush injuries wherein blood flow to the muscle is interrupted for a prolonged amount of time. Prevention of kidney dysfunction is paramount through the administration of IV fluids.[55] If rhabdomyolysis is diagnosed, treatment is aimed at prevention of subsequent kidney failure. Aggressive administration of intravenous fluids increases renal blood flow and decreases the concentration of nephrotoxic pigments.[55] Alkalinization of the urine and administration of diuretics have been studied, but their roles in the prevention or management of rhabdomyolysis are not firmly established.[55] Nursing management is directed toward achievement of fluid and electrolyte

balance. The patient should be assessed for hypernatremia, hyperosmolarity, acute kidney injury, and volume status.

Vascular Complications
Compartment Syndrome

Compartment syndrome is a condition in which increased pressure within a limited space compromises circulation, resulting in ischemia and necrosis of tissues within that space. Among those at high risk for the development of compartment syndrome are patients with lower extremity trauma, including fractures, penetrating trauma, vascular ruptures, massive tissue injuries, or venous obstruction. Clinical manifestations of compartment syndrome include obvious swelling and tightness of an extremity, paresis, and pain of the affected extremity. Diminished pulses and decreased capillary refill do not reliably identify compartment syndrome because they may be intact until after irreversible changes have occurred. Elevated intracompartmental pressures confirm the diagnosis. The treatment can consist of simple interventions, such as removing an occlusive dressing, to more complex interventions, including a fasciotomy.

Venous Thromboembolism

Despite improvements in the care of the trauma patient, venous thromboembolism (VTE), which includes both DVT and pulmonary emboli, remains an important cause of morbidity and mortality in the multiply injured trauma patient. Major trauma patients are at very high risk for VTE.[56] The factors that form the basis of VTE pathophysiology are blood stasis, injury to the intimal surface of the vessel, and hypercoagulopathy. Trauma patients are at risk for VTE because of endothelial injury, coagulopathy, and immobility.

Trauma patients are at the greatest risk for developing thromboembolism early in their hospitalization. Prevention is key. Routine thromboprophylaxis for the high-risk trauma patient includes use of low–molecular-weight heparin starting as soon as it is considered safe to do so and use of a mechanical method of prophylaxis, such as sequential compression devices.[56] For patients in whom the lower leg is inaccessible, foot pumps may act as an effective alternative to lower the rate of VTE.

Missed Injury

Nursing assessment of the multiply injured patient in the critical care unit may reveal missed diseases or missed injuries. Missed injuries have a reported incidence of 1.3% to 39% and are a cause of morbidity and mortality.[57] Missed disorders may include pre-existing undiagnosed medical illnesses such as endocrine disorders (diabetes, hypothyroidism), myocardial infarction, hypertension, decreased respiratory reserve, undiagnosed kidney failure, or malnutrition. Patients who have head injuries with a GCS of 8 or less and greater injury severity scores are more likely to have missed injuries or delayed diagnoses.[57]

Occasionally, injuries may not be diagnosed in the precritical care phases. Missed injuries are commonly discovered in the first 24 to 48 hours of the hospital stay during the routine

---

BOX 34-15 FACTORS CONTRIBUTING TO MISSED INJURIES

Hemodynamic Instability
- Shock states in the emergency department
- Aggressive resuscitation
- Emergent surgery taking precedence over thorough secondary surveys

Alterations in Consciousness
- Presence of drugs or alcohol intoxication confuses physical assessments and masks physical findings.
- Disoriented patients are challenging to assess.
- Agitation makes diagnostic testing challenging.
- Patients with altered consciousness cannot provide a history of the injury.

BOX 34-16 RISK FACTORS FOR FALLS IN OLDER ADULTS

Acute Illness
- Cerebrovascular accidents
- Dysrhythmias
- Syncope
- Diabetes

Cognitive Impairment
- Dementia

Neuromuscular Disorders
- Arthritis
- Lower extremity weakness
- Unstable gait

Medications
- Antidepressants
- Benzodiazepines
- Diuretics
- Phenothiazines

---

assessments of the trauma tertiary survey. Injuries are missed for a variety of reasons as summarized in Box 34-15. In the critical care unit, a missed injury may be suspected if the patient fails to show appropriate response to medical or surgical intervention. Change in the character of drainage from wounds or catheters may represent biliary or duodenal injuries. Hypotension and a falling hematocrit level despite aggressive fluid administration may indicate an expanding hematoma. As the patient begins to mobilize, small bone fractures and sprains may manifest. The critical care nurse must be alert to the possibility of a missed injury, especially when the patient does not appear to be responding appropriately to interventions. The physician must be notified immediately because potential complications of infection and hemorrhage may be life-threatening. Nurses play a key role in identifying missed injuries, particularly when patients regain consciousness and begin to increase their activity.

Multiple Organ Dysfunction Syndrome

MODS is a clinical syndrome of progressive dysfunction of organ systems. Trauma patients are at high risk for systemic inflammatory response syndrome (SIRS) and MODS. Organ dysfunction can be the result of primary MODS, which is caused by direct traumatic injury, as may occur with acute lung dysfunction because of pulmonary contusion. Organ dysfunction that occurs later in the trauma patient's critical care course, secondary MODS, results from uncontrolled systemic inflammation with resultant organ dysfunction. Trauma patients may experience primary and secondary MODS. Treatment is aimed at controlling or eliminating the source of inflammation, maintenance of oxygen delivery and consumption, and nutritional and metabolic support for individual organs (see Chapter 35).

SPECIAL CONSIDERATIONS

Meeting the Needs of Family Members and Significant Others

The impact of traumatic injury can be devastating for patients and for family members and significant others. They are faced with a crisis situation for which they have had little time to prepare. Trauma can precipitate a crisis within the family. Families may exhibit physical and sociocultural reactions and a combination of emotional reactions, including anger, fear, powerlessness, confusion, and mistrust. Recovery from traumatic injury can be long and frustrating for families. There may be many peaks and valleys of good days and bad days. During this time, the family may exhaust its social and financial support systems. Nurses should recognize this and facilitate supportive relationships for families.

A trend has evolved to move away from a paternalistic model of care to one that incorporates the family into all aspects of care, including resuscitation. Family members wish to remain close to their loved ones during these times, and there has been demonstrated benefit to the patient and the family in this model of care delivery.[58] One study demonstrated that family members present during trauma resuscitation suffered no ill psychologic effects and scored equivalent to those family members who were not present on anxiety, satisfaction, and well-being measures.[58] Regardless of the specific system of care delivery, the nurse ensures the family is supported during all aspects of care.

A valuable intervention is to bring families of trauma patients together in support groups. Trauma family support groups can offer sharing of experiences, expression of emotions, mutual support, sharing of coping strategies, and education about hospital and community services.

Trauma in the Older Patient

Trauma affects people of all ages. Older patients are predisposed to traumatic injuries because of the inevitable consequences of aging. The ability to react to or avoid environmental hazards is impaired because of age-related deterioration of the senses and changes in motor strength, postural stability, balance, and coordination (see Chapter 9).

Older persons experience most of the falls that result in injuries, and these falls are likely to occur from level surfaces or steps.[59] Factors that predispose older persons to falls are summarized in Box 34-16. Because many of the falls may be caused by an underlying medical condition (e.g., syncope, myocardial

BOX 34-17   FACTORS THAT PREDISPOSE OLDER ADULTS TO MOTOR VEHICLE CRASHES

- Alterations in visual and auditory acuity
- Deterioration in strength and slower reaction times
- Diminution of cerebral skills
- Diminution of motor skills
- Exacerbation of acute or chronic medical conditions
- Medications that may interfere with safe driving

infarction, dysrhythmias), management of the older patient who has fallen must include an evaluation of events and conditions immediately preceding the fall.

The exposure of older adults to MVC trauma is a consequence of the increasing growth of the older population and the growing number of older drivers and occupants of motor vehicles. Factors that predispose older adults to MVCs are summarized in Box 34-17. Many deaths of older individuals occur in crosswalks. Physiologic deterioration of cerebral and motor skills and alterations in visual and auditory acuity cause older pedestrians to walk directly into the path of oncoming vehicles.

Trauma in older adults can be associated with higher mortality rates, even when the injuries are less severe. Older adults have a higher complication rate and a higher mortality rate, starting at age 65 years, because of pre-existing medical conditions, decreased physiologic reserves, and decreased ability to compensate for severe injury.[60] Older patients who do survive traumatic injury are often faced with changes in their preinjury functional status. Relatively minor trauma can be the event that changes the lifestyle of an older person from one of relative independence to one that requires prolonged rehabilitation or skilled nursing care. Discharge planning early in the patient's hospitalization is necessary.

The concept of *limited physiologic reserve* in the older trauma patient highlights the key difference between the average younger trauma patient with normal physiologic reserve and the older patient with underlying physiologic derangements. Age-related changes that occur in virtually every organ system may not produce evidence of organ dysfunction in the resting state. However, the ability of organs to augment function in response to traumatic stress may be greatly compromised. Fluid resuscitation is an integral part of trauma resuscitation. Patients on chronic diuretic therapy may require more volume and potassium supplementation as a result of chronic volume and potassium depletion. The assessment and management of hypovolemic shock is more complex in the older trauma patient. Older adults have limited ability to increase their heart rate in response to blood loss, obscuring one of the earliest signs of hypovolemia—tachycardia.[9] Loss of physiologic reserve and the presence of pre-existing medical conditions are likely to produce further conflicting hemodynamic data. The older patient's lack of physiologic reserve makes it imperative that early nutritional support is initiated.

Many older adults take daily anticoagulants and/or antiplatelet medications to prevent thrombotic or embolic complications from preexisting medical conditions. Traumatic injury in conjunction with a prolonged International Normalized Ratio (INR) greatly increases the risk of major hemorrhage. It is essential that systemic anticoagulation be corrected as soon as possible after admission, and when head injury is suspected, a CT of the head is urgently obtained.[60]

Trauma protocols are well established for the management of young patients after injury. Clinicians increasingly are recognizing that these protocols must be individualized for the older trauma patient. The best outcomes for this patient population have been achieved through early, appropriate, aggressive trauma care, with admission to a trauma center with resources and protocols to provide excellent care to injured adults regardless of age.[60]

BOX 34-18   CASE STUDY

Patient with Trauma

Brief Patient History

Mr. G is a 21-year-old man. He was traveling in the back of a pickup truck that collided with another vehicle. He was ejected onto the side of the road and now is not awake and is barely breathing. He was intubated by emergency services, placed in a collar, and immobilized.

Clinical Assessment

Mr. G is admitted to the emergency department with minimal signs of external injury except for some small abrasions to the side of his face.

Diagnostic Procedures

Admission CT scan shows a large subdural hematoma.
  Radiography confirms appropriate placement of the endotracheal tube.
  Baseline vital signs are blood pressure (BP) 110/60, heart rate (HR) 108 (sinus tachycardia), respiratory rate (RR) 30, temperature (T) 98.3° F, O_2 saturation 88%, Glasgow Coma Scale 7.

Medical Diagnosis

Mr. G is diagnosed with subdural hematoma secondary to trauma.

Questions

1. What major outcomes do you expect to achieve for this patient?
2. What problems or risks must be managed to achieve these outcomes?
3. What interventions must be initiated to monitor, prevent, manage, or eliminate the problems and risks identified above?
4. What interventions should be initiated to promote optimal functioning, safety, and well-being of the patient?
5. What possible learning needs would you anticipate for this patient?
6. What cultural and age-related factors might have a bearing on the patient's plan of care?

SUMMARY

- Trauma is costly in lives lost and in dollars.
- Traumatic injuries may be caused by blunt or penetrating mechanisms.

Phases of Trauma Care

- Assessment of the trauma patient is performed in a systematic fashion, moving from the brief primary survey to the head-to-toe secondary survey to the very detailed tertiary survey.
- Resuscitation of the trauma patient involves hemostasis to control hemorrhage, goal-directed volume support to restore cellular oxygenation, maintenance of normothermia, and prevention and correction of acidosis and coagulopathy.

Specific Trauma Injuries

- Management of severe TBIs and SCIs focuses on the prevention of secondary injury by ensuring that healthy tissue remains intact through maintaining oxygen delivery to the brain and spinal cord.
- Airway compromise is a major focus of care for the patient who has sustained maxillofacial injuries.
- Rib fractures are a cause of morbidity and mortality and require that care be balanced between pain relief and respiratory sufficiency through the use of multimodal pain management.
- Pelvic fractures may result in tremendous volume loss, and the nurse must remain alert to the possibility of hemorrhagic shock.
- Complication prevention involves early enteral nutrition, DVT prophylaxis, and prevention of infection.

REFERENCES

1. Centers for Disease Control and Prevention. Preventing violence against women: program activities guide. http://www.cdc.gov/violenceprevention/pdf/IPV-SV_Program_Activities_Guide-a.pdf. Accessed November 2012.
2. Wu V, Huff H, Bhandari M. Pattern of physical injury associated with intimate partner violence in women presenting to the emergency department: A systematic review and meta-analysis. *Trauma, Violence, Abuse.* 2010;11(2):71.
3. The Joint Commission: Provision of Care Standards. https://e-dition.jcrinc.com/MainContent.aspx. Accessed November 26, 2012.
4. The Family Violence Prevention Fund. National Consensus Guidelines on Identifying and Responding to Domestic Violence Victimization in Healthcare Settings. http://www.futureswithoutviolence.org/section/our_work/health/_health_material/_jcaho Accessed November 2012.
5. US Dept of Transportation, National Highway Traffic Safety Administration (NHTSA). Traffic safety facts 2010: Alcohol-Impaired Driving, http://www-nrd.nhtsa.dot.gov/Pubs/811606.pdf. Accessed November 2012.
6. Centers for Disease Control and Prevention. Impaired Driving: Get the Facts. http://www.cdc.gov/motorvehiclesafety/impaired_driving/impaired-drv_factsheet.html. Accessed November 2012.
7. Committee on Trauma, American College of Surgeons. *Resources for Optimal Care of the Injured Patient.* Chicago: American College of Surgeons; 2006.
8. Neumann T, et al. Does the alcohol use disorders identification test–consumption identify the same patient population as the full 10-item Alcohol Use Disorders Identification Test? *J Subst Abuse Treat.* 2012;43:80.
9. American College of Surgeons. *Advanced Trauma Life Support.* 8th ed. Chicago: American College of Surgeons; 2008.
10. Hodgman EI, et al. Base deficit as a marker of survival after traumatic injury: consistent across changing patient populations and resuscitation paradigms. *J Trauma.* 2012;72(4):844.
11. Duchesne JC, et al. Damage control resuscitation: the new face of damage control. *J Trauma.* 2010;69(4):976.
12. Greera SE, et al. New developments in massive transfusion in trauma. *Curr Opin Anaesthesiol.* 2010;23:246.
13. Centers for Disease Control and Prevention, National Center on Injury Prevention and Control. Traumatic brain injury. http://www.cdc.gov/ncipc/tbi/TBI.htm. Accessed November 2012.
14. Centers for Disease Control and Prevention, National Center on Injury Prevention and Control. Traumatic brain injury. http://www.cdc.gov/traumaticbraininjury/pdf/BlueBook_factsheet-a.pdf. Accessed November 2012.
15. Spiotta AM, et al. Brain tissue oxygen–directed management and outcome in patients with severe traumatic brain injury. *J Neurosurg.* 2010;113:571.
16. Timmons SD. Current trends in neurotrauma care. *Crit Care Med.* 2010;38(9):S431.
17. Cooper JD, et al. Decompressive craniectomy in diffuse traumatic brain injury. *N Engl J Med.* 2010;364:1493.
18. Brain Trauma Foundation. Guidelines for the management of severe traumatic brain injury. *J Neurotrauma.* 2007;24(suppl 1):1.
19. Schroeppel TJ, et al. Beta-adrenergic blockade and traumatic brain injury: protective? *J Trauma.* 2010;69:776.
20. Giacino JT, et al. Placebo-controlled trial of amantadine for severe traumatic brain injury. *N Engl J Med.* 2012;366:819.
21. National Spinal Cord Injury Statistical Center. Spinal cord injury facts and figures at a glance, 2012. https://www.nscisc.uab.edu/PublicDocuments/fact_figures_docs/Facts%202012%20Feb%20Final.pdf. Accessed November 2012.
22. Como JJ, et al. Practice management guidelines for identification of cervical spine injuries following trauma: update from the Eastern Association for the Surgery of Trauma practice management guidelines committee. *J Trauma.* 2009;67:651.
23. Botelho RV, et al. Effectiveness of methylprednisolone in acute spinal cord injury: a systematic review of randomized controlled trials. *Rev Assoc Med Bras.* 2010;56(6):729.
24. Consortium for Spinal Cord Medicine. Early acute management in adults with spinal cord injury: a clinical practice guideline for health-care professionals. *J Spinal Cord Med.* 2008;31(4):403.
25. Kiraly L, Schreiber M. Management of the crushed chest. *Crit Care Med.* 2010;38(9):S469.

26. Battle CE, Hutchings H, Evans PA. Risk factors that predict mortality in patients with blunt chest wall trauma: a systematic review and meta-analysis. *Injury.* 2012;43:8.

27. Simon B, et al. Management of pulmonary contusion and flail chest: an Eastern Association for the Surgery of Trauma practice management guideline. *J Trauma Acute Care Surg.* 2012;73(5, Suppl 4):S351.

28. Kishore GSB, et al. Traumatic diaphragmatic hernia: Tertiary centre experience. *Hernia.* 2010;14:159.

29. Mowery NT, et al. Practice management guidelines for management of hemothorax and occult pneumothorax. *J Trauma.* 2011;70(2):510.

30. Press GM, Miller S. Utility of the cardiac component of FAST in blunt trauma. *J Emerg Med.* 2013;44(1):9.

31. Bock JS, Benitez M. Blunt cardiac injury. *Cardiol Clin.* 2012;30:545.

32. Neschis DG, Scalea TM, Flinn WR, Griffith BP. Blunt aortic injury. *N Engl J Med.* 2008;359:1708.

33. Kwolek CJ, Blazick E. Current Management of traumatic thoracic aortic injury. *Semin Vasc Surg.* 2011;23:215.

34. Biffl WL, Moore EE. Management guidelines for penetrating abdominal trauma. *Curr Opin Crit Care.* 2010;16:609.

35. Soyuncu S, et al. Accuracy of physical and ultrasonographic examinations by emergency physicians for the early diagnosis of intraabdominal haemorrhage in blunt abdominal trauma. *Injury.* 2007;38(5):564.

36. Moore CL, Copel JA. Point-of-care ultrasonography. *N Engl J Med.* 2011;364(8):749.

37. Diaz JJ, et al. The management of the open abdomen in trauma and emergency general surgery: Part 1—Damage control. *J Trauma.* 2010;68(6):1425.

38. De Waele JJ, De Laet I, Kirkpatrick AW, Hoste E. Intra-abdominal hypertension and abdominal compartment syndrome. *Am J Kidney Dis.* 2010;57(1):159.

39. Kozar RA, McNutt MK. Management of adult blunt hepatic trauma. *Curr Opin Crit Care.* 2010;16:596.

40. Stassen NA, et al. Selective nonoperative management of blunt splenic injury: an Eastern Association for the Surgery of Trauma practice management guideline. *J Trauma Acute Care Surg.* 2012;73(5, Suppl 4):S294.

41. Schnüriger B, et al. Serial white blood cell counts in trauma: Do they predict a hollow viscus injury? *J Trauma.* 2010;69:302.

42. Bjurlin MA, Fantus RJ, Mellett MM, Goble SM. Genitourinary injuries in pelvic fracture morbidity and mortality using the National Trauma Data Bank. *J Trauma.* 2010;67:1033.

43. Snyder KA, Veronese V. Genitourinary injuries and renal management. In: McQuillan KA, et al, eds. *Trauma Nursing: from Resuscitation Through Rehabilitation.* 4th ed. Philadelphia: Saunders; 2009.

44. Eastern Association of Surgeons in Trauma. Practice management guidelines for the management of genitourinary trauma, 2004. Available at http://www.east.org/resources/treatment-guidelines/genitourinary-trauma-management-of Accessed November 2012.

45. Stein DM, et al. Risk factors associated with pelvic fractures sustained in motor vehicle collisions involving newer vehicles. *J Trauma.* 2006;61:21.

46. Eckroth-Bernard K, Davis JW. Management of pelvic fractures. *Curr Opin Crit Care.* 2010;16:582.

47. Cullinane DC, et al. Eastern Association for the Surgery of Trauma Practice management guidelines for hemorrhage in pelvic fracture: update and systematic review. *J Trauma.* 2011;71:1850.

48. Cowley RA. The resuscitation and stabilization of major multiple trauma patients in a trauma center environment. *Clin Med.* 1976;83:16.

49. Trunkey DD. Trauma. *Sci Am.* 1983;249:28.

50. Gunst M, et al. Changing epidemiology of trauma deaths leads to a bimodal distribution. *Proc (Bayl Univ Med Cent).* 2010;23(4):349.

51. Eastern Association of Surgeons in Trauma. Practice management guidelines for nutritional support of the trauma patient, 2004. http://www.east.org/resources/treatment-guidelines/nutritional-support-in-trauma-patients. Accessed November 2012.

52. Chirag SV, et al. The impact of development of acute lung injury on hospital mortality in critically ill trauma patients. *Crit Care Med.* 2008;36:2309.

53. Alexander V, et al. Risk factors and outcome of transfusion-related acute lung injury in the critically ill: a nested case-control study. *Crit Care Med.* 2010;38(3):771.

54. Sara S, et al. Fat emboli syndrome in a nondisplaced tibia fracture. *J Orthop Trauma.* 2011;25(2):e27.

55. Bosch X, Poch E, Grau JM. Rhabdomyolysis and acute kidney injury. *N Engl J Med.* 2009;361:62.

56. Muntz JE, Michota FA. Prevention and management of venous thromboembolism in the surgical patient: options by surgery type and individual patient risk factors. *Am J Surg.* 2010;199:S11.

57. Pfeifer R, Pape HC. Missed injuries in trauma patients: a literature review. *Patient Saf Surg.* 2011;2:20.

58. Pasquale MA, et al. Family presence during trauma resuscitation: ready for primetime? *J Trauma.* 2010;69(5):1092.

59. Konstantinos S, et al. Ground level falls are associated with significant mortality in elderly patients. *J Trauma.* 2010;69(4):821.

60. Calland JF, et al. Evaluation and management of geriatric trauma: an Eastern Association for the Surgery of Trauma practice management guideline. *J Trauma Acute Care Surg.* 2012;73(5, Suppl 4):S345.

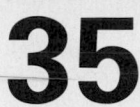

Shock, Sepsis, and Multiple Organ Dysfunction Syndrome

Beverly Carlson, Lorraine Fitzsimmons

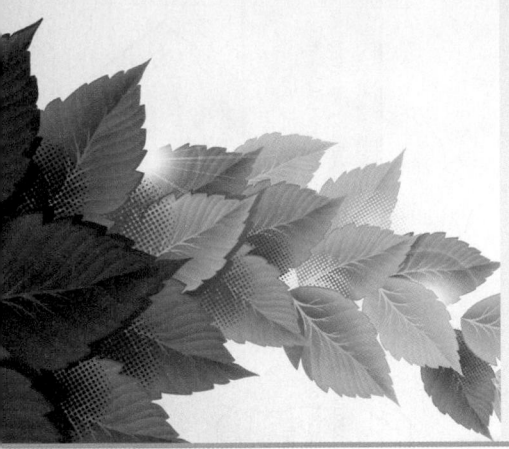

evolve WEBSITE

http://evolve.elsevier.com/Urden/criticalcare/

Evolve features:
- NCLEX Review Questions
- CCRN Review Questions
- PCCN Review Questions
- Mosby's Nursing Skills Procedures
- Animations
- Video Clips
- Glossary

Shock is an acute, widespread process of impaired tissue perfusion that results in cellular, metabolic, and hemodynamic alterations. Ineffective tissue perfusion occurs when an imbalance develops between cellular oxygen supply and cellular oxygen demand. This imbalance can occur for a variety of reasons and eventually results in cellular dysfunction and death. This chapter presents an overview of the general shock response, or shock syndrome, followed by a discussion of the various shock states. Information is also provided regarding the pathogenesis and clinical management of systemic inflammatory response (SIRS) and multiple organ dysfunction syndrome (MODS).

SHOCK SYNDROME

Description

Shock is a complex pathophysiologic process that often results in MODS and death. All types of shock involve ineffective tissue perfusion and acute circulatory failure. The shock syndrome is a pathway involving a variety of pathologic processes that may be categorized as four stages: initial, compensatory, progressive, and refractory. Progression through each stage varies with the patient's prior condition, duration of initiating event, response to therapy, and correction of underlying cause (Fig. 35-1).

Etiology

Shock can be classified as hypovolemic, cardiogenic, or distributive, depending on the pathophysiologic cause and hemodynamic profile. Hypovolemic shock results from a loss of circulating or intravascular volume. Cardiogenic shock results from the impaired ability of the heart to pump. Distributive shock results from maldistribution of circulating blood volume and can be further classified as septic, anaphylactic, or neurogenic. Septic shock is the result of microorganisms entering the body. Anaphylactic shock is the result of a severe antibody–antigen reaction. Neurogenic shock is the result of the loss of sympathetic tone.

Pathophysiology

During the initial stage, cardiac output (CO) is decreased, and tissue perfusion is threatened. Almost immediately, the compensatory stage begins as the body's homeostatic mechanisms attempt to maintain CO, blood pressure, and tissue perfusion. The compensatory mechanisms are mediated by the sympathetic nervous system (SNS) and consist of neural, hormonal, and chemical responses. The neural response includes an increase in heart rate and contractility, arterial and venous vasoconstriction, and shunting of blood to the vital organs. Hormonal compensation includes activation of the renin response and stimulation of the anterior pituitary and adrenal medulla. Activation of the renin response results in the production of angiotensin II, which causes vasoconstriction and the release of aldosterone and antidiuretic hormone (ADH), leading to sodium and water retention. Stimulation of the anterior pituitary results in the secretion of adrenocorticotropic hormone (ACTH), which stimulates the adrenal cortex to produce glucocorticoids, causing a rise in blood glucose levels. Stimulation of the adrenal medulla causes the release of epinephrine and norepinephrine, which further enhance the compensatory mechanisms.

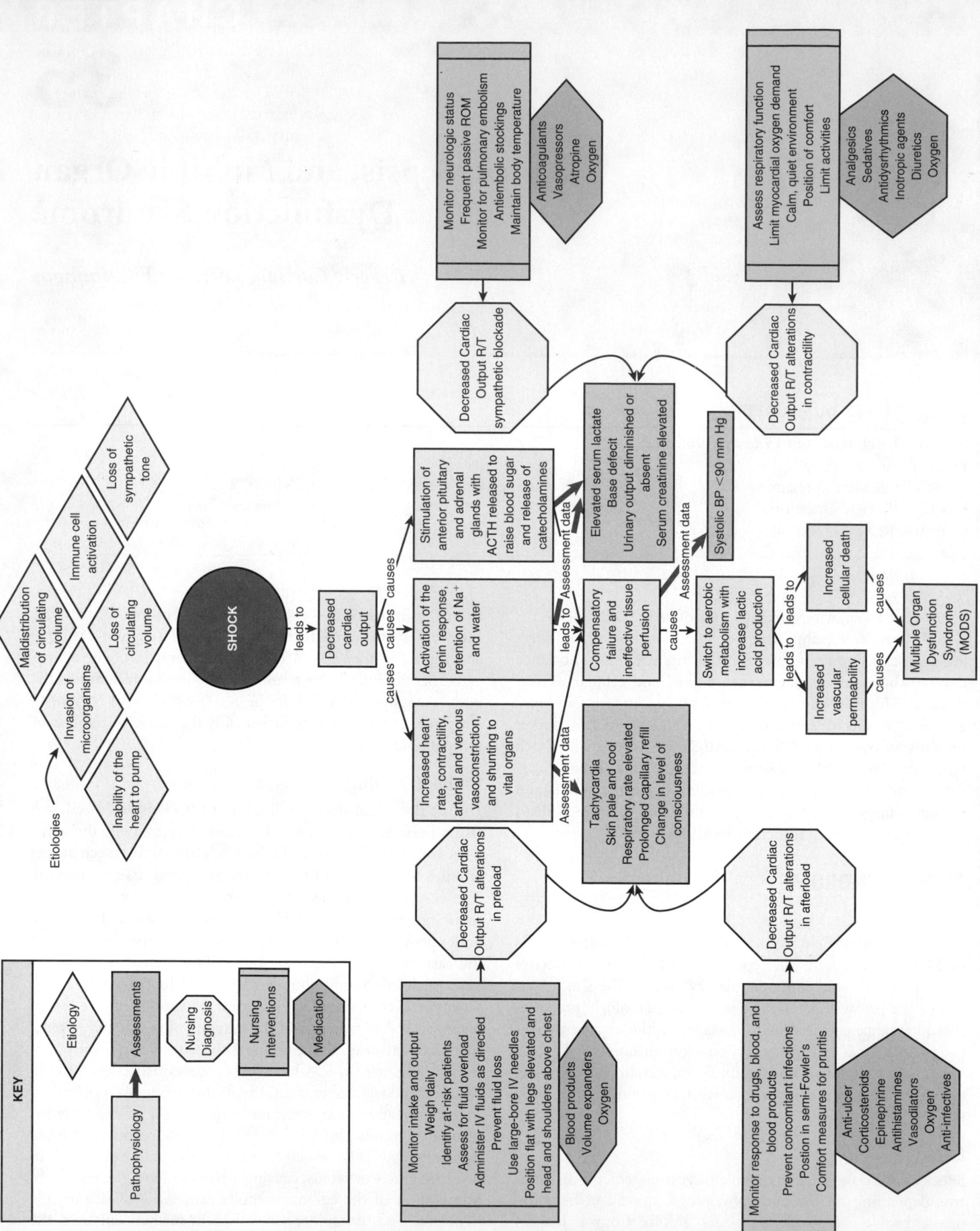

FIGURE 35-1   Concept Map for Shock. (Concept map illustration created by Elaine Bishop)

During the progressive stage, the compensatory mechanisms begin failing to meet tissue metabolic needs, and the shock cycle is perpetuated. As tissue perfusion becomes ineffective, the cells switch from aerobic to anaerobic metabolism to produce energy. Anaerobic metabolism produces small amounts of energy but large amounts of lactic acid, producing lactic acidemia. Vasodilation and increased vascular permeability from endothelial and epithelial hypoxia and inflammatory mediators results in intravascular hypovolemia, tissue edema, and further decline in tissue perfusion.[1-3] A systemic release of inflammatory mediators in response to tissue hypoxia, especially in gut tissue, produces microcirculatory impairment and derangement of cellular metabolism, facilitating progression of the shock cycle.[1-4] The patient is experiencing systemic inflammatory response syndrome (SIRS), and irreversible damage begins to occur. Some cells die as a result of apoptosis, an injury-activated, preprogrammed cellular suicide. Others die as the sodium–potassium pump in the cell membrane fails, causing the cell and its organelles to swell. Cellular energy production comes to a complete halt as the mitochondria swell and rupture. At this point, the problem becomes one of oxygen use instead of oxygen delivery. Even if the cell were to receive more oxygen, it would be unable to use it because of damage to the mitochondria. The cell's digestive organelles swell and leak destructive enzymes into the cell, accelerating cell death.[4]

Every system in the body is affected by this process (Box 35-1). Cardiac dysfunction develops as a result of the release of myocardial depressant cytokines.[1-3] Ventricular failure eventually occurs, further perpetuating the entire process. Central nervous system (CNS) dysfunction develops as a result of cerebral hypoperfusion, leading to failure of the SNS, cardiac and respiratory depression, and thermoregulatory failure. Endothelial injury from hypoxia and inflammatory cytokines and impaired blood flow result in microvascular thrombosis. Hematologic dysfunction occurs as a result of consumption of clotting factors, release of inflammatory cytokines, and dilutional thrombocytopenia. Disseminated intravascular coagulation (DIC) eventually may develop. Pulmonary dysfunction occurs as a result of increased pulmonary capillary membrane permeability, pulmonary microemboli, and pulmonary vasoconstriction. Ventilatory failure and acute respiratory distress syndrome (ARDS) develop. Renal dysfunction develops as a result of renal vasoconstriction and renal hypoperfusion, leading to acute kidney injury (AKI). Gastrointestinal dysfunction occurs as a result of splanchnic vasoconstriction and hypoperfusion and leads to failure of the gut organs. Disruption of the intestinal epithelium releases gram-negative bacteria into the system, which further perpetuates the entire shock syndrome.[5]

During the refractory stage, shock becomes unresponsive to therapy and is considered irreversible. As the individual organ systems die, MODS—defined as failure of two or more body systems—occurs. Death is the final outcome. Regardless of the etiologic factors, death occurs from ineffective tissue perfusion because of the failure of the circulation to meet the oxygen needs of the cell.[4]

Assessment and Diagnosis

The patient with a mean arterial blood pressure (MAP) less than 60 mm Hg or with evidence of global tissue hypoperfusion is considered to be in a shock state.[1,3] Because shock is a dynamic physiologic phenomenon, hypotension may occur late in the process or may normalize even when tissue perfusion is still inadequate.[6-9] Clinical manifestations vary according to the underlying cause of shock, the stage of the shock, and the patient's response to shock.

Compensatory mechanisms may produce normal hemodynamic values even when tissue perfusion is compromised.[3,5,8,10-11] Global indicators of systemic perfusion and oxygenation include serum lactate, arterial base deficit, serum bicarbonate, and central or mixed venous oxygen saturation levels. Inadequate cellular oxygenation with anaerobic metabolism and increased metabolic lactate production increase the serum lactate level.[8,12] The level and duration of this hyperlactatemia are predictive of morbidity and mortality,[7,10-12] and management guided by lactate levels has been effective in improving outcomes.[13-14] The base deficit derived from arterial blood gas (ABG) values also reflects global tissue acidosis and is useful to assess the severity of shock.[6,9-11] Studies have demonstrated serum bicarbonate to be an equivalent alternative to arterial base deficit in predicting mortality in surgical and trauma patients.[15-16] The use of mixed venous oxygen saturation (Svo_2) measured by means of a pulmonary artery catheter or central venous oxygen saturation ($Scvo_2$) measured with a central venous catheter allows assessment of the balance of oxygen delivery and oxygen consumption and the ratio of oxygen extraction.[3,17-19] After years of recommended use to guide the care of patients with severe sepsis, this measure of global oxygen balance is being evaluated for use in other critically ill populations.[17-21] Noninvasive indicators of regional tissue perfusion or oxygenation such as sublingual capnometry and subcutaneous or skeletal muscle tissue oxygen saturation (Sto_2) measured with near-infrared spectroscopy are also being evaluated.[3,8,19] The sections on different types of shock discuss clinical assessment and diagnosis of the patient in shock.

BOX 35-1   CONSEQUENCES OF SHOCK

Cardiovascular
- Ventricular failure
- Microvascular thrombosis

Neurologic
- Sympathetic nervous system dysfunction
- Cardiac and respiratory depression
- Thermoregulatory failure
- Coma

Pulmonary
- Acute lung failure (ALF)
- Acute respiratory distress syndrome (ARDS)

Renal
- Acute kidney injury (AKI)

Hematologic
- Disseminated intravascular coagulation (DIC)

Gastrointestinal
- Gastrointestinal tract failure
- Liver failure
- Pancreatic failure

Medical Management

The major focus of the treatment of shock is the improvement and preservation of tissue perfusion. Adequate tissue perfusion depends on an adequate supply of oxygen being transported to the tissues and the cell's ability to use it. Oxygen transport is influenced by pulmonary gas exchange, CO, and hemoglobin level. Oxygen use is influenced by the internal metabolic environment and mitochondrial function. Management of the patient in shock focuses on supporting oxygen delivery.[1,3]

Adequate pulmonary gas exchange is critical to oxygen transport. Establishing and maintaining an adequate airway are the first steps in ensuring adequate oxygenation. After the airway is patent, emphasis is placed on improving ventilation and oxygenation. Therapies include administration of supplemental oxygen and mechanical ventilatory support.

An adequate CO and hemoglobin level are crucial to oxygen transport. CO depends on heart rate, preload, afterload, and contractility. A variety of fluids and medications are used to manipulate these parameters. The types of fluids used include crystalloids and colloids. The categories of medications used include vasoconstrictors, vasodilators, positive inotropes, and antidysrhythmics.

Fluid administration is indicated for decreased preload related to intravascular volume depletion, and it can be accomplished by use of a crystalloid or colloid solution, or both. Crystalloids are balanced electrolyte solutions that may be hypotonic, isotonic, or hypertonic. Examples of crystalloid solutions used in shock situations are normal saline and lactated Ringer solution. Colloids are protein- or starch-containing solutions. Examples of colloid solutions are blood and blood components, such as albumin, and pharmaceutical plasma expanders, such as hetastarch, dextran, and mannitol.

The quantity and choice of fluid is a subject of debate and depends on the situation.[3,22-27] Excessive volume expansion, more than what increases preload and stroke volume (SV), worsens organ function and may produce coagulopathy, cytokine activation, and abdominal compartment syndrome.[3,24] Methods to measure preload responsiveness include respiratory or positional variation in pulse pressure, systolic pressure, and SV and are more accurate than central venous pressure (CVP).[3] Fluid resuscitation with normal saline or with albumin produces similar outcomes regardless of baseline serum albumin level.[26,28] Crystalloid solutions are inexpensive and effective. Advantages of colloids include faster restoration of intravascular volume and use of smaller amounts. Colloids are believed to stay in the intravascular space, unlike crystalloids, which readily leak into the extravascular space. Disadvantages include expense, allergic reactions, and difficulties in typing and cross-matching blood. Colloids also can leak out of damaged capillaries and cause a variety of additional problems, particularly in the lungs. Hypertonic or hyperoncotic fluids offer no additional benefit over isotonic crystalloids and are not recommended.[3,22,27,29-30]

Blood should be considered to augment oxygen transport if the patient's hemoglobin level is critically low, although what threshold value should be used is still undetermined.[3,5,31] Transfusion of stored red blood cells does not substantially increase oxygen consumption and has been associated with immunosuppression, infection, impairment of microcircula-

---

---

tory flow, increased pulmonary vascular resistance, coagulopathy, and increased mortality. Restrictive transfusion practice has demonstrated lower mortality.[3,5,17,31-32] Transfusion-related acute lung injury (TRALI) resulting from immune and nonimmune neutrophil activation has become the leading cause of transfusion-related death and may occur with transfusion of any plasma-containing blood or blood product.[32-35]

Vasoconstrictor agents are used to increase afterload by increasing the systemic vascular resistance (SVR) and improving the patient's blood pressure level. Vasodilator agents are used to decrease preload or afterload, or both, by decreasing venous return and SVR. Positive inotropic agents are used to increase contractility. Antidysrhythmic agents are used to influence heart rate. Box 35-2 provides examples of each of these agents.

Sodium bicarbonate is not recommended in the treatment of shock-related lactic acidosis.[17,36-37] No overall benefit has been found, and the risks associated with its use are significant. They include shifting of the oxyhemoglobin dissociation curve to the left, rebound increase in lactic acid production, development of hyperosmolar state, fluid overload resulting from excessive sodium, and rapid cellular electrolyte shifts.[36-37]

The critically ill patient should be started on enteral nutritional support therapy within 24 to 48 hours.[38] The type of nutritional supplementation initiated varies according to the cause of shock, and it should be tailored to the individual patient's needs, as indicated by the underlying condition, laboratory data, and treatment. When enteral feeding is contraindicated parental nutrition should be considered, though a delay of seven days is recommended for better outcomes.[38-41] Supplementation of enteral feeding with parenteral nutrition to increase caloric intake is a subject of debate but has not been shown to improve patient outcomes.[38,41-42] A delay of one week is recommended before consideration of this strategy.[38]

Glucose control to a target level of 140 to 180 mg/dL is recommended for all critically ill patients.[43-44] Benefits of glucose control in the critically ill include lower incidences of infection, renal failure, sepsis, and death.[43-46]

BOX 35-3   COLLABORATIVE MANAGEMENT

Shock

Support oxygen transport.
- Establish a patent airway.
- Initiate mechanical ventilation.
- Administer oxygen.
- Administer fluids (crystalloids, colloids, blood and other blood products).
- Administer vasoactive medications.
- Administer positive inotropic medications.
- Ensure sufficient hemoglobin and hematocrit.

Support oxygen use.
- Identify and correct cause of lactic acidosis.
- Ensure adequate organ and extremity perfusion.
- Initiate nutritional support therapy.

Identify underlying cause of shock and treat accordingly.
Provide comfort and emotional support.
Institute evidence-based practice protocols to prevent complications.
Assess response to therapy.
Prevent and maintain surveillance for complications.

Nursing Management

The nursing management of a patient in shock is a complex and challenging responsibility. It requires an in-depth understanding of the pathophysiology of the disease and the anticipated effects of each intervention, as well as a solid understanding of the nursing process. Later sections discuss specific interventions for the patient in shock.

The psychosocial needs of the patient and family dealing with shock are extremely important. These needs are based on situational, familial, and patient-centered variables. Nursing interventions for the psychosocial stress of critical illness include providing information on patient status, explaining procedures and routines, supporting the family, encouraging the expression of feelings, facilitating problem solving and shared decision making, individualizing visitation schedules, involving the family in the patient's care, and establishing contacts with necessary resources.[47] The consensus of all relevant professional organizations is that patients and families should be given the option of family presence during invasive procedures and resuscitation.[47-50]

Collaborative management of the patient with shock is outlined in Box 35-3.

HYPOVOLEMIC SHOCK

Description

Hypovolemic shock occurs from inadequate fluid volume in the intravascular space. The lack of adequate circulating volume leads to decreased tissue perfusion and initiation of the general shock response. Hypovolemic shock is the most commonly occurring form of shock (Fig. 35-2).

Etiology

Hypovolemic shock can result from absolute or relative hypovolemia. Absolute hypovolemia occurs when there is a loss of fluid from the intravascular space. This can result from an external loss of fluid from the body or from internal shifting of fluid from the intravascular space to the extravascular space. Fluid shifts can result from a loss of intravascular integrity, increased capillary membrane permeability, or decreased colloidal osmotic pressure. Relative hypovolemia occurs when vasodilation produces an increase in vascular capacitance relative to circulating volume (Box 35-4).

Pathophysiology

Hypovolemia results in a loss of circulating fluid volume. A decrease in circulating volume leads to a decrease in venous return, which results in a decrease in end-diastolic volume or preload. Preload is a major determinant of stroke volume (SV) and CO. A decrease in preload results in a decrease in SV and CO. The decrease in CO leads to inadequate cellular oxygen supply and ineffective tissue perfusion.

Assessment and Diagnosis

The clinical manifestations of hypovolemic shock depend on the severity of fluid loss and the patient's ability to compensate for it. Clinical classes developed by the American College of Surgeons to describe the levels of severity of hypovolemic shock in the trauma setting have been widely accepted, but a recent test of the validity of these classes suggests that modifications are necessary.[51] A simpler approach of classifying hypovolemic shock as mild, moderate, or severe is also commonly used. Class I, or mild shock, indicates a fluid volume loss up to 15% or an actual volume loss up to 750 mL. Compensatory mechanisms maintain CO, and the patient appears free of symptoms other than possibly slight anxiety.[1,5,51]

Class II hypovolemia occurs with a fluid volume loss of 15% to 30% or an actual volume loss of 750 to 1500 mL. As volume loss worsens, the patient moves from mild to moderate hypovolemic shock. Falling CO activates more intense compensatory responses. Anxiety increases.[1] The heart rate may increase to more than 100 beats/minute in response to increased SNS stimulation unless blocked by pre-existing beta-blocker therapy. The pulse pressure narrows as the diastolic blood pressure increases because of vasoconstriction. Postural hypotension develops.[1] The respiratory rate increases as blood loss worsens and ABG specimens drawn during this phase may reveal respiratory alkalosis, as evidenced by a low partial pressure of carbon dioxide ($Paco_2$). Urine output starts to decline to 20 to 30 mL/hour as renal perfusion decreases. The urine sodium level decreases, whereas urinary osmolality and specific gravity increase as the kidneys start to conserve sodium and water. The patient's skin becomes pale and cool with delayed capillary refill because of peripheral vasoconstriction. Jugular veins appear flat as a result of decreased venous return.[1,5]

Hypovolemic shock that is class III occurs with a fluid volume loss of 30% to 40% or an actual volume loss of 1500 to 2000 mL. This level of severity may produce the progressive stage of shock as compensatory mechanisms become overwhelmed and ineffective tissue perfusion develops. Blood pressure decreases, but often after tissue hypoperfusion is already significant.[6,9] The heart rate may increase to more than 120 beats/minute, and dysrhythmias may develop as

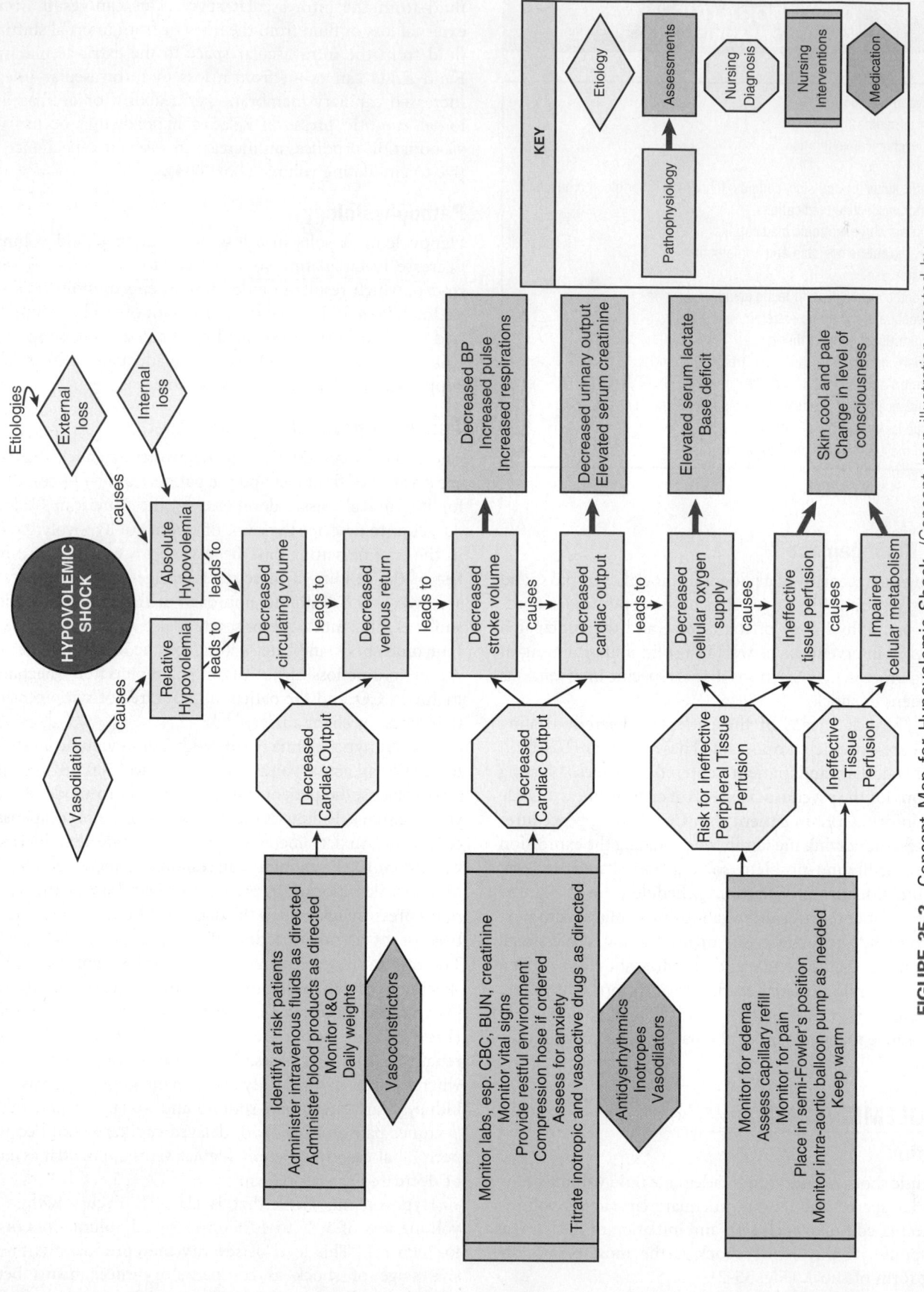

FIGURE 35-2 Concept Map for Hypovolemic Shock. (Concept map illustration created by Elaine Bishop Kennedy, EdD, RN.)

BOX 35-4 ETIOLOGIC FACTORS IN HYPOVOLEMIC SHOCK

Absolute Factors
- Loss of whole blood
  - Trauma or surgery
  - Gastrointestinal bleeding
- Loss of plasma
  - Thermal injuries
  - Large lesions
- Loss of other body fluids
  - Severe vomiting or diarrhea
  - Massive diuresis
  - Loss of intravascular integrity
  - Ruptured spleen
  - Long bone or pelvic fractures
  - Hemorrhagic pancreatitis
  - Hemothorax or hemoperitoneum
  - Arterial dissection or rupture

Relative Factors
- Vasodilation
  - SIRS/sepsis
  - Anaphylaxis
  - Loss of sympathetic stimulation
- Increased capillary membrane permeability
  - SIRS/sepsis
  - Anaphylaxis
  - Thermal injuries
- Decreased colloidal osmotic pressure
  - Severe sodium depletion
  - Hypopituitarism
  - Cirrhosis
  - Intestinal obstruction

◉ BOX 35-5 NURSING DIAGNOSES

Hypovolemic Shock

- Deficient Fluid Volume related to active blood loss, p. 1132
- Deficient Fluid Volume related to interstitial fluid shift, p. 1132
- Decreased Cardiac Output related to alterations in preload, p. 1128
- Imbalanced Nutrition: Less Than Body Requirements related to increased metabolic demands or lack of exogenous nutrients, p. 1143
- Risk for Infection, p. 1160
- Anxiety related to threat to biologic, psychologic, and/or social integrity, p. 1125
- Compromised Family Coping related to a critically ill family member, p. 1127

---

myocardial ischemia ensues. During this phase serum lactate levels increase and ABG values reveal metabolic acidosis evidenced by a low bicarbonate (HCO_3^-) and elevated base deficit. Decreased renal perfusion results in the development of oliguria. Blood urea nitrogen (BUN) and serum creatinine levels start to rise as the kidneys begin to fail. The patient's skin becomes ashen, cold, and clammy, with marked delayed capillary refill. The patient may appear confused as cerebral perfusion decreases.[1,5,51]

Class IV hypovolemic shock is severe shock and usually refractory in nature. It occurs with a fluid volume loss of greater than 40% or an actual volume loss of more than 2000 mL. As the compensatory mechanisms of the body become insufficient, tachycardia and hemodynamic instability worsen and hypotension ensues. Severe lactic acidosis is present. Peripheral pulses and capillary refill become absent because of marked peripheral vasoconstriction. The skin may appear cyanotic, mottled, and extremely diaphoretic. Organ failure occurs. Urine output ceases. The patient may be confused and agitated, eventually becoming unresponsive. Various clinical manifestations associated with failure of the different body systems will develop.[1,5]

Assessment of the hemodynamic parameters of a patient in hypovolemic shock varies by stage but commonly reveals a decreased CO and cardiac index (CI). Loss of circulating volume leads to a decrease in venous return to the heart, which results in a decrease in the preload of the right and left ventricles. This is evidenced by a decline in the CVP or right atrial pressure (RAP) and pulmonary artery occlusion pressure (PAOP). Vasoconstriction of the arterial system results in an increase in the afterload of the heart, as evidenced by an increase in the SVR. This vasoconstriction may produce inaccurate systolic and diastolic blood pressure values when measured by arterial catheter or noninvasive oscillometry. MAP is more accurate in this low-flow state.[18]

Medical Management

The major goals of therapy for the patient in hypovolemic shock are to correct the cause of the hypovolemia, restore tissue perfusion, and prevent complications. This approach includes identifying and stopping the source of fluid loss and administering fluid to replace circulating volume. Fluid administration can be accomplished with use of a crystalloid solution, a colloid solution, blood products, or a combination of fluids. The type of solution used depends on the type of fluid lost, the degree of hypovolemia, the severity of hypoperfusion, and the cause of hypovolemia.

Aggressive fluid resuscitation in trauma and surgical patients is the subject of great debate. The benefit of limited or hypotensive (systolic blood pressure 60 to 80 mm Hg or MAP 40 to 60 mm Hg) volume resuscitation in patients with uncontrolled hemorrhage is postulated to lessen bleeding and improve survival[22,52-54] and has been demonstrated in the preliminary results of a randomized controlled trial.[53] The type and amount of solutions used for fluid resuscitation and the rate of administration influence immune function, inflammatory mediator release, coagulation, and the incidence of cardiac, pulmonary, renal, and gastrointestinal complications.[3,22,24-25,27] Consensus on the optimal resuscitative strategy for hypovolemic shock is lacking and is likely situation specific.[18,22,24,52,54]

Nursing Management

Prevention of hypovolemic shock is one of the primary responsibilities of the nurse in the critical care area. Preventive measures include the identification of patients at risk and frequent assessment of the patient's fluid balance. Accurate monitoring of intake and output and daily weights are essential components of preventive nursing care. Early identification and treatment result in decreased mortality.

Management of the patient in hypovolemic shock requires continuous evaluation of intravascular volume, tissue perfusion, and response to therapy. The patient in hypovolemic shock may have any number of nursing diagnoses, depending on the progression of the process (Box 35-5). Nursing interventions include minimizing fluid loss, administering volume replacement, assessing response to therapy, providing comfort and emotional support, and preventing and maintaining surveillance for complications.

Measures to minimize fluid loss include limiting blood sampling, observing lines for accidental disconnection, and applying direct pressure to bleeding sites. Measures to facilitate the administration of volume replacement include insertion of large-bore peripheral intravenous catheters, rapid administration of prescribed fluids, and positioning the patient with the legs elevated, trunk flat, and head and shoulders above the chest. Monitoring the patient for clinical manifestations of fluid overload or complications related to fluid and blood product administration is essential for preventing further problems. It is also essential to monitor the patient for SIRS, which may occur for up to several days after resuscitation.[55]

CARDIOGENIC SHOCK

Description

Cardiogenic shock is the result of failure of the heart to effectively pump blood forward. It can occur with dysfunction of the right or the left ventricle, or both. The lack of adequate pumping function leads to decreased tissue perfusion and circulatory failure (Fig. 35-3). It occurs in approximately 5% to 8% of the patients with an ST-segment myocardial infarction (MI), and it is the leading cause of death of patients hospitalized with MI.[56-58] The mortality rate for cardiogenic shock has decreased with the advent of early revascularization therapy and is currently about 47% to 65%.[56-60]

Etiology

Cardiogenic shock can result from problems affecting the muscular function or the mechanical function of the heart or the cardiac rhythm.[57-59,61] The most common cause is acute MI resulting in the loss of 40% or more of the functional myocardium. It can occur with ST-elevation or non–ST-elevation MI.[57-59] The damage to the myocardium may occur after one massive MI (usually of the anterior wall), or it may be cumulative as a result of several smaller MIs or a small MI in a patient with pre-existing ventricular dysfunction.[56-57] Cardiomyopathy may cause cardiogenic shock as left ventricular function becomes unable to maintain adequate CO. Examples of problems affecting the mechanical function of the heart to fill and eject adequately include severe valvular disease; acute papillary muscle, chordal, or septal rupture; cardiac tamponade; and massive pulmonary embolus (Box 35-6).[57-59,61]

Pathophysiology

Cardiogenic shock results from the impaired ability of the ventricle to pump blood forward, which leads to a decrease in SV and an increase in the blood left in the ventricle at the end of systole. The decrease in SV results in a decrease in CO, which leads to decreased cellular oxygen supply and ineffective tissue perfusion. Typically, myocardial performance spirals downward as compensatory vasoconstriction increases myocardial afterload and low blood pressure worsens myocardial ischemia. As left ventricular contractility declines and ventricular compliance decreases, an increase in end-systolic volume results in blood backing up into the pulmonary system and the subsequent development of pulmonary edema. Pulmonary edema causes impaired gas exchange and decreased oxygenation of the arterial blood, which further impair tissue perfusion. In a substantial number of patients, the pathophysiology may follow a different course due to activation of inflammatory cytokines. A SIRS response results with systemic vasodilation and, possibly, normalization of the CO.[57-58,62] Whether this process contributes to the genesis or the outcome of cardiogenic shock is uncertain, but it is thought to be activated by acute MI and to facilitate development of sepsis.[57,62] Death due to cardiogenic shock results from cardiopulmonary collapse or multiple organ failure.[59]

Assessment and Diagnosis

A variety of clinical manifestations occur in the patient in cardiogenic shock, depending on etiologic factors, the patient's underlying medical status, and the severity of the shock state. Some clinical manifestations are caused by failure of the heart as a pump, whereas many are related to the overall shock response (Box 35-7).

Initially, clinical manifestations reflect the decline in CO. These signs and symptoms include systolic blood pressure less than 90 mm Hg or an acute drop in systolic or mean blood pressure of 30 mm Hg or more; decreased sensorium; cool, pale, moist skin; and urine output of less than 30 mL/hour.[57,59,63] The patient also may complain of chest pain. Tachycardia develops to compensate for the decrease in CO. A weak, thready pulse develops, and diminished S_1 and S_2 heart sounds may occur as a result of the decreased contractility. The respiratory rate increases to improve oxygenation. ABG values at this point indicate respiratory alkalosis, as evidenced by a decrease in $Paco_2$. Urinalysis findings demonstrate a decrease in urine sodium level and an increase in urine osmolality and specific gravity as the kidneys start to conserve sodium and water. Serum B-type natriuretic peptide (BNP) levels will likely be elevated.

As the left ventricle fails, auscultation of the lungs may disclose crackles and rhonchi, indicating the development of pulmonary edema. Hypoxemia occurs, as evidenced by a fall in Pao_2 and Sao_2 as measured by ABG values. Heart sounds may reveal an S_3 and S_4. Jugular venous distention is evident with right-sided failure. The patient also may experience dysrhythmias in response to tissue hypoxia, the underlying problem, and drug therapy.[58-59]

Assessment of the hemodynamic parameters of a patient in cardiogenic shock reveals a decreased CO with a CI less than 2.2 L/min/m² in the presence of an elevated PAOP of more than 15 mm Hg.[57,59,63] A proportional pulse pressure (systolic BP/pulse pressure) less than 25% is indicative of left ventricular failure and a CI less than 2.2 and may be useful when direct measurement of CI is unavailable.[64] Increased filling pressures are necessary to rule out hypovolemia as the cause of circulatory failure. The increase in PAOP reflects an increase in the left ventricular end-diastolic pressure (LVEDP) and left ventricular end-diastolic volume (LVEDV) resulting from decreased SV. With right ventricular failure, the RAP also increases. Compensatory vasoconstriction typically results in an increase in the afterload of the heart, as evidenced by an increase in the SVR, unless SIRS produces vasodilation and a normal or decreased SVR. Echocardiography confirms the diagnosis of cardiogenic shock, provides noninvasive estimates of PAOP and ejection fraction, and often clarifies etiologic factors.[57-59]

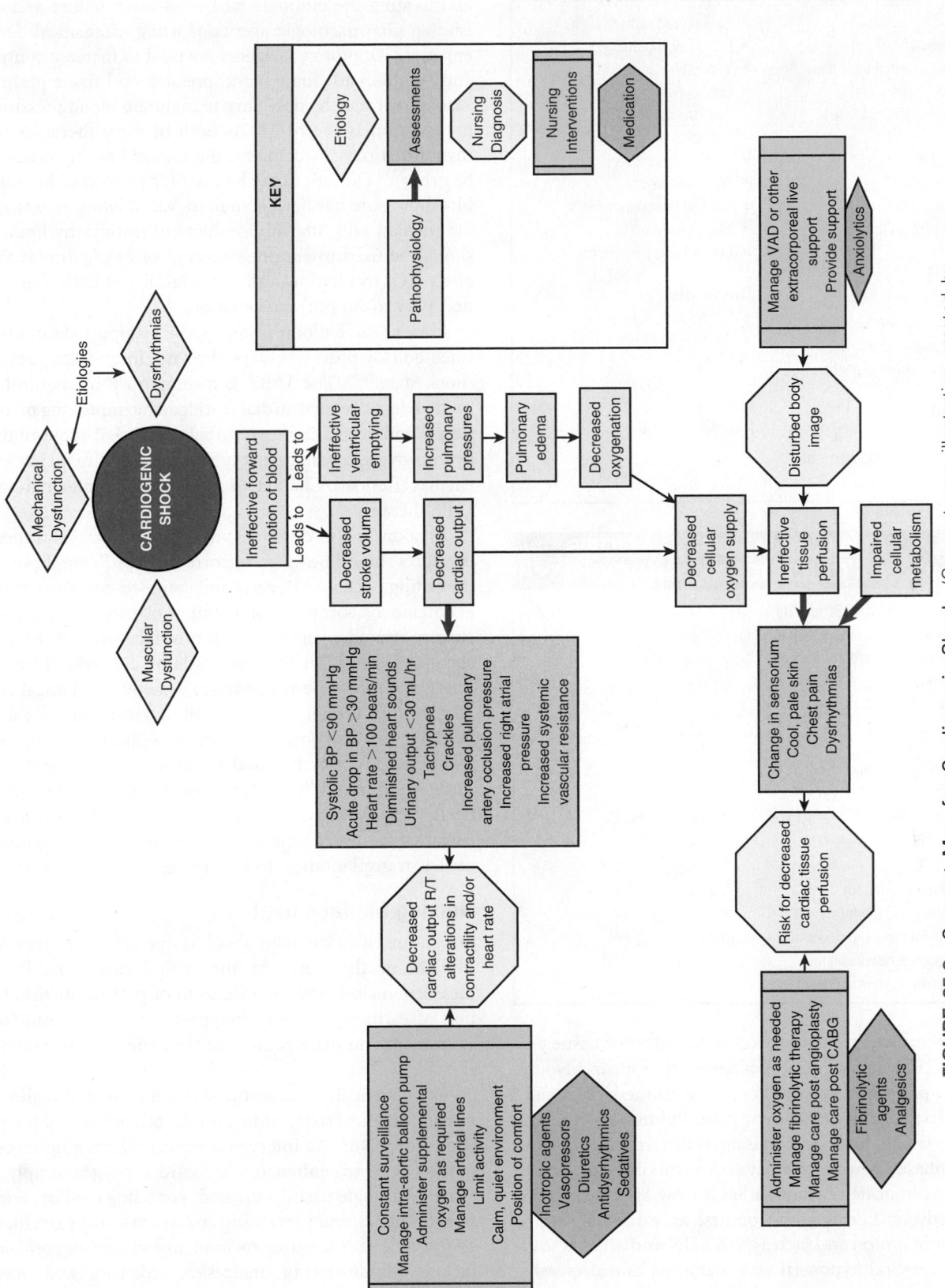

FIGURE 35-3 Concept Map for Cardiogenic Shock. (Concept map illustration created by Elaine Bishop Kennedy, EdD, RN.)

BOX 35-6 ETIOLOGIC FACTORS IN CARDIOGENIC SHOCK

Muscular
- Ischemic injury
  - Acute myocardial infarction
  - Cardiopulmonary arrest
- Acute decompensated heart failure
- Cardiomyopathy
- Acute myocarditis
- Myocardial contusion
- Prolonged cardiopulmonary bypass
- Septic shock
- Hemorrhagic shock
- Medications (beta-adrenergic blockers, calcium-channel antagonists, cytotoxic agents)

Mechanical
- Valvular dysfunction
- Papillary muscle dysfunction or rupture

- Septal wall rupture
- Free wall rupture
- Ventricular aneurysm
- Obstructive hypertrophic cardiomyopathy
- Intracardiac tumor
- Pulmonary embolus
- Atrial thrombus
- Cardiac tamponade
- Massive pulmonary embolus
- Constrictive pericarditis

Rhythmic
- Bradydysrhythmias
- Tachydysrhythmias

BOX 35-7 CLINICAL MANIFESTATIONS OF CARDIOGENIC SHOCK

- Systolic blood pressure <90 mm Hg
- Acute drop in blood pressure >30 mm Hg
- Heart rate >100 beats/min
- Weak, thready pulse
- Diminished heart sounds
- Change in sensorium
- Cool, pale, moist skin
- Urine output <30 mL/hr
- Chest pain
- Dysrhythmias
- Tachypnea
- Crackles
- Decreased cardiac output
- Cardiac index <2.2 L/min/m^2
- Increased pulmonary artery occlusion pressure
- Increased right atrial pressure
- Variable systemic vascular resistance

As compensatory mechanisms fail and ineffective tissue perfusion develops, other clinical manifestations appear. Myocardial ischemia progresses, as evidenced by continued increases in heart rate, dysrhythmias, and chest pain. Pulmonary function deteriorates, which leads to respiratory distress. ABG values during this phase reveal respiratory and metabolic acidosis and hypoxemia, as indicated by a high $Paco_2$, low HCO_3^-, and low Pao_2, respectively. Renal failure occurs, as exhibited by the development of anuria and increases in BUN and serum creatinine levels. Cerebral hypoperfusion manifests as a decreasing level of consciousness.

Medical Management

Treatment of the patient in cardiogenic shock requires an aggressive approach. The major goals of therapy are to treat the underlying cause, enhance the effectiveness of the pump, and improve tissue perfusion. This approach includes identifying and treating the etiologic factors of heart failure and administering pharmacologic agents or using mechanical devices to enhance CO. Inotropic agents are used to increase contractility and maintain adequate blood pressure and tissue perfusion. A vasopressor may be necessary to maintain blood pressure when hypotension is severe.[57-59] As both of these therapies increase myocardial oxygen demand, the lowest possible doses should be used.[57,59] Diuretics may be used for preload reduction. After blood pressure has been stabilized, vasodilating agents are used for preload and afterload reduction. Antidysrhythmic agents should be used to suppress or control dysrhythmias that can affect CO. Intubation and mechanical ventilation are usually necessary to support oxygenation.

Intra-aortic balloon pump (IABP) support should be instituted quickly if drug therapy does not immediately reverse the shock state.[57-58] The IABP is a temporary mechanical device used to decrease myocardial workload by improving myocardial supply and decreasing myocardial demand. It achieves this goal by improving coronary artery perfusion and reducing left ventricular afterload. Chapter 16 provides more information about IAPB therapy.

As soon as the cause of pump failure has been identified, measures should be taken to correct the problem if possible. In the setting of acute MI, early and complete revascularization by percutaneous coronary intervention or coronary artery bypass surgery provides significant survival benefit.[57-60] Fibrinolytic agents may be used in select patients. Procedural or surgical intervention may be necessary to remedy mechanical etiology. When conventional therapies fail, a ventricular assist device (VAD) or extracorporeal life support with a membrane oxygenator (ECMO) may be used to support the patient in acute cardiogenic shock.[57-59] These mechanical circulatory assist devices provide an external means to sustain effective organ perfusion, allowing time for the patient's ventricle to heal or for cardiac transplantation to take place.

Nursing Management

Prevention of cardiogenic shock is one of the primary responsibilities of the nurse in the critical care area. Preventive measures include the identification of patients at risk, facilitation of early reperfusion therapy for acute MI, and frequent assessment and management of the patient's cardiopulmonary status.

The patient in cardiogenic shock may have any number of nursing diagnoses, depending on the progression of the process (Box 35-8). Nursing interventions include limiting myocardial oxygen demand, enhancing myocardial oxygen supply, maintaining adequate tissue perfusion, providing comfort and emotional support, and preventing and maintaining surveillance for complications. Measures to limit myocardial oxygen demand include administering analgesics, sedatives, and agents to control afterload and dysrhythmias; positioning the patient for comfort; limiting activities; providing a calm and quiet environment and offering support to reduce anxiety; and teaching the patient about the condition. Measures to enhance myocardial oxygen supply include administering supplemental oxygen,

⊚ BOX 35-8 **NURSING DIAGNOSES**

Cardiogenic Shock

- Decreased Cardiac Output related to alterations in contractility, p. 1128
- Decreased Cardiac Output related to alterations in heart rate, p. 1128
- Imbalanced Nutrition: Less Than Body Requirements related to increased metabolic demands or lack of exogenous nutrients, p. 1143
- Risk for Infection, p. 1160
- Disturbed Body Image related to functional dependence on life-sustaining technology, p. 1136
- Compromised Family Coping related to a critically ill family member, p. 1127

monitoring the patient's respiratory status, administering prescribed medications, and managing device therapy.

Effective nursing management of cardiogenic shock requires precise monitoring and management of heart rate, preload, afterload, and contractility. This is accomplished through accurate measurement of hemodynamic variables and controlled administration of fluids and inotropic and vasoactive agents. Close assessment and management of respiratory function is also essential to maintain adequate oxygenation. Dysrhythmias are common and require immediate recognition and treatment.

Patients who require mechanical device therapy (IABP, LVAD, or ECMO) therapy need to be observed frequently for complications. Complications of cardiac mechanical assist devices may include infection, bleeding, thrombocytopenia, hemolysis, embolus, stroke, device malfunction, circulatory compromise of a cannulated extremity, SIRS, and sepsis.[63]

ANAPHYLACTIC SHOCK

Description

Anaphylactic shock, a type of distributive shock, is the result of an immediate hypersensitivity reaction. It is a life-threatening event that requires prompt intervention. The severe and systemic response leads to decreased tissue perfusion and initiation of the general shock response (Fig. 35-4).

Etiology

Anaphylaxis is a serious allergic reaction caused by an immunologic antibody–antigen response or nonimmunologic activation of mast cells and basophils.[65-69] A number of triggers have been identified that, when introduced by injection or ingestion or through the skin or respiratory tract, can cause a reaction. This list includes foods, food additives, diagnostic agents, biologic agents, environmental agents, medications, and venoms (Box 35-9).[67-69] Anaphylaxis can also be triggered by physical factors and can even be idiopathic in nature with no known trigger.[67-68] In the hospital environment, latex was once an extremely problematic antigen for patients and health care providers, but efforts to limit and prevent exposure have been highly successful.[68]

Immunologic anaphylactic reactions can be IgE-mediated or non–IgE-mediated responses. IgE is an antibody that is formed as part of the immune response. The first time an antigen enters the body, an antibody IgE, specific for the antigen, is formed. The antigen-specific IgE antibody is then stored by attachment to mast cells and basophils. This initial contact with the antigen is known as a *primary immune response*. The next time the antigen enters the body, the preformed IgE antibody reacts with it, and a secondary immune response occurs. This reaction triggers the release of biochemical mediators from the mast cells and basophils and initiates the cascade of events that precipitates anaphylactic shock.[66,68-69] Some immunologic anaphylactic reactions are non–IgE-mediated. These can be IgG mediated, occur as a result of direct activation of the mast cells, or be mediated by activation of the complement system.[68]

Nonimmunologic direct activation of the mast cells and basophils may occur with exercise or exposure to cold, heat, sunlight, ethanol, or medications. In some cases, multiple mechanisms contribute to the anaphylactic response.[68] The term *anaphylactoid reaction* was formerly used to denote all non–IgE-mediated reactions, but it is no longer recommended as there is no clinical distinction between the various mechanisms.[65,67-69]

Pathophysiology

Both immunologic and nonimmunologic activation of the mast cells and basophils result in the release of biochemical mediators. These mediators include histamine, tryptase, chymase, carboxypeptidase A3, platelet-activating factor (PAF), heparin, leukotrienes, prostaglandins, and cytokines such as IL-6, IL-33, and TNF-alpha, among others.[68-69] The activation of the biochemical mediators causes vasodilation; increased capillary permeability; laryngeal edema; bronchoconstriction; excessive mucus secretion; coronary vasoconstriction; inflammation; cutaneous reactions; and constriction of the smooth muscle in the intestinal wall, bladder, and uterus. Coronary vasoconstriction causes severe myocardial depression. Cutaneous reactions cause stimulation of nerve endings, followed by itching and pain.[68]

Peripheral vasodilation results in relative hypovolemia and decreased venous return. Increased capillary membrane permeability results in the loss of intravascular volume into the interstitial space, as much as 35% within 10 minutes, worsening the hypovolemic state.[67] Decreased venous return results in decreased end-diastolic volume and SV. The decline in SV leads to decreased CO and ineffective tissue perfusion. Death may result from airway obstruction or cardiovascular collapse, or both.[65-66,68,70]

Assessment and Diagnosis

Anaphylactic shock is a severe systemic reaction that can affect multiple organ systems. A variety of clinical manifestations occur in the patient in anaphylactic shock, depending on the extent of multisystem involvement. The symptoms usually start to appear within minutes of exposure to the antigen, but they may not occur for hours (Box 35-10).[65-66,68] Symptoms may also reappear after a 1- to 72-hour window of resolution in what is termed a biphasic *reaction.*[68,71-72] These late-phase reactions may be similar to the initial anaphylactic response, milder, or more severe.[72] In *protracted anaphylaxis*, symptoms may last up to 32 hours.[67]

The cutaneous effects may appear first and include pruritus, generalized erythema, urticaria, and angioedema. Commonly

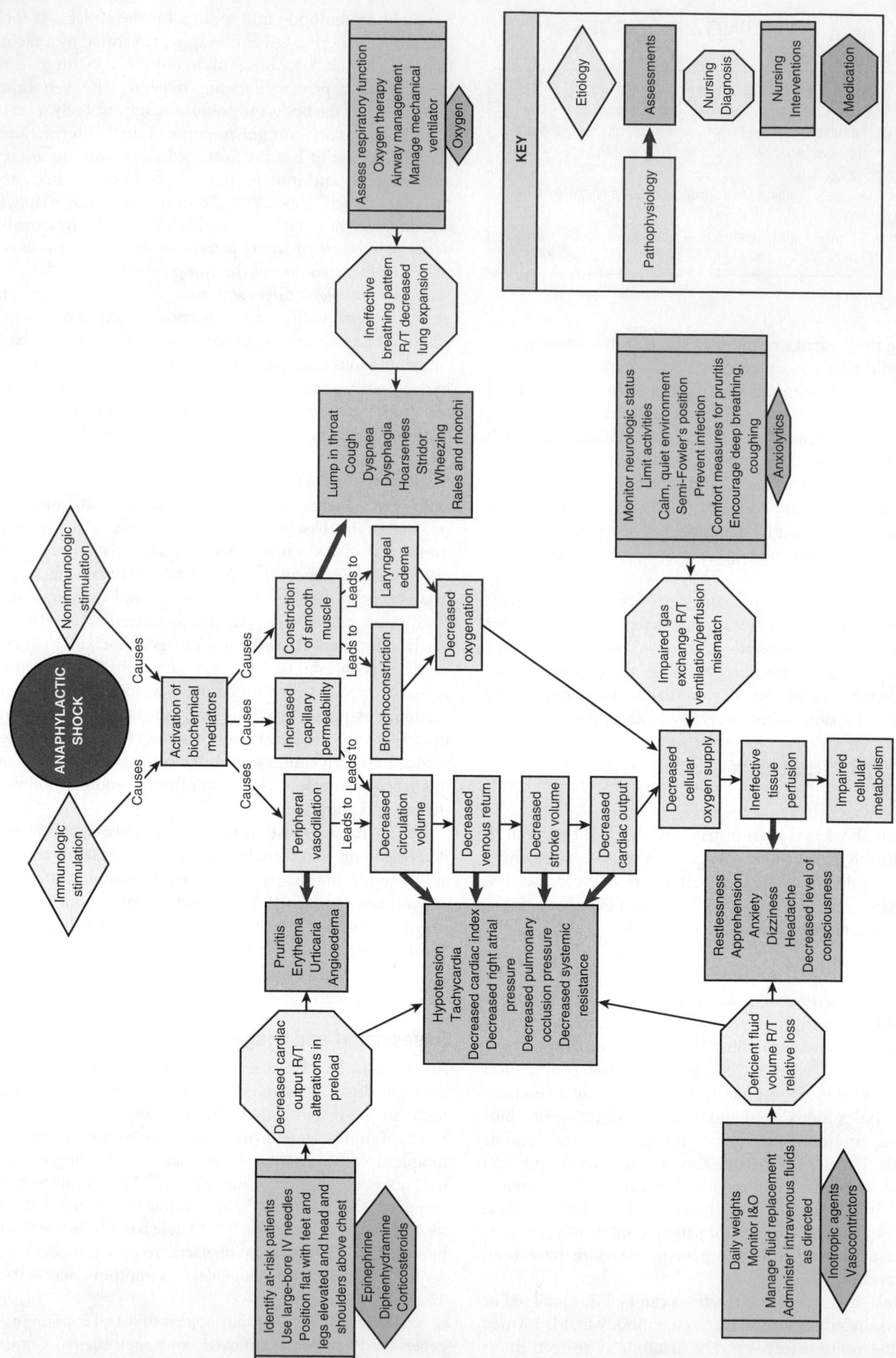

FIGURE 35-4 Concept Map for Anaphylactic Shock. (Concept map illustration created by Elaine Bishop Kennedy, EdD, RN.)

BOX 35-9 ETIOLOGIC FACTORS IN ANAPHYLACTIC SHOCK

Foods
- Eggs and milk
- Fish and shellfish
- Nuts and seeds
- Legumes and cereals
- Soy
- Wheat
- Strawberries
- Avocados
- Any

Food Additives
- Food coloring
- Preservatives

Diagnostic Agents
- Radiocontrast media
- Dehydrocholic acid (Decholin)
- Iopanoic acid (Telepaque)

Biologic Agents
- Blood and blood components
- Insulin and other hormones
- Gammaglobulin
- Seminal fluid
- Vaccines and antitoxins

Environmental Agents
- Pollens, molds, and spores
- Sunlight

- Cold or heat
- Animal dander
- Latex

Drugs
- Antibiotics
- Aspirin
- Nonsteroidal anti-inflammatory drugs
- Opioids
- Dextran
- Vitamins
- Muscle relaxants
- Neuromuscular blocking agents
- Barbiturates
- Nonbarbiturate hypnotics
- Protamine
- Infliximab (Remicade)
- Ethanol
- Other

Venoms
- Bees, hornets, yellow jackets, and wasps
- Snakes, jellyfish
- Deer flies
- Fire ants

Physical
- Exercise

BOX 35-10 CLINICAL MANIFESTATIONS OF ANAPHYLACTIC SHOCK

Cardiovascular
- Hypotension
- Tachycardia
- Bradycardia
- Chest pain

Respiratory
- Lump in throat
- Cough
- Dyspnea
- Dysphagia
- Hoarseness
- Stridor
- Wheezing
- Rhinitis
- Chest tightness

Cutaneous
- Pruritus
- Erythema
- Urticaria
- Angioedema
- Sense of warmth

Neurologic
- Restlessness
- Uneasiness

- Apprehension
- Anxiety
- Dizziness
- Headache
- Sense of impending doom
- Confusion
- Syncope or near syncope

Gastrointestinal
- Nausea
- Vomiting
- Diarrhea
- Cramping abdominal pain

Genitourinary
- Incontinence

Hemodynamic Parameters
- Decreased cardiac output (CO)
- Decreased cardiac index (CI)
- Decreased right atrial pressure (RAP)
- Decreased pulmonary occlusion pressure (PAOP)
- Decreased systemic vascular resistance (SVR)

seen on the face and in the oral cavity and lower pharynx, angioedema develops as a result of fluid leaking into the interstitial space. The patient may appear restless, uneasy, apprehensive, and anxious and may complain of being warm. Respiratory effects include the development of laryngeal edema, bronchoconstriction, and mucous plugs. Clinical manifestations of laryngeal edema include inspiratory stridor, hoarseness, a sensation of fullness or a lump in the throat, and dysphagia. Bronchoconstriction causes dyspnea, wheezing, and chest tightness.[68,70] Gastrointestinal and genitourinary manifestations, which may develop as a result of smooth muscle contraction, include vomiting, diarrhea, cramping, and abdominal pain.

Hypotension and reflex tachycardia may develop quickly. This occurs in response to massive vasodilation and rapid loss of circulating volume. Jugular veins appear flat as right ventricular end-diastolic volume is decreased. The eventual outcome is circulatory failure and ineffective tissue perfusion.[68,70] The patient's level of consciousness may deteriorate to unresponsiveness.

Assessment of the hemodynamic parameters of a patient in anaphylactic shock reveals a decreased CO and CI. Venous vasodilation and massive volume loss lead to a decrease in preload, which results in a decline in the RAP and PAOP. Vasodilation of the arterial system results in a decrease in the afterload of the heart, as evidenced by a decrease in the SVR. Box 35-11 outlines the clinical criteria for diagnosing anaphylaxis.

Medical Management

Treatment of anaphylactic shock requires an immediate and direct approach to prevent death. The goals of therapy are to remove the offending antigen, reverse the effects of the biochemical mediators, and promote adequate tissue perfusion. When the hypersensitivity reaction occurs as a result of administration of medications, dye, blood, or blood products, the infusion should be immediately discontinued. Often, it is not possible to remove the antigen because it is unknown or has already entered the patient's system.

Reversal of the effects of the biochemical mediators involves the preservation and support of the patient's airway, ventilation, and circulation. This is accomplished through oxygen therapy, intubation, mechanical ventilation, and administration of medications and fluids.

Epinephrine is the first-line treatment of choice for anaphylaxis and should be administered when initial signs and symptoms occur.[65,67] It promotes bronchodilation, vasoconstriction, and increased myocardial contractility and inhibits further release of biochemical mediators. In mild cases of anaphylaxis, 0.2 to 0.5 mg (0.3 to 0.5 mL) of a 1:1000 dilution of epinephrine is administered by intramuscular injection into the anterolateral thigh and repeated every 5 to 15 minutes until anaphylaxis is resolved.[65-68,70-71] Subcutaneous injection is no longer recommended.[71] For anaphylactic shock with hypotension, epinephrine is administered intravenously. The intravenous dose is 0.05 to 0.1 mg (1 mL) of a 1:10,000 dilution administered over 5 minutes.[70] If hypotension persists, a continuous infusion of

BOX 35-11 CLINICAL CRITERIA FOR DIAGNOSING ANAPHYLAXIS

Anaphylaxis is highly likely when one of the following three criteria is fulfilled:

1. Acute onset of an illness (minutes to several hours) with involvement of the skin or mucosal tissue, or both (e.g., generalized hives; pruritus or flushing; swollen lips, tongue, and uvula) *and at least one of the following:*

   a. Respiratory compromise (e.g., dyspnea, wheeze [bronchospasm], stridor, reduced peak expiratory flow, hypoxemia)

   b. Reduced blood pressure or associated symptoms of end-organ dysfunction (e.g., hypotonia [collapse], syncope, incontinence)

2. Two or more of the following that occur rapidly after exposure *to a likely allergen for that patient* (minutes to several hours):

   a. Involvement of the skin-mucosal tissue (e.g., generalized hives; pruritus or flushing; swollen lips, tongue, and uvula)

   b. Respiratory compromise (e.g., dyspnea, wheeze [bronchospasm], stridor, reduced peak expiratory flow, hypoxemia)

   c. Reduced blood pressure or associated symptoms of end-organ dysfunction (e.g., hypotonia [collapse], syncope, incontinence)

   d. Persistent gastrointestinal symptoms (e.g., crampy abdominal pain, vomiting)

3. Reduced blood pressure after exposure *to known allergen for that patient* (minutes to several hours):

   a. Infants and children: low systolic blood pressure (age-specific) or greater than 30% decrease in systolic blood pressure*

   b. Adults: systolic blood pressure of less than 90 mm Hg or greater than 30% decrease for the person's baseline

From Sampson HA, et al. Second symposium on the definition and management of anaphylaxis: summary report—second National Institute of Allergy and Infectious Disease/Food Allergy and Anaphylaxis Network symposium. *J Allergy Clin Immunol.* 2006;117:391.

*Low systolic blood pressure is defined as less than 70 mm Hg for children 1 month to 1 year old, less than (70 mm Hg + [2 × age]) for children 1 to 10 years old, and less than 90 mm Hg for children 11 to 17 years old.

epinephrine is recommended, administered at 1 to 4 mcg/min with titration up to 15 mcg/min as needed.[67,70] Patients receiving beta-blockers may have a limited response to epinephrine. Intravenous glucagon administered as a 20 to 30 mcg/kg bolus over 5 minutes followed by continuous infusion at 5 to 15 mcg/minute is recommended to treat bronchospasm and hypotension in these patients.[66-67,71]

Rapid volume replacement with crystalloid or colloid solutions is also used for patients with hypotension.[66-67,71] Up to 1 L in 5 to 10 minutes is suggested if needed to restore perfusion.[68] Vasopressors may be necessary to reverse the vasodilation and increase blood pressure.[65-66,68,71]

Several medications are used as second-line adjunctive therapy. Inhaled beta-adrenergic agents are used to treat bronchospasm unresponsive to epinephrine.[67-68,70] Diphenhydramine (Benadryl) given 1 to 2 mg/kg (25 to 50 mg) by a slow intravenous is used to block histamine response.[65,67,71] Ranitidine, given in conjunction with diphenhydramine at a dose of 1mL/kg intravenously over 10 to 15 minutes, has been found helpful.[65,67] Corticosteroids are not effective in the immediate treatment of acute anaphylaxis,[67,73] but may be given with the goal of preventing a prolonged or delayed reaction.[66,70-71]

BOX 35-12 NURSING DIAGNOSES

Anaphylactic Shock

- Deficient Fluid Volume related to relative loss, p. 1132
- Decreased Cardiac Output related to alterations in preload, p. 1128
- Decreased Cardiac Output related to alterations in afterload, p. 1128
- Ineffective Breathing Pattern related to decreased lung expansion, p. 1149
- Impaired Gas Exchange related to ventilation/perfusion mismatching or intrapulmonary shunting, p. 1144
- Imbalanced Nutrition: Less Than Body Requirements related to increased metabolic demands or lack of exogenous nutrients, p. 1143
- Risk for Infection, p. 1160
- Ineffective Coping related to situational crisis and personal vulnerability, p. 1150
- Compromised Family Coping related to a critically ill family member, p. 1127

Nursing Management

Prevention of anaphylactic shock is one of the primary responsibilities of the nurse in the critical care area. Preventive measures include the identification of patients at risk and cautious assessment of the patient's response to the administration of medications, blood, and blood products. A complete and accurate history of the patient's allergies is an essential component of preventive nursing care. In addition to a list of the allergies, a detailed description of the type of response for each one should be obtained.

The patient in anaphylactic shock may have any number of nursing diagnoses, depending on the progression of the process (Box 35-12). Nursing interventions include administering epinephrine, facilitating ventilation, administering volume replacement, providing comfort and emotional support, maintaining surveillance for recurrent reactions and preventing and maintaining surveillance for complications.

Measures to facilitate ventilation include positioning the patient to assist with breathing and instructing the patient to breathe slowly and deeply. Airway protection through prompt administration of prescribed medications is essential. Measures to facilitate the administration of volume replacement include inserting large-bore peripheral intravenous catheters; rapidly administering prescribed fluids; and positioning the patient in a supine position with the legs elevated. Measures to promote comfort include administering medications to relieve itching, and applying warm soaks to skin. Observing the patient for clinical manifestations of a delayed or recurrent reaction is critical. Patient education about how to avoid the precipitating allergen is essential for preventing future episodes of anaphylaxis. Education about how to recognize and respond to a future episode including self-administration of epinephrine is essential to prevent a future life-threatening event.

NEUROGENIC SHOCK

Description

Neurogenic shock, another type of distributive shock, is the result of the loss or suppression of sympathetic tone. The lack of sympathetic tone leads to decreased tissue perfusion and initiation of the general shock response (Fig. 35-5). Neurogenic shock is the most uncommon form of shock.

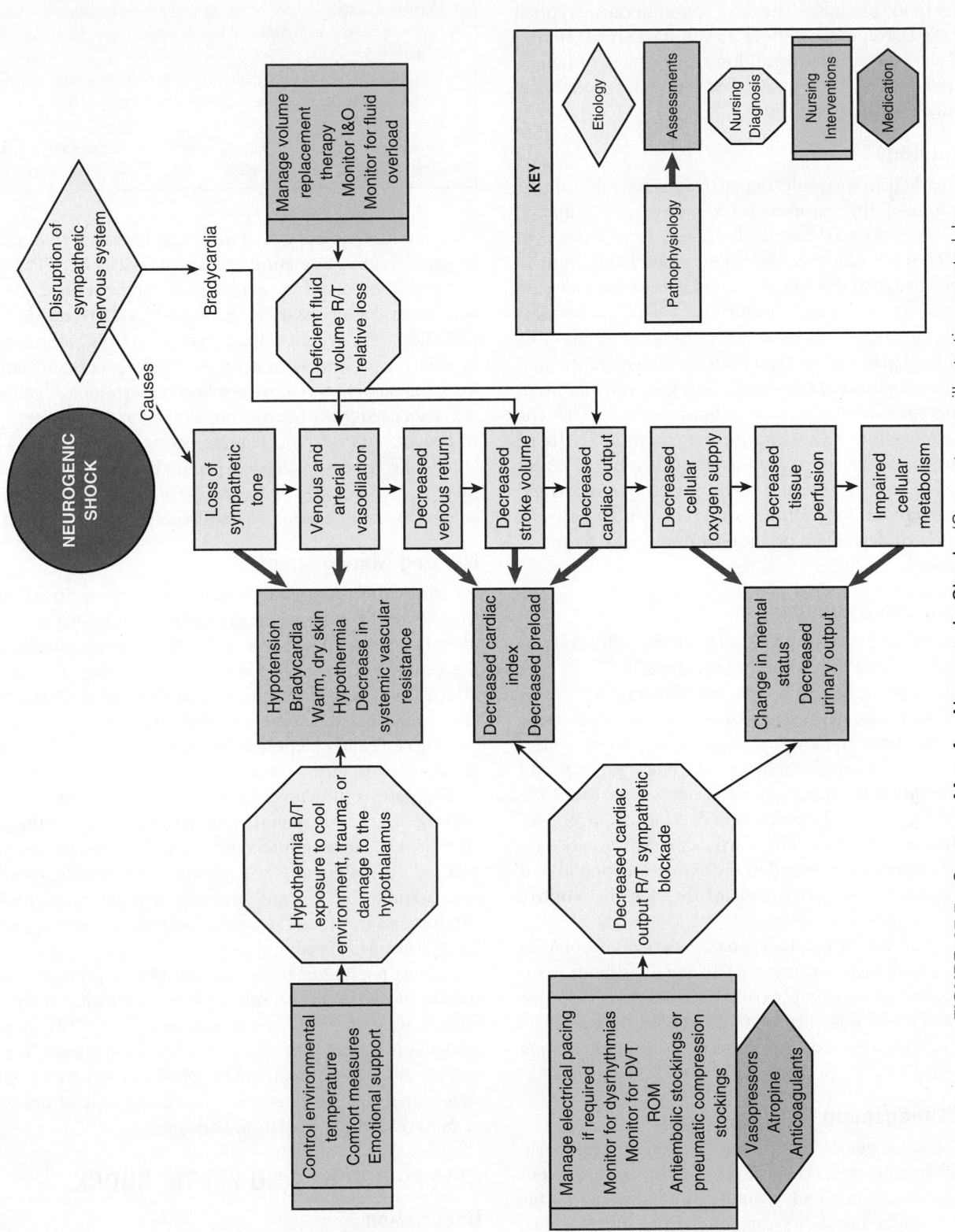

FIGURE 35-5 Concept Map for Neurogenic Shock. (Concept map illustration created by Elaine Bishop Kennedy, EdD, RN.)

Etiology

Neurogenic shock can be caused by anything that disrupts the SNS. The problem can occur as the result of interrupted impulse transmission or blockage of sympathetic outflow from the vasomotor center in the brain.[74-75] The most common cause is spinal cord injury (SCI). Neurogenic shock may mistakenly be referred to as *spinal shock*. The latter condition refers to loss of neurologic activity below the level of SCI, but it does not necessarily involve ineffective tissue perfusion.[74-76]

Pathophysiology

Loss of sympathetic tone results in massive peripheral vasodilation, inhibition of the baroreceptor response, and impaired thermoregulation. Arterial vasodilation leads to a decrease in SVR and a fall in blood pressure. Venous vasodilation leads to relative hypovolemia and pooling of blood in the venous circuit. The decreased venous return results in a decrease in end-diastolic volume or preload, causing a decrease in SV and CO. The fall in blood pressure and CO leads to inadequate or ineffective tissue perfusion. Loss of sympathetic tone and inhibition of the baroreceptor response result in bradycardia.[74-75,77-78] The slow heart rate worsens CO, which further compromises tissue perfusion. Impaired thermoregulation occurs because of loss of vasomotor tone in the cutaneous blood vessels that dilate and constrict to maintain body temperature. The patient becomes poikilothermic, or dependent on the environment for temperature regulation.

Assessment and Diagnosis

The patient in neurogenic shock characteristically presents with hypotension, bradycardia, and warm, dry skin.[74-75,78-79] The decreased blood pressure results from massive peripheral vasodilation. The decreased heart rate is caused by inhibition of the baroreceptor response and unopposed parasympathetic control of the heart.[74-75,78] Consensus on the specific blood pressure and heart rate thresholds for the diagnosis of neurogenic shock has not been established.[74-75] Hypothermia develops from uncontrolled peripheral heat loss. The warm, dry skin occurs as a consequence of pooling of blood in the extremities and loss of vasomotor control in surface vessels of the skin that control heat loss.

Assessment of the hemodynamic parameters of a patient in neurogenic shock reveals a decreased CO and CI. Venous vasodilation leads to a decrease in preload, which results in a decline in the RAP and PAOP. Vasodilation of the arterial system causes a decrease in the afterload of the heart, as evidenced by a decrease in the SVR.[75,78]

Medical Management

Treatment of neurogenic shock requires a careful approach. The goals of therapy are to treat or remove the cause, prevent cardiovascular instability, and promote optimal tissue perfusion. Cardiovascular instability can result from hypovolemia, bradycardia, and hypothermia. Specific treatments are aimed at preventing or correcting these problems as they occur.

Hypovolemia is treated with careful fluid resuscitation. The minimal amount of fluid is administered to ensure adequate tissue perfusion. Volume replacement is initiated for systolic blood pressure lower than 90 mm Hg or evidence of inadequate

BOX 35-13 NURSING DIAGNOSES

Neurogenic Shock

- Deficient Fluid Volume related to relative loss, p. 1132
- Decreased Cardiac Output related to sympathetic blockade, p. 1128
- Hypothermia related to exposure to cold environment, trauma, or damage to the hypothalamus, p. 1142
- Imbalanced Nutrition: Less Than Body Requirements related to increased metabolic demands or lack of exogenous nutrients, p. 1143
- Risk for Infection, p. 1160
- Anxiety related to threat to biologic, psychologic, or social integrity, p. 1125
- Compromised Family Coping related to a critically ill family member, p. 1127

tissue perfusion. Base deficit or lactate levels are recommended to guide fluid resuscitation in patients with SCI.[77] The patient is carefully observed for evidence of fluid overload. Vasopressors are used as necessary to maintain blood pressure and organ perfusion.[74,76-79] Higher than typical MAPs are commonly needed for patients with acute SCI to prevent cord ischemia, but optimal pressures have not been determined.[74,77] Bradycardia associated with neurogenic shock rarely requires specific treatment, but atropine, intravenous infusion of a beta-adrenergic agent, or electrical pacing can be used when necessary.[78,80] Hypothermia is treated with warming measures and environmental temperature regulation.

Nursing Management

Prevention of neurogenic shock is one of the primary responsibilities of the nurse in the critical care area. This includes the identification of patients at risk and constant assessment of the neurologic status. Vigilant immobilization of spinal cord injuries and slight elevation of the head of the patient's bed after spinal anesthesia are essential components of preventive nursing care. Early identification allows for early treatment and decreased mortality.

The patient in neurogenic shock may have any number of nursing diagnoses, depending on the progression of the process (Box 35-13). Nursing interventions include treating hypovolemia and maintaining tissue perfusion, maintaining normothermia, monitoring for and treating dysrhythmias, providing comfort and emotional support, and preventing and maintaining surveillance for complications.

Venous pooling in the lower extremities promotes the formation of deep vein thrombosis (DVT), which can result in a pulmonary embolism. All patients at risk for DVT should be started on prophylaxis therapy. DVT-prophylactic measures include monitoring of passive range-of-motion exercises, application of sequential pneumatic stockings, and administration of prescribed anticoagulation therapy.

SEVERE SEPSIS AND SEPTIC SHOCK

Description

Sepsis occurs when microorganisms invade the body and initiate a systemic inflammatory response. This host response often results in perfusion abnormalities with organ dysfunction (severe sepsis) and eventually hypotension (septic shock). The primary mechanism of this type of shock is the maldistribution of blood flow to the tissues (Fig. 35-6).[4] Severe sepsis is estimated to result in more than 700,000 hospitalizations annually in the United States, with an estimated hospital mortality rate of 23% to 50%.[81-84] It is the leading cause of in-hospital death and the eleventh leading cause of all deaths in the United States.[82,85]

Specific terms are used to describe the continuum of conditions that the patient with an infection may experience. In 1991 at the American College of Chest Physicians/Society of Critical Care Medicine (ACCP/SCCM) Consensus Conference, definitions were developed to describe and differentiate these conditions (Box 35-14).[86] These definitions were clarified and reinforced in subsequent conferences in 2001, 2004, and 2008.[17,87-88] This discussion focuses on severe sepsis and septic shock.

Etiology

Sepsis is caused by a wide variety of microorganisms, including gram-negative and gram-positive aerobes, anaerobes, fungi, and viruses. The source of these microorganisms varies. The respiratory system is the most common site of infection producing severe sepsis and septic shock, followed by the genitourinary and gastrointestinal systems.[82,83] Gram-positive bacteria are the predominant cause of sepsis.[83,89] Sepsis and septic shock are associated with a wide variety of intrinsic and extrinsic precipitating factors (Box 35-15). All of these factors interfere directly or indirectly with the body's anatomic and physiologic defense mechanisms. Several of the intrinsic factors are not modifiable or are very difficult to control. Several of the extrinsic factors may be required for diagnosis and management. All critically ill patients are therefore at risk for septic shock.

Pathophysiology

The syndrome encompassing severe sepsis and septic shock is a complex systemic response that is initiated when a microorganism enters the body and stimulates the inflammatory/immune system. In a host-pathogen interaction, both the invading organism and injured tissue release intracellular proteins activating neutrophils, monocytes, lymphocytes, macrophages, mast cells, and platelets as well as numerous plasma enzyme cascades (complement, kinin/kallikrein, coagulation, and fibrinolytic factors). When this reaction is localized, infection is contained and eradicated. But when the magnitude of the infectious insult is great or the patient is physiologically unable to generate an effective host response, containment fails.[90] The result is a systemic release of the pathogen, activated cells, and mediators, including cytokines, which initiate a chain of complex interactions leading to an uncontrolled SIRS.[90-94]

With systemic activation, a variety of physiologic and pathophysiologic events occur that affect clotting, the distribution of blood flow to the tissues and organs, capillary membrane permeability, and the metabolic state of the body. Subsequently, a systemic imbalance between cellular oxygen supply and demand develops that results in cellular hypoxia, damage, hibernation, and death.[5,91,93-94]

Hallmarks of severe sepsis are endothelial damage and coagulation dysfunction.[91-92,95-96] Tissue factor (TF) is released from endothelial cells and monocytes in response to stimulation by inflammatory cytokines.[91,95-97] Release of TF initiates the coagulation cascade, producing widespread microvascular thrombosis and further stimulation of the systemic inflammatory pathways.[91-92,95-97] Diffuse endothelial damage impairs endogenous anticlotting mechanisms.[91-92,95,97] Mediator-induced suppression of fibrinolysis slows clot breakdown. The result is DIC with eventual consumption of coagulation factors, bleeding, and hemorrhage.[92,96-97]

Significant alterations in cardiovascular hemodynamics are caused by the activation of inflammatory cytokines and endothelial damage.[90-92] Massive peripheral vasodilation results in the development of relative hypovolemia. Increased capillary permeability produces a loss of intravascular volume to the interstitium, which accentuates the reduction in preload and CO. These changes, coupled with the microvascular thrombosis, produce maldistribution of circulating blood volume, decreased tissue perfusion, and inadequate oxygen delivery to the cells. Microcirculatory shunting is a key feature of this distributive shock.[91,98] Impaired ventricular contractility results from cytokine activity.[5,91-92,96]

Activation of the central nervous and endocrine systems also occurs as part of the response to invading microorganisms. This activation leads to stimulation of the SNS and the release of ACTH. These events trigger the release of epinephrine, norepinephrine, glucocorticoids, aldosterone, glucagon, renin, and growth hormone, resulting in the development of a hypermetabolic state and contributing to vasoconstriction of the renal, pulmonary, and splanchnic beds. Selective vasoconstriction in the splanchnic bed may contribute to hypoperfusion of the gastrointestinal mucosal barrier, an area particularly vulnerable to the effects of inflammatory cytokines.[92,99] The resulting gut injury propagates the inflammatory response.[2,99]

Several metabolic alterations occur as a result of CNS, endocrine system, and cytokine activation. The hypermetabolic state increases energy expenditure and oxygen demand, and it contributes to cellular hypoxia. Lactic acid is produced as a result of increased metabolic lactate production and hypoxic anaerobic metabolism. Glucocorticoids, ACTH, epinephrine, glucagon, and growth hormone are all catabolic hormones that are released as part of this response. In conjunction with the inflammatory cytokines, these hormones stimulate catabolism of protein stores in the visceral organs and skeletal muscles to fuel glucose production in the liver, hyperglycemia, and insulin resistance.[94,100] The cytokines also stimulate the use of fats for energy production (lipolysis).[94,100-101]

Metabolic derangements in severe sepsis and septic shock include an inability of the cells to use oxygen even if blood flow is adequate. Mitochondrial dysfunction is thought to be the underlying mechanism.[91,94,101-102] This bioenergetic failure plays an important role in the development of tissue ischemia and multiple organ dysfunction.[91,94,101-102] These complex and interrelated pathophysiologic changes produce a pathologic imbalance between cellular oxygen demand and cellular oxygen supply and consumption.

The exaggerated systemic inflammatory response associated with severe sepsis and septic shock results in cell death via both ischemic necrosis and, to a large degree, apoptosis. Apoptosis is a programmed cell death or cellular suicide mediated by caspase-3, a cysteine protease, and affecting endothelial, gastrointestinal epithelial, and immune cells in particular.[91-92,94,96] Apoptosis of immune cells results in immunosuppression and

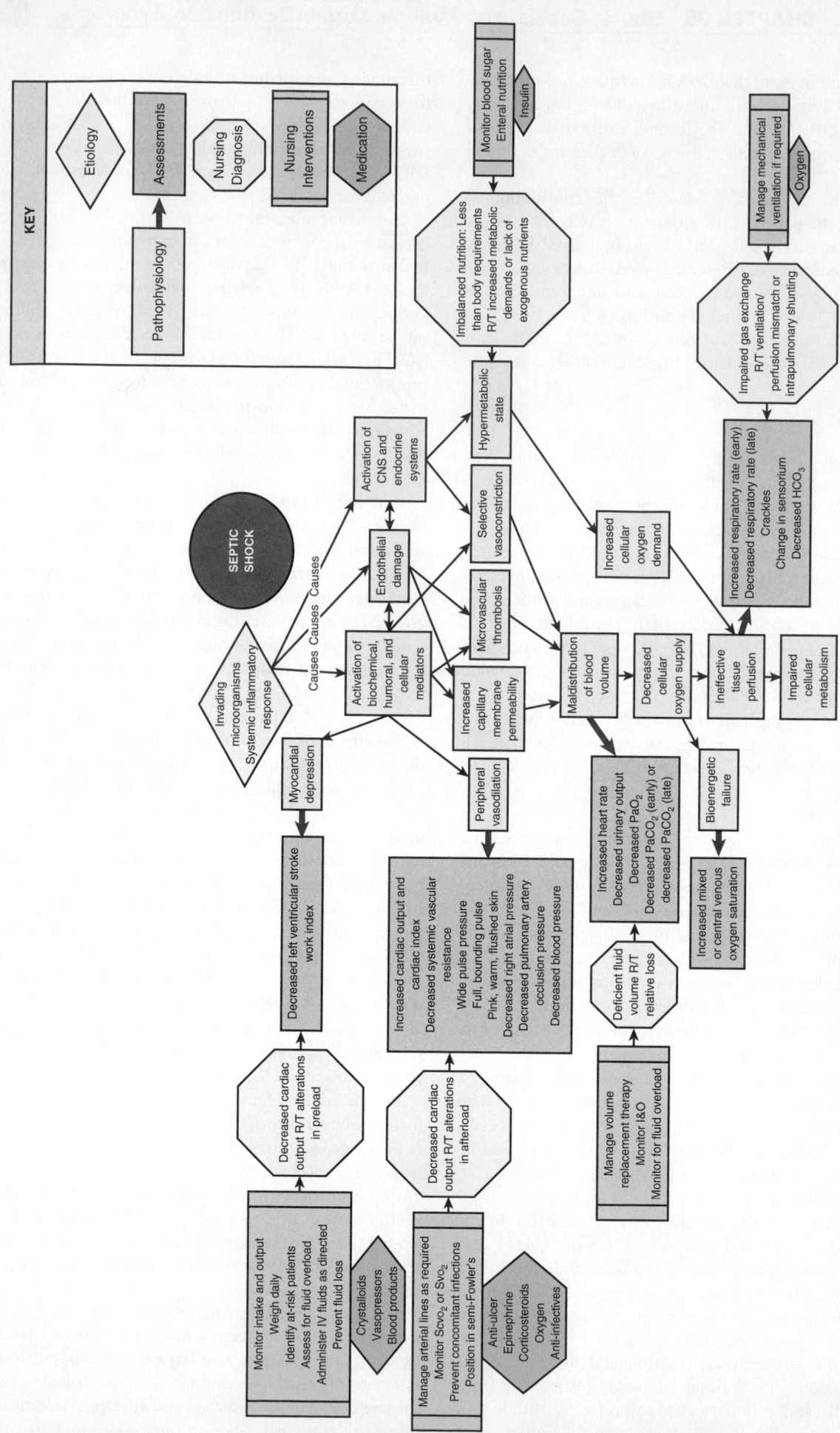

FIGURE 35-6 Concept Map for Septic Shock. (Concept map illustration created by Elaine Bishop Kennedy, EdD, RN.)

DEFINITIONS FOR SEPSIS AND ORGAN FAILURE

- *Infection:* Microbial phenomenon characterized by an inflammatory response to the presence of microorganisms or the invasion of normally sterile host tissue by those organisms.
- *Bacteremia:* Presence of viable bacteria in the blood.
- *Systemic inflammatory response syndrome (SIRS):* Systemic inflammatory response to a variety of severe clinical insults, manifested by two or more of the following conditions: 1) temperature >38° C or <36° C; 2) heart rate >90 beats/min; 3) respiratory rate >20 breaths/min or $PaCO_2$ <32 mm Hg; and 4) white blood cell count >12,000/mm³, <4000/mm³, or >10% immature (band) forms.
- *Sepsis:* Systemic response to infection, manifested by two or more of the following conditions as a result of infection: 1) temperature >38° C or <36° C; 2) heart rate >90 beats/min; 3) respiratory rate >20 breaths/min or $PaCO_2$ <32 mm Hg; and 4) white blood cell count >12,000/mm³, <4000/mm³, or >10% immature (band) forms.
- *Severe sepsis:* Sepsis associated with organ dysfunction, hypoperfusion, or hypotension. Hypoperfusion and perfusion abnormalities may include, but are not limited to, lactic acidosis, oliguria, or an acute alteration in mental status.
- *Septic shock:* Sepsis-induced shock with hypotension despite adequate fluid resuscitation, along with the presence of perfusion abnormalities that may include, but are not limited to, lactic acidosis, oliguria, or an acute alteration in mental status. Patients who are receiving inotropic or vasopressor agents may not be hypotensive at the time that perfusion abnormalities are measured.
- *Sepsis-induced hypotension:* A systolic blood pressure <90 mm Hg or a reduction of ≥40 mm Hg from baseline in the absence of other causes for hypotension.
- *Multiple organ dysfunction syndrome (MODS):* Altered organ function in an acutely ill patient such that homeostasis cannot be maintained without intervention.

Adapted from American College of Chest Physicians/Society of Critical Care Medicine Consensus Conference. Definitions for sepsis and organ failure and guidelines for the use of innovative therapies in sepsis. *Crit Care Med.* 1992;20:864.

PRECIPITATING FACTORS ASSOCIATED WITH SEPTIC SHOCK

Intrinsic Factors
- Extreme of age
- Coexisting diseases
  - Malignancies
  - Burns
  - Acquired immunodeficiency syndrome (AIDS)
  - Diabetes
  - Substance abuse
  - Dysfunction of one or more of the major body systems
- Malnutrition

Extrinsic Factors
- Invasive devices
- Medication therapy
- Fluid therapy
- Surgical and traumatic wounds
- Surgical and invasive diagnostic procedures
- Immunosuppressive therapy

---

secondary infection as well as release of immune cell toxins. Both ischemic necrosis and apoptosis stimulate further inflammation, propagating an ongoing cycle of infection, tissue injury, and SIRS.[90,96] If unabated, this situation ultimately results in MODS and death.

Assessment and Diagnosis

Effective treatment of severe sepsis and septic shock depends on timely recognition. The diagnosis of severe sepsis is based on the identification of three conditions: known or suspected infection, two or more of the clinical indications of the systemic inflammatory response, and evidence of at least one organ dysfunction. Clinical indications of systemic inflammatory response and sepsis were included in the original ACCP/SCCM consensus definitions and are listed in Box 35-14. The second consensus conference expanded this list to facilitate prompt clinical recognition (Box 35-16).[88]

Signs of individual organ dysfunction are discussed later in the chapter. The two most common organs to demonstrate dysfunction in severe sepsis are the cardiovascular system and the lungs. The patient with persistent hypotension requiring vasopressor therapy despite adequate volume resuscitation is demonstrating cardiovascular dysfunction. Pulmonary dysfunction is manifested by a PaO_2/FIO_2 (fraction of oxygen in inspired air) ratio of less than 300, indicating ARDS.[17,103] Signs indicating septic shock are hypotension despite adequate fluid resuscitation and the presence of perfusion abnormalities such as lactic acidosis, oliguria, or acute change in mentation.

The patient in severe sepsis or septic shock may present with a variety of clinical manifestations that may change dynamically as the condition progresses (Box 35-17). During the initial stage, massive vasodilation occurs in the venous and arterial beds. Dilation of the venous system leads to a decrease in venous return to the heart, which results in a decrease in the preload of the right and left ventricles. This is evidenced by a decline in the RAP and PAOP. Dilation of the arterial system results in a decrease in the afterload of the heart, as evidenced by a decrease in the SVR. The patient's skin becomes pink, warm, and flushed as a result of the massive vasodilation. Myocardial contractility is decreased, as evidenced by a decline in the left ventricular stroke work index (LVSWI) and ejection fraction.

The heart rate rises in response to increased SNS, metabolic, and adrenal gland stimulation. If circulating volume and preload are adequate, this results in a normal-to-high CO and CI despite impaired contractility. The pulse pressure widens as the diastolic blood pressure decreases because of the vasodilation, and the systolic blood pressure increases because of the elevated CO. A full, bounding pulse develops. The net result of these changes is a relatively normal blood pressure in severe sepsis. However, as the reduction in preload and afterload becomes overwhelming and contractility fails, hypotension ensues, resulting in septic shock.

In the lungs, ventilation/perfusion mismatching develops as a result of pulmonary vasoconstriction and the formation of pulmonary microemboli. Hypoxemia occurs, and the respiratory rate increases to compensate for the lack of oxygen. Crackles develop as increased pulmonary capillary membrane permeability leads to pulmonary edema.[103]

BOX 35-16 DIAGNOSTIC CRITERIA FOR SEPSIS

General Variables

Fever (>38.3° C)

Hypothermia (core temperature < 36° C)

Heart rate > 90/min^{-1} or more than two SD above the normal value for age

Tachypnea

Altered mental status

Significant edema or positive fluid balance (>20 mL/kg over 24 hr)

Hyperglycemia (plasma glucose > 140 mg/dL or 7.7 mmol/L) in the absence of diabetes

Inflammatory Variables

Leukocytosis (WBC count > 12,000 μL^{-1})

Leukopenia (WBC count < 4000 μL^{-1})

Normal WBC count with greater than 10% immature forms

Plasma C-reactive protein more than two SD above the normal value

Plasma procalcitonin more than two SD above the normal value

Hemodynamic Variables

Arterial hypotension (SBP < 90 mm Hg, MAP < 70 mm Hg, or an SBP decrease >40 mm Hg in adults or less than two SD below normal for age)

Organ Dysfunction Variables

Arterial hypoxemia (Pao$_2$/Fio$_2$ < 300)

Acute oliguria (urine output < 0.5 mL/kg/hr for at least 2 hrs despite adequate fluid resuscitation)

Creatinine increase > 0.5 mg/dL or 44.2 μmol/L

Coagulation abnormalities (INR > 1.5 or aPTT > 60 s)

Ileus (absent bowel sounds)

Thrombocytopenia (platelet count < 100,000 μL^{-1})

Hyperbilirubinemia (plasma total bilirubin > 4 mg/dL or 70 μmol/L)

Tissue Perfusion Variables

Hyperlactatemia (>1 mmol/L)

Decreased capillary refill or mottling

WBC, White blood cell; *SBP,* systolic blood pressure; *MAP,* mean arterial pressure; *INR,* international normalized ratio; *aPTT,* activated partial thromboplastin time.

Diagnostic criteria for sepsis in the pediatric population are signs and symptoms of inflammation plus infection with hyper- or hypothermia (rectal temperature >38.5° or <35° C), tachycardia (may be absent in hypothermic patients), and at least one of the following indications of altered organ function: altered mental status, hypoxemia, increased serum lactate level, or bounding pulses.

From Dellinger RP, Levy MM, Rhodes A, et al. Surviving Sepsis Campaign: international guidelines for management of severe sepsis and septic shock: 2012. *Crit Care Med.* 2013:41(2):585. Adapted from Levy MM, Fink MP, Marshall JC, et al: 2001 SCCM/ESICM/ACCP/ATS/SIS International Sepsis Definitions Conference. *Crit Care Med.* 2003; 31:1250–1256.

BOX 35-17 CLINICAL MANIFESTATIONS OF SEPTIC SHOCK

- Increased heart rate
- Decreased blood pressure
- Wide pulse pressure
- Full, bounding pulse
- Pink, warm, flushed skin
- Increased respiratory rate (early) or decreased respiratory rate (late)
- Crackles
- Change in sensorium
- Decreased urine output
- Increased temperature
- Increased cardiac output and cardiac index
- Decreased systemic vascular resistance
- Decreased right atrial pressure
- Decreased pulmonary artery occlusion pressure
- Decreased left ventricular stroke work index
- Decreased Pao$_2$
- Decreased Paco$_2$ (early) or increased Paco$_2$ (late)
- Decreased HCO$_3^-$
- Increased Svo$_2$ or Scvo$_2$

PaCO$_2$, Partial pressure of carbon dioxide; *PaO$_2$,* partial pressure of oxygen; *SCVO$_2$,* central venous oxygen saturation; *SVO$_2$,* mixed venous oxygen saturation.

The level of consciousness starts to change as a result of decreased cerebral perfusion, immune mediator activation, hyperthermia, and lactic acidosis. This septic encephalopathy is demonstrated by acute onset of impaired cognitive functioning, or delirium, which may fluctuate during its course.[104] The patient may appear disoriented, confused, combative, or lethargic.

ABG values initially reveal hypocarbia, hypoxemia, and metabolic acidosis. This is demonstrated by a low Pao$_2$, low Paco$_2$, and low HCO$_3^-$ level, respectively. The respiratory alkalosis is caused by the patient's increased respiratory rate. As pathologic pulmonary changes progress and the patient becomes fatigued, the effectiveness of respirations decreases and the Paco$_2$ increases, resulting in respiratory acidosis. The metabolic acidosis is the result of a lack of oxygen to the cells and the development of lactic acidemia. Serum lactate levels increase above 2 mmol/L because of anaerobic metabolism. The mixed venous oxygen saturation (Svo$_2$) may increase because of microcirculatory shunting or decrease because of inadequate oxygen delivery.[91,98] The white blood cell (WBC) count is elevated as part of the immune response to the invading microorganisms. The WBC differential count reveals an increase in immature neutrophils (shift to the left). This occurs because the body has to mobilize increasing numbers of WBCs to fight the infection. An elevated procalcitonin level is a valuable biomarker of significant bacterial infection and procalcitonin levels have been used in clinical trials to guide antibiotic therapy with positive outcomes.[91,105] Serum glucose levels increase as part of the hypermetabolic response and the development of insulin resistance. The patient's temperature is elevated in response to pyrogens released from the invading microorganisms, immune mediator activation, and increased metabolic activity. Urine output declines because of decreased perfusion of the kidneys. As impaired tissue perfusion develops, a variety of other clinical manifestations appear that indicate the development of MODS.

Medical Management

Treatment of the patient in severe sepsis or septic shock requires a multifaceted approach. The goals of treatment are to reverse the pathophysiologic responses, control the infection, and promote metabolic support. This approach includes supporting the cardiovascular system and enhancing tissue perfusion, identifying and treating the infection, limiting the systemic inflammatory response, restoring metabolic balance, and initiating nutritional therapy. Dysfunction of the individual organ systems

BOX 35-18 SEVERE SEPSIS BUNDLES

Sepsis Resuscitation Bundle

The goal is to perform all indicated tasks 100% of the time within the first 6 hours of identification of severe sepsis. The tasks are:

1. Measure serum lactate.
2. Obtain blood cultures prior to antibiotic administration.
3. Administer broad-spectrum antibiotic, within 3 hrs of ED admission and within 1 hour of non-ED admission.
4. In the event of hypotension and/or a serum lactate >4 mmol/L:
   a. Deliver an initial minimum of 20 mL/kg of crystalloid or an equivalent.
   b. Apply vasopressors for hypotension not responding to initial fluid resuscitation to maintain mean arterial pressure (MAP) >65 mm Hg.
5. In the event of persistent hypotension despite fluid resuscitation (septic shock) and/or lactate >4 mmol/L:
   a. Achieve a central venous pressure (CVP) of >8 mm Hg.
   b. Achieve a central venous oxygen saturation (ScvO$_2$) >70% or mixed venous oxygen saturation (SvO$_2$) >65%.

Sepsis Management Bundle

Efforts to accomplish these goals should begin immediately, but these items may be completed within 24 hours of presentation for patients with severe sepsis or septic shock.

1. Administer low-dose steroids for septic shock in accordance with a standardized ICU policy. If not administered, document why the patient did not qualify for low-dose steroids based upon the standardized protocol.
2. Initiate insulin therapy when blood glucose levels exceed 180 mg/dL and maintain a blood glucose of approximately 150 mg/dL.
3. Maintain a median inspiratory plateau pressure (IPP) <30 cm H$_2$O for mechanically ventilated patients.

From European Society of Intensive Care Medicine, International Sepsis Forum, and Society of Critical Care Medicine. Surviving Sepsis Campaign. http://www.survivingsepsis.org/Bundles/Pages/default.aspx. 2008.

must be prevented. Early treatment reduces mortality.[17,106-107] Guidelines for the management of severe sepsis and septic shock have been developed and updated under the auspices of the Surviving Sepsis Campaign (SSC), an international effort of more than 11 organizations to improve patient outcomes.[17,87] From these guidelines, a group ("bundle") of selected interventions was identified as having the most impact on patient outcomes (Box 35-18). The sepsis resuscitation bundle should be implemented within the first 6 hours, and the sepsis management bundle should be implemented within the first 24 hours. More information regarding these interventions is available at the SSC website (http://www.survivingsepsis.org).

The patient in severe sepsis or septic shock requires immediate resuscitation of the hypoperfused state. Specific interventions are aimed at increasing cellular oxygen supply and decreasing cellular oxygen demand. These treatments include administration of fluids, vasopressors, and positive inotropic agents. Early goal-directed therapy during the first 6 hours of resuscitation improves survival[84,106] and is recommended in the SSC guidelines.[17] This therapy includes aggressive fluid resuscitation to augment intravascular volume and increase preload until a CVP of 8 to 12 mm Hg (12 to 15 mm Hg in mechanically ventilated patients) is achieved. Crystalloids are the initial fluid of choice.[17] A fluid challenge for hypovolemia should be initiated with at least 1000 mL of crystalloids or 300 to 500 mL of colloids over 30 minutes. Vasopressors should be administered as necessary to maintain a MAP of at least 65 mm Hg. These agents reverse the massive peripheral vasodilation and increase SVR. Norepinephrine and dopamine have both been recommended as first-choice agents, but recent evidence strongly indicates superiority of norepinephrine in lowering mortality rates and a higher risk of dysrhythmias when dopamine is used.[108-109] Epinephrine is recommended as an alternative agent if response to norepinephrine is poor.[17] Arterial line placement is recommended for any patient requiring vasopressor therapy. Intermittent or continuous monitoring of central venous or mixed venous oxygen saturation (ScvO$_2$ or SvO$_2$) allows evaluation of the effectiveness of oxygen delivery. If the ScvO$_2$ is less than 70% or the SvO$_2$ is less than 65% after the CVP goal is achieved, administration of packed red cells to achieve a hematocrit of at least 30% or inotropic stimulation with dobutamine (administered to a maximum of 20 mcg/kg/minute) to counteract myocardial depression and maintain adequate CO is recommended to obtain this goal.[17,106] The dobutamine infusion should be reduced or discontinued if a tachycardia greater than 120 beats/minute develops.[106]

Intubation and mechanical ventilatory support are usually required to optimize oxygenation and ventilation for the patient in severe sepsis or septic shock. Ventilation with lower than traditional tidal volumes (6 versus 12 mL/kg) in patients with ARDS decreases mortality.[110] SSC guidelines recommend the goals of 6 mL/kg of predicted body weight and plateau pressures no more than 30 cm H$_2$O for patients with severe sepsis or septic shock with ARDS.[17] Increased PaCO$_2$ may result from this therapy and is acceptable if tolerated as evidenced by hemodynamic stability. Ventilator settings should include positive end-expiratory pressure (PEEP) and be adjusted to provide the patient with a PaO$_2$ greater than 70 mm Hg. Patients receiving mechanical ventilation should be maintained in a semirecumbent position with the head of the bed raised to 45 degrees to decrease the incidence of ventilator-associated pneumonia.[17] Prone positioning should be considered in the septic patient with ARDS requiring high levels of oxygen.[17] Sedation protocols using intermittent bolus or continuous infusion using a standardized sedation scale and specific goals are recommended for all patients requiring mechanical ventilation. Daily interruption of sedative infusions to allow wakefulness and re-evaluation of sedation needs reduce duration of mechanical ventilation and is recommended.[17] Neuromuscular blocking agents should be avoided, if possible, to prevent prolonged blockade after discontinuation.[17]

A key measure in the treatment of septic shock is finding and eradicating the cause of the infection. At least two blood cultures plus urine, sputum, and wound cultures should be obtained to find the location of the infection before antibiotic therapy is initiated.[17] Antibiotic therapy should be started within 1 hour of recognition of severe sepsis without delay for cultures.[17] Each hour of delay is associated with a substantial drop in the survival rate.[107] If the microorganism is unknown, anti-infective therapy with one or more agents known to be effective against likely pathogens should be initiated, with daily reassessment of the regimen. Combination therapy is recommended for known or suspected *Pseudomonas* infection and for neutropenic patients but should be limited to less than 3 to

5 days.[17] A specific source of infection should be established within 6 hours of presentation.[17] Surgical intervention to débride infected or necrotic tissue or to drain abscesses may be necessary to facilitate removal of the septic source.[17] Intravascular devices that may be the source of the infection should be removed after establishment of alternative vascular access.

Only one medication has been brought to market specifically for the treatment of severe sepsis and septic shock, recombinant human activated protein C (rhAPC), marketed as drotrecogin alfa [activated] under the trade name Xigris. This medication was recommended only for patients at high risk for death.[17] However, a Cochrane review found that none of the results of subsequent randomized clinical trials supported the beneficial findings in mortality demonstrated in the original trials used for drug approval both in the United States and Europe.[111] Following failure to show a survival benefit in a major clinical trial launched to reassess the medication, Xigris was voluntarily withdrawn from the market by the manufacturer in October 2011.[112-113] Studies of numerous other medications thought to block or alter the effects of immune mediators have failed to demonstrate effectiveness or have been associated with unacceptable adverse effects.[90,96]

Low-dose intravenous corticosteroids reduce mortality in a select group of catecholamine-dependent septic shock patients.[114-115] Therefore, intravenous hydrocortisone is recommended *only* for the patient in septic shock who remains hypotensive despite adequate fluid resuscitation and vasopressor therapy.[17,116] High doses of 300 mg/day or more may be harmful and should *not* be used.[17,116] Steroid therapy should be weaned when vasopressors are no longer required.

Continuous infusion of intravenous insulin is recommended by SSC guidelines when blood glucose level exceeds 180 mg/dL with a goal blood glucose level of approximately 150 mg/dL.[17,117] Glucose levels should be monitored every 1 to 2 hours until stable and then every 4 hours. Low glucose levels measured by capillary testing may be inaccurate in this population.[17] Platelets should be administered when counts are less than 5000/mm³ and red blood cell transfusions are recommended when the hemoglobin level is less than 7.0 g/dL to obtain a target value of 7 to 9 g/dL.[17] Stress ulcer prophylaxis using H₂-receptor antagonists or proton pump inhibitors and DVT prophylaxis are recommended for all patients with severe sepsis or septic shock. The SCCM guidelines recommend against the use of sodium bicarbonate for lactic acidemia if the pH is equal to or greater than 7.15.[17] Low-dose dopamine infusion for renal protection is not beneficial and should not be used.[17]

The initiation of nutritional therapy is critical in the management of the patient in severe sepsis or septic shock. The goal is to improve the patient's overall nutritional status, enhance immune function, and promote wound healing. A daily caloric intake of 20 to 30 kcal/kg of usual body weight is recommended for critically ill patients. The enteral route is strongly preferred. When compared to enteral nutrition, parenteral nutrition or a combination of both methods has been associated with higher mortality in patients with severe sepsis or septic shock.[118]

Sufficient protein needs to be provided because of the metabolic derangements that develop in the hypermetabolic state. A range of 1.2 to 2.0 g/kg actual body weight per day is recommended for patients with a body mass index (BMI) less than 30, with progressively larger amounts for those with higher BMI.[38] Specific nutritional therapies to reduce the inflammatory and hypermetabolic responses associated with sepsis, such as antioxidant supplementation and feeding with long-chain n-3 polyunsaturated fatty acids, are the source of much debate and evaluation.[100,119] Glutamine is considered by some to be an essential amino acid in critically ill patients and has the most empirical support,[91,119] but others may actually worsen outcomes. Current recommendations stress caution with any immune-modulating formulations in patients with severe sepsis.[38]

Nursing Management

Nursing recommendations to complement the SSC guidelines have recently been published and focus on infection prevention and transmission, early recognition and treatment of severe sepsis and septic shock and its progression, and supportive nursing care.[120] Prevention of severe sepsis and septic shock is one of the primary responsibilities of the nurse in the critical care area. These measures include the identification of patients at risk and reduction of their risk factors, including exposure to invading microorganisms. Hand washing, aseptic technique, and an understanding of evidence-based practice to reduce nosocomial infection in critically ill patients are essential components of preventive nursing care. Early identification allows for early treatment and decreases mortality. Figure 35-7 is a simple screening tool for identifying patients with severe sepsis. Subsequent continual observation to detect subtle changes that indicate the progression of the septic process is vitally important, as is evidence-based practice to prevent further infection. Immunosuppression is common as sepsis progresses,[96] and recent research has found that a resurgence in opportunistic infection in patients with severe sepsis and septic shock occurs in the later stages, more than 2 weeks after initial diagnosis and treatment.[121] Evidence-based practice to prevent complications of critical illness and prolonged bed rest are essential to prevent further compromise and negative short- and long-term outcomes. Ongoing mortality and impaired quality of life persist in the months and years after hospital discharge for survivors of sepsis.[122]

The patient in septic shock may have any number of nursing diagnoses, depending on the progression of the process (Box 35-19). Nursing interventions include early identification of sepsis syndrome; administering prescribed fluids, medications, and nutrition; providing comfort and emotional support; and preventing and maintaining surveillance for complications.

Evidence-based guidelines for the management of the patient with severe sepsis or septic shock are listed in the Box 35-20.

MULTIPLE ORGAN DYSFUNCTION SYNDROME

Description

Over the past two decades critical care professionals have witnessed the emergence of a new clinical syndrome, multiple organ dysfunction syndrome (MODS), in critically ill patients. MODS results from progressive physiologic failure of two or more separate organ systems in an acutely ill patient such that

Evaluation for Severe Sepsis Screening Tool

Instructions: Use this optional tool to screen patients for severe sepsis in the emergency department, on the wards, or in the ICU.

1. **Is the patient's history suggestive of a new infection?**

   ☐ Pneumonia, empyema
   ☐ Urinary tract infection
   ☐ Acute abdominal infection
   ☐ Meningitis
   ☐ Skin/soft tissue infection

   ☐ Bone/joint infection
   ☐ Wound infection
   ☐ Bloodstream catheter infection
   ☐ Endocarditis

   ☐ Implantable device infection
   ☐ Other _____

   ___ Yes ___ No

2. **Are any two of the following signs & symptoms of infection both present and new to the patient?** <u>Note:</u> laboratory values may have been obtained for inpatients but may not be available for outpatients.

   ☐ Hyperthermia > 38.3 °C (101.0 °F)
   ☐ Hypothermia < 36 °C (96.8 °F)
   ☐ Tachycardia > 90 bpm

   ☐ Tachypnea > 20 bpm
   ☐ Acutely altered mental status
   ☐ Leukocytosis (WBC count >12,000 mcg-1)

   ☐ Leukopenia (WBC count < 4000 mcg-1)
   ☐ Hyperglycemia (plasma glucose >120 mg/dL) in the absence of diabetes

   ___ Yes ___ No

   If the answer is yes to both either question 1 and 2, *suspicion of infection* **is present:**

   ✓ Obtain: **lactic acid, blood cultures,** CBC with differential, basic chemistry labs, bilirubin.
   ✓ At the physician's discretion obtain: UA, chest x-ray, amylase, lipase, ABG, CRP, CT scan.

3. **Are any of the following organ dysfunction criteria present at a site remote from the site of the infection that are not considered to be chronic conditions?** <u>Note:</u> the remote site stipulation is waived in the case of bilateral pulmonary infiltrates.

   ☐ SBP < 90 mmHg or MAP < 65 mmHg
   ☐ SBP decrease > 40 mm Hg from baseline
   ☐ Bilateral pulmonary infiltrates with a new (or increased) oxygen requirement to maintain SpO_2 > 90%
   ☐ Bilateral pulmonary infiltrates with PaO2/FiO2 ratio < 300
   ☐ Creatinine > 2.0 mg/dl (176.8 mmol/L) or Urine Output < 0.5 ml/kg/hour for > 2 hours
   ☐ Bilirubin > 2 mg/dl (34.2 mmol/L)
   ☐ Platelet count < 100,000
   ☐ Coagulopathy (INR > 1.5 or aPTT > 60 secs)
   ☐ Lactate > 2 mmol/L (18.0 mg/dl)

   ___ Yes ___ No

   If *suspicion of infection* **is present AND** *organ dysfunction* **is present, the patient meets the criteria for SEVERE SEPSIS and should be entered into the severe sepsis protocol.**

   Date: ___/___/___ (circle: dd/mm/yy or mm/dd/yy)   Time: ___:___ (24 hr. clock)

   Version 7.12.2005   © 2005 Surviving Sepsis Campaign and the Institute for Healthcare Improvement

FIGURE 35-7 Evaluation for Severe Sepsis Screening Tool. (Redrawn from the Institute for Healthcare Improvement, Cambridge, MA. Copyright 2005 Surviving Sepsis Campaign and the Institute for Healthcare Improvement.)

◎ BOX 35-19 **NURSING DIAGNOSES**

Septic Shock

- Deficient Fluid Volume related to relative loss, p. 1132
- Decreased Cardiac Output related to alterations in preload, p. 1128
- Decreased Cardiac Output related to alterations in afterload, p. 1128
- Decreased Cardiac Output related to alterations in contractility, p. 1128
- Impaired Gas Exchange related to ventilation/perfusion mismatching or intrapulmonary shunting, p. 1144

- Imbalanced Nutrition: Less Than Body Requirements related to increased metabolic demands or lack of exogenous nutrients, p. 1143
- Risk for Infection, p. 1160
- Anxiety related to threat to biologic, psychologic, or social integrity, p. 1125
- Compromised Family Coping related to a critically ill family member, p. 1127

BOX 35-20 **EVIDENCE-BASED PRACTICE**

Severe Sepsis and Septic Shock Management Guidelines

QSEN **A. Initial Resuscitation**

1. Protocolized, quantitative resuscitation of patients with sepsis-induced tissue hypoperfusion. Goals during first 6 hrs of resuscitation:

   a) Central venous pressure 8–12 mm Hg

   b) Mean arterial pressure (MAP) ≥ 65 mm Hg

   c) Urine output ≥ 0.5 mL/kg/hr

   d) Central venous (superior vena cava) or mixed venous oxygen saturation 70% or 65%, respectively (grade 1C).

2. In patients with elevated lactate levels, targeting resuscitation to normalize lactate (grade 2C).

B. Screening for Sepsis and Performance Improvement

1. Routine screening of potentially infected seriously ill patients for severe sepsis to allow earlier implementation of therapy (grade 1C).

2. Hospital–based performance improvement efforts in severe sepsis (UG).

C. Diagnosis

1. Cultures before antimicrobial therapy if delay is <45 min in the start of antimicrobial(s) (grade 1C). ≥2 sets of blood cultures (aerobic and anaerobic) with at least 1 drawn percutaneously and 1 drawn through each vascular access device, unless the device was inserted <48 hrs (grade 1C).

2. 1,3 beta-D-glucan assay (grade 2B), mannan and anti-mannan antibody assays (2C), if available and invasive candidiasis is in differential diagnosis.

3. Imaging studies to confirm a potential source of infection (UG).

D. Antimicrobial Therapy

1. Goal: IV antimicrobials within first hour of septic shock (grade 1B) and severe sepsis without septic shock (grade 1C).

2a. Initial empiric anti-infective therapy of drug(s) active against all likely pathogens and that penetrate in adequately into sepsis source tissues (grade 1B).

2b. Antimicrobial regimen reassessed daily for potential deescalation (grade 1B).

3. Low procalcitonin levels or similar biomarkers assist clinicians in discontinuation of therapy in patients who initially appeared septic, but have no subsequent evidence of infection (grade 2C).

4a. Combination therapy for neutropenic patients with severe sepsis (grade 2B) and for patients with difficult-to-treat, multidrugresistant bacterial pathogens (grade 2B). For patients with severe infections associated with respiratory failure and septic shock, combination therapy with an extended spectrum beta-lactam and either an aminoglycoside or a fluoroquinolone (for *P. aeruginosa* bacteremia) (grade 2B). A combination of beta-lactam and macrolide for patients with septic shock from bacteremic *Streptococcus pneumoniae* infections (grade 2B).

4b. Combination therapy should not be administered for >3–5 days. Deescalation to most appropriate single therapy should be performed as soon as the susceptibility profile is known (grade 2B).

5. Duration of therapy typically 7–10 days; longer courses may be appropriate in patients who have a slow clinical response, undrainable foci of infection, bacteremia with *S. aureus;* and some fungal and viral infections or immunologic deficiencies (grade 2C).

6. Antiviral therapy initiated as early as possible in patients with severe sepsis or septic shock of viral origin (grade 2C).

7. Antimicrobial agents should not be used in patients with severe inflammatory states determined to be of noninfectious cause (UG).

E. Source Control

1. Specific anatomical diagnosis and emergent source control should be diagnosed or excluded as rapidly as possible; source control intervention should be undertaken <12 hr after diagnosis, if feasible (grade 1C).

2. When source is potentially infected peripancreatic necrosis, definitive intervention is best delayed until after adequate demarcation of viable tissues (grade 2B).

3. For source control in severely septic patients, effective interventions associated with the least physiologic insult should be used (UG).

4. If IV access devices are possible sources, they should be removed promptly after other vascular access has been established (UG).

F. Infection Prevention

1a. Selective oral and digestive decontamination should be considered to reduce the incidence. of ventilator-associated pneumonia; this can be instituted in settings where it is effective (grade 2B).

1b. Oral chlorhexidine gluconate be used to reduce risk of ventilator-associated pneumonia in ICU patients with severe sepsis (grade 2B).

G. Fluid Therapy of Severe Sepsis

1. Crystalloids initially in resuscitation of severe sepsis and septic shock (grade 1B).

2. Against hydroxyethyl starches for resuscitation of severe sepsis and septic shock (grade 1B).

3. Albumin in resuscitation of severe sepsis and septic shock when patients require substantial crystalloids (grade 2C).

4. Initial fluid challenge (to a minimum of 30 mL/kg of crystalloids) in patients with sepsis-induced tissue hypoperfusion with suspicion of hypovolemia. More rapid administration and greater amounts may be needed in some (grade 1C).

5. Fluid challenge technique be applied wherein fluid administration is continued if there is hemodynamic improvement based on dynamic or static variables (UG).

H. Vasopressors

1. Vasopressor therapy initially to target mean arterial pressure (MAP) of 65 mm Hg (grade 1C).

2. Norepinephrine (NE) as first choice vasopressor (grade 1B).

3. Epinephrine (added to and potentially substituted for norepinephrine) when additional agent is needed to maintain adequate BP (grade 2B).

4. Vasopressin 0.03 units/minute can be added to NE to raise MAP or decrease NE dosage (UG).

5. Low dose vasopressin not recommended as the single initial vasopressor for treatment of sepsis-induced hypotension. Vasopressin doses >0.03-0.04 units/minute should be reserved for salvage therapy (UG).

6. Dopamine as an alternative to norepinephrine only in highly selected patients (grade 2C).

7. Phenylephrine not recommended in the treatment of septic shock except where (a) norepinephrine is associated with serious arrhythmias, (b) cardiac output is high and BP persistently low or (c) as salvage therapy when combined inotrope/vasopressor drugs and low dose vasopressin have failed to achieve MAP target (grade 1C).

8. Low-dose dopamine should not be used for renal protection (grade 1A).

9. All patients requiring vasopressors have an arterial catheter placed as soon as practical (UG).

I. Inotropic Therapy

1. A trial of dobutamine infusion up to 20 mcg/kg/min be administered or added to vasopressor (if in use) in the presence of (a) myocardial dysfunction, or (b) ongoing signs of hypoperfusion, despite adequate intravascular volume and adequate MAP (grade 1C).

2. Not using a strategy to increase cardiac index to predetermined supranormal levels (grade 1B).

J. Corticosteroids

1. Do not use IV hydrocortisone to treat adults if adequate fluid resuscitation and vasopressor therapy are able to restore hemodynamic stability. Otherwise, IV hydrocortisone alone at a dose of 200 mg per day (grade 2C) is suggested.

2. Do not use ACTH stimulation test to identify adults who should receive hydrocortisone (grade 2B).

3. If used, hydrocortisone tapered when vasopressors no longer required (grade 2D).

4. Do not use corticosteroids for treatment of sepsis without shock (grade 1D).

5. When hydrocortisone is given, use continuous flow (grade 2D).

K. Blood Product Administration

1. Once tissue hypoperfusion has resolved (in absence of extenuating circumstances), red blood cell transfusion is recommended only when Hgb decreases to <7.0 g/dL to target a Hgb concentration of 7.0 –9.0 g/dL in adults (grade 1B).

BOX 35-20   EVIDENCE-BASED PRACTICE

Severe Sepsis and Septic Shock Management Guidelines—cont'd

2. Do not use erythropoietin to treat anemia associated with severe sepsis (grade 1B).
3. Do not use fresh frozen plasma to correct laboratory clotting abnormalities in the absence of bleeding or planned invasive procedures (grade 2D).
4. Do not use antithrombin for treatment of severe sepsis and septic shock (grade 1B).
5. In patients with severe sepsis, administer platelets prophylactically when <10,000/mm^3 (10 x 10^9/L) in absence of apparent bleeding. Prophylactic platelet transfusion suggested when <20,000/mm^3 (20 x 10^9/L) if patient has significant risk of bleeding. Higher platelet counts (≥50,000/mm^3 [50 x 10^9/L]) advised for active bleeding, surgery, or invasive procedures (grade 2D).

L.   Immunoglobulins
1. Do not use IV immunoglobulins in adults with severe sepsis or septic shock (grade 2B).

M.   Selenium
1. Do not use IV selenium for treatment of severe sepsis (grade 2C).

N.   Mechanical Ventilation of Sepsis-Induced Acute Respiratory Distress Syndrome (ARDS)
1. Target tidal volume of 6 mL/kg predicted body weight in patients with sepsis-induced ARDS (grade 1A vs. 12 mL/kg).
2. Measure plateau pressures in patients with ARDS. Initial upper limit goal in a passively inflated lung is ≤30 cm H$_2$O (grade 1B).
3. Apply positive end-expiratory pressure (PEEP) to avoid alveolar collapse at end expiration (grade 1B).
4. Use strategies based on higher levels of PEEP for patients with sepsis-induced moderate or severe ARDS (grade 2C).
5. Use recruitment maneuvers in sepsis patients with severe refractory hypoxemia (grade 2C).
6. Use prone positioning in sepsis-induced ARDS patients with a Pao$_2$/Fio$_2$ ratio ≤100 mm Hg (grade 2B).
7. Maintain mechanically ventilated sepsis patients with head of bed elevated 30-45° to limit aspiration risk and prevent development of ventilator-associated pneumonia (grade 1B).
8. Use noninvasive mask ventilation (NIV) in that minority of sepsis-induced ARDS patients in whom the benefits of NIV have been carefully considered (grade 2B).
9. Put a weaning protocol in place. Mechanically ventilated patients with severe sepsis should undergo spontaneous breathing trials regularly to evaluate ability to discontinue mechanical ventilation when they: a) are arousable; b) are hemodynamically stable (without vasopressor agents); c) have no new potentially serious conditions; d) have low ventilator and end-expiratory pressure requirements; and e) have low Fio$_2$ requirements that can be met with a face mask or nasal cannula. If spontaneous breathing trial is successful, consider extubation (grade 1A).
10. Do not routinely use pulmonary artery catheter for patients with sepsis-induced ARDS (grade 1A).
11. Use a conservative fluid strategy for patients with established sepsis-induced ARDS who do not have evidence of tissue hypoperfusion (grade 1C).
12. In the absence of specific indications, do not use beta 2-agonists for treatment of sepsis-induced ARDS (grade 1B).

O.   Sedation, Analgesia, and Neuromuscular Blockade in Sepsis
1. Continuous or intermittent sedation should be minimized in mechanically ventilated sepsis patients, targeting specific titration endpoints (grade 1B).
2. Avoid neuromuscular blocking agents (NMBAs) if possible in septic patients *without ARDS* due to risk of prolonged neuromuscular blockade following discontinuation. If NMBAs must be maintained, use either intermittent bolus as required or continuous infusion with train-of-four monitoring (grade 1C).
3. Use a short course of NMBA ≤48 hours for patients *with* early sepsis-induced ARDS and Pao$_2$/Fio$_2$ < 150 mm Hg (grade 2C).

P.   Glucose Control
1. A protocolized approach to management in ICU patients with severe sepsis commencing insulin dosing when 2 consecutive blood glucose levels are >180 mg/dL. Approach should target an upper blood glucose ≤180 mg/dL (grade 1A).
2. Blood glucose values should be monitored every 1–2 hrs until glucose values and insulin infusion rates stabilize, then every 4 hr, thereafter (grade 1C).
3. Glucose levels obtained with point-of-care testing of capillary blood should be interpreted with caution (UG).

Q.   Renal Replacement Therapy
1. Continuous renal replacement therapies and intermittent hemodialysis are equivalent in severe sepsis and acute renal failure (grade 2B).
2. Use continuous therapies to facilitate management of fluid balance in hemodynamically unstable septic patients (grade 2D).

R.   Bicarbonate Therapy
1. Do not use sodium bicarbonate therapy for improving hemodynamics or reducing vasopressor requirements in patients with hypoperfusion-induced lactic acidemia with pH ≥7.15 (grade 2B).

S.   Deep Vein Thrombosis Prophylaxis
1. Patients with severe sepsis should receive daily pharmacoprophylaxis against venous thromboembolism (grade 1B). Accomplish with daily subcutaneous low-molecular weight heparin (LMWH) (grade 1B vs. twice daily UFH, grade 2C vs. three times daily UFH). If creatinine clearance <30 mL/min, use dalteparin (grade 1A) or another form of LMWH that has a low degree of renal metabolism (grade 2C) or UFH (grade 1A).
2. Treat patients with severe sepsis with combination of pharmacologic therapy and intermittent pneumatic compression devices if possible (grade 2C).
3. Do not use pharmacoprophylaxis in septic patients who have a contraindication for heparin use (grade 1B).Use mechanical prophylactic treatment (grade 2C), unless contraindicated. When risk decreases, start pharmacoprophylaxis (grade 2C).

T.   Stress Ulcer Prophylaxis
1. Give stress ulcer prophylaxis using H2 blocker or proton pump inhibitor to patients with severe sepsis/septic shock who have bleeding risk factors (grade 1B).
2. If used, proton pump inhibitors preferred over H2RA (grade 2D)
3. Patients without risk factors do not receive prophylaxis (grade 2B).

U.   Nutrition
1. Administer oral or enteral feedings rather than either complete fasting or provision of only IV glucose within the first 48 hours after diagnosis of severe sepsis/septic shock (grade 2C).
2. Avoid mandatory full caloric feeding in first week. Suggest low dose feeding, advancing only as tolerated (grade 2B).
3. Use IV glucose and enteral nutrition rather than total parenteral nutrition alone or parenteral nutrition in conjunction with enteral feeding in the first 7 days after diagnosis of severe sepsis/septic shock (grade 2B).
4. Use nutrition with no specific immunomodulating supplementation in patients with severe sepsis (grade 2C).

V.   Setting Goals of Care
1. Discuss goals and prognosis with patients and families (grade 1B).
2. Incorporate goals into treatment and end-of-life care planning (grade 1B).
3. Address goals as early as feasible, but no later than within 72 hours of ICU admission (grade 2C).

UG, Ungraded.
Data from Dellinger RP, Levy MM, Rhodes A, et al. Surviving Sepsis Campaign: international guidelines for management of severe sepsis and septic shock: 2012. *Crit Care Med.* 2013:41(2):580.

homeostasis cannot be maintained without intervention.[86] MODS is the major cause of death in patients cared for in critical care units. Mortality is closely linked to the number of organ systems involved. Dysfunction or failure of two or more organ systems is associated with an estimated mortality rate of 54%, which rises to 100% when five organ systems fail.[123] MODS survivors may develop generalized polyneuropathy and a chronic form of pulmonary disease from ARDS, complicating recovery. These patients often require prolonged, expensive rehabilitation.[124]

Trauma patients are particularly vulnerable to developing MODS because they often experience ischemia-reperfusion events resulting from hemorrhage, blunt trauma, or SNS-induced vasoconstriction.[125] Other high-risk patients include those who have experienced infection, a shock episode, various ischemia-reperfusion events, acute pancreatitis, sepsis, burns, aspiration, multiple blood transfusions, or surgical complications.[86] Patients age 65 years or older are at increased risk because of their decreased organ reserve and co-morbidities.[126]

Etiology

Organ dysfunction may be the direct consequence of an initial insult (Primary MODS) or can manifest latently and involve organs not directly affected in the initial insult (Secondary MODS). Patients can experience both Primary and Secondary MODS (Fig. 35-8). Primary MODS results from a well-defined insult in which organ dysfunction occurs early and is directly attributed to the insult itself. Direct insults initially cause localized inflammatory responses. Primary MODS accounts for only a small percentage of MODS cases. Examples of Primary MODS include the immediate consequences of post-traumatic pulmonary failure, thermal injuries, AKI, or invasive infections.[86] These cellular or microcirculatory insults may lead to a loss of critical organ function induced by failure of delivery of oxygen and substrates, coupled with the inability to remove end-products of metabolism. The inflammatory response in Primary MODS has a less apparent presentation and may resolve without long-term implications. However, Primary MODS may "prime" physiologic systems for a more a sustained exaggerated inflammatory response that leads to Secondary MODS.

Secondary MODS is a consequence of widespread sustained systemic inflammation that results in dysfunction of organs not involved in the initial insult. Secondary MODS develops latently after an initial insult.[86] The early impairment of organs normally involved in immunoregulatory function, such as the liver and the GI tract, intensifies the host response to the insult.[127] The initial insult may prime the inflammatory system in such a way that even a mild second insult (hit) may perpetuate a sustained hyperinflammatory response. This "two-hit hypothesis" has been increasingly recognized as an important contributor to morbidity and mortality in patients with Secondary MODS.[128]

SIRS and sepsis are common initiating events in the development of Secondary MODS. The systemic inflammatory response is an intense host response characterized by sustained generalized inflammation in organs remote from the initial insult. SIRS is widespread inflammation or clinical responses to inflammation that occur in patients suffering a variety of insults. Clinical conditions and manifestations associated with SIRS are listed in Box 35-21. These insults produce similar or identical systemic inflammatory responses, even in the absence of infection. The diagnostic criteria for SIRS has been previously addressed (Fig. 35-7). Manifestations of SIRS must represent an acute alteration from the patient's normal baseline and must not be related to other causes (e.g., neutropenia from chemotherapy). Organ dysfunction, such as ARDS, AKI, and MODS, is a complication of SIRS.[86,123] In epidemiologic studies, SIRS was found to occur in one third of all hospitalized patients, in 50% to 93% of all patients in critical care units, and in about 80% of all patients in surgical critical care units.[129-130]

When SIRS is a result of infection, the term *sepsis* is used. SIRS, sepsis, severe sepsis, and septic shock represent a hierarchical continuum of the inflammatory response to infection.[17] Infection and shock are the most common precipitating factors; however, any disease that induces a major inflammatory response can initiate the events that lead to MODS.

When inflammation is not contained locally, consequences occur systemically that lead to organ dysfunction, including intense, uncontrolled activation of inflammatory cells; direct damage of vascular endothelium; disruption of immune cell function; persistent hypermetabolism; and maldistribution of circulatory volume to organ systems. Inflammation becomes a systemic, self-perpetuating process that is inadequately controlled and results in organ dysfunction.[123]

During hypermetabolism, changes occur in cellular anabolic and catabolic function, resulting in autocatabolism. Autocatabolism manifests as a severe decrease in lean body mass, severe weight loss, anergy, and increased CO and VO_2 resulting from profound alterations in carbohydrate, protein, and fat metabolism.[123] Concurrently, GI, hepatic, and immunologic dysfunction may occur, which intensifies systemic inflammation.[131] Clinical consequences may affect gut function, wound healing, muscles wasting, host response, respiratory function, and continued promotion of the hypermetabolic response.

Not all patients develop MODS from SIRS. The development of MODS appears to be associated with failure to control the source of inflammation or infection, persistent hypoperfusion, flow-dependent oxygen consumption (VO_2), or the continued presence of necrotic tissue.[125]

Pathophysiology

Secondary MODS results from altered regulation of the patient's acute immune and inflammatory responses. Dysregulation, or failure to control the host inflammatory response, leads to the excessive production of inflammatory cells and biochemical mediators that cause widespread damage to vascular endothelium and organ damage.[123,132] The critically ill patient's compromised immune state also fosters an environment conducive to organ failure.

The definitive clinical course of secondary MODS has not been completely identified. Organ dysfunction may occur in a sequential or progressive pattern. Organ dysfunction may begin in the lungs, the most commonly affected major organ, and progress to the liver, gut, and kidneys. Cardiac and bone marrow dysfunction may follow. Neurologic and autonomic system impairment may occur and propagate the progression of organ

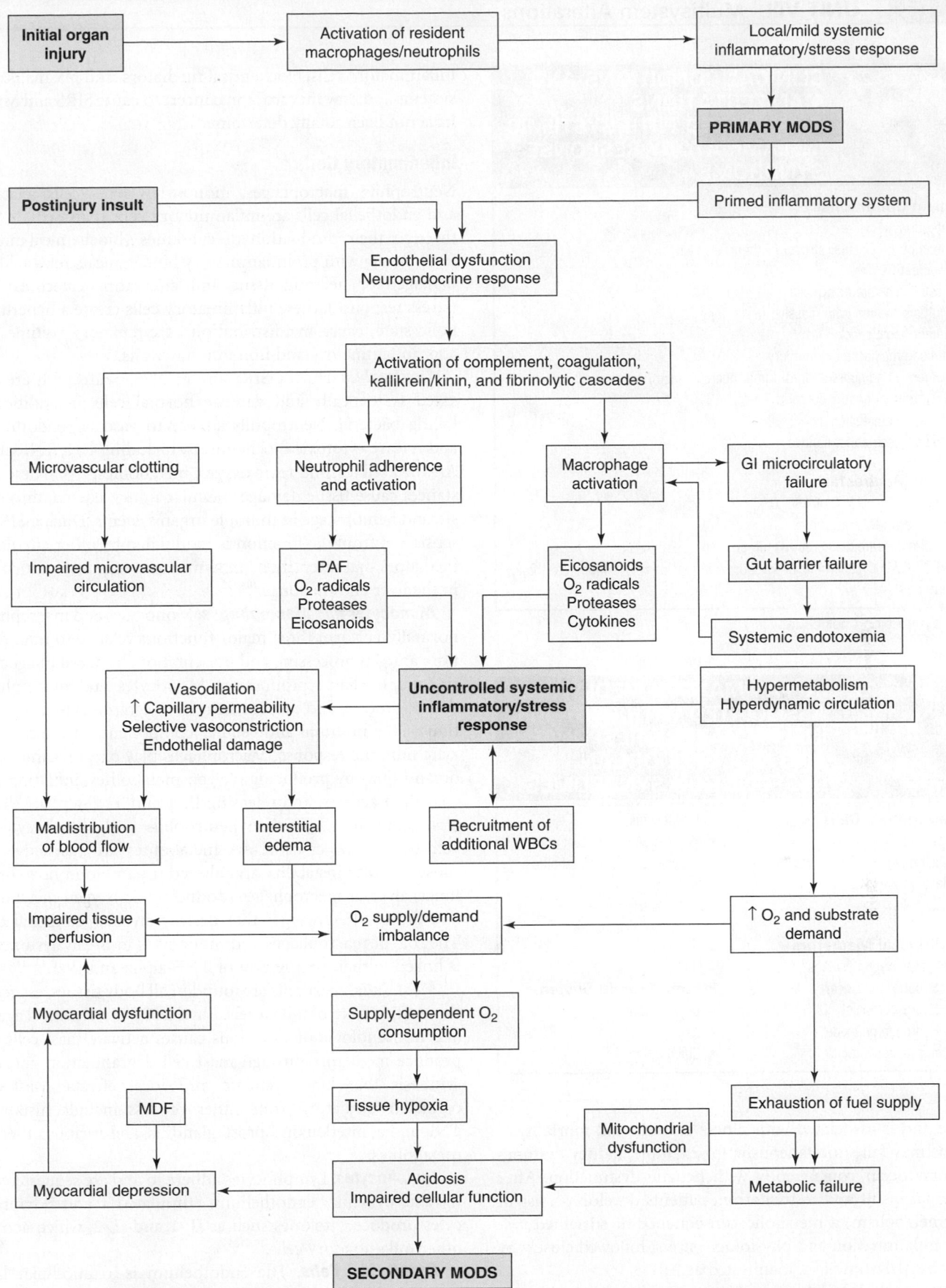

FIGURE 35-8 Pathogenesis of Multiple Organ Dysfunction Syndrome. *GI*, Gastrointestinal; *MDF*, myocardial depressant factor; *MODS*, multiple organ dysfunction syndrome; *PAF*, platelet activating factor; *WBCs*, white blood cells. (From Cheek DJ, Martin LL, Morris SE. Shock, multiple organ dysfunction syndrome, and burns in adults. In: McCance KL, Huether SE, eds. *Pathophysiology: The Biological Basis for Disease in Adults and Children*. 6th ed. St. Louis: Mosby; 2010.)

BOX 35-21   CLINICAL CONDITIONS AND MANIFESTATIONS ASSOCIATED WITH SYSTEMIC INFLAMMATORY RESPONSE SYNDROME

Clinical Conditions

- Infection
- Infection of vascular structures (heart and lungs)
- Pancreatitis
- Tissue ischemia or hypoxia
- Multiple trauma with massive tissue injury
- Hemorrhagic shock
- Immune-mediated organ injury
- Exogenous administration of tumor necrosis factor or other cytokines
- Aspiration of gastric contents
- Massive transfusion
- Host defense abnormalities

Clinical Manifestations

- Temperature >38° C or <36° C
- Heart rate >90 beats/min
- Respiratory rate >20 breaths/min or $PaCO_2$ <32 mm Hg
- WBC >12,000 cells/mm³ or <4000 cells/mm³ or >10% immature (band) forms

WBC, White blood cell count.

BOX 35-22   INFLAMMATORY MEDIATORS ASSOCIATED WITH SYSTEMIC INFLAMMATORY RESPONSE AND MULTIPLE ORGAN DYSFUNCTION SYNDROMES

Inflammatory Cells
- Neutrophils
- Macrophages or monocytes
- Mast lymphocytes
- Endothelial

Biochemical Mediators
- Reactive oxygen species
  - Superoxide radical
  - Hydroxyl radical
  - Hydrogen peroxide
- Tumor necrosis factor

- Interleukins
- Platelet activating factor
- Arachidonic acid metabolites
  - Prostaglandins
  - Leukotrienes
  - Thromboxanes
- Proteases

Plasma Protein Systems
- Complement
- Kinin
- Coagulation

failure and is associated with illness severity and mortality.[133] Organs may fail simultaneously; for example, kidney dysfunction may occur concurrently with hepatic dysfunction. After the initial insult and resuscitation, patients develop persistent hypermetabolism, a metabolic consequence of sustained systemic inflammation and physiologic stress, followed closely by pulmonary dysfunction, manifested as ARDS.

Certain cellular and biochemical activity evoke the inflammatory and immune responses implicated in SIRS and MODS. The mediators associated with SIRS and MODS can be classified as inflammatory cells, biochemical mediators, or plasma protein systems (Box 35-22). Activation of one mediator often leads to activation of another. The biologic activity of inflammatory cells, biochemical mediators, and plasma protein systems and how they work in concert to cause SIRS and MODS have not been totally determined.

Inflammatory Cells

Neutrophils, macrophages, monocytes, mast cells, platelets, and endothelial cells are inflammatory cells that mediate SIRS through their production of cytokines (biochemical mediators). Along with proinflammatory biochemicals released from damaged or necrotic tissue and circulating catecholamines (stress response), these inflammatory cells create a hypermetabolic state, cause maldistribution of circulatory volume, and alter inflammatory and immune functions.[132]

Neutrophils. During SIRS and MODS, neutrophils are activated systemically and damage normal cells in addition to killing bacteria. Neutrophils adhere to vascular endothelium and release cytotoxic biochemicals, including PAF, TNF-alpha, AA metabolites, and toxic oxygen metabolites.[123,132] These substances cause tissue damage, vascular injury, edema, thrombosis, and hemorrhage in multiple organ systems. During SIRS or sepsis, neutrophilic function is modulated by other circulating mediators that intensify its inflammatory response particularly in the liver and the lungs.[103,132]

Monocytes and Macrophages. Monocytes and macrophages normally perform three major functions relative to inflammation: antigen processing and presentation, bacterial phagocytosis, and mediator production. Monocytes and macrophages detect, process, and present antigen to lymphocytes for initiation of the humoral and cellular components of the lymphocytic immune response. Macrophages play a significant role in organ injury by producing oxygen metabolites, initiating procoagulant activity, and releasing IL-1 and TNF-alpha.[123] TNF-alpha and IL-1 stimulate neutrophils and lymphocytes to activate the AA cascade. AA metabolites are vasoactive and cause vascular instability and altered organ blood flow. In the lungs, alveolar macrophages produce toxic oxygen metabolites and proteolytic enzymes that destroy alveolar epithelial cells. The role of macrophages and monocytes in organ dysfunction is linked to their production of TNF-alpha and IL-1.[123,132]

Mast Cells. Mast cells are found in all body tissues, especially those adjacent to blood vessels. Physical injury, chemical agents, and immunologic or infectious causes activate mast cells and produce mediators through mast cell degranulation and new synthesis that have systemic and local effects. Mast–cell-regulated mediators from either process include histamine, TNF-alpha, interleukins, prostaglandins, and various other AA metabolites.[132]

Lymphocytes. Lymphocytes adhere to and are sequestered in the microvascular endothelium. Stimulated T and B lymphocytes produce cytokines such as IL-1 and IL-2, which activate other inflammatory cells.[103,123]

Endothelial Cells. The endothelium is a unicellular layer that lines the vascular system. Normally, little interaction occurs between the endothelium and leukocytes. However, during SIRS and MODS, endothelial cells become targets for leukocyte-derived mediators, and they become dysfunctional and release prothrombotic, proinflammatory, and vasoactive mediators. Endothelial damage results in the production of procoagulants such as TF, plasminogen-activating inhibitor (PAI), and prostacyclin (PGI₂), leading to the introduction of thrombin in the microvasculature. Endothelial cells manufacture chemotactic agents that attract neutrophils to areas of inflammation and endothelial injury. Collectively, these processes cause widespread endothelial destruction, intravascular coagulation, vascular instability, and permeability, which are key elements in SIRS and sepsis.[132,134]

Inflammatory mediators that cause endothelial damage include endotoxin, TNF-alpha, IL-1, and PAF. These mediators also recruit and activate neutrophils, activate complement, and perpetuate destruction of the endothelium. Endothelial cells produce and maintain a physiologic equilibrium between endothelin (the most potent vasoconstrictor known) and endothelial cell-derived relaxant factor (nitric oxide), a vasodilator.[132] An alteration in this balance leads to vascular instability, vasodilation, and the perfusion abnormalities commonly seen in patients with SIRS and MODS.[127,132,134]

Biochemical Mediators

Multiple biochemical inflammatory mediators play a role in SIRS and MODS, including proteases, TNF-alpha, interleukins, PAF, AA metabolites, and oxygen metabolites. TNF-alpha, IL-1, and IL-6 appear to be the most important cytokines associated with SIRS and MODS.[135-136]

Reactive Oxygen Species. Reactive oxygen species are produced in excessive amounts during critical illness and have been implicated in MODS.[137] Oxygen metabolites are normally produced as the result of many physiologic processes. However, the body has numerous antioxidant and enzyme systems to convert free oxygen radicals to nontoxic substances to prevent tissue injury. Excessive oxygen metabolites cause lipid peroxidation and damage to the cell membrane, activate the complement and coagulation cascades, and cause deoxyribonucleic acid (DNA) damage. Inflammatory neutrophils cause tissue injury by producing excessive numbers of reactive oxygen metabolites. Reperfusion organ injury is partially attributed to excessive oxygen metabolites. During reperfusion, severe tissue injury follows the massive production of oxygen free radicals. The organs most susceptible to injury include the small intestines, liver, lungs, heart, brain, stomach, muscle, and skin.[138]

Tumor Necrosis Factor-alpha. TNF-alpha is a polypeptide that is released from macrophages and lymphocytes in response to endotoxin, tissue injury, viral agents, and interleukins. When present in excessive amounts, TNF-alpha causes widespread destruction in most organ systems and is responsible for the pathophysiologic changes in SIRS and septic shock, including fever, hypotension, decreased organ perfusion, and increased capillary permeability.[139] TNF-alpha may precipitate organ injury by causing generalized endothelial injury, fibrin deposition, and a procoagulant state. TNF-alpha causes DIC; interstitial pneumonitis; AKI; and necrosis of the gastrointestinal tract, liver, and adrenal glands. TNF-alpha stimulates AA metabolism, the clotting cascade, and the production of PAF. Metabolically, excessive TNF-alpha causes hyperglycemia that progresses to hypoglycemia and hypertriglyceridemia. The destructive effects of TNF-alpha are exacerbated by AA metabolites and stress hormones.

Interleukins. Produced mainly by macrophages and lymphocytes, the interleukins are a class of cytokines that have biologic responses similar to that of TNF-alpha. More than 30 interleukins have been identified. Macrophages secrete substantial amounts of IL-1. IL-1 causes vascular congestion, capillary leakage, and increased coagulation, all of which are associated with SIRS and sepsis. IL-1 has profound vascular endothelial effects, stimulates the production of procoagulants by endothelial cells, increases catabolism of muscle tissue, and causes neutrophilia.[123,132]

Platelet-Activating Factor. PAF, a potent proinflammatory phospholipid, is released from inflammatory and immune cells in response to a multitude of factors or stimuli. PAF is released by platelets, mast cells, monocytes, macrophages, neutrophils, and endothelial cells. PAF has widespread effects on the heart, the vascular system, procoagulation, platelets, and the lungs. Effects of PAF include platelet aggregation, with resultant microvascular stasis and ischemia in the microvascular bed; platelet release of serotonin, which increases vascular permeability; and increased vasoconstriction from increased production of thromboxane A₂, an AA metabolite.[123]

Arachidonic Acid Metabolites. AA is a highly metabolic fatty acid that is a precursor of many biologically active substances known as *eicosanoids*. Lipid peroxidation of neutrophil cell membranes induces a release of these metabolites.[123] Select eicosanoids are implicated in the pathogenesis of SIRS and MODS. Eicosanoids contribute to organ failure by altering vascular reactivity and permeability and by fostering the accumulation and activation of inflammatory cells. Activation of the AA cascade by hypoxia, ischemia, endotoxin, catecholamines, and tissue injury produces metabolites from the cyclooxygenase and lipoxygenase pathways. AA metabolites produced through the cyclooxygenase pathway are called *prostaglandins* (PGs) and *thromboxanes* (TXs), whereas those from the lipoxygenase pathway are called *leukotrienes* (LTs). AA metabolites have profound effects on vasculature and cause vascular instability and maldistribution of blood flow. Some eicosanoids (e.g., PGH₂, TXA₂, LTD₄) are vasoconstrictors, and others (e.g., PGE₂, PGI₂) have potent vasodilatory properties. All LTs and TXA₂ enhance capillary membrane permeability and increase vascular leakage. TXA₂, PGH₂, and PGF₂ are potent platelet aggregators.[123]

Proteases. Proteases are proteolytic (protein-digesting) enzymes released from neutrophils. Proteases damage endothelium and contribute to vascular permeability and organ dysfunction.[123] One such protease, neutrophil elastase, damages lung tissue by inducing IL-8 production, attracting additional neutrophils, and stimulating mucus secretion.

Multiple clinical trials have been conducted in an attempt to stop or neutralize the sustained inflammatory response that causes organ dysfunction. These trials have included the use of corticosteroid therapy, antiendotoxin antibodies, antitumor necrosis factor monoclonal antibodies, interleukin-1 receptor antagonists, bradykinin antagonists, platelet activating factor antagonists, platelet activating factor receptor antagonists, phospholipase A2 inhibition, nitric oxide synthase inhibition, and antithrombin III. None of trials have demonstrated improved clinical outcomes in patients with sepsis and SIRS.[90]

Assessment and Diagnosis

Secondary MODS is a systemic disease with organ-specific manifestations. Organ dysfunction is influenced by numerous factors, including organ host defense function, response time to the injury, metabolic requirements, organ vasculature response to vasoactive medications, organ sensitivity to damage, and physiologic reserve. The responses of the gastrointestinal, hepatobiliary, cardiovascular, pulmonary, renal, and hematologic systems are discussed in the following paragraphs. Clinical manifestations of organ dysfunction are outlined in Box 35-23.

Gastrointestinal Dysfunction

The gastrointestinal tract plays an important role in MODS. Gastrointestinal organs normally have immunoregulatory functions, and the gastrointestinal tract contains about 70% to 80% of the immunologic tissue of the entire body. A normally functioning gastrointestinal tract prevents bacteria from entering the systemic circulation.[123] Normal gut flora and gut environment are altered in patients with severe SIRS. Healthy probiotics (e.g., *Bifidobacterium, Lacto bacillus*) are decreased in a SIRS state, and pathogenic organisms (e.g., *Staphylococcus, Pseudomonas*) proliferate.[131]

With microcirculatory failure to the gastrointestinal tract, the gut's barrier function may be lost, which leads to bacterial translocation, sustained inflammation, endogenous endotoxemia, and MODS.[123,132] Hypoperfusion and shocklike states damage the normal gastrointestinal mucosa barrier by decreasing mesenteric blood flow, leading to hypoperfusion of the villi, mucosal edema, ischemic necrosis, sloughing of the mucosa, and malabsorption. The gastrointestinal tract is extremely vulnerable to oxygen metabolite-induced reperfusion injury. Endothelial injury and gastrointestinal lesions occur in response

---

BOX 35-23 CLINICAL MANIFESTATIONS OF ORGAN DYSFUNCTION

Gastrointestinal
- Abdominal distention and ascites
- Intolerance to enteral feedings
- Paralytic ileus
- Upper or lower gastrointestinal bleeding
- Diarrhea
- Ischemic colitis
- Mucosal ulceration
- Decreased bowel sounds
- Bacterial overgrowth in stool

Liver
- Jaundice
- Hepatomegaly
- Increased serum bilirubin (hyperbilirubinemia)
- Increased liver enzymes
- Increased serum ammonia
- Decreased serum albumin
- Decreased serum transferrin

Gallbladder
- Right upper quadrant tenderness or pain
- Abdominal distention
- Unexplained fever
- Decreased bowel sounds

Metabolic and Nutritional
- Decreased lean body mass
- Muscle wasting
- Severe weight loss
- Negative nitrogen balance
- Hyperglycemia
- Hypertriglyceridemia
- Increased serum lactate
- Decreased serum albumin, serum transferrin, prealbumin
- Decreased retinol-binding protein

Immune
- Infection
- Decreased lymphocyte count
- Anergy

Pulmonary
- Tachypnea
- Acute lung injury pattern of respiratory failure (dyspnea, patchy infiltrates, refractory hypoxemia, respiratory acidosis, abnormal O_2 indexes)
- Pulmonary hypertension

Kidney
- Decreased glomerular filtration rate/creatinine clearance
- Increased serum creatinine, blood urea nitrogen levels
- Oliguria, anuria, or polyuria consistent with prerenal azotemia or acute kidney injury
- Urinary indexes consistent with prerenal azotemia or acute kidney injury
- Electrolyte imbalance

Cardiovascular
Hyperdynamic
- Decreased pulmonary capillary occlusion pressure
- Decreased systemic vascular resistance
- Decreased right atrial pressure
- Decreased left ventricular stroke work index
- Increased oxygen consumption
- Increased cardiac output, cardiac index, heart rate

Hypodynamic
- Increased systemic vascular resistance
- Increased right atrial pressure
- Increased left ventricular stroke work index
- Decreased oxygen delivery and consumption
- Decreased cardiac output and cardiac index

Central Nervous System
- Lethargy
- Altered level of consciousness
- Fever
- Hepatic encephalopathy

Coagulation or Hematologic
- Thrombocytopenia
- Disseminated intravascular coagulation

Modified from Cheek DJ, et al. Shock, multiple organ dysfunction syndrome, and burns in adults. In: McCance KL, et al, eds. *Pathophysiology: the Biologic Basis for Disease in Adults and Children.* 6th ed. St. Louis: Mosby; 2010.

to mediator-induced tissue damage. Ischemic events and the absence of feedings can disrupt the normal metabolism of the gastric or intestinal lumen and the normal protective function of the gut barrier.[119,127]

The translocation of gastrointestinal bacteria through a "leaky gut" into the systemic circulation initiates and perpetuates an inflammatory focus in the critically ill patient.[127] The gastrointestinal tract harbors organisms that present an inflammatory focus when carried from the gut via the intestinal lymphatics. After hemorrhagic shock, trauma, or a major burn injury, gut-released proinflammatory and tissue injurious factors may lead to acute lung injury, bone marrow failure, myocardial dysfunction, neutrophil activation, RBC injury, and endothelial cell activation and injury. These factors, released from the gut, and carried in the mesenteric lymphatics, are capable of causing a septic state and Secondary MODS. In summary, the "gut-lymph hypothesis" proposes that gut ischemia-reperfusion injury leads to loss of a gut protective barrier, bacterial translocation and a gut inflammatory response. Gut-derived inflammatory factors are carried in the mesenteric lymph leading to a septic state and distant organ failure and MODS.[2]

Lastly, the oropharynx of the critically ill patient also becomes colonized with potentially pathogenic organisms from the gastrointestinal tract. Pulmonary aspiration of colonized secretions presents an inflammatory focus that can contribute to concomitant pulmonary dysfunction.[140]

Hepatobiliary Dysfunction

The liver plays a vital role in host homeostasis related to the acute inflammatory response. The liver responds to sustained inflammation by selectively altering carbohydrate, fat, and protein metabolism. Consequently, hepatic dysfunction threatens the patient's survival. The liver normally controls the inflammatory response by several mechanisms. Kupffer cells, which are hepatic macrophages, detoxify substances that may normally induce systemic inflammation and vasoactive substances that cause hemodynamic instability. Failure to detoxify gram-negative bacteria causes endotoxemia, perpetuates SIRS, and may lead to MODS. The liver also produces proteins and antiproteases to control the inflammatory response; however, hepatic dysfunction limits this response.

Common causes of liver failure in critically ill patients are infection-related cholestasis and hepatocellular injury in response to toxins and to toxins themselves. In infection-related cholestasis, bacterial toxins and released cytokines affect the uptake and excretion of bilirubin leading to jaundice. In hepatocellular injury, endotoxins and bacteria are phagocytized by Kupffer cells that release hepatotoxic substances that cause cellular damage. Hepatic dysfunction may also occur with organ hypoperfusion, hemolysis, and with hepatotoxic medications. Measurements of liver enzymes, bilirubin, ammonia, and liver-produced proteins should be carefully monitored.[141]

The liver and gallbladder are extremely vulnerable to ischemic injury from organ hypoperfusion. Ischemic hepatitis occurs after a prolonged period of physiologic shock and is associated with centrilobular hepatocellular necrosis. The degree of hepatic damage is related directly to the severity and duration of the shock episode. Anoxic and reperfusion injuries damage hepatocytes and the vascular endothelium. Patients at high risk for ischemic hepatitis after a hypotensive event include those with a history of heart failure or cardiac dysrhythmias. Clinical manifestations of hepatic insufficiency are evident 1 to 2 days after the insult. Jaundice and transient elevations in serum transaminase and bilirubin levels occur. Hyperbilirubinemia results from hepatocyte anoxic injury and an increased production of bilirubin from hemoglobin catabolism. Ischemic hepatitis may resolve spontaneously or progress to acute liver failure. Although ischemic hepatitis is not a life-threatening complication, it can contribute to morbidity and mortality as a component of MODS. Acute liver failure is discussed further in Chapter 30.

Acalculous cholecystitis manifests 3 to 4 weeks after an insult. Its pathogenesis is unclear, but it may be related to ischemic reperfusion injury, PEEP greater than 5 cm H_2O, volume depletion, total parenteral nutrition (TPN), opioids, and cystic duct obstruction as a result of hyperviscous bile.[142] Visceral hypotension and vasoactive medication use may decrease perfusion of the gallbladder mucosa contributing to ischemia. Bacterial invasion may stimulate activation of factor XII and initiate the coagulation pathway.[142] Clinical manifestations of acalculous cholecystitis may mimic acute cholecystitis with gallstones. However, patients may demonstrate vague symptoms, including right upper quadrant pain and tenderness. Critical to the detection of acalculous cholecystitis is the recognition of abdominal distention, unexplained fever, loss of bowel sounds, and a sudden deterioration in the patient's condition. About 50% of patients with acalculous cholecystitis have gallbladder gangrene, and 10% have gallbladder perforation, requiring a cholecystectomy.[142]

Pulmonary Dysfunction

The lungs are frequent and early target organs for mediator-induced injury and are usually the first organs affected in the progression of SIRS to MODS.[143] ARDS is the pulmonary manifestation of MODS. Patients who develop MODS usually have pulmonary symptoms; however, not all patients with ARDS develop secondary MODS. ARDS patients who develop SIRS or sepsis concurrently with acute respiratory failure are at the greatest risk for MODS.[144]

ARDS associated with MODS usually occurs 24 to 72 hours after the initial insult. Patients initially exhibit a low-grade fever, tachycardia, dyspnea, and mental confusion. As dyspnea progresses, hypoxemia, and the work of breathing increase, intubation and mechanical ventilation are required. ARDS results in refractory hypoxemia caused by intrapulmonary shunting, decreased pulmonary compliance, and altered airway mechanics; there usually is radiographic evidence of noncardiogenic pulmonary edema.[145]

Mediators associated with ARDS include inflammatory cells such as polymorphonuclear cells, macrophages, monocytes, endothelial cells, and mast cells; and biochemical mediators such as AA metabolites, toxic oxygen metabolites, proteases, TNF, platelet activating factor (PAF), and interleukins. Intense mediator activity damages the pulmonary vascular endothelium and the alveolar epithelium, resulting in surfactant deficiency, mild pulmonary hypertension, and increased pulmonary capillary permeability leading to increased lung water (noncardiogenic pulmonary edema).[103,145] ARDS is discussed further in Chapter 20.

Kidney Dysfunction

Acute kidney injury (AKI) is a common manifestation of MODS. The kidney is highly vulnerable to hypoperfusion and reperfusion injury. Consequently, kidney ischemic-reperfusion injury may be a major cause of kidney dysfunction in MODS. Mechanisms of cellular death may differ in septic versus non–septic-induced AKI. Acute tubular apoptosis may occur in septic AKI, while nonseptic AKI may be associated with necrosis.[146]

The patient with AKI may demonstrate oliguria or anuria resulting from decreased renal perfusion and relative hypovolemia. Early oliguria is likely caused by decreases in renal perfusion related to shocklike states; late oliguria is typically a sign of evolving kidney injury and ischemia. Renal function may become refractory to diuretics, fluid challenges, and vasoactive medications. Prerenal oliguria may progress to AKI, necessitating continuous renal replacement therapies. The frequent use of nephrotoxic medications also intensifies the risk of AKI.

Early recognition of AKI is imperative. However, the lack of early and reliable biomarkers for AKI leads to a delay in initiating treatment. The instability of kidney function in the critically ill patient decreases the validity of measures that are based on creatinine assessment. An elevated serum creatinine level is usually a late sign, but it is typically accepted as the index for renal dysfunction. However, serum creatinine concentrations can vary for reasons other than renal function in organ failure patients and are rarely at a steady state.[146] It may be preferable to use either 8-, 12-, or 24-hr urinary creatinine clearance values to estimate GFR in critically ill patients especially when determining medication dosages.[141] Additional signs of kidney impairment may include decreased erythropoietin-induced anemia, vitamin D malabsorption, and altered fluid and electrolyte balance. AKI is discussed further in Chapter 27.

Cardiovascular and Hematologic System Dysfunction

The initial cardiovascular response in SIRS or sepsis is myocardial depression; decreased RAP and SVR; and increased venous capacitance, CO, and heart rate. Despite an increased CO, myocardial depression occurs and is accompanied by decreased SVR, increased heart rate, and ventricular dilation. These compensatory mechanisms help maintain CO during the early phase of SIRS or sepsis. An inability to increase CO in response to a low SVR may indicate myocardial failure or inadequate fluid resuscitation, and it is associated with increased mortality. VO_2 may be twice that of normal and may be flow dependent.[147]

As MODS progresses, heart failure develops. Cardiac dysfunction is characterized by ventricular dilation, decreased diastolic compliance, and decreased systolic contractile function. Cardiovascular function becomes vasopressor dependent. Heart failure may be caused by immune mediators, TNF-alpha, acidosis, or myocardial depressant factor, a substance secreted by the pancreas. Myocardial depression is exacerbated by myocardial hypoperfusion from a low CO state and persistent lactic acidosis. Cardiogenic shock and biventricular failure occur and lead to death.[147] Heart failure is discussed further in Chapter 15, and more information on cardiogenic shock can be found earlier in this chapter.

The most common manifestations of hematologic dysfunction in sepsis or MODS are thrombocytopenia, coagulation abnormalities, and anemia.[148] The most severe is coagulation system dysfunction manifesting as DIC. DIC is a complex, consumptive coagulopathy that occurs in patients with a variety of disorders, including sepsis, tissue injury, and shock; it is overstimulation of the normal coagulation process. DIC results simultaneously in microvascular clotting and hemorrhage in organ systems, leading to thrombosis and fibrinolysis in life-threatening proportions. Clotting factor derangement leads to further inflammation and further thrombosis. Microvascular damage leads to further organ injury. Cell injury and damage to the endothelium activate the intrinsic or extrinsic coagulation pathways.[97,134] Low platelet counts and elevated D-dimer concentrations and fibrinogen degradation products are clinical indicators of DIC. DIC is discussed further in Chapter 38.

Medical Management

The patient with MODS requires multidisciplinary collaboration in clinical management, including fluid resuscitation and hemodynamic support (when appropriate), prevention and treatment of infection, maintenance of tissue oxygenation, nutritional and metabolic support, comfort and emotional support, and support for individual organ function. The use of investigational therapies may be part of the patient's clinical management.

Identification and Treatment of Infection

Identification and treatment of the underlying source of inflammation or infection are important ways to reduce mortality. Medical and surgical intervention to remove sources of infection or contamination may limit the inflammatory response and improve chances of recovery. Surgical procedures such as early fracture stabilization, removal of infected organs or tissue, and burn excision are helpful. Appropriate antibiotics are needed if the cause cannot be removed by surgical débridement or incision and draining.[143]

Antibiotic management in septic patients with MODS remains a challenge.[141] Ulldemonlins and colleagues have provided antibiotic dosing recommendation for critically ill patients with MODS. They purport that tissue hypoperfusion during the early phases of sepsis/septic shock may lead to decreased antibiotic tissue concentrations. Therefore, "higher-than-standard" front-loading doses of *hydrophilic* antibiotics may be considered in the initial course of treatment because their volume of distribution will be significantly increased with tissue hypoperfusion. Hydrophilic antibiotics include beta-lactams, aminoglycosides, and glycopeptides. Hydrophilic antibiotics are cleared mostly by glomerular filtration and tubular secretion. Therefore, patients with renal dysfunction will require maintenance dose reductions or extended dosing intervals to prevent nephrotoxicity due to decreased drug elimination.[141]

Commonly administered *lipophilic* antibiotics include fluoroquinolones, lincosamides, and nitroimidazoles. As these antibiotics are cleared by the liver, kidney, or by both organs, attention to renal and hepatic function for initial and maintenance dosing is needed. In addition, total body weight, especially with obese patients, should be considered with front-loading administration of fluoroquinolones and lincosamides. Macrolides are *lipophilic* antibiotics and allow normal initial and maintenance dosing.

Underdosing of antibiotics may occur with tissue hypoperfusion and with decreased protein binding of highly bound antibiotics in patients with hepatic dysfunction. Overdosing may occur in patients with renal dysfunction due to decreased elimination of *hydrophilic* antibiotics and in hepatic dysfunction due to decreased metabolism of *lipophilic* antibiotics.

Other timely interventions, such as prevention of skin ulceration and early nutritional support, may improve outcomes. Regardless of the identification of potential risk factors, clinical markers, bacterial contaminants, and investigative approaches for detection and prevention, treatment remains largely supportive, and little improvement in the mortality rate has been appreciated.[90]

Maintenance of Tissue Oxygenation

Normally under steady state conditions, VO_2 is relatively constant and independent of oxygen delivery (DO_2) unless delivery becomes severely impaired. The relationship is called *supply-independent oxygen consumption*. Consequently a percentage of oxygen is not used (physiologic reserve). Patients with SIRS/MODS often develop supply-dependent oxygen consumption in which VO_2 becomes dependent on DO_2, rather than demand, at a normal or high DO_2. When VO_2 does not equal demand, a tissue oxygen debt develops, subjecting organs to failure.[143]

Hypoperfusion and resultant organ hypoxemia often occur in patients at high risk for MODS, subjecting essential organs to failure. Effective fluid resuscitation and early recognition of flow-dependent VO_2 is essential, and patients at risk for MODS require hemodynamic monitoring, frequent measurements or surrogate measurements of DO_2 and VO_2, and serum lactate levels to guide therapy. Serum lactate levels provide information regarding the severity of impaired perfusion and the presence of lactic acidosis and differ significantly in MODS survivors and nonsurvivors. Failure to maintain adequate oxygenation to vital organs results in organ dysfunction. Despite adequate DO_2, VO_2 may not meet the needs of the body during MODS.

Patients with ARDS, MODS, or SIRS frequently manifest supply-dependent oxygen consumption and are unable to use oxygen appropriately despite normal delivery.[143] Interventions that decrease oxygen demand and increase oxygen delivery are essential. Sedation, mechanical ventilation, rest, and temperature and pain control may be able to decrease oxygen demand.[133] Oxygen delivery maybe increased by maintaining normal hematocrit and Pao_2 levels, using PEEP, increasing preload or myocardial contractility to enhance CO, or reducing afterload to increase CO. Various methods of kinetic or prone therapies are available and may enhance alveolar recruitment, improve oxygenation delivery, and decrease other potential complications.

Nutritional and Metabolic Support

Hypermetabolism in SIRS or MODS results in profound weight loss, cachexia, and loss of organ function. The goal of nutritional support is the preservation of organ structure and function. Although nutritional support may not definitely alter the course of organ dysfunction, it prevents generalized nutritional deficiencies and preserves gut integrity. Enteral nutrition may exert a physiologic effect that down-regulates the systemic immune response and reduces oxidative stress.[149] The enteral route is preferable to parenteral support.[38] Enteral feedings are given distal to the pylorus to reduce the risk of pulmonary aspiration. Enteral feedings may limit bacterial translocation. In addition to early nutritional support, the pharmacologic properties of enteral feeding formulas may limit SIRS for selected critical care populations. Supplementation of enteral feedings with glutamine may be beneficial.[91,119,144] However, the optimum formulation of nutritional support and the use of immune-modulating supplements to improve outcomes in patients with or at risk for MODS continues to be the subject of much debate and study.[38,91,119] Nutritional support is discussed further in Chapter 8.

Nursing Management

Preventive measures include a multitude of assessment strategies to detect early organ manifestations of this syndrome. Patients who continue to experience sites of inflammation, septic foci, and inadequate tissue perfusion may be at higher risk. Hand hygiene, aseptic technique, and an understanding of how microorganisms can invade the body are essential components of preventive nursing care.

Nursing management of the patient with MODS incorporates a variety of nursing diagnoses (Box 35-24). Nursing interventions include preventing development of infection, facilitating oxygen delivery and limiting tissue oxygen demand, facilitating nutritional support, providing comfort and emotional support, and preventing and maintaining surveillance for complications.

◎ BOX 35-24 NURSING DIAGNOSES

Multiple Organ Dysfunction Syndrome

- Decreased Cardiac Output related to alterations in preload, p. 1128
- Decreased Cardiac Output related to alterations in afterload, p. 1128
- Decreased Cardiac Output related to alterations in contractility, p. 1128
- Impaired Gas Exchange related to ventilation/perfusion mismatching or intrapulmonary shunting, p. 1144
- Imbalanced Nutrition: Less Than Body Requirements related to increased metabolic demands or lack of exogenous nutrients, p. 1143
- Risk for Infection, p. 1160
- Acute Pain related to transmission and perception of cutaneous, visceral, muscular, or ischemic impulses, p. 1123
- Acute Confusion related to sensory overload, sensory deprivation, and sleep pattern disturbance, p. 1120
- Anxiety related to threat to biologic, psychologic, or social integrity, p. 1125
- Compromised Family Coping related to a critically ill family member, p. 1127

Patients are assessed closely for inflammation and infection. Subtle expressions of infection warrant investigation. Nursing measures include strict adherence to standards of practice to prevent infection. Practices related to infection control with invasive hemodynamic monitoring, urinary catheters, endotracheal tubes, intracranial pressure monitoring devices, TPN, and wound care must be stringent to prevent further infection. Prevention of a concomitant ventilator-associated pneumonia or aspiration pneumonia is a priority.[17,150]

Measures to limit tissue oxygen consumption include administering analgesics and sedatives, positioning the patient for comfort, limiting activities, offering support to reduce anxiety, providing a calm and quiet environment, and educating the patient and family about the condition. Measures to enhance tissue oxygen supply include administering supplemental oxygen, monitoring the patient's respiratory status, and administering prescribed fluids and medications.

Collaborative management of the patient with MODS is outlined in Box 35-25.

BOX 35-25　COLLABORATIVE MANAGEMENT

Multiple Organ Dysfunction Syndrome

- Support oxygen transport:
  - Establish a patent airway.
  - Initiate mechanical ventilation.
  - Administer oxygen.
  - Administer fluids (crystalloids, colloids, blood, and other blood products).
  - Administer vasoactive medications.
  - Administer positive inotropic medications.
  - Administer antidysrhythmic medications.
  - Ensure sufficient hemoglobin and hematocrit.
- Support oxygen use:
  - Identify and correct cause of lactic acidosis.
  - Ensure adequate organ and extremity perfusion.
- Decrease oxygen demand:
  - Administer sedation or paralytics.
  - Administer antipyretics and external cooling measures.
  - Administer pain medications.
- Identify the underlying cause of inflammation and treat accordingly:
  - Remove infected organs or tissue.
  - Administer antibiotics.
- Initiate nutritional support.
- Treat individual organ dysfunction:
  - Gastrointestinal
  - Hepatobiliary
  - Pulmonary
  - Renal
  - Cardiovascular
  - Coagulation system
- Prevent and maintain surveillance for complications, particularly infection.
- Provide comfort and emotional support.

BOX 35-26　INTERNET RESOURCES

- American Association of Critical-Care Nurses: **http://www.aacn.org/**
- Society of Critical Care Medicine: **http://www.sccm.org/**
- the heart.org: **http://www.theheart.org/**
- Trauma.org: **http://www.trauma.org/**
- The Food Allergy & Anaphylaxis Network: **http://www.foodallergy.org/**
- Anaphylaxis Campaign: **http://www.anaphylaxis.org.uk/**
- Neurogenic Shock Resource Blog: **http://www.neurogenicshock.net/**
- Surviving Sepsis Campaign: **http://www.survivingsepsis.org**
- Advances in Sepsis: **http://www.advancesinsepsis.com/**
- European Society of Intensive Care Medicine: **http://www.esicm.org/**
- International Sepsis Forum: **http://sepsisforum.org/**
- Survive Sepsis: **http://www.survivesepsis.org/**
- Sepsis Know From Day 1: **http://www.sepsisknowfromday1.com**
- American College of Physicians: **http://www.acponline.org/**
- American College of Surgeons: **http://www.facs.org/**
- American Medical Association: **http://www.ama-assn.org/**
- National Digestive Diseases Information Clearinghouse: **http://digestive.niddk.nih.gov/**
- National Institutes for Health: **http://www.nih.gov/**
- PubMed Health: **http://www.ncbi.nlm.nih.gov/pubmedhealth/**
- American Society for Parenteral and Enteral Nutrition: **http://www.nutritioncare.org/**

BOX 35-27　CASE STUDY

Patient with Systemic Inflammatory Response Syndrome

Brief Patient History

Mr. Z is a 38-year-old Hispanic construction worker who sustained a liver laceration after falling from a roof. He required an exploratory laparotomy for splenectomy and repair of the liver laceration 4 days earlier. His medical history reveals no chronic health problems, although he smokes 20 packs of cigarettes per year.

Clinical Assessment

Mr. Z is admitted to the medical intensive care unit from the telemetry unit with acute respiratory insufficiency and hypotension. He is using his accessory muscles to breathe. He is speaking Spanish. Mr. Z's abdomen is distended, and there are no bowel sounds. Small amounts of dark green drainage are visible in the nasogastric tube. There is no sign of redness or drainage around his surgical wound.

Diagnostic Procedures

Vital signs were as follows: blood pressure of 78/55 mm Hg, heart rate of 142 beats/min (sinus tachycardia), respiratory rate of 35 breaths/min, temperature of 103.1° F, and urine output of 20 mL over the past 8 hours. ABG values on a 100% non-rebreather mask were as follows: pH of 7.22, PaO_2 of 54 mm Hg, $PaCO_2$ of 69 mm Hg, HCO_3^- level of 18 mEq/L, and O_2 saturation of 88%. The chest radiograph revealed infiltrates in the right lower lobe. Laboratory data revealed a hemoglobin level of 9.8 g/dL, hematocrit of 25%, and WBC count of 18,000/mm³.

BOX 35-27 CASE STUDY

Patient with Systemic Inflammatory Response Syndrome—cont'd

Medical Diagnosis
Mr. Z is diagnosed with severe sepsis.

Questions
1. What major outcomes do you expect to achieve for this patient?
2. What problems or risks must be managed to achieve these outcomes?
3. What interventions must be initiated to monitor, prevent, manage, or eliminate the problems and risks identified?

4. What interventions should be initiated to promote optimal functioning, safety, and well-being of the patient?
5. What possible learning needs do you anticipate for this patient?
6. What cultural and age-related factors may have a bearing on the patient's plan of care?

SUMMARY

Shock

- Shock is an acute, widespread process of impaired tissue perfusion that occurs when an imbalance develops between cellular oxygen supply and cellular oxygen demand.
- Shock can be classified as hypovolemic, cardiogenic, or distributive (anaphylactic, neurogenic, and septic), depending on the pathophysiologic cause and hemodynamic profile.
- Shock evolves through four stages: initial, compensatory, progressive, and refractory.
- The patient with a MAP less than 60 mm Hg or with evidence of global tissue hypoperfusion is considered to be in a shock state.
- Management of the patient in shock focuses on supporting oxygen delivery.
- Prevention of shock is one of the primary responsibilities of the nurse in the critical care area.

Hypovolemic Shock

- Hypovolemic shock results from a loss of circulating or intravascular volume due to an absolute or relative fluid loss.
- Initial hemodynamic parameters include a decreased CO or CI, decreased CVP or PAOP, and increased SVR.
- Medical management focuses on identifying and stopping the source of fluid loss and administering fluid to replace circulating volume.
- Nursing interventions include minimizing fluid loss, administering volume replacement, assessing response to therapy, providing comfort and emotional support, and preventing and maintaining surveillance for complications.

Cardiogenic Shock

- Cardiogenic shock results from the impaired ability of the heart to pump due to problems affecting the muscular or mechanical function of the heart or dysrhythmias.
- Initial hemodynamic parameters include a decreased CO or CI, increased PAOP or CVP (or both), and increased SVR.
- Medical management focuses on identifying the etiologic factors of pump failure and administering pharmacologic agents to enhance CO.
- Nursing interventions include limiting myocardial oxygen demand, enhancing myocardial oxygen supply, maintaining

tissue perfusion, providing comfort and emotional support, and preventing and maintaining surveillance for complications.

Anaphylactic Shock

- Anaphylactic shock results from an immunologic antibody–antigen activation or nonimmunologic activation of mast cells and basophils and the release of biochemical mediators.
- Hemodynamic parameters include decreased CO or CI, decreased RAP or PAOP, and decreased SVR.
- Medical management focuses on removing the offending antigen, reversing the effects of the biochemical mediators, and promoting adequate tissue perfusion.
- Nursing interventions include administering epinephrine, facilitating ventilation, administering volume replacement, providing comfort and emotional support, and preventing and maintaining surveillance for recurrent reactions and complications.

Neurogenic Shock

- Neurogenic shock results from the loss of sympathetic tone due to interrupted impulse transmission or blockage of sympathetic outflow from the vasomotor center in the brain.
- Hemodynamic parameters include decreased CO or CI, decreased RAP or PAOP, decreased SVR, and decreased heart rate.
- Medical management focuses on preventing cardiovascular stability and promoting tissue perfusion.
- Nursing interventions include treating hypovolemia and maintaining tissue perfusion, maintaining normothermia, monitoring for and treating dysrhythmias, promoting comfort and emotional support, and preventing and maintaining surveillance for complications.

Septic Shock

- Septic shock results from the initiation of the systemic inflammatory response due to microorganisms entering the body.
- Hemodynamic parameters include decreased CO or CI, decreased RAP or PAOP, decreased SVR, and increased heart rate.

- Medical management focuses on reversing the pathophysiologic responses, controlling the infection, and promoting metabolic support.
- Nursing interventions include early identification of the sepsis syndrome, administering prescribed fluids, medications, and nutrition, promoting comfort and emotional support, and preventing and maintaining surveillance for complications.

Systemic Inflammatory Response

- The systemic inflammatory response is an intense host response characterized by generalized inflammation in organs remote from the initial insult.
- Consequences include uncontrolled activation of inflammatory cells, damage of vascular endothelium, disruption of immune cell function, hypermetabolism, and maldistribution of circulatory volume.

Multiple Organ Dysfunction Syndrome

- MODS results from progressive physiologic failure of two or more separate organ systems.
- Organ dysfunction is influenced by numerous factors, including organ host defense function, response time to the injury, metabolic requirements, organ vasculature response to vasoactive medications, and organ sensitivity to damage and physiologic reserve.
- Collaborative management focuses on fluid resuscitation and hemodynamic support, prevention and treatment of infection, maintenance of tissue oxygenation, nutritional and metabolic support, comfort and emotional support, and preservation of individual organ function.

REFERENCES

1. Maier RV. Approach to the patient with shock. In: Fauci AS, ed. *Harrison's Internal Medicine.* 17th ed. New York: McGraw-Hill; 2008.
2. Deitch EA, et al. Role of the gut in the development of injury and shock induced SIRS and MODS: the gut-lymph hypothesis, a review. *Front Biosci.* 2006;11:520.
3. Pieracci FM, et al. Current concepts in resuscitation. *J Intensive Care Med.* 2012;27:79.
4. Wilmot LA. Shock: early recognition and management. *J Emerg Nurs.* 2010;36:134.
5. Hameed SM, et al. Oxygen delivery. *Crit Care Med.* 2003;31(Suppl 12):S658.
6. Parks JK, et al. Systemic hypotension is a late marker of shock after trauma: a validation study of Advanced Trauma Life Support principles in a large national sample. *Am J Surg.* 2006;192:727.
7. Barbee RW, et al. Assessing shock resuscitation strategies by oxygen debt repayment. *Shock.* 2010;33:113.
8. Holley A, et al. Review article: part two: goal-directed resuscitation—which goals? Perfusion targets. *Emerg Med Australas.* 2012;24:127.
9. Martin JT, et al. Normal vital signs belie occult hypoperfusion in geriatric trauma patients. *Am Surg.* 2010;76:65.
10. Neville AL, et al. Mortality risk stratification in elderly trauma patients based on initial arterial lactate and base deficit levels. *Am Surg.* 2011;77:1337.
11. Vandromme MJ, et al. Lactate is a better predictor than systolic blood pressure for determining blood requirement and mortality: could prehospital measures improve trauma triage? *J Am Coll Surg.* 2010;210:861.
12. Jansen TC, et al. Blood lactate monitoring in critically ill patients: a systematic health technology assessment. *Crit Care Med.* 2009;37:2827.
13. Jansen TC, et al. Early lactate-guided therapy in intensive care unit patients: A multicenter, open-label, randomized controlled trial. *Am J Respir Crit Care Med.* 2010;182:752.
14. Jones AE, et al. Lactate clearance vs central venous oxygen saturation as goals of early sepsis therapy: a randomized clinical trial. *JAMA.* 2010;303:739.
15. FitzSullivan E, et al. Serum bicarbonate may replace the arterial base deficit in the trauma intensive care unit. *Am J Surg.* 2005;190:961.
16. Surbatovic M, et al. *Gen Physiol Biophys.* 2009;28(Spec No):271.
17. Dellinger RP, et al. Surviving Sepsis Campaign: international guidelines for management of severe sepsis and septic shock: 2012. *Crit Care Med.* 2013;41:580.
18. Holley A, et al. Review article: part one: goal-directed resuscitation—which goals? Haemodynamic targets. *Emer Med Australas.* 2012;24:14.
19. Nebout S, Pirracchio R. Should we monitor ScVO$_2$ in critically ill patients. *Cardiol Res Pract.* 2012;2012:370697.
20. Collaborative Study Group on Perioperative ScVO$_2$ Monitoring. Multicentre study on peri- and postoperative central venous oxygen saturation in high-risk surgical patients. *Crit Care.* 2006;10:R158.
21. Vallet B, et al. Physiologic transfusion triggers. *Best Tract Res Clin Anaesthesiol.* 2007;21:173.
22. Alam HB. Advances in resuscitation strategies. *Ing J Surg.* 2011;9:5.
23. Bunn F, Trivedi D. Colloid solutions for fluid resuscitation. *Cochrane Database Syst Rev.* 2012;(6):CD001319.
24. Cotton BA, et al. The cellular, metabolic, and systemic consequences of aggressive fluid resuscitation strategies. *Shock.* 2006;26:115.
25. Niemi TT, et al. Colloid solutions: a clinical update. *J Anesth.* 2010;24:913.
26. Perel P, Roberts I. Colloids versus crystalloids for fluid resuscitation in critically ill patients. *Cochrane Database Syst Rev.* 2011;(3):CD000567.
27. Reinhart K, et al. Consensus statement of the ESICM task force on colloid volume therapy in critically ill patients. *Intensive Care Med.* 2012;38:368.
28. SAFE Study Investigators. Effect of baseline serum albumin concentration on outcome of resuscitation with albumin or saline in patients in intensive care units: analysis of data from the saline versus albumin fluid evaluation (SAFE) study. *BMJ.* 2006;333:1044.
29. Bulger EM, et al. Out-of-hospital hypertonic resuscitation after traumatic hypovolemic shock. *Ann Surg.* 2011;253:431.

30. Patanwala AE, et al. Use of hypertonic saline injection in trauma. *Am J Health-Syst Pharm.* 2010;67:1920.

31. Carson JL, et al. Transfusion thresholds and other strategies for guiding allogenic red blood cell transfusion. *Cochrane Database Syst Rev.* 2012;(4):CD002042.

32. Dennison CA. Transfusion-related acute lung injury: a clinical challenge. *Dimens Crit Care Nurs.* 2008;27:1.

33. Federico A. Transfusion-related acute lung injury. *J Perianesth Nurs.* 2009;24:35.

34. Kopko PM. Transfusion-related acute lung injury. *J Infus Nurs.* 2010;33:32.

35. Murad MH, et al. The effect of plasma transfusion on morbidity and mortality: a systematic review and meta-analysis. *Transfusion.* 2010;50:1370.

36. Boyd JH, Walley KR. Is there a role for sodium bicarbonate in treating lactic acidosis from shock? *Curr Opin Crit Care.* 2008;14:379.

37. Rachoin JS, et al. Treatment of lactic acidosis: appropriate confusion. *J Hosp Med.* 2010;5:E1.

38. Martindale RG, et al. Guidelines for the provision and assessment of nutrition support therapy in the adult critically ill patient: Society of Critical Care Medicine and American Society for Parenteral and Enteral Nutrition: executive summary. *Crit Care Med.* 2009;37:1757.

39. Cahill NE, et al. When early eneral feeding is not possible in critically ill patients: results of a multicenter observational study. *J ParenterEnteral Nutr.* 2011;35:160.

40. Casaer MP, et al. Early versus late parenteral nutrition in critically ill adults. *N Engl J Med.* 2011;365:506.

41. Wenerman J. Combined enteral and parenteral nutrition. *Curr Opin Clin Nutr Metab Care.* 2012;15:161.

42. Kutsogiannis J, et al. Early use of supplemental parenteral nutrition in critically ill patients: results of an international multicenter observational study. *Crit Care Med.* 2011;39:2691.

43. American Diabetes Association. Standards of medical care in diabetes—2012. *Diabetes Care.* 2012;35(Suppl 1):S11.

44. Moghissi ES, et al. American Association of clinical endocrinologists and American diabetes association consensus statement on inpatient glycemic control. *Endocr Pract.* 2009;15:1.

45. Schetz M, et al. Tight blood glucose control is renoprotective in critically ill patients. *J Am Soc Nephrol.* 2008;19:571.

46. Wiener RS, et al. Benefits and risks of tight glucose control in critically ill adults: a meta-analysis. *JAMA.* 2008;300:933.

47. American Association of Critical-Care Nurses. Family presence during resuscitation and invasive procedures. http://www.aacn.org/WD/Practice/Docs/PracticeAlerts/Family%20Presence%2004-2010%20final.pdf. Accessed June 292012.

48. Davidson JE, et al. Clinical practice guidelines for support of the family in the patient-centered intensive care unit: American College of Critical Care Medicine Task force 2004-2005. *Crit Care Med.* 2007;35:605.

49. Egging D, et al. Emergency nursing resource: family presence during invasive procedures and resuscitation in the emergency department. *J Emerg Nurs.* 2011;37:469.

50. Morrison LJ, et al. Part 3: Ethics: 2010 American Heart Association Guidelines for Cardiopulmonary Resuscitation and Emergency Cardiovascular Care. *Circulation.* 2010;122(18 Suppl 3):S665.

51. Guly HR, et al. Vital signs and estimated blood loss in patients with major trauma: Testing the validity of the ATLS classification of hypovolaemic shock. *Resuscitation.* 2011;82:556.

52. Kwan I, et al. Timing and volume of fluid administration for patients with bleeding. *Cochrane Database Syst Rev.* 2009;(1):CD002245.

53. Morrison CA, et al. Hypotensive resuscitation strategy reduces transfusion requirements and severe postoperative coagulopathy in trauma patients with hemorrhagic shock: preliminary results of a randomized controlled trial. *J Trauma.* 2011;70:652.

54. Roppolo LP, et al. Intravenous fluid resuscitation for the trauma patient. *Curr Opin Crit Care.* 2010;16:283.

55. Szopinski J, et al. Microcirculatory responses to hypovolemic shock. *J Trauma.* 2011;71:1779.

56. Goldberg RJ, et al. Thirty-year trends (1975 to 2005) trends in the magnitude of, management of, and hospital death rates associated with cardiogenic shock in patients with acute myocardial infarction. *Circulation.* 2009;119:1211.

57. Reynolds HR, Hochman JS. Cardiogenic shock: current concepts and improving outcomes. *Circulation.* 2008;117:686.

58. Topalian S, et al. Cardiogenic shock. *Crit Care Med.* 2008;36(Suppl 1):S66.

59. Buerke M, et al. Pathophysiology, diagnosis, and treatment of infarction-related cardiogenic shock. *Herz.* 2011;36:73.

60. Hussain F, et al. The ability to achieve complete revascularization is associated with improved in-hospital survival in cardiogenic shock due to myocardial infarction: Manitoba cardiogenic SHOCK Registry investigators. *Catheter Cardiovasc Interv.* 2011;78:540.

61. Chatterjee K, et al. Analytic reviews: cardiogenic shock with preserved systolic function: a reminder. *J Intensive Care Med.* 2008;23:355.

62. Shpektor A. Cardiogenic shock: the role of inflammation. *Acute Card Care.* 2010;12:115.

63. Brown JL, et al. Short-term mechanical management of cardiogenic shock. *Curr Treat Options Cardiovasc Med.* 2011;13:343.

64. Stevenson LW, Perloff JK. The limited reliability of physical signs for estimating hemodynamics in chronic heart failure. *JAMA.* 1989;261:884.

65. Kemp SF, et al. Epinephrine: the drug of choice for anaphylaxis. A statement of the World Allergy Organization. *Allergy.* 2008;63:1061.

66. Kim H, Fischer D. Anaphylaxis, allergy. *Asthma Clin Immunol.* 2011;7(suppl 1):S6.

67. Lieberman P, et al. The diagnosis and management of anaphylaxis practice parameter: 2010 update. *J Allergy Clin Immunol.* 2010;126:477.

68. Simons FE. Anaphylaxis. *J Allergy Clin Immunol.* 2010; 125(2 suppl 2):S161.

69. Simons FE. Anaphylaxis: recent advances in assessment and treatment. *J Allergy Clin Immunol.* 2009;124:625.

70. American Heart Association. 2010 American Heart Association Guidelines for cardiopulmonary resuscitation and emergency cardiovascular care. Part 12.2: Cardiac arrest associated with anaphylaxis. *Circulation.* 2010;122(suppl 3):S832.

71. Sampson HA, et al. Second symposium on the definition and management of anaphylaxis: summary report—second National Institute of Allergy and Infectious Disease/Food Allergy and Anaphylaxis Network symposium. *J Allergy Clin Immunol.* 2006;117:391.

72. Tole JW, Lieberman P. Biphasic anaphylaxis: review of incidence, clinical predictors, and observation recommendations. *Immunol Allergy Clin N Am.* 2007;27:309.

73. Choo KJL, et al. Glucocorticoids for the treatment of anaphylaxis. *Cochrane Database Syst Rev.* 2012;(4):CD007596.

74. Furlan JC, Fehlings MG. Cardiovascular complications after acute spinal cord injury: pathophysiology, diagnosis, and management. *Neurosurg Focus.* 2008;25:1.

75. Guly HR, et al. The incidence of neurogenic shock in patients with isolated spinal cord injury in the emergency department. *Resuscitation.* 2008;76:57.

76. Krassioukov A, Claydon VE. The clinical problems in cardiovascular control following spinal cord injury: an overview. *Prog Brain Res.* 2006;152:223.

77. Consortium for Spinal Cord Medicine. Early acute management in adults with spinal cord injury: a clinical practice guideline for health-care professionals. http://www.pva.org/site/apps/ka/ec/product.asp?c=ajIRK9NJLcJ2E&b=6423003&en=8hIFLROvG7LOL1PyF6JLKYMJJlIQIXPAJfKRL8OQJvG&ProductID=895972. Accessed July 3, 2012.

78. Popa C, et al. Vascular dysfunctions following spinal cord injury. *J Med Life.* 2010;3:275.

79. Young WF. Shock. In: Stone CK, Humphries RL, eds. *Current Diagnosis & Treatment: Emergency Medicine.* 6th ed. New York: McGraw-Hill; 2008.

80. American Heart Association. 2010 American Heart Association Guidelines for cardiopulmonary resuscitation and emergency cardiovascular care. Part 8: Adult advanced cardiovascular resuscitation and emergency cardiovascular care. *Circulation.* 2010;122:S729.

81. Beale R, et al. Promoting global research excellence in severe sepsis (PROGRESS): lessons from an international sepsis registry. *Infection.* 2009;37:222.

82. Lagu T, et al. Hospitalizations, costs, and outcomes of severe sepsis in the United States 2003 to 2007. *Crit Care Med.* 2012;40:754.

83. Mann EA, et al. Comparison of mortality associated with sepsis in the burn, trauma, and general intensive care unit patient: a systematic review of the literature. *Shock.* 2012;37:4.

84. Sivayoham N, et al. Outcomes from implementing early goal-directed therapy for severe sepsis and septic shock: a 4-year observational cohort study. *Eur J Emerg Med.* 2012;19:235.

85. Murphy SL, et al. *Deaths: preliminary data for 2010. National Vital Statistics Reports; vol 60 no 4.* Hyattsville, MD: National Center for Health Statistics; 2012. http://www.cdc.gov/nchs/data/nvsr/nvsr60/nvsr60_04.pdf. Accessed April 15, 2012.

86. American College of Chest Physicians/Society of Critical Care Medicine Consensus Conference. Definitions for sepsis and organ failure and guidelines for the use of innovative therapies in sepsis. *Crit Care Med.* 1992;20:864.

87. Dellinger RP, et al. Surviving Sepsis Campaign guidelines for management of severe sepsis and septic shock. *Crit Care Med.* 2004;32:858.

88. Levy MM, et al. 2001 SCCM/ESICM/ACCP/ATS/SIS International Sepsis Definitions Conference. *Crit Care Med.* 2003;31:1250.

89. Seymour CW, et al. Marital status and the epidemiology and outcomes of sepsis. *Chest.* 2010;137:1289.

90. Fry DE. Sepsis, systemic inflammatory response, and multiple organ dysfunction: the mystery continues. *Am Surg.* 2012;78:1.

91. Cinel I, Dellinger RP. Advances in pathogenesis and management of sepsis. *Curr Opin Infect Dis.* 2007;20:345.

92. Nduka OO, Parrillo JE. The pathophysiology of septic shock. *Crit Care Nurs Clin N Am.* 2011;23:41.

93. Rivers EP, et al. The influence of early hemodynamic optimization on biomarker patterns of severe sepsis and septic shock. *Crit Care Med.* 2007;35:2016.

94. Singer M. Mitochondrial function in sepsis: acute phase versus multiple organ failure. *Crit Care Med.* 2007;35(suppl 9):S441.

95. Levi M, et al. Systemic versus localized coagulation activation contributing to organ failure in critically ill patients. *Semin Immunopathol.* 2012;34:167.

96. Stearns-Kurosawa DJ, et al. The pathogenesis of sepsis. *Annu Rev Pathol Mech Dis.* 2011;6:19.

97. Semeraro N, et al. Sepsis, thrombosis and organ dysfunction. *Thromb Res.* 2012;129:290.

98. Trzeciak S, et al. Early microcirculatory perfusion derangements in patients with severe sepsis and septic shock: relationship to hemodynamics, oxygen transport, and survival. *Ann Emerg Med.* 2007;49:88.

99. Vollmar B, Menger MD. Intestinal ischemia/reperfusion: microcirculatory pathology and functional consequences. *Langenbecks Arch Surg.* 2011;396:13.

100. Tappy L, Chiolero R. Substrate utilization in sepsis and multiple organ failure. *Crit Care Med.* 2007;35(suppl 9):S531.

101. Baumgart K, et al. Pathophysiology of tissue acidosis in septic shock: blocked microcirculation or impaired cellular respiration? *Crit Care Med.* 2008;36:640.

102. Garrabou G, et al. The effects of sepsis on mitochondria. *J Infect Dis.* 2012;205:392.

103. Perl M, et al. Pathogenesis of indirect (secondary) acute lung injury. *Expert Rev Respir Med.* 2011;5:115.

104. Jacob A, et al. Septic encephalopathy: inflammation in man and mouse. *Neurochem Int.* 2011;58:472.

105. Jensen JU, et al. Procalcitonin-guided interventions against infections to increase early appropriate antibiotics and improve survival in the intensive care unit: a randomized trial. *Crit Care Med.* 2011;39:2048.

106. Rivers E, et al. Early goal-directed therapy in the treatment of severe sepsis and septic shock. *N Engl J Med.* 2001;345:1368.

107. Kumar A, et al. Duration of hypotension before initiation of effective antimicrobial therapy is the critical determinant of survival in human septic shock. *Crit Care Med.* 2006;34:1589.

108. De Backer D, et al. Dopamine versus norepinephrine in the treatment of septic shock: a meta-analysis. *Crit Care Med.* 2012;40:725.

109. Vasu TS, et al. Norepinephrine or dopamine for septic shock: a systematic review of randomized clinical trials. *J Intensive Care Med.* 2012;27:172.

110. The Acute Respiratory Distress System Network. Ventilation with lower tidal volumes as compared with traditional tidal volumes for acute lung injury and the acute respiratory distress syndrome. *N Engl J Med.* 2000;342:1301.

111. Marti-Carvajal AJ, et al. Human recombinant activated protein C for severe sepsis. *Cochrane Database Syst Rev.* 2012;(3):CD004388.

112. Mullard A. Drug withdrawal sends critical care specialists back to basics. *Lancet.* 2011;378:1769.

113. FDA. FDA Drug Safety Communication. Voluntary market withdrawal of Xigis [drotrecogin alfa (activated)] due to failure to show a survival benefit. http://www.fda.gov/Drugs/DrugSafety/ucm277114.htm. Accessed October 25, 2011.

114. Annane D, et al. Effect of treatment with low doses of hydrocortisone and fludrocortisone on mortality in patients with septic shock. *JAMA.* 2002;288:862.

115. Annane D, et al. Corticosteroids for treating severe sepsis and septic shock. *Cochrane Database Syst Rev.* 2010;(12):CD002243.

116. Sprung CL, et al. Steroid therapy of septic shock. *Crit Care Nurs Clin N Am.* 2011;23:171.

117. Surviving Sepsis Campaign (SSC) Guidelines Committee Subgroup for Glucose Control. Surviving Sepsis Campaign Statement on Glucose Control in Severe Sepsis. http://www.survivingsepsis.org/About_the_Campaign/Documents/SSC%20Statement%20on%20Glucose%20Control%20in%20Severe%20Sepsis.pdf. Accessed June 12, 2009.

118. Elke G, et al. Current practice in nutritional support and its association with mortality in septic patients—results from a national, prospective, multicenter study. *Crit Care Med.* 2008;36:1762.

119. Beale RJ, et al. Early enteral supplementation with key pharmaconutrients improves Sequential Organ Failure Assessment score in critically ill patients with sepsis: outcome of a randomized, controlled, double-blind trial. *Crit Care Med.* 2008;36:131.

120. Aitken LM, et al. Nursing considerations to complement the surviving sepsis campaign guidelines. *Crit Care Med.* 2011;39:1800.

121. Otto GP, et al. The late phase of sepsis is characterized by an increased microbiological burden and death rate. *Crit Care.* 2011;15:R183.

122. Winters BD, et al. Long-term mortality and quality of life in sepsis: a systematic review. *Crit Care Med.* 2010;38:1276.

123. Cheek DJ, et al. Shock, multiple organ dysfunction syndrome, and burns in adults. In: McCance KL, et al, eds. *Pathophysiology: the Biologic Basis for Disease in Adults and Children.* 6th ed. St Louis: Mosby; 2010.

124. Garnacho-Martin J, et al. Effect of critical illness polyneuropathy on withdrawal from mechanical ventilation and length of stay in septic patients. *Crit Care Med.* 2005;33:349.

125. Cohn SM, et al. Tissue oxygen saturation predicts the development of organ dysfunction during traumatic shock resuscitation. *J Trauma.* 2007;62:44.

126. Epstein CD, et al. Oxygen transport and organ dysfunction in the older trauma patient. *Heart Lung.* 2002;31:315.

127. Clark JA, Coopersmith CM. Intestinal crosstalk: a new paradigm for understanding the gut as the "motor" of critical illness. *Shock.* 2007;28:384.

128. Tschoeke SK, et al. The early second hit in trauma management augments the proinflammatory immune response to multiple injuries. *J Trauma.* 2007;62:1396.

129. Dulhunty JM, et al. Does severe non-infectious SIRS differ from severe sepsis? Results from a multi-centre Australian and New Zealand intensive care unit study. *Intensive Care Med.* 2008;34:1654.

130. Sankoff J, et al. Validation of the Mortality in Emergency Department Sepsis (MEDS) score in patients with the systemic inflammatory response syndrome (SIRS). *Crit Care Med.* 2008;36:421.

131. Shimizu K, et al. Altered gut flora and environment in patients with severe SIRS. *J Trauma.* 2006;60:126.

132. Rote NS, Huether SE. Innate immunity: inflammation. In: McCance K, et al, eds. *Pathophysiology: the Biologic Basis for Disease in Adults and Children.* 6th ed. St. Louis: Mosby; 2010.

133. Schmidt H, et al. The alteration of autonomic function in multiple organ dysfunction syndrome. *Crit Care Clin.* 2008;24:149.

134. Gando S. Microvascular thrombosis and multiple organ dysfunction syndrome. *Crit Care Med.* 2010;38(Suppl 2):S35.

135. Shapiro N, et al. Sepsis syndromes. In: Marx J, ed. *Rosen's Emergency Medicine: Concepts and Clinical Practice.* 7th ed. Philadelphia: Mosby; 2009.

136. Bengmark S. Bioecologic control of inflammation and infection in critical illness. *Anesthesiol Clin.* 2006;24:299.

137. Abraham E, Singer M. Mechanisms of sepsis-induced organ dysfunction. *Crit Care Med.* 2007;35:2408.

138. Biesalski HK, McGregor GP. Antioxidant therapy in critical care—is the microcirculation the primary target? *Crit Care Med.* 2007;35:S577.

139. Menges T, et al. Sepsis syndrome and death in trauma patients are associated with variation in the gene encoding tumor necrosis factor. *Crit Care Med.* 2008;36:1456.

140. Marshall JC, et al. The gastrointestinal tract. The "undrained abscess" of multiple organ failure. *Ann Surg.* 1993;218:111.

141. Ulldemolins M, et al. Antibiotic dosing in multiple organ dysfunction syndrome. *Chest.* 2011;139:1210.

142. Barie PS, Eachempati SR. Acute acalculous cholecystitis. *Gastroenterol Clin North Am.* 2010;39:343.

143. Krau SD. Making sense of multiple organ dysfunction syndrome. *Crit Care Nurs Clin North Am.* 2007;19:87.

144. Vincent JL, Zambon M. Why do patients who have acute lung injury/acute respiratory distress syndrome die from multiple organ dysfunction syndrome? Implications for management. *Clin Chest Med.* 2006;27:725.

145. Crouser ED, Fahy RJ. Acute lung injury, pulmonary edema, and multiple system organ failure. In: Wilkins RL, et al, eds. *Egan's Fundamentals of Respiratory Care.* 9th ed. St. Louis: Mosby; 2009.

146. Honore PM, et al. Septic AKI in ICU patients, diagnosis, pathophysiology, and treatment type, dosing, and timing: a comprehensive review of recent and future developments. *Ann Intensive Care.* 2011;1:32.

147. Zanotti-Cavazzoni SL, Hollenberg SM. Cardiac dysfunction in severe sepsis and septic shock. *Curr Opin Crit Care.* 2009;15:392.

148. Dhainaut JF, et al. Dynamic evolution of coagulopathy in the first day of severe sepsis: relationship with mortality and organ failure. *Crit Care Med.* 2005;33:341.

149. McClave SA, Heyland DK. The physiologic response and associated clinical benefits from provision of early enteral nutrition. *Nutr Clin Pract.* 2009;24:305.

150. Villars PS. Multidisciplinary approach to VAP prevention. *Crit Care Nurse.* 2007;27(6):12.

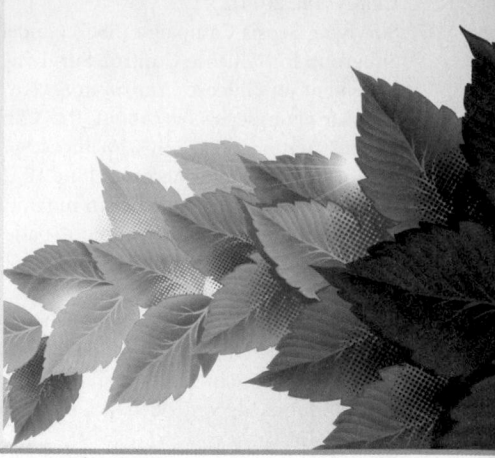

evolve WEBSITE

http://evolve.elsevier.com/Urden/criticalcare/

Evolve features:

- NCLEX Review Questions
- CCRN Review Questions
- PCCN Review Questions
- Mosby's Nursing Skills Procedures
- Animations
- Video Clips
- Glossary

Since the late 1980s, trends of burn incidence, hospitalization, and death have all decreased.[1,2] These decreases are attributed to fire and burn prevention education, management of burn patients in specialized burn centers, regulation of consumer products, and implementation of occupational safety standards. Many programs and organizations are dedicated to the prevention of burn injury. Societal changes involving decreased smoking and alcohol abuse, changes in home cooking practices, and reduced industrial employment also have contributed to the decline in burn incidence. However, in spite of a decline in overall burn incidence, because of an increase in child maltreatment (3.3 million referrals in 2010), burn injury as a result of physical abuse remains a differential diagnosis in pediatric burn patients.[3]

Burn injuries that require medical treatment annually number 450,000 per year.[2] Burn injuries requiring hospitalization total approximately 45,000 per year, and 55% of these patients are admitted to one of the 125 specialized burn centers in the United States.[2]

Great advances have been made in the care of burn patients. In the mid-twentieth century, burn shock claimed many patients' lives. If shock did not cause death, infection or respiratory insufficiency did. With improvements in fluid resuscitation, better critical care management, and the trend toward early excision and grafting, mortality rates have decreased. Focusing management on early eschar excision in patients with deeper, larger burns decreases wound sepsis, hypercatabolism, number of operations, and lengths of hospital stay.[4]

To provide comprehensive, holistic care to burn patients, close collaboration is required among members of the multidisciplinary team. The burn team comprises nurses, physicians, physical therapists, occupational therapists, recreational therapists, nutritionists, psychologists, social workers, family, and spiritual support staff members. The burn patient is characterized as the universal trauma model. The patient's response to a major burn injury is dramatic and involves multisystem alterations. Knowledge of local and systemic changes associated with patient needs is essential in providing care, which places extraordinary demands on the nurse in a burn practice who must be both a specialist and a broad-based generalist. The purpose of this chapter is to provide a basic understanding of the complexities of burn care and the patient's response to burn injury.

ANATOMY AND FUNCTIONS OF THE SKIN

The skin is the largest organ of the human body, ranging from 0.2 meter squared (m^2) in the newborn to more than 2 m^2 in the adult. The integumentary system consists of two major layers: (1) epidermis and (2) dermis (Fig. 36-1).

The outermost layer of the epidermis is 0.07 to 0.12 millimeters (mm) thick, with the deepest layer found on the soles of the feet and the palms of the hands. The epidermis is composed of dead, cornified cells that act as a tough protective barrier against the environment. It serves as a barrier to bacteria and moisture loss.[5] From the surface inward, its five layers are (1) stratum corneum, (2) stratum lucidum, (3) stratum granulosum, (4) stratum spinosum, and (5) stratum germinativum. The deepest layer of the epidermis contains fibronectin, which adheres the epidermis to the basement membrane. The epidermis regenerates every 2 to 3 weeks. The second, thicker layer, the dermis, is 1 to 2 mm thick and lies below the

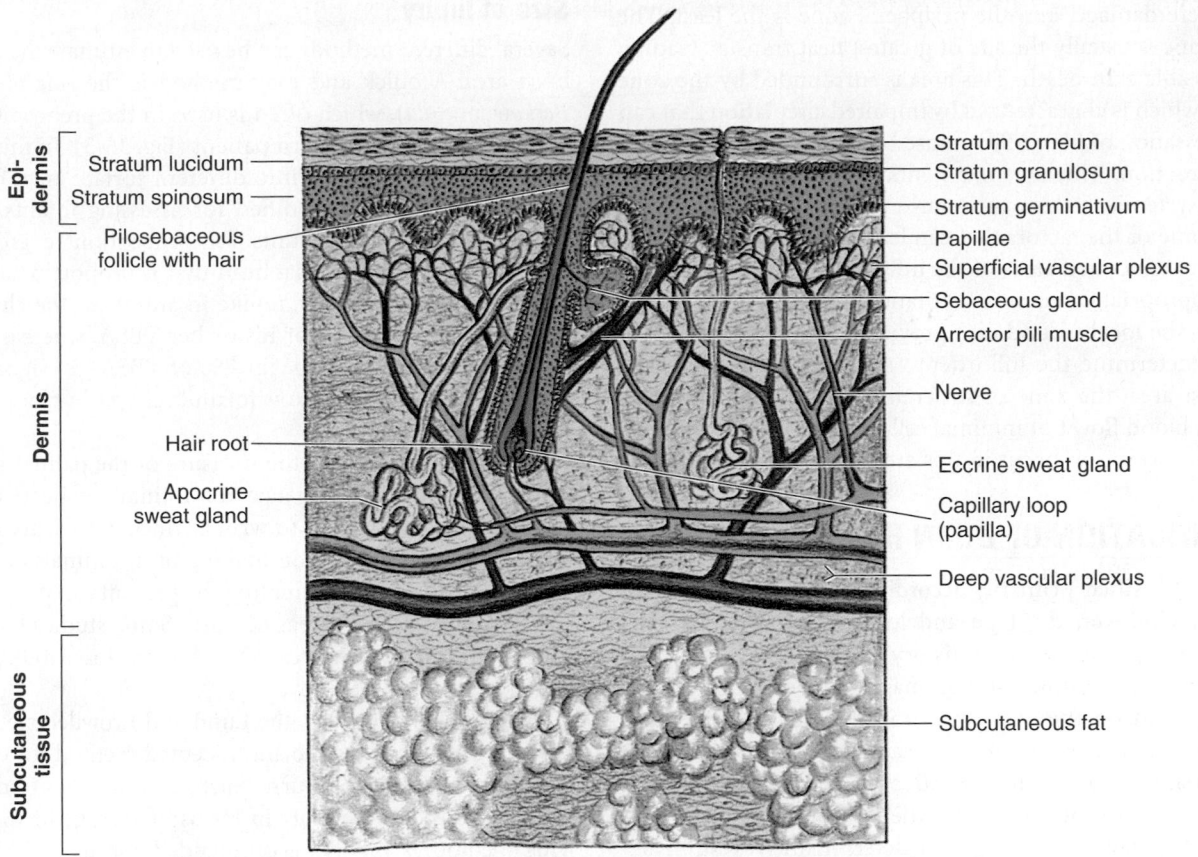

FIGURE 36-1 Anatomy of the Skin. (From Dains JE. Integumentary system. In: Thompson JM, et al, eds: *Mosby's Clinical Nursing*. 5th ed. St. Louis: Mosby; 2002.)

epidermis and regenerates continuously. The dermis is composed of two layers: (1) the more superficial, papillary layer next to the stratum germinativum and (2) the deeper, reticular layer. The dermis, composed primarily of connective tissue and collagenous fiber bundles made from fibroblasts, provides nutritional support to the epidermis. The dermis contains blood vessels; sweat and sebaceous glands; hair follicles; nerves to the skin and capillaries that nourish the avascular epidermis; and sensory fibers that detect pain, touch, and temperature. Mast cells in the connective tissue perform the functions of secretion, phagocytosis, and production of fibroblasts. Beneath the dermis is the hypodermis, which contains fat, smooth muscle, and areolar tissues. The hypodermis acts as a heat insulator, shock absorber, and nutritional depot.[6]

The skin provides functions crucial to human survival. They include maintenance of body temperature; a barrier to evaporative water loss; metabolic activity (vitamin D production); immunologic protection by preventing microbes from entering the body; protection against the environment through the sensations of touch, pressure, and pain; and overall cosmetic appearance.

PATHOPHYSIOLOGY AND ETIOLOGY OF BURN INJURY

A burn injury results in tissue loss or damage. Injury to tissue can be caused by exposure to thermal, electrical, chemical, or radiation sources. The temperature or causticity of the burning

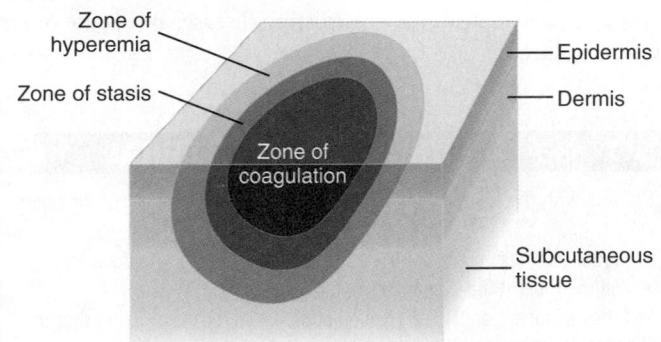

FIGURE 36-2 Zones of Burn Injury.

agent and duration of tissue contact with the source determine the extent of tissue injury. Tissue damage can occur at various temperatures, usually between 40° C (104° F) and 44° C (111.2° F). The burn wound itself is responsible for the local and systemic effects seen in the burned patient.[7] Tissue damage is caused by enzyme malfunction and denaturation of proteins. Prolonged exposure or higher temperatures can lead to cell necrosis and a process known as *protein coagulation*. The areas extending outward from this central area of injury sustain various degrees of damage and are identified by zones of injury.[8]

Zones of Injury

Three concentric zones are present in burn injury: (1) *zone of coagulation*, (2) *zone of stasis*, and (3) *zone of hyperemia* (Fig. 36-2). The central zone, or zone of coagulation, is the site of most severe damage, and the peripheral zone is the least. The central zone is usually the site of greatest heat transfer, leading to irreversible skin death. This area is surrounded by the zone of stasis, which is characterized by impaired circulation that can lead to cessation of blood flow caused by a pronounced inflammatory reaction. This area is potentially salvageable; however, local or systemic factors can convert it into a full-thickness injury. Some of the factors that can lead to deeper wound conversion are toxic mediators of the inflammatory process, infection, inappropriate volume resuscitation, malnutrition, chronic illness, or the local wound care provided. It may take 48 to 72 hours to determine the full extent of injury in this area. The outermost area, the zone of hyperemia, has vasodilation and increased blood flow but minimal cell involvement. Early spontaneous recovery can occur in this area.[7,8]

CLASSIFICATION OF BURN INJURY

Burns are classified primarily according to the size and depth of injury. However, the type and location of the burn and the patient's age and medical history are also significant considerations. Recognition of the magnitude of burn injury, which is based on the above-mentioned factors, is of crucial importance in the overall plan of care and in decisions concerning patient management and appropriate referral to a burn center (Box 36-1).[2] The patient's age, burn size, and inhalation injury are the cardinal determinants of survival.[9] A recent study of a large number of burn patients found the following factors to be the biggest predictors of patient mortality: age, percent total body surface area (TBSA), inhalation injury, coexistent trauma, pre-existing disease, and acute organ system failure.[9,10]

BOX 36-1   BURN CENTER REFERRAL

Patients with the following burn injuries are best treated in a certified burn center:

- Partial-thickness burns of 10% or more of the total body surface area
- Full-thickness (third-degree) burns in any age group
- Burns of face, hands, feet, genitalia, perineum, or major joints that may result in cosmetic or functional disability
- Electrical burns, including lightning injury
- Inhalation injury
- Chemical burns
- Burns in patients with pre-existing medical disorders that could complicate management, prolong recovery, or affect mortality (e.g., diabetes mellitus, symptomatic cardiopulmonary disease)
- Burn injury with concomitant trauma (such as fractures) in which the burn injury poses the greatest risk of morbidity or mortality. In such cases, if the trauma poses the greater immediate risk, the patient's condition may be stabilized initially in a trauma center before transfer to a burn center. Physician judgment will be necessary in above situations.
- Burned children in hospitals without qualified personnel or equipment for the care of children
- Burn injury in patients who will require special social, emotional, or long-term rehabilitative intervention

Modified from *American Burn Association.* Burn center referral criteria. Guidelines for the operation of burn centers. http://www.ameriburn.org. Accessed April 2012.

Size of Injury

Several different methods can be used to estimate the size of the burn area. A quick and easy method is the *rule of nines* (or *Berkow formula*), which often is used in the prehospital setting for initial triage of the burn patient (Fig. 36-3). In this method, the adult body is divided into different surface areas of 9% per area. This method is modified for assessing infants and very small children and accounts for proportionate growth. For example, a 1-year-old has a head that is proportionately larger than the rest of the body, unlike in adults, so the child's head would account for 19% of his or her TBSA, whereas the head of an adult would account for 7% of TBSA.[5] Designated burn centers have access to Berkow formula charts, but local hospitals may not.

Another method uses the measure of the palmar surface of the victim's hand as a gauge for estimating burn area. The palmar surface (fingertip to wrist), which represents 1% of the TBSA, also can be useful in making burn estimates in the prehospital setting or for estimating the percentage of involvement in small and scattered areas of burn. Some studies have shown the adult hand's TBSA is calculated to be closer to 0.8% versus 1% in a child.[5]

In the hospital setting, the Lund and Browder method (Fig. 36-4) is the most accurate and accepted method for determining the percentage of burn. Surface area measurements are assigned to each body part in terms of the age of the patient. This method is highly recommended for use with children younger than 10 years because it corrects for smaller surface areas of the lower extremities. It is also recommended for adult burn victims because of its accuracy.

Depth of Burn Injury

Traditionally, burn depth has been classified in degrees of injury based on the amount of injured epidermis, dermis, or both:

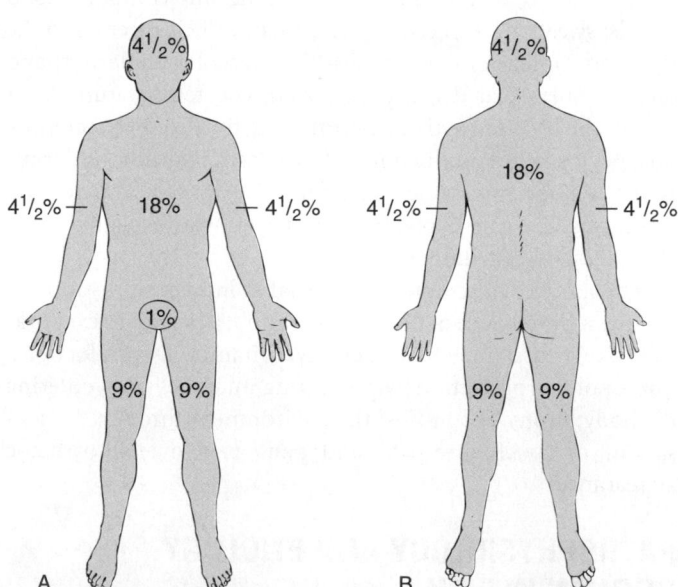

FIGURE 36-3 Estimation of adult burn injury: rule of nines. *A,* Anterior view; *B,* posterior view. (From Marx J, et al. *Rosen's Emergency Medicine Concepts and Clinical Practice.* 5th ed. St. Louis: Mosby; 2002.)

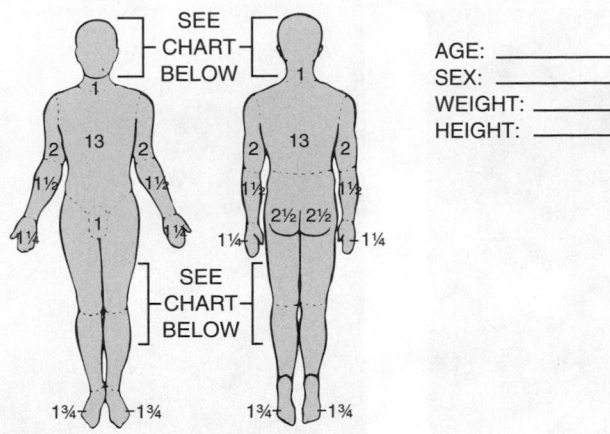

AGE: _____

SEX: _____

WEIGHT: _____

HEIGHT: _____

AREA	Inf.	1-4	5-9	10-14	15	Adult	Part.	Full	Total	Donor areas
HEAD	19	17	13	11	9	7				
NECK	2	2	2	2	2	2				
ANT. TRUNK	13	13	13	13	13	13				
POST. TRUNK	13	13	13	13	13	13				
R. BUTTOCK	2½	2½	2½	2½	2½	2½				
L. BUTTOCK	2½	2½	2½	2½	2½	2½				
GENITALIA	1	1	1	1	1	1				
R.U. ARM	4	4	4	4	4	4				
L.U. ARM	4	4	4	4	4	4				
R.L. ARM	3	3	3	3	3	3				
L.L. ARM	3	3	3	3	3	3				
R. HAND	2½	2½	2½	2½	2½	2½				
L. HAND	2½	2½	2½	2½	2½	2½				
R. THIGH	5½	6½	8	8½	9	9½				
L. THIGH	5½	6½	8	8½	9	9½				
R. LEG	5	5	5½	6	6½	7				
L. LEG	5	5	5½	6	6½	7				
R. FOOT	3½	3½	3½	3½	3½	3½				
L. FOOT	3½	3½	3½	3½	3½	3½				
						TOTAL				

FIGURE 36-4 The Lund and Browder Burn Estimate Diagram. (Modified from Cardona VD. *Trauma Nursing from Resuscitation Through Rehabilitation.* Philadelphia: Mosby; 1995.)

first-degree, second-degree, third-degree, or fourth-degree burns. However, these terms are not descriptive of the burn surface. The depth of the burn is defined by how much of the skin's two layers are destroyed by the heat source.[10]

Burns are classified as *superficial, partial-thickness, deep partial-thickness,* or *full-thickness burns.* These descriptions are based on the surface appearance of the wound. Superficial burns include first-degree burns. Partial-thickness wounds include various stages of second-degree burns, and full-thickness burns include third-degree burns. Four-degree burns extend through the skin to the subcutaneous fat, muscle, and even bone.[10] Some authorities further separate partial-thickness burns as *superficial, mid-partial,* or *deep-partial-thickness burns.* Wound assessment involves recognition of the depth of injury and the size of burn, and it can be challenging even for experienced caregivers. Because the management of burn wounds is closely tied to the correct assessment of wound severity, some newer strategies, other than observation, are being investigated. Some of these techniques have taken into account the presence of denatured collagen, wound edema, and altered blood flow.

One such technique is noncontact laser Doppler imaging, which can give a color perfusion map of the burn wound.[11] Other techniques of assessing burn depth include use of vital dyes, ultrasonography, thermography, and magnetic resonance imaging.[8] Research with these techniques is ongoing, but they are currently limited by their clinical usefulness at the bedside.

A *superficial (first-degree) burn* involves only the first two or three of the five layers of the epidermis. Erythema and mild discomfort characterize superficial partial-thickness wounds. Pain, the chief symptom, usually resolves in 48 to 72 hours. Common examples of these burn injuries are sunburns and minor steam burns such as those that may occur while cooking. These wounds usually heal in 2 to 7 days and do not require medical intervention aside from pain relief, management of pruritus (itching), and oral fluids. Swelling can be a common complication that may require intervention. Superficial burns are not included in the calculation of percent burn.

A *partial-thickness (second-degree) burn* involves all of the epidermis and part of underlying dermis.[5] These burns usually are caused by brief contact with flames, hot liquid, or exposure

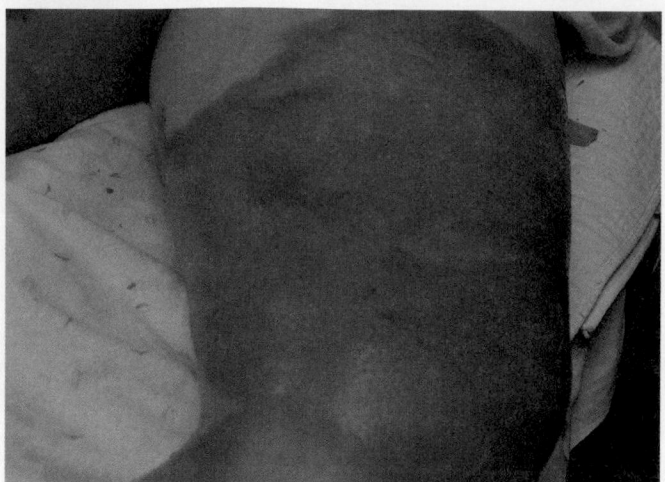

FIGURE 36-5 Partial-thickness burn to the left thigh.

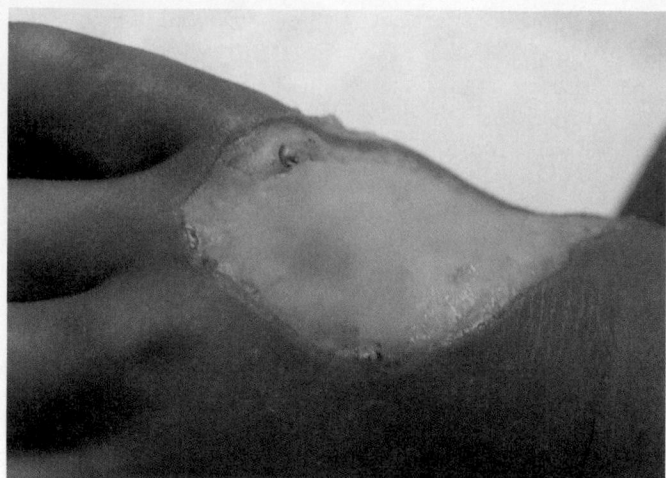

FIGURE 36-7 Full-thickness burn to the back of the hand.

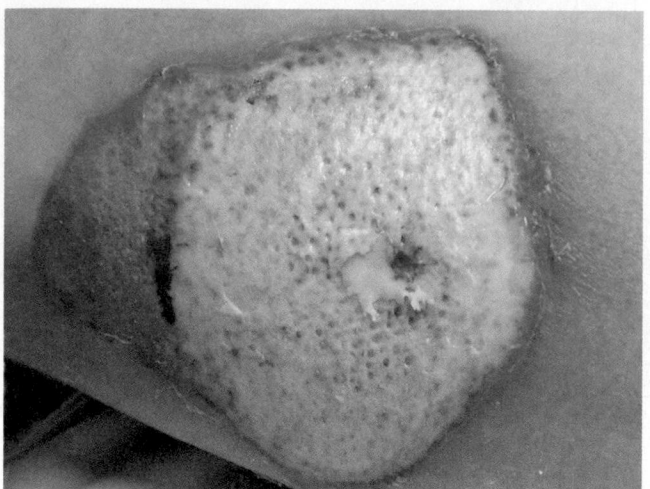

FIGURE 36-6 Deep partial-thickness thigh burn.

to dilute chemicals (Fig. 36-5). A light to bright red or mottled appearance characterizes superficial second-degree burns. These wounds may appear wet and weeping, may contain bullae, and are extremely painful and sensitive to air currents. These burns blanch painfully.[5] The microvessels that perfuse this area are injured, and permeability is increased, resulting in leakage of large amounts of plasma into the interstitium. This fluid lifts off the thin, damaged epidermis, causing blister formation. Despite the loss of the entire basal layer of the epidermis, a burn of this depth will heal in 7 to 21 days. Minimal scarring can be expected. Mid-dermal partial-thickness wounds commonly take 4 to 6 weeks to heal.

Deep-dermal partial-thickness (second-degree) burns involve the entire epidermal layer and deeper layers of the dermis.[5] These burns often result from contact with hot liquids or solids or with intense radiant energy. A deep-dermal partial-thickness burn usually is not characterized by blister formation. Only a modest plasma surface leakage occurs because of severe impairment in blood supply. The wound surface usually is red with patchy white areas that blanch with pressure. The appearance of the deep-dermal wound changes over time. Dermal necrosis and surface coagulated protein turn the wound from white to yellow (Fig. 36-6). These wounds have a prolonged healing

time. They can heal spontaneously as the epidermal elements germinate and migrate until the epidermal surface is restored, or they may require a skin substitute or surgical excision and grafting for wound closure. This process of healing by epithelialization can take up to 6 weeks. Left untreated, these wounds can heal primarily with unstable epithelium, late hypertrophic scarring, and marked contracture formation.[5] Partial-thickness injuries can become full-thickness injuries if they become infected, if blood supply is diminished, or if further trauma occurs to the site. The treatment of choice is surgical excision and skin grafting.

A *full-thickness (third-degree) burn* involves destruction of all the layers of the skin down to and including the subcutaneous tissue (Fig. 36-7). The subcutaneous tissue is composed of adipose tissue, includes the hair follicles and sweat glands, and is poorly vascularized. A full-thickness burn appears pale white or charred, red or brown, and leathery. The surface of the burn may be dry, and if the skin is broken, fat may be exposed. Full-thickness burns usually are painless and insensitive to palpation. Because all of the epithelial elements are destroyed, the wound will not heal by re-epithelialization. Wound closure of small full-thickness burns (<4 centimeters squared [cm^2] area) can be achieved with healing by contraction. All other full-thickness wounds require skin grafting for closure. Extensive full-thickness wounds leave the patient extremely susceptible to infections, fluid and electrolyte imbalances, alterations in thermoregulation, and metabolic disturbances.

The exact depth of many burn wounds cannot be clearly defined on the first inspection, and many burn wounds may contain superficial, mid-dermal, and deep-dermal wounds. A major difficulty is distinguishing deep-dermal partial-thickness from full-thickness injury. It is important to identify the depth of injury for appropriate treatment. Deep, partial-thickness wounds that will not heal within a relatively short time are treated with wound excision and grafting. Burn wounds can evolve over time, and they require frequent reassessment. Special consideration must always be given to very young and older patients because of their thin dermal layer. Older adults may also have reduced sensation and blood supply, causing them to be more susceptible to a full-thickness injury. Burn injuries in these age groups may be more severe than they initially appear.[12]

At the same time that assessment for wound depth occurs, the TBSA of the burn is calculated. This calculation provides the basis for determining the amount of fluid required for treatment. All burn wound surface area percentages, except for superficial burns, are used to calculate the patient's fluid requirements.

Types of Injury
Thermal Burns

The most common type of burn is a thermal burn caused by steam, scalds, contact with heat, and fire injuries. About 80% of burns in children are caused by scalds (i.e., contact with hot objects or liquids).[5] Toddlers are most often affected by scalding burns. Contact burns are also common. The length of time the hot object is in contact with the skin determines the depth of injury. Flame injuries are often associated with other trauma to the patient. The highest incidence of flame injuries are more common in patients older than 6 years of age.[5] Experimentation with lighters, lighter fluid, fire, firecrackers, and gasoline is more common in children age 6 to 16 years.[5] Contact and flame burns tend to be deep-dermal or full-thickness injuries.

Electrical Burns

Electrical and lightning injuries result in 1000 deaths per year in the United States. Electrical injuries count for 4% of burn patient admissions to burn centers.[2] Low-voltage (alternating) current or high-voltage (alternating or direct) current, which is greater than 1000 volts, can cause electrical burns.[4] Children have the highest incidence of electrical injury. These accidents occur as a result of insertion of an object into an outlet or by biting or sucking on an electrical cord. Pediatric electrical burns occur most often in the home, whereas in adults, electrical injuries occur in the workplace.[13] Common situations that may increase the risk for electrical injuries include occupational exposure and accidents involving household current.

Chemical Burns

Acid and alkali agents cause chemical burns. Alkali burns commonly result in more severe injuries compared with acid burns. Acid and alkali agents are found in many household and industrial substances such as liquid concrete. The concentration of the chemical agent and the duration of exposure are the key factors that determine the extent and depth of damage. Progression of injury from chemical burns to their complete depth may be delayed, and the full extent of the injury may not be apparent until up to 48 hours after injury. Time must not be wasted in looking for a specific neutralizing agent because the injury is related directly to the concentration of the chemical and the duration of the exposure, and the heat of neutralization can extend the injury. Hands are affected in approximately 70% of chemical burns, which are quite painful.

Radiation Burns

Burns associated with radiation exposure are uncommon. Radiation burns usually are localized and indicate high radiation doses to the affected area. Radiation burns may appear identical

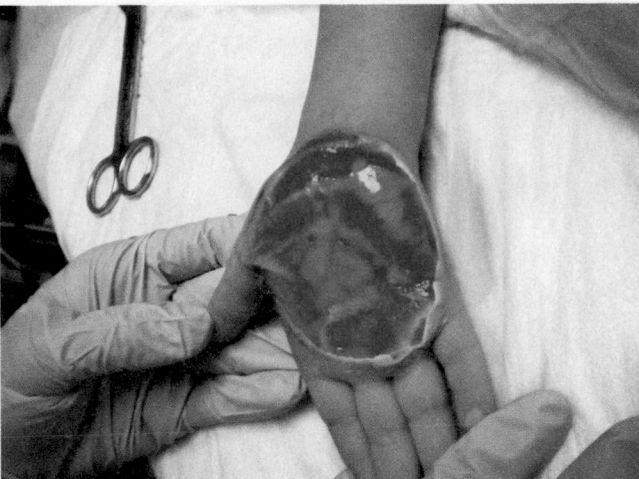

FIGURE 36-8 Partial-thickness contact palm burn.

to thermal burns.[14] The major difference is the time between exposure and clinical manifestation; it can be days to weeks, depending on the level of the radiation dose. Radiation injury can occur with exposure to industrial equipment such as accelerators and cyclotrons and to equipment used for medical treatment.

Location of Injury

Location of injury can be a determining factor in differentiating the level of care required. According to triage criteria from the American College of Surgeons, burns on the face, hands, feet, genitalia, major joints, and perineum are best treated in a burn center. These burns involve functional areas of the body and often require specialized intervention (Fig. 36-8). Injuries to these areas can result in significant long-term morbidity from impaired function and altered appearance.

Patient Age and History

Patient age and history are significant determinants of survival. Patients considered most at risk are those younger than 2 years and those older than 60 years. History of inhalation injury and electrical burns and all burns complicated by trauma and fractures (considered major injuries) significantly increase the risk for death. Obtaining the patient's medical history is important, particularly a history related to cardiac, pulmonary, or kidney dysfunction; diabetes; and central nervous system (CNS) disorders. In evaluating the pediatric patient, it is essential to obtain a thorough history, especially for the nonverbal patient. Attention should be paid to the description of the burn event to rule out nonaccidental trauma (Fig. 36-9). Social services such as child protective services and the police should be consulted if abuse or neglect is suspected.

Child Abuse

According to the U.S. Department of Health and Human Services Child Maltreatment 2010 report, 3.3 million referrals were made for child maltreatment, and of those, 436,321 were investigated and substantiated for abuse.[15] According to this report, 1560 children died from abuse and neglect. Child abuse or maltreatment should be a differential diagnosis when caring for

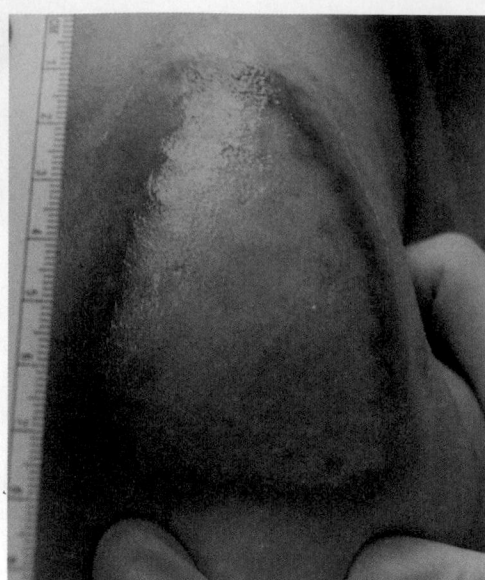

FIGURE 36-9 Partial-thickness iron burn to the right buttock from nonaccidental trauma.

children with burn injury, since greater than 15% of children suffering from maltreatment suffer from physical abuse.[15] Most often burns in children are accidental but are related to failure of the caregiver or parent to provide adequate supervision. However, the developmental age and size of the child are of key importance in ruling out accidental and nonaccidental burn injuries. The patterns of burns, that is, inflicted burns consistent with immersion or dunking, can be diagnostic of child abuse regardless of history.[16]

INITIAL EMERGENCY BURN MANAGEMENT

The goals of acute care of the patient with thermal injuries are to save life, minimize disability, and prepare the patient for definitive care. The burn injury may involve multiple organ systems, and the approach to the injured patient should be expeditious and methodical in identifying problems and establishing priorities of care.[17]

The resuscitation phase begins immediately after the burn insult has occurred; therefore, the nurse is concerned with patient management at the scene until admission to an appropriate medical facility. As with any major trauma, the first hour after injury is crucial; however, the first 24 to 36 hours after injury also are important in burn patient management. Management during this period has a major impact on the patient's survival and ultimate rehabilitation.

Obtaining a history regarding the nature of the injury is important in the management of the burn patient. Explosion of the water heater, propane gas, or grain elevator, and other types of explosions often throw the patient some distance and may result in concomitant orthopedic, neurologic, and internal trauma. It is valuable to know the specific agents involved if the burns are chemical. It also helps to know what substance was burned or inhaled and how long the patient was exposed to smoke or superheated air. A detailed patient history should include the mechanism of injury, patient's age, location and

size of burn, type and amount of fluid already administered, known allergies, status of tetanus immunization, and significant medical history. All rings, watches, and jewelry are removed from injured limbs to avoid a tourniquet effect when edema occurs as a result of fluid shifts and fluid resuscitation.

Airway Management

The first priority of emergency burn care is to secure and protect the airway. If there is any possibility of underlying cervical instability, cervical precautions must be initiated.[17] In patients with facial burns, exposure to fire in an enclosed space, or both, inhalation injury should be suspected. Carbon monoxide (CO) poisoning is associated with high mortality rates. Carboxyhemoglobin (HbCO) levels are obtained, and oxygen therapy is initiated. All patients with major burns or suspected inhalation injury are initially administered 100% oxygen.[17] The nurse should continue to observe the patient for clinical manifestations of impaired oxygenation such as tachypnea, agitation, anxiety, and upper airway obstruction (e.g., hoarseness, stridor, wheezing). Early intubation may save the life of the patient who has an inhalation injury because it may be impossible to perform this procedure later, when edema has obstructed the larynx. The need for frequent blood sampling and the benefit of continuous blood pressure monitoring may necessitate placement of an arterial line.

Respiratory Management

Circumferential, full-thickness burns to the chest wall can lead to restriction of chest wall expansion and decreased compliance. Decreased compliance requires higher ventilatory pressures to provide the patient with adequate tidal volumes. In the patient who has not undergone intubation, clinical manifestations of chest wall restriction include rapid, shallow respirations; poor chest wall excursion; and severe agitation. Arterial blood gas analysis reveals a decrease in oxygen tension and an increasing partial pressure of carbon dioxide ($Paco_2$) level. Patients receiving mechanical ventilation have increasing peak airway pressure values.

Escharotomies (burn eschar incisions) may be needed immediately to increase compliance and for improved ventilation. These incisions usually are made bilaterally along the anterior axillary lines and are connected by a transverse incision at the costal margin (Fig. 36-10).

Circulatory Management

The extent and depth of the burn are assessed. The extent of TBSA of the burn is calculated for estimation of fluid resuscitation requirements (Table 36-1); the Parkland formula is the most widely used method of calculation (see Box 36-5, Case Study: Patient with Burns at the end of the chapter). Burn shock is caused by the loss of fluid from the vascular compartment into the area of injury resulting in hypovolemia. The larger the percentage of burn area, the greater is the potential for development of shock. Lactated Ringer solution is infused through a large-bore cannula in a peripheral vein. Lactated Ringer solution, an isotonic crystalloid, is the resuscitation fluid used most often. Given in large amounts, it can restore cardiac output to normal in most patients. It is preferred over normal saline

TABLE 36-1   FORMULAS FOR FLUID REPLACEMENT OR RESUCITATION IN FIRST 24 HOURS

FLUID AND DOSE RATE	ABA CONSENSUS	PARKLAND	MODIFIED BROOKE	BROOKE	HYPERTONIC
Electrolyte solution	Ringer lactate	Ringer lactate	Ringer lactate	Ringer lactate	Hypertonic lactated saline (sodium, 250 mEq/L)
Dose: mL/kg/% burned*	2-4 50% of fluid over first 8 hr; 50% of fluid over next 16 hr	4	2	1.5	Rate based on urine output of 30-50 mL/hr

Examples using the ABA consensus formula: an 85-kg patient with 35% TBSA burn					
2 mL × 85 kg × 35% = 5950 mL in first 24 hours		3 mL × 85 × 35% = 8925 mL		4 mL × 85 × 35% = 11,900 mL	
2975 mL in first 8 hr = 372 mL/hr		4462 mL in first 8 hr = 558 mL/hr		5950 mL in first 8 hr = 744 mL/hr	
2975 mL in next 16 hr = 186 mL/hr		4462 mL in next 16 hr = 279 mL/hr		5950 mL in next 16 hr = 372 mL/hr	

*Adjust these rates to maintain a urine output >30 mL/hr in adults or 1 mL/kg/hr in children.
ABA, American Burn Association; *mEq/L*, milliequivalent per liter; *mL/hr*, milliliter per hour; *TBSA*, total body surface area.

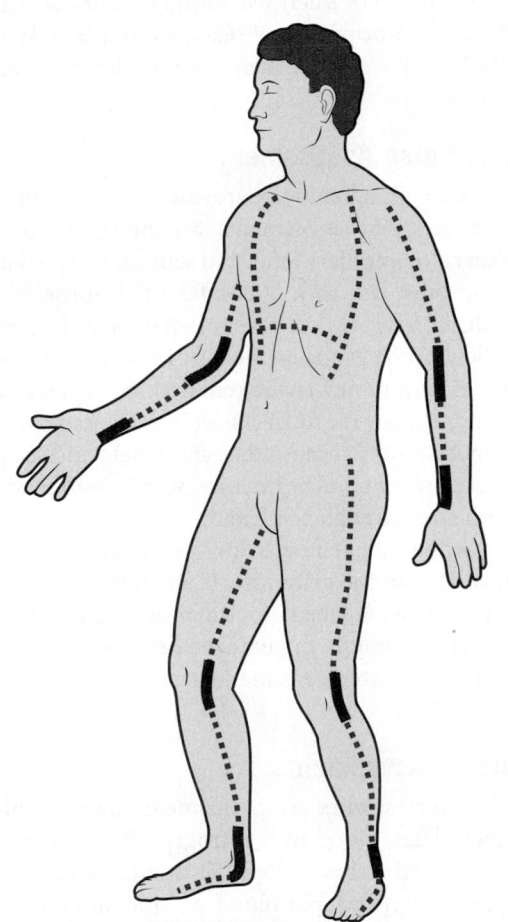

FIGURE 36-10 Preferred sites of escharotomy incisions. (From Carrougher GJ. *Burn Care and Therapy.* St. Louis: Mosby; 1998.)

because it most closely matches extracellular fluid. Because isotonic salt solutions generate no difference in osmotic pressure between plasma and the interstitial space, the entire extracellular space must be expanded to replace intravascular losses. Diuretics should not be given during the resuscitative phase of burn care.

According to the Parkland formula (see Table 36-1), half of the calculated amount of fluid is administered to the patient in the first 8 hours after injury; 25% is given in the second 8 hours, and 25% is given in the third 8 hours. It is important to remember that calculated fluid requirements are guidelines. Fluid resuscitation is a dynamic process. The rate of fluid administration is adjusted according to the individual's response, which is determined by monitoring urine output, heart rate, blood pressure, and level of consciousness. Meticulous attention to the patient's intake and output is imperative to ensure that he or she is appropriately resuscitated. Under-resuscitation may result in inadequate cardiac output, leading to inadequate organ perfusion and the potential for wound conversion from a partial-thickness to full-thickness injury. Over-resuscitation may lead to moderate to severe pulmonary edema, to excessive wound edema causing a decrease in perfusion of unburned tissue in the distal portions of the extremities, or to edema inhibiting perfusion of the zone of stasis, resulting in wound conversion.[11] Fluid requirements may be much higher than estimated by using the Parkland formula. The recommendations for these situations are included later in this chapter. For pediatric burn patients, add dextrose containing intravenous fluid at a maintenance rate along with Parkland resuscitation fluid. Pediatric patients need continuous dextrose infusions for vital organs.

Continuous monitoring with electrocardiograms (ECGs) should be used in patients with serious thermal burn injury and in the presence of electrical burns, inhalation injury, or associated traumatic injury. ECG lead placement may present a challenge with extensive burns, and nontraditional locations on nonburned skin should be selected instead.

Pathophysiology of Burn Shock

Burn injuries greater than 20% of TBSA can result in burn shock.[4] *Shock* is defined as inadequate cellular perfusion. Significant burn injury results in hypovolemic shock and tissue trauma. Both cause the production and release of several local and systemic mediators. Burn shock can occur even when hypovolemia is corrected.

The first component of burn shock is hypovolemic shock. At the cellular level, the burning agent produces dilation of the capillaries and small vessels, increasing the capillary permeability. Plasma seeps out into the surrounding tissue, producing blisters and edema. The type, duration, and intensity of the burn all affect the amount and extent of fluid loss. This progressive fluid loss in extensive burns results in significant intravascular fluid volume deficit. Edema occurs locally in the burn wound and systemically in unburned tissues. Edema formation is unique to thermal injury.

Burn edema has been attributed to several factors. Barrier property changes of the capillary wall occur by direct injury and indirect mediator-modulated changes. Increases in permeability of protein and water occur, resulting in edema. In most forms of shock, capillary pressure decreases as a result of arteriolar vasoconstriction. However, after burn injury, an increase in capillary pressure has been found in burned tissue in the first minutes to hours after injury, causing capillary leak for first 24 hours.[4] Coupled with this increase in capillary pressure is a negative interstitial hydrostatic pressure that occurs in the dermis layer of burned skin after thermal injury. This negative interstitial hydrostatic pressure represents an edema-generating mechanism that occurs for approximately 2 hours after injury. Plasma colloid osmotic pressure is decreased as a result of protein leakage into the extravascular space. Plasma is then further diluted with fluid resuscitation. The osmotic pressure is decreased, and further fluid extravasation can occur.

In addition to leaking capillaries, local and systemic mediators cause edema and the cardiovascular problems seen in burn patients. These mediators include histamine, prostaglandins, kinins, and oxygen radicals, they increase arteriolar vasodilation.[4] Manipulation of these mediators to stop the cascade of burn edema and burn shock is being researched.

The intravascular fluid changes combined with the action of inflammatory mediators and vasoconstricting mediators result in hemodynamic consequences in the burn patient. The hemodynamic alterations include decreased myocardial contractility and cardiac output despite adequate volume resuscitation, increased systemic vascular resistance (SVR), and increased pulmonary vascular resistance (PVR). Increased PVR can lead to pulmonary edema. Large but judicious volumes of resuscitation fluids are required to maintain the vascular volume during the first few hours after a large burn injury to provide optimal resuscitation. Early and full fluid resuscitation can prevent the complications of acute kidney injury, cardiovascular collapse, and death from shock. However, over-resuscitation increases edema formation, which can further impair tissue oxygen diffusion. The nurse must assess the patient's fluid status and response to resuscitation to obtain the optimal response.

Kidney Management

If fluid resuscitation is inadequate, acute kidney injury (AKI) may occur. An indwelling urinary catheter should be placed for burns greater than 15% to 20% of TBSA in the emergency department to monitor urine output and the effectiveness of fluid resuscitation. A catheter may be necessary if the burn extends into the perineal area because of the presence or development of edema. Urinary catheters with temperature probes should be used whenever possible. The nurse measures urine output hourly. Adequate urine output for adults is 0.5 to 1 milliliter per kilogram per hour (mL/kg/hr), or 30 to 50 mL/hr; in children, it is 1 mL/kg/hr.[4]

Gastrointestinal System Management

Patients with burns of more than 20% of TBSA are prone to gastric dilation as a result of paralytic ileus. Nasogastric or orogastric tubes are placed in these patients to prevent abdominal distention, emesis, and potential aspiration. This decrease in gastrointestinal (GI) function is caused by the effects of hypovolemia and the neurologic and endocrine response to injury. GI activity usually returns in 24 to 48 hours. Gastric prophylaxis with histamine blockers or sucralfate is initiated because burn patients are prone to *Curling stress ulcers*. These acute ulcerations of the duodenum are caused by sloughing of the gastric mucosa resulting from loss of plasma volume after severe burns. Enteral nutrition has been shown to be protective of gastric mucosal integrity and to improve intestinal flow, gastric motility, and intestinal blood flow in burned patients.[18] Enteral nutrition should be started as soon as possible. Severely burned patients can be safely fed within 6 hours of burn injury in the duodenum or jejunum.[18] Care should be taken to start enteral feeds for burn patients via nasoduodenal or nasojejunal tube promptly.

Extremity Pulse Assessment

Edema formation may cause neurovascular compromise to the extremities; frequent assessments are necessary to evaluate pulses, skin color, capillary refill, and sensation. Arterial circulation is at greatest risk with circumferential burns. If not corrected, reduced arterial flow causes ischemia and necrosis. The Doppler flow probe is one of the best ways to evaluate arterial pulses. An escharotomy may be required to restore arterial circulation and to allow for further swelling. The escharotomy can be performed at the bedside with a sterile field and scalpel. Care must be taken to avoid major nerves, vessels, and tendons. The incision extends through the length of the eschar, over joints, and down to the subcutaneous fat. The incision is placed laterally or medially on the extremity. If a single incision does not restore circulation, bilateral incisions are required (see Fig. 36-8). If escharotomy is required before the patient is transferred to a burn center, consultation with the receiving physician is advised.

Laboratory Assessment

Initial laboratory studies are performed: complete blood cell count, electrolytes, blood urea nitrogen (BUN), creatine, urinalysis, and blood screening. Special situations such as inhalation injury warrant arterial blood gas measurements, HbCO level determination, cultures, and alcohol and drug screens. A baseline assessment of nutritional status, including albumin and prealbumin, is helpful in monitoring future nutritional needs. An ECG is obtained for all patients with electrical burns or pre-existing heart disease.

Wound Care

After the wounds have been assessed, topical antimicrobial therapy is not a priority during emergency care. However, the wounds must be covered with clean, dry dressings or sheets. Every attempt must be made to keep the patient warm because of the high risk of hypothermia. The administration of tetanus prophylaxis is recommended for all burns covering more than

10% of the TBSA and for patients with a questionable immunization history.[10]

Burn Center Referral

After initial treatment and stabilization at an emergency department, referral to a burn center is considered (see Box 36-1). A burn center must be able to deliver all therapy required, including rehabilitation, and must perform personnel training and burn research.[17] Patients meeting the criteria for referral need the expertise of a multidisciplinary team. Referring hospitals must always contact the burn center in their region.[2] Providers in the field should cover the burns with clean, dry cloth until arrival at the burn center. Early communication between the initial provider and the burn center is encouraged by the American Burn Association (ABA).[19]

SPECIAL MANAGEMENT CONSIDERATIONS

Inhalation Injury

Inhalation injury can occur in the presence or absence of cutaneous injury. Inhalation injuries are strongly associated with burns sustained in a closed space, and they constitute the leading cause of fire-related deaths.[20] Inhalation injury appears in three basic forms, alone or in combination: CO poisoning, direct heat injury, and chemical damage. The three types of inhalation injury are CO poisoning, upper airway injury, and lower airway injury.

Immediate measures to save the life of the burn patient include management of the airway. The burn patient may exhibit few or no signs of airway distress; however, thermal injury to the airway must be anticipated if facial burns, singed eyebrows and nasal hair, carbon deposits in the oropharynx, and carbonaceous sputum are present or if the history suggests confinement in a burning environment. Any of these findings indicates acute inhalation injury and requires immediate and definitive care. To prevent the necessity of tracheostomy or cricothyrotomy, the use of early intubation and respiratory support must be considered before tracheal edema occurs. Inhalation injury predisposes the patient to the development of pneumonia and acute respiratory distress syndrome (ARDS).[20] Management of ARDS necessitates mechanical ventilatory support and, in extreme cases, high-frequency oscillatory ventilation or extracorporeal membrane oxygenation. The occurrence of inhalation injury with cutaneous burns increases the fluid requirements during resuscitation to a higher level than would be predicted by the cutaneous burn alone.

Carbon Monoxide Poisoning

Persons found dead at the scene of a fire, who may have few or no cutaneous thermal injuries, would have died of CO poisoning. CO is a colorless, odorless, and tasteless gas. Inhalation of CO, a byproduct of the incomplete combustion of carbon, results in its bonding to available hemoglobin, producing HbCO, which effectively decreases oxygen saturation of hemoglobin. The affinity of hemoglobin molecules for CO is approximately 200 to 250 times greater than that for oxygen.[9] HbCO binds poorly with oxygen, reducing the oxygen-carrying capacity of blood and causing hypoxemia. The shortage of oxygen at the tissue level is worsened by a shift to the left of the oxyhemoglobin dissociation curve, reflecting the fact that the oxygen in the hemoglobin is not readily given up to the cells.

Arterial oxygen saturation measurement is of limited value because oxygen saturation may be quite high despite dangerously low levels of oxygen content. Because the pulse oximeter cannot distinguish between oxyhemoglobin and HbCO, it is an unreliable predictor of tissue oxygenation during the initial stages of CO poisoning.[9] Arterial blood gas determinations and oxygen saturation are used to accurately assess the hemoglobin oxygen saturation level. A serum HbCO level is obtained the diagnosis. Normal HbCO levels are less than 2%. HbCO levels of 40% to 60% often produce unresponsiveness or obtundation; levels of 15% to 40% may result in various degrees of CNS dysfunction. Levels of 10% to 15%, which can be found in cigarette smokers, rarely produce serious symptoms but may cause a headache.

The major clinical manifestations of severe CO poisoning are related to the CNS and the heart. Symptoms associated with CO poisoning include headache, dizziness, nausea, vomiting, dyspnea, and confusion.[9] In severe cases, CO poisoning may lead to myocardial ischemia and CNS complications caused by lowered oxygen delivery and the already compromised circulatory system. Early signs of CO poisoning may include tachycardia, tachypnea, confusion, and lightheadedness. As the CO level rises, patients exhibit a decreased level of responsiveness, which may progress to unresponsiveness and respiratory failure.

The treatment of choice for CO poisoning is high-flow oxygen administered at 100% through a tight-fitting nonrebreathing mask or endotracheal intubation. The half-life of CO in the body is 4 hours at room air (21% oxygen), 2 hours at 40% oxygen, and 40 to 60 minutes at 100% oxygen.[9] The half-life of CO is 30 minutes in a hyperbaric oxygen chamber at three times atmospheric pressure. The use of hyperbaric oxygen is controversial in the care of the burn patient. Because of the rapid removal of CO with the administration of 100% oxygen, the time required to transport a patient who has received oxygen in the field should always be considered to avoid possible underestimation of inhalation injury.

Upper Airway Injury

Burns of the upper respiratory tract include those involving the pharynx, larynx, glottis, trachea, and larger bronchi. Injuries are caused by direct heat or by chemical inflammation and necrosis. Respiratory injury is most often confined to the upper airway. The heat exchange capability is so efficient that most heat absorption and damage occur in the pharynx and larynx above the true vocal cords.

Heat damage may be severe enough to cause upper airway obstruction at any time, beginning from moment of injury through the resuscitation period. Caution is taken for patients with severe hypovolemia because supraglottic edema may be delayed until fluid resuscitation is under way and third spacing occurs. Patients must be monitored for hoarseness, stridor, audible airflow turbulence, and the production of carbonaceous sputum. Maximal edema occurs 24 hours after injury with upper airway injuries, and these patients should be observed in the critical care unit for a minimum of 24 hours.[10]

The prediction of an upper airway obstruction is based on consideration of several variables: extent of injury to the face and neck, the presence of blisters on or redness of the posterior pharynx, signs of singed nasal hair, increased HbCO levels, increased rate and decreased depth of breathing, hoarseness, and stridor (which indicates a significant decrease in the diameter of the airway), increased amount of sputum, and the circumstances of the burn event (whether it occurred in an enclosed space or involved superheated gases or steam). Steam has a heat-carrying capacity many times that of dry air, and it is capable of overwhelming the extremely efficient heat-dissipating capabilities of the upper airway.

Intubation is recommended whenever airway patency is questionable, rather than delaying intubation until airway obstruction is so severe that intubation becomes a challenge. After the airway is secure, priority is given to minimizing airway edema, maintaining pulmonary hygiene, and treating bronchospasm. Elevating of the head of the bed to 30 degrees or higher decreases airway edema. Therapeutic deep breathing and coughing, early mobility, suctioning, and bronchodilators assist in mobilizing and removing secretions. Fiberoptic bronchoscopy may be required to remove secretions in some patients. Mechanical ventilatory support is necessary when respiratory fatigue or failure occurs. Precautions to prevent ventilator-associated pneumonia (VAP) should be implemented to avoid secondary infection.

Lower Airway Injury

Heated air rarely causes lower airway injury. If it does, it usually is associated with death at the scene. Lower airway injuries are typically caused by chemical damage to mucosal surfaces. Tracheobronchitis with severe spasm and wheezing may occur in the first minutes to hours after injury. Historically, the most accurate method of documenting lower airway injury is the xenon ventilation–perfusion lung scan. Prolonged retention or symmetry of washout of the radioisotope indicates pulmonary parenchymal injury on the side of the retained emissions. The onset of symptoms is unpredictable following smoke inhalation and patients at risk must be closely monitored for at least 24 to 48 hours after injury.[9]

Research into optimal ventilator management strategies for patients with inhalation injury is a high priority.[21] In addition to thermal damage, secondary effects from massive fluid resuscitation and high-volume, high-pressure ventilator settings can precipitate ARDS.[21] The use of lung protective ventilation with low tidal volumes, higher levels of positive end-expiratory pressure (PEEP), and plateau pressures maintained below 30 mm Hg are increasingly employed.[21] Intrabronchial surfactant and inhaled nitric are other last resorts in dealing with burn patients with inhalation injuries that have not responded to other means of ventilator support.[9] Benefits include decreased rates of pneumonia and increased survival.[22] Treatment of lower airway injury is largely symptomatic. As with upper airway injury management, aggressive pulmonary hygiene, removal of secretions, ventilatory support, and careful fluid resuscitation as to avoid exacerbating pulmonary edema and ARDS when caring for burn patients with lower airway inhalation injuries.[10]

Nonthermal Burns
Chemical Burns

Chemical burns can be caused by a variety of products. Acids, alkalis, and organic and inorganic compounds cause chemical burns. The acid or base quality determines the injurious nature of a product. The injury is caused by the pH of the product or by the concentration of the product. In the past, irrigation with neutralizing solutions was recommended to limit the extent and depth of chemical burns. This practice is no longer advocated because neutralizing agents may cause reactions that are exothermic (produce heat), thereby increasing the extent and depth of the burn. It also is possible that the neutralizing agent is neither immediately known nor available. Instead, large amounts of water should be used to flush the area. Clothing and shoes should be removed if they have been in contact with the chemical. Alkali burns of the eyes require continuous irrigation for many hours after the injury. Removal of contact lenses is necessary before irrigation.

Treatments for chemical burns vary. Phenol burns are first diluted, and then the skin is wiped quickly with polyethylene glycol or vegetable oil to decrease the severity of the burn. Areas exposed to hydrofluoric acid must be copiously irrigated with water; the burned area then can be treated with 2.5% calcium gluconate gel. The patient may need calcium gluconate supplements because the fluoride ion precipitates serum calcium, causing hypocalcemia. White phosphorus can ignite if kept dry, and these wounds must be covered with a moist dressing. After a tar or asphalt injury, the removal of tar or asphalt is best accomplished with the use of petroleum-containing distillates. One such product is Detachol (Ferndale Laboratories, Inc., Ferndale, MI). The solution can be placed directly on the wound and gently wiped off. Routine débridement of loose skin is initiated after tar removal. Topical antimicrobial therapy is then provided.

Electrical Burns

In electrical burns, the type and voltage of the circuit, resistance, pathway of transmission through the body, and duration of contact are considered in determining the amount of damage sustained. In these situations, the rescuer also may be injured if he or she becomes part of the electrical circuit. The rescuer must disconnect the electrical source to break the circuit or must know how to avoid becoming part of the circuit. The use of appropriately insulated equipment that diverts the circuit elsewhere is essential. Extreme caution must be used in the rescue of victims.

Electricity always travels toward the ground. The body conducts electrical current as a whole, as opposed to the earlier belief that it traveled most quickly through the nerves and circulatory system. Electrical burns often are much more serious than the surface appearance of the wound suggests.[22] As the electrical current passes through the body, it damages the inner tissues and may leave little evidence of a burn on the skin surface.

The electrical burn process can result in a profound alteration in acid–base balance and rhabdomyolysis resulting in myoglobinuria, which poses a serious threat to kidney function. Myoglobin is a normal constituent of muscle. With extensive muscle destruction, it is released into the circulatory system and filtered by the kidneys. It can be highly toxic and can lead to AKI. Fluid resuscitation for the electrical burn patient does not correlate with the Parkland formula, and the fluid is adjusted according to the patient's urine output. If myoglobin is present in the urine, a urine output greater than 100 mL/hr in adults and 2 mL/kg/hr in children is established until the urine is clear of all myoglobin pigment.[4,22]

If hemoglobinuria is identified, the clinician should assume that the patient has myoglobinuria and acidosis. Sodium bicarbonate may be administered to bring the pH level into the normal range, to correct a documented acidosis, or to alkalize urine to promote myoglobin excretion. Diuretics such as mannitol also may be administered intravenously until myoglobinuria resolves.[4] Sodium bicarbonate infusions and diuretic therapy are called *forced alkaline diuresis*. A baseline ECG and myocardial biomarker levels are obtained while the patient is in the emergency department. The following criteria are used for monitoring the cardiac status of burned patients:

- A history of loss of consciousness or cardiac arrest
- Documentation of cardiac dysrhythmia at the scene of the accident or in the emergency department
- Abnormal ECG findings on admission
- TBSA burns of more than 20%
- Very young age or advanced age
- Prior history of heart disease

Other burn patients may be admitted to nonmonitored settings and observed closely. Cardiac dysrhythmias must be treated promptly, and a protocol to rule out myocardial infarction must be followed.

BURN NURSING DIAGNOSES AND MANAGEMENT

The clinical course of a burn injury has three phases: (1) resuscitative, (2) acute care, and (3) rehabilitative. Each phase has a unique set of actual and potential problems. The resuscitative phase begins with initial hemodynamic response to the injury and lasts until capillary integrity is restored and the repletion of plasma volume by fluid replacement occurs. Spontaneous diuresis demonstrates that capillaries have regained their integrity. The acute phase begins with the onset of diuresis of fluid mobilized from the interstitial space and ends with the closure of the burn wound. The major focus of the acute phase is wound healing, wound closure, and prevention of infection. The rehabilitative phase begins when the patient is admitted to the hospital, with correction of functional deficits and scar management being major considerations. The rehabilitative phase may last months to years, depending on the severity of injury. The rehabilitation phase focuses on support for adequate wound healing, prevention of scarring and contractures, and psychologic support of the patient and the family.[23]

Resuscitation Phase

Life-threatening airway and breathing problems, cardiopulmonary instability, and hypovolemia characterize the resuscitation phase, or shock phase. Every organ is involved in the physiologic response that occurs with thermal injury of greater than 20%

of TBSA.[4] The magnitude of this pathophysiologic response is proportional to the extent of cutaneous injury. The goal of the resuscitation phase is to maintain vital organ function and perfusion. Emergent interventions for inhalation injury, airway management, and hypovolemia are concurrently addressed.

Oxygenation Alterations

Inhalation injuries have emerged as the most common cause of death in burn patients, whereas 40 to 50 years ago, burn shock and then burn sepsis accounted for most burn-related deaths. Early diagnosis of inhalation injury is essential to minimize complications and to decrease the mortality rate. Three oxygenation complications are associated with smoke inhalation during the resuscitation phase: (1) *CO poisoning*, (2) *upper airway obstruction*, and (3) *chemical pneumonitis*. Evaluation of a patient for inhalation injury includes physical assessment (e.g., singed facial hairs, mucosal burns of nose or mouth, carbonaceous sputum), arterial blood gas analysis, HbCO levels, chest radiography, flexible fiberoptic bronchoscopy, xenon 133 lung scan, and pulmonary function tests. Critical care nursing management includes the following:

- Assess breath sounds and the rate and quality of respirations.
- Administer oxygen, as prescribed.
- Monitor HbCO levels.
- Elevate the head of the bed, and implement VAP precautions.
- Assess and assist with pulmonary secretion suctioning.
- Observe for signs of airway obstruction (e.g., increased respiratory rate and heart rate, increased work of breathing, use of accessory muscles, stridor, wheezing, hoarseness, crackles).
- Prepare for endotracheal intubation and mechanical ventilation.
- Maintain accurate and timely documentation.

Impaired Gas Exchange. The most common pulmonary burn complication is CO poisoning. High-flow oxygen should be administered at 100% through a nonrebreathing mask or endotracheal intubation until the HbCO level is less than 10% to 15%.

Chemical pneumonitis is caused by inhalation of the byproducts of combustion of substances such as cotton, aldehydes, oxides of sulfur, and nitrogen. Burning polyvinylchloride yields at least 75 potentially toxic compounds, including hydrochloric acid and CO. Within days after a burn, ARDS commonly develops in patients with chemical pneumonitis. The primary clinical manifestation of ARDS is hypoxemia that is refractory to oxygen therapy. Early signs include increased pH, decreased $Paco_2$, and an increased respiratory rate. Ventilatory support with the use of PEEP is the treatment of choice.

Ineffective Airway Clearance. Laryngeal swelling and upper airway obstruction may occur at any time during the first 24 hours after the burn injury. Endotracheal intubation must be accomplished early because this simple procedure can become extremely difficult in the presence of laryngeal edema. Usually, enough time is available to intervene after obtaining the history and transporting the patient to the primary hospital. Edema may continue to develop for 72 hours after the burn incident.[4]

The patient who has not initially undergone intubation must be carefully monitored during this critical period. When prolonged ventilatory failure is expected as a result of severe inhalation, a tracheostomy is performed.

Extubation should occur only if the patient can meet extubation criteria: level of consciousness assessed as *awake*, intact cough and gag reflexes, inspiratory effort greater than −25 centimeter of water (cm H$_2$O) in adults, vital capacity of 10 mL/kg, and decreased volume and tenacity of the sputum. Resolution of airway edema can be assessed by deflating the endotracheal cuff and observing the patient's ability to breathe around the endotracheal tube.

Although uncommon, laryngospasm must be addressed. It usually is brought on by airway irritation from the inhalation of noxious agents.

Fluid Resuscitation

Current resuscitation protocols emphasize fluid delivery rates based on the extent of burn and the patient's weight. The patient's weight measured in kilograms must be obtained on admission to the hospital. The extent of the burn is calculated by using one of the methods previously described. Several formulas are available to guide fluid resuscitation and should be used to assist in the management of fluid replacement (see Table 36-1). The formulas differ primarily in terms of administration, volume, and sodium content. The actual amount of fluid given to any patient must be based on that individual's response.

The type of fluid used in resuscitation and at what point a switch should be made to a colloid solution are controversial topics. No clear-cut guidelines for resuscitation exist. The administration of crystalloid fluid (lactated Ringer solution) for the first 24 to 36 hours after the burn is the most common practice. Lactated Ringer solution is the crystalloid solution of choice because of its physiologic similarity to the composition of extracellular fluid. In the pediatric population, the addition of lactated Ringer solution with 5% dextrose (D$_5$LR) should be considered as maintenance fluid, especially in the first 24 hours. Assessment for secondary injuries that would affect the choice of fluid should be performed. Ideally, the capillary leak seals approximately 24 hours after the injury, making it possible to give colloid without leakage of protein into the interstitium. Colloid deficits are replaced in the next 24 hours with salt-free albumin or dextran at 0.3 to 1 mL/kg/% TBSA burn. In addition to colloid, maintenance fluids are given to replace evaporative losses, and the amount is adjusted according to the patient's serum electrolyte levels, urine output, weight, volume status, and clinical assessment.

Deficient Fluid Volume. Physiologic effects of the burn complicate the tissue damage that occurs after the burn insult. Coagulation factors are affected, protein is denatured, and cellular content is ionized. These factors, coupled with the dilation of capillaries and small vessels, lead to increased capillary permeability and fluid shifts from the intravascular space to the interstitial space. The lymphatic system, which normally carries away the increased interstitial fluid, may be damaged or overloaded and unable to function to its normal capacity.

In addition to the protein and electrolyte shift, an increased insensible water loss occurs. In the healthy adult, this loss is estimated to be 35 to 50 mL/hr. The burn patient's insensible water loss may be as much as 300 to 3000 mL/day. This increase may be related to temperature elevation, tracheostomy, and the size of the burn.

Burn shock is proportional to the extent and depth of injury. The loss of plasma begins almost immediately after the injury and reaches its peak within the first 48 hours. Desired clinical responses to fluid resuscitation include a urinary output of 0.5 to 1 mL/kg/hr, a heart rate lower than 120 beats per minute (beats/min), blood pressure in the normal to high range, a central venous pressure less than 12 cm H$_2$O or a pulmonary artery occlusion pressure (PAOP) less than 18 mm Hg, clear lung sounds, clear sensorium, and the absence of intestinal events such as nausea and paralytic ileus. Heart rate, blood pressure, and central venous pressure values are not always accurate or reliable predictors of successful fluid resuscitation.

Potassium and sodium, the two electrolytes of concern during the resuscitation period, must be monitored carefully. *Hyperkalemia* can occur during this phase because of (1) the release of potassium from damaged cells, (2) metabolic acidosis, and (3) impaired kidney function caused by hemoglobinuria, myoglobinuria, or decreased renal perfusion. The patient must be assessed for the clinical manifestations of hyperkalemia. Treatment includes correction of acidosis. During the resuscitation phase, using cation-exchange resins or intravenously administered insulin and hypertonic dextrose to transport potassium back into the cell is not recommended because of the unpredictable nature of fluid shifts that occur.

Hypokalemia can occur during the resuscitation phase because of the massive loss of fluids and electrolytes through the burn wounds or because of hemodilution. During the acute phase, it may be related to hemodilution; inadequate replacement; loss associated with diuresis, diarrhea, vomiting, nasogastric drainage, and long hydrotherapy sessions; or the shift of potassium from the intravascular space to the cell after the acidosis has been corrected. Nursing interventions include treating nausea and vomiting, limiting immersive hydrotherapy sessions to less than 30 minutes, preventing fluid volume excess, and judicious replacement of potassium.

Hyponatremia is not uncommon during the resuscitation phase because of the loss of sodium through the burn wound, the shift of fluid into the interstitial space, vomiting, nasogastric drainage, diarrhea, and the use of hypotonic salt solutions during the early phase of resuscitation. During this phase, it may be necessary to monitor serum sodium levels every 4 to 8 hours. Hyponatremia also may occur during the acute phase because of hemodilution and loss through the wound, lengthy hydrotherapy sessions, and excessive diuresis resulting from the fluid shift back into the intravascular space. Interventions are followed for treating nausea and vomiting, hydrotherapy sessions are limited, and intravenous replacement of sodium is considered. During diuresis, which occurs during the acute phase, restricting free water intake usually is the only required intervention to increase the serum sodium level.

Risk for Infection

Preventing infection in the burn patient is a true challenge and involves complex decision making. Considerable debate has been going on about the infection control precautions to use with burn patients. The burn wound is the most common source of infection in the burn patient. The loss of the protective mechanism of the skin and contamination from the patient's own bacterial flora can lead to bloodstream infections. Some centers advocate routine wound surveillance cultures and wound biopsy to identify infection early. Daily wound inspection for changes in appearance such as an increase in exudate, odor, or color is necessary to minimize the risk of bacteremia. Patients should not be treated with antibiotics prophylactically; rather, treatment should be tailored to positive culture results.[10]

Cross-contamination by direct contact is a significant source of infection and a subsequent cause of sepsis. Effective hand-washing technique cannot be overemphasized. Nurses must wash their hands and change gloves when moving from area to area on the same patient. For example, after changing the chest dressing, which may be contaminated with sputum from the tracheostomy, hands must be washed and gloves changed before the nurse moves to the legs. Gowns, gloves, and masks should be worn whenever contact with body fluids occurs. These garments also must be changed and hands washed before caring for a different patient. Maintaining patient-specific dressings and topical agents is recommended. Equipment such as thermometers, intravenous pumps, and stethoscopes should be designated for each patient or, when shared, should be cleaned with appropriate bactericidal cleansers between patients.

Whichever precautions are used, everyone coming in contact with the patient, including the patient's family and visitors, must be knowledgeable about the standard for infection control. These precautions should be strictly followed by all.

Tissue Perfusion
Ineffective Kidney Tissue Perfusion

Urinalysis to determine the myoglobin level may be performed soon after burn injury. Myoglobinuria can be detected grossly by the dark, port-wine color of the urine. Myoglobin is extremely toxic to the kidneys and can cause massive tubular destruction. It is best treated with rapid fluid administration and forced diuresis with diuretics such as mannitol, an osmotic diuretic. The goal is an hourly urine output that is at least double the general recommendations to flush the kidney tubules. All other diuretics are avoided because they will deplete the already compromised intravascular volume. Sodium bicarbonate is sometimes given intravenously to alkalinize the urine and assist in the elimination of heme pigments.

Maintaining and monitoring the renal system is vital in burn patient management. Impairment of the renal system may be related to hemoglobinuria, myoglobinuria, hypoperfusion, and hypovolemia. Urinary output must be monitored every hour for the first 48 to 72 hours, and specific gravity values can be used to determine the adequacy of hydration status and renal competency. The urine glucose concentration is monitored, as are urine sodium, creatinine, and BUN levels. Use of an indwelling urinary catheter is appropriate for the first 48 to 72 hours. Because of the tremendous risk of infection related to indwelling catheters, they are removed as soon as possible. However, leaving the catheter in place may be necessary if perineal burns are involved. Oliguria is usually related to inadequate fluid

resuscitation but may be associated with AKI. Other signs of kidney failure include increasing creatinine, BUN, phosphorus, and potassium levels; excessive fluid-weight gain; excessive edema; elevated blood pressure; lethargy; and confusion.

The presence of glucose in the urine causes osmotic diuresis. In this clinical situation, urine output is an unreliable estimate of volume status. Because of the increased loss of fluid through the kidneys, glucosuria may suggest the need for additional fluid beyond the original estimates.

Ineffective Cerebral Tissue Perfusion

The patient's neurologic status is assessed frequently during the first few days. Changes may be related to an associated head injury that occurred at the time of burn injury, hypoperfusion related to hypovolemia, hypoxemia associated with inadequate ventilation, CO poisoning, or electrolyte imbalances. Patients with electrical burns or major thermal burns may have peripheral neurologic injuries, which may not become evident for several days after the injury. The neurologic assessment includes use of the Glasgow Coma Scale (GCS). It is not unusual for the patient to be agitated, restless, and extremely anxious during the resuscitation phase of burn injury as a result of hypovolemia, pain, and the fear of disfigurement or death. However, the possibility of neurologic involvement must not be overlooked. Maintaining an adequate mean arterial pressure is essential to ensure adequate cerebral perfusion pressure.

Ineffective Peripheral Tissue Perfusion

Ineffective peripheral tissue perfusion results from third spacing of fluid during the resuscitation phase, which restricts blood flow to extremities. As hypovolemia ensues, vasoconstriction increases, which can be potentiated by the loss of body temperature. Peripheral tissue perfusion must be monitored carefully in all burn patients. Burned as well as unburned areas are carefully assessed for warmth, color, and peripheral pulses. Capillary refill time should be less than 3 seconds in unburned areas. Any clinical manifestation of diminished systemic tissue perfusion must be reported immediately. Nursing actions are taken to minimize any compromise of peripheral circulation. Close monitoring of appropriate fluid resuscitation and careful positioning of the patient are necessary to prevent compromised blood flow. Crossed legs, dependent positions, and pillows under the patient's knees should be avoided. Specialty mattresses and beds may be helpful to prevent secondary skin breakdown and assist with positioning and pulmonary toilet. The limbs should be elevated above the heart to decrease peripheral edema and enhance venous return. Assisted range-of-motion exercises can help to decrease edema.

Monitoring the peripheral circulation is crucial in the burn patient with circumferential, full-thickness burns of the extremities. The resulting edema may severely compromise the venous system and then the arterial system. Neurovascular integrity of extremities with circumferential burns must be assessed every hour for the first 24 to 48 hours using the six Ps: *pulselessness, pallor, pain, paresthesia, paralysis,* and *poikilothermy.* Careful, ongoing assessment is necessary, especially for patients who are intubated and may not be able to communicate pain or paresthesia. The use of a Doppler flowmeter may be necessary. Loss of pulses is a late sign of compromised vascular flow. If any changes are noticed, the physician must be notified immediately. Numbness and paresthesia may occur only 30 minutes before loss of pulses. Irreversible nerve ischemia resulting in loss of function may begin after 12 to 24 hours. An escharotomy may become necessary to allow the underlying tissue to expand. In deeper wounds, a fasciotomy, which involves incision into the fascia, may be necessary.

Ineffective Gastrointestinal Tissue Perfusion

Paralytic ileus is a common GI complication that can occur during resuscitation or when sepsis develops. The abdomen and bowel sounds should be assessed every 2 hours during the initial phase and every 4 hours thereafter. If clinical manifestations of a paralytic ileus occur, oral intake is withheld, and a nasogastric tube is inserted and placed on low to medium suction. Paralytic ileus can be related to hypokalemia, the sympathetic response to severe trauma, or decreased tissue perfusion related to hypovolemia.

A stress ulcer may develop as a result of decreased tissue perfusion to the GI tract, a change in the quantity or quality of mucus (which has a pH of 1), or an increase in gastric acid secretion resulting from the stress response. Gastric acid should be maintained above a pH of 5 through the administration of antacids, histamine blockers, or proton pump inhibitors to prevent the development of these ulcers. The patient should be carefully monitored for GI bleeding. All stools and gastric content are tested for occult blood. The patient should be observed for epigastric discomfort or fullness, decreased blood pressure, or increased pulse.

Invasive Monitoring. The decision to use invasive monitoring techniques requires careful consideration of the potential risk factors and how the data collected will influence the course of treatment. Invasive monitoring should be considered if treatment seems ineffective or if complicating factors such as severe respiratory involvement, major life-threatening injuries, head injuries, or pneumothorax occur. Patients with pre-existing medical conditions such as chronic obstructive pulmonary disease, acute heart failure, and kidney failure also may require invasive monitoring.

Invasive monitoring includes direct measurement of central venous pressure, pulmonary artery pressure, arterial pressure, core temperature, cardiac output, SVR, and PVR. The use of an arterial line is considered if serial and frequent arterial blood gas values are required for respiratory management or for hemodynamic instability requiring the titration of vasoactive drugs. Central venous catheters can be helpful in the early stages of fluid resuscitation to deliver the massive amount of fluids required. The physician selects the catheter insertion site based on burn location and the purpose of the catheter. It is preferable not to insert catheters through burned skin. It may be appropriate to use a multilumen catheter that can serve as a route for fluid resuscitation, maintenance fluids, antibiotic therapy, and vasoactive drugs. The risks involved include the increased chance of infection, potential for pneumothorax, and difficulty with insertion if hypovolemia is present.

Pulmonary artery catheters are placed only when necessary for optimal care. They may be essential to the survival of the septic patient despite the risks involved. Pulmonary artery catheters can provide data about PAOP, cardiac output, stroke volume, SVR and PVR, core temperature, and mixed venous oxygen saturation levels.

Centrally placed intravascular catheters require meticulous care. Strict guidelines should be established and monitored. Catheters are inserted under sterile conditions, and the dressings are changed under the same conditions. Because infection is such a major concern, all invasive catheters should be removed as early as possible.

Hypothermia. Thermoregulation maintenance is a nursing challenge. The patient with extensive burn injury is at high risk for hypothermia. Hypothermia is especially problematic during initial treatment, during hydrotherapy, and immediately after surgery. Heat is lost through open burn wounds by means of evaporation and radiation. The patient's core temperature should be maintained between 37.6° C (99.6° F) and 38.3° C (101° F).

Laboratory Assessment. Laboratory assessment is another important aspect of burn care. Because of the invasive nature of drawing blood, it is done only if absolutely indicated. Consideration should be given to the age of the patient, the size of the burn, the time since injury, and any underlying disease process.

White blood cell (WBC) counts usually are monitored for elevation, a sign of sepsis. It is not unusual, however, for the WBC count to fall below $5000/mm^3$ within 48 hours after injury. The value may drop even lower—$1500/mm^3$ to $2000/mm^3$—with the use of silver sulfadiazine. Hemoglobin and hematocrit data can be useful in the resuscitative phase to guide fluid administration. If surgical débridement is required, monitoring blood counts in the postoperative period is important. Serum chemistry information is helpful for ongoing assessment of kidney function and electrolyte balance. The myriad tests available should be used appropriately and as indicated by individual patient needs.

Acute Care Phase

The acute care phase of burn management begins after resuscitation and lasts until complete wound closure is achieved. The early postresuscitation phase is a period of transition from the shock phase to the hypermetabolic phase. Major cardiopulmonary and wound changes occur that substantially alter the manner of patient care from that given during resuscitation. Cardiopulmonary stability is optimal during this period because wound inflammation and infection have not developed. Hypermetabolic changes can be complicated with the onset of wound infection and sepsis. Early wound excision and skin grafting procedures, local wound care, nutritional support, and infection control characterize this phase.

Critical care nurses play a major role in promoting the healing process. Nurses, as skilled clinicians of the burn team, provide daily wound assessment, hydrotherapy, débridement, preoperative and postoperative management, and pain management.

Immediately after injury, the body responds by initiating a series of physiologic changes to restore skin integrity. These physiologic changes include the inflammatory phase, the proliferative phase, and the maturation phase.

Inflammatory Phase

The inflammatory phase begins immediately after injury. Vascular changes and cellular activity characterize this period. Changes in the severed vessels occur in an attempt to wall off the wound from the external environment. Platelets, activated as a result of vessel wall injury, aggregate; blood coagulation is initiated; and in larger vessels, smooth muscle tissue contraction occurs, resulting in a reduction in the diameter of the vessel lumen. These brief but important compensatory mechanisms protect the individual from excessive blood loss and increased exposure to bacterial contamination. As vasodilation occurs, vascular permeability and blood supply to the wound site increase. Clinically, this is observed as erythema and exudates.[24] Granulocytes invade the wound within 24 hours and initiate the phagocytosis of necrotic tissue and bacteria. Fibroblasts migrate to the wound and multiply, producing a bed of collagen. This phase of healing lasts from the moment of injury to day 3 to day 5.[25]

Proliferative Phase

The proliferative phase of healing occurs approximately 4 to 20 days after injury. The key cell in this phase of healing, the fibroblast, rapidly synthesizes collagen. Collagen synthesis provides the needed strength for a healing wound. Epithelial cells migrate across the wound bed. After these cells contact each other, the wound is covered. This process is known as *epithelialization*. The wound contraction process happens when specialized fibroblasts known as *myofibroblasts*, pull down the wound edges in an effort to close the wound.[24]

Maturation Phase

The maturation phase, or remodeling phase, of healing occurs from approximately 20 days after injury to longer than 1 year after injury. During this period, the wound develops tensile strength as collagen deposits form scar tissue. Regardless of how well collagen realigns itself, the tissue of the wound will never regain the degree of strength or intactness inherent in uninjured tissue.

Impaired Tissue Integrity

Management of the burn wound is the top priority after the resuscitation phase. The depth of the burn wound is the principal determinant of wound management. Expedient closure of the wounds decreases the potential for many complications such as fluid and electrolyte imbalances, loss of proteins and nitrogen, and infection. The major goal of burn wound care is wound closure. Initial débridement is done by removal of blisters and loose skin. The assessment of wound depth by the clinician guides the treatment based on whether the wound will close in a reasonable time with dressings or will require surgical débridement. The assessment of wound depth can be a difficult challenge. There are many alternative dressing regimens for wound closure that are temporary, semipermanent, or permanent. Several objectives must be met for optimal wound closure: control of infection through meticulous cleansing and débridement, promotion of re-epithelialization, and preparation of the wound for grafting and closure. Other goals are reduction of scarring and contracture formation and providing patient comfort with appropriate psychologic support and pharmacologic intervention.

Factors Affecting Healing of the Burn Wound

Sources of contamination include the patient's endogenous flora found on the skin, the upper respiratory tract, and the GI tract. Exogenous flora found in the patient care setting include bacteria carried by staff members and present in the environment. Patient-specific factors that predispose the patient to infection include age, diabetes, steroid therapy, extreme obesity, severe malnutrition, and infections in remote sites. Because wound healing and clinical infection are inflammatory responses, it is essential to differentiate between normal wound inflammation in the presence of colonization of microorganisms and that of invading organisms. Most burn wounds are colonized with bacteria and usually does not signify infection.[26] In diagnosing infection, the importance of microbiologic results must be evaluated in conjunction with clinical findings such as excessive erythema, edema, pain, and purulence. Clinical findings in conjunction with burn wound biopsy or culture results determine the diagnosis of wound infection. Other factors that affect wound healing are tissue hypoxia from low blood flow to the burn wound, presence of eschar that will require débridement, exudate on the wound that can be harmful to the granulating wound or consume oxygen in the wound, and trauma to the wound from daily dressing changes or lack of protection from the outside environment.

Wound Cleansing

A variety of equally appropriate methods can be used to cleanse burn wounds (e.g., sterile normal saline at the bedside, tap water in a hydrotherapy room). At some centers, a mild antimicrobial cleansing agent such as chlorhexidine (Hibiclens) is used. Wounds are gently cleansed with a gauze dressing or washcloth and patted dry before application of topical agents. Hydrotherapy facilitates the removal of debris and loose eschar. Daily cleansing and inspection of the wound and unburned skin are performed to assess for signs of healing and local infection. Wound care exposure is limited as much as feasible to prevent hypothermia and decrease exposure to bacteria. Measures to reduce pain and hypothermia are used. Patients must receive adequate premedication with analgesics, opiates, and sedatives.

Wound Care

Although many options for burn wound care are available, the basic principle of maintaining a moist wound environment while preventing wound infection is the standard of care. Benefits include preventing wound desiccation, optimal function of local wound growth factors and proteolytic enzymes to remove dead tissue, increased re-epithelialization and collagen synthesis, and decreased wound fluid loss. The most common regimen for burn wound care continues to involve the application of a topical antimicrobial agent, followed by a primary gauze dressing to absorb burn wound drainage and an outer layer to provide increased absorption, compression, and occlusion.[6]

Another method consists of covering the wound with a thin layer of gauze or nonadherent dressing that can be impregnated with a petroleum product, with or without a topical antimicrobial. This method is useful for less severe wounds when the amount of drainage has decreased and wound closure has almost been achieved.

Topical Antibiotic Therapy

Burn injuries destroy the function of the skin's protective mechanism, including that of sebaceous glands. Sebaceous glands normally secrete sebum, which contains fatty acids, including oleic acid. In addition to lubricating the skin, sebum is believed to help destroy some microorganisms, such as streptococci and some strains of staphylococci. Serum is lost from damaged capillaries, providing a rich nutritional medium for bacterial colonization. Topical antibiotic agents are used to control this colonization. Effective antibacterial agents should control colonization so that specimens for wound biopsy reveal fewer than 10^5 microorganisms per gram of tissue. More than 10^5 microorganisms per gram of tissue makes control of wound sepsis with topical antibiotics questionable. Oral or intravenous therapy may then be considered. Topical antibiotics selected must meet several criteria; side effects must be minimal; resistant strains must not develop with use; application must be easy and rapid; and use must be relatively economical. The most commonly used topical antibiotics are silver sulfadiazine (SSD), mafenide acetate cream (Sulfamylon), bacitracin ointment, and silver impregnated into the primary dressing (Table 36-2).

SSD (Silvadene cream) is a broad-spectrum antimicrobial agent with bactericidal action against many gram-negative and gram-positive bacteria associated with burn-wound infection. It is a thick white cream that is applied once or twice daily to a wound that has not been grafted, according to the burn unit protocol.[27] To provide antimicrobial benefit, sustained release of silver is necessary. This is achieved with moisture provided by the wound exudate that may give the SSD cream layer a yellow-gray pseudo-eschar.[27] The old SSD layer must be removed

prior to a new application.[27] The SSD cream removal is often painful for the patient, although reapplication of a new SSD layer is not. A common side effect of silver sulfadiazine is leukopenia resulting from bone marrow suppression, which may develop 24 to 72 hours after application. Rebound to normal leukocyte levels follows onset within 2 to 3 days, and it is not necessary to discontinue SSD use. SSD is indicated for use with partial and full-thickness wounds and is the most commonly used topical antimicrobial agent used to treat burn wounds.[6]

Mafenide acetate cream penetrates through burn eschar and is bacteriostatic against many gram-negative and gram-positive organisms.[27] Its use is limited because the application is uncomfortable for the patient as it creates a burning sensation, and it is rapidly absorbed, requiring dressing changes two or three times daily. It is used routinely for coverage of small wounds involving anatomic areas that contain cartilage such as the ears and nose.[27] Metabolic acidosis can result from the use of mafenide acetate. The patient must be observed closely for hyperventilation (see Table 36-2).

A 5% mafenide acetate solution is less painful on application than cream, and it is iso-osmolar and less desiccating to the burn wound. Gauze dressings are saturated with the solution and then applied over the burn wound and remoistened, as needed. The eschar penetration of the solution and the antimicrobial benefits are superior to SSD, but it does not provide fungal coverage.

Bacitracin ointment is a topical agent applied to superficial burns and facial burns. Bacitracin is effective against gram-positive organisms but not against gram-negative organisms or fungal organisms. It is not uncommon to get a yeast rash associated with repeated bacitracin usage.

Silver has long been used for the treatment of wounds because of its broad-spectrum bacteriostatic properties. The wound moisture activates the silver and releases it into the wound. An advantage of silver dressings is that the dressing does

TABLE 36-2   PHARMACOLOGIC MANAGEMENT

Topical Antimicrobial Agents

AGENT	ADVANTAGES	DISADVANTAGES	IMPLICATIONS
Silver sulfadiazine	Painless application Broad spectrum Easy application Rare sensitivities	May produce transient leukopenia by bone marrow suppression Minimal eschar penetration Some gram-negative resistance	Monitor white cell count Observe wounds for tunneling and subeschar infection Monitor culture reports
Mafenide acetate cream	Broad spectrum (esp. *Pseudomonas* coverage) Easy application Penetrates eschar	Painful application Rare acid–base imbalance Frequent sensitivities	Provide adequate analgesia Monitor arterial blood gases Observe for hyperventilation Observe for rashes
Bacitracin	Painless application Nonirritating Transparent Nontoxic	No eschar penetration No gram-negative or fungal coverage	
Pure silver	Painless application Broad spectrum, including fungus and resistant organisms Rare sensitivity Less frequent dressing changes	Keep moist with sterile water, not saline	Maintain dry linens No reported side effects

not need to be changed daily because of the sustained release of silver. Silver dressings should be used judicious and limited to 4 to 6 weeks despite the current absence of negative systemic or local consequences.[24]

A Cochrane systematic review of dressing products for superficial and partial thickness burn wounds reported a shorter wound healing time, fewer dressing changes and consequently fewer pain-experience opportunities with hydrocolloid dressings, antimicrobial dressings with silver as the active ingredient, silicon dressings, nylon polyurethane film and biosynthetic dressings compared with SSD cream.[28]

Wound Débridement

Eschar is the nonviable tissue that forms after the burn injury. This tissue has no blood supply, and polymorphonuclear leukocytes, antibodies, and systemic antibodies cannot reach these areas. Eschar provides an excellent medium for bacterial growth, and it is vital that loose eschar is débrided, as necessary. Débridement has two major aims: (1) removal of tissue contaminated by foreign bodies and bacteria, thereby protecting patients from invasive infection, and (2) removal of devitalized tissue. The three types of débridement are mechanical, enzymatic, and surgical.

Mechanical Débridement. Mechanical débridement involves the use of scissors and forceps to gently lift and trim loose, necrotic tissue (Fig. 36-11A and B). Only experienced nurses and physicians perform this procedure. Sterile gauze may be used in the form of a wet-to-dry or wet-to-wet dressing to further débride the wound bed.

Enzymatic Débridement. Enzymatic débridement involves the topical application of proteolytic substances to the wound bed. These agents are useful in softening eschar and dissolving devitalized tissue. They promote the separation of eschar, which can lead to earlier wound closure.

Surgical Débridement. An experienced surgeon performs surgical débridement in the operating room. The goal of débridement is to remove nonviable tissue down to bleeding viable tissue with an electric dermatome or surgical knife.

Skin Substitutes

To assist in wound closure, many temporary and permanent skin substitute dressings have gained popularity throughout the United States. A wide variety of products are available. Each dressing has specific indications for use. Temporary substitutes are designed for placement on partial-thickness or clean, excised wounds, and permanent substitutes provide a permanent skin replacement.

Skin substitutes must possess properties that mimic the native epidermis and dermis. They are made from a variety of synthetic materials such as nylon, polyurethane, or solid silicone polymers. Skin barrier substitutes must possess several properties to accomplish their desired effect as a temporary wound covering to protect the granulating tissue and to preserve a clean, viable wound surface for future autografting (Box 36-2). The most important property of these materials is adherence so that the skin substitute can simulate the function of the skin. Adherence must be uniform to prevent fluid accumulation beneath the surface of the substitute, which can lead to bacterial proliferation.

For application of skin substitutes, the wound must be clean, and ideally, it should have a bacterial count of less than 10^5 organisms per gram of tissue. The burn wound must be free from eschar, and hemostasis must exist. Eschar and blood provide an excellent medium for bacterial proliferation, and the presence of blood may interfere with adherence. The surface is cleaned and rinsed with saline solution, and the skin barrier substitutes must be applied according to established procedures using sterile techniques.

Definitive Burn Wound Closure

The primary goal of burn wound management is wound closure during the acute phase. Full-thickness (third-degree) burns are most often treated by excision and grafting.[29] Some deep partial burns that have a prolonged healing time may also benefit from excision and grafting. If a burn wound does not heal

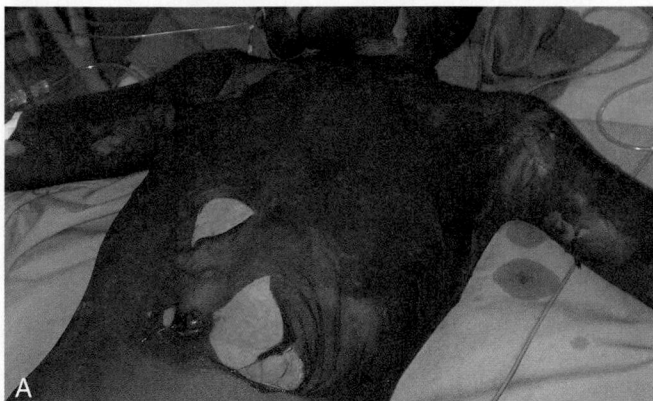
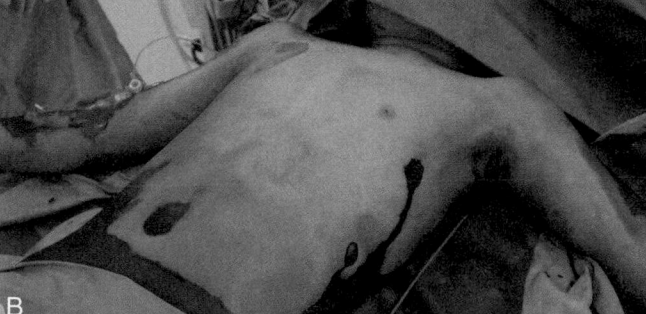

FIGURE 36-11 Anterior trunk and bilateral arm burn. *A,* Before mechanical débridement; *B,* after mechanical débridement.

BOX 36-2 IDEAL PROPERTIES OF SKIN SUBSTITUTES

- Adherence
- Decreased pain
- Easy application and removal
- Intact bacterial barrier
- Shelf storage capability
- Inexpensive in relation to alternatives
- Nonantigenic
- Similar to normal skin in transport of water vapor
- Elastic and durable
- Hemostatic
- Decreased protein and electrolyte loss
- Enhanced natural healing processes

TABLE 36-3 TYPES OF GRAFTS

GRAFT	USE	ADVANTAGES	DISADVANTAGES
Autograft	Provides permanent coverage of burn wounds Used in sheets or meshed form	Permanent coverage Nonantigenic Least expensive Meshing allows a small amount of tissue to cover a large area	Lack of available donor sites, which may delay wound coverage Donor sites are painful partial-thickness wounds Must be done in surgical suite
Homograft (allograft)	Temporary wound coverage	Can be placed at bedside or in operating room Allows for vascularization over deep wound Provides better control over bacterial growth than xenograft	Possibility of disease transmission Antigenic; body rejects in approximately 2 weeks Not readily available to all burn centers Expensive Requires rigorous quality controls

in 10 to 14 days, excision should be undertaken to improve functional and cosmetic results, decrease infection risk, decrease in-hospital time, and to reduce the cost of burn care.[6,29] Surgical débridement may begin as early as 3 to 5 days after the burn insult, as soon as hemodynamic stability has been achieved.[27] Some physicians operate within 24 hours of admission if the patient is hemodynamically stable. To minimize contraction, burn wounds over joint surfaces should be excised and grafted as soon as possible.[30] Typically, excision procedures are limited to 20% of the body surface or 2 hours of operating time. In patients with massive burns, excision procedures are commonly staged, requiring the patient to return to the operating room every 2 to 3 days until all wounds have been excised. This technique helps avoid excessive transfusions and limits the physiologic stress.[27] Table 36-3 reviews advantages and disadvantages of different graft types.

Autograft

An autograft is a skin graft harvested from a healthy, uninjured donor site on the burn patient and then placed over the patient's burn wound to provide permanent coverage of the wound. Autografts are the only grafts that provide permanent wound coverage. Preferred sites for obtaining these grafts are the thighs, back, and abdomen; however, grafts can be harvested from almost anywhere on the body.[9] Autografting with the patient's own skin from a donor site is the preferred choice for wound closure. However, with large TBSA burns, availability of donor sites can be problematic. When an autograft is not available, many alternate methods are used to achieve this goal. Creative attempts have been initiated to establish a skin substitute that permanently closes the wound in a cosmetically and functionally acceptable fashion. Skin substitutes can be used until the patient's own skin is available for harvesting. Previously used and healed donor sites can be used again in later return visits to the operating room.[29]

Surgical excision is performed to mechanically remove necrotic tissue from the burn wound; it may be performed tangentially or fascially. Tangential excision involves sequentially excising the eschar down to bleeding, viable tissue and then placing a split-thickness skin graft over the wound. Fascial excision is used when the wounds are deep and the fat does not appear viable.[29] Sheets of the patient's epidermis and a partial layer of the dermis are harvested with use of a dermatome. These grafts are referred to as *split-thickness skin grafts* and can

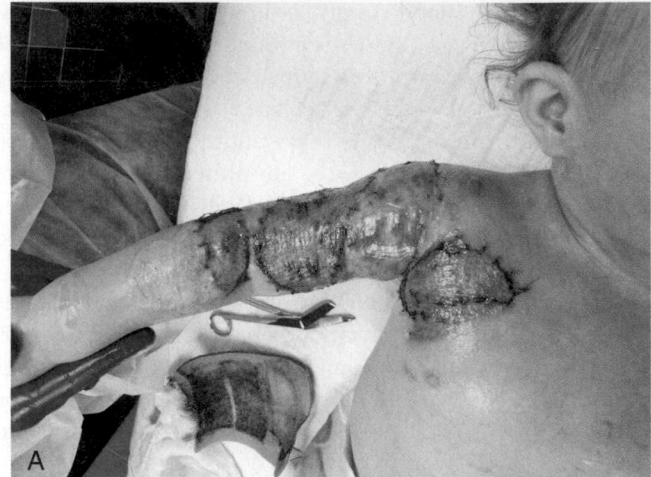

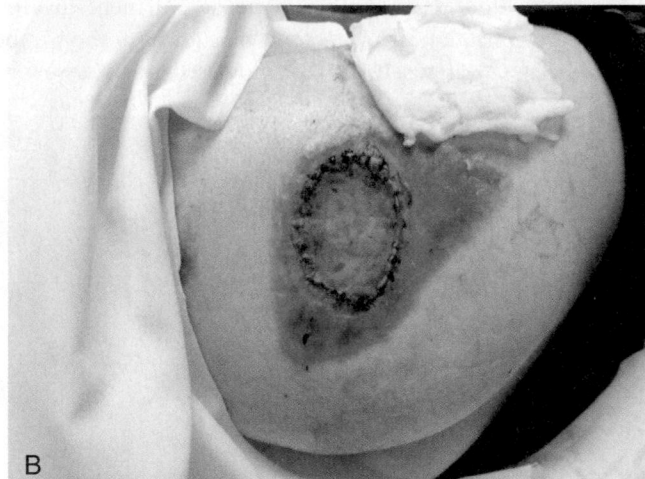

FIGURE 36-12 *A,* Split-thickness skin graft. *B,* Sheet graft to left buttock.

be applied to the wound bed as a sheet or in meshed form (Fig. 36-12). The split-thickness skin grafts harvested are approximately twelve thousandths of an inch thick. The split-thickness skin graft can be meshed 1.5:1 to 4:1 in a mesher and then placed on the wounds.[6] The size of the mesh is based on the areas requiring grafting and the availability of donor skin. This meshing prevents serum accumulation under the graft and permits coverage of a surface area larger than its original surface. Grafts that are placed on the face, neck, lower portions of the arms, and hands are sheet grafts, when possible. Grafts that are meshed can cover more area but may not produce the cosmetic appearance desired, and therefore, they are usually placed on areas covered by clothing.

The grafts can be secured with sutures, fibrin glue, or staples. The choice of dressing that is placed over the graft varies widely based on physician and institution preference. One choice is fine mesh gauze impregnated with an emollient. It is placed over the graft, covered with a heavy gauze dressing, and secured to the patient with or without a splint, depending on the anatomic area of the graft. A vacuum-assisted closure device provides a safe and effective method for securing split-thickness skin grafts, and it is associated with improved graft survival.[31] Negative wound pressure therapy can be used to secure the graft in place. Trained nursing professionals or physicians remove the dressings on postoperative day 3 to 5 for assessment of adherence and graft survival. Nurses, in collaboration with the multidisciplinary team, provide proper positioning, splinting, and pain management in the postoperative period. Great care must be taken not to disturb the graft. Mobilization of the graft area usually occurs around the first dressing change on postoperative day 3 to 5, according to the surgeon's preference.

Care of the donor site is equally important because it represents a wound similar to that of a partial-thickness injury. Donor sites can be covered with many different types of dressings. These dressings should not be removed forcibly because this would interfere with the re-epithelialization process and cause considerable pain.

Biosynthetic Skin Substitutes

Skin substitutes include homografts (allografts) and heterografts (xenografts). *Homograft skin* can be obtained from live or deceased donors (cadaver skin). The homograft is harvested from cadaver skin and, with advances in cryopreservation, can be frozen and stored in a tissue bank. Because it is possible to transmit disease through the application of a homograft, tissue banks must adhere to strict guidelines. Before application, homograft skin is tested for a variety of transmissible diseases, including the human immunodeficiency virus and hepatitis B surface antigens. Homograft skin can be applied as a biologic dressing for débridement at the bedside or as temporary wound coverage on excised burn wounds. Vascular ingrowth occurs, and the homograft seals the wound and protects it from bacterial invasion; however, it is rejected approximately 2 weeks after its application. Homografts must be handled and applied very carefully. The grafts can be dressed with a nonadherent agent that usually is not changed for 24 to 48 hours.

Disadvantages include the homograft antigenicity, lack of accessibility, difficulties with storage and quality control, expense of procurement, and possibility of disease transmission from the donor. Homografts are harvested during the first 4 hours after death, and they are taken from the abdomen, thighs, and back. Homografts usually are available only in centers in which the rigorous processing procedure can be achieved. These centers usually have skin and tissue bank facilities. Procurement of the allograft is much the same as for any other donated organ.

The *xenograft* (heterograft) is a graft transferred between two different species to provide temporary wound coverage. The most common and widely accepted xenograft is pigskin (porcine skin). Pigskin is available in frozen and shelf forms, with each type having a much longer storage life than an allograft. Depending on how the pigskin was prepared, it can have a shelf life of 1 month to 1 year. The pigskin is packaged in a variety of ways and in various sizes. It can be treated with silver sulfadiazine and can be meshed or nonmeshed. Pigskin can be used for temporary coverage of full-thickness and partial-thickness wounds, burn wounds, and donor sites. It meets many of the ideal skin substitute properties mentioned previously. It has two disadvantages: (1) it is antigenic, and (2) it has the potential for being digested by the wound collagenase, possibly leading to infection.

After the pigskin is in place, it may be dressed with antibacterial-impregnated dressings or other forms of dressings. Pigskin usually is removed or dissolves because of lack of blood supply in 5 to 7 days. If sloughing or purulent drainage occurs, the xenograft is removed (see Table 36-3).

Synthetic Skin

The lack of available donor sites for major burn injury often delays wound closure.[32] In an effort to minimize infection and to promote healing, many attempts have been made to develop skin substitutes that will seal the wound in a functional and cosmetically acceptable fashion.[32] Integra has become a very popular dermal substitute with its ultrathin layer of epidermal autograft used successfully. Integra is intended to be placed on freshly excised, full-thickness burns, and the outer silicone membrane replaced with an ultrathin epithelial autograft 2 to 3 weeks later.[33] Integra can also lead to more superficial donor sites.[34] A technique that involves the growth and subsequent graft placement of cultured epithelial autograft (CEA) has also become an adjunct to the treatment of burn wounds. A complex process that allows for separation of keratinocytes is performed. The CEA is grown over a period of 2 to 3 weeks to achieve a graft size of 25 cm². This represents an expansion of 50 to 70 times the original specimen. These confluent sheets of cultured epithelial cells are attached to a gauze backing and placed on the wound. The published results reveal that graft acceptance is unpredictable because the CEA lacks dermis. Even when grafts take initially, graft loss can occur later. Compared with other methods, the CEA also is more fragile, and the technique is quite costly. This therapy is being recommended as an adjunct for traditional split-thickness skin graft, and it continues to be investigated and combined with newer dermal skin substitutes.

Imbalanced Nutrition: Less Than Body Requirements

The basal metabolic rate of a burn patient may be elevated 40% to 100% above the normal rate, depending on the amount of TBSA involved. The metabolic rate is influenced by the amount of protein and albumin lost through the wounds, the catabolic response associated with stress, associated injuries, fluid loss, fever, infection, immobility, gender, and the height and weight of the patient before the injury.[31] A 10% loss of total body mass leads to immune dysfunction; 20% leads to decreased wound healing; 30% leads to severe infections; and a 40% loss leads to death. Severely burned, catabolic patients can lose up to 25% of total body mass after acute severe burn injury.[18]

The goal in nutritional management of the burn patient is to provide adequate calories to enhance wound healing. To achieve this goal, nutritional support and a reduction of energy demand are imperative. Every effort should be made to reduce the release of catecholamines, which increase metabolic rate. Pain, fear, anxiety, and cold stimulate release of catecholamine stores. Appropriate interventions for each of these stimuli must be performed. Examples of nonpharmacologic interventions include early excision and burn wound closure, elevation of the environmental temperature to thermal neutrality (31.5° C ± 0.7° C), and high-carbohydrate, high-protein feeds.

Because of the increased nutritional needs of the burn patient, oral feedings are usually inadequate, and supplemental enteral feedings are necessary. Caloric requirements are calculated on the basis of the size of the burn; the age, height, and weight of the patient; and stress factors. Protein and caloric requirements for the burn patient are elevated by a negative nitrogen balance. The daily protein requirement may increase to two to four times the normal 0.8 g/kg of body weight. Carbohydrates and fat are used for energy and to spare proteins required for wound healing. Daily caloric intake can be 2 to 20 times higher than normal. Vitamins and minerals usually are given in doses higher than normal. Serum albumin, prealbumin, iron, zinc, calcium, phosphate, and potassium values are monitored, and supplements given as indicated by results.[31]

Pain Management

Burn injuries are very painful. Pain management must be addressed early and frequently reassessed. Pain is an individualized and subjective phenomenon, and it has physiologic and psychologic components. Pain results from the acute burn injury and throughout the phases of healing. Background pain is related to the physiologic changes associated with the burn injury and includes the damage or exposure of the nerve endings within partial-thickness burns and donor sites. Range of motion of the affected limbs and routine activities contribute to background pain. Breakthrough pain is described as episodes of pain more severe than background pain, and it is not relieved by routine pain medications. Procedural pain includes pain caused by interventions such as daily wound care, arterial punctures, physical and occupational therapy, and the use of splints.[35] *Pruritus* (itch) may replace pain as a stressful symptom in the rehabilitation phase.

Initially after burn injury, narcotics are administered intravenously in small doses and titrated to effect. The constant background pain may be addressed with the use of a patient-controlled analgesia device. After hemodynamic stability has occurred and GI function has returned, oral narcotics can be useful. Intramuscular or subcutaneous injections must not be administered because absorption by these routes is unpredictable because of the fluid shifts that occur with burn injury. Additional premedication and analgesics are necessary during therapeutic procedures. The use of acetaminophen and nonsteroidal anti-inflammatory drugs can be useful in patients who are not at risk for bleeding. Anxiolytics and antidepressants also should be considered and used appropriately. The nurse must be flexible with dosing and should assess the effectiveness of medication by using a numerical or visual analog scale. The nurse should assure the patient that pain control issues will be continually addressed.

Pain continues even after healing; some patients describe the itching, tingling, and paresthesias as being as uncomfortable as the initial injury.[35] Paresthesias are abnormal neurologic sensations of numbness, tingling, or burning that can last 1 year or more after injury. Inadequate pain management is an issue in many burn units because of the fear of opioid side effects and opioid addiction and the lack of pain evaluation or treatment protocols.

Loss of control, forced dependence, loneliness, and separation from home and family can contribute to anxiety, which heightens the patient's perception of pain. The patient's fears abound in thoughts of disfigurement and loss of love, function, and job. The psychologic experience or subjective component may be related to past experiences, anxiety, and altered coping mechanisms. Attention to the psychologic component of the patient's pain may lead to useful strategies that decrease perceived pain. If possible, past experiences with pain, hospitalization, and successful coping strategies should be explored. Pain is a psychologic and physical experience that accumulates over time and becomes part of the individual's deepest psychology.

Nonpharmacologic techniques such as imagery, hypnosis, and distraction and methods adapted from some of the popular childbirth techniques can be effective in reducing anxiety and the pain experience. Giving the patient some management control also can reduce anxiety and the perception of pain. The perception of pain often is increased in the patient who is anxious and lacks control of the situation.[29]

Treatment strategies need to be individualized. Failure to adequately treat pain can increase burn hypermetabolism, result in loss of confidence between the burn team and patient, and lead to the development of psychiatric disorders. The nurse should assess and discuss on a regular basis the patient's psychologic status and avoid using psychotropics for analgesia and narcotics for anxiety and depression.

Rehabilitation Phase

The rehabilitation phase is one of recuperation and healing physically and emotionally. The patient is not acutely ill but may or may not be ready for discharge. This phase can last several years. Psychologic rehabilitation is equally important in the burn patient. The patient may require extensive reconstructive surgery. Psychologically, the patient focuses on attaining specific personal goals related to achieving as much preburn function as possible.[23] Minor and major accomplishments must be praised. This phase is characterized by scar management techniques and by physical and occupational therapies.

The burn team and the patient prepare for the transition to the outside world. The use of group therapy is a valuable tool used at many burn centers. Patients, family members, and health care providers express ideas and feelings. Often, burn patients establish priorities and make realistic decisions about their lives. Staff intervention during this phase is primarily one of support.

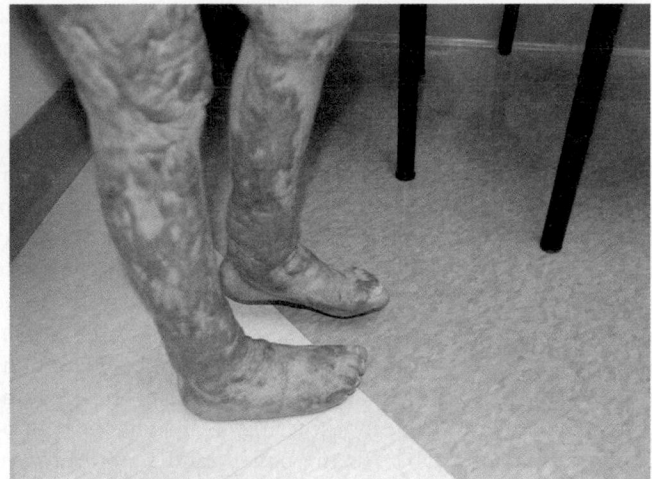

FIGURE 36-13 Severe contracture to bilateral lower extremities.

Impaired Physical Mobility

Tremendous advances have been made in the physical care of the burn patient. The survival rate of patients with full-thickness burns greater than 40% of TBSA has increased significantly. Survival of patients with burns greater than 90% of TBSA is not impossible. As patients with larger and deeper burns survive, the challenge to maintain their optimal mobility and cosmetic appearance has been met with increased success. Despite the advances in other areas of burn care, contractures still develop after a burn injury. A contracture is the shortening of a scar over a joint surface and is the primary cause of functional deficits in the burn patient (Fig. 36-13). Contractures develop because of a variety of factors: the extent, depth, location, and configuration of the burn; the position of comfort the patient most frequently assumes; the relative underlying muscle strength; and the patient's motivation and compliance. The affected body parts should be positioned to prevent long-term deformity. Frequent change of position also is important and may need to be performed as often as every hour. Burn patients are at greater risk for pressure sores than the general hospital population.

Splints can be used to prevent or correct contracture or to immobilize joints after grafting. If splints are used, they must be checked daily for proper fit and effectiveness. Splints that are used to immobilize body parts after grafting must be left on at all times, except to assess the graft site for pressure points during every shift. Splints to correct severe contracture may be off for 2 hours per shift to allow burn care and range-of-motion exercises.

Active exercise is encouraged and is preferred, although active-assisted or gentle-passive exercises also may be an important part of the rehabilitation program. Active exercise maintains muscle mass, aids in restoring protein structures within the muscle tissue, aids in venous and lymphatic return, and reduces the risk of pulmonary embolus and deep vein thrombosis. The patient's tolerance must be carefully evaluated. The number of repetitions of an exercise is proportional to the degree of anticipated contracture and the patient's tolerance. Anticipation of the patient's pain also must be carefully

considered. Before range-of-motion exercises and activities of daily living are performed, the need for pain medication must be assessed.[12] Nursing diagnoses for the burn patient are summarized in the Nursing Diagnoses features on the three phases of burn injury (Box 36-3 and Box 36-4).

Scar Management

Another concern in burn wound healing is the prevention or reduction of scarring. A person's skin response to a burn injury can be barely noticeable such as slight color change or lead to cosmetic disfigurement and dysfunction. The goal of scar management is to minimize scarring, and it is important to inform the patient that the tissue may not return to the preburn texture or appearance. Hypertrophic scars are red, raised, and lack elasticity, and they are painful and itchy.[24] Deep partial and full-thickness burns are at the highest risk for scar tissue development because of their depth and increased risk of infection. Areas of the skin that required skin grafting also leave a visible scar (Fig. 36-14). Scar maturation occurs 6 months to 2 years from the time of the injury. One method to reduce scar formation is timely application of uniform pressure. Hypertrophic scarring can be controlled with the use of tubular support bandages. They are readily available for immediate use during the wait for the commercial manufacture of the customized elastic pressure garment for long-term use, which can take up to 3 or 4 weeks. Custom-made elastic pressure garments are worn for 6 months to 1 year, if needed (Fig. 36-15). These garments reduce scar blood flow and may provide force

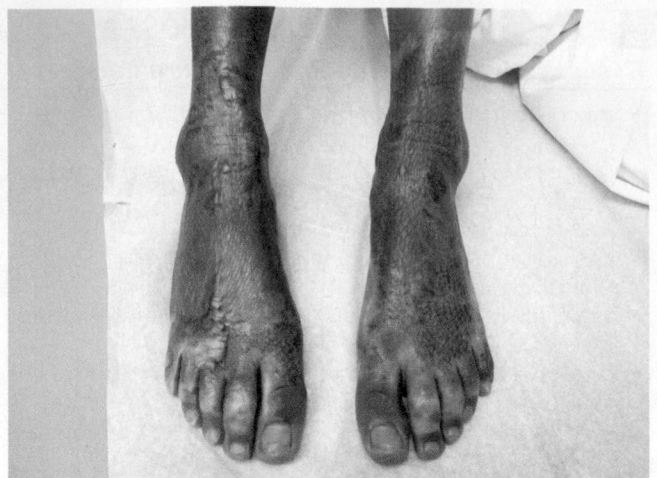

FIGURE 36-14 Healed split-thickness skin graft to bilateral feet.

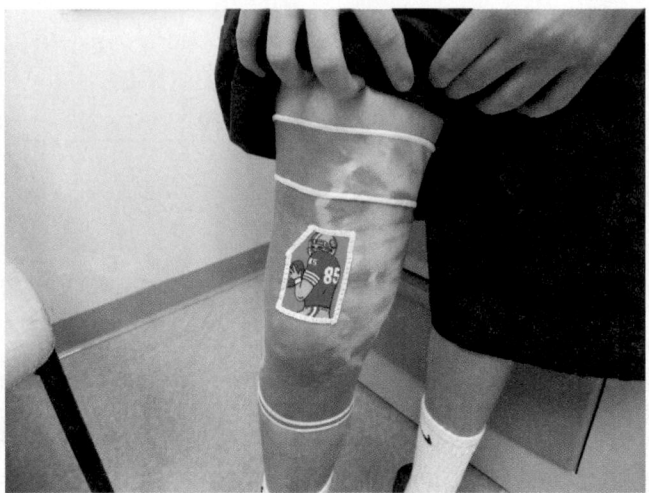

FIGURE 36-15 Compression garment to right leg.

that helps developing collagen to organize.[23] Although compression therapy is one of the main prophylaxis and treatment of burn scars, its mechanism is not totally understood.[36] It is important to assess for pressure points under the garment as weight is gained and as growth occurs. It is necessary to assess the garment for elasticity over time because elasticity decreases with washing.

Additional approaches to reduce scarring are scar massage, high-SPF sun protection, silicone gel sheeting and steroid treatment. Scar massage works by stretching the scar and providing moisture and is most helpful in preventing contractures. Sun protection over the healed burn may decrease the long-term pigment change to the injured area. Silicone gel sheets are used alone over the scar or in conjunction with compression to soften the scar by maintaining scar hydration and tension reduction. Injectable or topical steroids are used for treatment of hypertrophic scars; however, they have some side effects that may make them undesirable. Corticosteroid injections inhibit fibroblast growth and enhance collagen breakdown leading to a flatter and softer scar.[24] Topical steroid treatment poses less risk, however has been found to be less effective. If less invasive

techniques have been unsuccessful for troublesome scars that cause pain or inhibit full range of motion, surgical excision may be recommended by the physician.

Itching

Pruritus is common in the maturing burn wound. One study reported itching as the most common skin-related problem described by 94% of patients.[37] For 6 to 8 weeks, a mild, non–alcohol-based skin cream is applied every 4 hours to healed areas to lubricate the skin until natural lubrication occurs. Patients can be relieved of this discomfort by the administration of an antipruritic agent such as diphenhydramine hydrochloride, doxepin hydrochloride (5%), or hydroxyzine and by the application of moisturizing creams. Itching can be extremely uncomfortable for the patient and should be continually assessed.

Multidisciplinary Care

A multidisciplinary approach to burn treatment is integral in providing quality care. This approach involves considering all aspects of patient's care when treatment decisions are made.[38] The burn team should work together to address all needs of the patient and the family. The team should meet frequently to review patient care and maximize patient and family support. The multidisciplinary team includes, but is not limited to, physicians, nurses, social work, nutrition, physical and occupational therapy, respiratory therapy, psychology, pain service, child life services, and utilization review.

Outpatient Burn Care

Outpatient burn care must be considered for minor burns. It is cost effective and removes the potential for a wound infection by endemic, drug-resistant microorganisms within the hospital environment. The hospital environment also changes many of the self-care routines such as diet, family contact, hygiene, and coping mechanisms. However, patients considered for outpatient burn care must be screened carefully. Nursing evaluation of the patient, the family, or both, includes consideration of motivation, willingness to participate in care, ability to understand and perform the necessary procedures, potential aversions to wound care or dressing changes, and reliability of transportation. The transition to outpatient care must also include physical and occupational therapy needs and involve exercises designed to accelerate return to activities of daily living such as work, school, or both.

A clean, synthetic antimicrobial agent can be applied to help reduce dressing change frequency. Home health nurses are helpful in monitoring these patients. If epithelialization of these wounds has not occurred in 2 to 3 weeks, use of primary excision and grafting must be considered.

Support of the Burn Patient

Burn injuries are physically and psychologically traumatic and life altering for the patient. The patient's preburn level of emotional functioning can greatly affect the course of recover.[39] The family of the burn patient is also affected, and their needs should be remembered during the healing process. Often, guilt is associated with burn injuries, especially when the victim is a child. It is important for the clinical providers to support the burn patient in all aspects. As health care providers, we heal and support the patient throughout the hospital stay but often forget that the survivor's biggest challenges may still lie ahead after hospitalization. Many survivors have stated that they wish they could take the hospital staff home with them to help them transition into the community.[40]

Many resources are available to help burn survivors cope after they are home and should be provided by the hospital team during their inpatient stay. Psychologic distress occurs in as many as 34% of burn patients and persists in severity long after discharge.[9] Research has shown that many patients have difficulty returning to work and desire a coordinator during the rehabilitation process to assess work capacity.[41] Programs are available to help with such issues as social and school re-entry, support for sexual considerations, and dealing with scars. These resources are needed at different times of the recovery process.[40] The clinical team and the community must collaborate to improve burn survivor transition and support.

STRESSORS OF BURN NURSING

Burn units can be interesting in that they offer the fast-paced, high-technology atmosphere of any critical care setting; the complexity of advanced nursing management; and the dynamics of an interdisciplinary, collaborative model of practice. However, all of these elements combined contribute to a potentially stressful work environment for the nurse. The physical environment can be a difficult one for a variety of reasons. The amount of equipment necessary to maintain the patient can be overwhelming and can limit the workspace dramatically. The temperature of the room usually is kept at approximately 85° F and can become much warmer, depending on the amount of equipment in the room. The various odors in the room may be very unpleasant. Noise levels within a unit also are distressing. Self-care and care of other nurses and staff are issues just as important as the care of the patient and the family. The decision to specialize in burn nursing, therefore, requires careful consideration.

BOX 36-5 CASE STUDY

Patient with Burns

Brief Patient History

Ms. J is a 40-year-old victim of a car crash. She was found conscious at the scene and pulled out of a burning car to safety by a passerby. The paramedics at the scene reported her as awake but disorientated and anxious. She is otherwise healthy and is the mother of a 5-year-old child, who was also rescued at the scene with no injuries.

Clinical Assessment

Ms. J is sent from the emergency department to your trauma unit. She is intubated and sedated on arrival. She has partial-thickness burns covering her face, including her nose, lips, and neck. She has areas of partial-thickness and full-thickness burns to both her hands and to her chest and left leg. Her breath sounds are auscultated as present bilaterally, but she is wheezing, and her sputum has a dark carbon appearance. She has a triple-lumen catheter in her right femoral vein with good blood return to all ports.

Diagnostic Procedures

Ms. J has a HbCO level of 3.4% and arterial blood gas values as follows: pH of 7.27, $PaCO_2$ of 29 mm Hg, PaO_2 of 313 mm Hg, HCO_3^- of 14 mEq/L (mmol/L),

and O_2 saturation of 88% on 100% FIO_2. Her serum cyanide level is 45 mmol/L. The chest radiograph obtained on arrival in the emergency department was normal. Her blood pressure is 85/50 mm Hg, heart rate is 136 beats/min (sinus tachycardia), respiratory rate is 14 breaths/min, and temperature is 96.3° F.

Medical Diagnosis

Ms. J is diagnosed with burns covering 40% of TBSA, inhalation injury, and cyanide toxicity.

Questions

1. What major outcomes do you expect to achieve for this patient?
2. What problems or risks must be managed to achieve these outcomes?
3. What interventions must be initiated to monitor, prevent, manage, or eliminate the problems and risks identified?
4. What interventions should be initiated to promote optimal functioning, safety, and well-being of the patient?
5. What possible learning needs do you anticipate for this patient?
6. What cultural and age-related factors may have a bearing on the patient's plan of care?

SUMMARY

- Burn care is highly complex, and decisions regarding appropriate management of burn injuries are best managed by certified burn centers, where the most accurate burn size estimates can be made.
- Burn size, types of injury, location of the burn, and the patient's age and history are all determinants of survival.
- Size and depth of burns are divided into four main categories: (1) superficial (first-degree) burns, which are injuries to epidermis; (2) partial-thickness (second-degree) burns, which involve the epidermis and dermis of the skin; (3) deep-dermal, partial thickness (second-degree) burns, which involve the entire epidermal layer of the skin and part

of the dermis; and (4) full-thickness (third-degree) burns, which involve destruction of skin layers from the epidermis down to and including the subcutaneous tissue.

- Accurate fluid resuscitation of a burn patient for more severe burn injuries (>10% of TBSA) is crucial to prevent acute kidney injury that may result in acute kidney failure, cardiovascular collapse, and death from burn shock. The Parkland formula is a guide for determining resuscitation fluid (Ringer lactate) volume.
- Careful assessment of the burn patient's intake and output is critical to achieve the optimal patient response to fluid resuscitation.

- After the resuscitative phase of burn patients, the acute care phase of wound healing, wound closure, and prevention of infection begins. This hypermetabolic phase can be complicated by wound infection and sepsis.
- The gold standard of burn wound care includes the application of a topical antimicrobial agent, followed by a gauze dressing to absorb excess drainage, with an outer layer to provide increased absorption, compression, and occlusion. Silver dressings have shown positive results in the prevention of bacterial growth without silver toxicity.

- The rehabilitative phase of the burn patient care starts from admission of the burn-injured patient and may last years, depending on future surgical procedures, therapy needs, contracture prevention, and psychologic or emotional needs of the patient.
- All of the multidisciplinary needs of burn-injured patients must be addressed for them to be able to perform in and feel accepted back into society.

REFERENCES

1. Lancaster BA, et al. National Burn Repository 2006: a ten year review. *J Burn Care Res*. 2007;28(5):635.
2. American Burn Association. Fact sheet. http://www.ameriburn.org. 2011. Accessed April 2012.
3. National and state child abuse and neglect statistics. http://www.childwelfare.gov. 2010. Accessed April 2012.
4. Pham T, et al. Thermal and electrical injuries. *Surg Clin North Am*. 2007;87(1):185.
5. Lloyd E, et al. Outpatient burns: prevention and care. *Am Fam Physician*. 2012;85(1):25.
6. Edlich R, et al. Burns, thermal. http://emedicine.medscape.com/article/1278244-overview. 2008. Accessed May 2009.
7. Demling RH, et al. Burn wound module. Part IV. *Burn wound: histological assessment (Zones of Injury)*. http://www.burnsurgery.org. Accessed May 2009.
8. Singer AJ, et al. Management of local burn wounds in the ED. *Am J Emerg Med*. 2007;25(6):667.
9. Brunicardi FC, et al. *Schwartz's Principles of Surgery*. 9th ed. New York: McGraw-Hill Companies, Inc.; 2010.
10. Tintinalli JE, et al. *Tintinalli's Emergency Medicine: A Comprehensive Study Guide*. 7th ed. New York: McGraw-Hill Companies, Inc.; 2011.
11. Gomez R, Cancio LC. Management of burn wounds in the emergency department. *Emerg Med Clin North Am*. 2007;25(1):135.
12. Davidge K, Fish J. Classification of burn depth. *Geriatr Aging*. 2008;11(5):270.
13. Chen EH, Sareen A. Do children require ECG evaluation and inpatient telemetry after household electrical exposures? *Ann Emerg Med*. 2007;49(1):64.
14. McPhee SJ, et al. *Current Medical Diagnosis and Treatment*. 51st ed. New York: McGraw-Hill Companies; 2012.
15. U.S. Department of Health & Human Services. Child Maltreatment Report 2010. http://www.acf.hhs.gov/programs/cb/pubs/cm10. 2010. Accessed April 2012.
16. Legano L, et al. Child abuse and neglect. *Curr Prob Pediatr Adolesc Health Care*. 2009;39(2):31.e1.
17. Prem SC, et al. Initial evaluation and management of the burn patient. http://emedicine.medscape.com/article/435402-overview. 2008. Accessed May 2009.
18. Williams F, et al. What, how, and how much should patients with burns be fed? *Surg Clin North Am*. 2011;91(3):609.
19. White CE, Renz E. Advances in surgical care: management of severe burn injury. *Crit Care Med*. 2008;36(7):S318.
20. Endorf FW, Gamelli RL. Inhalation injury, pulmonary perturbations, and fluid resuscitation. *J Burn Care Res*. 2007;28(1):80.
21. Dries DJ. Key questions in ventilator management of the burn-injured patient. *J Burn Care Res*. 2009;30(1):128.
22. Pham TN, Gibran NS. Thermal and electrical injuries. *Surg Clin North Am*. 2007;87(1):185.
23. Blakeney PE, et al. Psychosocial care of persons with severe burns. *Burns*. 2008;34(4):433.
24. Bryant R, Nix D. *Acute and Chronic Wounds: Current Management Concepts*. 3rd ed. St. Louis: Mosby; 2007.
25. Stipcevic T, Piljac A, Piljac G. Enhanced healing of fullthickness burn wounds using rhamnolipid. *Burns*. 2007;32(1):24.
26. Greenhalgh D. Topical antimicrobial agents for burn wounds. *Clin Plastic Surg*. 2009;36(4):597.
27. Connor-Ballard PA. Understanding and managing burn pain: Part 2. *Am J Nurs*. 2009;109(5):54.
28. Wasiak J, Cleland H, Campbell F. Dressings for superficial and partial thickness burns. *Cochrane Datab System Rev 2008*. 2008;Issue 4. Art. No.: CD002106.
29. Orgill DP. Excision and skin grafting of thermal burns. *N Engl J Med*. 2009;360(9):893.
30. Mosier MJ, et al. Surgical Excision of the Burn Wound. *Clinics in Plastic Surgery*. 2009;36(4):619.
31. Wolf SE. The year in burns 2007. *Burns*. 2008;34(8):1059.
32. Sheridan R. Closure of the excised burn wound: autografts, semipermanent skin substitutes, and permanent skin substitutes. *Clin Plastic Surg*. 2009;36(4):643.
33. Demling RH, et al. Burn wound module, part III: managing the burn wound. http://www.burnsurgery.org. Accessed May 2009.
34. Stipcevic T, Piljac A, Piljac G. Enhanced healing of full thickness burn wounds using rhamnolipid. *Burns*. 2007;32(1):24.
35. Summer GJ, et al. Burn injury pain: the continuing challenge. *J Pain*. 2007;8(7):533.
36. Meyer T. Pressure-related analysis of compression therapy after burn injuries in children. *Zentralbl Chir*. 2008;133(4):386.
37. Walker K, et al. Management of post-burn itching and dryness. *J Burn Care Rehab*. 2000;21:S240.
38. Al-Mousaw A, et al. Burn teams and burn centers: the importance of a comprehensive team approach to burn care. *Clin Plastic Surg*. 2009;36(4):547 .
39. Wiechman S. Psychosocial recovery, pain, and itch after burn injuries. *Phys Med Rehab Clin North Am*. 2011;22(2):327.
40. Acton AR, et al. The burn survivor perspective. *J Burn Care Res*. 2007;28(4):615.
41. Oster C. Return to work after burn injury: burn-injured individual's perception of barriers and facilitators. *Burn Care Res*. 2010;31(4):540.

Organ Donation and Transplantation

Jamie D. Blazek, Christine Hartley, Mary E. Lough,
Mary Martel, Teresa J. Shafer, Schawnté Williams-Taylor

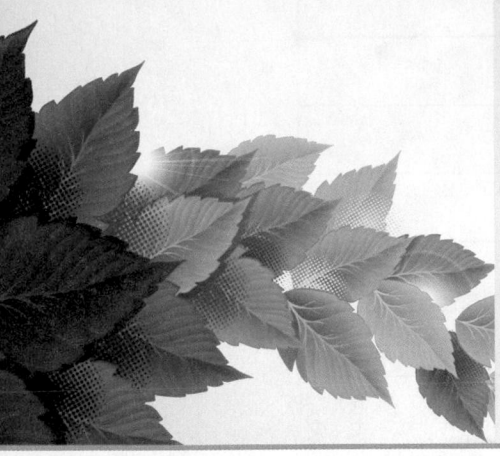

evolve WEBSITE

http://evolve.elsevier.com/Urden/criticalcare/

Evolve features:
- NCLEX Review Questions
- CCRN Review Questions
- PCCN Review Questions
- Mosby's Nursing Skills Procedures
- Animations
- Video Clips
- Glossary

Organ transplantation provides the only opportunity for patients with end-stage organ disease to have an enhanced quality of life and an extended survival. Organ transplantation is accepted as the preferred and often only treatment option for end-stage organ disease. Success rates in patients treated—as well as increases in organ donation from the general public—have improved as the field of organ donation and transplantation has evolved. Such evolution came as a result of increased cultural acceptance of brain death, donation, and transplantation; legal and political efforts to facilitate organ donation; improved procurement and allocation processes; advances in organ preservation, organ recovery, and surgical techniques in transplantation, immunology, immunosuppression; and management of infectious diseases.[1]

Nationwide, more than 114,241 people are waiting for a lifesaving or life-enhancing organ transplant. In 2011, the Organ Procurement Transplant Network (OPTN) reported 14,147 donors, of which 8128 were deceased donors and 6019 were living donors (Fig. 37-1). The categories of organ donors are described in Table 37-1. Total transplants performed in 2011 numbered 28,535. This is encouraging although insufficient, as one patient is added to a transplant waiting list every 10 minutes.[2]

Ongoing collaboration between organ procurement organizations, transplant centers, and critical care nurses, physicians, and other health care workers is necessary to have a significant impact in saving lives through organ and tissue donation and transplantation.

ORGAN DONATION

Role of the Critical Care Nurse in Organ Donation

The critical care nurse is an essential member of the team in the donation process, linking the hospital to the *organ procurement organization* (OPO), physicians, and families of potential donors. The Centers for Medicare & Medicaid Services (CMS) guidelines, The Joint Commission standards, and hospital policies require that patients meeting criteria for imminent death and cardiac death be referred to an OPO in a timely manner.[3] Once the notification has been made, nurses must follow the established donation policies for their hospital in accordance with federal guidelines and state laws. Hospitals will already have worked with their federally designated OPO to develop their hospital policy to ensure that it meets these regulations and laws.

Continued hemodynamic support is necessary during the process of brain death declaration. Patients progressing to brain death undergo many physiologic changes that can compromise the viability of organs for transplantation. Ensuring that oxygenation and perfusion of the organs is maintained, as well as electrolyte and acid–base balance, preserves the opportunity for donation.

Collaboration between the nurse and the OPO staff is necessary to protect the right of the patient, who may already have made the decision to donate by indicating his or her wishes on a state registry. Failing that, the family can make the decision about donation. After declaration of death, the family is

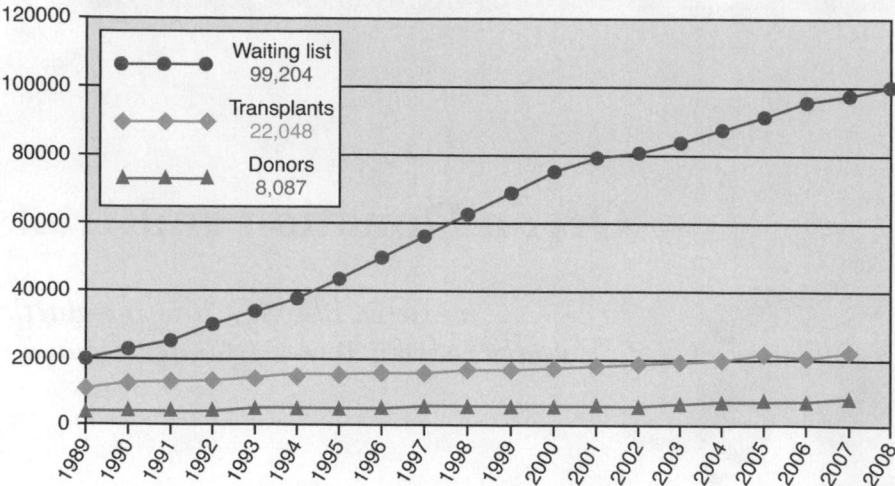

FIGURE 37-1 Growth in U.S. organ transplant waiting list outpaces growth in deceased organ donors. (From *Department of Health and Human Services. Organ Procurement Transplantation Network*. Collaborative scorecard. Data for period: September 2009-August 2010. https://www.healthcarecommunities.org.)

TABLE 37-1	CATEGORIES OF ORGAN DONORS
DONOR	**DEFINITION**
Brain-Dead Donor	Donor declared dead by neurologic criteria for brain death
Donation After Cardiac Death (DCD)	Donor declared dead by circulatory criteria for death
Living Related Donor	Living family member related by blood who donates a kidney, portion of the liver, pancreas, intestine, or lung to another family member
Living, Unrelated Donor (Directed/Nondirected)	Living individual not related to a patient requiring a transplant who donates a kidney, portion of the liver, pancreas, intestine or lung to another individual. The donor may be anonymous or altruistic

From *United Network for Organ Sharing website*. http://www.unos.org/donation. Accessed May 7, 2012.

informed about the opportunity for donation. The goal of medical management of the patient shifts toward optimal preservation of organ function so that the organs are suitable for transplant. It is at this point that the OPO assumes the care of the donor, providing direction for medical management.

After death of the patient, nurses advocates for their patient by ensuring the patient's donation decision is honored or—if the patient had not made such a decision during his or her lifetime—upholding the family's right to be offered the opportunity to donate organs and tissues.[4] Once authorization (*formerly known as "consent"*) is obtained, the OPO coordinator and nurse collaborate on management of the donor according to established donor management protocols. Such protocols include managing fluid and electrolyte imbalances secondary to brain death. It is not uncommon for patients to have a low circulating volume or high serum sodium levels, since hypertonic sodium may have been administered to prevent brain

herniation. The donor management phase corrects deficits in the patient's physiologic status in order to provide optimal organ function prior to surgical recovery and preservation. Nursing care shifts from cerebral protective strategies to aggressive donor management along with continued support of the family.[5]

The critical care nurse monitors and records vital signs, intake and output, and oxygenation status; draws labs; and assists with line insertions and multiple diagnostic assessments, such as chest radiographs, bronchoscopies, electrocardiograms, or echocardiograms, to evaluate organ function. This donor management phase of the donation process starts following brain death and continues until the patient is taken to the operating room and organs are recovered.

A recent study of hospital donation practices and their impact on organ donation outcomes revealed gaps in knowledge of organ donation, brain death, referral criteria, and at times, a poor relationship between the hospital and OPO.[6] It is important that nurses are knowledgeable about the organ donation process. Nurses must assess their own beliefs that pertain to organ donation since the attitude of the nurse and care given to the family can impact the outcome of the donation.

Organ Procurement Organization as Part of the Health Care Team

Nurses, physicians, nurses, respiratory therapists, social workers, and other health care disciplines practice in the hospital because that is where the patients are. OPO staff practice in hospitals because that is where the potential donors are. The 2003 Organ Donation Breakthrough Collaborative helped break down many of the silos that exist in providing care to patients by various health care professionals.[7-9]

Gone are the days when hospitals and hospitals staff considered donation a "nice-to-do," and "add-on" in terms of care. The federal government has made clear the responsibility placed on hospitals to actively engage and work through the donation process with OPOs, caring for the donor while the OPO is leading and managing the donor assessment, obtaining authorization, and facilitating the recovery process.

Because only OPO staff or trained designated requestors can make the request for donation, they are part of the health care team. In one of the largest donor family studies in the nation, a primary finding was that speaking to an OPO staff member was one of the few variables highly associated with authorization (versus nonauthorization) for donation.[10] A successful donation environment is dependent on a deep, close, and open relationship with a hospital's designated OPO. The OPO should be called before the patient has died when death is imminent. This requirement is established by federal regulation, by state law, and is practiced by the vast majority of hospitals and critical care units as policy and best practice.[3]

National Donation and Transplantation Laws

Organ transplantation is the only medical and surgical therapy that is regulated entirely by law. From donation to transplantation, the federal government—and to some extent the state governments—monitor the administrative and financial aspects of this process. These regulations ensure that organs are shared on a fair and equitable basis. In addition, the responsibilities and functions of health care professionals are sanctioned and safeguarded by these laws so that their responsibilities may be discharged with assurance and protection medically, legally, and ethically. The major laws are listed in Table 37-2.

The Uniform Anatomical Gift Act

The *Uniform Anatomical Gift Act* (UAGA) of 1968 established the legal framework for organ and tissue donation and donor designation, as well as the priority of legal next-of-kin for authorization in the absence of donor designation. It required that the physician pronouncing or certifying death may not in any way participate in the procedures for removing or transplanting anatomical gifts. It also protects health care professionals from liability associated with donation. The act was later amended to require hospitals to establish agreements with an OPO to coordinate recovery. It prohibits the sale or purchase of organs or tissues. This act clarifies who can provide authorization for donation in the absence of known donor wishes.[11]

Uniform Determination of Death Act

The *Uniform Determination of Death Act* (UDDA) of 1981 states that an individual who has sustained either 1) irreversible cessation of circulatory and respiratory functions, or 2) irreversible cessation of all functions of the entire brain, including the brainstem, is dead. A determination of death must be made in accordance with accepted medical standards. Most states have adopted similarly worded Determination of Death Acts in their state statutes.

National Organ Transplant Act (NOTA) (1984)

The *National Organ Transplant Act* of 1984 mandated the establishment of the national Organ Procurement and Transplantation Network (OPTN). The United Network for Organ Sharing (UNOS) administers the national contract to operate the OPTN and houses the database that contains the list of waiting recipients nationwide and by which all donor and recipient matches are determined. This act also made it illegal to buy or sell organs and tissues.

Omnibus Budget Reconciliation Act

This federal mandate required OPOs to coordinate the recovery and transplantation process at local levels and requires hospitals to be affiliated with a federally mandated OPO. There is only one designated OPO per service area. This act gave families the right to know about organ and tissue donation by mandating that all hospitals participating in the CMS reimbursement program institute a "required request" policy to ensure that families of potential donors are made aware of the option of organ or tissue donation and their option to decline. Hospitals must have a signed agreement with an OPO, tissue bank, and eye bank.[3]

Medical Examiner State Laws

Medical examiner laws encourage or require the release of organs for transplantation. In some states, medical examiners or justices of the peace cannot deny organ donation, under any circumstances. In other states, they cannot deny organ donation unless they are physically present at the donation surgery viewing the organ(s). In situations such as these, the medical examiner or justice of the peace may request a biopsy while in surgery. These state laws were passed to provide protection for recipients waiting at centers, so that every possible organ that can be recovered is being recovered to save a life (see Table 37-2).

Overview of the Donation Process

CMS requires hospitals to notify their respective OPOs of all deaths, including patients meeting imminent death criteria and

TABLE 37-2	NATIONAL DONATION AND TRANSPLANTATION LAWS	
LAWS	**TYPE**	**FIRST ENACTED**
Uniform Anatomical Gift Act (UAGA)	State law	1968; Revised in 1987 and 2006
National Organ Transplant Act (NOTA)	Federal law	1984
Uniform Determination of Death Act (UDDA)	State laws	1980
Hospital Conditions of Participation—Organ Donation; Centers for Medicare and Medicaid Services (CMS)	Federal regulation	1998
Medical Examiner Laws Restricting Ability of Medical Examiner or Coroner to deny organ donation	State laws	Various years by state
Omnibus Budget Reconciliation Act (OBRA)	Federal law	1986

From *Organ Procurement and Transplantation Network* (OPTN). http://www.organdonor.gov/legislation/timeline.html. Accessed May 7, 2012.

TABLE 37-3 ORGAN AND TISSUE DONOR REFERRALS TO THE ORGAN PROCUREMENT ORGANIZATION

ORGAN REFERRAL		TISSUE REFERRAL
BRAIN DEATH	**DONATION AFTER CARDIAC DEATH (DCD)**	**CARDIAC ARREST**
Irreversible, nonsurvivable brain injury	Irreversible, nonsurvivable brain injury	Patient may or may not have sustained a brain injury
Patient currently maintained on a ventilator	Patient currently maintained on a ventilator	Patient is not currently on a ventilator
Tests performed to confirm brain death (e.g., clinical exam, apnea test)	Any ventilator-dependent patient whose plans are to forgo life-sustaining treatment	No cardiac or respiratory activity
First person authorization/authorizing agent gives authorization for donation	Patient has not progressed to brain death	First person authorization/Authorizing agent gives authorization for donation
Patient maintained in critical care unit while donation evaluation and work-up is completed	Family decides to withdraw life-sustaining therapies	May donate tissue and corneas (bone, heart valves, skin, etc.)
To operating room for organ recovery	Family authorizes donation	
Organ donors may also donate tissue and corneas	Patient is extubated, circulator arrest within 60-90 minutes, rapid recovery of organs in operating room Organ donors may also donate tissue and corneas	

Developed by staff at *LifeGift.* Corporate headquarters Houston, TX.

cardiac death to increase the potential for organ, tissue, and eye donation. Table 37-3 lists the types of organ donor referrals made to the OPO. All patients meeting imminent death criteria must be referred within the agreed-upon time (usually within 1 hour) of meeting criteria. All cardiac deaths must be referred, irrespective of age, medical condition, or cause of death.[3] The nurse or hospital designee makes the initial call to the OPO to provide demographic information, admitting diagnosis, and current neurologic status of the patient. Most OPOs have either in-house staff or on-call coordinators who will respond to the initial referral call from the hospital. Once onsite the OPO coordinator will communicate with the bedside nurse and physicians involved in the care of the patient to obtain information about the patient's present hospital course, past medical history, and the plan of care.

Determining medical suitability is solely the responsibility of the OPO. Speaking to the family about donation is also the responsibility of the OPO, unless designated requestors at the hospital have been trained to do so.[3]

Types of Referrals

Imminent death referrals include patients with severe acute brain injury who 1) require mechanical ventilation; 2) are in a critical care unit or emergency department; and 3) have clinical findings consistent with a low Glasgow Coma Score (GCS) typically 5 or less; patients for whom physicians are evaluating the diagnosis of brain death or have ordered that life-sustaining therapies be withdrawn, pursuant to the family's decision.[9]

Donation After Brain Death

Patients meeting the imminent death referral criteria may be or become brain dead (discussed later in chapter), resulting in *donation after brain death* (DBD) donation. Patients not meeting all necessary criteria for brain death but having an

unsurvivable injury resulting in withdrawal of life support and subsequent cardiac arrest can be donation after cardiac death organ donors.

Donation After Cardiac Death

Donation after cardiac death (DCD), also known as *donation after circulatory death determination* (DCDD), donors are those patients who are not brain dead but who have suffered an irreversible neurologic brain injury, are ventilator dependent, and the family has made a decision to withdraw life-sustaining support. Patients with high spinal cord injuries as well as others dependent on mechanical ventilation may be candidates for DCDD. Organs are recovered after cardiac asystole and a 3- to 5-minute wait period. Cardiac asystole must occur within 60 to 90 minutes for organ donation to occur.

Cardiac death referrals provide the opportunity for patients to be tissue and eye donors after cardiac asystole. Because of the relatively rare occurrence of brain death or withdrawal of treatment, many more deceased patients have the opportunity to donate tissue and eyes. Other transplantable tissues include bone, skin, fascia, cartilage, tendons, ligaments, saphenous veins, heart valves, eyes and/or corneas.

Donor Evaluation

Once the initial call is made to the OPO an organ coordinator will contact the critical care nurse and request specific information regarding the patient's age; sex; race; neurologic, ventilatory, and hemodynamic status; as well as the hospital's plan of care. Once on site, the OPO coordinator will assess the patient and review the medical records, history of the current hospitalization, and major procedures—surgeries, therapies, current medications, past medical history, laboratory values specific to each organ, pulmonary status, systemic infection, diagnostic reports, and the hemodynamic status of the patient.[12] The time between brain death declaration and organ procurement is often marked by significant instability. During this time, optimal medical management is crucial to ensure post-transplant graft survival.

If the patient is not brain dead or there are no plans to withdraw support/decelerate care, the OPO coordinator will collaborate with the critical care nurse on a follow-up plan for ongoing evaluation. The OPO will continue to follow the patient until the patient meets neurologic criteria for brain death, death is declared, or there is a plan to withdraw life-sustaining support. Many patients referred to the OPO do not become donors because they do not meet brain death criteria or there are no plans to withdraw support as the patient's status may improve. Patients declared dead by neurologic criteria constitute only 1% of total deaths in the United States.[13]

Brain Death

Brain death is the irreversible cessation of all brain functions including the brainstem. The clinical diagnosis of brain death is based on guidelines established by the American Academy of Neurology. The practice of brain death declaration varies based on hospital policy and state legislation. Neurologists, neurosurgeons, intensivists, and anesthesiologists usually perform the brain death evaluation. Prior to establishing brain death certain conditions must be confirmed, including the cause and the irreversibility of coma and confounding factors such as:

- Absence of severe hypothermia, defined as a core temperature of 32° C or less
- Absence of hypotension, defined as a systolic blood pressure of 90 mm Hg or less
- Absence of evidence of drug intoxication or poisoning, defined by a careful history, calculation of clearance, and if needed, a normal drug screen
- Absence of recent or current administration of neuromuscular-blocking medications, defined by the presence of four twitches with maximal ulnar nerve stimulation by a train of four peripheral nerve stimulation as shown in Figure 21-17 in Chapter 21
- Absence of electrolyte, acid–base or endocrine dysfunction, as defined by severe acidosis and marked deviation from normal values

Confirmatory Tests

Additional confirmatory testing for the determination of brain death may include cerebral angiography, electroencephalography, transcranial Doppler, and cerebral scintigraphy although these diagnostic procedures are not required (Box 37-1). The bedside clinical examination has three components: 1) absence of cerebral motor reflexes; 2) absence of brainstem reflexes; and 3) absence of respiratory drive.

Cerebral Motor Responses. Cerebral motor responses to pain in all extremities are absent in brain death. These motor responses can be stimulated by the application of pressure to the nail beds or supraorbital ridge. Some motor responses may occur spontaneously during the apnea testing because of the presence of hypoxia or hypotension and are considered

---

BOX 37-1 CONFIRMATORY TESTS IN BRAIN DEATH

Cerebral Angiography
- Contrast medium under high pressure in both anterior and posterior circulation injections
- No intracerebral filling at the level of the carotid or vertebral artery entry to the skull
- Patent external carotid circulation
- Possible delayed filling of the superior longitudinal sinus

Electroencephalography
- Minimum of eight scalp electrodes
- Electrode dependencies should be between 100 and 10,000
- Integrity of the entire recording system should be tested
- Electrode distances should be at least 10 cm
- Sensitivity should be increased to at least 2 microV for 30 minutes with inclusion of appropriate calibrations
- High-frequency filter setting should be at 30 Hz, and low-frequency setting should not be below 1 Hz
- There should be no electroencephalographic reactivity to intense somatosensory or audiovisual stimuli

Transcranial Doppler Ultrasonography
- Bilateral insonation
- The probe is placed at the temporal bone above the zygomatic arch or the vertebrobasilar arteries through the suboccipital transcranial window
- The abnormalities should include a lack of diastolic or reverberating flow, small systolic peaks in early systole, and a lack of flow found by the investigator who previously demonstrated normal velocities

Cerebral Scintigraphy (Technetium Tc 99m Hexametazime)
- Injection of isotope within 30 minutes of reconstitution
- Static image of 500,000 counts at several time intervals: immediately, between 30 and 60 minutes, and at 2 hours
- Correct intravenous injection needs to be confirmed with additional liver images demonstrating uptake (optional)

This information is based on the American Academy of Neurology Guidelines. From Wijdicks EFM. The clinical diagnosis of brain death. In: *The Comatose Patient*. New York: Oxford University Press; 2008.

---

spinal cord reflexes. These may also be elicited in the presence of respiratory acidosis and can include spontaneous flexion and muscle stretch reflexes in the arms and legs that can resemble grasping movements. It is important to determine whether the patient has been given any neuromuscular blocking medications that may induce pharmacologic motor weakness.

Brainstem Reflexes. Brainstem reflexes that will be tested include pupillary signs, ocular movements, facial sensory and motor responses, and pharyngeal and tracheal reflexes.

Pupillary Reflexes. Pupillary signs are evaluated by absence of the light reflex, which is consistent with brain death. Most often the pupils are round, oval, or irregularly shaped, although dilated pupils may remain even after brain death has occurred. This dilation may exist if the sympathetic cervical pathways to the pupillary dilator muscle are intact. Medications do not normally alter pupil response, although the application of topical medications or severe trauma to the eye may affect pupil reactivity.[14]

Oculocephalic Reflex. Ocular movements are lost with brain death. The oculocephalic *reflex* also described as *doll's eyes* involves fast turning of the head to both sides. In brain death this should not generate any eye movements. Neck movements should be avoided in patients with a traumatic brain injury.

Oculovestibular Reflex. Because the oculovestibular reflex is tested using iced water or normal saline, it is sometimes called *cold calorics*. The head of the bed is elevated 30 degrees and approximately 50 mL of ice water or normal saline is injected into the ear, and no movement of the eye toward the side of the stimulus should be present. It is recommended that the patient be observed for up to 1 minute following each ear irrigation and 5 minutes should be allowed before testing the opposite ear. Medications that can influence the vestibulo-ocular reflex include sedatives, aminoglycosides, tricyclic antidepressants, anticholinergics, and anti-seizure agents.

Corneal and Jaw Reflexes. Facial sensory and motor responses are elicited by testing for corneal and jaw reflexes. Stroking a cotton-tipped swab gently across the cornea tests the corneal reflexes. Grimacing in response to pain can be elicited by applying deep pressure to the nail beds, to the supraorbital ridge, or the temporomandibular joint. Severe trauma within these areas could inhibit interpretation of facial brainstem reflexes.[14]

Gag and Cough Reflexes. Pharyngeal and tracheal reflexes are absent in patients with brain death. The gag reflex can be evaluated by stimulating the posterior part of the pharynx with a tongue blade. The cough reflex can be tested with bronchial suctioning.[14]

Apnea Testing. The loss of brainstem function results in the loss of centrally controlled breathing with resultant apnea. The respiratory neurons are controlled by cerebral chemoreceptors that sense changes in the partial pressure of carbon dioxide ($PaCO_2$) and pH of the cerebrospinal fluid that accurately reflect changes in plasma $PaCO_2$.

Guidelines for determination of death recommend achieving $PaCO_2$ levels greater than 60 mm Hg for maximal stimulation of brainstem respiratory centers. Prerequisites and the procedure for apnea testing are outlined in Box 37-2. The prerequisites that should be addressed prior to the apnea test are to prevent cardiac dysrhythmias, hypotension, and decreased oxygen saturation. If any of these conditions occur during the apnea test, the test should be aborted and confirmatory testing should be performed (see Box 37-1). In cases where a patient is a CO_2 retainer or the clinical examination is not reliable due to head trauma, confirmatory testing is necessary. Confirmatory testing is mandatory in children.

Donation After Cardiac Death

As stated above, *donation after cardiac death* (DCD) is also known as *donation after circulatory death determination* (DCDD). DCDD is based on the cessation of circulatory and respiratory functions.[15] Previously, DCD donors were known as non–heart-beating donors or asystolic donors. Patients who do not meet brain death criteria, but have an unsurvivable condition, such as a catastrophic neurologic injury, high spinal cord

---

BOX 37-2　APNEA TEST

Prerequisites
1. Normothermia
2. Systolic blood pressure ≥90 mm Hg
3. Euvolemia
4. Eucapnia
5. Normoxemia

Procedure
- A pulse oximeter is connected to the patient to monitor the O_2 saturation
- Preoxygenation for 10 minutes with FiO_2 of 100%
- Reduce ventilation frequency to 10 breaths per minute and reduce PEEP to 5 cm H_2O
- If pulse oximetry oxygen saturation remains more than 90%, obtain baseline arterial blood gas, including $PaCO_2$, pH, bicarbonate and base excess
- Disconnect the ventilator
- Place a cannula at the level of the carina and deliver 100% O_2 6 liters/min
- Observe closely for respiratory movements for 8-10 minutes. Respiration is defined as abdominal or chest excursions that produce adequate tidal volumes
- Abort if blood pressure remains less than 90 mm Hg systolic or declining despite increasing vasopressors
- Abort if oxygen saturation is less than 80% for 2 minutes or drops steadily (consider retry with T-piece and CPAP)
- If no breathing drive is observed, measure arterial PaO_2, $PaCO_2$, and pH after approximately 8 minutes
- If respiratory movements are absent and $PaCO_2$ is ≥60 mm Hg (or 20 mm Hg increase in $PaCO_2$ over a baseline normal $PaCO_2$) the apnea test result is positive (i.e., it supports the clinical diagnosis of brain death)
- If the patient breathes, repeat test a few hours later

From Wijdicks EFM. The clinical diagnosis of brain death. In: *The Comatose Patient*. New York: Oxford University Press; 2008.

---

injury, or a medical condition requiring mechanical ventilation, are candidates for DCD. Before the enactment of brain death laws in the 1970s, all organ donors were DCD donors. Interest in DCD has increased due to 1) family interest in organ donation when neurologic criteria for brain death have not been met, and 2) the continued national demand for organs.[16,17]

Controlled Donation After Cardiac Death

DCD donors are classified as controlled and uncontrolled DCD donors. *Controlled DCD* occurs when the family has made a decision to withdraw life-sustaining support and death is declared at the time of circulatory arrest. In controlled DCD, families, health care providers, and OPO staff are involved in the timing and planning of the time when support will be withdrawn.[14]

Uncontrolled Donation After Cardiac Death

Uncontrolled DCD describes a situation in which cardiac arrest has occurred and resuscitation efforts are determined to be futile. The uncontrolled DCD process is rapid as the patient is undergoing cardiopulmonary resuscitation. After authorization from the family, the patient is taken to the operating room for immediate recovery of organs, primarily kidneys.[18]

DCD is an opportunity to increase the number of organs available for transplantation. Five-year organ survival rates in kidney and pancreas recipients from DCD donors and brain-dead donors are similar.[19] Liver transplant grafts from DCD donors can encounter complications secondary to *ischemic cholangiopathy* (damage to the bile ducts from an impaired blood supply); consequently many transplant centers have changed their criteria for acceptance of DCD donors based on the age of the donor.[20] DCD lung donor outcomes are favorable to those of brain-dead lung donors.[21]

Authorization for Donation

"Presumed Consent" is the donation law existing in many European countries. This is a system in which one is deemed a donor unless the person has taken action not to be a donor. That is not the law in the United States. The United States retains a voluntary system, often referred to as "opting-in." The architecture of U.S. organ donation law, also termed "Gift Law," is the Uniform Anatomical Gift Act (UAGA), which is enacted in all 50 states.

The OPO coordinator is an advocate for the donor/donor family and potential recipients. Many factors are important in working with potential donor families. The nurse and OPO coordinator are important in providing a safe, comfortable environment for families in a position to make decisions about donation.[22] Assessing the needs of the family is crucial to the outcome of the donation conversation. Timing of the conversation is also important. Donation does not consist of simply asking the family if they wish to donate.[15] The critical care nurse should inform the family that an expert member of the health care team is available to provide information and answer their questions about donation.[26]

Many myths and misconceptions surround organ donation. Common misconceptions from families surround religious beliefs, cultural milieus, and concerns about possible body disfigurement, concern about the ability to have an open casket funeral, and costs to family.[23] Another common misperception is that hospital staff will not attempt to save the life of their loved one if they believe the patient could be a donor.[23] These misperceptions must be debunked with the family. Finally, research has shown the manner in which the donation request is made is the main factor in a family's ultimate decision regardless of pre-existing attitudes.[24] Many families report that donation has helped their healing in the grieving process and say that donation represents something positive in their loss.[24]

Donor Management

The donor management phase includes ongoing collaboration between the OPO coordinator and OPO medical director, critical care nurse, intensivist, respiratory therapist, and transplant professionals to ensure optimal preservation of organ function for organ recovery and transplantation.[25]

Standing orders for the care of an organ donor are provided by the OPO. These encompass required testing and screening of donors as well as parameters for continued medical management of the cadaveric donor, as listed in Box 37-3. The goals of donor management are to maximize oxygenation and provide optimal organ perfusion to maintain the viability of organs for transplantation as listed in Table 37-4.

BOX 37-3 STANDARD DONOR CARE PROTOCOLS

The Organ Procurement Organization (OPO) coordinator should write orders to initiate standard donor care.

1. Transfer care to [Name of OPO]
2. Discontinue all prior orders
3. Blood pressure, heart rate, temperature, urine output, central venous pressure (CVP) (if central venous catheter present), pulmonary artery occlusion pressure (PAOP) (if pulmonary artery [PA] catheter present) every 1 hour
4. Reorder mechanical ventilator parameters as previously set
5. Maintain head of bed at 30-40 degrees elevation
6. Continue routine pulmonary suctioning and side-to-side body positioning
7. Warming blanket to maintain body temp above 36.5° C
8. Maintain sequential compression devices (SCDs)
9. Continue chest tube suction or water seal as previously ordered (if present)
10. Nasogastric (orogastric) tube to low intermittent suction (if present)
11. Intravenous fluid: D5 0.45% saline plus 20 meq KCl per liter at 75 mL/ hour
12. Call OPO coordinator if: MAP <70 mm Hg; systolic pressure >170 mm Hg; heart rate <60 or >130 bpm; temp <36.5° C or >37.8° C; urine output <75 or >250 mL/hr; CVP or PAOP <8 or >18 mm Hg
13. Medications:
    Pantoprazole 40 mg IV every 24 hours, first dose now
    Artificial tears every 1 hour and PRN to prevent corneal drying

Albuterol and Atrovent unit dose per aerosol every 4 hours
Antibiotics previously ordered continued at same dose and frequency
Vasoactive medication infusions (dopamine, norepinephrine) at previously ordered concentrations and infusion rates

14. Review all medications previously ordered. Most anticonvulsants, pain medications, laxatives, gastrointestinal motility agents, eye drops, antihypertensives, antinausea agents, subcutaneous heparin, osmotic agents (mannitol), and diuretics are unnecessary during donor care and will be discontinued automatically with order number 2 above. Review any other medications in question with MD
15. Send electrolytes, magnesium, ionized calcium, CBC, platelets, glucose, blood urea nitrogen (BUN), creatinine, phosphorous, arterial blood gas (ABG), prothrombin time (PT)/international normalized ratio (INR), partial thromboplastin time (PTT), STAT and repeat every 4 hours
16. Send blood for type and screen with above blood draw (if not previously done)
17. Finger-stick blood glucose every 2 hours—call OPO coordinator if blood glucose <90 or >180 mg/dL
18. Electrocardiogram STAT
19. Radiography STAT-Indication: initial donor evaluation
20. Add other orders for specific organ evaluation as indicated

The above order set provides a "safety net" of call orders so that the coordinator is alerted to significant changes in donor status. It also prescribes the foundation for ongoing monitoring of physiologic and laboratory variables.

Modified from Powner DJ, O'Connor KJ. Adult clinical donor care. In: LaPointe-Rudow D, Ohler L, Shafer TJ, eds. *A Clinician's Guide to Donation and Transplantation.* Lenexa, KS: Applied Measurement Professionals; 2006.

TABLE 37-4	DONOR MANAGEMENT CLINICAL PARAMETERS
PARAMETER	**CLINICAL GOAL**
1. Mean Arterial Pressure (MAP)	60-110 mm Hg
2. Central Venous Pressure (CVP)	4-12 mm Hg
3. Ejection Fraction (EF)	>50%
4. Vasopressors	One low-dose vasopressor
5. Arterial Blood Gas pH	7.3-7.5
6. PaO_2 : FiO_2 (P : F ratio)	>300 on PEEP of 5
7. Serum Na^+	<155 mEq/L
8. Blood Glucose	<150 mg/dL
9. Urine Output (averaged over 4 hours)	>0.5 mL/kg/hr

Patients with critical neurologic impairment present with many clinical challenges including: hypotension—81%, diabetes insipidus—65%, disseminated intravascular coagulation (DIC)—28%, cardiac arrhythmias—25%, pulmonary edema—18%, and metabolic acidosis—11%. There is increasing evidence that control of these pathophysiologic changes by active clinical management increases the number and quality of organs available for transplantation, which ultimately impacts the potential recipient.[26,27]

Further assessment of the donor by the OPO coordinator includes screening for any transmissible diseases, including serologic tests for infectious diseases, such as human immunodeficiency virus (HIV), hepatitis, syphilis, cytomegalovirus (CMV), and Epstein-Barr virus (EBV). The OPO coordinator will conduct a medical social history questionnaire with the authorizing person(s) or others who can provide information on the donor's past medical and social history. The questionnaire is comprised of standard questions about the donor's past behavioral, medical, social, and sexual health. These questions have been approved by UNOS, the Food and Drug Administration (FDA), and other accrediting agencies for organ and tissue donation.

Organ Allocation

The Organ Procurement and Transplantation Network (OPTN) is responsible for operating the national database, which lists all patients waiting for an organ transplant in the United States. The United Network for Organ Sharing (UNOS) manages the national list. The OPO coordinator will access the UNOS computer to generate a donor-specific list of potential recipients from the national list. Potential recipients are matched with the donor based on blood type, height, weight, HLA (human leukocytic antigen), distance from the donor, waiting time on the list, and severity of illness. The national system in place for organ allocation is fair and equitable for those requiring a transplant. The list does not reference race, gender, or socioeconomic status. Organs are offered electronically to the transplant team of the first person on the list. If the organ is refused for any reason, the transplant hospital of the next patient on the list is contacted. The process

continues until a match is made. Once a patient is selected and contacted and all testing is complete, surgery is scheduled and the transplant takes place.

Role of the Medical Examiner/Coroner in Organ and Tissue Donation

Medical examiners and coroners play a vital role in organ and tissue donation. They are responsible for investigating and determining the cause and manner of deaths that occur in cases falling within their jurisdiction. Deaths falling within the jurisdiction of medical examiners and coroners include those that occur from unexpected and violent circumstances, and in many states, any pediatric death under age 6. These cases are the very same cases that make up the majority of potential organ donors. Thus, organ and tissue donation and medical examiner/coroner activities directly intersect. The medical examiner/coroner must review these cases and release them in a timely manner in order for donation to occur.

Organ Recovery

Once all recipients have been identified, the OPO coordinator schedules the operating room time and coordinates the surgical recovery teams' arrival for organ retrieval. The OPO coordinator and critical care nurse coordinate the transport, collaborating with OR staff and anesthesiology. The nurse ensures the donor is connected to a transport monitor; oxygen and emergency medications must be available. In the operating room, hemodynamic support and continued medical management is coordinated between the OPO staff, anesthesiologist, and the recovery surgeons.

Organs are flushed with preservative solution containing electrolytes and nutrients. The organs are then removed from the donor, examined individually in a sterile basin, and packed in sterile containers for transport. For heart, heart and lung, and lungs, transport is immediate. For the pancreas and liver, time to transplant ranges from 6 to 20 hours. For kidneys, approximately 24 hours may elapse before transplantation takes place. Tissue typing is primarily carried out between kidney and pancreas donors and recipients; less frequently between heart, heart and lung, and single-lung donor and recipient.

Tissue Donation

Families have the opportunity to enhance and save many lives through tissue and eye donation. This donation could impact the lives of 60 to 80 individuals awaiting tissue transplantation. There are approximately 40,000 tissue donors per year and an estimated 1,000,000 Americans receive tissue transplants each year, from sight-saving corneas to hip replacements, bone repair, and heart valves.[9] Patients who have reached cardiac death are able to donate tissues if deemed medically suitable by the OPO. After the authorization process, if tissue recovery is going to be delayed, it is imperative that the body of the donor is cooled. The American Association of Tissue Banks (AATB) standards require that tissue be recovered within 24 hours of cardiac death provided the body has received sufficient cooling.

The recovery of tissue is performed in an operating room suite using sterile technique. OPO-trained specialists perform the recovery and bring the necessary supplies required for tissue recovery; hospital operating room staff is not needed for tissue recovery.[12]

Organ Donation Summary

Organ and tissue donation saves lives. Critical care nurses are in a unique position to impact the lives of many patients, those who are able to give the gift of life and those awaiting a lifesaving transplant. Nurses collaborate closely with the OPO to honor the wishes of patients and their families. Nursing care does not stop when a patient meets the criteria to become an organ donor. Provision of expert nursing care, compassion, and support of families facing end-of-life decisions are part of daily practice.

IMMUNOLOGY OF TRANSPLANT REJECTION

Organ transplantation has become a commonly practiced procedure for end-stage heart, lung, liver, kidney, and pancreatic disease. Major advances have been made in organ procurement and preservation; surgical techniques; and prevention, identification, and treatment of rejection. Ultimately the long-term success of transplantation depends on the immune system's tolerance for the transplanted graft. Virtually every cell in the human body carries distinctive molecules that enable the immune system to distinguish self from nonself. An intact immune system will recognize and eliminate any foreign biologic material recognized as nonself. Only suppression or down regulation of the normal immune response can achieve tolerance of the transplanted organ. To understand the principles of immunosuppressive therapy, it is important to have some understanding of the cells of the immune system, the immune response, and the process of organ rejection.

Immune Mechanism

Whenever the body is confronted with any substance that is nonself, a *primary immune response* is elicited. There are three phases of any primary immune response: 1) recognition of the substance as nonself; 2) proliferation of immunocompetent cells; and 3) action against the foreign substance (effector phase). During the primary response, immunologic memory is established, and any subsequent encounter with the same substance induces a more rapid and intense immune response. Subsequent encounters are called *secondary immune responses.*

An *antigen* is a substance that is capable of eliciting an immune response. Each cell has antigens on its surface that are determined by a series of linked genes known as the *major histocompatibility complex* (MHC). If tissue from one person is transplanted into a genetically different person, the antigens on the transplanted tissue cells are immediately recognized as nonself, and rejection occurs. MHC determines the antigens to which the immune system should respond. The human MHC

is called *human leukocyte antigen* (HLA), because these markers were first discovered on lymphocytes.

HLA antigens are divided into two classes. *Class I antigens* consist of HLA-A, HLA-B, HLA-C, and HLA-D loci and are expressed on the plasma membranes of all nucleated cells. *Class II antigens* consist of HLA-DR, HLA-DQ, and HLA-DP loci and are expressed on activated immune cells.[28] Because of the potential for millions of different arrangements of these antigens, the chances of finding a donor organ with the same genes as a recipient are almost nil unless the donor and recipient are identical twins.

Cells of the Immune System

The immune system contains a variety of cells responsible for general defense as well as very specific immune responses. When a particular antigen (foreign protein) appears, those cells are stimulated to multiply and mount a response. Immune cells are originally produced in the bone marrow as stem cells; their descendants become lymphocytes or phagocytes (Fig. 37-2).

The two major classes of lymphocytes are *B cells* and *T cells*. B cells remain in the bone marrow to complete their maturation. T cells migrate to the thymus gland and mature there. In the thymus, T cells acquire the ability to distinguish self from nonself. After they have matured, some B and T cells are stored in the lymph nodes, whereas others circulate in the blood and lymphatic systems.

Humoral Immunity

Humoral immunity is mediated by B cells, which are responsible for the production of antibody or immunoglobulin. When a B cell encounters an antigen to which it is specifically coded to respond, the B cell enlarges, divides, and differentiates into a *plasma cell*. It is the plasma cell that actually produces and secretes antigen-specific *antibody* (Fig. 37-3). After exposure to an antigen, the immune system retains a memory of that antigen. Subsequent exposure stimulates the B cell memory cells, resulting in a rapid mobilization of antibody-secreting cells. Antibodies work in several ways, but their primary purpose is to mark an antigen for destruction by the immune system. Other antibodies are capable of neutralizing toxins produced by bacteria, or they can trigger the release of serum proteins known as *complement.*

Cell-Mediated Immunity

T cells provide cell-mediated immunity. Approximately 65% to 80% of all lymphocytes are T cells, of which there are three basic types: *cytotoxic T cells, helper T cells,* and *suppressor T cells.*

Cytotoxic T Cells. Cytotoxic T cells are cells responsible for killing invading cells. Their primary role is to rid the body of cells that have become infected, have been transformed by cancer, or are nonself (e.g., transplanted tissue). They are also called *T8* or *CD8 lymphocytes,* referring to a marker that distinguishes cytotoxic T cells from other T cells. Cytotoxic T cells are activated by macrophages that present the foreign antigen to immature cytotoxic T cells. With the assistance of helper T cells and their release of chemical mediators, the cytotoxic T cells

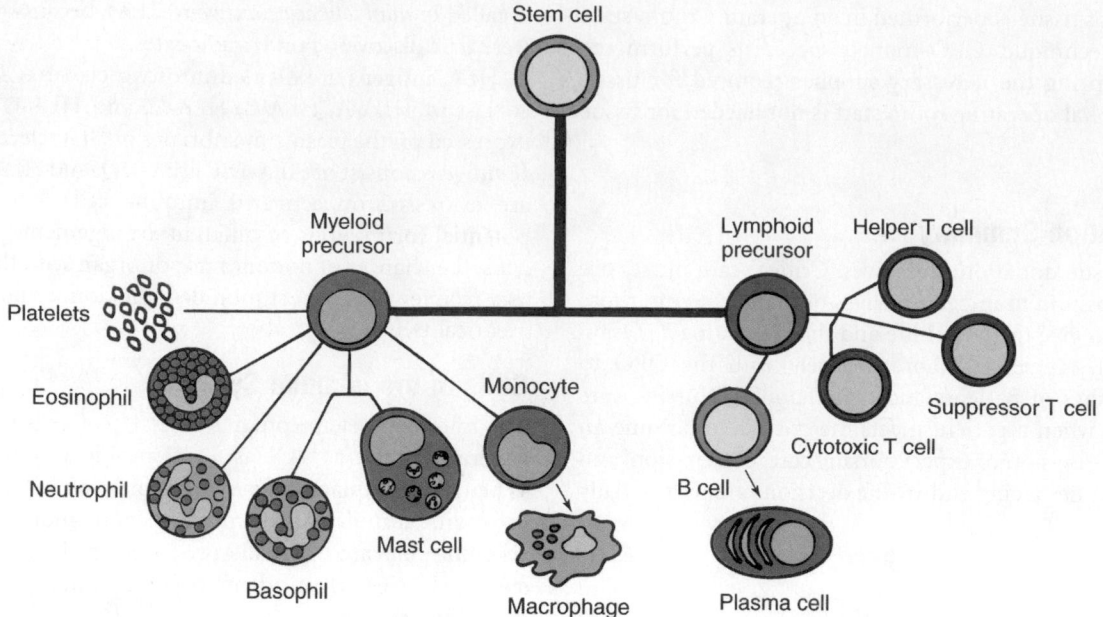

FIGURE 37-2 All cells of the immune system originate from stem cells in the bone marrow. (From Schindler LW. *Understanding the immune system*. NIH publication no. 92-529. Bethesda, MD: Department of Health and Human Services; 1991.)

mature and kill foreign cells that carry that specific antigen (Fig. 37-4).

Helper T Cells. Helper T cells up-regulate the immune response by stimulating B cells to differentiate into plasma cells and begin antibody production, by activating cytotoxic T cells, and by stimulating natural killer (NK) cells and macrophages. Helper T cells are identified by surface glycoproteins known as CD4 or T4 markers. Figure 37-5 illustrates the process responsible for activating helper T cells. *Macrophages* present processed antigen to the immature helper T cells. With the assistance of chemical mediators (interleukins) released by the macrophages, the helper T cells mature and begin to activate other cells of the immune system previously described.

Suppressor T Cells. A third type of T cell is the suppressor T cell. These cells suppress, or down-regulate, the immune response. They play an important role in keeping the immune response controlled and in turning off the response after the antigenic threat is no longer present.

Other Immune System Defenses

T and B cells work with other parts of the immune system, notably NK cells, phagocytic cells, and complement, to enhance the immune response.

Natural Killer Cells. NK cells are another type of lymphocyte. They are not targeted for any specific antigen but will attack and destroy any cell that is identified as nonself. NK cells contain granules filled with potent chemicals that are released when they bind to the targeted nonself cell. These chemicals are capable of lysing the cell membrane and causing the cell's death. NK cells can also cause tissue inflammation through the release of proinflammatory cytokines.[29]

Phagocytes. Phagocytes are a major category of immune cells capable of destroying foreign cells. Critical phagocytes include monocytes, macrophages, neutrophils, eosinophils, and

basophils. Table 37-5 outlines the primary functions of these cells. Macrophages are vitally important to the immune response because of their role in "presenting" antigens to the helper and cytotoxic T cells. This presentation alerts T cells to the presence of antigen. Macrophages also produce chemical regulators, or interleukins, that stimulate the maturation of helper and cytotoxic T cells.

Complement. An important system in the immune response is complement. Complement consists of a series of 25 proteins that when activated develop into powerful enzymes capable of lysing alien cell walls. Complement is triggered by the presence of antibody bound to a foreign cell or antigen (antigen–antibody complex). Complement also stimulates basophils, attracts neutrophils, and coats foreign cells to make them more attractive to phagocytes. The latter action is called *opsonization*.

Graft Rejection

Rejection of any transplanted organ occurs when the transplanted tissue is recognized as nonself by the immune system. Cellular-mediated rejection occurs when HLA class I antigens, displayed on cells of the donor organ, activate helper T cells that promote the expansion of cytotoxic T cells and recruit macrophages into the transplanted tissue. NK cells also begin to attack any cell with foreign HLA class I antigens. As a result, the transplanted organ becomes infiltrated with these cells, which proceed to destroy the foreign graft tissue.

At the same time, antibody-mediated or humoral-mediated rejection occurs as antigen–antibody complexes form. These complexes are present in the transplanted organ and release complement that is capable of cell destruction. Complement plays a role in recruiting basophils and tissue-destroying neutrophils to the site. Antibody also coats the foreign cells, making them more attractive to macrophages.

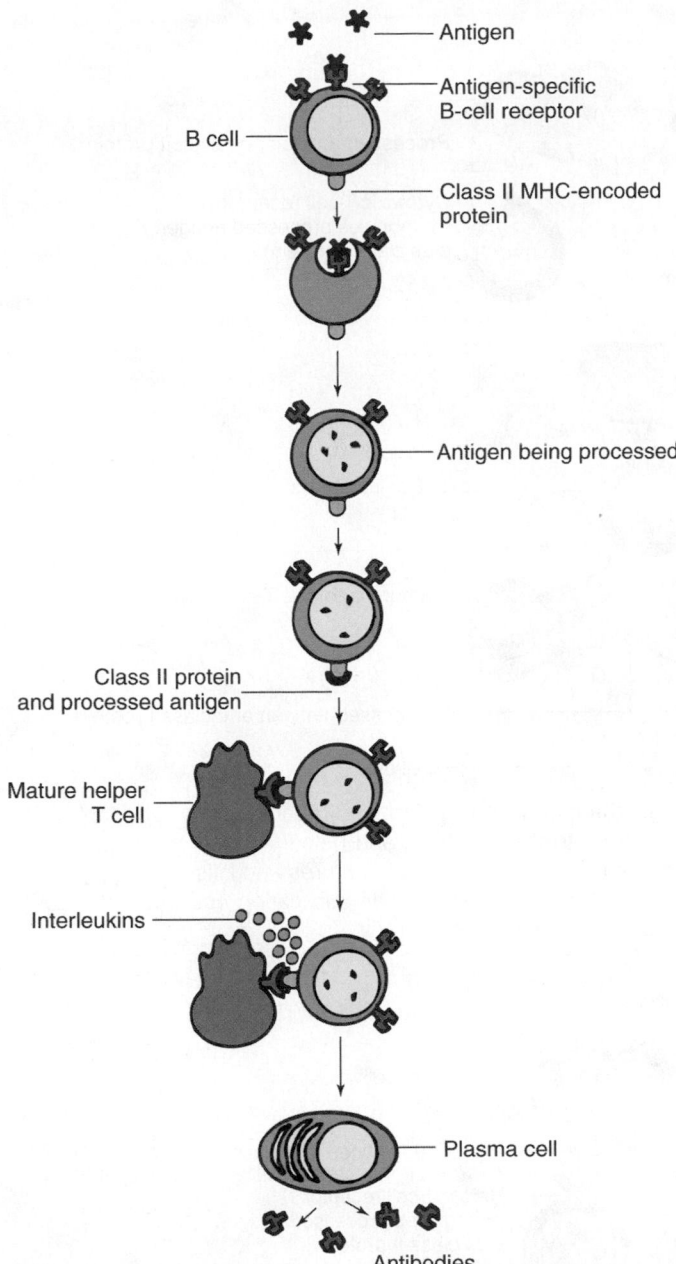

FIGURE 37-3 Foreign antigen is processed by the B cell and displayed with its major histocompatibility complex (MHC) class II antigen (protein), which attracts helper T cells. The release of interleukins by the helper T cell stimulates differentiation of the B cell into a plasma cell, which begins to produce antibody. (From Schindler LW. *Understanding the Immune System*. NIH publication no. 92-529. Bethesda, MD: Department of Health and Human Services; 1991.)

Graft rejection can occur at different time intervals and has different injury patterns. The three types of rejection patterns are hyperacute rejection, acute rejection, and chronic rejection.

Hyperacute Rejection

Hyperacute rejection is a humoral-mediated response, which occurs within hours after transplantation and results in immediate graft failure. The rapid immune response is caused by the presence of preformed reactive antibodies as a consequence of previous exposure to antigens. Presensitization can be the result of previous blood transfusions, multiple pregnancies, or previous organ transplantation.[28] Left ventricular assist devices, which are used as a bridge to eventual heart transplantation, can also sensitize potential recipients because of the physical properties of the device itself, activation of the immune system, and increased production of antibodies.[29,30] Transplantation of an organ from a donor with an incompatible blood type can have the same effect. Hyperacute rejection is prevented by testing for the presence of preformed antibodies in the recipient and by selecting donors with compatible blood types.

Acute Rejection

Acute rejection tends to occur weeks to months after transplantation but can occur at any time. Class I or II antigens on the cells of the transplanted graft activate a cellular-mediated response.

Chronic Rejection

Chronic rejection occurs at varying times after transplantation and progresses for years until it leads to ultimate failure of the transplanted organ. Chronic rejection is the result of both humoral-mediated and cellular-mediated immune responses. Chronic inflammation results in diffuse scarring of tissue and stenosis of the organ's vasculature, eventually leading to ischemia and necrosis of tissue.

Immunosuppressive Therapy

Immunosuppression protocols vary among institutions and according to the type of organ transplanted. The primary goal of immunosuppressive therapies is to suppress the activity of helper and cytotoxic T cells. In general, most protocols combine high-dose corticosteroids with a *calcineurin inhibitor* such as cyclosporine or with tacrolimus in addition to mycophenolate mofetil, sirolimus, or occasionally azathioprine. These *"triple-drug"* regimens are designed to prevent rejection while reducing the toxicity of the individual medications. In addition to these primary agents, cytolytic therapy is often used in an attempt to induce graft tolerance and prevent early rejection. Cytolytic agents include antilymphocyte globulins, antithymocyte globulins, and OKT3 monoclonal antibody (discussed later). Table 37-6 summarizes immunosuppressive medications. Absolute care must be taken to monitor the effectiveness of medication therapy and to minimize unnecessarily high doses of these agents, which could predispose patients to greater risks for infection, malignancy, or other toxic effects.

Corticosteroids

Corticosteroids—intravenous methylprednisolone (Solu-Medrol) and oral prednisone—have complex and diverse effects on the immune system. They are used for maintenance therapy and to treat acute rejection. The anti-inflammatory actions of steroids provide important protection of the transplanted organ against permanent damage from the body's natural immune response. As maintenance therapy, steroids impair the sensitivity of T cells to antigen, decrease the proliferation of sensitized

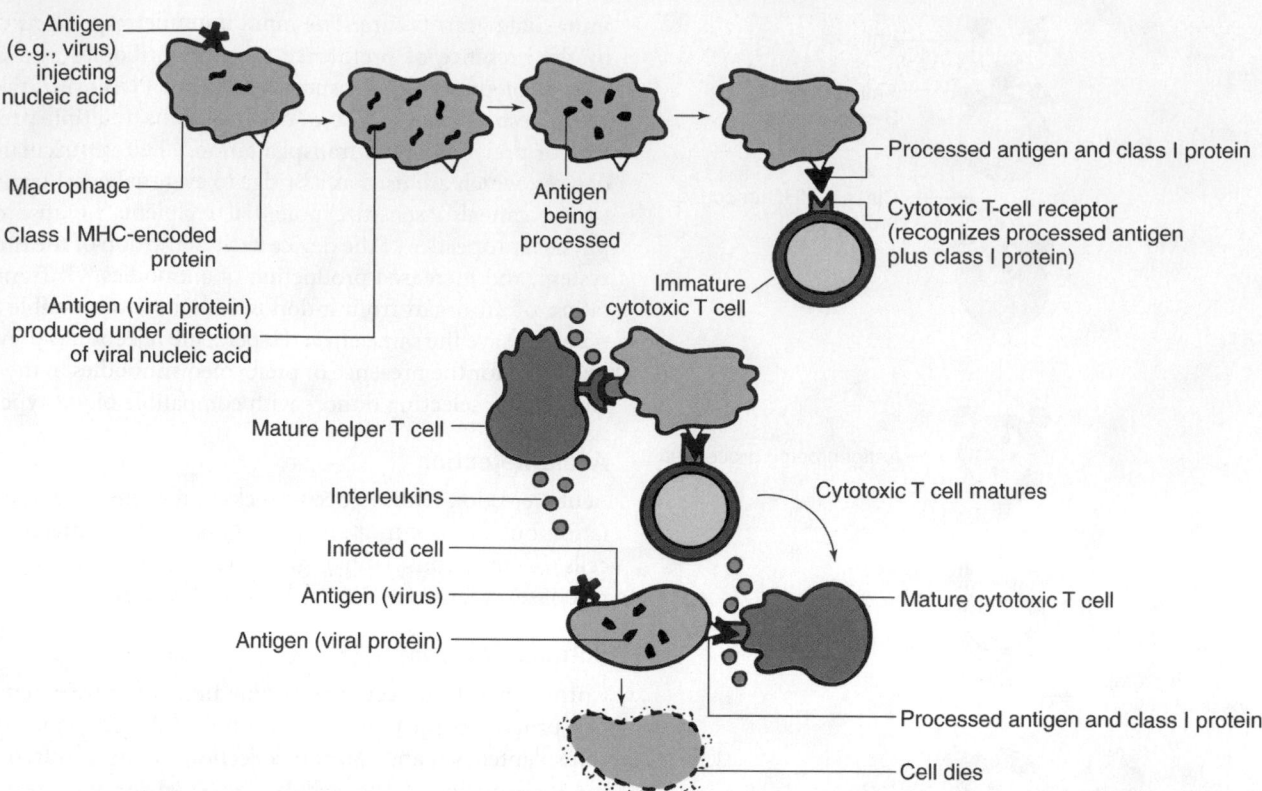

FIGURE 37-4 The macrophage presents the processed antigen from the foreign organism on the major histocompatibility complex (MHC) class I protein to the cytotoxic and helper T cells. Aided by the release of interleukins from the helper T cell, the cytotoxic T cell matures and kills the foreign cell. (From Schindler LW. *Understanding the Immune System*. NIH publication no. 92-529. Bethesda, MD: Department of Health and Human Services; 1991.)

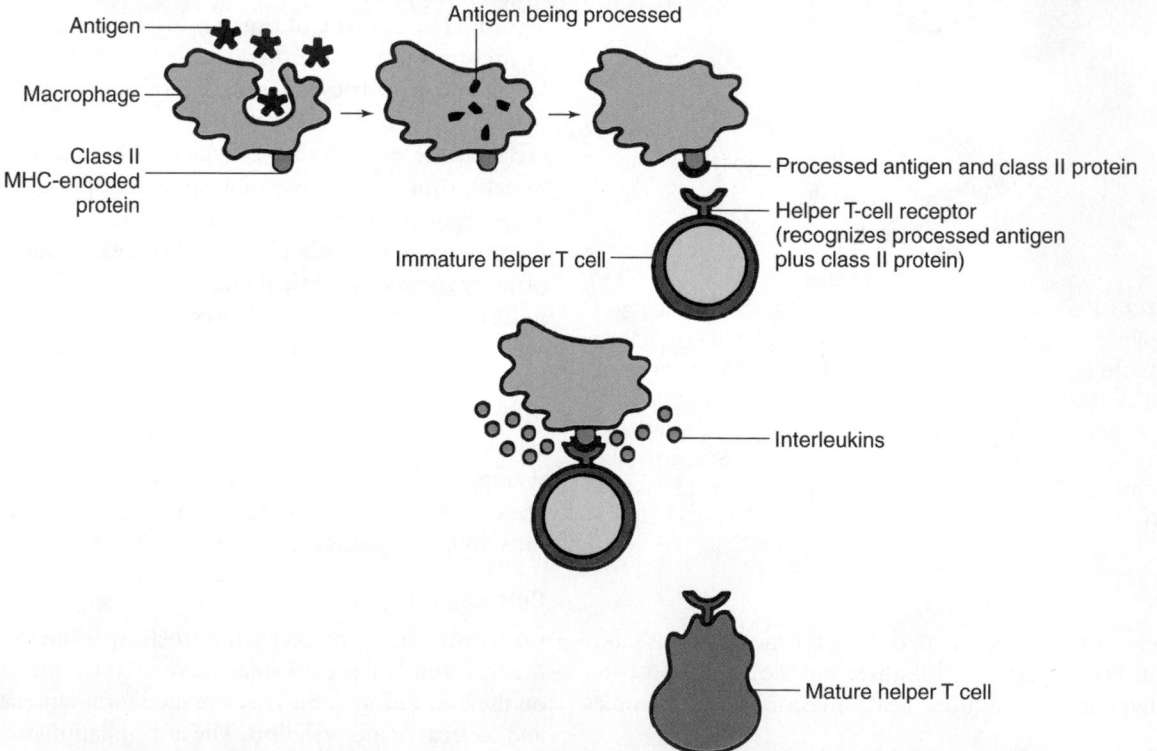

FIGURE 37-5 The helper T cell is activated by the presence of processed antigen in combination with the major histocompatibility complex (MHC) class II antigen (protein) on the surface of a macrophage. It matures with the stimulus from interleukins. (From Schindler LW. *Understanding the Immune System*. NIH publication no. 92-529. Bethesda MD: Department of Health and Human Services; 1991.)

TABLE 37-5 PHAGOCYTES AND THEIR FUNCTIONS

PHAGOCYTE	FUNCTION
Monocytes	Migrate from blood tissues to become macrophages Act as scavenger cells in tissues Present antigen to T cells
Macrophages	Secrete enzymes, complement proteins, and immune regulatory factors (cytokines) Activated by lymphokines
Neutrophils	Contain granules capable of destroying alien organisms Key role in inflammatory reactions
Eosinophils	Contain granules capable of destroying alien organisms Weaker phagocyte
Basophils	Contain granules capable of destroying alien organisms Key role in allergic reaction

T cells, and impair the production of interleukins. Steroids also decrease macrophage mobility.

Unfortunately chronic steroid therapy is associated with numerous adverse effects and predisposes the patient to an increased risk of infection (see Table 37-6). A primary goal of corticosteroid therapy is to titrate the medication dose to as low a level as possible. An ideal therapeutic regimen would allow for elimination of the medication altogether. Chronic use of corticosteroids is associated with painful osteoporosis, avascular necrosis of joints, fragile skin that is easily traumatized, poor wound healing, susceptibility to skin cancers, steroid-induced acne, insulin resistance, and problems with obesity.

Cyclosporine

Cyclosporine belongs to a class of immunosuppressants called calcineurin inhibitors. Its primary mechanism of action is to

TABLE 37-6 PHARMACOLOGIC MANAGEMENT

Organ Transplantation

MEDICATION	DOSAGE*	ACTION	SPECIAL CONSIDERATIONS
Azathioprine	Titrate to WBC count of 3000-6000 cells/mm³	Inhibits purine synthesis	Monitor for bone marrow depression
Cyclosporine gelatin (Neoral),‡ oral solution and capsules	Therapeutic range: 100-400 ng/mL Standard dose ranges for specific organs:† Liver, 14-18 mg/kg/day Kidney, 10-14 mg/kg/day, tapered to 5-10 mg/kg/day Heart, 4-6 mg/kg/day	Suppresses T lymphocytes	Hold for elevated levels Monitor for nephrotoxicity, HTN, hepatotoxicity, tremors, and seizures Monitor for medications that exhibit nephrotoxic synergy (e.g., gentamicin, tobramycin, vancomycin, amphotericin B, ketoconazole, cimetidine, ranitidine)
Muromonab-CD3 (Orthoclone OKT3)	5 mg/day for 5-7 days (less in some centers)	Suppresses circulating T lymphocytes	Monitor for reactions For initial doses, pretreat with: Acetaminophen (Tylenol) Diphenhydramine (Benadryl) Hydrocortisone, 50 mg
Mycophenolate mofetil (CellCept)	2-3 g/day†	Similar to azathioprine but less toxic to bone marrow	Increased blood level concentrations when used with other medications excreted through the kidney tubules
Prednisone	1 mg/kg/day, tapered to 0.3 mg/kg/day or off, if tolerated	Suppresses inflammatory response	Tapered to as low a dose as tolerated; dose is increased with rejection
Rabbit antithymocyte globulin (Thymoglobulin, RATG)	1.5 mg/kg for 1-7 days May be given once daily initially then every other day	Suppresses circulating T lymphocytes	Used in lung transplantation for induction therapy Used as rescue therapy for other transplantation procedures Monitor for reactions Pretreatment may be used
Sirolimus (Rapamycin, Rapamune)	10 mg/day, tapered to trough level of 12-20 mg/mL (depending on organ and center)	Blocks ability of cytokines to activate T and B lymphocytes	Synergistic effects when used with cyclosporine or tacrolimus Monitor for thrombocytopenia Used in place of azathioprine or mycophenolate mofetil
Tacrolimus (Prograf, FK506)	0.1-0.3 mg/kg/day† Therapeutic range: 5-20 mg/mL	Inhibition of interleukin release	Nephrotoxicity with high doses Hyperkalemia

*These dosage ranges are general guidelines. Significant variations in dosages occur based on institutional practices, other medications being used in combination, type of transplantation, and patient response to the medications.
†Daily dose is divided and administered 12 hours apart.
‡The cyclosporine preparations Neoral and Sandimmune are not bioequivalent and cannot be used interchangeably; Gengraf and Neoral are bioequivalent.
HTN, Hypertension; *WBC*, white blood cell.

suppress the activation of T lymphocytes, which inhibits the production of interleukin-2 (IL-2).[31] Because cyclosporine is specifically targeted to T cells, the patient's immune system is not completely impaired, and some ability to protect the body from infection is preserved.

Three preparations of cyclosporine are available. The first preparation to arrive on the market was Sandimmune (Novartis), followed by Neoral (Novartis). Neoral has demonstrated greater bioavailability and medication exposure than Sandimmune, with no significantly greater adverse events.[32,33] Neoral and Sandimmune are not bioequivalent and cannot be used interchangeably. Gengraf (Abbott Laboratories) is the latest form of cyclosporine to be introduced to the market. Gengraf is bioequivalent to Neoral, and because it is a generic formulation, it is less costly. Gengraf is also better tolerated by patients, who report that it is easier to swallow, tastes better, and has less impact on breath and body odor.[34] The most common side effects of cyclosporine are hypertension, hyperlipidemia, hirsutism, gingival hyperplasia, nephrotoxicity, hepatotoxicity, and seizures.[31]

Tacrolimus

Tacrolimus (Prograf, FK506) was first approved for use in clinical trials for liver transplant recipients in 1989. Tacrolimus is a calcineurin inhibitor with similar activity to cyclosporine in that it also impairs T-cell activation by inhibiting the formation of IL-2.[31] Tacrolimus is used in place of cyclosporine in the immunosuppressive regimen of some transplant programs because of its more favorable side effect profile. Tacrolimus is less likely than cyclosporine to cause hyperlipidemia, hypertension, and hirsutism.[31] The most common side effects of tacrolimus are diabetes mellitus,[35] electrolyte imbalances (hyperkalemia, hypophosphatemia, hypomagnesemia), nephrotoxicity, and tremor.[31]

Several studies comparing cyclosporine to tacrolimus as a primary immunosuppressant in kidney and liver transplant recipients have found tacrolimus to be superior in improving patient survival, graft survival, and in preventing acute rejection. Similar studies in heart transplant and lung transplant recipients showed comparable survival between the two medications but lower incidences of acute rejection in patients receiving tacrolimus.[36-39]

Azathioprine

Azathioprine (Imuran) is an antimetabolite that interferes with purine synthesis, which is necessary for the production of antibodies and for the synthesis of nucleic acids in rapidly proliferating cells, such as the cells of the immune system. Azathioprine is used as a maintenance medication to prevent the activation and rapid proliferation of T cells responding to an antigen. A common adverse effect is suppression of other rapidly proliferating cells; this results in leukopenia, thrombocytopenia, and anemia. The dose of the medication is adjusted to keep the white blood cell count between 3000 and 5000 cells/mm[3], thereby protecting the patient from an increased risk of infection. The actual minimum acceptable white blood cell count varies with institutional preferences and the type of organ transplanted. Many centers have abandoned the use of azathioprine in favor of mycophenolate mofetil.

Mycophenolate Mofetil

Mycophenolate mofetil (CellCept) is a derivative of mycophenolic acid. Mycophenolic acid is a selective inhibitor of the enzyme inosine monophosphate dehydrogenase, which is crucial in the pathway for purine synthesis. Because this pathway is responsible for signaling lymphocyte proliferation, mycophenolate mofetil is a potent inhibitor of T and B lymphocyte proliferation.[40] This inhibition also disrupts antibody formation and the generation of cytotoxic T cells, effectively suppressing cellular-mediated and humoral-mediated immunity. The mechanism of action is similar to that of azathioprine except that mycophenolate mofetil selectively inhibits T and B cells.

The use of mycophenolate mofetil in heart transplant recipients was associated with significant reduction in mortality and graft loss, as well as a significant reduction in severe rejection requiring treatment.[41,42] Its use was also associated with delayed progression of coronary artery intimal thickening, a type of proliferative arteriopathy associated with chronic rejection in heart transplant recipients.[43] Side effects consist mainly of gastrointestinal symptoms such as nausea, vomiting, diarrhea, gastritis, and anorexia.[44] Leukopenia is sometimes seen, although not to the same extent as with azathioprine.

The gastrointestinal side effects of mycophenolate mofetil are sometimes difficult to tolerate for patients and can lead to dose interruptions or omissions. A newer and better-tolerated enteric-coated formulation of mycophenolate, mycophenolate sodium, is now available; this is helpful for patients who do not tolerate the traditional mycophenolate mofetil formulation. Several studies have shown that mycophenolate sodium is therapeutically similar and has a comparable safety profile to mycophenolate mofetil.[45-47]

Sirolimus

Sirolimus (Rapamycin, Rapamune) is a newer immunosuppressive agent that is also a macrolide antibiotic known for its powerful antifungal properties. Whereas cyclosporine and tacrolimus inhibit cytokine production, the mechanism of action of sirolimus is to block the effect of cytokines on the proliferation of lymphoid cells (T and B lymphocytes) by inhibiting a protein (mTOR) that is essential for cytokine-driven T-cell proliferation.[48-50] This class of medications are known as *proliferation signal inhibitors*. Several large clinical trials in kidney transplant recipients found fewer cases of rejection among patients who received sirolimus compared to those who received azathioprine or placebo.[51] Studies have also shown that heart transplant recipients treated with sirolimus have lower rates of rejection and fewer total episodes of rejection, all without increased rates of infection.[50-52]

Sirolimus also inhibits the proliferation of nonlymphoid cells such as endothelial and smooth muscle cells, as well as fibroblasts.[50] Studies have shown that sirolimus slows the progression of graft vasculopathy in heart transplant recipients.[53,54] However, the fibroblasts and endothelial cells that are inhibited by sirolimus are also responsible for wound healing. Several studies found a significant increase in the incidence of impaired wound healing among heart transplant recipients who received sirolimus compared with other immunosuppressants such as azathioprine or mycophenolate mofetil.[55-57] Many centers are now delaying the introduction of sirolimus into the immunosuppressant regimen until the recipient is several months from transplantation and has had the opportunity to heal any surgical wounds. Another immunosuppressant agent is often substituted for sirolimus for several weeks to months before any scheduled surgical procedure, to lessen the risk of delayed wound healing. Other primary side effects of this medication include hyperlipidemia and myelosuppression.[58-60] Most of the myelosuppressive effect is directed at platelets, and severe thrombocytopenias can result, making it necessary to discontinue the medication.

Although dosages vary among institutions, several administer a loading dose followed by a maintenance dose to achieve serum levels between 5 and 15 ng/mL. Because of its prolonged half-life, sirolimus is administered once daily. Sirolimus has also been shown to have synergistic effects when combined with cyclosporine and tacrolimus, which can result in a lower dose requirement for these medications. Because cyclosporine and tacrolimus can be nephrotoxic, lower doses of these two medications can be advantageous.[49,59] Sirolimus also specifically interacts with cyclosporine and must be administered 4 hours after cyclosporine.

Everolimus

Everolimus is an analogue of sirolimus with a shorter half-life and more rapid time to steady state. Everolimus is also more convenient to administer in that, unlike sirolimus, it can be given concomitantly with cyclosporine.[60-62] Like sirolimus, everolimus is a proliferation signal inhibitor and works by blocking IL-2 receptor signal transduction in activated lymphocytes.[63,64] Several studies have found that the synergistic effect of everolimus and calcineurin inhibitors such as cyclosporine and tacrolimus allows for lower doses of those medications to be used.[65] Lower doses of calcineurin inhibitors have been shown to be beneficial in improving kidney function in transplant recipients.[66] Several trials have been conducted to study the safety and efficacy of everolimus in calcineurin inhibitor-free regimens.[66-68]

Side effects of sirolimus and everolimus are similar: both can cause hypertension, hypercholesterolemia, hypertriglyceridemia, thrombocytopenia, edema, acne, rash, and mouth sores.[31]

Induction Therapy

Induction therapy involves the intraoperative and/or postoperative use of an immunosuppressive agent for a limited period of time. The purpose of induction therapy is to induce tolerance to the transplanted graft. It is used by some, but not all, transplant centers, as there is ongoing debate regarding the need for and effectiveness of induction therapy. According to the 2010 Annual Report from the Scientific Registry of Transplant Recipients (SRTR), approximately 54% of heart transplant recipients, 61% of lung transplant recipients, 84% of kidney recipients, and 26% of liver recipients receive induction therapy.[69]

Antilymphocyte Preparations

Muromonab-CD3 (Orthoclone OKT3) was one of the first medications introduced to target distinct subpopulations of T cells. It is a monoclonal antibody produced in mice to specifically target cells with the T3 surface antigen found on mature T cells. Orthoclone OKT3 removes these cells from circulation by forming antibody–antigen complexes. Orthoclone OKT3 also interferes with T-cell recognition of foreign antigen, which renders the T cells incapable of responding.[31] OKT3 can be used as induction therapy or to treat and reverse severe rejection.

Because OKT3 is an animal protein, antibodies against it develop in some patients. Its initial adverse effects are caused by the massive destruction of T cells, which leads to cytokine release syndrome, resulting in fever, rigors, and pulmonary edema. Reactions usually subside with subsequent doses. As the T-cell population declines, the severity of the reaction diminishes. The severity of reactions can be minimized by pretreatment of patients with acetaminophen and diphenhydramine for the initial doses. A dose of 50 mg of hydrocortisone is often given with the first dose of Orthoclone OKT3. A greater concern regarding the use of Orthoclone OKT3 is the increased incidence of lymphoma in patients who have received this medication. Incidence varies from center to center, probably related to the length of therapy in the different protocols.

Antithymocyte Preparations

Antithymocyte preparations are made by injecting human thymocytes into an animal, usually a horse, rabbit, or goat. The animal produces antibody in response to the foreign human antigen. Antibody to human thymocytes can then be extracted from the serum of the animal. Antithymocyte medications cause depletion of T cells by promoting T-cell clearance from the circulation and modulation of T-cell activation.[31] Depending on the protocol of the institution, antithymocyte preparations may be administered as induction therapy or to treat acute rejection. As with Orthoclone OKT3, patients are subject to reactions caused by the release of pyrogens during the massive T-cell lysis and by the foreign animal protein contained in the preparation.

Antilymphocyte and antithymocyte preparations are *cytolytic* medications. Use of cytolytic medications has been associated with an increased incidence of malignancy,[30] most likely caused by the suppression of cytotoxic T cells, which normally play an important role in identifying and eliminating malignant cells. For that reason, many centers use these medications only to reverse rejections that are unresponsive to conventional treatment with increased corticosteroids. However, a short (3-day) course of antihuman thymocyte immunoglobulin has been successfully used for induction therapy, with a demonstrated lower rate of early rejection and absence of a long-term cancer-promoting effect at 5 and 10 years of follow-up.[70]

Interleukin-2 Receptor Antagonists

Basiliximab is currently the only interleukin-2 receptor antagonist available in the United States. IL-2Ra are antibodies to a receptor found on activated T lymphocytes. As discussed earlier, IL-2 mediates the activation of T lymphocytes; IL-2Ra competitively antagonizes this function.[71] IL-2Ra are generally better tolerated than other induction agents, with fewer incidences of fever, leukopenia, thrombocytopenia, and other adverse reactions.[71]

Alemtuzumab (Campath 1H)

Campath 1H is a humanized antibody targeted against the CD52 antigen that is present on the surface of lymphocytes; it causes depletion of peripheral lymphocytes, monocytes, and NK cells. Campath is used in the treatment of chronic lymphocytic leukemia and is being investigated for use in transplantation.[72-74] Campath has been used most frequently with kidney transplant recipients. Early studies are promising and show that use of alemtuzumab may be associated with low incidence of acute rejection. However, there have been no large randomized clinical trials comparing its use with other induction agents.[75]

HEART TRANSPLANTATION

The first human heart transplantation was performed at the University of Cape Town, South Africa, in 1967 by Christian Barnard; the patient survived 18 days. In 1968, Shumway and colleagues performed the first successful heart transplant in the United States, at Stanford University. The number of heart transplantation procedures grew dramatically for the first few years and then rapidly declined because of poor results. Over time, technologic pharmaceutical, and surgical advancements contributed to increased survival. These included the development of the endomyocardial biopsy to detect allograft rejection, the introduction of T–cell-specific agents such as rabbit antithymocyte globulin, the ability of laboratories to measure specific T cells (rosette counts) in the blood, and the introduction of the immunosuppressive medication cyclosporine (previously described). Over 53,000 heart transplants have been performed in the United States since 1988.[76]

Indications and Selection

Heart transplantation is deemed necessary for an individual who suffers from cardiac disease if the symptoms of heart failure can no longer be managed with conventional medical therapy, if there are no surgical options offering more favorable long-term outcomes, and if the individual's short-term prognosis is poor without transplantation.[77] The most common conditions necessitating heart transplantation are nonischemic cardiomyopathies of various origins (idiopathic, viral, valvular) and ischemic cardiomyopathy, or coronary artery disease.[78] Other, less common etiologic factors include severe heart failure resulting from chemotherapy, radiation treatment, myocardial tumor, and complex congenital defects. Many centers grade the severity of heart failure by the classification developed by the New York Heart Association (NYHA) (Table 37-7), which is based on the amount of exertion required to cause symptoms. Most patients who need a heart transplant are categorized as NYHA class III to IV.

In addition to satisfying medical criteria, patients generally are evaluated for the presence of familial or social support, absence of chemical dependence, and commitment to adhering

TABLE 37-7 NEW YORK HEART ASSOCIATION CLASS AND PHYSICAL MANIFESTATION OF HEART FAILURE

NYHA CLASS	PHYSICAL MANIFESTATION
I	No limitation of physical activity; no dyspnea, fatigue, or palpitations with ordinary activity
II	Slight limitation of physical activity; patients have fatigue, palpitations, and dyspnea with ordinary physical activity but are comfortable at rest
III	Marked limitation of activity; less than ordinary physical activity results in symptoms, but patients are comfortable at rest
IV	Symptoms are present at rest, and any physical exertion exacerbates the symptoms

BOX 37-4 HEART TRANSPLANTATION CONTRAINDICATIONS

Medical Contraindication

ABSOLUTE
- Elevated pulmonary artery pressures
- Irreversible severe renal, hepatic, or pulmonary disease
- Kidney dysfunction
- Chronic liver dysfunction
- Recent or unresolved pulmonary infarction
- Active uncontrolled infection
- Active malignancy or recent malignancy with high risk of recurrence

RELATIVE
- Advanced age (>70 years of age)
- Diabetes mellitus with end-organ damage and/or poor glycemic control
- Obesity
- Severe cachexia or malnutrition
- Systemic disease with a high probability of recurrence in the transplanted heart
- Severe peripheral vascular disease or cerebrovascular disease
- History of multiple prior sternotomies
- High level of allosensitization

Psychosocial Contraindications

ABSOLUTE
- Inadequate social support system
- Illicit substance use
- Alcohol dependence
- Nicotine abuse
- Active psychotic symptoms
- Dementia
- History of multiple suicide attempts

RELATIVE
- Inadequate social support system
- Illicit substance use
- Alcohol dependence
- Nicotine abuse
- Active psychotic symptoms
- Dementia
- History of multiple suicide attempts

to a strict lifelong medical regimen and follow-up. Specific contraindications to heart transplantation are listed in Box 37-4. Heart transplant recipients range from neonates to patients in their 60s, with upper age limits varying among transplant institutions. Advanced age was once considered an absolute contraindication to transplantation, but it is now considered a relative contraindication, based on the findings of several studies that demonstrated excellent survival in carefully selected older recipients.[79,80]

Pre-existing malignancy, once considered an absolute contraindication because of the potential for recurring cancer or development of second cancers resulting from therapeutic immunosuppression, is now considered only a relative contraindication if the potential recipient has been free of malignancy for a specific number of years and if there are no signs of metastasis. Severe liver and kidney dysfunction that is not thought to be reversible by an increase in cardiac output is also a contraindication for transplantation. However, combined organ transplants such as heart and kidney or heart and liver transplant can be considered for certain individuals.[81] Diabetes mellitus is not an absolute contraindication if the hyperglycemia is adequately treated and there is no sign of end-organ damage such as nephropathy, neuropathy, or retinopathy. If the patient has an active infection, transplantation is delayed until the infection has cleared. Recent pulmonary infarctions increase the risk for postoperative infection and complicate oxygenation and ventilation; a recent history of infarction often precludes transplantation.

Distribution of organs is strictly regulated by a regional, state, and national network organized and managed by UNOS and contracted by the federal government. Heart transplant candidates are prioritized based on medical urgency, which is determined by the patient's need for inotropic support with invasive hemodynamic monitoring, mechanical ventilation, or mechanical assist devices. Patients who require this degree of assistance are listed as status 1A or 1B; all other heart transplantation candidates are listed as status 2 (Table 37-8).

In addition to candidate status, other variables such as blood type will impact the length of time a candidate will await a transplant. For example, blood type O candidates may wait longer on the list if organs are allocated to non-O recipients. There is also some regional variability that can affect median wait times. The states of New York and Vermont are within the same region and average a median waiting time of 308 days on the waiting list for blood type O candidates. In contrast, the region encompassing California, Nevada, Arizona, New Mexico, and Utah have a median waiting time of 124 days for blood type O candidates.[82] This variability is due to population density of the regions as well as the number of transplant centers within each region, which can often compete for the same donors.

Heart Transplantation Surgical Procedure
Biatrial Technique

The standard surgical procedure for orthotopic heart transplantation (OHT) was originally developed by Lower and Shumway in 1960.[83] A standard median sternotomy is used, the great vessels are cannulated, and cardiopulmonary bypass is instituted after anticoagulation and standard hypothermia are achieved. The donor heart is prepared by interconnecting the pulmonary veins to form a single left atrial cuff and by trimming the aorta and pulmonary artery to fit the recipient's anatomy. All of the recipient's heart is removed except the posterior walls of the atria that contain the orifices of the pulmonary veins and vena cava. Four major anastomoses are performed between the donor heart and the recipient's native atrial remnant: in order, they are those of the right and left atria, the aorta, and the pulmonary artery (Fig. 37-6). The native atrial remnant remains innervated by the parasympathetic and sympathetic nerve fibers from the autonomic nervous system. The donor heart, however, is denervated, resulting in a faster resting heart rate of 90 to 100 beats/min. The rate of the transplanted heart is the normal intrinsic rate generated by the donor sinoatrial (SA) node located in the right atrium.

Although it was long regarded as the gold standard for heart transplantation, the standard biatrial technique had disadvantages related to the large atrial cavities. The loss of normal atrial anatomy increased the risk of mitral and tricuspid valve

STATUS	DEFINITION
TABLE 37-8	**CLASSIFICATION OF HEART TRANSPLANT CANDIDATES**
1A	Admitted to the listing transplant center hospital and has at least one of the following devices or therapies in place: • Mechanical circulatory support such as left and/or right ventricular assist device (may be listed for 30 days at any point after being implanted) • Total artificial heart • Intra-aortic balloon pump • Extracorporeal membrane oxygenator (ECMO) • Mechanical circulatory support with objective medical evidence of significant device-related complications such as thromboembolism, device infection, mechanical failure or life-threatening ventricular arrhythmias • Continuous mechanical ventilation • Continuous infusion of a single high-dose intravenous inotrope or multiple intravenous inotropes, in addition to continuous hemodynamic monitoring of left ventricular filling pressures
1B	At least one of the following devices or therapies in place: • Left and/or right ventricular assist device implanted • Continuous infusion of intravenous inotropes
2	A candidate who does not meet the criteria for Status 1A or 1B

Modified from *Health Resources and Services Administration.* Organ distribution allocation of thoracic organs. http://optn.transplant.hrsa.gov/policiesAndBylaws/policies.asp. Accessed May 24, 2012.

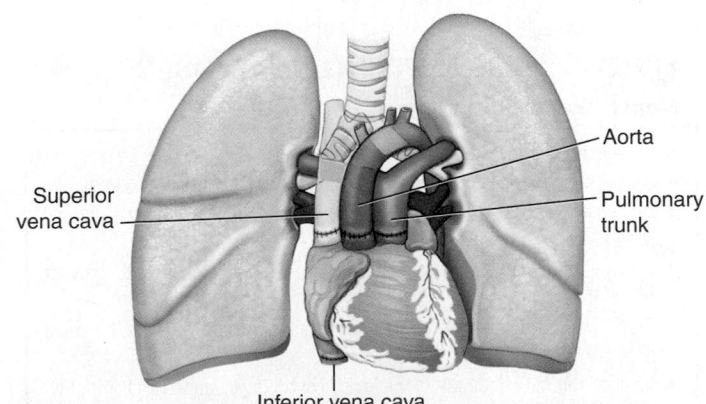

Superior vena cava

Inferior vena cava

Aorta

Pulmonary trunk

FIGURE 37-6 Surgical procedure for heart transplantation.

regurgitation, atrial septal aneurysm, atrial thrombus formation, and tachydysrhythmias.

Bicaval Technique

The bicaval technique, an alternative to the standard surgical approach, was originally reported by Sievers and associates in 1991 and is now the most commonly used method for OHT.[84] The anastomotic sites of the bicaval technique include the left atrial cuff, which contains the orifices of pulmonary veins, the superior and inferior vena cava, as well as the aorta and the main pulmonary artery (Figure 37-6). This technique leaves the recipient with more anatomically normal atria. Benefits of the bicaval technique include preserved SA node function with decreased incidence of atrial dysrhythmias, and mitral and tricuspid regurgitation.[85]

Postoperative Medical and Nursing Management

Immediate postoperative management of the heart transplant recipient is similar to that of patients undergoing other heart surgery procedures. Nursing care of the transplant recipient involves several nursing diagnoses, as listed in Box 37-5. The most frequently used diagnosis is decreased cardiac output. Possible causes for a decrease in cardiac output include right-heart dysfunction, dysrhythmias, hypothermia, myocardial depression, tamponade, and rejection.

Variables that influence myocardial performance include prolonged ischemic time (time from excision of the donor heart to removal of the aortic cross-clamp after implantation into the recipient), reperfusion injury, and hypothermia. Dysrhythmias may occur as a result of myocardial irritation, local ischemia, edema around the atrial suture line, and disruption of the SA nodal blood supply.

An electrocardiogram abnormality unique to the transplanted heart is the presence of a second P wave, which is generated by the native SA node that has been left in the atrial cuff. Because this impulse does not cross the suture line, it is capable of conducting only through the remnant of the native recipient atria. This impulse is not seen in hearts transplanted with use of the bicaval technique, because the native right atrium and its SA node are removed.

Isoproterenol, a powerful beta-adrenergic agonist, is sometimes used in the postoperative period for chronotropic (heart rate) support. Its chronotropic and vasodilator properties effectively sustain the heart rate, increase cardiac output, and decrease pulmonary vascular resistance (PVR). PVR may be increased as a result of pre-existing left ventricular failure and may be a cause of transient right ventricular dysfunction in the newly transplanted heart. Dopamine and epinephrine are often used for inotropic support in the postoperative period. However, the use of inotropic and chronotropic medications is highly individualized based on institutional preference. Generally speaking, inotropic medications are gradually discontinued over 24 to 48 hours as tolerated by the patient, and the need for isoproterenol decreases as the heart begins to maintain its normal intrinsic rate of approximately 100 beats/min. Temporary pacing is required only occasionally, and fewer than 10% of transplant recipients require a permanent pacemaker implant.

Cardiac tamponade does not occur with greater frequency in heart transplantation compared with other heart surgeries, but it may be more difficult to detect as a result of an enlarged pericardial sac due to long-standing cardiomyopathy.

Signs and Symptoms of Rejection

The occurrence of hyperacute rejection in heart transplants is uniformly fatal unless emergency hemodynamic support such as extracorporeal membrane oxygenation (ECMO) is initiated until retransplantation can be performed. Signs and symptoms of hyperacute rejection are not subtle. The donor heart will become cyanotic and graft failure and hemodynamic collapse occur within minutes. Thankfully, careful ABO matching and advances in antibody screening have made hyperacute rejection a rare occurrence.

Acute cellular rejection in heart transplant recipients can occur at any time, although it is most likely to occur during the first 3 to 6 months after transplantation. Box 37-6 lists the signs and symptoms of rejection.

BOX 37-6 SIGNS AND SYMPTOMS OF HEART TRANSPLANT REJECTION

R	Rub (pericardial friction)
E	ECG voltage decreased
J	JVD
E	Edema (peripheral, sudden onset)
C	Cardiac dysrhythmias (atrial, brady)
T	Tiredness
I	Intolerance of exercise
O	Onset of low-grade fever
N	New S3 or S4
E	Enlarged cardiac silhouette
P	Pulmonary crackles, wheezes
I	Increased weight
S	SOB
O	Onset of hypotension
D	Disturbance in mood
E	Echo findings (systolic function, LV mass/thickness)

From Cupples SA. Heart transplantation. In: Cupples SA, Ohler L, eds. *Transplantation Nursing Secrets*. Philadelphia: Hanley & Belfus; 2003.

◎ BOX 37-5 NURSING DIAGNOSES

Heart Transplantation

- Decreased Cardiac Output related to alterations in preload, p. 1128
- Decreased Cardiac Output related to alterations in afterload, p. 1128
- Decreased Cardiac Output related to alterations in heart rate or rhythm, p. 1128
- Risk for Infection: Immunosuppressive medications required to prevent rejection of transplanted organ, p. 1160
- Disturbed Body Image related to actual change in body structure, function, or appearance, p. 1136
- Anxiety related to threat to biologic, psychologic, and social integrity, p. 1125

TABLE 37-9 STANDARDIZED CARDIAC BIOPSY GRADING

GRADE	NOMENCLATURE
0R	No rejection
1R, mild	Interstitial and/or perivascular infiltrate with up to 1 focus of myocyte damage
2R, moderate	Two or more foci of infiltrate with associated myocyte damage
3R, severe	Diffuse infiltrate with multifocal myocyte damage, +/− edema, +/− hemorrhage, +/− vasculitis

Rejection Surveillance

Diagnosis of heart transplant rejection is determined by fluoroscopic or echocardiography-guided endomyocardial biopsy. A bioptome is percutaneously inserted through the right internal jugular vein and advanced through the right atrium to the right ventricle. The femoral, subclavian, and left internal jugular veins are alternate sites for venous access although the right internal jugular vein provides the most direct access. Endomyocardial tissue is obtained from the interventricular septum. The samples are microscopically evaluated for interstitial and perivascular infiltration. Heart biopsies are graded according to the severity of the interstitial infiltration of lymphocytes. The standardized cardiac biopsy grading scale ranges from mild to severe (Table 37-9).[86]

The frequency of surveillance biopsies varies from center to center. Generally speaking, biopsies occur more frequently in the first few weeks and months after transplant and become less frequent as time goes on. Many centers halt routine biopsies after 2 to 5 years and rely instead on clinical assessment to determine the need for biopsy. A major but rare complication of biopsy is ventricular perforation, which can result in cardiac tamponade. Pneumothorax is another potential complication of endomyocardial biopsy and may result from perforation of the visceral pleura during cannulation of the jugular vein; its clinical manifestations are a sudden onset of sharp pain in the affected side and dyspnea.

Despite the invasive nature and potential for complications around endomyocardial biopsies, it remains the gold standard of rejection surveillance in heart transplantation. Alternative methods for noninvasive monitoring with comparable sensitivity and specificity remain elusive although some progress has been made with the development of the *AlloMap* test. This blood test measures the genes expressed by activated T cells as a marker of possible rejection. Though it has yet to be widely accepted, some heart transplant programs are utilizing the test as a trigger for performing endomyocardial biopsy. If the AlloMap indicates increased T-cell gene expression, patients will undergo a biopsy in order to rule out rejection.[87,88]

Treatment of acute rejection episodes may require intravenously administered corticosteroids. Recurrence of acute rejection is managed with various pharmacologic agents, depending on the patient's clinical condition and institutional preference. Strategies include augmenting current maintenance immunosuppression or switching to alternatives such as tacrolimus, mycophenolate mofetil, or rapamycin. Other agents used for recurrent rejection include polyclonal antibodies, such as antilymphocyte globulin or antithymocyte globulin.

Salvage therapy for persistent rejection that has not responded to conventional immunosuppression includes multiple steroid boluses, anti–T-cell antibodies, or total lymphoid irradiation in which low-dose ionizing radiation is used to treat the lymphoid tissue.

Infection Surveillance

Infection surveillance is a high priority for the immunocompromised person. It is well known that immunosuppression predisposes the patient to infection by a multitude of opportunistic pathogens that cannot easily be prevented with infection control. Development of infection is encountered most often in the early postoperative period, when immunosuppression is maximized. Infection is one of the leading causes of death during this period (up to 2 years after surgery).[78] Great care must be taken to use aseptic technique for all intravenous line and dressing changes. Centers differ widely in their protective practices regarding the transplant recipient. Some use reverse isolation, whereas others put transplant recipients in rooms with other patients and simply use standard precautions.

Development of fever is aggressively investigated, with systematic blood, wound, and respiratory tract cultures; chest radiographs; and observation. Because steroids are known to suppress the body's inflammatory reaction, an elevated temperature generally is considered significant when it reaches 38° C (100.4° F). Nurses must be suspicious of any new productive cough, dry cough, change in type of secretions, or change in chest roentgenogram findings.

Cytomegalovirus (CMV) is a particular threat to transplant recipients. CMV is a herpes virus that can produce latent infection that persists throughout life. Between 50% and 80% of adults in the United States are infected with CMV by age 40 years.[89] CMV can be transmitted through organ and blood product donation. Transplantation from a CMV-seropositive donor to a CMV-seronegative recipient poses the highest risk to the recipient for acquiring a primary infection. The antiviral agent ganciclovir can inhibit viral replication and ameliorate symptoms and is used in the prophylaxis and treatment of CMV infections. CMV immune globulin can be administered for both prevention of primary CMV disease and for treatment of CMV disease.[90]

Patient Education

Thorough, effective, and ongoing education of patients and their caregivers is vital to successful long-term outcomes after heart transplantation. The education process begins before the transplant and continues throughout the patient's life. Many members of the health care team provide education about posttransplant care, including nurses, transplant coordinators, pharmacists, dieticians, physical therapists, occupational therapists, and other health professionals. Patients and caregivers are taught about transplant medications, self-monitoring for signs of infection and rejection, safety precautions, and are provided with guidelines for maintaining a heart-healthy diet and

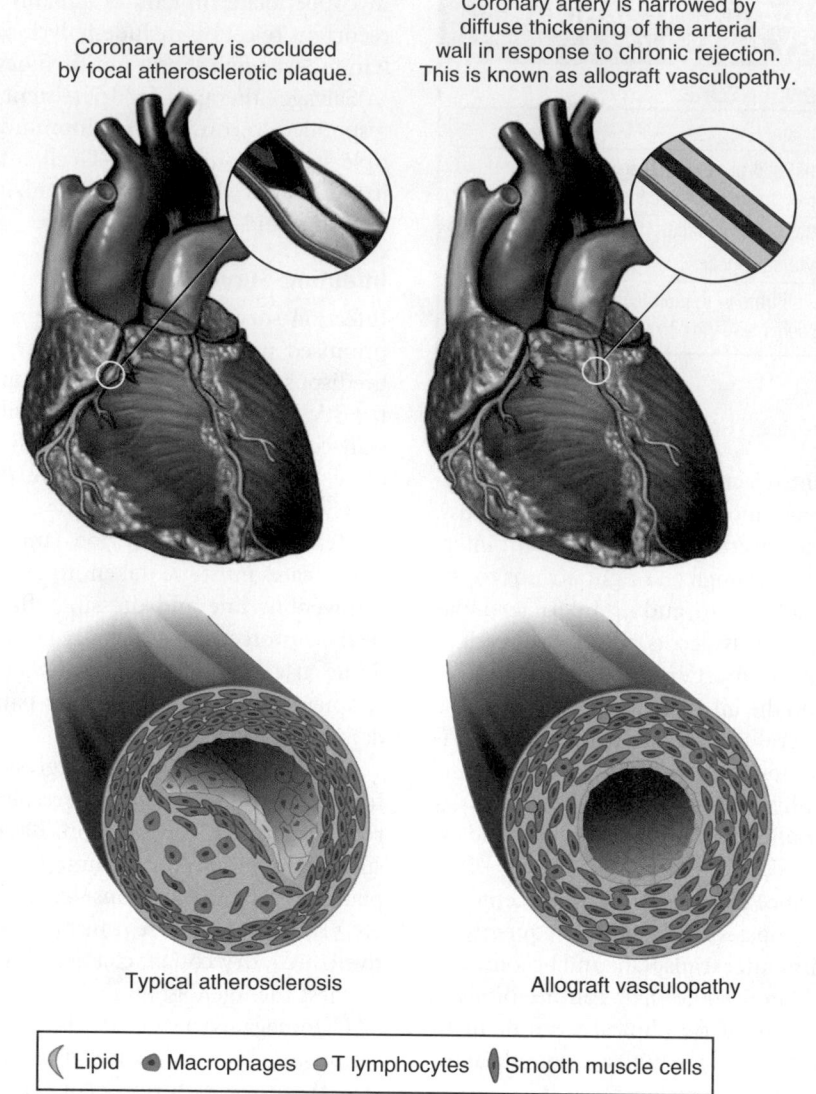

Coronary artery is occluded by focal atherosclerotic plaque.

Coronary artery is narrowed by diffuse thickening of the arterial wall in response to chronic rejection. This is known as allograft vasculopathy.

Typical atherosclerosis

Allograft vasculopathy

(Lipid ● Macrophages ● T lymphocytes (Smooth muscle cells

FIGURE 37-7 Allograft vasculopathy compared with typical atherosclerosis.

increasing physical activity. Patients may be required to check their blood glucose, blood pressure, temperature, and daily weight at home. At first, frequent clinic visits are needed to monitor progress and adjust medications. A schedule is established for routine laboratory tests and clinic visits to ensure long-term success of the transplant.

Long-Term Considerations

Chronic immunosuppression results in significant morbidity. Steroid administration can result in osteoporosis, avascular necrosis of joints, fragile skin, and obesity. Cyclosporine can cause kidney damage, excessive hair growth, gingival hyperplasia, tremor, and hypertension necessitating pharmacologic control. Azathioprine can be hepatotoxic (see Table 37-7). Concomitant use of these immunosuppressants also leaves patients more susceptible to malignancies and late infections.

Graft vasculopathy, or coronary artery disease in the transplanted heart, is thought to develop as a result of chronic rejection and is a major cause of late morbidity and mortality.[78] It is a diffuse and rapidly progressive type of coronary disease that causes concentric narrowing of the coronary arteries. Because the lesions are discrete, they are not amenable to interventions such as angioplasty or bypass grafting. The pathophysiology is completely different from typical atherosclerotic coronary artery disease as illustrated in Figure 37-7.

Patients with denervated hearts cannot feel anginal pain, although reinnervation of transplanted hearts can occur over time. Graft vasculopathy can cause ischemic injury, heart failure, or sudden death. The disease is recognized initially by angiographic screening and later in the course of the disease by silent infarctions on the ECG. Patients may have the disease and demonstrate no clinical sequelae. Many transplant programs have initiated baseline and annual angiographic studies to look for the development and progression of graft vasculopathy. Proliferation signal inhibitor medications such as sirolimus and everolimus are sometimes used as prophylaxis against graft vasculopathy or to slow its progression. However, the only definitive treatment for advanced graft vasculopathy is retransplantation.

In general, heart transplant recipients report improvement in their quality of life.[91-93] At 5 years post-transplant, 90% report no activity limitations,[78] and 29% are employed.[94] The 1-, 5-, and 10-year patient survival rates are 89%, 75%, and 56%, respectively.[95] Leading causes of mortality 3 to 5 years after transplantation are malignancy (18.5%), graft vasculopathy (14%), and graft failure (14.7%).[78]

Unfortunately, donor hearts continue to be a limited resource, As of May 17, 2012, there were 3188 people registered on the heart transplant waiting list.[95] Yet only 402 heart transplants have been performed from January 1, 2012 to May 17, 2012.

HEART–LUNG TRANSPLANTATION

Prior to the first human heart–lung en bloc transplant in 1981, the technique of heart–lung transplantation (HLT) was perfected in dogs in the 1940s and primates in the 1970s with good success. This was in part due to improvements in immunosuppressant medications (described earlier in the chapter) that prevented rejection. The advances in heart transplantation management such as antithymocyte globulin, endomyocardial biopsy, and cyclosporine improved morbidity and mortality, provided the foundation for cardiopulmonary transplantation. Bruce Reitz and colleagues performed the first heart–lung transplant at Stanford University in 1981 for a 45-year-old woman with end-stage primary pulmonary hypertension (PPH) who survived for more than 5 years.[96,97]

Today, HLT remains a viable option for those suffering from end-stage cardiopulmonary failure such as congenital cardiac anomalies with pulmonary hypertension, PPH with irreversible right-heart failure, and primary parenchymal lung disease with severe right-sided heart failure.

Indications and Selection

HLT is a viable option for patients suffering from end-stage cardiopulmonary failure. HLT was performed for the following end-stage cardiopulmonary and pulmonary diseases in the United States between 1982 and 2010: congenital heart disease 36%; idiopathic pulmonary arterial hypertension 28%; cystic fibrosis (CF) 14%; chronic obstructive pulmonary disease (COPD)/alpha-1 antitrypsin deficiency 6%; other conditions (including lymphangioleiomyomatosis [LAM], obliterative bronchiolitis [OB], cancer, sarcoidosis, bronchiectasis) 6%; acquired heart disease 5%; idiopathic pulmonary fibrosis (IPF) 4%, and retransplantation 2%.[98] Box 37-7 lists indications for heart–lung, single-lung, and double-lung transplantation. While there are general standards that all centers adhere to in the candidate selection process, relative contraindications vary case-by-case in most centers. Box 37-8 lists absolute and relative contraindications for heart–lung, single-, and double-lung transplantation.

Any patient with end-stage cardiopulmonary or pulmonary disease who has exhausted medical management with the

---

BOX 37-7 INDICATIONS FOR HEART–LUNG AND LUNG TRANSPLANT

Pulmonary Vascular Disease
Primary pulmonary hypertension
Eisenmenger syndrome
Cardiomyopathy with pulmonary hypertension

Restrictive Lung Disease
Idiopathic pulmonary fibrosis
Sarcoidosis
Asbestosis
Histiocytosis X
Bronchiolitis obliterans organizing pneumonia (BOOP)
Desquamative interstitial pneumonitis

Obstructive Lung Disease
Emphysema—idiopathic
Emphysema—alpha-1 antitrypsin deficiency
Cystic fibrosis
Bronchiectasis
Bronchopulmonary dysplasia
Idiopathic and post-transplant obliterative bronchiolitis
Lymphangioleiomyomatosis

---

capacity for full rehabilitation may be considered for transplantation. Desperate clinical situations are not in themselves indications for transplantation. Patients are assessed with regard to the "transplant window." The patient must be terminally ill to require a transplant, but also maintain the strength and stamina to survive the long wait, complex surgery, and rigorous rehabilitation post-transplant.

Heart–Lung Transplant Surgical Procedure

Suitable donors are required for the success of a heart–lung transplant. All potential donors are brain dead from an event that leads to donor ventilator dependence to keep potential organs viable. Lungs are at risk for pulmonary edema, embolism, infectious processes, and atelectasis. Besides these risks, underlying donor pathology and chest trauma also determine whether donor organs are suitable for placement.

Lung tissue has a relatively short preservation time, generally 4 to 6 hours, leading to procurement distance limits. Donors must first meet brain-death criteria, be free of cardiopulmonary pathology, and have preserved lung function with no evidence of infection or malignancy. Donors with a history of smoking may be accepted if they meet the above criteria.

To overcome the shortage of donor lungs, marginal donor lungs—those that do not meet all criteria—may be accepted. Although most donors are under the age of 55, older donors may be taken if they meet all other criteria. Lung fields must be clear on radiologic findings with arterial oxygenation greater than 100 mm Hg on 40% inspired oxygen. A 100% oxygen challenge must show a Pao$_2$ greater than 300 mm Hg.[99-102]

The donor and potential recipients are matched for ABO compatibility and organ size. Chest circumference, wall

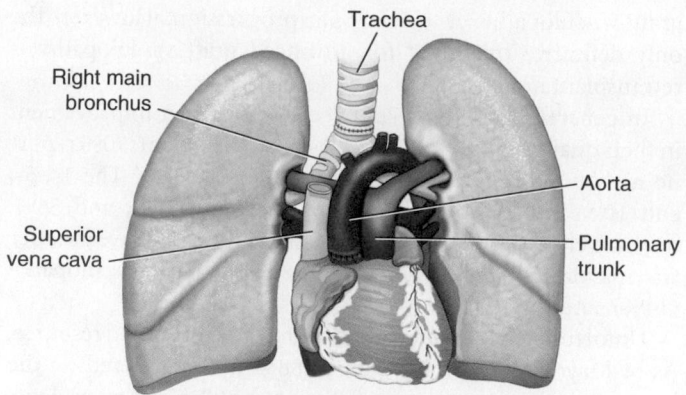

FIGURE 37-8   Heart Lung transplant en bloc surgical procedure; incisions in the trachea and aorta are shown. The heart is attached to a remnant atrial cuff which contains the openings of the superior and inferior vena cava and pulmonary veins (not shown).

dimensions, and height- and weight-adjusted lung volumes are assessed. A donor with slightly smaller lungs than the recipient helps prevent postoperative compression atelectasis. Finally, inspection of the donor organs while procuring is essential for assessing lesions and trauma, which may impact transplant outcomes.[99-102]

During procurement, a sternotomy is made to inspect the heart and lungs. Once it is determined that the organs are suitable, the heart and lungs are mobilized. Prostaglandins are administered into the pulmonary artery.[103] The donor heart is then flushed with cold cardioplegia solution while the donor lungs are flushed with cold modified Collins solution, Perfadex, or University of Wisconsin (UW) solution. Once the heart and lungs are perfused, they are removed and placed in cold electrolyte solution for transport using sterile technique.[103]

Cardiopulmonary bypass is used for the recipient operation. The phrenic nerves and bronchial artery circulation are preserved and maintained to prevent bleeding complications in the postoperative period. The heart–lung en bloc is placed with the tracheal anastomosis performed first, followed by the atrial anastomosis and then the aortic anastomosis. The donor trachea is kept short due to limited vascular blood supply in the area (Fig. 37-8).

Postoperative Management

Immediately following surgery, the heart–lung transplant recipient is admitted to the critical care unit and monitored for general hemodynamic stability, oxygenation, bleeding, ischemic reperfusion injury, acute rejection, infection, deep vein thrombosis, pulmonary emboli, and multiorgan function.

Ventilation

Ventilation settings are determined partially by the underlying disease process and patient progression. Regular suctioning of secretions is crucial to maintain airway clearance. Extubation is performed after satisfactory gas exchange and lung mechanics are accomplished and most patients are extubated within 24 to 48 hours. Evaluation for graft dysfunction, reperfusion injury, gas trapping, and phrenic nerve injury is ongoing. Early mobilization after extubation is essential for improved pulmonary toilet and helps prevent reintubation. Bronchoscopy is used to assess for potential complications such as stenosis, dehiscence, infection, rejection, and assessing the anastomosis.[100]

Fluids

Care must be maintained when managing fluids in the early postoperative period. The lungs are extremely sensitive to volume overload. Pulmonary artery occlusion pressure (PAOP) and daily weight are used to determine volume status and the need for diuretics. Over-diuresis results in hypotension and prerenal azotemia.[99,100] Most patients are maintained on low-dose dopamine for the first 24 to 48 hours for inotropic support and kidney vasodilation. Epinephrine may also be used for inotropic support. Prostaglandin E$_1$ (PGE$_1$)

and nitroprusside provide pulmonary and systemic vasodilation.[99,100] Nitric oxide, a potent vasodilator, has been found useful in decreasing pulmonary artery pressures and improving oxygenation.[100]

Pleural Drainage

Pleural drainage must be observed and documented, and careful attention should be paid to signs of active bleeding from the mediastinal and pleural chest tubes. Frank blood of more than 100 mL per hour over 3 hours should be a concern in those with normal coagulation. Exploratory surgery of the chest may be required to find the source of bleeding. Once chest tube drainage produces less than 200 mL in 24 hours without a noted air leak, chest tubes can be removed.[100]

Ischemia-Reperfusion Injury

Reperfusion injury, also called primary graft dysfunction (PGD) in the clinical setting, usually occurs within the first 72 hours after transplantation and is typified by nonspecific alveolar damage with pulmonary infiltrates on radiography, hypoxemia, lung edema with poor pulmonary compliance, and normal or low left atrial filling pressures.[99,100] Severe cases require ventilation, moderate levels of positive end-expiratory pressure (PEEP) and Fio_2, pharmacologic therapy, and perhaps nitric oxide or ECMO.[100]

Rejection Surveillance

Rejection is diagnosed by transbronchial biopsy of the lung or endomyocardial biopsy of the heart. Whether the episode of rejection is cellular or antibody mediated, the symptoms of rejection are the same. Shortness of breath, cough, fever, fatigue, wheezes, crackles, and drop in lung function noted on pulmonary function tests are all potential signs of rejection but can also be present with infection.[99] Most centers perform surveillance bronchoscopies at 1 month, 3 months, 6 months, and 1 year post heart–lung or lung transplant for early diagnosis and treatment of a rejection episode.[104]

Rejection of the lung is often followed by rejection of the heart. Heart biopsy is not recommended after 4 to 6 months post-transplant, only with symptoms of heart failure, left ventricular, or biventricular dysfunction on echocardiography. Rejection of the lungs can be detected by a decline in lung function on pulmonary function tests with a decrease in forced expiratory volume in 1 second (FEV_1) greater than 10%, and a decrease in forced vital capacity (FVC) greater than 10%. The patient may also desaturate on exercise oximetry.

Spirometry has been shown to have a sensitivity of greater than 60% for detecting infection or rejection grade A2 and higher, but it cannot differentiate between the two. The ability to detect rejection diminishes even further in single-lung transplants due to the impact of native lung dysfunction hindering the results.[104] Pulmonary function testing should be used as an adjunct to clinical evaluation and biopsy, not solely to diagnose acute lung rejection.[104] Some centers treat patients empirically with high doses of steroids, normally methylprednisolone (Solu-Medrol) 10 mg/kg intravenously daily for three consecutive days. Severe grades of rejection may also warrant the use of rabbit antithymocyte globulin (RATG). Table 37-10 depicts pulmonary grading of lung rejection.[104]

Humoral rejection is mediated by antibody and complement. It can occur immediately after transplantation (hyperacute) or

TABLE 37-10	PATHOLOGIC GRADING OF LUNG REJECTION			
CATEGORY		**GRADE**	**MEANING**	**APPEARANCE**
A: Acute rejection		0	None	Normal lung parenchyma
		1	Minimal	Inconspicuous small mononuclear perivascular infiltrates
		2	Mild	More frequent, more obvious, perivascular infiltrates, eosinophils may be present
		3	Moderate	Dense perivascular infiltrates, extension into interstitial space, can involve endothelialitis, eosinophils, and neutrophils
		4	Severe	Diffuse perivascular, interstitial, and air-space infiltrates with lung injury Neutrophils may be present
B: Airway inflammation		0	None	No evidence of bronchiolar inflammation
		1R	Low grade	Infrequent, scattered, or single-layer mononuclear cells in bronchiolar submucosa
		2R	High grade	Larger infiltrates of larger and activated lymphocytes in bronchiolar submucosa Can involve eosinophils and plasmacytoid cells
		X	Ungradable	No bronchiolar tissue available
C: Chronic airway rejection—obliterative bronchiolitis		0	Absent	If present describes intraluminal airway obliteration with fibrous connective tissue
		1	Present	
D: Chronic vascular rejection—accelerated graft vascular sclerosis			Not graded	Fibrointimal thickening of arteries and poor cellular hyaline sclerosis of veins Usually requires open lung biopsy for diagnosis

Modified from Martinu T, Chen DF, Palmer SM. Acute rejection and humoral sensitization in lung transplant recipients. *Proc Am Thorac Soc.* 2009;6(1):54.

months later. Antibodies are either preformed antibodies or represent antidonor antibodies that develop after transplantation. Blood testing for donor-specific antibodies provides a method for determining whether a recipient has built antibodies specific to the donor after transplant. Treatment for antibody-mediated rejection warrants high dose steroids, plasmapheresis, immunoglobulin, and Rituxan. Intractable rejection can be treated with monoclonal or polyclonal antibodies, total lymphoid irradiation, or methotrexate.

Infection

Infectious complications are one of the most common causes of morbidity and mortality following HLT. Direct exposure to microbes, denervation of the graft with impaired cough reflex, impaired lymphatic drainage, infections transferred from the donor, infection from the native lung in single-lung transplants, and immunosuppression all contribute to infection risk.[105] Evidence of infection after HLT can be found in blood cultures, sputum, urine, and while performing a bronchoscopy with bronchoalveolar lavage (BAL). Bronchoscopies with lavage are done prior to extubation while assessing anastomotic patency and during routine surveillance. Bronchial lavage washings are sent for cultures to assess for bacteria, fungi, and viruses.[99]

Antimicrobial prophylaxis for *Pneumocystis jiroveci* with sulfamethoxazole and trimethoprim is utilized in most centers due to successful prevention of this bacterium with additional antimicrobial effects against *Toxoplasma gondii* and *Nocardia* species. There are many other bacterial colonizers and infections seen after heart–lung and lung transplant but no widely used prophylaxis.[105]

Candida and *Aspergillus* species infections remain the most common fungal infections in transplant patients. Prophylactic antifungal medications are used by many centers but there is no clear data as to optimal treatment or duration.[106]

CMV is the most common viral infection in transplant recipients (described earlier in chapter). CMV may occur within the first few months after transplantation and may occur later on. Universal prophylaxis and pre-emptive therapy are the main measures taken to prevent occurrence. CMV infection occurs in 25% to 50% of heart transplant recipients but is highest in lung transplant recipients, with a reported incidence of 54% to 92% in those not taking prophylactic antiviral medications.[107] Intravenous ganciclovir followed by oral Valcyte are the primary prophylactic antiviral medications to prevent CMV infection.

Other common viruses after transplant include respiratory syncytial virus, influenza, adenovirus, human metapneumovirus, and parainfluenza. These are not treated prophylactically but as they occur. Nevertheless, they still pose a threat to recipient health and may lead to allograft injury over time.[99]

Immunosuppression

Immunosuppressive therapy begins with the induction phase, perioperatively and immediately after transplantation, followed by maintenance therapy that continues for the life of the allograft. As noted earlier in this chapter, induction medication regimes are different from maintenance medications and their

use varies by transplant center. Maintenance immunosuppression is the key to prevention of acute and chronic rejections throughout the life of the graft. Most centers utilize a three-medication regimen consisting of a calcineurin inhibitor, antimetabolite, and corticosteroid.[99]

Patient Education

Patient education begins during the evaluation process and continues after transplant. Primary caregivers must be part of the learning experience to ensure understanding of the entire process from selection through post-transplantation. Transplant pharmacology, signs and symptoms of infection and rejection, and follow-up requirements are all part of the discussion during pre- and post-transplant teaching.

Long-Term Considerations
Bronchiolitis Obliterans Syndrome

Chronic rejection—*bronchiolitis obliterans syndrome* (BOS)—is the primary cause of morbidity and mortality after heart–lung and lung transplantation.[108] BOS is defined as an irreversible decline in FEV_1 after excluding other causes of allograft dysfunction.[108]

Factors such as acute cellular rejection and lymphocytic bronchiolitis are known to be associated with BOS. Non–alloimmune factors such as primary graft dysfunction, infections, airway ischemia, and gastroesophageal reflux may also trigger an inflammatory response that initiates an alloimmune response.[108] Therefore, the balancing act with immunosuppression dosage to prevent rejection and infection is a careful art. Investigation of patient gastrointestinal complaints should be done promptly to avoid aspiration risk leading to allograft damage. Currently, there is no cure for chronic rejection; however, researchers are trying to find interventions to slow the process and eliminate BOS. Table 37-11 depicts the BOS classification system.

Co-morbidities

There are a number of morbidities that develop over time in the transplant population: hypertension and hyperlipidemia from calcineurin inhibitor medications, diabetes mellitus from

TABLE 37-11	BRONCHIOLITIS OBLITERANS SYNDROME (BOS) CLASSIFICATION SYSTEM	
STAGE	**DESCRIPTION**	
BOS 0	FEV_1 >90% of baseline and $FEF_{25\%-75\%}$ >75% of baseline	
BOS 0	$pFEV_1$ 81%-90% of baseline and/or $FEF_{25\%-75\%}$ ≤75% of baseline	
BOS 1	FEV_1 66%-80% of baseline	
BOS 2	FEV_1 51%-65% of baseline	
BOS 3	FEV_1 ≤50% of baseline	
	BOS 0 p = potential BOS; $FEF_{25\%-75\%}$ = forced expiratory flow, midexpiratory phase	

Modified from Ahmad S, Shlobin OA, Nathan SD. Pulmonary complications of lung transplantation. *Chest*. 2011;139(2):402.

corticosteroids and calcineurin inhibitors, kidney disease from calcineurin inhibitors, cancers such as skin cancer, and post-transplant lymphoproliferative disease (PTLD) from immuno-suppressive agents. Most 5-year survivors have one or more of these morbidities.[98,100]

Although the success rate for HLT is not at the level of other organs, HLT still remains a viable option for those with cardiopulmonary end-stage disease. The survival rate for adult heart–lung transplants as reported by the International Society for Heart and Lung Transplantation (ISHLT) for 3303 recipients from January 1982 to June 2009 listed 1-year survival at 67.9%, 3-year survival at 57.2%, and 5-year patient survival at 49.7%.[98]

SINGLE-LUNG AND DOUBLE-LUNG TRANSPLANTATION

Single-Lung Transplantation Indications

Lung transplantation is a viable option for those with end-stage pulmonary disease without end-stage cardiac disease. COPD and restrictive lung diseases such as IPF, CF, and PPH are the main diseases warranting a lung transplant. Lung transplantation is considered when life expectancy is no more than 36 months despite maximum medical management with disease symptoms classified as New York Heart Association (NYHA) class III or IV.[109]

COPD remains the predominant reason for lung transplantation, with IPF following as the second indication, and CF as the third.[109] Suitable donor lungs are a scarce resource; consequently single- versus double-lung transplant surgery is always a major topic for discussion in the transplant community. Single-lung transplantation benefits two recipients from one donor. Some advantages of a single-lung transplant include shorter extubation time, less need for cardiopulmonary bypass, and a shorter hospitalization. However, quality of life and success rates of double-lung transplants have made double-lung transplantation the preferred method of surgery.[99]

Lung hyperinflation is a common complication following single-lung transplantation.[103] Graft compression by the hyper-inflated native lung can cause mediastinal shift and respiratory failure. Lobectomy and lung volume reduction surgery are two methods to prevent graft compression leading to decreased ventilation of the allograft. The native lung can also be a source of infections or problematic for a pneumothorax.

Single-Lung Transplant Surgical Procedure

The lung with the worst function is chosen for excision. If both lungs are equally in function, the right lung is chosen for explantation with a new donor lung inserted to avoid maneuvering around the heart. A thoracotomy incision is made anteriorly or posteriorly at the fourth or fifth intercostal space. Alternatively, a sternotomy incision can be used. The lung is collapsed while the blood vessels are tied off. The lung is then removed at the bronchus. Next, the donor lung is placed and the blood vessels are attached. Finally the implanted lung is inflated and the incision is closed.[103] Figure 37-9 shows the surgical procedure for single-lung transplantation.

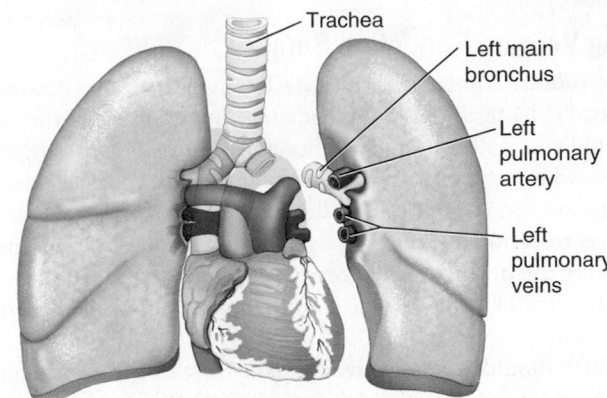

FIGURE 37-9 Single lung transplantation procedure shows where incisions will be for the left main bronchus, the left pulmonary artery and the left pulmonary veins.

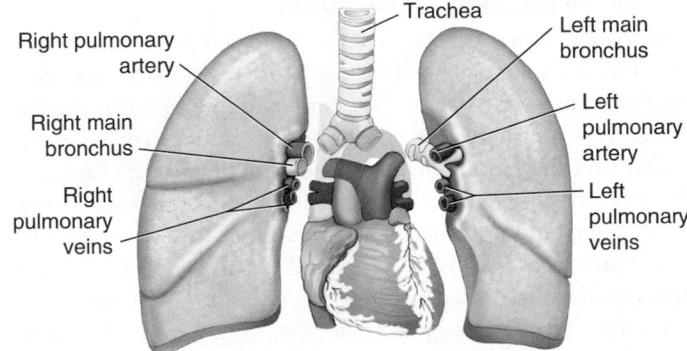

FIGURE 37-10 Simultaneous double-lung transplantation procedure where both lungs are sequentially replaced, shows where incisions will occur between the right and left pulmonary veins, the right and left pulmonary arteries, and the right and left bronchi.

Double-Lung Transplantation Surgical Procedure

Double-lung transplantation is the preferred surgical procedure for patients with CF or bronchiectasis given the significance of infections in both lungs, which would remain in the native lung if both lungs were not transplanted. A double lung transplant can be performed sequentially (Figure 37-10) or simultaneously, also known as en bloc[109] (Figure 37-8). Bilateral lung transplant is increasingly selected over single-lung transplant.[110,111]

A transverse thoracosternotomy, clamshell incision, or median sternotomy are the incisional approaches used in double-lung transplant surgery. The first lung is collapsed and the blood vessel is tied off and cut at the corresponding bronchi. The new lung is then placed and the vessels reattached. The same process is done for the second lung to be placed. Patients may be placed on cardiopulmonary bypass during the surgery in patients with pulmonary hypertension to avoid right-heart failure.[103] Figure 37-10 shows the surgical procedure for a double-lung transplant.

Lung Volume Reduction Surgery

Lung volume reduction surgery (LVRS) is one option that may be available to those with end-stage lung disease with co-morbidities. LVRS may be indicated in patients with emphysema who have relative or absolute contraindications to transplant. The technique involves reducing the lung volume by wedge resection of the emphysematous tissue.[103] LVRS may decrease the mismatch between the hyperinflated lungs and the chest cavity. This may lead to elastic recoil and improved expiratory flow.

LVRS should be considered for patients with chronic medical conditions such as active hepatitis B, hepatitis C with biopsy proven liver disease, HIV infection, and organ system dysfunction. Conditions that make patients ineligible for transplant may be acceptable for LVRS, including limited stage non-small cell cancer with resection, lack of family support, psychiatric conditions, or a history of poor compliance.[99,112]

Living Donor Lung Transplantation

Living lobar lung transplant was introduced at the University of Southern California in 1993 for patients who were too ill to wait for cadaveric organs. Two donors are required to donate either a right or left lower lobe of their own lung. The recipient must meet the requirements for cadaveric lung transplant and be wait-listed.[99] The risk of complication or death is higher than in cadaveric donor transplants since it involves two healthy living donors as well as the recipient.[99] Postsurgery, donor lung function has been shown to decline over time. FVC has been shown to decrease by 17%, while total lung capacity has been shown to decrease by 16% within the first year after donation.[99] Recipient pulmonary function, exercise capacity, and freedom from bronchiolitis obliterans were equal to those who received cadaveric lungs. However, survival rates after 3 months were significantly lower, possibly due to more serious illness before transplant in the living lobar group.[99]

Postoperative Management

Postoperative management for lung transplant recipients is similar to heart–lung transplants. Ventilation, hemodynamic monitoring, fluid management, drainage, immunosuppression, ischemic reperfusion injury, rejection, and infection are monitored in the same way. Typically, single-lung transplant recipients have an easier time weaning off the ventilator and have shorter hospitalizations.[99] Ventilation issues may warrant a bronchoscopy while the patient is still intubated. Airway complications such as partial anastomotic dehiscence and stenosis are common and are diagnosed by bronchoscopy. Airway dehiscence is treated by reoperation or close observation and supportive care, while stenosis may require a stent placement in the affected airway.

Aggressive postoperative pulmonary toilet is essential to promote airway clearance because surgical denervation of the lungs diminishes the cough reflex after surgery. Ischemia-reperfusion injury and disrupted pulmonary lymphatics can increase vascular permeability, leading to interstitial edema. Other potential postoperative complications are dysrhythmias, deep vein thrombosis, pulmonary emboli, and pneumothorax, all of which are prevalent in the early postoperative period.

Patient Education

Patient and caregiver education begins prior to transplant in the evaluation period and continues through the life of the patient. Similarly to HLT, information is provided about signs and symptoms of infection and rejection, as well as follow-up care.

Long-Term Considerations

BOS is the histopathologic finding of chronic lung rejection, which at 1, 3, and 5 years affects 10%, 27%, and 50%, respectively, of lung transplant recipients.[113] Acute rejection, infectious episodes, cancer, hypertension, diabetes mellitus, kidney dysfunction, gastrointestinal disturbances, and psychosocial issues are all very common problems both short-term and long-term after transplantation and need to be addressed regularly.[114]

LIVER TRANSPLANTATION

Liver transplantation was first attempted in canine models in the 1950s. The outcomes were unsuccessful because of technical complications, infection, and graft failure. The effort to improve surgical technique continued, and successful liver transplantation in dogs was achieved several years later. In 1963, Starzl and colleagues performed the first human liver transplant, although the patient died intraoperatively. Starzl subsequently performed the first successful human liver transplantation in 1967 in a patient with malignant hepatoma.[115] The patient survived 1 year before succumbing to recurrent disease. Patient 1-year survival rates in the late 1960s and throughout the 1970s remained at less than 50% despite continued improvements in the surgical techniques. These early attempts were hindered by the difficulty of the surgery, poor methods of organ preservation, and inadequate immunosuppression.

Clinical trials of cyclosporine began in 1979 and revolutionized liver transplantation. One-year survival rates in the early 1980s increased to 70% and higher. This prompted the National Institutes of Health to declare that liver transplantation was no longer experimental but rather an accepted therapeutic modality for patients with end-stage liver disease.[116] This position statement resulted in an increase in the number of liver transplant centers worldwide and in the number of liver transplantations performed. Fewer than 200 liver transplantations were performed in the United States in 1983. But over 6500 were performed in 2011, including deceased and living donors combined. By 2008, adjusted patient survival rate after liver transplantation was 95% at 3 months, 89% at 1 year, and 74% at 5 years.[117]

Indications and Selection

Liver transplantation must be considered for any patient who suffers from irreversible acute or chronic liver disease that is progressive and for which there is no therapy of established

BOX 37-9 END-STAGE LIVER DISEASES COMMONLY TREATED WITH LIVER TRANSPLANTATION

Cholestatic Liver Diseases
- Biliary atresia
- Primary sclerosing cholangitis
- Primary biliary cirrhosis

Chronic Hepatocellular Diseases
- Viral hepatitis (types A, B, C, D, E)
- Alcoholic liver disease (Laennec disease)
- Autoimmune hepatitis
- Cryptogenic cirrhosis
- Medication-induced liver disease

Vascular Diseases
- Budd-Chiari syndrome
- Veno-occlusive disease

Acute and Subacute Liver Failure
- Viral hepatitis (types A, B, C, D, E)
- Medication-induced liver failure (acetaminophen, isoniazid overdoses)
- Fulminant Wilson disease

Inborn Metabolic Disorders
- Wilson disease
- Alpha-1 antitrypsin deficiency
- Hemochromatosis
- Tyrosinemia
- Glycogen storage disease, types I and II

Primary Hepatic Malignancies
- Hepatocellular carcinoma
- Hemangioendothelioma
- Hepatoblastoma

BOX 37-10 CONTRAINDICATIONS TO LIVER TRANSPLANTATION

ABSOLUTE CONTRAINDICATIONS	RELATIVE CONTRAINDICATIONS
• Brain death	• Physiologic age
• Metastatic malignancy	• Advanced renal disease
• Extrahepatic malignancy	• Multiple hepatic malignancies
• Active drug or alcohol abuse	• Moderate cardiopulmonary disease
• Advanced cardiopulmonary disease	• Peripheral vascular disease
• Acquired immunodeficiency syndrome	• Psychosocial behaviors indicating noncompliance with medical regimens
• Extrahepatic sepsis	• Human immunodeficiency virus infection

- Those who would not be likely to survive major surgery
- Those who would not survive the effects of long-term immunosuppression
- Those who have a disease that is likely to recur quickly and fatally after transplantation
- Those who are not willing to comply with long-term and sometimes difficult and demanding medical regimens

The absolute contraindications listed in Box 37-10 fall under these four specific categories. Having one relative contraindication may not rule out transplantation, but having several predicts poor outcome. Chronologic age is less important than physiologic age. Reports of transplantation in older patients describe favorable results.[120,121] UNOS reports that 745 patients age 65 years or older received a liver transplant in 2011.[117] Certain diseases can recur after transplantation, including viral hepatitis, sclerosing cholangitis, and biliary malignancies.[122,123] In the case of viral hepatitis, serologic indicators of viral replication are monitored closely. In the presence of aggressively replicating virus and in certain malignancies, it is in the patient's best interest not to proceed to transplantation, because it would actually hasten death. Multicenter protocols are important in evaluating the outcomes of transplantations in patients with diseases that recur. The decision to offer liver transplantation to any patient must be based on evaluation criteria, which vary among institutions and which are modified as advances in technical ability, immunosuppression, and perioperative management continue.

Recipient Evaluation

The candidate for liver transplantation undergoes a thorough evaluation to determine the cause and severity of the liver disease, to establish the need for transplantation rather than other interventions, and to identify objective indications and contraindications. Evaluation begins with a carefully elicited patient history (Box 37-11). A comprehensive approach includes laboratory, radiographic, and diagnostic testing and multidisciplinary consultations (Box 37-12). Not every patient undergoes every test and consultation. Careful history taking and a good physical examination direct the initial diagnostic testing. For instance, a patient with a past history of malignancy would undergo extensive testing to rule out metastases, whereas a patient with acute liver failure may have a more abbreviated

efficacy. Diseases of the liver may be categorized as chronic, vascular, fulminant or subfulminant, inborn errors of metabolism, and hepatic malignancies. Box 37-9 lists the most common diseases seen in patients who undergo liver transplantation. In the United States, the single most common indication for liver transplantation in adults is chronic viral hepatitis C. Biliary atresia and metabolic disorders account for more than 70% of the diseases leading to transplantation in the pediatric population.[118]

Candidate selection is an important aspect of transplantation. Given the shortage of available organs, the transplantation team must have reasonable assurance of a successful outcome. The timing of transplantation is of utmost importance. The patient must not be so ill as to be unable to survive the surgery, yet must be experiencing deterioration in the quality of life. Body mass index (BMI) plays a role in post-transplantation survival. Patients who are underweight (BMI less than 20) or morbidly obese (BMI greater than 40) are at greater risk for death after transplantation.[119] In general, liver transplantation is not to be offered to persons in the following groups:

workup that is focused on determining the cause and potential for hepatic recovery.

During the workup, the candidate's support systems are evaluated by the entire transplantation team, which includes the surgeon, the hepatologist, the clinical transplantation nurse coordinator, the social worker, the dietitian, and the financial counselor. Other services, such as cardiology, nephrology, psychiatry, gynecology, anesthesia, infectious disease, endocrinology, hematology, rheumatology, and oral surgery or dentistry, may also be included in the evaluation. Ideally, all immunizations are brought up to date in an attempt to minimize postoperative infections. The patient and family receive education regarding the evaluation, waiting list, surgery, postoperative

management including immunosuppression, and long-term follow-up. At the conclusion of the evaluation, one of several outcomes is possible: 1) the patient is a transplant candidate; 2) the patient is not a candidate; or 3) the patient may be a candidate sometime in the future if certain criteria are met. These criteria may be of a physical nature (e.g., it is too early in the disease process to list now, in which case the patient will be re-evaluated at set intervals), or they may be of a psychosocial nature (e.g., the patient must attend a formal alcohol or drug rehabilitation program or undergo treatment of depression).

After candidacy has been determined and the patient is ready for transplantation, the candidate is entered into the national computer system operated by UNOS. Objective criteria are used to place a patient on the waiting list. These data are used in a formula to determine the patient's liver disease score, which is directly associated with risk of death within 3 months (the higher the score, the higher the risk of death).

Model for End-Stage Liver Disease Formula. The Model for End-Stage Liver Disease (MELD) formula is used in all U.S. transplant centers to calculate risk of 3-month mortality in patients 12 years old or older.[124] The MELD objective criteria include serum total bilirubin, serum creatinine, prothrombin time, international normalized ratio, and whether the patient has undergone hemodialysis at least twice in the past 2 weeks.

Pediatric End-Stage Liver Disease Formula. The Pediatric End-Stage Liver Disease (PELD) formula is used to calculate risk of 3-month mortality for patients 11 years old or younger.[124] The PELD objective criteria include date of birth, gender, weight, height, serum albumin, serum total bilirubin, prothrombin time, and international normalized ratio.

BOX 37-11   PRETRANSPLANTATION HISTORY FOR A PATIENT WITH END-STAGE LIVER DISEASE

- Risk factors for viral hepatitis: transfusions, intravenous drug abuse, tattoos, other parenteral exposure
- Family history of liver disease
- Associated disorders: hypothyroidism, osteoporosis, infertility, arthritis
- Onset, duration, and description of symptoms and complications: jaundice, lethargy, bleeding disorders, pruritus, confusion, ascites, edema, melenic stools, abdominal pain, bone pain or fractures, chronic diarrhea, gynecomastia (in men), amenorrhea (in women)
- Current and past medical history: hospitalizations, surgeries
- Social history: exposure to alcohol, drugs, toxins, tobacco products
- Status of immunizations

BOX 37-12   SAMPLE EVALUATION BEFORE LIVER TRANSPLANTATION

Laboratory Tests
- Liver function profile: transaminases (AST, ALT, GGT), alkaline phosphatase, bilirubin, albumin, prothrombin time, partial thromboplastin time, clotting factors, cholesterol, triglycerides
- Kidney function profile with electrolytes: blood urea nitrogen, creatinine, sodium, potassium, carbon dioxide, chloride
- Hematology: CBC, reticulocytes, ESR
- Thyroid function: T_3RIA; T_4RIA; thyroid-stimulating hormone; T_4 and T_3 uptake
- Serology studies for hepatic viruses and other infectious diseases: viral hepatitis (A, B, C, D, E); cytomegalovirus, Epstein-Barr virus, herpesvirus I and II, parvovirus, HIV; RPR
- Blood type and antibody screen
- Immunologic profiles: antinuclear antibody, antimitochondrial antibody, antismooth muscle antibody, immunoglobulins (A, G, M)
- Nutritional profiles: vitamin levels (A, D, E, B_{12}, folate); iron studies with ferritin
- Tumor markers: alpha-fetoprotein, CEA, PSA,
- Miscellaneous: ceruloplasmin, alpha-1 antitrypsin level and phenotype

Urine
- 24-hour protein and electrolytes, cultures, creatinine clearance, urinalysis, copper

Stool
- Ova, cysts, parasites, occult blood, 48-hour fecal fat, cultures

Gastrointestinal Workup
- Endoscopy, colonoscopy, endoscopic retrograde cholangiopancreatography, liver biopsy

Pulmonary Profile
- Arterial blood gases, pulmonary function studies

Radiographic and Diagnostic Tests
- Chest radiograph, ultrasound studies of liver including vascular studies

Optional Tests
- Doppler studies; sinus radiography; computed tomography (abdomen, chest, head); electrocardiography; echocardiography; cardiac stress test; cardiac catheterization; mammography; peripheral vascular studies; carotid ultrasonography; abdominal angiography; percutaneous cholangiography; bone mineral density

ALT, Alanine aminotransferase; *AST*, aspartate transaminase; *CBC*, complete blood cell count; *CEA*, carcinoembryonic agents; *ESR*, erythrocyte sedimentation rate; *GGT*, gamma-glutamyltransferase; *HIV*, human immunodeficiency virus; *PSA*, prostate-specific antigen; *RPR*, rapid plasma reagin; *T_3RIA*; serum triiodothyronine (T_3) radioimmunoassay; *T_4RIA*, serum triiodothyronine (T_4) radioimmunoassay.

Placement on the waiting list is determined by blood type, weight, and patient urgency. Patients with acute liver failure are considered to be in most urgent need and are placed as status 1 at the top of the list. Patients with chronic end-stage liver disease are prioritized by their MELD or PELD scores below all status 1 patients. Those with higher scores are placed higher on the list. The duration of waiting time is used only as a tie-breaker for patients with equal scores. Requests may be made to the UNOS regional review board to assign a higher-than-calculated score for a patient with special problems that are not addressed by the use of only objective criteria, such as children with intractable pruritus. Patients who have hepatocellular carcinoma that meet specific tumor criteria are automatically given a MELD score of 20 because the risk of metastasis outside the liver within 3 months is high.[125] Once metastasis occurs the patient is no longer deemed a transplant candidate.

The frequency of recalculation of the MELD score is determined by the score itself. MELD scores greater than 25, between 19 and 24, and between 11 and 18 are evaluated every 7, 30, and 90 days, respectively.[124] A score of less than 10 is recalculated yearly,[124] barring any exacerbation of the liver disease or patient condition.

Next, one of the most difficult phases begins: the waiting period. It is not possible to anticipate when an appropriate organ will become available. The patient may feel that his or her life is being put "on hold." Because of the shortage of donors, it is not uncommon for patients in critical care units to die while awaiting transplantation; this is especially true for pediatric recipients. And knowing that another person must die so that he or she may live can cause feelings of guilt as the patient hopes for a liver to become available. Patients with end-stage liver disease know that the only alternative to transplantation is death. By understanding the basic social processes that patients experience while awaiting transplantation, nurses can facilitate health-promotion activities.[126] It is important for the patient and family to receive ongoing psychosocial assessment and to attend pretransplantation support groups, which are available at most transplant centers.

Pretransplantation Phase

The patient with end-stage liver disease who is awaiting a transplant may pose one of the greatest care challenges in the critical care unit. Hepatic encephalopathy, coagulopathies, portal hypertension, severe fluid and electrolyte imbalances, heart failure, pulmonary compromise, and kidney failure are not uncommon. Frequent mental status assessments are important in determining the patient's continued candidacy for transplantation. Hepatic encephalopathy may improve with the administration of antibiotics and laxatives, or the patient may proceed to stage IV coma. Later stages of hepatic encephalopathy may be clinically indistinguishable from cerebral hemorrhage. Diagnostic studies may be needed to evaluate the possibility of an intracranial bleed. Some centers use intracranial pressure monitoring catheters with these patients. The head of the patient's bed is maintained at 30 to 45 degrees to avoid even slight increases in intracranial pressure. Protection of the airway is especially important in an encephalopathic patient who is not intubated. In these circumstances, if hematemesis or vomiting occurs, intubation and use of paralytic agents may be necessary to protect the patient's airway.

Patients who have chronic liver disease are malnourished due to poor dietary intake and impaired digestion, absorption, and metabolism of nutrients. They require supplements of the fat-soluble vitamins (A, D, E, and K). Recommended dietary intake for patients with chronic liver disease includes 35 to 40 kcal/kg/d and 1.2 to 1.5 g/kg/d of protein utilizing ideal body weight for those with ascites and actual body weight for those without ascites.[127]

Consequences of portal hypertension must be corrected. Gastrointestinal hemorrhage from varices may respond to administration of propranolol or to procedures such as banding and sclerotherapy. Portal hypertension may be reduced by transjugular intrahepatic portosystemic shunting (TIPS) in interventional radiology. Rarely, the patient may need to undergo surgical intervention with a vascular shunt created between the portacaval system and the mesangial, splenic, or renal vascular system. But surgically created vascular shunts are usually not considered in patients who are transplant candidates. Patients with massive ascites usually have total body fluid overload but are intravascularly contracted and require sodium restriction and administration of colloidal fluids (e.g., albumin) along with diuretics. Careful documentation of fluid intake and output, daily weight determinations, and frequent measurement of vital signs are needed to monitor fluid status. Ascites can interfere with lung expansion and can compromise oxygenation. Patients with large, distended abdomens also find adequate oral nutrition difficult. Use of diuretics to control ascites is common but can compromise kidney function or worsen hepatorenal syndrome. *Paracentesis* (removal of ascites) may be required for intractable ascites. However, frequent large-volume paracentesis procedures can contribute to kidney and heart compromise related to fluid volume shifts.

Spontaneous bacterial peritonitis can be manifested in the patient with end-stage liver disease by an acute decline in the liver and kidney function accompanied by fever, abdominal pain, and hepatic encephalopathy. The paracentesis fluid shows increased white blood cells, with or without a positive culture. Patients are treated aggressively with antibiotics and are temporarily deferred from transplantation during treatment for and recovery from bacterial peritonitis.

Determining Donor Suitability

The two criteria necessary for matching a donor liver to a recipient are blood type and body size. HLA tissue typing is not used in the matching of donor livers, because it has not been shown to affect patient outcomes significantly. Donors are carefully screened for infectious diseases and metastatic carcinomas, because these can be transmitted to the recipient. The transplant center is notified by the regional OPO that a liver is available. If the organ is accepted, a member of the transplant team contacts the patient.

In very urgent situations, the donor blood type (e.g., type O) may not be compatible with that of the recipient (e.g., type A). Despite this ABO incompatibility, liver transplants can occur in urgent situations and can be successful. There may be some early postoperative complications, such as mild hemolysis, higher incidence of acute cellular rejection, and increased post-operative hepatic vascular and biliary complications, but innovative use of immunosuppressive regimens and plasmapheresis have improved graft survival of patients with recipient–donor ABO incompatibility.[128]

Extended-criteria donor livers, such as from DCD donors, livers with a cold ischemia time longer than 12 hours, or those from donors older than 60 years are expanding the donor pool and shortening waiting times.[129]

After a donor liver becomes available, it is necessary to expedite the preoperative preparation of the recipient. The use of newer preservation solutions has allowed for longer cold ischemia time (i.e., the length of time from when the organ is removed from the donor, flushed, and packed in ice for storage until the time when it is transplanted).

Living Donor Liver Transplantation

Since 1985, approximately 23,000 people have died while registered and awaiting a liver from a deceased donor. Many liver transplant centers in the United States now offer *living donor liver transplantation* (LDLT). The peak number of LDLT procedures occurred in 2006. In 2009 only 2.9% of transplanted livers were from living donors.[117] Living liver donation is more common in pediatric liver transplantation.[117]

LDLT began in 1989 with adult-to-child donations, commonly from a parent to his or her infant. The left lateral hepatic lobe is resected, leaving the donor with the larger mass of liver remaining. In such cases, the risks to the healthy donor are thought to be outweighed by the benefits of having a healthy child.[130] Adult-to-adult LDLT donation began in the 1990s. The whole left hepatic lobe or right hepatic lobe is resected, taking 30% to 60% of the liver mass from the living donor.

Living Liver Donor Complications. Complications for the donor after partial hepatectomy can be graded I-IV.[131,132] Grade I complications are not life-threatening and do not result in permanent disability. Grade II complications require medications or transfusion. Grade III can be potentially life-threatening and require invasive therapy such as a return to the operating room. Grade IV leads to disability or death. Most living liver donor complications are grade I-II, such as urinary tract infection, rash, dysrhythmia, wound infection, pulmonary emboli, pleural effusion, postoperative bleeding, bile leak, or biliary stricture.[131,132] The more serious grade III and IV complications that have been reported for the liver donor include pleural effusions requiring chest tubes, bleeding requiring surgery, biliary complications requiring surgery, wound dehiscence, hepatic artery thrombosis, intra-abdominal abscess, splenectomy, perforated gastric ulcer, deep vein thrombosis, and death.[133] By 2008, there had been 33 deaths among living liver donors reported in the United States and Europe.[134] Living donors must undergo a rigorous evaluation to determine eligibility to donate. This includes both physical health and psychosocial assessments. During this evaluation the mass of the liver is measured and the volume that can be safely removed is determined. The volume of liver that can safely be removed must be of sufficient mass so as to be able to support the recipient adequately.

Donor Advocate. Each center that performs living donor procedures must have a *donor advocate* that is not a member of the transplant team. The donor advocate is involved in all phases of the procedure to ensure donor safety and well-being. Postoperative care of the living liver donor is similar to any patient who has undergone a liver resection. Critical care nurses play an important role in caring for these donors and must be vigilant in assessing for complications and initiating early interventions.

Liver Transplantation Surgical Procedure

Liver transplantation surgery is lengthy and technically difficult, often lasting 4 to 12 hours. The patient is taken to the operating room for anesthesia induction, insertion of large-bore intravenous catheters that allow high-volume fluid infusion, and insertion of a pulmonary artery catheter for hemodynamic monitoring. Continuous renal replacement therapy (CRRT) may be continued or initiated in the operating room. The patient is positioned on the operating room table in such a way as to minimize pressure that could cause ischemia and chronic injury to tissue and peripheral nerves. Liver transplantation surgery can be divided into three stages: 1) recipient hepatectomy; 2) vascular anastomoses with donor liver; and 3) biliary anastomosis.

Recipient Hepatectomy

Stage 1 is the longest and most difficult part of the surgery, because it involves removal of the native liver. It is complicated even more by coagulopathies, adhesions, portal hypertension, and venous collaterals. Before completion of this stage, the patient may be placed on venovenous bypass (Fig. 37-11), although not all patients require this procedure. A centrifugal pump cycles the blood out through iliac and portal vein cannulas and returns it to the central circulation through the axillary or subclavian vein. Advances in surgical techniques, anesthesia, and fluid management have shortened the length of surgery enough to warrant elimination of venovenous bypass in many cases.

Vascular Anastomoses with a Donor Liver

Stage 2 comprises the four vascular anastomoses: suprahepatic inferior vena cava, infrahepatic vena cava, hepatic artery, and portal vein. Many variations and adaptations, such as vascular patches, may be used, depending on the anatomy of the donor and recipient. If venovenous bypass is used, it is removed after the infrahepatic vena cava anastomosis and before the hepatic artery anastomosis.

Biliary Anastomosis

Stage 3 can be achieved by *choledochojejunostomy* (bile duct to jejunum) or by *choledochocholedochostomy* (bile duct to bile duct). Choledochojejunostomy is performed in patients with diseased bile ducts, such as those with biliary atresia or sclerosing cholangitis. It is also known as a *Roux-en-Y* procedure and is shown in Figure 37-12. The choledochocholedochostomy is performed in patients who have a healthy and intact common bile duct and is shown in Figure 37-13. The patient returns from surgery with, or without, an external stent or T-tube that is connected to a bag into which bile drains. Patients who do not have external biliary tubes may have an internal stent inserted

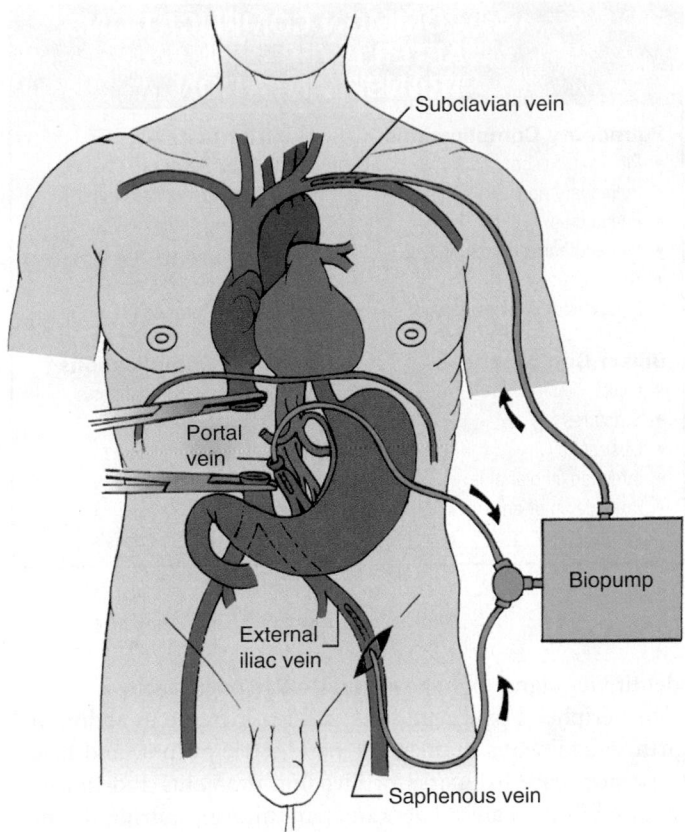

FIGURE 37-11 Venovenous bypass during removal of the native liver. The portal and iliac veins are cannulated, and blood is circulated by a centrifugal pump to the subclavian vein.

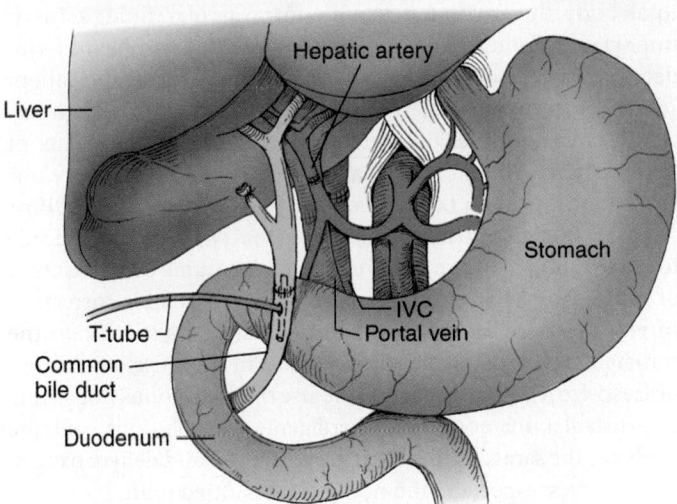

FIGURE 37-13 Choledochocholedochostomy procedure. *IVC,* Inferior vena cava.

BOX 37-13 NURSING DIAGNOSES

Liver Transplantation

- Risk for Infection: Immunosuppressive medications required to prevent rejection of the transplanted liver, p. 1160
- Imbalanced Nutrition: Less Than Body Requirements related to lack of exogenous nutrients or increased metabolic demand, p. 1143
- Deficient Fluid Volume related to absolute loss, p. 1132
- Disturbed Body Image related to actual change in body structure, function, or appearance, p. 1136
- Anxiety related to threat to biologic, psychologic, and social integrity, p. 1125

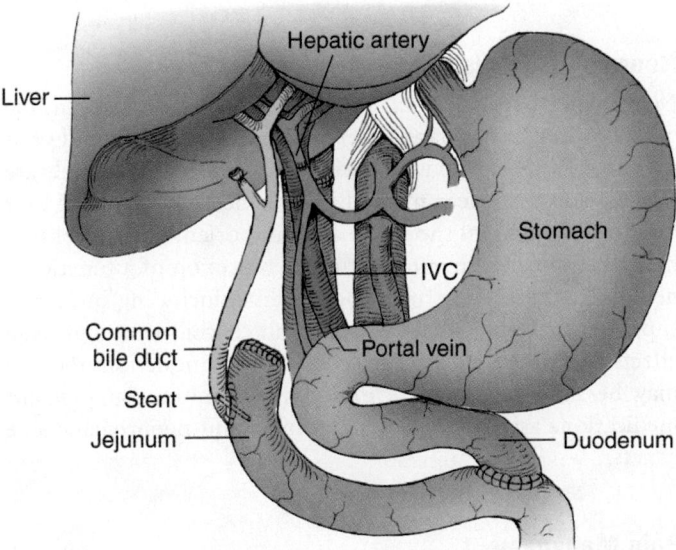

FIGURE 37-12 Roux-en-Y procedure (choledochojejunostomy). *IVC,* Inferior vena cava.

in the bile duct across the biliary anastomosis. Eventually, the internal stent moves and is passed with the stool. Sometimes the internal biliary stent must be removed by an endoscopic procedure.

Postoperative Medical and Nursing Management

The common nursing diagnoses associated with liver transplantation are listed in Box 37-13. After surgery, some patients are extubated before they arrive in the critical care unit, but most arrive unreversed from anesthesia and remain intubated for 12 to 24 hours. Immediate goals include: 1) re-establishment of normal body temperature; 2) hemodynamic stabilization; and 3) maintenance of an effective airway. Postoperative hypothermia is common after orthotopic liver transplantation (OLT). The critical care nurse must achieve rewarming safely by the use of methods such as warming blankets, heating lamps, and head covers.

Hemodynamics

Hemodynamic stabilization is a particular challenge, because the patient may arrive hypervolemic, euvolemic, or hypovolemic and may be hypertensive or hypotensive. Assessment of total body fluids compared with intravascular fluid status is important. Because of inherent presurgical problems with decreased serum albumin, some centers tend to keep the patient "dry." Hypervolemia often results in third spacing, with resultant ascites and a leaking wound. Accurate measurements of hemodynamic function, such as arterial blood pressure, peripheral blood pressure, central venous pressure (CVP), PAOP or "wedge" pressure, urinary output, patency of drains, and bile totals are assessed frequently to evaluate volume status. Choice of replacement fluids and pharmacologic agents for correction of volume and blood pressure abnormalities is specific to the transplant center. These protocols vary in their use of albumin or fresh-frozen plasma, and in the use of intravenous dopamine or prostaglandin, as well as other agents and solutions. Still, the goals are the same: optimize tissue perfusion and deliver oxygen to all tissues, especially the newly transplanted graft.

Electrolytes

Electrolyte abnormalities can occur after liver transplantation. Disturbances in potassium and magnesium levels are common. High serum levels of electrolytes are usually associated with acute kidney injury; low levels can be the result of medication side effects (e.g., diuretic therapy). The presence of hypernatremia or hyponatremia complicates the correction of volume status and fluid replacement. Calcineurin inhibitors can cause hypomagnesemia, which will lower seizure thresholds. Since these medications can also cause seizures, careful monitoring and replacement of magnesium is important.

Pulmonary Management

Ventilatory support of the patient is maintained until the anesthetic agent has been metabolized and cleared by the new liver and the patient awakens. Frequent measurement of arterial blood gas levels, continuous pulse oximetry, and assessment of breath sounds are needed. The patient may require changes in ventilatory settings, suctioning to remove secretions, or administration of pharmacologic agents to correct acid–base imbalances. Pulmonary complications are common, as listed in Box 37-14. While the patient is on ventilatory support, pneumonia can be avoided by maintaining the head of bed elevated at 30 degrees, turning the patient frequently, providing good oral care, and brushing the patient's teeth. After extubation, patients must be encouraged to perform incentive spirometry exercises and to turn, cough, and deep breathe frequently to help prevent atelectasis and pneumonia. Respiratory treatments with bronchodilators, prophylactic antimicrobials, and chest physiotherapy also may be used. Early mobilization and physical therapy are encouraged.

Coagulopathy Risk

Management of coagulopathies is important in the early postoperative phase. Characterization and careful measurement of drain lines and drainage from incisions are needed along with other nursing assessments of blood loss, such as

---

BOX 37-14   COMMON COMPLICATIONS AFTER LIVER TRANSPLANTATION

Pulmonary Complications
- Pleural effusion
- Pulmonary edema
- Pneumonia
- Pneumothorax or hemothorax
- Atelectasis
- Paralysis of right diaphragm

Biliary Complications
- Leaks
- Strictures
- Obstruction
- Infection (cholangitis)
- Breakdown of anastomosis

Gastrointestinal Complications
- Bleeding and ulceration
- Gastrointestinal infections (cytomegalovirus, *Candida*, *Clostridium difficile*)
- Bowel perforations

Vascular Complications
- Hepatic artery thrombosis
- Portal vein thrombosis
- Vena caval thrombosis
- Peripheral and central line sepsis
- Hepatic vein thrombosis

---

identifying signs of hypovolemia, tachypnea, tachycardia, or poor peripheral oxygenation. A sudden increase in abdominal girth, sanguineous drainage or nasogastric output, and black, tarry stools are hallmarks of bleeding problems and must be reported immediately. Laboratory monitoring during the first 24 hours after surgery is necessary to assess blood loss and coagulopathies and includes hematocrit, hemoglobin, platelet count, prothrombin time, partial thromboplastin time, fibrinogen, and fibrin split products. Reversal of coagulopathies is done judiciously, with consideration for the potential to thrombose newly anastomosed blood vessels in the liver. Blood products such as platelets, fresh-frozen plasma, and specific factors can be given along with pharmacologic agents such as vitamin K.

Neurologic Status

Neurologic assessment of the patient is important in the early postoperative phase to determine mental status and graft function. Patients who were encephalopathic preoperatively are usually slower to clear mentally. Nevertheless, with good liver function, the patient should be alert and oriented within 1 to 2 days; the improved mental status is a reflection of a functional new liver. Certain pharmacologic agents, including immunosuppressants, can cause peripheral and central neurologic side effects that may alter neurologic status. Induction therapy may be used to delay the initiation of immunosuppressant medications associated with neurologic and nephrogenic side effects.

Pain Management

The critical care nurse must always be aware of the potential for intracranial bleeds in a patient who has coagulopathies, serum sodium imbalances, and hemodynamic instability. All of these conditions can interfere with pain management, because the pharmacologic agents used for pain can mask deterioration in mental status. Medications to relieve pain are administered, but other nonpharmacologic nursing interventions also must be used.

Glucose Control

Glucose control after liver transplant can be altered by steroid administration, graft function, calcineurin inhibitors, and pre-existing diabetes. Intensive blood glucose control (less than 150 mg/dL) during liver transplantation surgery has been associated with a significant decrease in the infection rate at 30 days and in the mortality rate at 1 year.[135] Perioperative hyperglycemia has been associated with increased risk of liver allograft rejection in a retrospective study.[136] Low serum glucose in the absence of insulin administration can indicate primary nonfunction of the liver allograft.

Kidney Function

Kidney function can be altered by several mechanisms after liver transplantation, including cyclosporine or tacrolimus administration, acute kidney injury, intrinsic kidney disease, and poor liver function. Patients are managed with attention to fluid and electrolyte imbalances, by avoidance of nephrotoxic medications, and occasionally with ultrafiltration, CRRT, or intermittent hemodialysis. With good liver function, kidney function usually improves. However, certain immunosuppressive agents and antimicrobials can deleteriously affect the kidney. Adjustments in dose or avoidance of use must be balanced with assessment of kidney and liver function. Daily monitoring of cyclosporine or tacrolimus serum levels is vital to determining adequate immunosuppression, and daily serum creatinine levels are necessary to monitor for acute kidney injury. As the patient's condition continues to improve, the frequency of laboratory testing may decrease.

Infection Risk

Immunosuppressive therapy places the transplant recipient at an increased risk for infection. Infectious complications are common and continue to be the leading cause of death among OLT patients.[137,138] The potential for infection is greatest when patients receive high doses of immunosuppressants. All persons who come into contact with the transplant recipient throughout the hospitalization must practice good hand-washing techniques and standard precautions to prevent the transmission of infection. Infections are treated with appropriate antimicrobials specific to the invading organism. Prophylactic therapies are commonly used as well.[137,138] Removal of central lines, arterial lines, urinary catheters, and drains is accomplished as early as is safe for the patient to avoid line-associated infections.

Bile Drains

Careful attention to any external biliary drain line is important. If the patient has an external biliary drain, the critical care nurse documents color, character, and amount of drainage and reports

any changes. Biliary complications and other complications can occur after liver transplantation (see Box 37-14).

Nutrition

The nasogastric tube is removed when its output is minimal, bowel sounds have returned, and the patient is extubated. The patient who undergoes a Roux-en-Y biliary anastomosis will keep the nasogastric tube longer since postoperative ileus is more common. If oral nutrition is delayed longer than several days, total parenteral nutrition may be started. Consultation with a nutritionist (dietitian) should be sought. Prealbumin levels may be measured to assess nutritional status. Otherwise, nutrition may begin orally or through a feeding tube as soon as the patient is extubated. When bowel function returns, the diet is advanced as tolerated.

Liver Function Tests

The standard laboratory biomarkers used to monitor graft function are serum aspartate aminotransferase (AST), alanine aminotransferase (ALT), alkaline phosphatase, and gamma-glutamyltransferase (GGT); serum bilirubin; and prothrombin time. The serum levels of these markers are measured frequently during the first few postoperative days. These levels may continue to rise for a few days before peaking and subsequently falling. As liver function improves, the frequency of laboratory testing decreases.

Liver Graft Nonfunction

The patient with suspected primary nonfunction of a liver graft demonstrates: 1) hemodynamic instability; 2) progressive deterioration of kidney function; 3) coagulopathies and abnormal serum liver function laboratory tests; 4) hypoglycemia; 5) continued ventilatory dependence; and 6) an inability to awaken from anesthesia. Continued nonfunction of the graft necessitates relisting the patient for another donor liver. Early signs of optimal graft function include improving kidney function, mental alertness, a high to normal serum glucose concentration, and early extubation. The serum ALT, AST, GGT, and alkaline phosphatase levels may peak on the third or fourth day but later should decrease. The serum bilirubin concentration may take a week before beginning to fall, and there may be a mild elevation when the external biliary drainage tube is clamped or after a blood transfusion.

Rejection Surveillance

Acute rejection is a cellular-mediated event and should be suspected if the serum liver enzymes, especially AST and ALT, become elevated compared with previous levels. This can be followed by elevations in total bilirubin. Such elevations usually precede any other sign of acute rejection of the liver allograft. Sometimes, the patient also exhibits fever, a drop in bile output (if a T-tube is still connected to a drainage bag), and a change in the color and viscosity of the bile. At first the patient may not have any other physical symptoms, but eventually late signs of rejection may occur, including jaundice, malaise, dark urine, and clay-colored stools. Certain infections, such as CMV, can also cause liver function test values to increase.

Rejection is suspected when liver function test values increase, but other reasons for these elevations need to be ruled out. Mechanical and vascular complications are ruled out by Doppler ultrasonography and angiography. Endoscopic retrograde cholangiopancreatography, hepatobiliary iminodiacetic acid (HIDA) scanning, or transhepatic cholangiography may reveal biliary obstruction or leakage. A liver biopsy may be indicated to determine cause of liver dysfunction if the other tests are inconclusive. Acute rejection can occur at any time after transplantation, but most commonly it occurs during the first few months and even as early as the first week after surgery. Most liver transplant recipients experience at least one acute rejection episode. Treatment of acute rejection requires increasing immunosuppression. Immunosuppressant protocols vary from center to center and are usually successful at reversing acute rejection.

Chronic rejection is both a humoral and cellular event and is progressive over time and nonreversible. It results in destruction and loss of bile ducts. It is sometimes treated with plasmapheresis to remove circulating antibodies along with pharmacologic immunotherapies that bind B cells. Chronic rejection in a liver transplant recipient usually requires retransplantation if the patient is still a candidate.

Transfer Out of Critical Care

After the patient is stable and the transplanted liver is functional, central venous catheters and arterial lines are removed. The urinary catheter is removed as soon as the patient is awake enough to be continent. Drain lines are removed as drainage outputs become minimal. As the patient begins to participate in self-care, plans are made for transfer out of the critical care unit to the transplant step-down nursing unit.

On the transplant medical–surgical unit, laboratory data and vital signs continue to be monitored on a routine basis. Self-care is promoted. Increasing levels of physical therapy are encouraged, diet is advanced, and much of the nurse's interventions are directed toward teaching the patient and family.

Patient Education

Considerable attention is focused on patient education and discharge planning. Discharge booklets are helpful in the education process. It is important for the patient to learn how to self-administer medications, monitor vital signs, care for the incision and the T-tube (if present), prevent infections, follow safe living practices, and identify problems that must promptly receive medical attention.[139] Because it is not uncommon for patients to be discharged within 2 weeks after OLT, it is important for discharge instructions to begin as soon as the patient is mentally alert. Patients discharged early may require home health nurse referrals to assist with follow-up of incision care, intravenous therapies, and other procedures. Education must be provided about rejection surveillance, signs and symptoms

of infection, lifestyle changes as needed, long-term medication considerations, and the follow-up visit schedule.

Long-Term Follow-Up

Liver transplant patients who do not live in the same city in which their surgery was performed usually remain in the immediate area of the transplant center after discharge before returning home. During this period, they may be monitored by a home health nurse and be seen in clinic several times a week by the transplant team. Continued serologic testing is performed to monitor graft function, to determine blood levels of certain immunosuppressive agents, and to identify postoperative complications. Although many of these complications can be managed successfully in the outpatient setting, readmissions do occur. Because rejections, readmissions, grieving for the donor, and pharmacologic side effects can create anxiety for the family and the patient, they are encouraged to attend transplantation support groups if offered by the center. After patients return home, they are encouraged to resume a close relationship with their local primary care physician and gastroenterologist.

With the proliferation in the number of liver transplantations being performed, it is not unreasonable for recipients to be admitted to a nontertiary care hospital for management of some long-term post-transplantation complications. Even nurses who work for hospitals that do not perform transplants may have the opportunity to care for these patients. Nurses in these settings must also become knowledgeable about the signs and symptoms of rejection, administration of immunosuppressant medications, monitoring of immunosuppressant levels, and medication-to-medication interactions with the immunosuppressants. Every transplant patient has a coordinator who follows the patient at the transplant center. The transplant coordinator is also available for consultation with community health care providers who have questions about transplant patients.

Liver transplant patients need long-term follow-up surveillance for hypertension, kidney failure, obesity, dyslipidemias, biliary and infectious complications, and malignancies. Early intervention affects the quality and length of life. Behavior modifications and therapeutic lifestyle changes should be frequently reinforced to positively affect long-term health. Financial concerns are a major source of stress in this patient population.[140] Many transplant recipients suffered from chronic liver disease before their surgery. They often were disabled for some time and already have experienced financial stressors related to illness. As these patients live longer with liver transplants, issues of insurability, continued disability, and even the ability to obtain work will have to be addressed.[140]

Transplantation offers hope for survival, but at considerable expense. Many insurance providers, including Medicare, provide partial reimbursement for liver transplant procedures. The costs to patients can be staggering.[140] Transplant centers must find innovative ways to control rising costs because of decreasing reimbursements, complexity of patient care, and increasing patient loads. Close management of post-transplant complications and avoidance of rehospitalization is important in reducing costs. Advanced practice nurses who work in transplant centers offer an effective economic model in the delivery of safe patient care.[141]

The Future

Clinical trials are in process to identify new medications and define improved treatment protocols. With increasing choices of therapies, medications will be selected for patients after other immunosuppressive therapies have failed or severe side effects have occurred. Studies on tolerance and chimerism also may influence future immunosuppressive protocols.[142] As recipients spend more time on the waiting list, improved methods of medical management of end-stage liver disease and bridges to transplantation become increasingly necessary, including transarterial chemoembolization (TACE) of hepatocellular cancer, and transjugular intrahepatic portosystemic shunts (TIPS).[143]

A limiting factor in liver transplantation continues to be the shortage of organ donors (see Fig. 37-1).[129,143] Attention is being focused on ways to increase the number and availability of donor organs. This includes reduced-size organs, split-liver technique (in which one liver is divided and transplanted into two recipients), and living liver donors. Expanded criteria for deceased liver donors can include donation after cardiac death, advanced donor age, steatosis, hepatitis C positive allografts, human T-cell lymphotrophic virus-positive allografts, hepatitis B-core antibody positive allografts, donors with active infections, and high-risk donors.[129] Studies are exploring the roles of xenografts and bioartificial liver devices that can support the patient who is awaiting a homograft.[143] Recipient selection criteria also will continue to be redefined for diseases and conditions such as hepatic malignancies,[144] HIV positivity,[144,145] and alcoholism.[146] As recipients live longer and healthier lives, reproduction and pregnancy after transplantation will become more common.[147] These and other factors will influence the future of liver transplantation.

KIDNEY TRANSPLANTATION

The first successful kidney transplantation was performed in 1954 in Boston. Today, it is the treatment of choice for patients with end-stage kidney disease. It allows the recipient to lead a much less restricted lifestyle and provides a more cost-effective treatment method than long-term dialysis. Advances in the study of the immune system and the development of new immunosuppressant medications have allowed for increased graft survival rates for deceased donor and living donor kidney transplants.

In the early years of transplantation, large doses of oral steroids were the immunosuppressant of choice for preventing graft rejection. Large doses or prolonged use of oral steroids can cause severe osteoporosis, decreased wound healing, and many of the symptoms of Cushing syndrome. In the 1970s, cyclosporine was added to the list of immunosuppressive medications used to prevent rejection. Cyclosporin represented a breakthrough in immunosuppression, and graft survival rates soared.[31] Transplant centers use a combination of immunosuppressive medications to prevent rejection, in an attempt to lower the doses of each agent so that the associated side effects can be minimized.

In 2009, a total of 16,830 kidney transplantations were performed in the United States. However, 84,614 patients were listed with the Scientific Registry of Transplant Recipients (SRTR) awaiting a donor kidney.[148] Discovery of new medications and finding ways to increase the number of donor organs recovered are two of the challenges that the transplantation community faces.

Indications and Selection

Many disease processes can lead to end-stage kidney disease. For this reason, potential recipients must undergo numerous laboratory tests and some noninvasive physical testing before they can be approved as candidates (Box 37-15). Because after transplantation the patient's immune system will be purposely and controllably compromised, there are several contraindications to kidney transplantation (Box 37-16). If any of these risk factors is present, the patient's risk is determined to be too high for transplantation and the immunosuppressant regimen that follows. The alternative for such a patient is to decrease or eliminate the risk factors that can be controlled and be re-evaluated at a later date. If the candidate is unwilling to eliminate controllable high-risk behaviors, the only alternative for survival is to remain on dialysis.

BOX 37-15 **EVALUATION BEFORE KIDNEY TRANSPLANTATION**

- Chem 24 panel; human leukocyte antigen tissue typing; prothrombin time; partial thromboplastin time; complete blood count with differential; platelet count; human immunodeficiency virus; hepatitis; cytomegalovirus; Epstein-Barr virus; lipid profile; urine for analysis, culture, and sensitivities; 24-hour urine for creatinine clearance and protein (if patient still produces urine); dialysate fluid for culture and sensitivity (if patient is undergoing continuous ambulatory peritoneal dialysis)
- Kidney ultrasonography or spiral computed tomography; chest radiography (posteroanterior and lateral views); electrocardiography; stress test and cardiac catheterization (if indicated); weight management (if indicated); colonoscopy (if >55 years old); mammography (for women >35 years old); venography (for patients with diabetes)
- Consultants: psychologist or psychiatrist, urologist, transplantation surgeon or transplantation nephrologist, social worker, dietitian, chaplain, financial counselor

---

BOX 37-16 **CONTRAINDICATIONS TO KIDNEY TRANSPLANTATION**

- Malignancy during the past 3 years
- Active infectious process
- Advanced cardiopulmonary disease
- High risk for surgery
- Nonadherence to current medical regimen
- Recreational drug use
- Other serious contributing disease processes

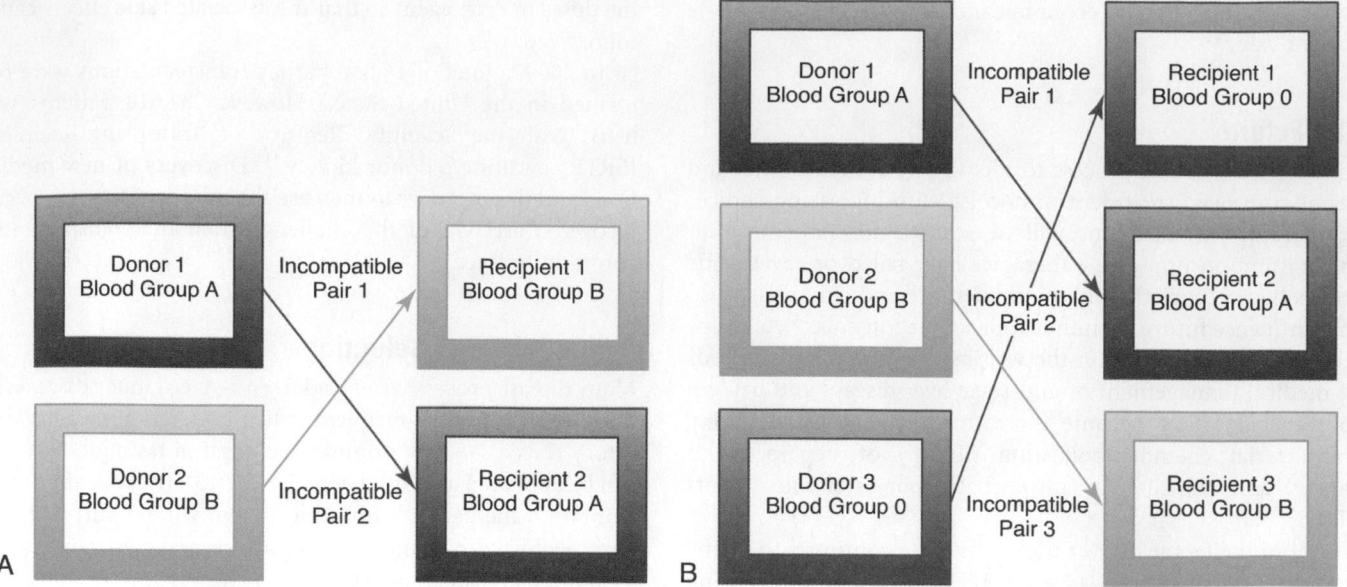

FIGURE 37-14 *Kidney paired donation* (KPD) is an option for the person who wants to donate a kidney to a family member, but does not have a compatible blood type with the intended recipient. With this option, donors can participate in a donation exchange with another living donor–recipient pair, as shown in *A*. There could also be a three-way living donor exchange, as shown in *B*.

Deceased Kidney Donation

Most kidneys transplanted in the United States come from a deceased donor who meets the criteria for brain death or cardiac death (described earlier in the chapter). Because of the shortage of donor organs, candidates are typically on the deceased donor waiting list for 3 to 5 years before their transplant.[148] Donor and recipient are matched by ABO blood type. A simplified description of the current organ allocation criteria is described below.

The first priority for a deceased donor kidney is to candidates who are listed for a kidney and a simultaneous non-kidney organ (pancreas, heart, or liver) transplant.[149] Second priority is given to candidates who have a perfect human leukocyte antigen (HLA) match with the donor kidney, because this optimizes graft survival. The third priority is by local geographic region.[149] Organ allocation is managed not by the transplant center but through the OPTN/UNOS registry (described in the beginning of the chapter).[149]

Deceased kidney donors are further classified as: 1) *standard criteria donor* (SCD) kidneys, delineated by donor age, whether younger than 35 years, or older than 35 years; 2) *expanded criteria donor* (ECD) kidneys; and 3) donation after cardiac death (DCD) donor kidneys.[149] There were 11,765 deceased donor transplants performed in the United States in 2009; 16% of these were ECD donors.[148]

Living Kidney Donation

The first successful kidney transplant was a living donor transplant between identical twins in 1954. In most cases today, the living donor is related to the recipient. There were 5065 living donor kidney transplants performed in the United States in 2009.[148]

Living Kidney Paired Donation. An innovative new option is *kidney paired donation* (KPD). A person may want to donate one of his or her kidneys to a family member but their blood type is not compatible with the intended recipient. In this situation they could participate in a donation exchange with another living donor–recipient pair as shown in Figure 37-14A. This could also be a three-way living donor exchange as shown in Figure 37-14B.[150] Several other variations have also been used involving a "chain" of donor-to-recipient transplants.[151-153]

Kidney Transplantation Surgical Procedure

When the kidney to be transplanted is procured from the donor—whether living or deceased—the ureter, renal vein, and renal artery are dissected, leaving as much length as possible.

Living Donor Kidney Transplantation

If the donor is living, the procurement is typically by laparoscopic nephrectomy. Open surgical kidney removal is rare today. After the kidney is secured, it is flushed with a cold electrolyte preservative solution until the venous return is clear.[154] This usually requires 100 to 200 mL of solution.[154] The kidney is then transported to operating room to be transplanted.

Deceased Donor Kidney Transplantation Surgery

If the kidney is from a deceased donor, it is flushed with a cold electrolyte preservative solution and simultaneously cooled externally as quickly as possible. It can be transported on a kidney perfusion machine or packed in an iced preservation solution. After it is procured and placed in the hypothermic solution, it can be maintained for 48 to 72 hours before it must be transplanted.[154] Most transplant centers attempt to

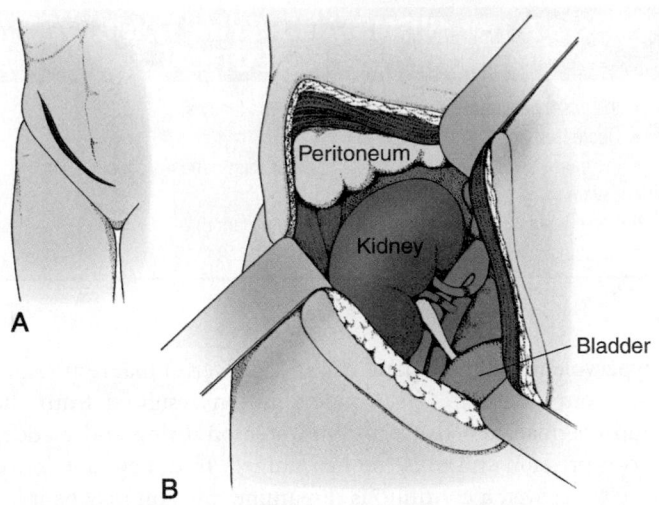

FIGURE 37-15 Placement of the renal graft into the iliac fossa. *A*, The incision in the right side of the abdomen is used for graft implantation in the right iliac fossa. *B*, The iliac vessels are exposed. (Modified from Smith SL. *AACN Tissue and Organ Transplantation: Implications for Professional Nursing Practice.* St. Louis: Mosby; 1990.)

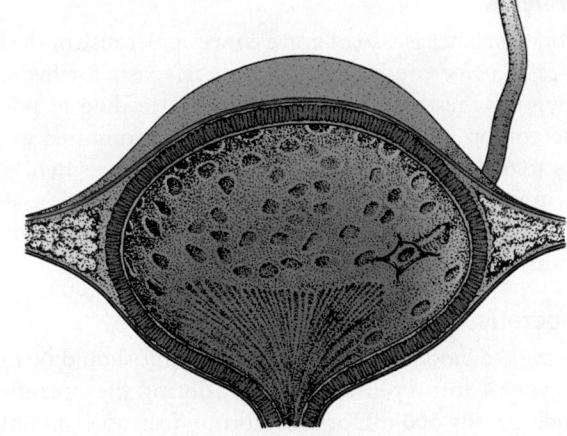

FIGURE 37-16 Ureteroneocystostomy reconstruction of the urinary tract. The donor ureter is passed through a posterior bladder wall tunnel and anastomosed to the bladder mucosa. (From Smith SL. *AACN Tissue and Organ Transplantation: Implications for Professional Nursing Practice.* St. Louis: Mosby; 1990.)

transplant the organ within 24 hours after procurement, to avoid cold ischemic injury and acute kidney injury.[154] At the time of procurement, the kidney is assessed in situ for color, shape, and form. It is palpated to determine firmness, and often a biopsy is taken to rule out undiagnosed kidney dysfunction.

Recipient Surgery

The patient is anesthetized in the usual manner, and a urinary catheter is placed. A curvilinear incision is made 3 to 4 cm above the symphysis pubis and extended to the iliac crest (Fig. 37-15A). The kidney is to be placed in the extraperitoneal space of the right or left iliac fossa. The muscles and fascia are divided and retracted medially to expose the iliac vessels. The renal artery is anastomosed to the external iliac artery, using an end-to-side or an end-to-end anastomosis, and the vein is sutured to the common iliac vein in a similar manner (Fig. 37-15B).[154]

After the revascularization procedures are completed, the ureteral anastomosis is performed. The most common method used is *ureteroneocystostomy*. During this procedure, an incision is made in the dome of the recipient's bladder. The donor ureter is tunneled through the recipient's mucosal layer and sutured (end-to-side) to the mucosal opening (Fig. 37-16).[154] If the patient has a history of bladder surgeries, augmentations, or infections, a *ureteroureterostomy* can be done, in which the donor ureter is anastomosed to the recipient's ureter. If the patient has a history of ureteral reflux in his or her native kidneys, the *ureteroneocystostomy* is the procedure of choice. Tunneling of the ureter prevents reflux into the transplanted kidney with every bladder contraction.[154]

During the surgery, a CVP ranging from 8 to 16 mm Hg must be maintained, and a systolic blood pressure at least as high as the patient's baseline value should be maintained to ensure adequate perfusion of the transplanted kidney.

BOX 37-17 NURSING DIAGNOSES

Kidney Transplantation

- Deficient Fluid Volume related to absolute loss, p. 1132
- Risk for Ineffective Renal Perfusion related to decreased blood flow to the kidney, p. 1159
- Risk for Infection: Immunosuppressive medications to prevent rejection of the transplanted kidney, p. 1160
- Disturbed Body Image related to actual change in body structure, function, or appearance, p. 1136
- Anxiety related to threat to biologic, psychologic, and social integrity, p. 1125

Postoperative Medical Management and Nursing Care

After the transplantation is completed and the patient is stable and ready for discharge from the recovery room, most transplant centers admit the patient directly to the organ transplantation unit or to the critical care unit. Serious complications can occur in the immediate postoperative period, and sound knowledge base of medical/surgical nursing, kidney function, anatomy, and immunosuppressive medications is imperative. Relevant nursing diagnoses are listed in Box 37-17.

Fluid Status

If the transplanted organ is working well, the patient's fluid status, as monitored by observations of CVP, weight, and vital signs, must be regulated very closely. Adequate hydration is an absolute necessity for continued graft function in the immediate postoperative period. Hypovolemia can lead to compromised blood flow to the kidney, acute kidney injury, and possible graft failure. The new kidney will be producing large amounts of urine, and fluid replacement, usually maintained in a 1:1 ratio, must be sustained.

Electrolytes

Electrolyte balance is also of grave concern. Because of the large volumes of urine produced, the potential exists for hypokalemia, hypomagnesemia, and hypocalcemia, leading to possible cardiac compromise. Electrolytes must be monitored at least every 4 to 6 hours and replaced as necessary. Assessment of the blood urea nitrogen and the creatinine concentration also is necessary every 4 to 6 hours to monitor graft function and determine the need for dialysis.

Postoperative Complications

The complete blood count and platelet count should be monitored every 4 to 6 hours. Blood loss during the operation is minimal, usually 500 mL or less. Abrupt decreases or continuously falling counts may indicate hemorrhage at an anastomosis site, which requires a return to the operating room for repair. Even with minimal blood loss during surgery, transfusion of blood products after the surgery is often necessary. Frequent observation and assessment of the surgical incision are needed to evaluate for drainage and swelling. Urine output volume and color should be monitored at least every 30 minutes. The bladder anastomosis is fragile, and it is not uncommon for clots to occlude the catheter. The bladder must remain decompressed for several days to promote proper healing. If clots occlude the end of the catheter, gentle irrigation or aspiration may be necessary. If the clot cannot be dislodged or aspirated out, it may be necessary to change the catheter. Painful bladder spasms also can occur, and opiates, usually in the form of a belladonna and opium suppository, may be required to relax the bladder.

Immunosuppression

Initiation of induction immunosuppressant therapy begins at the time of transplantation, usually in the form of a polyclonal antithymocyte/antilymphocyte intravenous compound or an intravenous monoclonal antibody compound. These compounds remove the lymphocytes from the patient's system, preventing rejection and suppressing the immune system until oral medications can be safely administered and blood levels are sufficient to allow discontinuation of the intravenous agent. Because the patient is now immunocompromised, strict aseptic technique is required to prevent infection.

Infection Risk

Thorough hand washing, aseptic dressing changes, discontinuation of any unnecessary invasive lines, and limiting the number of visitors are necessary protective measures. Because of the patient's immunocompromised status, subtle changes in the temperature, white blood cell count, or wound drainage can signal an active infection. Patients also are susceptible to infection by opportunistic native organisms such as *Candida*, pneumocystis pneumonia, CMV, Epstein-Barr virus, and herpes simplex virus.

Kidney Graft Nonfunction

If the kidney is not functioning in the immediate postoperative period, the patient's fluid status must be monitored very closely.

BOX 37-18 SIGNS AND SYMPTOMS OF KIDNEY REJECTION

- Increased tenderness over the transplanted kidney site
- Decreased urine output
- Increased serum creatinine levels, greater than patient's baseline level
- Fever
- Rapid weight gain (4-6 pounds in a 24-hour period)
- Swelling, usually in the hands and feet

Hypervolemia in these patients may be so great that respiratory compromise occurs. Electrolyte dilution resulting from the fluid overload is a concern. Output monitoring and bladder decompression still must be maintained. If kidney function is slow to recover, a continuous dopamine infusion may be initiated at a rate of 3 mcg/kg/min to increase urine output. Close observation of blood pressure is necessary to observe for potentially serious hypertension that would require medical management. If significant fluid overload or respiratory compromise occurs, oxygen therapy and dialysis treatments may be necessary for several days.

Preparation for Discharge Home

The average length of stay in the hospital after uncomplicated kidney transplantation is 5 to 7 days. During the first few days, the patient must learn the self-care routines essential for graft survival. Medication regimens are complex and most centers initiate a self-medication program at the patient's bedside as a training tool. Patients are taught the signs and symptoms of infection and graft rejection (Box 37-18), the protocols of the transplant clinic, and new dietary limitations. Frequent transplant clinic visits to check the functioning of the organ and to adjust down the doses of immunosuppressant medications are necessary for the first few months after transplantation.

Long-Term Considerations

Rejection of the transplanted kidney is an ongoing concern for all of these patients. The graft function is monitored closely, and if rejection is suspected, a biopsy is performed. If the biopsy reveals acute rejection, rescue therapy is initiated. This therapy can be in the form of high-dose intravenous steroids for mild rejection or intravenous monoclonal antibody for moderate to severe rejection. If the biopsy reveals chronic rejection, the oral immunosuppressant medications are increased or returned to the higher doses used immediately after transplantation. No two patients' immune systems are exactly alike, and the immunosuppressant medication regimen required to prevent rejection must be tailored to each patient individually. The goal is to create a balance among medications that allows the patient to fight off most infections but avoid rejection of the transplanted organ.

Patient adherence to the medical regimen that is required to maintain a transplanted organ is a major concern. Adequate education of the patient and family as to the importance of taking the medications as instructed is of paramount importance. Patients are reluctant to take the medications appropriately if they are experiencing severe side effects. Decreasing the dose of the medications can often alleviate these symptoms but may lead to a rejection episode.

Patients often have financial concerns. A 1-month supply of medications can cost more than $1200, and paying for the medications over the long term is a great burden for some patients. The federal government helps to pay for the immunosuppressant medications for 36 months after transplantation.

PANCREAS TRANSPLANTATION

One of the most common causes of chronic kidney disease is Type 1 diabetes mellitus. Despite meticulous glycemic control, dietary restrictions, healthy exercise programs, and advances in disease-modifying medication regimens, many patients with type 1 diabetes mellitus develop chronic kidney disease requiring long-term dialysis treatments. Pancreas transplantation offers the opportunity of normal glucose control without the use of exogenous insulin. The first pancreas transplantation procedures were performed in 1966, with little success.[155] Advances in immunosuppressive medications, diagnosis of rejection, management of the exocrine secretions, and improved surgical techniques have dramatically improved the success rate of pancreas transplantation. Most (70%) pancreas transplantation occurs simultaneously with another organ, usually kidneys.[156] A total of 1170 pancreas transplantations were performed in 2009; all were from deceased donors.[156] The advances in immunosuppressant medications and in the diagnosis of rejection have resulted in 1-year simultaneous kidney–pancreas transplant survival of 86% and 1-year survival for pancreas transplant alone of 76%.[156]

Indications and Selection

Patients who are selected for pancreas transplantation must undergo a thorough evaluation similar to that for other transplantation candidates (Box 37-19). The disease processes involved in diabetes mellitus and their effects on all major body systems require that special care be taken to ensure the candidate is in the best possible condition before transplantation. Severe and often life-threatening complications can occur

BOX 37-19   EVALUATION BEFORE PANCREAS TRANSPLANTATION

- Blood chemistries, tissue typing, and viral studies similar to those for kidney transplantation candidates
- Complete cardiovascular workup, including cardiac catheterization
- Complete vascular studies, particularly of the lower extremities, to ensure proper vascularization of the graft
- Nerve conduction studies to evaluate for neuropathy
- Urologic and bladder function studies
- Consultations as required for all transplantation candidates

after transplantation if the major body systems have not been properly evaluated beforehand. As with other organ transplants, organ allocation is managed through the OPTN/UNOS registry.[149]

Pancreas Transplantation Surgical Procedure

The surgical techniques for pancreas transplantation are diverse, and different programs use different methods. The principles are consistent, however, and all include these three precepts:

1. Provide adequate arterial blood flow to the pancreas and duodenal segment
2. Provide adequate venous outflow from the pancreas
3. Provide management of the pancreatic exocrine secretions

The cold-ischemia time of the pancreas before implantation should be minimized as pancreas allografts do not tolerate cold ischemia as well as kidney allografts do. Ideally, the pancreas should be revascularized within 24 hours from the time of cross-clamping.

The abdomen is entered through a midline incision. The pancreas graft is transplanted into the right iliac fossa, with the head of the pancreas placed downward into the pelvis.[155] Most transplantation centers place both organs on the right side, although some put the pancreas on the right and the kidney on the left. The native pancreas is not removed.[157]

Arterial and Venous Revascularization

Arterial flow to the pancreas graft is provided from the recipient's iliac artery (Fig. 37-17). Venous outflow from the transplanted graft can be via an anastomosis to the portal vein

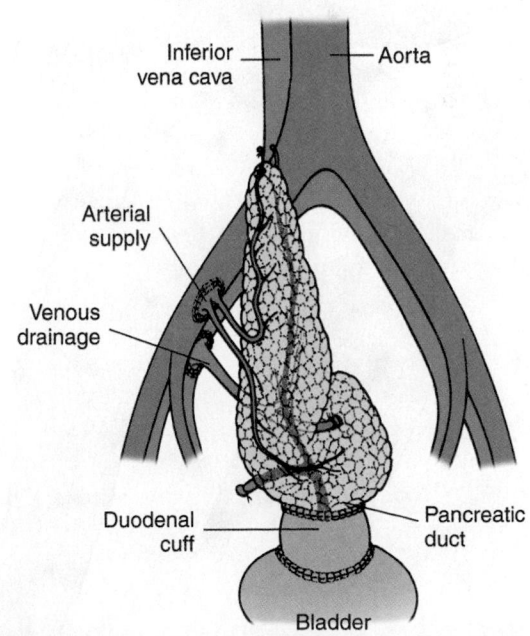

FIGURE 37-17 Exocrine management by urinary diversion. (Modified from Smith SL. *AACN Tissue and Organ Transplantation: Implications for Professional Nursing Practice.* St. Louis: Mosby; 1990.)

or to the iliac vein.[155] The iliac vein is more commonly used,[155] and graft outcomes and survival are similar with both venous anastomosis methods.[158]

Exocrine Drainage

The exocrine drainage of the pancreas presents one of the most challenging aspects of the transplantation procedure. The head of the pancreas is positioned to drain downward into either the bowel or the bladder, depending on the surgical technique that is used.

Enteric Exocrine Drainage. Enteric drainage is the draining of pancreatic exocrine secretions into the bowel. The pancreas and a segment of the donor duodenum are transplanted onto the recipient's small bowel. All of the enzymes drain into the bowel and are excreted with the stool. Exocrine drainage into the duodenum most closely approximates normal physiology. Unfortunately, complications with the side-to-side anastomosis can cause peritonitis. To decrease this risk, a roux-en-Y duodenojejunostomy is constructed (Fig. 37-18).[155] One disadvantage of enteric drainage is that it is not possible to monitor pancreatic enzymes as a direct measure of pancreatic

function. Nevertheless, enteric drainage is more commonly used.[155]

Bladder Exocrine Drainage. Bladder drainage is the draining of pancreatic exocrine secretions into the bladder (see Fig. 37-15). A major advantage of this method is that direct monitoring of graft function is possible by measuring urinary amylase. A decrease in urinary amylase precedes irreversible hyperglycemia associated with acute cellular rejection of the transplanted pancreas.[155] The disadvantage of bladder exocrine drainage is that it is associated with genitourinary complications such as recurrent urinary tract infections, prostatitis, urethritis, and hematuria. Other complications include urinary bicarbonate loss and metabolic acidodis.[155] Surgical conversion to enteric drainage is required in 30% of pancreas transplant patients within 5 years and 50% of patients within 15 years.[155]

Postoperative Medical Management and Nursing Care

After surgery, the patient is taken to the critical care unit. Even though these patients now have a functioning pancreas, they are at high risk for surgical complications because of the long-term effects of diabetes. Oxygenation, hemodynamics, and cardiac status must be monitored closely. If simultaneous kidney–pancreas transplantation is performed, fluid and electrolyte management is indicated, including intravenous fluid replacement, monitoring of intake and output, and measurements of potassium, blood urea nitrogen, and creatinine levels. A nasogastric tube is usually placed and remains for 24 to 48 hours after surgery. A continuous insulin drip may be used to prevent hyperglycemia until the new pancreas graft is fully functional. Frequent blood glucose monitoring is essential for patient safety while the continuous insulin infusion is in place.

The same aseptic techniques used for kidney transplant recipients are used for pancreas transplant recipients. An increased potential for urinary catheter occlusion exists for pancreas recipients who have undergone a urinary diversion procedure. The exocrine pancreatic enzymes make the urine more viscous, and may irritate the anastomosis site on the bladder, causing an increased risk of bleeding. The same gentle aspiration techniques described earlier can be used to clear out the clots. Continuous bladder irrigation may be necessary to keep the catheter patent. Relevant Nursing Diagnoses are listed in Box 37-20.

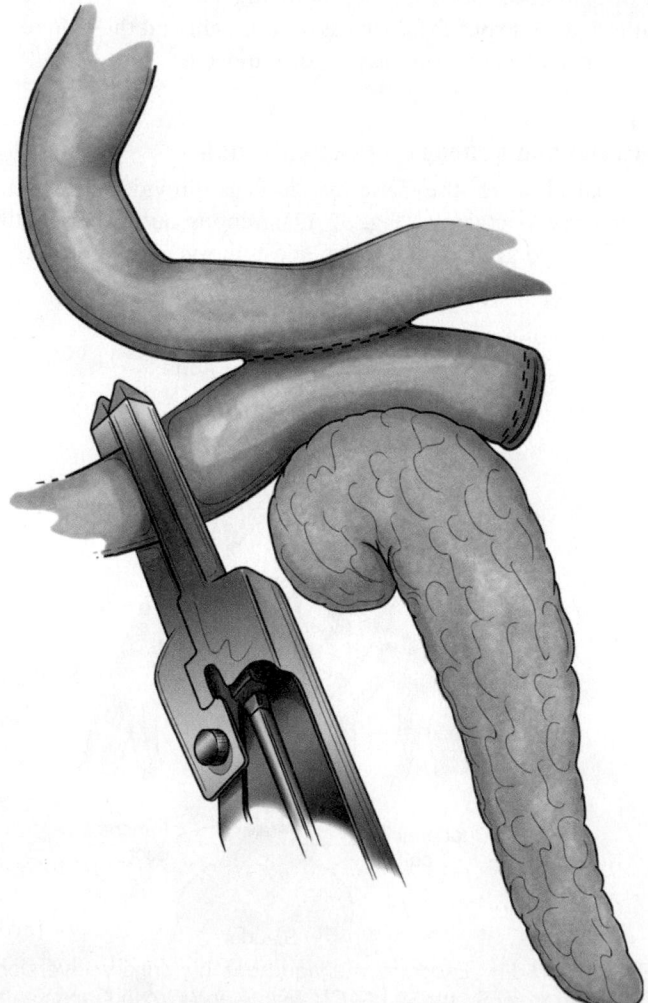

FIGURE 37-18 Exocrine management by bowel diversion. A segment of the donor bowel remains attached to minimize handling of pancreas.

◎ BOX 37-20   NURSING DIAGNOSES

Pancreas Transplantation

- Risk for Infection: Immunosuppressive medications required to prevent rejection of pancreas, p. 1160
- Imbalanced Nutrition: Less Than Body Requirements related to lack of exogenous nutrients and increased metabolic demand, p. 1143
- Disturbed Body Image related to actual change in body structure, function, or appearance, p. 1136
- Anxiety related to threat to biologic, psychologic, and social integrity, p. 1125
- Activity Intolerance related to prolonged immobility or deconditioning, p. 1119

Long-Term Considerations

Rejection in this patient population can be very difficult to detect. Serum amylase levels after pancreas-only transplantation are not effective in monitoring graft function, and blood glucose levels become elevated only in the late stages of rejection. Urine amylase levels in patients with the urinary diversion are an effective means of monitoring for rejection. If kidney transplantation has been performed simultaneously, an increase in the serum creatinine level is predictive of rejection. Because of the fragility of pancreas tissue, a pancreas biopsy is rarely performed. However, a kidney biopsy specimen may be obtained to determine rejection and treatment options. Treatment of pancreas rejection is the same as for all other types of organ rejection.

Adherence to the medication regimen is always a concern. It is very important that the patient take the immunosuppressants as prescribed by the physician. Patients with functional pancreas grafts continue to need glucose monitoring at home but often forget to continue this practice after they no longer require insulin. Continued monitoring with frequent clinic visits is required for several months after pancreas transplantation.

Islet Cell Transplantation

Islet cell transplantation continues to be investigational. One major emphasis is to reduce the number of donor pancreases required from 2 to 4 per recipient down to a single donor per recipient.[159] This would simultaneously increase the number of potential donor pancreas islets and decrease recipient exposure to the multiple HLA antigens associated with multiple donors.[159]

BOX 37-21 CASE STUDY

Patient with a Transplant

Brief Patient History

Mr. V is a 42-year-old man with chronic viral hepatitis C. He has a Model for End-Stage Liver Disease (MELD) score greater than 25. Mr. V is in acute fulminant liver failure and is on the waiting list to receive a liver transplant. Mr. V was hospitalized 2 weeks ago with ascites, hepatorenal syndrome, and hepatic encephalopathy. He has been treated with diuretics, antibiotics, and laxatives. Before transplantation, he remained in the intermediate care unit and was not intubated. He is now undergoing liver transplantation.

Clinical Assessment

Mr. V is admitted to the critical care unit from the operating room after receiving an orthotopic liver transplant. He is intubated and sedated. Mr. V moves all extremities but does not follow commands. He has a nasogastric tube, pulmonary artery catheter, arterial line, urinary catheter, abdominal drain (draining bright red blood), and external biliary drain in place. Continuous renal replacement therapy (CRRT) is in progress.

Diagnostic Procedures

Baseline vital signs include the following: blood pressure of 100/60 mm Hg, heart rate of 118 beats/min (sinus tachycardia), respiratory rate of 20 breaths/min, temperature of 98.3° F, and O_2 saturation of 98%.
Urine output was 75 mL/hr and is now 15 mL/hr. Central venous pressure is 14 mm Hg, pulmonary artery pressure is 30/16 mm Hg, pulmonary artery occlusion pressure (wedge pressure) is 18 mm Hg, and intra-abdominal pressure is greater than 25 mm Hg.
His current laboratory values include the following:
White blood cell count: 3100 cells/mm³
Hematocrit: 25.3%

Hemoglobin: 8.6 g/dL
Platelet count: 47,000/microliter
Aspartate aminotransferase: 315 U/L
Aminotransferase: 230 U/L
Alkaline phosphatase: 380 U/L
Gamma-glutamyltransferase: 1040 U/L
Total bilirubin: 12.5 mg/dL
Prothrombin time: 21.3 seconds
International normalized ratio: 2.5
Partial thromboplastin time: 69.9 seconds
Blood urea nitrogen: 39 mg/dL
Serum creatinine: 1.4 mg/dL
Potassium: 3.8 mEq/L (mmol/L)

Medical Diagnosis

Mr. V is diagnosed with intra-abdominal hypertension and abdominal compartment syndrome.

Questions

1. What major outcomes do you expect to achieve for this patient?
2. What problems or risks must be managed to achieve these outcomes?
3. What interventions must be initiated to monitor, prevent, manage, or eliminate the problems and risks identified?
4. What interventions should be initiated to promote optimal functioning, safety, and well-being of the patient?
5. What possible learning needs do you anticipate for this patient?
6. What cultural and age-related factors may have a bearing on the patient's plan of care?

SUMMARY

Organ Donation

- The fields of organ donation and solid organ transplantation have made dramatic progress in the past 50 years. There is every reason to believe that this trajectory will continue. As transplantation becomes more widespread, more nurses will encounter patients who have undergone solid organ transplantation. Even more likely is that critical care nurses will assist with the care of a potential organ donor.

Knowledge of the rationales for care is essential to delivering safe and high-quality patient care.
- There are 58 OPOs in the United States, Puerto Rico, Guam, and Bermuda. They are nonprofit corporations that provide organ donation services to a designated regional area.
- There are many more individuals listed for transplants than the number of donor organs available.

- The recipient of an organ transplant is required to adhere to a strict regimen of immunosuppressive medications to avoid rejection of the organ by the recipient's own immune system, which recognizes the foreign graft as nonself. The immunosuppressants increase vulnerability to infection. The goal is to create a balance among medications that allows the patient to fight off most infections but avoid rejection of the transplanted organ.

Heart Transplantation

- The transplanted heart must come from a deceased donor. Immediate postoperative management of the heart transplant recipient is similar to that for patients undergoing other heart surgery procedures.

Lung Transplantation

- Transplanted lungs come from a deceased donor. Lungs have a limited ischemic time of about 4 hours, which limits the geographic area for donor procurement, and relatively few are available for donation.

Liver Transplantation

- Liver transplants may come from a deceased donor or from a living donor who donates a section of the liver. Before transplantation, the severity of liver disease and level of placement on the transplantation waiting list is determined by the MELD score for anyone older than 12 years. The postoperative course is highly variable. Many liver transplant recipients were encephalopathic before transplantation and may have a complicated course afterward. Other patients who have a lower MELD score and receive a functional liver may recover very quickly and should be alert and oriented within 1 to 2 days.

Kidney Transplantation

- Kidney transplants come from a deceased donor or from a living donor who donates one kidney. Postoperative management of fluid status is vital to ensure that the kidney is functional and to avoid volume overload. The bladder must remain decompressed by a urinary catheter for several days to promote effective healing.

Pancreas Transplantation

- Pancreas transplantation is usually performed in tandem with kidney transplantation, because most recipients have type 1 diabetes mellitus that has caused their kidneys to fail.

REFERENCES

1. Linden PK. History of solid organ transplantation and organ donation. *Crit Care Clin.* 2009;1(25):165.
2. Organ Procurement and Transplantation Network. http://optn.transplant.hrsa.gov. Accessed May 7, 2012.
3. Federal Register/Vol. 63, No. 119/Monday, June 22, 1998/Rules and Regulations. 33856-33875;US Department of Health and Human Services; Health Care Financing Administration 42 CFR Part 482 [HCFA-3005 F] RIN: 0938-AI95.
4. Tamburri LM. The role of critical care nurse in the organ donation breakthrough collaborative. *Crit Care Nurse.* 2006;2(26):20.
5. Walton-Tanner. Maximizing organ donation through aggressive donor management. *Am Nurse Today.* 2011;6:2.
6. Siminoff LA, Traino HM. Improving donation outcomes: hospital development and the rapid assessment of hospital procurement barriers in donation. *Prog Transplant.* 2009;19(2):180.
7. Shafer TJ, et al. U.S. organ donation breatkthrough collaborative increases organ donation. *Crit Care Nurse Q.* 2008;51(3):190.
8. Shafer TJ, et al. Organ donation breakthrough collaborative: increasing organ donation through system redesign. *Crit Care Nurse.* 2006;26(2):44.
9. Shafer TJ, et al. The organ donation breakthrough collaborative. In: LaPointe-Rudow D, Ohler L, Shafer TJ, eds. *A Clinician's Guide to Donation and Transplantation.* Lenexa, KS: Applied Measurement Professionals, Inc; 2006:711.
10. Siminoff LA, et al. Factors influencing families' consent for donation of solid organs for transplantation. *JAMA.* 2001;286(1):71.
11. *Revised Uniform Anatomical Gift Act; 2006.* National Conference of Commissioners on Uniform State Law, July 7-14, 2006.
12. Shafer TJ. The forensic nurse examiner and organ donation: a partnership for life. In: Lynch V, ed. *Forensic Nursing.* St. Louis: Mosby; 2006.
13. Rushton CH. Donation after cardiac death: ethical implications and implementation strategies. *AACN Adv Crit Care Nurse.* 2006;17(3):345.
14. Wijdicks EFM. The clinical diagnosis of brain death. In: *The Comatose Patient.* New York: Oxford University Press, Inc. 2008:102-103.
15. Bernat JL, et al. The circulatory-respiratory determination of death in organ donation. *Crit Care Med.* 2010;38(3):963.
16. Non-Heart Beating Organ Transplantation, Practice and Protocols, Institute of Medicine, Committee on Non-Heart-Beating Transplantation II: The Scientific and Ethical Basis for Practice and Protocol. Division of Healthcare Services Institute of Medicine. Washington, DC: National Academy of Sciences; 2000:9.
17. Sills P, et al. Donation after cardiac death: lessons learned. *J Trauma Nurs.* 2007;14(1):47.
18. Edwards J, et al. Maximizing organ donation opportunities through donation after cardiac death. In: LaPointe-Rudow D, Ohler L, Shafer TJ, eds. *A Clinician's Guide to Donation and Transplantation.* Lenexa, KS: Applied Measurement Professionals, Inc. 2006:878.
19. Pine JK, et al. Comparable outcomes in donation after cardiac death and donation after brainstem death: a matched analysis of renal transplants. *Transplant Proc.* 2010;42(10):3947.
20. Reich DJ, Hong JC. Current status of donation after cardiac death liver transplantation. *Curr Opin Organ Transplant.* 2010;15(3):316.

21. De Oliveira NC, et al. Lung transplantation with donation after cardiac death donors: long-term follow-up in a single center. *J Thorac Cardiovasc Surg.* 2010;139(5):1306.

22. Siminoff LA, et al. Requesting organ donation: effective communication. In: LaPointe-Rudow D, Ohler L, Shafer TJ, eds. *A Clinician's Guide to Donation and Transplantation.* Lenexa, KS: Applied Measurement Professionals, Inc; 2006:878.

23. Anker AE, Feely TH. Why families decline donation: the perspective of the organ procurement coordinators. *Prog Transplant.* 2010;20(3):239.

24. Strouder DB, et al. Family, faith and friends: how organ donor families heal. *Prog Transplant.* 2009;19(4):358.

25. Wood K, et al. Care of the potential organ donor. *N Engl J Med.* 2004;351:2730.

26. Haddon R, et al. Brain Death and Management of the Organ Donor. In: Albert RK, ed. Critical Care Medicine. Philadelphia, PA: Mosby; 2006.

27. McKeown DW, et al. Management of the heartbeating brain-dead organ donor. *Br J Anaesth.* 2012;108(suppl 1):96.

28. Van Gelder FEL, Ohler L. Basics in transplant immunology. In: Ohler L, Cupples S, eds. *Core Curriculum for Transplant Nurses.* Philadelphia: Mosby; 2008.

29. Kroemer A, et al. The innate natural killer cells in transplant rejection and tolerance induction. *Curr Opin Organ Transplant.* 2008;13:339.

30. Schuster M, et al. B-cell activation and allosensitization after left ventricular assist device implantation is due to T-cell activation and CD40 ligand expression. *Human Immunol.* 2002;63:211.

31. Costello A, Pearson GJ. Transplant pharmacology. In: Ohler L, Cupples S, eds. *Core Curriculum for Transplant Nurses.* Philadelphia: Mosby; 2008.

32. White M, et al. Pharmacokinetic, hemodynamic, and metabolic effects of cyclosporine Sandimmune versus the microemulsion Neoral in heart transplant recipients. *J Heart Lung Transplant.* 1997;16:787.

33. Meulle EA, et al. Pharmacokinetics and tolerability of a microemulsion formulation of cyclosporine in renal allograft recipients: a concentration controlled comparison with the commercial formulation. *Transplantation.* 1994;57:1178.

34. Steinberg SM, et al. Randomized, open label preference study of two cyclosporine capsule formulations (USP modified) in stable solid-organ transplant recipients. *Clin Ther.* 2003;25(7):2037.

35. Vincenti F, et al. Results of an international randomized trial comparing glucose metabolism disorders and outcome with cyclosporine versus tacrolimus. *Am J Transplant.* 2007;7:1506.

36. Ye F, et al. Tacrolimus versus cyclosporine microemulsion for heart transplant recipients: a meta-analysis. *J Heart Lung Transplantation.* 2009;28(1):58.

37. Fan Y, et al. Tacrolimus versus cyclosporine for adult lung transplant recipients: a meta-analysis. *Transplant Proc.* 2009;41:1821.

38. Webster AC, et al. Tacrolimus versus cyclosporin as primary immunosuppression for kidney transplant recipients. *Cochrane Database Syst Rev.* 2005;(4):CD003961.

39. Haddad E, et al. Cyclosporine versus tacrolimus for liver transplanted patients. *Cochrane Database Syst Rev.* 2006;(4):CD008852.

40. Bullingham RE, et al. Clinical pharmacokinetics of mycophenolate mofetil. *Clin Pharmacokinet.* 1998;34:429.

41. Kobashigawa JA, et al. A randomized active-controlled trial of mycophenolate mofetil in heart transplant recipients. mycophenolate mofetil investigators. *Transplantation.* 1998;66:4.

42. Eisen HJ, et al. Three year results of a randomized double blind controlled trial of mycophenolate mofetil versus azathioprine in cardiac transplant recipients. *J Heart Lung Transplant.* 2005;24:5.

43. Kobashigawa JA, et al. Mycophenolate mofetil reduces intimal thickness by intravascular ultrasound after heart transplant: reanalysis of the multicenter trial. *Am J Transplant.* 2006;6:5.

44. Behrend M. Adverse gastrointestinal effects of mycophenolate mofetil. *Drug Safety.* 2001;24:645.

45. Budde K, et al. Enteric coated mycophenolate sodium can be safely administered in maintenance renal transplant patients: results of a 1 year study. *Am J Transplant.* 2004;4:237.

46. Salvadori M, et al. Enteric coated mycophenolate sodium is therapeutically equivalent to mycophenolate mofetil in de novo renal transplant patients. *Am J Transplant.* 2004;4:231.

47. Kobashigawa JA, et al. Similar efficacy and safety of enteric coated mycophenolate sodium compared with mycophenolate mofetil in de novo heart transplant recipients: results of a 12 month single blind randomized parallel group multicenter study. *J Heart Lung Transplant.* 2006;25:935.

48. Ingle GT, et al. Sirolimus: continuing the evolution of transplant immunosuppression. *Ann Pharmacother.* 2000;34:1044.

49. McAlister VC, et al. Sirolimus-tacrolimus combination immunosuppression. *Lancet.* 2000;355:376.

50. Radovancevic B, Vrtovec B. Sirolimus therapy in cardiac transplantation. *Transplant Proc.* 2003;35:171S.

51. Machado PG, et al. An open-label randomized trial of the safety and efficacy of sirolimus vs. azathioprine in living related renal allograft recipients receiving cyclosporine and prednisone combination. *Clin Transplant.* 2004;18(1):28.

52. Keogh A, et al. Sirolimus in de novo heart transplant recipients reduces acute rejection and prevents coronary artery disease at 2 years: a randomized clinical trial. *Circulation.* 2004;110:2694.

53. Mancini D, et al. Use of rapamycin slows progression of cardiac transplantation vasculopathy. *Circulation.* 2003;108:48.

54. Eisen H, et al. Everolimus for the prevention of allograft rejection and vasculopathy in cardiac transplant recipients. *N Engl J Med.* 2003;349:847.

55. Keogh A, et al. Sirolimus in de novo heart transplant recipients reduces acute rejection and prevents coronary artery disease at 2 years: a randomized clinical trial. *Circulation.* 2004;110:2694.

56. Kobashigawa JA, et al. Tacrolimus with mycophenolate mofetil (MMF) or sirolimus vs. cyclosporine with MMF in cardiac transplant patients: 1-year report. *Am J Transplant.* 2006;6:1377.

57. Kuppahally S, et al. Wound healing complications with de novo sirolimus versus mycophenolate mofetil-based regimen in cardiac transplant recipients. *Am J Transplant.* 2006;6:986.

58. Kahan BD, et al. Immunosuppressive effects and safety of a sirolimus/cyclosporine combination regime for renal transplantation. *Transplantation.* 1998;66:1040.

59. Watson CJE, et al. Sirolimus: a potent new immunosuppressant for liver transplantation. *Transplantation.* 1999;67:505.

60. Pascual J. Everolimus (Certican) in renal transplantation: a review of clinical trial data, current usage and future directions. *Transplant Rev.* 2006;20:1.

61. Gurk-Turner C, et al. A comprehensive review of everolimus clinical reports: a new mammalian target of rapaycin inhibitor. *Transplantation.* 2012;94(7):659.

62. MacDonald A, et al. Clinical pharmacokinetics and therapeutic drug monitoring of sirolimus. *Clin Ther.* 2000;22:B101.

63. Böhler T, et al. Pharmacodynamic effects of everolimus on anti-CD3 antibody-stimulated T-lymphocyte proliferation and interleukin-10 synthesis in stable kidney-transplant patients. *Cytokine.* 2008;42:306.

64. Valantine H, et al. From clinical trials to clinical practice: an overview of Certican (everolimus) in heart transplantation. *J Heart Lung Transplant.* 2005;24:S185.

65. Pascual J. Concentration controlled everolimus (Certican): combination with reduced dose calcineurin inhibitors. *Transplantation.* 2005;79:S76.

66. Vitko S, et al. Everolimus (Certican) 12 months safety and efficacy versus mycophenolate mofetil in de novo renal transplant recipients. *Transplantation.* 2004;78:1532.

67. Chapman HR, et al. Proliferation signal inhibitors in transplantation: questions at the cutting edge of everolimus therapy. *Transplant Proc.* 2007;39:2937.

68. Rothenburger M, et al. Calcineurin inhibitor free immunosuppression using everolimus (Certican) in maintenance heart transplant recipients: 6 months follow up. *J Heart Lung Transplant.* 2007;26:250.

69. Scientific Registry of Transplant Recipients. OPTN/SRTR Annual Report. http://www.srtr.org/annual_reports/2010/109a_dh.htm. Accessed May 23, 2012.

70. Van Gelder T, et al. A randomized trial comparing safety and efficacy of OKT3 and a monoclonal anti-interleukin-2 receptor antibody (BT563) in the prevention of acute rejection after heart transplantation. *Transplantation.* 1996;62:51.

71. Webster A, et al. Interleukin 2 receptor antagonists for renal transplant recipients: a meta-analysis of randomized trials. *Transplantation.* 2004;77:166.

72. Kirk AD, et al. Results from a human renal allograft tolerance trial evaluating the humanized CD52-specific monoclonal antibody alemtuzumab (CAMPATH-1H). *Transplantation.* 2003;76:120.

73. Knechtle SJ, et al. Campath-1H induction plus rapamycin monotherapy for renal transplantation: results of a pilot study. *Am J Transplant.* 2003;3:722.

74. Morgan RD, et al. Alemtuzumab Induction therapy in kidney transplantation: a systematic review and meta-analysis. *Transplantation.* 2012. (Epub ahead of print.)

75. Weissenbacker A, et al. Alemtuzumab in solid organ transplantation and in composite tissue allotransplantation. *Immunotherapy.* 2010;2(6):783.

76. Health Resources and Services Administration. Transplants in the US by Region. http://optn.transplant.hrsa.gov/latestData/rptData.asp. Accessed December 7, 2012.

77. Hartley C, et al. Heart transplantation. In: Ohler L, Cupples S, eds. *Core Curriculum for Transplant Nurses.* Philadelphia: Mosby Elsevier; 2008.

78. Stehlik J, et al. Registry of the International Society for Heart and Lung Transplantation: twenty-seventh official adult heart transplant report—2010. *J Heart Lung Transplant.* 2010;29(10):1089.

79. Aliabadi AZ, et al. Immunosuppressive therapy in older cardiac transplant patients. *Drugs Aging.* 2007;24:913.

80. Weiss ES, et al. Outcomes in patients older than 60 years of age undergoing orthotopic heart transplantation: an analysis of the UNOS database. *J Heart Lung Transplant.* 2008;27(2):184.

81. Cannon RM, et al. A review of the United States experience with combined heart-liver transplantation. *Transplant Internat.* 2012;25:1223.

82. Health Resources and Services Administration. Regional Data. http://optn.transplant.hrsa.gov/latestData/stateData.asp?type=region. Accessed May 23, 2012.

83. Lower RR, Shumway NE. Studies on the orthotopic homotransplantations of the canine heart. *Surg Forum.* 1960;11:18.

84. Sievers HH, et al. An alternative technique for orthotopic cardiac transplantation with preservation of the normal anatomy of the right atrium. *Thorac Cardiovasc.* 1991;39:70.

85. Schnoor M, et al. Bicaval versus standard technique in orthotopic heart transplantation: a systematic review and meta-analysis. *J Thorac Cardiovasc Surg.* 2007;134(5):1322.

86. Stewart S, et al. Revision of the 1990 working formulation for the standardization of nomenclature in the diagnosis of heart rejection. *J Heart Lung Transplant.* 2005;24:1710.

87. Pham MX, et al. Molecular testing for long-term rejection surveillance in heart transplant recipients: design of the invasive monitoring attenuation through gene expression (IMAGE) trial. *J Heart Lung Transplant.* 2007;26(8):808.

88. Pham MX, et al. Gene-expression profiling for rejection surveillance after cardiac transplantation. *New Engl J Med.* 2010;362:1890.

89. Centers for Disease Control and Prevention. Cytomegalovirus (CMV) and Congenital CMV Infection. http://www.cdc.gov/cmv/index.html. Accessed May 25, 2012.

90. Bonaros N, et al. CMV-hyperimmune globulin for preventing cytomegalovirus infection and disease in solid organ transplant recipients: a meta-analysis. *Clin Transplant.* 2008;22(1):89.

91. Decampli WM, et al. Characteristics of patients surviving more than ten years after cardiac transplantation. *J Thorac Cardiovasc Surg.* 1995;109:1103.

92. Lough ME, et al. Impact of symptom frequency and symptom distress on self-reported quality of life in heart transplant recipients. *Heart Lung.* 1987;16:193.

93. Evans RW, et al. *The National Heart Transplantation Study: Final Report.* Seattle: Batelle Human Affairs Research Centers; 1984.

94. White-Williams C, et al. Factors associated with work status at 5 and 10 years after heart transplantation. *Clin Transplant.* 2011;25:E599.

95. Scientific Registry of Transplant Recipients. OPTN/SRTR Annual Report. http://www.srtr.org/annual_reports/2010/data_tables.htm#XI. Accessed May 25, 2012.

96. Reitz B. The first successful combined heart-lung transplantation. *J Thorac Cardiovasc Surg.* 2011;141(4):867.

97. Deuse T, et al. Review of heart-lung transplantation at Stanford. *Ann Thorac Surg.* 2010;90:329.

98. The International Society for Heart Lung Transplantation; 2011. *J Heart Lung Transplant.* 2011;30(10):1071-1132. http://www.ishlt.org/registries/slides.asp?slides=heartLungRegistry. Accessed April 21, 2012.

99. Lynch JP III, Ross DJ. *Lung & Heart-Lung Transplantation.* New York: 2006.

100. Stuart FP, et al. *Organ Transplantation.* 2nd ed. Georgetown, TX: 2003:280.

101. Snell GI, Westall GP. Selection and management of the lung donor. *Clin Chest Med.* 2011;32:223.

102. Naik PN, Angel LF. Special issues in the management and selection of the donor for lung transplantation. *Semin Immunopathol.* 2011;33:201.

103. Boasquevisque CHR, et al. Surgical techniques: lung transplant and lung volume reduction. *Proc Am Thorac Soc.* 2009;6:66.

104. Martinu T, et al. Acute allograft rejection: cellular and humoral processes. *Clin Chest Med.* 2011;32:295.

105. Remund KF, et al. Infections relevant to lung transplantation. *Proc Amer Thorac Soc.* 2009;6(1):94.

106. Solea A, Salavert M. Fungal infections after lung transplantation. *Transplant Rev.* 2008;22:89.

107. Kotton CN. Management of cytomegalovirus infection in solid organ transplantation. *Nat Rev Nephrol.* 2010;6:711.

108. Ahmad S, et al. Pulmonary complication of lung transplantation. *Chest.* 2011;139(2):402.

109. The International Society for Heart Lung Transplantation Registry. *J Heart Lung Transplant.* 2007;26:782.

110. The U.S. Organ Procurement and Transplantation Network and the Scientific Registry of Transplant Recipients. 2010 OPTN / SRTR Annual Report: Transplant Data 2000-2009. http://srtr.transplant.hrsa.gov/annual_reports/2010/pdf/06_lung_11.pdf. Accessed April 21, 2012.

111. Braun AT, Melo CA. Cystic fibrosis lung transplantation. *Curr Opin Pulm Med.* 2011;17:467.

112. Patel N, et al. Lung transplantation and lung volume reduction surgery versus transplantation in chronic obstructive pulmonary disease. *Proc Am Thorac Soc.* 2008;5(4):447.

113. Knoop C, Estenne M. Chronic allograft dysfunction. *Clin Chest Med.* 2011;32:311.

114. Bhorade SM, et al. Lung transplant considerations for the community pulmonologist. *Transplant Network Amer Coll Chest Phys.* 2007. http://accpstorage.org/networks/LungTX.pdf. Accessed April 14, 2012.

115. Starzl TE, et al. Orthotopic homotransplantation of the human liver. *Ann Surg.* 1968;168(3):392.

116. National Institutes of Health. National Institutes of Health Consensus Development Conference Statement: liver transplantation—June 20-23, 1983. *Hepatology.* 1984;4(1S):107S.

117. Scientific Registry of Transplant Recipients. Annual Report on Liver Transplantation. http://srtr.transplant.hrsa.gov/annual_reports/2010/pdf/03_liver_11.pdf. Accessed December 15, 2012.

118. Kamath BM, Olthoff KM. Liver transplantation in children: Update 2010. *Ped Clin North Am.* 2010;57(2).

119. Pelletier SJ, et al. Effect of body mass index on the survival benefit of liver transplantation. *Liver Transplant.* 2007;13(12):1678.

120. Lipschutz GS, Busuttil RW. Liver transplantation in those of advancing age: the case for transplantation. *Liver Transplant.* 2007;13(10):1355.

121. Cappell M. Breaking the age barrier for liver transplantation. *Gastroenterol Nurs.* 2009;31(4):301.

122. Rosen CB, et al. Liver transplantation for cholangiocarcinoma. *Transplant Internat.* 2010;23(7):692.

123. Nissen N. Emerging role of transplantation for primary liver cancer. *Cancer J.* 2010;10(2):88.

124. United network for Organ Sharing (UNOS) MELD/PELD Calculator. http://www.unos.org/docs/MELD_PELD_Calculator_Documentation.pdf. Accessed March 23, 2012.

125. Abrams P, Marsh J. Current approach to hepatocellular carcinoma. *Surg Clin North Am.* 2010;98(4):803.

126. Kendall K, O'Dell M. Psychosocial issues in transplantation. In: Ohler L, Cupples S, eds. *Core Curriculum for Transplant Nurses.* St. Louis: Mosby; 2008.

127. Zhao V, Ziegler T. Nutritional support in end-stage liver disease. *Critical Care Nurs Clin North Am.* 2010;22(3):369.

128. Urbani L. The role of immunomodulation in ABO-incompatible adult liver transplant recipients. *J Clin Apher.* 2008;23(2):55.

129. Haring T, O'Mahoney C, Goss J. Extended criteria donors in liver transplantation. *Clin Liver Dis.* 2011;15(4):879.

130. Tan H, Marcos A, Shapiro R. *Living Donor Transplantation.* New York: Informa Health Care USA, Inc; 2009.

131. Adcock L, et al. Adult living liver donors have excellent long term medical outcomes: The University of Toronto Liver Transplant Experience. *Amer J Transplant.* 2010;10:364.

132. Lapointe-Rudow D, Goldstein MJ. Critical care management of the liver transplant recipient. *Crit Care Nurs Q.* 2008;31(3):232.

133. Ghobrial RM, et al. Donor morbidity after living donation for liver transplantation. *Gastroenterology.* 2008;135(2):468.

134. Ringe B, Strong R. The dilemma of living related liver death: to report or not to report. *Transplantation.* 2008;85(6):790-793.

135. Ammori JB, et al. Effect of intraoperative hyperglycemia during liver transplantation. *J Surg Res.* 2007;140(2):227.

136. Wallia A, et al. Post-transplant hyperglycemia is associated with increased risk of liver allograft rejection. *Transplantation.* 2010;89(2):222.

137. Kumar D, Humar A, eds. *The AST Handbook of Transplant Infections.* Hoboken, NJ: Blackwell Publishing; 2011.

138. Grogan T. Liver transplantation: issues and nursing care requirements. *Crit Care Nurs Clin North Am.* 2011;23(3):443.

139. Ford E, John E. Patient education for the transplant recipient. In: Ohler L, Cupples S, eds. *Core Curriculum for Transplant Nurses.* St. Louis: Mosby; 2008:51.

140. Kendall K, O'Dell M. Psychosocial issues in transplantation. In: Ohler L, Cupples S, eds. *Core Curriculum for Transplant Nurses.* St. Louis: Mosby; 2008:629.

141. Hoch D, Maynard E, Whiting J. Billing and reimbursement for advanced practice in solid organ transplantation. *Prog Transplant.* 2011;21(4):274.

142. Levitsky J. Operational tolerance: past lessons and future prospects. *Liver Transplant.* 2011;17(3):222.

143. Grogan TA. Liver transplantation: nursing care issues. *Crit Care Nurs Clin North Am.* 2011;23(3):443.

144. Murray K, Carithers R. AASLD practice guidelines: evaluation of the patient for liver transplantation. *Hepatology.* 2005;41(6).

145. Skagen C, Lucey M, Said A. Liver transplantation: an update 2009. *Curr Opin Gastroenterol.* 2009;25(3):202.

146. Bramstedt KA. Alcohol abstinence criteria for living liver donors and their organ recipients. *Curr Opin Organ Transpl.* 2008;132:207.

147. Bonanno C, Dove L. Pregnancy after liver transplantation. *Semin Perinatol.* 2007;31(6):348.

148. Organ Procurement and Transplantation Network and Scientific Registry of Transplant Recipients. OPTN/SRTR 2010 Annual Data Report. Department of Health and Human Services, Health Resources and Services Administration, Healthcare Systems Bureau, Division of Transplantation; 2011. http://srtr.transplant.hrsa.gov/annual_reports/2010/pdf/01_kidney_11.pdf. Accessed December 12, 2012.

149. Smith JM, et al. Kidney, pancreas and liver allocation and distribution in the United States. *Amer J Transplant.* 2012;12:3191.

150. Gentry SE, et al. Kidney paired donation: fundamentals, limitations, and expansions. *Am J Kid Dis.* 2010;57(1):144.

151. Hanto RL, et al. The development of a successful multiregional kidney paired donation program. *Transplantation.* 2008;86:1744.

152. Melcher ML, et al. Chain transplantation: initial experience of a large multicenter program. *Amer J Transplant.* 2012;12:2429.

153. Leeser DB, et al. Living donor kidney paired donation transplantation: experience as a founding member center

of the National Kidney Registry. *Clin Transplant.* 2012;26: E213.

154. Forsythe LR, ed. *Transplantation: a Companion to Specialist Surgical Practice.* 3rd ed. Philadelphia: Elsevier; 2005.

155. Dhanireddy KK. Pancreas transplantation. *Gastroenterol Clin N Am.* 2012;41:133.

156. Organ Procurement and Transplantation Network and Scientific Registry of Transplant Recipients. *OPTN/SRTR 2010 Annual Data Report.* Department of Health and Human Services, Health Resources and Services Administration, Healthcare Systems Bureau, Division of Transplantation; 2011.

http://srtr.transplant.hrsa.gov/annual_reports/2010/pdf/02_pancreas_11.pdf. Accessed December 14, 2012.

157. Blakely MD, et al. Pancreas and kidney-pancreas transplantation. In: Ohler L, Cupples S, eds. *Core Curriculum for Transplant Nurses.* Philadelphia: Mosby; 2008.

158. Bazerbachi F, et al. Portal venous versus systemic venous drainage of pancreas grafts: impact on long-term results. *Amer J Transplant.* 2012;12:226.

159. Shapiro AMJ. Strategies toward single-donor islets of Langerhans transplantation. *Curr Opin Organ Transplant.* 2011;16:627.

Hematologic Disorders and Oncologic Emergencies

Mary Russell, Carol Suarez

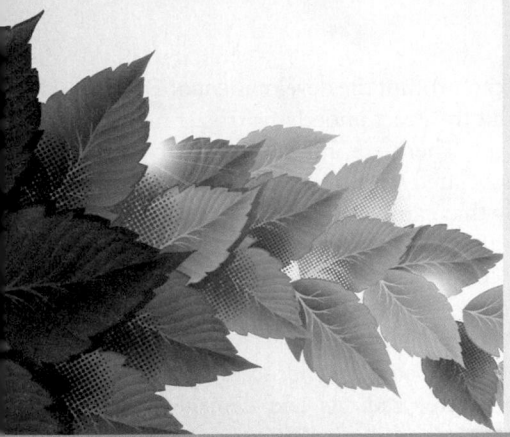

Understanding the pathology of a disease, the areas of assessment on which to focus, and the usual medical management allows the critical care nurse to more accurately anticipate and plan nursing interventions. This chapter focuses on hematologic and oncologic disorders commonly seen in the critical care environment.

OVERVIEW OF COAGULATION AND FIBRINOLYSIS

Hemostasis, the ability of the body to control bleeding and clotting, is an intricate balancing act between the coagulation mechanism and fibrinolysis. Four major actions are involved in achieving hemostasis: 1) local vasoconstriction to reduce blood flow; 2) platelet aggregation at the injury site and formation of a platelet plug; 3) formation of a fibrin mesh to strengthen the plug; and 4) dissolution of the clot after tissue repair is complete.[1] Disruption of the normal hemostatic balance can result in devastating hemorrhagic or thrombotic conditions.

Coagulation Mechanism

The coagulation mechanism consists of 13 factors that work together through a series of feedback loops to achieve hemostasis (Table 38-1 and Fig. 38-1). Depending on the initial triggering event, the extrinsic or intrinsic coagulation pathway is initiated.[1,2] The extrinsic pathway begins when vascular injury occurs, resulting in release of tissue factor and activation of coagulation factor VII. The intrinsic pathway is activated when the damaged subendothelium comes into direct contact with circulating blood. In this contact phase, proteins activate

additional coagulation factors (XII, XI, IX, and VIII).[1] At this point, the two pathways converge into a common pathway, and prothrombin and fibrinogen are converted to their active forms, resulting in clot formation.[3,4]

Clot Formation

Platelets are activated by the arrival of thrombin at the site of injury (Fig. 38-2). Local platelets change shape, become sticky, and begin to aggregate along the vessel wall. Activated platelets undergo degranulation, releasing several factors to assist in clot formation. Serotonin and histamine, two potent vasoconstrictors, help limit blood loss while the clot is forming. The prostaglandin thromboxane A_2 (TXA_2) contributes to vasoconstriction and promotes further platelet degranulation. Adenosine diphosphate (ADP) recruits platelets by increasing adherence and degranulation,[2,3] and the process continues.

At the convergence of the intrinsic and extrinsic pathways, factor X is converted into its active form, thereby enabling the conversion of prothrombin to thrombin. Thrombin then converts fibrinogen to fibrin. Strands of fibrin form and radiate around the newly formed clot, essentially creating a net in which platelets, red blood cells (RBCs), and white blood cells (WBCs) are trapped.[1] The clot is further secured to the site as platelet actomyosin causes it to contract and consolidate.[2]

Regulatory Mechanisms

Under normal conditions, feedback systems prevent the coagulation process from spinning out of control. Prostacyclin I_2 (PGI_2) is a prostaglandin released from damaged endothelial cells. It counteracts the effects of TXA_2, serotonin, and

TABLE 38-1	COAGULATION FACTORS AND COMMON NAMES
FACTOR	**COMMON NAME**
I	Fibrinogen
II	Prothrombin
III	Tissue factor
IV	Calcium
V	Proaccelerin
VI	Accelerin
VII	Proconvertin
VIII	Antihemophilic
IX	Christmas factor
X	Stuart
XI	Plasma thromboplastin antecedent
XII	Hageman factor
XIII	Fibrin stabilizing factor

histamine through vasodilation and inhibition of platelet degranulation.[1-3] Another means of regulating clot formation is through inhibition of enzymes necessary for activation of coagulation factors along the intrinsic and extrinsic pathways, preventing the conversion of prothrombin to thrombin. The most important of these regulators is antithrombin III; however, protein C and protein S also play a role in thrombin inhibition.[5]

Fibrinolysis

The process of fibrinolysis promotes dissolution and remolding of the clot to promote repair of the vessel wall and maintain flow through the vessel lumen (Fig. 38-2D). Fibrinolysis begins as soon as the fibrin clot is formed. Circulating plasminogen, a precursor to the powerful enzyme plasmin, binds to fibrin and is trapped within the newly formed clot. The injured epithelial wall releases tissue-type plasminogen activator (tPA), which converts plasminogen to its active state, plasmin. The plasmin begins to digest the fibrin, rapidly breaking down the clot.[2,4] When fibrin is broken down, the fibrin degradation products released act as anticoagulants.

DISSEMINATED INTRAVASCULAR COAGULATION

Description

Disseminated intravascular coagulation (DIC) is a syndrome that arises as a complication of other serious or life-threatening conditions. Although DIC is not seen often, it can seriously hamper diagnostic and treatment efforts for the critically ill patient. An understanding of the etiologic and pathophysiologic mechanisms of DIC can assist in anticipating the syndrome's occurrence, recognizing its signs and symptoms, and prompting intervention. Also known as consumptive *coagulopathy*, DIC is characterized by bleeding and thrombosis, both of which result from depletion of clotting factors, platelets, and

RBCs. If not treated quickly, DIC will progress to multiple organ failure and death.[6]

Etiology

Many clinical events can prompt the development of DIC in the critically ill patient, but the exact underlying trigger may not be identifiable (Box 38-1). There are, however, some commonly known conditions associated with the development of DIC.

Sepsis, particularly that caused by gram-negative organisms, can be identified as the culprit in as many as 20% of cases, making it the most common cause of DIC. In this instance, endotoxins serve as a trigger for activation of tissue factor and the extrinsic coagulation pathway. Metabolic acidosis and hypoperfusion associated with shock syndromes can result in increased formation of free radicals and damage to tissues. Tissue factor is activated, resulting in DIC. Massive trauma or burns are frequently associated with DIC. Direct tissue damage activates the extrinsic coagulation pathway, and damage to endothelial surfaces activates the intrinsic pathway.[3] Obstetric emergencies, such as abruptio placenta, retained placenta, or incomplete abortion, are also associated with the development of DIC. Tissue factor is concentrated in the placenta, and damage or disruption of this structure can activate coagulation pathways, resulting in coagulopathy.[7]

Pathophysiology

Regardless of the cause, the common thread in the development of DIC is damage to the endothelium that results in activation of the coagulation mechanism (Fig. 38-3).[1] The extrinsic coagulation pathway plays a major role in the development of DIC. Direct damage to the endothelium results in the release of tissue factor and activation of this pathway. The secondary surge of thrombin formation as a result of activation of the intrinsic coagulation pathway leads to the massive disruption of the delicate balance that is hemostasis. Excessive thrombin formation results in rapid consumption of coagulation factors and depletion of regulatory substances—protein C, protein S, and antithrombin.[5] With no checks and balances, thrombi continue to form along damaged epithelial walls, resulting in occlusion of the vessels. As occlusion reaches a critical level, tissue ischemia ensues, leading to further tissue damage and perpetuating the process. Eventually, end-organ function is affected by the ischemia, and failure is evident.[1]

In response to the formation of clots, the fibrinolytic system is activated. As plasmin breaks down the fibrin clots, fibrin split products are released, and they act as anticoagulants.[3,7] Coupled with depletion of circulating clotting factors, activation of fibrinolysis results in excessive bleeding. The end result is shock and further tissue ischemia that aggravate end-organ dysfunction and failure. Death is imminent if this destructive cycle is not interrupted.[8]

Assessment and Diagnosis

Favorable outcomes for patients with DIC depend on accurate and timely diagnosis of the condition. Realization of the role underlying pathology plays, recognition of clinical manifestations, and assessment of appropriate laboratory values are key steps in this process.

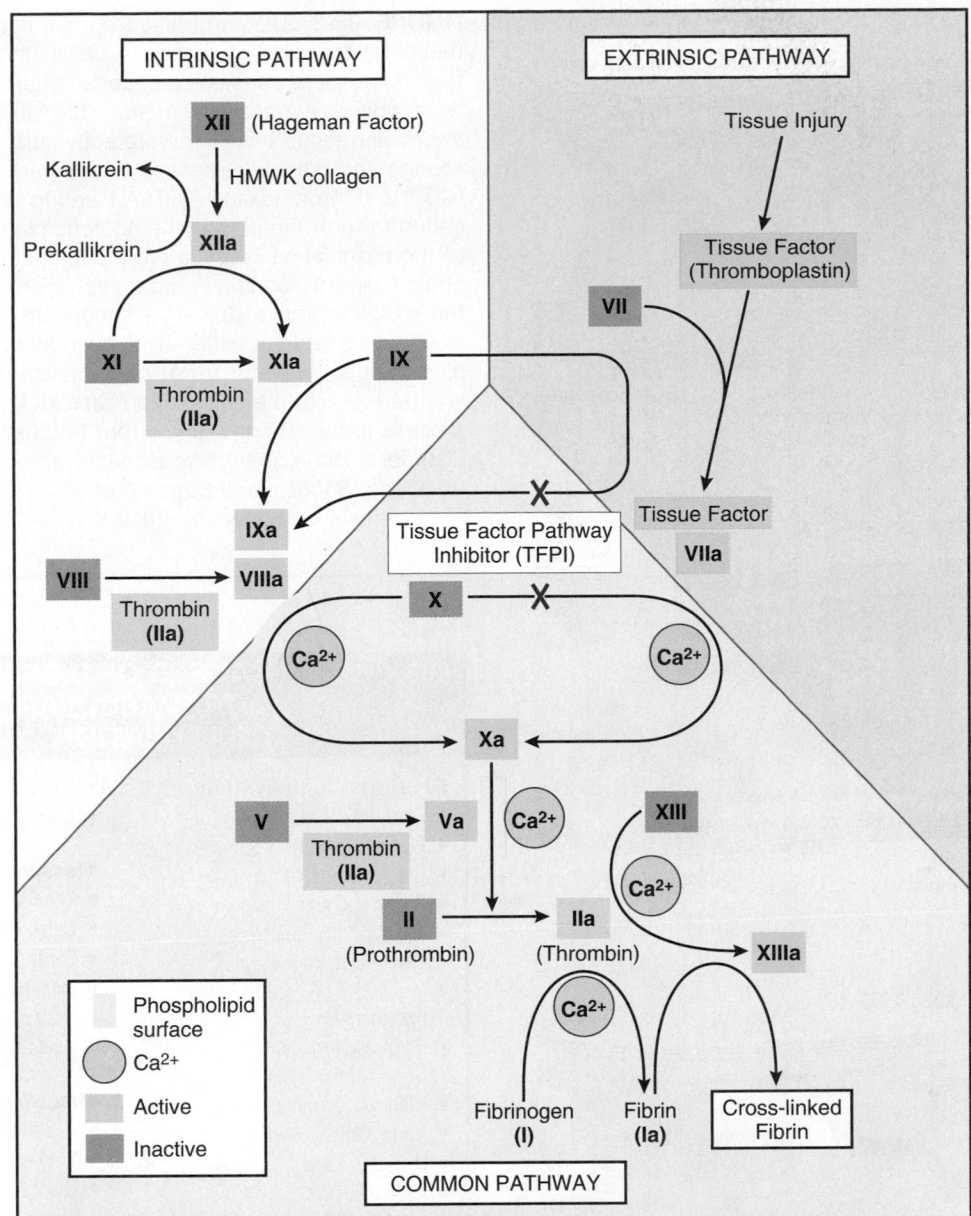

FIGURE 38-1 The coagulation cascade. Factor IX can be activated either by factor XIa or factor VIIa; in lab tests, activation is predominantly dependent on factor XIa of the intrinsic pathway. Factors in red boxes represent inactive molecules; activated factors are indicated with a lower case "a" and a green box. Note also the multiple points where thrombin (factor IIa; light blue boxes) contributes to coagulation through positive feedback loops. The red Xs denote points of action of tissue factor pathway inhibitor (TFPI), which inhibits the activation of factors X and IX by factor VIIa. *HMWK*, High–molecular-weight kininogen; *PL*, phospholipid. (From Mitchell RN. Hemodynamic disorders, thromboembolic disease, and shock. In: Kumar V, et al, eds. *Robbins and Cotran Pathologic Basis of Disease.* 8th ed. Philadelphia: Saunders; 2010.)

Clinical Manifestations

Clinical manifestations are related to the two primary pathophysiologic mechanisms of DIC: the formation of thrombi and bleeding. Thrombi in peripheral capillaries can lead to cyanosis, particularly in the fingers, toes, ears, and nose. In severe, untreated cases, this peripheral ischemia may progress to gangrene.[3,6] As the condition progresses, ischemia worsens, and end organs are affected. The result of this more central ischemia can be respiratory insufficiency and failure, acute kidney injury,

bowel infarction, and ischemic stroke. The tissue damage that results perpetuates the anomalies of DIC.[3]

As coagulation factors are depleted, bleeding from intravenous and other puncture sites is observed. Ecchymoses may result from even routine interventions such as the use of a manual blood pressure cuff, bathing, or turning.[3,6] Bloody drainage may also occur from surgical sites, drains, and urinary catheters. With progression of DIC, the patient is at risk for severe gastrointestinal or subarachnoid hemorrhage.[3,6]

A. VASOCONSTRICTION

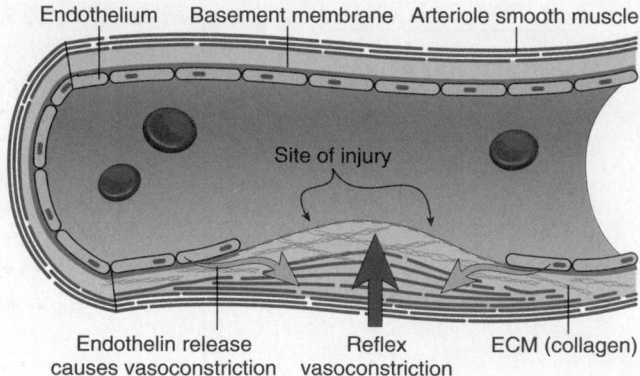

B. PRIMARY HEMOSTASIS

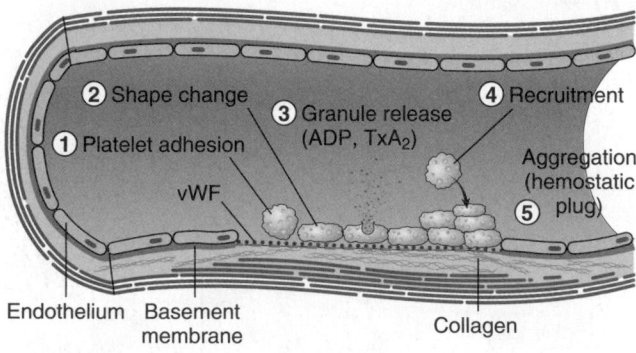

C. SECONDARY HEMOSTASIS

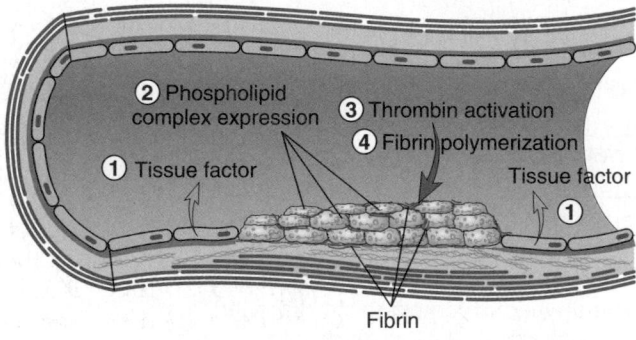

D. THROMBUS AND ANTITHROMBOTIC EVENTS

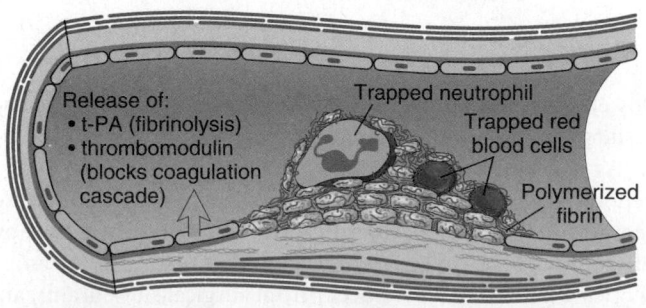

FIGURE 38-2 Diagrammatic representation of the normal hemostatic process. *A,* After vascular injury, local neurohumoral factors induce a transient vasoconstriction. *B,* Platelets adhere to exposed extracellular matrix (ECM) by means of von Willebrand factor (vWF) and are activated, undergoing a shape change and granule release. Released adenosine diphosphate (ADP) and thromboxane A₂ (TxA₂) lead to further platelet aggregation to form the primary hemostatic plug. *C,* Local activation of the coagulation cascade (involving tissue factor and platelet phospholipids) results in fibrin polymerization, "cementing" the platelets into a definitive secondary hemostatic plug. *D,* Counterregulatory mechanisms, such as release of tissue-type plasminogen activator (t-PA) (fibrinolytic) and thrombomodulin (interfering with the coagulation cascade), limit the hemostatic process to the site of injury. (From Mitchell RN. Hemodynamic disorders, thromboembolic disease, and shock. In: Kumar V, et al, eds. *Robbins and Cotran Pathologic Basis of Disease.* 8th ed. Philadelphia: Saunders; 2010.)

BOX 38-1 CAUSES OF DISSEMINATED INTRAVASCULAR COAGULATION

Obstetric Complications
- Abruptio placenta
- Placenta previa
- Retained dead fetus
- Septic abortion
- Amniotic fluid embolism
- Toxemia of pregnancy

Infections
- Gram-negative sepsis
- Gram-positive sepsis
- Meningococcemia
- Rocky Mountain spotted fever
- Histoplasmosis
- Aspergillosis
- Malaria

Neoplasms
- Carcinomas of pancreas, prostate, lung, and stomach
- Acute promyelocytic leukemia

- Tumor lysis syndrome
- Chemotherapy

Massive Tissue Injury
- Traumatic
- Crush injuries
- Burns
- Extensive surgery
- Heat stroke
- Acute transplant rejection

Miscellaneous
- Acute intravascular hemolysis
- Snakebite
- Giant hemangioma
- Shock
- Heat stroke
- Vasculitis
- Aortic aneurysm
- Liver disease
- Cardiac arrest

Modified from Cotran RS, et al. *Robbins Pathologic Basis of Disease.* 6th ed. Philadelphia: Saunders; 1999.

Table 38-2 lists many of the common signs and symptoms of DIC.

Laboratory Findings

Laboratory tests used to diagnose DIC essentially assess the four basic characteristics of this syndrome: 1) increased coagulant activity; 2) increased fibrinolytic activity; 3) impaired regulatory function; and 4) end-organ failure.[3]

Continuous activation of the coagulation pathways results in consumption of coagulation factors. Because of this, the prothrombin time (PT), the activated partial thromboplastin time

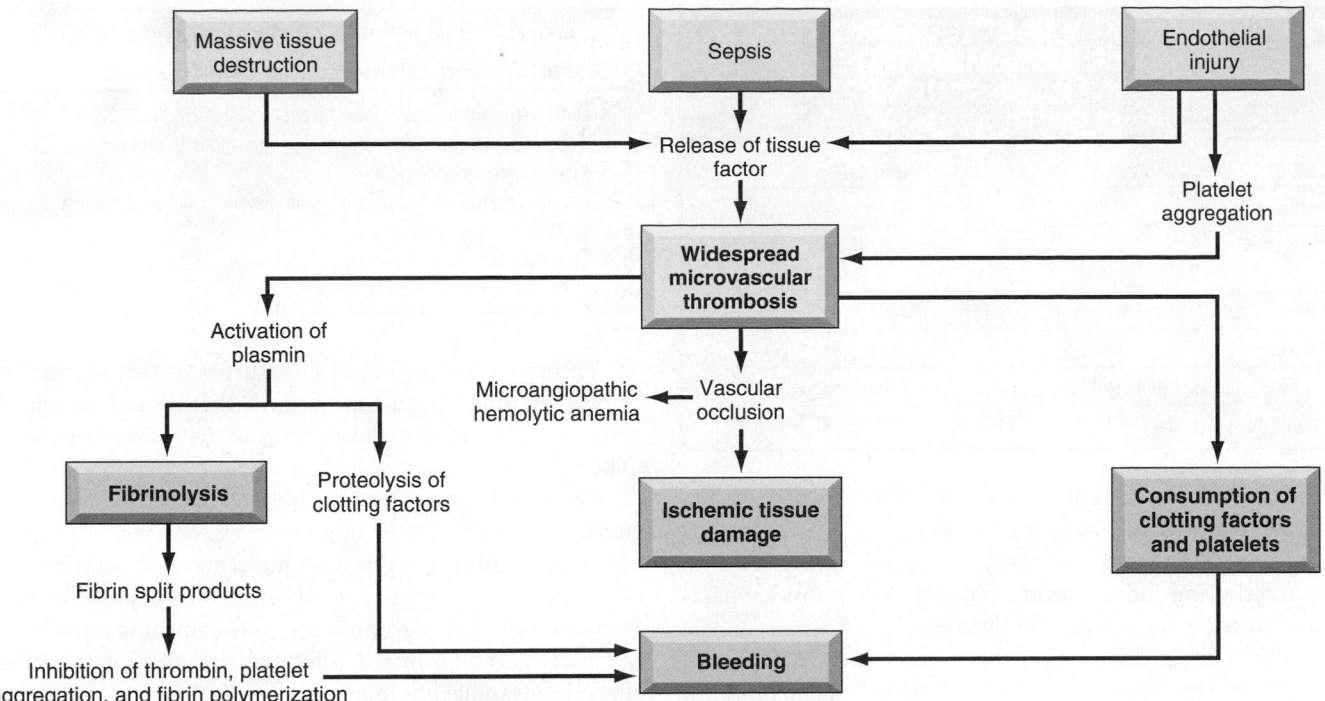

FIGURE 38-3 Pathophysiology of disseminated intravascular coagulation. (From Kumar V, et al. Red blood cell and bleeding disorders. In: Kumar V, et al, eds. *Robbins and Cotran Pathologic Basis of Disease.* 8th ed. Philadelphia: Saunders; 2010.)

TABLE 38-2	COMMON SIGNS AND SYMPTOMS OF DISSEMINATED INTRAVASCULAR COAGULATION	
SYSTEM	**SIGNS RELATED TO HEMORRHAGE**	**SIGNS RELATED TO THROMBI**
Integumentary	Bleeding from gums, venipunctures, and old surgical sites; epistaxis; ecchymoses	Peripheral cyanosis, gangrene
Cardiopulmonary	Hemoptysis	Dysrhythmias, chest pain, acute myocardial infarction, pulmonary embolus, respiratory failure
Renal	Hematuria	Oliguria, acute kidney injury, renal failure
Gastrointestinal	Abdominal distention, hemorrhage	Diarrhea, constipation, bowel infarct
Neurologic	Subarachnoid hemorrhage	Altered level of consciousness, ischemic stroke

formation in small vessels narrows the vessel lumen, forcing RBCs to squeeze through. The resulting damage and fragmentation of these cells can be seen on microscopic examination of blood samples. Damaged, fragmented RBCs are called *schistocytes.*[3,6]

In response to the excess clotting activity, the fibrinolytic process accelerates, and levels of byproducts increase. This is reflected in markedly elevated levels of fibrin degradation products. Another key laboratory test used to evaluate the degree of clot dissolution—and therefore the severity of the coagulopathy—is the D-dimer level.[1] D-dimers exclusively indicate clot degradation because, unlike fibrin degradation products, which also result from the breakdown of free circulating fibrin, D-dimers result only from dissolution of clots.[3] With progression of the coagulopathy, normal regulatory mechanisms are disrupted, as reflected in decreasing levels of inhibitory factors such as protein C, factor V, and antithrombin III.[3,6,9]

Unchecked DIC resulting in occlusion of vessels and tissue ischemia leads to end-organ dysfunction. Respiratory failure, indicated by abnormal arterial blood gas (ABG) levels; liver failure, indicated by increasing liver enzymes; and renal impairment, indicated by rising blood urea nitrogen (BUN) and creatinine levels are common findings in advanced DIC.[9]

No single laboratory study can confirm the diagnosis of DIC, but several key results are strong indicators of the condition (Table 38-3). The International Society of Thrombosis and Hemostasis emphasizes early detection of DIC through observation of abnormal trends in laboratory values.[5]

Medical Management

Without question, the primary intervention in DIC is prevention. Being aware of the conditions that commonly contribute

(aPTT), and the international normalized ratio (INR) values are elevated. Although the platelet count may fall within normal ranges, serial examination reveals a declining trend in values. An unexpected drop of at least 50% in the platelet count, particularly in the presence of known contributing factors and associated signs and symptoms, strongly indicates DIC.[1] Fibrinogen levels drop as more and more clots are formed. Thrombus

TABLE 38-3 KEY LABORATORY STUDIES IN DISSEMINATED INTRAVASCULAR COAGULATION

TEST	VALUE
Prothrombin time (PT)	>12.5 sec
Platelets	<50,000/mm³, or at least 50% drop from baseline
Activated partial thromboplastin time (aPTT)	>40 sec
D-dimer	>250 ng/mL
Fibrin degradation products (FDP)	>40 mg/mL
Fibrinogen	<100 mg/dL

BOX 38-2 NURSING DIAGNOSES

Disseminated Intravascular Coagulation

- Deficient Fluid Volume related to active blood loss, p. 1132
- Decreased Cardiac Output related to alterations in preload, p. 1128
- Risk for Infection, p. 1160
- Anxiety related to threat to biologic, psychologic, and/or social integrity, p. 1125
- Compromised Family Coping related to a critically ill family member, p. 1127

to the development of DIC and treating them vigorously and without delay provide the best defense against this devastating condition.[3,6,7,9] After DIC is identified, maintaining organ perfusion and slowing consumption of coagulation factors are paramount to achieving a favorable outcome.[1,3]

Multiple organ dysfunction syndrome (MODS) frequently results from DIC and exacerbates the underlying pathology.[8] It is essential to prevent end-organ ischemia and damage by supporting blood pressure and circulating volume. Administration of intravenous fluids and inotropic agents and, if overt hemorrhaging is evident, infusion of packed RBCs are appropriate interventions to replace blood volume and essential, oxygen-carrying RBCs.

In the presence of severe platelet depletion (less than 50,000/mm³) and severe hemorrhage, platelet transfusions are often indicated.[5,6] However, caution must be used when administering platelets because antiplatelet antibodies may be formed. These antibodies may become activated during future platelet transfusions and elicit DIC.[3]

Replacement of clotting factors in the patient with DIC is thought by some authorities to perpetuate the coagulopathy; however, there is little scientific evidence to support this theory.[1] Fibrinogen levels less than 100 mg/dL indicate the appropriateness of administering cryoprecipitate. A prolonged PT indicates the need for fresh-frozen plasma.[3,5,6]

Slowing consumption of coagulation factors by inhibiting the processes involved in clot formation is another strategy used in treating DIC. The use of heparin, particularly low–molecular-weight heparin (LMWH), to prevent formation of future clots is controversial.[6] It is contraindicated in patients with DIC associated with recent surgery or with gastrointestinal or central nervous system (CNS) bleeding. However, heparin has been beneficial in obstetric emergencies such as retained placenta or incomplete abortion, severe arterial occlusions, or MODS caused by microemboli.[3,6] Inhibitors such as aminocaproic acid may be used in conjunction with heparin.[3,6]

The use of recombinant activated protein C is gaining popularity in treating DIC, especially in the setting of severe sepsis. Activated protein C acts as an anticoagulant and works to restore normal inhibition of coagulation pathways. However, it has been associated with an increased incidence of intracerebral bleeding and must be used with caution in patients with severely decreased platelets.[3,5]

Thrombin production in DIC surpasses that of antithrombins and other regulatory factors that would normally be present to inactivate thrombin and its subsequent actions. The use of antithrombin III has recently been approved in the United States. Ongoing research is yielding mixed results in the treatment of DIC.[5] One interesting area of research is the use of protease inhibitors. Protease molecules normally inhibit the conversion of fibrinogen to fibrin in the coagulation mechanism, but in DIC, this inhibitory mechanism is impaired. The introduction of protease inhibitors by intravenous infusion may be advantageous in arresting DIC.[3]

Nursing Management

Nursing management of the patient with DIC incorporates a variety of nursing diagnoses (Box 38-2). Assessment and monitoring are the primary weapons in the critical care nurse's arsenal against DIC. Knowing the diseases and conditions that are most often associated with DIC and understanding the pathophysiologic mechanisms involved enables the critical care nurse to anticipate its development and intervene quickly. Nursing interventions include supporting the patient's vital functions, initiating bleeding precautions, providing comfort and emotional support, and maintaining surveillance for complications.

Supporting Patient's Vital Functions

Frequent assessments should include parameters for neurologic status, renal function, cardiopulmonary function, and skin integrity that indicate impaired tissue or organ perfusion. Particular parameters to include are mental status, BUN and creatine levels, urine output, vital signs, hemodynamic values, cardiac rhythm, arterial blood gas and pulse oximetry values, skin breakdown, ecchymoses, or hematomas.[6]

The critical care nurse must recognize and support the patient's vital physiologic functions. Administration of intravenous fluids, blood products, and inotropic agents to provide adequate hemodynamic support and tissue oxygenation is essential in preventing or combating end-organ damage. Close monitoring of vital signs, hemodynamic parameters, intake and output, and appropriate laboratory values assists the critical care nurse in administering and titrating appropriate agents.[3]

Initiating Bleeding Precautions

Awareness of the patient's bleeding potential necessitates adjustments to normal nursing interventions (Box 38-3). The nurse avoids unnecessary venipunctures that may result in bleeding, bruising, or hematomas by drawing blood from and

BOX 38-3 NIC

Bleeding Precautions

Definition

Reduction of stimuli that may induce bleeding or hemorrhage in at-risk patients

Activities

Monitor the patient closely for hemorrhage

Note hemoglobin/hematocrit levels before and after blood loss, as indicated

Monitor for signs and symptoms of persistent bleeding (e.g., check all secretions for frank or occult blood)

Monitor coagulation studies, including prothrombin time (PT), partial thromboplastin time (PTT), fibrinogen, fibrin degradation/split products, and platelet counts, as appropriate

Monitor orthostatic vital signs, including blood pressure

Maintain bed rest during active bleeding

Administer blood products (e.g., platelets, fresh-frozen plasma), as appropriate

Protect the patient from trauma, which may cause bleeding

Avoid injections (IV, IM, or SQ), as appropriate

Instruct the ambulating patient to wear shoes

Use soft toothbrush or toothettes for oral care

Use electric razor, instead of straight-edge, for shaving

Tell patient to avoid invasive procedures; if they are necessary, monitor closely for bleeding

Coordinate timing of invasive procedures with platelet or fresh-frozen plasma transfusions, if appropriate

Refrain from inserting objects into a bleeding orifice

Avoid taking rectal temperatures

Avoid lifting heavy objects

Administer mediations (e.g., antacids), as appropriate

Instruct patient to avoid aspirin and other anticoagulants

Instruct patient to increase intake of foods rich in vitamin K

Use therapeutic mattress to minimize skin trauma

Avoid constipation (e.g., encourage fluid intake and stool softeners), as appropriate

Instruct the patient and/or family on signs of bleeding and appropriate actions (e.g., notify the nurse), should bleeding occur

From Bulechek GM, et al. *Nursing Interventions Classification (NIC)*. 6th ed. St. Louis: Mosby; 2013.
IM, Intramuscular; *IV*, intravenous; *SQ*, subcutaneous.

BOX 38-4 COLLABORATIVE MANAGEMENT

Disseminated Intravascular Coagulation

- Identify and eliminate the underlying cause.
- Provide hemodynamic support to prevent end-organ ischemia.
  - Intravenous fluids
  - Positive inotropic agents
- Administer blood and blood components.
  - Fresh-frozen plasma
  - Platelets
  - Cryoprecipitate
  - Antithrombin III
- Administer medications.
  - Heparin
  - Aminocaproic acid
  - Protein C
  - Antithrombin III
- Initiate bleeding precautions.
- Maintain surveillance for complications.
  - Hypovolemic shock
  - Peripheral ischemia
  - Central ischemia
  - Multiple organ dysfunction syndrome (MODS)
- Provide comfort and emotional support.

administering medications through existing arterial or venous lines. The use of manual or automatic blood pressure cuffs is avoided whenever possible. If tracheal or oral suctioning is necessary, the use of low-level suction is recommended.[6] Meticulous skin care is advised, keeping the skin moist and using specialty mattresses and beds as appropriate to prevent breakdown. Gentle care should be used when bathing or turning the patient to prevent bruising or hematoma formation.

Providing Comfort and Emotional Support

The development of DIC in the already critically ill patient can be stressful for the patient and his or her significant others. It is imperative to provide psychosocial support throughout this crisis. Calm reassurance and uncomplicated explanations of the care the patient is receiving can help to allay much of the anxiety experienced. The critical care nurse must answer all questions and provide information in terms best understood by all parties. The use of an interpreter when English is not the primary language can enhance understanding and help avoid misconceptions. Providing spiritual support as requested may also be of assistance.

Collaborative management of the patient with DIC is outlined in Box 38-4.

THROMBOCYTOPENIA

Description

Thrombocytopenia is defined as a platelet count less than 140,000/mm^3.[10,11] Similar to DIC, thrombocytopenia often results from another underlying condition that affects the platelet count. Thrombocytopenia is more common in women than in men, affecting adults most often between the ages of 20 and 50 years.[12,13]

Etiology

Onset of thrombocytopenia often follows a viral infection, pregnancy, administration of certain medications (e.g., heparin, thiazide diuretics, chemotherapeutic agents), malignancies, splenomegaly, blood transfusions, or alcoholism.[12] Regardless of the precipitating condition, the development of thrombocytopenia occurs by means of one of four mechanisms: 1) decreased platelet production; 2) increased platelet destruction; 3) splenic sequestration of platelets; and 4) platelet dilution.[10] The most common form of thrombocytopenia seen in the critical care unit is immune thrombocytopenic purpura (ITP).[11]

Pathophysiology

In ITP, lymphocytes produce antibodies that begin to destroy existing platelets. The cause of this autoimmune response is unknown.[13] With insufficient platelets available, the normal coagulation pathways are disrupted. Inadequate hemostasis

TABLE 38-4 **IDIOPATHIC THROMBOCYTOPENIA PURPURA: SIGNS, SYMPTOMS, AND LABORATORY DATA**

SYSTEM OR STUDY	SIGNS AND SYMPTOMS
Integumentary	Petechial hemorrhage of lower extremities, ecchymoses, gingival bleeding, spontaneous epistaxis
Neurologic	Sudden, severe headache; nausea and vomiting; seizures; focal neurologic deficits; decreased level of consciousness
Renal	Hematuria
Gastrointestinal	Hematemesis, melena, hematochezia
Other	Heavy menses in women, retinal hemorrhage
Laboratory	Decreased platelet count, often <30,000 mm³

BOX 38-5 **NURSING DIAGNOSES**

Immune Thrombocytopenia Purpura

- Deficient Fluid Volume related to active blood loss, p. 1134
- Powerlessness related to lack of control over the current situation and/or disease progression, p. 1152
- Disturbed Body Image related to actual change in body structure, function, or appearance, p. 1136

BOX 38-6 **COLLABORATIVE MANAGEMENT**

Immune Thrombocytopenia Purpura

- Administer medications.
  - Glucocorticoids
  - Intravenous immunoglobulin
- Prepare patient for splenectomy if unresponsive to medication therapy.
- Administer platelets.
- Initiate bleeding precautions.
- Maintain surveillance for complications.
  - Intracranial or other major hemorrhage
  - Severe blood loss
- Provide comfort and emotional support.

ensues, and bleeding results. Although life-threatening gastrointestinal or intracerebral bleeding can occur, the bleeding seen in ITP does not result in deep visceral hemorrhage and hematoma.[10]

Assessment and Diagnosis

ITP is characterized by the gradual onset of signs and symptoms.[13] The diagnosis is primarily based on findings in the patient's history and physical examination.

Clinical Manifestations

Petechial hemorrhages, which manifest as small red spots primarily on legs and oral mucosa, are most indicative of a platelet disorder, unlike larger hematomas, which are most commonly associated with coagulation disorders.[11] Bruising unrelated to trauma is another common sign of ITP.[12] The signs and symptoms of ITP are listed in Table 38-4.

Unusual bleeding is a hallmark of ITP. Excessive bleeding from the gums after dental work, spontaneous epistaxis, blood in the urine or stool, and in women, unusually heavy menses are typical features of ITP. Rarely, retinal hemorrhage or intracerebral bleeding may be observed.[13,14]

Laboratory Findings

A complete blood cell count reveals a severely diminished platelet count, often falling below 30,000/mm³ for a patient with ITP.[14] However, the numbers of RBCs and WBCs, the hemoglobin level, results of coagulation studies, and bleeding times are normal.[14]

Medical Management

In most cases, ITP resolves spontaneously, and treatment is not necessary. In mild cases in which diminished platelets counts result in symptoms, administration of oral corticosteroids is appropriate.[10,13] Platelet counts will increase to normal levels with 2 to 6 weeks, and dosages can then be tapered.

In patients exhibiting life-threatening hemorrhage, rapid intervention is necessary. Administration of intravenous

immunoglobulin suppresses the platelet-destroying antibody response. This therapy is extremely expensive and is reserved for the most severe manifestations of ITP.[13] High-dose methylprednisolone can be given intravenously and is very effective in treating ITP.[11] Platelet transfusion is recommended after administration of intravenous immunoglobulin or methylprednisolone. When steroid therapy fails to arrest the condition, surgical removal of the spleen is considered.[13,14]

Nursing Management

Nursing management of the patient with ITP incorporates a variety of nursing diagnoses (Box 38-5). Nursing interventions include supporting the patient's vital functions, initiating bleeding precautions (see Box 38-3), providing comfort and emotional support, and maintaining surveillance for complications.

Recognizing potential hazards and providing a safe care environment is of utmost concern. For example, padding bed rails can protect the patient from bruising. Substituting sponge-tipped oral care devices for firm-bristled toothbrushes can help minimize mucosal trauma and bleeding, and the patient is instructed on how to blow the nose gently to avoid instigating epistaxis. When shaving patients, use an electric razor to reduce the risk of laceration associated with a blade. Venipuncture and intramuscular injections are avoided. In the event venipuncture is required, prolonged pressure on the site may be necessary to arrest bleeding. The critical care nurse must carefully administer prescribed medications, monitor for adverse effects of platelet transfusions, and monitor for complicating or contributing factors, such as hemorrhage and infection.

Collaborative management of the patient with ITP is outlined in Box 38-6.

HEPARIN-INDUCED THROMBOCYTOPENIA

Description

Another form of thrombocytopenia seen in critical care patients is heparin-induced thrombocytopenia (HIT). There are two distinct types of HIT. The most common form is non–immune-mediated HIT, formally known as type 1 HIT.[15] Seen in up to 30% of patients receiving heparin therapy, this nonautoimmune condition manifests within a few days of initiation of therapy. Platelet depletion is moderate, counts are usually less than 100,000/mm³, and the condition is transient, often resolving spontaneously. Discontinuation of heparin is not required. The second form is type 2 HIT, or immune-mediated HIT,[15] which is less commonly encountered but has more severe consequences.[10,16,17] This discussion is limited to immune-mediated HIT.

Etiology

Immune-mediated HIT is a response to the administration of heparin therapy. It has been observed in 0.5% to 5% of patients treated with unfractionated heparin and has occurred after exposure to LMWH, although to a lesser degree.[15] The disorder is characterized by severe thrombocytopenia during heparin therapy. Diagnostically it is identified by a platelet count less than 50,000/mm³ or at least a 50% decrease from the baseline platelet count from the initiation of therapy. Onset usually occurs 5 to 14 days from the first exposure to heparin, but the onset can occur within hours of a re-exposure to heparin.[10,16-18] Depending on the source of the disorder, reported mortality rates are as high as 30%.[15]

Pathophysiology

The thrombocytopenia that occurs with immune-mediated HIT is related to the formation of heparin-antibody complexes. These complexes release a substance known as platelet factor 4 (PF4). PF4 attracts heparin molecules, forming immunogenic complexes that adhere to platelet and endothelial surfaces (Fig. 38-4). Activation of platelets stimulates the release of thrombin and the subsequent formation of platelet clumps.[10]

Patients with immune-mediated HIT are at greater risk for thrombosis than bleeding. Vessel occlusion can result in the need for limb amputation, stroke, acute myocardial infarction, and even death.[10,16-18] The resultant formation of fibrin-platelet-rich thrombi is the primary characteristic of HIT that distinguishes it from other forms of thrombocytopenia and gives rise to its more descriptive name: white clot syndrome.[16]

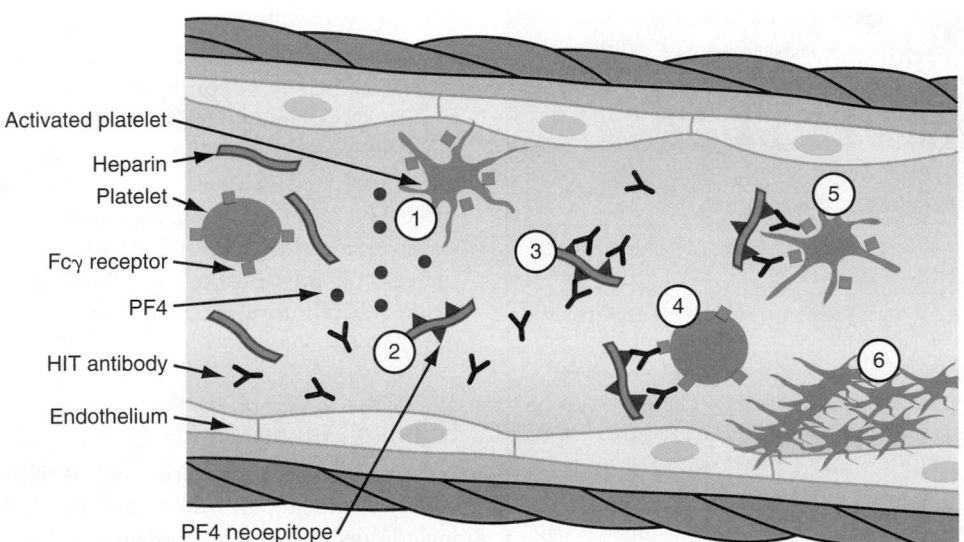

FIGURE 38-4 Pathogenesis of heparin-induced thrombocytopenia (HIT). *(1)* Activated platelets release procoagulant proteins from α-granules, including platelet factor 4 (PF4). Administered heparin binds PF4 *(2)*, which undergoes a conformation change and expresses a new antigen (neoepitope). Individuals with HIT produce an immunoglobulin G (IgG) antibody that specifically reacts *(3)* with multiple identical neoepitopes on the heparin-PF4 complex. The reaction forms heparin-PF4-IgG immune complexes. Platelets express FcγRIIa receptors (Fcγ receptor) that react *(4)* with the Fc portion of IgG in immune complexes. Cross-linking of Fc receptors *(5)* results in FcγRIIa-dependent platelet activation. The activated platelets mediate a series of events that lead to further activation of the coagulation cascade, resulting in thrombin generation. Further release of PF4 from newly activated platelets leads to a cycle of continuing platelet activation and *(6)* formation of a primary clot. The reaction can be enhanced by the release of platelet-derived microparticles that are rich in surface phosphatidylserine and increase activation of coagulation and by the binding of heparin-PF4 complexes and HIT-IgG to the vascular endothelium (not shown.) (From Rote NS, McCance KL. Alterations of leukocyte, lymphoid, and hemostatic function. In: McCance KL et al, eds. *Pathophysiology: The Biologic Basis for Disease in Adults and Children.* 6th ed. St. Louis: Mosby; 2010.)

Assessment and Diagnosis

HIT can be associated with severe consequences. Rapid recognition of risk factors and subsequent development of signs and symptoms is essential in treating this condition.

Clinical Manifestations

Common signs and symptoms are listed in Table 38-5. The clinical manifestations of HIT are related to the formation of thrombi and subsequent vessel occlusion.[15] Most thrombotic events are venous, although venous and arterial thrombosis can occur. Thrombotic events typically include deep vein thrombosis, pulmonary embolism, limb ischemia thrombosis, thrombotic stroke, and myocardial infarction.[15,18] The presence of blanching and the loss of peripheral pulses, sensation, or motor function in a limb indicate peripheral vascular thrombi. Neurologic signs and symptoms such as confusion, headache, and impaired speech can signal the onset of cerebral artery occlusion and stroke. Acute myocardial infarction may be heralded by dyspnea, chest pain, pallor, and alterations in blood pressure. Thrombi in the pulmonary vasculature may be evidenced by pleuritic pain, rales, and dyspnea.[10,16]

Laboratory Findings

The key indicator for identifying HIT is the platelet count. General consensus in the literature considers a platelet count of less than 100,000/mm³ or a sudden drop of 50% from the patient's baseline after initiation of heparin therapy to strongly indicate HIT.[16-18]

Two types of assays have become available to assist in confirming the diagnosis of HIT: activation assays, based on platelet aggregation or the release of granular contents such as serotonin, and assays that identify the HIT antigen. Activation assays are highly sensitive in detecting the presence of HIT. The most common assay used is heparin-induced platelet aggregation (HIPA). Serotonin release assay (SRA) is used by a few institutions. The enzyme-linked immunosorbent assay (ELISA) identifies the presence of the HIT antigen.[16]

Medical Management

Early identification is critical to managing the effects of immune-mediated HIT. Current guidelines suggest that for high-risk patients platelet count monitoring be performed every 2 or 3 days from day 4 to day 14.[19] When a decrease in the platelet count is detected, heparin therapy should be discontinued immediately, and the patient should be tested for the presence of heparin antibodies.[10,17-19] If the original indication for heparin still exists or new thromboses occur, an alternative form of anticoagulation is usually necessary.[19]

Direct Thrombin Inhibitors

Direct thrombin inhibitors (DTIs) are being used with increasing frequency to treat HIT. DTIs bind directly to the thrombin molecule, thereby inhibiting its action.[18] Two such medications for use in the United States are lepirudin and argatroban. Warfarin, although commonly used to treat deep vein thrombosis, is not indicated as a sole agent in treating HIT because of its prolonged onset of action. Studies have shown that the use of warfarin without concomitant use of DTIs can significantly increase the incidence of thrombosis in patients with HIT.[15-18] Comparative information on these medications is provided in Table 38-6.

Nursing Management

Nursing management of the patient with HIT incorporates a variety of nursing diagnoses (Box 38-7). Nursing interventions include decreasing the incidence of heparin exposure, maintaining surveillance for complications, providing comfort and emotional support, and educating the patient and family. The critical care nurse plays a pivotal role in prevention and detection of HIT. Initial assessment is crucial to identifying those patients at risk for HIT. Ascertaining a medical history that includes previous heparin therapy, deep vein thrombosis, or cardiovascular surgery that included the use of cardiopulmonary bypass can alert the nurse to potential problems.

Decreasing the Incidence of Heparin Exposure

Ensuring that all heparin has been removed from the patient's hemodynamic pressure monitoring system, avoiding the use of heparin-coated catheters, and discontinuing heparin flushes to maintain the patency of other intravenous lines are essential elements of nursing management.

TABLE 38-5	HEPARIN-INDUCED THROMBOCYTOPENIA: SIGNS, SYMPTOMS, AND LABORATORY DATA
SYSTEM OR STUDY	**SIGNS AND SYMPTOMS**
Cardiac	Chest pain, diaphoresis, pallor, alterations in blood pressure, dysrhythmias
Vascular	Arterial: pain, pallor, pulselessness, paresthesia, paralysis Venous: pain, tenderness, unilateral leg swelling, warmth, erythema, a palpable cord, pain on passive dorsiflexion of the foot, and spontaneous maintenance of the relaxed foot in abnormal plantar flexion (Homans sign)
Pulmonary	Dyspnea, pleuritic pain, rales, chest pain, chest wall tenderness, back pain, shoulder pain, upper abdominal pain, syncope, hemoptysis, shortness of breath, wheezing
Renal	Thirst, decreased urine output, dizziness, orthostatic hypotension
Gastrointestinal	Abdominal pain, vomiting, bloody diarrhea, abnormal bowel sounds
Neurologic	Confusion, headache, impaired speech patterns, hemiparesis or hemiplegia, vision disturbances, dysarthria, aphasia, ataxia, vertigo, nystagmus, sudden decrease in consciousness
Laboratory	Platelets <50,000/mm³ or sudden drop of 30%-50% from baseline; positive results for HIPA, SRA, ELISA

ELISA, Enzyme-linked immunosorbent assay; *HIPA*, heparin-induced platelet aggregation; *SRA*, serotonin release assay.

TABLE 38-6 PHARMACOLOGIC MANAGEMENT

Heparin-Induced Thrombocytopenia

MEDICATION	DOSAGE	ACTION	SPECIAL CONSIDERATIONS
Lepirudin (Refludan)	Loading dose: 0.4 mg/kg IV bolus IV infusion: 0.15 mg/kg/hr	Used to inhibit free and clot-bound thrombin; a recombinant form of leech-derived hirudin	Monitor aPTT; maintain INR 1.5-2.5 times normal Reduce dosage in patients with known or suspected renal insufficiency Side effects include bleeding Can develop antilepirudin antibodies that enhance anticoagulant effect
Argatroban	Loading dose: None IV infusion: 2 mcg/kg/min not to exceed 10 mcg/kg/min	Used to inhibit thrombin	Obtain baseline aPTT 2 hr after therapy started Monitor aPTT; maintain INR 1.5-3.0 times initial baseline Reduce dosage in patients with known or suspected hepatic impairment
Bivalirudin	Loading dose: 0.75 mg/kg IV bolus IV infusion: 1.75-2.0 mg/kg/hr	Used to inhibit thrombin	Monitor aPTT, maintain INR 1.5-2.5 times initial baseline Adjust dose in presence of renal failure

aPTT, Activated partial thromboplastin time; *INR,* international normalized ratio; *IV,* intravenous.

BOX 38-7 NURSING DIAGNOSES

Heparin-Induced Thrombocytopenia

- Risk for Decreased Cardiac Tissue Perfusion, p. 1155
- Risk for Ineffective Peripheral Tissue Perfusion, p. 1158
- Risk for Ineffective Renal Tissue Perfusion, p. 1159
- Risk for Ineffective Gastrointestinal Tissue Perfusion, p. 1157
- Risk for Ineffective Cerebral Tissue Perfusion, p. 1156
- Powerlessness related to lack of control over the current situation or disease progression, p. 1152
- Deficient Knowledge related to lack of previous exposure to information, p. 1134 (see Box 38-8, Patient Education for Heparin-Induced Thrombocytopenia)

BOX 38-8 PATIENT EDUCATION

Heparin-Induced Thrombocytopenia

- Pathophysiology of disease
- Purpose of heparin
- Measures to avoid future exposure to heparin
- Identify different types of heparin (unfractionated and low–molecular-weight forms)
- Encourage purchase of medical alert bracelet or similar type of warning device
- Tell any new health care provider about the heparin allergy and previous reaction

BOX 38-9 COLLABORATIVE MANAGEMENT

Heparin-Induced Thrombocytopenia

- Stop all heparin exposure.
  - Unfractionated and low–molecular-weight heparin by any route
  - Heparin flushes
  - Heparin-coated vascular access devices
- Begin therapy with an alternative anticoagulant.
  - Lepirudin
  - Argatroban
- Maintain surveillance for complications.
  - Deep vein thrombosis
  - Pulmonary emboli
  - Acute limb ischemia
  - Ischemic stroke
  - Acute myocardial infarction
- Administer antifibrinolytic therapy (as indicated) if thrombosis occurs.
- Prepare patient for surgical embolectomy (as indicated) if thrombosis occurs.
- Provide comfort and emotional support.

Maintaining Surveillance for Complications

Patients with HIT remain at high risk for thrombotic complications for several days or weeks after cessation of heparin. Vigilant monitoring, early recognition of signs and symptoms, deep vein thrombosis prevention strategies, and prompt notification of the physician are key roles of the critical care nurse.

Educating the Patient and Family

Prevention of subsequent episodes in patients sensitized to heparin incudes education of the patient and family (Box 38-8).

Education should include measures to avoid future exposure to heparin. The use of medical alert bracelets and listing heparin allergies in the medical record are necessary to avoid this serious complication in the future.

Collaborative management of the patient with HIT is outlined in Box 38-9.

SICKLE CELL ANEMIA

Description

Sickle cell anemia (SCA) is a disease passed down through families in which RBCs form an abnormal sickle or crescent shape. RBCs carry oxygen to the body and are normally shaped like a disk.[1] The sickle-shaped cells have a shortened life span; are unable to carry adequate oxygen to tissues, and due to their shape become trapped in the vasculature; and can cause severe pain, increased risk of infection, and life-threatening complications.[20]

Etiology

SCA is an autosomal recessive genetic disorder. An individual with normal hemoglobin has two copies of hemoglobin A (Hb A) gene. An individual with SCA has two copies of hemoglobin S (Hb S) gene. Individuals who have one gene for Hb S and one gene for Hb A are known as "carriers" of the sickle cell trait (Hb AS). When two "carriers" have a child, there is a 25% chance that they will have a child with SCA (Hb SS), a 50% chance of having a child with sickle cell trait (Hb AS), and a 25% chance of having a child with entirely normal hemoglobin (Hb AA).[21,22]

This genetic trait is primarily found in people of West African descent. The disease has also been linked to persons of sole European or Middle Eastern ancestry; however, this is extremely rare. The disease is not prevalent in persons of Asian or Pacific Islander descent.[21]

SCA is usually diagnosed during the first few years of life due to manifestation of initial symptoms. Prenatal screening is now available for at-risk couples.[22] This consists of DNA analysis from fetal cells. This should be offered as part of their prenatal counseling. There are more than 40 states that undergo universal neonatal screening for hemoglobinopathies.[22]

Pathophysiology

Sickle cell disease (SCD) is a chronic inflammatory condition characterized by hemolysis and vasoocclusion. The cause of SCA is a mutation in the genetic sequence in the beta chain gene of the hemoglobin. This results in a sequence of the replacement of valine with glutamic acid at the N-terminal amino acid position 6 of the protein chain.[21,22] This substitution leads to the production of hemoglobin S.

Normal RBCs contain hemoglobin that are flexible, biconcave disks. When deoxygenated, RBCs containing predominantly Hb S distort into a crescent or sickle shape. In this form the hemoglobin becomes is rigid and friable, causing vasoocclusion in the small vessels of the circulatory system. This tends to happen during times of physiologic stress, such as physical overexertion, muscle tissue ischemia, dehydration, infection, or extreme temperatures.[22] Even though these conditions have a tendency to exacerbate the condition, the majority of the sickling events have no identifying cause.[21]

The RBCs become lodged in the vasculature and the microcirculation causing stasis and obstruction of blood flow and damage to the surrounding organs, tissue ischemia, infarction, and if not corrected eventually, necrosis (Fig. 38-5).[22] In addition, hemolysis of the RBCs occurs, resulting in anemia.

Assessment and Diagnosis

SCA can be associated with severe consequences. Rapid recognition of signs and symptoms is essential in treating this condition.

Clinical Manifestations

There are a variety of clinical manifestations associated with SCA (Fig. 38-6). The patient may present with a low-grade fever,

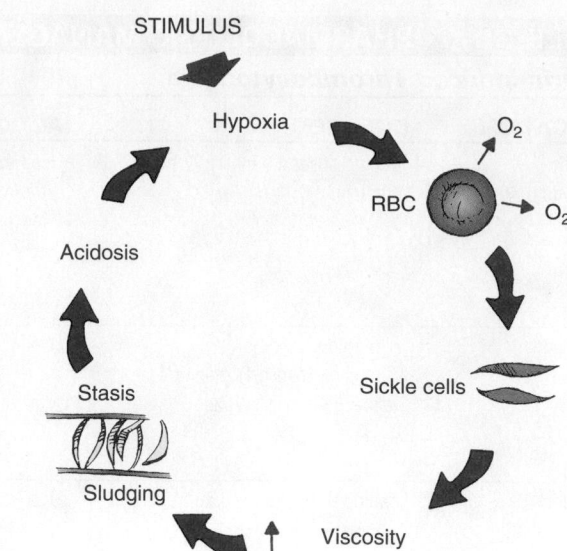

FIGURE 38-5 Cycle causing vasoocclusive episodes in sickle cell anemia. (From Hockenberry M, Coody D, eds. *Pediatric Oncology and Hematology: Perspectives on Care.* St. Louis: Mosby; 1986.)

bone or joint pain, pinpoint pupils, inability to follow commands, photophobia, tachycardia, tachypnea, decreased respiratory excursion, hepatomegaly, nonpalpable spleen, and pretibial ulcers.[23]

Laboratory Studies

Initial laboratory studies include a complete blood count (CBC), a peripheral blood smear, and a quantitative hemoglobin electrophoresis. Sickle cells constitute 5% to 10% of the blood smear. The elevated reticulocyte count (greater than 10%) is characteristically accompanied by the presence of Howell-Jolly bodies. Howell-Jolly bodies are small remnants of nuclear material from hemolyzed erythrocytes reflective of hyposplenia or autoinfarction, and target cells (an erythrocyte with a deeply stained core surrounded by a lighter-stained margin; it resembles a target with a bull's eye).[22] Typically an elevated WBC count occurs during and following a crisis. Other tests might include an indirect bilirubin level, which will be elevated following hemolysis. The haptoglobin level will be low or absent because it cannot be replaced quickly enough after severe hemolysis. Haptoglobin, a glycoprotein, exists to bind free hemoglobin that is released from hemolyzed erythrocytes.[22]

Medical Management

SCA is not a curable disease; however, there are treatment options available for management of symptoms and complications. Bone marrow transplant offers a cure in limited number of cases.[20] Medical interventions are aimed at preventing infections, managing pain, transfusing RBCs, and administering hydroxyurea. Patients with chronic disease are more effective managed through a multidisciplinary approach.[20] It is also important to look at other issues that may exacerbate the patient disease process such as diet, poor housing, inadequate housing, lack of education, poor access to services, and poor lifestyle choices.

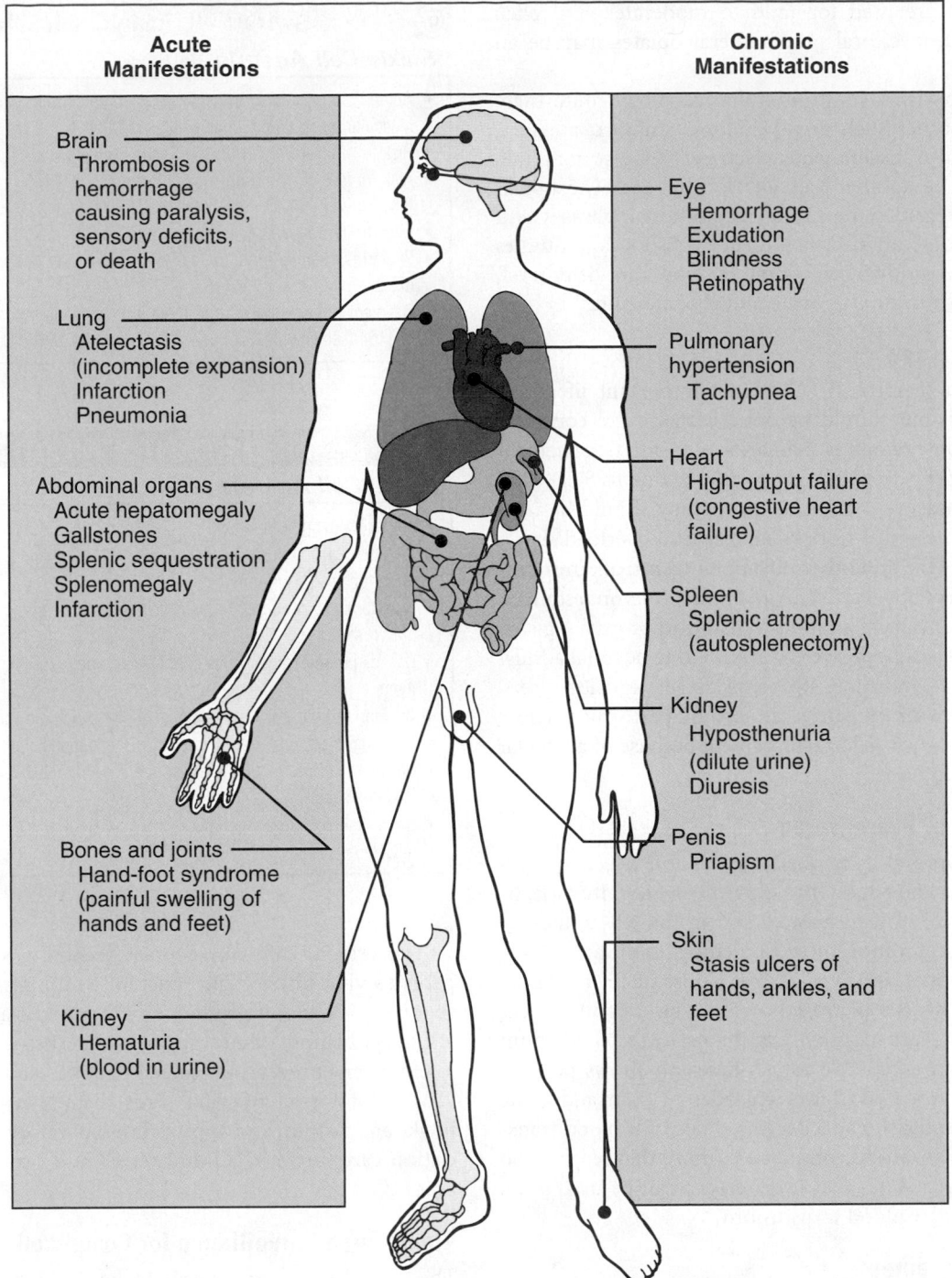

Acute Manifestations

Brain
  Thrombosis or
  hemorrhage
  causing paralysis,
  sensory deficits,
  or death

Lung
  Atelectasis
  (incomplete expansion)
  Infarction
  Pneumonia

Abdominal organs
  Acute hepatomegaly
  Gallstones
  Splenic sequestration
  Splenomegaly
  Infarction

Bones and joints
  Hand-foot syndrome
  (painful swelling of
  hands and feet)

Kidney
  Hematuria
  (blood in urine)

Chronic Manifestations

Eye
  Hemorrhage
  Exudation
  Blindness
  Retinopathy

Pulmonary
hypertension
  Tachypnea

Heart
  High-output failure
  (congestive heart
  failure)

Spleen
  Splenic atrophy
  (autosplenectomy)

Kidney
  Hyposthenuria
  (dilute urine)
  Diuresis

Penis
  Priapism

Skin
  Stasis ulcers of
  hands, ankles, and
  feet

FIGURE 38-6 Clinical Manifestations of Sickle Cell Disease. (From Kline NE. Alterations of hematologic function in children. In: McCance KL, et al, eds. *Pathophysiology: The Biologic Basis for Disease in Adults and Children.* 6th ed. St. Louis: Mosby; 2010.)

Prevent Infection

Both children and adults with SCA are more prone to infection and have a more difficult time fighting off infection.[23] This can result in damage to the spleen from constant sickling of the RBCs. Damage to the spleen can prevent the destruction of bacteria in the blood. Prophylactic administration of oral antibiotics starting at 2 months old can decrease the chances of a pneumococcal infection and early death. Proper vaccinations against pneumococcal infections, meningitis, hepatitis, and influenza are important to prevent future infections.[23]

Pain Management

Pain associated with SCA can be acute or chronic in nature. The most common type of pain associated with SCA is vasoocclusive pain. It is commonly treated with an anti-inflammatory and opioid or non-opioid analgesics.[23,24] The pain associated with SCA can vary enormously; therefore, a number of different approaches may be required. The medication of choice should be influenced by the patient's history of analgesia use. Some patients may have extremely intricate medication regimes.[23] Paracetamol and nonsteroidal anti-inflammatory drugs (NSAIDs) are used for mild to moderate pain relief. If this is not effective, oral or parenteral opiates may be an alternative.[23,24]

For those who wish to try the nonpharmacologic route, there are other approaches such as psychologic support, massage, acupuncture, and transcutaneous electrical nerve stimulation. Distraction can be another valuable tool to use. The use of television, video games, repeating inspirational phrases and mental calculations can also be a form of distraction. Studies suggested that cognitive behavioral therapy can help teach patients coping strategies for acute and chronic pain.[23]

Transfusion Therapy

RBC transfusion therapy in SCD is an important lifesaving treatment option but should be done with careful consideration. Transfusion therapy is primarily used for treatment of patients who are experiencing complications due to SCD or as an emergency measure.[24] Transfusion therapy should be used with extreme caution due to risks such as iron overload, exposure to hepatitis, HIV and other infectious agents, alloimmunization, induction of hyperviscosity, and limitations on resources. The indication for having a blood transfusion or exchange are recurrent painful vasoocclusive crises with long hospital admissions, acute chest syndrome, stroke, priapism, and leg ulcers. Blood transfusions or exchange can also be performed before major operations, such as hip replacement because of avascular necrosis of the hip bone.[23]

Administration of Hydroxyurea

Hydroxyurea is an oral agent that is a safe and effective treatment for children and adults that suffer from SCA. It works by increasing the level of fetal hemoglobin in the RBCs, thereby reducing the concentration of sickle hemoglobin and sickling itself.[23] The patient is usually started at a dose of 15 mg/kg PO once a day. The dose is increased by 5 mg/kg every 12 weeks until 35 mg/kg is reached, providing the patient's blood count remains within an acceptable range. Research shows patients receiving hydroxyurea had lower episodes of pain and acute chest syndrome and also had a decreased need for blood transfusion and hospitalizations compared to those that received no treatment. Research states that hydroxyurea can be used as an alternative to regular blood transfusions.[24]

Nursing Management

Nursing management of the patient with SCA incorporates a variety of nursing diagnoses (Box 38-10). Nursing interventions include supporting the patient's vital functions, providing comfort and emotional support, maintaining surveillance for complications, and educating the patient and family.

Supporting Patient's Vital Functions

Frequent assessments should include parameters for neurologic status, renal function, cardiopulmonary function, and skin integrity that indicate impaired tissue or organ perfusion. Particular parameters to include are mental status, BUN and creatine levels, urine output, vital signs, hemodynamic values, cardiac rhythm, arterial blood gas and pulse oximetry values, skin breakdown, ecchymoses, or hematomas.[24]

◎ BOX 38-10 NURSING DIAGNOSES

Sickle Cell Anemia

- Acute Pain related to transmission and perception of cutaneous, visceral, muscular, or ischemic impulses, p. 1123
- Risk for Ineffective Peripheral Tissue Perfusion, p. 1158
- Risk for Ineffective Renal Tissue Perfusion, p. 1159
- Risk for Ineffective Gastrointestinal Tissue Perfusion, p. 1157
- Risk for Ineffective Cerebral Tissue Perfusion, p. 1156
- Powerlessness related to lack of control over the current situation or disease progression, p. 1152
- Deficient Knowledge related to lack of previous exposure to information, p. 1134 (see Box 38-11, Patient Education for Sickle Cell Anemia)

BOX 38-11 PATIENT EDUCATION

Sickle Cell Anemia

- Pathophysiology of disease
- Precipitating factor modification
- Importance of taking medications
- Maintenance of adequate hydration (especially during febrile periods and hot weather)
- Use of pharmacologic and nonpharmacologic methods of pain management
- Avoidance of situations that can precipitate condition such as extreme cold
- Smoking cessation and avoidance of secondhand smoke
- Get plenty of rest and relaxation and avoid exhaustive exercise
- Genetic screening
- Encourage purchase of medical alert bracelet or similar type of warning device

---

The critical care nurse must recognize and support the patient's vital physiologic functions. Administration of intravenous fluids, blood products, and inotropic agents to provide adequate hemodynamic support and tissue oxygenation is essential in preventing or combating end-organ damage. Close monitoring of vital signs, hemodynamic parameters, intake and output, and appropriate laboratory values assists the critical care nurse in administering and titrating appropriate agents.[24]

Maintaining Surveillance for Complications

The critical care nurse needs to be vigilant for signs of life-threatening complications such as septicemia, acute myocardial infarction, priapism, ischemic stroke, and shock.[20] If there are any significant concerns these must be reported immediately. Other issues that may arise are dehydration, hypoxia, infection, skin and tissue viability, and decreased hemoglobin levels.

Educating the Patient and Family

Even though there is no cure for SCA, the focus of care is prevention. Early in the patient's hospital stay, the patient and family should be taught about SCA, its etiologies, and its treatment (Box 38-11). Patient and family education focuses on measures to help prevent painful reoccurring episodes. If the patient smokes, he or she should be encouraged to stop smoking and be referred to a smoking cessation program. In addition, the importance of continuous medical follow-up should be stressed. While research continues to try to find a cure, nurses must continue to be sensitive to the effects of the disease on the patient and the family as well as the need to be culturally sensitive.[20]

Collaborative management of the patient with SCA is outlined in Box 38-12.

BOX 38-12 COLLABORATIVE MANAGEMENT

Sickle Cell Anemia

- Prevent infection
  - Prophylactic antibiotics
  - Vaccinations
- Manage pain
  - Pharmacologic management
  - Nonpharmacologic management
- Administration of blood
- Administration of hydroxyurea
- Maintain surveillance for complications
  - Septicemia
  - Acute kidney injury
  - Acute myocardial infarction
  - Acute limb ischemia
  - Ischemic stroke
  - Anemia
- Provide comfort and emotional support

TUMOR LYSIS SYNDROME

Description

Tumor lysis syndrome (TLS) refers to a variety of metabolic disturbances that may be seen with the treatment of cancer. A potentially lethal complication of various forms of cancer treatment, TLS occurs when large numbers of neoplastic cells are rapidly killed, resulting in the release of large amounts of potassium, phosphate, and uric acid into the systemic circulation. It is most commonly seen in patients with lymphoma, leukemia, or multiple metastatic conditions.[25]

Etiology

Although most often associated with the use of chemotherapeutic medications, biologic agents, and irradiation used in the treatment of malignant disorders, TLS can in rare instances occur spontaneously. The development of TLS has been linked to other pathophysiologic conditions such as elevated WBC counts, large tumors, multiple organ involvement by malignancy, and renal insufficiency.[25]

Pathophysiology

The primary mechanism involved in the development of TLS is the destruction of massive numbers of malignant cells by chemotherapy or radiation therapy (Fig. 38-7). Massive destruction of cells releases large amounts of potassium, phosphorus, and nucleic acids, leading to severe metabolic disturbances such as hyperuricemia, hyperkalemia, hyperphosphatemia, and hypocalcemia (Table 38-7). Vomiting, diarrhea, and other insensible fluid losses from fever or tachypnea also contribute

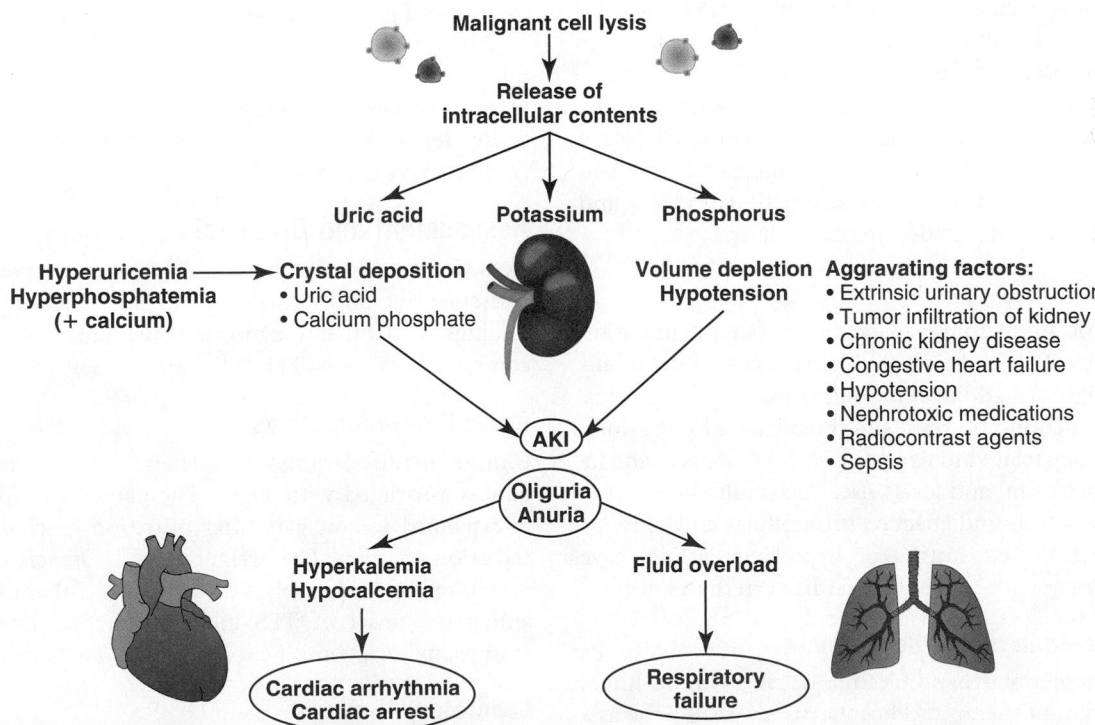

FIGURE 38-7 Metabolic abnormalities in tumor lysis syndrome and clinical consequences. *AKI,* Acute kidney injury. (From Abu-Alfa AK, Younes A. Tumor lysis syndrome and acute kidney injury: evaluation, prevention and management. *Am J Kidney Dis.* 2010;55[5 suppl 3]:S1.)

TABLE 38-7   ELECTROLYTE ABNORMALITIES ENCOUNTERED IN TUMOR LYSIS SYNDROME AND THEIR CLINICAL CONSEQUENCES

ELECTROLYTE	PATHOPHYSIOLOGY	CLINICAL CONSEQUENCE	TREATMENT OPTIONS
Potassium	Rapid expulsion of intracellular K^+ into the circulation due to cell lysis	Adverse skeletal and cardiac manifestations (e.g., ventricular dysrhythmias, weakness, paresthesias)	Insulin/glucose, sodium bicarbonate, inhaled beta-agonist, K^+-binding resins, dialysis, calcium gluconate
Phosphate	Release of intracellular PO_4^- due to cell lysis		
May be compounded by renal dysfunction	Muscle cramps, tetany, dysrhythmias, seizures	Dialysis, phosphate binders	
Calcium	Precipitation of the calcium phosphate complex because of the rapid increase in the phosphorous concentration	Muscle cramps, tetany, dysrhythmias, seizures, renal failure (acute nephrocalcinosis)	Calcium gluconate (treatment should be reserved for those with neuromuscular irritability)
Uric acid	Cell lysis leads to increased levels of purine nucleic acids into the circulation that are metabolized to uric acid	Renal failure (uric acid nephropathy)	Hydration, dialysis, xanthine oxidase inhibitors, alkalization of urine, urate oxidase

From Davidson MB, et al. Pathophysiology, clinical consequences, and treatment of tumor lysis syndrome. *Am J Med.* 2004;116:546.

to these electrolyte disturbances.[25] Death of patients with TLS is most often caused by complications of renal failure or cardiac arrest.[25-27]

Hyperuricemia

Hyperuricemia occurs 48 to 72 hours after the initiation of anticancer therapy.[25] Tumor cells undergo rapid growth and development, and large amounts of nucleic acids are present within them. When therapy is initiated, tumor cell destruction releases nucleic acids, which are metabolized into uric acid. Metabolic acidosis ensues, resulting in crystallization of the uric acid in the distal tubules of the kidney and leading to obstruction of urine flow. Glomerular filtration rates drop as the kidneys are unable to clear the increasing amounts of uric acid. Consequently, acute kidney injury eventually occurs.[28] Acute kidney injury is discussed further in Chapter 27.

Hyperuricemia associated with TLS can be potentiated by several other factors, including elevated uric acid levels before the initiation of therapy. Other causes of increased uric acid production are elevated WBC counts, destruction of WBCs, and enlargement of the lymph nodes, spleen, or liver.[25]

Hyperkalemia

Hyperkalemia occurs within 6 to 72 hours after the initiation of chemotherapy. This is the most deleterious of all the manifestations of TLS.[25] In addition to the release of nucleic acids, tumor cell destruction also results in the release of potassium. Renal insufficiency related to hyperuricemia prevents adequate excretion of potassium, and levels rise. The resultant hyperkalemia may have a profound effect on intracellular and extracellular fluid levels.[29] Left untreated, hyperkalemia can have devastating consequences, including cardiac arrest and death.[25]

Hyperphosphatemia and Hypocalcemia

Hyperphosphatemia and hypocalcemia occur 24 to 48 hours after the initiation of therapy.[25] Phosphorus levels also rise as a consequence of tumor cell destruction. Calcium ions then bind with the excess phosphorus, creating calcium phosphate salts and bringing about hypocalcemia. These salts precipitate in the

TABLE 38-8   COMMON FINDINGS IN TUMOR LYSIS SYNDROME

DIAGNOSTIC PARAMETER	FINDINGS
Clinical	Weight gain, edema, diarrhea, lethargy, muscle cramps, nausea and vomiting, paresthesia, weakness, oliguria, uremia, seizures
Laboratory	↑ Potassium, phosphorus, uric acid, BUN, Cr ↓ Calcium, creatinine clearance, pH, bicarbonate, $PaCO_2$
Diagnostic	Positive Chvostek and Trousseau signs, hyperactive deep tendon reflexes, dysrhythmias, ECG changes

BUN, Blood urea nitrogen; *Cr*, creatinine; *ECG*, electrocardiogram; *$PaCO_2$*, partial pressure of carbon dioxide; ↑ increased; ↓ decreased.

kidney tubules, worsening renal insufficiency. Hypocalcemia causes tetany and cardiac dysrhythmias, which can result in cardiac arrest and death.[28,29]

Assessment and Diagnosis

Detection and recognition of TLS is accomplished through assessment of clinical manifestations, evaluation of laboratory findings, and other diagnostic tests. Table 38-8 summarizes common findings in TLS.[25,27]

Clinical Manifestations

Clinical manifestations are related to the metabolic disturbances associated with TLS.[27] The patient's history reveals an unexplained weight gain after initiation of chemotherapy or radiation therapy. The weight gain is associated with fluid retention due to electrolyte disturbances. Other early signs heralding the onset of TLS include diarrhea, lethargy, muscle cramps, nausea, vomiting, paresthesias, and weakness.[26]

Laboratory Findings

Laboratory findings demonstrate electrolyte disturbances such as elevated potassium and phosphorus levels and a decreased calcium level. Uric acid levels are increased. Elevated levels of

BUN and creatinine and a decreased creatinine clearance also indicate TLS. Metabolic acidosis is confirmed by the presence of decreased pH, bicarbonate levels, and partial pressure of carbon dioxide ($Paco_2$) on arterial blood gas measurements.[26]

Other Diagnostic Tests

Physical examination reveals positive Chvostek and Trousseau signs related to hypocalcemia. Hyperactive deep tendon reflexes indicate hyperkalemia and hypocalcemia.[27] Potassium and calcium disturbances result in changes that can be seen on the electrocardiogram (ECG), such as peaked or inverted T waves, altered QT intervals, widened QRS complexes, and dysrhythmias.[25]

Medical Management

Medical interventions are aimed at maintaining adequate hydration, treating metabolic imbalances, and preventing life-threatening complications (see Table 38-7).[26,29]

Adequate Hydration

Administration of intravenous fluids may be necessary early in the course of treatment if inadequate hydration exists. The administration of isotonic saline (0.9% normal saline) reduces serum concentrations of uric acid, phosphate, and potassium.[27] The use of nonthiazide diuretics to maintain adequate urine output may be required. If renal failure occurs, hemodialysis should be considered.[27]

Metabolic Imbalances

Electrolytes and arterial blood gases are closely monitored. Dietary restrictions of potassium and phosphorus may be necessary. The goals in treating hyperuricemia are to inhibit uric acid formation and to increase renal clearance.[29] This can be accomplished through the administration of sodium bicarbonate to increase the pH of the urine to above 7.0, which increases the solubility of uric acid, preventing subsequent crystallization. Allopurinol administration can also inhibit uric acid formation.[27]

Life-Threatening Complications

If potassium levels rise dangerously, Kayexalate (sodium polystyrene sulfonate) may be given orally, or if the patient is unable to tolerate oral medications due to nausea and vomiting, rectal instillation may be used. If the patient is oliguric, glucose and insulin infusions may be given to facilitate lowering the potassium levels. A 10% solution of calcium gluconate may be administered to stabilize cardiac tissue membranes to prevent life-threatening dysrhythmias.[30] Phosphorus-binding antacids can be used for treating hyperphosphatemia. Stool softeners may be necessary to treat the constipation often associated with the administration of these antacids. Calcium gluconate may be required to replace calcium, but it should be used judiciously.[25]

Nursing Management

Nursing management of the patient with TLS incorporates a variety of nursing diagnoses (Box 38-13). Nursing interventions include monitoring fluid and electrolytes, providing comfort

---

BOX 38-13 NURSING DIAGNOSES

Tumor Lysis Syndrome

- Excess Fluid Volume related to renal dysfunction, p. 1139
- Decreased Cardiac Output related to alterations in contractility, p. 1128
- Anxiety related to threat to biologic, psychologic, and/or social integrity, p. 1125
- Ineffective Coping related to a situational crisis and personal vulnerability, p. 1150

BOX 38-14 COLLABORATIVE MANAGEMENT

Tumor Lysis Syndrome

- Facilitate adequate renal function.
  - Volume hydration with 0.9% normal saline
  - Nonthiazide diuretics
- Treat hyperkalemia.
  - Kayexalate
  - Glucose and insulin
- Treat hyperuricemia.
  - Sodium bicarbonate
  - Allopurinol
- Treat hyperphosphatemia.
  - Dietary restrictions
  - Phosphorus-binding antacids
- Treat hypocalcemia.
  - Calcium gluconate
- Maintain surveillance for complications.
  - Acute kidney injury
  - Cardiac dysrhythmias
- Provide comfort and emotional support.

---

and emotional support, maintaining surveillance for complications, and education the patient and family.

Monitoring Fluid and Electrolytes

Assessment and continued monitoring of the patient is an important role of the critical care nurse when caring for the patient with TLS. Recognizing critical laboratory changes or development of symptoms and notifying the physician in a timely manner are essential. Insertion of a urinary catheter and maintenance of the intravenous line site are necessary to ensure adequate intake and output. Vital signs should be monitored frequently, and weight should be monitored daily.

Maintaining Surveillance for Complications

Nursing interventions are aimed at preventing complications. Seizure precautions should be instituted, especially if calcium levels are disrupted. Insertion of a nasogastric tube is appropriate if nausea or vomiting occurs. Dietary adjustments are necessary, such as potassium and phosphorus restrictions in the presence of elevated serum levels and providing additional fiber to combat the constipation associated with the administration of antacids.[30]

Educating the Patient and Family

Education of the patient and family is a primary role of the critical care nurse. All treatments and interventions should be explained before carrying them out, and questions should be answered at a level understandable to the patient and family. Before discharge, potential risk factors and identification of early signs and symptoms should be reviewed.

Collaborative management of the patient with TLS is outlined in Box 38-14.

ANEMIA OF CRITICAL ILLNESS

Etiology

Anemia of critical illness (ACI) is a hospital-acquired disorder commonly seen in critically ill patients. It is the result of inflammation, iron deficiency, trauma, surgery, gastrointestinal bleeding, and iatrogenic blood loss from diagnostic testing. Inflammation causes decreased RBC production and increased destruction of RBCs by macrophages. Frequent phlebotomy, coagulopathies, and nutritional deficits are just a few reasons for this increasing problem.[31,32] Studies have shown that as many as 50% of transfusions administered in the critical care unit are related to hospital-acquired anemia.[33] For these reasons, research has been focused on determining ways to minimize iatrogenic blood losses, improve blood salvage techniques, and develop alternatives to traditional blood transfusion therapy.

Blood Conservation Strategies

As more patients and clinicians opt for the limited use of blood products, strategies for conserving blood and preventing unnecessary loss become an important part of the critical care nurse's standard of care. These strategies include minimizing blood loss, managing oxygen delivery and consumption, stimulating production of RBCs, and understanding transfusion safety and alternative agents.[34,35]

Minimizing Blood Loss

Frequent blood draws in the critically ill patient have been associated with the development of anemia. Blood losses correspond to actual volume of samples and discards when drawing from venous access lines. Critical care nurses can be instrumental in significantly decreasing blood loss in this arena. The use of pediatric collection tubes and point-of-care testing are techniques that yield valid diagnostic results but require smaller blood samples. Closed-loop vascular devices that retain the sterility of the potential discard and allow its return to the patient are also being used.[36] Noninvasive monitoring devices such as pulse oximetry and capnography can reduce the need for arterial blood gas analysis.

The critical care nurse plays a key role in preventing and managing hemorrhagic blood loss in the critically ill patient. Control of hypertension, which can contribute to significant hemorrhage, can be accomplished through fluid management and the administration of antihypertensive and vasodilatory medications as needed.[37] Blood salvage devices can be employed to collect shed blood and return it to the patient.[35] Several pharmacologic agents can assist in achieving hemostasis and can prevent further blood loss. Desmopressin is a potent vasoconstrictor that also affects clotting factor VIII.[35] Aminocaproic acid (Amicar) inhibits activation of plasminogen.[35] All of these agents and devices work to control bleeding.

Managing Oxygen Delivery and Consumption

Illness-related stress, blood loss from surgery, infection, pain, and anxiety contribute to the higher than normal demand for oxygen by the critically ill patient.[32] Monitoring pulse oximetry is useful in identifying activities and interventions that can contribute to the imbalance between supply and demand. Supplemental oxygen therapy assists in maintaining available oxygen supplies. Promoting a restful environment through modulation of nursing care activities and providing pain and sedation control can assist in decreasing the demand for oxygen. It is important to monitor cardiac output and other hemodynamic parameters to manage interventions that optimize oxygen delivery. Administration of fluids and inotropic agents optimizes blood pressure and cardiac output, and vasodilators are used to decrease afterload and improve efficiency of cardiovascular function.[35]

Stimulating Production of Red Blood Cells

Insufficient erythropoiesis can contribute to anemia in the critically ill patient. The administration of epoetin alpha can stimulate the production of RBCs, reducing the need for transfusions. Iron preparations such as ferrous sulfate, iron sucrose, or iron gluconate may be administered to provide necessary iron stores for the increased erythropoiesis.[38]

Encouraging Safer Transfusions and Alternative Agents

Finding ways to decrease the risks associated with blood transfusions and make the blood supply safer for patients is a high priority. Better, more sensitive screening tests, irradiation, and removal of leukocytes are a few of the current methods in use. Plasma expanders manufactured from nonhuman sources are also available. Autologous transfusions, for which the patient donates his or her own blood before a surgical procedure or other anticipated need, has also been a common practice for many years. Recombinant DNA technology is being used to develop safe alternatives to blood transfusions. The use of blood from other species is being researched in the quest to provide safe and effective products for use in severe anemia.[35]

BOX 38-15 CASE STUDY

Patient with Hematologic Disorders and Oncologic Emergencies

Brief Patient History

Mr. L is an otherwise healthy, 23-year-old African American man who presents with a week-long history of diarrhea, nausea, and vomiting after attending a barbecue last weekend.

Clinical Assessment

Mr. L is admitted to the critical care unit from the emergency department with hypotension, fever, and leukocytosis.

Diagnostic Procedures

His vital signs are as follows: blood pressure of 65/42 mm Hg, heart rate of 145 beats/min (sinus tachycardia), respiratory rate of 35 breaths/min, and temperature of 102.4° F. His white blood cell count is 25,000/mm³ with 15% bands, lactate level is 7 mmol/L, prothrombin time is 25 seconds, and platelet count is 22,000/mm³. Blood cultures reveal gram-negative bacilli.

Patient with Hematologic Disorders and Oncologic Emergencies—cont'd

Medical Diagnosis

Mr. L is diagnosed with severe sepsis and disseminated intravascular coagulation.

Questions

1. What major outcomes do you expect to achieve for this patient?
2. What problems or risks must be managed to achieve these outcomes?

3. What interventions must be initiated to monitor, prevent, manage, or eliminate the problems and risks identified?
4. What interventions should be initiated to promote optimal functioning, safety, and well-being of the patient?
5. What possible learning needs do you anticipate for this patient?
6. What cultural and age-related factors may have a bearing on the patient's plan of care?

SUMMARY

Coagulation and Fibrinolysis

- Hemostasis is the ability of the body to control bleeding and clotting.
- Four actions are involved in achieving hemostasis: local vasoconstriction to reduce blood flow; platelet aggregation at the injury site and formation of a platelet plug; formation of a fibrin mesh to strengthen the plug; and dissolution of the clot after tissue repair.

Disseminated Intravascular Coagulation

- DIC is characterized by bleeding and thrombosis, which result from depletion of clotting factors, platelets, and RBCs and, if left untreated, will result in death.
- Medical management focuses on identification of the underlying cause, provision of hemodynamic support to preserve end-organ function, and administration of blood, blood components, and medications to interrupt the process.
- Nursing actions include initiating bleeding precautions, providing comfort and emotional support, and maintaining surveillance for complications (e.g., hypovolemic shock, ischemia, multiple organ dysfunction syndrome).

Idiopathic Thrombocytopenia Purpura

- Idiopathic thrombocytopenia purpura is caused by an autoimmune response that results in the destruction of existing platelets.
- Medical management focuses on administration of glucocorticoids, immunoglobulin, and platelets.
- Nursing actions include initiating bleeding precautions, providing comfort and emotional support, and maintaining surveillance for complications (e.g., intracranial hemorrhage, severe blood loss).

Heparin-Induced Thrombocytopenia

- There are two forms of heparin-induced thrombocytopenia: type 1 and type 2. Type 1 is more common, milder, and transient. Type 2 is the result of an autoimmune response to the administration of heparin and is more severe than type 1.
- Medical management focuses discontinuation of all heparin, initiation of anticoagulation with an alternative anticoagulant, and treatment of thrombosis.

- Nursing actions include providing comfort and emotional support and maintaining surveillance for complications (e.g., deep vein thrombosis, pulmonary emboli, limb ischemia, ischemic stroke, acute myocardial infarction).

Sickle Cell Anemia

- Sickle cell anemia (SCA) is a disease passed down through families in which red blood cells form an abnormal sickle or crescent shape.
- Medical management focuses on prevention of infection, management of pain, and administration of red blood cells and hydroxyurea.
- Nursing actions include supporting the patient's vital functions, providing comfort and emotional support, maintaining surveillance for complications (e.g., ischemic stroke, acute myocardial infarction, acute limb ischemia, acute kidney injury), and educating the patient and family.

Tumor Lysis Syndrome

- Tumor lysis syndrome occurs when a large number of neoplastic cells are rapidly killed, resulting in the release of large amounts of potassium, phosphate, and uric acid in the systemic circulation.
- Medical management focuses on preservation of renal function and treatment of electrolyte disorders (hyperkalemia, hyperuricemia, hyperphosphatemia, and hypocalcemia).
- Nursing actions include providing comfort and emotional support and maintaining surveillance for complications (e.g., acute kidney injury, dysrhythmias).

Hospital-Acquired Anemia

- Anemia of critical illness occurs as a result of inflammation, iron deficiency, trauma, surgery, gastrointestinal bleeding, and from iatrogenic blood loss from diagnostic testing.
- Blood conservation strategies include minimizing blood loss, managing oxygen delivery and consumption, and stimulating production of RBCs.

REFERENCES

1. Rote NL, McCance KL. Structure and function of the hematologic system. In: McCance KL, et al, eds. *Pathophysiology: The Biologic Basis for Disease in Adults and Children*. 6th ed. St. Louis: Mosby; 2010.
2. Furie B, Furie BC. Mechanisms of thrombus formation. *N Engl J Med*. 2008;359:938.
3. Levi M, van der Poll T. Disseminated intravascular coagulation: a review for the internist. *Intern Emerg Med*. Epub ahead of print. Sept 27, 2012.
4. Holroyd EW, Simari RD. Interdependent biological systems, multi-functional molecules: the evolving role of tissue factor pathway inhibitor beyond anti-coagulation. *Throm Res*. 2010;125(suppl 1):S57.
5. Castoldi E, Hackeng TM. Regulation of coagulation by protein S. *Curr Opin Hematol*. 2008;15:529.
6. Kitchens CS. Thrombocytopenia and thrombosis in disseminated intravascular coagulation (DIC). *Hematology Am Soc Hematol Educ Program*. 2009;2009:240.
7. Levi M. Disseminated intravascular coagulation. *Crit Care Med*. 2007;35:2191.
8. Gando S. Microvascular thrombosis and multiple organ dysfunction. *Crit Care Med*. 2010;38(suppl 2):S35.
9. Blaisdell FW. Causes, prevention, and treatment of intravascular coagulation and disseminated intravascular coagulation. *J Trauma Acute Care Surg*. 2012;72:1719.
10. Marques MB. Thrombotic thrombocytopenic purpura and heparin-induced thrombocytopenia: two unique causes of life-threatening thrombocytopenia. *Clin Lab Med*. 2009;29:321.
11. Battistelli S, et al. Heparin-induced thrombocytopenia in surgical patients. *Am J Surg*. 2010;199:43.
12. Noonan K. Introduction to B-cell disorders. *Clin J Oncol Nurs*. 2007;11:3.
13. McCrae K. Immune thrombocytopenia: no longer "idiopathic." *Cleve Clin J Med*. 2011;758:358.
14. Liebman HA, Pullarkat V. Diagnosis and management of immune thrombocytopenia in the era of thrombopoietic mimetics. *Hematol Am Soc Hematol Educ Program*. 2011;2011:384.
15. Shantsila E, et al. Heparin-induced thrombocytopenia. A contemporary clinical approach to diagnosis and management. *Chest*. 2009;135:1651.
16. Warkentin TE. Heparin-induced thrombocytopenia. *Hematol Oncol Clin North Am*. 2007;21:589.
17. Selleng K, et al. Heparin-induced thrombocytopenia in intensive care patients. *Crit Care Med*. 2007;35:1165.
18. Donavan JL, et al. An overview of heparin-induced thrombocytopenia. *J Pharm Pract*. 2010;23:226.
19. Linkins LA, et al. Treatment and prevention of heparin-induced thrombocytopenia: Antithrombotic Therapy and Prevention of Thrombosis, 9th ed: American College of Chest Physicians Evidence-Based Clinical Practice Guidelines. *Chest*. 2012;141(2 Suppl):e495S.
20. De D. Acute nursing care and management of patients with sickle cell. *Br J Nurs*. 2012;17:818.
21. Pack-Mabien A, Haynes J Jr. A primary care provider's guide to preventive and acute care management of adults and children with sickle cell disease. *J Am Acad Nurse Pract*. 2009;21:250.
22. Porter B, et al. Hematologic and immune problems. In: Dunphy L, et al, eds. *Primary Care: The Art and Science of Advanced Practice Nursing*. 2nd ed. Philadelphia: FA Davis; 2007.
23. Addis G. Sickle cell disease, part 1: Understanding the condition. *Br J Nurs*. 2010;5:231.
24. Brown M. Managing the acutely ill adult with sickle cell disease. *Br J Nurs*. 2012;21:90.
25. Robison J. Metabolic emergencies: tumor lysis syndrome. In: Newton S, et al, eds. *Oncology Nursing Advisor: A Comprehensive Guide to Clinical Practice*. St. Louis: Mosby; 2009.
26. Tosi P, et al. Consensus conferences on the management of tumor lysis syndrome. *Haemtologica*. 2008;93:1877.
27. Behl D, et al. Oncologic emergencies. *Crit Care Clin*. 2010; 26:181.
28. Shelton BK. Tumor lysis syndrome. In: Chernecky CC, Murphy-Ende K, eds. *Acute Care Oncology*. 2nd ed. St. Louis: Mosby; 2009.
29. Abu-Alfa AK, Younes A. Tumor lysis syndrome and acute kidney injury: evaluation, prevention and management. *Am J Kidney Dis*. 2010;55(5 suppl 3):S1.
30. Myers JS. Complications of cancer and cancer treatment. In: Langhorne ME, et al, eds. *Oncology Nursing*. 5th ed. St. Louis: Mosby; 2007.
31. Brophy DF, et al. An epidemiological study of anemia and renal dysfunction in patients admitted to ICUs across the United States. *Anemia*. Epub ahead of print. Aug 14, 2012.
32. Prakash D. Anemia in the ICU: anemia of chronic disease versus anemia of acute illness. *Crit Care Clin*. 2012;28:333.
33. Collins TA. Packed red blood cell transfusions in critically ill patients. *Crit Care Nurse*. 2011;31:24.
34. Thomas J, Martinez A. Blood conservation in the critically ill. *Am J Health Syst Pharm*. 2007;64:S11.
35. Tinmouth AT, et al. Blood conservation strategies to reduce the need for red blood cell transfusion in critically ill patients. *CMAJ*. 2008;178:49.
36. Mukhopadhyay A, et al. The use of blood conservation device to reduce red blood cell transfusion requirements: a before and after study. *Crit Care*. 2010;14:R7.
37. Cannon-Diehl MR. Transfusion in the critically ill: does it affect outcome? *Crit Care Nurs Q*. 2010;33:324.
38. Shermock KM, et al. Erythropoietic agents for anemia of critical illness. *Am J Health Syst Pharm*. 2008;65:540.

The Obstetric Patient

Susie Hutchins

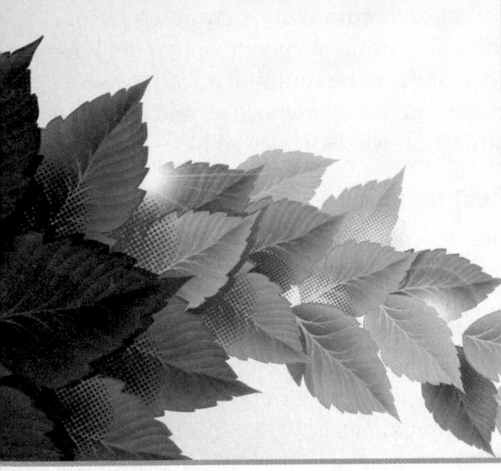

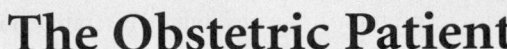

evolve WEBSITE

http://evolve.elsevier.com/Urden/criticalcare/

Evolve features:

- NCLEX Review Questions
- CCRN Review Questions
- PCCN Review Questions

- Mosby's Nursing Skills Procedures
- Animations

- Video Clips
- Glossary

Innovations in technology and advances in treatment options have placed the worlds of critical care and obstetrics on a pathway of collaboration and sometimes of conflict. Traditionally, the two specialties have been separated, in part because of the typical normalcy and health-oriented approach of obstetrics and the crisis and illness orientation of critical care. Pregnancy alters the function of virtually every organ system, and the baseline state and patient response to physiologic changes are very different in the pregnant patient. Fetal considerations often are important in designing and leading the clinical approach to the critically ill woman. Many common conditions in pregnancy require special medical care with associated complications that have the potential for serious maternal morbidity and mortality.

In 2010, the maternal mortality rate of the United States was 21 deaths per 100,000 live births, compared with 12 per 100,000 in 1990. This represents a total of about 840 women who died from maternal causes in 2010.[1] Some of this increase observed over the past decades may have been caused by changes in the coding and classification of maternal deaths. An alarming trend in maternal mortality in the United States is race-specific pregnancy-related mortality rates. Analysis of rates has demonstrated that compared with white women, African American women have 2.7 times the risk of dying as a result of childbirth and that the maternal mortality rate among Hispanic women was about 0.8% less than that of white women.[2] At the global level, the World Health Organization (WHO), The United Nations Children's Fund, the United Nations Population Fund and the World Bank assessed trends in maternal mortality rate from the period 1990-2010 and revealed that the number of women dying of pregnancy- and childbirth-related complications has almost halved in 20 years. The WHO's fifth Millennium Development Goal (MDG) aims to improve maternal health with a target of reducing maternal death by 75% in the period 1990-2015. The resulting findings were that the percentage reductions for 10 countries have already achieved the MDG by 2010, 11 countries are "on track" of achieving this goal, 50 countries are "making progress," 14 countries have made "insufficient progress," and 11 countries are characterized as having made "no progress" and are likely to miss the MDG target unless accelerated interventions are put in place.[1]

It is important to recognize that critical care obstetrics encompasses two distinct populations: 1) women with preexisting disease who become pregnant and 2) women with normal pregnancies who become compromised by critical illness or injury. The two priorities for the pregnant critically ill woman are: 1) supporting fetal growth and development and 2) optimizing maternal and family experiences.

It is impossible to discuss in one chapter every aspect of management of the critically ill obstetric patient. Instead, the focus is to provide a synopsis of the more commonly seen conditions or concerns in the realm of critical care obstetrics and to emphasize the collaborative nature of this emerging field, recognizing that the manifestations and management of many critical illnesses are typically identical in pregnant and nonpregnant patients, although the data value changes associated with pregnancy must be considered. Nursing management, unless unique to the critically ill obstetric patient, is not detailed here.

RISKS TO FETAL DEVELOPMENT

Factors that influence embryonic and fetal development may be intrinsic or extrinsic in nature. Intrinsic factors such as chromosomal abnormalities and congenital anomalies account for 25% of all birth defects. Extrinsic factors, also known as *teratogens*, account for those remaining.[3] A teratogen is any chemical, substance, or exposure that may cause any form of birth defects in a developing fetus. This would include medicines, radiation, and agents of infection. It is important to remember that the effects of teratogens depend on maternal and fetal genotypes, the stage of development when exposure occurs, and the dose and duration of the exposure of the agent.[3] Exposure to ionizing radiation is usually not a concern until more than a cumulative 100 to 200 milligrays (mGy; 10 to 20 rads) have been exceeded, but some experts recommend caution in the first 25 weeks because of fetal organogenesis and central nervous system development.[4-5] At doses less than 0.05 gray (Gy), no evidence of an increased risk of fetal anomalies, intellectual disability, growth restriction, or pregnancy loss from ionizing radiation is present. A small increased risk of childhood cancer, 1 in 2000 versus the 1 in 3000 background rate, may exist.[4]

Medication use in critically ill obstetric patients requires analysis of the risk–benefit ratio. It is important to consider the influence that drug exposure could have on the developing fetus, but often, the benefit may outweigh the potential fetal risk when all factors are considered.[6] Also, fetal and newborn outcomes may be dependent on timely maternal stabilization on potential harmful medication. Critical ill obstetric patients may be reluctant to take medication during pregnancy because of the possibility or perceived possibility of the adverse effects on the fetus. The U.S. Food and Drug Administration (FDA) placed medications into risk categories regarding use during pregnancy along with potential effects on the growing fetus. Box 39-1 describes the FDA labeling with regard to a drug's risk to a fetus.[6-7] (As of February 2011, the FDA proposed major revisions to prescription drug labeling to more completely inform the use of medicines during pregnancy and breastfeeding. They are presently in the writing and clearance process.[8])

BOX 39-1 FDA CATEGORIES OF LABELING FOR DRUG USE IN PREGNANCY

- *Category A:* Controlled studies in women fail to demonstrate risk to the fetus in the first 12 weeks. Possibility of fetal harm is remote.
- *Category B:* Animal studies do not indicate a risk to the fetus. Well-controlled studies with pregnant mothers fail to demonstrate a risk to the fetus.
- *Category C:* Studies have shown teratogenic effects in animal studies. No controlled studies in women have been conducted.
- *Category D:* Evidence of fetal risk exists, but benefits in life-threatening or serious disease may make it acceptable despite risks.
- *Category X:* Studies demonstrate fetal abnormalities, or evidence of risk from human experience exists. The risk clearly outweighs the benefit.

Data from Briggs G, et al. *Drugs in Pregnancy and Lactation.* 9th ed. Baltimore: Williams & Wilkins; 2011; Riordan J, Auerbach K. *Breastfeeding and Human Lactation.* 3rd ed. Boston: Jones & Bartlett; 2005.

Perinatal Infection

Infections—bacterial, viral, and protozoan—may pose a serious threat to the health and safety of the pregnant woman and her fetus or newborn. Several of the more common infections along with the adverse maternal and fetal consequences and perinatal management of each infection will be reviewed here.

Group B Streptococcal Infection

During the 1970s, group B *Streptococcus* (GBS) was recognized as the leading infectious cause of neonatal sepsis and mortality and remains so today.[9] The prevalence of neonatal infection is approximately 0.4 per 1000 live births, and approximately 1300 cases of neonatal streptococcal septicemia occur each year in the United States.[10] Mortality is higher among preterm infants, with case fatality rates of approximately 20% and as high as 30% among those less than 33 weeks' gestation, compared with 2% to 3% among full-term infants.[11]

Maternal colonization may be intermittent, transient, or chronic, and it is likely that nearly every woman is colonized by GBS at some time. Most women are asymptomatic, but in symptomatic women, GBS is responsible for considerable maternal morbidity from infections such as pyelonephritis, chorioamnionitis, postpartum endometrioses, sepsis, wound infections and, in rare instances, meningitis.[9]

In the infant, GBS may result in unexpected intrapartum stillbirth.[12] Early-onset neonatal infection results almost exclusively from vertical transmission from a colonized mother to her infant and is often characterized by signs of serious illness, including respiratory distress, apnea, and shock. Late-onset disease occurs 1 week or more after birth. These infants often develop meningitis. Long-term neurologic complications are common in survivors of both types of GBS.[9]

At the present time, the standard for diagnosis of GBS infection is bacteriologic culture using the Todd-Hewitt broth or selective blood agar. The specimen for culture should be obtained from the lower vagina, perineum, and anus using a simple cotton swab.[13] Prevention of early onset neonatal GBS infection is based on the guidelines from the Centers for Disease Control and Prevention (CDC), which were published in 1996 and updated in 2010.[14]

Cytomegalovirus Infection

Cytomegalovirus (CMV) is a deoxyribonucleic acid (DNA) virus belonging to the herpes simplex virus (HSV) group. It causes both congenital and acquired disorders. The significance of this virus in pregnancy is related to its ability to be transmitted by asymptomatic women across the placenta to the fetus or by the cervical route during birth.[15] Although the virus is usually innocuous in adults and children, it may be fatal to the fetus. The virus is passed between humans by close contact such as during kissing, breastfeeding, and sexual intercourse.[15] The diagnosis of CMV infection can be confirmed by isolation of the virus in tissue culture, with the highest concentrations of virus typically in the urine, seminal fluid, saliva, and breast milk. About 50% to 80% of adult women in the United States have serologic evidence of past CMV infection. The overall risk of congenital infection is greatest when maternal infection occurs in the third trimester, but the probability of severe fetal injury is highest when maternal infection develops in the first trimester.[16]

Although 85% to 90% of infected fetuses will be asymptomatic at birth, the remaining 10% to 15% will have abnormalities of varying severity.[16] Mortality rate among the symptomatic infants is 20% to 30%, and 90% of the these survivors have significant neurologic complications. The most common severe neonatal infections are hepatosplenomegaly, intracranial calcification, growth restriction, microcephaly, chorioretinitis, hearing loss, thrombocytopenia, hyperbilirubinemia, and intellectual disability. The virus may be identified in amniotic fluid by culture or polymerase chain reaction (PCR); however, mere identification of the virus does not necessarily delineate the severity of the fetal injury.[17] Ultrasonographic findings may include fetal hydrops, growth restriction, hydramnios, cardiomegaly, and fetal ascites.

Currently, no effective therapies are available to manage this infection. A recent placebo-controlled, randomized, double-blind trail evaluated a CMV vaccine and showed that it has the potential to decrease cases of maternal and congenital CMV infection.[18] Ideally, preventive measures should be employed to ensure that women do not contract CMV infection during pregnancy. One simple measure is encouraging women to use careful hand-washing techniques.

Toxoplasmosis

Toxoplasmosis is caused by the protozoan *Toxoplasma gondii* (*T. gondii*), with both farm animals, especially cattle, pigs, and sheep, and domestic cats playing an important role in the life cycle of the *Toxoplasma* organism. Cats are the usual host for the protozoan, and the infective oocytes are passed in feces and subsequently ingested by grazing farm animals. The organism disseminates throughout the animal's body, ultimately forming cysts in brain tissue and muscle. Cats acquire the organism through ingestion of undercooked or uncooked meat, possibly infected rodents. Human infection occurs when infected, undercooked meat is ingested or when food has been contaminated by cat feces.[19]

In the United States, congenital toxoplasmosis is found to occur in 0.8 per 10,000 live births annually, and in Europe, it is estimated to be 10 cases per 10,000 live births.[12] It is innocuous in most adults, resembling a minor viral illness, but it affects the fetus profoundly, creating long-term sequelae if the mother contracted the disease shortly before or during pregnancy.[19]

Maternal infection occurring in the first trimester typically results in more severe fetal damage and often ends in spontaneous abortion. The fetal infection occurring during the last month of pregnancy results in infants being born without any clinical signs of infections, although 50% will become symptomatic if left untreated.[12,16] Severe neonatal disorders associated with congenital infection include convulsions, coma, microcephaly, and hydrocephalus, causing many infant to die soon after birth. Survivors often have visual, hearing, and intellectual impairment.[20]

The goal is to identify the woman at risk and to treat the disease promptly if diagnosed. Diagnosis is made by serologic testing, including the immunoglobulin M (IgM) and IgG fluorescent antibody test.[20] PCR for *T. gondii* DNA in amniotic fluid is the best way to diagnose fetal infection, with ultrasonography revealing findings such as ascites, ventriculomegaly, microcephaly, and growth restriction.[20] If fetal infection is suspected, pyrimethamine, sulfadiazine, or folinic acid should be given to the mother after the 18th week of pregnancy.[12]

Rubella

Rubella is one of the most teratogenic of all viruses. Although it presents as a mild illness in most children and adults, rubella infection in the fetus can have overwhelming consequences. Estimates suggest that in the United States up to 10% of women are susceptible to rubella.[12]

The period of greatest risk for the teratogenic effects of rubella on the fetus is during the first trimester, when maternal infection results in up to 80% of maternal–fetal transmission.[12] Defects are rare when infection develops after 20 weeks' gestation.[21] Infants born with congenital rubella syndrome are infectious and should be isolated at birth. Prognosis of these infants is poor, with 10% to 20% of the affected infants dying during the first year of life. Rubella syndrome manifests in the newborn most commonly as congenital cataract, sensorineural deafness, and congenial heart defects. Mental retardation and cerebral palsy may become evident in infancy. Diagnosis is made when these conditions and an elevated rubella IgM antibody titer are present at birth.[21]

The best therapy for rubella is prevention. Vaccination with live, attenuated vaccines should be given to all women of childbearing age who are susceptible and prior to pregnancy. Although no fetal infection has resulted from immunization of a pregnant woman, pregnancy should be avoided for 1 month after immunization. Testing for immunity involves the serology test of hemagglutination inhibition (HAI); the presence of a 1 : 18 titer or greater is evidence of immunity, and less than 1 : 8 indicates susceptibility to rubella. If pregnant when diagnosed as being "nonimmune," the immunization should be administered in the postpartum period.[22]

Herpes Simplex Virus

HSV is a DNA virus with two principle strains: 1) HSV-I and 2) HSV-II. HSV is estimated to infect 1 in 6 people between the ages of 14 and 49 years (16.2%) in the United States.[23] The incidence of neonatal herpes infection is 1 per 3500 live births.[22] A primary herpes simplex infection may increase the risk of spontaneous abortion when infection occurs in the first trimester, whereas preterm labor, intrauterine growth restriction (IUGR), and neonatal infection are greater risks if the infection occurs late in the second trimester or early in the third trimester. If a primary lesion develops close to the time of labor, the risk of transmission is 30% to 60% for a vaginal birth.[21] Exposure of the newborn to a recurrent lesion drops the risk of transmission to between 2% and 5%.[24] The most likely mechanism of infection is exposure of the neonate to the viruses in the lower genital tract during the process of vaginal delivery; therefore, in a woman with either a primary or secondary outbreak of genital herpes during labor, the preferred method of delivery is by cesarean section. An estimated number of 1500 to 2000 newborns contact herpes each year, with 85% resulting from viral transmission near the time of birth from asymptomatic women.[21]

Neonatal HSV infection may take the form of disseminated mucocutaneous eruption, central nervous system (CNS) infection, or disseminated visceral infection. Approximately 30% of infants with disseminated disease die despite antiviral therapy, and 40% of the survivors have severe neurologic damage. Many times, the infected infant is asymptomatic at birth, with symptoms occurring any time after birth and up to 4 weeks of age.[16] These symptoms include jaundice, fever, seizures, vesicular skin lesion, and poor feeding. CNS symptoms generally occur during the second or third week. All infants who have neonatal herpes should be evaluated and treated with acyclovir.[25]

Any woman who is planning a pregnancy and who might have been exposed to the herpesvirus should have type specific serology testing to determine her risk of acquiring HSV. If she has HSV and has experienced recurrent outbreaks during pregnancy, antiviral therapy (with acyclovir, famciclovir, and valacyclovir) is recommended after 36 weeks' gestation to reduce the need for a cesarean section.[24] Currently, no evidence of any adverse fetal effects exists in relation to exposure to these antiviral drugs used in HSV treatment during any trimester.[26]

Parvovirus is caused by the DNA organism, the B19 parvovirus. It causes erythema infectiosum, or "fifth disease," in children and a mild disease in adults that produces a characteristic "slapped cheek" rash but a potential extremely serious fetal outcome. Although the risk of fetal morbidity is low, fetal infection is associated with spontaneous abortion, fetal hydrops, and stillbirth. Severe effects occur most frequently with maternal infection before 20 weeks' gestation.[27] The major concern for the fetus is nonimmune hydrops and fetal anemia, which, if left untreated, may result in death. If hydrops and fetal anemia are diagnosed, intrauterine fetal transfusion may reduce the mortality from about 50% to 18%.[27] Fetal death may occur at 4 to 12 weeks after infection; therefore, fetal surveillance should be maintained from 8 to 12 weeks. In fetuses who survive the infection, long-term development appears to be normal. Nonimmune women with school-age children are more likely to acquire parvovirus, and serologic evaluation should be performed if the pregnant woman has been exposed to a child diagnosed with fifth disease.[28]

Prematurity

The condition or illness in a critically ill mother may justify an early termination of pregnancy to prevent serious complications in or death of the patient. Depending on the duration of gestation, a severely premature infant may result. Technologic advances, improvements in maternal–fetal diagnostics, and aggressive neonatal interventions have improved the survival of extremely low-birth-weight infants. Research has placed minimal viability parameters between 23 and 24 weeks' gestation and fetal weight between 500 and 1000 g (0.5 and 1 kg).[22] Critical care clinicians may encounter situations in which extrauterine viability, fetal outcomes, and maternal stability are uncertain. Clinical decisions must be made in light of the maternal–fetal risk–benefit ratio. Personal, cultural, spiritual, and social beliefs regarding viability may affect the clinical decision-making process. Parental and family beliefs and desires may conflict with those of the health care team. When confronting the dilemma of viability, the parameters of gestational age, fetal weight, parental desires, and maternal–fetal mortality must be considered.

PHYSIOLOGIC ALTERATIONS IN PREGNANCY

During pregnancy, the woman's body undergoes profound physiologic changes. These changes are necessary to maintain the pregnancy and to allow for fetal growth and development. The changes are so dramatic that they would probably be considered pathologic in the nonpregnant woman. Adaptations occur in nearly every organ system, beginning during the first week of gestation and continuing until up to 6 weeks after delivery. The only system in which no documented characteristic changes occur is the nervous system. Boxes 39-2 and 39-3 and Tables 39-1 to 39-4 summarize the various systems and alterations during pregnancy.[12,22,23,29] Understanding the physiologic adaptations is important to the management of the critically ill pregnant woman. More detailed information can be found in textbooks dedicated to obstetric issues.

BOX 39-2   PRIMARY FUNCTIONS AND IMPLICATIONS OF ESTROGEN AND PROGESTERONE

Functions and Effects of Estrogen
- Promote growth and function of the uterus
- Cause uterine musculature hypertrophy and hyperplasia
- Increase blood supply to uteroplacental unit
- Promote breast (ductal, alveolar, nipple) development
- Increase pliability of connective tissue
  - Relax pelvic joints and ligaments
  - Allow cervical softening
- Promote sodium and water retention
- Produce psychologic changes leading to emotional lability
- Decrease gastric secretion of hydrochloric acid and pepsin
- Increase sensitivity to carbon dioxide (CO_2) levels in the blood
- Produce integumentary changes
  - Hyperpigmentation
  - Striae gravida
- Affect blood component concentrations
  - Increase fibrinogen (factor 1) concentration
  - Decrease plasma protein concentration
  - Cause leukocytosis

Functions and Effects of Progesterone
- Decrease maternal smooth muscle contractility
  - Uterus: prevent contractility
  - Gastrointestinal tract: contribute to nausea, heartburn, and constipation
  - Renal system: contribute to urinary dilation leading to urinary stasis
  - Vascular system: dilate vessels and contribute to peripheral edema
- Produce metabolic effects
  - Reset hypothalamus up approximately 0.2° C (0.5° F)
  - Promote fat storage
- Stimulate respiratory center to decrease CO_2 retention
- Stimulate secretion of sodium in the urine, thereby stimulating aldosterone production
- Promote breast development and inhibit the action of prolactin

BOX 39-3 INDICATIONS FOR HEMODYNAMIC MONITORING IN PREGNANCY

- Severe pregnancy-induced hypertension with persistent oliguria or pulmonary edema
- Massive hemorrhage or volume replacement needs
- Adult respiratory distress syndrome
- Shock of unknown cause
- Sepsis with oliguria or refractory hypotension
- Cardiovascular decompression during intrapartum or intraoperative periods
- Chronic disease during labor or intraoperatively (New York Heart Association class III or IV cardiac disease)
- Pulmonary edema, oliguria, or heart failure refractory to treatment or of unknown cause

TABLE 39-1 POSITIONAL CARDIAC OUTPUT CHANGES IN PREGNANCY

MATERNAL POSITION	CARDIAC OUTPUT (L/min)
Knee-chest	6.9 (± 2.1)
Right lateral	6.8 (± 1.3)
Left lateral	6.6 (± 1.4)
Sitting	6.2 (± 0.0)
Supine	6.0 (± 0.4)
Standing	5.4 (± 2.0)

TABLE 39-2 HEMODYNAMIC CHANGES ASSOCIATED WITH TERM PREGNANCY

PARAMETER	PREGNANCY NORMAL VALUE	CHANGE
Mean arterial pressure (mm Hg)	90 ± 6	No significant change
Central venous pressure (mm Hg)	8 ± 2	No significant change
Pulmonary artery occlusion pressure (mm Hg)	4 ± 3	No significant change
Heart rate (beats/min)	83 ± 10	Increase 17%
Cardiac output (L/min)	6.2 ± 1.0	Increase 43%
Systemic vascular resistance (dyn · sec · cm⁻⁵)	1210 ± 266	Decrease 21%
Pulmonary vascular resistance (dyn · sec · cm⁻⁵)	78 ± 22	Decrease 34%
Serum colloid oncotic pressure (mm Hg)	18 ± 1.5	Decrease 14%
Left ventricular stroke work index (g-m/m²)	48 ± 6	No significant change

TABLE 39-3 PHYSIOLOGIC ADAPTATION OF THE GASTROINTESTINAL SYSTEM DURING PREGNANCY

GASTROINTESTINAL FUNCTION CHANGE	PRESUMED CAUSE
Heartburn	Progesterone and estrogen; size of gravid uterus impeding gastroesophageal junction
Bleeding gums	Hyperemia
Constipation	Progesterone, causing decreased motility and intestinal secretion, enhanced water absorption
Hemorrhoids	Hyperemia, pelvic congestion, obstruction of venous return
"Morning sickness" or nausea	Increased levels of estrogen and human chorionic gonadotropin (hCG)
Risk for aspiration	Displacement of lower esophageal sphincter and reduced gastric motility
Gallstones	Decreased gallbladder activity, impaired emptying

TABLE 39-4 RENAL PHYSIOLOGIC CHANGES IN PREGNANCY

PARAMETER	PERCENT CHANGE	NORMAL LEVELS IN PREGNANCY
Renal blood flow	Increase 25%-50%	1250-1500 mL/min
Glomerular filtration rate	Increase 50%	140-170 mL/min
Renal plasma flow	Increase 35%	700-900 mL/min

PHYSIOLOGIC CHANGES DURING LABOR AND DELIVERY

Labor and delivery bring additional stresses to the maternal system, especially as a result of the pain and anxiety associated with labor. The most dramatic requirements are for the cardiopulmonary system. During labor, uterine contractions produce cyclic auto-transfusions of approximately 300 to 500 milliliters (mL). Immediately after birth, cardiac output peaks, with an 80% increase over prelabor values.[12] This occurs because of the contracted uterus shunting its blood, sudden removal of fetal supply demands, and resolution of vena cava compression. Table 39-5 summarizes the cardiac output changes in labor and delivery.[12,23,29]

Normal blood loss from a vaginal birth is typically 500 mL; blood loss from cesarean deliveries usually is 1000 mL. Clinical estimates tend to underestimate actual blood loss by up to 50%.[30] The cardiopulmonary changes occurring during labor and delivery are of significant concern because they occur over a short period and because maternal decompensation may occur.

In summary, maternal physiology is profoundly and rapidly affected by pregnancy. Adaptations begin early in the pregnancy and continue through the postpartum period, gradually returning to prepregnant states over 6 weeks. Understanding the

TABLE 39-5 CARDIAC OUTPUT CHANGES IN LABOR AND DELIVERY

STAGE OF LABOR OR DELIVERY	CHANGE IN CARDIAC OUTPUT
Early first stage of labor	↑ 15% plus additional 15% with each contraction
Last first state of labor	↑ 30% plus additional 15% with each contraction
Second stage of labor	↑ 45% plus additional 15% with each contraction
First 5 minutes postpartum	↑ 80% secondary to auto-transfusion
First hour postpartum	↑ 25%

physiologic stresses uniquely presented during pregnancy allows the clinician to provide comprehensive care to the pregnant woman experiencing critical illness or injury.

CARDIAC DISORDERS IN PREGNANCY

Cardiac disease ranks fourth after pregnancy-induced hypertension, hemorrhage, and infection as a cause of maternal mortality.[31] Several factors have to be taken into consideration in the care of the pregnant woman with cardiac disease. Cardiac disease during pregnancy may be a result of pre-existing conditions such as congenital diseases, or it may be a result of primary cardiac disease arising prior to or during pregnancy. The woman with heart disease has decreased cardiac reserve, making it more difficulty for her heart to accommodate the higher workload of pregnancy. Thus, prepregnancy counseling is highly recommended for women with known cardiac disease. Counseling would include determining the New York Heart Association (NYHA) functional class, which is especially useful for pregnant women with structural heart disease, and determining the maternal and fetal risks associated with the pregnancy (Box 39-4).[29,32] Major fetal risks include fetal development of congenital heart disease, prematurity, IUGR, and intrauterine fetal demise (IUFD).

The method and timing of delivery are decided primarily by obstetric considerations, taking into account the woman's ability to tolerate the labor process and associated physiologic changes. Selection of anesthesia techniques involves weighing the risks and benefits of the procedures. As a general rule, most patients tolerate epidural anesthesia more favorably than they tolerate general anesthesia (see Chapter 42).

Congenital Cardiac Disorders

Congenital heart defects have become a more common finding in pregnant women, as improved surgical techniques have enabled females born with heart defects to live to childbearing age. When surgical repair can be accomplished with no remaining evidence of organic heart disease, pregnancy may be undertaken with confidence. When congenital heart disease is associated with cyanosis, whether the defect was originally uncorrected or the correction failed to relieve the cyanosis, the woman should be counseled about risks to both herself and to her fetus. Of equal concern in pregnant women with congenital

BOX 39-4 MATERNAL MORTALITY RISKS

Group 1: Mortality <1%
- Atrial septal defect
- Ventricular septal defect
- Patent ductus arteriosus
- Pulmonic tricuspid disease
- Tetralogy of Fallot, corrected
- Bioprosthetic valve
- Mitral stenosis, NYHA classes I and II

Group 2: Mortality 5%-15%
Group 2A
- Mitral stenosis, NYHA classes III and IV
- Aortic stenosis
- Coarctation of aorta, without valvular involvement
- Tetralogy of Fallot, uncorrected
- Previous myocardial infarction
- Marfan syndrome with normal aorta

Group 2B
- Mitral stenosis with atrial fibrillation
- Artificial valve

Group 3: Mortality 25%-50%
- Pulmonary hypertension
- Coarctation of aorta, with valvular involvement
- Marfan syndrome with aortic involvement

NYHA, New York Heart Association.

heart disease is the risk of fetal congenital cardiac anomalies, which is approximately 5%. During the antepartum period, serial ultrasonography should be performed to access the fetus for appropriate interval growth.[33]

Atrial Septal Defect

Atrial septal defect (ASD) is the most common congenital anomaly seen during pregnancy, and most women with ASD tolerate pregnancy, labor, and delivery without complications. The decrease in systemic vascular resistance (SVR) lessens the degree of left-to-right shunt, whereas the hypervolemic state may slightly worsen the shunt and increase right ventricular workload. The most common complications seen with ASD are dysrhythmias, heart failure, and thromboembolism.[34]

Ventricular Septal Defect

The outcome for the pregnant woman with ventricular septal defect (VSD) and resultant left-to-right shunt depends on the size of the defect, with larger defects producing a less favorable prognosis. The majority of VSDs are diagnosed and repaired before the women reaches childbearing age. In the absence of significant symptoms and pulmonary hypertension, pregnancy is typically well tolerated. Therapy is aimed at early recognition and treatments of signs of heart failure.[35] Common complications include tachycardia, heart failure, and pulmonary hypertension.

Patent Ductus Arteriosus

During pregnancy patent ductus arteriosus (PDA) is an unusual finding, as it is generally detected and closed during the newborn period. Patients who present with a PDA during pregnancy, usually tolerate the hemodynamic stress of labor and delivery without difficulty. Precautions against the risks of infective endocarditis and thromboembolism may be taken. Severe PDA may produce large left-to-right shunts, causing acute heart failure or pulmonary hypertension that is associated with significant maternal mortality.[30]

Tetralogy of Fallot

Tetralogy of Fallot (ToF) is the most common cyanotic heart defect in individuals who survive to adulthood.[36] The four primary lesions associated with ToF include: 1) VSD, 2) overriding aorta, 3) right ventricular hypertrophy, and 4) pulmonary stenosis. Women with corrected ToF generally can tolerate pregnancy well. Although rare, if the congenital anomalies are not corrected, the maternal mortality rate and fetal complications increase significantly.[36] Cardiopulmonary function must be maximized by measures that include treatment of dysrhythmias and use of prophylaxis for endocarditis. Considerations during labor and delivery include maintenance of adequate preload and blood pressure.

Coarctation of the Aorta

Coarctation of the aorta may occur in isolation or, most often, in combination with valvular or septal anomalies. Patients with uncomplicated coarctation of the aorta who are relatively asymptomatic (NYHA class I or II) have demonstrated good prognosis and minimal risk of complications or death.[12] Assessment of the aortic gradient may also be useful in predicting pregnancy outcome in patients with coarctation of the aorta. In general, aortic gradients across the site of coarctation that are less than 20 mm Hg are associated with good maternal and fetal outcomes.[34] Intrapartum management focuses on the prevention of hypertension to avoid aortic wall stress. Careful management of fluid balance and left ventricular function must occur to prevent CHF and to promote adequate perfusion.

Eisenmenger Syndrome

Eisenmenger syndrome is not a single congenital defect but a complication that may be the result of other cardiac lesions that cause left-to-right shunting. This syndrome is more likely to occur with VDS or ASD because of the high pressure and high flow associated with these defects. This shunting may result in progressive pulmonary hypertension, leading to shunt reversal or bidirectional shunting.[37] Regardless of the cause, the risk of sudden death because of pulmonary hypertension in pregnancy is 40%, which has remained unchanged for the past 50 years. Avoidance or termination of pregnancy is commonly recommended. If pregnancy is continued, therapeutic management is directed at avoidance of pulmonary vasoconstrictors, thromboembolism, and hypotension; maintenance of adequate preload and oxygenation; fetal surveillance; and reduction of stress at the time of delivery.[37]

Acquired Cardiac Disorders

Special consideration must be given to physical assessment during the antepartum period. Normal physiologic changes such as murmur development or shortness of breath may mask symptoms of cardiac disease or make diagnosis more challenging.

Mitral Stenosis

The presence of a stenotic mitral valve is the most common rheumatic valve disease of pregnancy. The primary concern with mitral stenosis during pregnancy is the impedance to ventricular filling, which produces a relatively fixed cardiac output. Additional risks include thromboembolism, heart failure, and arrhythmias, especially atrial fibrillation. Cardiac output in the face of mitral stenosis is determined by two primary factors: 1) length of diastolic filling and 2) left ventricular preload. The length of diastolic filling may be negatively affected because of the increased pulse rate during a normal pregnancy. Discomfort or anxiety associated with labor may produce a tachycardic state, which may drastically impede ventricular filling, producing an even lower cardiac output, with resultant heart failure and pulmonary edema. As pregnancy is a hypercoagulable state, thrombi may rapidly form, and fibrillation may dislodge the thrombi and cause arterial embolism. Thus, prophylactic anticoagulation should be considered in this subset of women.[38,39]

Maintenance and management of left ventricular preload is the second important consideration in mitral stenosis. Patients may require high-normal or slightly elevated left ventricular filling pressures to maintain adequate flow across the stenotic mitral valve. It is especially important to assess the patient's fluid status. Caution must be exercised when employing therapies that decrease preload, for example, diuresis or epidural anesthesia.[38] Invasive hemodynamic monitoring may be indicated to carefully tailor therapy.

In the immediate postpartum period, careful monitoring is essential because of the massive fluid shifts and large increases in cardiac output. Authorities recommend that optimal predelivery pulmonary artery occlusion pressures be maintained at 14 mm Hg or less to accommodate the increase in occlusion pressure of up to 16 mm Hg that may be associated in the immediate postpartum period.[38]

Aortic Stenosis

Aortic stenosis often is accompanied by other valvular disease, especially disease affecting the mitral valve. The hallmark of aortic stenosis is decreased left ventricular ejection.[12] Mild aortic stenosis is usually well tolerated during pregnancy because of the natural hypervolemic state. Significant aortic stenosis can produce left ventricular hypertrophy and dilation. Thromboembolic prophylaxis is recommended. Critical to successful management is maintenance of cardiac output through prevention of hypovolemia, especially at the time of delivery. The maintenance of adequate cardiac output and oxygen transport is vital in the clinical management of pregnant women with aortic stenosis. Any factor that diminishes venous return or produces hypotension worsens the effects of aortic stenosis and significantly reduces cardiac output. Heart failure occurs in less than 10% of patients with severe aortic stenosis and arrhythmias in 3% to 25%.[40] Mortality is now rare if careful management is provided.

Marfan Syndrome

Marfan syndrome is an autosomal dominant disorder of connective tissue, in which serious cardiovascular involvement, usually dissection or rupture of the aorta, may occur. Prognosis is based on aortic root and wall involvement, with most authorities citing 40 millimeters (mm) as maximal root diameter, after which significant increases in mortality occur.[39,41] Prevention of tachydysrhythmias and hypertension is recommended, along with endocarditis prophylaxis. Beta-blockade therapy may be initiated for cardiac rate control and to decrease pressure on the weakened aortic wall. Goals of management include maintenance of cardiac output to meet physiologic needs without producing undue stress on the aortic wall, use of regional anesthesia, and avoidance of Valsalva maneuver by shortening the second stage of labor. Careful blood pressure maintenance is essential. Differential diagnosis of chest and back pain is essential, along with recognition of other signs of aortic dissection. Because of its inheritance pattern there is a 50% risk that the disease will be transmitted to the infant.[41]

Peripartum Cardiomyopathy

Peripartum cardiomyopathy (PPCM) is a type left ventricle dysfunction of unknown origin that occurs in the last month of pregnancy and up to 5 months after delivery in women with no previous history of heart disease. Thus, PPCM is a diagnosis of exclusion. Occurring in 1 in 3000 to 4000 live births, it is a relatively rare but serious condition. Early report suggested a mortality rate of nearly 50%, but more recent studies indicate a 0% to 5% rate in the United States.[42,43] Controversy regarding exact causes of peripartum cardiomyopathy continues, as symptoms that are often attributable to viral and immune sources, chronic hypertension, mitral stenosis, obesity, and myocarditis have all been proposed.[43] The definitive diagnosis of PPCM depends on the echocardiographic identification of new-onset heart failure during a limited period toward the end of pregnancy or in the months following delivery.[40,43,44]

Symptoms are identical to those of classic heart failure, but treatment depends on the pregnancy status of the patient. Women who present with PPCM during pregnancy require joint cardiac and obstetric care, but as soon as the baby is born and the patient is hemodynamically stable, standard therapy for heart failure may be applied.[40] This would include treatment of diuretics, digoxin, beta-blockade, and afterload reduction. Angiotensin-converting enzyme (ACE) inhibitors, angiotensin receptor blockers (ARBs), and renin inhibitors are contraindicated during pregnancy because of fetotoxicity but may be used once the infant is born.[40,44] Once the bleeding has been stopped after delivery, anticoagulation is commonly employed to prevent thromboembolism and the formation of left ventricular thrombus, which is associated with a worse prognosis.[44] The clinical course of peripartum cardiomyopathy is quite variable, but 50% to 60% of patients show clinical recovery within the first 6 months after delivery.[45] The prognosis of PPCM is positively related to the recovery of ventricular function. Medical therapy as outlined in the American College of Cardiology Foundation and American Heart Association (ACCF/AHA) guidelines should be continued when a woman

does not recover function.[44] Subsequent pregnancy carries a recurrence risk for PPCM of 30% to 50%.[40]

Ischemic Cardiac Disease
Acute Myocardial Infarction

Although acute myocardial infarction (AMI) during pregnancy is rare, pregnancy has been shown to increase the risk of AMI three- to fourfold.[46] With the continuing trend of childbearing at older ages and advances in reproductive technology enabling many older women to conceive, it may be expected that the occurrence of AMI will increase. Mortality rates from an AMI during pregnancy range from 37% to 50%, depending on the timing of the myocardial event.[47] However, the majority of AMI in pregnancy is not related to atherosclerosis; about 50% of ischemic heart disease in pregnancy is linked to idiopathic dissections of the coronary arteries.[40] Other reported conditions that contribute to AMI risk are eclampsia, thrombophilia, postpartum infections, and severe postpartum hemorrhage.[40] Increased mortality is associated with many factors, including occurrence of the event during the third trimester, multigravidas older than 33 years, cesarean section, and delivery occurring within 2 weeks of infarction.[47]

Clinical diagnostics are similar to those for standard AMI detection, although diagnosis must be made with consideration of the normal physiologic cardiovascular changes. Coronary angiography with the possibility of coronary intervention is preferred to thrombolysis, as it will also diagnose coronary artery dissection.[47]

Treatment of AMI during pregnancy is focused on restoring myocardial blood flow and balancing myocardial oxygen supply and demand.[47] Management may include percutaneous coronary intervention; nitrate therapy, beta-blockade therapy, or both; cardiac monitoring; oxygen therapy; management of pain and anxiety; and afterload reduction. Again ACE inhibitors, ARBs, and renin inhibitors are not indicated during pregnancy.[40] Coronary angiograms, angioplasty, bypass surgery, and intra-aortic balloon pumps all have been successfully used during pregnancy. Special consideration is given to the maternal physiologic demands required during the labor and delivery processes. Operative delivery interventions, such as forceps or cesarean section, may be necessary (see "Myocardial Infarction" in Chapter 15).

Prior Myocardial Infarction

The outcome in the pregnant woman with prior myocardial damage depends on many factors. The length of time between the myocardial event and delivery is especially important.[47] Increased myocardial oxygen demands during pregnancy must be considered, and therapy is usually supportive in nature. Careful attention to preload is essential to prevent burdening the heart and producing congestive failure (see "Heart Failure" in Chapter 15).

Cardiac Arrest in Pregnancy

The occurrence of cardiopulmonary arrest during pregnancy is uncommon. Successful management of the pregnant patient in cardiac arrest requires integration of physiologic changes present during pregnancy and adaptations for those from standard resuscitative guidelines. Fetal outcomes are directly related to the mother's condition and well-being. The interrelationship between fetal and maternal well-being may present unique ethical dilemmas for health care providers and family members. Causes of obstetric and nonobstetric cardiopulmonary arrest during pregnancy are summarized in Table 39-6.

Basic Cardiac Life Support. The AHA recommendations include only minor deviations from usual life support procedures.[48] The facilitation of venous return is critically important. This is accomplished by performing chest compressions slightly above the center of the sternum and lateral displacement of the uterus through manual manipulation or through the use of a wedge under the woman's hip, as this will improve venous return by decreasing compression of the vena cava by the gravid uterus.[48] Physiologic adaptations in pregnancy place the woman at greater risk for complications from cardiopulmonary resuscitation (CPR) such as fractured ribs and sternum, hemothorax, hemopericardium, and internal organ damage. Specific organs of concern include the uterus, spleen, and liver.

Advanced Cardiac Life Support. The AHA recommends that the standard resuscitation algorithm be followed for advanced cardiac life support (ACLS), with a few modifications to compensate for the altered anatomy and physiology of pregnancy.[49] The airway should be secured early with effective preoxygenation, and cricoid pressure should be applied both to aid in intubation and to prevent aspiration. As pregnancy progresses, edema of the oropharynx increases, thus necessitating the use of a smaller endotracheal tube than in a nonpregnant woman.[49] Careful attention to confirmation of tube placement and oxygenation is important because of the enhanced oxygen demands during pregnancy.

Standard ACLS recommendations should be followed for administration of resuscitation medications. Use of lower extremity sites or the femoral vein for venous access should be avoided because of the potential of the gravid uterus to impede venous return.[49] Epinephrine may decrease uteroplacental perfusion because of its vasoconstrictive nature; however, the benefits outweigh the risks of administration. Lidocaine crosses the placenta but in therapeutic levels does not have adverse fetal or uteroplacental effects. If maternal toxicity occurs, fetal cardiac and CNS depression may occur. No contraindications exist for use of atropine in pregnancy. Administration of sodium bicarbonate is to be undertaken cautiously. Maternal acidosis increases uteroplacental adrenergic reactivity and must be avoided, although maternal alkalosis may impair oxygen exchange to the fetus. Electrical therapies such as defibrillation, cardioversion, and pacing are not contraindicated in pregnancy, but all fetal monitoring devices should be removed because a theoretical risk of the scalp electrode arcing and electrocuting the infant does exist.

Evaluation of fetal tolerance of the mother's condition is essential during cardiopulmonary arrest. Fetal hypoxia may develop because of decreased uteroplacental perfusion. Fetal gestational age is a prime consideration when determining course of action. Before 24 weeks' gestation, resuscitative efforts are focused primarily on maternal outcome. After the 24th week of gestation, evaluation includes maternal and fetal responses to resuscitative efforts. Emergent cesarean section may be undertaken for fetal distress or to improve maternal status, although consideration also must be given to the stress that cesarean section produces. In late pregnancy, survival of the infant is directly proportional to the time interval between death of the mother and delivery of the infant. Infant viability is best if delivery occurs within 5 minutes of cardiac arrest.[47, 49]

HYPERTENSIVE DISEASE

Hypertensive disease is present in up to 5% of pregnant women.[50] Hypertension is defined as systolic blood pressure of 140 mm Hg or greater, or diastolic blood pressure of 90 mm Hg or greater, or both.[50] It is the second leading cause of death in childbearing women, and it contributes to high rates of newborn morbidity and mortality.[12,51,52] Maternal complications include pathologic compromise of the cardiovascular, pulmonary, renal, neurologic, and hepatic systems (Table 39-7).[52-54] Understanding of hypertensive disease in pregnancy is based on: 1) a classification according to manifestations and time of onset in relation to gestation; 2) the fact that pregnancy could induce hypertension in women without a history of high blood pressure; and 3) the fact that elevated blood pressure in pregnancy could occur without the presence of generalized edema or proteinuria (transient hypertension).[53] Proper diagnosis of

TABLE 39-6	OBSTETRIC AND NONOBSTETRIC CAUSES OF CARDIAC ARREST IN PREGNANCY	
OBSTETRIC CAUSES	**NONOBSTETRIC CAUSES**	
Hemorrhage (17%)	Pulmonary embolism (19%)	
Pregnancy-induced hypertension (16%)	Infection or sepsis (13%)	
Idiopathic peripartum cardiomyopathy (8%)	Stroke (5%)	
Anesthetic complications (2%)	Myocardial infarction	
Amniotic fluid embolism	Trauma	

From Campbell T, Sanson T. Cardiac arrest and pregnancy. *J Emerg Trauma Shock.* 2009;2(1):34.

TABLE 39-7	COMPLICATIONS OF HYPERTENSIVE DISEASE IN PREGNANCY
BODY SYSTEM	**COMPLICATION**
Cardiovascular	Dysrhythmias, acute heart failure, severe hypertension
Pulmonary	Pulmonary edema, acute airway obstruction
Renal	Oliguria, renal failure, acute kidney injury
Neurologic	Cerebral edema, eclampsia, cerebral hemorrhage, coma
Hepatic	Necrosis, rupture, periportal and subcapsular hemorrhage
Hematologic	Disseminated intravascular coagulation (DIC), hemolysis thrombocytopenia

hypertensive complications is critical and requires in-depth knowledge of disease pathophysiology to prevent or decrease the risk of maternal or fetal compromise.

Classification of Hypertension

The National Institutes of Health Working Group on High Blood Pressure has endorsed the classification and terminology of the American Congress of Obstetricians and Gynecologists (ACOG; 2012) for hypertensive disease in pregnancy.[50,52] These definitions have proved useful in establishing consistent guidelines for pregnancy management:[55]

   I. *Chronic hypertension* is hypertension before conception or diagnosed before 20 weeks' gestation.
  II. *Preeclampsia and eclampsia* constitute a systemic syndrome of hypertensive disease, with proteinuria diagnosed after 20 weeks' gestation. Eclampsia indicates the additional presence of convulsions.
 III. *Preeclampsia superimposed on chronic hypertension* may occur before 20 weeks' gestation or have a sudden onset.
  IV. *Gestational hypertension* is hypertension without proteinuria after 20 weeks' gestation.

Preeclampsia and Eclampsia

Preeclampsia is the most common hypertensive disorder of pregnancy. It is estimated that 50,000 women die from preeclampsia each year worldwide. Among women with chronic hypertension, 22% to 25% will develop this complication.[56,57] Preeclampsia is a syndrome that affects both mother and fetus. It is clinically defined as an increase in blood pressure after 20 weeks' gestation, accompanied by proteinuria in a previously normotensive woman.[57,58] Eclampsia is the occurrence of a seizure in a woman with preeclampsia who has no other cause for seizure.

Preeclampsia has been called a "disease of theories" because true mechanisms behind the pathogenesis remain unclear. It is a multisystem disorder unique to humans and therefore difficult to study in laboratory animals, which creates an obstacle to discovering its exact etiology.[58]

One of the key features of preeclampsia involves the failure of uterine spiral arteries to transform from thick-walled muscular vessels to saclike flaccid vessels, exaggerated inflammatory response, and inappropriate endothelial-cell activation.[59] Characteristics of preeclampsia include widespread arteriolar vasospasms resulting in decreased perfusion to virtually all organs, including the placenta; a decrease in plasma volume; activation of coagulation cascade; and alteration in glomerular capillary endothelium. These generalized cyclic vasospasms lead to tissue ischemia and eventually end-organ dysfunction (Fig. 39-1).[54]

One of the more common problems related to preeclampsia is pulmonary edema caused by increased capillary permeability.

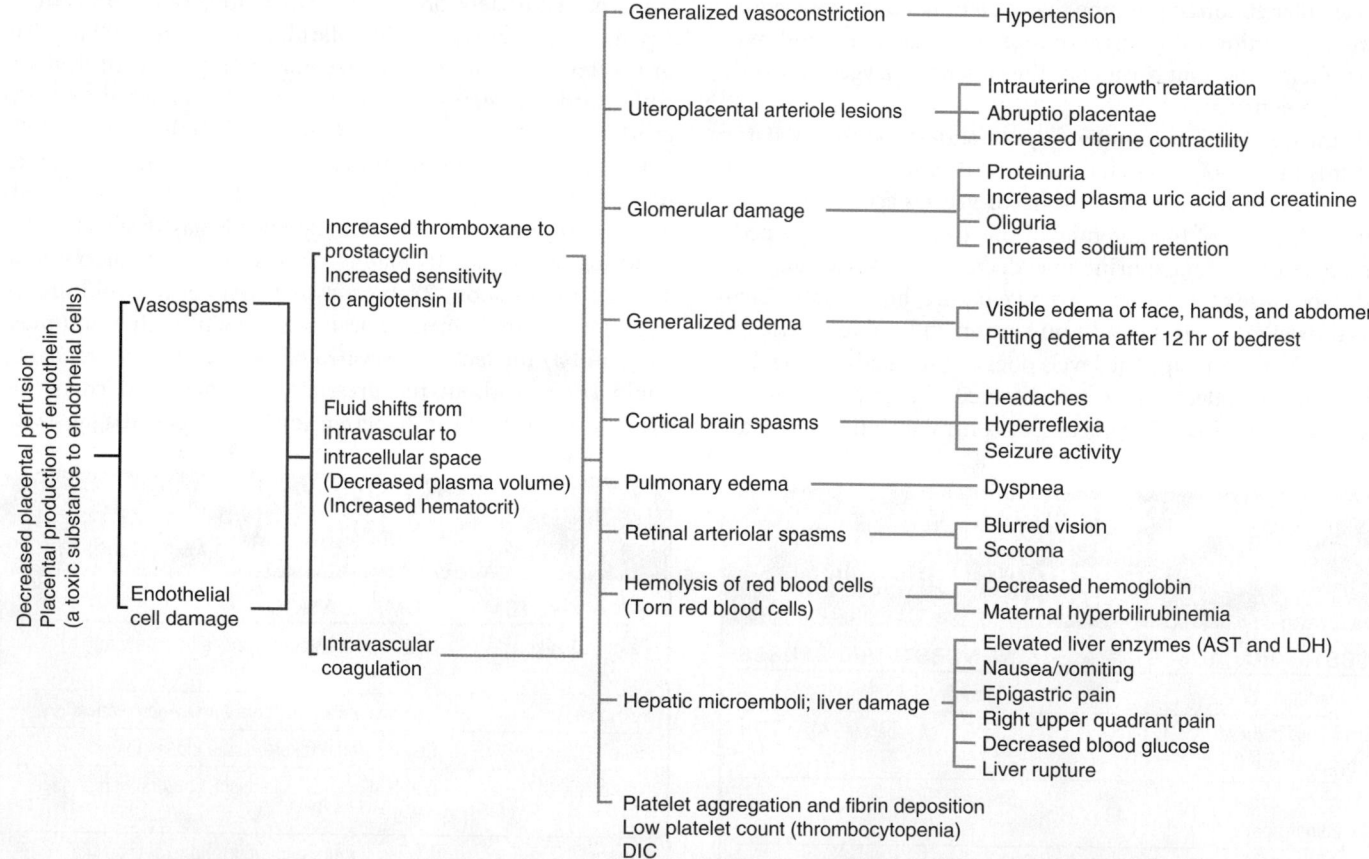

FIGURE 39-1 Pathophysiologic changes of pregnancy-induced hypertension. *AST*, Aspartate aminotransferase (SGOT); *DIC*, disseminated intravascular coagulation; *LDH*, lactate dehydrogenase. (From Gilbert E. *Manual of High Risk Pregnancy and Delivery*. 5th ed. St. Louis: Mosby; 2011.)

Thrombocytopenia complicates severe preeclampsia in about 7% to 11% of women.[59,60] Abruptio placentae and the release of procoagulants such as thromboplastin may result in acute disseminated intravascular coagulation (DIC). Women who develop preeclampsia are more sensitive to pressor agents, and this response has been linked to the ratio between prostaglandins, prostacyclin, and thromboxane. Prostacyclin is decreased in preeclampsia, allowing the potent vasoconstrictor and platelet-aggregating effects of thromboxane to dominate. No effective intervention seems to be available, although low-dose aspirin may lead to modest risk reduction of the disease.[59]

New research suggests pathogenesis related to imbalance between circulating antiangiogenesis-related factors.[61,62] These antiangiogenic factors produce systemic endothelial dysfunction, resulting in hypertension, proteinuria, and other systemic expressions of preeclampsia. The molecular basis for placental misuse of these pathogenic factors remains unknown, and the role of angiogenic proteins in early placental vascular development and trophoblast invasion is just beginning to be explored. Widespread systemic vascular dysfunction and microangiopathy is demonstrated in the mother but not in the fetus.[61,62] With preeclampsia, decreased production of nitric oxide, which is a potent vasodilator and important regulator of maternal blood pressure, also occurs.

Hyperhomocysteinemia may play role in the etiology or pathophysiology of preeclampsia.[63] Mild elevations of homocysteine have been found in women with normal blood pressures who go on to develop preeclampsia. Once preeclampsia is established, homocysteine levels are considerably increased. It is unclear whether the increased levels of homocysteine caused the disease or if they reflect the metabolic alterations resulting from preeclampsia. Deficiencies of vitamin B_6, vitamin B_{12}, or folic acid may cause a rise in homocysteine. In one study in which approximately 4000 women received folic acid supplements, the results demonstrated a decrease in plasma homocysteine and a reduced risk of preeclampsia.[63]

Intracerebral hemorrhage is a rare complication, but it is the most common cause of death in women with severe preeclampsia and eclampsia, being fatal in 50% to 60% of the cases. Infants of women with preeclampsia tend to be small for gestational age because of IUGR. In addition, the maternal condition may warrant early termination of pregnancy, which leads to a severely premature infant. Placental abruption secondary to hypertension may result in fetal hypoxia or death.[57,58]

The treatment goals of severe preeclampsia are to prevent seizures, decrease arterial spasms, and effect prompt delivery of the fetus. Magnesium sulfate ($MgSO_4$) is the standard treatment for the prevention and control of seizures in women with preeclampsia or eclampsia. Serum magnesium levels of 4 to 7 milliequivalent per liter (mEq/L) are thought to be therapeutic for prevention of seizure activity. A loading dose of 4 to 6 grams (g) is given by infusion pump over 15 to 20 minutes, followed by a maintenance infusion of 2 to 3 gram per hour (g/hr).[12]

Control of eclamptic seizures is accomplished through administration of 4 to 6 g of intravenous $MgSO_4$ over 5 to 10 minutes. This bolus is followed by a continuous infusion of 2 to 3 g/hr. If a patient has a recurrent seizure, another bolus of 2 to 4 g may be given over 3 to 5 minutes. Sodium amobarbitol

I, benzodiazepines, or phenytoin may be used for treating seizures that are not responsive to $MgSO_4$.[51,64] The use of multiple agents to decrease eclamptic seizures should be avoided, unless necessary.

Severe hypertension must be addressed after magnesium infusions. Antihypertensive agents need to be used to keep diastolic blood pressure between 90 and 100 mm Hg. The main drugs used to achieve this are hydralazine hydrochloride or labetalol.[51,64] Diuretics are used only in the setting of pulmonary edema. The placenta plays a central role in the development of the disease, for which the only known cure is delivery of the fetus and removal of the placenta.

Hemolysis, Elevated Liver Enzymes, and Low Platelet Syndrome

Hemolysis, elevated liver enzymes, and low platelet (HELLP) syndrome affects 2% to 20% of patients with severe preeclampsia or eclampsia.[56,65] Maternal mortality ranges from 3.5% to 24%, whereas perinatal mortality ranges from 10% to 60%.[53] Approximately 10% to 15% of pregnant patients with HELLP syndrome do not have elevated proteinuria of hypertensive disease.[58,66,67] The clinical manifestations of HELLP syndrome, which include nausea, vomiting, malaise, flulike symptoms, and epigastric pain, may suggest a multitude of other clinical diagnoses. Misdiagnosis is common and may result in a delay of correct treatment. HELLP syndrome may be confused with acute renal disease, gastroenteritis, hepatitis, gallbladder disease, pyelonephritis, or thrombotic thrombocytopenic purpura.[23] Any pregnant woman demonstrating clinical manifestations and showing hemolysis, elevated liver enzymes, and low platelets must be diagnosed with HELLP syndrome. Complications of HELLP syndrome include abruptio placentae, liver hematoma, DIC, pulmonary edema, liver rupture, and acute kidney injury.[12,58]

Collaborative management for patients with severe preeclampsia or eclampsia or with HELLP syndrome is based on stabilization of the mother and the fetus. Continuous assessment of the cardiovascular, renal, central nervous, and pulmonary systems provides early indications of worsening maternal condition. Fetal surveillance may include continuous fetal monitoring, biophysical profile, and fetal lung maturity testing. Delivery of the fetus may be indicated because of the maternal condition or fetal compromise. The goal of the health care team is to accurately monitor ongoing organ system dysfunction and prevent further damage leading to end-organ failure and maternal–fetal mortality.

DISSEMINATED INTRAVASCULAR COAGULATION

DIC is not a separate clinical entity; rather, it is an effect of other disease processes. The obstetric causes of DIC include abruptio placentae, preeclampsia or eclampsia, dead fetus syndrome, septic abortion, and amniotic fluid embolus. In DIC, fibrinogen levels and platelet counts are usually decreased, whereas prothrombin time (PT) and partial thromboplastin time (PTT) are normal to prolonged.[68] The pathophysiologic mechanisms of DIC are summarized in Table 39-8.[12,53] Primary treatment goals

TABLE 39-8	**CONDITIONS ASSOCIATED WITH DISSEMINATED INTRAVASCULAR COAGULATION**	
OBSTETRIC	**OBSTETRIC OR NONOBSTETRIC**	**NONOBSTETRIC**
Abruptio placentae	Prolonged shock, any cause	Malignancy
Amniotic fluid embolism	Transfusion-incompatible blood	Extensive surgery
Eclampsia, preeclampsia	Septicemia: bacterial fungal, viral	Collagen vascular disease
Abortion	Septic abortion	Central nervous system trauma
Dead fetus syndrome	Severe chorioamnionitis	Allergic reactions
Hydatidiform mole		Burns
Retained placenta		Vascular malformations
Uterine rupture		Pancreatitis
Maternal hemorrhage		

include identification of the underlying disorder, removal of the trigger or initiating event, and volume replacement, including blood component therapy. Secondary treatment may include anticoagulation therapy. Heparin therapy remains controversial.

Abruptio Placentae

Because abruptio placentae is the most common obstetric cause of DIC, evaluating the results of coagulation tests is imperative. Of mothers experiencing abruption, 20% have a significant clotting defect, with 25% of this group experiencing postpartum hemorrhage.[66] Supportive treatment to decrease risk of DIC includes a type and cross-matching for blood transfusions, clotting mechanism evaluation, and the administration of intravenous fluids.[68] If DIC is established, the basic element of treatment is the removal of blood clots from the uterus, blood component therapy, and fluid volume resuscitation.

Dead Fetus Syndrome

Prolonged retention of a dead fetus may lead to development of DIC, also called *consumption coagulopathy*, in the mother. After the release of thromboplastin from the degenerating fetal tissues into the maternal bloodstream, the extrinsic clotting system is activated, triggering the formation of multiple tiny blood clots. Fibrinogen and factor V and VII are subsequently depleted and the woman begins to display symptoms of DIC. Fibrinogen levels begin a linear descent 3 to 4 weeks after the death of the fetus and continue to decrease in the absence of appropriate medical intervention.[23] Because of the risk of DIC, the once common practice of waiting for the onset of labor has largely been abandoned in recent years.[69]

Septic Abortion

Although septic abortion is a well-documented cause of obstetric DIC, because of the legalization of abortion, a large reduction in the number of cases of septic abortion has occurred.[23] Bacterial endotoxins are the most likely initiating mechanism. The clinical findings of gram-negative septic shock are applicable to this condition. The severity of the disease correlates well with the degree of coagulopathy. Aggressive antibiotic therapy and evacuation of the uterus are the frontline therapies for patients who are hemodynamically stable.

SHOCK

Shock is defined as tissue hypoxia resulting from decreased perfusion secondary to decreased intravascular volume. Because pregnancy is a hyperdynamic, low-resistance state with increased oxygen delivery and consumption requirements, the management of shock in the pregnant patient necessitates an approach that is different from that for the nonpregnant patient. Normal physiologic adaptations that occur during pregnancy may alter ranges in vital signs and laboratory values, which may mislead the practitioner and complicate timely diagnosis and early treatment. Frequently, the clinician may be obtaining data from and managing two patients—the mother and the fetus.

Causes of hemorrhagic shock unique to pregnancy include abruptio placentae, ectopic pregnancy, placenta previa, and postpartum hemorrhage.[12,23] Postpartum hemorrhage may be attributed to uterine atony, genital tract lacerations, hematoma formation, retained placenta, and uterine prolapse. Unique causes of septic shock in the pregnant patient include chorioamnionitis, septic abortion, and postpartum pyelonephritis.[12] Cardiogenic shock is most frequently a result of the presence of severe valve disease. Regardless of the cause, whether specific to pregnancy or not, the occurrence of shock requires aggressive intervention with treatment of the underlying cause.

Management of shock in pregnancy focuses on optimizing maternal stability in an effort to provide the most stable uterine environment. Clinical judgments include assessment of the risks and benefits of therapeutic interventions and fetal viability. Consideration must be given to the potential vasoconstrictive nature of some pharmacotherapeutics and the potential for uteroplacental insufficiency.

PULMONARY DYSFUNCTION

Oxygen consumption increases by approximately 15% to 25% throughout pregnancy.[23] To meet these needs for additional oxygen, ventilatory changes (Fig. 39-2) must occur. Pulmonary dysfunction carries clinical significance because of the normally slightly hyperoxygenated condition associated with the physiologic changes in pregnancy. As a result of normal cardiorespiratory changes that occur during pregnancy, the pregnant woman has very limited cardiopulmonary reserve. It is, therefore, relatively easy for her to demonstrate pulmonary decompensation in the presence of any respiratory compromise.

Compromise of respiratory function places the mother and the fetus at risk. Maternal hypoxia may be the end result of several conditions, including pneumonia, asthma, cystic fibrosis, trauma, acute respiratory distress syndrome (ARDS), and pulmonary embolism. Contributing factors (e.g., smoking, drug use, pre-existing disease states), manifestations, and

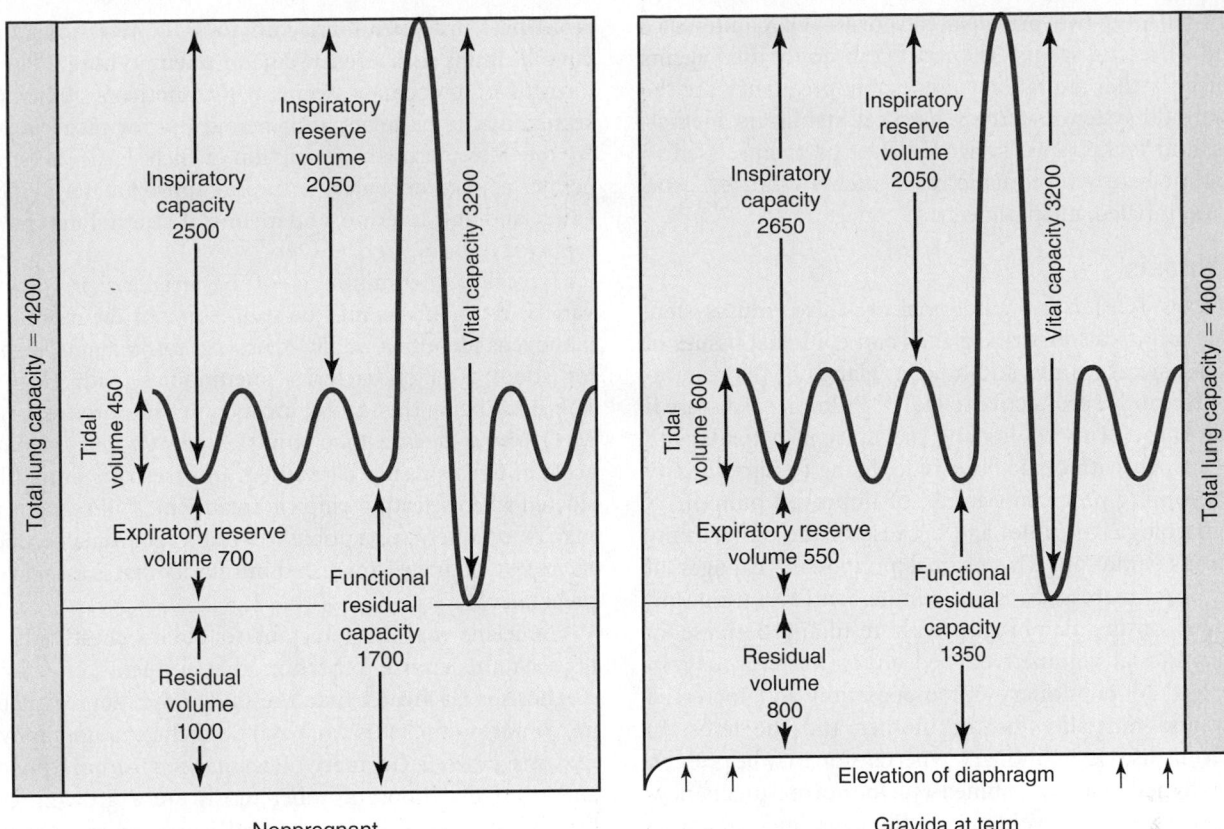

FIGURE 39-2 Pulmonary volumes and capacities (in milliliters) during pregnancy, labor, and the postpartum period. (From Bonica JJ. *Principles and Practice of Obstetric Analgesia and Anesthesia*. Philadelphia: FA Davis; 1967.)

management differ very little from those seen in the nonpregnant individual. Common to these respiratory disorders is the issue of maternal–fetal hypoxia. Sufficient fetal oxygenation requires a maternal arterial oxygen tension (Pao_2) greater than 70 mm Hg, which corresponds to an oxygen saturation of 95%.[70] Hyperventilation, shortness of breath, and dyspnea are commonly seen in pregnancy and must be differentiated from the usual maternal complaints.

Asthma

Although asthma is an increasingly common chronic pulmonary complication in women in the reproductive age group, the management strategies do not differ significantly in pregnant women with asthma from women who are not.[71] Patients who may not be compliant with medical regimens while pregnant for fear of fetal harm should be reassured that, although poorly controlled asthma greatly increases pregnancy risk, well-controlled asthma does not appear to affect pregnancy adversely.[72,73] Poorly controlled asthma during pregnancy has been associated with an increased incidence of pneumonia (more than 60% of pneumonias that arise during pregnancy occur in women with asthma), hyperemesis gravidarum, gastroesophageal reflux disease, preeclampsia, chronic hypertension, preterm labor or birth, perinatal mortality, spontaneous abortion, complicated labor, and low birth weight.[74,75] The literature indicates that maternal and fetal outcomes are related to the severity of the disease and the degree of control achieved with medical management.

It is estimated that approximately one third of patients will experience no change in asthma symptoms, one third will see improvement, and one third will have worsening of symptoms. The peak incidence of asthma exacerbation occurs during the second and early third trimesters; exacerbations during labor are rare because of the natural occurring increase of endogenous epinephrine and steroids.[73,75] The lessening of asthma symptoms during pregnancy is the result of smooth muscle relaxation caused by progesterone. Decreased cell-mediated immunity and an increased level of corticosteroids may assist in diminishing the inflammatory response. Cyclic adenosine monophosphate (cAMP) levels are increased and aid in maintaining an ongoing energy supply to cells.

Factors that may contribute to exacerbation of asthma symptoms include nasal congestion, decreased functional residual volume, anxiety, noncompliance with medical regimens, stress, exercise, exposure to allergens, environmental irritants, respiratory infections, sinusitis, and smoking.[73-75] The decrease in cell-mediated immunity may predispose the mother to viral infections.

Management recommendations include use of a peak flow meter twice per day to assist in objectively measuring maternal pulmonary function. A decrease in peak expiratory flow rate (PEFR) of more than 20% of the patient's personal best requires a call the to the physician; a decrease to of greater than 50% of the patient's personal best signals the need for a visit to the emergency department and the need for rapid assessment and intervention.[73,75] Pharmacologic agents used to treat asthma in pregnancy fall into two principal categories: 1) maintenance agents and 2) rescue agents. The most commonly used agents in this category that are safe for use during pregnancy are the inhaled steroids, systemic steroids, mast cell stabilizers, methylxanthines, and leukotriene antagonist. Rescue agents, used to provide immediate symptomatic relief, include inhaled beta-agonists and inhaled anticholinergics.[6,72-74]

Cystic Fibrosis

Cystic fibrosis (CF) is an autosomal recessive, multisystem disease that affects the exocrine glands and epithelial tissues of the pancreas, sweat glands, and mucous glands of the respiratory, digestive, and reproductive tracts.[74,76] Pulmonary disease is the leading cause of morbidity and mortality in patients with CF. More women with cystic fibrosis are living to reproductive age and becoming pregnant because of improved pulmonary and pharmacologic therapies and because of the opportunity of lung transplantation. The normal pulmonary changes of pregnancy (e.g., increased resting minute ventilation; upward displacement of the diaphragm, with resultant decrease in functional residual volume; widened alveolar-arterial oxygen gradient) lead to pulmonary decompensation and increased morbidity and mortality for the mother and the fetus. In advanced lung disease, pulmonary hypertension may be present. Pulmonary hypertension, combined with the normal pregnancy-related increase in blood volume and the consequent inability to increase cardiac output, may lead to uteroplacental insufficiency and cardiovascular collapse, especially during labor and delivery.[74] Management recommendations include ongoing cardiopulmonary assessment (chest radiography, pulmonary function studies, saturation of peripheral oxygen [SpO_2] monitoring, arterial blood gas determinations, pulmonary artery pressure monitoring), bronchial drainage and chest physiotherapy, ongoing replacement of pancreatic enzymes and supplementation of nutrition, and antibiotic administration for persistently present organisms such as *Pseudomonas aeruginosa* and *Burkholderia cepacia*.[66,74-75] Historically, mothers with CF have poor pregnancy outcomes; however, more recent reports suggest that in women with milder disease, pregnancy outcome may be favorable. Additionally, the patient should receive genetic counseling on the risk of her children being affected by CF.[77]

Pneumonia

Pneumonia is one of the leading causes of infection-related death in the United States and remains a leading cause of maternal and fetal morbidity and mortality.[78,79] Although data suggest that infants born to mother whose pregnancies have been complicated by pneumonia are more likely to be born preterm and to have a lower birth weight, care must be taken to balance treatment to serve both the mother and the fetus.[80] Exacerbations are more common in the second and third trimesters, and they are often associated with other maternal disease processes. Prior respiratory disease, concurrent illness, human immunodeficiency virus (HIV) infection, drug or tobacco use, aspiration, and anemia have been linked with an increased maternal risk of pneumonia.[78,79]

Pregnancy itself appears to be an independent risk factor for major complications of pneumonia. Of pregnant women suffering from pneumonia, up to 40% may undergo major complications such as empyema or pneumothorax. Physiologic changes of pregnancy decrease the mother's ability to clear secretions and place her at increased risk for gastric aspiration. In the fetus, growth restriction, which leads to small-for-gestational-age neonates, occurs in approximately 12% of the cases; and intrauterine and neonatal death rates have been reported to be as high as 12%.[78]

Typically, pneumonia is of bacterial origin; however, a variety of organisms may be seen. Some of the more common pathogens identified are *Streptococcus pneumoniae*, responsible for about 50% of bacterial pneumonias, with *Haemophilus influenzae* being the second most common causative organism. *Mycoplasma pneumoniae* and *Chlamydia pneumoniae* may account for a substantial number of cases and should be considered when selecting empiric treatment.[12,66] Pregnant women may be uniquely susceptible to viral pneumonia secondary to the reduction in cell-mediated immunity that is associated with pregnancy.[80]

Clinicians may be reluctant to obtain chest radiographs; however, the hazard, to both mother and fetus, of delaying the diagnosis is far greater than the small dose (approximately 300 microrads) to the fetus from standard chest radiography. *Pneumocystis jirovecii* (formerly *Pneumocystis carinii*) pneumonia and resistant strains of tuberculosis are a growing concern, because many women who are HIV positive or have acquired immunodeficiency syndrome (AIDS) are in their reproductive years.[78,81]

Acute Respiratory Distress Syndrome

ARDS in pregnancy is often the result of a variety of conditions, including aspiration, preeclampsia, abruptio placentae, postpartum hemorrhage, massive blood transfusions, sepsis, amniotic fluid embolism (AFE), and certain drugs such as tocolytics and aspirin, which lead to the development of pulmonary edema (noncardiogenic).

An important presenting symptom is dyspnea, especially if it is associated with a degree of anxiety or tachypnea. As this evolves, pulmonary function rapidly deteriorates over a 24-hour period. Symptoms include coughing, wheezing, diffuse crackles, pulmonary infiltrates or pleural effusion on the chest radiograph, and a deteriorating PaO_2 with increasing fractional inspired oxygen (FiO_2) demands and declining PF ratio.[81] Pulmonary compliance may decrease from the normal average of 75 milliliters per centimeters of water (mL/cm H_2O) to 20 mL/cm H_2O in severe ARDS.[12] In all suspected cases of ARDS, additional laboratory tests and examinations must be completed to differentiate this syndrome from other causes such as fluid overload and heart failure, which may sometimes be seen in the last trimester.

Management of Respiratory Failure

Management of maternal hypoxia includes restoration and maintenance of the hypervolemic state without inducing fluid overload and further compromising cardiopulmonary function. Because colloidal osmotic pressure is decreased, great care must be taken to prevent the development of pulmonary edema when providing fluid replacement therapy. Oxygen is administered at a high flow rate by mask to achieve an optimal Pao_2 greater than 100 mm Hg and an Spo_2 greater than 95%. Noninvasive mechanical ventilation should be used with caution because of the risk of gastric aspiration. If intubation is required, placement of an orotracheal tube is more desirable than a nasotracheal tube because of hyperemic nasal passageways. If nasotracheal intubation is required, the smallest tube possible that still allows adequate ventilation is used. Gastric decompression is instituted with a small-bore nasogastric or orogastric tube.[66,79] Precautions must be taken to maintain the maternal $Paco_2$ of 28 to 32 mm Hg because respiratory alkalosis may lead to decreased uterine blood flow. Pulmonary compliance should be routinely assessed to evaluate the effectiveness of interventions. Pharmacologic therapies must consider maternal–fetal risk and benefits. Table 39-9 summarizes common medications used in pulmonary dysfunction and obstetric concerns regarding their use.[71,74,75]

Pulmonary Embolism

Venous thromboembolism (VTE), including pulmonary embolism (PE), results from a variety of causes, many of which are related to the physiologic changes in pregnancy. Deep vein thrombosis (DVT) during pregnancy is far more common in the left leg than in the right leg. In one study of 60 pregnant women with a first episode of VTE, 58 had isolated left lower extremity DVTs, 2 had bilateral DVTs, and no isolated right lower extremity DVTs occurred.[82] This unusual distribution has been attributed to increased venous stasis in the left leg related to compression of the left iliac vein by the right iliac artery, combined with compression of the inferior vena cava by the gravid uterus itself. Pelvic vein DVT is also more likely in pregnancy, making the diagnosis more difficult.

Other factors to be considered include the increasing frequency of long-term bed rest for high-risk multiple pregnancies, preterm labor, maternal age older than 35 years, obesity, smoking, cancer, surgery, and a history of VTE or PE.[83-86]

Pulmonary embolism remains a leading cause of maternal mortality and accounts for 20% of pregnancy-related deaths.[82] The greatest risk for developing PE is in the immediate postpartum period, especially if a cesarean section was performed. Two thirds of the patients who die of PE do so within 30 minutes of the initial event. Unfortunately, physiologic changes associated with pregnancy may obscure the diagnosis of VTE during pregnancy. Assessment, management, and complications associated with PE are essentially no different from those in the nonpregnant woman; however, differential diagnosis of amniotic fluid embolism (AFE) must be considered.[83] If DVT or PE is diagnosed, anticoagulation should be initiated. Either

TABLE 39-9	COMMON MEDICATIONS USED IN PULMONARY DYSFUNCTION DURING PREGNANCY
MEDICATION	**CONSIDERATIONS**
Antibiotics	Cephalosporins, erythromycin are generally well tolerated. Tetracyclines and quinolones should be avoided. Vancomycin and aminoglycosides may lead to fetal toxicity. Acyclovir improves maternal morbidity and appears to improve fetal outcomes.
Inhaled corticosteroids	Beclomethasone generally considered safe.
Systemic corticosteroids	Documentation of decreased birth weights and increase in small-for-date babies. Most drug is metabolized by placental enzymes before entering the fetal circulation. Small amount of steroid may cross into breast milk, but breastfeeding is still considered safe.
Mast cell stabilizers	Cromolyn and nedocromil are generally considered safe. They are not associated with increased risks to the fetus.
Beta-adrenergic agonists	Epinephrine and isoproterenol may contribute to maternal–fetal tachycardia.
	Albuterol and terbutaline have fewer side effects and may have the additional benefit of tocolytic actions.
Leukotriene receptor antagonists	They appear to be safe for the management of chronic, mild to moderate asthma.
Inhaled anticholinergics	Ipratropium is beneficial for acute asthma attack. They probably are safe for the fetus because they are poorly absorbed by bronchial mucosa, decreasing the risk of fetal exposure.
Theophylline	It is not commonly used because of maternal side effects. It is recommended that serum levels be maintained between 5 and 12 mg/mL to prevent complications of toxicity.
Analgesics	Morphine and meperidine should be avoided in active labor because they can worsen bronchospasm They will cross the placenta and should be considered when completing a fetal assessment Fentanyl may be a better agent to use. Epidural analgesia is considered safe.
Beta-mimetic tocolytics	These are contraindicated because they may worsen maternal lung damage.
Labor induction	Oxytocin is the drug of choice. Prostaglandin F_2 should be avoided because it is a bronchoconstrictor.
Neuromuscular blockade	It can be administered safely as long as peripheral nerve testing is conducted to monitor drug dosages. These agents will cross the placenta, which should be considered when assessing fetal activity.

(unfractionated) heparin or low–molecular-weight heparin is an acceptable treatment for acute VTE. Both have risks and benefits, but both may be used safely during pregnancy. Intravenous heparin is the treatment of choice surrounding delivery because of its short half-life. Because of the risk of adverse effects on the fetus, warfarin is not generally used until the postpartum period.[87,88] A vena cava filter may be implanted, but a suprarenal position is selected to prevent restriction of venous blood coming from the left ovary and draining into the left renal vein.

Amniotic Fluid Embolism

A potentially disastrous complication involving cardiopulmonary collapse in the pregnant woman is amniotic fluid embolism (AFE), also known as anaphylactoid syndrome of pregnancy (ASP).[89] ASP, or AFE, is rare. Most studies indicate that the incidence rate is between 1 and 12 cases per 100,000 deliveries.[89,90] The maternal mortality rate from AFE has been reported to be anywhere from 10% to 90%, although more recent data from large unselected populations suggest that overall mortality rates may be closer to 20%.[91] Those who survive generally have a poor outcome, with as many as 85% suffering significant neurologic injury from cerebral hypoxia.[89,90] It is one of the leading causes of maternal mortality.

The most common precipitating factors associated with the syndrome are a large fetus, multiparity, premature separation of the placenta, induction of labor, tumultuous labor, and small tears in the endocervical veins that may occur during normal labor.[79,89,91,92] An increased risk also was noted in older, ethnic-minority women.[91] Placental abruption is seen in almost half the cases, with fetal death having occurred before the event.[92] Figure 39-3 presents the pathophysiology of AFE.[93]

A patient with AFE may present with sudden onset of agitation and dyspnea, followed by symptomatic hypoxia,

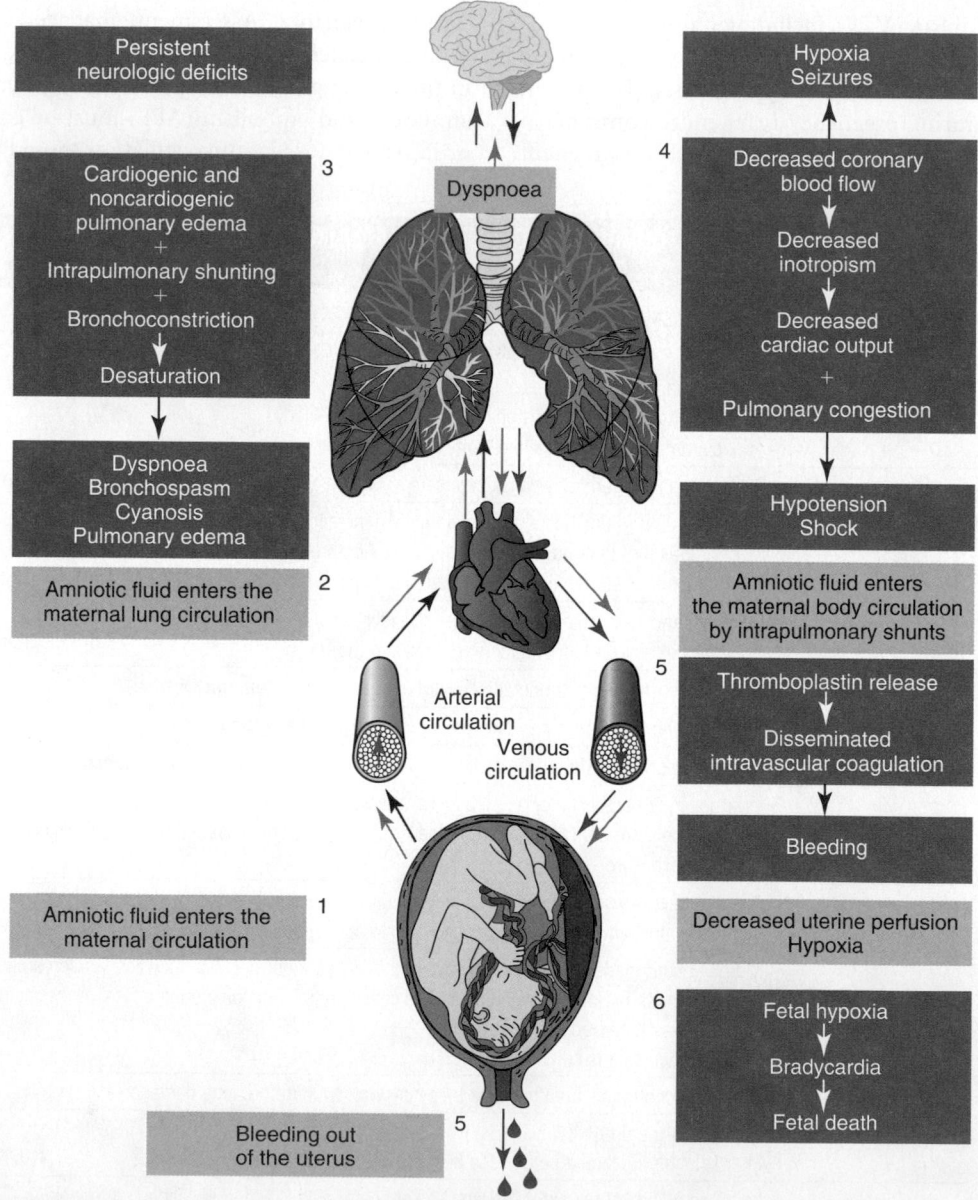

FIGURE 39-3 Pathophysiology of the amniotic fluid embolism. (From Gei G, Hankins GDV. Amniotic fluid embolism: an update. *Contemp Ob Gyn.* 2000;45:53.)

hypotension, and later DIC. Signs and symptoms of shock out of proportion to blood loss and altered mental status may also be observed. Chest pain and bronchospasm are uncommon. In a small percentage of patients, a grand mal seizure may be the initial symptom. More than 25% to 50% of patients die within the first hour, 80% die within the first 9 hours, and 40% of survivors develop DIC.[79,92] The fetal mortality rate is 21%.[92]

No specific diagnostic test exists for ASP, although the presence of fetal squamous cells, lanugo, vernix caseosa, meconium, and mucin in blood aspirated from the pulmonary artery indicates a possibility of its occurrence; however, this debris has been reported even in blood samples obtained from normal pregnant women.[79,91] Testing should be done to rule out DIC. Chest radiography may show pulmonary edema, effusions, and cardiac enlargement. Electrocardiography (ECG) may show tachycardia, nonspecific ST-wave changes, and right ventricular strain. Lung scans may indicate perfusion defects.

Management consists of maintaining oxygenation and supporting cardiac function. Supportive therapy consists of maintenance of blood pressure through aggressive volume replacement and inotropic support, intubation and mechanical ventilation, and blood component therapy for hemorrhage.[79,89] Other therapies such as low-dose heparin, bronchodilators, and steroids may be used.

TRAUMA

Trauma is the leading nonobstetric cause of death among pregnant women; the rate has been estimated to be about 6% to 7%, although a precise number is difficult to obtain because injuries may range from minor to life threatening.[94,95] Motor vehicle accidents (MVAs) are the leading cause of maternal blunt trauma and account for 55% to 82% of maternal trauma.[96] Blunt abdominal trauma is associated with a 3% to 38% incidence of fetal mortality. Direct fetal injury is not usually seen with blunt trauma because of the absorption of forces by the uterus, placenta, and amniotic fluid. Fetal injury and death are more indirect results of maternal shock and death. When the mother survives, abruption is the next leading cause of fetal mortality, followed by uterine rupture.[96]

With domestic violence or intimate partner violence (IPV), rates are estimated to be 4% to 17%; exact rates are unknown because of underreporting and differences in methods of data collection. Injuries associated with domestic violence include defensive wounds; multiple blunt trauma injuries; penetrating injuries: bruises in various stages of healing; injuries to the face, neck, and especially the abdomen; and uterine rupture.[97-100] It may be difficult to differentiate between damage occurring as a result of an accidental fall and that resulting from being pushed or struck; therefore, the patient should be carefully interviewed. Reports of violence were more likely to be associated with alcohol consumption, drugs, inadequate prenatal care (contributing to low birth weight), and a history of a fetal death and previous induced or spontaneous abortion.[101] The attacks may also become increasingly violent and include knife wounds, gunshot wounds, and homicide.[102] Additionally, if IPV is suspected as the cause of maternal injury, appropriate reporting and referrals should be initiated without delay.

Burn injuries during pregnancy may be caused by exposure to a thermal, chemical, or electrical source. The severity of total body surface area (TBSA) of thermal injury in the mother correlates with deteriorating fetal outcomes related to prolonged hypotension, inadequate volume resuscitation, sepsis, hypernatremia, and carbon monoxide exposure.[94,103,104] The best chance of fetal survival is maternal survival.

Approximately 10% of traumatic injuries occur in the first trimester, 40% in the second trimester, and 50% in the third trimester.[103] As women continue to work late into their pregnancies and become involved in higher-risk activities, the type and severity of injuries may begin to increase. Most mechanisms that produce injuries in pregnant patients are no different from those that injure nonpregnant women.

Some types of fall injuries may be associated with the stage of pregnancy. In the first trimester, fall injuries may result from fainting from fatigue, hypoglycemia, and normal physiologic changes. At this stage, the fetus is usually well protected from external trauma because the uterus is located within the pelvis and is protected by bony structures. In the second and third trimesters, as the enlarging uterus expands out of the pelvis, maternal abdominal organs are displaced upward and laterally. Some protection is provided to the maternal abdominal organs because the uterus and fetus now occupy much of the abdominal cavity; however, the growing fetus becomes more vulnerable to injury. Hyperventilation and fainting are common as the fetus grows and places greater metabolic demands on the mother. By the third trimester, the fetus has begun to settle into the pelvis in preparation for birth. As relaxin secretion increases, the end effect of relaxed pelvis ligaments may lead to lordosis and pelvic tilt. This produces a change in gait and in the center of gravity and balance, which, again, may increase the risk of falls.[12] Normal physiologic changes associated with pregnancy may mask assessment findings and thus affect decisions about interventions that are provided (Table 39-10).[101,103]

Types of Injuries
Cardiovascular Injuries

Manifestations related to cardiovascular injury may be masked because of normal physiologic changes in pregnancy. The hypervolemic, low systemic-resistance state and increased heart rate that occur during pregnancy may mask shock because significant blood volume may have been lost before the classic manifestations are seen.[12] Therefore, tachycardia and hypotension in the pregnant trauma patient are clinically significant findings that require careful evaluation and should not be solely attributed to pregnancy. Because of venous congestion of the lower extremities, leg wounds may bleed more vigorously than expected.[105]

Pulmonary Injuries

The pregnant patient has diminished oxygen reserves and decreased blood buffering capacity. This leaves the pregnant trauma patient vulnerable to hypoxemia and less able to compensate when acidemia ensues. During pregnancy, as the uterus grows, the maternal diaphragm is displaced 4 cm above its normal location. This change in location must be considered if placement of a chest tube is necessary to avoid injury to the

TABLE 39-10 INITIAL ASSESSMENT AND MANAGEMENT OF OBSTETRIC TRAUMA

ASSESSMENT	MANAGEMENT, RATIONALE, OR PURPOSE
Primary Survey *Airway* *Signs of Obstruction* Same as for nonpregnant patient	Remove visible debris with caution because of increased hyperemia of nasal or oral area. Decrease risk of aspiration (because of enlarged uterus and effects of progesterone) by lateral tilt or by inserting an NGT or OGT. Emergency cricoid thyrotomy or tracheotomy, if performed, is done above usual site because of upward displacement of thoracic structures.
Breathing *Signs of Ineffective Respiration* Same as for nonpregnant patient with exception of the following: SpO_2 <95 PaO_2 <100 mm Hg $PaCO_2$ >30 mm Hg pH <7.40 Tidal volume <800 mL Labored respirations RR <20 breaths/min or >24 beats/min	100% oxygen by mask because passages tend to be hyperemic and a tendency for breathing through mouth exists. Elevate head of bed, if possible, to decrease pressure on thoracic structures caused by elevated diaphragm. Oral intubation using smaller size (5.5 to 7.0 French) endotracheal tubes to reduce risk of bleeding caused by increased vascularity of area. Gastric decompression with OGT (or small NGT if patient does not tolerate OGT placement) because prone to ileus and gastric reflux. Physiologic monitoring (RR, SpO_2, $ETCO_2$). Obtain ABGs, chest radiograph. Emergent needle decompression or chest tube insertion for hemopneumothorax; may need to reassess entry point because of upward or outward displacement of thorax.
Circulation *Signs of Ineffective Circulation* Same as for nonpregnant patient with exception of the following: Systolic blood pressure <110 mm Hg	Diagnostic peritoneal lavage may be performed; open technique is usually preferred. Assess for possible placental abruption. Normally hypervolemic skin is warm and slightly moist because of progesterone and may mask signs of hypoperfusion.
Mean arterial pressure <80 mm Hg Central venous pressure <6 mm Hg Pale, moist, cool skin	Central venous catheter or large-bore IV access to upper extremity sites because of potential for impeded venous return from lower extremities. Fluid resuscitation. LR is recommended because it has the potential to metabolize into bicarbonate through intrinsic body pathways; do not administer blood products through same IV line. With 0.9 NS, can administer blood products through line; may decrease risk of developing maternal alkalosis (compared with LR). O-negative blood may be given until type and cross-matching are done. Replace 3 mL per 1 mL of blood lost to compensate for hypervolemia associated with pregnancy. Use caution because of increased risk of pulmonary edema caused by decreased colloidal osmotic pressure. May apply MAST, but *do not* inflate abdominal compartment. Tilt the patient to her side, even if on a back board, to maximize venous return.
Secondary Survey *Focused Obstetric History* Gestational age	Keep the mother alive.
Single versus multiple pregnancy	Keep the baby where it is.
Number of pregnancies, live births, abortions	Perform vaginal examination to determine fetal presentation, status of amniotic membrane, and presence of fetal parts or umbilical cord in vagina.
Name of obstetrician	Avoid manipulating cord because of risk of spasms.
Rh factor	Emergent delivery; vaginal versus cesarean; live versus perimortem.
Prenatal complications	
Past vaginal drainage, bleeding, clots	
Past abdominal pain or uterine contractions	

TABLE 39-10 INITIAL ASSESSMENT AND MANAGEMENT OF OBSTETRIC TRAUMA—cont'd

ASSESSMENT	MANAGEMENT, RATIONALE, OR PURPOSE
Maternal Studies	
Unexpected Diagnostic Study Results	
CBC WBC >18,000/mm³	Insert a urinary Foley catheter with caution because of the risk of bleeding caused by increased pelvic vascularity; consider using a smaller size of catheter.
RBC <6,500,000/mm³ Hg <12 g/dL	Consider significance of positive toxicity results. Is the fetus at risk for issues such as drug withdrawal or fetal alcohol syndrome?
Hct <32% Platelets <200,000/mm³	Hct and Hg values that are below those identified may put the mother and fetus at risk for hypoxia.
Fibrinogen >400 mg/dL Chemistries: BUN <9 mg/dL Creatinine >0.5 mg/dL Na⁺ slightly increased Glucose slightly decreased	Use caution when performing a rectal examination to assist in determining fetal position or traumatic damage; pelvic vascular congestion contributes to development of hemorrhoids and predisposes the mother to bleeding from this site. Obtain radiologic studies, as needed; however, implement measures to decrease risk to fetus. Left axis deviation may be seen on the 12-lead electrocardiogram as a normal variant.
Fetal Studies	
Signs of Fetal Distress	
Fetal heart rate <100-110	Ultrasound to evaluate fetus.
Nonreassuring patterns on fetal monitor Fundal height not appropriate for gestational age	Assess fundal height, firmness, contractions every 30 min. Fetal monitoring (with pocket Doppler, ultrasonography, or fetal monitor) as allowed based on interventions provided to mother. Differentiate uterine pain or contractions from other sources of abdominal pain.
Vaginal drainage, bleeding, clots present	Administer tocolytics, as needed. L/S ratio and presence of PG to determine fetal lung maturity.
Abdominal pain, uterine firmness or contractions present	Kleihauer-Betke result indicates a break in the integrity of placental circulation if fetal cells are present.
Amniocentesis:	
Presence of RBCs	
L/S ratio and presence of PG	
Kleihauer-Betke test to detect presence of fetal blood in maternal bloodstream	
Tertiary Survey	
Aspect of Care	
Administer "follow-up meds"	Prophylactic measures: Choose broad-spectrum antibiotics, nonteratogenic agents. Tetanus toxoid does not cross placenta. Rh-negative mothers: May become Rh immunized within 72 hr. Administer Rh immune globulin (300 mcg/15 mL of fetal blood or 30 mL of whole blood) if possibility of mother having received Rh-positive blood. Breach in integrity of the placenta of an Rh-positive fetus as evidenced by positive Kleihauer-Betke test result.

ABGs, Arterial blood gas determinations; *BUN*, blood urea nitrogen; *CBC*, complete blood cell count; *ETCO₂*, end tidal CO; *Hct*, hematocrit; *Hg*, hemoglobin; *IV*, intravenous; *LR*, lactated Ringer solution; *L/S*, lecithin-to-sphingomyelin ratio; *MAST*, military antishock trousers; *Na⁺*, sodium ion; *NGT*, nasogastric tube; *NS*, normal saline; *OGT*, orogastric tube; *PG*, phosphatidyl glycerol; *RBC*, red blood cell; *RR*, respiration rate; *WBC*, white blood cell.

diaphragm. The insertion point during pregnancy is usually between the third and fourth intercostal spaces.[106]

Neurologic Injuries

Spinal cord injury (SCI) in pregnancy may be acute (result of recent trauma) or may be chronic (from pre-existing damage). Initial management of acute SCI is the same as for nonpregnant patients, including the administration of steroids. Adequate uterine perfusion may be evaluated by observing for a reassuring fetal heart rate tracing and lack of uterine contractions.[107] Patients with SCI, similar to pregnant women, are at high risk for DVT, which necessitates the provision of prophylactic anticoagulation. Disruption of autonomic nervous system activity is not associated with labor dysfunction; therefore, vaginal delivery with a SCI is possible. Patients with injuries above T6 are at risk to developing autonomic dysreflexia reaction

(ADR) and may require assisted vaginal delivery or a cesarean section.[107-109] Uterine sensory nerves enter the spinal cord at T11 to L1; women with SCI above T10 are, therefore, unable to feel uterine contractions.[108] They must rely on fetal monitoring of contractions or uterine palpation, and symptoms such as shortness of breath and abdominal spasms to determine labor. Of most importance is that autonomic dysreflexia often occurs with uterine contractions at time of labor and delivery. Proper anesthesia or antihypertensives may treat the problem but immediate delivery of the baby and placenta is vital.[109]

If SCI is severe, irreversible traumatic brain injury (TBI) or maternal brain death occurs, the fetus may remain viable and continue to develop in utero. The issue of pregnancy maintenance in an irreversibly brain-damaged or brain-dead mother remains a controversial ethical issue.

Abdominal and Pelvic Injuries

As stated earlier, MVAs are the primary cause of blunt trauma during pregnancy. Failure to wear seat belts or the improper use of seat belts increases the likelihood of abdominal injury, causes excessive maternal bleeding, and thus increases the risk of fetal death. The engorgement of pelvic vasculature increases the risk of retroperitoneal hemorrhage after lower abdominal trauma.[96] Because the uterus displaces maternal abdominal structures, the traditional assessment findings and sites of referred pain may be altered. Peritoneal signs such as tenderness, rigidity, and rebound tenderness are unreliable indicators because of stretching of the abdominal wall. All of these factors may contribute to delayed detection of abdominal injuries. Splenic injuries are seen more commonly in the third trimester, and damage with blood loss may be seen after relatively mild trauma from vascular engorgement.

Penetrating abdominal injuries are also seen, with gunshot and stab wounds being the most common causes of a penetrating injury.[102] Mortality rates following gunshot or stab wounds are lower in pregnant women because of the anatomic changes that occur related to the growing uterus. In contrast, the fetal mortality rate ranges from 40% to 70% and generally results from either direct fetal injury from the object of penetration or from preterm delivery following the injury.[102]

Blunt abdominal trauma may also be one of the more common types of injury from IPV during pregnancy. The abuser tends to focus the attacks on the abdomen, breasts, and genitalia, the "swim suit" area. The effects of this violence may include placental abruption and uterine injury.[102]

Reproductive System Injuries

Until 12 weeks' gestation, the uterus is a pelvic organ. As the uterus enlarges, it may assist in protecting other organs, but it becomes more vulnerable to injury. Direct trauma to the uterus or placenta reverses protective hemostasis by releasing an increased concentration of placental thromboplastin, a plasminogen activator, from the myometrium. The uteroplacental bed functions as a dilated, passive, low-resistance system that lacks autoregulation and, therefore, has few or no compensatory mechanisms.[12]

Abruptio placentae, commonly seen with blunt abdominal trauma and pelvic fractures, may occur immediately, within 48 hours, or up to 5 days after injury.[102] Uterine damage or rupture is rare, but if it occurs, it is commonly at the fundus or the site of a previous cesarean section and usually results in fetal death. Even if no identifiable damage is present after trauma, the risk for premature rupture of membranes (PROM), premature labor, fetal or maternal hemorrhage, or fetal damage or demise is increased. It is recommended that pregnant patients with trauma be admitted to the hospital for 24 to 48 hours of fetal monitoring because latent injuries or the need for tocolytics may be present.[105,106]

Fetal Injuries

The fetus is usually well cushioned by the amniotic fluid, the gravid uterus, and the abdominal wall, which distribute the force of injury. In most cases of minor trauma, the fetus survives intact. The most common cause of fetal death in maternal trauma is maternal death. The second leading cause of fetal death is placental abruption.[12] Although not common, fetal death may occur even in the absence of significant maternal injury. During the third trimester, direct fetal injury is more common, as the uterine wall has thinned and the amniotic fluid may have decreased and is thus unable to absorb the impact. Additionally, the fetal head may be engaged in the pelvis; a resulting pelvic trauma may lead to a skull fracture in the fetus. Potential predictors of fetal demise vary, depending on the study. Increased maternal injury severity score (ISS), increased maternal hypoxia and acidemia, need for blood replacement, and presence of DIC have been associated with increased fetal mortality rates.[96]

POSTPARTUM HEMORRHAGE

Postpartum hemorrhage (PPH) is the leading cause of maternal mortality. All women beyond 20 weeks' pregnancy are at risk for PPH and its complications. The direct pregnancy-related maternal mortality rate in the United States is approximately 7 to 10 women per 100,000 live births. National statistics suggest that approximately 8% of these deaths are caused by PPH.[110]

Risk Factors and Causes

PPH is best defined, and diagnosed clinically, as excessive bleeding that makes the patient symptomatic (pallor, lightheadedness, weakness, palpitations, diaphoresis, restlessness, confusion, air hunger, syncope), results in signs of hypovolemia (hypotension, tachycardia, oliguria, low oxygen saturation of less than 95%), or both.[111] Other definitions that have been suggested have been problematic. The most common definition of PPH is estimated blood loss of greater than 500 mL after vaginal birth or greater than 1000 mL after cesarean delivery. The inadequacy of this definition was illustrated in studies that assessed blood loss using various objective methods; also, clinicians were likely to underestimate the volume of blood lost.[112]

Another classic definition of PPH is a 10% decline in postpartum hemoglobin concentration from antepartum levels. However, this is not a clinically useful definition, as rapid blood loss may trigger a medical emergency prior to observation of a fall in hemoglobin concentration; also, laboratory changes that are not correlated with events that endanger the patient should not be used to define a medical emergency.[112] In a recent randomized trial, increased risk of PPH was associated with infant's birth weight, labor induction and augmentation, chorioamnionitis, $MgSO_4$ use, and previous PPH.[111]

PPH has many potential causes. As a way of remembering the causes of PPH, several sources have suggested using the "4 T's" as a mnemonic: 1) tone, 2) tissue, 3) trauma, and 4) thrombosis.[113] *Tone* refers to uterine atony, which is, by far, the most common cause of PPH. Overdistension of the uterus, fatigue caused by prolonged labor or rapid forceful labor, and inhibition of contractions by drugs constitute major risk factor for atony. *Tissue* would include retained placenta or failure of complete separation of the placenta, which occurs with placenta accreta. Any damage to the genital tract during delivery would constitute trauma. *Trauma* would also include cesarean delivery, uterine rupture, and cervical or vaginal sidewall lacerations. With *thrombosis*, the abnormities may be pre-existing or acquired. Thrombocytopenia may be related to a pre-existing disease such as idiopathic thrombocytopenic purpura or acquired secondary to HELLP syndrome, abruptio placentae, DIC, or sepsis.[114]

Prevention

Research suggests that active management of the third stage of labor reduces the incidence and severity of PPH.[115] Active management consist of a uterine-contracting medication (preferably oxytocin) immediately on delivery of the baby, early cord clamping and cutting, and gentle cord traction with uterine countertraction when the uterus is well contracted (Brandt-Andrews maneuver). One research demonstrated that early administration of oxytocin (before placental delivery) did not increase the rate of retained placenta, as initially suspected. Plus, the trial showed trends toward a benefit for early administration of oxytocin, including a 25% reduction in PPH and a 50% reduction in the need for transfusion.[115]

Rapid recognition and diagnosis of PPH is essential to successful management. Resuscitative measures and the diagnosis and treatment of the underlying cause must occur quickly before complication of severe hypovolemia develops.

BOX 39-5 CASE STUDY

Patient with Obstetric Issues

Brief Patient History

Mrs. S is 33 years old, G_2P_1. She delivered a term baby boy by cesarean section this morning. Mrs. S has experienced chills, malaise, and abdominal pain since the operation, and she has been given morphine for pain relief but is still complaining of abdominal pain.

Clinical Assessment

Mrs. S is admitted to the critical care unit with hypotension, tachypnea, and tachycardia. She is lethargic, curled up in bed, and groaning. She does not follow commands or answer questions. No urine output has occurred over the last 4 hours, and when a urinary catheter is placed, only 10 mL of dark amber urine has accumulated.

Diagnostic Procedures

Her admission vital signs are as follows: blood pressure of 60/35 mm Hg, heart rate of 145 beats/min (sinus tachycardia), respiratory rate of 30 breaths/min, temperature of 97.5°F, hemoglobin level of 5 g/dL, and platelet level of 30,000/μL. Ultrasound reveals a large fluid collection in the abdomen.

Medical Diagnosis

Mrs. S is diagnosed with an intra-abdominal bleed.

Questions

1. What major outcomes do you expect to achieve for this patient?
2. What problems or risks must be managed to achieve these outcomes?
3. What interventions must be initiated to monitor, prevent, manage, or eliminate the problems and risks identified?
4. What interventions should be initiated to promote optimal functioning, safety, and well-being of the patient?
5. What possible learning needs do you anticipate for this patient?
6. What cultural and age-related factors may have a bearing on the patient's plan of care?

SUMMARY

- Optimal care for the critically ill obstetric patient or one who has sustained injuries requires persistent application of physiologic changes of pregnancy to normal adult values.
- Symptoms of serious disorders may be altered because of the pregnant state.
- Understanding the intricate maternal–fetal relationship provides practitioners with a focus of maintaining maternal stability to enhance uteroplacental perfusion and an optimal in utero environment.
- All potential therapeutic and pharmacologic interventions must be weighed in light of the risk–benefit ratio to maternal–infant status.

- Critical situations may bring personal, cultural, social, spiritual, and ethical values into conflict.
- Determining the appropriate environment may be challenging. Some institutions have created dedicated obstetric intensive care units, whereas others provide care in the obstetric care unit or critical care unit.
- Decision making must be done in collaboration with family and health care team members, and all options should be considered.
- The key factor is collaboration among specialties to optimize maternal–fetal outcomes and facilitate the family experience.

REFERENCES

1. WHO/UNICEF/UNFPA/World Bank. *Trends in Maternal Mortality: 1990-2010*. Geneva: World Health Organization; 2012.

2. Xu K, Kochanek K, Murphy S, Tejada-Vera B. *Deaths: Final data for 2007. National Vital Statistics Report;* 58:19. Hyattsville, MD: National Center for Health Statistics; 2010.

3. Niebyl J. Teratology and drugs in pregnancy. In: Scott JR, et al, eds. *Danforth's Obstetrics and Gynecology*. 10th ed. Philadelphia: Lippincott; 2008.

4. Austin LM, Frush DP. Compendium of national guidelines for imaging the pregnant patient. *AJR Am J Roentgenol.* 2011;197:737.

5. McCollough C, et al. Radiation exposure and pregnancy: when should we be concerned? *Radiographics.* 2007;24:909.

6. Briggs G, et al. *Drugs in Pregnancy and Lactation*. 9th ed. Baltimore: Williams & Wilkins; 2011.

7. Riordan J, Auerbach K. *Breastfeeding and Human Lactation*. 3rd ed. Boston: Jones & Bartlett; 2005.

8. *U.S. Federal Drug Administration*. Pregnancy and lactation labeling. Available at http://www.fda.gov/Drugs/DevelopmentApprovalProcess/DevelopmentResources/Labeling/ucm093307.htm. Accessed April 28, 2012.

9. Hollier L. *Group B Streptococcus. ACOG, Infectious Disease in Obstetrics and Gynecology: A Systematic Approach to Management*, 2009, Washington, D.C.

10. *Centers for Disease Control and Prevention*. Active Bacterial Core Surveillance Report, Emerging Infections Program Network, Group B Streptococcus, 2008. Atlanta, GA: US Department of Health and Human Services, CDC; 2009. Available at http://www.cdc.gov/abcs/reports-findings/survreports/gbs08.html.

11. Centers for Disease Control and Prevention. Trends in perinatal group B streptococcal disease—United States, 2000-2006. *MMWR.* 2009;58:109.

12. Cunningham FG, et al. *Williams Obstetrics*. 23th ed. New York: McGraw-Hill; 2010.

13. Meyn LA, Krohn MA, Hillier SL. Rectal colonization by group B Streptococcus as a predictor of vaginal colonization. *Am J Obstet Gynecol.* 2009;201:76.

14. Center for Disease Control and Prevention. Prevention of perinatal group B streptococcal disease: revised guidelines from CDC. *MMWR.* 2010;59(RR-10):1-36.

15. Sheffield JS, Boppana SB. Cytomegalovirus infection in pregnancy. 2012. UpToDate.com. Accessed April 20, 2012.

16. Johnson KE. Overview of TORCH infections, 2011, UpToDate.com. Accessed April 14, 2012.

17. Demmler-Harrison GJ. Cytomegalovirus. In: Feigin RD, Cherry JD, Demmler-Harrison GJ, Kaplan SL, eds. *Feigin and Cherry's Textbook of Pediatric Infectious Diseases*. 6th ed. Philadelphia: Saunders; 2009.

18. Pass RR, et al. Vaccine prevention of maternal cytomegalovirus infection. *New Engl J Med.* 2009;360(12):1191.

19. Pappas G, Roussos N, Falagas ME. Toxoplasmosis snapshots: global status of Toxoplasma gondii seroprevalence and implications for pregnancy and congenital toxoplasmosis. *Int J Parasitol.* 2009;39(12):1385.

20. Toxoplasmosis snapshots: global status of *Toxoplasma gondii* seroprevalence and implications for pregnancy and congenital toxoplasmosis. *Int J for Parasitology.* 2009;39:1385.

21. American College of Obstetricians and Gynecologists. *Perinatal Viral and Parasitic Infections. ACOG Practice Bulletin no 20*. Washington, DC: ACOG; 2008.

22. American Academy of Pediatrics & American College of Obstetricians and Gynecologists. Antepartum care. In *Guidelines for Perinatal Care*. Elk Grove Village, IL: Author; 2007.

23. Davidson M, London M, Ladewig P. *Old's Maternal-Newborn Nursing and Women's Health Across the Lifespan*. 9th ed. Upper Saddle River, NJ: Pearson Prentice Hall; 2012.

24. *Centers for Disease Control and Prevention (CDC)*. CDC analysis of national herpes prevalence. www.cdc.gov/std/Herpers/herpes-NHANES-2010.htm. Accessed April 14, 2012.

25. Society of Obstetricians & Gynecologists of Canada, Guidelines for the management of herpes simplex virus in pregnancy. No. 208. *Inter J Gynecol Obstetr.* 2008;104:167.

26. *Centers for Disease Control and Prevention*. Genital herpes simplex. www2a.cdc.gov/stdtraining/ready-to-use/manuals/HSV/hsv-notes-2009.pdf. Accessed April 23, 2012.

27. Kriebs JM. Understanding Herpes simplex virus transmission diagnosis, and considerations in pregnancy management. *J Midwifery Womens Health.* 2008;53(3):202.

28. Tolfvenstam T, Broliden K. Parvovirus B19 infection. *Semin Fetal Neonatal Med.* 2009;14:218.

29. Monga M, Creasy R. Cardiovascular and renal adaptation to pregnancy. In: Creasy R, Resnik R, Iams JD, eds. *Creasy and Resnik: Maternal-Fetal Medicine, Principle and Practice*. 5th ed. Philadelphia: Saunders; 2004.

30. Oyelese Y, Ananth CV. Postpartum hemorrhage. Epidemiology, risk factors and causes. *Clin Obstet Gynecol.* 2010;53(1):147.

31. Curry R, Swan L, Steer PJ. Cardiac disease in pregnancy. *Curr Opin Obstetrics Gynecol.* 2009;21:508.

32. Criteria Committee of the New York Heart Association. *Nomenclature and Criteria for Diagnosis of Disease of the Heart and Great Vessels*. 9th ed. Boston: Little, Brown; 1994.

33. Foley MR. Cardiac disease. In: Dildy GA, et al, eds. *Critical Care Obstetrics*. 4th ed. Maiden, MA: Blackwell Publishing; 2004.

34. Hameed AB, Sklansky MS. Pregnancy: maternal and fetal heart disease. *Curr Problems Cardiol.* 2007;32:419.

35. Shabetai R. Cardiac disease. In: Creasy RK, et al, eds. *Creasy and Resnik's Maternal-fetal Medicine: Principles and Practice*. 6th ed. Elsevier; 2009.

36. Bashore TG. Adult congenital heart disease: Right ventricular outflow tract lesions. *Circulation.* 2007;115:1933.

37. Makaryus AN, Forouzesh A, Johnson M. Pregnancy in the patient with Eisenmenger's syndrome. *Mt Sinai J Med.* 2006;73(7):1033.

38. Vasu S, Stergiopoulos K. Valvular heart disease in pregnancy. *Hellenic J Cardiol.* 2009;50:498.

39. Rutherford JD, Hands M. Pregnancy with preexisting heart disease. In: Douglas PS, ed. *Cardiovascular Health and Disease in Women*. Philadelphia: Saunders; 1993.

40. Regitz-Zagroske V, et al. ESC guidleines on the management of cardiovascular diseases during pregnancy. The task force on the management of cardiovascular diseses during pregnancy of the eruopena society of Cardiology (ESC). *Eur Heart J.* 2011;32:3147.

41. Pacini L, et al. Maternal complication of pregnancy in marfan syndrome. *Inter J Cardiol.* 2009;136(2):156.

42. Ramaraj R, Sorrell VL. Peripartum cardiomyopathy: causes, diagnosis, and treatment. *Cleveland Clin J Med.* 2009;76(5):289.

43. Brar S, et al: Incidence, mortality, and racial differences in peripartum cardiomyopathy. *Am J Cardiol,* DOI: 10. 1016/j.amjcard.2007.02.092.

44. Johnshon-Coyle L, Jensen L, Sobey A. Peripartum cardiomyopsthy: review and proactice guidelines. *Am J Crit Care.* 2012;21(2):89.

45. Abboud J, et al. Peripartum cardiomyopathy: a comprehensive review. *Internat J Cardiol.* 2007;118(3)L 295.

46. Roth A, Elkayam U. Acute myocardial infarction associated with pregnancy. *J Am Coll Cardiol.* 2008;52:171.

47. James AH, et al. Acute myocardial infarction in pregnancy: a United States population-based study. *Circulation.* 2006;113(12):1564.

48. American Heart Association. 2010 American Heart Association guidelines for cardiopulmonary resuscitation and emergency cardiovascular care. *Circulation.* 2010;112(suppl IV):IV150.

49. American Heart Association. 2010 American Heart Association guidelines for advanced cardiac life support. *Circulation.* 2010;172.

50. American College of Obstetricians and Gynecologists. Chronic hypertension in pregnancy, ACOG practice bulletin no 125. *Obstet Gynecol.* 2012;119:396.

51. Habli M, Sabai B. Hypertensive disorders of pregnancy. In: Gibbs RS, et al, eds. *Danforth's Obstetrics and Gynecology.* 10th ed. Philadelphia: Lippincott, Williams & Wilkins; 2008.

52. National High Blood Pressure Education Working Group on High Blood Pressure in Pregnancy. Report of the National High Blood Pressure Education Working Group on High Blood Pressure in Pregnancy. *Am J Obstet Gynecol.* 2000;183(1):S1.

53. Clark S, et al. *Handbook of Critical Care Obstetrics: The Fetus and Mother.* 3rd ed. Boston: Blackwell Publishing Co; 2007.

54. Gilbert E. *Manual of High Risk Pregnancy and Delivery.* 5th ed. St Louis: Mosby; 2011.

55. Leeman L, Fontaine P. Hypertensive disorders of pregnancy. *Am Fam Physician.* 2008;78(1):93.

56. American College of Obstetricians and Gynecologists. *Diagnosis and management of preeclampsia and eclampsia, ACOG practice bulletin no 33.* Washington, DC: ACOG; 2008.

57. Chappell LC, et al. Adverse perinatal outcomes and risk factors for preeclampsia in women with chronic hypertension. A prospective study. *Hypertension.* 2008;51(4):354.

58. Martin D. HELLP syndrome A-Z: Facing an obstetric emergency. In: Davidson M, et al, eds. *Old's Maternal-Newborn Nursing and Women's Health Across The Lifespan.* 9th ed. Upper Saddle River, NJ: Pearson Prentice Hall; 2012.

59. Barton JR, Sibai BM. Prediction and prevention of recurrent preeclampsia. *Obstet Gynecol.* 2008;11(2):359.

60. Ghulmiyyah LM, Sibai BM. Managing an eclamptic seizure and its aftermath. *Contemporary OB/GYN.* 2006;51(3):54.

61. Karumanchi SA, Lindheimer MD. Preeclampsia pathogenesis: triple A rating-autoantibodies and antiangiogenic factors. *Hypertension.* 2008;51(4):991.

62. Wang A, Rana S, Karumanch SA. Preeclampsia: the role of angiogenic factors in its pathogenesis. *Physiology.* 2009;24(3):147.

63. Wen SW, et al. Folic acid supplementation in early second trimester and the risk of preeclampsia. *Am J Obstet Gynecol.* 2008;198(1):45.

64. Ross MG, et al. Eclampsia. http://emedicine.medscape.com/article/253960-overview #a3. Accessed July 20, 2012.

65. Hay JE. Liver disease in pregnancy. *Hepatology.* 2008;47(3):1067.

66. Clark S. Critical care obstetric. In: Gibbs RS, et al, eds. *Danforth's Obstetrics and Gynecology.* 10th ed. Philadelphia: Lippincott, Williams & Wilkins; 2008.

67. Airoldi J, Weinstein L. Clinical significance of proteinuria in pregnancy. In: Davidson M, et al, eds. *Old's Maternal-Newborn Nursing & Women's Health Across the Lifespan.* 9th ed. Upper Saddle River, NJ: Pearson Prentice Hall; 2012.

68. Creasy RD, et al. *Creasy & Resnik's Maternal-Fetal Medicine. Principles and Practice.* 6th ed. Philadelphia: Saunders; 2009.

69. Lindsey JL. Evaluation of fetal death, 2010. http://emedicine.medscape.com/article/259165-overview. Accessed April 18, 2012.

70. Cole DE, et al. Acute respiratory distress syndrome in pregnancy. *Crit Care Med.* 2005;33:S269.

71. Powrie R. Respiratory disease. In: James D, et al, eds. *High Risk Pregnancy: Management Options.* 4th ed. Philadelphia: Saunders; 2010.

72. Schatz M, et al. National Heart, Lung and Blood Institute: the relationship of asthma medication use in perinatal outcomes. *J Allergy Clin Immunol.* 2004;113:1040.

73. Montoro M. Pulmonary disorders in pregnancy. In: DeCherney A, et al, eds. *Current Diagnosis and Treatment Obstetrics and Gynecology.* 10th ed. New York: McGraw-Hill; 2007.

74. Schatz M. Asthma. In: Queenan J, ed. *Management of High-Risk Pregnancies.* 5th ed. Malden, MA: Blackwell Publishing; 2007.

75. Whitty J, Dombrowski M. Respiratory diseases in pregnancy. In: Gabbe S, ed. *Obstetrics: Normal and Problem Pregnancies.* 5th ed. Philadelphia: Churchill Livingstone Elsevier; 2007.

76. O'Sullivan BP, Freedman SD. Cystic fibrosis. *Lancet.* 2009;373:1891.

77. Katkin JP. Cystic fibrosis: Clinical manifestations and diagnosis. http://www.uptodate.com/hme/index.html. Accessed April 17, 2012.

78. Smith SE, Osborne K. What are the risks of pneumonia in pregnancy? http://www.wisegeek.com/what-are-the-risks-of-pneumonia-in-pregnncy.htm. Accessed July 22, 2012.

79. American Lung Association. Trends in pneumonia and influenza morbidity and mortality. *American Lung Asssociation Research and Progam Services Edpidemiology and Statistics Unit April 2010.* Author.

80. Graves C. Pneumonia in pregnancy. *Clin Obstet Gynecol.* 2010;53(2):329.

81. Goldberg J, Smith R. Critical care obstetrics. In: DeCherney A, et al, eds. *Current Diagnosis and Treatment Obstetrics and Gynecology.* 10th ed. New York: McGraw-Hill; 2007.

82. Schwartz DR, Malhotra A, Weinberger SE. *Deep vein thrombosis and pulmonary embolism in pregnancy: epidemiology, pathogenesis, and diagnosis,* 2012. http://UpToDate.com. Accessed April 28, 2012.

83. Laros R. Thromboembolic disease. In: Creasy R, Resnik R, eds. *Creasy & Resnik's Maternal-Fetal Medicine. Principles and Practice.* 6th ed. Philadelphia: Saunders; 2009.

84. Pettker C, Lockwood C. Thromboembolic disorders. In: Gabbe S, et al, eds. *Obstetrics: Normal and Problem Pregnancies.* 5th ed. Philadelphia: Churchill Livingstone; 2007.

85. Pettker C, Lockwood C. Pathophysiology and diagnosis of thromboembolic disorders in pregnancy. In: Queenan J, et al, eds. *Management of High-Risk Pregnancies.* 5th ed. Malden, MA: Blackwell Publishing; 2007.

86. Shaughnessy K. Massive pulmonary embolism. *Crit Care Nurs.* 2007;27(1):39.

87. Schwartz DR, Malhotra A, Weinberger SE. Deep vein thrombosis and pulmonary embolism in pregnancy: Treatment. Literature review current through Jun 2012. http://www.uptodate.com/hme/index.html. Accessed July 20, 2012.

88. Cooney M. Heparin-induced thrombocytopenia: advances in diagnosis and treatment. *Crit Care Nurs.* 2006;26(6):30.

89. Stafford I, Sheffield J. Amniotic fluid embolism. *Obstet Gynecol Clin North Am.* 2007;34:545.

90. Baldisseri MR, Manaker S, Lockwood C. Amniotic fluid embolism syndrome. http://UpToDate.com. Accessed July 22, 2012.

91. Knight M, et al. Incidence and risk factors for amniotic-fluid embolism. *Obstet Gynecol.* 2010;115:910.

92. Dildy GA, Clark SL. Anaphylactoid syndrome of pregnancy (amniotic fluid embolism). In: Dildy GA, ed. *Critical Care Obstetrics.* 4th ed. Malden, MA: Blackwell Scientific; 2003.

93. Gei G, Hankins GDV. Amniotic fluid embolism: an update. *Contemp Ob/Gyn.* 2000;45(53):66.

94. El Kady D. Perinatal outcomes of traumatic injures during pregnancy. *Clin Obstet Gynecol.* 2007;50(3):582.

95. Tweedale C. Trauma during pregnancy. *Crit Care Nurs Q.* 2006;29(1):53-67.

96. El-Kady D, et al. Trauma during pregnancy: an analysis of maternal and fetal outcomes in a large population. *Am J Obstet Gynecol.* 2004;190(6):1661.

97. American College of Obstetricians and Gynecologists (ACOG). *Intimate Partner Violence and Domestic Violence. Special Issues in Women's Health.* Washington, DC: ACOG; 2005.

98. Sillman J. Diagnosing, screening, and counseling for domestic violence, 2011. http://UpToDate.com. Accessed April 30, 2012.

99. Lu M, et al. Domestic violence and sexual assault. In: DeCherney A, et al, eds. *Current Diagnosis and Treatment Obstetrics and Gynecology.* 10th ed. New York: McGraw-Hill; 2007.

100. Gunter J. Intimate Partner Violence. *Obstet Gynecol Clin North Am.* 2007;34:367.

101. American College of Obstetricians and Gynecologists (ACOG). *Screening Tools: Domestic Violence.* Washington, DC: ACOG; 2008.

102. Chambliss L. Intimate partner violence and its implication for pregnancy. *Clin Obstet Gynecol.* 2008;51(2):385.

103. Muench MV, Canterino JC. Trauma in pregnancy. *Obstet Gynecol Clin North Am.* 2007;34:555.

104. Kennedy BB, Baird SM, Troiano NH. Burn injuries and pregnancy. *J Perinat Neonat Nurs.* 2008;22(1):21.

105. Bobrowski R. Trauma. In: James D, et al, eds. *High Risk Pregnancy: Management Options.* 3rd ed. Philadelphia: Elsevier Saunders; 2006.

106. Cusick S, Tibbles C. Trauma in pregnancy. *Emerg Med Clin North Am.* 2007;25:861.

107. Ghidini A, Healey A, Andreani M, Simonson MR. Pregnancy and women with spinal cord injuries. *Obstetr Gynecol Surv.* 2009;64(3):141.

108. American College of Obstetricians and Gynecologists. *Obstetric management of patients with spinal cord injuries,* ACOG committee opinion 275. Washington, DC: ACOG; 2002.

109. Carhuapoma F, et al. Neurologic disorders. In: James D, et al, eds. *High Risk Pregnancy: Management Options.* 3rd ed. Philadelphia: Saunders; 2006.

110. Berg CJ, et al. Pregnancy-related mortality in the United States, 1998-2005. *Obstet Gynecol.* 2010;116(6):1302.

111. Jacobs AJ, Lockwood CJ. Overview of postpartum hemorrhage. http://UpToDate.com. Accessed July 22, 2012.

112. Prata N, Gerdts C. Measurement of postpartum blood loss. *BMJ.* 2010;340:555.

113. Society of Obstetrics and Gynecology of Canada. Postpartum hemorrhage. In: *ALARM Manual.* 15th ed. 2008.

114. James AH, et al. Von Willebrand disease and other bleeding disorders in women: Consensus on diagnosis and management from an international expert panel. *Am J Obstet Gynecol.* 2009;6(24):45.

115. Prendiville WJ, Elbourne D, McDonald S. Active versus expectant management in the third stage of labor. *Cochrane Database Syst Rev.* 2009;(3):CD000007.

The Pediatric Patient

Cynthia A. Lewis

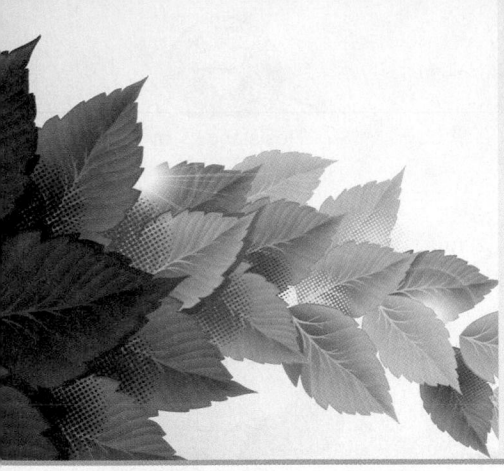

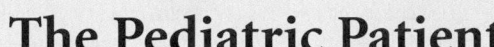

Some of the developmental and physiologic differences between adults and children, older than 1 month, are discussed in this chapter. Although children may experience medical conditions similar to those of adults, they are assessed and managed differently. During periods of stress, children may maintain physiologic stability for a period, but they may then decompensate quickly. Children are *not* small adults. Box 40-1 describes the differences between children and adults. Many of the laboratory values, medications, blood product dosages and methods of administration, and other therapeutic modalities for children are different from those used with adults.

Regardless of the anticipated outcome, admission to a critical care unit is stressful for families. Critical care nurses who successfully deal with pediatric patients see the child and the family as an integral unit and are perceptive to the needs of the entire family.[1] Knowledge of normal growth and development and the ability to assess the child's developmental level are important for working with children and their parents. Nurses who take care of pediatric patients can conceptualize using a developmental perspective as the ideal norm.[1] The developmental stages include the different age groups: infancy (0 to 12 months), toddlers (1 to 3 years), preschoolers (3 to 5 years), school-age children (6 to 12 years), and adolescents (12 to 18 years).

Even though some critically ill children may be managed in adult critical care units, in certain situations, children need the services of various pediatric subspecialists or pediatric intensivists, and they must be transferred to a tertiary care pediatric critical care unit (PICU). This also is true for pediatric trauma patients. The risk of death is significantly lower for patients receiving care in a facility with a designated trauma center.[2] Conditions that may require transfer to a hospital with a PICU include the need for high-frequency ventilation, extracorporeal membrane oxygenation (ECMO), or cardiac surgery and treatment for some neurologic conditions that require intracranial pressure monitoring. Transfer is also considered for children who do not respond to treatment.

RESPIRATORY SYSTEM

Anatomy and Physiology
Upper Airway

The upper airway of the infant and child is different from that of the adult. The epiglottis is located at the level of the cervical spine. It is located at C1 in the newborn, at C3 in the older infant, and at C4 to C5 in the adult.

The infant's epiglottis is large and floppy, and because of its high placement, it may press against the pharyngeal soft palate on inspiration. The infant's tongue is large relative to its head size. The tongue fills most of the oral cavity. Because of this anatomy, the infant usually is an obligate nose breather until 4 to 6 months of age, after which the larynx descends with growth.[1] Oral breathing is a very complex process for an infant, and it never occurs alone. Oronasal breathing is possible, but only up to 30% to 40% of ventilation may be provided orally. During sleep, oronasal breathing may occur spontaneously and last for about 20 seconds.

The larynx of the infant and young child, unlike that of the adult, is a funnel-shaped structure, with the narrowest portion at the cricoid ring.[3] The larynx is pliable because the cartilage

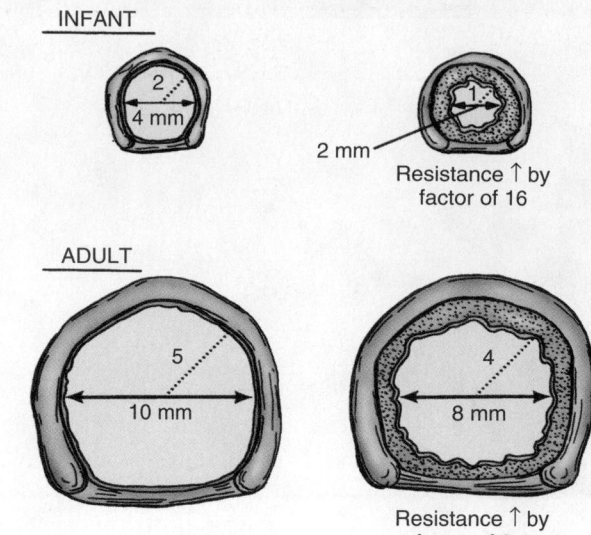

FIGURE 40-1 Effects of edema on airway resistance are shown by proportional increases in airflow resistance with 1 millimeter (mm) of circumferential edema in the infant versus the adult. (From Hazinski MF. Children are different. In: Hazinski MF, ed. *Nursing Care of the Critically Ill Child*. 3rd ed. St. Louis: Elsevier; 2013.)

is less developed, making it easier to collapse on inspiration or expiration. With changes in intrathoracic pressure, collapse may occur even with crying.[3] By age 8 to 10 years, the larynx has grown cylindrical, has assumed the narrowest portion at the glottic opening, and has increased in length, width, and internal diameter. By age 12 years, the diameter has grown to 1.8 cm.

The submucosal layer of the larynx is also looser in the infant and young child, and fluid accumulates more easily in that space. Within the airway's relatively rigid confines, any accumulation of fluid encroaches into the airway space. Along with a shorter and narrower airway, any decrease in airway radius leads to an exponential increase in airflow resistance, which increases the work of breathing. Turbulent airflow, as occurs with crying, doubles the already increased airflow resistance.[4] Figure 40-1 illustrates the changes in airway diameter and airflow resistance with obstruction from edema in an adult and in an infant. The infant or child with an abnormally small jaw and low-set ears should be considered as having a potentially difficult airway to manage and must have a consultation with an anesthesiologist if airway management is required.

Lower Airway

Alveolar collapse is more likely in the infant and young child because of the smaller alveolar size. Infants and young children are at greater risk for ventilation–perfusion mismatch and atelectasis without this collateral ventilation.

Infants and children have a higher metabolic rate compared with adults; therefore, oxygen consumption per kilogram is higher. Hypoxemia develops more rapidly in the context of respiratory compromise in young children than in adults.[3]

Chest Mechanics

The respiratory structure and mechanics of infants and young children are very different from those of mature adults. In the infant and young child, the chest wall is more compliant because the bones are smaller and more cartilaginous. The ribs are more horizontally placed, providing less of a bellowing action on inspiration. Accessory muscles are less developed, and the external intercostals do not contribute to pulling the ribs up on inspiration. The diaphragm is the principal muscle for inspiration. The diaphragm is more horizontal in the chest of the infant and tends to pull the lower ribs inward on inspiration.[5] Because of these mechanics, the infant and the toddler depend almost totally on diaphragmatic contraction for lung expansion. Anything that impedes diaphragmatic contractions may result in respiratory compromise. The intercostal muscles are inadequately developed before school age, and they are unlikely to help with effective ventilation if the diaphragm is impaired.[3] With any decrease in lung compliance, as with lung disease, diaphragmatic contractions, which cause decreased intrathoracic pressure, produce intercostal and substernal retractions rather than inflation of the lungs.[5] The greater the chest wall retractions, the more the diaphragm must contract to offset the changes in intrathoracic pressure to generate an adequate tidal volume for the child. The compliant chest wall of the infant or the young child should expand easily outward with positive-pressure ventilation. If the chest wall does not expand bilaterally during the positive-pressure ventilation, either the ventilation effort is inadequate or the airway is obstructed.[3]

Assessment and Oxygen Devices

The infant or child usually experiences respiratory failure more often than primary heart failure. Unlike the older adult, who may have underlying cardiovascular disease, the infant and the child tend to demonstrate bradycardia and apnea in cardiopulmonary failure and not ventricular dysrhythmias.[4] For the infant or child who is conscious and needs supplemental oxygen, the

TABLE 40-1	CLINICAL INDICATORS FOR THE INFANT OR CHILD AT RISK FOR RESPIRATORY FAILURE	
ASSESSMENT AREA	**PHYSICAL FINDINGS**	**DISCUSSION POINTS**
Respiratory rate	Infant: >60/min	Tachypnea usually first sign of distress in an infant; fatigue is a common contributing factor in respiratory failure
	Child: >40/min	
	Slow or irregular	Late signs: apnea, gasping or agonal respirations
Mechanics	Retractions (intercostal, supraclavicular, substernal)	
	Paradoxic movements (chest in and abdomen out)	
	Signs of diaphragm fatigue, respiratory alternans	
	Grunting	Closing of the glottis to create "auto-PEEP" to keep alveoli open at end-expiration
	Stridor	Sign of upper airway obstruction
	Wheezing	Sign of lower airway obstruction
Air entry	Changes in pitch rather than volume of breath sounds	Chest expansion sometimes is barely perceptible in a normal, spontaneously breathing infant. The small, thin chest wall causes breath sounds from any area of the lungs to be easily referred throughout the chest, even over fluid or atelectasis. Listen for bilateral breath sounds high in the axillae because these are the two most separated points
Color or temperature	Central coolness, pallor, or cyanosis	Peripheral changes may be normal in the infant or child
Heart rate	<5 years: <60 or >180 beats/min	The infant and child have a limited ability to increase stroke volume; therefore, with hypoxemia, the heart rate increases to improve cardiac output. If bradycardia occurs with cardiorespiratory distress, arrest may be imminent
	5-10 years: <60 or >160 beats/min	
	>10 years: <50 or >140 beats/min	
Neurologic status	Infant: hypotonia	Sign of hypoxia for infants
	Child: irritability	An early sign of hypoxia, often manifested as a decreased responsiveness to parents or to pain
	Decreased level of consciousness	

PEEP, Positive end-expiratory pressure.
Based on data from Kline-Tilford A, et al. Pulmonary disorders. In: Hazinski MF, ed. *Nursing Care of the Critically Ill Child.* 3rd ed. St. Louis: Elsevier; 2013.

device of comfort must be selected.[3] Minimizing anxiety and fear in the child is paramount to decrease the work of breathing. Table 40-1 outlines the assessment areas for the pediatric patient at risk for respiratory failure.[3]

Airway Positioning

Knowledge of childhood anatomy is necessary to establish a patent airway. The infant or toddler younger than 2 years of age, because of the large occiput, needs to have a small roll or towel placed under the upper shoulders, with the jaw slightly extended into a "sniffing" position.[4] Optimal positioning of the head should assist in maintenance of a patent airway or help when bag-mask ventilation is required.[4] This head positioning displaces the tongue and lines up the posterior pharynx and tracheal opening for a clear airway. For the infant younger than 6 months, correct head positioning still may not prevent the large tongue from falling back into the posterior pharynx. Oral airways must not be used unless the infant is unconscious because the airway tip may stimulate laryngospasm as a result of the higher placement of the larynx. Side-lying placement, with the neck in a neutral position, should be attempted.[3] The older child needs to have a folded towel placed under the head, with the neck in an extended position to maintain a patent airway.[3] Figure 40-2 illustrates proper head positioning for the infant and the child. The conscious child must be allowed to assume a position of choice for airway maintenance.

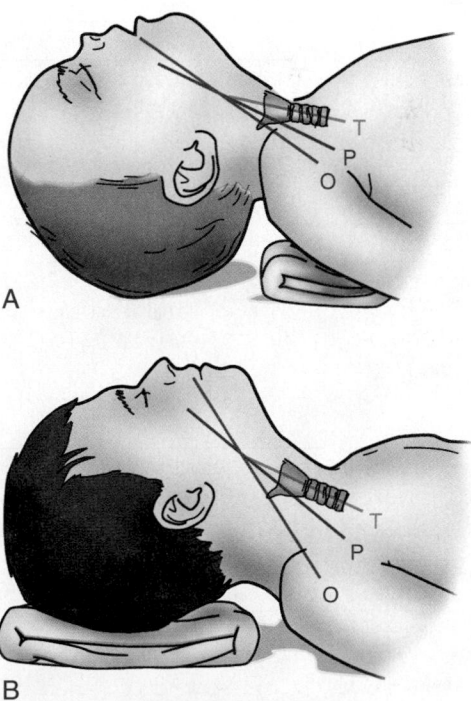

FIGURE 40-2 Correct airway positioning for ventilation is shown for an infant *(A)* and a child *(B)*. Better airflow is provided with a straight alignment of the oropharynx *(O)*, pharynx *(P)*, and trachea *(T)*.[54]

Supplemental Oxygen Devices

Many of the oxygen devices used for adults also are used for children. Some additions include oxygen hoods for infants up to 1 year old. The hoods are clear plastic boxes that envelop the head and allow full vision of the head and access to the body. Other oxygen devices include oxygen tents, which are used less often, and oxygen "blow-by," which uses oxygen tubing to blow oxygen approximately 2 to 3 inches from the child's face. Because of the unpredictability of the actual oxygen percentage that is delivered, the child should never be left unattended with blow-by as an oxygen delivery method. Oxygen masks may aggravate the child and often are not well tolerated because of the snug fit of the mask to ensure adequate delivery of oxygen.[6] One option in older infants and children is to use a nasal prong or cannula.[6] This method allows the child to talk and eat without a facial obstruction.

The appropriate device for oxygen delivery is determined by the patient's age, size, and inspiratory flow rate (tidal volume milliliter per second [mL/s]), and the fraction of inspired oxygen (Fio_2) needed.[7] Oxygen delivery devices may be divided into two different classes: low-flow devices and high-flow devices. Low-flow (variable performance) devices are unable to deliver an oxygen flow rate sufficient to supply the patient's inspiratory flow rate. This allows the child to entrain room air with supplemental oxygen on inspiration. The Fio_2 the child receives depends on the patient's respiratory rate and tidal volume. High-flow (fixed performance) devices may deliver an oxygen flow rate that meets or exceeds the child's inspiratory flow rate. This allows a higher Fio_2 to be consistently delivered.[7] Nursing care for a child receiving supplemental oxygen delivery should include monitoring and recording the type of oxygen delivery device, the liter flow (liters per minute [L/min]), the Fio_2, and the patient's response to the oxygen therapy.

An adult-sized, self-inflating resuscitation bag may be carefully used on an infant, provided only the force needed to cause appropriate chest expansion is used.[3] In general, two types of manual resuscitation bags are used: the self-inflating bag and the flow-dependent bag. Self-inflating bags do not require a gas source to provide ventilation, but flow-dependent bags do require a gas flow.[7] Resuscitation bag sizes, along with other supplemental oxygen devices and oxygen administration, are summarized in Table 40-2. Leaf-flap outlet valves should be avoided when a self-inflating bag is used to assist spontaneous

TABLE 40-2	SUPPLEMENTAL OXYGEN DEVICES AND OXYGEN ADMINISTRATION IN INFANTS AND CHILDREN	
DEVICE	**ADMINISTRATION**	**DISCUSSION POINTS**
Nasal cannula	Infant	Minute volume, inspiratory/expiratory times, and amount of mouth breathing affects infant fraction of inspired oxygen (Fio_2) by a nasal cannula differently from an adult given the same gas flow and oxygen (O_2) percent
	Child	Low-flow O_2 devices are inaccurate for Fio_2 delivery. Titrate to patient's O_2 saturation readings
Oxygen hood	10-15 L/min = nearly 100% O_2	Use with infants <1 year old
Oxygen blow-by	10-15 L/min	Better tolerated than oxygen masks
		Short-term method of O_2 delivery
		Titrated to child's O_2 saturation
		Allows child or parent to hold tubing
Simple mask	0.4-0.5 Fio_2	Entrains room air. Fio_2 does not correlate with high flow rates
Nonrebreather mask	0.9-0.95 Fio_2	No entrainment of room air. O_2 flow is determined by child's minute ventilation
Self-inflating resuscitation bag	Infant	Do not use bags with leaf-flap outlet valves or with spring-loaded PEEP valves
	<3 mo old: 0.25-L bag	
	3 mo–4 yr old: 0.5-L bag	
	Child	
	5-10 yr old: 1-L bag	
	>10 yr old: 1.5-L bag	
Flow-inflating resuscitation bag	Spontaneously breathing	Set the O_2 flow rate at a level necessary to achieve the desired level of ventilation
	Flow rate 3 × minute ventilation	
	Not spontaneously breathing	
	8-10 L/min flow rate	
Peak inspiratory pressure	≤20-30 cm H_2O	
Ventilatory mask size	<6 mo old: 0	Fit and placement on face same as for adult
	6 mo-3 yr old: 1	
	3-6 yr old: 2	
	>6 years old: 3	

PEEP, Positive end-expiratory pressure.
Based on data from Kuch B. Respiratory monitoring and support. In: Hazinski MF, ed. *Nursing Care of the Critically Ill Child.* 3rd ed. St. Louis: Elsevier; 2013:1007.

ventilation in an infant because the infant cannot generate enough negative inspiratory pressure to open the valve.[3] Resuscitation bags equipped with spring-loaded, positive end-expiratory pressure (PEEP) valves to provide continuous positive airway pressure (CPAP) must not be used with the spontaneously breathing child for the same reason previously discussed.[3] Flow-inflating bags have no flow valves that require opening on inspiration and, therefore, may be used to provide supplemental oxygen, PEEP, or CPAP to the spontaneously breathing infant or child.[3] Pressure manometers may be attached to these bags to measure peak inspiratory pressure. Ventilatory masks are measured in the child, as in the adult, from the bridge of the nose to the point before the end of the chin. Using a correctly sized mask for the infant or child is critical for adequate oxygenation and ventilation of the patient.

Endotracheal Intubation

Procedure

Endotracheal tube (ETT) placement and management for the pediatric patient is an important intervention to maintain airway in a patient with respiratory failure.[4] Preoxygenation of the child before intubation is very important. Bag-mask ventilation is an effective way to assist the child's ventilation. Attempts for intubation should to be no longer than approximately 30 seconds per attempt to prevent deterioration in heart rate or the child's appearance. Box 40-2 provides formulas as a guideline for ETT measurements in the pediatric patient. It is important to ensure that pediatric emergency equipment of the correct size is used. Many facilities are using length-based or color-coded resuscitation tapes such as the Broselow system.[4,8] This tape gives an estimate of the child's body weight based on the crown-to-heel length and may be used to determine the appropriate size of resuscitation equipment and medication dosages for the child. Figure 40-3 provides an illustration of a Broselow tape.

When correctly placed, the tip of the ETT should be 1 to 2 cm above the carina, no higher than the first rib.[3] After the child is intubated, bilateral breath sounds should be assessed high in the axillae along with bilateral chest expansion. The easy transmission of sounds in the chest of the child may be mistaken for breath sounds in the event of accidental esophageal intubation. Initial confirmation of the tube placement after assessment of bilateral breath sounds and adequate chest expansion is made with the use of the colorimetric carbon dioxide (CO_2) detector. This device detects the delivery of CO_2 after six breaths. Additional confirmation of the correct placement of the endotracheal tube must be obtained by using a capnography waveform.[4] This is a very reliable indicator of exhaled CO_2 and tracheal tube placement because a perfusing cardiac rhythm is needed to deliver CO_2 to the lungs. During a cardiac arrest, CO_2 may not be present, and CO_2 may not be detected even if the ETT is in the correct location. Re-expansion of the bulb of the esophageal detector device indicates tracheal tube placement.[9] A chest radiograph is obtained once the endotracheal tube is taped in place to confirm proper tube depth and the position.

ETT dislodgement may occur more easily in the infant or young child and cause acute deterioration of the patient's condition. The tip of the ETT is pulled upward with neck extension or when the head is turned completely to the side. Conversely, the ETT moves downward with neck flexion. With the trachea of the young child being short, an ETT placed higher or lower may become dislodged or intubate the bronchus. ETT obstruction may occur with high placement, neck flexion, or head rotation, which may cause the bevel of the ETT to press against the tracheal wall, occluding the lumen. Secretions and mucous plugs may more easily occlude the lumen of a small-diameter ETT. The assessment of the tube by the bedside nurse is critical in the evaluation of proper functioning of the child's ETT.

The nurse and the respiratory therapist must ensure that the child's ETT remains patent and in correct placement to maintain correct oxygenation and ventilation. Causes of acute deterioration in the intubated pediatric patient may be recalled by using the mnemonic DOPE[3]:

D: displacement of the tube
O: obstruction of the tube
P: pneumothorax (or other air leak)
E: equipment failure

Suction equipment and a bag-valve mask need to be readily available for resuscitation if any of the above intubation complications occurs.

Securing Endotracheal and Nasotracheal Tubes

The small infant or child has less facial area for tape adherence for securing the tubes. A method with a low incidence of accidental extubation uses two pieces of cloth tape, split halfway down the middle, creating a "Y" shape (Figure 40-4). The skin of the child is more fragile than that of an adult. Cloth tape may be irritating to the child's skin. A soft foam dressing (i.e., Mepilex) may be applied to the cheeks, with the securing tape attached on top of the dressing. Breath sounds should be auscultated before and after taping or re-taping of the tubing to ensure that the ETT position has not changed.[3] Commercially manufactured devices to secure ETTs are available, but these are limited in infant and pediatric sizes. No single method of securing a tube has been identified as superior for minimizing ETT dislodgement.[9]

BOX 40-2 ENDOTRACHEAL TUBE MEASUREMENT

Size

- For infants and toddlers: size based on aged 1 to 2 = 3.5 mm
- For children >2 years old: (age in years + 16) ÷ 4
- For any age: compare the circumference of the child's little finger with the external diameter size of the endotracheal tube (ETT)
- Cuffed tube: external diameter one-half size smaller than appropriate-sized uncuffed tube

Depth of Insertion

- From the teeth to midtrachea: internal diameter of ETT × 3

Cuff Pressure

- Allow for a slight air glottic leak

Modified from Hazinski MF. *Nursing Care of the Critically Ill Child.* 3rd ed. St. Louis: Elsevier; 2013.

Equipment	GRAY* 3-5 kg	PINK Small Infant 6-7 kg	RED Infant 8-9 kg	PURPLE Toddler 10-11 kg	YELLOW Small Child 12-14 kg	WHITE Child 15-18 kg	BLUE Child 19-23 kg	ORANGE Large Child 24-29 kg	GREEN Adult 30-36 kg
Resuscitation bag		Infant/child	Infant/child	Child	Child	Child	Child	Child	Adult
Oxygen mask (NRB)		Pediatric	Pediatric	Pediatric	Pediatric	Pediatric	Pediatric	Pediatric	Pediatric/adult
Oral airway (mm)		50	50	60	60	60	70	80	80
Laryngoscope blade (size)		1 Straight	1 Straight	1 Straight	2 Straight	2 Straight	2 Straight or curved	2 Straight or curved	3 Straight or curved
ET tube (mm)†		3.5 Uncuffed 3.0 Cuffed	3.5 Uncuffed 3.0 Cuffed	4.0 Uncuffed 3.5 Cuffed	4.5 Uncuffed 4.0 Cuffed	5.0 Uncuffed 4.5 Cuffed	5.5 Uncuffed 5.0 Cuffed	6.0 Cuffed	6.5 Cuffed
ET tube insertion length (cm)	3 kg 9-9.5 4 kg 9.5-10 5 kg 10-10.5	10.5-11	10.5-11	11-12	13.5	14-15	16.5	17-18	18.5-19.5
Suction catheter (F)	8	8	8	10	10	10	10	10	10-12
BP cuff	Neonatal #5/infant	Infant/child	Infant/child	Child	Child	Child	Child	Child	Small adult
IV catheter (ga)		22-24	22-24	20-24	18-22	18-22	18-20	18-20	16-20
IO (ga)		18/15	18/15	15	15	15	15	15	15
NG tube (F)		5-8	5-8	8-10	10	10	12-14	14-18	16-18
Urinary catheter (F)	5	8	8	8-10	10	10-12	10-12	12	12
Chest tube (F)		10-12	10-12	16-20	20-24	20-24	24-32	28-32	32-38

FIGURE 40-3 Broselow pediatric color-coded resuscitation tape. *BP,* Blood pressure; *ET,* endotracheal; *F,* French; *IO,* intraosseous; *IV,* intravenous; *NG,* nasogastric; *NRB,* nonrebreathing.

*For Gray column, use Pink or Red equipment sizes if no size is listed.

†Per 2010 AHA Guidelines, in the hospital, cuffed or uncuffed tubes may be used. (Adapted from Broselow Pediatric Emergency Tap. Distributed by Armstrong Medical Industries. Lincolnshire, IL. Copyright 2007 Vital Signs, Inc. All rights reserved).

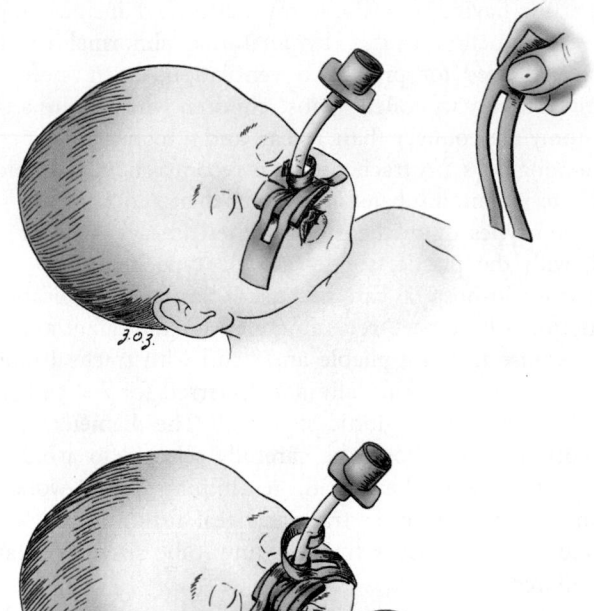

FIGURE 40-4 Securing an endotracheal tube with split taping. (Modified from Kline-Tilford A, et al. Pulmonary disorders. In: Hazinski MF, ed. *Nursing Care of the Critically Ill Child*. 3rd ed. St. Louis: Elsevier; 2013.)

BOX 40-3	CHARACTERISTICS OF A PEDIATRIC VENTILATOR

SPECIFICATIONS	VISUAL INDICATORS
• Volume, pressure or time cycled, mixed modes of ventilation • Assist/control, CPAP (continuous positive airway pressure), PSV (pressure support ventilation), SIMV (synchronized intermittent mandatory ventilation) • Tidal volume range of 20-450 mL/breath (minute ventilation of 0.4-0.6 L/min) • Respiratory rate of 1-1000/min (high frequency ventilation capability is also desirable) • Variable inspiratory flow of 0. 5-40 L/min • Variable inspiratory/expiratory flow ratios • Adjustable peak inspiratory pressure of 10-80 cm H_2O • Adequate humidification • Provision for positive end-expiratory pressure (PEEP)/CPAP	• Proximal airway pressure (patent airway) • Proximal airway temperature (patent airway) • Fraction of inspired oxygen (FiO_2) (high and low) • Inspiratory/expiratory times • Flow rate (L/min) • Tidal volume • Minute ventilation

Alarms
- High and low pressure
- Apnea
- Loss of PEEP
- Power failure/disconnect
- Loss of air/oxygen
- High temperature
- Failure to cycle
- Output jacks to allow ventilator alarms to be connected to a remote alarm in nursing stations

Modified from Kuch B. Respiratory monitoring and support. In: Hazinski MF, ed. *Nursing Care of the Critically Ill Child*. 3rd ed. St. Louis: Elsevier; 2013.

Mechanical Ventilation

Many types of unconventional mechanical ventilation (e.g., high-frequency, oscillation, jet ventilation) are used, but for most infants and children, standard means of positive-pressure ventilation support use volume or pressure-controlled ventilators. The type of ventilation chosen depends on the child's size, minute ventilation requirements, and lung compliance. Newer ventilators have flow and pressure triggers that are sensitive enough to ventilate infants and children.[10]

For the older child, noncontinuous-flow, volume-limited ventilation in synchronized intermittent mandatory ventilation (SIMV) mode is used most often. Pressure support ventilation is also used in the child in conjunction with other modes to assist with spontaneous breathing, especially during the weaning process. Currently used ventilators have flow triggering designed for infants. Some type of synchronized ventilation mode is used almost exclusively for the ventilation of infants and children. Box 40-3 outlines what the characteristics are for the ideal pediatric ventilator for the infant and child.[11]

Ventilator–patient asynchrony may have several causes. The Hering-Breuer reflex is a vagal reflex in which the child's sensing of positive lung inflation sets off immediate expiration, and lung deflation stimulates inspiration. Apnea, or active expiration during the ventilator's inspiratory cycle, also may cause asynchrony. The use of adult ventilators not appropriately adapted for the infant or child may cause asynchrony. In the small child, decreased tidal volume and increased respiratory rates occur to cope with respiratory compromise. Adult ventilators may not sense rapidly enough, if at all, any spontaneous respiratory efforts, which leads to increased work of breathing in the child.

Asynchrony may lead to poor oxygenation or volutrauma. Significant asynchrony may require sedation, alone or with neuromuscular blockade. Criteria for weaning and extubation are much more extensive for the adult than for the child, but some guidelines exist for these procedures. SIMV with pressure support ventilation (PSV) is used to wean from positive-pressure ventilation. PSV allows the child to have greater control over breathing, and asynchrony is not a problem. Table 40-3 outlines the indicators for initiating weaning and extubation.[9,10] Supplemental oxygen may be supplied after extubation by a nasal cannula, ventilation mask, or oxygen hood. Noninvasive ventilation devices such as nasal or facial CPAP may be an option for the patient, but if the child cannot be managed on these options, reintubation may be necessary.

Extubation Complications

A postextubation croup may occur in the small child. Manifestations arising from airway edema include hoarseness, stridor, or a crowing cough that begins immediately or up to 3 hours after extubation. Initial treatment consists of keeping the child calm. Procedures must be withheld, if possible, and crying must be prevented to avoid increasing airway resistance. Supplemental humidified oxygen should be administered to the child immediately after extubation and a cool mist continued to be provided. More severe symptoms may be treated with racemic epinephrine and with intravenous or inhaled steroid therapy. Intubation equipment and personnel qualified to intubate should be available after extubation, in case the patient requires reintubation.

Tracheostomies

Over the past three decades, tracheostomy has become an increasingly common procedure in children. The primary reasons for having a tracheotomy performed include upper airway obstruction caused by anatomic abnormalities, the anticipated need for prolonged ventilation, or the need for effective pulmonary toilet.[12] Most children who require a tracheostomy are younger than 1 year, and a higher incidence is seen among boys.[12] A tracheotomy is recommended if an older child is to remain intubated for longer than 2 to 3 weeks.

Several types of tracheostomy tubes are available for the child, with the plastic, single-cannula type being the most popular for in-hospital care because it has few complications. Silastic tubes have been recommended for the infant and the child because they are pliable and bend with tracheal movement. Uncuffed tubes usually are preferred for the pediatric patient to prevent subglottic stenosis.[13] The diameter of the tracheostomy tube should be carefully selected to avoid any damage to the tracheal wall, to minimize the work of breathing, and to promote translaryngeal airflow, when possible. Table 40-4 describes tracheostomy tube sizes for infants and children.

Complications with a tracheostomy may be categorized as those occurring early or late. Early complications may occur intraoperatively and up to the first tracheostomy tube change. Studies have shown that a cannula obstruction is the most common early complication.[12] Late complications may occur after the first tube change. Some of the most significant late complications include recurrent tracheitis, accidental decannulation, cannula obstruction, subglottic stenosis, suprastomal obstruction, and tracheal ulceration.[13]

If accidental decannulation occurs in a new tracheostomy, replacing the tube may be a difficult procedure. However, in the child who has had a long-term tracheostomy, reinserting a tracheal tube after accidental decannulation should be relatively easy because the stoma is well established. An extra tracheostomy tube and obturator of the child's size and an additional tube that is a half size smaller should be kept at the bedside in case of emergency. Tracheomalacia may cause the development

---

TABLE 40-3	INDICATORS FOR INITIATING WEANING OF THE PEDIATRIC PATIENT

- Achievement of baseline mental status
- Presence of cough and gag reflexes
- Absence of a fever
- Spontaneous respiratory effort
- Normal acid–base balance
- Oxyhemoglobin saturation $\geq$90% or Pao$_2$ $\geq$60 mm Hg (in the absence of cyanotic heart disease)
- Fraction of inspired oxygen (Fio$_2$) <0.5
- Positive end-expiratory pressure (PEEP) <7 cm H$_2$O
- Partial pressure of carbon dioxide (Paco$_2$) <mm Hg
- Stable hemodynamically
- Stable ventilation support for $\geq$24 hours
- No plans that will require significant sedation or operative procedures in the next 12 hours

From Kline-Tilford A, et al. Pulmonary disorders. In: Hazinski MF, ed. *Nursing Care of the Critically Ill Child*. 3rd ed. St. Louis: Elsevier; 2013:483.

TABLE 40-4	GUIDELINES FOR INTUBATION EQUIPMENT AND TRACHEOSTOMY TUBES FOR PEDIATRICS

	EQUIPMENT CHOICES BASED ON AGE AND WEIGHT							
	3 mo	6 mo	1 yr	3 yr	6 yr	8 yr	12 yr	16 yr
FACTORS	**6 kg**	**8 kg**	**10 kg**	**15 kg**	**20 kg**	**25 kg**	**40 kg**	**60 kg**
ETT size (mm)	3.0-3.5	3.5-4.0	4.0-4.5	4.5-5.0	5.0-5.5	6.0 c/u	7.0 c	7.0-8.0 c
Laryngoscope blade	0-1 s	0-1 s	1 s	2 s	2 s	2 s/c	3 s/c	3 s/c
Stylet (Fr)	6	6	6	6	14	14	14	14
Suction catheter (Fr)*	6-8	8	8	8-10	10	10-12	12-14	12-14
Shiley Tracheostomy								
Shiley size (mm)	0	1	1-12	4	4	4	6	6
Internal diameter (mm iD)	3.4	3.7	3.7-4.1	5	5	5	7	7
Length (cm)	4	4.1	4.1-4.2	4.6	4.6	4.6	6.7	6.7

*Catheter size twice the internal diameter size of any tracheal tube.
cm, Centimeter; *c/u*, cuffed or uncuffed; *ETT*, endotracheal tube; *Fr*, French; *ID*, internal diameter; *mm*, millimeter; *s/c*, straight or curved.
Based on data from Kuch B. Respiratory monitoring and support. In: Hazinski MF, ed. *Nursing Care of the Critically Ill Child*. 3rd ed. St. Louis: Elsevier; 2013:1007.

of cricoid cartilage collapse, resulting in upper airway obstruction after the tube is no longer in place. In some cases, an airway can be re-established only surgically. In other children, an ETT that is a size smaller may be inserted into the stoma; otherwise, the child may have to be orally or nasally intubated.

Bronchiolitis

Bronchiolitis is one of the diseases that primarily affects the very young infant and is the most common disease in infants and children less than 2 years of age.[14] *Bronchiolitis* is a term used to describe a condition that affects the lower respiratory tract and results in obstruction of the small airways. Although this disease has a relatively low mortality rate (200-500 deaths per year), it is the most frequent cause of hospitalization in the infant population.[14] However, bronchiolitis is one of the most common diagnoses in children who present in the critical care unit with respiratory failure.[15] The disease is characterized by mucosal edema, inflammation, increased mucus production, and sloughing of epithelial cells. This leads to obstruction of the bronchioles, resulting in hypoxemia and hypercapnia.[14] Widespread fine end-inspiratory crackles and an expiratory wheeze are heard on auscultation. This clinical pattern may be seen during the first year of life, with most hospital admissions occurring within the first 6 months of life.[14] Respiratory syncytial virus (RSV) is the most common cause of viral bronchiolitis, and it infects almost all children by the age of 2 years.[16] The peak incidence for viral bronchiolitis occurs during midwinter and into early spring. RSV is highly contagious and may be spread by close contact through droplets. Meticulous hand washing by clinical staff is the most important step to prevent hospital-acquired infections in other patients or staff members.[17]

Pathophysiology

RSV infection has an overall low mortality rate, but the mortality rate is 37% among infected infants with congenital heart disease. In children less than 2 years of age, up to 40% of RSV infections may progress to lower respiratory infections.[14] Those with cystic fibrosis or bronchopulmonary dysplasia or who are immunocompromised are also at greater risk for more serious disease and for occurrence beyond 1 year of age. The chance of recovery from RSV may be excellent, but reactive airway disease residual effects may be seen several years after infection.[18] RSV involves inflammation of respiratory epithelium, which leads to necrosis. The epithelium is replaced with nonciliated tissue. Submucosal edema forms with lymphocytic infiltrates and other alveolar debris. Obstruction occurs from mucous secretions and debris not being cleared because of the lack of ciliated epithelium. Pathologic pulmonary dynamics involve lung hyperinflation almost two times the normal. Obstruction occurs in a patchy distribution with complete obstruction, leading to atelectasis and partial obstruction, which results in hyperinflation. Inspiratory resistance and expiratory resistance are present, along with ventilation–perfusion mismatch, which leads to hypoxemia and some degree of CO_2 retention. The probable mechanism in addition to the ventilation–perfusion mismatch is hypoventilation, which results from a marked increase in the work of breathing in the infant.[18]

Clinical Assessment

The first symptoms to appear are those of an upper respiratory tract infection—sneezing and rhinorrhea. In many cases, a family member has had a respiratory illness. After 2 to 3 days, respiratory distress ensues with increased respirations, coughing, nasal flaring, chest retractions, wheezing, irritability, and feeding difficulties. Fever and lung rhonchi may or may not occur. After bronchiolar obstruction has occurred, these patients present with increased work of breathing. This may lead to muscle fatigue and respiratory failure if the work of breathing exceeds the capacity of the patient's respiratory muscles. Infants tolerate respiratory loads poorly and are susceptible to fatigue because of the immature pattern of their muscle fibers.[19]

Treatment

The overall treatment goal with bronchiolitis is supportive. Oxygen continues to be the primary therapy to decrease the work of breathing and oxygen demands. Depending on the severity of illness, the infant may receive supplemental humidified oxygen by mask, nasal CPAP (despite lung hyperinflation), or mechanical ventilation.[5,20] RSV causes airway obstruction, and no therapy has demonstrated an ability to rapidly reduce this obstruction.

Suctioning of the airways will be required to help alleviate the signs and symptoms of airway obstruction from mucous secretions. The mucus will be thick and initially cause the infant to be suctioned frequently. Inhaled beta$_2$-agonists, anticholinergic agents, and corticosteroids during the acute or recovery phase have been tried with various degrees of success.[14] The use of a clinical pathway for bronchiolitis has been shown to be effective in the literature. A decrease in the use of therapies such as bronchodilators, glucocorticoids, antibiotics, and chest physiotherapy, and a decrease in admission rates and length of stays have occurred in association with the use of a bronchiolitis clinical pathway.[14]

The current recommendation from the American Academy of Pediatrics for the prevention of RSV is the administration of the monoclonal antibody palivizumab (Synagis, MedImmune). Clinicians may administer palivizumab prophylactically to selected infants and children with chronic lung disease or a history of prematurity (<35 weeks' gestation) or with congenital heart disease.[17] Palivizumab is administered in 5 monthly doses during the RSV season, usually beginning in November or December, at a dose of 15 milligrams per kilogram (mg/kg) per dose administered intramuscularly.[17]

Status Asthmaticus
Pathophysiology

Asthma is a chronic inflammatory disorder of the airways, in which many cells and cellular elements, including mast cells, eosinophils, T lymphocytes, neutrophils, and epithelial cells, play a role.[21] An acute asthma exacerbation is an event of progressive wheezing, cough, chest tightness, shortness of breath, or a combination of all these symptoms. Asthma is identified as the disease with a triad of physiologic processes, airway inflammation, edema, and airway hyperactivity. Inflammation has been recognized as the primary underlying cause in the pathogenesis of this disease.[21] The treatment for asthma is aimed at decreasing and reducing airway inflammation.

The universal feature of the inflammatory response in asthma includes the activation and infiltration of the airway by cells. The early phase in the inflammation reaction is caused by a trigger, and this may be different with each child. The immediate response to this trigger is bronchospasm and smooth muscle contraction caused by the mediators from the various inflammatory cells in the airway. If this early phase is not responsive to beta$_2$-agonists, a late phase will occur about 6 to 9 hours after the initial exposure to the trigger.[21] This will lead to increased release of the mediator cells in the airway and produce cellular infiltration, airway edema, mucus secretions, bronchospasm, and smooth muscle contraction. Without treatment, atelectasis and mucous plugging may occur in the child.

Clinical Assessment

Assessing severe asthma in the infant is different compared with that in the older child because of the anatomic and physiologic differences between them. Physiologic changes may progress rapidly to respiratory failure in the infant. Table 40-5 outlines

guidelines for classifying the severity of an asthma exacerbation. A moderate asthma episode requires hospitalization with close monitoring. In a severe event, the child may only able to speak in short phrases or not at all. The position of comfort or degree of agitation should be noted; sitting upright and unable to lie down indicates severe distress.[22] A severe episode requires critical care, with intubation and ventilation equipment readily available.[5]

Treatment

Standard treatment for the pediatric patient who has asthma includes receiving oxygen, beta-adrenergic therapy, corticosteroids, and anticholinergic medications, as indicated.[5,21] Pharmacologic therapy is based on the concept of reducing airway inflammation. Beta-adrenergic agonists are the first-line agents in the treatment of asthma. Beta-agonist medications that are selective for beta$_2$-receptors on airway smooth muscle (e.g., albuterol, levalbuterol) are preferred to avoid the stimulation of the beta$_1$-cardiac receptors.[21] These medications are given by nebulation intermittently or continuously. Anticholinergic medications in conjunction with beta-agonists improve

---

TABLE 40-5   GUIDELINES FOR ASSESSING SEVERE ASTHMA IN INFANTS AND CHILDREN

ASSESSMENT AREA	PHYSICAL FINDINGS		DISCUSSION POINTS
	INFANT	CHILD	
Respiratory rate	Increase of >50% above normal	Can range from normal to >95th percentile for age	Sleeping rates in infants and resting rates in children are good measures of obstruction; awake or activity rates are too variable.
Level of consciousness	Decreased	May be decreased	Assess response to parents and pain.
Accessory muscle use	Retractions in less-than-severe states	Severe intercostal, tracheosternal, and sternocleidomastoid retractions and nasal flaring	In infants, compliant chest wall produces retractions earlier in course. In children, retractions and flaring correlate well with degree of obstruction and with PEF <50% of predicted for age.
Color	Pallor, grayness, or cyanosis	Possible cyanosis	
Dyspnea		Can speak only single words or short phrases; cannot count to 10 in one breath	Drowsy or confused.
Quality of cry	Softer and shorter as FEV$_1$ decreases		
Oxygen saturation	<90% in less-than-severe states	<90% on room air	Infants have greater ventilation–perfusion mismatch. In children, hypoxemia correlates well with degree of obstruction.
Auscultation (Breath sounds)	Wheezing; then becoming inaudible because of decreased air movement	Same as in infant	Presence and volume of wheezing is the least sensitive predictor of obstruction.
PaCO$_2$	If >50 mm Hg or if rising 5-10 mm Hg/hr, consider mechanical ventilation	Can range from <40 mm Hg with respiratory distress to >40 mm Hg as air movement significantly decreases	PaCO$_2$ is best measure of ventilation in infants. A continually rising PaCO$_2$ of >40 mm Hg in a child occurs when PEF is <20% of predicted for age. Hypercapnia develops more readily in young children than adults.
PEF	≥70%		It is not needed in cases of severe asthmatic exacerbation. This is used after asthma is under control.
Feeding/sucking ability	Decreased or absent		

FEV$_1$, Forced expiratory volume over 1 second; PaCO$_2$, partial pressure of carbon dioxide; PEF, peak expiratory flow.
Based on data from Gomez M, Felauer A. Asthma. In: Reuter-Rice K, et al, eds. *Pediatric Acute Care: A Guide for Interprofessional Practice.* Burlington, MA: Jones & Bartlett Learning, 2012; Marcoux K: Current management of status asthmaticus in the pediatric ICU. *Crit Care Nurs Clin North Am.* 2005;17:463.

pulmonary function in children, especially school-age patients.[21] These medications may decrease bronchomotor tone and secretions. The most commonly administered inhaled anticholinergic is ipratropium bromide. This medication works synergistically with beta-agonists to improve and prolong bronchodilation. Ipratropium bromide should be administered with albuterol in a nebulizer and not given alone. Corticosteroids are also an important part of the treatment for airway inflammation. Corticosteroids may be administered enterally or parenterally. Both methods are equally efficacious in the treatment of asthma.[21] The peak effect for corticosteroids is virtually the same with either route. Treatment for asthma does not have to be held up because of a lack of intravenous access in the pediatric patient. The corticosteroid of choice is a glucocorticoid (e.g., prednisone, prednisolone, methylprednisolone). Intravenous magnesium sulfate is administered to pediatric patients as an adjunct therapy, as it provides smooth muscle relaxation to patients with severe or life-threatening asthma events.[22] Magnesium is a physiologic calcium antagonist, which has a direct effect on the calcium uptake in the muscle, causing smooth muscle relaxation.[5] Magnesium sulfate (12 to 50 mg/kg) is administered intravenously, usually over 20 minutes.[23]

Critical care management of the child with status asthmaticus involves humidified oxygen to maintain an oxygen saturation of more than 95%, combined with the pharmacologic therapies. Heliox is a mixture of 80% helium and 20% oxygen, which makes this mixture lighter than air. Administration of heliox is effective in decreasing airway resistance and in decreasing the work of breathing. The use of heliox does not appear to have adverse effects, and its administration may improve the status of the child.[21] The use of noninvasive positive-pressure ventilation by means of nasal prongs or a facemask may avoid the need for intubation. Some of the indications for considering mechanical ventilation are respiratory muscle fatigue, markedly diminished or absent breath sounds, pulsus paradoxus greater than 20 to 40 mm Hg, deterioration in mental status, and partial pressure of oxygen (Pao_2) less than 70 mm Hg on 100% Fio_2.[21] The child and family should be informed of the management approach and plan of care. Pediatric patients, who have status asthmaticus, if properly and effectively treated, may return to their usual state of health but will require close follow-up by their pediatrician or pulmonologist.[21]

Apparent Life-Threatening Event
Pathophysiology

An apparent life-threatening event (ALTE) is an episode that is characterized by a combination of apnea, change in skin color, marked changes in muscle tone, and choking or gagging, as defined by the National institutes of Health Consensus Development Conference on infant Apnea in 1986.[24] An ALTE is an apneic event, which is combined with pallor or cyanosis and a loss of muscle tone that requires vigorous stimulation all the way to full cardiopulmonary resuscitation (CPR).[25] Many abnormalities have been found through detailed investigation and reported in the literature. They include relationships among gastroesophageal reflux disease (GERD), apnea, and sleep-related impairment of respiratory control when the infant sleeps in the prone position.[25]

In one study, GERD was documented in 55% of the infants with ALTE.[25] The next highest documented condition (30%) related to ALTE was chronic gastric volvulus.[25] Chronic gastric volvulus is a condition in which all or part of the stomach has rotated over the physiologic range. In infants, this condition may occur easily because of weak ligaments around the stomach. This may cause a large amount of gas to accumulate and push the stomach upward, resulting in worsening of the volvulus and causing vomiting and apnea.[25] Vagally induced fainting spells may occur in specific circumstances such as after vomiting, feeding, crying, bathing, and pain. Vagal overstimulation is probably an underestimated condition in ALTE infants.[25]

Some of the infants with ALTE requiring resuscitation ultimately pass away, and their condition may be classified as sudden infant death syndrome (SIDS), raising the possibility that ALTE and SIDS are the same disease.[26] Although some similarities exist in clinical presentations, ALTE and SIDS should not be considered different manifestations of the same disease process. ALTE and SIDS are disorders of the first year of life; each event occurs at different ages, with ALTE manifesting 10 weeks earlier than SIDS on average.[26]

Monitoring

One of most widely used diagnostic tests for ALTE is the use of a continuous recording of cardiorespiratory patterns, a pneumocardiogram.[25] The four channels monitor heart rate, respiratory rate, nasal airflow, and oxygen saturation. Some infants who have normal results may still have subsequent apneic episodes. The critical care nurse is a major source of support for families in terms of education, observation of the infant's status, and immediate intervention during an apneic episode. The appropriately sized resuscitation equipment should be available at the bedside of these infants.

Treatment

Episodes of apnea must first be treated with gentle shaking of the infant or tapping the bottoms of the infant's feet while observing for return of effective respirations. Slight extension of the neck to reopen the airway may be attempted. If recovery does not occur, manual ventilation with bag and mask at the infant's normal respiratory rate for age should be performed. This manual ventilation should continue until the infant's normal respiratory pattern and heart rate return. For frequent episodes (i.e., more than two to three per hour) or for those who require prolonged manual ventilation, other treatments include prone positioning, rocker beds, recurrent cutaneous stimulation, nasal CPAP, or a switch to continuous gavage feedings to help control symptoms of GERD. Treatment may also include the use of respiratory stimulant drugs such as theophylline or caffeine.[25] The therapeutic ranges are 6 to 13 microgram per milliliter (mcg/mL) of theophylline and 10 to 20 mcg/mL of caffeine.

Discharge Education

These infants are sent home with a continuous home monitor until they have gone at least 3 months without an ALTE requiring intervention. Topics for discharge education for parents need to include the following: 1) Attend a CPR class prior to discharge; 2) ensure that the infant will reside in a smoke-free environment; 3) have a firm mattress for the infant for sleeping; 4) breastfeed the infant, if possible; 5) avoid overheating the infant; 6) do not permit bed linens to cover infant's face; and 7) if a "blue spell" is noted, seek immediate medical attention.[27]

CARDIOVASCULAR SYSTEM

Anatomy and Physiology

The differences in cardiovascular function between children and adults are related to early physical development and the presence or absence of congenital cardiac disease. Congenital heart defects (CHDs) occur during the embryologic development of the heart, whereas acquired defects occur after birth. Most fetal cardiac development occurs between the fourth and seventh weeks of fetal life. The heart is most susceptible to teratogenic influences at this time.[3] About 90% of CHDs are caused by a genetic predisposition and an adverse response to environmental teratogens during cardiac development. Environmental factors alone account for only about 1% of all CHDs. Approximately 5% to 8 % of CHDs are associated with genetic anomalies or syndromes.[3] Although more than 35 well-recognized cardiac defects have been documented, the most common is ventricular septal defect (VSD).

The design of fetal circulation allows prenatal needs to be met and permits the modifications at birth that support the postnatal circulation.[3] Before the child is born, the lungs are essentially nonfunctional, the liver is partially functional, and the brain requires the highest oxygen concentration. The structures that support fetal circulation and bypass the lungs and liver are the foramen ovale, ductus arteriosus, ductus venosus, umbilical arteries, and umbilical vein (Fig. 40-5). After the child is born, the lungs and liver begin normal function, and the structures of fetal circulation are no longer needed. The foramen ovale closes, and the ductus arteriosus, the ductus venosus, and the umbilical vessels become ligaments (Fig. 40-6). During fetal life, the patency of the ductus arteriosus is controlled by the low oxygen content and exogenous prostaglandins. Postnatally, hypoxia maintains patency of the ductus arteriosus. Before repair of some congenital defects, it is essential that the ductus arteriosus remain open and that the newborn receive a pulmonary vasodilator such as a prostaglandin E_1 (PGE$_1$) continuous intravenous drip.[28] The appropriate use of this medication is to infuse for the shortest time at the lowest dose, which is consistent with good patient care. The use of PGE$_1$ greater than 120 hours has been associated with antral hyperplasia or gastric outlet obstruction.[23] At birth, pulmonary resistance is high but quickly falls to 80% and reaches adult levels in the first few weeks of life if the ductus closes normally.[3] In newborns, hypoxia, acidosis, and hypothermia may result in pulmonary vasoconstriction. This may lead to right-to-left (pulmonary-to-systemic) shunting of blood through the ductus arteriosus and foramen ovale. Treatment includes oxygenation, mechanical ventilation with hyperventilation to produce alkalosis, and sedation while maintaining the temperature of the infant.

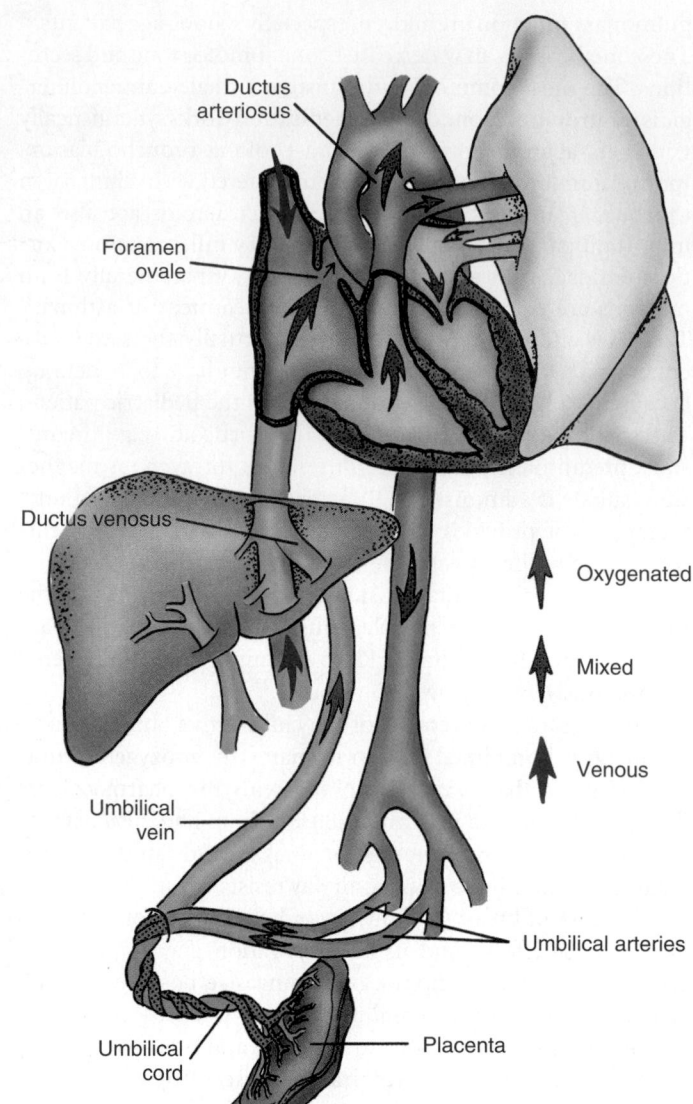

FIGURE 40-5 In the fetal circulation, blood is oxygenated in the placenta, which is a less-efficient oxygenator than the lungs are. The oxygenated blood enters the fetus through the umbilical vein and enters the ductus venosus, bypassing the hepatic circulation and flowing into the inferior vena cava. When this blood reaches the right atrium, it is diverted by the crista dividens toward the atrial septum and flows through the foramen ovale into the left atrium. The blood then passes through the left ventricle and ascending aorta to perfuse the head and upper extremities. This pathway allows the best-oxygenated blood from the placenta to perfuse the fetal brain. Venous blood from the head and upper extremities returns to the fetal heart through the superior vena cava, enters the right atrium and ventricle, and flows into the pulmonary artery. Because pulmonary vascular resistance is high, this blood is diverted through the ductus arteriosus into the descending aorta. Ultimately, much of this blood returns to the placenta through the umbilical arteries. (Modified from Rummell M. Fetal development of the heart and great vessels. In: Hazinski MF, ed. *Nursing Care of the Critically Ill Child.* 2nd ed. St. Louis: Elsevier; 2013.)

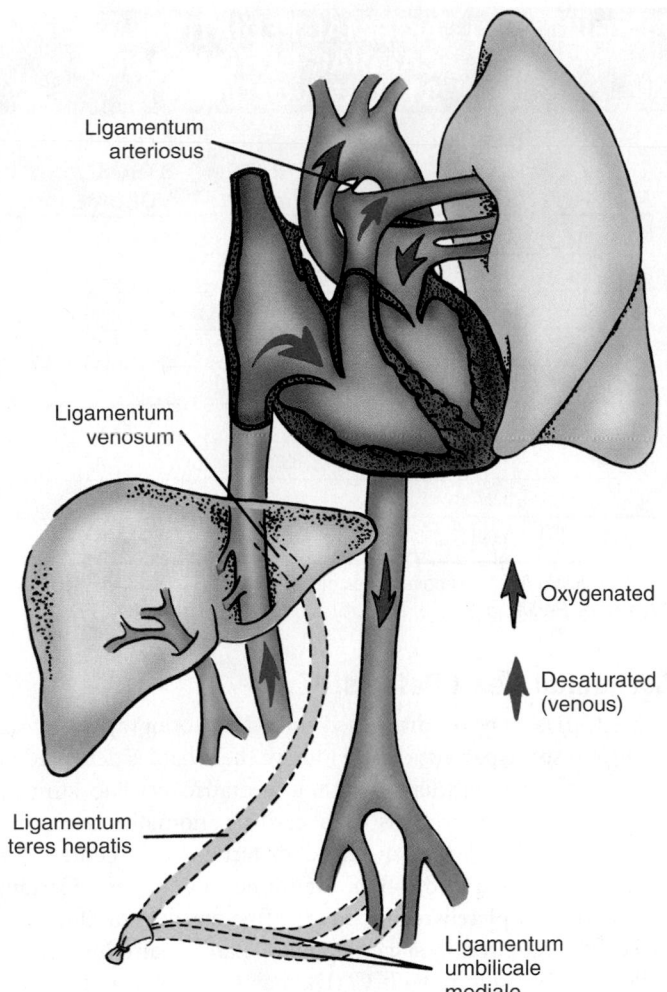

FIGURE 40-6 In the postnatal circulation, blood is oxygenated in the lungs, and pulmonary vascular resistance is low. Systemic venous (desaturated) blood returns to the heart through the superior and inferior vena cavae. This blood then flows through the right atrium and right ventricle, into the pulmonary artery, and ultimately into the pulmonary circulation. Oxygenated blood from the lungs returns to the left atrium through the pulmonary veins. This blood passes into the left ventricle and flows into the aorta and systemic arteries to perfuse the body. (Modified from Rummell M. Fetal development of the heart and great vessels. In: Hazinski MF, ed. *Nursing Care of the Critically Ill Child.* 2nd ed. St. Louis: Elsevier; 2013.)

TABLE 40-6	NORMAL HEART RATES IN CHILDREN	
AGE	AWAKE HEART RATE (per minute)	SLEEPING HEART RATE (per minute)
Neonate	100-205	90-160
Infant (6 mo)	100-180	90-160
Toddler	98-140	80-120
Preschooler	80-120	65-100
School-age child	75-118	58-90
Adolescent	60-100	50-90

From Hazinski MF. *Nursing Care of the Critically Ill Child.* 3rd ed. St. Louis: Elsevier; 2013.

TABLE 40-7	NORMAL BLOOD PRESSURES IN CHILDREN		
AGE	SYSTOLIC PRESSURE (mm Hg)*	DIASTOLIC PRESSURE (mm Hg)*	MEAN ARTERIAL PRESSURE (mm Hg)*
Birth (12 hr, <1000 g)	39-59	16-36	28-42
Birth (12 hr, 3 kg)	60-76	31-45	48-57
Neonate (96 hr)	67-84	35-53	45-60
Infant (1-12 months)	72-104	37-56	50-62
Toddler (1-2 yr)	86-106	42-63	49-62
Preschool (3-5 yr)	89-112	46-72	58-69
School age (7 yr)	97-115	57-76	66-72
Preadolescent (10-12 yr)	102-120	61-80	71-79
Adolescent (15 yr)	110-131	64-83	73-84

*Blood pressure ranges are taken from the following sources. *Neonate:* Versmold H et al: Aortic blood pressure during the first 12 hours of life in infants with birth weight 610-4220 g. *Pediatrics* 1981;67:107. Tenth through ninetieth percentile ranges are used. *Others:* Horan MJ, chairman: Task Force on Blood Pressure Control in Children, report of the Second Task Force on Blood Pressure in Children. *Pediatrics* 1987;79:1. Fiftieth through ninetieth percentile ranges are indicated.
Modified from Hazinski MF. *Nursing Care of the Critically Ill Child.* 3rd ed. St. Louis: Elsevier; 2013.

Assessment

Assessment of the cardiovascular system in the child requires the complete health history, including birth history and physical assessment. As the pediatric database is completed for the child with cardiac disease, the parents may report any of the following: poor feeding with fatigue noticed during feeding, diaphoresis with feeding, weight loss or inability to gain weight, respiratory problems (e.g., dyspnea, tachypnea), frequent respiratory infections, cyanosis, and fatigue during play. Heart rate and blood pressure should be within normal range for age (Tables 40-6 and 40-7). Measurement of blood pressure is the most important diagnostic tool in the detection of hypertension in the child.[29] On admission, blood pressure readings should be obtained on all four extremities. If the readings are greater in the upper extremities than in the lower ones, the child may have a coarctation of the aorta. Thigh blood pressure readings are equal to the upper extremity readings until a child is 1 year old.[29] Selection of the correct blood pressure cuff size is considered one of the most important factors when measuring blood pressure.[30] The heart should be auscultated for extra heart sounds and murmurs. Auscultation may be the most important action in obtaining important information about the diagnosis of acyanotic heart disease. Conversely, auscultation is rarely diagnostic in children with cyanotic CHDs, in which the heart murmur is often absent.[29] Murmurs are heard because of turbulent flow through an abnormal opening or obstructed area. Systolic murmurs are heard between S_1 and S_2. Midsystolic ejection murmurs start after S_1 and end before S_2, usually with a crescendo–decrescendo sound.[31] Diastolic murmurs are heard

TABLE 40-8   CALCULATION OF CIRCULATING BLOOD VOLUME

AGE GROUP	BLOOD VOLUME (mL/kg)
Neonates	80-85
Infants	75-80
Children	70-75
Adults	65-70

From Hazinski MF. *Nursing Care of the Critically Ill Child.* 3rd ed. St. Louis: Elsevier; 2013.

TABLE 40-9   NORMAL PEDIATRIC CARDIAC OUTPUT AND STROKE VOLUME

AGE	CARDIAC OUTPUT (L/min)	HEART RATE (beats/min)	NORMAL STROKE VOLUME (mL)
Newborn	0.7-0.8	145	5
6 mo	1.0-1.6	120	10
1 yr	1.3-1.5	115	13
2 yr	1.5-2.0	115	18
4 yr	2.3-2.375	105	27
5 yr	2.5-3.0	95	31
8 yr	3.4-3.6	83	42
10 yr	3.8-4.0	75	50
15 yr	5.0-6.0	70	85

From Hazinski MF. Cardiovascular disorders. In: Hazinski MF, ed. *Manual of Pediatric Critical Care.* St. Louis: Mosby; 1999:112.

after S_2 heart sounds. To further monitor perfusion, central and pedal pulses, skin temperature and color, and capillary refill are evaluated hourly. Urine output must be at least 1 milliliter per kilogram per hour (mL/kg/hr).

Hemodynamic Monitoring

Hemodynamic monitoring may be indicated in the critically ill pediatric patient. Issues with monitoring are related to the smaller size of the pediatric patient; fluid overload and blood loss are concerns. To accurately monitor intake, all fluid used for intravascular hemodynamic monitoring lines must be given by volume infusion pumps. Heparinized fluid is given in each line and only small volumes of blood should be drawn for laboratory tests. Each medical facility that cares for pediatric patients should have institutional policies on the amount of blood to draw for each test. All flush volumes are recorded as intake, an accurate record is kept of the amount of blood lost, and the child periodically receives replacement, if appropriate. Table 40-8 describes pediatric circulating blood volumes for children at different ages.

When continuously monitoring the blood pressure in the child, the arterial reading is preferred when arterial blood sampling or vasoactive medications are in use.[31] A 4- or 5-French (Fr) pulmonary artery catheter is used for the child. The child's vessel must be large enough to accept the 4-Fr catheter to initiate pulmonary artery monitoring. Because the smaller catheters have smaller balloons, the clinician should refer to the catheter for the specific balloon volume. To limit fluid intake, smaller volumes (usually 3 or 5 mL) of injectant are used for cardiac output studies. Table 40-9 provides cardiac output and stroke volume values. Left atrial pressure (LAP), central venous pressure (CVP), and pulmonary artery pressure (PAP) in the child are comparable with adult values. Hemodynamic parameters are related to the body surface area of the child. The normal cardiac index for children is 3.5 to 5.5 liters per minute per meter squared (L/min/m²), which is higher than that for adults. The stroke volume in adults and children is influenced by cardiac preload, ventricular contractility, afterload, and compliance. Subtle differences exist between pediatric and adult ventricular functions. The principles of treatment for shock and the manipulation of stroke volume are the same in all age groups.[3] When evaluating hemodynamic parameters, the numbers should always be related to the clinical condition of the child. If the numbers do not correlate, the calibration and zeroing of the monitoring equipment should be re-evaluated.

Congenital Heart Defects

Some CHDs may be diagnosed with ultrasonography before birth, and some parents decide to have these babies delivered at a tertiary center affiliated with a pediatric cardiac surgery program. Other newborns with cardiac anomalies are diagnosed after birth and transferred to tertiary care centers for further evaluation and, often, for immediate surgery. Certain defects are completely repaired in the first few days of life, other defects are repaired in stages, and some are repaired when the child is older. Infants with CHDs may develop complications after discharge after a surgical procedure or while waiting for surgery, and they may be admitted to an adult critical care unit. Examples of postoperative surgical complications in the pediatric cardiac patient are wound infection, pericardial effusion, pleural effusion, and cardiac dysrhythmia.

A useful classification system for CHDs is based on the hemodynamic pathophysiology or movements involved in the circulation of blood. The four defining pathophysiologic characteristics are: 1) increased pulmonary blood flow, 2) decreased pulmonary blood flow, 3) mixed blood flow, and 4) obstruction of the flow of blood out of the heart.[31] This classification system is outlined in Figure 40-7.

Using this hemodynamic classification system, the clinical characteristics of each CHD are more uniform and presentable. Cardiac defects that allow the blood to flow from a high-pressure left side of the child's heart to the lower-pressure right side (i.e., left-to-right shunt) cause an increase in pulmonary blood flow and congestive heart failure (CHF). Obstructive defects impede blood flow out of the ventricles. Obstructions on the left side of the heart results in CHF, whereas obstructions on the right side cause cyanosis. The pediatric patient with mixed lesions presents with variable clinical symptoms that depend on the degree of mixing of the pulmonary blood, hypoxemia, and CHF.[31]

Two major clinical conditions may be seen in a child with a cardiac defect with altered hemodynamics. These conditions are CHF and hypoxemia.[31] Critical care nurses play a critical role

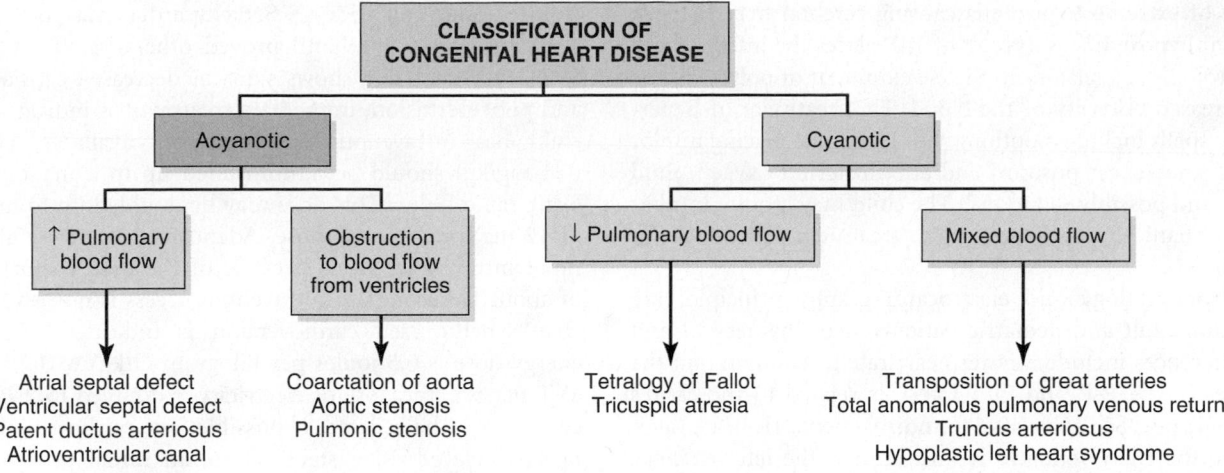

FIGURE 40-7 Comparison of acyanotic-cyanotic and hemodynamic classification systems of congenital heart disease. (From Delany A, et al. The child with cardiovascular dysfunction. In: Hockenberry MF, Wilson D, eds. *Wong's Nursing Care of Infants and Children.* 9th ed. St. Louis: Mosby; 2011.)

with the pediatric patient in early identification and supportive management of these conditions.

CHF is a clinical syndrome in which the heart is unable to pump enough blood to the body to meet its needs, to dispose of systemic or pulmonary venous return adequately, or a combination of both.[29] Common causes of CHF are volume or pressure overload, congenital or acquired heart disease, and myocardial diseases. The most common cause of CHF in infancy is a CHD. Beyond infancy, myocardial dysfunctions have various causes.[29] Symptoms of CHF are related to responses of impaired cardiac function, pulmonary venous congestion, and systemic venous congestion. Infants may exhibit a change in responsiveness and may be lethargic or irritable, have tachypnea with feedings, have poor weight gain, and have a cold sweat on the forehead.[29] Tachycardia is a common and early sign of CHF. Older children may complain of dyspnea, especially with activity, or early fatigue and exhibit puffy eyelids or swollen feet. Crackles and wheezing may be auscultated in the infant.[29] During an abdominal assessment, the liver may be palpated, but hepatomegaly may be absent in early CHF. In children younger than 5 years, the liver is normally palpated at the costal margin to 1 cm below. Cardiomegaly is almost always present in patients with CHF. Chest radiography is more reliable than a physical examination for determining cardiomegaly.[29]

Treatment of CHF consists of eliminating the underlying causes and getting control of the heart failure state.[29] The three major classes of medications commonly used to treat CHF in children are: 1) inotropic agents, 2) diuretics, and 3) afterload reducers. Rapid-acting inotropic agents such as dopamine, dobutamine, or milrinone are used in the critically ill child.[29] Diuretics remain the principal therapeutic agent to control pulmonary and systemic venous congestion. Diuretic therapy alters the patient's serum electrolyte levels. Hypokalemia is a common problem and needs to be monitored. Digoxin is the inotropic medication of choice for CHF in pediatric patients. The pediatric dosage of digoxin is much larger than an adult dosage on the basis of body weight. Pharmacokinetic studies indicate that pediatric patients require a larger dose of digoxin compared

with adults to attain a comparable serum level.[29] When the child is receiving digoxin, the nurse should observe for signs of digitalis toxicity. Digoxin toxicity is best detected by monitoring the child's electrocardiogram (ECG), not serum levels for the first 3 to 5 days after digitalization.[29] Any cardiac dysrhythmia or conduction disturbance in the absence of other clinical signs may indicate digoxin toxicity. Hypokalemia, hypomagnesemia, and hypocalcemia may aggravate digoxin cardiotoxicity even in the presence of a normal digoxin level. The therapeutic range of serum digoxin for treating CHF is 0.8 to 2 nanogram per milliliter (ng/mL).

Hypoxemia

Cyanosis is a bluish discoloration of the skin and mucous membranes, and it is observed in children with certain congenital heart defects.[29] Cyanosis is visible when hemoglobin is reduced by 5 g per 100 mL of blood.[29] Cyanosis associated with desaturation of arterial blood is called *central cyanosis*. Peripheral cyanosis is a condition in which cyanosis exists, but the child has a normal arterial oxygen saturation.[29]

Cyanosis may have a number of causes. Central cyanosis may result from cyanotic CHD, lung disease, or central nervous system (CNS) depression. Differentiation of cardiac cyanosis from cyanosis caused by pulmonary disease is essential for proper medical management. Hyperoxitest helps distinguish the source of the infant's cyanosis by assessing the infant's arterial Po_2 response to the inhalation of 100% oxygen.[29] With pulmonary disease, the arterial Po_2 usually rises to a level greater than 100 mm Hg. If a significant intracardiac right-to-left shunt exists, the arterial Po_2 does not exceed 100 mm Hg, with a rise of usually not more than 10 to 30 mm Hg.[29]

Some children with CHD manifest hypercyanotic spells. This is most common in children with tetralogy of Fallot (ToF). These episodes often are called *Tet spells*. These spells rarely are seen before 2 months of age, occur most often during the first year of life, and occur more often in the morning. During these episodes, the child becomes highly cyanotic, hypoxic, and tachypneic and may lose consciousness or develop seizures because of extreme hypoxemia causing cerebral hypoxia. The persistent hypoxemia as a result of ToF places the infant at risk for neurologic sequelae from the development of polycythemia and increased viscosity of the blood. The treatment of hypercyanotic spells includes soothing the child while placing him or her in a knee-chest position and administering oxygen, fluid boluses, and possibly sedation.[31] The child may require intubation, mechanical ventilation, and treatment of metabolic acidosis.

Electrophysiology and electrocardiography principles are similar for adult and pediatric patients (see Chapters 12 and 14). Differences include a faster heart rate in children and the variances in the P-R and Q-T intervals related to the child's rapid heart rate. See Table 40-6 for normal pediatric heart rates. At birth, the right ventricle is thicker than the left ventricle. Right ventricular dominance of the newborn period is replaced by left ventricular dominance in childhood and in adulthood. Anatomic changes are most rapid in the first month, and by age 6 months, the left ventricle is dominant. With increasing age, the heart rate decreases, and the P-R interval, QRS duration, and Q-T interval increase.

In the pediatric patient, monitoring of respiratory rate and oxygen saturation is done concurrently with cardiac monitoring. It is important to recognize the manifestations of impending respiratory failure in the pediatric patient because respiratory failure precedes heart failure and potential cardiac arrest. ECG monitoring electrodes are placed along the nipple line on the chest to facilitate monitoring of cardiac rate and rhythm and respiratory rate. To capture and diagnose transient events such as a dysrhythmia or conduction disorders, the best method is to use a 24-hour Holter monitor. The Holter monitor has an extremely valuable role in the assessment of high-risk patients, both postoperatively and with cardiomyopathy. However, in children with palpitations, syncope, and chest pain, the Holter monitor does not yield as much data.[32]

Dysrhythmias may result from many different causes. Some of these include CHD, surgical correction, hypoxia, electrolyte or acid–base imbalances, drug toxicity, or myocardial injury.[3] Dysrhythmias may be symptomatic or asymptomatic, but they have the potential to deteriorate into a symptomatic condition for the child. The three most common types of clinically significant pediatric dysrhythmias are: 1) bradyarrhythmias, 2) tachyarrhythmias, and 3) those that produce cardiac collapse or loss of pulses.[3,4] Hypoxia and heart block are the most common causes of bradyarrhythmias. Supraventricular tachycardia (SVT) is probably the most common form of pediatric tachyarrhythmias. Sinus tachycardia is not considered a dysrhythmia; it is the most efficient method of increasing cardiac output and the chief method of increasing cardiac output in a child. Tachycardia is normally observed in a child who is febrile, scared, or stressed. However, a heart rate that goes to extremely high rates, such as greater than 220 beats per minute (beats/min), may actually reduce the child's cardiac output.[3]

Supraventricular Tachycardia

The most common symptomatic tachyarrhythmia in children is SVT. P waves may or may not be seen, and the rate often exceeds 220 beats/min. Wide-QRS SVT is uncommon in children, and any wide-QRS tachycardia must be treated as ventricular in origin until proved otherwise. If the child in SVT is unstable and shows signs of decreased cardiac output and poor perfusion, immediate treatment is indicated.[4] If the child has intravenous access readily available, adenosine (0.1 mg/kg) should be administered up to a maximum of a 6-mg rapid bolus. This dose may be doubled up to maximum of 12 mg for a second dose. Adenosine should be given as a rapid intravenous bolus because of the drug's short half-life of about 10 seconds. If intravenous access is not readily available, synchronized cardioversion is indicated.[4] The initial energy dose is 0.5 joules per kilogram (J/kg) to 1 J/kg. If the SVT persists, the dose of electricity is doubled to 2 J/kg.[4] The child should be sedated, if possible, but cardioversion should not be delayed. In a stable child, an initial procedure may include vagal maneuvers, but these should never delay synchronized cardioversion. Consultation with a pediatric cardiologist is advised. If additional treatment is needed, amiodarone (5 mg/kg given intravenously over 20 to 60 minutes) or procainamide (15 mg/kg given intravenously over 30 to 60 minutes) should be considered. These medications should not routinely be given together.[4]

Bradycardias

Bradycardia may result from hypoxia, acidosis, or hypothermia. Bradycardia is defined as a cardiac rate less than 100 beats/min for an infant and less than 60 beats/min for a child.[3] Treatment initially includes adequate oxygenation and ventilation for the pediatric patient. If the bradycardia continues to cause cardiopulmonary compromise despite oxygenation and ventilation, compressions are started for a heart rate of less than 60 beats/min. If the bradycardia continues, the nurse should plan to administer epinephrine (0.01 mg/kg, 1:10,000 concentration) given intravenously or intraosseously) or through the ETT (0.1 mg/kg, 1:1000 concentration). Epinephrine may be repeated every 3 to 5 minutes. The intravenous or intraosseous route is preferred to medications given through the ETT.[4] If increased vagal tone or a primary atrioventricular block is the cause of the bradycardia, atropine (0.02 mg/kg) may be given. This dose may be repeated (minimum dose 0.1 mg to maximum dose of 1 mg for a child and 2 mg for an adolescent).[4] If additional treatment is indicated, consider cardiac pacing. If the child's rhythm develops into pulseless arrest, then proceed to the pulseless arrest resuscitation procedure.

Shock in Infants and Children

Shock is a critical condition that results from inadequate delivery of oxygen and nutrients to the tissues to meet the metabolic demand.[3] Shock frequently is the end result of severe dehydration, hemorrhage, progressive heart failure, or sepsis. The treatment goal for a child in shock is to prevent end-organ injury and stop the progression from cardiopulmonary failure to cardiac arrest. Shock is typically classified by etiologic mechanism. These classifications include hypovolemic, distributive or septic, cardiogenic, or obstructive.[4]

Shock may be present in a pediatric patient with normal or abnormal blood pressure. The blood pressure reading may be used to further classify the shock as compensated or hypotensive shock.[4] Compensated shock describes a child with signs of poor perfusion but normal blood pressure. The systolic reading may be normal, but the diastolic pressure may not be normal because of increased systemic vascular resistance with a narrowing pulse pressure.[4] In hypotensive shock, the blood pressure is low, and cardiopulmonary failure may be imminent.[3]

Hypovolemic Shock

Hypovolemic shock is the most common cause of shock in children worldwide.[4] Fluid loss from diarrhea is the leading cause of hypovolemic shock.[4] Causes of volume loss that may lead to hypovolemic shock include diarrhea, hemorrhage, vomiting, inadequate fluid intake, osmotic diuresis, third space losses, and burns.[4] The treatment for hypovolemic shock is fluid resuscitation. Pediatric patients with hypovolemic shock need to receive the appropriate volume of fluid within the first hour of resuscitation to have the best chance of survival and recovery. Fluid resuscitation should start with rapid infusion of isotonic crystalloid in boluses of 20 mL/kg.[4] With severe fluid losses, the child may require up to two to three fluid boluses initially. If blood replacement is required, packed red cells should be considered, starting with 10 mL/kg. The child must be closely monitored and reassessed after each fluid bolus for effectiveness of the fluid resuscitation on end-organ perfusion.

Cardiogenic Shock

Cardiogenic shock is a condition of inadequate tissue perfusion resulting from myocardial dysfunction. This dysfunction may be the result of pump failure, congenital heart disease, or a rhythm abnormalilty.[4] Cardiogenic shock is characterized by decreased cardiac output, marked tachycardia, and a high systemic vascular output. The child has decreased urine output (<0.5 to 1 mL/kg/hr) and changes in mental status as end-organ perfusion is affected. Crackles may be heard on lung auscultation, and frothy sputum may be present. Often, it is increased respiratory effort that distinguishes cardiogenic shock from hypovolemic shock.[4]

The main treatment objectives are to improve the effectiveness of cardiac function and overall cardiac output by increasing the efficiency of ventricular emptying.[4,31] Many children with cardiogenic shock have a high preload and do not require additional fluids. However, if the child's history is consistent with fluid loss, a fluid bolus of 5 to 10 mL/kg may be cautiously given. Frequent assessments of the child's respiratory function should be performed in anticipation of respiratory failure. Supplemental oxygen should be given, but the nurse should be prepared to assist with ventilation with intubation and helping to establish a central venous access in the child.[4] This approach allows for the measurement of the central venous pressure and provides access for fluid and medication infusion.

Typical pharmacologic support of a child with cardiogenic shock includes the use of diuretics and vasodilators. Diuretics are indicated when the child has evidence of pulmonary edema. The vasodilators are given as a continuous infusion. Milrinone is the preferred medication for cardiogenic shock (loading dose 50 mcg/kg, followed by an infusion at 0.25 to 0.75 mcg/kg/min).[4]

Laboratory studies should be obtained to assess the impact of the shock on the end-organ function. No single laboratory test is specific for cardiogenic shock. Consultation with a pediatric cardiologist should be initiated at the earliest opportunity to help facilitate a diagnosis (using the ECG), guide the therapy, and possibly transfer of the patient for additional care or surgery with a pediatric specialist.[4]

Distributive Shock, Sepsis, and Septic Shock

Septic shock is the most common form of distributive shock. This condition is caused by infectious agents or their endotoxins, which stimulate the child's immune system and trigger release or activation of inflammatory mediators. Septic shock in children typically evolves along a continuum from a systemic inflammatory response in the early stages to septic shock in the later ones.[4] The child exhibits manifestations of systemic inflammatory response syndrome (SIRS) with severe sepsis or septic shock. The infant or child may have a temperature elevation, a low temperature, or temperature instability. Along with level of consciousness changes, the child may be irritable, restless, or lethargic. Urine output is decreased, the skin may be warm or mottled, and peripheral pulses may be strong and bounding. The child does not feed well, and decreased fluid intake may precipitate dehydration. Blood pressure is maintained within normal limits from activation of the body's compensatory mechanisms. Parents may remark that the child "does not seem right" or "something is different" with the child. It is important to listen to the parents' assessment of the child's status.

Treatment of SIRS consists of early identification and goal-directed resuscitation. Treatment includes administration of oxygen, providing support ventilation, monitoring vital signs, initiating aggressive fluid boluses, and obtaining laboratory work, which includes blood cultures prior to administration of antibiotics. Other laboratory work to consider is performing a CBC with differential, lactate concentration, and venous blood gas sample. However, the most effective treatment of SIRS is prevention. Hand washing before and after patient contact is essential. Sterile technique is maintained during suctioning, while managing invasive lines, and during dressing changes and wound care.

Severe sepsis or septic shock is diagnosed when perfusion decreases and the child becomes hypotensive. If the child is receiving inotropic agents, the blood pressure may be normal, but a change occurs in perfusion. The patient exhibits metabolic acidosis and hypoxemia. This may require intubation, mechanical ventilation, sedation, fluids, and vasopressor medications. Complications of septic shock include acute respiratory distress syndrome, acute kidney injury, disseminated intravascular coagulation, and multiple organ dysfunction syndrome (MODS). Figure 35-6 in Chapter 35 presents a concept map of septic shock that depicts the process from etiology through treatment.

Obstructive Shock

Obstructive shock is a condition of impaired cardiac output caused by some physical obstruction of blood flow. The physiology of the clinical symptoms varies according to the cause of the obstruction.[4] Four types of obstructive shock occur in children.

One type of obstructive shock is caused by a *cardiac tamponade*.[4] This occurs when fluid, blood, or air accumulates in the pericardial space around the heart. This condition is seen after cardiac surgery or a penetrating cardiac injury. Symptoms of a cardiac tamponade include muffled or distant heart sounds, distended neck veins, or pulses paradoxus (i.e., decrease in systolic blood pressure by more than 10 mm Hg during inspiration). The treatment is supportive and includes fluids, adequate oxygenation and ventilation, vasopressors, and a possible pericardiocentesis.[4]

A second type of obstructive shock is caused by a *tension pneumothorax*,[4] which is caused by entry of air into the pleural space. This is most often seen in a pediatric patient when chest trauma has occurred or when an intubated child on positive-pressure ventilation deteriorates suddenly. The signs and symptoms include diminished breath sounds on the affected side, distended neck veins, tracheal deviation, and a rapid deteriorating clinical condition of the child that may result in bradycardia, hypotension, and hypoxemia. The treatment is immediate needle decompression over the third rib at the midclavicular line. The decompression should lead to an escaping of air. The decompression should be followed by an insertion of a chest tube.

A third but rare cause of obstructive shock is caused by a *massive pulmonary embolism*,[4] which results from partial or total obstruction of the pulmonary artery. The symptoms include signs of cyanosis, hypotension, and right heart failure. Treatment includes adequate oxygenation and ventilation, and fluid therapy is administered if the patient is poorly perfused. Additional diagnostic tests and medications such as fibrinolytic agents may be required.

A fourth type of obstructive shock is caused by a *ductal-dependent congenital heart lesion*.[4] Because systemic circulation is supported by the right side of the heart through the ductus arteriosus, these lesions are called *ductal-dependent lesions*. The affected infant shows signs of severe shock, CHF, hypotension, poor perfusion, lethargy, and acidosis. The infant is treated with prostaglandin E_1 (PGE_1) to maintain the patency of the ductus arteriosus.

Cardiopulmonary Arrest

The pediatric patient must be assessed for manifestations of respiratory failure and shock, as failure to recognize these problems may result in the development of cardiopulmonary failure and respiratory or cardiac arrest. In the pediatric patient, respiratory arrest usually precedes cardiac arrest. In an arrest situation, oxygen is administered, and an airway established and maintained (see "Assessment and Oxygen Devices"). In the event of a cardiac arrest, compressions are started, and an intravenous or intraosseous line is established. Intraosseous placement is recommended as an alternative means to deliver intravenous fluids and medications in children of all ages when vascular access is not obtained within 90 seconds or after three attempts. Intraosseous access often is achieved in 30 to 60 seconds and is the preferred route over the endotracheal route for medications. Any medication or fluid that is administered

by a peripheral intravenous line may be given by the intraosseous route.[4] The preferred site is the broad, flat portion of the anteromedial surface of the tibia approximately 1 to 2 cm below the tibial tuberosity. Other interventions are based on the cardiac rhythm and the cause of the arrest.

Pulseless arrest includes the following dysrhythmias: asystole, ventricular fibrillation (VF), pulseless ventricular tachycardia (VT), and pulseless electrical activity (PEA).[4] Treatment of asystole starts with cardiopulmonary resuscitation (CPR; rate of 15 compressions to two breaths with two rescuers), airway maintenance with oxygenation, attachment to a monitor or defibrillator, and obtaining intravenous or intraosseous access. After an advanced airway is in place, chest compressions may continue without pauses for breaths. A child requires 8 to 10 breaths per minute. The next step in the treatment algorithm depends on whether the rhythm is shockable.[4] The rhythms of VF or VT are shockable. On a manual defibrillator, the initial dose of electricity is 2 J/kg. Immediately after the shock, compressions are resumed for 2 minutes (five cycles). The compressions support the heart while it is in a recovery state, even if a perfusion rhythm has returned.[4] If the VT or VF persists, another shock is administered at 4 J/kg, compressions are resumed, and epinephrine is given. The first dose of epinephrine is 0.01 mg/kg (1:10,000 at 0.1 mL/kg) given intravenously or intraosseously; if given endotracheally, the dose is 0.1 mg/kg (1:1,000 at 0.1 mL/kg). Subsequent doses may be given every 3 to 5 minutes. Maximum dosage is 1 mg (1 mL). After 2 minutes of CPR, the patient's rhythm should be checked. If the VT or VF rhythm continues, the patient is defibrillated again at 4 J/kg, compressions are resumed immediately, and an antiarrhythmic medication such as amiodarone (5 mg/kg) is given intravenously or intraosseously.

If the rhythm is not shockable, as in asystole or PEA, the first action after starting CPR is to give the epinephrine at the same dose listed previously. After five cycles or 2 minutes of CPR, the patient's rhythm is checked, and if asystole or PEA persists, CPR and dosing with epinephrine every 3 to 5 minutes are continued. The treatment needs to include reversible causes which include hypovolemia, hypoxia, hydrogen ion (acidosis), hypoglycemia, hypokalemia or hyperkalemia, hypothermia, tension pneumothorax, tamponade, toxins, and thrombosis (pulmonary or coronary).

The primary goals of postresuscitation management of the pediatric patient include the following:[4]
1. Optimization of the cardiopulmonary function to restore and maintain vital organ perfusion and function, especially the brain
2. Prevention of any secondary organ injury
3. Identification and treatment of the cause of any acute illnesses
4. Initiation of measures to help improve long-term, neurologically intact survival of the child

The nurse should assess the patient using a systematic approach. In addition to primary assessments, the approach should include review of the patient's history, a thorough physical examination, the use of invasive and noninvasive monitoring techniques, and use of appropriate laboratory testing.[4]

NERVOUS SYSTEM

Anatomy

The nervous system grows rapidly before birth, and growth continues during infancy and childhood. Compared with the adult, an infant or toddler's head size is proportionally larger than the rest of the body. When infants fall, the head usually leads, and a significant head injury may occur.[3] The skull is more flexible because the skull bones are not fused and are separated by spaces called *fontanels*. The anterior fontanel is the junction of the coronal, sagittal, and frontal sutures, whereas the posterior fontanel is the junction of the parietal and occipital bones. By age 3 months, the posterior fontanel is usually closed, and the anterior fontanel is closed by age 20 months.

The brain of a young child has a high water content and contains less myelin compared with the brain of an adult. This makes the child's brain more homogeneous and less compartmentalized.[3] Shear hemorrhages and diffuse brain injuries are more common in children than in adults.

Spinal cord injuries are less common in children than in adults because the spine of the child is elastic and the vertebrae less likely to fracture. In children with head injuries or multisystem trauma, spinal cord injuries should always be suspected until ruled out.[3]

Physiology

Cerebral blood flow and oxygen consumption are increased in childhood in relation to increased metabolic needs. Hyperemia, tissue hypoxia, and acidosis result in cerebral arterial dilation and increased cerebral blood flow. Hyperventilation decreases cerebral blood flow, but severe hypercarbia may result in decreased oxygen consumption and use. The normal cerebral perfusion pressure (CPP) values in children are unknown. It is thought, that CPP should be in the range of 40 to 60 mm Hg, but this figure may vary because perfusion is determined by blood flow and not by blood pressure.[3] CPP must be maintained at a level to maintain blood flow. A patient with a normal CPP does not necessarily have effective cerebral perfusion.

Assessment

Cognitive function cannot be evaluated until the preschool and early childhood years, but level of consciousness, movement, and pupils can be evaluated in the pediatric patient. The Glasgow Coma Scale (GCS) is used for older children and has been modified for use in infants and younger children (Table 40-10). Survival and recovery of a patient with a GCS score of 5 to 8 are better for children than for adults.[3] Evaluation of reflexes in children is comparable with that in adults, with a couple of exceptions. Although a positive Babinski reflex is an abnormal response in an adult, this response is normal in the child until age 1 year.[6] In the first few months of life, grasp is reflexive in the infant. With severe neurologic disease or injury, grasp may revert to a reflex as opposed to a purposeful response, and the grasp response may not indicate improvement of the child's neurologic status.

The pediatric patient's responsiveness should be evaluated in relation to the child's age, clinical condition, and changes in responsiveness over time. Infants and children should always respond to their parents or caregivers and to a painful stimulus.

TABLE 40-10   MODIFIED GLASGOW COMA SCALE FOR INFANTS AND CHILDREN

	CHILD	INFANT	SCORE
Eye opening	Spontaneous	Spontaneous	4
	To verbal stimuli	To verbal stimuli	3
	To pain only	To pain only	2
	No response	No response	1
Verbal response	Oriented, appropriate	Coos and babbles	5
	Confused	Irritable cries	4
	Inappropriate words	Cries to pain	3
	Incomprehensible words or nonspecific sounds	Moans to pain	2
	No response	No response	1
Motor response	Obeys command (e.g., child holds up two fingers, wiggles toes, or sticks out tongue)	Moves spontaneously and purposefully	6
	Localizes painful stimulus (e.g., child reaches for hand that is rubbing sternum or pinching trapezius)	Withdraws to touch	5
	Withdraws in response to pain (e.g., child adducts each extremity when medial aspect is pinched)	Withdraws in response to pain	4
	Flexion in response to pain (e.g., decorticate posturing when sternum is rubbed or trapezius muscle pinched)	Decorticate posturing (abnormal flexion) in response to pain	3
	Extension in response to pain (i.e., decerebrate posturing when sternum rubbed or trapezius pinched)	Decerebrate posturing (abnormal extension) in response to pain	2
	No response (flaccid)	No response (flaccid)	1

Data from Tasker RC. Head and spinal cord trauma. In Nichols DG, ed. *Rodgers Textbook of Pediatric Intensive Care*. 4th ed. Philadelphia: Lippincott Williams & Wilkins, 2008; Originally proposed in Morray JP, et al. Coma scale for use in brain-injured children. *Crit Care Med.* 1984;12:1018.
Modifications in parentheses from Milonovich L, Eichler V. Neurological disorders. In: Hazinski MF, ed. *Nursing Care of the Critically Ill Child*. 3rd ed. St Louis: Elsevier; 2013:587.

A decrease in the responsiveness is abnormal and should be investigated.[3] If the child is older than 2 years, the ability to follow commands may be assessed by asking him or her to hold up two fingers or wiggle the toes. This action is not accomplished by a reflex action.

When a child is unconscious, the most important component of the GCS to assess is the motor function.[3] The patient's central and peripheral responses to a painful stimulus need to be assessed. A central stimulus is applied to the head and trunk, above the nipple line. The peripheral stimulus may be assessed at the medial aspect of each extremity. The patient's best response is the one that is recorded for the GCS score.

Signs of increased intracranial pressure (ICP) in pediatric patients include a change in responsiveness, a deterioration in the ability to follow commands, a change in the response to pain, and pupil dilation with light stimulation.[3] The Cushing triad sign of an increased ICP may only be observed during cerebral herniation and should not be used as an early indicator or ICP. If any neurologic deterioration is detected in the pediatric patient, a complete neurologic assessment is required, including the child's vital signs and consultation with the patient's physician.

Seizures

Seizures are brief manifestations of the brain's electrical system that result from cortical neuronal discharge. Regardless of the etiology, the basic mechanism of a seizure is the same. Abnormal electrical discharge may arise from central areas of the brain that may affect consciousness. This activity may be restricted to one area of the cerebral cortex or spread to other portions of the brain. Seizures are the most commonly observed neurologic deficit in children and may occur with a variety of CNS conditions (Box 40-4). At least 8% of the general population will experience one or more seizures in their lifetime, and approximately 1% will develop epilepsy, involving recurring seizures.[33] The incidence of causative factors that are associated with seizures in children is related to the child's age. In infants, the most common factors are related to birth traumas (i.e., anoxia, congenital defects, and intracranial bleeds).[33] Acute infections are a common cause in late infancy and early childhood but uncommon in the child who is in middle childhood. In children who are older than 3 years, the most common cause of seizures is idiopathic epilepsy.[33] As children enter adolescence, hormonal and metabolic changes may alter the seizure threshold. The child who is in an unconscious state must be evaluated for a history of seizures because unconsciousness may be the result of a postictal state.

Many different types of seizures exist, and each has unique clinical manifestations. Seizures may be classified in three major groups: 1) partial seizures, 2) generalized seizures, and 3) unclassified epileptic seizures.[33] Partial seizures have a local onset and involve a relative small part of the brain. Manifestation of this type of seizure depends on which part of the brain is involved. The initial event may provide the best clue for assessing the type of seizure and the location. Generalized seizures involve both hemispheres of the brain without a focal onset. Loss of consciousness and motor impairment occur from this type of seizure. Unlike the partial seizure, no aura exists,

BOX 40-4 CAUSES OF SEIZURES IN CHILDREN

NONRECURRENT (ACUTE)

- Febrile episodes
- Intracranial infection
- Intracranial hemorrhage
- Space-occupying lesions (cyst, tumor)
- Acute cerebral edema
- Anoxia
- Toxins:
  - Drugs
  - Tetanus
  - Lead (encephalopathy)
  - *Shigella, Salmonella*
- Metabolic alterations:
  - Hypocalcemia
  - Hypoglycemia
  - Hyponatremia or hypernatremia
  - Hypomagnesemia
  - Alkalosis
  - Disorders of amino acid metabolism
  - Deficiency states
  - Hyperbilirubinemia

RECURRENT (CHRONIC)

- Idiopathic epilepsy
- Epilepsy resulting from:
  - Trauma
  - Hemorrhage
  - Anoxia
  - Infections
  - Toxins
  - Degenerative phenomena
  - Congenital defects
  - Parasitic brain disease
  - Hypoglycemic injury
- Epilepsy—sensory stimulus
- Epilepsy—stimulating states:
  - Narcolepsy and catalepsy
  - Psychogenic causes
  - Tetany from hypocalcemia, alkalosis
- Hypoglycemic states:
  - Hyperinsulinism
  - Hypopituitarism
  - Adrenocortical insufficiency
  - Hepatic disorders
- Uremia
- Allergy
- Cardiovascular dysfunction or syncopal episodes
- Migraine

Modified from Schultz R, Hockenberry M. The child with cerebral dysfunction. In: Hockenberry MJ, Wilson D, eds. *Wong's Nursing Care of Infants and Children*. 9th ed. St. Louis: Mosby: 2011.

and the seizure may occur at any time of the day or night, with different lengths of time between seizures.[33] Unclassified epileptic seizures are events for which insufficient information is available to classify them. In addition to seizures, several types of epileptic syndromes display a group of signs and symptoms that characterize a certain condition.

Clinical manifestations of seizures may be subtler in the infant because of immaturity of the CNS. Some common behaviors seen with subtle seizures include: 1) tonic horizontal deviations of the eyes with or without nystagmoid jerking; 2) repetitive blinking or fluttering of the eyelashes; 3) drooling, sucking, or tongue thrusting; and 4) swimming or rowing movements of the arms with occasional bicycling movements of the legs. Apnea may also occur, and the respiratory status of the infant must be closely monitored. Seizures must be differentiated from jitteriness in infants. With jitteriness, the predominant type of movement is tremors characterized by alternating rhythmic movements of equal rate and magnitude. Jitteriness and seizures may be observed in the infant with asphyxia, hypoglycemia, or hypocalcemia. Laboratory studies may help determine the metabolic status of the infant.

Nursing management of seizures includes providing a safe environment for the child, monitoring respiratory status and perfusion, assessing for the cause of the seizure, determining methods to prevent additional seizures, and documenting the seizure activity. Children admitted to the critical care unit may require intubation for respiratory complications of seizures, for the sedative effects of anticonvulsants, or for status epilepticus. Anticonvulsant therapy may be indicated for prolonged or recurrent seizures. The primary therapy for seizure disorders is administration of the appropriate antiepileptic medication or a combination of medications to provide the desired effort without causing undesirable side efforts. Phenobarbital, phenytoin (Dilantin), levetiracetam (Keppra), fosphenytoin, and benzodiazepines (lorazepam, diazepam) are some medications that may be used for the child with seizures.[33]

Status Epilepticus

Status epilepticus is a medical emergency that requires immediate intervention to prevent possible brain injury or death.[33] This condition is characterized by two or more unprovoked seizures that may be caused by a variety of pathologic processes in the brain.[33] Causes may include high fever, meningitis, encephalitis, metabolic disorders, and abrupt cessation of anticonvulsant medications. Cerebral blood flow, metabolic requirements, and oxygen needs all increase when a seizure occurs. An electroencephalogram (EEG) is required to confirm status epilepticus in patients in a deep coma or with pharmacologic paralysis. The goal of treatment is to control the seizures or reduce their frequency and severity and to discover the correct the cause of the seizures. This will allow the child live as normal a life as possible. Treatment includes short-term administration of anticonvulsant medications such as diazepam, lorazepam, or midazolam. The critical care nurse should assess and evaluate the child to ensure that the patient has a patent airway, adequate ventilation effort, and adequate oxygenation and systemic perfusion. Clinical documentation should contain the patient's neurologic assessment, including the seizure manifestation and duration.

Bacterial Meningitis

Meningitis is an acute inflammation of the meninges, the outer covering of the brain and spinal cord, and cerebral spinal fluid (CSF). The pathogens usually come from a distant site and colonize. They enter the bloodstream, producing sepsis, and they then invade the meninges.[34] The highest incidence is found among children younger than age 1 year. Meningococcal meningitis is readily transmitted by droplet infection from nasopharyngeal secretions. The risk of transmission increases with the number of contacts. This may occur most frequently in school-age children or adolescents.[33]

The causes of meningitis may be septic (bacterial or fungal) or aseptic (viral), but the information in this section pertains only to bacterial meningitis. Common causative organisms are *Haemophilus influenzae*, type B; *Streptococcus pneumoniae*; and *Neisseria meningitides*. Other causative organisms are beta-hemolytic streptococci, *Staphylococcus aureus, Escherichia coli, Pseudomonas,* and *Listeria monocytogenes. S. pneumoniae* remains the most common cause of bacterial meningitis in children between 3 to 10 years of age despite appropriate treatment.[33] Invasion of microorganisms triggers a response that causes inflammation, production of purulent exudates, white blood cell accumulation, and various degrees of tissue damage.[33] The brain becomes hyperemic and edematous. The entire surface of the brain is covered in purulent exudates, and this may obstruct the flow of CSF, leading to the development of hydrocephalus.

The clinical manifestations of bacterial meningitis include fever, chills, headache, vomiting, irritability or lethargy, photophobia, nuchal rigidity, and a positive Kernig (pain with extension of the legs) or Brudzinski sign (flexion of the neck stimulates flexion at the knees and hips). One of the most dramatic and serious complications usually associated with meningococcal infection is meningococcal sepsis or meningococcemia. When the onset is severe and sudden, it is known as *Waterhouse-Friderichsen syndrome*. This syndrome is characterized by overwhelming septic shock, disseminated intravascular coagulation, massive bilateral adrenal hemorrhage, and pupura.[33] Meningococcemia requires emergency treatment and critical care because of the high mortality rate.[33] The late stages of this disease may produce increased ICP and cardiovascular collapse. Symptoms in infants are less specific and may include lethargy, vomiting, bulging fontanels, hypothermia or hyperthermia, diarrhea, and poor feeding.

CSF analysis is the standard for diagnosing bacterial meningitis obtained by a lumbar puncture. The CSF studies show an elevated white blood cell (WBC) count, increased protein level, decreased glucose concentration, and positive results from the Gram stain and culture of the organism. CSF may look cloudy or turbid. The child with meningitis is isolated during initial antibiotic treatment and for 24 hours after appropriate antibacterial therapy is started. The appropriate antibiotic therapy is continued for 10 to 14 days. The administration of dexamethasone is recommended in children with *H. influenzae* to prevent hearing loss.[34]

Nursing management must include early recognition and immediate start of therapies to prevent possible disabilities. Initial management includes use of isolation precautions, initiation of antibiotic therapy, maintenance of ventilation and hydration, reduction of increased ICP, management of systemic shock, control of seizures and temperature, and provision of family education and support.[33] The sudden nature of the illness makes emotional support of the child and parents extremely important. Parents frequently feel guilty for not having suspected the seriousness of this disease. They should be kept informed about their child's progress and all procedures and results.[33] The complications of bacterial meningitis may include the development of hearing loss, hydrocephalus, loss of digits or parts of extremities, and possible death. The long-term effect on infants manifests as communicating hydrocephalus, whereas in the older child, the effects are related to the inflammatory process or vasculitis associated with the disease. Hearing impairment is the most common sequela of this disease.[33] Evaluation of the child's hearing for possible hearing loss is needed for at least 6 months following the infection.

Head Trauma

Unintentional injury is the leading cause of death in children between ages 1 and 17 years. The number of children in this age range dying of their injuries is higher compared with the total number of pediatric patients dying of the next nine leading causes.[2] Current evidence suggests that most injured children are not being treated in pediatric trauma centers. About 47% of pediatric trauma care occurs in nontrauma centers.[35] The best outcome after pediatric trauma occurs when the clinical team is prepared and knowledgeable about the unique aspects of the injured child.[8] Much of the anxiety of taking care of injured pediatric patients are eliminated by having instruments, equipment, and medication dosages carefully precalculated. One effective practice in many centers is the use of the Broselow tape that is colored coded for specific weight groups of infants and children (see Fig. 40-3).

Head trauma in the pediatric patient results from closed head injuries resulting from motor vehicle accidents, bicycle crashes, falls, or child abuse.[36] During infancy and childhood, children tend to have heads that are proportionally larger compared with the remainder of their bodies. As a result, a child may be propelled head first in unrestrained crashes, causing acceleration–deceleration injuries when their heads hit objects. Child abuse resulting from blunt trauma to the head or from shaking is the leading cause of head injury among infants and young children.[36]

Traumatic brain injury (TBI) is the leading cause of childhood death and disability in developing nations. In the United States, 435,000 children visit the emergency room each year because of head trauma; and of these patients, 37,000 require hospitalization.[37] Morbidity and mortality associated with head trauma are attributed to injury suffered in two distinct phases: the *primary* phase and the *secondary* phase. The primary phase of injury occurs at the moment of impact, when the mechanical forces cause direct disruption of the brain parenchyma. Primary injuries may be focal or diffuse in nature. Examples of focal brain injuries include intracranial contusion, extra-axial hemorrhage (epidural, subdural, or subarachnoid hemorrhage). Diffuse brain injury is typically produced by acceleration or deceleration forces that result in shear trauma at the interface of the white and gray matter.[37]

The secondary phase of injury comprises sequelae of local and systematic events triggered by the primary injury. The three basic mechanisms leading to secondary brain injury are ischemia, energy failure, and excitotoxicity resulting in cell death.[37] Other factors that may contribute to secondary brain injury include axonal injury and death, cerebral edema, and ICP abnormalities.[37]

Head injuries are classified on the basis of the GCS score for the patient: mild injuries with a score of 13 to 15 on the GCS, which may be associated with symptoms such as brief loss of consciousness, disorientation, headache, or vomiting; moderate TBI with a score of 9 to 12 on the GCS; and severe TBI with a score of less than 8 on the GCS. Patients with moderate or severe TBI typically have more significant symptoms compared with those seen with mild TBI and also abnormal brain imaging. Children with severe TBI need to be admitted to a critical care unit for aggressive management and treatment of increased ICP.[36] Several studies on children with severe TBI have reported that an ICP greater than 20 mm Hg is associated with a poor outcome.[37] Thus, therapy should be directed to maintain ICP below this level. Treatment goals include measures to ensure adequate cerebral oxygenation and prevention of secondary brain injury. The child's plan of care includes providing optimal ventilation and oxygenation, maintenance of a normal partial pressure of carbon dioxide (Pco_2), maintenance of a normal ICP with monitoring and interventions, and maintenance of adequate systemic and cerebral perfusion pressures.[36]

Complications of head injuries include hemorrhage, infections, cerebral bleeding, cerebral edema, seizures, and brain herniation. Treatment is based on the clinical signs in the patient. Treatment for epidural hematoma is surgical intervention. Subdural hematomas are more common in children, and treatment of a subdural hematoma may also be surgical intervention for large hematomas associated with increased ICP.[3]

Children, especially infants, are at risk for seizures after severe head injury. The child admitted to the critical care unit with a TBI must be constantly monitored for cerebral edema and signs of increased ICP. Two other potential complications of head injury—diabetes insipidus and syndrome of inappropriate antidiuretic hormone (SIADH)—are discussed in Chapter 33.

Nursing interventions include precise neurologic assessment, which includes use of GCS scores and monitoring for signs of increased ICP. The psychologic impact of injury on a child cannot be underestimated. Studies have shown that 60% of injured children have post-traumatic stress disorder (PTSD) symptoms immediately after the injury. Thirty-eight percent of children continue to have symptoms 18 months after their injury.[8] Children who survive severe head injuries often require extended rehabilitation services to improve long-term outcomes. The pediatric rehabilitation team should be involved in the care of the child even while the child is in the critical care unit.

Working with the family of the child with a head injury is challenging. Information given to the parents must be accurate and consistent. The parents may be guilt-ridden, especially if they feel they could have prevented the injury. Parents are encouraged to interact with the child soothingly and gently, even if the child cannot respond. Reading books, making a tape of home activities, and bringing familiar toys or stuffed animals to the child are ways to involve the family in the care of the child.

If the child is not expected to survive, the parents should be informed. The child should be evaluated for brain death and possible organ donation. Before the tests begin, the parents are offered the opportunity to spend time with the child. If brain death has been determined, the parents are informed of the test results. Parents may be asked to participate in deciding when, not if, to discontinue support. If the decision has been made to discontinue the critical care treatment, the priorities for the critical care nurse include providing comfort and dignity for the child and the family.[38] The most important aspects of care for the families at this time are to show a genuinely caring attitude, to extend kindness and understanding, and to be present with them.[38] Parents must always be approached in a sensitive and compassionate manner. The critical care nurse is typically the member of the team who is closest to the family and the best person to help the family members get ready for the death of the child. Special circumstances such as the impending arrival of additional family members may influence the timing of the decision. Parents must be allowed to spend as much time as they desire with the child to see that everything possible has been done for their child.

GASTROINTESTINAL SYSTEM, FLUIDS, AND NUTRITION

Anatomy and Physiology

Coordination of sucking, swallowing, esophageal peristalsis, and breathing is established just after birth. Infant sucking, which is also a reflex, may be nutritive or nonnutritive. Non-nutritive sucking involves no swallowing; occurs at a rapid rate; has self-soothing capacities, which may also be used with the intubated infant; and affects the postprandial process. Nutritive sucking involves moving food from the mouth through the small intestines. It involves bursts of about 10 to 30 sucks, interspersed with one to four swallows. The quality of nutritive sucking is one of several indicators of illness in the infant. Sucking involves a considerable amount of motor activity, and when changes in oxygen demand and consumption occur during illness, the infant fatigues more readily, and sucking becomes weaker or even abates.

After birth, growth and maintenance of the small intestine require nutritional components and the stimulation that comes from having food in the gut lumen. The intestinal tracts of infants and young children are larger in relation to body weight than is the case with adults' intestinal tracts. Sodium and water conservation, which occurs in the large intestine, is an immature process in the infant. For the first 2 years of life, gut immunity is lower, and mucosal binding for bacterial toxins is greater. With these differences in immunity, sensitivity, and greater potential for fluid loss, the infant and the toddler have greater morbidity and mortality rates associated with enteric infections compared with the adult.[3]

Assessment and Treatment

The child's fluid requirements involve replacing output and insensible losses and extra fluid for the production of new intracellular and extracellular fluid during growth. Fluid maintenance for the child with normal renal and cardiac status may be calculated using several formulas, but these account only for basal metabolic needs and growth. The amount of fluid given to a pediatric patient must be determined by the child's clinical condition, fluid balance, and insensible water losses.[3] Table 40-11 provides guidelines for normal fluid and electrolyte maintenance for the infant and the child. Box 40-5 provides adjustments to fluid maintenance based on level of activity or increased metabolic rate associated with disease.

Pediatric patients with fluid volume deficit may present with vomiting and diarrhea. When considering fluid requirements, the bedside nurse assesses the pediatric patient for signs and symptoms of dehydration. The degree of dehydration may be classified as mild, moderate, or severe:[3]

- *Mild dehydration:* The child is restless, thirsty, and alert; has a normal pulse rate and strength; and has normal blood pressure, respiratory rate, and fontanels. The skin readily retracts when pinched; mucous membranes are moist; and urine output is normal. Dehydration accounts for

TABLE 40-11	NORMAL FLUID AND ELECTROLYTE MAINTENANCE FOR INFANTS AND CHILDREN[52]	
COMPONENT	**WEIGHT OF INFANT OR CHILD**	**TOTAL AMOUNT**
Fluids	1-10 kg	100 mL/kg/day (may be increased to 150 mL/kg for caloric requirements)
	11-20 kg	1000 mL + 50 mL/each kg over 10 kg
	>20 kg	1500 mL + 25 mL/each kg over 20 kg or 100 mL/100 kcal/day can be used for children of any weight or 1500 mL/m²/day can be used for children >10 g
Sodium		2-4 mEq/kg/day
Potassium		1-2 mEq/kg/day
Hourly fluid maintenance	1-10 kg	4 mL/kg/hr
	11-20 kg	40 mL + 2 mL/kg over 10 kg
	>20 kg	60 mL + 1 mL/kg over 20 kg

BOX 40-5	ADJUSTMENTS TO FLUID MAINTENANCE

- Fever or hypothermia: increases or decreases 0.42 milliliter per kilogram (mL/kg) for each degree greater or less than 37°C.
- Tachypnea: increases 25% to 30%
- Humidified mechanical ventilation: decreases 12%
- Activity of noncritically ill, resting child: increases 10%
- Restless or active child: increases 30%
- Diaphoresis: increases 10% to 25%
- High-humidity environment: decreases 25% to 40%

Modified from Hazinski MF. *Nursing Care of the Critically Ill Child.* 3rd ed. St. Louis: Elsevier; 2013.

approximately 4% to 5% body weight loss in infants or 3% in children or adolescents.

- *Moderate dehydration:* The child is thirsty, restless, lethargic, and irritable; has a rapid or weak pulse; has respirations that may be deep and the rate may be rapid; has a sunken fontanel; and has normal or low blood pressure. The skin retracts slowly when pinched; mucous membranes are dry; and urine is dark and the amount reduced. Dehydration accounts for approximately 10% of body weight loss in infants and 5% to 7% in children and adolescents.

- *Severe dehydration:* The child is drowsy, limp, cold, and sweaty, and extremities may be cyanotic; has a rapid or feeble pulse that is sometimes difficult to palpate; and has respirations that are deep and a rate that is rapid; signs of hypotensive shock. The fontanel is very sunken; urine is not excreted for several hours, and no tears are evident; and the eyes are very sunken. Dehydration accounts for approximately 15% body weight loss in infants and 7% to 9% loss in children and adolescents.

Fluid and electrolyte requirements are based on the patient's history, degree of dehydration, and presenting symptoms. The infant and the child need more calories per body weight compared with the adult for energy expenditure because of growth. Critical illness has a major impact on the nutritional status of a child. If a child is in a critical care unit for longer than 5 to 7 days, the chances of developing a serious nutritional deficiency increases significantly.[39] Suboptimal nutritional intake may result in malnutrition as well as poor recovery and outcomes. Nutritional support after the initial nutritional assessment is an essential aspect of care for the child. Critical care nurses play an important role in the feeding of critically ill children. Many procedures such as placing feeding tubes, checking gastric retentions, performing mouth care, and administering enteral or parenteral nutrition are within the nursing domain.[39]

Parenteral Nutrition

Providing needed calories in the face of fluid restrictions is a significant problem for the infant or child who is critically ill if the intestinal tract is nonfunctional. One method that may provide the necessary nutrition is parenteral nutrition. This form of nutrition is given by the intravascular route, and although it does not provide greater nutrition compared with enteral feedings, it may give sufficient support until enteral route for feeding is possible.[3] Table 40-12 outlines daily dextrose, lipid, and amino acid amounts; administration rates; and intravenous line concentration limits for the infant or child

receiving total parenteral nutrition (TPN). The TPN solution should be tailored to account for the unique needs of each patient. Determination of the child's individual nutrient requirements may vary, depending on such factors as age, weight, organ dysfunction, disease state, metabolic condition, body composition, and current medications.[40]

Dextrose solutions initially are titrated up gradually over several days to reach desired caloric levels to prevent hyperglycemia and to allow adjustment of endogenous insulin secretions. Intravenous administration of fat emulsion may be started at the same time as the administration of amino acid and dextrose solution. The rate of infusion of the fat emulsion is increased in a stepwise manner.[41] The required route for parenteral nutrition solution containing final concentrations exceeding 10% dextrose should be administered through a central venous catheter.[42] This catheter is inserted with the catheter tip residing in the lower one third of the superior vena cava or above the level of the diaphragm in the inferior vena cava. The four types of central venous catheters used in the pediatric patient are: 1) peripherally inserted central catheter (PICC), 2) nontunneled venous device (port), 3) tunneled venous device, and 4) totally implanted venous device. The administration of parenteral nutrition requires close attention to the administration, nutritional requirements and monitoring, and patient assessments. Daily assessment of the catheter site is a component of the central line bundle known to decrease risk of infection.[42]

TABLE 40-12 **TOTAL PARENTERAL NUTRITION ADMINISTRATION FOR TERM INFANTS AND CHILDREN**

PER 24 HOURS	INFANTS AND CHILDREN			ADOLESCENTS
	10 kg	10-20 kg	20 kg	
Fluids (mL/kg)	100-125	1000 mL: add 50 mL/kg for each extra kg >10 kg		1500 mL: add 20-25 mL for each extra kg >20 kg
Calories (kcal/kg)	75-90	75-90	>40	30-60
Protein (g/kg) Max peripheral: 2 g/kg/day Max central: 3.5 g/kg/day	2-2.5	1.5-2.5	1.5-2.5	1-2
Dextrose (%) Max peripheral: 10%-12.5% Max central: 30%	5-30	5-30	5-30	5-30
Fat (g/kg/day)	1-3	1-3	1-3	1-3
	INFANTS AND CHILDREN (>2.5 kg and <11 yr)			CHILDREN AND ADULTS (>11 yr)
Vitamins (mL/day) MVI-peds (vit K = 0.2 mg/5 mL) MVI-13 (vit K = 0.15 mg/10 mL)	5 mL/day			10 mL/day
Heparin*	0-0.5 unit/mL			0-0.5 unit/mL
Levocarnitine†	>30 days = 5 mg/kg/day			> 30 days = 1-5 mg/kg/day

*Recommended for slow infusion rates.
†Prematurity or TPN dependent.
MVI, Multiple vitamins for infusion; *PN*, parenteral nutrition; *TPN*, total parenteral nutrition.
Based on the guidelines from American Society for Parenteral and Enteral Nutrition. Modified from Ratz N. Parenteral nutrition. In: Reuter-Rice K, et al, eds. *Pediatric Acute Care: A Guide for Interprofessional Practice.* Burlington, MA: Jones & Bartlett Learning; 2012.

Enteral Nutrition

The enteral route is important for providing nutrition to a child.[39] Its advantages are convenience, safety, and low cost. The enteral route also is important in maintaining gastrointestinal mucosal integrity and immunologic function.[39]

Many different formulas based on age, host factors, and nutritional requirements are available for the infant or child. Amounts for formula feeds are based on needed kilocalories per kilogram per day (kcal/kg/day) and tolerance for each child and the clinical condition. For the full-term infant younger than 1 year, cow's milk (Enfamil, Similac) or soy-based formulas (Isomil, ProSobee) are most commonly given. Standard dilution for infant formulas is 20 kcal/ounce.[43] Human breast milk is highly recommended for feedings for infants. Feedings designed specifically for children between 1 and 6 years old include infant formulas, pediatric follow-up formulas, pediatric enteral formulas, various homemade and pureed feedings, and commercial adult formulas.[43] Adult formulas may be given to children older than 6 years. Osmolite and Isocal are preferred for their isotonicity and caloric and protein content.

Continuous gavage feedings have advantages over bolus feedings. The risk for aspiration is less, particularly for the infant with reflux. In practice, the individual child's tolerance ultimately dictates the method on how the formula is delivered. Feeding pumps are typically used to control the rate of continuous drip-feeding. The important features of the enteral pump for use with children is the ability to provide low delivery rates (<5 mL/hr) and to advance in small increments (1 to 5 mL/hr).[43]

Gastric and duodenal or jejunal feeding tubes are used to administer enteral feeds in the critically ill child.[39] Gastric feeding tubes can be placed easily at the bedside by the nurse. Determining the insertion length of a nasogastric tube in the child has traditionally been the same as that in the adult—naris to ear to xyphoid process. However, this measurement may not always allow for all the side holes of a feeding tube to be in the stomach. Measuring to a point between the xyphoid and the umbilicus is a safer method. Table 40-13 provides guidelines for gavage feeding tube sizes and feeding rates for infants and children. Nasoduodenal or transpyloric tubes are recommended to reduce the risk of aspiration in the presence of delayed gastric emptying or reflux. These tubes also ensure the delivery of enteral feeds to the main sites of nutrient absorption. Gastric retention, diarrhea, and abdominal distention may limit the use of enteral nutrition. Parenteral nutrition should be considered when it is impossible to obtain enteral access or when enteral nutrition cannot meet the child's nutritional requirements.[39]

Both overfeeding and underfeeding may have deleterious effects on the hospitalized child. Overfeeding places additional stress on organ systems and may increase the risk of mortality and morbidity.[44] Underfeeding is common in hospitals, and it is caused by inappropriate delivery of nutrition because of intermittent holds on feeds, NPO (nothing by mouth) time for procedures, and fluid restriction. This may result in weight loss or poor weight gain.[44] Refeeding syndrome may occur when previously malnourished patients are aggressively fed. This condition results in metabolic disturbances. Oral, enteral, and parental nutrition should be initiated and slowly advanced in patients deemed to be at risk for this problem.[44]

PAIN MANAGEMENT

The past 20 years of research has witnessed remarkable growth in pediatric pain management. Research has proven that infants and children do feel pain; when they are not treated, morbidity and mortality rates and hyperalgesia are increased. A negative impact may occur on development of the infant or child. *Pain* is defined as an unpleasant sensory and emotional experience associated with actual or potential tissue damage or described in terms of such damage.[45]

Physiology and Pharmacokinetics

Neurotransmitters and peripheral and central neural pathways for pain transmission are developed and are functional before birth, and they continue to mature during the first 2 years of life. After age 2 years, the perception of pain is the same for adults and children, but the psychosocial and behavioral expressions of the responses to pain change with the child's growth and developmental stage.[3] The nerve tracks to the brain are myelinated by 30 weeks' gestation, and the thalamocortical tracks are myelinated by 37 weeks' gestation, indicating that neonates are able to perceive all forms of pain. No perfect guide exists for providing analgesia to a pediatric patient. Children may demonstrate a wide variety in the medications needed, the duration and dosing requirements, and the responses to the medications.[3] Each child must be monitored for his or her response to the pain therapy.

The physiologic effects of untreated pain in the child may result in the following:

TABLE 40-13	GUIDELINES FOR GAVAGE FEEDING IN INFANTS AND CHILDREN[53]				
PARAMETERS	**AGE AND SIZE DETERMINATIONS**				
Age	3 mo	6 mo	2 yr	5 yr	10 yr
Tube size	6 Fr	8 Fr	10 Fr	12 Fr	14 Fr
METHOD	**INITIAL VOLUME AND RATE**			**ADVANCEMENT VOLUME AND RATE**	
Bolus	2-5 mL/kg every 3-4 hr over 20 min			2-5 mL/kg every other feeding	
Continuous	1-2 mL/kg/hr; initial volume not to exceed 55 mL/hr regardless of child's weight			1-2 mL/kg every 8-12 hr	

Fr, French.

- Hyperglycemia from decreased insulin secretion with breakdown of carbohydrate and fat stores
- Metabolic acidosis from increased use of fat
- Increased corticosteroids, growth hormone, and catecholamines
- Increased pulmonary vascular resistance
- Hypoxemia

Assessment

Pain assessment is the key to effective pain management. Many of the factors that influence an adult's pain also influence a child's pain. One difference is the influence of parental anxiety and behavior regarding their child's overall experience of pain. Although most of the pain research has involved procedural pain, it is important to be cognizant of the acute and chronic pain and distress associated with the critical care unit and its repetitive procedures.

The child may not spontaneously express his or her need for pain treatment. Staff members must be vigilant and actively explore a child's level of pain whenever the potential for pain exists. A child's verbal statement of pain is the most reliable indicator in acute pain management. However, this approach may not be possible with the preverbal child, the child who cannot comprehend the request to symbolically identify pain, or the child who has a significantly altered level of consciousness. For the child up to age 3 years, behavioral scales are used as the primary source for pain assessment, and physiologic parameters are used as secondary sources. One such tool is the face, legs, activity, crying, and consolability (FLACC) postoperative pain scale.

For the child at least 6 years old, self-reports are the primary assessment tool, with behavioral scales used as secondary sources. For the child 3 to 6 years old, self-reports may be used, but with a caveat. Many self-report scales have been tested as effective with this age group, but the young child 3 to 4 years old may have difficulty using them. Cognitive ability may not be advanced enough, or the child might have regressed in cognitive ability because of the illness. The child's rating may indicate a mood state rather than pain. Within this age group, self-reports and behavioral scales may need to be used together to get a true picture of the child's pain. One of the most valuable clues to pain relief is a change in behavior and vital signs after the administration of pain medication.

Parents often are the primary source of information about how their child exhibits pain. Parents are sensitive to changes in the child's behavior and often want to be involved in efforts for the child's pain relief. Encouraging parents to be involved gives them a sense of control and helping. Parents usually know what comfort measures to take with their children when they are in pain. For most children, having the supportive presence of their parents provides the most comfort. (See Chapter 9 for a discussion of pain-rating scales.)

Treatment of Pain

Some general principles are applied to the management of pain in children:

- *Prevention of pain:* If pain can be anticipated, pain should be treated prophylactically.

- *Adequate assessment:* Developmentally appropriate assessment tools are available.
- *Multimodal approach:* Analgesics; physical strategies such as massage, acupuncture, and hot or cold therapies; and behavioral, cognitive, and psychologic approaches are available.
- *Parental involvement:* Parents are the best source of information about their child. They should be taught different strategies to help their child cope with the pain.
- *Non-noxious routes:* The route of administration of analgesia should be as painless as possible.
- *Pain control during procedures:* Inadequate pain control during procedures may create an atmosphere of anxiety and increased pain during subsequent procedures.

Nonsteroidal Anti-inflammatory Drugs

Nonsteroidal anti-inflammatory drugs (NSAIDs) are effective for the management of mild to moderate pain, and they may be used in combination with opioids. They have superior anti-inflammatory properties compared with aspirin or acetaminophen.[3] The drawbacks to NSAIDs is that a ceiling effect exists and they affect the gastric mucosa, decrease platelet aggregation, and cause peptic ulcer formation and hepatic dysfunction. It is recommended that an H_2-receptor blocker be given concurrently for prolonged use of these medications.[23] The use of NSAIDs should be avoided in children with a history of severe renal disease, dehydration, or heart failure.[23] Examples of NSAIDs commonly used are ibuprofen and ketorolac (1 mg/kg given intravenously). Ketorolac is the only NSAID that is approved for parenteral use by the U.S. Food and Drug Administration.[46]

Opioid Analgesics

Narcotic analgesics are the single most important class of medications for the relief of moderate to severe pain. Administration of narcotics requires decisions about the route of administration of the medication, the choice of narcotic, and the method of administration.

The most commonly used narcotics for the child are morphine (0.02 to 0.1 mg/kg given intravenously), fentanyl (0.5 to 1.5 mcg/kg given intravenously), and hydromorphone (0.005 to 0.2 mg/kg given intravenously). Methadone (0.1 mg/kg) is an extremely long-acting narcotic, but it is not used as commonly for acute pain control. This medication is used for weaning from iatrogenic narcotic dependency or for chronic pain control.[3] Meperidine (0.75 mg/kg) is not a medication of choice because it decreases cardiac output and causes tachycardia. The medication's metabolite lowers the child's seizure threshold, causing hyperexcitability with multiple dosing. Opioids are given by intravenous push (IVP), continuous infusion, patient-controlled analgesia (PCA), or epidurals. Table 40-14 outlines standard dosages of morphine, fentanyl, and hydromorphone for the infant and child. Ketorolac in combination with morphine PCA in children has provided a very effective combination of analgesia.[46]

Naloxone is an opioid antagonist that is required if the child becomes unresponsive after receiving narcotics, the respirations become shallow and less than eight per minute, and the pupils become pinpoint. The initial dose is 1 to 2 mcg/kg/dose given

TABLE 40-14 OPIOID DOSAGES FOR INFANTS AND CHILDREN

AGENT	AGE	DOSAGE
Morphine		
Intravenous push (IVP)	<6 mo >6 mo	0.03-0.05 mg/kg/dose 0.1 mg/kg/dose
Continuous infusion		0.025-0.01 mg/kg/hr; max 0.2 mg/kg/hr
Patient-controlled analgesia (PCA)		0.005-0.02 mg/kg/hr continuous + (0.04 mg/kg/dose) boluses
Epidural		0.03-0.1 mg/kg bolus every 6-12 hr
Fentanyl		
Intravenous (short procedure)		2-3 mcg/kg/dose (if sedation used: 1-2 mcg/kg/dose)
Continuous infusion (intubated)		1-5 mcg/kg/hr, max 20 mcg/kg/hr
Epidural		0.2-2 mcg/kg/hr, possibly with bupivacaine
Hydromorphone		
Intravenous (short procedure)		8-15 mcg/kg, every 3-6 hours for pain
Patient controlled analgesia (PCA)		1-4 mcg/kg/hour continuous plus 8 mcg/kg/dose, every 10 minutes up to three doses
Epidural		With bupivacaine 0.1% or ropivacaine 0.1% 0.5-4 mcg/kg/hour With bupivacaine 0.125% 0.5-3 mcg/kg/hour

From *Lexi-Comp Online Formulary.* http://www.crlonline.com/crlsql/servlet/crlonline. Accessed July 2012.

intravenously over 2 minutes. The patient will need to be observed for the response to the medication. If patient is not responsive, the medication is continued until a total dose of 10 mcg/kg/dose has been given.[23]

Topical Anesthetics

The use of topical analgesic ointments reduces the local pain of procedures such as suturing or venipuncture and reduces the child's anticipated pain and anxiety over the upcoming procedure. The use of these agents has been expanded to include pain reduction for lumbar punctures or bone marrow aspiration. Some of the ointments take approximately 10 to 60 minutes to be effective. ElaMax is a topical formulation of 4% lidocaine that is encapsulated by liposomes, which create lipid solubility and allow transdermal medication delivery. ElaMax provides anesthesia in about 30 minutes.[23] A transdermal patch, Synera, containing lidocaine and tetracaine, may also be used on children older than age 3 years.[23] Lidocaine iontophoresis allows active transdermal delivery of lidocaine under the influence of a low-level electric current. It is available as Numby Stuff. Numby provides topical anesthesia to the child in as little as 10 minutes.

Nonpharmacologic Management of Pain

Nonpharmacologic techniques should be used to supplement, not replace, the use of pain medications. Some of the nonpharmacologic interventions that may be used in children include distraction, relaxation, guided imagery, and cutaneous stimulation. The use of these techniques may decrease the perceived threat of pain, provide a sense of control, enhance the child's comfort, and promote rest or sleep. These nonpharmacologic techniques are safe, noninvasive, and usually inexpensive, and most are independent nursing functions.

Oral sucrose is a valuable analgesic option for neonates undergoing brief procedural painful procedure. It has a rapid onset of effects and short-lived action thought to be mediated by the release of endogenous brain opioids. Use of the sugar has a low risk, and it is simple to administer to the neonate.[47]

PSYCHOSOCIAL ISSUES OF THE CHILD AND FAMILY

An unplanned admission of a child to a critical care unit, including those with illnesses or injuries, is a traumatic event for parents and for the child. In a crisis situation, parents may feel overwhelmed and become focused solely on the physiologic well-being of their child. If the child is conscious, he or she desperately needs the continual physical presence and emotional support of the parents; however, this is a time when it may be very difficult for the parents to help their child emotionally. Critical care nurses encounter the child and family at a very emotionally vulnerable time. Parents may view the nurses and physicians as their lifeline, controlling the needs and the life of their child.[3] One of the common complaints of families and patients is the lack of accuracy, clarity, and consistency of the information that is presented to them. Family members indicate a willingness and desire that bad news be empathetically communicated.[48] The critical care nurse needs to be knowledgeable about childhood cognitive and emotional development and about family dynamics to assist the child and the family through this health crisis. The following sections address some common issues that hospitalized children and their families face during hospitalization.

The Ill Child's Experience of Critical Illness

The term *family-centered care* defines the focus of care for a child because the nursing care of a child not only involves the child but the family as a whole. Family-centered care supports the child's family by prioritizing the family members' needs and values and empowering the family unit.[49] Two basic concepts in family-centered care are *enabling* and *empowering*. The critical care staff enable families by creating opportunities and means for family members to be present during examinations and procedures.[37] Empowerment describes the interaction of the staff members with the families in a way that allows the families to maintain control or acquire a sense of control over their lives.

The emotional reactions of the child to hospitalization depend on the type and quantity of stress produced by the illness itself, the hospitalization experience, and the notions that the child has about the situation. The final outcome is influenced by the child's age and level of development. A child in the critical care unit experiences significant stress, and the important question is whether the child's capacity to cope physically or emotionally in an age-appropriate fashion is exceeded.

Three elements help a child cope successfully with a crisis: 1) a resilient personality, 2) a supportive family, and 3) an outside support system.[3] The critical care health team members serve as the outside support system, applying the family-centered concept as they reinforce and strengthen the coping efforts of the child and family. Nurses must take every opportunity to reassure the parents that they are an integral part of their child's care and recovery. When children were asked who or what helped the most while they were in the pediatric critical care unit, 43% stated their nurses were the most helpful and 29% said that it was their families.[50] This is not a surprising finding considering that the critical care nurse has the most contact with the child in the critical care unit and provides most of the care to the child.[50]

The child who is critically ill needs the physical presence of the parents (or primary caretaker) at the bedside. Young children are most frightened by the separation from parents. Unrestricted visitation (i.e., 24 hr/day) for parents is imperative. The parents are the most reassuring persons in the child's eyes and are needed psychologically by the child to believe that he or she will not be abandoned, left to be unsafe, or left in pain and distress. Anxiety and fear are easily heightened when the child recognizes scary words or fills in ambiguities heard with his or her own distorted interpretations. For the child who is very ill and prostrate, anxieties may fester within, unknown to staff members. Every member of the health care team should have an understanding of the five phases of development of logical thought—infancy, toddlerhood, preschool age, school age, and adolescence—to communicate effectively with a child and should understand the basis of a child's perceptions, fears, and misunderstandings.[3]

The *infant* and the primary caregiver bond and develop the ability to take cues from one another. Oral gratification is very important to infants and may provide them comfort. Touch is also important; infants need to be caressed, cuddled, and comforted by being held close to the body. A major source of fear for the young infant is separation from parents. The critical care environment disrupts the infant's normal sleep cycle and feeding routines and may provide noxious and sometimes painful stimuli. Sleep deprivation or sensory overload may be interpreted as irritability or lethargy.[3]

Toddlers are at high risk for emotional sequelae related to the experiences of hospitalization and separation from parents. The critical care unit may be very frightening because of all the unfamiliar faces routines, sights, and sounds.[3] Any procedure that is painful may be perceived as punishment. If possible, parents should remain with the toddler as much as possible for comfort. Parents should not be asked to participate in painful procedures but should be there to comfort the child afterward. Most of a toddler's time is spent in play. Passive play such as music, mobiles, toys that make sounds, and movies may be used in a critical care environment and involve the family members.

The *preschool-age child* can tolerate brief separations from parents and is less upset by strangers compared with the toddler. The major fears of this age group include bodily injury and mutilation, loss of control, the unknown, the dark, and being left alone. This anxiety may be lessened by telling the child that his parents or nurse are close by. The coping style a preschooler uses often is apparent when the child is hospitalized. Withdrawal, projection, aggression, or regression may be observed behaviors.[3] Sleeping is one type of activity that children may use to maintain control when in an environment that allows them very little control.[50] Play is an important aspect of care for a child, and it may help the preschooler cope with the anger and fear about procedures. Preschool children are very verbal, and health care workers may forget how vulnerable and immature these children are.

For the *school-age child*, these years are ones of accomplishment and tremendous intellectual growth. The major crisis of the school years is the resolution of the balance between assuming new knowledge and skills. However, this may cause a sense of inferiority if attempts at tasks or goals are met with repeated failure. This age group enters a period of concrete operational thought. The school-age child may become accustomed to brief separations from family members but takes comfort and strength from their presence. The hospitalized school-age child is forced to depend on others for basic personal care and hygiene, and this may create stress. The health care team must respect the child's privacy and modesty and enable the child to make some choices with regard to personal care.[3] In addition to the child's parents; members of the child's peer group play an important role in providing comfort and support.

Adolescence is a time of great physical and psychologic change. Critical illness or injury may cause a crisis for children in this age group. The major threats of hospitalization for adolescents are loss of control and of identity, change in body appearance or image, and separation from their peer group.[3] It is hard for adolescents to be surrounded by strangers who are discussing their personal information. While hospitalized, the adolescent may use a variety of coping strategies, such as denial, regression, withdrawal, intellectualization, projection, and displacement.[3] The critical care staff should support the adolescent's attempt to master the situation and help to provide support. Questions should be answered honestly, and any misconceptions should be clarified. The adolescent should be allowed to be an integral part of the decision making about his or her care and to make choices, when possible. The patient should be allowed to maintain contact with his or her peer group if possible. The nurse should teach the adolescent coping techniques such as relaxation, deep breathing, and the use of imagery.[3]

Parents' Experience of a Child's Critical Illness

When their child is admitted to the critical care unit, parents may experience a staged response not unlike the grief process.[3] With a sudden illness or injury, the initial emotions may be shock, disbelief, and denial. These feelings may last for a few hours or a few days. Parents may question the diagnosis or want to prove the physician wrong. The situation may feel unreal, as if it were not happening to them. It may be difficult to grasp the totality of what has happened to their child. They may feel paralyzed and not know what they should do next. The parents may find it difficult to remember and process explanations given to them about what is happening with their child. This is usually a defense against pain. Forgetting may result in some parents feeling that staff members do not explain much to them. Other parents may feel that this is a sign of their own inadequacy. Explanations about their child's condition may have to be given in small amounts of information with compassion and repetition. Some parents may appear to be competent and composed during the height of the crisis, but this should not be interpreted as their being less stressed or anxious.

Parents need to be reunited with their child, if this is their wish, as soon as they have been prepared about what to expect. However, parents may be afraid to see their child. Changes in their child's appearance and in the child's emotional reactions will be very upsetting to parents. If the child is conscious and relatively alert, the parents need to be informed that their child may show some form of regressive behavior such as withdrawal or anger, which is to be expected given the stress of the situation and the degree of illness or injury. Parents also may feel frightened about touching or talking to their child, believing that this may harm the child. They must be reassured that they can do this and that if they have any concerns, staff members will be present in the room to help them.

Intense anxiety may make parents question whether their reactions are normal. They wonder how other parents feel or behave. They may be extremely frightened by the intensity of their feelings and may wonder whether they are going to have a breakdown. These feelings are common in a crisis, and parents need to hear that their feelings are understandable. Some parents may behave with hostility toward staff or family members. Some may behave quite rigidly, visiting only briefly or not asking questions in an attempt to maintain composure.

Anger is an emotion that usually takes its toll after the crisis period, usually with longer critical care unit stays. Destructive anger occurs when parents seek justification for their anger by blaming others for their child's condition. They are unreasonably critical of the health care team and may make complaints about the child's care as a manifestation of the anger. Parents may become depressed as they realize the severity of their child's condition. At this time, parents should be given an opportunity to express their feelings and participate in activities such as bathing the child.

The critical care nurse can assist the parents by clarifying information and by helping them support their child.[3] During crises, communication with the parents must be frequent and clear. Key elements to effective communication include communication at frequent, predictable intervals; use of consistent, understandable terminology; provision of opportunities for parents to ask questions and express opinions; and assistance of support personnel.[3] The primary focus in decision making should be the interests of the child.[48]

Critical care nurses who provide direct care to the child and parents have the greatest degree of contact with the family. In addition to the nurse's role in psychologic assessment and intervention, other support staff members should be available to assist the family. The creation of an ethical working environment in the critical care unit is a necessary precondition for addressing ethical issues raised by specific parent situations.[48] Clinical nurse specialists assess parental worries and concerns and, based on the assessment, help the parents to make plans to address their concerns.[51] Social workers provide the family with support and advocacy during their time of crisis. Many critical care units also have access to child life specialists, chaplains, discharge planners, and ethicists to assist in providing psychosocial support to the families. Concern for the psychosocial and developmental well-being of the pediatric patients and their families is the primary focus of the child life specialist.[49] An important role of the critical care nurse is to mobilize and introduce the families to the support staff available in their institutions for their support. The case study below discusses some of these concepts.

BOX 40-6 CASE STUDY

The Pediatric Patient

Brief Patient History
A 2-month-old infant is admitted directly to the critical care unit with a history of vomiting and diarrhea over the past 24 hours. The mother reports that the infant was irritable yesterday but is more lethargic today. The infant has had three wet diapers over the past 24 hours, and the urine appears dark. She continues not to tolerate any formula or Pedialyte.

Clinical Assessment
Physical assessment reveals the following—weight: 6.84 kg (weight 1 week prior: 7.6 kg), temperature: 38.5° C; pulse: 180; respiratory rate: 46-50; BP: 60/43; pulse oximetry: 93%. The infant's lips and mucous membranes are dry and tacky. Her fontanel is sunken. Extremities are cool and mottled, nail beds are dusky, and capillary refill is 4 seconds. Pulses are rapid and weak both centrally and peripherally. The infant is lethargic.

Diagnostic Procedures
The infant is placed on oxygen, and intravenous (IV) access is attained. A point-of-care testing glucose reveals a blood sugar of 60 milligram per deciliter (mg/dL).

Medical Diagnosis
This infant presents in the critical care unit with a diagnosis of hypovolemic, hypotensive shock.

Questions
1. For the bedside nurse, what is the priority in caring for this infant?
2. What category of shock applies to this situation?
3. Describe the pathophysiology of hypovolemic shock in the pediatric patient.
4. What are the two goals of therapy?
5. What level of dehydration does this infant appear to suffer?
6. Describe how and when to treat hypoglycemia in infants.
7. What is the fluid of choice to treat the volume deficit?
8. After the infant has received the initial volume replacement of two normal saline boluses, the infant is arousable. Vital signs are as follows: pulse: 160; BP: 70/40, capillary refill is 3 seconds; blood glucose is 80 mg/dL. What is the next step in the treatment of the infant's hypovolemic shock?

SUMMARY

- Children are physically, physiologically, and emotionally immature, and they are different from adults.
- Complete respiratory failure may develop rapidly in a child when respiratory distress is present.
- In infants and children, most cardiac arrests result from progressive respiratory failure, shock, or both.
- Bradycardia is an ominous sign in the seriously ill or injured child.
- Hypotension is typically only a late sign of hypotensive shock in children.

- Head injury is a primary insult to the child. Patient outcomes will be compromised if secondary insults such as hypotension or hypoxemia occur.
- Most children in the critical care unit experience pain and anxiety, and they should be treated accordingly.
- The concept of family-centered care recognizes that the family is the one constant in a child's life.

REFERENCES

1. Mullen J, Frances M. Caring for critically ill children and their families. In: Slota M, ed. *Core Curriculum for Pediatric Critical Care Nursing.* 2nd ed. St. Louis: Mosby; 2006.
2. Guice K, et al. Traumatic injury and children: a national assessment. *J Trauma.* 2007;36:S68.
3. Hazinski MF. Children are different. In: Hazinski MF, ed. *Nursing Care of the Critically Ill Child.* 3rd ed. St. Louis: Elsevier; 2013:1.
4. *American Heart Association.* Pediatric Advanced Life Support. Dallas; 2011. http://www.heart.org/cpr.
5. Grant M, Webster H. Pulmonary system. In: Slota M, ed. *Core Curriculum for Pediatric Critical Care Nursing.* 2nd ed. St. Louis: Mosby; 2006.
6. Wilson D. The child with disturbance of oxygen and carbon dioxide. In: Hockenberry M, et al, eds. *Wong's nursing care of infants and children.* 9th ed. St. Louis: Mosby; 2011.
7. Slota M. Bioinstrumentation: principles and techniques. In: Hazinski MF, ed. *Nursing Care of the Critically Ill Child.* 3rd ed. St. Louis: Elsevier; 2013:961.
8. Knudson M, McGrath J. Improving outcomes in pediatric trauma care: essential characteristics of the trauma center. *J Trauma.* 2007;63:S140.
9. Kline-Tilford A, et al. Pulmonary disorders. In: Hazinski MF, ed. *Nursing Care of the Critically Ill Child.* 3rd ed. St. Louis: Elsevier; 2013:483.
10. Kacmarek R, et al. *The Essentials of Respiratory Care.* 4th ed. St Louis: Mosby; 2005.
11. Kuch B. Respiratory monitoring and support. In: Hazinski MF, ed. *Nursing Care of the Critically Ill Child.* 3rd ed. St. Louis: Elsevier; 2013:1007.
12. Amin R. Chronic respiratory failure. In: Chernick V, et al, eds. *Kendig's Disorders of the Respiratory Tract in Children.* 7th ed. Philadelphia: WB Saunders; 2006.
13. Frankel L, Kache S. Mechanical ventilation. In: Kliegman R, et al, eds. *Nelson's Textbook of Pediatrics.* 18th ed. Philadelphia: WB Saunders; 2007.
14. Zentz S. Care of infants and children with bronchiolitis: a systematic review. *J Pediatr Nurs.* 2011;26:519.
15. Langley J, Bradley J. Defining pneumonia in critically ill infants and children. *Pediatr Crit Care Med.* 2005;6:S9.
16. Mansbach J, et al. US outpatient office visits for bronchiolitis, 1993-2004. *Ambul Pediatr.* 2007;7:304.
17. American Academy of Pediatrics Subcommittee on Diagnosis and Management of Bronchiolitis. Diagnosis and management of bronchiolitis. *Pediatrics.* 2006;118:1774.
18. Wohl M. Bronchiolitis. In: Chernick V, et al, eds. *Kendig's Disorders of the Respiratory Tract in Children.* 7th ed. Philadelphia: WB Saunders; 2006.
19. Cambonie G, et al. Clinical effects of Heliox administration for acute bronchiolitis in young infants. *Chest.* 2006;129:676.
20. Buckmaster A, et al. Continuous positive airway pressure therapy for infants with respiratory distress in nontertiary care centers: a randomized controlled trial. *Pediatrics.* 2007;120:509.
21. Marcoux K. Current management of status asthmaticus in the pediatric ICU. *Crit Care Nurs Clin North Am.* 2005;17:463.
22. Gomez M, Felauer A. Asthma. In: Reuter-Rice K, et al, eds. *Pediatric Acute Care: A Guide for Interprofessional Practice.* Burlington, MA: Jones & Bartlett Learning; 2012.
23. Lexi-Comp Online Formulary. http://www.crlonline.com/crlsql/servlet/crlonline. Accessed on July 2012.
24. National Institutes of Health. Consensus Development Conference on Infantile Apnea and Home Monitoring, consensus statement. *Pediatrics.* 1987;17:292.
25. Wilson D. Health Problems during infancy. In: Hockenberry M, et al, eds. *Wong's Nursing Care of Infants and Children.* 9th ed. St. Louis: Mosby; 2011.
26. Kiechl-Kohlendorfer U, et al. Epidemiology of apparent life threatening events. *Arch Dis Child.* 2005;90:297.
27. Chaiken J. In: Reuter-Rice K, et al, eds. *Pediatric Acute Care: A Guide for Interprofessional Practice.* Burlington, MA: Jones & Bartlett Learning; 2012:1012.
28. Ibsen L, Ungerleider R. Perioperative management of patient with congenital heart disease: a multidisciplinary approach. In: Nichols D, et al, eds. *Critical Heart Disease in Infants and Children.* 2nd ed. Philadelphia: Mosby; 2006.
29. Park M. *Pediatric Cardiology for Practitioners.* 5th ed. Philadelphia: Mosby; 2008.
30. Schell K. Evidence-based practice: noninvasive blood pressure measurement in children. *Pediatr Nursing.* 2006;23:263.
31. Callow L, Suddaby E. Cardiovascular system. In: Slota M, ed. *Core Curriculum for Pediatric Critical Care Nursing.* 2nd ed. St Louis: WB Saunders; 2006.
32. Hegazy R, Lotfy W. The value of Holter Monitoring in the assessment of pediatric patients. *Indian Pacing Electrophysiol J.* 2007;7(4):204.
33. Schultz R, Hockenberry M. The child with cerebral dysfunction. In: Hockenberry MJ, et al, eds. *Wong's Nursing Care of Infants and Children.* 9th ed. St. Louis: Mosby; 2011.
34. Vernon-Levett P. Neurologic system. In: Slota M, ed. *Core Curriculum for Pediatric Critical Care Nursing.* 2nd ed. St. Louis: WB Saunders; 2006.

35. Ochoa C, et al. Prior studies comparing outcomes from trauma care at children's hospitals versus adult hospitals. *J Trauma.* 2007;63:S87.

36. Pasek TA, Etzel KA. Multisystem issues. In: Slota M, ed. *Core Curriculum for Pediatric Critical Care Nursing.* 2nd ed. St. Louis: Saunders; 2006.

37. O'Brien N. Traumatic brain injury. In: Reuter-Rice K, et al, eds. *Pediatric Acute Care: A Guide for Interprofessional Practice.* Burlington, MA: Jones & Bartlett Learning; 2012.

38. Smith J, Martin S. Caring practice: providing developmentally supportive care. In: Curley M, Maloney-Harmon P, eds. *Critical Care Nursing of Infants and Children.* 2nd ed. Philadelphia: WB Saunders; 2001.

39. Ista E, Joosten K. Nutritional assessment and enteral support of critically ill children. *Crit Care Nurs Clin North Am.* 2005;17:385.

40. Ratz N. Parental Nutrition. In: Reuter-Rice K, et al, eds. *Pediatric Acute Care: A Guide for Interprofessional Practice.* Burlington, MA: Jones & Bartlett Learning; 2012.

41. Shuman R, Phillips S. Parental nutrition indications, administration, and monitoring. In: Baker S, et al, eds. *Pediatric Nutrition Support.* Sudbury, MA: Jones & Bartlett; 2007.

42. Infusion Nursing Standards of Practice. *J Infus Nurs.* 2011;34(1S):S102.

43. Nevin-Filino N, Miller M. Enteral nutrition. In: Samour P, King K, eds. *Handbook of Pediatric Nutrition.* 3rd ed. Sudbury, MA: Jones & Bartlett; 2003.

44. Fuchs S. Physiology and diagnostics. In: Reuter-Rice K, et al, eds. *Pediatric Acute Care: A Guide for Interprofessional Practice.* Burlington, MA: Jones & Bartlett Learning; 2012.

45. The International Association for the Study of Pain (IASP). http://www.iasppain.org/AM/Template.cfm?Section=Pain_Definitions&Template=/CM/HTMLDisplay.cfm&ContentID=1728. Accessed March, 2009.

46. Drain C. *Perianesthesia Nursing: A Critical Care Approach.* 4th ed. St. Louis: WB Saunders; 2003.

47. Paske T, et al. Hospitalized infants who hurt: a sweet solution with oral sucrose. *Crit Care Nurse.* 2012;32(1):61.

48. Perkin R. Ethical issues in pediatric critical care. In: Hazinski MF, ed. *Nursing Care of the Critically Ill Child.* 3rd ed. St. Louis: Elsevier; 2013:1071.

49. Pike M, Enright K. Child life: developmental considerations. In: Reuter-Rice K, et al, eds. *Pediatric Acute Care: A Guide for Interprofessional Practice.* Burlington, MA: Jones & Bartlett Learning; 2012.

50. Board R. School-age children's perceptions of their PICU hospitalization. *Pediatr Nurse.* 2005;31:166.

51. McNelis A, et al. Concerns with needs of children with epilepsy and their parents. *Clin Nurse Spec.* 2007;21:195.

52. Milonovich L, Eichler V. Neurological disorders. In: Hazinski MF, ed. *Nursing Care of the Critically Ill Child.* 3rd ed. St. Louis: Elsevier; 2013:587.

53. Pietsch J, Chung D. Care of the child with burns. In Hazinski MF, ed. *Nursing Care of the Critically Ill Child.* 3rd ed. St. Louis: Elsevier; 2013:921.

54. Coté CJ, Todres ID. The pediatric airway. In: Coté CJ, et al, eds. *A Practice of Anesthesia for Infants and Children.* 2nd ed. Philadelphia: WB Saunders Co; 1993:55.

The Older Adult Patient

Fiona Winterbottom

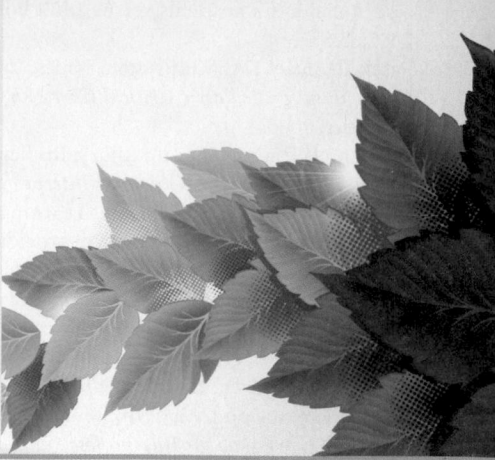

evolve WEBSITE

http://evolve.elsevier.com/Urden/criticalcare/

Evolve Features:

- NCLEX Review Questions
- CCRN Review Questions
- PCCN Review Questions
- Mosby's Nursing Skills Procedures
- Animations
- Video Clips
- Glossary

OVERVIEW

Senescence, or aging, is characterized by several physiologic changes. Incidence of disease and chronic conditions increases in older adults, although physiologic decline occurs independently of disease and is responsible for development of symptoms at an earlier stage of disease in older adults than in their younger counterparts.[1] Changes in physiologic function are important to consider when caring for older adult patients. Various physiologic changes that occur with aging warrant special physical examination techniques.[2] Clinicians must distinguish between changes in health caused by physiologic or pathologic processes. Comprehensive physiologic, psychologic, and environmental nursing assessment of the older adult and significant others/family members is vital in critical care and subsequent coordination of care.[3] The purpose of this chapter is to familiarize the critical care nurse with literature and research on care of the critically ill older adult.

Health Care Statistics

The senescent population is increasing worldwide. In 2009 there were approximately 39.6 million American residents over the age of 65. Average life expectancy in 2009 was 84 years.[4] In 2030 the number of Americans older than 65 years will be close to 70 million.[2] Demographic shifts and overall population increases have resulted in changes in provision and reimbursement of health care delivery and services. Medicare and Medicaid have become major payers of hospital services, creating challenges for health care providers and organizations.[5]

In 2008 the Medicare program had 45 million enrollees and expenditures of $468 billion, which was a $36 billion increase

over 2007.[4] The Patient Protection and Affordable Care Act (PPACA) is estimated to increase coverage to an additional 32 million uninsured individuals by 2014.[5] Health care services rendered to persons age 65 and over in 2007 included 289.7 million ambulatory visits, 13.9 million hospital in-patient care discharges, 1.3 million nursing home residents, 1 million home health patients, and 868,100 hospice discharges.[4] Patients older than 65 years currently account for 42% to 52% of admissions to critical care units and almost 60% of all critical care unit days.[2] Recent estimates of critical care costs account for 4% of national health expenditures, or approximately $81.7 billion.[6]

Health Conditions and the Older Adult

Health conditions experienced by older persons include hypertension (64% to 80%), heart disease (31% to 46%), cancer (17% to 23%), and diabetes (27%). Causes of mortality in persons over age 65 include heart disease (28%), cancer (22%), stroke (7%), chronic lower respiratory diseases (6%), and Alzheimer's disease (4%).[4] All mortality rates declined between 1997 and 2007 except Alzheimer's disease, which increased more than 50%.[7] Many of these conditions result in admission to critical care units; therefore critical care nurses need to understand key components in caring for older adult patients.

CARDIOVASCULAR SYSTEM

Age-Related Changes of the Cardiovascular System

Advancing age has many effects on the cardiovascular system (Table 41-1). Age-related anatomic and cellular changes in the myocardium and peripheral vasculature have significant impact

TABLE 41-1 AGE-RELATED CARDIOVASCULAR CHANGES

PHYSIOLOGIC ALTERATION	MECHANISM	PATHOLOGIC CHANGE
Cardiovascular Structural Remodeling		
↑ Vascular intimal thickness	↑ Migration of and ↑ matrix production by VSMC Possible derivation of intimal cells from other sources	Early stages of atherosclerosis
↑ Vascular stiffness	Elastin fragmentation ↑ Elastase activity ↑ Collagen production by VSMC and ↑ cross-linking of collagen Altered growth factor regulation/tissue repair mechanisms	Systolic hypertension LV wall thickening Stroke Atherosclerosis
↑ LV wall thickness	↑ LV myocyte size with altered Ca²⁺ handling ↑ Myocyte number (necrotic and apoptotic death) Altered growth factor regulation Focal matrix collagen deposition	Retarded early diastolic cardiac filling ↑ Cardiac filling pressure Lower threshold for dyspnea ↑ Likelihood of heart failure with relatively normal systolic function
↑ Left atrial size	↑ Left atrial pressure/volume	↑ Prevalence of lone atrial fibrillation and other atrial arrhythmias
Cardiovascular Functional Changes		
Altered regulation of vascular tone	↓ NO production/effects	Vascular stiffening; hypertension Early atherosclerosis
Reduced threshold for cell Ca²⁺ overload	Changes in gene expression of proteins that regulate Ca²⁺ handling; ↑ PUFA ration in cardiac membranes	Lower threshold for atrial and ventricular arrhythmia Increases myocyte death Increased fibrosis
↑ Cardiovascular reserve		Lower threshold for increased severity of heart failure
Reduced physical activity	Learned lifestyle	Exaggerated age changes in some aspects of cardiovascular structure and function. Negative impact on atherosclerotic vascular disease, hypertension, and heart failure

Adapted from Strait JB, Lakatta EG. Aging-associated cardiovascular changes and their relationship to heart failure. *Heart Failures Clinic.* 2012;8(1):143.
LV, Left ventricular; *PUFA,* polyunsaturated fatty acids; *VSMC,* vascular smooth muscle cells.

on the critically ill older adult.[2] Age is a major risk factor for cardiovascular disease in older adults, leading to more cardiovascular events in this population when admitted to the critical care unit.[8] Cardiac and arterial system changes include atherosclerosis, hypertension, myocardial infarction, and stroke. Pathologic alterations of aging include hypertrophy, altered left ventricular (LV) function, increased arterial stiffness, and impaired endothelial function.[8]

Age-Related Changes in Electrocardiogram

Changes in the electrocardiogram (ECG) include decreased R-wave and S-wave amplitude, increased P-R interval, and increased Q-T duration reflective of prolonged rate of relaxation (Table 41-2).[9] The QRS axis shifts leftward with age, perhaps due to increased LV wall thickness or hypertrophy.[9] Intrinsic heart rate decreases with age in the deficiency of parasympathetic influences; however, increases in atrial and ventricular arrhythmias increase in prevalence.[9] Cardiac dysrhythmias include atrial fibrillation, paroxysmal supraventricular tachycardia, with the most common dysrhythmia of premature ventricular contraction (PVC).[9] Reports show that 3% to 4% of patients older than 60 years of age experience atrial fibrillation[9]; incidence may be as high 10% in octogenarians.[8]

TABLE 41-2 AGE-RELATED CHANGES IN RESTING ELECTROCARDIOGRAPHIC VARIABLES

ECG VARIABLE	CHANGE WITH AGE
R–R internal	No change
P-wave duration	Minor increase
PR interval	Increase
QRS duration	No change
QRS axis	Leftward shift
QRS voltage	Decrease
QT interval	Minor increase
T-wave voltage	Decrease

Modified from Strait JB, Lakatta EG. Aging-associated cardiovascular changes. *Heart Failure Clin.* 2012;8:143.

A study of healthy geriatric patients with 24-hour ambulatory ECG recordings showed that 13% to 50% experienced paroxysmal supraventricular tachycardia in frequency with exercise.[9] Older individuals also have a high prevalence of left ventricular hypertrophy (LVH), which predisposes them to ventricular arrhythmias and sudden death. Atrial fibrillation is thought to be related to increased arterial stiffness, reduced LV compliance and rate control, and anticoagulation is recommended for most patients.[10] Age-associated cardiac conduction changes (even if asymptomatic) are predictive of future cardiac morbidity and mortality older adults.[9]

Age-Related Changes in Myocardial Structure and Function

Collagen is the principal noncontractile protein occupying the cardiac interstitium. Since myocardial collagen content increases with age, increased myocardial collagen content renders the myocardium less compliant and may be responsible for increased loading of blood vessels.[11] Slipping of myocytes can adversely affect diastolic filling, and structural changes that occur in the walls of blood vessels can lead to increased systolic blood pressure (SBP).[11] Collagen type I is more plentiful in the aging heart than the young heart, which contains more collagen type III. Collagen type I is less distensible than type III collagen, and both have different physical and mechanical properties.[11] Consequently, the left ventricle must develop a higher filling pressure for a given increase in ventricular volume. Decreased LV compliance may be evident in the older adult by the presence of an S_4 heart sound.[12]

Myocardial Infarction and Heart Failure

Chronic heart failure (CHF) affects approximately 5.7 million people in the United States of America and may be a contributing cause of death in 282,000 individuals per year, at a predicted cost of $39 billion annually.[13] Approximately 50% of heart failure (HF) cases are found within the 6% of U.S. population older than age 75.[9] Incidence of myocardial infarction (MI) in the Framingham Heart Study demonstrated that the rate of MI doubles for men and increases more than five-fold in women from the age group of 55 to 64 years to the age group of 85 to 94 years.[13] Similar results were seen in the Atherosclerosis Risk in Communities (ARIC) surveillance study.[13] Critical care nurses should recognize that older adult patients are not only more likely than young patients to experience an MI, but are more likely to die from an MI.

MI is one of the most common causes of CHF leading to HF via an intricate process known as left ventricular (LV) remodeling.[13] Age-associated changes in arterial structure and function cause large vessels to become less distensible, leading to prolonged systolic contraction, lengthened diastolic relaxation, increased myocardial oxygen demand, and diminished organ perfusion.[9] Additionally, atherosclerotic coronary arteries may limit blood flow to the myocardium, creating a higher risk of developing myocardial ischemia or infarction. MI in older adults is often associated with ST-segment depression rather than ST elevation. Sensation of chest pain may be altered and may be less intense and of shorter duration.[2] Other atypical symptomatology may include dyspnea, confusion, and failure to thrive, which results in unrecognized signs and symptoms of cardiac problems and delays in diagnosis and treatment.[2]

The aging heart undergoes a modest degree of hypertrophy and thickening of the LV wall without significant changes in LV cavity size.[9] Increase in LV wall thickness is primarily due to

growth in muscle cell size, which can lead to delayed early diastolic filling and increased cardiac pressures.[9] The early diastolic filling period and isovolumic phase of myocardial relaxation are prolonged in the older adult human myocardium. These changes may suggest diastolic dysfunction, but do not translate into decreases in end-diastolic volume or stroke volume.[9] Myocardial contraction is dependent on intracellular levels of free calcium and the sensitivity of the contractile proteins for calcium.[9] The senescent myocardium may have a lower threshold for atrial and ventricular arrhythmias due to changes in gene expression of proteins that regulate calcium.[9] Prolonged duration of contraction (systole) is caused in part by a slowed or delayed rate of myocardial relaxation. This may be an adaptive mechanism to preserve contractile function compromised by age-related increases in afterload.[9]

Age-Related Changes in Left Ventricular Function During Exercise

Aging is associated with a decline in exercise performance due to many physiologic variables. Cardiac performance is dependent on the heart's ability to increase and maintain cardiac output (CO), allowing oxygen delivery to the peripheral tissues. During exercise CO is increased by several mechanisms, the most important of which are increased heart rate, increased inotropic state of the myocardium, and decreased aortic impedance.[9] The Baltimore Longitudinal Study of Aging reported that older adults' diminished ability to exercise was not related to a difference in CO response.[9] Maximal heart rate achieved during exercise is attenuated in older adults; however, decreased heart rate response is accompanied by increased LV end-diastolic volume. As adults age, there is a progressive decline in VO_{2max}, which begins in the second decade of life and falls by roughly 10% per decade.

In summary, an older individual's ability to exercise may be limited by reduction in cardiac reserve, increased vascular afterload, arterial-ventricular load mismatching, pulmonary function, reduced intrinsic myocardial contractility, impaired autonomic regulation, and physical deconditioning.[9]

Peripheral Vascular System

The aging effects on the peripheral vascular system are revealed in a gradual but linear rise in SBP up until age 80 years when values tend to plateau.[2] Diastolic blood pressure (BP) is less affected by age and generally remains the same or decreases.[2] Important determinants of SBP include vascular compliance and blood volume within the system. Endothelial function and compliance of the vasculature is determined by cell type and tissue composition. In older adults, the intimal layer of the large and distal arteries thickens due to an increase in smooth muscle cells and connective tissue.[8] This gradual decrease in arterial compliance, or "stiffening of the arteries," is sometimes referred to as arteriosclerosis. Arteriosclerotic changes are also accompanied by changes caused by atherosclerosis. Atherosclerosis is the accumulation of lipoproteins and fibrinous products such as platelets, macrophages, and leukocytes within a vessel.[8] Arteriosclerotic and atherosclerotic processes cause arteries to become progressively less distensible and alter the vascular pressure-volume relationship. These changes are clinically significant because small changes in intravascular volume are accompanied by disproportionate increases in SBP, leading to increases in afterload and development of concentric (pressure-induced) ventricular hypertrophy in the older adult.[8]

Improved cardiovascular care has led to delay of cardiovascular disease; however, monitoring of cardiovascular risk factors such as cholesterol, BP, and obesity is now needed in the older adult population.[14] Lipoprotein levels increase with advancing age, adding to risk factors for development and progression of atherosclerosis. Serum lipoproteins are particles that contain various amounts of cholesterol, triglycerides, phospholipids, and apoproteins. The classification of lipoproteins is based on their size and relative concentration of cholesterol, triglycerides, and apoproteins. The five principal serum lipoproteins are chylomicrons, low-density lipoproteins (LDLs), very-low-density lipoproteins (VLDLs), intermediate-density lipoproteins (IDLs), and high-density lipoproteins (HDLs). Lipoprotein (Lp) (a) is composed of an LDL-like particle that in elevated levels has been implicated as a strong risk factor for coronary heart disease (CHD) and stroke.[15] Timely identification of high-risk individuals with high Lp(a) may allow for therapy such as statins to reduce LDL cholesterol to guideline-recommended levels.[15]

Another condition that may warrant attention in persons older than 65 years is metabolic syndrome. Metabolic syndrome is characterized by a group of risk factors, including abdominal obesity, high triglycerides, low HDLs, small LDLs, elevated BP, proinflammatory, prothrombotic states, and high plasma insulin (insulin resistance).[14] Metabolic syndrome has been reported to increase cardiovascular and mortality risk in middle-aged populations due to glucose metabolism and insulin resistance that is linked to cholesterol metabolism.[14] Reduction of risk associated with diabetes and metabolic syndrome may be modulated by manipulation of cholesterol absorption, leading to fewer events and improved survival in older adult cardiovascular patients.[14]

Hypertension

The population is aging, with hypertension affecting most individuals older than 65 years of age.[10] Pathophysiology of hypertension in older adults results from changes in arterial structure and function that decrease distensibility of large vessels, reduce forward circulation flow, increase pulse wave velocity, cause late SBP augmentation, and increase myocardial oxygen demand, all of which limit organ perfusion.[10] Older adults with poor BP control have an increased risk of cerebrovascular disease (CVD), coronary artery disease (CAD), disorders of LV structure and function, aortic and peripheral arterial disease, chronic kidney disease (CKD), ophthalmologic disorders, and quality of life (QOL) issues.[10] Secondary issues related to hypertension include renal artery stenosis, obstructive sleep apnea, primary aldosteronism, and thyroid disorders. Older adult patients with higher baseline SBP or longer duration of hypertension often experience autonomic dysfunction, microvascular damage, and CKD related to reduced renal tubular mass, fewer transport pathways for potassium excretion, and hyperkalemia.[10] Glomerulosclerosis and interstitial fibrosis lead to progressive renal dysfunction and reduction in GFR, increased intracellular sodium, reduced

sodium–calcium exchange, and volume expansion.[10] Older adults generally have contracted intravascular volumes and impaired baroreflexes, which may be exacerbated by diuretics, sodium, and water depletion, causing orthostatic hypotension. Volume overload is commonly due to excessive salt intake, inadequate kidney function, or insufficient diuretic therapy. An age-related decline in plasma renin activity, tubular function, and glomerular filtration rate affects overall sodium and water homeostasis.[2]

Management Recommendations. Risk stratification tools like the Framingham Risk Score can be used to predict MI, stroke, or CVD.[10] Evaluation of older adult patients with known or suspected hypertension should include identification of reversible and/or treatable causes, evaluation of organ damage, assessment for other risk factors, and identification of treatment barriers. Recommended laboratory testing for hypertensive patients includes urinalysis, serum chemistries, lipid profile, blood glucose testing (including hemoglobin A1c), and ECG/echocardiography.[10]

Treatment of cardiovascular risk factors in older adults includes aggressive treatment of dyslipidemia with lipid-lowering medication, control of blood glucose, and lifestyle modification. There should be consideration that QOL issues such as cognitive function, physical activity, and sexual function are reduced by aging and disease.[10] Drug treatment is recommended for older adult hypertensive patients with attention to alterations in medication distribution and disposal, changes in homeostatic CV control, and QOL factors. Lifestyle modification may be the only treatment necessary for milder forms of hypertension in older adults. Smoking cessation, weight reduction, increased physical activity, and sodium restriction result in greater benefit in older individuals than in young adults.[10]

Pharmacologic Management of Uncomplicated Hypertension. Antihypertensive treatment in older adults should be started at the lowest dose and gradually increased to the maximum dose needed to achieve an SBP 140 mm Hg. A second medication from another class should be added if the initial therapeutic response does not achieve an SBP 140 mm Hg. A third medication from another class can be added after maximum doses of two classes of medications are reached. Recommended initial medications include thiazide diuretics (hydrochlorothiazide), calcium antagonists (diltiazem, nicardipine), angiotensin-converting enzyme inhibitors (captopril, lisinopril), angiotensin-receptor blockers (losartan), and beta-blockers (metoprolol, carvedilol).[10]

Refer to cardiovascular chapter for more information on cardiac medications.

Pharmacologic Management of Complicated Hypertension. Older adult patients who have CAD, hypertension, stable angina, or previous MI should be prescribed a beta-blocker such as metroprolol for initial therapy. A long-acting calcium antagonist (CA) such as verapamil may be added to initial therapy if the BP remains elevated or if angina persists. An angiotensin-converting enzyme inhibitor (ACEI) such as benzapril is indicated if LV ejection fraction is reduced and/or if HF is present. Verapamil and diltiazem are not recommended if significant LV systolic dysfunction or conduction system disease is present.[10]

A BP of 130/80 mm Hg should be targeted in patients with HF and CAD.[10] Older adult patients with hypertension and systolic HF should receive a diuretic, beta-blocker, ACEI, and aldosterone antagonist. Limited studies support use of ARBs and ACEIs in the presence of chronic renal dysfunction. Older, black hypertensive patients with HF may benefit from a regimen including isosorbide dinitrate and hydralazine. Older adult patients with hypertension and asymptomatic LV systolic dysfunction should be treated with ACEIs and beta-blockers. Because HF may improve in hypertensive older adult patients with renal artery stenosis after renal revascularization, this should be considered when HF patients are refractory to conventional management of hypertension. Older adults with diabetes mellitus, hypertension, and nephropathy should be treated initially with ACEIs or ARBs. In older adults with prediabetes/metabolic syndrome, attempts should be made to reduce BP using lifestyle modification. If medications are needed, thiazide diuretics increase risk for incident diabetes mellitus and hyperglycemia.[10]

Medication regimens for hypertensive older adult patients with CKD include angiotensin-converting enzyme inhibitors or angiotensin-receptor blockers (ARBs). ACEIs should be considered for patients with nondiabetic nephropathy and ACEIs or ARBs are indicated if proteinuria is present. Older adult patients with hypertension and diabetes mellitus have a higher mortality risk than similarly aged nondiabetic controls.[10] Hypertension and HF are both associated with a more pronounced decline in renal function in older age. With the recognition of early renal dysfunction, more patients should benefit from aggressive therapy.[10]

Age-Related Changes in Baroreceptor Function

Baroreceptors are mechanoreceptors that respond to stretch and other changes in the blood vessel wall. They are located at the bifurcation of the common carotid artery and the aortic arch.[16] Impulses arising in the baroreceptor region project to the vasomotor center (nucleus of tractus solitarius) in the medulla. Abrupt changes in BP caused by increases in peripheral resistance, CO, or blood volume are sensed by baroreceptors, resulting in an increase in impulse frequency to the vasomotor center within the medulla. This increase inhibits vasoconstrictor impulses arising from the vasoconstrictor region within the medulla, resulting in a decrease in heart rate and peripheral vasodilation returning BP to within normal limits.[16] The baroreflex can be tested by measuring heart rate response (i.e., increase or decrease in heart rate) after administration of a pressor or a depressor agent and by changing the patient's position from lying to standing. Baroreflex-mediated tachycardia response to depressor agents is also attenuated in older adults. There are several reports of attenuation in heart rate response of older adults after changes in position.[16] When an individual changes position from supine to standing, distribution of blood volume changes, resulting in a reduction in CO and BP. This is known as orthostatic hypotension.[16] Simultaneously baroreceptors increase heart rate and maintain BP by increasing CO. The baroreceptor-reflex response also mediates changes in peripheral resistance and force of myocardial contraction, which offsets the drop in BP. Prevalence of orthostatic hypotension is greater in geriatric patients; therefore, judicious use of antihypertensive medications is recommended.[16]

Cardiac Medication Considerations in Older Adults

Treatment with medication should be considered when non-pharmacologic interventions are unsuccessful. Medication therapy for hypertension should target a SBP of 140 mm Hg to 145 mm Hg and diastolic of greater than 95 mm Hg in patients older than 80 years of age.[10] Heart rate control can be managed with beta-blockers and calcium channel blockers. Amiodarone can be used for conversion and maintenance of sinus rhythm with atrial fibrillation.[10] Aging increases the risk of major hemorrhage in patients with atrial fibrillation, with or without warfarin therapy.[10] Anticoagulation therapy can be complicated by polypharmacy, simultaneous use of antiplatelet medications, uncontrolled hypertension, and poorly controlled anticoagulation therapy.[17] Ventricular dysrhythmias are best managed with cardiac-resynchronization therapy and pharmacologic therapy in patients with advanced HF.[18] Cardiac resynchronization therapy (CRT) is a type of pacemaker or pacemaker/defibrillator that resynchronizes the contractions of the heart's ventricles by sending electrical impulses to the heart muscle, assisting blood flow and vascular remodeling. CRT has become an established therapy for advanced heart failure LV reverse remodeling, with significant reduction in LV volumes and improvement in LVEF.[18]

Combination pharmacologic therapy in older adult patients provides opportunity for enhanced efficacy, avoidance of adverse effects, enhanced convenience, and compliance.[17] Older adult patients will often discontinue or take medications inappropriately, resulting in failure to reach recommended targets and outcomes.[17] The average older adult patient takes six prescription medications; therefore, daily polypharmacy, nonadherence, and potential medication interactions are important concerns.[17] Nonadherence to medication regimens may be due to competing health problems, socioeconomic status, treatment complexity, side effects, and cost of medications.[19] Clinical and fiscal consequences of medication nonadherence can lead to increased hospital readmissions and adverse medical events.[19] Assessing factors that affect medication adherence such as literacy, eyesight, understanding of directions, education level, severity of disease, and comorbid conditions may assist in understanding barriers to compliance.[17] Patient management is most effective when intraprofessional health care teams collaborate to achieve and maintain goals. Novel opportunities for therapeutic management and compliance include smart phones, telemedicine, and computerized technologies. Other collaborative efforts include effective communication with local pharmacies, medication reconciliation at discharge, follow-up discharge phone calls, and timely provider handoff.

PULMONARY SYSTEM

Many changes in the pulmonary system that occur with aging are reflected in tests of pulmonary function and include changes in compliance of the chest wall, in static elastic recoil of the lung, and in strength of respiratory muscles.[20] Progressive changes due to age should not alter the older adult's ability to breathe effortlessly; however, factors such as repeated exposure

TABLE 41-3 AGE-RELATED CHANGES IN COMMONLY PERFORMED PULMONARY FUNCTION TESTS

PULMONARY FUNCTION TEST	DESCRIPTION	STANDARD LUNG VOLUME AND CAPACITY (mL)	AGE-RELATED CHANGE (mL)
Total lung capacity (TLC)	Vital capacity plus residual volume	6000	No change
Vital capacity (VC)	Amount of air exhaled after a maximal inspiration	5000	↓ 3750
Tidal volume (VT)	Amount of air inhaled or exhaled with each breath	500	No change
Residual volume (RV)	Amount of air left in lungs after forced exhalation	1200	↓ 1800
Inspiratory reserve volume (IRV)	Amount of air that can be forcefully inhaled after inspiring a normal V_T	3100	↓ 2800
Expiratory reserve volume (ERV)	Amount of air that can be forcefully exhaled after expiring a normal V_T	1200	↓ 1000
Forced expiratory volume in 1 second (FEV₁)	Volume exhaled in the first second of a single forced expiratory volume; expressed as a percentage of the forced vital capacity	80%	↓ 75%

TABLE 41-4 PROGRESSIVE CHANGES IN ARTERIAL OXYGEN TENSION AND CARBON DIOXIDE TENSION

AGE GROUP (YR)	Pao_2 (mm Hg)	$Paco_2$ (mm Hg)
≤30	94	39
31-40	87	38
41-50	84	40
51-60	81	39
>60	74	40

Data from Sorbini CA, et al. Arterial oxygen tension in relation to age in healthy subjects. *Respiration*. 1968;25:3.
$Paco_2$, Carbon dioxide tension; Pao_2, arterial oxygen tension.

to environmental pollutants and frequent pulmonary infections may accelerate age-related changes. Changes in tests of pulmonary function are listed in Tables 41-3 and 41-4.

Thoracic Wall and Respiratory Muscles

The aging thorax has a greater anterior–posterior diameter than in younger adults and there is some degree of dorsal kyphosis due to osteoporosis.[20] Rib mobility declines because of contractures of intercostal muscles and calcification of costal cartilage. Progressive decreases in chest wall compliance and changes in the shape of the thorax change chest wall mechanics and lead to deterioration in respiratory function (Fig. 41-1).[20] Strength of the diaphragm and intercostal muscles decreases with age. The diaphragm is the most important inspiratory muscle because its movement accounts for 75% of change in intrathoracic volume during quiet respiration. Other factors, such as an increase in abdominal girth and change in posture, also decrease thoracic excursion. Respiratory muscle function is affected by skeletal muscle and peripheral muscle strength.[20] During aging, skeletal muscle progressively atrophies and its energy metabolism decreases, which may partially explain the declining strength of the respiratory muscles.[20] Handgrip strength testing can be a simple and useful measurement in assessment of

muscle function.[20] Respiratory muscle performance is impaired concomitantly by the age-related geometric modifications of the rib cage, decreased chest wall compliance, and increase in functional residual capacity (FRC) resulting from decreased elastic recoil of the lung. Changes in chest wall compliance lead to a greater contribution to breathing from the diaphragm and abdominal muscles and a lesser contribution from thoracic muscles.[20] These anatomic changes are reflected by an increase in residual volume and decrease in vital capacity (see Table 41-3). Age-related decline in chest wall compliance of the respiratory system is 20% less in a 60-year-old subject compared with a 20-year-old.[20] Table 41-5 summarizes age-related changes in the chest.

Maximum inspiratory and expiratory pressures may decrease by as much as 50% because of decline in respiratory muscle strength, resulting in a decrease in thoracic wall excursion.[2] The age-related reductions in maximal inspiratory pressure and maximal expiratory pressure are likely a consequence of impaired respiratory mechanics and sarcopenia.[21] Sarcopenia describes reduced muscle mass and function, which may be related to decreased muscle protein synthesis, increased muscle proteolysis, motor neuron loss, and increased muscle fat content.[21] Respiratory muscle strength is related to nutritional status, often deficient in older adults.[20] Additionally, prevalence of vertebral fractures increases with age, particularly in women.[20] The accessory inspiratory muscles (sternocleidomastoid, scalene, and trapezius) facilitate inspiration during exercise. Reports have described that ventilatory muscle strength improved after older adult men and women received ventilatory muscle training.[2]

There is an age-associated decrease in effectiveness of the cough reflex and decrease in ciliary responsiveness and motion that predisposes older adult patients to aspiration and hospital-acquired infections.[2] These changes emphasize the importance of dysphagia screening, deep breathing, and coughing for the older patient in the critical care unit.

Age-associated changes in pulmonary function do not alter the older adult's ability to breathe effortlessly, although a decrease in respiratory muscle strength may be a limiting factor

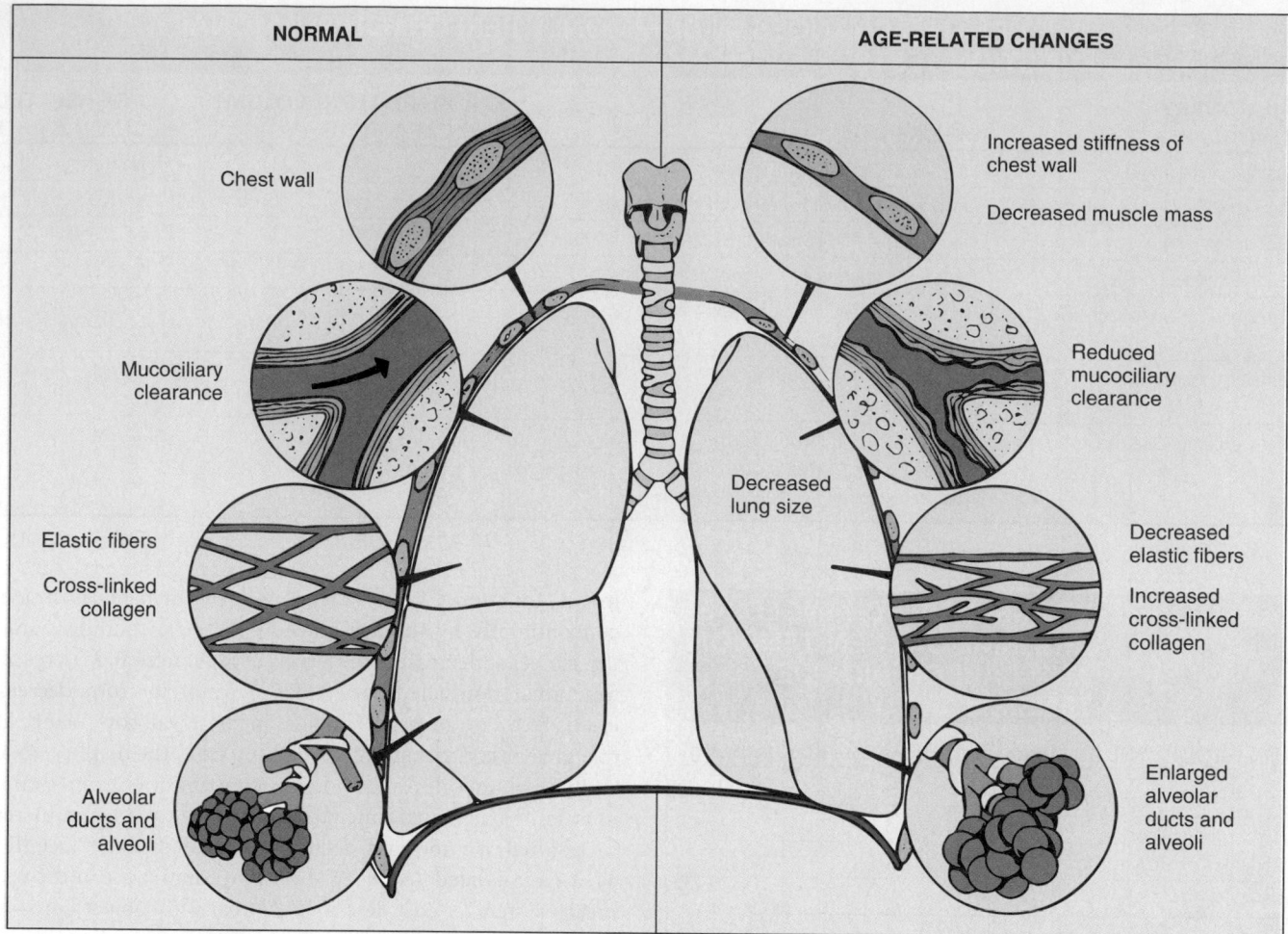

| NORMAL | AGE-RELATED CHANGES |

Chest wall

Increased stiffness of chest wall

Decreased muscle mass

Mucociliary clearance

Reduced mucociliary clearance

Decreased lung size

Elastic fibers

Cross-linked collagen

Decreased elastic fibers

Increased cross-linked collagen

Alveolar ducts and alveoli

Enlarged alveolar ducts and alveoli

FIGURE 41-1 Age-related changes occur in the respiratory system. With advancing age, the compliance of the chest wall and lung tissue changes. There is also a reduced clearance of mucus by the cilia that line the pulmonary tree and an enlargement of the alveolar ducts and alveoli.

during exercise. The application of conventional quality control standards to objective assessment of pulmonary function in older subjects may prove difficult because of mood alterations, fatigability, lack of cooperation, or cognitive impairment.[21]

Pulmonary Gas Exchange

A diminished recoil of the lung occurs with aging, causing increased lung volume, distention of the alveolar spaces, and a decrease in surface area of airspace occurs starting in the third decade of life.[20] Reduced lung elasticity results from changes in the ratio of elastic to support tissue that occur with advancing age.[22]

Ventilation and diffusion depend on numerous factors, including lung surface area. Displacement of inhaled air volume away from the alveoli limits the surface area available for gas exchange. This may in part explain the progressive and linear decrease in pulmonary diffusion capacity, which depends on surface area and capillary blood volume.[22] There are reports that capillary blood volume and surface area also decrease with advancing age. Changes in pulmonary circulation result in a ventilation/perfusion (V/Q) mismatch.[21] V/Q mismatch leads to a decline in arterial oxygen tension of approximately 0.3 mm Hg per year from the age of 30 years.[2] The typical Pao$_2$

for healthy persons older than 65 years is approximately 89 mm Hg, compared with 100 mm Hg for younger adults aged 18 to 24 years.[21] Age-related changes in ventilation and arterial tension for carbon dioxide (Paco$_2$) occur across the adult life span. Total minute ventilation (V$_E$) must increase with advancing age to maintain arterial tension for carbon dioxide (Paco$_2$). Paco$_2$ is largely dependent on the V$_E$, which is the sum of alveolar ventilation (V$_A$) and dead space ventilation. V/Q inequality may exist with decreased diffusion capacity of the lung for carbon monoxide and the transfer capacity of oxygen across the alveolar–capillary interface.[21] The impact of exposure to air and inhaled pollutants creates a challenge in differentiating the true impact of normal physiologic aging from that of environmental exposure.[20]

Control of ventilatory responses to hypoxia and hypercapnia falls by 50% and 40%, respectively, in the older adult.[2] This may be due to declining chemoreceptor function.[5] Decreases in Pao$_2$ could be the result of an increase in closing volume in dependent lung zones during resting tidal breathing in older subjects.[22a,22b] Consequently, dependent lung zones may be ventilated intermittently, leading to regional differences. Alterations in blood volume and vascular resistance within the pulmonary circulation may also contribute to V/Q mismatching.

TABLE 41-5 AGE-RELATED CHANGES IN THE CHEST

Frame

Soft tissues	• Hypotonia and muscular hypertrophy • Distribution • Reduction of fat
Ribs	• Decalcification • Depletion
Vertebrae	• Cartilaginous calcification • Decalcification • Kyphoscoliosis • Arthrosis • Deformation
Diaphragm	• Widening of the hiatuses • Parietal anterior/posterior modifications • "Bell" chest • Vertebral interior/posterior modifications • "Barrel" chest

Mediastinum

Heart	• Coronary arteriosclerosis • Increase in adipose tissue • Muscular hypertrophism • Thickening of the endocardium • Rheumatic-like valvular margins
Aorta	• Arteriosclerosis • Ectasia • Lengthening
Trachea	Parietal malacia
Pulmonary arteries	Arteriosclerosis

Lung

Macroscopically	• Increase in support tissue • Enlargement of the distal airspaces • Reduction of capillary bed • Possible terminal bronchiolitis
Microscopically	• Increase in collagen • Modification of elastin

Adapted from Bonomo L, et al. Aging and the respiratory system. *Radiologic Clin North Am.* 2008;46(4).

Important considerations for critical care nurses with regard to older adult patients includes recognition of decreased respiratory reserve and more rapid decompensation than in younger patients.[2] Other factors, such as exposure to environmental pollutants and chronic pulmonary disease, have an impact on the ability to compensate for respiratory conditions or wean from mechanical ventilation.[2]

Lung Volumes and Capacities

Pulmonary function studies may be the best way to assess respiratory impairment in older adults, because muscle strength, ventilator control, and gaseous exchange may impair respiratory mechanics.[21] Dynamic lung volumes and flow rates depend on resistance of airways and chest wall compliance and are limited by collapse of small airways during forced expiration. Age-related changes in respiratory mechanics lead to airflow restrictions, which are reflected in decreased 1-second forced expiratory volume (FEV_1).[21] Maximal expiratory flow rate and maximal midexpiratory flow rate are also decreased.[21] Age-related decrease in dynamic lung volume is probably caused by decreased chest wall compliance, small airways closure during forced expiration, and decreased strength of expiratory muscles. Breathing exercises generate lung volumes of forced vital capacity (FVC), which is an untimed lung volume and FEV_1, which is a timed lung volume. These spirometry tests can assist in assessing restrictive respiratory patterns.[21] Reduced timed lung volume is exhibited in chronic obstructive pulmonary disease (COPD), asthma, bronchiectasis, and cystic fibrosis.[21] Other conditions that display reductions in the timed and untimed lung volumes include kyphosis, scoliosis, myasthenia gravis, diaphragmatic paralysis, pleural effusions or fibrosis, and pulmonary hypertension.[21]

Older individuals are less able to protect against environmental injury and infection of the respiratory system. Decreases in T-cell function, decline in mucociliary clearance, and a decrease swallowing ability with loss of cough reflex can increase frequency and severity of pneumonia in older adults. Poor dentition, nutrition, and oral hygiene also play a role in the incidence of oropharyngeal colonization with gram-negative bacteria and aspiration pneumonia.[2] Noncritical conditions of the respiratory system such as bronchitis, emphysema, COPD, and lung cancer should also be assessed in older adults, as pathology and normal aging processes are often difficult to differentiate.[21]

RENAL SYSTEM

Acute kidney injury (AKI) is common in critically ill patients, with a prevalence ranging from 2% to 25%.[23] Age places patients at a higher risk of developing AKI and end-stage renal disease. Aging produces changes in renal structure and function that begin at approximately 25 years of age.[2] Between the ages of 25 and 85 years, approximately 40% of nephrons become sclerotic and others hypertrophy.[2] Sclerosis of the glomeruli is accompanied by atrophy of afferent and efferent arterioles, leading to a fall in renal blood flow of approximately 50%.[2] Decrease in number and size of nephrons begins in the cortical regions and progresses toward the medullary portions of the kidney.[2] This decrease in number of nephrons corresponds to a 20% decrease in weight of the kidney between 40 and 80 years of age. Initially, this loss of nephrons does not appreciably alter renal function because of the large renal reserve and simultaneous decrease in lean muscle mass.[2] The kidney contains approximately 2 to 3 million nephrons, more than is needed to maintain adequate fluid and acid–base homeostasis. Over time, the geriatric patient also loses this renal reserve.[2]

The RIFLE (risk, injury, failure, loss, and end-stage) classification has been used to detect changes and predict prognosis of renal function.[23] The age of 76 years has been found to be an important marker for RIFLE predictability and mortality in geriatric patients.[23]

Fluid Filtration

Glomerular filtration rate (GFR) is the volume of fluid traversing the glomerular membrane in a given period. GFR declines approximately 45% by age 80 years and is reflected as decreased creatinine clearance (CrCl).[2] GFR is usually estimated by collecting a 24-hour urine sample to measure creatinine excretion. Endogenous creatinine is a metabolic byproduct of muscle metabolism that is excreted by the kidney and is not reabsorbed. With advancing age, muscle mass decreases, thereby reducing the renal load of serum concentration of creatinine. In the geriatric patient, neither the creatinine excreted nor the plasma creatinine level may reflect changes in GFR. In older adults, the Cockcroft-Gault equation often is used to assess CrCl and GFR (in milliliters per minute), because it incorporates the serum creatinine concentration, body weight (in kilograms), age (in years), and gender as variables.[2] The Cockcroft-Gault equation for males is CrCl = (140 − Age)/72 × Serum creatinine × Weight. For females, this calculated value is multiplied by 0.85.

Renal tubular function is an important regulator of water and solute excretion and depends on permeability of glomerular capillaries, surface area available for filtration, and balance of pressure gradients between the glomerular capillaries and Bowman space.[2] Decreased GFR in older adults is most likely caused by decreased nephron number and reduced renal blood flow. Even though remaining nephrons adapt to loss of nephrons by glomerular hyperfiltration and increased solute load per nephron, the reduced GFR predisposes older adults to dehydration, adverse drug reactions, drug-induced renal failure, and acid–base imbalance.[2] Some medications are excreted unchanged in the urine, whereas other medications have active or nephrotoxic metabolites.

The senescent kidney is more susceptible to injury by hypotensive episodes because of age-related decreases in renal blood flow and reduced pressure gradient across afferent arterioles. Blood urea nitrogen (BUN) and serum creatinine levels can be normal or decreased in older adults (Box 41-1). The ability of the renal tubules to regulate fluid and acid–base balance decreases with age.[2] These functions are governed by the amount of sodium and water delivered to the tubules and overall acid–base balance. Age-related changes in tubular function become apparent when extreme changes occur in body fluid composition or acid–base balance. For example, with systemic acidosis the rate and amount of total acid excretion (i.e., bicarbonate, titratable acid, and ammonium) are reduced. This predisposes the older adult patient to metabolic acidosis, volume depletion, and hyperchloremia.

There is a diminished ability of the senescent kidney to excrete free water load, conserve water during periods of dehydration, and conserve sodium during periods of low salt intake.[2] Dehydration becomes a problem as the aging kidney's capacity to conserve sodium and excrete hydrogen ions decreases. The body does not compensate for nonrenal losses of sodium and water by the usual mechanisms of sodium retention, urinary concentration, and thirst. This may be due to decline in activity of the reticular activating system (RAS), decreased end-organ responsiveness to antidiuretic hormone, and changes in osmoreceptor function in the hypothalamus. Other extrarenal mechanisms such as the sympathetic nervous system are also important in homeostasis and maintaining BP in response to changes in body position. Decreased activity and responsiveness of the senescent kidney to the sympathetic

---

BOX 41-1 EFFECTS OF AGING ON VARIOUS LABORATORY VALUES

Values That Do Not Change with Age
- Hemoglobin, hematocrit
- Platelet count
- White blood cell count with differential
- Serum electrolytes
- Coagulation profile
- Liver function tests
- Thyroid function tests
- NC or ↓ Blood urea nitrogen
- NC or ↓ Creatinine

Values That Change with Age but Have Little Clinical Significance
- ↓ Calcium
- ↑ Uric acid

Values That Change with Age and Have Clinical Significance
- ↓ Erythrocyte sedimentation rate
- ↓ Arterial oxygen pressure
- ↑ Blood glucose
- ↓ or ↑ Serum lipid profile
- ↓ Albumin

From Duthie EH, Abbasi AA. Laboratory testing: current recommendations for older adults. *Geriatrics.* 1991;46:41. *NC,* No change; ↓ decreased; ↑ increased.

---

nervous system and renin–angiotensin–aldosterone system are important in integrating overall fluid homeostasis and maintaining BP in response to changes in body position.[2]

GASTROINTESTINAL SYSTEM

The gastrointestinal tract is made up of an epithelium, mucosal immune system, numerous bacteria, and the enteric nervous system.[24] The gut is complex and plays a key role in homeostasis. Age-related gastrointestinal changes occur in the processes of swallowing, motility, and absorption.[24] Swallowing may be difficult for older adults because of incomplete mastication of food within the oral cavity.[24] The result of deteriorating dentition, diminished lubrication (from salivary dysfunction), ill-fitting dentures, and incomplete mastication can put the older adult patient at risk for aspiration.[2] The number and velocity of peristaltic contractions in the older adult's esophagus decreases, and the number of nonperistaltic contractions increases.[24] These changes in esophageal motility are referred to as *presbyesophagus.* The changes may predispose patients to erosion of the esophageal wall (i.e., recurrent esophagitis), because food remains in the esophagus longer. Bed rest and reclining in a supine position for prolonged periods can cause esophageal reflux, which also can lead to esophagitis. The aging process also produces thinning of smooth muscle within the gastric mucosa.[24]

The epithelial layer of gastric mucosa, which contains the chief and parietal cells, undergoes a modest degree of atrophy resulting in hyposecretion of pepsin and acid, respectively.[24]

Gastritis-induced achlorhydria (decreased acid secretion) is prevalent in older adults. Mucin secretion from mucus cells decreases, thereby altering the protective function of the gastric mucosal (bicarbonate) barrier. Because of this, the stomach wall is more susceptible to acid injury, increasing incidence of gastric ulcerations.[24] It remains unknown whether changes in gastric acid secretion are a result of age-related changes or a disease process such as gastritis. Most duodenal and gastric ulcers arise because of the presence of *Helicobacter pylori*. Ulcers can also be promoted by the use of nonsteroidal anti-inflammatory drugs. The combination of *H. pylori* and medication effects can be a significant risk for gastrointestinal bleeding in critically ill older adults.[24]

Aging alters taste, smell, and gastric motility. Dysphagia and alterations in motor and sensory function can lead to silent aspiration and delay in gastric emptying that may contribute to postprandial hypotension and maldigestion. The gag reflex has been reported to be absent in 40% of healthy older adults and reports have revealed a reduction in esophageal peristalsis, increase in nonpropulsive contractions, and reduction in lower esophageal sphincter pressure.[25]

Few age-related changes have been noted in sensory and motor function of the small bowel; however, aging is linked to weakening of colonic muscles and altered rectal sensation. Structure and function of the pelvic floor and anorectum may contribute to constipation, fecal incontinence, and diverticulosis encountered in older adults.[25]

Although most vitamins and minerals are normally absorbed, calcium absorption is reduced, fat-soluble vitamin A is increased, and there is the potential for impaired absorption of vitamin D, B_{12}, and folic acid.[26] Thinning of intestinal lining, decreased mucus production, weaker intestinal muscles, and medications mobility may increase risks of constipation and fecal impaction in older adult patients.[26]

Pre-existing malnutrition can be problematic in the older hospitalized critically ill patient but can be avoided by early management of nutrition and dietary consultation during the critical care admission process. The problem of malnutrition may be undetected, which increases the risk of adverse outcomes such as increased morbidity and mortality.[2] Careful nutritional assessment is essential for determining older patients' nutritional status and planning adequate nutritional care to prevent malnutrition and propagation of critical illness in older adults.[25]

Age-Related Changes in the Liver

Mortality ascribed to liver disease may increase four-fold in adults aged 45 to 85 years.[27] Liver disease can also shorten potential lifespan in individuals under 75 years of age with a similar magnitude to that of COPD.[27] Compromised hepatic function in older adults decreases hepatocyte numbers, liver weight, hepatic volume, and perfusion.[27]

Structural changes in liver morphology and cell structure include increased volume of the dense body compartment (secondary lysosomes, residual bodies, or lipofuscin), loss of smooth-surfaced endoplasmic reticulum, diminished bile acid secretion, and increased biliary cholesterol.[27] Another age-related alteration in hepatocellular structure includes increased hepatocyte polyploidy (organisms containing more than two paired sets of chromosomes).[27] Effects of aging on hepatocyte structure may be due to increased oxidative stress and older adults' reduced capacity to eliminate superoxide radicals as efficiently as younger individuals. The liver has many complex functions, including carbohydrate storage, ketone body formation, reduction and conjugation of adrenal and gonadal steroid hormones, synthesis of plasma proteins, deamination of amino acids, synthesis and storage of cholesterol, urea formation, and detoxification of toxins and medications. Age-related changes in hepatic function include a reduction in synthesis of cholesterol, total bile acid pool, and bile acid from cholesterol. There is also a reduced capacity of the liver for regeneration in response to injury compared with a younger population. Despite these age-related changes, liver function is not appreciably affected.[27]

Tests of liver function, such as serum bilirubin, alkaline phosphatase, and aspartate aminotransferase (AST) levels are unaltered with advancing age. First-pass clearance of medications may be reduced due to decreases in total liver blood flow. The most important age-related change in liver function decreases the liver's capacity to metabolize medications.[27] Although clinical tests of liver function do not reflect this change in metabolism, it is well recognized that medication side effects and toxic effects occur more frequently in older adults than in young adults. Polypharmacy is cited as a common cause of adverse medication reactions in the older adult population.[27] Reduced medication-metabolizing capacity is caused by a decline in activity of the medication-metabolizing enzyme system, microsomal ethanol oxidizing system, and decrease in total liver blood flow.[27] Medications that depend on the cytochrome P450 group of liver enzymes are most affected because age-associated changes cause as much as a 50% decline in enzymatic function.[27]

A clinically significant age-related change is decline in the rate of hepatic regeneration following partial liver resection (hepatectomy) or injury.[28] The rate of liver regeneration (hepatocyte proliferation) following injury is decreased in older adults, which may enhance the progress of hepatic diseases and compromise liver transplantation in older adults.[27] Liver transplantation is a complex issue, since some evidence reports that livers from older donors may be less viable than those from young donors. Recipient age should also be a consideration, since post-transplant mortality increases by 15% between 55 and 75 years of age. The impact of age is modest with respect to recipient and graft survival, at least during the first few post-transplantation years, as both recipient and graft survival rates decline in older adult patients receiving livers from older donors by only 10% to 15% over the first 3 post-transplant years.[28]

Age, Disease, and the Liver

Although there are no specific age-related liver diseases, the percentage of older adults will increase over the next twenty years, leading to development of new conditions and options for treatment.[29] Some liver diseases are more frequently seen in older adults, including chronic hepatitis C virus (HCV) and hepatocellular carcinoma. Clinical management of liver disease in older adults may differ in several aspects from those of younger adults, for example, offering antiviral treatment to patients with chronic HCV to decrease risk of hepatocellular carcinoma.[29] End-stage liver disease will increase over the coming years with augmented numbers of individuals with decompensated liver disease and hepatocellular carcinomas.

Older adults infected with hepatitis B virus (HBV) often develop a subclinical hepatitis with a low rate of HBV clearance, perhaps due to impaired immunologic status.[29] These individuals appear healthy, but are highly infective chronic HBV surface antigen carriers. Persons with chronic hepatitis and/or cirrhosis are usually inactive, progress slowly, and do not reach old age, due to progressive disease.[29]

HCV infection is the most important clinical form of chronic hepatitis in older adults. Prevalence of antibodies against HCV increases with advancing age. Prior to this decade, estimates of subjects over 65 years of age infected with HCV ranged from 5.2% to 42.1%.[29] HCV infection has been linked to blood transfusions and nondisposable syringes. Advancing age is associated with more severe histologic damage and increased risk for progression to cirrhosis. Additionally, factors such as alcohol, medications, or metabolic alteration can affect the severity of hepatic damage and disease in older adults.[29]

Alcohol consumption and subsequent liver disease is common in old age. Reports suggest that 5% to 15% of older adults over 65 years of age have alcohol-related problems.[29] Individuals with alcoholic hepatitis and underlying alcoholic cirrhosis have the highest mortality. Hepatocellular carcinoma is the most common complication of liver cirrhosis affecting older adults, with incidence rates tripling between 1975 and 2005.[29]

In conclusion, aging and liver impairment may decrease liver regeneration related to hepatocyte proliferation, increase residual bodies or lipofuscin in hepatocytes, and create inability to eliminate cellular waste products that compromise normal cell activity. Furthermore, lifestyle, age, hepatocyte telomere shortening, and hepatic injury and disease can affect individual outcomes.[28]

CENTRAL NERVOUS SYSTEM

Cognitive Functioning and Aging

Cognitive functioning has become one of the greatest threats of old age, with more than 50% of older adults over the age of 85 years affected by Alzheimer's disease.[30] Structural and neurophysiologic changes occur in the brain with aging; however, it is not clear which changes are a normal process of aging or pathology of neurogenic disorders.[30] Cognitive function involves transforming, synthesizing, storing, and retrieving sensory input in addition to perception, attention, thinking, memory, and problem solving. Neuropsychologic assessment of older adults can be achieved with psychometric and clinical neuropsychologic assessment and standardized testing. Cognitive profile information can be helpful in differentiating between normal aging, mild cognitive impairment, early dementia, depression, mental health issues, and progressive neurologic disease. An assessment may also be useful following a stroke—or in conditions such as Parkinson disease—to assist in decision making about ability to drive or about the extent to which the individual has capacity to make specific decisions (medical

treatment, financial affairs, or self-care).[31] The rate at which complex tasks are completed may diminish; however, this is not synonymous with cognitive impairment, as deterioration of cognitive functioning is not a normal expectation of the aging process. Some slight memory dysfunction is common with increasing age, but significant decline may represent a change in individual need and may be a result of acute or chronic conditions. Acute mental status changes due to infection, metabolic imbalances, or medications are usually reversible after identification and treatment.

Delirium is a frequent complication in critical care but is often unrecognized in the hospitalized older adult.[32] Delirium is characterized by acute changes in mental status from baseline, inattention, and disorganized thinking or changes in level of consciousness. Cost estimates for care associated with delirium including postcare range from $38 to $152 billion annually.[32] Delirium is discussed further in another section of this book.

Postoperative cognitive dysfunction (POCD) is an acute and short-term disorder of cognition, memory, and attention that may be seen in critical care. Distinction should be made between etiologic factors and this syndrome. A study of Long-term Postoperative Cognitive Dysfunction in the Elderly (ISPOCD1) found that POCD was present in 26% of patients 1 week after surgery and in 9.9% 3 months after surgery, compared with 3.4% and 2.8% of controls.[2] Increasing age, duration of anesthesia, postoperative infections, and respiratory complications were risk factors for early POCD. Only age was a risk factor for prolonged POCD. POCD after cardiac surgery in older adults, with an incidence of up to 80% at discharge and 50% at 6 weeks. In some cases, neurocognitive decline lasted up to 5 years following some cardiac surgeries. Cardiopulmonary bypass appears to be a factor in short- and long-term POCD.[2]

Delusions and hallucinations may be present in delirium but are also evident in other psychiatric disorders. Long-term chronic impairment develops from more organic causes, such as those associated with neurodegenerative dementias (e.g., Alzheimer's disease) or nonneurodegenerative types (e.g., multi-infarct dementia, traumatic brain injury). Although dementia is pathology-based there is an increased incidence associated with advanced age, especially in those older than 85 years.[30] Alzheimer's disease is identified by amyloid-containing neuritic plaques and intraneuronal neurofibrillary tangles in various areas of the cortex.[30] Alzheimer's disease is characterized initially by progressive short-term memory loss, and later by long-term memory loss. Marked decline in memory leaves individuals functionally impaired and physically dependent. In contrast, non-neurodegenerative dementias, such as multi-infarct types, present as fixed deficits associated with the area of brain injury. In contrast to Alzheimer's type of dementia, cognitive impairment may be associated with significant impairment following stroke rather than over time.[31]

Baseline dementia, stress of surgery or acute illness, and hospitalization can cause cognitive decline and significantly increase risk for delirium in older adults. Sensory perception decreases with age, resulting in difficulties for the older patient in unfamiliar surroundings such as hospitals. Immobility and deprivation of vision and hearing increase the likelihood of dehydration, anorexia, confusion, depression, and disorientation.[2]

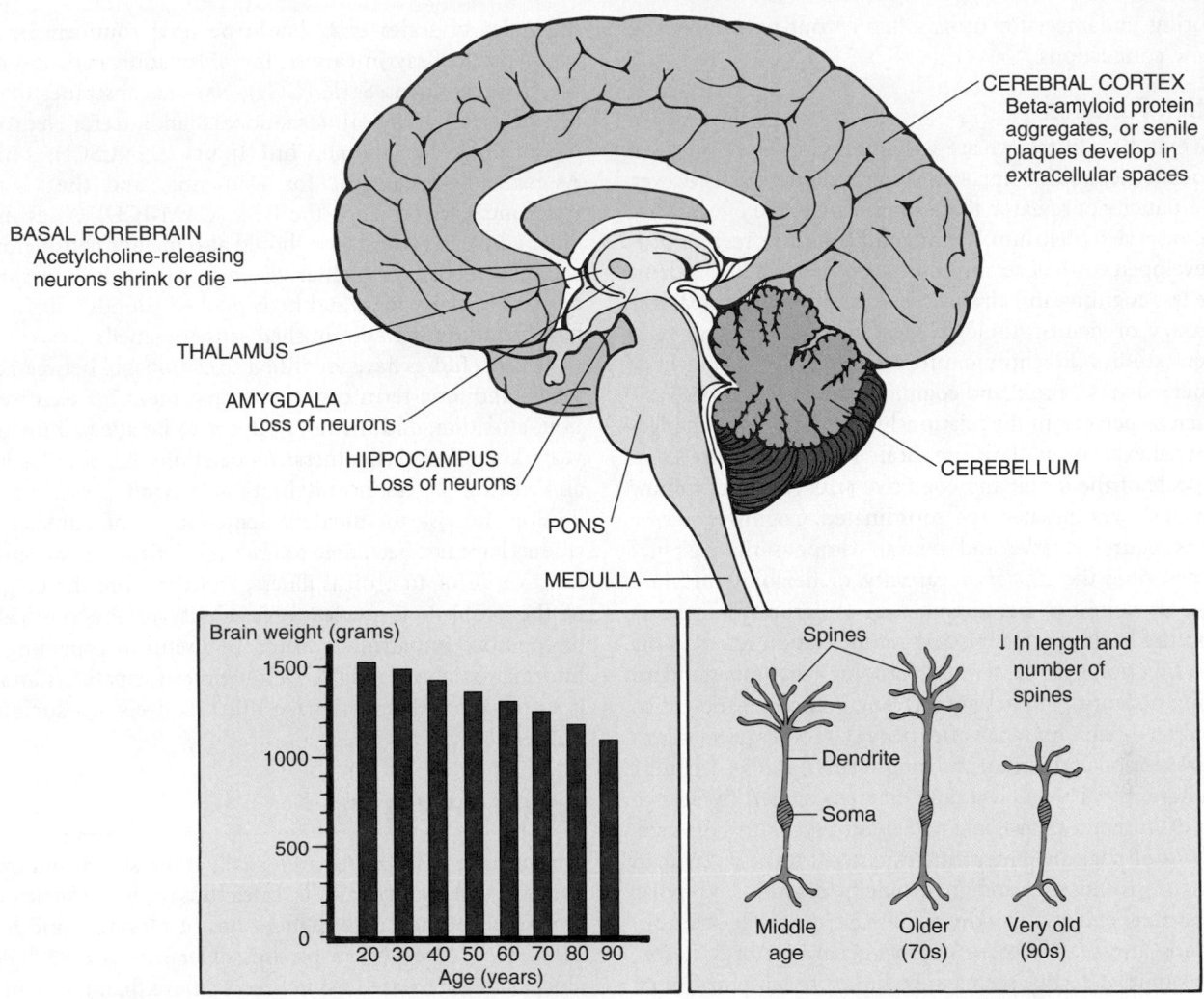

FIGURE 41-2 Summary of age-related changes in the brain. (From Selkoe DJ. Aging brain, aging mind. *Sci Am.* 1992;267:134.)

Structure and Morphology

The brain decreases approximately 20% in size between 25 and 95 years of age (Fig. 41-2).[33] Reduced brain weight may be related to the overall decrease in the number of neurons that occurs with advancing age. Neurons are lost from the hippocampus, amygdala, cerebellum, and from areas of the brainstem such as the locus ceruleus, dorsal motor nucleus of the vagus, and substantia nigra. Conversely, very few neurons disappear from the hypothalamus with advancing age.[30] Portions of the cerebral cortex atrophy, predominantly the frontal and temporal cortical association areas (the superior frontal gyrus and superior temporal gyrus, respectively).[30] Cerebral blood flow (CBF) and brain weight decrease with advancing age, most likely due to reduction in neuron number and metabolic needs of cerebral tissue.[33] CBF is also influenced by age-related changes in BP, barometric response to positional change, and severity of CVD. Accompanying the loss of neurons are changes in ultrastructure and intracellular structures of the neuron. The neuron is composed of a cell body, dendrite, and axon. Dendrites are long, spiny processes that extend out from the cell body. Dendrite spines decrease in number with age; the length of dendritic spines increases in middle and late old age, then decreases after

late old age (older than 90 years).[33] Shrinking of large neurons and degenerative changes occurring in cell bodies and axons of some acetylcholine-secreting neurons have been reported. These changes may explain alterations in processing and receiving of information.[33]

Lipofuscins, neuritic plaques, and neurofibrillary bodies appear within the cytoplasm of the neuron.[34] Lipofuscins, or age pigments, are granules containing a dark, fluorescent pigment and derive from lipid-rich membranes that have been partially disintegrated and oxidized. It is still not clear whether lipofuscin accumulation is harmful to the brain.[34] Neuritic, or senile, plaques are aggregates of beta-amyloid protein that accumulate in the brain of normal senescent persons. Neuritic plaques are found in the hippocampus, cerebral cortex, and other brain regions.[34] Neurofibrillary tangles, which are bundles of helically wound protein filaments, occur in the hippocampus with advancing age in healthy persons. They are present in larger numbers in persons with neuropathologic disorders such as Alzheimer's disease and may affect neuronal signaling.[34] Synaptogenesis or synaptic regeneration still occurs after partial nerve degeneration but at a slower rate in the older brain. After a nerve fiber is damaged, neighboring undamaged neurons often sprout new fibers and form new connections.[35]

Cognitive Function

Cognitive and brain reserve are well studied in the context of age-associated cognitive impairment and dementia. However, there is a paucity of research that examines the role of cognitive or brain reserve in delirium.[36] Brain and cognitive reserve concepts developed from observations that some individuals demonstrate less cognitive impairment than others with comparable brain injury or neuropathology. Most research on reserve is based on studies in chronic progressive disorders such as Alzheimer's disease. Brain and cognitive reserve describes variability across persons in the relationship of pathologic changes with clinical expression of disease. Brain reserve refers to structural aspects of the brain, and cognitive reserve relates to how cognitive tasks are initiated and coordinated. Cognitive reserve comprises neural reserve and neural compensation. Neural reserve describes the efficiency, capacity, or flexibility of brain networks or cognitive paradigms that underlie task performance in the healthy brain. Neural compensation refers to the ability to function optimally when pathology disrupts standard processing networks. Studies are ongoing to assess if these processes are modifiable and may offer benefit to older populations for the prevention of delirium and long-term cognitive decline.[36]

Cognitive impairment is a core element shared by a large number of different neurologic and neuropsychiatric diseases. Some form of cognitive impairment appears to be a factor in many neuropsychiatric and neurologic disorders (bipolar disease, stroke, epilepsy, Parkinson disease, multiple sclerosis, Alzheimer's disease, and other neurodegenerative brain disorders).[37] Cognitive decline seems to be linked to temporofrontal functional deficiency, which is expressed as deficient auditory discrimination and orienting.[37] New electrophysiologic technology is known as mismatch negativity (MMN). MMN abnormality is closely associated with cognitive change and decline occurring in a number of different neurologic and neuropsychiatric illnesses as well as in normal aging, providing ability to measure cognitive decline.[37]

Central Nervous System Assessment

Central nervous system assessment includes mental status, level of consciousness, memory, and ability to communicate. In the critical care unit, parameters may be altered by hypoxia, electrolyte imbalances, or various medications.

Neurologic examination of the geriatric patient always includes assessment of muscle strength, reflexes, sensation, and cranial nerves.[30] There may be changes in fine and gross motor skills and handgrip strength, leading to decreased ability to perform fine motor activities. Age diminishes the geriatric patient's vibratory sense in the lower extremities. Reflexes are slowed as a result of neuronal loss. Neurologic deficits may alter the patient's ability to perform self-care, including ability to follow instructions and interpret patient-teaching instructions.[30]

Several standardized neurologic assessments are available for use in critical care.[38] Most can be used for all critical care patients to accurately and consistently define patient status.

Examples of scales that should be used routinely in critical care—particularly in care of the older adult patient—include the Glasgow Coma Scale (GCS), National Institutes of Health Stroke Scale (NIHSS), International Standards for Neurological Classification of Spinal Cord Injury (ISNCSCI), Mini-Cog Assessment Instrument for Dementia, and the Confusion Assessment Method for the ICU (CAM-ICU). Assessment of older adults in critical care should also include consideration of age-related changes such as vision impairment,[38] hearing deficits (particularly low- and high-pitched sounds), slight loss of taste/dentition, and diminished sense of smell.

Recent studies have identified a relationship between critical illness and long-term cognitive impairment.[39] Executive function, attention, and memory appear to be affected for up to 6 years after a critical illness. Associations between acute care and critical illness hospitalizations permit greater cognitive decline and risk for incident dementia.[39] Unfortunately, most studies have not been able to objectively demonstrate cognitive function prior to critical illness, and therefore the magnitude of the problem is unclear. The ability to prognosticate risk of cognitive impairment would be useful in providing better information about long-term outcomes for patients and families and allow them to make difficult decisions surrounding critical illness.[39]

IMMUNE SYSTEM

Infections in older adults are usually more severe and frequent than those in younger adults. Infections in the geriatric population are associated with higher rates of mortality and hospital admissions, especially in persons older than age 85.[40] Persons older than age 65 are hospitalized at more than three times the rate of persons of all ages.[40] Since persons older than 65 years are the fastest growing segment of the population, more critical care services will be required during the next decade if treatment patterns remain unchanged. Alterations in immune function, increase in comorbidities, and greater frailty render older adults more susceptible to infections. Common infections in the older adult are associated with bacterial pneumonia, urinary tract infection, intra-abdominal infections, gram-negative bacteremia, and decubitus ulcers.[40] Increased susceptibility to infection may be due to cell-mediated and humoral-mediated immunity and breakdown in physical barriers, such as the skin and oral mucosa.

Cell-Mediated and Humoral-Mediated Immunity

Immune system function depends on many cell types with distinct functions. T cells are the primary effector of cell-mediated immunity, whereas bone marrow-derived B cells produce antibodies that are effector cells of humoral-mediated immunity. Cell-mediated immunity declines and T-cell function decreases with aging despite the total number of T cells remaining unchanged.[41] Older adults show deficiencies in the ability to produce appropriate defensive immune responses to pathogens and vaccines, contributing to increased vulnerability to infections and bacterial pathogens. Defects in T-cell function are often found in protective immunity at the cellular and humoral levels. Furthermore, evidence suggests that T cells from older

TABLE 41-6 AGE-RELATED CHANGES IN THE INTEGUMENTARY SYSTEM

SKIN PROBLEM	UNDERLYING MECHANISMS	NURSING INTERVENTIONS
Delayed wound healing	↓ Vascular supply to dermis ↓ Connective tissue layer ↓ Subcutaneous tissue layer Impaired inflammatory response ↓ New connective tissue proliferation	Use nonrestrictive dressings Weigh patient daily Support nutritional needs
Thermoregulation	↓ Subcutaneous tissue layer ↓ Number of capillary arterioles supplying skin ↓ Number of eccrine (sweat glands)	Monitor room temperature
Pressure ulcers	↓ Flattening of capillary bed ↓ Thinning of epidermis	Reposition patient every 2 hr Use pressure-relieving devices
IV infiltrations	↓ Connective tissue layer Vascular fragility	Monitor peripheral IV site hourly Discontinue IV administration at first sign of infiltration
Diminished skin turgor	↓ Connective tissue layer ↓ Eccrine and sebaceous gland activity	Bathe patient with tepid water Avoid use of deodorant soap

adult donors are generally slower and of lower amplitude than responses of T cells from younger individuals. Defects in cytoskeletal motors, hyperglycosylation of T-cell surface macromolecules, and changes in dynamics of membrane microdomains may offer opportunity for effective methods to rectify the age-related defects in protective cellular immunity, and those affect responses to vaccines, infectious agents, and perhaps neoplasia.[41]

Older patients may not be more likely to contract an infectious illness, but impaired ability of bone marrow to increase neutrophil production in response to infection may cause eradication to be slower. Older adult patients with major infections often have normal white blood cell counts, but the differential count usually shows a large proportion of immature forms. Infections in the older adult may present as acute mental status changes, anorexia, urinary incontinence, falls, or generalized weakness.[40] These may be signs of a urinary tract infection or pneumonia—two common infections in older adults—or may be signs of severe sepsis and septic shock.

INTEGUMENTARY AND MUSCULOSKELETAL SYSTEMS

Skin disorders are common in older adults and prevalence is dependent on the patient's clinical environment.[42] Older adult conditions of the skin include seborrheic keratosis, xerosis, and Campbell de Morgan spots.[42] Since the aging population is increasing, incidences of skin diseases will also increase. Older adults are vulnerable to a wide variety of dermatologic conditions resulting from degenerative and metabolic changes occurring throughout the skin layers.[42] Dermatologic changes can be considered in the categories of intrinsic and extrinsic aging.[42] Intrinsic aging refers to the skin's natural, metabolic aging process where the skin's upper layers become thin and blood flow is decreased, which leads to a reduced ability to nourish and repair cells. Extrinsic influences describe metabolic reactions to environmental factors such as solar radiation/sun exposure that leads to a decline in dermatologic integrity and skin that easily sags, breaks, bruises, and itches.[42] Seborrheic

keratosis and xerosis are common skin diseases affecting older adults; however, infectious skin conditions such as scabies are also frequently seen. Melanoma or skin cancer is a concern in older adult populations.[42]

Alterations in collagen structure reduce overall skin elasticity and reductions in immune function degrade the skin's ability to protect against bacterial assault.[42] The loss of elastic and connective tissue causes skin to wrinkle. The underlying structures such as veins and muscles are more visible because of skin transparency. Table 41-6 summarizes age-related changes in the skin and associated nursing interventions. Ecchymotic areas may be seen because of decreased protective subcutaneous tissue layers, increased capillary fragility, and flattening of the capillary bed, predisposing older adults to developing ecchymoses. Medications and physiologic factors may result in augmented bleeding tendency and appearance of ecchymotic areas; nevertheless, consideration should be given to the possibility of older adult abuse if ecchymosis is widespread or in unusual areas.

The skin is the largest organ of the body and is constantly exposed to environmental insult, which affects healing potential and leads to acute and chronic wounds. Nearly 1 million Americans develop chronic wounds, with annual prevalence of 10% to 35% in frail older adults.[43] Partial thickness skin injuries (skin tears) are caused by flattening and loss of cohesiveness of rete ridges and rete pegs of intact skin to the dermal layer. Decreased cytokine and growth factor production, reduced cytokine receptors, and increased number of senescent cells result in a diminished inflammatory response, when compared to skin of younger persons.[43] Cellular senescence is characterized by reduction of cell proliferative ability by shortening of telomeres (specialized structures on the ends of chromosomes) and increase in auto-fluorescent deposits, resulting in termination of cell division (also called replicative *senescence*).[43] Cellular senescence is particularly important with breaks in skin integrity/wounds. Critical care nurses should recognize these issues related to wound healing when caring for patients with pressure ulcers, venous ulcers, and surgical wounds. Additionally, impaired wound healing is affected by disease conditions, comorbidities, environment, genetic factors, and the aging process.[43]

Musculoskeletal changes in the older adult include a decrease in lean body mass, body composition, and energy expenditure.[2] There is an increase in body fat, a decrease in lean muscle mass, and a decline in muscle strength due to selective loss of muscle fibers by up to 40% at age 80 years. Inadequate nutrition, particularly high-quality protein, also affects muscle mass in older adults. Energy expenditure decreases with age, with resting energy expenditure decreasing by as much as 15%.[2] Oxygen consumption and energy expenditure after acute illness or injury are approximately 20% to 25% less in patients over 65 years than in younger patients. In light of this, it is recommended that nutritional support should begin within 24 hours of admission to the critical care unit.[2]

Low bone mineral density (BMD) is a risk factor for osteoporotic fractures.[44] Dual-energy x-ray absorptiometry (DXA) is the "gold standard" for measuring BMD and fracture prediction. The fracture risk assessment tool (FRAX) is also used as a gained estimator of hip fracture probability.[44] Bone demineralization affects both men and women as they age but occurs more often in women than in men. Bone demineralization refers to an increase in osteoblast and osteoclast activity, which decreases calcium absorption into bone. Mineral loss (calcium and phosphorus) with a decrease in bone mass is referred to as osteoporosis.[44] Osteoporosis produces bones that are more "porous" or fragile. With extensive bone demineralization, an older adult patient may sustain multiple fractures. There is an accelerated incidence of osteoporosis in women, which occurs after onset of menopause (possibly due to decreased estrogen). Decreased intake of dietary calcium, immobility, excess glucocorticoid secretion, and smoking all contribute to development of osteoporosis. Physical signs of deformities associated with osteoporosis, such as kyphosis or scoliosis, may place limitations on physical mobility or lead to gait instability. Fractures, particularly hip fractures, are especially devastating in older adults, leading to diminished QOL and increase morbidity and mortality. Risk assessment in critical care should consider these musculoskeletal issues when caring for and mobilizing patients.

Other complications of critical illness include polyneuropathy and myopathy. Many critical care unit survivors report limitations in physical function and activities of daily living (ADLs).[45] Impairment in ADLs was reported in virtually all critical care unit survivors assessed in the first week after discharge from the critical care unit. Functionality may improve with time; however impairments still occur in 50% of critical care unit survivors in the first year after illness and are more prevalent in mechanically ventilated patients.[45]

Older adults have an increased likelihood of developing new or worsening disability after hospitalization.[46] Hospitalization-associated disability occurs in almost 30% of older adults for up to 1 year after discharge, with less than 50% regaining pre-illness functional ability.[45] The number of older adults affected by hospitalization-associated disability increases to more than 70% in those ventilated for more than 48 hours. Many older adults who require nursing home placement do not experience long-term survival.[45] Hospital-associated disability is usually due to a combination of factors, including comorbid diseases, cognitive impairment, depression, immobility, polypharmacy, and lack of social support.[45]

PHARMACOLOGIC THERAPY IN OLDER ADULTS

Many benefits of modern advancements in pharmacologic therapy are offset by adverse medication effects, interactions, and therapeutic failure.[48] Adverse drug effects and medication interactions may be related to pharmacokinetics or the manner in which the body absorbs, distributes, metabolizes, and excretes a medication.[48] The aging process is associated with changes in gastric acid secretion, which can alter ionization or solubility of a medication and hence its absorption[48a,48b] (Table 41-7). Medication distribution depends on body composition and on

TABLE 41-7 AGE-RELATED CHANGES IN PHARMACOKINETICS

PHARMACOKINETIC PARAMETER	DEFINITION	AGE-RELATED CHANGES
Absorption	Receptor-coupled or diffusional uptake of medication into tissue	Decreased absorptive surface area of small intestine Decreased splanchnic blood flow Increased gastric acid pH Decreased gastrointestinal motility
Distribution	Theoretic space (tissue) or body compartment into which free form of medication distributes	Decreased lean body mass and total body water Increased total body fat Decreased serum albumin level Increased alpha$_1$-acid glycoprotein
Metabolism	Chemical change in medication that renders it active or inactive	Decreased liver mass Decreased activity of microsomal medication-metabolizing enzyme system Decreased total liver blood flow
Excretion	Removal of medication through an eliminating organ, often the kidney; some medications are excreted in bile or feces, in saliva, or through the lungs	Decreased renal blood flow and glomerular filtration rate Decreased distal renal tubular secretory function

Data from Gilman AG, et al, eds. *Goodman and Gilman's the Pharmacological Basis of Therapeutics.* 8th ed. London: Pergamon Press; 1990; Vestal RE, Cusack BJ. Pharmacology and aging. In: Schneider EL, Rowe JW, eds. *Handbook of the Biology of Aging,* San Diego: Academic Press; 1990.

physiochemical medication properties. With advancing age, fat content increases, lean body mass decreases, and total body water decreases, which can alter medication disposition.[43] For example, because of the increase in the ratio of body fat content to body weight, lipophilic medication have a greater volume of distribution per body weight in older adults compared with younger adults. Other age-related factors affecting medication disposition are listed in Table 41-7.

The senescent liver and kidneys are less able to metabolize and excrete medications, leading to changes in absorption rates, time to peak plasma concentration, and clearance. Examples include high dosing regimens of diuretics to facilitate diuresis.[10] Increased risk of metabolic acidosis then occurs, since high diuretic doses increase competition for organic acid transport pathways at the proximal tubule. Using the example of diuretics, bioavailability between agents may also be variable. For instance, bumetanide has a fairly consistent bioavailability in advanced age, whereas that of furosemide varies from 20% to 80%.[10]

Similarly, other medications associated with management of common disorders seen in critically ill patients—such as digoxin, angiotensin II-converting enzyme (ACE) inhibitors, and angiotensin II-receptor blockers (ARBs)[10]—have delayed excretion, increased serum concentration, and more prolonged duration of action because their excretion parallels GFR, which decreases with age. Table 41-7 describes age-related changes in medication pharmacokinetics.

Pharmacodynamics refers to the pharmacologic or physiologic response to a medication that occurs after the medication interacts with its receptor on the plasma membrane. Chronotropic and inotropic effects of beta-adrenergic agonists appear to decrease in older adults.[10] Age may produce no change in heparin-stimulated increases in partial thromboplastin time, whereas the effects of warfarin (Coumadin) are very susceptible to medication interactions. Table 41-8 presents cardiac medication considerations for older adults.

The Critical Care Safety Study found that 61% of adverse events in the critical care unit were associated with medications.[49] Annual costs related to adverse pharmacologic events have been estimated to be $76.6 billion to ambulatory care, $20 billion to hospitals, and $4 billion to nursing home facilities.[48] Medications most often associated with errors were cardiovascular medications (24%), anticoagulants (20%), and anti-infective agents (13%).[48] Insulin and hypoglycemic agents are also responsible for hospital readmissions.[48] The Beers Criteria is a list of medications that was developed to avoid inappropriate medication prescribing in adults aged 65 years and over. (Visit this website for more information: http://www.dcri.duke.edu/ccge/curtis/beers.html.)[48] Table 41-9 lists potentially inappropriate symptom management medications for older adults.

HOSPITAL-ASSOCIATED RISK FACTORS FOR OLDER ADULTS

Multiple concurrent chronic illnesses produce systemic stressors that diminish immune function. Critical care nurses must be aware that exacerbation of pre-existing illness such as diabetes or emphysema may manifest before infection is suspected. Invasive devices such as central lines or chest tubes may threaten

suppressed immune systems. Nutritional deficiencies are a common problem in older adults. Inadequate protein intake can develop from prolonged anorexia and cognitive impairment associated with a shrinkage of lymphoid tissue, diminishing T-cell functioning and decreased cell-mediated immunity.[49] Inadequate emptying of urine because of bed rest, obstruction, or side effects from anticholinergic medications can result in stagnation of urine and recurrent urinary tract infections. Long-term placement of urinary catheters is a significant source of bacteria; however, treatment with antibiotic therapy is not indicated unless the patient becomes symptomatic with anorexia or cognitive impairment or has a history of a chronic illness, such as diabetes or COPD.

LONG-TERM COMPLICATIONS OF CRITICAL CARE

Improved critical care outcomes have led to an increase in survivors of critical illness and additional challenges related to long-term complications of critical care. Mortality post-critical care ranges from 26% to 63% in the first year, with mortality risk factors dependent on age, comorbidity, and critical care severity of illness.[45] Medical costs are incurred during initial hospitalizations with 40% requiring ongoing medical care for up to 2 years related to rehabilitation and readmissions increasing utilization of long-term acute care three-fold between 1997 and 2006.[45] Post-critical care unit conditions create an additional burden for patients and their families for years after critical care unit discharge.[45] Post-critical care unit issues include depression, lifestyle disruption, employment problems, mobility dysfunction, and cognitive impairment.[46]

Critical care nursing now involves prevention and management of long-term complications of critical care.[47] Critical care nurses have an essential role in multidisciplinary collaboration and assessment of older patients. Nurses gather vital information about patient needs, implement key nursing interventions, and recommend specialty service consults to improve long-term clinical outcomes.

Coordination of critical care interventions can decrease negative physical, functional, and cognitive long-term outcomes associated with critical illness.[47] Noise reduction and medication management can enhance orientation, decrease delirium, and improve long-term consequences of critical care. Early mobility protocols, avoidance of restraints, and removal of indwelling catheters can decrease infection risks and improve rehabilitative care. Physical and occupational therapy can assist with mobility and ADLs. Daily reviews of medical care, medications, nutrition, and emphasis on discharge needs of patients and caregivers can expedite recovery and improve outcomes.[50] Evidence supports utilization of care bundles to improve process of care.[50] Bundles such as Awakening and Breathing Coordination, Delirium Monitoring and Management, and Early Mobility (ABCDE) standardize care through algorithms.[50] Intraprofessional teams pair sedation protocols and daily awakening for ventilator management; use the Confusion Assessment Method-ICU (CAM-ICU) or the Intensive Care Delirium Screening Checklist (ICDSC) for delirium screening, and mobilize patients based on individual physiologic stability and

TABLE 41-8 CARDIAC MEDICATION CONSIDERATIONS IN OLDER ADULTS

MEDICATION	CLINICAL CONSIDERATIONS
Thiazide diuretics • Hydrochlorothiazide (HCTZ) • Chlorthalidone • Bendrofluazide	Recommended for initial hypertensive therapy • ↓ peripheral vascular resistance • ↓ intravascular volume • ↓ BP • Generally well tolerated in older adults • ↓ CV, cerebrovascular, renal adverse outcomes • May exacerbate arrhythmias, hyperuricemia, glucose intolerance, and dyslipidemia
Nonthiazide diuretics • Indapamide-sulfonamide diuretic	• Increases blood glucose • Does not increase uric acid • Can cause potassium independent prolongation of the QT interval
• Furosemide-loop diuretic	• Increases glucose • May cause headaches, fever, anemia • May cause electrolyte disturbances
Mineralocorticoid antagonists • Spironolactone/eplerenone	Useful in hypertension when combined with other agents • Causes potassium retention • Not associated with adverse metabolic effects
Beta-blockers • Metoprolol	Indicated for older adult patients with • Hypertension CAD, HF • Certain arrhythmias • Migraine headaches • Senile tremor
Calcium antagonists (CAs) • Phenylalkylamines-verapamil • Benzothiazepines-diltiazem • Dihydropyridines-nicardipine	• Variable effects on heart muscle, sinus node function, atrioventricular conduction, peripheral arteries, and coronary circulation • Effective in older adult patients with hypertension due to increasing arterial stiffness, decreased vascular angina and supraventricular arrhythmias, compliance, and diastolic dysfunction
Angiotensin-converting enzyme inhibitors (ACEIs) • Captopril (Capoten) • Enalapril (Vasotec) • Lisinopril (Prinivil, Zestril)	Blocks conversion of angiotensin I to angiotensin II in tissue and plasma • Lowers peripheral vascular resistance and BP without reflex stimulation of heart rate and contractility ACEIs reduce morbidity and mortality in patients with • HF, reduced systolic function, post-MI • Retard progression of diabetic renal disease and hypertensive nephrosclerosis
Angiotensin-receptor blockers (ARBs) • Losartan (Cozaar) • Valsartan (Diovan)	Selectively block AT1-receptor subtype to • Reduce BP • Protect the kidney • Reduce mortality and morbidity in HF patients ARBs are considered first line and as an alternative to ACEI in older adult hypertensive patients with diabetes mellitus, hypertension, and HF who cannot tolerate ACEIs
Direct renin inhibitors • Aliskiren	• Effective for BP lowering without dose-related increases in adverse events in older adult patients • May be used in combination therapy
Nonspecific vasodilators • Hydralazine • Minoxidil	Fourth-line antihypertensive due to unfavorable side effects • Tachycardia • Fluid accumulation and atrial arrhythmias (minoxidil) used as part of combination regimens • Centrally acting agents (e.g., clonidine) are not first-line treatments in older adults because of sedation and/or bradycardia • Abrupt discontinuation leads to increased BP and heart rate, which may aggravate ischemia and/or HF • These agents should not be considered in noncompliant patients but may be used as part of a combination regimen if needed after several other agents are deployed
Centrally acting agents • Clonidine	• Not first-line treatments in older adults because of sedation and/or bradycardia • Abrupt discontinuation leads to increased BP and HR

Adapted from Aronow WS, Fleg JL, Pepine CJ, et al. ACCF/AHA 2011 expert consensus document on hypertension in the elderly: a report of the American College of Cardiology Foundation Task Force on Clinical Expert Consensus Documents. *J Am Coll Cardiol.* 2011;57:2037.

TABLE 41-9 POTENTIALLY INAPPROPRIATE SYMPTOM MANAGEMENT MEDICATIONS FOR OLDER ADULTS

MEDICATION	POSSIBLE SIDE EFFECT
Nonsteroidal Anti-Inflammatory Drugs (NSAIDs)[‡]	
Indomethacin	Central nervous system (CNS) effects (highest of all NSAIDs)*
Ketorolac	Asymptomatic gastrointestinal conditions (ulcers*)
Aspirin (>325 mg)	Asymptomatic gastrointestinal conditions (ulcers*)
Naproxen	Gastrointestinal bleeding*; renal failure*; high blood pressure*; heart failure*
Opioids	
Meperidine	Intense side-effect profile for adverse effects, especially CNS effects (seizures) Most critical in individuals with renal compromise*
Morphine, hydromorphone, fentanyl	Intense side-effect profile at higher doses, especially CNS effects (such as somnolence, respiratory depression, and delirium)*
Adjuvant Medications	
Muscle relaxants (methocarbamol, carisoprodol, chlorzoxazone, metaxalone, cyclobenzaprine, baclofen)	Anticholinergic effects*[†]; sedation*; weakness*; cognitive impairment*
Tricyclic antidepressants (amitriptyline and amitriptyline compounds)	Strong anticholinergic effects*[†]; may lead to ataxia, impaired psychomotor function, syncope, falls; cardiac arrhythmias (QT interval changes)*; may produce polyuria or lead to urinary incontinence*; may exacerbate chronic constipation
Doxepin	Cardiac arrhythmias*; may produce polyuria or lead to urinary incontinence*; may exacerbate chronic constipation
Antihistamines (diphenhydramine, hydroxyzine, promethazine)	Potent anticholinergic properties*[†] May lead to confusion and sedation
Benzodiazepines	Increased sensitivity at higher doses with prolonged sedation and increased risk for falls
Short acting (lorazepam ≥3 mg, oxazepam ≥60 mg, alprazolam ≥2 mg)	May produce or exacerbate depression; smaller doses may be both effective and safer
Long acting (diazepam)	CNS effects*; may cause or exacerbate respiratory depression in chronic obstructive pulmonary disease*; may produce polyuria or lead to urinary incontinence*
Selective serotonin reuptake inhibitor antidepressants (fluoxetine, citalopram, paroxetine, sertraline)	May produce CNS stimulation, sleep disturbances, and increasing agitation*; may exacerbate or cause syndrome of inappropriate secretion of antidiuretic hormone or hyponatremia
Decongestants	High level of CNS stimulation, which may lead to insomnia*
CNS stimulants (methylphenidate)	Altered CNS function, leading to cognitive impairment*; appetite-suppressing effect*

Based on data from Fick DM, et al. Updating the Beers criteria for potentially inappropriate medication use in older adults: results of a U.S. consensus panel of experts. *Arch Intern Med.* 2003;163(22):2716; Laroche ML, Charmes JP, Merle L. Potentially inappropriate medications in the elderly: a French consensus panel. *Eur J Clinical Pharmacol.* 2007;63(8),725.
*High-severity rating.
[†]Anticholinergic effects include some of the following symptoms: blurred vision, constipation, drowsiness, sedation, dry mouth, tachycardia, urinary retention, confusion, disorientation, memory impairment, dizziness, nausea, nervousness, agitation, anxiety, facial flushing, weakness, and delirium.
[‡]May cause or exacerbate gastric or duodenal ulcers, prolonged clotting time and international normalized ratio, and decreased platelet function.

readiness.[51] These strategies allow for optimal patient progression along the continuum of care.

Care Transitions

Transitions of care and provider hand-off within one episode of care are difficult for older adults, resulting in multiple touch points and increasing fragmentation of care due to incomplete transfer of information between health care providers.[52] Families and informal caregivers of vulnerable older adults often become the messengers between providers. Older adults without family frequently remain in higher levels of care for extended time periods, reducing bed availability for others. Several

models exist for a new nursing role known as a *navigator.* Navigators combine the role of nurse, social worker, and case manager to assist high-risk older patients through transitions of care. The navigation role may offer opportunity for vulnerable populations and older adults to safely navigate the complex continuum of care while assisting with economic and clinical outcomes.[52]

Palliative Care and End of Life in Critical Care

In 2001, 17% of U.S. deaths occurred in critical care units, with 47% of hospital deaths preceded by a critical care unit stay.[53] Almost three-quarters of all deaths in the United States occur among persons 65 years of age and over, accounting for about 1.8 million deaths in 2007.[53] During the past decade, overall death rates have declined by 8% for this age group. Older adult deaths account for 42% to 52% of admissions to critical care units and for almost 60% of all critical care unit days.[2] Because of this, palliative care is a necessary part of critical care nursing.

Palliative care is frequently misconstrued as synonymous with withdrawal of life support in the critical care unit. Palliative care is focused on the relief of suffering, in all of its dimensions, throughout the course of a patient's illness. Palliative care teams offer specialized medical care for people with serious illnesses. Palliative care teams focus on providing patients with relief from symptoms, pain, and stress of serious illness irrespective of diagnosis. The goal is to improve QOL for both the patient and the family. (Visit this website for more information: http://www.getpalliativecare.org.) Palliative care teams can assist with pain/symptom assessment, social/spiritual assessment, understanding of illness/prognosis, treatment options, identification of patient-centered goals of care, and transition of care postdischarge.[54]

Compassionate end-of-life care in accordance with patient wishes is an essential component of critical care. Studies have found that performance of specific evidence-based care processes are essential components of high-quality critical care but these specific practices are inconsistent and infrequent.[55] Recommendations include use of care and communication bundles. These bundles provide daily goals of care to be performed on specified days. For example, day 1 interventions include identification of a decision-maker, advance directives, and resuscitation preferences. On day 1 families are also provided with information and patients symptoms are managed. Day 3 interventions include support from social work or spiritual support and consideration of plans for a family meeting. Critical care nurses must be skilled in end of-life care just as in clinical competency. Team collaboration promotes clear communication and goal alignment for patients and families.[56]

CONCLUSION

Older adults require more intense observation and consideration in critical care units because they are less adaptable to stress and illness. Table 41-10 summarizes the major changes in various systems with clinical considerations.[2] As shown in Figure 41-3, many physiologic changes occur with advancing age, and each change may render a particular system less adaptable to stress. Changes in one system may affect another system in the presence of disease. The inability to adapt poses a significant risk for functional decline after discharge. Older adults at greatest risk include those with poor nutritional status or cognitive dysfunction and those who required assistance with at least two ADLs before admission. To provide the best care and prevent iatrogenic complications, the critical care nurse must consider all physiologic and psychologic factors that affect the older adult patient.

TABLE 41-10	PHYSIOLOGIC CHANGES OF AGING AND THEIR RELATIONSHIP TO SYMPTOM MANAGEMENT CHANGE	
AGE-RELATED EFFECT	**CLINICAL CONSIDERATIONS**
Skin	
Decreased cutaneous layers and thinned subcutaneous tissue	Can increase risk for effects of anorexia and cachexia
Decreased blood vessels	May alter absorption of transdermal medications May decrease ability to use intravenous route for symptom management
Decreased nerves	May alter pain sensation
Decreased elasticity	Increases risk for skin tears
Bones	
Altered calcium metabolism leading to bone loss	Increases risk for bone instability with metastatic bone disease
Tooth loss	Increases risk for malnutrition during therapy and subsequent nutrition-related symptoms such as anemia, mucous membrane and skin breakdown, and electrolyte disturbances
Soft Tissue	
Muscle atrophy	Decreases strength and endurance, which may increase fatigue
Nervous system slowing	Decreases fine motor control, which may have an impact on implementing symptom management strategies
Increased body fat	May have an impact on medication metabolism

TABLE 41-10 PHYSIOLOGIC CHANGES OF AGING AND THEIR RELATIONSHIP TO SYMPTOM MANAGEMENT CHANGE—cont'd

AGE-RELATED EFFECT	CLINICAL CONSIDERATIONS
Sensory Loss	
Hearing	May have an impact on communication of patient education information for symptom management
Vision	May have an impact on communication of patient education information for symptom management
Smell	May have an impact on successful treatment of anorexia or cachexia
Hematology and Immunology	
Decreased bone marrow reserve	May have delayed response to infection and anemia
Anemia related to decreased intrinsic factor production and decreased iron metabolism	May contribute to cancer-related fatigue
Increased clotting caused by increased platelet adhesion	May contribute to perfusion issues and lead to vague, non–cancer-related symptoms
Circulation	
Enlargement of heart; slowing of electrical activity; and changes in collagen in arteries, causing stiffness and thickening	Caution should be used with symptom management medications that may affect cardiac function, such as medications used for treating neuropathic pain
Pulmonary	
Decreased oxygen and carbon dioxide exchange because of decreased elasticity of lung tissue and alveoli enlargement	Caution should be used with medications that have a direct effect on pulmonary functioning, such as benzodiazepines or opioids
Decreased cough reflex and ciliary function	May increase risk of decreased airway clearance
Gastrointestinal	
Decline in small intestinal absorption of vitamins D and B_{12} and folic acid	Increases risk for developing anemia and bone loss
Thinning of intestinal lining, decreased mucus production, and weaker intestinal muscles	Increases risk for constipation
Diminished liver function because of circulatory and metabolic changes	May have an impact on medication metabolism by slowing drug metabolism and leading to increased medication toxicity
Urinary	
Decreased renal perfusion beginning at age 40 years	Increases risk for developing drug toxicity, especially with nonsteroidal anti-inflammatory medications and diuretics
Decreased number of nephrons and glomeruli with decreased glomerular filtration rate	May increase risk for dehydration or fluid overload
Decreased adaptability of kidneys to handle stress	Altered potassium regulation
Decreased bladder capacity and tone Decreased tone of pelvic floor	May lead to urinary incontinence
Enlargement of prostate	Eventually leads to lower urinary tract symptoms
Cognitive	
Decrease in short-term memory	May decrease ability to remember details of symptom onset, duration, and treatment

Based on data from Lacasse C. Polypharmacy and symptom management in older adults. *Clin J Oncology Nurs.* 2010;15(1):27. doi: 10.1188/11. CJON. 27-30; Aldwin CM, Gilmer DF. *Health, Illness, and Optimal Aging.* Thousand Oaks, CA: Sage; 2004; Tabloski PA. *Gerontological Nursing.* Upper Saddle River, NJ: Pearson Prentice Hall; 2006.

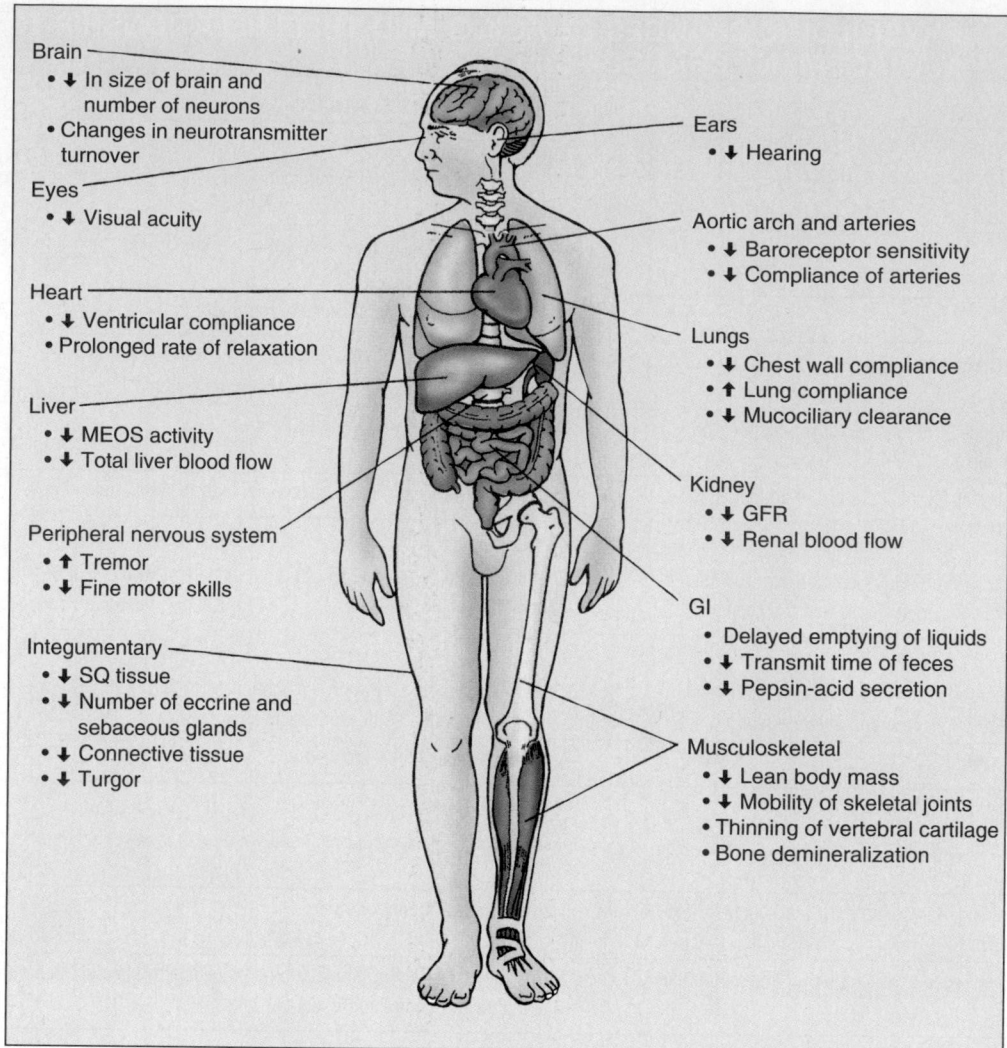

FIGURE 41-3   Summary of the physiologic changes that occur in all systems and that the critical care nurse must consider in caring for the older adult patient in the critical care unit. *GFR*, Glomerular filtration rate; *GI*, gastrointestinal; *MEOS*, microsomal enzyme oxidative system; *SQ*, subcutaneous.

BOX 41-2   CASE STUDY

Older Patient with Gastrointestinal Bleeding and Delirium

Brief Patient History

Ms. Jones is an 85-year-old woman with a long history of diabetes treated with insulin. Over the past week, Ms. Jones has experienced fatigue, nausea, and vomiting. She is very dizzy and weak.

Clinical Assessment

Ms. Jones is admitted to the critical care unit from the emergency department. Nursing assessment findings show limits in eyesight and poor nutritional intake. She has experienced some left shoulder pain and general aches.

Diagnostic Procedures

Ms. Jones's admission laboratory work reveals a blood glucose of level of 350 and ketones. Baseline vital signs include the following: blood pressure of 85/60 mm Hg, heart rate of 100 beats/min (atrial fibrillation), respiratory rate of 30 breaths/min, and temperature of 99.3° F, ST depression on ECG.

Medical Diagnosis

Ms. Jones is diagnosed with ketoacidosis and non–ST segment myocardial infarction.

Questions

1. What major outcomes do you expect to achieve for this patient?
2. What problems or risks must be managed to achieve these outcomes?
3. What interventions must be initiated to monitor, prevent, manage, or eliminate the problems and risks identified?
4. What interventions should be initiated to promote optimal functioning, safety, and well-being of the patient?
5. What possible learning needs do you anticipate for this patient?
6. What cultural and age-related factors may have a bearing on the patient's plan of care?

SUMMARY

Cardiovascular System

- Aorta and other arteries become stiff and less pliable, leading to increased workload on the heart to perfuse tissue.
- Systolic and diastolic pressures increase, along with an increase in systemic vascular resistance and a decrease in cardiac output.
- There is a loss of capacity in the myocardium and arterial system and decreased ability to respond and recover from periods of physiologic and psychologic stress.

Pulmonary System

- Lung tissue stiffens.
- Diffusion of gases is impaired by 8% per year after age 65 years.
- There is a decrease in vital capacity and maximal breathing capacity.

Renal System

- Decreased renal blood flow leads to a decrease in glomerular filtration and decreased renal tubule function.
- There is decreased elimination of physiologic substances (i.e., BUN and creatinine).
- The older adult is predisposed to developing metabolic acidosis, volume depletion, and hyperchloremia.

Gastrointestinal System

- Gastric emptying, splenic blood flow, and gastrointestinal motility are decreased; gastrointestinal pH and thinning or reduction of the absorptive surface of the gut are increased.

- *H. pylori* infection and medication effects increase the risk for gastrointestinal bleeding.
- Absorption rates are decreased.

Central Nervous System

- There are changes in gyral function, formation of neurofibrillary tangles, a decrease in brain volume, and increase in size of cerebral ventricles.
- Senile plaque formation increases.
- There are changes in neurotransmitter synthesis and function, and there is degeneration of the blood–brain barrier.

Immune System

- The number of gamma/delta and helper T cells increases, suppressor/cytotoxic T lymphocytes decrease, germinal centers of lymph nodes decrease, and plasma cells and lymphocytes in the bone marrow increase.
- Cell surface characteristics of lymphocytes change.
- Humoral immune and antibody responses are impaired.

Pharmacokinetics and Pharmacodynamics

- Loading and maintenance doses of certain medications should be reduced.
- Reduced clearance of medications by the kidneys from dehydration may be reversible by rehydration.
- Liver and kidney function tests need to be repeated at regular intervals or when new medications are added.
- Nonessential medications should be limited, and patients should be monitored for toxic effects associated with new medications.

REFERENCES

1. Resnick NM, et al. Geriatric medicine. In: Kasper D, et al, eds. *Harrison's Principles of Internal Medicine*. 16th ed. New York: McGraw-Hill; 2005.
2. Marik P. Management of the critically ill geriatric patient. In: O'Donnell JM, Nacul FE, eds. *Surgical Intensive Care Medicine*. 2nd ed. New York: Springer Science; 2010.
3. Armstrong J, Mitchell E. Comprehensive nursing assessment in care of older people. *Nurs Older People*. 2008;20(1):36.
4. *Centers for Disease Control and Prevention*. FastStats. http://www.cdc.gov/nchs/fastats/older_americans.htm. Accessed April 20, 2012.
5. Feldstein PJ. *Health Policy Issues: An Economic Perspective*. 5th ed. Chicago: Health Care Administration Press; 2011.
6. Halpern NA, Pastores SM. Critical care medicine in the United States 2000-2005: An analysis of bed numbers, occupancy rates, payer mix, and costs. *Crit Care Med*. 2010;38(1):65.
7. Xu JQ, Kochanek KD, Murphy SL, Tejada-Vera B. Deaths: Final data for 2007. National Vital Statistics Reports. 58(19). Hyattsville, MD: National Center for Health Statistics; 2010. http://www.cdc.gov/nchs/data/nvsr/nvsr58/nvsr58_19.pdf. Accessed May, 2012.
8. North BJ. The intersection between aging and cardiovascular disease. *Circ Res*. 2012;110(8):1097. doi. 10.1161/CIRCRESAHA.111.246876.
9. Strait J, et al. Aging-associated cardiovascular changes and their relationship to heart failure. *Heart Failures Clin*. 2012;8(1):143.
10. Aronow WS, et al. ACCF/AHA 2011 Expert Consensus Document on Hypertension in the Elderly: A Report of the American College of Cardiology Foundation Task Force on Clinical Expert Consensus Documents. *J Am Coll Cardiol*. 2011;57(20):2037.
11. Gazoti Debassa CR, Messiano Maifrino LB, Rodrigues de Souza R. Age related changes of the collagen network of the human heart. *Mech Ageing Dev*. 2001;122(2001):1049.
12. Francis GS, et al. Pathophysiology of heart failure. In: Fuster V, et al, eds. *Hurst's the Heart*. 12th ed. New York: McGraw-Hill; 2008.
13. Shih H, et al. The aging heart and post-infarction left ventricular remodeling. *JACC*. 2010;57(1):9.
14. Strandberg TE, et al. Cholesterol and glucose metabolism and recurrent cardiovascular events among the elderly: a prospective study. *J Am Coll Cardiol*. 2006;48(4):708.
15. Nenseter MS. Lipoprotein(a) levels in coronary heart disease-susceptible and -resistant patients with familial hypercholesterolemia. *Atherosclerosis*. 2011;216(2):426.
16. Hajjar I. Postural blood pressure changes and orthostatic hypotension in elderly patients: impact of antihypertensive medications. *Drugs Aging*. 2005;22(1):55.
17. Cooney D, Pascuzzi K. Polypharmacy in the elderly Focus on drug interactions and adherence in hypertension. *Clin Geriatr Med*. 2009;25:221. doi:10.1016/j.cger.2009.01.005.

18. Moss AJ, et al. Cardiacresynchronization therapy for the prevention of heart failure events. *N Engl J Med.* 2009;361:1.

19. Resnick B, Pacala JT. 2012 Beers criteria. *J Am Geriatr Soc.* 2012;60(4):612. doi: 10.1111/j.1532-5415.2012.03921.x.

20. Janssens JP. Aging of the respiratory system: impact on pulmonary function tests and adaptation to exertion. *Clin Chest Med.* 2005;26(30).

21. Fragoso CAV, Gill TM. Respiratory impairment and the aging lung: a novel paradigm for assessing pulmonary function. *J Gerontol A Biol Sci Med Sci.* 2011;67A(3):264. doi: 10.1093/gerona/glr198.

22. Bonomo L, et al. Aging and the respiratory system. *Radiol Clin North Am.* 2008;46(4).

22a. LeBlanc P, et al. Effects of age and body position on "airway closure" in man. *J Appl Physiol.* 1970;28:448.

22b. Holland J, et al. Regional distribution of pulmonary ventilation and perfusion in elderly subjects. *J Clin Invest.* 1968;47:81.

23. Chao CT, et al. Advanced age affects the outcome-predictive power of RIFLE classification in geriatric patients with acute kidney injury. *Kidney Internat.* 2012;80:1222. doi:10.1038/.

24. Clark JA, Coopersmith CM. Intestinal crosstalk: a new paradigm for understanding the gut as the "motor" of critical illness. *Shock.* 2007;28:384.

25. Bitar K, et al. Aging and gastrointestinal neuromuscular function: insights from within and outside the gut. *Neurogastroenterol Motil.* 2011;23:490.

26. Lacasse C. Polypharmacy and symptom management in older adults. *Clin J Oncol Nurs.* 2010;15(1):27. doi: 10.1188/11.CJON.27-30.

27. Schmucker DL. Age-related changes in liver structure and function: Implications for disease? *Exper Gerontol.* 2005;40:650. doi:10.1016/j.exger.2005.06.009.

28. Schmucker DL, Sanchez H. Liver regeneration and aging: a current perspective. *Curr Gerontol Geriatr Res.* 2011. Article ID 526379. doi:10.1155/2011/526379.

29. Floreani A. Liver disorders in the elderly. *Best Pract Res Clin Gastroenterol.* 2009;23:909.

30. Bishop NA, Lu T, Yankner BA. Neural mechanisms of ageing and cognitive decline. *Nature.* 2010;464:529.

31. Clare L. Neuropsychological assessment. In: Abou-Saleh MT, Katona C, Kumar A, eds. *Principles and Practice of Geriatric Psychiatry.* 3rd ed. London: John Wiley & Sons; 2011.

32. Rice KL, et al. Nurses' recognition of delirium in the hospitalized older adult. *Clin Nurse Specialist.* 2011;25(6):299. doi: 10.1097/NUR.0b013e318234897b.

33. Quinn J, Kaye J. The neurology of aging. *Neurologist.* 2001;7:98.

34. Selkoe DJ. Aging brain, aging mind. *Sci Am.* 1992;267:134.

35. Gottstein U, Held K. Effects of aging on cerebral circulation and metabolism in man. *Acta Neurol Scand Suppl.* 1979;72:54.

36. Jones RN, et al. Aging, brain disease, and reserve: implications for delirium. *Am J Geriatr Psychiatry.* 2010;18(2):117.

37. Naatanen R, et al. The mismatch negativity: an index of cognitive decline in neuropsychiatric and neurological diseases and in ageing. *Brain.* 2011;134:3435. doi:10.1093/brain/awr064.

38. Mink J. The neurologic assessment toolbox: key assessments at critical times. *Nurs 2012 Crit Care.* 2012;7(3):12.

39. Ehlenbach WJ, et al. Association between acute care and critical illness hospitalization and cognitive function in older adults. *JAMA.* 2010;303(8):763.

40. Htwe TH, et al. Infection in the elderly. *Infect Dis Clin North Am.* 2007;21(3):711.

41. Akha AAS, Miller RA. Signal transduction in the aging immune system. *Curr Opin Immunol.* 2005;17(5):486.

42. Smith DR, Leggat PA. Prevalence of skin disease among the elderly in different clinical environments. *Austral J Ageing.* 2005;24(2):71.

43. Pittman J. Effect of aging on wound healing current concepts. *J WOCN.* 2007;34:412.

44. Black DM, Rosen CJ. Following the bone density trail: a clinical perspective. *J Clin Endocrinol Metabol.* 2012;97(4):1176. doi: 10.1210/jc.2012-1528.

45. Desai SV, Law TJ, Needham DM. Long-term complications of critical care. *Crit Care Med.* 2011;39(2):371.

46. Gill TM, Allore HG, Gahbauer EA, Murphy TE. Change in disability after hospitalization or restricted activity in older persons. *JAMA.* 2010;304(17):1919.

47. Covinsky KE, Pierluissi E, Johnston CB. Hospitalization-associated disability. *JAMA.* 2011;306(16):1783.

48. Fick DM, et al. Updating the Beers criteria for potentially inappropriate medication use in older adults: results of a US consensus panel of experts. *Arch Intern Med.* 2003;163(2716).

48a. Guay DRP, et al. The pharmacology of aging. In: Tallis RC, Rillit HM, eds. *Brocklehurst's Textbook of Geriatric Medicine and Gerontology.* 6th ed. London: Churchill Livingstone; 2003.

48b. Yuen GJ. Altered pharmacokinetics in the elderly. *Clin Geriatric Med.* 1990;6:257.

49. Rothschild JM, et al. The critical care safety study: the incidence and nature of adverse events and serious errors in intensive care. *Crit Care Med.* 2005;33:1694.

50. Balas M, et al. Critical care nurses' role in implementing the "ABCDE bundle" into practice. *Crit Care Nurse.* 2012;32(2):35. doi:10.4037/ccn2012229.

51. Pandharipande P, Banerjee A, McGrane S, Ely EW. Liberation and animation for ventilated ICU patients: the ABCDE bundle for the back-end of critical care. *Crit Care.* 2010;14(3):157.

52. Manderson B, et al. Navigation roles support chronically ill older adults through healthcare transitions: a systematic review of the literature. *Health Soc Care Community.* 2012;20(2):113. doi: 10.1111/j.1365-2524.2011.01032.x.

53. Wunsch H, et al. Use of intensive care services during terminal hospitalizations in England and the United States. *Am J Respir Crit Care Med.* 2009;180(9):875.

54. Frost DW, Cook DJ, Heyland DK. Patient and healthcare professional factors influencing end-of-life decision-making during critical illness: a systematic review. *Crit Care Med.* 2011;39(5):1134.

55. Penrod JD, Pronovost PJ, Livote EE. Meeting standards of high-quality intensive care unit palliative care: clinical performance and predictors. *Crit Care Med.* 2012;40(4):1105. doi: 10.1097/CCM.0b013e3182374a50.

56. Lamas D, Rosenbaum L. Freedom from the tyranny of choice—teaching the end-of-life conversion. *New England Journal of Medicine.* 2012;366(18):1655. doi: 10.1056/NEJMp1201202.

The Perianesthesia Patient

Denise O'Brien

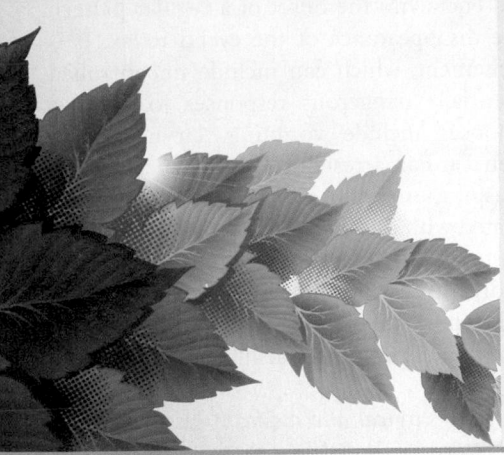

Advances in anesthetic agents and monitoring have resulted in more precise and safer delivery of anesthetic agents. Caring for the critically ill patient who is emerging from anesthesia requires diligent monitoring of the patient's physical and psychologic status to prevent potential complications that may occur as a result of the anesthetic agents or techniques. To provide safe and competent patient care, the critical care nurse needs knowledge of anesthetic agents and techniques and the physiologic and psychologic responses of patients who receive anesthesia.[1,2]

SELECTION OF ANESTHESIA

The complex structure of the anesthetic agents, combined with potential medication interactions and the patient's physical condition, can make it difficult to predict the patient's response when emerging from anesthesia. Knowledge of the general principles of anesthesia prepares the nurse for the most commonly expected outcomes.[2,3] The American Society of Anesthesiologists' physical status classification is widely accepted as a method of preoperative patient evaluation.[4] It guides communication of clinical conditions and predicts risks for anesthesia (Box 42-1). Preoperative evaluation allows the anesthesia care provider to individualize and modify care for patients at high risk for surgery.[4]

The type of anesthesia used for surgery may be local, regional, or general. Local and regional anesthetics eliminate the sensation of pain to a specific part of the body without loss of protective reflexes or consciousness. Many patients also receive intravenous sedation with benzodiazepines to relieve anxiety, provide amnesia, and promote relaxation. Local anesthesia with sedation may be defined as moderate or *procedural* sedation. Another term used is *monitored anesthesia care*. Depending on the sedation given and the patient's response, the level of consciousness can range from light to deep. Further information on sedation is provided in Chapter 10. Regional anesthesia includes peripheral and central neuraxial (spinal, epidural, caudal) blocks. The blocks include single injection and continuous infusion techniques, typically used for postoperative or postprocedural analgesia. Spinal anesthesia involves injecting local anesthetic into cerebrospinal fluid contained within the subarachnoid space, below L1 in the adult and L3 in the child.[5] Epidural anesthesia involves injecting the epidural space, which lies within the vertebral canal but outside the dural sac, with local anesthetics. Epidurals may be performed at all levels of the neuraxis. Spinal and epidural anesthesia cause sensory and motor anesthesia. The advantages of epidural over spinal anesthesia are a decreased incidence of spinal headache, less incidence of systemic hypotension, ability to provide a segmental sensory block, and increased ability to provide postoperative pain management.[6]

General anesthesia is a controlled, reversible state of unconsciousness: the patient is not arousable, there is partial or complete loss of protective reflexes, and the airway and ventilation needs to be continuously monitored and maintained. An endotracheal tube is commonly used for airway maintenance for general anesthesia, although a laryngeal mask airway (LMA) may also be used.[7]

Several factors influence the choice of anesthetic agent and the mode of delivery, including age and coexisting diseases, site of surgery, position of patient during surgery, status of surgery (i.e. elective, emergent), duration of the procedure, the skills of the anesthesia care provider and surgeon, and patient preference.[8]

GENERAL ANESTHESIA

The goals of general anesthesia are analgesia, amnesia/hypnosis, suppression of autonomic and sensory reflexes, and skeletal muscle relaxation.[9] Stages of anesthesia, defined by Guedel around World War I, were initially used to identify the patient's physiologic state and monitor anesthetic depth. These stages are less relevant today due to technologic advances in monitoring and anesthetic agents with faster onset and elimination, limiting the usefulness of the classic signs and symptoms associated with the stages to assessment and care of the patient after surgery.[10]

Stage I, commonly called the *stage of analgesia*, begins with the initiation of an anesthetic agent and ends with the loss of consciousness. This stage has been described as the lightest level of anesthesia and represents mild sensory and mental depression. Patients can open their eyes on command, breathe normally, and maintain protective reflexes. The patient's pain threshold is not appreciably lowered during this stage.

Stage II, also called the *stage of delirium*, begins with the loss of consciousness and ends with the onset of a regular pattern of breathing and the disappearance of the eyelid reflex. It is characterized by excitement, which can include uncontrolled movement and potentially dangerous responses to noxious stimuli. Other responses include vomiting, laryngospasm, tachycardia, and even cardiac arrest. If vomiting occurs, the patient is at risk for aspiration because of the loss of protective reflexes that is associated with this stage of anesthesia. With the use of newer and faster-acting anesthetic agents, this stage is passed through rapidly, decreasing the risk of complications. The use of propofol, etomidate, or short-acting barbiturates during the induction of anesthesia also facilitates rapid transition through stage II.

Stage III is the *stage of surgical anesthesia*. It lasts from the onset of a regular pattern of breathing to the cessation of breathing. This is the goal for anesthesia, because the response to surgical incision is absent. Patients experience a depression in all elements of nervous system function (i.e., sensory depression, loss of recall, reflex depression, and some skeletal muscle relaxation). Each anesthetic agent affects the patient's clinical signs differently; therefore, monitoring the effects of anesthesia depends on the specific properties of each agent.

Stage IV is considered the *stage of overdose* and occurs when the patient receives too much anesthesia. In this stage, the patient shows signs of circulatory failure, and full cardiovascular and pulmonary support must be provided.

During general anesthesia, the goal is to keep the patient insensate, immobile, and safe. Recall or awareness during surgery can occur when the depth of anesthesia is inadequate (Box 42-2). Excessive anesthesia may stress the patient and increase emergence and recovery time. The level of anesthesia is monitored by continual assessment of the patient's clinical presentation. Basic anesthetic monitoring standards adopted by the American Society of Anesthesiologists (ASA) mandate the use of pulse oximetry, capnography, an oxygen analyzer, disconnect alarms, body temperature measurements, and a visual display of an electrocardiogram (ECG) during the

---

BOX 42-1 AMERICAN SOCIETY OF ANESTHESIOLOGISTS' PHYSICAL STATUS CLASSIFICATION

- Category 1: Normal, healthy patient
- Category 2: Patient with mild systemic disease
- Category 3: Patient with severe systemic disease (e.g., hypertension, diabetes)
- Category 4: Patient with severe systemic disease that is a threat to life
- Category 5: Patient with high morbidity
- Category 6: Brain death

⚡ BOX 42-2 PATIENT SAFETY ALERT

Preventing and Managing the Impact of Anesthesia Awareness

QSEN Anesthesia awareness, also called unintended intraoperative awareness, occurs under general anesthesia when a patient becomes cognizant of some or all events during a procedure and has direct recall of those events. Because of the routine use of neuromuscular blocking agents (paralytics) during general anesthesia, the patient is often unable to communicate with the surgical team when this occurs.

The frequency of anesthesia awareness has been found in multiple studies to range between 0.1% and 0.2% of all patients undergoing general anesthesia.[1-3] General anesthesia is administered to 21 million patients annually in the United States, so 20,000 to 40,000 cases of anesthesia awareness occur each year. Patients experiencing awareness report auditory recollections (48%), sensations of not being able to breathe (48%), and pain (28%).[1] More than 50% experience mental distress after surgery, including an indeterminate number with post-traumatic stress syndrome.[2,3] Some patients describe these occurrences as their "worst hospital experience," and some determine to never again undergo surgery.

The incidence of awareness is reported to be greater in patients for whom the dose of general anesthetic must be smaller and carefully titrated to decrease significant side effects, such as a patient who is hemodynamically unstable. Procedures typically identified as falling into this category are some cardiac, obstetric, and major trauma cases.[4] Factors contributing to the risk of anesthesia awareness include the increasing use of intravenous delivery of anesthesia, as opposed to inhalation, and the premature lightening of anesthesia at the end of procedures to facilitate operating room turnover.

Monitoring of patients under general anesthesia to prevent anesthesia awareness can be challenging. Despite a variety of available monitoring methods, awareness is difficult to recognize while it is occurring. Typical indicators of physiologic and motor response, such as high blood pressure, fast heart rate, movement, and hemodynamic changes, are often masked by the use of paralytic agents to achieve necessary muscle relaxation during the procedure, as well as the concurrent administration of other medications necessary to the patient's management, such as beta-blockers or calcium channel blockers.

⚡ BOX 42-2   PATIENT SAFETY ALERT

Preventing and Managing the Impact of Anesthesia Awareness—cont'd

To overcome the limitations of current methods to detect anesthesia awareness, new methods are being developed that are less affected by the medications typically used during general anesthesia. These devices measure brain activity rather than physiologic responses. These electroencephalography devices (also called level-of-consciousness, sedation-level, or anesthesia-depth monitors) include the Bispectral Index (BIS), spectral edge frequency (SEF), and median frequency (MF) monitors. These devices may have a role in preventing and detecting anesthesia awareness in patients with the highest risk, thereby ameliorating the impact of anesthesia awareness. A body of evidence has not yet accumulated to precisely define the role of these devices in detecting and preventing anesthesia awareness; The Joint Commission expects additional studies on these subjects to emerge. In its review of the BIS monitor, the U.S. Food and Drug Administration determined that "Use of BIS monitoring to help guide anesthetic administration may be associated with the reduction of the incidence of awareness with recall in adults during general anesthesia and sedation."

The anesthesia professional must often balance the psychologic risks of anesthesia awareness against the physiologic risks of excessive anesthesia for many critical medical conditions. The Joint Commission has asked the American Society of Anesthesiologists (ASA) and the American Association of Nurse Anesthetists (AANA) to address the adequacy of current monitoring practices regarding anesthesia levels, including those practices that involve little or no technologic support. The ASA recommends in its 2006 practice advisory that intraoperative monitoring include clinical (e.g., purposeful or reflex movement), conventional monitors (e.g., end-tidal anesthetic analyzer, HR, BP), and brain function monitoring on a case-by-case basis.[5] Multimodal monitoring is suggested rather than reliance on any single monitor.

Reducing the Risk of Anesthesia Awareness

The ASA and the AANA provide guidelines for administering and monitoring anesthesia. Specific recommendations for the prevention of awareness were addressed in the February 2000 issue of *Anesthesiology*[4]:

- Consider premedication with amnesic medications (e.g., benzodiazepines, scopolamine), particularly when light anesthesia is anticipated.
- Administer more than a "sleep dose" of induction agents if they will be followed immediately by tracheal intubation. Avoid muscle paralysis unless absolutely necessary and, even then, avoid total paralysis (by using only the amount clinically required).
- Conduct periodic maintenance of the anesthesia machine and its vaporizers, and meticulously check the machine and its ventilator before administering anesthesia.
- Be alert to patients taking beta-blockers, calcium channel blockers, or other medications that can mask physiologic responses to inadequate anesthesia.

Managing the Impact of Anesthesia Awareness

Anesthesia awareness cannot always be prevented. Health care practitioners must be prepared to acknowledge and manage the occurrence of anesthesia awareness with compassion and diligence. The following practices are suggested when patients report awareness[4]:

- Interview the patient after the procedure, taking a detailed account of his or her experience and including it in the patient's chart.
- Apologize to the patient if anesthesia awareness occurred.
- Assure the patient of the credibility of his or her account, and sympathize with the patient's suffering.

- Explain what happened and its reasons (e.g., the necessity to administer light anesthesia in the presence of significant cardiovascular instability).
- Offer the patient psychologic or psychiatric support, including referral to a psychiatrist or psychologist.
- Notify the patient's surgeon, nurse, and other key personnel about the incident and the subsequent interview with the patient.

Surgical team members should also be educated about anesthesia awareness and its management.

Joint Commission Recommendations

Anesthesia awareness is underrecognized and undertreated in health care organizations. The Joint Commission recommends that health care organizations performing procedures under general anesthesia take the following steps to help prevent and manage anesthesia awareness:

1. Develop and implement an anesthesia awareness policy that addresses the following:
   - Education of clinical staff about anesthesia awareness and how to manage patients who have experienced awareness.
   - Identification of patients at proportionately higher risk for an awareness experience and discussion with such patients, before surgery, of the potential for anesthesia awareness.
   - The effective application of available anesthesia monitoring techniques, including timely maintenance of anesthesia equipment.
   - Appropriate postoperative follow-up of all patients who have undergone general anesthesia, including children.
   - The identification, management, and, if appropriate, referral of patients who have experienced awareness.
2. Ensure access to necessary counseling or other support for patients who are experiencing post-traumatic stress syndrome or other mental distress.

References

1. Sebel PS, Bowdle TA, Ghoneim MM, et al. The incidence of awareness during anesthesia: a multicenter United States study. *Anesth Analg.* 2004;99(3):833.
2. Lennmarken C, Sandin R. Neuromonitoring for awareness during surgery. *Lancet.* 2004;363(9423):1747.
3. Osterman JE, Hopper J, Heran WJ, et al. Awareness under anesthesia and the development of posttraumatic stress disorder. *Gen Hosp Psychiatry.* 2001;23(4):198.
4. Ghoneim MM. Awareness during anesthesia. *Anesthesiology.* 2000;92(2):597.
5. Practice advisory for intraoperative awareness and brain function monitoring: A report by the American Society of Anesthesiologists Task Force on Intraoperative Awareness. *Anesthesiology.* 2006;104:847.

Bibliography

Ekman A, Lindholm ML, Lennmarken C, et al. Reduction in the incidence of awareness using BIS monitoring. *Acta Anaesthesiol Scand.* 2004;48(1):20.

Liska JM. *Silenced screams: surviving anesthetic awareness during surgery—a true-life account.* Park Ridge, IL: AANA Publishing, Council for Public Interest in Anesthesia; 2002.

Myles PS, Leslie K, McNeil J, et al. Bispectral index monitoring to prevent awareness during anaesthesia: the B-Aware randomised controlled trial. *Lancet.* 2004;363(9423):1757.

Modified from *The Joint Commission*. Sentinel event alert. Issue 32. October 6, 2004. http://www.jointcommission.org/SentinelEvents/SentinelEventAlert/sea_32.htm. Accessed September 2012.

intraoperative period in all patients undergoing anesthesia.[11] The standard may be exceeded as warranted by the patient's condition and additional monitors used. External monitoring devices used to assess levels of anesthesia include lower esophageal contractility, heart rate variability, surface electromyogram, spontaneous electroencephalographic activity monitors, and evoked potentials.

ANESTHETIC AGENTS

Typically two or more anesthetic agents are used in combination to achieve the desired level of anesthesia. To anticipate the patient's response, it is important for the nurse to have knowledge of the anesthetic agents that are used and their usual physiologic effects.[2] The characteristics of ideal anesthetic agents and adjuncts are listed in Box 42-3.

Inhalation Agents

Inhalation agents are used for induction and maintenance of anesthesia or, in combination with other anesthetic agents, to maintain surgical anesthesia. They can be classified as volatile

---

BOX 42-3 CHARACTERISTICS OF IDEAL ANESTHETIC AGENTS AND ADJUNCTS

- Rapid onset of action
- Controllable duration of action
- Identifiable levels of depth
- Technically easy to administer
- No untoward effects on hemodynamic status
- No toxic metabolites
- Predictable elimination
- High specificity of action
- High margin of safety
- Useful with all ages
- Cost-effective
- Rapid emergence

---

or gaseous. Volatile agents are further classified as halogenated hydrocarbons or ethers, are liquid at room temperature, and have a boiling point of 20° C. Gaseous agents are gases at room temperature. Inhaled anesthetics are delivered through the respiratory tract and are absorbed into the circulation through the alveoli. The effects of inhalation agents depend on alveolar ventilation, the ventilation-perfusion ratio, co-administered gases, gas flow, and the physicochemical properties of the gas. Their exact mechanism of action is unknown, but all cause central nervous system (CNS) depression and a state of unconsciousness that is deep enough to allow surgery. Table 42-1 lists the inhalation anesthetics presently used and their chief characteristics, effects, and nursing implications.[10]

Intravenous Anesthetics

Because inhalation anesthetics can produce adverse effects such as vasodilation, hypotension, dysrhythmias, and myocardial depression, other medications and methods of delivery have been sought to provide general anesthesia. Intravenous anesthetics are commonly used in the perioperative period. Intravenous anesthetics are grouped by their primary pharmacologic action as nonopioid or opioid intravenous agents.[12-14] The nonopioid agents are further divided into the barbiturates, nonbarbiturates, and sedatives. These medications can be administered by intermittent intravenous push dosing to induce anesthesia or by continuous intravenous drip to maintain anesthesia.

Nonopioid Intravenous Anesthetics

Gamma-aminobutyric acid (GABA) is an inhibitory neurotransmitter. The nonopioid medications appear to interact with GABA in the brain. Activation of the GABA receptors inhibits the postsynaptic neurons and results in a loss of consciousness. Barbiturates bind to GABA postsynaptic receptors, inhibiting neuronal activity and causing a loss of consciousness. Sedatives such as benzodiazepines potentiate the action of GABA, leading to inhibition of neuronal activity. Nonbarbiturate induction agents, such as etomidate, antagonize the

---

TABLE 42-1 INHALATION ANESTHETICS

MEDICATION	CHARACTERISTICS	EFFECTS	CONSIDERATIONS
Nitrous oxide	Light anesthetic; inorganic gas; nontoxic, nonirritating; carrier for other inhalation agents; always given with oxygen	Anesthetic and analgesic; minimal pulmonary, cardiac, or CNS effects; increases intracranial pressure; amnesia	Eliminated by ventilation; postoperative nausea and vomiting; diffusion hypoxia; mild myocardial depression
Isoflurane (Forane)	Pungent, ether-like odor; low potential for toxicity; volatile agent	Higher cardiovascular stability; potentiates muscle relaxants	Mild depression of spontaneous ventilation; may trigger malignant hyperthermia; postoperative shivering; fewer dysrhythmias noted
Desflurane (Suprane)	Strong, pungent odor; rapid onset; volatile agent; requires warmed vaporizer for administration	Minimal metabolism; respiratory depression; cardiovascular depression; no lingering analgesia	Observe for breath holding; coughing and laryngospasm; may trigger malignant hyperthermia; needs immediate postoperative analgesia
Sevoflurane (Ultane)	Nonirritating to airway; volatile agent; choice for pediatric anesthetic	Minimal airway irritation; rapid elimination; great precision and control over anesthetic depth; decreases SVR	May trigger malignant hyperthermia; observe for breath holding; needs immediate postoperative analgesia

CNS, Central nervous system; *SVR,* systemic vascular resistance.

muscarinic receptors in the CNS and work as opioid agonists, resulting in a hypnotic state and loss of consciousness. Table 42-2 presents the nonopioid intravenous anesthetics and their effects and nursing considerations.[12]

Benzodiazepine Antagonists

Flumazenil (Romazicon) reverses the sedative, amnesic, respiratory depressant, and muscle-relaxant effects of benzodiazepines.[14] This medication is specific for the benzodiazepine receptors and does not reverse the effects of barbiturates or opiates. It should be used with caution in patients who have a history of seizures or chronic benzodiazepine use, as it can precipitate seizures. Because flumazenil has a shorter duration of action than most of the benzodiazepines, the risk of resedation can occur after the initial dose starts to wear off, especially when high doses of benzodiazepines are administered. The patient must be monitored for resedation and other residual effects. If the patient develops signs of resedation, flumazenil is repeated at 20-minute intervals. Flumazenil has proved to be a valuable asset in the care of the patient who has received an excessive dose of a benzodiazepine such as midazolam or lorazepam. Consequently, flumazenil is very useful intraoperatively, postoperatively, and in the critical care unit.

Opioid Intravenous Anesthetics

Intravenous opioid anesthetics play an important role in clinical anesthesia care. These medications enhance the effectiveness of inhalation agents by providing the analgesic portion of the anesthetic process. Intravenous opioids blunt the sympathetic response to painful stimuli during anesthesia. The use of opioids allows for reduction in the concentration of the inhalation agent to be administered, increasing safety. Opioids bind to specific receptors and produce a morphine-like or opioid agonist effect. Opioids are used to manage acute and chronic pain and are administered for general anesthesia, sedation, and pain relief during regional anesthesia; they are important in all phases of the perioperative experience. Table 42-3 presents a summary of clinical uses and nursing implications for the most frequently used opioids.[13]

Opioid Antagonists

Opioid antagonists are used to reverse the effects of opioids, particularly respiratory depression, restoring spontaneous ventilation in patients who are breathing inadequately. The medication of choice in perianesthesia care is naloxone (Narcan). Naloxone competes with and displaces the opioid on the receptor site; it therefore reverses respiratory depressant and analgesic effects of opioids. Naloxone is diluted and then titrated to the patient's response, minimizing the risk of rapid reversal and subsequent adverse effects. The onset of action is 1 to 2 minutes and the duration of action is 1 to 4 hours. If adequate reversal has not been achieved after 3 to 5 minutes, naloxone administration is repeated until reversal is complete.[15]

If long-acting opioids are used, the patient must be monitored for respiratory insufficiency, because the depressant effects of the opioids may return. Often, a low-dose, continuous intravenous drip of naloxone proves effective. Close monitoring of vital signs is critical. Monitor the patient for increased blood pressure, which may occur in response to pain following large doses of naloxone. In addition, tachycardia, nausea, vomiting, or diaphoresis may occur if the reversal is too rapid. Naloxone must be used with caution in patients with cardiac irritability and in patients who are physically dependent on opioids, because reversal may precipitate an acute withdrawal syndrome.

Neuromuscular Blocking Agents

Neuromuscular blocking agents (NMBAs), or muscle relaxants, interrupt the transmission of impulses from the nerve to the muscle, causing a decrease in muscle activity. Decreasing muscle activity allows the surgeon to operate in a quiet field and decreases the need for deep anesthesia. These medications have contributed greatly to clinical anesthesia care. Use of NMBAs is not limited to the operating room; they are used to facilitate endotracheal intubation, to terminate laryngospasm, to eliminate chest wall rigidity that may occur after the rapid injection of potent opioids, and to facilitate mechanical ventilation by producing total paralysis of the respiratory muscles.[15]

NMBAs cause paralysis of the respiratory muscles, and the patient receiving these agents requires ventilatory support with a handheld bag-valve-mask device or a mechanical ventilator. NMBAs do not have analgesic, amnesic, anxiolytic, or sedative effects. The paralyzed patient is not able to communicate his or her needs; NMBAs must be used in combination with other medications to prevent pain and provide sedation.

Skeletal muscle contraction occurs when acetylcholine is released from the motor neuron and binds to receptor sites on the muscle fiber (i.e., neuromuscular junction), resulting in depolarization. Skeletal muscle relaxation occurs when the release of acetylcholine ceases and any residual acetylcholine is destroyed by the enzyme acetylcholinesterase, resulting in repolarization. NMBAs interfere with the relationship between acetylcholine and the receptor. There are two general categories of skeletal muscle relaxants: nondepolarizing and depolarizing.

Depolarizing agents compete with acetylcholine at the neuromuscular junction, causing the muscle to depolarize and inhibiting repolarization. The muscle stays in a prolonged depolarized state, and movement is inhibited. The principal depolarizing skeletal muscle agent is succinylcholine (Anectine). After succinylcholine attaches to the receptor, a brief period of depolarization occurs, which is manifested by transient muscular fasciculations. Succinylcholine has a rapid onset, 60 to 90 seconds, and a short duration of action, 5 to 10 minutes. It is frequently used to facilitate intubation. Succinylcholine cannot be pharmacologically reversed.

Nondepolarizing NMBAs are typically longer-acting agents than depolarizing agents. Nondepolarizing agents do not cause initial muscle contraction or depolarization. They compete with and block the uptake of acetylcholine at the muscle receptor site and prevent repolarization. Sustained muscle relaxation occurs, and voluntary control of skeletal muscle contraction is weakened or lost.

Table 42-4 presents a pharmacologic overview of the commonly used skeletal muscle relaxants.[16] A number of factors can potentiate or antagonize the effects of nondepolarizing NMBAs; these factors are listed in Box 42-4.[17]

TABLE 42-2   NONOPIOID INTRAVENOUS ANESTHETICS

MEDICATION	CHARACTERISTICS	EFFECTS	CONSIDERATIONS
Barbiturates			
Sodium thiopental* (Pentothal)	Good patient acceptance; quick onset; very brief duration; no analgesia	CNS depression; spontaneous ventilation arrested; loss of laryngeal reflexes; causes histamine release (vasodilation, hypotension, and flushing)	IV administration painful; may cause myoclonus, coughing, and hiccoughs; increased risk of aspiration
Methohexital (Brevital)	Similar to thiopental but three times as potent; no analgesia; hepatic metabolism; ultra-fast onset of action	Similar to thiopental; lowers seizure threshold (epileptiform)	Similar to thiopental
Nonbarbiturates			
Etomidate (Amidate)	Agent of choice in patients with cardiovascular dysfunction	Heart rate and cardiac output remain constant; minimal negative inotropic effects; suppression of adrenal function up to 5-8 hours after a single dose	May cause nausea and vomiting; burns when given IV; may cause myoclonus, laryngospasm, cough, and hiccoughs; no analgesic effects
Propofol (Diprivan)	No analgesic effect; avoid in patients with coronary stenosis, ischemia, or hypovolemia; antiemetic properties; hepatic metabolism	Minimal residual CNS effects; myocardial depressant; may decrease blood pressure 20%-25%	Rapid emergence may hasten pain awareness; low incidence of postoperative side effects; pain on administration; dose reduction in older adults, patients with cardiac disease and hypovolemia; long-term or high-dose infusions can result in hypertriglyceridemia; contraindicated in patients allergic to soybean oil, egg lecithin, or glycerol
Dissociative Anesthetic			
Ketamine (Ketalar)	Profound analgesia and unconsciousness; provides amnesia; may be used alone, may be given IV, IM, or PO	Produces cardiovascular and respiratory stimulation; may increase blood pressure and heart rate 10%-50%; increases intracranial pressure	Monitor for and prevent emergent reactions; minimize stimulation of the patient during emergence; titrate pain medications; benzodiazepines or dexmedetomidine may help reduce agitation during emergence
Butyrophenones			
Haloperidol (Haldol)	Limited use in anesthesia because of long duration; antipsychotic; antiemetic	—	High incidence of extrapyramidal reactions Potential for torsade de pointes due to prolongation of QT interval
Droperidol (Inapsine)	Major tranquilizer; works with CNS as dopamine antagonist; hepatic metabolism; used in low doses for antiemetic prophylaxis	Prevents and treats nausea and vomiting; in higher doses acts as neuroleptic, causing amnesia or indifference to surroundings; adrenergic blocker, causing extrapyramidal muscle movements, hypotension, and peripheral vasodilation	Postanesthetic dysphoria (internalized overwhelming fear); effects last longer than those of opioids (rare in low doses); prolongs QT interval
Benzodiazepines			
Diazepam (Valium)	Rapid onset; long half-life; anterograde amnesic; effective anxiolysis; renal excretion	—	Titrate opioid medications and monitor for respiratory depression; used orally as premedicant
Midazolam (Versed)	Rapid onset; short duration; potent amnesic; effective anxiolysis; hepatic metabolism	—	Reduce dose in older adults, debilitated, use cautiously in patients with myocardial ischemia, COPD, and hepatic disease; titrate opioid medications; monitor for respiratory depression
Lorazepam (Ativan)	Slow onset of action; long duration; anticonvulsant action; hepatic metabolism; renal excretion; no active metabolites	Pronounced sedation; minimal cardiovascular effects	Poor IV compatibility; titrate opioid medications and monitor for respiratory depression; watch for orthostatic hypotension

*Unavailable in United States since January 2011.

CNS, Central nervous system; *COPD,* chronic obstructive pulmonary disease; *IM,* intramuscular; *IV,* intravenous; *PO,* per os (orally).

Neuromuscular Blocking Agent Antagonists

The pharmacologic actions of nondepolarizing NMBAs can be reversed by anticholinesterase medications such as neostigmine (Prostigmin). These medications increase the amount of acetylcholine available at the receptor sites by preventing its destruction by acetylcholinesterase. This promotes more effective competition of acetylcholine with the nondepolarizing skeletal muscle relaxant that is occupying the receptor sites. Because of the increased availability and mobilization of the acetylcholine, the concentration gradient favors acetylcholine and the removal of the nondepolarizing agent from the receptors, resulting in the return of normal skeletal muscle depolarization and contraction.[18] These medications also produce undesired side effects by increasing the level of acetylcholine at receptor sites in the heart, the lungs, the eyes, and gastrointestinal tract, which can lead to bradycardia, bronchospasm, miosis, and increased peristalsis and secretion. To prevent or minimize these effects, anticholinergic agents such as atropine or glycopyrrolate (Robinul) are given with the anticholinesterase agent. Table 42-5 outlines the common NMBA reversal agents used in anesthesia and their nursing implications.[18]

PERIANESTHESIA ASSESSMENT AND CARE

The goal of management in the immediate postoperative period is the recognition and immediate treatment of any problems, to eliminate or lessen complications that may occur. This requires the collaborative effort of the nurse, the anesthesiologist, and

TABLE 42-3 OPIOID ADJUNCTIVE AGENTS*

CLINICAL USES	IMPLICATIONS	CONSIDERATIONS
Preoperative sedation	Monitor for hypotension	Keep naloxone (Narcan) available
Induction of anesthesia	Monitor for bradycardia	Keep resuscitation equipment available
Maintenance of anesthesia	Monitor for respiratory depression	Respiratory depressant effect may outlast analgesia
Postoperative pain management	May cause nausea and vomiting	

*Agents include alfentanil (Alfenta), fentanyl (Sublimaze), ketorolac (Toradol), morphine, sufentanil (Sufenta), remifentanil (Ultiva), and hydromorphone (Dilaudid).

BOX 42-4 FACTORS INFLUENCING NEUROMUSCULAR BLOCKADE

Potentiating Factors
- Hypocalcemia
- Hypokalemia
- Hyponatremia
- Hypermagnesemia
- Acidosis
- Hypothermia
- Antibiotics (gentamicin, tobramycin, amikacin, kanamycin, neomycin, polymyxin B, clindamycin, tetracyclines, piperacillin, streptomycin)
- Antidysrhythmics (procainamide, lidocaine, quinidine)
- Beta-adrenergic blockers
- Calcium channel blockers
- Diuretics (furosemide, thiazides)
- Droperidol
- Inhalation agents
- Local anesthetics
- Cyclosporine
- Lithium
- Dantrolene
- Etomidate
- Hepatobiliary disease
- Renal failure
- Neuromuscular diseases

Antagonizing Factors
- Phenytoin
- Carbamazepine
- Aminophylline
- Theophylline
- Sympathomimetic agents
- Corticosteroids
- Azathioprine

TABLE 42-4 NEUROMUSCULAR BLOCKING AGENTS*

CHARACTERISTICS	IMPLICATIONS	
	DEPOLARIZING	**NONDEPOLARIZING**
Compete with acetylcholine at the myoneural junction	Nonreversible	Reversible with time and anticholinesterases
	Use cautiously in patients with neuromuscular disease, such as myasthenia gravis or muscular dystrophy; contraindicated for pediatric use except in emergencies	Use cautiously in patients with hepatic or renal disease, obesity, asthma, or COPD
Shorter-acting agents are most appropriate for anesthesia	Adverse effects include bradycardia, tachycardia, ventricular dysrhythmias, asystole, hypertension, hyperkalemia	Adverse effects include tachycardia, hypertension, hypotension, bronchospasm, and flushing
Provide surgical relaxation Facilitate intubation	Increases intraocular, intracranial, and intragastric pressure	
Assist in ventilatory support	Precipitates muscle fasciculations and pain Prolongs respiratory depression Histamine release causes hypotension Use cautiously in patients with head injury, cerebral edema, trauma, burns, electrolyte imbalances, and renal or hepatic disease Monitor for clinical signs of malignant hyperthermia	

*Long-acting agents include pancuronium (Pavulon); intermediate-acting agents include atracurium (Tracrium), vecuronium (Norcuron), and cisatracurium (Nimbex); short-acting agents include rocuronium (Zemuron) and succinylcholine (Anectine), which is a depolarizing agent.

TABLE 42-5 NMBA REVERSAL AGENTS

MEDICATION	CHARACTERISTICS	EFFECTS	CONSIDERATIONS
Anticholinesterase			
Neostigmine (Prostigmin)	Binds with cholinesterase and inactivates it Preserves endogenous anticholinesterase More effective in antagonizing intense blocks than pyridostigmine or edrophonium	Antidote for nondepolarizing NMBAs Prevents postoperative distention and urinary retention Muscarinic effects cause bradycardia, bronchoconstriction, peripheral vasodilation, and coronary vasoconstriction	Does not cross blood–brain barrier Lasts 30-90 min May be given with atropine and glycopyrrolate to decrease muscarinic effects; most commonly given with glycopyrrolate Use cautiously in patients with asthma or coronary artery disease
Pyridostigmine (Regonol)	Analogue of neostigmine with fewer adverse effects Only 20% as potent as neostigmine Rapid onset of action (5-15 min)	Antidote for nondepolarizing NMBAs Muscarinic effects less severe than those of neostigmine	Longer half-life Lasts 120 min May be given with atropine and glycopyrrolate Use cautiously in patients with asthma, peptic ulcer, epilepsy, or pregnancy
Edrophonium (Tensilon)	Cholinergic Short-acting anticholinesterase	Parasympathetic effects: GI: salivation, dysphasia, nausea, vomiting, increased peristalsis CV: bradycardia, cardiac dysrhythmias, hypotension RESP: increased pharyngeal and tracheobronchial secretions EENT: lacrimation, miosis, diplopia	Must be given with atropine Very rapid onset but brief duration of action Use cautiously in presence of asthma, peptic ulcer, or bradycardia
Anticholinergic			
Atropine	Anticholinergic Antimuscarinic Chronotropic stimulator in event of bradycardia	Preanesthetic medication to prevent or reduce respiratory tract secretions Restoration of cardiac rate during anesthesia Antidote for cholinesterase inhibitors Causes decreased sweating and predisposition to heat prostration	Crosses blood–brain barrier Ensures adequate hydration Provides temperature control to prevent hyperpyrexia
Glycopyrrolate (Robinul)	Similar to atropine Longer duration	Less incidence of dysrhythmias Slow increase in heart rate Protection against peripheral muscarinic effects of neostigmine and pyridostigmine	Does not cross blood–brain barrier Contraindicated in presence of glaucoma, peptic ulcer, or COPD

COPD, Chronic obstructive pulmonary disease; *CV,* cardiovascular; *EENT,* eyes, ears, nose, and throat; *GI,* gastrointestinal; *NMBA,* neuromuscular blocking agent; *RESP,* respiratory.

the surgeon. Physical assessment of the postanesthesia patient begins immediately on admission to the unit. This initial assessment focuses on airway, ventilation, and circulation (heart rate, rhythm, and blood pressure). Following the brief initial assessment, the nurse admitting the patient receives a verbal report from the anesthesia care provider and surgeon. The report includes information about the patient's general condition, significant past history or co-morbidities, the operation performed, the type of anesthesia administered, estimated blood loss, total intake and output during surgery, and any problems or complications encountered in the operating room.[19]

Assessment of the cardiopulmonary system is the immediate priority. The patient's airway is assessed to ensure that it is patent, with or without adjuncts, and the patient's breathing pattern is evaluated to ensure that it is unlabored. The patient's blood pressure, pulse, rate of respiration, oxygen saturation level, and temperature are measured and recorded. All dressings and drains are quickly inspected for integrity and gross bleeding. After these initial observations have been made, it is essential to systematically assess the patient's total condition.

Respiratory Function

Because patients have experienced some interference with their respiratory system, postanesthesia maintenance of adequate gas exchange is a crucial aspect of care in the immediate postoperative period. Oxygen administration may be used in the immediate postoperative phase. Any change in respiratory function must be detected early so that appropriate measures can be taken to ensure adequate oxygenation and ventilation. Respiratory function is evaluated by using physical assessment skills: inspection, palpation, percussion, and auscultation. Several preexisting conditions can increase the probability that ventilatory support will be needed in the postoperative period. These include pre-existing pulmonary disease, thoracic or upper abdominal surgery, history of smoking, recent significant opioid administration, and low oxygen saturation before surgery.

Pulse oximetry, a noninvasive technique, measures oxygen saturation of functional hemoglobin. Pulse oximetry can be used to identify hypoxemia, and its use should be standard on all postoperative patients. If the patient is intubated and mechanically ventilated, capnography can be used to assess for adequate ventilation. Arterial blood gas measurements are appropriate to definitively confirm abnormal pulse oximetry or capnography values. Normal pulse oximetry values are 97% to 99%; however, preanesthetic baseline values must be noted. Some patients normally have lower saturation values on room air for a variety of reasons, and attempting to maintain higher oxygen saturation levels may result in prolonged oxygen therapy.[20]

For spontaneously breathing patients, supplemental oxygen may be needed, typically using nasal cannula (prongs) or simple facemask. Surgery and anesthesia often interrupt the normal functioning of the nose, so humidification or nebulization with oxygen delivery may be needed. Humidifiers convert water from the liquid to the gaseous state, whereas nebulizers produce tiny water particles. This is especially helpful at higher flow rates.[21]

Patients may require mechanical ventilation following anesthesia. Various modes, such as positive end-expiratory pressure (PEEP), continuous positive airway pressure (CPAP), and synchronized intermittent mandatory ventilation (SIMV), are used to improve the respiratory status of the patient.[21]

Stir-Up Regimen

A significant aspect of perianesthesia nursing management is the stir-up regimen.[22] The regimen is aimed at the prevention of complications, primarily atelectasis and venous stasis. The stir-up regimen consists of five major activities—deep-breathing exercises, coughing, positioning, mobilization, and pain management.

Deep-Breathing Exercises. The major factor contributing to postoperative pulmonary complications is low lung volumes resulting from a shallow, monotonous, sighless breathing pattern caused by general anesthesia, opioids, and pain. The patient must be stimulated to take three or four deep breaths every 5 to 10 minutes. Full lung expansion is important, and every effort must be made to enhance the patient's ability to accomplish it.

The sustained maximal inspiration (SMI) maneuver is a method to enhance the lung volumes of postoperative patients.[22] The SMI maneuver consists of having the patient inhale as close to lung capacity as possible and, at the peak of inspiration, hold that volume for 3 to 5 seconds before exhaling it. This maneuver is more effective than simple deep breathing in preventing reduced lung volumes in the immediate postanesthesia periods. If the patient's vital capacity is inadequate or if anesthesia respiratory depression is prolonged, deep breathing and the SMI maneuver may be augmented with a manual resuscitation bag connected to an oxygen source or with an intermittent positive-pressure breathing apparatus.

Incentive spirometry is used to assist with preventing and treating atelectasis, promoting normal lung expansion, and improving oxygenation. Incentive spirometry devices allow patients visual feedback and observation of inspiratory volume. Instruction and practice before surgery provide patients with the opportunity to master the device and establish their baseline levels before anesthetic and surgical interventions.

Coughing. A purposeful cough is the most effective method to clear the air passages of obstructive secretions.[22] For the patient recovering from anesthesia, the cascade cough is the most effective coughing maneuver. Instruct the patient to take

a rapid, deep inhalation. This will increase the volume of air in the lungs and dilate the airways, allowing air to pass behind the retained secretions. On exhalation, have the patient perform multiple coughs. With each cough the length of the airways increases, enhancing the effectiveness of the cough.

Coughing is most effective with the patient sitting upright. Splinting of incisions and adequate analgesia facilitate coughing. If the patient is unable to sit upright, place the patient in a side-lying position with hips and knees flexed, or in a semi-Fowler's position with the head and arms supported with pillows and the knees flexed. This positioning decreases abdominal tension and allows maximal movement of the diaphragm, improving the effectiveness of the cough.

Between cascade cough maneuvers, the patient is encouraged to inhale and close the glottis. This dilates the airways, increases intrathoracic pressure, and compresses the smaller airways, pushing the secretions toward the larger airways where they can be expectorated in succeeding cough maneuvers.

When a large amount of secretions accumulates in the patient's lungs and cannot be handled effectively by coughing, suctioning must be instituted. Suctioning is not without complications and should be done only when necessary and not routinely

Positioning. Ideally, patients recovering from anesthesia are positioned in a semiprone, side-lying position if possible. The semiprone position promotes maintenance of a patent airway, prevents aspiration, and permits optimal ventilation of the lower lung lobes. Frequent repositioning of patients (at least every hour) from side to side is essential for the prevention of atelectasis and venous stasis. Patients are encouraged to turn and change positions as soon as possible. Positioning changes may be limited by the operative procedure or special needs of the patient.

Mobilization. To prevent venous stasis, patients must be encouraged to move their legs and arms rhythmically, flexing and extending their extremities. Mobilization and flexion of the muscles aids venous return, improves cardiac output (CO), and prevents venous stasis and the formation of deep vein thrombosis.

Pain Management. Adequate analgesia is a major consideration in the recovering patient. Without it, it is difficult to implement the first four interventions of the stir-up regimen. Poorly controlled pain can have serious consequences in terms of hemodynamic responses to catecholamines and physical limitations on respiratory function. On the other hand, the medications used to control pain may in themselves have deleterious effects on hemodynamic and respiratory function. Opioids depress the cough reflex, ciliary activity, and the respiratory center in the brain and should not be used indiscriminately. However, if the patient refuses to deep breathe, cough, or move because of pain, he or she is at risk for postoperative respiratory and embolic complications.

Pain accelerates the cardiovascular system by activating the sympathetic nervous system and the adrenal system. Normally, this causes an increase in heart rate and blood pressure. However, anesthesia and some cardiac medications can blunt the sympathetic response; asking the patient his or her pain level is the most valid method of assessing pain levels (see Chapter 9). It has been suggested that pain, especially at upper abdominal and thoracic sites, decreases or eliminates the normal sighing (yawning) mechanism. The absence of an appropriate sigh leads to reduced lung volumes and, ultimately, to atelectasis and pneumonia. Appropriate pain relief in these patients reduces the postoperative incidence of atelectasis and pneumonia.[23]

After the assessment has been completed and it has been determined that the patient is experiencing acute postoperative pain, certain interventions are suggested. If the patient has received an inhalation anesthetic, such as isoflurane, and demonstrates manifestations of acute pain, relief is instituted early in the postanesthetic period. Similarly, patients undergoing a nitrous oxide–opioid technique are medicated early in the immediate postoperative period, particularly if the intraoperative opioids were of short duration. If medications such as sufentanil and morphine were used intraoperatively, opioids must be administered with caution to avoid respiratory depression as a result of the synergistic action of the intraoperative and postoperative opioid agonists. Because of the synergistic effects of the medications, it may be necessary to decrease the amount of opioids administered during the first 24 hours after administration of anesthesia, but this decision must always be based on the patient's report of pain and clinical status.[24-27]

Cardiovascular Function

Evaluation of the cardiovascular system involves assessment of the heart, circulating blood, and the arteriovenous system. These three basic components control CO. Because tissue perfusion depends on a satisfactory CO, most of the assessment is aimed at evaluating this component.[28]

In most patients, the nurse uses physical assessment skills to evaluate cardiovascular function.[29] The patient's overall condition is observed, especially skin color and turgor. Peripheral cyanosis, edema, jugular venous distention, shortness of breath, and many other findings may be indicative of cardiovascular problems. All operative and access sites are checked for bleeding, and the amount of blood lost during surgery and the patient's most recent hemoglobin level are noted.

The patient's blood pressure must be assessed and correlated to the preoperative assessment, intraoperative course, and anesthetic course. The major component of systolic pressure is stroke volume, and the major component of diastolic pressure is systemic vascular resistance (SVR). Changes in the patient's systolic or diastolic pressure or narrowing of the pulse pressure may indicate cardiovascular compromise.[29] Peripheral pulses are assessed bilaterally. The rate, character, and any irregularities are documented and reported to the physician if clinically indicated.[29] Electrocardiographic (ECG) monitoring is also essential in the immediate postoperative recovery period. Dysrhythmias of any type may occur at any time and in any patient during the postoperative period.[29,30]

Two components of CO are heart rate and stroke volume. If CO is compromised, one of the first compensatory responses is an increase in heart rate, followed by peripheral vasoconstriction. Medications such as beta-blockers and angiotensin-converting enzyme inhibitors, as well as anesthetic agents, can impair the patient's ability to initiate that response. The nurse must be aware of the patient's preoperative medications and

the impact they may have in the initial phase of recovery. Hemodynamic monitoring is commonly used with higher-acuity patients in the postanesthesia recovery period. Hemodynamic monitoring is usually accomplished by a pulmonary artery catheter and arterial blood pressure monitoring.

Central Nervous System Function

Assessment of the CNS in the immediate postanesthesia period typically involves gross evaluation of behavior, level of consciousness, intellectual performance, and emotional status. Anesthetic agents are usually reversed before the patient leaves the operating room, and the nurse should anticipate that the patient will be responsive. However, even if anesthesia is not reversed, most patients can respond within 60 to 90 minutes from time of admission to the unit.[31] Perioperative stroke can occur in up to 7% of patients following noncardiac and non-neurosurgical procedures.[32] As a result of this risk, the nurse caring for the postanesthesia patient following general anesthesia should complete a neurologic assessment that includes stroke assessment (facial symmetry, vocalization to assess for slurred speech, strength, and movement of extremities), and pupillary check. In addition, Glasgow coma scale assessment may be completed. For patients who have undergone neurosurgical procedures, a more detailed assessment of the CNS is necessary.

Occasionally, a patient becomes agitated and thrashes about; this behavior when extreme is referred to as *emergence delirium*. It occurs more often in children, older adults, and patients with histories of drug dependency or psychiatric disorder.[30] Emergence delirium also tends to occur more commonly in patients who have undergone breast and abdominal procedures and procedures of longer duration.[33]

Thermal Balance

Measurement of the patient's body temperature in the immediate postanesthesia recovery period is particularly important. Factors influencing the body temperature include type of anesthesia, preoperative medication, age of patient, site and temperature of intravenous fluids, body surface exposure, temperature of irrigation solutions, temperature of the ambient air, and vasoconstriction (from blood loss or anesthetic agents). Hypothermia (temperature less than 36°C) and hyperthermia (temperature greater than 38°C) are associated with physiologic alterations that may interfere with recovery.[34]

The body maintains its temperature in a narrow range, between 36°C and 38°C. This is accomplished by a balance of heat production and heat loss that is controlled by the thermoregulation mechanisms in the CNS. These mechanisms receive input from various thermoreceptors located in the skin, nose, oral cavity, thoracic viscera, and spinal cord. They then send sensory information in hierarchic order to the spinal cord, the reticular formation, and the primary control center in the hypothalamic region of the brain.[35]

The central temperature controls maintain body temperature through physiologic and behavioral responses. The physiologic thermoregulatory responses consist of sweating, shivering, and alterations in peripheral vasomotor tone. These responses fine-control the regulatory process of body temperature; heat is conserved by vasoconstriction and lost by vasodilation and sweating. The physiologic responses also can lower the metabolic rate to decrease heat production or increase muscle tone and shivering to increase heat production. Behavioral thermoregulation is accomplished by subjective feelings of discomfort or comfort. For example, in a hot environment a person seeks air conditioning, and in a cold environment a person seeks heat. Behavioral thermoregulation is a stronger response mechanism, but it cannot fine-tune body temperature as the physiologic responses can.[35]

Fluid and Electrolyte Balance

Evaluation of a patient's fluid and electrolyte status involves total body assessment. Imbalances readily occur in the postoperative patient because of a number of factors, including restriction of food and fluids preoperatively, fluid loss during surgery, and stress. The normal body response to stress, surgery, trauma, and anesthesia is to release the antidiuretic hormone responsible for the retention of water and sodium. Postanesthesia patients often have abnormal avenues of fluid loss after surgery.

Each patient must be evaluated to determine his or her baseline requirements and the fluid needed to replace abnormal losses. Most patients in the immediate postanesthesia recovery period receive intravenous fluids. It is important to know what fluids, if any, are to follow and whether the infusion is to be discontinued. All intravenous sites are checked regularly for signs of extravasation, phlebitis, and infection.

Oral intake is prohibited after anesthesia until the patient regains laryngeal and pharyngeal reflexes. These reflexes are demonstrated by the patient's ability to gag and swallow effectively. The management of postoperative nausea and vomiting (PONV) remains critical.

Normal output in the average adult results from urinary output and insensible losses, including evaporation of water from the skin and exhalation during respiration.[36]

A lower-than-normal urinary output can be expected in the immediate postanesthesia recovery period as a result of the body's normal reaction to stress and anesthetics. External losses from vomiting, nasogastric tubes, T-tubes, and wound drainage are assessed and monitored. Accurate measurement and recording of all intake and output is vital in the assessment of the patient's fluid and electrolyte status.[36]

In the surgical patient, intravenous access to the circulatory system is necessary for the administration of anesthesia, resuscitation medications, blood and blood products, and fluid and electrolyte solutions. Postoperative parenteral fluid requirements vary with the patient's preoperative status and with the surgical procedure. Disease processes, tissue injuries, and operative procedures greatly influence the physiology of fluids and electrolytes in the body.

In deciding the type of fluid to use in the postanesthesia recovery period, the clinician can differentiate between crystalloids and colloids, between maintenance and replacement fluids, and among fluids of differing tonicity. Because of the large variety of fluid solutions, some general guidelines are recommended in clinical practice.[36] Crystalloids are typically used as maintenance fluids to compensate for insensible fluid losses and as replacement fluids to correct body fluid deficits

(i.e., treatment of specific fluid and electrolyte disturbances). Maintenance fluid requirements are calculated according to body weight and are used to replace insensible losses from the lungs, skin, urine, and feces. Adults typically require 1.5 to 2 mL/kg/hour. When crystalloids are used to replace blood loss, the replacement factor is 3 mL of crystalloid for each 1 mL of blood loss.[37] Isotonic solutions, 0.9% normal saline, or lactated Ringer solution are usually administered in the immediate postoperative period. Colloids typically are used for fluid replacement associated with severe hypotension or shock resuscitation. In general, they do not leave the intravascular space and therefore require lower infusion volumes to achieve volume replacement.

The goal of fluid therapy in the immediate postanesthesia recovery period is the restoration of blood volume and tissue perfusion. Recovery after surgery is a dynamic process, and fluid reassessment is conducted periodically. Fluid challenges may be necessary in the hypovolemic patient or in the patient with clinical manifestations of hypoperfusion. The decision of whether to use crystalloids or colloids for fluid resuscitation is complex, controversial, and often determined by physician preference. Either can meet the replacement needs of the patient and achieve the desired outcome when administered appropriately. As with any therapeutic intervention, complications can occur with fluid administration, and the patient should be monitored closely.

Blood and blood components are reserved for specific patient situations.[37] Red blood cells are indicated to increase oxygen-carrying capacity in patients with anemia. Platelets are used to treat bleeding associated with deficiencies in platelet number or function. Fresh-frozen plasma is transfused to increase clotting factor levels in patients with demonstrated deficiencies. A good understanding of the fluid types available, a systematic approach to evaluating fluid depletion, and awareness of the indications for blood component therapy allow the nurse to make appropriate decisions when implementing fluid therapy in the immediate postanesthesia period.

Psychosocial Status

Assessment of the patient's psychosocial and emotional well-being is an important component of perianesthesia care. As with any other assessment, this must be made in the context of the whole patient. Almost all patients experience a degree of anxiety about anesthesia and the surgical procedure and a fear of postoperative pain.[38] The physical manifestations include increased heart rate and blood pressure; pale, cool skin; increased respiratory rate; increased muscle tone; restlessness; agitation; and dilated pupils.

Other Nursing Considerations

In the postanesthesia care unit (PACU), assessment and nursing care are based on the complexity and acuity of the patient's condition.[39] Concerns surround the use of the PACU as an overflow unit for critically ill patients.[40] Issues surrounding these concerns are competencies of staff; adequacy of equipment, medications, supplies, and technology; and appropriate nurse staffing. Refer to Box 42-5 for guidelines for the overflow of critical care patients into the PACU.[40]

BOX 42-5 A JOINT POSITION STATEMENT ON ICU OVERFLOW PATIENTS

Developed by ASPAN, AACN, and ASA's Anesthesia Care Team Committee and Committee on Critical Care Medicine and Trauma Medicine

Issue

A phase I postanesthesia care unit (PACU) is a critical care area providing postanesthesia nursing care for patients immediately after operative and invasive procedures, before discharge to the phase II ambulatory setting, the inpatient surgical unit, and the intensive care unit.

Perianesthesia nurses have identified concerns regarding the increasing use of the phase I PACU for the care of surgical and nonsurgical intensive care unit (ICU) patients when ICU beds are not available in the facility.

Purpose

As professional societies involved in the provision of care for operative and invasive procedures and critically ill patients, the American Society of PeriAnesthesia Nurses (ASPAN), the American Association of Critical-Care Nurses (AACN), and the American Society of Anesthesiologists (ASA) collaborated to develop criteria for the purposes of maintaining quality care in the PACU, ensuring quality care for the ICU patient, and promoting the safe practice of perianesthesia nursing and critical care nursing.

ASPAN exists to promote quality and cost-effective care for patients, their families, and the community through public and professional education, research, and standards of practice. ASPAN has the responsibility for defining the practice of perianesthesia nursing. An integral part of this responsibility involves identifying the educational requirements and competencies essential to perianesthesia practice and recommending acceptable staffing requirements for the perianesthesia environment.

AACN was established to provide the highest quality resources to maximize nurses' contributions to care for critically ill patients and their families. AACN provides and inspires leadership to develop standards and guidelines that establish work and care environments that are respectful, healing, and humane.

ASA was established to raise and maintain the standard of the medical practice of anesthesiology and improve the care of the patient during anesthesia and recovery, and ASA is involved in the provision of critical care medicine in the ICU.

Background

In response to concerns expressed by perianesthesia nurses around the country, the ASPAN Standards and Guidelines Committee conducted a review of current literature and perianesthesia nursing practice to identify issues related to the care of critically ill surgical and nonsurgical patients in phase I PACUs during times when all other ICU beds are full. The review identified the following trends:

1. Staffing requirements identified for phase I PACUs may be exceeded during times when PACUs are being utilized for ICU overflow patients.[1]
2. The phase I PACU nurse may be required to provide care to a surgical or nonsurgical ICU patient despite a lack of proper training and the required valid care competencies.[1]
3. Phase I PACUs may be unable to receive patients normally admitted from the operating room when staff are caring for ICU overflow patients.[1]
4. Because the need to send ICU overflow patients to the phase I PACU does not occur regularly, the PACU and hospital management may not be properly prepared to deal with the admission and discharge of phase I PACU and ICU patients.[1]

Statement

When it is necessary to admit ICU overflow patients or to prolong the stay of the surgical ICU patient in the phase I PACU, ASPAN, AACN, and ASA recommend that the following criteria be met:

1. It must be recognized that the primary responsibility for the phase I PACU is to provide the optimal standard of care to the postanesthesia patient and to effectively maintain the flow of the surgery schedule.
2. Appropriate staffing requirements should be met to maintain safe, competent nursing care of the postanesthesia patient and the ICU patient.[2] Staffing criteria for the ICU patient should be consistent with ICU guidelines and based on individual patient acuity and needs.[3]
3. Phase I PACUs are by their nature critical care units, and PACU staff should meet the competencies required for the care of the critically ill patient. These competencies include, but are not limited to, ventilator management, hemodynamic monitoring, and medication administration, as appropriate to the patient population.
4. Management should develop and implement a comprehensive resource utilization plan with ongoing assessment that supports the staffing needs for PACU and ICU patients when the need for overflow admission arises.[3]
5. Management should have a multidisciplinary plan to address appropriate utilization of ICU beds. Admission and discharge criteria should be used to evaluate the necessity for critical care and to determine the priority for admissions.[3]

Expected Actions

ASPAN, AACN, and the ASA committees (Anesthesia Care Team, Critical Care Medicine, and Trauma Medicine) recognize the complexity of caring for patients in a dynamic health care environment where reduced availability of resources and expanding roles for the registered nurse have an impact on patient care. We encourage all members to actively pursue the education and development of competencies required for the care of the critically ill patient in the perianesthesia environment. We also encourage members to actively identify strategies for collaboration and problem solving to address complex staffing issues.

This information and position is to be shared with all individuals, organizations, and institutions involved in the care of the critically ill patient in the perianesthesia environment.

Approval Statement

This statement was recommended by a vote of the ASPAN Board of Directors on April 14, 2000 in Kansas City, Missouri, and approved by a vote of the ASPAN Representative Assembly on April 16, 2000 in Kansas City, Missouri.

This position statement was reviewed and updated at the October 2009 meeting of the Standards and Guidelines Committee in Batesville, Indiana.

References

1. Johannes MS. A new dimension of the PACU: The dilemma of the ICU overflow patient. *J Post Anesth Nurs.* 1994;9:297.
2. American Society of PeriAnesthesia Nurses. Resource 2: patient classification/recommended staffing guidelines in the *Standards of Perianesthesia Nursing Practice.* Thorofare, NJ: ASPAN; 1998.
3. Medina J. *Staffing Blueprint: Constructing Your Staffing Solutions.* Alisa Viejo, CA: AACN; 1999.

Bibliography

AACN standards for establishing and sustaining healthy work environments: a journey to excellence. *Am J Crit Care.* 2005;3(14):187.

Hegeedus M. Taking the fear out of postanesthesia care in the intensive care unit. *Dimens Crit Care Nurs.* 2003;6(22):237.

Kiekkas P, et al. Workload of postanesthesia care unit nurses and intensive care overflow. *Brit J Nurs.* 2005;8(14):434.

Odom-Forren J. The PACU as Critical Care Unit. *J PeriAnesth Nurs.* 2003; 6(18):431.

Schweizer A, et al. Opening of a new postanesthesia care unit: impact on critical care utilization and complications following major vascular and thoracic surgery. *J Clin Anesth.* 2002;14:486.

Sullivan E. Teamwork and collaboration. *J PeriAnesth Nurs.* 2002;17:334.

Weissman C. The enhanced postoperative care system. *J Clin Anesth.* 2005;(17):314.

From *American Society of Perianesthesia Nurses.* A joint position statement on ICU overflow patients developed by ASPAN, AACN, and ASA's Anesthesia Care Team Committee and Committee on Critical Care Medicine and Trauma Medicine. http://www.aspan.org/Portals/6/docs/ClinicalPractice/PositionStatement/1012/Pos_Stmt_5_Joint_ICUOverflow.pdf. Accessed September 2012.

General Comfort Management

Postanesthesia care includes general comfort and safety measures.[22] Whenever patients are recovering, at least two nurses (one of whom is a registered nurse competent in Phase I perianesthesia nursing) must always be present in the same room or unit for safety.[41] Patients should not be left alone, especially when unconscious and emerging from anesthesia. Side rails should be in the up position and locked when care is not being provided. Wheel locks prevent sliding of the bed.

General physical measures such as cleaning and comfort measures are important to the total well-being of postanesthesia patients and are often overlooked. Following the initial assessment and when safe, the skin should be cleansed of preparation solutions and electrodes or sensors that are not in use should be removed. Repositioning in an alternative position from the operative position may prevent future complaints of discomfort for patients who have undergone lengthy operative procedures. While repositioning, patient movement and deep breathing may help prevent atelectasis, promote circulation, and prevent pressure ulcers from developing on skin surfaces.

Oral care is comforting to the patient who has had no oral intake and has received drying medications. Ice chips and small sips of water or juice may be offered to patients who can tolerate fluids. A non–petroleum-based ointment is applied to the lips after oral care to prevent drying and cracking.

Patients often complain of being cold when returning from the operating suite. This is a result of the effects of anesthesia and premedications and the cool atmosphere of the operating suite. The normothermic patient may shiver or complain of feeling cold, so warm blankets may provide psychologic comfort. Blankets of any type must not, however, obscure the intravenous lines, arterial lines, or other monitoring apparatus from the direct view of the attending nurse. The patient's temperature must be monitored closely to avoid overheating.

In addition to the physical comfort measures, psychologic comfort should be provided. Reorientation, especially to time and place, is important to the postanesthesia patient, as is constant reassurance that the procedure has been completed and the patient is now recovering. The nurse's presence at the bedside or gentle touch may also be comforting to the patient.

MANAGEMENT OF POSTANESTHESIA PROBLEMS AND EMERGENCIES

In the immediate postoperative period, significant physiologic changes occur as the patient emerges from the effects of anesthesia. Factors that influence the development of problems are listed in Box 42-6.[42]

Respiratory Complications and Emergencies

Respiratory complications occur with some regularity in the postanesthesia period. All general anesthetic agents and opioid analgesic medications have respiratory depressant effects. Acute pain also impairs the ability to breathe deeply. Most respiratory complications are related to upper airway obstruction, although other problems can occur, including acute respiratory failure, aspiration, pulmonary edema, and respiratory arrest.[30]

BOX 42-6   FACTORS INFLUENCING THE DEVELOPMENT OF POSTOPERATIVE PROBLEMS

- Intraoperative complications
- Type of anesthetic technique
- Patient co-morbidities and pre-existing diseases
- Preoperative condition of patient
- Length and type of surgery
- Urgency of surgery
- Poorly controlled pain
- Other medications administered intraoperatively
- Changes in fluid status and electrolyte balance
- Alterations in body temperature

Airway Obstruction

Relaxed nasal or oropharyngeal muscles, rigid neck muscles, or secretions in the upper respiratory tract can cause obstruction of the airway. Soft tissue obstruction occurs when the pharynx is blocked and air cannot flow in and out. The most common cause of soft tissue obstruction is the tongue. Clinical manifestations of an airway obstruction include snoring, stridor, flaring of the nostrils, retractions at the intercostal spaces and the suprasternal notch, abnormal use of accessory muscles, asynchronous movements of the chest and abdomen, increased pulse rate, decreased oxygen saturation level, and decreased breath sounds.[43]

Management of an airway obstruction begins with immediate recognition. Stimulation may be all that is necessary to relieve the obstruction and obtain a patent airway. With the nonreactive patient, the head tilt–chin lift maneuver or elevation of the mandible at its angles (jaw thrust) can be used to displace the tongue and open the airway. If patency of the airway cannot be achieved by either of these methods, an oropharyngeal or nasopharyngeal airway is inserted. A nasopharyngeal airway is usually better tolerated, although it can occasionally cause nasal bleeding. Oropharyngeal airways should be used only for an unconscious patients, because they can cause gagging, vomiting, and laryngospasm in the awake patient. The patient can also be turned on his or her side to a lateral position, which facilitates displacement of the tongue and drainage of secretions. If the obstruction is still unrelieved, positive-pressure mask ventilation, intubation, tracheotomy, or cricothyrotomy may be required.[4,30,43]

Laryngeal Edema

Laryngeal edema is defined as swelling of the laryngeal tissue. This edema can cause various degrees of airway obstruction. Manifestations include stridor, retraction, hoarseness, and a crouplike cough. Apprehension and restlessness may be present in the awake patient.

Management consists of placing the patient in the upright position; using cool, humidified oxygen; and administering nebulized racemic epinephrine. If the laryngeal edema is a result of an allergic reaction, the reaction must be managed with epinephrine, bronchodilators, and antihistamines. Reintubation is performed only if the patient's symptoms cannot be controlled by an inhalation treatment within 30 minutes, if hypercarbia persists, or if the patient appears to be in respiratory distress. If reintubation is done, the endotracheal tube must be at least one size smaller than the previous tube used, and an air leak must be present around the cuff.[30,43]

Laryngospasm

Laryngospasm is caused by reflex contractions of the pharyngeal muscles, which results in spasms of the vocal cords and the inability of the patient to take a breath. The spasms may result in partial or complete airway obstruction. Involvement of the intrinsic laryngeal muscles causes a reflex closure of the glottis, which results in an incomplete obstruction. Involvement of the extrinsic muscles causes a reflex closure of the larynx, which results in a complete airway obstruction. Signs and symptoms of laryngospasm include dyspnea, hypoxia, hypoventilation, absence of breath sounds, and hypercarbia. Crowing sounds may be heard if the spasm is incomplete. The chest does not expand normally, and a rocking motion of the chest wall that stimulates abdominal breathing may be present. The patient panics if awake.

Several factors can help identify the patient at risk for a laryngospasm. Preoperatively, risks include a history of asthma, chronic obstructive pulmonary disease (COPD), or smoking. Intraoperatively, risks include the use of an endotracheal tube, anesthetic agents, "light" anesthesia, multiple attempts at intubation, and surgical airway manipulation. After surgery, risks include coughing, "bucking" on the endotracheal tube, repeated suctioning, and excessive secretions in the nasopharyngeal area. Laryngospasm may also be precipitated by irritants and foreign bodies.

Laryngospasm is an emergency that requires an immediate response; otherwise, the patient may rapidly deteriorate. Management is initiated by removing the stimulus, along with any irritants such as secretions, blood, or an artificial airway that is too long. The patient's head must be hyperextended and positive-pressure mask ventilation instituted on 100% oxygen. The anesthesiologist is notified immediately. If complete obstruction is unrelieved by positive-pressure ventilations, a small dose of succinylcholine (10 to 20 mg) may be needed to relax the vocal cords to allow for ventilation. Positive-pressure mask ventilation is continued until full muscle function has resumed. Endotracheal intubation is required if the laryngospasm persists or if refractory hypoxemia develops, even though it may cause further irritation of the airways. Medications that may be used in the treatment of laryngospasm include lidocaine, steroids, and atropine.

After the spasm, the patient continues to receive supplemental oxygen until stable. It is also important at that time for the nurse to reassure the patient that the spasm has resolved. The patient's feelings of being unable to breathe during laryngospasm are intense, and emotional support from the nurse is imperative.[30,44]

Bronchospasm

Bronchospasm is a lower airway obstruction that is characterized by spasmodic contractions of the bronchial tubes. Bronchial airway constriction is a result of an increase in smooth muscle tone in the airways, and bronchospasms develop when the smooth muscles constrict and obstruct the airway. Inflammation has also been recognized as a fundamental component of bronchospasms.

Bronchiolar constriction may be centrally generated, as in asthma, or it may be a local response to airway irritation. Manifestations include wheezing; noisy, shallow respirations; chest retractions; and use of accessory muscles. The patient can exhibit shortness of breath, coughing, and a prolonged expiratory phase of respiration. Hypertension and tachycardia may be present. The patient's level of consciousness may range from lethargy to extreme anxiety.

Patients who smoke and those with chronic bronchitis have essentially irritable airways that react to stimulation. A preoperative history of asthma, a recent upper respiratory infection, severe emphysema, pulmonary fibrosis, and radiation pneumonitis are indicators of a greater risk of bronchospasm. Stimuli that may produce a bronchospasm postoperatively include secretions, vomitus, and blood. Patients who have had laryngoscopy, bronchoscopy, or other surgical stimulation are also at increased risk of bronchospasm. Some medications are also thought to predispose the patient to bronchoconstriction resulting from cholinomimetic stimulation; these medications include physostigmine, neostigmine, edrophonium, and barbiturates. Other histamine-releasing medications, such as tubocurarine, morphine, metocurine, and atracurium, may potentially foster bronchospasm.

Bronchospasm is treated initially by removal of any possible irritants or medications. The first line of therapy consists of inhaled bronchodilators. These inhalants cause fewer cardiovascular side effects than systemically administered medications. Common inhalant medications used are albuterol, metaproterenol, and beclomethasone. Systemic bronchodilators and anti-inflammatory agents may also be required at times. Epinephrine is occasionally needed as a continuous infusion. Intravenous methylprednisolone manages the inflammatory aspect of bronchospasm. Cholinergics have been given by nebulizer to decrease secretions.[30,44]

Noncardiogenic Pulmonary Edema

Pulmonary edema may be defined simply as increased total lung water. Fluid can accumulate in the interstitial spaces or in the alveoli as the result of cardiogenic or pulmonary capillary processes. Noncardiogenic pulmonary edema, also known as postobstructive pulmonary edema, in the postanesthesia recovery period can result from pulmonary aspiration, blood transfusion reaction, allergic medication reaction, upper airway obstruction, or sepsis.[45] The most common causative factor seems to be an upper airway obstruction, usually laryngospasm. Often, a short episode of airway obstruction occurred in the operating room. Noncardiogenic pulmonary edema has also been reported after the administration of naloxone to patients who have received general anesthesia. Reversal of the analgesics causes a rise in the level of adrenal catecholamines, which can lead to pulmonary hypertension and probably increased pulmonary vascular permeability.

During laryngospasm, the patient is inhaling against a closed glottis. This generates an increase in negative intrathoracic pressure. A tremendous subatmospheric transpulmonary pressure gradient is created that causes transudation, or leakage of fluid, from the pulmonary capillaries into the interstitium.

Management consists of maintenance of an unobstructed airway and supplemental oxygen to correct hypoxemia. Those patients who cannot maintain adequate oxygenation with a mask may require the use of CPAP or even mechanical ventilation with PEEP. The use of PEEP or CPAP improves hypoxemia by restoring the functional residual capacity (FRC). Vigorous pulmonary toilet and the use of hemodynamic monitoring may be required if the patient's blood pressure is labile and fluid balance is difficult to maintain. Morphine can be titrated to relieve anxiety. Corticosteroid therapy can be used to decrease laryngeal edema and stabilize the pulmonary membrane. Noncardiogenic pulmonary edema occurs rapidly and requires early assessment and immediate intervention.

Aspiration

Aspiration can be defined as the passage of regurgitated gastric contents or other foreign materials into the trachea and down to the smaller air units. It can occur during the period of reduced protective airway reflexes. The most common and most severe form of aspiration is the aspiration of gastric contents. The gastric acid in gastric contents damages the alveolar and capillary endothelial cells. Fluid rich with protein leaks into the interstitium and alveoli. This results in atelectasis and consolidation. Pulmonary compliance and FRC are decreased, and airway resistance and intrapulmonary shunting are increased, with hypoxemia resulting.

If aspiration is suspected, management begins with lowering the patient's head, if possible. The patient is positioned to the side or the head is turned to the side to permit gravity to pull secretions from the trachea. Management centers on promoting tissue oxygenation by maintaining arterial oxygenation by means of CPAP and supplemental oxygen. Positive-pressure ventilation by mask can be applied if the patient is awake and can protect his or her airway or by an endotracheal tube if the patient cannot tolerate the mask or requires higher levels of airway pressure.[30,44]

Hypoxemia

Administration of oxygen by facemask or nasal cannula to recovering patients may be needed to prevent hypoxemia in the postoperative patient, based on oxygen saturation levels that may be assessed by noninvasively by pulse oximetry. Respiratory depressant effects of residual agents may result in a shallow breathing pattern with an increased ratio of dead space to tidal volume. This is even more evident in patients after upper abdominal surgery, and the reduction in the effective ventilation can have serious effects on oxygenation.[42]

The most common cause of hypoxemia is ventilation perfusion mismatching. Atelectasis often occurs as a result of bronchial obstruction by secretions or blood. Reduction in FRC is caused by the effects of anesthesia and, in the case of upper abdominal surgery, by the surgical procedure. When FRC falls below closing capacity, dependent alveoli occlude, leading to increased mismatching. Impairment of hypoxic pulmonary vasoconstriction by inhalation agents and some vasoactive medications potentiates this effect.[30]

Hypoventilation

Central respiratory depression is caused by all anesthetic agents. This may lead to significant hypoventilation and hypercarbia. Impaired respiratory muscle function, particularly after upper abdominal surgery, may contribute to the problem of carbon dioxide elimination. Incomplete reversal of neuromuscular blockade must also be considered. Other contributory factors may include tight dressings and body casts, obesity, and gastric dilation. Increased carbon dioxide production may occur as a result of shivering or sepsis. This leads to hypercarbia in patients who are unable to increase ventilation enough to compensate.

Hypercarbia resulting from postoperative hypoventilation may cause hypertension and tachycardia, increasing the risk of myocardial ischemia in susceptible individuals. Hypoventilation, by itself or in combination with the other factors previously discussed, can cause hypoxemia. Very high levels of carbon dioxide may have sedative effects. Evaluation of suspected hypoventilation requires measurement of arterial blood gases. Capnographic monitoring may be especially useful in patients at high risk for hypoxemia.[30]

Careful titration of opioid antagonists, such as naloxone, may be effective in improving ventilation without compromising pain relief. Planning ahead to provide adequate postoperative analgesia is essential for maintaining ventilation, particularly in patients undergoing abdominal or thoracic procedures. Placing obese patients in a semi-Fowler's position and relieving the effects of tight dressings and casts can also be important. Hypoventilation that cannot be improved sufficiently by noninvasive means requires intubation and mechanical ventilation until the patient can maintain adequate ventilation.[44]

Cardiovascular Problems and Emergencies

In the immediate postoperative period, cardiovascular complications causing an alteration in CO can occur. These include anesthetic effects on cardiac function, myocardial dysfunction, dysrhythmias, hypertension, and hypotension. These conditions may occur individually or in combination.[30,46]

Effects of Anesthesia on Cardiac Function

In the immediate postoperative period, the residual effects of anesthetic agents and their adjuncts must be considered in the evaluation of a patient who has cardiac dysfunction. Volatile anesthetic agents such as sevoflurane and isoflurane can cause a dose-related reduction in myocardial function. The actions of these agents may be observed for several hours after the conclusion of surgery.[4] Nitrous oxide is an inhalation agent that demonstrates insignificant cardiac depression. However, the combined action of opioids given during emergence from nitrous oxide can result in marked cardiovascular depression.[3]

Therapy directed toward mitigating the myocardial depressant effects of inhalation anesthetic agents primarily focuses on increasing preload. Elevation of the legs and a crystalloid fluid bolus are commonly sufficient treatment, but ephedrine or other positive inotropic agents may be needed.[24]

Individually, most opioids and benzodiazepines only moderately depress cardiac function. Opioids reduce the sympathetic response and enhance vagal and parasympathetic tone. This results in vasodilation and a decrease in SVR. Benzodiazepines also cause vasodilation and a decrease in the SVR. Used in combination, these medications can have a significant effect on the cardiovascular system. Specifically, the overall reaction may include a lowered SVR, heart rate, ventricular contractility, catecholamine level, baroreceptor reflex, CO, and blood pressure. Aggressive administration of crystalloid solutions may be required to counteract these effects. High-dose opioids combined with vecuronium produce a negative inotropic and chronotropic effect. Patients may require short-term vascular support until these medications dissipate.[30,47]

Barbiturates depress the activity of the vasomotor center, causing peripheral vasodilation and hypotension. These actions are dose related and are more marked in the presence of underlying cardiovascular disease. Ketamine has a direct myocardial depressant effect that is usually counterbalanced by its indirect effect on the autonomic nervous system to increase heart rate and blood pressure. In patients who are unable to mount a sympathetic response to stress, ketamine causes a net decrease in CO. Propofol causes a dose-dependent decrease in blood pressure primarily because of a decrease in SVR. This must be considered when caring for patients who are hypovolemic or have minimal cardiac reserves.[44,48]

Local anesthetic agents can cause cardiovascular toxicity if inadvertently injected into the systemic circulation or if an excessive dosage of the agent is used. Decreased myocardial contractility, reduced SVR, and diminished CO have resulted from these agents. Cardiovascular compromise appears to occur in a dose-related fashion. Management of the cardiovascular complications associated with local anesthetic agents includes measures to increase preload, namely elevation of legs and fluid administration. In refractory cases, ephedrine may also be needed.[4,30]

Myocardial Dysfunction

During the immediate postoperative period, the causes of myocardial depression include pathologic processes and aberrant physiologic states, in addition to anesthetic side effects. These processes may occur alone or in combination and may be particularly hazardous in the presence of underlying cardiac disease.

Myocardial ischemia results from an imbalance of oxygen supply and demand. Commonly, ischemia results from a decrease in myocardial blood flow caused by atherosclerosis, vasospasm, or hypotension. In the postoperative period, the stress of surgery and the actions of certain anesthetic agents can increase myocardial ischemia.[30,46]

Dysrhythmias

In the immediate postanesthetic period, patients are predisposed to a variety of cardiac dysrhythmias. The most common dysrhythmias are sinus tachycardia, sinus bradycardia, premature ventricular contractions, supraventricular tachydysrhythmias, and ventricular tachycardia. A variety of causes can result in dysrhythmias, including circulatory instability, pre-existing heart disease, an increase in vagal tone, medications, pain, electrolytic disturbances, and hypoxemia.[49]

Accurate interpretation and identification of the dysrhythmia are essential, because therapeutic intervention is based on diagnosis. Appropriate skin preparation and lead placement are extremely important to ensure a clear, readable tracing that is free from artifact. Additional 12-lead ECG capabilities should be used if an interpretation cannot be made from tracings obtained with bedside monitoring.

The hemodynamic effects of the dysrhythmia also should be thoroughly assessed. The clinical presentation of the dysrhythmia determines the severity of underlying cardiac disease and the type of treatment. Tachydysrhythmias shorten diastolic filling time and interfere with coronary artery perfusion. These two effects, coupled with an increase in myocardial oxygen consumption, may produce cardiac decompensation. Bradycardia can produce a clinically significant decrease in CO if stroke volume is limited by underlying cardiac disease or if the venous return is reduced. The cause of the rhythm disturbance should be considered.[48]

General anesthesia lowers the dysrhythmia threshold of the myocardium. Inhalation agents sensitize the myocardium to catecholamines and depress sinoatrial (SA) and atrioventricular (AV) nodal function. Junctional rhythms and premature ventricular contractions are the most common dysrhythmias. Ketamine produces sympathetic stimulation, resulting in tachycardia and hypertension. Succinylcholine stimulates the cholinergic receptors, enhancing vagal tone, and it can produce sinus bradycardia or junctional escape rhythms. Opioids may cause bradycardia because of direct stimulation of the vagus nerve.

Endogenous catecholamine levels in postoperative patients are elevated because of the pain and stress of surgery. Increased catecholamine levels increase sinus and AV node rates, as well as atrial and ventricular irritability. The direct result is tachydysrhythmias and atrial or ventricular premature contractions.[30,46,48]

Postoperative Hypertension

Hypertension is not an unusual occurrence in the immediate postoperative period. The diagnosis of hypertension must be considered in the context of an elevated blood pressure in relation to the patient's preoperative and intraoperative blood pressure range. Most commonly, postoperative hypertension is related to fluid overload, heightened sympathetic nervous system activity, or pre-existing hypertension. Postoperative hypertension, even as a transient episode, can have significant cardiovascular and intracranial consequences, so aggressive diagnosis and treatment are indicated.

Increased sympathetic tone in the immediate postoperative period may result from the stress of surgery, postoperative pain, anxiety, or restlessness during emergence from anesthesia, bladder or bowel distention, or hypothermia. Stimulation of the autonomic nervous system can occur because of hypoxia or hypercarbia. These factors can occur alone or in combination.

Pain is one of the most common sources of increased sympathetic tone. Administering adequate amounts of analgesics, repositioning the patient for comfort, providing reassurance, and limiting environmental stimuli can contribute to alleviating postoperative pain and to lowering blood pressure.

Hypothermia and shivering also contribute to postoperative hypertension and are easily treated with warm blankets, active warming devices, and warm intravenous fluids. Bladder distention contributes to postoperative hypertension and must be alleviated. Placement of a urinary catheter may be needed. Hypoxia and hypercarbia must also be treated.

Pharmacologic treatment of postoperative hypertension includes the use of vasodilators, adrenergic inhibitors, and calcium channel blockers. The use of these agents is necessary when hypertension persists despite conservative measures previously mentioned.[30,46]

Postoperative Hypotension

Maintenance of blood pressure depends on adequate preload, myocardial contractility, and afterload. The most common cause of hypotension is intravascular volume depletion caused by inadequate replacement of blood loss, third space fluid loss, insensible loss, and urinary output. Pulmonary embolism may also reduce preload by blocking flow of blood to the left side of the heart. Reduced myocardial contractility may be a result of the effects of anesthetic medications, myocardial ischemia, or dysrhythmias. Reduced afterload in the form of low SVR may occur as a result of sepsis, hyperthermia, sympathectomy, or large arteriovenous shunts, as seen in chronic liver failure.

Prolonged hypotension can lead to serious ischemic organ damage. Prompt treatment is essential. If the underlying cause is not immediately apparent, the first treatment is an attempt to increase preload by elevating the patient's legs and infusing fluids. Examination of the ECG monitor for dysrhythmias or evidence of ischemia may help guide therapy. The lungs are examined for evidence of pulmonary edema or tension pneumothorax. Vasopressors may be administered to maintain perfusion while additional monitoring modalities are evaluated and established. Insertion of a central venous catheter allows measurement of right ventricular filling pressure and may be used to guide fluid administration in patients with normal myocardial function. In the presence of left ventricular dysfunction or when the cause remains unclear, a pulmonary artery catheter may be inserted to guide therapy through evaluation of left-sided filling pressure, CO, and SVR. The use of additional fluids, inotropic agents, or vasoconstrictor or vasodilator medications is determined by these measurements.[49]

Thermoregulatory Problems and Emergencies

Patients recovering from anesthesia usually experience some form of thermoregulatory imbalance (i.e., a core body temperature that is outside the normothermic range of 36°C to 38°C). Hypothermia and hyperthermia can occur in the postoperative patient. Management of these alterations is important, because they are associated with other physiologic alterations that may interfere with recovery.

Hypothermia

Hypothermia is a common occurrence intraoperatively and postoperatively, because the conditions associated with surgery and anesthesia typically inhibit the body's heat-generating mechanisms and favor its heat-loss mechanisms.[50] Hypothermia occurs when systemic heat loss lowers core body temperature below 36°C. Causes include wound and skin exposure, respiratory gas exchange, fluid and blood administration, use of mechanical warming or cooling devices, chemical reactions, alterations in body temperature regulation, and disease states. Clinical manifestations of hypothermia include bluish tint to the skin (peripheral cyanosis); shivering and an increase in metabolic rate (early sign); dysrhythmias; and a decrease in metabolic rate (late sign), oxygen consumption, muscle tone, heart rate, and level of consciousness.[35]

Hypothermia has several adverse effects, including discomfort, vasoconstriction, and shivering. It depresses the myocardium and increases susceptibility to ventricular dysrhythmias. Significant hypothermia slows metabolic processes, leading to reduced medication biotransformation and impaired renal transport. This may prolong medication effects and delay emergence.[35,50]

Shivering

Shivering may be a result of the compensatory response to hypothermia or the effects of anesthetic agents, and it can produce an increase in the metabolic rate. Under these conditions, increased oxygen consumption and greater carbon dioxide production can increase the ventilatory requirements. If these requirements are not met, the $Paco_2$ increases and the Pao_2 can decrease, especially if any significant intrapulmonary shunting coexists. The demand for blood flow by the diaphragm can increase sharply, requiring CO and myocardial workload to increase and causing an increase in myocardial oxygen consumption. This can result in myocardial ischemia, particularly in older adult patients and patients with coronary artery disease.[35,50]

Vasoconstriction, a particularly deleterious consequence of postoperative hypothermia, may be responsible for unexplained hypertension in the postanesthesia period. Because vasoconstriction can increase SVR and myocardial workload, the potential for myocardial ischemia exists. Vasoconstriction can mask hypovolemia, and sudden reductions in blood pressure can occur as the patient warms and vasodilates.[51] Delayed medication clearance as a consequence of hypothermia is particularly significant in older adult patients who may already have impaired medication-clearing mechanisms and a decreased metabolic rate. For example, the maximal rate of renal excretion of a medication can decline by 10% for every 0.6°C drop in body temperature. Older adult hypothermic patients are more likely to have residual paralysis because of muscle relaxants that are difficult to reverse pharmacologically.[52]

Management of the hypothermic patient is directed toward the restoration of normothermia. Rewarming prevents the thermoregulatory responses to cold, such as shivering. Management depends on the degree of temperature loss. If the patient's body temperature is between 36°C and 37°C, the patient can simply be covered with warmed blankets, and heat lamps can be used to keep the patient adequately warm. If the patient's body temperature is less than 36°C, rapid rewarming is required to decrease the possible complications of hypothermia and the postanesthesia recovery time. Convective warming devices provide a safe and effective means of rewarming the patient.[34] In patients with a normal metabolic rate, a setting of "low" or "medium" increases the mean body temperature by about 1°C per hour. A "high" setting increases the mean body temperature by about 1.5°C per hour.[4] Other methods of rewarming are thermal mattresses, fluid and blood warming, and environmental warming. Supplemental oxygen may be needed to meet the increased metabolic demand in shivering patients. Patients who are shivering may respond to a small dose of meperidine (Demerol).[51]

Hyperthermia

By definition, hyperthermia occurs at any core body temperature above normal. Severe, clinically significant hyperthermia results when core temperature exceeds 40°C. Although it is not as common perioperatively as hypothermia, hyperthermia is nevertheless a serious complication of surgery. Postoperative temperature elevations may be caused by accidental overwarming of the patient during surgery, infection, sepsis, or transfusion reactions. Because an elevated temperature increases oxygen demand and, subsequently, the ventilatory and cardiac workload, a hyperthermia patient with poor cardiac reserve suffers serious consequences.[53]

Postoperative fever must be distinguished from other hyperthermic syndromes. A fundamental difference exists between fever and specific hyperthermic states. In non–fever-related hyperthermic states, body temperature rises above normal despite the body's heat-dissipating mechanisms (e.g., vasodilation, sweating). Excessive heat gain from internal or external factors exceeds the body's cooling capabilities, with a consequent rise in body temperature.[2,4]

In contrast, fever results from a resetting to a higher temperature from the normal set point. Until the body reaches its new set point temperature, heat-generating mechanisms (i.e., vasoconstriction and shivering) are activated. After the new set point temperature is reached, there is an equilibrium between heat generation and heat loss. Unlike hyperthermia, with fever there is no physiologic activity to bring body temperature back to normal. Factors that can contribute to raising core body temperature and fever during the perioperative period are listed in Box 42-7.[50]

BOX 42-7 FACTORS INFLUENCING TEMPERATURE AND FEVER

CAUSES OF ELEVATED CORE TEMPERATURE

- Blood transfusion
- Medication-induced fever
- Overuse of techniques to prevent hypothermia
- Hypothalamic injury
- Malignant hyperthermia
- Warm environment
- Use of anticholinergics
- Endocrine disorders
- Neurogenic hyperthermia

CAUSES OF POSTOPERATIVE FEVER

- Atelectasis
- Wound infection
- Abscess formation
- Fat emboli after bone trauma
- Medication reactions
- Malignancy
- Silent aspiration
- Dehydration
- Blood transfusion reaction
- Central nervous system damage
- Urinary tract infections
- Phlebitis, deep vein thrombosis
- Pulmonary emboli

Primary therapy for hyperthermia includes cooling and decreasing thermogenesis. Cooling by evaporative or direct external methods has proved effective. This includes ice packs, a cool environment, and cooling blankets. Gastric and bladder lavage have also proved effective. Although physical cooling is an appropriate therapy for other hyperthermias, attempts to cool a febrile patient may be resisted by the thermoregulatory system. Consequently, the first course of action is to restore normothermia with the use of antipyretic medications. Antipyretics are useful because they have the ability to prevent prostaglandin synthesis in the hypothalamus. Measures to manage the febrile patient include using antipyretics (as indicated), providing a sponge bath with tepid water, keeping the environment cool, using a cooling blanket for sustained fever, and monitoring fluid and electrolyte balance as fluid needs increase during fever. The possibility of malignant hyperthermia (MH) must always be considered.[53]

Malignant Hyperthermia

Malignant hyperthermia is a genetically determined condition. MH is precipitated by certain general inhalation anesthetics, depolarizing skeletal muscle relaxants, local anesthetics, and stress in susceptible patients. The incidence of MH ranges from 1 in 15,000 in children to 1 in 50,000 in adults. The onset of MH usually occurs during induction of anesthesia but may occur within the first few hours of recovery from anesthesia.[3] Because successful management of MH depends on early assessment and prompt intervention, the nurse must be knowledgeable about the pathophysiology and treatment of this syndrome.

Identification before anesthesia of patients who may be susceptible to MH is of major therapeutic importance.[54] Patient history or genealogy going back two generations may be positive. Physical examination may reveal myopathies such as cryptorchidism, pectus carinatum, kyphosis, lordosis, ptosis, or hypoplastic mandible. Electromyographic changes are seen in fewer than half of MH-susceptible patients.

The most definitive test for detecting MH susceptibility is a biopsy of skeletal muscle.[54] Samples are obtained from the quadriceps muscles and are subjected to isometric contractor testing. The skeletal muscle of the MH-susceptible patient has an increased isometric tension when exposed to caffeine or halothane. Genetic testing for the presence of a ryanodine mutation that predicts MH susceptibility may ultimately replace the invasive diagnostic tests.[3]

When a susceptible patient is exposed to a triggering agent for MH, such as isoflurane, the clinical features are produced by an excess of calcium ions in the myoplasm. With an elevated calcium ion concentration in the myoplasm, skeletal muscle contraction is intense and prolonged, leading to a hypermetabolic state of acid and heat production. More specifically, heat is produced by the accelerated and continued synthesis and use of adenosine triphosphate (ATP) during glycolysis. The metabolic byproduct of glycolysis, lactic acid, is transported to the liver and then back to the metabolically active muscle, where the cycle repeats. Respiratory acidosis and metabolic acidosis develop because of this hypermetabolic state, and symptoms such as tachycardia, tachypnea, ventricular dysrhythmias, and

BOX 42-8	SIGNS AND SYMPTOMS OF MALIGNANT HYPERTHERMIA

- Muscle rigidity
- Increased CO_2 production (hypercapnia)
- Rhabdomyolysis
- Marked temperature elevation (hyperthermia)
- Tachycardia
- Tachypnea
- Metabolic acidosis
- Respiratory acidosis
- Hyperkalemia
- Myoglobinuria
- Elevated creatine phosphokinase
- Ventricular dysrhythmias
- Cyanosis
- Skin mottling
- Hot, flushed skin
- Rigidity
- Profuse sweating
- Unstable blood pressure

Modified from Odom-Forren J. *Drain's Perianesthesia Nursing: a Critical Care Approach.* 6th ed. St. Louis: Elsevier; 2013.

BOX 42-9	ENVIRONMENTAL AND PHARMACOLOGIC TRIGGERS OF MALIGNANT HYPERTHERMIA

Environmental Stimuli
- Extremely hot and humid weather
- Strenuous and prolonged exercise

Pharmacologic Agents
- Isoflurane
- Sevoflurane
- Desflurane
- Succinylcholine

Modified from Odom-Forren J. *Drain's Perianesthesia Nursing: a Critical Care Approach.* 6th ed. St. Louis: Elsevier; 2013.

unstable blood pressure appear. Because of intense vasoconstriction, the skin is mottled and cyanotic.[55] Box 42-8 lists the clinical manifestations of MH.

Elevated body temperature can actually be a late sign of MH. For this reason, the nurse must not prolong the assessment of the patient on the assumption that the patient's temperature must be significantly elevated before intervention is attempted. After the patient's temperature begins to rise, it may increase at a rate of 1°C every 3 to 5 minutes and may approach levels as high as 46°C.[30]

Muscle rigidity occurs in about 75% of the patients who experience MH. This is especially true in MH-susceptible patients after the administration of succinylcholine. Muscle rigidity may be so severe that the nurse cannot open the patient's mouth to insert an airway. The onset of skeletal muscle rigidity after the administration of succinylcholine could be a sign of impending development of MH.[53,55]

Various environmental and pharmacologic agents can stimulate an acute episode of MH (Box 42-9).[54] Fatigue, emotional upset, or very hot and humid weather can trigger a waking febrile episode. The anesthetic agents that may trigger MH seem to affect the sarcoplasmic reticulum. Because of their widespread use, volatile anesthetic agents (e.g., isoflurane) and succinylcholine are the most common triggering agents. In MH-susceptible patients and in patients who have had an

episode of MH in the operating room, all possible triggering agents must be stringently avoided. As another precaution, because emotional upsets trigger MH, nurses must provide a stress-free environment for the MH-susceptible patient.

The cornerstone of successful management of MH is early detection. If the patient develops acute MH, all inhalation anesthetics are stopped, the patient is hyperventilated with 100% oxygen, and dantrolene is given. To be administered, dantrolene must be diluted with sterile water. Cooling measures, such as administering cold intravenous fluids, packing the patient in ice, and irrigating body cavities (e.g., stomach, bladder) with cold fluids, are initiated as needed based on the patient's temperature. Accurate intake and output records are essential because large amounts of fluids and diuretics are given. Laboratory tests, such as complete blood cell counts (CBC) and coagulation studies, are closely scrutinized for signs of bleeding or the onset of disseminated intravascular clotting. Ongoing ECG and temperature monitoring are also essential. It is recommended that all emergency medications be available on a special cart in the operating room or in the PACU.

Neurologic Problems and Emergencies

Almost all patients exhibit some level of arousal within 15 minutes after anesthesia is completed.[3] Although many factors are known to prolong anesthetic effects, most reports of delayed emergence and emergence delirium are anecdotal.

Delayed Emergence

Delayed awakening after general anesthesia occurs occasionally, and is defined as a failure to regain consciousness within 20 to 30 minutes after the anesthetic ends.[56] It can usually be attributed to prolonged action of anesthetic medications, metabolic causes, or neurologic injury.[30] In most cases, prolonged sedation is the result of residual general anesthetic. Hypoventilation resulting from a high concentration of inhaled anesthetic limits exhalation of the agent and prolongs its retention. Opioids used as adjunct therapy may contribute to hypercarbia and sedation as well. Hypothermia, advanced age, hepatic dysfunction, and renal disease may contribute to prolonged recovery from anesthetics by heightening sensitivity or delaying elimination, or both. The use of premedication may also prolong recovery, especially if opioids or benzodiazepines, particularly lorazepam, are used.[57]

In addition to experiencing a slowing elimination of potent inhalation anesthetic, the hypoventilating patient may develop hypoxia and hypercapnia. The hypercapnia may cause significant narcosis and may potentiate the depressive effects of the anesthetics. In the diabetic patient, fasting or excessive insulin may cause electrolyte abnormalities, leading to unconsciousness, or even coma.[56]

Severe electrolyte disturbances are most commonly seen after excessive water absorption during transurethral prostate surgery. The subsequent dilution hyponatremia may manifest as sedation, coma, or hemiparesis. Dilution hyponatremia may also be seen after the inappropriate release of antidiuretic hormone. Hypocalcemia after parathyroid surgery may result in delayed awakening. High magnesium levels after prolonged administration of magnesium sulfate to the eclamptic or pre-eclamptic patient may also result in prolonged postoperative sedation and in muscle weakness after cesarean section under general anesthesia.[36]

Neurologic injury and subsequent unconsciousness may be the result of an unsuspected cerebral vascular accident. Intracranial hemorrhage may result from hypertensive responses to anesthetic agents or surgical manipulations, especially in the patient receiving anticoagulant therapy. Paradoxic air emboli may cross a patent foramen ovale in the presence of a right-to-left shunt. Direct emboli from cardiac valves, intracardiac thrombi, and atherosclerotic vessels may also be a threat. Fat emboli can occur after massive long-bone or tissue damage and may not appear until during or after surgical manipulation or reduction of the fracture. Deliberate, induced hypotension in normal patients is not usually associated with neurologic damage. However, uncontrolled intraoperative hypotension may result in ischemia, especially in the patient with hypertension or carotid occlusive disease.[57]

The successful management of delayed arousal depends on careful consideration of the differential diagnosis. A thorough review of the patient's preoperative medical condition and the intraoperative course (surgical and anesthetic) usually points to a cause. If the cause of the sedation is not immediately obvious, the first consideration must be assessing the patient's oxygenation and ensuring adequate gas exchange. Pulse oximetry, end-tidal carbon dioxide measurement, and arterial blood gas analysis can give an estimate of any ventilatory depression and rule out ongoing hypoxia and hypercarbia factors.[57,58]

If the cause is thought to be residual inhalation anesthetic, maintenance of adequate ventilation should be sufficient treatment. Residual opioids can be reversed by naloxone, and anticholinergic CNS depression can be reversed by physostigmine. The benzodiazepine antagonist flumazenil has been shown to directly antagonize the CNS sedative and amnesic effects of the benzodiazepines.[4]

Body temperature is measured, and warming is instituted if hypothermia exists. Serum electrolytes and magnesium and calcium levels are checked if ion disturbance is suspected. Blood for a serum glucose assay may also be drawn, but the simple fingerstick glucose determination is faster and accurate enough to exclude hypoglycemia from consideration if the result is normal. Other laboratory tests may be useful if hepatic or renal disease is being considered. Unless perioperative events point specifically to it, neurologic injury is usually a diagnosis of exclusion. If other causes of prolonged arousal have been excluded, a thorough neurologic consultation is obtained.[57]

Emergence Delirium

Most patients emerge from general anesthesia in a calm, tranquil manner. Some patients, however, emerge in a state of excitement, a condition characterized by restlessness, disorientation, crying, moaning, or irrational talking. In the extreme form of excitement, which is referred to as *emergence delirium*, the patient screams, shouts, and thrashes about wildly. This condition is seen most frequently after tonsillectomy, thyroid surgery, circumcision, hysterectomy, and perineal and abdominal wall procedures.[30,58]

Hypoxia with resulting air hunger and hypercarbia may appear as restlessness, disorientation, slurred speech, and agitation. Hyponatremia, hypochloremia, and acid–base changes can all be seen during the immediate postoperative period and can be the cause of mental confusion. Pain is a common cause of restlessness and is frequently seen postoperatively. Urinary bladder and gastric distention, which can cause considerable discomfort, are easily overlooked.[30,58]

Medication reactions are commonly implicated as the cause of postoperative agitation. Such reactions are less common than they once were, because the use of offending medications is less prevalent. The most frequently implicated medications are the anticholinergics, most notably scopolamine and atropine. They have been shown to have CNS-toxic effects that can include psychotic behavior, delirium, and motor disturbance. Ketamine is also associated with a high incidence of unpleasant agitation. Neuroleptic medications such as droperidol, especially in rarely used high doses, may be associated with development of dyskinesia and involuntary muscle activity and with postoperative confusion.[57]

The patient's state of apprehension or anxiety can have a marked effect on emergence agitation; it is especially notable in apprehensive patients and, conversely, in those who are seemingly unconcerned about forthcoming major surgery. Factors such as fear of disfigurement (e.g., caused by cancer surgery) and feelings of suffocation also increase the likelihood of emergence excitement. Young patients tend to have an increased incidence of postoperative excitation, as do patients undergoing emergency procedures. Several psychiatric factors have been shown to increase the incidence of postoperative delirium, including a history of alcoholism, insomnia, depression, or debility.[30,58]

If emergence delirium occurs, the patient's status is thoroughly evaluated. Management includes determining a cause, initiating specific therapy, and protecting patients from injuring themselves. When the nurse encounters a restless, confused postoperative patient, the first measure is to ensure that the agitation is not the result of hypoxia. Presuming pain to be the cause of agitation in a hypoxic patient and treating the excitement with opioids or sedatives can have disastrous consequences. Hypoxia must be quickly excluded from the differential diagnosis by pulse oximetry or arterial blood gas determination, or both.[2,59]

Hyponatremia may be suspected in the confused patient after prostate surgery, especially if the surgery was prolonged. A serum electrolyte determination can confirm the diagnosis. The treatment usually consists of fluid restriction and, rarely, hypertonic saline administration. Severe acid–base disturbances can be diagnosed and therapy directed by arterial blood gas determination. If pain appears to be the diagnosis after exclusion of hypoxia, intravenous opioids may be administered in small increments. The CNS effects of the anticholinergics are usually dramatically reversed by the administration of physostigmine. The incidence of hallucinations with ketamine may be decreased by benzodiazepine administration. Gastric distention may be relieved by nasogastric aspiration, and urinary bladder distention is easily treated with catheterization.[4]

When dealing with perioperative anxiety, the best treatment is prevention. Some patients need reassurance that they will not experience intraoperative awareness and will receive pain medication, if needed, on awakening.

Occasionally, the nurse is faced with a restless postoperative patient who does not seem to be getting relief from opioid administration. Small intravenous doses of a short-acting benzodiazepine such as midazolam may be warranted. The anxiolytics are administered in reduced doses, because their respiratory depressant effects are cumulative with those of existing opioids, sedatives, and residual general anesthetics. If overt psychotic behavior is apparent despite adequate treatment, psychiatric consultation should be obtained.[58]

The patient's respiratory function and airway patency are checked first, because restlessness is a well-known manifestation of hypoxia. Other causes of emergence delirium include a full bladder, cramped or sore muscles and joints from prolonged abnormal positioning on the operating table, pain, incomplete reversal of NMBAs, withdrawal from alcohol and other medications, acid–base disturbances, and electrolyte abnormalities. The restless patient requires constant, careful observation. Gentle physical restraint may be required to prevent injury. Several nurses or other personnel may be needed. If hypoxia, pain, and a full bladder are ruled out, a change in positioning may have a quieting effect.[2]

Nausea and Vomiting

Nausea and vomiting, although usually not life-threatening, are probably the most unpleasant and lasting memories many patients have of their anesthesia.[60] Although the incidence has decreased in recent years, nausea and vomiting still result in significant postoperative morbidity and patient discomfort. Nausea is described as a subjective, unpleasant mental experience that usually leads to vomiting. Retching is the rhythmic muscular activity that usually precedes vomiting. Vomiting is defined as the forceful expulsion of gastrointestinal contents through the mouth.[61]

Decidedly unpleasant, vomiting can also be significant.[62] The physical exertion may increase postoperative bleeding and disrupt delicate suture lines. Tearing or rupture of the esophagus is probably rare but must be a concern in patients with a history of esophageal pathology. Aspiration of emesis is a life-threatening complication in a patient whose airway-protective reflexes are blunted by residual anesthetic or sedative medications or damaged by surgical activity. If the vomiting is protracted, dangerous hypokalemia, hypochloremia, hyponatremia, and dehydration may develop. Nausea and vomiting are also the leading causes of unexpected hospitalization after surgery.[61,63]

Risk factors most strongly associated with postoperative nausea and vomiting include female gender, history of PONV, history of motion sickness (subjective as reported by patient), nonsmoker, postoperative use/administration of opioids, use of volatile anesthetics, and use of nitrous oxide.[64] Age, duration of surgery, and type of surgery are supported as risk factors by weak or conflicting evidence.

The most effective treatment of postoperative nausea and vomiting is prevention.[62] Several maneuvers merit mention as being fairly simple to perform and effective in their usefulness. Avoidance of gastric insufflation is paramount. Swallowing of blood should be prevented during oral, pharyngeal, or nasal surgery. If distention is suspected, it should be decompressed intraoperatively.[4,52] A nasogastric tube is placed to empty fluid and gases from the stomach, but its presence may trigger gagging and subsequent vomiting. An oral airway may elicit the same response in a partially conscious patient and is removed at the first signs of gagging to prevent vomiting and subsequent aspiration.[65]

Many medications have been shown to possess antiemetic qualities, and prophylactic antiemetics and combination medications have been shown to be effective in decreasing or preventing postoperative nausea and vomiting. Available antiemetics include anticholinergics, phenothiazines, antihistamines, butyrophenones, and antidopaminergics. Complementary therapies, including acupuncture and aromatherapy with peppermint oil, have also been shown to be effective in relieving symptoms.[66] It is important to remember the supportive care of the nauseated and vomiting patient. If vomiting is severe, electrolyte replacement must be considered. Prolonged vomiting may result in hypovolemia. Intravenous fluids may need to be increased to compensate for fluid losses. Decreased opioid doses may be needed to reduce the risk of nausea and vomiting; adding nonopioids, such as nonsteroidal anti-inflammatory drugs (NSAIDs) or acetaminophen, may allow for adequate analgesia with less risk of nausea.[67]

BOX 42-10 **INTERNET RESOURCES**

American Association of Critical-Care Nurses: **http://www.aacn.org**
American Association of Nurse Anesthetists: **http://www.aana.com**
American College of Surgeons: **http://www.facs.org**
American Society for Pain Management Nursing: **http://www.aspmn.org**
American Society of Anesthesiologists: **http://www.asahq.org**
American Society of PeriAnesthesia Nurses: **http://www.aspan.org**
British Anaesthetic and Recovery Nurses Association:
   http://www.barna.co.uk

Malignant Hyperthermia Association of the United States:
   http://www.mhaus.org
National Association of PeriAnesthesia Nurses of Canada:
   http://www.napanc.org
National Institutes for Health: **http://www.nih.gov**
PubMed Health: **http://www.ncbi.nlm.nih.gov/pubmedhealth**
Society for Critical Care Medicine: **http://www.sccm.org**

BOX 42-11   CASE STUDY

Patient with Complex Perianesthesia Management

Brief Patient History

Ms. C is a 60-year-old, bilingual Hispanic woman. She has a history of colon cancer with metastasis, and she has been taking the equivalent of 400 mg of morphine each day for the past 2 weeks in order to effectively manage her pain. Ms. C is a recovering alcoholic and opioid addict but has been "clean" for 6 years. Other significant medical history includes hypertension, which has been controlled for the past 2 years with lisinopril 10 mg daily. She has undergone a colon resection with general anesthesia (combination of inhalation and intravenous opioid and nonopioid agents), which took several hours to complete. Her vital signs were stable throughout the surgical procedure. Ms. C received a total of 20 mg of morphine during the 4 hours she was in the postanesthesia care unit (PACU).

Clinical Assessment

Ms. C is admitted to the surgical critical care unit from the PACU because of difficulty in controlling her hypertension. She is somnolent but arousable to painful stimuli; however, she states in Spanish that she is having abdominal pain. Ms. C's skin is warm and dry; her breaths are being taken through her nose, but respirations are slow and shallow.

Diagnostic Procedures

Ms. C's baseline vital signs are: blood pressure (BP), 190/92; heart rate (HR), 120 (sinus tachycardia); respiratory rate (RR), 14; temperature (T), 36.5° C; chest x-ray, right lower lobe atelectasis; hemoglobin, 9; hematocrit, 27; pulse oximetry O_2 saturation, 80% on 100% O_2 via nonrebreather mask; end-tidal CO_2, 70 mm Hg. Ms. C reports that her pain is an 8 out of 10. Riker Sedation-Agitation Scale is 2.

Medical Diagnosis

Ms. C is diagnosed with respiratory depression and hypoxemia secondary to opioid analgesia.

Questions

1. What major outcomes do you expect to achieve for this patient?
2. What problems or risks must be managed to achieve these outcomes?
3. What interventions must be initiated to monitor, prevent, manage, or eliminate the problems and risks identified above?
4. What interventions should be initiated to promote optimal functioning, safety, and well-being of the patient?
5. What possible learning needs would you anticipate for this patient?
6. What cultural and age-related factors might have a bearing on the patient's plan of care?

SUMMARY

Selection of Anesthesia

- The type of anesthesia used for surgery may be local, regional, or general.
- Local and regional anesthetics eliminate the sensation of pain to a specific part of the body without loss of protective reflexes or consciousness.
- General anesthesia is a controlled state of unconsciousness; the patient is not arousable, there is partial or complete loss of protective reflexes, and the airway needs to be continuously monitored and maintained.

Perianesthesia Assessment and Care

- Caring for the critically ill patient who is emerging from anesthesia requires monitoring of the patient's physical and psychologic status to prevent potential complications that may occur as a result of anesthesia or surgical procedures.
- Knowledge of the preoperative history is important in evaluating and managing postoperative care.
- Communication and hand-off among the anesthesia care provider, the perioperative nurse, and the registered nurse caring for the patient in the immediate postoperative period is important for continuity and safe patient care.
- The goal of patient management in the immediate postoperative period is recognition and immediate treatment of any problems to eliminate or lessen complications.

- Assessment of the cardiopulmonary system is the immediate priority.
- The stir-up regimen is probably the most important aspect of perianesthesia nursing management and consists of five major activities: deep-breathing exercises, coughing, positioning, mobilization, and pain management.

Management of Postanesthesia Problems and Emergencies

- The most frequent complications include respiratory compromise, hypovolemia, hypothermia, and cardiac dysrhythmias.
- The most common adverse reaction is postoperative nausea and vomiting.
- The most lethal complication is malignant hyperthermia.
- Respiratory issues include upper airway obstruction, laryngeal edema, laryngospasm, bronchospasm, acute respiratory failure, aspiration, pulmonary edema, and respiratory arrest.
- Pain management is a priority; inadequate analgesia can interfere with respiratory function and adequate ventilation, affect hemodynamic status, and have a prolonged psychologic impact.

REFERENCES

1. Krenzischek DA, et al. Patient safety: perianesthesia nursing's essential role in safe practice. *J Perianesth Nurs*. 2007;22:385.
2. Cartwright SMI, Andrews SM. Perianesthesia nursing as a specialty. In: Odom-Forren J, ed. *Drain's Perianesthesia Nursing: A Critical Care Approach*. 6th ed. St. Louis: Elsevier; 2013.
3. Barash PG, et al. *Handbook of Clinical Anesthesia*. 6th ed. Philadelphia: Lippincott Williams & Wilkins; 2006.
4. Fleisher LA. Risk of anesthesia. In: Miller RD, et al, eds. *Miller's Anesthesia*. 7th ed. New York: Churchill Livingstone; 2009.
5. Duke J. *Anesthesia Secrets*. 4th ed. Philadelphia: Elsevier; 2011.
6. Drasner K, Larson MD. Spinal and epidural anesthesia. In: Miller RD, Pardo Jr MC, eds. *Basics of Anesthesia*. 6th ed. St. Louis: Elsevier; 2011.
7. Henderson J. Airway management in the adult. In: Miller RD, et al, eds. *Miller's Anesthesia*. 7th ed. New York: Churchill Livingstone; 2009.
8. Miller RD. Choice of anesthetic technique. In: Miller RD, Pardo Jr MC, eds. *Basics of Anesthesia*. 6th ed. St. Louis: Elsevier; 2011.
9. Pazdernik TL, Kerecsen L. Anesthetics. In: Paxdernik TL, Kercsen L, eds. *Rapid Review of Pharmacology*. 3rd ed. St. Louis: Elsevier; 2010.
10. Drain CB. Inhalation anesthesia. In: Odom-Forren J, ed. *Drain's Perianesthesia Nursing: A Critical Care Approach*. 6th ed. St. Louis: Elsevier; 2013.
11. de Silva A. Anesthetic monitoring. In: Miller RD, Pardo Jr MC, eds. *Basics of Anesthesia*. 6th ed. St. Louis: Elsevier; 2011.
12. Drain CB. Nonopioid intravenous anesthetics. In: Odom-Forren J, ed. *Drain's Perianesthesia Nursing: A Critical Care Approach*. 6th ed. St. Louis: Elsevier; 2013.
13. Drain CB. Opioid intravenous anesthetics. In: Odom-Forren J, ed. *Drain's Perianesthesia Nursing: A Critical Care Approach*. 6th ed. St. Louis: Elsevier; 2013.
14. Reves JG, et al. Intravenous anesthetics. In: Miller RD, et al, eds. *Miller's Anesthesia*. 7th ed. New York: Churchill Livingstone; 2009.
15. Nazareno AR, Gahart BL. *Intravenous Medications: A Handbook for Nurses and Health Professionals*. 29th ed. St. Louis: Elsevier; 2013.
16. Drain CB. Neuromuscular blocking agents. In: Odom-Forren J, ed. *Drain's Perianesthesia Nursing: A Critical Care Approach*. 6th ed. St. Louis: Elsevier; 2013.
17. Wilson J, et al. Residual neuromuscular blockade in critical care. *Crit Care Nurse*. 2012; 32(3):e1.
18. Naguib M, Lien CA. Pharmacology of muscle relaxants and their antagonists. In: Miller RD, et al, eds. *Miller's Anesthesia*. 7th ed. New York: Churchill Livingstone; 2009.
19. American Society of PeriAnesthesia Nurses. Practice recommendation 6: safe transfer of care. *Perianesthesia Nursing Standards and Practice Recommendations 2010-2012*. Cherry Hill, NJ: American Society of PeriAnesthesia Nurses; 2010.
20. Schutz SL. Oxygen saturation monitoring by pulse oximetry. In: Wiegand DLM, ed. *AACN Procedure Manual for Critical Care*. 6th ed. Philadelphia: Elsevier; 2011.
21. Watson CB. Respiratory complications associated with anesthesia. *Anesthesiol Clin North Am*. 2002;20:513.
22. O'Brien D. Patient education and care of the perianesthesia patient. In: Odom-Forren J, ed. *Drain's Perianesthesia Nursing: A Critical Care Approach*. 6th ed. St. Louis: Elsevier; 2013.
23. Dunwoody CJ, et al. Assessment, physiological monitoring, and consequences of inadequately treated acute pain. *Pain Manag Nurs*. 2008;9(suppl 1):S11.
24. Cohen SP, Raja SN. Pain. In: Goldman L, Schafer AI, eds. *Goldman's Cecil Medicine*. 24th ed. St. Louis: Elsevier; 2011.
25. Aubrun F, et al. Relationships between measurement of pain using visual analog score and morphine requirements during postoperative intravenous morphine titration. *Anesthesiology*. 2003;98:1415.
26. Golembiewski JA. Morphine and hydromorphone for postoperative analgesia: focus on safety. *J PeriAnesth Nurs*. 2003;18:120.
27. Polomano RC, et al. Perspective on pain management in the 21st century. *Pain Manag Nurs*. 2008;9(suppl 1):3.
28. Sun LS, Schwarzenberger JC. Cardiac physiology. In: Miller RD, et al, eds. *Miller's Anesthesia*. 7th ed. New York: Churchill Livingstone; 2009.
29. Schick L, Windle PE. *Perianesthesia Nursing Core Curriculum*. 2nd ed. St. Louis: Elsevier; 2010.
30. O'Brien D. Postanesthesia care complications. In: Odom-Forren J, ed. *Drain's Perianesthesia Nursing: A Critical Care Approach*. 6th ed. St. Louis: Elsevier; 2013.
31. Brown EN, et al. General anesthesia, sleep, and coma. *N Engl J Med*. 2010;363:2638.
32. Ng JLW, et al. Perioperative stroke in noncardiac, nonneurosurgical surgery. *Anesthesiology*. 2011;115:879.
33. Lepousé C, et al. Emergence delirium in adults in the post-anaesthesia care unit. *Br J Anaesth*. 2006;96:747.
34. Hooper VD, et al. ASPAN's evidence-based clinical practice guideline for the promotion of perioperative normothermia: second edition. *J PeriAnesth Nurs*. 2010;25:346.
35. AORN Recommended Practice Committee. Recommended practices for the prevention of unplanned perioperative hypothermia. *AORN J*. 2007;85:972.
36. Kaye AD, Riopelle JM. Intravascular fluid and electrolyte physiology. In: Miller RD, et al, eds. *Miller's Anesthesia*. 7th ed. New York: Churchill Livingstone; 2009.
37. Malina DP. Fluid and electrolytes. In: Odom-Forren J, ed. *Drain's Perianesthesia Nursing: A Critical Care Approach*. 6th ed. St. Louis: Elsevier; 2013.
38. Rosén S, et al. Calm or not calm: the question of anxiety in the perianesthesia patient. *J PeriAnesth Nurs*. 2008;23:237.
39. Kiekkas P, et al. Nursing activities and use of time in the postanesthesia care unit. *J PeriAnesth Nurs*. 2005;20:311.
40. American Society of PeriAnesthesia Nurses. Position statement 5: A joint position statement on ICU overflow patients developed by ASPAN, AACN, and ASA's Anesthesia Care Team Committee and Committee on Critical Care Medicine and Trauma Medicine. http://www.aspan.org/Portals/6/docs/ClinicalPractice/PositionStatement/1012/Pos_Stmt_5_Joint_ICUOverflow.pdf. Accessed September 12, 2012.
41. American Society of PeriAnesthesia Nurses. *Perianesthesia Nursing Standards and Practice Recommendations 2010-2012*. Cherry Hill, NJ: ASPAN; 2010.
42. Litwack K. *Post Anesthesia Care Nursing*. 2nd ed. St. Louis: Mosby; 1995.
43. Wright SM. Assessment and management of the airway. In: Odom-Forren J, ed. *Drain's Perianesthesia Nursing: A Critical Care Approach*. 6th ed. St. Louis: Elsevier; 2013.
44. Odom JL. Airway emergencies in the post anesthesia care unit. *Nurs Clin North Am*. 1993;28:483.
45. Udeshi A, et al. Postobstructive pulmonary edema. *J Crit Care*. 2010;25:508.
46. Weitz HH. Perioperative cardiac complications. *Med Clin North Am*. 2001;85:1151.

47. Mokhlesi B, Corbridge T. Toxicology in the critically ill patient. *Clin Chest Med.* 2003;24:689.

48. Sloan SB, Weitz HH. Postoperative arrhythmias and conduction disorders. *Med Clin North Am.* 2001;85:1171.

49. Nicholau D. Postanesthesia recovery. In: Miller RD, Pardo Jr MC, eds. *Basics of Anesthesia.* 6th ed. St. Louis: Elsevier; 2011.

50. Kurz A. Thermal care in the perioperative period. *Best Pract Res Clin Anaesthesiol.* 2008;22:39.

51. De Witte J, Sessler DI. Perioperative shivering: physiology and pharmacology. *Anesthesiology.* 2002;96:467.

52. Hildebrand F, et al. Pathophysiologic changes and effects of hypothermia on outcome in elective surgery and trauma patients. *Am J Surg.* 2004;187:363.

53. McHenry CR, et al. Recognition, management, and prevention of specific operating room catastrophes. *J Am Coll Surg.* 2004;198:810.

54. Rosenberg H, et al. Malignant hyperthermia. *Orphanet J Rare Dis.* 2007;2:21.

55. Hommertzheim R, Steinke EE. Malignant hyperthermia: the perioperative nurse's role. *AORN J.* 2006;83:149.

56. McClain DA. Delayed emergence. In: Atlee JL, ed. *Complications in Anesthesia.* 2nd ed. St. Louis: Saunders; 2006.

57. Mecca RS. Coma and delayed emergence. In: Lobato EB, et al, eds. *Complications in Anesthesiology.* 4th ed. Philadelphia: Lippincott Williams & Wilkins; 2008.

58. O'Brien D. Acute postoperative delirium: definitions, incidence, recognition, and interventions. *J Perianesth Nurs.* 2002;17:384.

59. Hagberg CA. *Benumof's Airway Management.* 2nd ed. Philadelphia: Mosby; 2007.

60. Chandrakantan A, Glass PS. Multimodal therapies for postoperative nausea and vomiting, and pain. *Br J Anaesth.* 2011;107(1 Suppl):i27.

61. Ho K-Y, Gan TJ. Postoperative nausea and vomiting. In: Lobato EB, et al, eds. *Complications in Anesthesiology.* 4th ed. Philadelphia: Lippincott Williams & Wilkins; 2008.

62. Kranke P, Eberhart LH. Possibilities and limitations in the pharmacological management of postoperative nausea and vomiting. *Eur J Anaesthesiol.* 2011;28:758.

63. Gan TJ, et al. Society for ambulatory anesthesia guidelines for the management of postoperative nausea and vomiting. *Anesth Analg.* 2007;105:1615.

64. American Society of PeriAnesthesia Nurses PONV/PDNV Strategic Work Team. ASPAN'S evidence-based clinical practice guideline for the prevention and/or management of PONV/PDNV. *J PeriAnesth Nurs.* 2006;21:230.

65. Odom-Forren J, et al. Evidence-based interventions for post discharge nausea and vomiting: a review of the literature. *J Perianesth Nurs.* 2006;21:411.

66. Mamaril ME, et al. Prevention and management of postoperative nausea and vomiting: a look at complementary techniques. *J Perianesth Nurs.* 2006;21:404.

67. Pasero C, McCaffery M. *Pain Assessment and Pharmacologic Management.* St. Louis: Elsevier; 2011.

Nursing Management Plans of Care

⊚ NURSING MANAGEMENT PLAN

Activity Intolerance

Definition: Insufficient physiologic or psychologic energy to endure or complete required or desired daily activities

Activity Intolerance Related to Cardiopulmonary Dysfunction

Defining Characteristics
- Chest pain with activity
- Electrocardiographic changes with activity
- Heart rate is >15 beats/min above baseline with activity for patients on beta-blockers or calcium channel blockers
- Heart rate remains elevated above baseline 5 minutes after activity
- Breathlessness with activity
- SpO_2 <92% with activity
- Postural hypotension when moving from supine to upright position
- Patient reports fatigue with activity

Outcome Criteria
- Heart rate is <20 beats/min above baseline with activity and is <10 beats/min above baseline with activity for patients on beta-blockers or calcium channel blockers.
- Heart rate returns to baseline 5 minutes after activity.
- Chest pain with activity is absent.
- Patient reports tolerance to activity.

Nursing Interventions and Rationale
1. Encourage active or passive range-of-motion exercises while the patient is in bed *to keep joints flexible and muscles stretched.*
2. Teach patient to refrain from holding breath while performing exercises and *to avoid the Valsalva maneuver.*
3. Encourage performance of muscle-toning exercises at least three times daily, *because a toned muscle uses less oxygen when performing work than an untoned muscle.*
4. Progress ambulation *to increase tolerance to activity.*
5. Teach patient to take pulse *to determine activity tolerance:* Take pulse for a full minute before exercise and then for 10 seconds and multiply by 6 at exercise peak.
6. Consult with physician regarding the administration of fluids to ensure that the patient is hydrated to 24-hour fluid requirements per body surface area (BSA) *to increase preload and thereby increase stroke volume and cardiac output.*

Activity Intolerance Related to Prolonged Immobility or Deconditioning

Defining Characteristics
- Decrease in systolic blood pressure is >20 mm Hg
- Increase in heart rate is >20 beats/min with postural change
- Syncope with postural change
- Patient reports lightheadedness with postural change

Outcome Criteria
- Decrease in systolic blood pressure is <10 mm Hg.
- Increase in heart rate is <10 beats/min with postural change.
- Syncope or lightheadedness is absent with postural change.
- Absence of hypoxemia
- Patient reports tolerance to activity.

Nursing Interventions and Rationale
1. Collaborate with physician regarding patient's activity level and the need for physical therapy *to ensure patient's safety.*
2. Collaborate with physical therapist to develop progressive activity plan for patient *to return to prior level of function.*

For Patient on Bed Rest
1. Instruct the patient how to perform straight-leg raises, dorsiflexion or plantar flexion, and quadriceps-setting and gluteal-setting exercises *to increase muscular and vascular tone.*
2. Reposition patient incrementally *to avoid syncope:*
   a. Head of bed to 45 degrees and hold until symptom free
   b. Head of bed to 90 degrees and hold until symptom free
   c. Dangle until symptom free
   d. Stand until symptom free and ambulate

For Patient on Ventilator
1. Collaborate with physician, respiratory care practitioner, and physical therapist regarding patient's eligibility for early progressive mobility *to ensure patient is ready and able to participate*.
2. Initiate early progressive mobility program when patient is ready *to limit the effects of prolonged immobility.*
   a. Elevation of the head of the bed
   b. Turn patient every 2 hours
   c. Perform passive range of motion at least 3 times/day
   d. Progress patient to active range of motion when ready
   e. Place bed in chair position to position patient in upright/leg-down position
   f. Initiate bed mobility activities such as sitting on the edge of the bed (dangling)
   g. Initiate transfer training
   h. Implement pre-gait activities such as standing at the side of the bed and marching in place
   i. Progress patient to ambulation
3. Monitor patient's response to activity and discontinue activity if patient shows signs of intolerance *to ensure patient safety:*
   a. Hypoxemia
   b. Hypotension
   c. Dysrhythmias or electrocardiographic changes

◉ NURSING MANAGEMENT PLAN

Acute Confusion

Definition: Abrupt onset of reversible disturbances of consciousness, attention, cognition, and perception that develop over a short period of time

Acute Confusion Related to Sensory Overload, Sensory Deprivation, and Sleep Pattern Disturbance

Defining Characteristics

Early Symptoms

- Sudden onset of global cognitive function impairment (hours to days)
- Restlessness, agitation, and combative behavior
- Drowsiness (can lead to loss of consciousness)
- Slurring of speech, inappropriate statements or "word salad," mumbling, or inappropriate gestures
- Short attention span (needs questions repeated); inability to learn new material
- Disordered sleep/wake cycle
- Disorientation to person, time, place, and situation
- Difficulty in separating dreams from reality (may experience bizarre dreams or nightmares)
- Anger at staff for continued questions about his or her orientation

Later Symptoms

- Symptoms that tend to fluctuate throughout the day and night
- Continuations of early symptoms, which may be more frequent or of longer duration
- Illusions
- Hallucinations
- Extreme agitation (e.g., attempts to climb out of bed, pull out catheters, rip off dressings)
- Calling out in loud voice, swearing, or attempting to bite or hit people who approach patient

Nursing Interventions and Rationale

1. Determine and document the patient's dominant spoken language, his or her literacy, and the languages in which he or she is literate. *Sometimes, people are not literate in their spoken language, or, less commonly, they are literate only in their second language.*
2. Determine and document patient's premorbid degree of orientation, cognitive capabilities, and any sensory/perceptual deficits.

For Sensory Overload

1. Initiate each nurse/patient encounter by calling the patient by name and identifying yourself by name. *This fosters reality orientation and assists the patient in filtering irrelevant or impersonal conversation.*
2. Assess the patient's immediate physical environment from his or her viewpoint, and explain equipment, its sounds, and its therapeutic purpose. Demonstrate audible and visual alarms, and explain possible alarm conditions. *This decreases alienation of the patient from the technologic environment and reduces the inherent sense of fear and urgency accompanying alarm conditions.*
3. Provide preparatory sensory information by explaining procedures in relation to the sensations the patient will experience, including duration of sensations. *Preparatory sensory information enhances learning and lessens anticipatory anxiety.*
4. Limit noise levels. *Audible alarms cannot and must not be silenced, and many critical but noisy activities must take place in the critical care area. It has been shown, however, that noise levels produced by clinical personnel exceed those levels designated as acceptable and are often greater than those generated by technologic devices.*
   a. Keep staff conversations soft enough that they are inaudible to the patient whenever possible.

b. Assume that everything said at or around a patient's bedside is intended for that patient's awareness and that it will be interpreted as pertaining to him or her. *As in the discussion that follows, conversations about the patient but not to him or her foster depersonalization and delusions of reference.*
   c. Enforce nighttime noise limits.
5. Readjust alarm limits on physiologic monitoring devices as the patient's condition changes (improves or deteriorates) *to lessen unnecessary alarm states.*
6. Consider use of headphones and digital music player with patient's favorite and/or subliminal or classical music. *This can effectively filter out assaultive noise of the critical care environment and supplant it with familiar, soothing sounds and rhythms.*
7. Modify lighting. *Day and night cycles need to be simulated with environmental lighting.*
   a. Never turn on overhead fluorescent lights abruptly without warning the patient, assisting him or her out of the supine position, and/or shielding his or her eyes with gauze or a face cloth. *Continuous bright lighting sustains anxiety and promotes circadian rhythm desynchronization.*
8. Shield patients from viewing urgent and emergent events in the critical care unit. *Resuscitation efforts, albeit difficult to conceal, engender fear in the patient and a sense of instability and vulnerability (e.g., "I'm next").*
   a. When such an event occurs, elicit the patient's cognitive and emotional reaction; *thoughts, impressions, and feelings need to be shared and misconceptions clarified.*
9. Ensure patients' privacy, modesty, and dignity. *Physical exposure and nudity, although they seemingly pale in importance compared with priorities such as physiologic assessment and stabilization, are primal indignities for all individuals.*
   a. Keep the patient minimally exposed. When it becomes necessary to expose the patient, verbally apologize for this necessity. *To be naked is to feel vulnerable; to be vulnerable is to feel fearful.*

For Sensory Deprivation

1. Provide reality orientation in four spheres (personal, place, time, and situation) at more frequent intervals than when testing.
   a. Convey this information in the context of routine conversation. *Sample statements*: "Mr. Clark, this is Tuesday morning and you're in University Hospital. Your heart surgery was yesterday morning, and you're doing well. My name is Joe, and I'm your nurse today." *The patient is made to feel patronized by repetitions such as, "Do you know where you are?" Given the effects of general anesthesia, opioid analgesics, sedatives, and sleep, it is expected that some degree of disorientation will exist normally.*
2. Ensure the patient's visual access to a calendar.
3. Apprise the patient of daily news events and the weather.
4. Touch patients for the express purpose of communicating caring. Hold their hands, stroke their brows, and rub the skin on an aspect of the arms. *Touch is the universal language of caring. In the setting of critical care, in which there is considerable physical body manipulation, it is useful and important to contrast assaultive touch with comforting touch. Touch can be used as a technique for distraction from painful stimuli when used in conjunction with uncomfortable procedures.* (NOTE: See later discussion of the use of touch in management of the patient experiencing hallucinations.)
5. Foster liberal visitation by family and significant others. Encourage significant others to touch the patient as consistent with their individual comfort level and cultural norms.

NURSING MANAGEMENT PLAN

Acute Confusion—cont'd

6. Structure and identify opportunities for the patient to exercise decision-making skills, however small. *Although not so designated, patients with sensory alterations also experience a type of cognitive deprivation.*

7. Assist patients to find meaning in their experiences. *Patients need to find meaning and to identify their roles in the experience of critical illness and critical care.*
   a. Explain the therapeutic purpose of all they are asked to do for themselves and all that is done with them and for them.
   b. Avoid statements such as, "Will you turn to that side for me?" or "I need you to swallow this medication." *These statements implicitly convey that the maneuver has some value for the nurses instead of the patients.*
   c. Similarly, use "thank you" judiciously. *This simple salutation, when used indiscriminately, suggests something was done to benefit the nurses, not the patients.*

For Hallucinations

1. Approach the patient with a calm, matter-of-fact demeanor. *The goal of this interaction is for the nurse to demonstrate external control. This helps decrease the anxiety and fear that generally accompany hallucinations and allows the patient to feel safe. Anxiety is transferable.*

2. Address the patient by name. *This is a useful presentation of reality because self-identity is the last sphere of orientation to vanish.*

3. In responding to the patient's description of the hallucination, do not deny, argue, or attempt to disprove the existence of the perceived event. Statements such as, "There are no voices coming from that air vent" or "Look, I'm brushing my hand across the wall, and there are no bugs" confuse the patient further, *because the hallucination, although frightening, is his or her perceived reality.*

4. Express to the patient that your experiences are dissimilar, and acknowledge how frightening his or hers must be. *Sample statements:* "I don't hear (see, etc.) what you do, but I know how frightening such an experience must be to you. I'm Joe, your nurse, and I'm going to stay with you until the voices (visions, etc.) go away." *Validating the patient's feelings demonstrates acceptance and sensitivity to the experience and promotes trust.*

5. Remain with any patient who is experiencing a hallucination. *Feelings of fear and anxiety often accelerate when a patient is left alone. He or she needs someone to represent a nonthreatening reality.*

6. Do not explore the content of the hallucination with the patient by asking about its nature or character. *The nurse is the patient's link with reality. Pursuit of a detailed description of a hallucination may signify to the patient that the nurse accepts his or her sensory distortion as factual. This may further confuse the patient and distance him or her more from reality.*
   a. Ascertain that the voices are not telling the patient to harm himself or herself, by asking simply and concretely, "What are the voices saying?" *The nurse can help bridge the gap between the patient's misperception and reality by addressing the feelings (e.g., fear, anxiety) and/or meanings (e.g., danger, death) engendered by the hallucination.*
   b. Determine how the misperception affects the patient emotionally, acknowledge those feelings, and use a calm, controlled, matter-of-fact approach to provide the trust and comfort the patient needs to tolerate this frightening experience. *In other words, the nurse should deal with the intent more than the content of the hallucination. The resultant decrease in anxiety will enable the patient to focus more accurately on his or her immediate environment.*

7. Talk concretely with the patient about things that are really happening. *Sample statements:* "How does your chest incision feel this afternoon, Mr. Clark?" "Your sister Kate was here to see you, but you were sleeping. She went down to the cafeteria and will be back." "Your secretions are a little easier for you to cough up today." *Interpretation of reality-based stimuli by the nurse encourages the patient to focus on actual circumstances and discourages a preoccupation with sensory misperceptions.*

8. Distract the patient by changing the topic. *This tactic is useful in situations of escalating anxiety and confusion or when all else fails. Topics need to consist of basic themes that are universally understood and culturally congruent, such as music, food, or weather or topics of special interest to the patient, such as hobbies, crafts, or sports.*
   a. Avoid topics that evoke strong emotions, such as politics, religion, or sexuality. *This is especially true of the patient with reality distortions; sometimes, hallucinations and delusions are expressions of repressed conflicts associated with religious, sexual, or aggressive issues. Pursuit of such subjects could increase confusion and anxiety.*

9. Avoid the use of touch as an intervention strategy for any patient who demonstrates escalating anxiety or paranoid, suspicious, or mistrustful thoughts. *While touch can therefore be useful in the management of patients with sensory alterations, however, for patients experiencing hallucinations (as well as delusions and illusions), touch can be readily misinterpreted as aggression or pain, and it can actually provide the basis for a tactile illusion.*

10. For auditory hallucinations:
    a. *Patient behaviors:* Head cocked as if listening to an unseen presence; lips moving.
    b. *Therapeutic nurse responses:* "Mr. Clark, you appear to be listening to something." If the patient acknowledges voices: "I don't hear any voices, but I know this is troubling you. The voices will go away. Nothing is going to harm you. I'm Joe, your nurse, and I'll be here with you."
    c. *Nontherapeutic nurse responses:* "Tell me about your conversations with these voices." "To whom do these voices belong—anyone you know?"

11. For visual hallucinations:
    a. *Patient behaviors:* Staring into space as if focused on an unseen object; startled movements and anxious facial expression.
    b. *Therapeutic nurse responses:* "Mr. Clark, something seems to be troubling you. Tell me what it is." If patient states he visualizes people, images, or the devil in his environment and implies a sense of danger, respond, "There are only nurses and doctors here, Mr. Clark. I know this must be upsetting, but these images will go away. We're here with you in the hospital. Nothing will happen to you."
    c. *Nontherapeutic nurse responses:* "Describe the people you see. What are they wearing?" "What does the devil mean in your life? What about God?"

For Delusions

1. Explain all unseen noises, voices, and activity simply and clearly. *They readily feed a delusional system. Sample statements:* "That is Dr. Smith. He's come to see you and other patients here in the hospital." "The voices and activity you hear are from the bedside of the patient behind this curtain. He's being helped by one of the nurses."

Continued

◎ NURSING MANAGEMENT PLAN

Acute Confusion—cont'd

2. Avoid the "negative challenge" of the patient's delusions (e.g., "Nobody here stole your belongings" or "Doctors and nurses do not harm people"). Similarly, avoid defending the referents of the patient's belief: "Nurses are good" and "Doctors mean well." *A delusion is a belief, albeit false, that cannot be changed with logic. To attempt this change is to challenge the patient's belief system and thereby escalate his or her anxiety, further blurring the boundaries between reality and the patient's internally based "logic."*

3. For the patient with persecutory delusions who refuses food, fluids, or medications because of a belief that he or she has been poisoned or the medications are tainted, permit the refusal unless it is a life-threatening event. Try again in 20 minutes; allow the patient to choose an alternative selection of food or to read the label on the unit's medication. *Coercion, show of force, or engagement in complicated, logical justifications will only heighten the patient's suspiciousness and possibly reinforce the delusional belief. When the patient feels more in control, he or she need not rely on the "paradoxical" quality of the delusion to equip him or her with a false sense of power. His or her power instead is derived from making reality-based decisions.*

4. Staff members should be particularly careful not to engage in unnecessary laughter or whispering within view of the delusional patient. *The delusional patient is hypervigilant, scanning the environment for evidence to corroborate or confirm his or her belief that staff members are colluding against him or her; laughter and whispers easily suggest this belief, this delusion of reference. This rationale also pertains to the patient experiencing hallucinations and/or illusions.*

5. Observe the principles detailed in the third intervention in *For Hallucinations* section.

For Illusions

1. Interpret a reality-based stimulus for the patient in a calm, matter-of-fact manner. *Seen and unseen noises, voices, activity, and people can provide the stimulus for a sensory misinterpretation, an illusion.*

2. Minimize stimulation in the patient's immediate environment. *Nursing interventions detailed previously under "Sensory Overload" are especially relevant here.*

3. Address the feeling and meaning associated with the experience, not the content of the sensory misinterpretation.
   a. *Patient behaviors*: Eyes darting, startled movements, frightened facial expression. "I know who you are. You're the devil come to take me to hell."
   b. *Therapeutic nurse responses*: "I'm Joe, your nurse. I know this experience is troubling for you. You're in the hospital, and no one here will harm you."
   c. Nontherapeutic nurse responses: "There are no such things as devils and angels." "Do you think the devil would be dressed in white?" *The first nontherapeutic nurse response carries a parental tone (i.e., "You know better than that."), infantilizing the patient and adding to his or her feelings of powerlessness over the environment. The second nontherapeutic response reflects obvious logic, which is not in the patient's sensory domain; it cannot be processed and only adds to his or her confused state.*

4. Observe the principles detailed in the fifth intervention of the *For Hallucinations* section.

◎ NURSING MANAGEMENT PLAN

Acute Pain

Definition: Unpleasant sensory and emotional experience arising from actual or potential tissue damage or described in terms of such damage (International Association for the Study of Pain); sudden or slow onset of any intensity from mild to severe with an anticipated or predictable end and a duration of less than 6 months

Acute Pain Related to Transmission and Perception of Cutaneous, Visceral, Muscular, or Ischemic Impulses

Defining Characteristics

Subjective
- Patient verbalizes presence of pain
- Patient rates pain on a scale of 1 to 10 using a visual analog scale

Objective
- Increase in blood pressure, heart rate, and respiratory rate
- Pupillary dilation
- Diaphoresis, pallor
- Skeletal muscle reactions (e.g., grimacing, clenching fists, writhing, pacing, guarding or splinting of affected part)
- Apprehension, fearful appearance
- May not exhibit any physiologic change

Outcome Criteria
- Patient verbalizes that pain is reduced to a tolerable level or is totally relieved.
- Patient's pain rating is lower on a scale of 1 to 10.
- Blood pressure, heart rate, and respiratory rate return to baseline 5 minutes after administration of an intravenous opioid analgesic or 20 minutes after administration of intramuscular opioid analgesic.

Nursing Interventions and Rationale
1. Modify variables that heighten the patient's experience of pain.
   a. Explain to the patient that frequent, detailed, and seemingly repetitive assessments will be conducted to allow the nurse to better understand the patient's pain experience, not because the existence of pain is in question.
   b. Explain the factors responsible for pain production in the individual. Estimate the expected duration of the pain if possible.
   c. Explain diagnostic and therapeutic procedures to the patient in relation to sensations the patient should expect to feel.
   d. Reduce the patient's fear of addiction by explaining the difference between drug tolerance and drug addiction. *Drug tolerance is a physiologic phenomenon in which a medication begins to lose effectiveness after repeated doses; drug dependence is a psychologic phenomenon in which opioids are used regularly for emotional, not medical, reasons.*
   e. Instruct the patient to ask for pain medication when pain is beginning and not to wait until it is intolerable.
   f. Explain that the physician will be consulted if pain relief is inadequate with the present medication.
   g. Instruct patient in the importance of adequate rest, especially when it reduces pain *to maintain strength and coping abilities and to reduce stress.*
2. Collaborate with physician regarding pharmacologic interventions.
   - **For postoperative or posttraumatic cutaneous, muscular, or visceral pain,** perform the following:
     a. Medicate with an opioid analgesic to break the pain cycles as long as level of consciousness and vital signs are stable: check patient's previous response to similar dosage and opioids.

   (1) Given a physician order for a range of doses of an opioid analgesic, start with the lowest dose *to evaluate the patient's individual response to medication.*
   b. Continuous pain requires continuous analgesia.
     (1) Establish optimal analgesic dose that brings optimal pain relief.
     (2) Offer pain medication at prescribed regular intervals rather than making patient ask for it *to maintain more steady blood levels.*
     (3) Consider waking patient to avoid loss of opiate blood levels during sleep.
   c. If administering medication on as-necessary (PRN) basis, give it when the patient's pain is just beginning, rather than at its peak.
     (1) Advise patient to intercept pain, not endure it, or several hours and higher doses of opioid analgesics may be necessary to relieve pain, leading to a cycle of undermedication and pain alternating with overmedication and drug toxicity.
   d. Perform rehabilitation exercises (turn, deep breathe, leg exercises, ambulate) shortly before peak of drug effect *because this will be the optimal time for the patient to increase activity with the least risk of increasing pain.*
   e. When making the transition from one drug to another or from intramuscular or intravenous to oral medication, use an equianalgesic chart. *Equianalgesic means approximately the same pain relief. The patient's response should be closely monitored to determine if the right analgesic choice was made.*
   f. To assess effectiveness of pain medication, do the following:
     (1) Reevaluate pain 5 minutes after intravenous and 20 minutes after intramuscular medication administration, observe patient's behavior, and ask patient to rate pain on a scale of 1 to 10.
     (2) Collaborate with the physician to add or delete other medications that potentiate the action of analgesics, such as antiemetics, hypnotics, sedatives, or muscle relaxants.
     (3) Observe for indicators of undertreatment: report of pain not relieved; observed restlessness, sleeplessness, irritability, and anorexia; decreased activity level.
     (4) Observe for indicators of overtreatment: hypotension or bradycardia; respiratory rate <10/min; excessive sedation.
   g. If patient-controlled analgesia (PCA) is used, perform the following:
     (1) Instruct the patient on what the drug is, the dose, and how often it can be self-administered by pushing the button to activate the PCA machine. For example, "When you have pain, instead of asking the nurse to bring medication, push the button that activates the machine and a small dose of the pain medicine will be injected into your IV line. You can keep your pain under control by administering additional medicine as soon as your pain begins to return or increases. Push the button before undertaking a painful activity, such as ambulation. Try to balance your pain relief against sleepiness, and don't activate the machine if you start to feel sleepy. If your pain medicine seems to stop working despite pushing the button several times, call the nurse to check your IV. If you are not receiving adequate pain relief, the nurse will call your doctor."
     (2) Monitor vital signs, especially blood pressure and respiratory rate, every hour for the first 4 hours, and assess postural heart rate and blood pressure before initial ambulation.
     (3) Monitor respiratory rate every 2 hours while patient is on patient-controlled analgesia.

Continued

NURSING MANAGEMENT PLAN

Acute Pain—cont'd

(4) If patient's respiratory rate decrease to <10/min or if patient is overly sedated, anticipate administration of naloxone.

h. If epidural opioid analgesia is used, do the following:

(1) Keep patient's head elevated 30 to 45 degrees after injection **to prevent respiratory depressant effects.**

(2) Observe closely for respiratory depression up to 24 hours after injection. Monitor respiratory rate every 15 minutes for 1 hour; every 30 minutes for 7 hours; and every hour for the remaining 16 hours.

(3) Assess for adequate cough reflex.

(4) Avoid use of other central nervous system depressants, such as sedatives.

(5) Observe for reports of pruritus, nausea, and vomiting.

(6) Anticipate administration of naloxone for respiratory depression (and smaller doses of naloxone for pruritus).

(7) Assess for and treat urinary retention.

(8) Assess epidural catheter site for local infection. Keep the catheter taped securely **to prevent catheter migration.**

- For peripheral vascular ischemic pain (hypothetic vascular occlusion of leg), do the following:

a. Correctly identify and differentiate ischemic pain from other types of pain. **(NOTE: Ischemic pain is usually a burning, aching pain made worse by exercise and lessened or relieved by rest. Eventually, the pain occurs at rest. Coldness and pallor of extremity may be noted, especially if the limb is elevated above the heart level. Rubor and mottling of the skin may be evident from prolonged tissue anoxia and inability of damaged vessels to constrict. Eventually, cyanosis and gangrenous tissue will be evident. Chronic ischemia leads to visible changes in the limb, such as flaking skin, brittle nails and hair, leg ulcers, and cellulitis.)**

b. Administer pain medications, and evaluate their effectiveness as previously described. **Remember that the pain of ischemia is chronic and continuous and can make the patient irritable and depressed.**

c. Treat the cause of the ischemic pain, and institute measures **to increase circulation to the affected part.**

3. Initiate nonpharmacologic interventions.

a. Treat contributing factors; provide explanations (see second at beginning of this nursing management plan).

b. Apply comfort measures.

(1) Use relaxation techniques, such as back rubs, massage, warm baths, music, and aromatherapy.

(a) Use blankets and pillows to support the painful part and reduce muscle tension.

(b) Encourage slow, rhythmic breathing.

(2) Encourage progressive muscle relaxation techniques.

(a) Instruct patient to inhale and tense (tighten) specific muscle groups and then relax the muscles as exhalation occurs.

(b) Suggest an order for performing the tension and relaxation cycle (e.g., start with facial muscles and move down body, ending with toes).

(3) Encourage guided imagery.

(a) Ask patient to recall an experienced image that is very pleasurable and relaxing and involves at least two senses.

(b) Have patient begin with rhythmic breathing and progressive relaxation and then travel mentally to the scene.

(c) Have patient slowly experience the scene (e.g., how it looks, sounds, smells, feels).

(d) Ask patient to practice this imagery in private.

(e) Instruct patient to end the imagery by counting to three and saying, "Now I'm relaxed." If the person does not end the imagery and falls asleep, the purpose of the technique is defeated.

◉ NURSING MANAGEMENT PLAN

Anxiety

Definition: Vague uneasy feeling of discomfort or dread accompanied by an autonomic response (the source often nonspecific or unknown to the individual); a feeling of apprehension caused by anticipation of danger. It is an alerting signal that warns of impending danger and enables the individual to take measures to deal with threat.

Anxiety Related to Threat to Biologic, Psychologic, or Social Integrity

Defining Characteristics

Subjective

- Verbalizes increased muscle tension
- Expresses frequent sensation of tingling in hands and feet
- Relates continuous feeling of apprehension
- Expresses preoccupation with a sense of impending doom
- Reports difficulty falling asleep
- Repeatedly expresses concerns about changes in health status and outcome of illness

Objective

- Psychomotor agitation (fidgeting, jitteriness, restlessness)
- Tightened, wrinkled brow
- Strained (worried) facial expression
- Hypervigilance (scans environment)
- Startles easily
- Distractibility
- Sweaty palms
- Fragmented sleep patterns
- Tachycardia
- Tachypnea

Outcome Criteria

- Patient effectively uses learned relaxation strategies.
- Patient demonstrates significant decrease in psychomotor agitation.
- Patient verbalizes reduction in tingling sensations in hands and feet.
- Patient is able to focus on the tasks at hand.
- Patient expresses positive, future-based plans to family and staff.
- Patient's heart rate and rhythm remain within limits commensurate with physiologic status.

Nursing Interventions and Rationale

1. Instruct the patient in the following simple, effective relaxation strategies:
   a. If not contraindicated for cardiovascular reasons, tense and relax all muscles progressively from toes to head. *Progressive toe-to-head relaxation releases the muscular tension that may be a stress-related effect resulting from the threat or change in the patient's health status and outcome of illness.*
   b. Perform slow deep-breathing exercises. *Deep-breathing exercises provide slow, rhythmic, controlled breathing patterns that relax the patient and distract him or her from the effects of his or her illness and hospitalization.*
   c. Focus on a single object or person in the environment. *Focusing on a single object or person helps the patient dismiss myriad*

disorienting stimuli from his or her visual-perceptual field, which can have a dizzying, distorted effect. A clear sensorium allows him or her to feel more in control of his or her environment.
   d. Listen to soothing music or relaxation tapes with eyes closed. *Music or words expressed in soft, low tones tend to produce soothing, relaxing effects that counteract or inhibit escalating anxiety and provide respites from the patient's situational crisis. Closed eyes eliminate distracting visual stimuli and promote a more restful environment.*

2. Actively listen to and accept the patient's concerns regarding the threats from his or her illness, outcome, and hospitalization. *Active listening and unconditional acceptance validate the patient as a worthwhile individual and assure him or her that his or her concerns, no matter how great, will be addressed. Knowledge that he or she has an avenue for ventilation will assuage anxiety.*

3. Help the patient distinguish between realistic concerns and exaggerated fears through clear, simple explanations. *Sample statements*: "Your lab results show that you're doing okay right now." "The shortness of breath you're experiencing is not unusual." "The pain you described is expected, and this medication will relieve it." *A patient who is informed about his or her progress and is reassured about expected symptoms and management of care will be better equipped to maintain a more realistic perspective of his or her illness and its outcome. Anxiety emanating from imagined or exaggerated fears will likely be assuaged or averted.*

4. Provide simple clarification of environmental events and stimuli that are not related to the patient's illness and care. *Sample statements*: "That loud noise is coming from a machine that is helping another patient." "The visitor behind the curtain is crying because she's had an upsetting day." "That gurney is here to take another patient to x-ray." *Clarification of events and stimuli that are unrelated to the patient helps to disengage him or her from the extant anxiety-provoking situations surrounding him or her, avoiding further anxiety and apprehension.*

5. Assist the patient in focusing on building on prior coping strategies to deal with the effects of his or her illness and care. *Sample statements*: "What methods have helped you get through difficult times in the past?" "How can we help you use those methods now?" (See the nursing management plan for Ineffective Coping for interventions that assist patients to use coping strategies effectively.) *Use of previously successful coping strategies in conjunction with newly learned techniques arms the patient with an arsenal of weapons against anxiety, providing him or her with greater control over the situational crisis and decreased feelings of doom and despair.*

6. Give the patient permission to deny or suppress the effects of his or her illness and hospitalization with which he or she cannot cope or control. *Sample statements*: "It's perfectly okay to ignore things you can't handle right now." "How can we help ease your mind during this time?" "What are some things or tasks that may help distract you?" *Adaptive denial can be helpful in reducing feelings of anxiety in patients with life-threatening illness.*

◎ NURSING MANAGEMENT PLAN

Autonomic Dysreflexia

Definition: Life-threatening, uninhibited sympathetic response of the nervous system to a noxious stimulus after a spinal cord injury at T7 or above

Autonomic Dysreflexia Related to Excessive Autonomic Response to Noxious Stimuli

Defining Characteristics

- Paroxysmal hypertension (sudden increase in both systolic and diastolic blood pressure >20 mm Hg above patient's normal blood pressure); for many spinal cord injury patients, a normal blood pressure may be only 90/60 mm Hg
- Pounding headache
- Bradycardia (may be a relative slowing so the heart rate may still appear with in the normal range)
- Profuse sweating (above the level of the injury) especially in the face, neck, and shoulders
- Pilomotor erection (goose bumps) above the level of the injury
- Cardiac dysrhythmias (atrial fibrillation; premature ventricular contractions; and atrioventricular conduction abnormalities)
- Flushing of the skin (above the level of the injury) especially in the face, neck, and shoulders
- Blurred vision
- Appearance of spots in the visual fields
- Nasal congestion
- Feelings of apprehension or anxiety

Outcome Criteria

- Blood pressure returns to patient's baseline level.
- Heart rate and rhythm returns to patient's baseline level.
- Absence of headache
- Absence of sweating, flushing, and piloerection above level of injury
- Absence of visual disturbances and nasal congestion
- Absence of feelings of apprehension or anxiety

Nursing Interventions and Rationale

1. Place the patient on cardiac monitor, and assess for bradycardia or other dysrhythmias. *Disturbances of cardiac rate and rhythm can occur because of autonomic dysfunction associated with dysreflexia.*
2. Check the patient's blood pressure every 3 to 5 minutes *as blood pressure may fluctuate very quickly.*
3. Sit the patient upright and lower their legs if possible *to decrease venous return and blood pressure.*
4. Loosen any clothing or constrictive devices *to decrease venous return and blood pressure.*
5. Investigate for and remove instigating cause of dysreflexia:

a. Bladder
   (1) If indwelling catheter not in place, catheterize patient immediately.
      (a) Prior to inserting the catheter, instill 2% lidocaine jelly into the urethra and wait 2 minutes, if possible.
      (b) Drain 500 mL of urine, and recheck BP.
      (c) If BP still elevated, drain another 500 mL of urine.
      (d) If BP declines after the bladder is empty, serial BP must be monitored closely because the bladder can go into severe contractions causing hypertension to recur.
   (2) If indwelling catheter is in place, check the catheter and tubing for kinks, folds, constrictions, or obstructions, and for correct placement. If problem is found, correct it immediately.
   (3) If catheter is plugged, irrigate it gently with no more than 10-15 mL of sterile normal saline solution at body temperature.
   (4) If unable to irrigate catheter, remove it and prepare to reinsert a new catheter: proceed with its lubrication, drainage, and observation as outlined above.
   (5) Avoid manually compressing or tapping on the bladder.
b. Bowel: if systolic blood pressure is >150 mm Hg, proceed to no. 6 prior to checking for a fecal impaction.
   (1) With a gloved hand, instill a topical anesthetic agent (2% lidocaine jelly), generously into the rectum *to decrease flow of impulses from bowel.*
   (2) Wait 2 minutes if possible *for sensation in area to decrease.*
   (3) With a gloved hand, insert a lubricated finger into the rectum and check for the presence of stool.
   (4) If stool is felt, gently remove, if possible.
c. Skin
   (1) Loosen clothing or bed linens as indicated.
   (2) Inspect skin for pimples, boils, pressure ulcers, and ingrown toenails, and treat as indicated.
6. If symptoms of dysreflexia do not subside, collaborate with physician regarding the administration of antihypertensive medications (e.g., nifedipine [immediate-release form], nitrates [sodium nitroprusside, isosorbide dinitrate, or nitroglycerin ointment], hydralazine, mecamylamine, diazoxide, phenoxybenzamine, captopril, prazosin).
   a. Administer medications, and monitor their effectiveness.
   b. Assess blood pressure and heart rate.
7. Instruct patient about causes, symptoms, treatment, and prevention of dysreflexia.
8. Encourage patient to carry medical bracelet or informational card to present to medical personnel in the event dysreflexia may be developing.

NURSING MANAGEMENT PLAN

Compromised Family Coping

Definition: Usually, supportive primary person (family member or close friend) provides insufficient, ineffective, or compromised support, comfort, assistance, or encouragement that may be needed by the patient to manage or master adaptive tasks related to his or her health challenge.

Compromised Family Coping Related to Critically Ill Family Member

Defining Characteristics

- Disruption of usual family functions and roles
- Inability to accept or deal with crisis situation; use of defense mechanisms (e.g., denial, anger); unrealistic expectations of patient's outcome and care provided; judgmental toward health care providers
- Nonrecognition that family is in state of crisis
- Inappropriate emotional outbursts; arguments among family and with others; inability to respond to each other's feelings or support each other
- Misinterpretation of information; short attention span with repeated questions about information already provided; members not sharing information with each other
- Inability to make decisions regarding changes in family structure or about course of care for ill member; noncooperation among family members
- Expressions of grief, hopelessness, powerlessness, and isolation; do not seek or respond to support services
- Hesitancy to spend time with ill person in the critical care unit, or inappropriate behavior when visiting (may upset patient)
- Neglect of own personal health; fatigue, apathy; refusal of offers for respite time

Outcome Criteria

- The family will express an understanding of course/prognosis of illness, therapies, and alternative measures.
- The family will diminish or resolve conflicts and cooperate in decision making.
- The family will develop trust and mutual support for each member and form a cohesive unit.
- The family will support ill person in making decisions (if capable) or respect prior wishes regarding provision of health care.
- Family efforts will be directed toward a purpose and readjust to changes in life patterns and role function. Members will accept responsibility for changes.
- The family will identify and use effective coping strategies.
- The family will identify and use available resources as needed to facilitate resolution of the crisis.
- The family will have a sense of control and confidence in meeting personal and collective needs.

Nursing Interventions and Rationale

1. Identify family's perception of the crisis situation. *All initial nursing interventions should be directed toward resolving the crisis situation. Understanding and using family theory principles will facilitate this process and individualize care.*
   a. Determine family structure; roles' developmental phase; and ethnic, cultural, and belief factors that may affect communication with family and the plan of care.
   b. Identify strengths of the family.

2. Provide honest and accurate information in language persons can understand. Give updated information as appropriate. Listen! *This facilitates open communication among family and health care providers, projects a caring attitude and concern for them and patient, and assists family in making decisions and being involved with the plan and goals of care.*
3. Encourage liberal visitation with patient.
   a. Before the visit, prepare family members for what they will observe in a technical environment. *This prevents a strong emotional reaction to an unfamiliar and frightening situation.*
      (1) Inform them about patient's appearance, behaviors (etc.) that may be distressing to them.
      (2) Explain the etiology of patient responses to stimuli (e.g., pain, trauma, surgery, medication), and explain that these behaviors are being monitored and are usually temporary.
   b. Encourage them to touch the patient and let the patient know of their presence.
4. Identify and support effective coping behaviors. *This aids in the family's sense of control and resolution of helplessness/powerlessness.*
5. Observe for signs of fatigue and the need for emotional/spiritual support and respite from hospital waiting routine. *This provides support and comfort, facilitates hope, resolves sense of isolation, gives sense of security, and diminishes guilt feeling for attending to personal needs.*
   a. Encourage family to verbalize feelings.
   b. Provide information on available resources.
   c. Alert interdisciplinary team members (social, psychologic, spiritual) to family needs.
   d. Provide pager device (if available), or obtain phone numbers when family leaves the hospital premises.
6. Instruct family in simple caregiving techniques, and encourage participation in patient's care. *This facilitates giving a sense of normalcy to the experience, self-confidence, and assurance that good care is being provided.*
7. Serve as advocate for patient and family. Teach family how to negotiate with the health care delivery system, and include them in health care team conferences when appropriate. *This facilitates informed decision making, promotes control and satisfaction, and permits mutual goal-setting.*
8. Consider nonbiologic or nonlegal family relationships. Encourage contact with patient and participation in care. *This facilitates holistic care and support of emotional ties and demonstrates respect for the family unit and relationships.*
9. Provide emotional support and compassion when patient's condition worsens or deteriorates. *The use of touch and expression of concern for the patient and family convey comfort and trust in the health care provider and respect and assurance that the family's loved one will receive appropriate care and attention.*

NURSING MANAGEMENT PLAN

Decreased Cardiac Output

Definition: Inadequate blood pumped by the heart to meet the metabolic demands of the body

Decreased Cardiac Output Related to Alterations in Preload

Defining Characteristics
- Cardiac output is <4.0 L/min
- Cardiac index is <2.5 L/min/m^2
- Heart rate is >100 beats/min
- Urine output is <30 mL/hr or 0.5 mL/kg/hr
- Decreased mentation, restlessness, agitation, confusion
- Diminished peripheral pulses
- Blue, gray, or dark purple tint to tongue and sublingual area
- Systolic blood pressure is <90 mm Hg
- Subjective complaints of fatigue

Reduced Preload
- Right atrial pressure is <2 mm Hg
- Pulmonary artery occlusion pressure is <6 mm Hg

Excessive Preload
- Right atrial pressure is >8 mm Hg
- Pulmonary artery occlusion pressure is >12 mm Hg

Outcome Criteria
- Cardiac output is 4-8 L/min.
- Cardiac index is 2.5-4 L/min/m^2.
- Right atrial pressure is 2-8 mm Hg.
- Pulmonary artery occlusion pressure is 6-12 mg Hg.

Nursing Interventions and Rationale
1. Collaborate with physician regarding the administration of oxygen to maintain an SpO$_2$ >92% **to prevent tissue hypoxia.**
2. Maintain surveillance for signs of decreased tissue perfusion and acidosis **to facilitate the early identification and treatment of complications.**
3. Monitor fluid balance and daily weights to facilitate regulation of the patient's fluid balance.

For Reduced Preload Resulting from Volume Loss
1. Collaborate with physician regarding the administration of crystalloids, colloids, blood, and blood products **to increase circulating volume.**
2. Limit blood sampling, observe intravenous lines for accidental disconnection, apply direct pressure to bleeding sites, and maintain normal body temperature **to minimize fluid loss.**
3. Position patient with legs elevated, trunk flat, and head and shoulders above the chest **to enhance venous return.**
4. Encourage oral fluids (as appropriate), administer free water with tube feedings, and replace fluids that are lost through wound or tube drainage **to promote adequate fluid intake.**
5. Maintain surveillance for signs of fluid volume excess and adverse effects of blood and blood product administration **to facilitate the early identification and treatment of complications.**

For Reduced Preload Resulting from Venous Dilation
1. Collaborate with physician regarding the administration of vasoconstrictors **to increase venous return.**
2. Maintain surveillance for adverse effects of vasoconstrictor therapy **to facilitate the early identification and treatment of complications.**

3. If patient is hyperthermic, administer tepid bath, hypothermia blanket, and/or ice bags to axilla and groin **to decrease temperature and promote vasoconstriction.**

For Excessive Preload Resulting from Volume Overload
1. Collaborate with physician regarding the administration of the following:
   a. Diuretics to remove excessive fluid.
   b. Vasodilators to decrease venous return.
   c. Inotropes to increase myocardial contractility.
2. Restrict fluid intake and double concentrate intravenous drips **to minimize fluid intake.**
3. Position patient in semi-Fowler's or high-Fowler's position **to reduce venous return.**
4. Maintain surveillance for signs of fluid volume deficit and adverse effects of diuretic, vasodilator, and inotropic therapies **to facilitate the early identification and treatment of complications.**

For Excessive Preload Resulting from Venous Constriction
1. Collaborate with physician regarding the administration of vasodilators **to promote venous dilation.**
2. Maintain surveillance for adverse effects of vasodilator therapy **to facilitate the early identification and treatment of complications.**
3. If patient is hypothermic, wrap him or her in warm blankets or administer hyperthermia blanket **to increase temperature and promote vasodilation.**

Decreased Cardiac Output Related to Alterations in Afterload

Defining Characteristics
- Cardiac output is <4 L/min
- Cardiac index is <2.5 L/min/m^2
- Heart rate is >100 beats/min
- Urine output is <30 mL/hr
- Decreased mentation, restlessness, agitation, confusion
- Diminished peripheral pulses
- Blue, gray, or dark purple tint to tongue and sublingual area
- Systolic blood pressure is <90 mm Hg
- Subjective complaints of fatigue

Reduced Afterload
- Pulmonary vascular resistance is <100 dyn·sec·cm^{-5}
- Systemic vascular resistance is <800 dyn·sec·cm^{-5}

Excessive Afterload
- Pulmonary vascular resistance is >250 dyn·sec·cm^{-5}
- Systemic vascular resistance is >1200 dyn·sec·cm^{-5}

Outcome Criteria
- Cardiac output is 4-8 L/min.
- Cardiac index is 2.5-4 L/min/m^2.
- Pulmonary vascular resistance is 80-250 dyn·sec·cm^{-5}.
- Systemic vascular resistance is 800-1200 dyn·sec·cm^{-5}.

Nursing Interventions and Rationale
1. Collaborate with physician regarding the administration of oxygen to maintain an SpO$_2$ >92% **to prevent tissue hypoxia.**
2. Maintain surveillance for signs of decreased tissue perfusion and acidosis **to facilitate the early identification and treatment of complications.**

NURSING MANAGEMENT PLAN

Decreased Cardiac Output—cont'd

For Reduced Afterload

1. Collaborate with physician regarding the administration of vasoconstrictors *to promote arterial vasoconstriction and prevent relative hypovolemia.* If decreased preload is present, implement nursing management plan for Decreased Cardiac Output Related to Alterations in Preload.
2. Maintain surveillance for adverse effects of vasoconstrictor therapy *to facilitate the early identification and treatment of complications.*
3. If patient is hyperthermic, administer tepid bath, hypothermia blanket, and/or ice bags to axilla and groin *to decrease temperature and promote vasoconstriction.*

For Excessive Afterload

1. Collaborate with physician regarding the administration of vasodilators *to promote arterial vasodilation.*
2. Collaborate with physician regarding initiation of intraaortic balloon pump *to facilitate afterload reduction.*
3. Promote rest and relaxation and decrease environmental stimulation *to minimize sympathetic stimulation.*
4. Maintain surveillance for adverse effects of vasodilator therapy *to facilitate the early identification and treatment of complications.*
5. If patient is hypothermic, wrap patient in warm blankets or administer hyperthermia blanket *to increase temperature and promote vasodilation.*
6. If patient is in pain, treat pain *to reduce sympathetic stimulation.* Implement nursing management plan for Acute Pain Related to Transmission and Perception of Cutaneous, Visceral, Muscular, or Ischemic Impulses.

Decreased Cardiac Output Related to Alterations in Contractility

Defining Characteristics

- Cardiac output is <4 L/min
- Cardiac index is <2.5 L/min/m²
- Heart rate is >100 beats/min
- Urine output is <30 mL/hr
- Decreased mentation, restlessness, agitation, confusion
- Diminished peripheral pulses
- Blue, gray, or dark purple tint to tongue and sublingual area
- Systolic blood pressure is <90 mm Hg
- Subjective complaints of fatigue
- Right ventricular stroke work index is <7 g/m²/beat
- Left ventricular stroke work index is <35 g/m²/beat

Outcome Criteria

- Cardiac output is 4-8 L/min.
- Cardiac index is 2.5-4 L/min/m².
- Right ventricular stroke work index is 7-12 g/m²/beat.
- Left ventricular stroke work index is 35-85 g/m²/beat.

Nursing Interventions and Rationale

1. Collaborate with physician regarding the administration of oxygen to maintain an SpO₂ >92% *to prevent tissue hypoxia.*
2. Maintain surveillance for signs of decreased tissue perfusion and acidosis *to facilitate the early identification and treatment of complications.*
3. Ensure preload is optimized. If preload is reduced or excessive, implement nursing management plan for Decreased Cardiac Output Related to Alterations in Preload.
4. Ensure afterload is optimized. If afterload is reduced or excessive, implement nursing management plan for Decreased Cardiac Output Related to Alterations in Afterload.

5. Ensure electrolytes are optimized. Collaborate with physician regarding the administration of electrolyte replacement therapy *to enhance cellular ionic environment.*
6. Collaborate with physician regarding the administration of inotropes *to enhance myocardial contractility.*
7. Monitor ST segment continuously *to determine changes in myocardial tissue perfusion.* If myocardial ischemia is present, implement nursing management plan for Ineffective Cardiopulmonary Tissue Perfusion.

Decreased Cardiac Output Related to Alterations in Heart Rate or Rhythm

Defining Characteristics

- Cardiac output is <4 L/min
- Cardiac index is <2.5 L/min/m²
- Heart rate is >100 beats/min or <60 beats/min
- Urine output is <30 mL/hr or 0.5 mL/kg/hr
- Decreased mentation, restlessness, agitation, confusion
- Diminished peripheral pulses
- Blue, gray, or dark purple tint to tongue and sublingual area
- Systolic blood pressure is <90 mm Hg
- Subjective complaints of fatigue
- Dysrhythmias

Outcome Criteria

- Cardiac output is 4-8 L/min.
- Cardiac index is 2.5-4 L/min/m².
- Absence of dysrhythmias or return to baseline.
- Heart rate is >60 beats/min or <100 beats/min.

Nursing Interventions and Rationale

1. Collaborate with physician regarding the administration of oxygen to maintain an SpO₂ >92% *to prevent tissue hypoxia.*
2. Ensure electrolytes are optimized. Collaborate with physician regarding the administration of electrolyte therapy *to enhance cellular ionic environment and avoid precipitation of dysrhythmias.*
3. Collaborate with physician and pharmacist regarding patient's current medications and their effect on heart rate and rhythm *to identify any prodysrhythmic or bradycardic side effects.*
4. Maintain surveillance for signs of decreased tissue perfusion and acidosis *to facilitate the early identification and treatment of complications.* .
5. Monitor ST segment continuously *to determine changes in myocardial tissue perfusion.* If myocardial ischemia is present, implement nursing management plan for Altered Cardiopulmonary Tissue Perfusion.

For Lethal Dysrhythmias or Asystole

1. Initiate Advanced Cardiac Life Support interventions and notify physician immediately.

For Nonlethal Dysrhythmias

1. Collaborate with physician regarding administration of antidysrhythmic therapy, synchronized cardioversion, and/or overdrive pacing *to control dysrhythmias.*
2. Maintain surveillance for adverse effects of antidysrhythmic therapy *to facilitate the early identification and treatment of complications.*

For Heart Rate <60 Beats/Min

1. Collaborate with physician regarding the initiation of temporary pacing *to increase heart rate.*

Continued

NURSING MANAGEMENT PLAN

Decreased Cardiac Output—cont'd

Decreased Cardiac Output Related to Sympathetic Blockade

Defining Characteristics

- Decreased cardiac output and cardiac index
- Systolic blood pressure is <90 mm Hg or below patient's baseline
- Decreased right atrial pressure and pulmonary artery occlusion pressure
- Decreased systemic vascular resistance
- Bradycardia
- Cardiac dysrhythmias
- Postural hypotension

Outcome Criteria

- Cardiac output and cardiac index are within normal limits.
- Systolic blood pressure is >90 mm Hg or returns to baseline.
- Right atrial pressure and pulmonary artery occlusion pressure are within normal limits.
- Systemic vascular resistance is within normal limits.
- Sinus rhythm is present.
- Dysrhythmias are absent.
- Fainting or dizziness with position change is absent.

Nursing Interventions and Rationale

1. Implement measures to prevent episodes of postural hypertension:
   a. Change patient's position slowly **to allow the cardiovascular system time to compensate.**
   b. Apply pneumatic compression stockings **to promote venous return.**
   c. Perform range-of-motion exercises every 2 hours **to prevent venous pooling.**
   d. Collaborate with the physician and physical therapist regarding the use of a tilt table **to progress the patient from supine to upright position.**
2. Collaborate with the physician regarding the administration of the following:
   a. Crystalloids and/or colloids to increase the patient's circulating volume, **which increases stroke volume and subsequently cardiac output.**
   b. Vasopressors if fluids are ineffective to constrict the patient's vascular system, **which increases resistance and subsequently blood pressure.**
3. Monitor cardiac rhythm for bradycardia and/or dysrhythmias, **which can further decrease cardiac output.**
4. Avoid any activity that can stimulate the vagal response **because bradycardia can result.**
5. Treat symptomatic bradycardia and symptomatic dysrhythmias according to unit's emergency protocol or advanced cardiac life support (ACLS) guidelines.

NURSING MANAGEMENT PLAN

Decreased Intracranial Adaptive Capacity

Definition: Intracranial fluid dynamic mechanisms that normally compensate for increases in intracranial volumes are compromised, resulting in repeated disproportionate increases in intracranial pressure (ICP) in response to a variety of noxious and non-noxious stimuli.

Decreased Intracranial Adaptive Capacity Related to Failure of Normal Intracranial Compensatory Mechanisms

Defining Characteristics

- Intracranial pressure is >15 mm Hg, sustained for 15-30 minutes
- Headache
- Vomiting, with or without nausea
- Seizures
- Decrease in Glasgow Coma Scale score of 2 or more points from baseline
- Alteration in level of consciousness, ranging from restlessness to coma
- Change in orientation: disoriented to time and/or place and/or person
- Difficulty or inability to follow simple commands
- Increasing systolic blood pressure of more than 20 mm Hg with widening pulse pressure
- Bradycardia
- Irregular respiratory pattern (e.g., Cheyne-Stokes, central neurogenic hyperventilation, ataxic, apneustic)
- Change in response to painful stimuli (e.g., purposeful to inappropriate or absent response)
- Signs of impending brain herniation:
  - Hemiparesis or hemiplegia
  - Hemisensory changes
  - Unequal pupil size (1 mm or more difference)
  - Failure of pupil to react to light
  - Disconjugate gaze and inability to move one eye beyond midline if third, fourth, or sixth cranial nerves involved
  - Loss of oculocephalic or oculovestibular reflexes
  - Possible decorticate or decerebrate posturing

Outcome Criteria

- Intracranial pressure is <15 mm Hg.
- Cerebral perfusion pressure is >60 mm Hg.
- Clinical signs of increased intracranial pressure are absent.

Nursing Interventions and Rationale

1. Maintain adequate cerebral perfusion pressure.
   a. Collaborate with physician regarding the administration of volume expanders, vasopressors, or antihypertensives **to maintain the patient's blood pressure within normal range.**
   b. Implement measures to reduce intracranial pressure.
      (1) Elevate head of bed 30-45 degrees **to facilitate venous return.**
      (2) Maintain head and neck in neutral plan (avoid flexion, extension, or lateral rotation) **to enhance venous drainage from the head.**
      (3) Avoid extreme hip flexion.
      (4) Collaborate with the physician regarding the administration of steroids, osmotic agents, and diuretics and need for drainage of cerebrospinal fluid if a ventriculostomy is in place.
      (5) Assist patient to turn and move self in bed (instruct patient to exhale while turning or pushing up in bed) **to avoid isometric contractions and Valsalva maneuver.**
2. Maintain patent airway and adequate ventilation and supply oxygen **to prevent hypoxemia and hypercarbia.**
3. Monitor arterial blood gas values and maintain PaO_2 >80 mm Hg, $PaCO_2$ >35 mm Hg, and pH at 7.35-7.45 **to prevent cerebral vasodilation.**
4. Avoid suctioning beyond 10 seconds at a time; hyperoxygenate and hyperventilate before and after suctioning **to avoid hypoxia.**
5. Plan patient care activities and nursing interventions around patient's intracranial pressure response. Avoid unnecessary additional disturbances, and allow patient up to 1 hour of rest between activities as frequently as possible. **Studies have shown the direct correlation between nursing care activities and increases in intracranial pressure.**
6. Maintain normothermia with external cooling or heating measures as necessary. Wrap hands, feet, and male genitalia in soft towels before cooling measures **to prevent shivering and frostbite.**
7. With physician's collaboration, control seizures with prophylactic and PRN anticonvulsants. **Seizures can greatly increase the cerebral metabolic rate.**
8. Collaborate with the physician regarding the administration of sedatives, barbiturates, or paralyzing agents **to reduce cerebral metabolic rate.**
9. Counsel family members to maintain calm atmosphere and avoid disturbing topics of conversation (e.g., patient condition, pain, prognosis, family crisis, financial difficulties).
10. If signs of impending brain herniation are present, implement the following:
    a. Notify the physician at once.
    b. Ensure that head of bed is elevated 45 degrees and that patient's head is in neutral plane.
    c. Administer mainline intravenous infusion slowly to keep-open rate.
    d. Drain cerebrospinal fluid as ordered if a ventriculostomy is in place.
    e. Prepare to administer osmotic agents and/or diuretics.
    f. Prepare patient for emergency computed tomography head scan and/or emergency surgery.

⊚ NURSING MANAGEMENT PLAN

Deficient Fluid Volume

Definition: Decreased intravascular, interstitial, and/or intracellular fluid. This refers to dehydration, water loss alone without a change in sodium concentration.

Deficient Fluid Volume Related to Absolute Loss
Defining Characteristics
- Cardiac output is <4 L/min
- Cardiac index is <2.2 L/min
- Pulmonary artery occlusion pressure is <6 mm Hg
- Right atrial pressure is <2 mm Hg
- Tachycardia
- Narrowed pulse pressure
- Systolic blood pressure is <100 mm Hg
- Urinary output is <30 mL/hr
- Pale, cool, moist skin
- Apprehensiveness

Outcome Criteria
- Cardiac output is >4 L/min, and cardiac index is >2.2 L/min.
- Pulmonary artery occlusion pressure is >6 mm Hg or returns to baseline level.
- Right atrial pressure is >2 mm Hg or returns to baseline level.
- Heart rate is normal or returns to baseline level.
- Systolic blood pressure is >90 mm Hg.
- Urinary output is >30 mL/hr.

Nursing Interventions and Rationale
1. Secure airway and administer oxygen to maintain SpO_2 >92%.
2. Place patient in supine position with legs elevated *to increase preload.* For patient with head injury, consider using low-Fowler's position with legs elevated.
3. For fluid repletion, use the 3:1 rule, replacing three parts of fluid for every unit of blood lost.
4. Administer crystalloid solutions using the fluid challenge technique: infuse precise boluses of fluid (usually 5-20 mL/min) over 10-minute periods; monitor hemodynamic pressures serially *to determine successful challenging.* If the pulmonary artery occlusion pressure elevates more than 7 mm Hg above beginning level, the infusion should be stopped. If the pulmonary artery occlusion pressure rises only to 3 mm Hg above baseline or falls, another fluid challenge should be administered.
5. Replete fluids first before considering use of vasopressors, *because vasopressors increase myocardial oxygen consumption out of proportion to the reestablishment of coronary perfusion in the early phases of treatment.*
6. When blood replacement is indicated, replace it with fresh packed red cells and fresh frozen plasma *to keep clotting factors intact.*
7. Move or reposition patient minimally to decrease or limit tissue oxygen demands.
8. Evaluate patient's anxiety level, and intervene through patient education or sedation *to decrease tissue oxygen demands.*
9. Maintain surveillance for signs and symptoms of fluid overload.

Deficient Fluid Volume Related to Decreased Secretion of Antidiuretic Hormone (ADH)
Defining Characteristics
- Confusion and lethargy
- Decreased skin turgor
- Thirst
- Weight loss over short period
- Decreased pulmonary artery occlusion pressure
- Decreased right atrial pressure
- Urinary output is >6 L/day
- Serum sodium is >148 mEq/L
- Serum osmolality is >295 mOsm/kg
- Urine osmolality is <100 mOsm/kg
- Urine specific gravity is <1.005

Outcome Criteria
- Weight returns to baseline.
- Urinary output is >30 mL/hr and <200 mL/hr.
- Serum osmolality is 280-295 mOsm/kg.
- Urine specific gravity is 1.010-1.030.

Nursing Interventions and Rationale
1. Record intake and output every hour, noting color and clarity of urine *because color and clarity are an indication of urine concentration.*
2. Monitor cardiac rhythm continuously for dysrhythmias *caused by electrolyte imbalance.*
3. Collaborate with physician regarding administration of vasopressin or desmopressin *to replace ADH.*
    a. Monitor patient for adverse effects of medications (e.g., headache, chest pain, abdominal pain) *caused by vasoconstriction.*
    b. Report adverse effects to physician immediately.
4. Collaborate with physician regarding intravenous fluid and electrolyte replacement therapy *to restore fluid balance, correct dehydration, and maintain electrolyte balance.*
    a. Administer hypotonic saline *to replace free water deficit.*
5. Provide oral fluids low in sodium such as water, coffee, tea, or orange juice *to decrease sodium intake.*
6. Weigh patient daily (at same time, in same amount of clothing, and preferably with same scale) *to ensure accuracy of readings.*
7. Reposition patient every 2 hours to prevent skin integrity issues caused by dehydration.
8. Provide mouth care every 4 hours to prevent breakdown of oral mucous membranes.
9. Collaborate with physician regarding administration of medications to prevent constipation *caused by dehydration.*
10. Maintain surveillance for symptoms of hypernatremia (muscle twitching, irritability, seizures), hypovolemic shock (hypotension, tachycardia, decreased CVP and PAOP), and deep vein thrombosis (calf pain, tenderness, swelling).

Deficient Fluid Volume Related to Relative Loss
Defining Characteristics
- Pulmonary artery occlusion pressure is <6 mm Hg
- Right atrial pressure is <2 mm Hg
- Tachycardia
- Narrowed pulse pressure
- Systolic blood pressure is <100 mm Hg
- Urinary output is <30 mL/hr
- Increased hematocrit level

Outcome Criteria
- Pulmonary artery occlusion pressure is >6 mm Hg or returns to baseline level.

NURSING MANAGEMENT PLAN

Deficient Fluid Volume—cont'd

- Right atrial pressure is >2 mm Hg or returns to baseline level.
- Systolic blood pressure is >90 mm Hg.
- Urinary output is >30 mL/hr.
- Hematocrit level is normal.

Nursing Interventions and Rationale

1. Collaborate with the physician regarding the administration of intravenous fluid replacements (usually normal saline solution or lactated Ringer solution) at a rate sufficient to maintain urinary output >30 mL/hr. Colloid solutions are avoided in the initial phases (but can be used later) because of the possibility of increased edema formation *as a result of the increased capillary permeability.*

⊚ NURSING MANAGEMENT PLAN

Deficient Knowledge

Definition: Absence or deficiency of cognitive information related to a specific topic

Deficient Knowledge Related to Cognitive or Perceptual Learning Limitations

Defining Characteristics

- Verbalized statement of inadequate knowledge of skills
- Verbalization of inadequate recall of information
- Verbalization of inadequate understanding of information
- Evidence of inaccurate follow-through of instructions
- Inadequate demonstration of a skill
- Lack of compliance with prescribed behavior

Outcome Criteria

- Patient participates actively in necessary and prescribed health behaviors.
- Patient verbalizes adequate knowledge or demonstrates adequate skills.

Nursing Interventions and Rationale

1. Determine specific cause of patient's cognitive or perceptual limitation.
2. Provide uninterrupted rest period before teaching session to decrease fatigue and encourage optimal state for learning and retention.
3. Manipulate environment as much as possible to provide quiet and uninterrupted learning sessions.
   a. Ensure that lights are bright enough to see teaching aids but not too bright.
   b. Schedule care and medications to allow uninterrupted teaching periods.
   c. Move patient to quiet, private room for teaching if possible.
4. Adapt teaching sessions and materials to patient's and family's levels of education and ability to understand.
   a. Provide printed material appropriate to reading level.
   b. Use terminology understood by the patient.
   c. Provide printed materials in patient's primary language if possible.
   d. Use interpreters during teaching sessions *when necessary.*
5. Teach only present-tense focus during periods of sensory overload.
6. Determine potential effects of medications on ability to retain or recall information. Avoid teaching critical content while patient is taking sedatives, analgesics, or other medications that affect memory.
7. Reinforce new skills and information in several teaching sessions. Use several senses when possible in teaching session (e.g., see a film, hear a discussion, read printed information, demonstrate skills related to self-injection of insulin).
8. Reduce patient's anxiety.
   a. Listen attentively, and encourage verbalization of feelings.
   b. Answer questions as they arise in a clear and succinct manner.
   c. Elicit patient's concerns, and address those issues first.
   d. Give only correct and relevant information.
   e. Continually assess response to teaching session, and discontinue if anxiety increases or physical condition becomes unstable.
   f. Provide nonthreatening information before more anxiety-producing information is presented.
   g. Plan for several teaching sessions so information can be divided into small, manageable packages.

Deficient Knowledge Related to Lack of Previous Exposure to Information

Defining Characteristics

- Verbalized statement of inadequate knowledge or skills
- New diagnosis or health problem requiring self-management or care
- Lack of prior formal or informal education about the specific health problem

- Demonstration of inappropriate behaviors related to management of health problem

Outcome Criteria

- Patient verbalizes adequate knowledge about or performs skills related to disease process, its causes, factors related to onset of symptoms, and self-management of disease or health problem.
- Patient actively participates in health behaviors required for performance of a procedure or in those behaviors enhancing recovery from illness and preventing recurrence or complications.

Nursing Interventions and Rationale

1. Determine existing level of knowledge or skill.
2. Assess factors that affect the knowledge deficit:
   a. Learning needs, including patient's priorities and the necessary knowledge and skills for safety.
   b. Learning ability of patient, including language skills, level of education, ability to read, preferred learning style.
   c. Physical ability to perform prescribed skills or procedures; consider effect of limitations imposed by treatment such as bed rest, restriction of movement by intravenous or other equipment, or effect of sedatives or analgesics.
   d. Psychologic effect of stage of adaptation to disease.
   e. Activity tolerance and ability to concentrate.
   f. Motivation to learn new skills or gain new knowledge.
3. Reduce or limit barriers to learning:
   a. Provide consistent nurse–patient contact to encourage development of trusting and therapeutic relationship.
   b. Structure environment to enhance learning and control unnecessary noise or interruptions.
   c. Individualize teaching plan to fit patient's current physical and psychologic status.
   d. Delay teaching until patient is ready to learn.
   e. Conduct teaching sessions during period of day when patient is most alert and receptive.
   f. Meet patient's immediate learning needs as they arise (e.g., give brief explanation of procedures when they are performed).
4. Promote active participation in the teaching plan by the patient and family:
   a. Solicit input during development of plan.
   b. Develop mutually acceptable goals and outcomes.
   c. Solicit expression of feelings and emotions related to new responsibilities.
   d. Encourage questions.
5. Conduct teaching sessions, using the most appropriate teaching methods.
6. Use the "teach-back" method **to confirm that you have explained to the patient what they need to know in a manner that the patient understands.**
   a. Use simple lay language, explain the concept or demonstrate the process to the patient/caregiver.
      (1) Avoid technical terms to avoid misunderstandings.
      (2) If the patient/caregiver has limited English proficiency, use a professional translator to reduce miscommunication.
   b. Ask the patient/caregiver to repeat in his or her own words how he or she understands the concept explained. If a process was demonstrated to the patient, ask the patient/caregiver to demonstrate it independent of assistance.
   c. Identify and correct misunderstandings of or incorrect procedures by the patient/caregiver.

NURSING MANAGEMENT PLAN

Deficient Knowledge—cont'd

d. Ask the patient/caregiver to demonstrate his or her understanding or procedural ability again *to ensure the above-noted misunderstandings are now corrected.*

e. Repeat steps until convinced the patient/caregiver comprehends the concept or possesses the ability to perform the procedure accurately and safely.

7. Provide written materials that enhance health literacy:

a. Limit content to one or two key objectives. Don't provide too much information or try to cover everything at once.

b. Limit content to what patients really need to know. Avoid information overload.

c. Use only words that are well known to individuals without medical training.

d. Make certain content is appropriate for age and culture of the target audience.

e. Write at or below the 6th-grade level.

f. Use one- or two-syllable words.

g. Use short paragraphs.

h. Use active voice.

i. Avoid all but the most simple tables and graphs. Clear explanations (legends) should be placed adjacent to the table or graph, and also in the text.

j. Use large font (minimum 12 point) with serifs. (Serif text has the little horizontal lines that you see at the bottoms of letters like f, x, n, and others.)

k. Don't use more than two or three font styles on a page. *Consistency in appearance is important.*

l. Use upper- and lower-case text. ALL UPPER-CASE TEXT IS HARD TO READ.

m. Ensure a good amount of empty space on the page. Don't clutter the page with text or pictures.

n. Use headings and subheadings to separate blocks of text.

o. Bulleted lists are preferable to blocks of text in paragraphs.

p. Illustrations are useful if they depict common, easy-to-recognize objects. Images of people, places, and things should be age appropriate and culturally appropriate to the target audience. Avoid complex anatomical diagrams.

8. Initiate referrals for follow-up if necessary:

a. Health educators

b. Home health care

c. Rehabilitation programs

d. Social services

9. Evaluate effectiveness of teaching plan, based on patient's ability to meet preset goals and objectives *to determine need for further teaching.*

◎ NURSING MANAGEMENT PLAN

Disturbed Body Image

Definition: Confusion in mental picture of one's physical self

Disturbed Body Image Related to Actual Change in Body Structure, Function, or Appearance

Defining Characteristics

- Actual change in appearance, structure, or function
- Avoidance of looking at body part
- Avoidance of touching body part
- Hiding or overexposing body part (intentional or unintentional)
- Trauma to nonfunctioning part
- Change in ability to estimate spatial relationship of body to environment
- Verbalization of the following:
  - Fear of rejection or reaction by others
  - Negative feeling about body
  - Preoccupation with change or loss
  - Refusal to participate in or to accept responsibility for self-care of altered body part
- Personalization of part or loss with a name
- Depersonalization of part or loss by use of impersonal pronouns
- Refusal to verify actual change

Outcome Criteria

- Patient verbalizes the specific meaning of the change to him or her.
- Patient requests appropriate information about self-care.
- Patient completes personal hygiene and grooming daily with or without help.
- Patient interacts freely with family or other visitors.
- Patient participates in the discussions and conferences related to planning his or her medical and nursing management in the critical care unit and transfer from the unit.
- Patient talks with trained visitors (support-group representatives) at least twice about his or her loss.

Nursing Interventions and Rationale

1. Evaluate patient's mental, physical, and emotional state; recognize assets, strengths, response to illness, coping mechanisms, past experience with stress, and support system.
2. Appraise the response of family and significant others. *Body image is derived from the "reflected appraisals" of family and significant others.*
3. Determine the patient's goals and readiness for learning.
4. Provide the necessary information to help the patient and family adapt to the change. Clarify misconceptions about future limitations.
5. Permit and encourage the patient to express the significance of the loss or change; note nonverbal behavior responses.
6. Allow and encourage the patient's expression of anxiety. *Anxiety is the most predominant emotional response to a body image disturbance.*
7. Recognize and accept the use of denial as an adaptive defense mechanism when used early and temporarily.
8. Recognize maladaptive denial as that which interferes with the patient's progress and/or alienates support systems. Use confrontation.
9. Provide an opportunity for the patient to discuss sexual concerns.
10. Touch the affected body part *to provide the patient with sensory information about altered body structure and/or function.*
11. Encourage and provide movement of altered body part *to establish kinesthetic feedback. This enables the person to know his or her body as it now exists.*
12. Prepare the patient to look at the body part. Call the body part by its anatomic name (e.g., stump, stoma, limb) as opposed to "it" or "she." *The use of impersonal pronouns increases a sense of fantasy and depersonalization of the body part.*
13. Allow the patient to experience excellence in some aspect of physical functioning—walking, turning, deep breathing, healing, self-care—and point out progress and accomplishment. *This helps to balance the patient's sense of dysfunction with function.*
14. Avoid false reassurance. Acknowledge the difficulty of incorporating the altered body part or function into one's body image. *This evidences the nurse's sensitivity and promotes trust.*
15. Talk with the patient about his or her life, generativity, and accomplishments. *Patients with disturbances in body image frequently see themselves in a distortedly "narrow" sense. Encouraging a wider focus of themselves and their life reduces this distortion.*
16. Help the patient explore realistic alternatives.
17. Recognize that incorporating a body change into one's body image takes time. Avoid setting unrealistic expectations and *thereby inadvertently reinforcing a low self-esteem.*
18. Suggest the use of additional resources such as trained visitors who have mastered situations similar to those of the patient.
    a. Refer the patient to a psychiatric nurse, psychologist, or psychiatrist if needed.

Disturbed Body Image Related to Functional Dependence on Life-Sustaining Technology

Defining Characteristics

- Actual change in function requiring permanent or temporary replacement
- Refusal to verify actual loss
- Verbalization of the following: feelings of helplessness, hopelessness, powerlessness, fear of failure to wean from technology

Outcome Criteria

- Patient verifies actual change in function.
- Patient does not refuse or fight technologic intervention.
- Patient verbalizes acceptance of expected change in lifestyle.

Nursing Interventions and Rationale

1. Evaluate patient's response to the technologic intervention.
2. Assess responses of family and significant others. *Body image is derived from the "reflected appraisals" of family and significant others.*
3. Provide information needed by patient and family.
4. Promote trust, security, comfort, and privacy.
5. Recognize anxiety. Allow and encourage its expression. *Anxiety is the most predominant emotion accompanying body image alterations.* Implement nursing management plan for Anxiety Related to Threat to Biologic, Psychologic, or Social Integrity.
6. Assist patient to recognize his or her own functioning and performance in the face of technology. For example, assist patient to distinguish spontaneous breaths from mechanically delivered breaths. *The activity will assist in weaning patient from the ventilator when feasible. To establish realistic, accurate body boundaries, a patient needs help to separate himself or herself from the technology that is supporting his or her functioning. Any participation or function on the part of the patient during periods of dependency is helpful in preventing and/ or resolving an alteration in body image.*
7. Plan for discontinuation of the treatment (e.g., weaning from ventilator). Explain procedure that will be followed, and be present during its initiation.
8. Plan for transfer from the critical care environment.
9. Document care, ensuring an up-to-date management plan is available to all involved caregivers.

NURSING MANAGEMENT PLAN

Disturbed Sleep Pattern

Definition: Time-limited disruption of sleep amount and quality due to external factors

Disturbed Sleep Pattern Related to Fragmented Sleep

Defining Characteristics

- Decreased sleep during one block of sleep time
- Daytime sleepiness
- Decreased sleep
  - Less than one half of normal total sleep time
  - Decreased slow-wave or rapid-eye-movement (REM) sleep
- Anxiety
- Fatigue
- Restlessness
- Disorientation and hallucinations
- Combativeness
- Frequent awakenings

Outcome Criteria

- Patient's total sleep time approximates patient's normal.
- Patient can complete sleep cycles of 90 minutes without interruption.
- Patient has no delusions or hallucinations.
- Patient has reality-based thought content.

Nursing Interventions and Rationale

1. Assess normal sleep pattern on admission and any history of sleep disturbance or chronic illness that may affect sleep or sedative/hypnotic use.
   a. Promote normal sleep activity while patient is in critical care unit.
   b. Assess sleep effectiveness by asking patient how his or her sleep in the hospital compares with sleep at home.
2. Promote comfort, relaxation, and a sense of well-being.
   a. Treat pain; change, smooth, or refresh bed linens at bedtime; and provide oral hygiene.
   b. Eliminate stressful situations before bedtime.
   c. Use relaxation techniques, imagery, music, massage, or warm blankets.
   d. Have a close family member sit beside the bed and provide the patient with his or her own garments or coverings.
   e. Provide quiet or background noise of the television or music (patient preference) *to best promote sleep.*
   f. Provide a comfortable room temperature.
3. Minimize noise, particularly that of the staff and noisy equipment.
   a. Reduce the level of environmental stimuli.
   b. Dim the lights at night.
4. Foods containing tryptophan (e.g., milk, turkey) may be appropriate *because these promote sleep.*
5. Plan nap times to assist in approximating the patient's normal 24-hour sleep time.
6. Minimize awakenings *to allow for at least 90-minute sleep cycles.*
   a. Continually assess the need to awaken the patient, particularly at night. Distinguish between essential and nonessential nursing tasks.
   b. Organize nursing management to allow for maximal amount of uninterrupted sleep while ensuring close monitoring of the patient's condition. Whenever possible, monitor physiologic parameters without waking the patient.
   c. Coordinate awakenings with other departments, such as laboratory and radiography, *to minimize sleep interruptions.*
7. Be aware of the effects of commonly used medications on sleep. *Many sedative and hypnotic medications decrease REM sleep.*
   a. Use sedative and analgesic medications that minimally disrupt sleep to complement comfort measures, with dosages reduced gradually as the medication is no longer necessary.
   b. Do not abruptly withdraw REM-suppressing medications *because this can result in REM rebound.*
8. Document amount of uninterrupted sleep per shift, especially sleep episodes lasting longer than 2 hours. *Sleep pattern disturbance is diagnosed, treated, and resolved more efficiently when formally documented in this manner.*

◎ NURSING MANAGEMENT PLAN

Dysfunctional Ventilatory Weaning Response

Definition: Inability to adjust to lowered levels of mechanical ventilator support that interrupts and prolongs the weaning process

Dysfunctional Ventilatory Weaning Response (DVWR) Related to Physical, Psychosocial, or Situational Factors

Defining Characteristics

Mild DVWR

- Responds to lowered levels of mechanical ventilator support with:
  - Restlessness
  - Slightly increased respiratory rate from baseline
  - Expressed feelings of increased need for oxygen, breathing discomfort, fatigue, warmth
  - Queries about possible machine malfunction
  - Increased concentration on breathing

Moderate DVWR

- Responds to lowered levels of mechanical ventilator support with:
  - Slight baseline increase in blood pressure is <20 mm Hg
  - Slight baseline increase in heart rate is <20 beats/min
  - Baseline increase in respiratory rate is <5 breaths/min
  - Hypervigilance to activities
  - Inability to respond to coaching
  - Inability to cooperate
  - Apprehension
  - Diaphoresis
  - Eye widening ("wide-eyed look")
  - Decreased air entry on auscultation
  - Color changes: pale, slight cyanosis
  - Slight respiratory accessory muscle use

Severe DVWR

- Responds to lowered levels of mechanical ventilator support with:
  - Agitation
  - Deterioration in arterial blood gases from current baseline
  - Baseline increase in blood pressure is >20 mm Hg
  - Baseline increase in heart rate is >20 beats/min
  - Respiratory rate increases significantly from baseline
  - Profuse diaphoresis
  - Full respiratory accessory muscle use
  - Shallow, gasping breaths
  - Paradoxic abdominal breathing
  - Discoordinated breathing with the ventilator
  - Decreased level of consciousness
  - Adventitious breath sounds, audible airway secretions
  - Cyanosis

Outcome Criteria

- Airway is clear.
- Underlying disorder is resolving.
- Patient is rested, and pain is controlled.
- Nutritional status is adequate.
- Patient has feelings of perceived control, situational security, and trust in the nurses.
- Patient is able to adapt to selected levels of ventilator support without undue fatigue.

Nursing Interventions and Rationale

1. Communicate interest and concern for the patient's well-being, and demonstrate confidence in ability to manage weaning process **to instill trust in the patient.**

2. Use normalizing strategies (e.g., grooming, dressing, mobilizing, social conversation) **to reinforce the patient's self-esteem and feeling of identity.**
3. Identify parameters of the patient's usual functioning before the weaning process begins **to facilitate early identification of problems.**
4. Identify the patient's strengths and resources that can be mobilized **to enhance the patient's coping and maximize weaning effort.**
5. Note concerns that adversely affect the patient's comfort and confidence, and manage them discreetly **to facilitate the patient's ease.**
6. Praise successful activities, encourage a positive outlook, and review the patient's positive progress **to increase the patient's perceived self-efficacy.**
7. Inform the patient of his or her situation and weaning progress **to permit the patient as much control as possible.**
8. Teach the patient about the weaning process and how he or she can participate in the process.
9. Negotiate daily weaning goals with the patient **to gain cooperation.**
10. Position the patient with the head of the bed elevated **to optimize respiratory efforts.**
11. Coach the patient in breath control by regular demonstrations of slow, deep, rhythmic patterns of breathing **to assist with dyspnea.**
12. Remain visible in the room and reassure the patient that help is immediately available if needed **to reduce the patient's anxiety and fearfulness.**
13. Encourage the patient to view weaning trials as a form of training, regardless of whether the weaning goal is achieved **to avoid discouragement.**
14. Encourage the patient to maintain emotional calmness by reassuring, being present, comforting, talking down if emotionally aroused, and reinforcing the idea that he or she can and will succeed.
15. Monitor the patient's status frequently **to avoid undue fatigue and anxiety.**
16. Provide regular periods of rest by reducing activities, maintaining or increasing ventilator support, and providing oxygen as needed before fatigue advances.
17. Provide distraction (e.g., visitors, radio, television, conversation) when the patient's concentration starts to create tension and increases anxiety.
18. Ensure adequate nutritional support, sufficient rest and sleep time, and sedation or pain control **to promote the patient's optimal physical and emotional comfort.**
19. Start weaning early in the day **when the patient is most rested.**
20. Restrict unnecessary activities and visitors who do not cooperate with weaning strategies **to minimize energy demands on the patient during the weaning process.**
21. Coordinate necessary activities to promote adequate time for rest and relaxation. Implement the nursing management plan for Activity Intolerance Related to Prolonged Immobility or Deconditioning.
22. Monitor the patient's underlying disease process **to ensure it is stabilized and under control.**
23. Advocate for additional resources (e.g., sedation, analgesia, rest) needed by the patient **to maximize comfort status.**
24. Develop and adhere to an individualized plan of care **to promote the patient's feelings of control.**

NURSING MANAGEMENT PLAN

Excess Fluid Volume

Definition: Increased isotonic fluid retention

Excess Fluid Volume Related to Increased Secretion of Antidiuretic Hormone (ADH)

Defining Characteristics

- Headache
- Decreased sensorium
- Weight gain over short period
- Intake greater than output
- Increased pulmonary artery occlusion pressure
- Increased right atrial pressure
- Urine output is <30 mL/hr
- Serum sodium is <120 mEq/L
- Serum osmolality is <275 mOsm/kg
- Urine osmolality greater than serum osmolality
- Urine sodium is >200 mEq/L
- Urine specific gravity is >1.03

Outcome Criteria

- Weight returns to baseline.
- Urine output is >30 mL/hr.
- Serum sodium is 135-145 mEq/L.
- Urine specific gravity is 1.005-1030.

Nursing Interventions and Rationale

1. Monitor cardiac rhythm continuously for dysrhythmias **caused by electrolyte imbalance.**
2. Restrict patient's fluids to 500 mL less than output per day **to decrease fluid retention.**
3. Provide patient chilled beverages high in sodium content such as tomato juice or broth **to increase sodium intake.**
4. Collaborate with physician regarding administration of demeclocycline, lithium, and/or opioid agonists **to inhibit renal response to ADH.**
5. Collaborate with physician regarding administration of hypertonic saline and furosemide **for rapid correction of severe sodium deficit and diuresis of free water.**
   a. Administer hypertonic saline at a rate of 1-2 mL/kg/hr until the patient's serum sodium is increased no greater than 1-2 mEq/L/hr.
6. Weigh patient daily (at same time, in same amount of clothing, and preferably with same scale) **to ensure accuracy of readings.**
7. Provide frequent mouth care to prevent breakdown of oral mucous membranes.
8. Initiate seizure precautions because patient is at high risk as a result of hyponatremia.
   a. Pad side rails of bed to protect patient from injury.
   b. Remove any objects from immediate environment that could injure patient in the event of a seizure.
   c. Keep appropriate-size oral airway at bedside to assist with airway management after the seizure.
9. Collaborate with physician regarding administration of medications to prevent constipation **caused by decreased fluid intake and immobility.**
10. Maintain surveillance for symptoms of hyponatremia (e.g., headache, abdominal cramps, weakness) and congestive heart failure (e.g., dyspnea, rales, increased central venous pressure, and pulmonary artery occlusion pressure).

Excess Fluid Volume Related to Renal Dysfunction

Defining Characteristics

- Weight gain that occurs during a 24- to 48-hour period
- Dependent pitting edema
- Ascites in severe cases
- Fluid crackles on lung auscultation
- Exertional dyspnea
- Oliguria or anuria
- Hypertension
- Engorged neck veins
- Decrease in urinary osmolality as renal failure progresses
- Right atrial pressure is >8 mm Hg
- Pulmonary artery occlusion pressure is >12 mm Hg

Outcome Criteria

- Weight returns to baseline.
- Edema or ascites is absent or reduced to baseline.
- Lungs are clear to auscultation.
- Exertional dyspnea is absent.
- Blood pressure returns to baseline.
- Heart rate returns to baseline.
- Neck veins are flat.
- Mucous membranes are moist.

Nursing Interventions and Rationale

1. Promote skin integrity of edematous areas by frequent repositioning and elevation of areas where possible. Avoid massaging pressure points or reddened areas of skin **because this results in further tissue trauma.**
2. Plan patient care to provide rest periods **to not heighten exertional dyspnea.**
3. Weigh patient daily (at same time, in same amount of clothing, and preferably with same scale).
4. Instruct the patient about the correlation between fluid intake and weight gain, using commonly understood fluid measurements; for example, ingesting 4 cups (1000 mL) of fluid results in an approximate 2-pound weight gain in the anuric patient.

◉ NURSING MANAGEMENT PLAN

Hyperthermia

Definition: Body temperature elevated above normal range

Hyperthermia Related to Increased Metabolic Rate
Defining Characteristics
- Increased body temperature above normal range
- Seizures
- Flushed skin
- Increased respiratory rate
- Tachycardia
- Skin warm to touch
- Diaphoresis

Outcome Criteria
- Temperature is within normal range.
- Respiratory rate and heart rate are within patient's baseline range.
- Skin is warm and dry.

Nursing Interventions and Rationale
1. Monitor temperature every 15 minutes to 1 hour until within normal range and stable and then every 4 hours *to maintain close surveillance for temperature fluctuations and evaluate effectiveness of interventions.*
   a. Use temperature taken from pulmonary artery catheter or bladder catheter if available *because these methods closely reflect core body temperature.*
   b. Use tympanic membrane temperature if core body temperature devices are unavailable.
   c. Use rectal temperature if none of the methods listed above are available.
2. Collaborate with physician regarding administration of antithyroid medications *to block the synthesis and release of thyroid hormone.*
3. Collaborate with physician regarding the use of cooling blanket *to facilitate heat loss by conduction.*
   a. Wrap hands, feet, and genitalia to protect them from maceration during cooling and decrease chance of shivering.
   b. Avoid rapidly cooling the patient and overcooling the patient because this initiates the heat-conserving response (i.e., shivering).
4. Place ice packs in patient's groin and axilla *to facilitate heat loss by conduction.*
5. Maintain patient on bedrest *to decrease the effects of activity on the patient's metabolic rate.*
6. Provide tepid sponge baths *to facilitate heat loss by evaporation.*
7. Decrease the patient's room temperature *to facilitate radiant heat loss.*
8. Place fan near patient to circulate cool air *to facilitate heat loss by convection.*
9. Provide patient with nonrestrictive gown and lightweight bed coverings *to allow heat to escape from the patient's trunk.*
10. Collaborate with physician and respiratory care practitioner on the administration of oxygen to maintain SpO_2 >90% *because patient has increased oxygen consumption resulting from an increased metabolic rate.*
11. Collaborate with physician regarding use of antipyretic medications *to facilitate patient comfort.*
12. Collaborate with physician regarding use of intravenous and oral fluids *to maintain adequate hydration of the patient.*

Hyperthermia Related to Pharmacogenic Hypermetabolism (Malignant Hyperthermia)
Defining Characteristics
Early Signs
- Blood pressure is >140/90 mm Hg
- Profuse diaphoresis
- Heart rate is >100 beats/min
- Masseter and general skeletal muscle rigidity and fasciculations
- Tachypnea
- Decreased level of consciousness
- Increased end-tidal carbon dioxide pressure ($PETCO_2$)

Late Signs
- Increasing core body temperature up to 42° to 43° C (107.6° to 109.4° F)
- Hot skin
- Systolic blood pressure is <90 mm Hg
- Heart rate is >100 beats/min and ventricular dysrhythmias
- Cardiac index is >4.0 L/min/m²
- Pulmonary artery occlusion pressure is >12 mm Hg
- Continued skeletal muscle rigidity and fasciculations
- PaO_2 is <80 mm Hg
- Respiratory and metabolic acidosis
- Fixed, dilated pupils
- Seizures, coma, or decerebrate posturing
- Urinary output is <30 mL/hr; urine color reddish brown (myoglobinuria)
- Prolonged bleeding (disseminated intravascular coagulation [DIC])

Outcome Criteria
- Core body temperature is below 38.3° C (101° F).
- Muscle rigidity and fasciculations are absent.
- Patient is alert and oriented.
- Pupils are normoreactive.

Nursing Interventions and Rationale
1. Obtain the emergency kit for malignant hyperthermia. *It is recommended that health care institutions have an emergency malignant hyperthermia kit available that contains the items mentioned in the following plan.* Call the malignant hyperthermia hotline for more information (1-800-644-9737).
2. Collaborate with the physician to implement measure to rapidly decrease metabolism:
   a. Administer dantrolene (Dantrium) at a dose of 2.5 mg/kg rapidly through a large-bore intravenous (IV) line, *which relaxes skeletal muscles by reducing the release of calcium from the sarcoplasmic reticulum.*
   b. Observe for infiltration of dantrolene into surrounding tissues. *Dantrolene is very alkaline and irritating to tissues.*
3. Collaborate with the physician to initiate cooling measures:
   a. Administer cold IV solutions (IV bag has been submerged in ice bath before solution is administered).
   b. Provide cool-water sponge bath.
   c. Apply cooling blanket until temperature is within 1° to 3° F of desired level *to avoid "overshoot," in which excessive cooling lowers the body temperature below the desired range.*
   d. Institute iced saline lavages of stomach, rectum, and bladder.
   e. Monitor core temperature continuously *to avoid overcooling.*

◎ NURSING MANAGEMENT PLAN

Hyperthermia—cont'd

4. Collaborate with physician to implement interventions to reverse metabolic and respiratory acidosis:
   a. Administer sodium bicarbonate at a dose of 1-2 mEq/kg IV as necessary *to treat metabolic acidosis and hyperkalemia.*
   b. Hyperventilate patient with 100% oxygen; then ventilate with 15-20 mL/kg tidal volume at 15-20 breaths/min.
   c. Assess arterial blood gas values frequently, and make ventilatory adjustments as necessary *to remedy hypoxemia and hypercarbia.*
5. Collaborate with physician to provide adequate nutrients to the tissues, and correct electrolyte imbalances:
   a. Administer 50% dextrose and regular insulin *to increase glucose uptake into liver to meet hypermetabolic needs of body and enhance the movement of potassium from extracellular fluid back into the cells.*
   b. Administer calcium chloride at a dose of 10 mg/kg IV or calcium gluconate at a dose of 10-50 mg/kg *for life-threatening hyperkalemia.*
   c. Monitor serum electrolytes *to assess efficacy of previously mentioned action.*
   d. Monitor blood urea nitrogen (BUN) and creatinine levels *to evaluate for renal failure.*
   e. Monitor serum enzyme levels, particularly creatine phosphokinase (CPK) elevations *for indication of degree of muscle hyperactivity.*
6. Collaborate with physician to correct cardiovascular instability and dysrhythmias:
   a. Titrate vasoactive and inotropic drips per protocol to desired systemic blood pressure, pulmonary artery occlusion pressure, and/or pulmonary artery diastolic pressure.
   b. Follow critical care emergency standing orders about the administration of antidysrhythmic agents.
   c. Do not administer calcium channel blockers *as they may cause hyperkalemia and cardiac arrest in the presence of dantrolene.*
7. Collaborate with physician to maintain a high urinary output (>50 mL/hr):
   a. Administer osmotic agents (mannitol) *for excretion of excess fluid load and to increase urinary output to prevent renal failure.*
   b. Administer diuretics (furosemide) *to enhance secretion of myoglobin, potassium, sodium, and magnesium.*
   c. Administer supplemental potassium chloride as indicated by serum potassium levels.
   d. Administer steroids (e.g., Solu-Cortef) *for its mineralocorticoid effect of potassium excretion, to increase glomerular filtration rate, and to reduce cerebral edema.*
8. Maintain surveillance for hematologic abnormalities:
   a. Monitor coagulation studies *for indications of DIC and for efficacy of heparin therapy.*
   b. Assess stool, urinary, and nasogastric (NG) drainage for occult blood.
9. Weigh patient daily (at same time, in same amount of clothing, and preferably with same scale) *to assist in assessment of hydration status.*

NURSING MANAGEMENT PLAN

Hypothermia

Definition: Body temperature below normal range

Hypothermia Related to Decreased Metabolic Rate
Defining Characteristics
- Reduction in body temperature below normal range
- Shivering
- Pallor
- Piloerection
- Hypertension
- Skin cool to touch
- Tachycardia
- Decreased capillary refill

Outcome Criteria
- Temperature is within normal range.
- Heart rate is within patient's baseline range.
- Skin is warm and dry.
- Capillary refill is normal.

Nursing Interventions and Rationale
1. Monitor temperature every 15 minutes to 1 hour until within normal range and stable and then every 4 hours *to maintain close surveillance for temperature fluctuations and evaluate effectiveness of interventions.*
   a. Use temperature taken from pulmonary artery catheter or bladder catheter if available *because these methods closely reflect core body temperature.*
   b. Use tympanic membrane temperature *if core body temperature devices are unavailable.*
   c. Use rectal temperature if none of the methods listed above are available.
2. Collaborate with physician regarding administration of thyroid medications *to replace lacking thyroid hormone.*
3. Collaborate with physician regarding the use of fluid-filled heating blanket *to facilitate rewarming by conduction.*
4. Initiate forced air-warming therapy *to facilitate convective heat gain.*
5. Provide patient with warm blankets *to facilitate heat transfer to the patient.*
6. Increase the patient's room temperature *to decrease radiant heat loss.*
7. Replace wet patient gown and bed linen promptly *to decrease evaporative heat loss.*
8. Warm intravenous fluids and blood products *to facilitate rewarming by conduction.*

Hypothermia Related to Exposure to Cold Environment, Trauma, or Damage to the Hypothalamus
Defining Characteristics
- Core body temperature below 35° C (95° F)
- Skin cold to touch
- Slurred speech, incoordination
- At temperature below 33° C (91.4° F):
  - Cardiac dysrhythmias (atrial fibrillation, bradycardia)
  - Cyanosis
  - Respiratory alkalosis
- At temperatures below 32° C (89.6° F):
  - Shivering replaced by muscle rigidity
  - Hypotension
  - Dilated pupils

- At temperatures below 28° to 29° C (82.4° to 84.2° F):
  - Absent deep tendon reflexes
  - 3-4 breaths/min to apnea
  - Ventricular fibrillation possible
- At temperatures below 26° to 27° C (78.8° to 80.6° F):
  - Coma
  - Flaccid muscles
  - Fixed, dilated pupils
  - Ventricular fibrillation to cardiac standstill
  - Apnea

Outcome Criteria
- Core body temperature is greater than 35° C (95° F).
- Patient is alert and oriented.
- Cardiac dysrhythmias are absent.
- Acid–base balance is normal.
- Pupils are normoreactive.

Nursing Interventions and Rationale
1. Monitor core body temperature continuously.
2. Collaborate with the physician regarding the need for intubation and mechanical ventilation.
   a. Heated air or oxygen can be added *to help rewarm the body core.*
   b. Do not hyperventilate the hypothermic patient *because carbon dioxide production is low and this action may induce severe alkalosis and precipitate ventricular fibrillation.*
3. Maintain cardiopulmonary resuscitation and advanced cardiac life support (ACLS) until core body temperature is up to at least 29.5° C (85.1° F) before determining that patients cannot be resuscitated. *Electrical defibrillation is usually successful in terminating ventricular fibrillation if the temperature is greater than 28° C (82.4° F).*
4. Administer cardiac resuscitation drugs sparingly *because as the body warms, peripheral vasodilation occurs. Drugs that remain in the periphery are suddenly released, leading to a bolus effect that may cause fatal dysrhythmias.*
5. Monitor arterial blood gas values *to direct further therapy, and ensure that the pH, PaO$_2$, and PaCO$_2$ are corrected for temperature.*
6. Rewarm patient rapidly *because the pathophysiologic changes associated with chronic hypothermia have not had time to evolve.*
   a. Institute rapid, active rewarming by immersion in warm water (38° to 43° C) (100.4° to 109.4° F).
   b. Apply thermal blanket at 36.6° to 37.7° C (97.9° to 99.9° F). Some researchers suggest rewarming only the torso or trunk first, leaving the extremities exposed to room temperature. *This is done to prevent early peripheral vasodilation with abrupt redistribution of intravascular volume. This also prevents colder blood trapped in the extremities from returning to the body core before the heart is rewarmed.*
   c. Perform rapid core rewarming with heated (37° to 43° C; 98.6° to 109.4° F) intravenous infusion, hemodialysis, peritoneal dialysis, and colonic or gastric irrigation fluids.
7. Monitor peripheral circulation *because gangrene of the fingers and toes is a common complication of accidental hypothermia.*

◎ NURSING MANAGEMENT PLAN

Imbalanced Nutrition: Less Than Body Requirements

Definition: Intake of nutrients insufficient to meet metabolic needs

Imbalanced Nutrition: Less Than Body Requirements Related to Lack of Exogenous Nutrients and Increased Metabolic Demand

Defining Characteristics

- Unplanned weight loss of 20% of body weight within the past 6 months
- Serum albumin is <3.5 g/dL
- Total lymphocytes are <1500/mm^3
- Anergy
- Negative nitrogen balance
- Fatigue; lack of energy and endurance
- Nonhealing wounds
- Daily caloric intake less than estimated nutritional requirements
- Presence of factors known to increase nutritional requirements (e.g., sepsis, trauma, multiple organ dysfunction syndrome)
- Maintenance of nothing by mouth (NPO) status for >7-10 days
- Long-term use of 5% dextrose intravenously
- Documentation of suboptimal calorie counts
- Drug or nutrient interaction that might decrease oral intake (e.g., chronic use of bronchodilators, laxatives, anticonvulsives, diuretics, antacids, opioids)
- Physical problems with chewing, swallowing, choking, and salivation and presence of altered taste, anorexia, nausea, vomiting, diarrhea, or constipation

Outcome Criteria

- Patient exhibits stabilization of weight loss or weight gain of one-half pound daily.
- Serum albumin is >3.5 g/dL.
- Total lymphocytes are <1500/mm^3.
- Patient has positive response to cutaneous skin antigen testing.
- Patient is in positive nitrogen balance.
- Wound healing is evident.
- Daily caloric intake equals estimated nutritional requirements.
- Increased ambulation and endurance are evident.

Nursing Interventions and Rationale

1. Inquire if patient has any food allergies and food preferences **to ensure the food provided to the patient is not contraindicated.**
2. Monitor patient's caloric intake and weight daily **to ensure adequacy of nutritional interventions.**
3. Collaborate with dietitian regarding patient's nutritional and caloric needs **to determine the appropriateness of the patient's diet to meet those needs.**
4. Monitor patient for signs of nutritional deficiencies **to facilitate evaluation of extent of nutritional deficient.**
5. Provide patient with oral care before eating **to ensure optimal consumption of diet.**
6. Assist patient to eat as appropriate **to ensure optimal consumption of diet.**
7. Collaborate with physician and dietitian regarding the administration of parenteral and enteral nutrition as needed.

NURSING MANAGEMENT PLAN

Impaired Gas Exchange

Definition: Excess or deficit in oxygenation and/or carbon dioxide elimination at the alveolar–capillary membrane

Impaired Gas Exchange Related to Alveolar Hypoventilation

Defining Characteristics

- Abnormal arterial blood gas values (decreased PaO_2, increased $PaCO_2$, decreased pH, decreased SaO_2)
- Somnolence
- Neurobehavioral changes (e.g., restlessness, irritability, confusion)
- Tachycardia or dysrhythmias
- Central cyanosis

Outcome Criteria

- Arterial blood gas values are within patient's baseline.
- Central cyanosis is absent.

Nursing Interventions and Rationale

1. Initiate continuous pulse oximetry or monitor SpO_2 every hour.
2. Collaborate with physician and respiratory care practitioner on the administration of oxygen to maintain an SpO_2 >90%.
   a. Administer supplemental oxygen by an appropriate oxygen-delivery device *to increase driving pressure of oxygen in the alveoli.*
   b. If supplemental oxygen alone is not effective, administer high-flow oxygen via high-flow nasal cannula, or BiPAP via noninvasive ventilation (NIV) or positive end-expiratory pressure (PEEP) via invasive mechanical ventilation *to open collapsed alveoli and increase the surface area for gas exchange.*
3. Prevent hypoventilation.
   a. Position patient in high-Fowler's position or semi-Fowler's position *to promote diaphragmatic descent and maximal inhalation.*
   b. Assist with deep-breathing exercises and/or incentive spirometry with sustained maximal inspiration 5-10 times/hr *to help reinflate collapsed portions of the lung.* See the nursing management plan for Ineffective Breathing Pattern Related to Decreased Lung Expansion for further instructions.
   c. Treat pain, if present, *to prevent hypoventilation and atelectasis.* Implement the nursing management plan for Acute Pain Related to Transmission and Perception of Cutaneous, Visceral, Muscular, or Ischemic Impulses.
4. Assist physician with intubation and initiation of mechanical ventilation as indicated.

Impaired Gas Exchange Related to Ventilation/Perfusion Mismatching or Intrapulmonary Shunting

Defining Characteristics

- Abnormal arterial blood gas values (decreased PaO_2, decreased SaO_2)
- Somnolence
- Neurobehavioral changes (restlessness, irritability, confusion)
- Central cyanosis

Outcome Criteria

- ABG values are within patient's baseline.
- Central cyanosis is absent.

Nursing Interventions and Rationale

1. Initiate continuous pulse oximetry, or monitor SpO_2 every hour.
2. Collaborate with physician and respiratory care practitioner on the administration of oxygen to maintain an SpO_2 >90%.
   a. Administer supplemental oxygen by an appropriate oxygen-delivery device *to increase driving pressure of oxygen in the alveoli.*
   b. If supplemental oxygen alone is not effective, administer high-flow oxygen via high-flow nasal cannula, or BiPAP via noninvasive ventilation (NIV) or positive end-expiratory pressure (PEEP) via invasive mechanical ventilation *to open collapsed alveoli and increase the surface area for gas exchange.*
3. Position patient to optimize ventilation/perfusion matching.
   a. For patient with unilateral lung disease, position with the good lung down *because gravity will improve perfusion to this area, and this will best match ventilation with perfusion.*
   b. For patient with bilateral lung disease, position with the right lung down *because this lung is larger than the left and affords a greater area for ventilation and perfusion,* or change position every 2 hours, favoring positions that improve oxygenation.
   c. For patient with diffuse bilateral disease, collaborate with the physician regarding the use of prone positioning *to encourage perfusion to the anterior region of the lungs, which are usually less damaged than the posterior region.*
   d. Avoid any position that seriously compromises oxygenation status.
4. Perform procedures only as needed and provide adequate rest and recovery time in between *to prevent desaturation.*
5. Collaborate with the physician regarding the administration of the following:
   a. Sedatives *to decrease ventilator asynchrony and facilitate patient's sense of control.*
   b. Neuromuscular blocking agents *to prevent ventilator asynchrony and decrease oxygen demand.*
   c. Analgesics *to treat pain if present.* Implement the nursing management plan for Acute Pain Related to Transmission and Perception of Cutaneous, Visceral, Muscular, or Ischemic Impulses.
6. Evaluate patient for the presence of secretions. If present, implement the nursing management plan for Ineffective Airway Clearance Related to Excessive Secretions or Abnormal Viscosity of Mucus.

NURSING MANAGEMENT PLAN

Impaired Spontaneous Ventilation

Definition: Decreased energy reserves result in an individual's inability to maintain breathing adequate to support life.

Impaired Spontaneous Ventilation Related to Respiratory Muscle Fatigue or Metabolic Factors

Defining Characteristics
- Dyspnea and apprehension
- Increased metabolic rate
- Increased restlessness
- Increased use of accessory muscles
- Decreased tidal volume
- Increased heart rate
- Abnormal arterial blood gas values (decreased PaO_2, increased $PaCO_2$, decreased pH, decreased SaO_2)
- Decreased cooperation

Outcome Criteria
- Metabolic rate and heart rate are within patient's baseline.
- Patient experiences eupnea.
- ABG values are within patient's baseline.

Nursing Interventions and Rationale
1. Collaborate with the physician regarding the application of pressure support to the ventilator *to assist patient in overcoming the work of breathing imposed by the ventilator and endotracheal tube.*
2. Carefully snip excess length from the proximal end of the endotracheal *tube to decrease dead space and thereby decrease the work of breathing.*
3. Collaborate with the physician and dietitian to ensure that at least 50% of the diet's nonprotein caloric source is in the form of fat rather than carbohydrates *to prevent excess carbon dioxide production.*
4. Collaborate with the physician and respiratory care practitioner regarding the best method of weaning for individual *patients because each situation is different and a variety of weaning options are available.*

   a. Consider initiating daily spontaneous awakening trial ("sedation vacation") and spontaneous breathing trial.
   b. Monitor patient for signs of weaning intolerance.
5. Collaborate with the physician and physical therapist regarding a progressive ambulation and conditioning plan *to promote overall muscle conditioning and respiratory muscle functioning.* Implement the nursing management plan for Activity Intolerance Related to Prolonged Immobility or Deconditioning.
6. Determine the most effective means of communication for the patient *to promote independence and reduce anxiety.*
7. Develop a daily schedule and post it in patient's room *to coordinate care and facilitate patient's involvement in the plan.*
8. Treat pain, if present, *to prevent respiratory splinting and hypoventilation.* Implement the nursing management plan for Acute Pain Related to Transmission and Perception of Cutaneous, Visceral, Muscular, or Ischemic Impulses.
9. Ensure that patient receives at least 2- to 4-hr intervals of uninterrupted sleep in a quiet, dark room. Collaborate with the physician and respiratory care practitioner regarding the use of full ventilatory support at night *to provide respiratory muscle rest.*
10. Place patient in semi-Fowler's position or in a chair at the bedside *for best use of ventilatory muscles and to facilitate diaphragmatic descent.*
11. Explain the weaning procedure to the patient before the trial *so that patient will understand what to expect and how to participate.*
12. Monitor patient during the weaning trial for evidence of respiratory muscle fatigue *to avoid overtiring the patient.*
13. Collaborate with physician and occupational therapist to provide diversional activities during the weaning trial *to reduce the patient's anxiety.*
14. Collaborate with physician and respiratory care practitioner regarding the removal of the ventilator and artificial airway *when patient has been successfully weaned.*

◎ NURSING MANAGEMENT PLAN

Impaired Swallowing

Definition: Abnormal functioning of the swallowing mechanism associated with deficits in oral, pharyngeal, or esophageal structure or function

Impaired Swallowing Related to Neuromuscular Impairment, Fatigue, and Limited Awareness

Defining Characteristics

- Evidence of difficulty swallowing:
  - Drooling
  - Difficulty handling oral secretions
  - Absence of gag, cough, and/or swallow reflex
  - Moist, wet, gurgling voice quality
  - Decreased tongue and mouth movements
  - Presence of dysarthria
- Difficulty handling solid foods:
  - Uncoordinated chewing or swallowing
  - Stasis of food in the oral cavity
  - Wet-sounding voice or change in voice quality
  - Sneezing, coughing, or choking with eating
  - Delay in swallowing of more than 5 seconds
  - Change in respiratory patterns
- Difficulty handling liquids:
  - Momentary loss of voice or change in voice quality
  - Nasal regurgitation of liquids
  - Coughing with drinking
- Evidence of aspiration:
  - Hypoxemia
  - Productive cough
  - Frothy sputum
  - Wheezing, crackles, or rhonchi
  - Temperature elevation

Outcome Criteria

- Evidence of swallowing difficulties is absent.
- Evidence of aspiration is absent.

Nursing Interventions and Rationale

1. Collaborate with physician and speech therapist regarding swallowing evaluation and rehabilitation program *to decrease the incidence of aspiration.*
2. Collaborate with physician and dietitian regarding a nutritional assessment and nutritional plan *to ensure that the patient is receiving enough nutrition.*
3. Place the patient in an upright position with the head midline and the chin slightly down *to keep food in the anterior portion of the mouth and to prevent it from falling over the base of the tongue into the open airway.*
4. Provide patient with single-textured soft foods (e.g., cream cereals) that maintain their shape *because these foods require minimal oral manipulation.*
5. Avoid particulate foods (e.g., hamburger) and foods containing more than one texture (e.g., stew) *because these foods require more chewing and oral manipulation.*
6. Avoid dry foods (e.g., popcorn, rice, crackers) and sticky foods (e.g., peanut butter, bananas) *because these foods are difficult to manipulate orally.*
7. Provide patient with thick liquids (e.g., fruit nectar, yogurt) *because thick liquids are more easily controlled in the mouth.*
8. Thicken thin liquids (e.g., water, juice) with a thickening preparation or avoid them *because thin liquids are easily aspirated.*
9. Place foods in the uninvolved side of the mouth *because oral sensitivity and function are greatest in this area.*
10. Avoid the use of straws *because they can deposit the liquid too far back in the mouth for the patient to handle.*
11. Serve foods and liquids at room temperature *because the patient may be overly sensitive to heat or cold.*
12. Offer solids and liquids at different times *to avoid swallowing solids before being properly chewed.*
13. Provide oral hygiene after meals *to clear food particles from the mouth that could be aspirated.*
14. Collaborate with physician and pharmacist regarding oral medication administration *to adjust medication regimen to prevent aspiration and choking and to ensure all prescribed medications are swallowed.*
15. Crush tablets (if appropriate) and mix with food that is easily formed into a bolus, use thickened liquid medications (if available), and/or embed small capsules into food *to facilitate oral medication administration.*
16. Inspect mouth for residue after all medication administration *to ensure medication has been swallowed.*
17. Educate patient and family on the swallowing problem, rehabilitation program, and emergency measures for choking.

NURSING MANAGEMENT PLAN

Impaired Verbal Communication

Definition: Decreased, delayed, or absent ability to receive, process, transmit, and use a system of symbols

Impaired Verbal Communication Related to Cerebral Speech Center Injury

Defining Characteristics

- Inappropriate or absent speech or responses to questions
- Inability to speak spontaneously
- Inability to understand spoken words
- Inability to follow commands appropriately through gestures
- Difficulty or inability to understand written language
- Difficulty or inability to express ideas in writing
- Difficulty or inability to name objects

Outcome Criterion

- Patient is able to make basic needs known.

Nursing Interventions and Rationale

1. Consult with physician and speech pathologist *to determine the extent of the patient's communication deficit (e.g., whether fluent, nonfluent, or global aphasia is involved).*
2. Have the speech therapist post a list of appropriate ways to communicate with the patient in the patient's room *so that all nursing personnel can be consistent in their efforts.*
3. Assess the patient's ability to comprehend, speak, read, and write.
   a. Ask questions that can be answered with "yes" or "no." If a patient answers "yes" to a question, ask the opposite (e.g., "Are you hot?" "Yes." "Are you cold?" "Yes."). *This may help determine whether the patient understands what is being said.*
   b. Ask simple, short questions, and use gestures, pantomime, and facial expressions to give the patient additional clues.
   c. Stand in the patient's line of vision, giving a good view of your face and hands.
   d. Have the patient try to write with a pad and pencil. Offer pictures and alphabet letters at which to point.
   e. Make flash cards with pictures or words depicting frequently used phrases (e.g., glass of water, bedpan).
4. Maintain an uncluttered environment, and decrease external distractions *to enhance communication.*
5. Maintain a relaxed and calm manner, and explain all diagnostic, therapeutic, and comfort measures before initiating them.
6. Do not shout or speak in a loud voice. *Hearing loss is not a factor in aphasia, and shouting will not help.*
7. Have only one person talk at a time. *It is more difficult for the patient to follow a multisided conversation.*
8. Use direct eye contact, and speak directly to the patient in unhurried, short phrases.
9. Give one-step commands and directions, and provide cues through pictures and gestures.

10. Try to ask questions that can be answered with a "yes" or a "no," and avoid topics that are controversial, emotional, abstract, or lengthy.
11. Listen to the patient in an unhurried manner, and wait for his or her attempt to communicate.
    a. Expect a time lag from when you ask the patient something until the patient responds.
    b. Accept the patient's statement of essential words without expecting complete sentences.
    c. Avoid finishing the sentence for the patient if possible.
    d. Wait approximately 30 seconds before providing the word the patient may be attempting to find (except when the patient is very frustrated and needs something quickly, such as a bedpan).
    e. Rephrase the patient's message aloud *to validate it.*
    f. Do not pretend to understand the patient's message if you do not.
12. Encourage the patient to speak slowly in short phrases and to say each word clearly.
13. Ask the patient to write the message, if able, or draw pictures if only verbal communication is affected.
14. Observe the patient's nonverbal clues for validation (e.g., answers "yes" but shakes head "no").
15. When handing an object to the patient, state what it is *because hearing language spoken is necessary to stimulate language development.*
16. Explain what has happened to the patient, and offer reassurance about the plan of care.
17. Verbally address the problem of frustration over the inability to communicate, and explain that both the nurse and the patient need patience.
18. Maintain a calm, positive manner, and offer reassurance (e.g., "I know this is very hard for you, but it will get better if we work on it together").
19. Talk to the patient as an adult. Be respectful, and avoid talking down to the patient.
20. Do not discuss the patient's condition or hold conversations in the patient's presence without including him or her in the discussion. *This may be the reason some aphasic patients develop paranoid thoughts.*
21. Do not exhibit disapproval of emotional utterances or spontaneous use of profanity; instead, offer calm, quiet reassurance.
22. If the patient makes an error in speech, do not reprimand or scold but try to compliment the patient by saying, "That was a good try."
23. Delay conversation if the patient is tired. *The symptoms of aphasia worsen if the patient is fatigued, anxious, or upset.*
24. Be prepared for emotional outbursts and tears from patients who have more difficulty in expressing themselves than with understanding. *The patient may become depressed, refuse treatment and food, ignore relatives, and push objects away.* Comfort the patient with statements such as, "I know it's frustrating and you feel sad, but you are not alone. Other people who have had strokes have felt the way you do. We will be here to help you get through this."

◎ NURSING MANAGEMENT PLAN

Ineffective Airway Clearance

Definition: Inability to clear secretions or obstructions from the respiratory tract to maintain a clear airway

Ineffective Airway Clearance Related to Excessive Secretions or Abnormal Viscosity of Mucus

Defining Characteristics
- Abnormal breath sounds (displaced normal sounds, adventitious sounds, diminished or absent sounds)
- Ineffective cough with or without sputum
- Tachypnea, dyspnea
- Verbal reports of inability to clear airway

Outcome Criteria
- Cough produces thin mucus.
- Lungs are clear to auscultation.
- Respiratory rate, depth, and rhythm return to baseline.

Nursing Interventions and Rationale
1. Assess sputum for color, consistency, and amount.
2. Assess for clinical manifestations of pneumonia.
3. Provide for maximal thoracic expansion by repositioning, deep breathing, splinting, and pain management **to avoid hypoventilation and atelectasis.** If hypoventilation is present, implement the nursing management plan for Ineffective Breathing Pattern Related to Decreased Lung Expansion.
4. Maintain adequate hydration by administering oral and intravenous fluids (as ordered) **to thin secretions and facilitate airway clearance.**
5. Provide humidification to airways by an oxygen-delivery device or artificial airway **to thin secretions and facilitate airway clearance.**
6. Administer bland aerosol every 4 hours **to facilitate expectoration of sputum.**
7. Collaborate with the physician regarding the administration of the following:
   a. Bronchodilators **to treat or prevent bronchospasms and facilitate expectoration of mucus.**
   b. Mucolytics and expectorants **to enhance mobilization and removal of secretions.**
   c. Antibiotics **to treat infection.**
8. Assist with directed coughing exercises **to facilitate expectoration of secretions.** If patient is unable to perform cascade cough, consider using huff cough (patients with hyperactive airways), end-expiratory cough

(patient with secretions in distal airway), or augmented cough (patient with weakened abdominal muscle).
   a. Cascade cough—instruct patient to do the following:
      (1) Take a deep breath, and hold it for 1-3 seconds.
      (2) Cough out forcefully several times until all air is exhaled.
      (3) Inhale slowly through the nose.
      (4) Repeat once.
      (5) Rest, and then repeat as necessary.
   b. Huff cough—instruct patient to do the following:
      (1) Take a deep breath, and hold it for 1-3 seconds.
      (2) Say the word "huff" while coughing out several times until air is exhaled.
      (3) Inhale slowly through the nose.
      (4) Repeat as necessary.
   c. End-expiratory cough—instruct patient to do the following:
      (1) Take a deep breath, and hold it for 1-3 seconds.
      (2) Exhale slowly.
      (3) At the end of exhalation, cough once.
      (4) Inhale slowly through the nose.
      (5) Repeat as necessary, or follow with cascade cough.
   d. Augmented cough—instruct patient to do the following:
      (1) Take a deep breath, and hold it for 1-3 seconds.
      (2) Perform one or more of the following maneuvers to increase intraabdominal pressure:
         (a) Tighten knees and buttocks.
         (b) Bend forward at the waist.
         (c) Place a hand flat on the upper abdomen just under the xiphoid process and press in and up abruptly during coughing.
         (d) Keep hands on the chest wall and press inward with each cough.
      (3) Inhale slowly through the nose.
      (4) Rest and repeat as necessary.
9. Suction nasotracheally or endotracheally as necessary **to assist with secretion removal.**
10. Reposition patient at least every 2 hours or use kinetic therapy **to mobilize and prevent stasis of secretions.**
11. Allow rest periods between coughing sessions, suctioning, or any other demanding activities **to promote energy conservation.**

◎ NURSING MANAGEMENT PLAN

Ineffective Breathing Pattern

Definition: Inspiration and/or expiration that does not provide adequate ventilation

Ineffective Breathing Pattern Related to Decreased Lung Expansion
Defining Characteristics
- Abnormal respiratory patterns (hypoventilation, hyperventilation, tachypnea, bradypnea, obstructive breathing)
- Abnormal arterial blood gas values (increased $PaCO_2$, decreased pH)
- Unequal chest movement
- Shortness of breath, dyspnea

Outcome Criteria
- Respiratory rate, rhythm, and depth return to baseline.
- Minimal or absent use of accessory muscles.
- Chest expands symmetrically.
- Arterial blood gas values return to baseline.

Nursing Interventions and Rationale
1. Treat pain, if present, *to prevent hypoventilation and atelectasis.* Implement the nursing management plan for Acute Pain Related to Transmission and Perception of Cutaneous, Visceral, Muscular, or Ischemic Impulses.
2. Position patient in high-Fowler's or semi-Fowler's position *to promote diaphragmatic descent and maximal inhalation.*
3. Assist with deep-breathing exercises and incentive spirometry with sustained maximal inspiration 5-10 times/hr *to help reinflate collapsed portions of the lung.*
   a. Deep breathing—instruct patient to do the following:
      (1) Sit up straight or lean forward slightly while sitting on edge of bed or chair (if possible).
      (2) Take in a slow, deep breath.
      (3) Pause slightly, or hold breath for at least 3 seconds.
      (4) Exhale slowly.
      (5) Rest, and repeat.
   b. Incentive spirometry—instruct patient to do the following:
      (1) Exhale normally.
      (2) Place lips around the mouthpiece, and close mouth tightly around it.
      (3) Inhale slowly and as deeply as possible, noting the maximal volume of air inspired.
      (4) Hold maximal inhalation for 3 seconds.
      (5) Take the mouthpiece out of mouth, and slowly exhale.
      (6) Rest, and repeat.
4. Assist physician with intubation and initiation of mechanical ventilation as indicated.

Ineffective Breathing Pattern Related to Musculoskeletal Fatigue or Neuromuscular Impairment
Defining Characteristics
- Unequal chest movement
- Shortness of breath, dyspnea
- Use of accessory muscles
- Tachypnea
- Thoracoabdominal asynchrony
- Abnormal arterial blood gas values (increased $PaCO_2$, decreased pH)
- Nasal flaring
- Assumption of 3-point position

Outcome Criteria
- Respiratory rate, rhythm, and depth return to baseline.
- Use of accessory muscles is minimal or absent.
- Chest expands symmetrically.
- Arterial blood gas values return to baseline.

Nursing Interventions and Rationale
1. Prevent unnecessary exertion *to limit drain on patient's ventilatory reserve.*
2. Instruct patient in energy-saving techniques *to conserve patient's ventilatory reserve.*
3. Assist with pursed-lip and diaphragmatic breathing techniques *to facilitate diaphragmatic descent and improved ventilation.*
   a. Diaphragmatic breathing—instruct the patient to do the following:
      (1) Sit in the upright position.
      (2) Place one hand on the abdomen just above the waist and the other on the upper chest.
      (3) Breathe in through the nose, and feel the lower hand push out; the upper hand should not move.
      (4) Breathe out through pursed lips, and feel the lower hand move in.
4. Position patient in high-Fowler's or semi-Fowler's position *to promote diaphragmatic descent and maximal inhalation.*
5. Assist physician with intubation and initiation of mechanical ventilation as indicated.

⊚ NURSING MANAGEMENT PLAN

Ineffective Coping

Definition: Inability to form a valid appraisal of the stressors, inadequate choices of practiced responses, and/or inability to use available resources

Ineffective Coping Related to Situational Crisis and Personal Vulnerability

Defining Characteristics
- Verbalization of inability to cope. *Sample statements*: "I can't take this anymore." "I don't know how to deal with this."
- Ineffective problem solving (problem lumping). *Sample statements*: "I have to eliminate salt from my diet. They tell me I can no longer mow the lawn. This hospitalization is costing a mint. What about my kids' future? Who's going to change the oil in the car? This is an incredible amount of time away from work."
- Ineffective use of coping mechanisms
  - Projection: blames others for illness or pain
  - Displacement: directs anger and/or aggression toward family
    - *Sample statements*: "Get out of here. Leave me alone."
    - Cursing, shouting, or demanding attention; striking out or throwing objects
  - Denial: of severity of illness and need for treatment
- Noncompliance. *Examples*: activity restriction; refusal to allow treatment or to take medications
- Suicidal thoughts (verbalizes desire to end life)
- Self-directed aggression. *Examples*: disconnects or attempts to disconnect life-sustaining equipment; deliberately tries to harm self
- Failure to progress from dependent to more independent state (refusal or resistance to care for self)

Outcome Criteria
- Patient verbalizes beginning ability to cope with illness, pain, and hospitalization. *Sample statements*: "I'm trying to do the best I can." "I want to help myself get better."
- Patient demonstrates effective problem solving (lists and prioritizes problems from most to least urgent).
- Patient uses effective behavioral strategies to manage the stress of illness and care.
- Patient demonstrates interest or involvement in illness or environment. *Examples*: patient does the following:
  - Requests medications when anticipating pain
  - Questions course of treatment, progress, and prognosis
  - Asks for clarification of environmental stimuli and events
  - Seeks out supportive individuals in his or her environment
  - Uses coping mechanisms and strategies more effectively to manage situational crisis
  - Demonstrates significant reduction in impulsive, angry, or aggressive outbursts (projection, shouting, cursing) directed toward family
  - Verbalizes future-based plans, with cessation of self-directed aggressive acts and suicidal thoughts
  - Willingly complies with treatment regimen
  - Begins to participate in self-care

Nursing Interventions and Rationale
1. Actively listen and respond to patient's verbal and behavioral expressions. *Active listening signifies unconditional respect and acceptance for the patient as a worthwhile individual. It builds trust and rapport, guides the nurse toward problem areas, encourages the patient to express concerns, and promotes compliance.*
2. Offer effective coping strategies to help the patient better tolerate the stressors related to his or her illness and care. Give permission to vent feelings in a safe setting. *Sample statements:* "I don't blame you for feeling angry or frustrated." "Others who are ill like you have expressed similar feelings." "I will listen to anything you want to share with me." "We don't have to talk; I'd like to sit here with you." "It's perfectly okay to cry." *Individuals who are provided with opportunities to express their feelings will be better able to release pent-up emotions and derive a greater sense of relief and comfort. They are less likely to resort to overly impulsive, aggressive acts, which may harm self or others.*
3. Inform the family of the patient's need to displace anger occasionally but that you will be working with the patient to help him or her release his or her feelings in a more constructive, effective way. *Family members who are well informed are better equipped to cope with their loved one's emotional anguish and outbursts. They are less likely to waste energy on feelings of guilt, fear, anger, or despair and can use their strength to help the patient in more constructive ways. The knowledge that their loved one is being cared for emotionally as well as physically provides family members with a greater sense of comfort and understanding. They will feel nurtured and respected by the nurse's attempt to include them in the process.*
4. With the patient, list and number problems from the most to least urgent. Assist him or her in finding immediate solutions for most urgent problems; postpone those that can wait; delegate some to family members; and help him or her to acknowledge problems that are beyond his or her control. *Listing and numbering problems in an organized fashion helps to break them down into more manageable "pieces" so that the patient is better able to identify solutions for those that are solvable and to suppress those that are less relevant or not amenable to interventions.*
5. Identify individuals in the patient's environment who best help him or her to cope, and identify those who do not. Validate your observations with the patient. *Sample statements:* "I notice you seemed more relaxed during your daughter's visit." "After the clergy left, you were able to sleep a bit longer than usual; would you like to see him more often?" "Your grandson was a bit upset today; I'll be glad to talk to him if you like." *Supportive persons can invoke a calming effect on the patient's physiologic and psychologic states. Conversely, well-meaning but nonsupportive individuals can have a deleterious effect on the patient's ability to cope and must be carefully screened and counseled by the nurse.*
6. Teach the patient effective cognitive strategies to help him or her better manage the stress of critical illness and care. Help him or her construct pleasant thoughts, situations, or images that can simultaneously inhibit unpleasant realities. Examples: a day at the beach, a walk in the park, drinking a glass of wine, or being with a loved one. *Pleasant thoughts and images constructed during critical illness and care tend to inhibit or reduce the intensity of the unpleasant, stressful effects of the experience.*
7. Assist the patient in using coping mechanisms more effectively so he or she can better manage his or her situational crisis.
   a. Suppression of problems beyond his or her control
   b. Compensation for illness and its effects; focusing on his or her strengths, interests, family, and spiritual beliefs
   c. Adaptive displacement of anger, fear, or frustration through healthy, verbal expressions to staff. *Effective use of coping mechanisms helps to assuage the patient's painful feelings in a safe setting. The patient is strengthened and need not resort to the use of more ineffective defenses to eliminate anxiety.*
8. Initiate a suicidal assessment if the patient verbalizes the desire to die, states that life is not worth living, or exhibits self-directed aggression.

⊚ NURSING MANAGEMENT PLAN

Ineffective Coping—cont'd

Sample statement: "We know that this is a bad time for you. You're saying repeatedly that you want to die. Are you planning to harm yourself?" If the response is "yes," remain with the patient, alert staff members, and provide for psychiatric consultation as soon as possible. Continue to express concern to the patient and protect him or her from harm. *Suicidal thoughts as a result of ineffective coping or exhaustion of coping devices are not an uncommon occurrence in critically ill patients. If the mood state is distressing enough, a patient may seek relief by attempting a self-destructive act. Although the patient may not imminently have the energy to succeed in his or her attempt, voicing a specific plan* *signifies a depressed mood state and depletion of coping strategies. Immediate intervention is needed, because the attempt may be successful when the patient's energy is restored.*

9. Encourage the patient to participate in self-care activities and treatment regimen in accordance with his or her level of progress. Offer praise for his or her efforts toward self-care. *Patients who take an active role in their own treatment and progress are less apt to feel like helpless or powerless victims. This greater sense of control over their illness and environment will guide them more swiftly toward becoming as independent as possible.*

◎ NURSING MANAGEMENT PLAN

Powerlessness

Definition: Perception that one's own action cannot significantly affect an outcome; a perceived lack of control over a current situation or immediate happening

Powerlessness Related to Lack of Control over Current Situation or Disease Progression

Defining Characteristics

Severe

- Verbal expressions of having no control or influence over situation
- Verbal expressions of having no control or influence over outcome
- Verbal expressions of having no control over self-care
- Depression over physical deterioration that occurs despite patient's compliance with regiments
- Apathy

Moderate

- Nonparticipation in care or decision making when opportunities are provided
- Expressions of dissatisfaction and frustration about inability to perform previous tasks and/or activities
- Lack of progress monitoring
- Expressions of doubt about role performance
- Reluctance to express true feelings, fearing alienation from caregivers
- Passivity
- Inability to seek information about care
- Dependence on others that may result in irritability, resentment, anger, and guilt
- No defense of self-care practices when challenged

Low

- Passivity

Outcome Criteria

- Patient verbalizes increased control over situation by wanting to do things his or her way.
- Patient actively participates in planning care.
- Patient requests needed information.
- Patient chooses to participate in self-care activities.
- Patient monitors progress.

Nursing Interventions and Rationale

1. Evaluate the patient's feelings and perception of the reasons for lack of power and sense of helplessness.
2. Determine as far as possible the patient's usual response to limited control situations. Determine through ongoing assessment the patient's usual locus of control (i.e., believes that influence over his or her life is exerted by luck, fate, powerful persons [external locus of control] or that influence is exerted through personal choices, self-effort, self-determination [internal locus of control]).
3. Support patient's physical control of the environment by involving him or her in care activities; knock before entering room if appropriate; ask permission before moving personal belongings. Inform the patient that, although an activity may not be to his or her liking, it is necessary. *This gives the patient permission to express dissatisfaction with the environment and the regimen.*
4. Personalize the patient's care using his or her preferred name. *This supports the patient's psychologic control.*
5. Provide therapeutic rationale for all the patient is asked to do for himself or herself and for all that is being done for and with him or her. Reinforce the physician's explanations; clarify misconceptions about the illness situation and treatment plans. *This supports the patient's cognitive control.*
6. Include the patient in care planning by encouraging participation and allowing choices wherever possible (e.g., timing of personal care activities; deciding when pain medicines are needed). Point out situations in which no choices exist.
7. Provide opportunities for the patient to exert influence over himself or herself and his or her body, thereby affecting an outcome. For example, share with the patient the nurse's assessment of his or her breath sounds and explain that they can be improved by self-initiated deep-breathing exercises. *Feedback that the patient has been successful in helping clear his or her lungs reinforces the influence he or she does retain.*
8. Encourage family to permit patient to do as much independently as possible *to foster perception of personal power.*
9. Assist the patient to establish realistic short-term and long-term goals. *Setting unrealistic or unattainable goals inadvertently reinforces the patient's perception of powerlessness.*
10. Document care to provide for continuity *so that the patient can maintain appropriate control over the environment.*
11. Assist the patient to regain strength and activity tolerance as appropriate, *increasing a sense of control and self-reliance.*
12. Increase the sensitivity of the health team members and significant others to the patient's sense of powerlessness. Use power over the patient carefully. Use the words *must, should,* and *have to* with caution *because they communicate coercive powers and imply that the objects of "musts" and "shoulds" are of benefit to the nurse instead of the patient.*
13. Plan with the patient for transfer from the critical care unit to the intermediate unit and eventually to home.

NURSING MANAGEMENT PLAN

Relocation Stress Syndrome

Definition: Physiologic and/or psychologic disturbances after transfer from one environment to another

Relocation Stress Syndrome Related to Transfer Out of the Critical Care Unit

Defining Characteristics

- Alienation
- Aloneness
- Anger
- Anxiety
- Concern over relocation
- Dependency
- Depression
- Fear of an unknown environment
- Frustration
- Increased illness
- Increased physical symptoms
- Increased verbalization of needs
- Insecurity
- Loneliness
- Loss of identify
- Loss of self-esteem
- Loss of self-worth
- Move from critical care unit to another environment
- Pessimism
- Sleep disturbance
- Unwillingness to move
- Withdrawal
- Worry

Outcome Criteria

- Patient will express willingness to move to new environment.
- Absence of anxiety

Nursing Interventions and Rationale

1. Initiate pretransfer teaching as soon as appropriate during the patient's stay in the critical care unit **to ease the transition from critical care to the next environment.** Teaching should focus on the differences in the environment and the care they would receive.
2. Provide the patient and family written information regarding the transfer (if available) **to enhance effectiveness of teaching.**
3. Help the patient see that progress is being made **in preparation for transfer.** Each time a tube is removed or a treatment frequency is decreased, reinforce with the patient and family that the patient is progressing.
4. Remove monitoring and supportive equipment from the patient's room when no longer needed **to allow the patient to experience the loss of technology while still in the critical care unit.**
5. Encourage patient and family to discuss concerns regarding relocation.
6. Assist patient and family members to develop and maintain a positive perception of the transfer.
7. Arrange for the patient's family to have a tour of the new unit **as a means of familiarizing them with the unit before the patient's transfer.**

◎ NURSING MANAGEMENT PLAN

Risk for Aspiration

Definition: At risk for entry of gastrointestinal secretions, oropharyngeal secretions, solids, or fluids into tracheobronchial passages

Risk Factors

- Impaired laryngeal sensation or reflex
  - Reduced level of consciousness
  - Extubation
- Impaired pharyngeal peristalsis or tongue function
  - Neuromuscular dysfunction
  - Central nervous system dysfunction
  - Head or neck injury
- Impaired laryngeal closure or elevation
  - Laryngeal nerve dysfunction
  - Artificial airways
  - Gastrointestinal tubes
- Increased gastric volume
  - Delayed gastric emptying
  - Enteral feedings
  - Medication administration
- Increased intragastric pressure
- Upper abdominal surgery
  - Obesity
  - Pregnancy
  - Ascites
- Decreased lower esophageal sphincter pressure
  - Increased gastric acidity
  - Gastrointestinal tubes
- Decreased antegrade esophageal propulsion
  - Trendelenburg or supine position
  - Esophageal dysmotility
  - Esophageal structural defects or lesions

Outcome Criteria

- Breath sounds are normal, or there is no change in patient's baseline breath sounds.
- Arterial blood gas values remain within patient's baseline.
- There is no evidence of gastric contents in lung secretions.

Nursing Interventions and Rationale

1. Assess gastrointestinal function **to rule out hypoactive peristalsis and abdominal distention.**
2. Position patient with head of bed elevated 30 degrees **to prevent gastric reflux through gravity.** If head elevation is contraindicated, position patient in right lateral decubitus position **to facilitate passage of gastric contents across the pylorus.**
3. Maintain patency and functioning of nasogastric suction apparatus **to prevent accumulation of gastric contents.**
4. Provide frequent and scrupulous mouth care **to prevent colonization of the oropharynx with bacteria and inoculation of the lower airways.**
5. Ensure that the endotracheal or tracheostomy cuff is properly inflated **to limit aspiration of oropharyngeal secretions.**
6. Treat nausea promptly; collaborate with physician on an order for antiemetic **to prevent vomiting and resultant aspiration.**

Additional Interventions for Patient Receiving Continuous or Intermittent Enteral Tube Feedings

7. Position patient with head of bed elevated 45 degrees **to prevent gastric reflux.** If a head-down position becomes necessary at any time, interrupt the feeding 30 minutes before the position change.
8. Check placement of feeding tube by auscultation or radiographically at regular intervals (e.g., before administering intermittent feedings and after position changes, suctioning, coughing episodes, or vomiting) **to ensure proper placement of the tube.**
9. Monitor patient for signs of delayed gastric emptying **to decrease potential for vomiting and aspiration.**
    a. For large-bore tubes, check residuals of tube feedings before intermittent feedings and every 4 hours during continuous feedings. Consider withholding feedings for residuals greater than 150% of the hourly rate (continuous feeding) or greater than 50% of the previous feeding (intermittent feeding).
    b. For small-bore tubes, observe abdomen for distention, palpate abdomen for hardness or tautness, and auscultate abdomen for bowel sounds.

NURSING MANAGEMENT PLAN

Risk for Decreased Cardiac Tissue Perfusion

Definition: At risk for a decrease in cardiac (coronary) circulation that may compromise health

Risk Factors

- Hypovolemia
- Hypoxemia
- Hypertension
- Hypotension
- Vasoconstriction
- Vasodilation
- Embolism
- Stenosis
- Coronary artery disease
- Trauma
- Cardiac tamponade

Outcome Criteria

- Systolic blood pressure is >90 mm Hg.
- Mean arterial pressure is >60 mm Hg.
- Heart rate is <100 beats/min.
- Pulmonary artery pressures are within normal limits or back to baseline.
- Cardiac index is >2.2 L/min/m^2.
- Urine output is >0.5 mL/kg/hr or >30 mL/hr.
- 12-lead ECG is normalized without new Q waves.
- Chest pain is absent.
- CK-MB enzymes, troponin I, and myoglobin levels are within normal range.

Nursing Interventions and Rationale

1. Collaborate with the physician regarding the administration of fibrinolytic therapy or the preparation of the patient for percutaneous coronary intervention (PCI) *to restore myocardial blood flow.*
2. Collaborate with physician regarding the administration of oxygen at 2 L/min to achieve SpO$_2$ >90% *to maximize myocardial oxygen supply.*
3. Collaborate with physician regarding the administration of sublingual nitroglycerin and/or intravenous nitroglycerine infusion *to augment coronary blood flow and reduce cardiac work by decreasing preload and afterload.*

   a. Do not administer nitrates to patients who have taken phosphodiesterase inhibitors for erectile dysfunction within the last 24 or 48 hours (depending the medication) *as severe hypotension may occur.*
4. Collaborate with physician regarding the administration of morphine *to control pain.*
5. Collaborate with the physician regarding the administration of aspirin, antiplatelet therapy, and heparin *to prevent recurrent thrombosis and inhibit platelet function.*
6. Collaborate with the physician regarding the administration of beta-blockers *to decrease myocardial oxygen demand and prevent recurrent ischemia.*
7. Collaborate with the physician regarding the administration of angiotensin-converting enzyme (ACE) inhibitors *to block the conversion of angiotensin I to angiotensin II, a potent vasoconstrictor.*
8. Maintain the patient on bed rest with bedside commode privileges *to minimize myocardial oxygen demand.*
9. Monitor patient's hemodynamic and cardiac rhythm status:

   a. Select cardiac monitoring leads based on infarct location and rhythm to obtain the best rhythm for monitoring.

   b. Evaluate cardiac rhythm for presence of dysrhythmias, which are common complications of myocardial ischemia.

   c. Collaborate with physician regarding the administration of antidysrhythmic medications.

   d. Assess serum electrolytes (potassium and magnesium) and arterial blood gases.

   e. Collaborate with physician regarding the administration of electrolytes to correct any imbalances.

   f. Monitor ST segment continuously to determine changes in myocardial tissue perfusion.

   g. Monitor patient's blood pressure at least every hour as many conditions (e.g., drugs, dysrhythmias, myocardial ischemia) may cause hypotension (systolic blood pressure <90 mm Hg).

   h. Treat symptomatic dysrhythmias according to unit's emergency protocol or advanced cardiac life support (ACLS) guidelines.
10. Instruct patient to avoid the Valsalva maneuver as forced expiration against a closed glottis causes sudden and intense changes in systolic blood pressure and heart rate.

◎ NURSING MANAGEMENT PLAN

Risk for Ineffective Cerebral Tissue Perfusion

Definition: At risk for a decrease in cerebral tissue circulation that may compromise health

Risk Factors
- Hypovolemia
- Hypoxemia
- Hypertension
- Hypotension
- Vasoconstriction
- Vasodilation
- Embolism
- Stenosis
- Hemorrhage
- Vascular disease
- Trauma

Outcome Criteria
- Patient is oriented to time, place, person, and situation.
- Pupils are equal and normoreactive.
- Blood pressure is within baseline or ordered parameters.
- Motor function is bilaterally equal.
- Headache, nausea, and vomiting are absent.
- Patient verbalizes importance of and displays compliance with reduced activity.
- Absence of neurologic deficits.

Nursing Interventions and Rationale
For Ischemia

1. Collaborate with physician regarding the administration of fibrinolytic therapy **to facilitate lysis of the clot and restoration of blood flow to affected area.**
2. Monitor the patient for alterations in blood pressure, oxygenation, temperature, rhythm, and glucose levels.
3. Collaborate with physician regarding the administration vasodilators for hypertension **to maintain the patient's blood pressure within desired range.** Use caution in lowering blood pressure **as hypotension decreases cerebral blood flow.**
   a. Patients receiving fibrinolytic therapy—keep systolic blood pressure <185 mm Hg and diastolic blood pressure <110 mm Hg.
   b. Patients not receiving fibrinolytic therapy—keep systolic blood pressure <220 mm Hg and diastolic blood pressure <120 mm Hg.
4. Collaborate with physician regarding the administration of intravenous fluids and vasoconstrictors for hypotension **as hypotension decreases cerebral blood flow.**
5. Collaborate with physician regarding the administration of oxygen to maintain SpO$_2$ >95% **to prevent hypoxemia and potential worsening of the neurologic injury.**
6. Collaborate with physician regarding administration of acetaminophen for elevated temperature **because hyperthermia is associated with increased morbidity in the stroke patient.**
7. Collaborate with the physician regarding the treatment of dysrhythmias **due to increased sympathetic nervous system stimulation.**
8. Collaborate with the physician regarding the administration of insulin for hyperglycemia **as elevated blood glucose has been linked to an increase in the area of infarct.**
9. Collaborate with the speech therapist regarding the patient's ability to swallow before initiating oral feedings **to ensure patient is not at risk for aspirating.**
10. Collaborate with the physical therapist to assess the patient's ability to ambulate safely **to ensure the patient is not at risk for falling** and ability to perform activities of daily living **to facilitate discharge home.**
11. Maintain surveillance for complications such as increased intracranial pressure, seizures, and acute lung failure.
12. Collaborate with the physician and rehabilitation specialist regarding the patient's need for rehabilitation **to maximize the patient's independence.**

For Hemorrhage
1. Assess for indicators of increased intracranial pressure and brain herniation (see the nursing management plan for Decreased Intracranial Adaptive Capacity Related to Failure of Normal Intracranial Compensatory Mechanism).
2. Collaborate with the physician regarding the administration of anticonvulsant medications **to prevent the onset of seizures or to control seizures.**
3. Collaborate with physician regarding the administration vasodilators for hypertension **to avoid further bleeding.** Use caution in lowering blood pressure **as hypotension decreases cerebral blood flow.**
   a. If systolic blood pressure is >200 mm Hg or mean arterial pressure is >150 mm Hg, aggressive reduction in blood pressure is indicated.
   b. If systolic blood pressure is >180 mm Hg or mean arterial pressure is >130 mm Hg in the presence of increased intracranial pressure, cautious reduction in pressure is indicated maintaining cerebral perfusion pressure >60-80 mm Hg.
   c. If systolic blood pressure is >180 mm Hg or mean arterial pressure is >130 mm Hg in the absence of elevated intracranial pressure, reduction in blood pressure is indicated with a target of 160/90 mm Hg.
4. Collaborate with the physician regarding the administration of insulin for hyperglycemia **as elevated blood glucose has been linked to an increase in the area of infarct.**
5. Collaborate with physician regarding administration of acetaminophen for elevated temperature **because hyperthermia is associated with increased morbidity in the stroke patient.**
6. Initiate precautions **to prevent rebleeding.**
   a. Ensure bed rest in a quiet environment **to lessen external stimuli.**
   b. Maintain a darkened room to lessen symptoms of photophobia.
   c. Restrict visitors, and instruct them to keep conversation as nonstressful as possible.
   d. Administer sedatives as prescribed **to reduce anxiety to promote rest.**
   e. Administer analgesics as prescribed **to relieve or lessen headache.**
   f. Provide a soft, high-fiber diet and stool softeners to prevent constipation, which can lead to straining and increased risk of rebleeding.
   g. Assist with activities of daily living (feeding, bathing, dressing, toileting).
   h. Avoid any activity that could lead to increased intracranial pressure; ensure that patient does not flex hips beyond 90 degrees and avoids neck hyperflexion, hyperextension, or lateral hyperrotation **that could impede jugular venous return.**
7. Collaborate with the physical therapist to assess the patient's ability to ambulate safely **to ensure the patient is not at risk for falling** and ability to perform activities of daily living **to facilitate discharge home.**
8. Collaborate with the physician and rehabilitation specialist regarding the patient's need for rehabilitation **to maximize the patient's independence.**

NURSING MANAGEMENT PLAN

Risk for Ineffective Gastrointestinal Perfusion

Definition: At risk for decrease in gastrointestinal circulation that may compromise health

Risk Factors

- Hypovolemia
- Hypoxemia
- Hypertension
- Hypotension
- Vasoconstriction
- Vasodilation
- Embolism
- Stenosis
- Vascular disease
- Trauma

Outcome Criteria

- Normal bowel sounds
- Absence of abdominal pain, distention, and guarding
- Vital signs at baseline

Nursing Interventions and Rationales

1. Collaborate with physician regarding the administration of crystalloids, colloids, blood, and blood products **to maintain adequate circulating volume.** Implement the nursing management plan for Deficit Fluid Volume Related to Absolute Loss.
2. Collaborate with physician regarding pain management. Implement the nursing management plan for Acute Pain Related to Transmission and Perception of Cutaneous, Visceral, Muscular, or Ischemic Impulses.
3. Collaborate with physician regarding the administration of oxygen to maintain $SpO_2 > 92\%$ **to prevent hypoxemia and potential worsening of the gastrointestinal injury.**
4. Collaborate with physician regarding the administration of electrolyte replacement therapy **to maintain adequate electrolyte balance.**
5. Collaborate with dietitian regarding administration of nutrition **because patient will be unable to eat.** Implement the nursing management plan for Imbalanced Nutrition: Less Than Body Requirements.
6. Maintain surveillance for complications such as gastrointestinal hemorrhage, hypovolemic shock, and septic shock.
7. Collaborate with physician regarding preparation for surgery **to remove infarcted bowel.**

◎ NURSING MANAGEMENT PLAN

Risk for Ineffective Peripheral Tissue Perfusion

Definition: At risk for a decrease in blood circulation to the periphery that may compromise health

Ineffective Peripheral Tissue Perfusion
Risk Factors
- Hypovolemia
- Hypoxemia
- Hypertension
- Hypotension
- Vasoconstriction
- Vasodilation
- Embolism
- Stenosis
- Iatrogenic (arterial catheters, intraaortic balloon pump catheters)
- Vascular disease
- Trauma

Outcome Criteria
- Peripheral pulses are full and equal bilaterally.
- Capillary refill is equal bilaterally.
- Ischemic pain is absent.
- Skin temperature is equal in both extremities.
- Skin is pink and warm in both extremities.
- Paresthesias are absent.

Nursing Interventions and Rationale
1. Collaborate with physician regarding the administration of antiplatelet, anti-coagulant, and/or fibrinolytic therapy.
2. Collaborate with physician regarding pain management. Implement the nursing management plan for Acute Pain Related to Transmission and Perception of Cutaneous, Visceral, Muscular, or Ischemic Impulses.
3. Ensure patient is adequately hydrated **to decrease blood viscosity.**
4. Maintain affected extremity in dependent position if possible **to enhance blood flow.**
5. Keep affected extremity warm and protect it from injury. **Do not apply heat directly to the affected extremity because this can result in injury.**
6. Maintain surveillance for pain, pallor, pulselessness, paresthesia, paralysis, and poikilothermia **as indicators of abrupt change in blood flow.**
7. Maintain surveillance for tissue breakdown and arterial ulcers **as indicators of injury.**
8. Prepare patient for possible surgery or interventional procedure to restore blood flow.

NURSING MANAGEMENT PLAN

Risk for Ineffective Renal Perfusion

Definition: At risk for a decrease in blood circulation to the kidney that may compromise health

Risk Factors

- Hypovolemia
- Hypoxemia
- Hypertension
- Hypotension
- Vasoconstriction
- Vasodilation
- Embolism
- Stenosis
- Nephrotoxic medications
- Vascular disease
- Trauma

Outcome Criteria

- Electrolytes are within normal range.
- Serum creatinine and BUN are within normal range.
- Normal acid–base balance.
- Urinary output is within normal limits, or patient is stable on dialysis.
- Hemoglobin and hematocrit values are stable.

Nursing Interventions and Rationale

1. Monitor intake and output, urine output, and patient weight.
2. Collaborate with physician regarding the administration of crystalloids, colloids, blood, and blood products **to increase circulating volume and maintain mean arterial pressure >70 mm Hg.**
3. Collaborate with physician regarding the administration of inotropes **to enhance myocardial contractility and increase cardiac index to >2.5 L/min.**
4. Collaborate with physician regarding the administration of diuretics to the oliguric patient **to flush out cellular debris and increase urine output.**
5. Minimize the patient's exposure to nephrotoxic medications **to decrease damage to kidneys.**
6. Monitor blood levels of drugs cleared by kidneys **to avoid accumulation.**
7. Monitor patient for signs of electrolyte imbalance **due to impaired electrolyte regulation.**
8. Maintain surveillance for signs and symptoms of fluid overload.
9. Monitor patient's clinical status and response to dialysis therapy **to ensure the patient is receiving safe and effective dialytic therapy.**

NURSING MANAGEMENT PLAN

Risk for Infection

Definition: At increased risk for being invaded by pathogenic organisms

Risk Factors

- Inadequate primary defenses (e.g., broken skin, traumatized tissue, decreased ciliary action, stasis of body fluids, change in pH secretions, altered peristalsis)
- Inadequate secondary defenses (e.g., decreased hemoglobin, leukopenia, suppressed inflammatory or immune response)
- Immunocompromise
- Inadequate acquired immunity
- Tissue destruction and increased environmental exposure
- Chronic disease
- Invasive procedures
- Malnutrition
- Pharmacologic agents (e.g., antibiotics, steroids)

Outcome Criteria

- Total lymphocyte count is >1000/mm^3.
- White blood cell count is within normal limits.
- Temperature is within normal limits.
- Blood, urine, wound, and sputum culture results are negative.

Nursing Interventions and Rationale

1. Perform proper hand hygiene before and after patient care **to reduce the transmission of microorganisms.**
2. Use appropriate personal protective equipment in accordance with CDC guidelines.
   a. Ensure physician uses maximum barrier precautions when inserting lines.
      (1) Ensure sterile gloves, gown, and mask are worn.
      (2) Drape patient completely with a sterile sheet.
3. Use aseptic technique for insertion and manipulation of invasive monitoring devices, intravenous (IV) lines, and urinary drainage catheters **to maintain sterility of environment.**
   a. Ensure physician uses maximum barrier precautions when inserting lines.
      (1) Ensure sterile gloves, gown, and mask are worn.
      (2) Drape patient completely with a sterile sheet.
4. Stabilize all invasive lines and catheters **to avoid unintentional manipulation and contamination.**
5. Use aseptic technique for dressing changes **to prevent contamination of wounds or insertion sites.**
6. Change any line placed under emergent conditions within 24 hours **because aseptic technique is usually breached during an emergency.**
7. Collaborate with the physician to change any dressing that is saturated with blood or drainage **because these are mediums for microorganism growth.**
8. Minimize use of stopcocks and maintain caps on all stopcock ports **to reduce the ports of entry for microorganisms.**
9. Avoid the use of nasogastric tubes, nasotracheal tubes, and nasopharyngeal suctioning in the patient with a suspected cerebrospinal fluid leak **to decrease the incidence of central nervous system infection.**
10. Change ventilator circuits with humidifiers when visibly soiled or mechanically malfunction **to avoid introducing microorganisms into the system.** Do not change routinely.
11. Provide the patient with a clean manual resuscitation bag **to avoid cross-contamination between patients.**
12. Provide oral care to patient with artificial airway or unresponsive patient every 2-4 hours and PRN **to decrease the incidence of hospital-acquired pulmonary infections.**

a. Swab mouth and moisten lips every 4 hours.
b. Brush teeth with in-line suction toothbrush every 12 hours. Rinse or swab patient's mouth with chlorhexidine after brushing.
c. Suction subglottic secretions (secretions pooling above the cuff of the endotracheal [ET] or tracheostomy tube) every 12 hours and before repositioning the tube or deflation of the cuff.
d. Provide lip balm to keep patient's lips moistened PRN.
e. Provide mouth moisturizer to keep patient's mouth moistened PRN.

13. Cleanse in-line suction catheters with sterile saline according to the manufacturer's instructions **to avoid accumulation of secretions within the catheter.**
14. Maintain the head of the bed elevated at 30 to 45 degrees in patients with an artificial airway **to decrease the incidence of aspiration.**
15. Use disposable sterile scissors, forceps, and hemostats **to reduce the transmission of microorganisms.**
16. Maintain a closed urinary drainage system **to decrease incidence of urinary infections.**
17. Keep the urinary drainage tubing and bag below the level of the patient's bladder **to prevent the backflow of urine.**
18. Assess the urinary drainage tubing for kinks **to prevent stasis of urine.**
19. Protect all access device sites from potential sources of contamination (nasogastric reflux, draining wounds, ostomies, sputum).
20. Refrigerate parenteral nutrition solutions and opened enteral nutrition formulas **to inhibit bacterial growth.**
21. Maintain daily surveillance of invasive devices for signs and symptoms of infection.
22. Notify physician of elevated temperature or if any signs or symptoms of infection are present.

Additional Interventions for Patient Receiving Immunosuppressive Drugs

23. Obtain blood, urine, and sputum cultures for temperature elevations >38° C (100.4° F) **inasmuch as elevation likely is caused by bacteremia or bladder or pulmonary infection.**
24. Auscultate breath sounds at least every 6 hours. **Pulmonary infection is the most common type of infection, and changes in breath sounds might be an early indication.**
25. Inspect wounds at least every 8 hours for redness, swelling, and/or drainage, **which may indicate infection.**
26. Inspect overall skin integrity and oral mucosa for signs of breakdown, **which place the patient at risk for infection.**
27. Notify physician of new-onset cough. **Even a nonproductive cough may indicate pulmonary infection.**
28. Monitor white blood cell count daily, and report leukocytosis or sudden development of leukopenia, **which may indicate an infectious process.**
29. Protect patient from exposure to any staff or family member with contagious lesion (e.g., herpes simplex) or respiratory infections.
30. Collaborate with dietitian regarding the patient's nutritional status and need for augmentation of nutritional intake as necessary **to prevent debilitation and increased susceptibility to infection.**
31. Collaborate with physician to remove invasive lines and catheters as soon as possible **to decrease potential portals of entry.**
32. Teach patient the clinical manifestations of infection. **A knowledgeable patient will seek medical attention promptly, which will result in earlier treatment and a decreased risk that infection will become life threatening.**

NURSING MANAGEMENT PLAN

Situational Low Self-Esteem

Definition: Development of a negative perception of self-worth in response to a current situation

Situational Low Self-Esteem Related to Feelings of Guilt about Physical Deterioration

Defining Characteristics

- Inability to accept positive reinforcement
- Lack of follow-through
- Nonparticipation in therapy
- Not taking responsibility for self-care (i.e., self-neglect)
- Self-destructive behavior
- Lack of eye contact

Outcome Criteria

- Patient verbalizes feelings of self-worth.
- Patient maintains positive relationships with significant others.
- Patient manifests active interest in appearance by completing personal grooming daily.

Nursing Interventions and Rationale

1. Evaluate the meaning of health-related situation. How does the patient feel about himself or herself, the diagnosis, and the treatment? How does the present fit into the larger context of his or her life?
2. Assess the patient's emotional level, interpersonal relationships, and feeling about himself or herself. Recognize the patient's uniqueness (e.g., how the hair is worn, preference for name used).
3. Help the patient discover and verbalize feelings and understand the crisis by listening and providing information.
4. Assist the patient to identify strengths and positive qualities that increase the sense of self-worth. Focus on past experiences of accomplishment and competency. Help the patient with positive self-reinforcement. Reinforce the obvious love and affection of family and significant others.
5. Assess coping techniques that have been helpful in the past. Help the patient decide how to handle negative or incongruent feedback about the situation.
6. Encourage visits from family and significant others. Facilitate interactions, and ensure privacy. Help family members entering the critical care unit by explaining what they will see. Increase visitors' comfort with equipment; offer chairs and other courtesies.
7. Encourage the patient to pursue interest in individual or social activities, even though difficult in the critical care unit.
8. Reflect caring, concern, empathy, respect, and unconditional acceptance in nurse–patient relationships.
9. Remember that for the patient the nurse is a significant other who provides important appraisals of the patient and who can facilitate the change process.
10. Help the family support the patient's self-esteem.
11. Provide for continuity of nurse assignment to ensure consistent contacts that can *facilitate support of the patient's self-esteem.*

◎ NURSING MANAGEMENT PLAN

Unilateral Neglect

Definition: Impairment in sensory and motor response, mental representation and spatial attention of the body, and the corresponding environment characterized by inattention to one side and over-attention to the opposite side. Left-side neglect is more severe and persistent than right-side neglect.

Unilateral Neglect Related to Perceptual Disruption
Defining Characteristics
- Neglect of involved body parts and/or extrapersonal space
- Denial of existence of the affected limb or side of body
- Denial of hemiplegia or other motor and sensory deficits
- Left homonymous hemianopia
- Difficulty with spatial–perceptual tasks
- Left hemiplegia

Outcome Criteria
- Patient is safe and free from injury.
- Patient is able to identify safety hazards in the environment.
- Patient recognizes disability and describes physical deficits present (e.g., paralysis, weakness, numbness).
- Patient demonstrates ability to scan the visual field to compensate for loss of function or sensation in affected limbs.

Nursing Interventions and Rationale
1. Adapt environment to patient's deficits *to maintain patient safety.*
   a. Position the patient's bed with the unaffected side facing the door.
   b. Approach and speak to the patient from the unaffected side. If the patient must be approached from the affected side, announce your presence as soon as entering the room *to avoid startling the patient.*
   c. Position the call light, bedside stand, and personal items on the patient's unaffected side.
   d. If the patient will be assisted out of bed, simplify the environment *to eliminate hazards* by removing unnecessary furniture and equipment.
   e. Provide frequent reorientation of the patient to the environment.
   f. Observe the patient closely, and anticipate his or her needs. *In spite of repeated explanation, the patient may have difficulty retaining information about the deficits.*
   g. When patient is in bed, elevate his or her affected arm on a pillow *to prevent dependent edema and support the hand in a position of function.*
2. Assist the patient to recognize the perceptual defect.
   a. Encourage the patient to wear any prescriptive corrective glasses or hearing aids *to facilitate communication.*
   b. Instruct the patient to turn the head past midline *to view the environment on the affected side.*
   c. Encourage patient to look at the affected side and to stroke the limbs with the unaffected hand. Encourage handling of the affected limbs *to reinforce awareness of the affected side.*
   d. Instruct the patient to look for the affected extremity when performing simple tasks *to know where it is at all times.*
   e. After pointing to them, have the patient name the affected parts.
   f. Encourage the patient to use self-exercises (e.g., lifting the affected arm with the unaffected hand).
   g. If the patient is unable to discriminate between the concepts of *right* and *left*, use descriptive adjectives such as "the weak arm," "the affected leg," or "the good arm" to refer to the body. Use gestures, not just words, to indicate right and left.
3. Collaborate with the patient, physician, and rehabilitation team *to design and implement a beginning rehabilitation program for use during the critical care unit stay.*
   a. Use adaptive equipment (braces, splints, slings) as appropriate.
   b. Teach the patient the individual components of any activity separately, and then proceed to integrate the component parts into a completed activity.
   c. Instruct the patient to attend to the affected side, if able, and to assist with the bath or other tasks.
   d. Use tactile stimulation to reintroduce the arm or leg to the patient. Rub the affected parts with different textured materials to stimulate sensations (e.g., warm, cold, rough, soft).
   e. Encourage activities that require the patient to turn the head toward the affected side, and retrain the patient to scan the affected side and environment visually.
   f. If the patient is allowed out of bed, cue him or her with reminders to scan visually when ambulating. Assist and remain in constant attendance *because the patient may have difficulty maintaining correct posture, balance, and locomotion.* There may be vertical–horizontal perceptual problems, with the patient leaning to the affected side to align with the perceived vertical. Provide sitting, standing, and balancing exercises before getting the patient out of bed.
4. Assist patient with oral feedings.
   a. Avoid giving patient any very hot food items that could cause injury.
   b. Place the patient in an upright sitting position if possible.
   c. Encourage the patient to feed himself or herself; if necessary, guide the patient's hand to the mouth.
   d. If the patient is able to feed himself or herself, place one dish at a time in front of the patient. When the patient is finished with the first, add another dish. Tell the patient what he or she is eating.
   e. Initially, place food in patient's visual field; then gradually move the food out of the field of vision and teach the patient to scan the entire visual field.
   f. When the patient has learned to visually scan the environment, offer a tray of food with various dishes.
   g. Instruct the patient to take small bites of food and to place the food in the unaffected side of the mouth.
   h. Teach the patient to sweep out pockets of food with the tongue after every bite *to eliminate retained food in the affected side of the mouth.*
   i. After meals or oral medications, check the patient's oral cavity for pockets of retained material.
5. Initiate patient and family health teaching.
   a. Assess to ensure that the patient and the family understand the nature of the neurologic deficits and the purpose of the rehabilitation plan.
   b. Teach the proper application and use of any adaptive equipment.
   c. Teach the importance of maintaining a safe environment, and point out potential environmental hazards.
   d. Instruct family members how to facilitate relearning techniques (e.g., cueing, scanning visual fields).

APPENDIX

B

Physiologic Formulas for Critical Care

HEMODYNAMIC FORMULAS

Mean (Systemic) Arterial Pressure (MAP)

$$MAP = \frac{(Diastolic \times 2) + (Systolic \times 1)}{3}$$

Systemic Vascular Resistance (SVR)

$$\frac{MAP - RAP}{CO} = SVR \text{ in units}$$

Normal range is 10-18 units.

$$\frac{MAP - RAP}{CO} \times 80 = SVR \text{ in dyn} \cdot sec \cdot cm^{-5}$$

Normal range is 800-1400 dyn·sec·cm^{-5}.

Systemic Vascular Resistance Index (SVRI)

$$\frac{MAP - RAP}{CO} \times 80 = SVR \text{ in dyn} \cdot sec \cdot cm^{-5}/m^2$$

Normal range is 2000-2400 dyn·sec·cm^{-5}/m^2.

Pulmonary Vascular Resistance (PVR)

$$\frac{PAP \text{ mean} - RAP}{CO} = PVR \text{ in units}$$

Normal range is 1.2-3 units.

$$\frac{PAP \text{ mean} - RAP}{CO} \times 80 = PVR \text{ in dyn} \cdot sec \cdot cm^{-5}$$

Normal range is 100-250 dyn·sec·cm^{-5}.

Pulmonary Vascular Resistance Index (PVRI)

$$\frac{PAP \text{ mean} - PAOP}{CI} \times 80 = PVR \text{ in dyn} \cdot sec \cdot cm^{-5}/m^2$$

Normal range is 225-315 dyn·sec·cm^{-5}/m^2.

CI, Cardiac index; *CO*, cardiac output; *PAOP*, pulmonary arterial occlusion pressure (wedge pressure); *PAP*, pulmonary arterial pressure; *RAP*, right atrial pressure.

Left Cardiac Work Index (LCWI)

Step 1. MAP × CO × 0.0136 = LCW

Step 2. $\frac{LCW}{BSA} = LCWI$

Normal range is 3.4-4.2 kg-m/m^2.

Left Ventricular Stroke Work Index (LVSWI)

Step 1. MAP × SV × 0.0136 = LVSW

Step 2. $\frac{LVSW}{BSA} = LVSWI$

Normal range is 50-62 g-m/m^2.

Right Cardiac Work Index (RCWI)

Step 1. PAP mean × CO × 0.0136 = RCW

Step 2. $\frac{RCW}{BSA} = RCWI$

Normal range is 0.54-0.66 kg-m/m^2.

Right Ventricular Stroke Work Index (RVSWI)

Step 1. PAP mean × SV × 0.0136 = RVSW

Step 2. $\frac{RVSW}{BSA} = RVSWI$

Normal range is 7.9-9.7 g-m/m^2.

Corrected QT Interval (QTc)

$$\frac{QT}{\sqrt{(RR \text{ interval})}} = QTc$$

Body Surface Area (BSA)

Many hemodynamic formulas can be indexed or adjusted to body size by use of a BSA nomogram (Fig. B-1). To calculate BSA:

1. Obtain height and weight.
2. Mark height on the left scale and weight on the right scale.

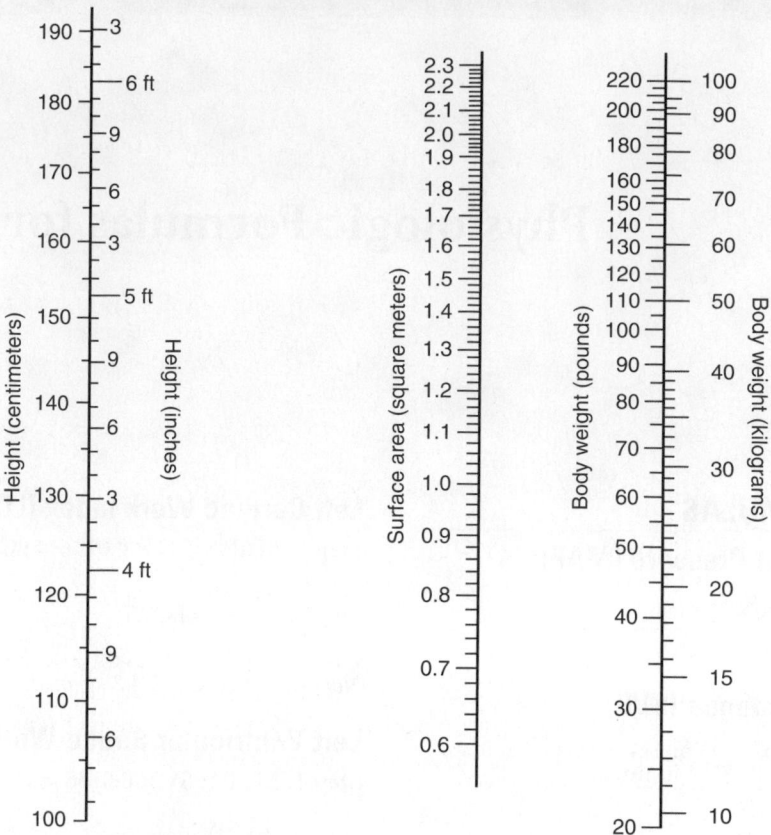

FIGURE B-1   Body surface area (BSA) nomogram.

3. Draw a straight line between the two points marked on the nomogram.

The number where the line crosses the middle scale is the BSA value.

PULMONARY FORMULAS

Shunt Equation (Qs/Qt)

$$\frac{Qs}{Qt} = \frac{Cco_2 - Cao_2}{Cco_2 - Cvo_2}$$

Cco_2 = Pulmonary capillary oxygen content (calculated value)
Cao_2 = Arterial oxygen content (calculated value)
Cvo_2 = Venous oxygen content (calculated value)
Normal range is less than 5%.

Pulmonary Capillary Oxygen Content (Cco₂)

$$Cco_2 = (Hgb \times 1.34 \times Sco_2) + (Pco_2 \times 0.003)$$

Hgb = hemoglobin (measured via laboratory sample or arterial blood gas)
Sco_2 = Pulmonary capillary oxygen saturation
Pco_2 = Partial pressure of oxygen in capillary blood
Normal range is greater than 19 mL/dL.

Arterial Oxygen Content (CO₂)

$$Cao_2 = (Hgb \times 1.34 \times Sao_2) + (0.003 \times Pao_2)$$

Hgb = Hemoglobin (measured via laboratory sample or arterial blood gas)

Sao_2 = Arterial oxygen saturation (measured via arterial blood gas)
Pao_2 = Partial pressure of oxygen in arterial blood (measured via arterial blood gas)
Normal range is 17 to 20 mL/dL.

Venous Oxygen Content (Cvo₂)

$$Cvo_2 = (Hgb \times 1.34 \times Svo_2) + (0.003 \times Pvo_2)$$

Hgb = Hemoglobin (measured via laboratory sample or arterial blood gas)
Svo_2 = Mixed venous oxygen saturation (measured via mixed venous blood gas)
Pvo_2 = Partial pressure of oxygen in mixed venous blood (measured via mixed venous blood gas)
Normal range is 12 to 15 mL/dL.

Alveolar Pressure of Oxygen (PAO₂)

$$CAO_2 = FIO_2 \times (Pb - PH_2O) - Paco_2 / RQ$$

FIO_2 = Fraction of inspired oxygen (obtained from oxygen settings)
Pb = Barometric pressure (assumed to be 760 mm Hg at sea level)
PH_2O = Water pressure in the lungs (assumed to be 47 mm Hg)
$Paco_2$ = Partial pressure of carbon dioxide in arterial blood (measured via arterial blood gas)
RQ = Respiratory quotient (assumed to be 0.8)
Normal range is 60 to 100 mm Hg.

Arterial/Inspired Oxygen Ratio

$$PaO_2/FiO_2 \ ratio = \frac{PaO_2}{FiO_2}$$

Pao_2 = Partial pressure of oxygen in arterial blood (measured via arterial blood gas)
Fio_2 = Fraction of inspired oxygen (obtained from oxygen settings)
Normal range is greater than 300.

Arterial/Alveolar Oxygen Ratio

$$PaO_2/PAO_2 = \frac{PaO_2}{PAO_2}$$

Pao_2 = Partial pressure of oxygen in arterial blood (measured via arterial blood gas)
Pao_2 = Partial pressure of oxygen in alveoli (calculated value)
Normal range is greater than 0.75 (75%).

Alveolar-Arterial Gradient

$$P(A\text{-}a)O_2 = PAO_2 - PaO_2$$

Pao_2 = Partial pressure of oxygen in alveoli (calculated value)
Pao_2 = Partial pressure of oxygen in arterial blood (measured via arterial blood gas)
Normal range is 25 to 65 mm Hg.

Dead Space Equation (Vd/Vt)

$$Vd = \frac{PaCO_2 - PETCO_2}{VTPaCO_2}$$

$Paco_2$ = Partial pressure of carbon dioxide in arterial blood (measured via arterial blood gas)
$Petco_2$ = Partial pressure of carbon dioxide in exhaled gas (measured via end-tidal CO_2 monitor)
Normal range is 0.2 to 0.4 (20% to 40%).

Static Compliance (C$_{ST}$)

This value is calculated for mechanically ventilated patients.

$$C_{ST} = \frac{VT}{PP} - PEEP$$

VT = Tidal volume (obtained from ventilator)
PP = Plateau pressure (measured via ventilator)
$PEEP$ = Positive end-expiratory pressure (obtained from ventilator)
Normal value is 60 to 100 mL/cm H$_2$O.

Dynamic Compliance (C$_{DY}$)

Also called *characteristic*, this value is calculated for mechanically ventilated patients.

$$C_{DY} = \frac{VT}{PIP} - PEEP$$

VT = Tidal volume (obtained from ventilator)
PIP = Peak inspiratory pressure (obtained from ventilator)

$PEEP$ = Positive end-expiratory pressure (obtained from ventilator)
Normal value is: 40 to 80 mL/cm H$_2$O.

NEUROLOGIC FORMULAS

Cerebral Perfusion Pressure (CPP)

$$CCP = MAP - ICP$$

MAP = Mean arterial pressure (measured via arterial line or blood pressure cuff)
ICP = Intracranial pressure (measured via ICP monitoring device)
Normal range is 60 to 150 mm Hg.

Arteriojugular Oxygen Difference (AjDO$_2$)

$$AjDO_2 = (SaO_2 - SjvO_2) \times 1.34 \times Hgb$$

Sao_2 = Arterial oxygen saturation (measured via arterial blood gas)
$Sjvo_2$ = Jugular venous oxygen saturation (measured via jugular blood gas or jugular venous catheter)
Hgb = Hemoglobin (measured via laboratory sample or arterial blood gas)
Normal range is 5 to 7.5 mL/dL.

ENDOCRINE FORMULAS

Serum Osmolality

$$Serum \ osmolality = 2(Na^+ + K^+) + \frac{Glucose}{18} + \frac{BUN}{2.8}$$

Na^+ = Sodium
K^+ = Potassium
BUN = Blood urea nitrogen
Normal range is 275 to 295 mOsm/kg of water.

Fluid Volume Deficit in Liters

$$Fluid \ volume \ deficit = \frac{0.6(kg/weight) \times (Na^+ - 140)}{140}$$

Na^+ = Sodium

KIDNEY FORMULAS

Anion Gap

$$[Na^+] - ([Cl^-] + [HCO_3^-])$$

Normal range is 8 to 16 mEq.

Clearance

$$Clearance = U \times \frac{(V)}{(P)}$$

U = Concentration of substance in urine
V = Time
P = Concentration of substance in plasma
Normal range depends on substance measured.

NUTRITIONAL FORMULAS

Resting Metabolic Rate (RMR)
PSU 2003b (Penn State Equation)

When indirect calorimetry is not available, the Penn State Equation is the best equation to use to estimate resting metabolic rate (RMR) in critically ill patients of any age with BMI below 30 or critically ill patients who are younger than 60 years old with BMI over 30. This equation was validated in 2009 by the Academy of Nutrition and Dietetics Evidence Analysis Library.[1]

$$RMR = Mifflin\ RMR\ (0.96) + V_E(31) + T_{max}(167) - 6212*$$

PSU 2010 (Modified Penn State Equation)

For a subset of obese critically ill patients aged 60 years and older, a modified Penn State Equation (PSU 2010) is recommended to estimate RMR. Validated in 2010 by the Academy of Nutrition and Dietetics Evidence Analysis Library.[2]

$$RMR = Mifflin\ RMR\ (0.71) + V_E(64) + T_{max}(85) - 3085*$$

*Where:

Mifflin RMR = Resting metabolic rate as calculated by the MSJ equation

V_E = Minute ventilation in liters per minute (L/min)

T_{max} = Maximum temperature in degrees Celsius

Mifflin-St. Jeor Equation

In non-critically ill populations, the Mifflin-St. Jeor equation performed the best when predicting RMR in non-obese and obese populations, 20 to 82 years of age.[3]

> **Men:** Mifflin RMR
> $= (9.99 \times weight) + (6.25 \times height) - (4.92 \times age) + 5$

> **Women:** Mifflin RMR
> $= (9.99 \times weight) + (6.25 \times height) - (4.92 \times age) - 161$

Mifflin-St. Jeor equation uses weight in kg, height in cm, age in years.

Caloric and Protein Needs[4]
Estimating Caloric Needs

Step 1. Calculate resting metabolic rate (RMR) using the appropriate equation from above. This is the energy needed for basic life processes, such as respiratory function and maintenance of body temperature.

Step 2. Multiply by an appropriate stress factor to meet the needs of the ill or injured patient (see the following table). If the patient has more than one stressor (e.g., burn and pneumonia), use only the stress factor for the highest level of stress.

Estimating Protein Needs

Protein needs vary with the degree of malnutrition and stress (see the following table).

TYPE OF STRESS	MULTIPLY THE VALUE FROM STEP 2 BY
Fever	1 + 0.13/1°C above normal (or 0.07/1°F)
Pneumonia	1.2
Major injury	1.3
Severe sepsis, burn of 15%-30% of BSA	1.5
Burn of 31%-49% of BSA content (calculated value)	1.5-2.0
Burn ≥50% of BSA	1.8-2.1

BSA, Body surface area.

CONDITION	MULTIPLY DESIRABLE BODY WEIGHT (kg) BY
Healthy individual or well-nourished elective surgery patient	0.8-1.0 g protein
Malnourished or catabolic state (e.g., sepsis, major injury)	1.2 to 2+ g protein
Burns	
15%-30% BSA	1.5 g protein
31%-49% BSA	1.5-2.0 g protein
50% or greater BSA	2.0-2.5 g protein

BSA, Body surface area.

Example of a Calculation of Calorie and Protein Needs

A 28-year-old woman has a fracture of the left femur and burns to 40% of her BSA after a motor vehicle crash. Her height is 1.65 m (5 ft 5 in), and her weight is 59.1 kg (130 lb).

Energy Needs

1. $RMR = (9.99 \times 59.1\ kg) + (6.25 \times 165\ cm) - (4.92 \times 28\ years) - 161 = 1323$ calories/day
2. Energy needs for injury = 1323 calories × 1.75 = 2315 calories/day

Protein Needs

Protein needs = 59.1 kg × 1.75 g = 103 g/day

REFERENCES

1. *Academy of Nutrition and Dietetics.* Evidence Analysis Library. If indirect calorimetry is unavailable or impractical, what is the best way to estimate resting metabolic rate (RMR) in non-obese adult critically ill patients? http://www.adaevidencelibrary.com. Accessed April 24, 2012.
2. *Academy of Nutrition and Dietetics.* Evidence Analysis Library. If indirect calorimetry is unavailable or impractical, what is the best way to estimate resting metabolic rate (RMR) in obese adult critically ill patients? http://www.adaevidencelibrary.com. Accessed April 24, 2012.
3. *Academy of Nutrition and Dietetics.* Evidence Analysis Library. Estimating RMR with predictive equations: what does the evidence tell us? http://www.adaevidencelibrary.com. Accessed April 24, 2012.
4. Data from Deitch EA. *Crit Care Clin.* 1995;11:735; Owen OE, et al. *Am J Clin Nutr.* 1986;4:1; Owen OE, et al. *Am J Clin Nutr.* 1987;46:875; Garrel DR, Jobin N, de Jonge LH. *Nutr Clin Pract.* 1996;11:99.

Note: Page numbers followed by f, t, and b indicate figures, tables, and boxes, respectively.

SPECIAL FEATURES